ANTIMICROBIAL AGENTS
AND
CHEMOTHERAPY

VOLUME 11

WASHINGTON, D C 20006

1977

ANTIMICROBIAL AGENTS AND CHEMOTHERAPY

VOLUME 11 ● 1977

Antimicrobial Agents and Chemotherapy, an interdisciplinary publication of the American Society for Microbiology, 1913 I St., N.W., Washington, D.C. 20006, is devoted to the dissemination of knowledge relating to all aspects of antimicrobial agents and chemotherapy, including cancer chemotherapy. *Antimicrobial Agents and Chemotherapy* is published monthly, and the twelve numbers are divided into two volumes per year. The nonmember subscription price is $60 per year. The member subscription price is $14 per year. Single copies are $6. Correspondence relating to subscriptions, reprints, defective copies, availability of back issues, lost or late proofs, disposition of submitted manuscripts, and general editorial matters should be directed to the ASM Publications Office, 1913 I St., N.W., Washington, D.C. 20006 (area 202 833-9680).

Second class postage paid at Washington, D.C. 20006, and at additional mailing offices.
Made in the United States of America.

Volume 11

Contents for January

Number 1

Biosynthesis; Chemistry; Mechanisms of Action and Resistance

Lysis of Enterobacteria by Cefoxitin, Cefuroxime, and Cephalothin. C. S. GOODWIN* AND JOYCE P. HILL 26

Production of Megacins C and Cx: Presumptive Evidence of Extrachromosomal Control. HELEN D. DONOGHUE 34

Effect of Atebrin on Bacterial Membrane Adenosine Triphosphatases in Relation to the Divalent Cation Used as Substrate and/or Activator. JOSÉ CARREIRA AND EMILIO MUÑOZ* 38

Mechanisms of Gentamicin Resistance in *Staphylococcus aureus*. J. E. DOWDING* 47

Inactivation of Lipid-Containing Viruses by Long-Chain Alcohols. WALLACE SNIPES,* STANLEY PERSON, GREGORY KELLER, WILLIAM TAYLOR, AND ALEX KEITH 98

L-Glyceraldehyde 3-Phosphate, a Bactericidal Agent. CHU-TAY TANG, ROBERT ENGEL, AND BURTON E. TROPP* 147

Comparison of the Binding Properties of Two 6β-Amidinopenicillanic Acid Derivatives That Differ in Their Physiological Effects on *Escherichia coli*. BRIAN G. SPRATT 161

Nalidixic Acid-Induced Protein Alterations in *Escherichia coli*. LEE CHAO 167

Bactericidal Effects of Combinations of Ampicillin with Anti-R-Plasmid Compounds on *Salmonella typhimurium* R1^{+}. FRED E. HAHN* AND JENNIE CIAK 176

Physiological Effects and Microbial Susceptibility

Comparative In Vitro Activity of Pirbenicillin, Ticarcillin, and Carbenicillin Against *Pseudomonas aeruginosa*. TAKEO MURAKAWA AND L. D. SABATH* 1

Susceptibility of Three Groups of *Staphylococcus aureus* to Newer Antimicrobial Agents. GEORGE W. JORDAN* AND PAUL D. HOEPRICH 7

Temperature-Sensitive R Plasmid Obtained from Naturally Isolated Drug-Resistant *Vibrio cholerae* (Biotype El Tor). TAKESHI YOKOTA* AND SHOGO KUWAHARA 13

Bioassay Method for Polyene Antibiotics Based on the Measurement of Rubidium Efflux from Rubidium-Loaded Yeast Cells. R. F. COSGROVE AND J. E. FAIRBROTHER 31

Microassay for Amphotericin B. ROBERT M. BANNATYNE,* ROSE CHEUNG, AND HANNA R. DEVLIN 44

In Vitro Studies with Netilmicin Compared with Amikacin, Gentamicin, and Tobramycin. VIJAY DHAWAN, EUGENE MARSO, WILLIAM J. MARTIN, AND LOWELL S. YOUNG* 64

Mezlocillin: In Vitro Studies of a New Broad-Spectrum Penicillin. GERALD P. BODEY* AND THERESA PAN 74

Cefoxitin Activity Against Multiply Antibiotic-Resistant *Klebsiella pneumoniae*. ROGER T. JACKSON,* FRANK E. THOMAS, AND ROBERT H. ALFORD 84

Comparative In Vitro Activity of Nafcillin, Oxacillin, and Methicillin in Combination with Gentamicin and Tobramycin Against Enterococci. CHATRCHAI WATANAKUNAKORN* AND CHERYL GLOTZBECKER 88

Rapid Method for Determining the Minimum Inhibitory Concentration of Ampicillin for *Haemophilus influenzae*. RAYMOND RYAN AND RICHARD C. TILTON* . 114

* Asterisk refers to person to whom inquiries regarding the paper should be addressed.

Antimicrobial Activity In Vitro of Netilmicin and Comparison with Sisomicin, Gentamicin, and Tobramycin. BURT R. MEYERS AND SHALOM Z. HIRSCHMAN* 118

In Vitro Activity of Netilmicin, Gentamicin, and Amikacin. ROBERT J. KANTOR AND CARL W. NORDEN* 126

Beta-Lactamase Activity in Strains of *Bacteroides melaninogenicus* and *Bacteroides oralis*. A. A. SALYERS,* J. WONG, AND T. D. WILKINS 142

Effects of Amphotericin B on Macrophages and Their Precursor Cells. HSIU-SAN LIN,* GERALD MEDOFF, AND GEORGE S. KOBAYASHI 154

Susceptibility of *Propionibacterium acnes* to Seventeen Antibiotics. WEN LAN LOU WANG,* E. DALE EVERETT, MARCIA JOHNSON, AND EVELYN DEAN 171

Pharmacology and Therapeutics

Therapy of Murine Aspergillosis with Amphotericin B in Combination with Rifampin or 5-Fluorocytosine. JULIO ARROYO, GERALD MEDOFF,* AND GEORGE S. KOBAYASHI 21

Laboratory Evaluation of FR10024, a New Cephalosporin Derivative. MINORU NISHIDA,* TAKEO MURAKAWA, TOSHIAKI KAMIMURA, NAOHIKO OKADA, SHIGEMI FUKADA, HIROSHI SAKAMOTO, SHOJI NAKAMOTI, YOSHIKO YOKOTA, AND YOKO KONO 51

Interferon Induction in Cynomolgus and Rhesus Monkeys After Repeated Doses of a Modified Polyriboinosinic-Polyribocytidylic Acid Complex. M. L. SAMMONS, E. L. STEPHEN,* H. B. LEVY, S. BARON, AND D. E. HILMAS 80

Evaluation of Various Analogues of Tilorone Hydrochloride against Venezuelan Equine Encephalitis Virus in Mice. RALPH W. KUEHNE,* WALLACE L. PANNIER, AND EDWARD L. STEPHEN 92

Rapid Analysis of Cefazolin in Serum by High-Pressure Liquid Chromatography. JOHN S. WOLD 105

Comparative Penetration of Amikacin, Gentamicin, and Penicillin G into Exudate Fluid in Experimental Sterile Peritonitis. ROB ROY MACGREGOR 110

Inhibition of Multiplication of *Mycobacterium leprae* by Polyinosinic-Polycytidylic Acid. LOUIS LEVY AND THOMAS C. MERIGAN* 122

Pharmacokinetics of Amoxicillin: Dose Dependence After Intravenous, Oral, and Intramuscular Administration. DANIEL A. SPYKER,* RAYMOND J. RUGLOSKI, ROBERT L. VANN, AND WILLIAM M. O'BRIEN 132

Stability of Cephalosporins in Horse Serum. M. A. FOGLESONG 174

Errata

New Method for Detecting In Vitro Inactivation of Penicillins by *Haemophilus influenzae* and *Staphylococcus aureus*. WIE-SHING LEE* AND LOUIS KOMARMY 178

Antibiotic Resistance Among Coliform and Fecal Coliform Bacteria Isolated from Sewage, Seawater, and Marine Shellfish. MARYLYN D. COOKE 178

Antibiotic Resistance Among Coliform and Fecal Coliform Bacteria Isolated from the Freshwater Mussel *Hydridella menziesii*. MARYLYN D. COOKE 178

Inhibition of *Neisseria gonorrhoeae* by a Bacteriocin from *Pseudomonas aeruginosa*. STEPHEN A. MORSE,* PATRICK VAUGHAN, DEANNE JOHNSON, AND BARBARA H. IGLEWSKI 178

Volume 11

Contents for February

Number 2

Biosynthesis; Chemistry; Mechanisms of Action and Resistance

Synthesis of Vaccinia Viral Antigens in HeLa Cells in the Presence of Isatin Beta-Thiosemicarbazone. EHUD KATZ* AND HAYA FELIX 202

Requirements of Glucose and Incubation Under Static Conditions for Optimal Colicin E_1 Induction. ATSUCHI NAKAZAWA,* NOBUO SUZUKI, AND TERUMI TAMADA 219

Prevention of 5-Fluorouracil-Caused Growth Inhibition in *Sordaria fimicola*. HOWARD F. SCHOEN* AND JOHN BERECH, JR. 234

Changes in Superhelical Density of Closed Circular Deoxyribonucleic Acid by Intercalation of Anti-R-Plasmid Drugs and Primaquine. RICHARD G. ALLISON AND FRED E. HAHN* 251

Development of a Chemically Defined Medium for the Synthesis of Actinomycin D by *Streptomyces parvulus*. W. KENNETH WILLIAMS AND EDWARD KATZ* 281

Relationship Between the Physicochemical Nature of Human Interferon, the Cell Induced, and the Inducing Agent. THOMAS C. CESARIO,* PATRICIA J. SCHRYER, AND JEREMIAH G. TILLES 291

Lethal and Mutagenic Effects of 5-Iodouracil on Bacteriophage T4*td*8*r*II. DANIEL M. BYRD* AND WILLIAM H. PRUSOFF 312

Tetracycline Inhibits Propagation of Deoxyribonucleic Acid Replication and Alters Membrane Properties. MARTIN L. PATO 318

Transfer of a Plasmid-Specified Beta-Lactamase Gene from *Haemophilus influenzae*. J. R. SAUNDERS* AND R. B. SYKES 339

Comparison of Colicins B-K260 and D-CA23: Purification and Characterization of the Colicins and Examination of Colicin Immunity in the Producing Strains. ANTHONY P. PUGSLEY* AND PETER REEVES 345

Physiological Effects and Microbial Susceptibility

Drug Resistance and R Factors in *Salmonella typhi* Isolated in Korea. DOKI CHUN,* SUNG YONG SEOL, DONG TAEK CHO, AND RYONBIN TAK 209

Microdilution Transfer Plate Technique for Determining In Vitro Synergy of Antimicrobial Agents. PAULA F. DOUGHERTY, DAVID W. YOTTER, AND THOMAS R. MATTHEWS* 225

Effects of Purines and Pyrimidines on the Fungistatic Activity of 5-Fluorocytosine in *Aspergillus* Species. GERALD E. WAGNER AND SMITH SHADOMY* 229

In Vitro Activity of Ticarcillin Against Anaerobic Bacteria Compared with That of Carbenicillin and Penicillin. IRA ROY, VINH BACH, AND HARAGOPAL THADEPALLI* 258

Simple, Direct Broth-Disk Method for Antibiotic Susceptibility Testing of *Ureaplasma urealyticum*. MONIEK S. SPAEPEN AND RUTH B. KUNDSIN* 267

Evaluation of the Performance Parameters of a Prediluted, Quantitative Susceptibility Test Device. RICHARD C. TILTON* AND HENRY D. ISENBERG 271

Amphotericin B Susceptibility Testing of Yeasts with a Bactec Radiometric System. ROY L. HOPFER* AND DIETER GROSCHEL. 277

Hemagglutination Inhibition Assay for Gentamicin. W. A. MAHON,* RHODA I. FELDMAN, AND GEORGE H. SCHERR 359

In Vitro Activity of Netilmicin. J. A. SMITH, J.R. MORGAN,* AND M. MOGYOROS 362

Bioassay for Miconazole. ANA ESPINEL-INGROFF, S. SHADOMY,* AND JOHN F. FISHER 365

Pharmacology and Therapeutics

Emergence of Gentmicin-Resistant *Klebsiella* in a General Hospital. R. P. RENNIE* AND I. B. R. DUNCAN 179

Pharmacological and Clinical Study of Bacampicillin in Acute Peritonsillitis—a Comparison with Ampicillin. HANS O. HALLANDER,* ANDERS FLODSTRÖM, AND JAN SJÖVALL 185

Antiviral Activities of Acyl Derivatives of 2,2′-Anhydro-1-β-D-arabinofuranosylcytosine and 1-β-D-arabinofuranosylcytosine in Cell Culture. KOSABURA SATO,* AKIO NOMURA, AND JOHN G. MOFFATT 191

Comparative Study of the Antiviral Activity of Acyl Derivatives of 2,2′-Anhydro-1-D-arabinofuranosylcytosine and Other Nucleosides Against Encephalitis in Mice. SHINYA NISHIYAMA, KOSABURO SATO,* TOSHIHIKO YAMANAKA, AND JOHN G. MOFFATT 198

Pharmacokinetics of Amikacin During Hemodialysis and Peritoneal Dialysis. LISBETH REGEUR, HANNE COLDING,* HERLUF JENSEN, AND JENS P. KAMPMANN 214

Antimicrobial Prophylaxis for Catheter-Associated Bacteriuria. MICHAEL R. BRITT,* RICHARD A. GARIBALDI, WILLIAM A. MILLER, RICHARD M. HEBERSTON, AND JOHN P. BURKE 240

Bone Marrow Toxicity Associated with 5-Fluorocytosine Therapy. CAROL A. KAUFMAN* AND PETER T. FRAME 244

Pharmacokinetics of Cefamandole in Patients with Renal Failure. BURT R. MEYERS AND SHALOM Z. HIRSCHMAN* 248

Pharmacokinetics of Cefamandole in Patients with Normal and Impaired Renal Function. HANS-EBERHARD MELLIN, PETER G. WELLING, AND PAUL O. MADSEN* 262

Combined Antiviral Effects of Interferon, Adenine Arabinoside, Hypoxanthine Arabinoside, and Adenine Arabinoside-5′-Monophosphate in Human Fibroblast Cultures. YVONNE J. BRYSON AND L. H. KRONENBERG* 299

Experimental Herpes Simplex Virus Type 1 Encephalitis: Treatment with 5-Trifluoromethyl-2′-Deoxyuridine. D. W. CLOUGH* AND J. RODNEY PARKHURST 307

Cefadroxil, a New Broad-Spectrum Cephalosporin. R. E. BUCK* AND K. E. PRICE 324

Comparative Human Oral Clinical Pharmacology of Cefadroxil, Cephalexin, and Cephradine. MORRIS PFEFFER,* ANDRE JACKSON, JOSE XIMENES, AND HAIRO PERCHE DE MENEZES 331

Antimicrobial Activity of Cefamandole Against *Salmonella typhi*. SHALOM Z. HIRSCHMAN,* BURT R. MEYERS, AND ALBERT MILLER 369

Errata

Laboratory Evaluation of BL-S786, a Cephalosporin with Broad-Spectrum Antibacterial Activity. F. LEITNER,* M. MISIEK, T. A. PURSIANO, R. E. BUCK, D. R. CHISHOLM, R. D. DEREGIS, Y. H. TSAI, AND K. E. Price 372

Effect of Long-Term Therapies with Penicillin and Sulfadiazine on *Streptococcus mutans* and Lactobacilli in Dental Plaque. H. G. WELD AND H. J. SANDHAM* 372

R Plasmids in *Streptococcus agalactiae* (Group B). THEA HORODNICEANU,* D. H. BOUANCHAUD, G. BIETH, AND Y. A. CHABBERT 372

Anitmicrobial Susceptibility Testing of Yeasts: a Turbidimetric Technique Independent of Inoculum Size. JOHN N. GALGIANI* AND DAVID A. STEVENS 372

Volume 11

Contents for March

Number 3

Biosynthesis; Chemistry; Mechanisms of Action and Resistance

Cairomycin B, a New Antibiotic. IBRAHIM R. SHIMI,* NADIA ABEDALLAH, AND SHADIA FATHY 313

Plasmid-Mediated Chloramphenicol Resistance in *Haemophilus influenzae*. V. VAN KLINGEREN,* J. D. A. VAN EMBDEN, AND M. DESSENS-KROON 383

Effect of Penicillin on Streptomycin Production by *Streptomyces griseus*. G. BARABAS* AND G. SZABO 392

Gardimycin, a New Antibiotic Inhibiting Peptidoglycan Synthesis. SERGIO SOMMA, WILMA MERATI, AND FRANCESCO PARENTI 396

Antibiotic Metabolites from a Murine Pseudomonad. STEPHEN J. WRATTEN, MARGARET S. WOLFE, RAYMOND J. ANDERSON, AND D. JOHN FAULKNER* 411

Chemically Defined Antimicrobial Susceptibility Test Medium for *Pseudomonas aeruginosa*. J. H. JORGENSEN,* J. C. LEE, AND P. M. JONES 415

Resistance Plasmid Transfer by *Seratia marcescens* in Urine. DENNIS R. SCHABERG,* ANITA K. HIGHSMITH, AND INA K. WACHSMUTH 449

Comparison of the Actions of 5-Fluorouracil and Ftorafur (NSC 148958) in *Escherichia coli*. PRISCILLA P. SAUNDERS* AND LIAN-YU CHAO 451

Terminal Stages in the Biosynthesis of Tylosin. E. T. SENO,* R. L. PIEPER, AND F. M. HUBER 455

Effects of 2-Deoxy-D-Glucose and 3-Deazauridine Individually and in Combination on the Replication of Japanese B Encephalitis Virus. DANIEL R. WOODMAN* AND JIMMY C. WILLIAMS 475

Inhibition of Initiation, Elongation, and Termination of Eukaryotic Protein Synthesis by Trichothecene Fungal Toxins. ERIC CUNDIFFE AND JULIAN E. Davies* 491

Cytochemical and Biochemical Studies of Yeasts After In Vitro Exposure to Miconazole. SONJA DE NOLLIN,* H. VAN BELLE, F. GOOSSENS, F. THONÉ, AND M. BORGERS 500

Mobilization of Morganocin 174 Plasmid and Kinetics of Morganocin Production in *Proteus* and *Escherichia coli* Hosts. J. A. WILLIAMS 514

Inhibition of Cellular and Viral Protein Synthesis by 3-Methyleneoxindole. SERGIO L. ABREU AND JEAN LUCAS-LENARD* 521

Plasmid-Mediated Beta-Lactamase Production in *Neisseria gonorrhoeae*. LYNN P. ELWELL,* MARILYN ROBERTS, LEONARD W. MAYER, AND STANLEY FALKOW 528

Effect of Ethambutol on the Viable Cell Count in *Mycobacterium smegmatis*. JAMES O. KILBURN* AND JOSEPH GREENBERG 534

Comparison of the Effects of Mecillinam and 6-Aminopenicillanic Acid on *Proteus mirabilis*, *Escherichia coli*, and *Staphylococcus aureus*. VICTOR LORIAN* AND BARBARA ATKINSON 541

Characterization of an R-Plasmid Associated with Ampicillin Resistance in *Shigella dysenteriae* Type 1. JORGE H. CROSA,* JORGE OLARTE, LEONARDO J. MATA, LINDA K. LULTROP, AND MARIA E. PENARANDA 553

Ampicillin-Induced Morphological Alterations of *Haemophilus influenzae* Type B. G. H. LUGINBUHL* AND RICHARD D. KLEIN 559

Action of the *N*-Trifluroacetyl Analogue of D-Chloramphenicol. K. B. FREEMAN 563

Microbial Formation of 4-Thiouracil. L. DOLAK,* W. T. SOKOLSKI, S. MIZAK, D. W. STROMAN, AND O. K. SEBEK 569

Stimulation of Interferon Production in Mice and Spleen Leukocytes by Analogues of BL-20803. PAUL SIMINIOFF* AND R. R. CRENSHAW 571

Physiological Effects and Microbial Susceptibility

Bacteriostatic and Bactericidal Activities of Selected Beta-Lactam Antibiotics Studied on Agar Plates. GOHTA MASUDA,* SUSUMU TOMIOKA, HIROSHI UCHICA, AND MITSUTO HASEGAWA 376

Antibacterial Activity of Netilmicin, a New Aminoglycoside Antibiotic, Compared with That of Centamicin. IAN PHILLIPS,* ANNE SMITH, AND KEVIN SHANNON 402

Pirbenicillin: Comparison with Carbenicillin and BL-P1654, Alone and with Gentamicin, Against *Pseudomonas aeruginosa*. CARLOS E. LOPEZ, HAROLD C. STANDIFORD,* BEVERLY A. TATEM, FRANK M. CALIA, STEPHEN C. SCHIMPFF, MERRILL J. SNYDER, AND RICHARD B. HORNICK 441

Comparison of In Vitro Activity of Cephalexin, Cephradine, and Cefaclor. NANCY J. BILL AND JOHN A. WASHINGTON II* 470

Antimicrobial Susceptibilities of *Yersinia enterocolitica* Biotype 4, Serotype O:3. M. I. MARKS,* S. SORGER, AND S. HAMMERBERG 566

Cerulenin-Inhibited Cells of *Staphylococcus aureus* Resume Growth When Supplemented with Either a Saturated or an Unsaturated Fatty Acid. ROBERT A. ALTENBERN 574

Pharmacology and Therapeutics

Changing Patterns of Plasmid-Mediated Drug Resistance During Tetracycline Therapy. J. K. MØLLER,* A. LETH BAK, A. STENDERUP, H. ZACHARIAE, AND H. AFZELIUS 388

In Vivo Effects of Josamycin, Erythromycin, and Placebo Therapy on Nasal Carriage of *Staphylococcus aureus*. SAMUEL Z. WILSON,* R. RUSSEL MARTIN, AND MARGARET PUTMAN 407

Comparative Trial of Carbenicillin and Ampicillin Therapy for Purulent Meningitis. G. D. OVERTURF,* E. A. STEINBERG, A. E. UNDERMAN, J. WILKINS, J. M. LEEDOM, A. W. MATHIES, JR., AND P. F. WEHRLE 420

Cefoxitin: Clinical Evaluation in 38 Patients. PETER N. R. HESELTINE,* DAVID F. BUSCH, RICHARD D. MEYER, AND SYDNEY M. FINEGOLD 427

Chemotherapy of an Experimental *Bacteroides fragilis* Infection in Mice. CLAY B. WALKER,* DORRIT NITZAN, AND TRACY D. WILKINS 435

Bioavailability of Tetracycline and Deoxycycline in Fasted and Nonfasted Subjects. PETER G. WELLING,* PATRICIA A. KOCH, CURTIS C. LAU, AND WILLIAM A. CRAIG 462

Comparative Growth Rates of Selected Anaerobic Species in Four Commonly Used Broth Media. WILLIAM SOTTILE II AND R. J. ZABRANSKY* 482

Volume 11

Contents for April

Number 4

Biosynthesis; Chemistry; Mechanismns of Action and Resistance

R Plasmids from Asian Strains of *Vibrio cholerae*. R. W. HEDGES,* N. J. PEARSON, F. O'GRADY, AND J. L. VIALARD 585

Pseudomonas aeruginosa Strain Isolated in France That Carries a Plasmid Determining Carbenicillin Resistance. Y. MICHEL-BRIAND,* VILMA A. STANISICH, AND M. JOUVENOT 589

Penicillin Resistance and Penicillinase Production in Clinical Isolates of *Bacteroides melaninogenicus*. PATRICK R. MURRAY* AND JON E. ROSENBLATT ... 605

Influence of Antioxidants on the Bioactivity of Amphotericin B. FRED A. ANDREWS,* WILLIAM H. BEGGS, AND GEORGE A. SAROSI ... 615

Plasmid-Mediated Aminoglycoside Phosphotransferase of Broad Substrate Range That Phosphorylates Amikacin. PATRICE COURVALIN AND JULIAN DAVIES* 619

Growth Inhibition of *Escherichia coli* W by D-Norvalyl-D-Alanine: an Analogue of D-Alanine in Position 4 of the Peptide Subunit of Peptidoglycan. F. C. NEUHAUS,* S. GOYER, AND D. W. NEUHAUS ... 638

Macrolide Resistance in *Staphylococcus aureus*: Induction of Macrolide-Resistant Protein Synthesis. NORRIS E. ALLEN ... 661

Macrolide Resistance in *Staphylococcus aureus*: Inducers of Macrolide Resistance. NORRIS E. ALLEN ... 669

Bacteriocin Production by Strains of *Bacteroides* Isolated from Human Feces and the Role of These Strains in the Bacterial Ecology of the Colon. S. J. BOOTH,* J. K. JOHNSON, AND T. D. WILKINS ... 718

Cefoxitin Resistance to Beta-Lactamase: a Major Factor for Susceptibility of *Bacteroides fragilis* to the Antibiotic. GARY DARLAND* AND JEROME BIRNBAUM . 725

Bactericidal Factor Produced by *Haemophilus influenzae* b: Partial Purification of the Factor and Transfer of Its Genetic Determinant. RICHARD A. VENEZIA,* P. M. MATUSIAK, AND R. G. ROBERTSON ... 735

Effects of Ionenes on Interferon Induction by Poly(Inosinic Acid)·Poly(Cytidylic Acid). BOREK JANIK,* ERIK DE CLERCQ, AND RONALD G. SOMMER ... 756

Physiological Effects and Microbial Susceptibility

In Vitro Activity of Cinoxacin, Ampicillin, and Chloramphenicol Against *Shigella* and Nontyphoid *Salmonella*. ETHAN RUBINSTEIN* AND BRACHA SHAINBERG 577

Susceptibility of Anaerobic Bacteria to Metronidazole, Ornidazole, and Tinidazole and Routine Susceptibility Testing by Standardized Methods. JÜRG WÜST . 631

Susceptibility of Clinical Isolates of Cytomegalovirus to Human Interferon. BOSKO POSTIC* AND JOHN N. DOWLING ... 656

Measurement of Polyene Antibiotic-Mediated Erythrocyte Damage by Release of Hemoglobin and Radioactive Chromium. E. B. SIEGEL ... 675

Comparative Susceptibility of Anaerobic Bacteria to Ticarcillin, Cefoxitin, Metronidazole, and Related Antimicrobial Agents. DAVID K. HENDERSON, ANTHONY W. CHOW,* AND LUCIEN B. GUZE ... 679

Susceptibility of *Clostridium perfringens* Isolated from Human Infections to Twenty Antibiotics. JOSEPH D. SCHWARTZMAN,* L. BARTH RELLER, AND WEN-LAN L. WANG ... 695

Cefazaflur, a New Parenteral Cephalosporin: In Vitro Studies. GEORGE W. COUNTS,* DAVID GREGORY, DELORES ZELZNIK, AND MARVIN TURCK ... 708

Evaluation of the In Vitro Antifungal Activity of Allicin. YASUO YAMADA* AND KEIZŌ AZUMA ... 743

Evaluation of the Autobac 1 Susceptibility Testing System in a Clinical Diagnostic Laboratory. MIGUEL MOGYOROS, JOHN R. MORGAN, AND JOHN A. SMITH* . 750

Mutagenicity and Antibacterial Activity of Hydroxamic Acids. CHING YUNG WANG* AND LANFORD H. LEE ... 753

Mycobacterium chelonei Infection: Successful Treatment Based on a Radiometric Susceptibility Test. JULIO ARROYO AND GERALD MEDOFF* ... 763

^{125}I Radioimmunoassay of Netilmicin. PAUL STEVENS,* LOWELL S. YOUNG, AND WILLIAM L. HEWITT ... 768

Pharmacology and Therapeutics

Effects of Antibiotics on Chemotaxis of Human Leukocytes. ARNE FORSGREN* AND DAVID SCHMELING 580

Penetration of Cefazolin, Cephaloridine, and Cefamandole into Interstitial Fluid in Rabbits. CLAUDE CARBON, ALAIN CONTREPOIS, NILS BRION, AND SUZANNE LAMOTTE-BARRILLON* 594

Comparative Activity of Ampicillin and Cefuroxime Against Three Types of *Haemophilus influenzae*. R. B. SYKES,* A. GRIFFITHS, AND D. M. RYAN 599

Netilmicin and Gentamicin: Comparative Pharmacology in Humans. LOUISE J. RIFF* AND GAIL MORESCHI 609

Therapeutic Evaluation of Minocycline and Tetracyline for Mixed Anaerobic Infection in Mice. GALE B. HILL 625

Therapy of Antimicrobial-Resistant Typhoid Fever. THOMAS BUTLER,* NGUYEN NGOC LINH, AND KEITH ARNOLD 645

Assay of Gentamicin in Serum by High-Pressure Liquid Chromatography. JOHN P. ANHALT 651

Indirect Mouse Model for the Evaluation of Potential Antiviral Compounds: Results with Venezuelan Equine Encephalomyelitis. RALPH W. KUEHNE,* WALLACE L. PANNIER, AND EDWARD L. STEPHEN 683

Tobramycin: Maternal-Fetal Pharmacology. BETTY BERNARD,* SALVADOR J. GARCIA-CAZARES, CHARLES A. BALLARD, LAURI D. THRUPP, ALLEN W. MATHIES, AND PAUL F. WEHRLE 688

Levels of Carbenicillin, Ticarcillin, Cephalothin, Cefazolin, Cefamandole, Gentamicin, Tobramycin, and Amikacin in Human Serum and Interstitial Fluid. JAMES S. TAN* AND SARA JANE SALSTROM 698

Chemotherapy of Genital Herpes Simplex Virus Type 2 Infections of Female Hamsters. HAROLD E. RENIS 701

Side Effects of Minocycline: a Double-Blind Study. W. LEE FANNING, DIETER W. GUMP,* AND ROBERT A. SOFFERMAN 712

Distribution of Sodium Cefazolin in Serum, Muscle, Bone Marrow, and Bone of Normal Rabbits. D. J. PITKIN, C. SACHS, I. ZAJAC, AND P. ACTOR* 760

Efficacy of 5,6-Dihydro-5-Azathymidine Against Cutaneous Herpes Simplex Virus in Hairless Mice. GERALD E. UNDERWOOD AND SHELDON D. WEED* 765

Erratum

Preparation of Isolated Intestinal Villi Useful for Studying Hydrolysis Rates of Penicillin and Cephalosporin Esters. WALTER E. WRIGHT AND VERLE D. LINE 771

Volume 11 **Contents for May** **Number 5**

Biosynthesis: Chemistry; Mechanisms of Action and Resistance

Permeability Barrier to Rifampin in Mycobacteria. J. HUI, N. GORDON, AND R. KAJIOKA* 773

Beta-Lactamases Produced by a *Pseudomonas aeruginosa* Strain Highly Resistant to Carbenicillin. ROGER LABIA,* MARLENE GUIONIE, JEAN-MICHEL MASSON, ALAIN PHILLIPPON, AND MICHEL BARTHELEMY 785

Amphotericin B and Filipin Effects on L and HeLa Cells: Dose Response. JANINA

KOTELR-BRAJTBURG, GERALD MEDOFF,* DAVID SCHLESSINGER, AND GEORGE S. KOBAYASHI ... 803

Clavulanic Acid, a Beta-Lactamase-Inhibiting Beta-Lactam from *Streptomyces clavuligerus*. C. READING AND M. COLE* ... 852

Aggregation-Dependent Changes in Susceptibility of *Dictyostelium discoideum*. EDWARD F. ROSSOMANDO,* MARY ANN HESLA, MARY ANN HEITZ, AND BARBARA MALDONADO ... 858

Inducible Resistance to D-Cycloserine in *Bacillus subtilis* 168. VIRGINIA L. CLARK AND FRANK E. YOUNG* ... 871

D-Cycloserine-Induced Alterations in the Transport of D-Alanine and Glycine in *Bacillus subtilis* 168. VIRGINIA L. CLARK AND FRANK E. YOUNG* ... 877

Energy Coupling Factor as Target of Colicin K: Characterization of a Colicin K-Insensitive *ecf* Mutant of *Escherichia coli*. JEN-SHIANG HONG,* LYNNE HAGGERTY, AND MICHAEL A. LIEBERMAN ... 881

Tolerant Response of *Streptococcus sanguis* to Beta-Lactams and Other Cell Wall Inhibitor. DIANE HORNE AND ALEXANDER TOMASZ* ... 888

Unusual Susceptibility of *Erwinia amylovora* to Antibacterial Agents in Relation to the Barrier Function of its Cell Envelope. ARUN K. CHATTERJEE, RICHARD F. BUSS, AND MORTIMER P. STARR* ... 897

Extreme Sensitivity of Staphylococcal Enterotoxin B and C Production to Inhibition by Cerulenin. ROBERT A. ALTENBERN ... 906

Phosphonoacetic Acid-Resistant Mutants of Herpes Simplex Virus: Effect of Phosphonoacetic Acid on Virus Replication and In Vitro Deoxyribonucleic Acid Synthesis in Isolated Nuclei. YECHIEL BECKER,* YAEL ASHER, YAFFA COHEN, EYNAT WEINBERG-ZAHLERING, AND JOSEPH SHLOMAI ... 919

Physiological Effects and Microbial Susceptibility

In Vitro Activity of Netilimicin Compared with Gentamicin, Tobramycin, Amikacin, and Kanamycin. THEODORE C. EICKHOFF* AND JOSEPHINE M. EHRET ... 791

Inhibition of Herpes Simplex Virus Strains Isolated from Herpetic Keratitis by Polyinosinic Acid-Polycytidylic Acid. OFIRE SMETANA, EMAULE EYLAN,* AND MIRIAM WEINBERG ... 797

Synergistic Action of Erythromycin and Cefamandole Against *Bacteroides fragilis* subsp. *fragilis*. R. S. GRIFFITH,* G. L. BRIER, AND J. D. WOLNY ... 813

Antimicrobial Susceptibility of *Haemophilus parainfluenzae*. JOAN B. MAYO AND LAURENCE R. McCARTHY* ... 844

Rapid Microbiological Assay for Chlorhydroxyquinoline That Uses a Cryogenically Stored Inoculum. R. F. COSGROVE* ... 848

Azlocillin: In Vitro Studies of a New Semisynthetic Penicillin. DOROTHY STEWART AND GERALD P. BODEY* ... 865

Susceptibility of Anaerobic Bacteria to Cefoxitin and Related Compounds. VINH TOAN BACH, IRA ROY, AND HARAGOPAL THADEPALLI* ... 912

Gas Chromatographic Determination of 5-Fluorocytosine: a Modified Extraction Method. SIOK-HIU WEE AND JOHN P. ANHALT* ... 914

Semiautomated Turbidimetric Bioassay for the Ionophore A23187. JACK E. WESTHEAD* ... 916

Pharmacology and Therapeutics

Amoxicillin Therapy of Acute Urinary Infections in Adults. A. R. RONALD,* F. JAGDIS, G. HARDING, S. HOBAN, P. MUIR, AND M. GURWITH ... 780

Effect of Probenecid on the Blood Levels and Urinary Excretion of Cefamandole. R. S. GRIFFITH,* H. R. BLACK, G. L. BRIER, AND J. D. WOLNY 809

Antimicrobial Therapy of Experimental Group B Streptococcal Infection in Mice. A. DEVEIKIS,* V. SCHAUF, M. MIZEN, AND L. RIFF 817

Renal Pharmacology of Netilmicin. PETER J. S. CHIU,* GEORGE H. MILLER, ARTHUR D. BROWN, JAMES F. LONG, AND J. ALLAN WAITZ 821

Activities of Various 4-Aminoquinolines Against Infections with Chloroquine-Resistant Strains of *Plasmodium falciparum*. L. H. SCHMIDT,* DENNIS VAUGHN, DONNA MUELLER, RUTH CROSBY, AND REBECCA HAMILTON 826

Cephradine: Penetration into Cerebrospinal Fluid and Effects of Its Administration into the Cerebral Ventricles of Cats. SAMI I. HARIK,* KAMAL F. AKL, AND MARWAN UWADAH 909

Volume 11 Contents for June Number 6

Biosynthesis; Chemistry; Mechanisms of Action and Resistance

Drug Resistance in Group D Streptococci of Clinical and Nonclinical Origin: Prevalence, Transferability, and Plasmid Properties. J. D. A. VAN EMBDEN,* H. W. B. ENGEL, AND B. VAN KLINGEREN 925

Beta-Lactamase-Directed Barrier for Penicillins of *Escherichia coli* Carrying R Plasmids. TATSUO YAMAMOTO AND TAKESHI YOKOTA* 936

Inhibition of Influenza Virus Ribonucleic Acid Polymerase by Ribavirin Triphosphate. BERTIL ERIKSSON, ERIK HELGSTRAND, NILS GUNNAR JOHANSSON, ALF LARSSON, ALFONS MISIORNY, JAN OLOF NORÉN, LENNART PHILLIPSON, KJELL STENBERG, GÖRAN STENING, STIG STRIDH, AND BO OBERG* 946

Cyclic Adenylic Acid-Dependent and -Independent Production of Chloramphenicol Acetyltransferase in *Escherichia coli* Carrying R Plasmids. TAKESHI YOKOTA, RIE KUWAHARA, SUMIKO HAGIWARA, AND SHOGO KUWAHARA* 952

Inhibition of Amino Acid Transport in *Escherichia coli* by Some Beta-Lactam Antibiotics. SCOTT V. ANDERSON AND CLAIRE M. BERG* 968

Altered Surface Properties of *Escherichia coli* Associated with a Specific Amino Acid Change in the S12 Ribosomal Protein of Streptomycin-Resistant Mutants. SIDNEY PESTKA,* HARRY WALTER, AND LAWRENCE G. WAYNE 978

Evaluation of Three Newer Methods for Investigating Protein Interactions of Penicillin G. LANCE R. PETERSON,* DALE N. GERDING, HORACE H. ZINNEMAN, AND BARBARA A. MOORE 993

Mercury Resistance and R Plasmids in *Escherichia coli* Isolated from Clinical Lesions in Japan. HIDEOMI NAKAHARA, TOMOAKI ISHIKAWA, YASUNAGA SARAI, ISAMU KONDO, HIROYUKI KOZUKUE,* AND SUSUMU MITSUHASHI 999

Transfer of Beta-Lactamase Genes of *Neisseria gonorrhoeae* by Conjugation. LINDA A. KIRVEN* AND CLYDE THORNSBERRY 1004

Novel Actinomycins Formed by Biosynthetic Incorporation of *cis* and *trans*-4-Methylproline. E. KATZ,* W. K. WILLIAMS, K. T. MASON, AND A. B. MAUGER 1056

Induction of Bacteriocins from *Clostridium perfringens* by Treatment with Mitomycin C. D. E. MAHONY 1067

Production of an Antibiotic by an Organism from Human Feces. WALLACE J. IGLEWSKI 1084

Rapid Penicillinase Paper Strip Test for Detection of Beta-Lactamase-Producing *Haemophilus influenzae* and *Neisseria gonorrhoeae*. JAMES H. JORGENSEN,* JEAN C. LEE, AND GARY A. ALEXANDER 1087

Physiological Effects and Microbial Susceptibility

Bactericidal Activity of Macromomycin, an Antitumor Antibiotic. FRANCIS L. A. BUCKMIRE* AND JEFFREY L. WINKELHAKE 1010

In Vitro Studies of Netilimicin, a New Aminoglycoside Antibiotic. DOROTHY STEWART, GERALD P. BODEY,* AND BARBARA LEBLANC 1017

Manner and Meaning of Susceptibility Testing of Ampicillin-Resistant *Haemophilus influenzae*. BARRY M. GRAY, CAROL A. HUBBELL, AND HUGH C. DILLION, JR.* 1021

Five-Hour Minimal Inhibitory Concentration Test of Four Antimicrobial Agents for *Pseudomonas aeruginosa*. W. J. BROWN* AND R. L. SAUTTER 1064

In Vitro Antibiotic Susceptibility of Salmonellae. FACELUCIA BARROS, OKSANA M. KORZENIOWSKI, MERLE A. SANDE,* KATIA MARTINS, LUIZ CARLOS SANTOS, AND HEONIR ROCHA 1071

Double-Osmotic-Shock Procedure to Prepare Gentamicin Adenine Mononucleotide Transferase for the Enzymatic Assay of Gentamicin. J. DANKERT* AND J. WOLTJES 1074

Effect of Anaerobiosis on Antimicrobial Susceptibility of Staphylococci. LIZZIE J. HARRELL AND JAMES B. EVANS* 1077

Incidence and Elimination of R Plasmids in *Vibrio cholerae*. SUJATA G. DASTIDAR, ROMA PODDAR, RANAJIT KUMAR, AND A. N. CHAKRABARTY* 1079

Pharmacology and Therapeutics

Penetration of Cefamandole into Spinal Fluid. EVAN A. STEINBERG,* GARY D. OVERTURF, LARRY J. BARAFF, AND JEANETTE WILKINS 933

Mechanism of Accumulation of the Protein Antibiotic Neocarzinostatin in Bladder Tissue: Intravenous Administration, Urinary Excretion, and Absorption into Bladder Tissue. HIROSHI MAEDA,* SADAAKI SAKAMOTO, AND JIRO OGATA 941

Synergy Between Ticarcillin and Tobramycin Against *Pseudomonas aeruginosa* and *Enterobacteriaceae* In Vitro and In Vivo. K. R. COMBER, M. J. BASKER, CHRISTINE D. OSBORNE, AND R. SUTHERLAND* 956

Nafcillin Entry into Human Cerebrospinal Fluid. BYRON E. FOSSIECK, JR.,* JAMES G. KANE, CARLOS R. DIAZ, AND RICHARD H. PARKER 965

Distribution of Gentamicin and Amikacin in Rabbit Tissue. MARGARET L. KORNGUTH* AND CALVIN M. KUNIN 974

Comparative Interferon-Inducing and Antiviral Properties of 2-Amino-5-Bromo-6-Methyl-4-Pyrimidinol (U-25,166), Tilorone Hydrochloride, and Polyinosinic-Polycytidylic Acid. DALE A. STRINGFELLOW 984

Absorption of Orally Administered Nafcillin in Normal Healthy Volunteers. CHATRCHAI WATANAKUNAKORN 1007

Effects of Gestational Age, Birth Weight, and Hypoxemia on Pharmacokinetics of Amikacin in Serum of Infants. MARTIN G. MYERS,* ROBERT J. ROBERTS, AND NAJWA J. MIRHIJ 1027

Penetration of Cefazolin into Pleural Fluid. DONALD R. COLE* AND JUANITO PUNG 1033

In Vitro Synergism Between Carbenicillin and Aminoglycosidic Aminocyclitols Against *Acinetobacter calcoaceticus* var. *anitratus*. RICHARD H. GLEW,* ROBERT C. MOELLERING, JR., AND KAREN R. BUETTNER 1036

Exudate Levels and Bactericidal Activity of Cefazolin in a New Local Infection System Using Rat Granuloma Pouches. MINORU NISHIDA* and TAKEO MURAKAWA 1042

Uniform Susceptibility of Various Strains of *Coccidioides immitis* to Amphotericin B. M. S. COLLINS AND D. PAPPAGIANIS* 1049

Response of Influenza Virus-Infected Mice to Selected Doses of Ribavirin Administered Intraperitoneally or by Aerosol. R. F. BERENDT,* J. S. WALKER, J. W. DOMINIK, AND E. L. STEPHEN 1069

Distribution of Amikacin in Serum, Muscle, and Fat in Children After a Single Intramuscular Injection. F. DASCHNER,* E. REISS, AND JÜRGEN ENGERT .. 1081

Erratum

Microassay for Amphotericin B. ROBERT M. BANNATYNE, ROSE CHUENG, AND HANNA R. DEVLIN 1089

Antimicrobial Agents and Chemotherapy, Jan. 1977, p. 1–6 Vol. 11, No. 1

Comparative In Vitro Activity of Pirbenicillin, Ticarcillin, and Carbenicillin Against *Pseudomonas aeruginosa*

TAKEO MURAKAWA AND L. D. SABATH*

Section on Infectious Diseases, Department of Medicine, University of Minnesota Medical School, Minneapolis, Minnesota 55455

Received for publication 29 March 1976

Pirbenicillin, a semisynthetic penicillin, showed greater in vitro activity against 68 recent isolates of *Pseudomonas aeruginosa* than did ticarcillin or carbenicillin. The median minimum inhibitory concentration of each of these three compounds, respectively, was 3.1, 12.5, and 25 μg/ml when a 10^{-4} dilution of an overnight culture (about 10^5 colony-forming units [CFU]/ml) was used as inoculum, but these differences were less striking when larger inocula were used: at 10^7 CFU/ml these values were 6.25, 12.5, and 50 μg/ml, and at 10^8 to 10^9 CFU/ml these values were 50, 50, and 100 μg/ml. All three compounds showed greater inhibitory activity at pH 6 than at pH 8. This pH effect was greatest with pirbenicillin, for 6.25 μg of pirbenicillin per ml inhibited 7, 11, and 57% of the strains at pH 6, 7, and 8, respectively; these values were 4, 4, and 11% with ticarcillin and 0, 0, and 7% with carbenicillin. At sufficient inhibitory concentrations, the rates of bacterial killing of the three compounds were similar. The observed differences in anti-pseudomonad activity were not due to differences in stability to pseudomonad β-lactamases, but all three compounds were more stable than were cefazolin, cephaloridine, and benzylpenicillin.

Pirbenicillin is a relatively new semisynthetic penicillin with a spectrum of action similar to that of carbenicillin and ticarcillin (9a; Lopez et al., personal communication). The molecular weight of pirbenicillin is 533.36 and its formula is shown in Fig. 1. Its major potential clinical usefulness would appear to be related to its activity against *Pseudomonas aeruginosa*. The purpose of this communication is to report the comparative in vitro activities of these three related compounds against *P. aeruginosa*, with special attention to the effect of inoculum, pH of the medium, and susceptibility to β-lactamase.

MATERIALS AND METHODS

Antibiotics. All antibiotics were gifts from the suppliers: pirbenicillin, carbenicillin, and benzylpenicillin from Pfizer, Inc.; ticarcillin and cloxacillin from Beecham Pharmaceuticals, Inc.; cephaloridine and cefazolin from Eli Lilly Laboratories for Clinical Research.

Organisms. Sixty-eight recent clinical isolates of *P. aeruginosa* were studied. These were supplied by D. Blazevic from material submitted to the Diagnostic Microbiology Laboratory at the University of Minnesota Hospitals during late 1975.

Variation in inoculum. Dilutions of overnight (18-h) cultures in Trypticase soy broth (TSB) (BBL) were made in sterile 0.9% saline.

Susceptibility testing. The inocula replicator of Steers et al. (12) was used to apply the indicated dilutions of 18-h cultures to brain heart infusion agar containing various concentrations of each antibiotic studied. The plates were incubated for 24 h at 37°C and read; the minimal inhibitory concentration (MIC) was defined as the lowest amount in a plate that permitted no more than five colonies (usually there were none) to grow. For tests of the effect of pH on the MIC, the pH of the test medium was adjusted to 6, 7, or 8, after autoclaving, by the addition of concentrated H_2SO_4 or 10% NaOH, using a pH meter.

Rate of killing. Cultures were grown 18 h in TSB at 37°C and diluted with 0.9% saline to give approximately 10^7 viable cells per ml. Samples (0.5 ml) of diluted culture were inoculated into sterile tubes containing various concentrations of antibiotic in 4.5 ml of brain heart infusion broth and incubated at 37°C. At 2, 4, and 6 h after the start of incubation cultures were sampled and an *Escherichia coli* β-lactamase solution (which destroyed residual antibiotics in 5 min at 37°C) was added to each sample. The remaining viable organisms were then enumerated by performing colony counts; 10-fold dilutions in 0.9% saline were made, and 0.1 ml of each dilution was spread over the surface of heart infusion agar plates, which were incubated 18 to 24 h at 37°C before counting.

β-lactamase activity. One milliliter of 18-h pseudomonas culture in TSB was added to 1 ml of antibiotic solution (500 μg/ml) in 1/15 M phosphate buffer (pH 7.0), and the mixture was incubated at

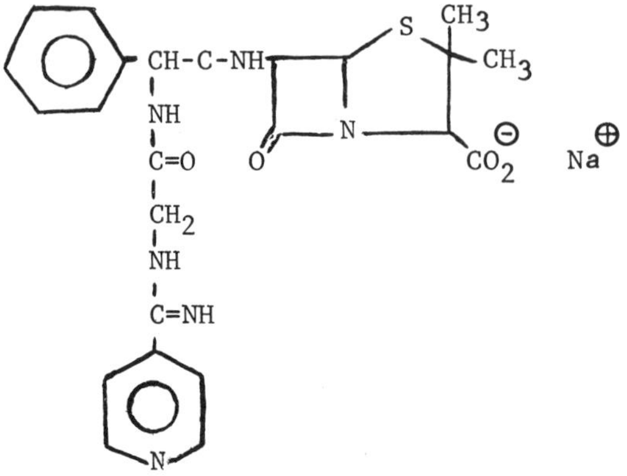

FIG. 1. *Structural formula of pirbenicillin.*

37°C for 3 h. Then 2 ml of 95% ethanol was added to stop the reaction. The residual activity was determined by a disk method using antibiotic medium no. 5 of Grove and Randall in the assay plates and *Bacillus subtilis* ATCC 6633 as the test organism. Enzyme activity was detected by reduction in antibiotic activity in this assay, compared with a control of 500 μg/ml in buffer to which sterile TSB (without organisms and β-lactamase) had been added.

Preparation of *E. coli* β-lactamase. An overnight culture of *E. coli* (a clinical isolate identified by Analylab Products Inc. criteria) in heart infusion broth was centrifuged at 16,000 × *g* for 5 min to collect cells, which were suspended in 1/15 M pH 7 Sorenson phosphate buffer, and disrupted in 2 min with a Bronwill Biosonik III sonicator at an intensity of 50. After removing the cell debris at 16,000 × *g* for 20 min, the soluble fraction was chromatographed on a Sephadex G-100 column, and the active fraction was collected.

Preparation of β-lactamase from *P. aeruginosa*. Test strains were cultured in 500 ml of heart infusion broth at 37°C for 20 h in a Lab-Line Orbit Environ platform shaker incubator. Before incubation, 50 mg of ampicillin (100 μg/ml) was added to the culture broth to induce the production of β-lactamase. A cell suspension in 30 ml of 1/15 M phosphate buffer, pH 7.0, was prepared after centrifugation at 10,000 × *g* for 15 min. The samples were disrupted for 3 min at 0°C in a Mullard ultrasonic disintegrator. The sonic extracts were centrifuged at 10,000 × *g* for 30 min at 4°C and the supernatant was used as crude β-lactamase for estimation of substrate profiles.

Substrate profiles. Substrate profiles of β-lactamases from *P. aeruginosa* were determined with benzylpenicillin, pirbenicillin, carbenicillin, ticarcillin, cloxacillin, cephaloridine, and cefazolin as substrates, using crude preparations of enzyme. The profiles were calculated against an arbitrary value of 100 for the rate of hydrolysis of penicillin G. The hydrolysis of each antibiotic was determined as described above (β-lactamase activity), using the crude enzyme instead of culture broth.

RESULTS

The comparative activities of three penicillins against 68 clinical isolates of *P. aeruginosa* are shown in Fig. 2a-c). With all three inocula, the relative activities of the three antibiotics maintained the same order: pirbenicillin most active, ticarcillin next, and carbenicillin least active. These differences were smallest with the undiluted inoculum (10^8 to 10^9 colony-forming units [CFU]/ml) and greatest with the lightest inoculum (10^{-4} dilution of 18-h culture, about 10^5 CFU/ml). The median MIC of pirbenicillin for the 68 strains with this lightest inoculum was 3.1 μg/ml, whereas with ticarcillin it was 12.5 μg/ml and with carbenicillin it was 25 μg/ml. However, with heavier inocula (10^{-2} dilution of 18-h cultures, about 10^7 CFU/ml) the median MIC values were 6.25, 12.5, and 50 μg/ml, respectively. With undiluted cultures (10^8 to 10^9 CFU/ml), the difference between pirbenicillin, ticarcillin, and carbenicillin was minimal, with median MICs of 50, 50, and 100 μg/ml, respectively (Fig. 2a).

The effect of pH on antibiotic susceptibility was determined using a 10^{-1} dilution (10^7 to 10^8 CFU/ml) of 18-h cultures of 28 of the strains. The results (Fig. 3) indicate that all three compounds were more active at pH 6 than at pH 8. The increased anti-pseudomonad activity was most striking with pirbenicillin, for at pH 8 only 25% of the strains were inhibited by 6.25 μg/ml, whereas at pH 7 and pH 6 the proportion inhibited by 6.25 μg/ml was 43% and 57%, respectively. The increase in activity with ticarcillin and carbenicillin related to lower pH was less marked: with ticarcillin the proportion of strains inhibited by 6.25 μg/ml was 4, 4, and 11%, and with carbenicillin these values were 0, 0, and 7% and pH 8, pH 7, and pH 6, respectively.

The rate of killing of *P. aeruginosa* by the three antibiotics was almost identical when their concentrations were clearly above the MIC (Fig. 4); with each antibiotic there was a 2-log decrease in viable bacterial count over 6 h.

However, when the killing rate was observed at various antibiotic concentrations (Fig. 5), it was quite apparent that pirbenicillin caused greater decreases in the viable count at lower antibiotic concentrations (5 and 10 μg/ml) than did the other two antibiotics. This was apparent at 2 h and became more pronounced at 4 and 6 h, at which times there were actual increases in the viable counts in the presence of ticarcillin or carbenicillin. At antibiotic concentrations of 50 μg and above there was no appreciable difference in killing rates of these three antibiotics. There were minimal increases in killing

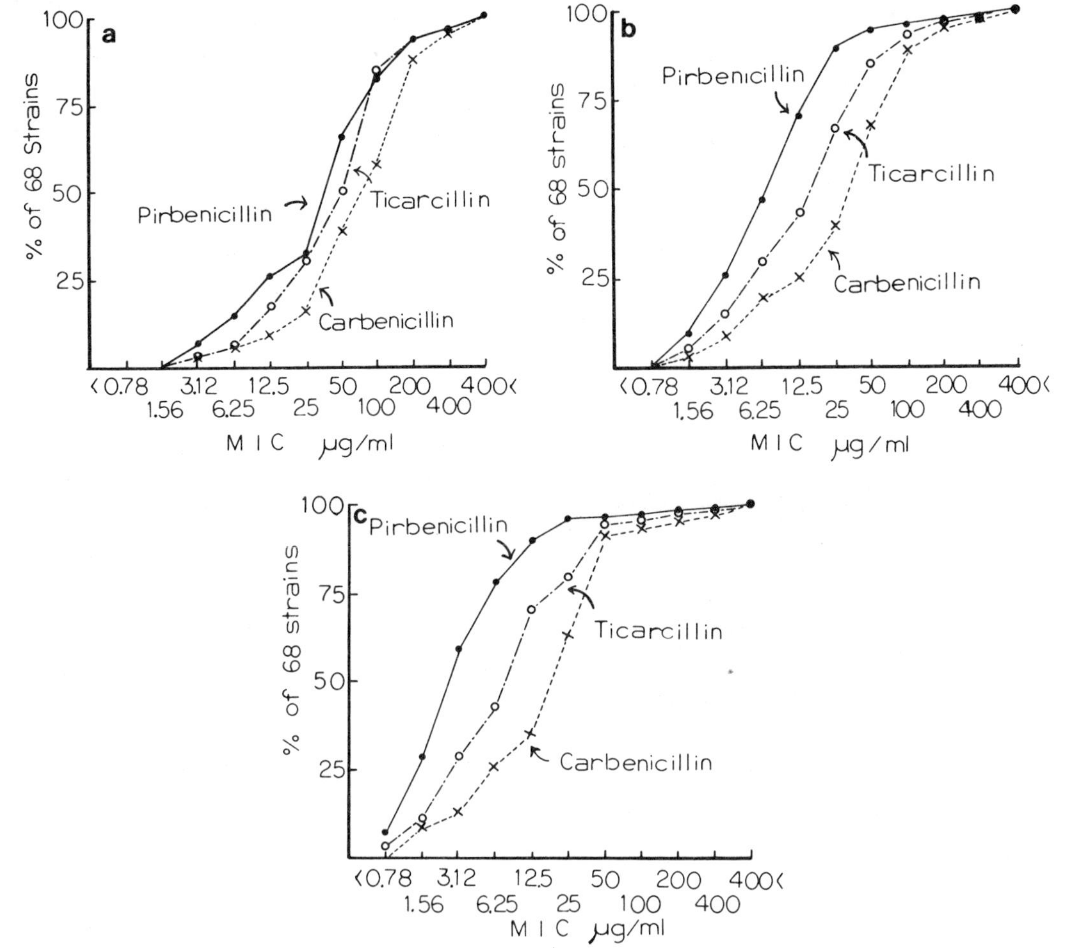

FIG. 2. *Effect of inoculum on proportion of 68 strains of P. aeruginosa inhibited by various concentrations of pirbenicillin, ticarcillin and carbenicillin. (a) Undiluted overnight culture (about 10^8 to 10^9 CFU/ml); (b) 10^{-2} dilution (about 10^7 CFU/ml); (c) 10^{-4} dilution of overnight culture (about 10^5 CFU/ml). Test performed in brain heart infusion agar using Steers replica inoculator.*

rates as the concentration of each antibiotic was increased from 50 to 500 μg/ml. Ten of the 68 strains were tested for their ability (i.e., of their culture supernatants) to inactivate pirbenicillin, ticarcillin, and carbenicillin; there were only relatively minimal differences in the stabilities of these three penicillins to the 10 culture supernatants (Table 1). With three of the strains, no decrease in antibiotic concentration was observed during the 3-h incubation with any of the antibiotics. Of the remaining seven strains, four showed slightly greater inactivation of carbenicillin than the others, and in two instances slightly more pirbenicillin was inactivated than the others.

When sonic extracts of two of these ten strains were prepared and used as crude β-lactamase (Table 2), their relative activities against pirbenicillin, ticarcillin, and carbenicillin were very similar to the β-lactamase activity observed in culture supernatants (Table 1) of these same strains. These two crude β-lactamase preparations showed no activity when cloxacillin was used as a substrate, but they hydrolyzed benzylpenicillin 12 to 75 times as readily as pirbenicillin, ticarcillin, and carbenicillin. The two cephalosporins tested as substrates were hydrolyzed one and one-half to four times more readily than was benzylpenicillin. The β-lactamases from both strains hydrolyzed cefazolin more readily than cephaloridine.

DISCUSSION

These results show that pirbenicillin had greater anti-pseudomonad activity than did ti-

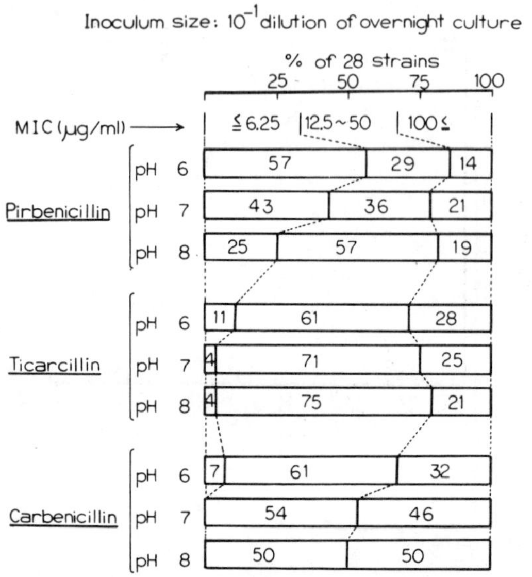

FIG. 3. *Effect of pH on the activity of three penicillins against 28 strains of P. aeruginosa. Each horizontal bar represents 100% of the 28 strains tested against the indicated antibiotic at the pH shown on the left. The numbers written within each section of the horizontal bars (two or three sections per bar) indicate the percentage of the test strains with MIC values of 6.25 or less µg/ml, 12.5 to 50 µg/ml, and 100 µg or more per ml, respectively (reading from left to right). The vertical lines within each horizontal bar delineate the sections and are connected by dotted lines which, projected to the top of the figure, indicate which of the three MIC groups each section represents. The activity of ticarcillin was least affected by pH; pirbenicillin's activity was enhanced by low pH more than the others and was greater than that of the others at each pH tested.*

TABLE 1. *Inactivation of three penicillins by culture supernatants of 10 strains of P. aeruginosa*

Strain no.[a]	% of antibiotic inactivated[b]		
	Pirbenicillin	Ticarcillin	Carbenicillin
1	15	23	28
2	13	8	15
4	0	0	0
7	19	11	16
8	0	0	0
11	28	36	23
14	5	3	8
15	11	9	7
16	16	5	32
20	0	0	0

[a] Strain number of recent clinical isolates in collection of Infectious Diseases Section.

[b] Percent inactivated is in relation to amount of penicillin G inactivated by same preparation. See text for details of enzyme preparation and methodology for detecting antibiotic inactivation.

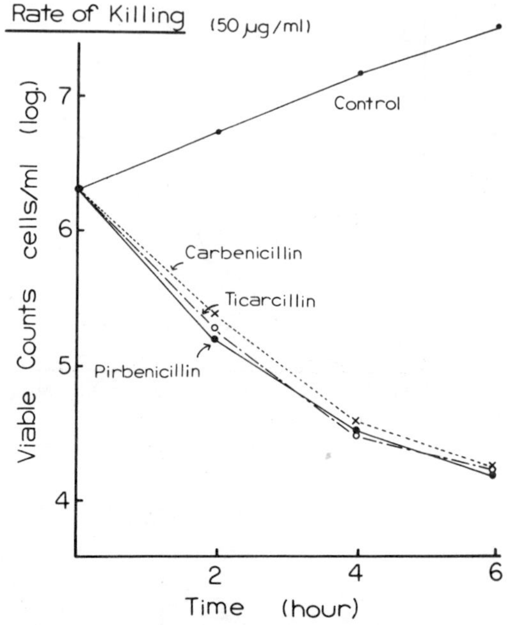

FIG. 4. *Rate of killing of P. aeruginosa 16 by three penicillins, each at 50 µg/ml, in Trypticase soy broth.*

TABLE 2. *Substrate profiles: susceptibility of seven β-lactam antibiotics to β-lactamase from two strains of P. aeruginosa*

Substrate	Relative activity[a]	
	Strain no. 11[b]	Strain no. 16[b]
Pirbenicillin	7.1	3.5
Ticarcillin	8.7	1.4
Carbenicillin	6.8	8.2
Penicillin G	100	100
Cloxacillin	0	0
Cefazolin	343	428
Cephaloridine	181	150

[a] Activity relative to the rate of hydrolysis with penicillin G as substrate.

[b] Strain number as in Table 1.

carcillin and carbenicillin. The fact the differences in activity were greatest with the lightest inocula tested and relatively minimal with heavy inocula would suggest the possibility that pirbenicillin might be less stable to β-lactamase produced by pseudomonas. However, only minimal differences in rates of hydrolysis of these three antibiotics were noted with pseudomonas β-lactamase, indicating this is not the reason for the inoculum-related differences in relative activities.

The fact that the relative activities of the β-lactamases obtained from strains 11 and 16 (Tables 1 and 2) were the same, whether observed

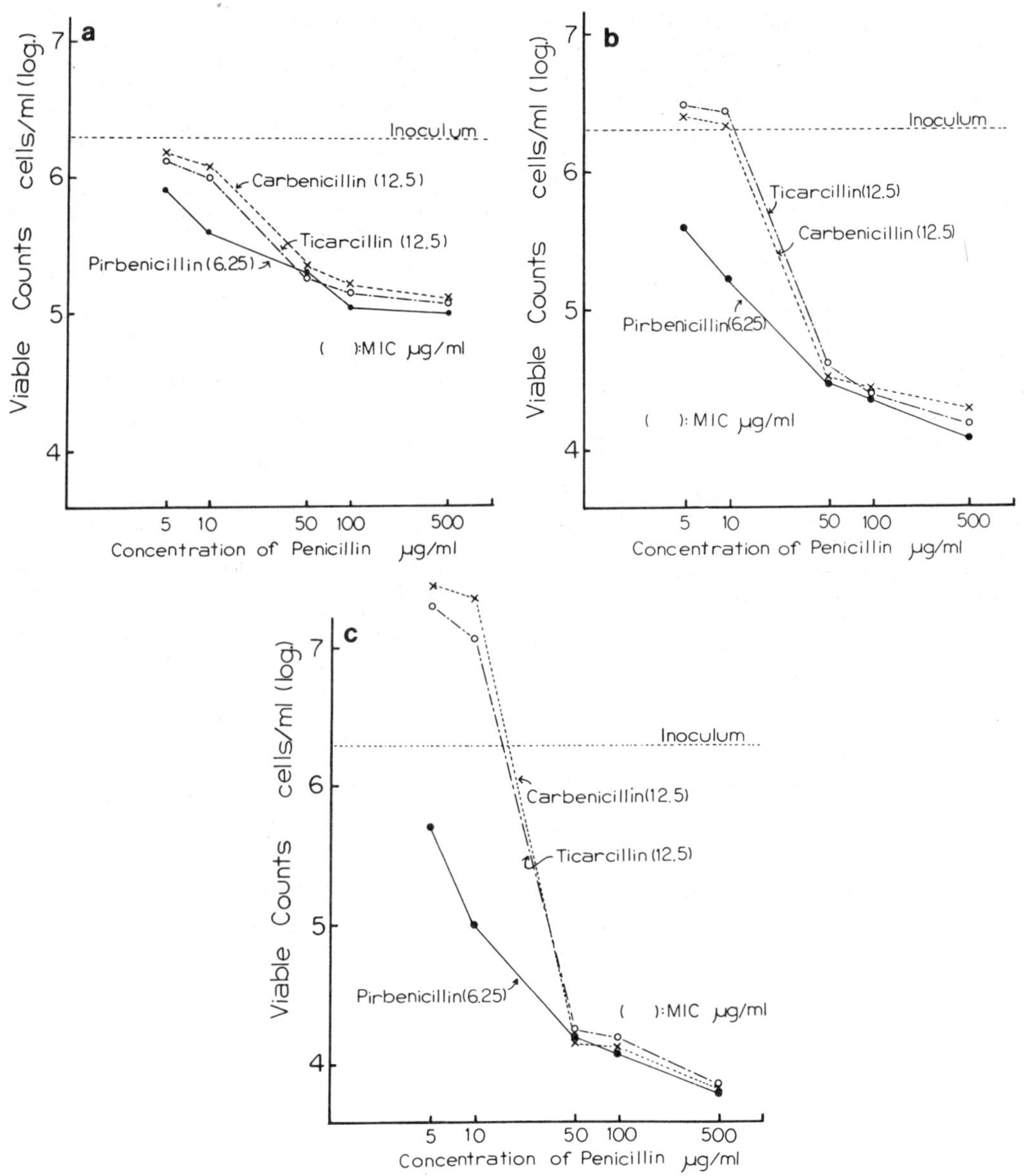

FIG. 5a-c. *Effect of concentration of three penicillins on viable counts of P. aeruginosa 16 at 2 h (a), 4 h (b), and 6 h (c) in Trypticase soy broth.*

in culture supernatants (Table 1) or in sonic extracts of cell suspension (Table 2), indicates the cell-associated and extracellular enzymes in each case are probably the same. This identity of activity of extracellular and cell-associated β-lactamase activity has been reported previously (11).

The fact that pirbenicillin was considerably more active at pH 6 than the other two antibiotics tested would suggest that in acid environments (e.g., foci of infection) this compound might be more active against *P. aeruginosa* than the other two compounds. Obviously, this would have to be studied in experimental infections.

The differences in the rates of killing at the lowest antibiotic concentrations tested most likely reflect the fact that pirbenicillin had a lower MIC (6.25 µg/ml) for this strain than did ticarcillin and carbenicillin (both 12.5 µg/ml). The fact that even a 10-fold increase in antibiotic concentration (to 500 µg/ml) did not decrease the killing rate indicates that no "paradoxic effect" could be demonstrated with this *P. aeruginosa*. This is in sharp contrast to the early observations of Kirby (8), Eriksen (5), and Eagle and Musselman (4), who noted with *Staphylococcus aureus* that increasing the benzylpenicillin concentration above the MIC decreased the rate of killing.

A potential clinical usefulness for pirbenicillin seems possible in view of some of the findings reported here. Certainly *P. aeruginosa* accounts for a large proportion of gram-negative infections, perhaps 10 to 15% of them (1, 3, 6). Carbenicillin, the first semisynthetic penicillin with significant activity against *P. aeruginosa* (10), has been widely used in this country. The high doses (often to 30 g/day) used have probably been responsible for some of the adverse effects noted: sodium overload, bleeding diatheses, and hypokalemia (2, 7, 9). It seems reasonable that a semisynthetic penicillin with greater activity than carbenicillin might be efficacious in lower doses and thus might be so used with fewer of these untoward effects. The in vitro activity of pirbenicillin demonstrated here raises the possibility that it might be such a compound.

ACKNOWLEDGMENTS

This work was supported in part by a grant from Pfizer, Inc. We thank Dianne Welter for technical assistance, and the suppliers mentioned for gifts of antibiotics.

LITERATURE CITED

1. **Altemeier, W. A., J. C. Todd, and W. W. Inge.** 1967. Gram-negative septicemia: a growing threat. Ann. Surg. 166:530–542.
2. **Brown, C. H., E. A. Natelson, W. Bradshaw, T. W. Williams, and C. P. Alfrey.** 1974. The hemostatic defect produced by carbenicillin. N. Engl. J. Med. 291:265–270.
3. **Dupont, H. L., and W. W. Spink.** 1969. Infection due to gram-negative organisms; an analysis of 860 patients with bacteremia at the University of Minnesota Medical Center, 1958–1966. Medicine 48:307–332.
4. **Eagle, H., and A. D. Musselman.** 1948. The rate of bactericidal action of penicillin *in vitro* as a function of its concentration, and its paradoxically reduced activity at high concentrations against certain organisms. J. Exp. Med. 88:99–131.
5. **Eriksen, K. R.** 1946. Some studies on the lytic action of penicillin on staphylococci and pneumococci. Acta Pathol. Microbiol. Scand. 23:221–228.
6. **Freid, M. A., and K. L. Vosti.** 1968. The importance of underlying disease in patients with gram-negative bacteria. Arch. Intern. Med. 73:179–187.
7. **Hoffman, T. A., and W. E. Bullock.** 1970. Carbenicillin therapy of pseudomonas and other gram-negative bacillary infections. Ann. Intern. Med. 73:178–187.
8. **Kirby, W. M. M.** 1945. Bacteriostatic and lytic actions of penicillin on sensitive and resistant staphylococci. J. Clin. Invest. 24:165–169.
9. **Klastersky, J., B. Vanderkelen, D. Daneau, and M. Mathieu.** 1973. Carbenicillin and hypokalemia. Ann. Intern. Med. 78:774–775.

9a. **Retsema, J. A., A. R. English, and J. E. Lynch.** 1976. Laboratory studies with a new broad-spectrum penicillin, pirbenicillin. Antimicrob. Agents Chemother. 9:975–982.

10. **Rolinson, G. N., and R. Sutherland.** 1968. Carbenicillin, a new semisynthetic penicillin active against *Pseudomonas aeruginosa*, p. 608–613. Antimicrob. Agents Chemother. 1967.
11. **Sabath, L. D., M. Jago, and E. P. Abraham.** 1965. Cephalosporinase and penicillinase activities of a β-lactamase from *Pseudomonas pyocyanea*. Biochem. J. 96:739–752.
12. **Steers, E., E. L. Foltz, and B. S. Graves.** 1959. Inocula replicating apparatus for routine testing of bacterial susceptibility to antibiotics. Antibiot. Chemother. 9:307–311.

ANTIMICROBIAL AGENTS AND CHEMOTHERAPY, Jan. 1977, p. 7-12 Vol. 11, No. 1

Susceptibility of Three Groups of *Staphylococcus aureus* to Newer Antimicrobial Agents

GEORGE W. JORDAN* AND PAUL D. HOEPRICH

Section of Infectious and Immunologic Diseases, Sacramento Medical Center, University of California at Davis, Davis, California 95616

Received for publication 27 May 1976

Because of the need for non-β-lactam antimicrobics with antistaphylococcal activity, 14 antimicrobics (3 penicillinase-resistant penicillins, 7 aminocyclitols [5 new], 2 macrolides [1 new], clindamycin, and a new polysaccharide, everninomicin) were tested in vitro for activity against 22 penicillin-susceptible, 51 penicillin-resistant, and 47 methicillin-resistant strains of *Staphylococcus aureus*. Gentamicin, tobramycin, sisomicin, and verdamicin inhibited almost all strains at concentrations less than 1 μg/ml. The methicillin-resistant strains were as susceptible as other strains to the aminocyclitols and everninomicin. In contrast, many of the methicillin-resistant strains were also resistant to erythromycin, rosamicin, and clindamycin at attainable serum concentrations. The use of the bacterial synthetic amino acid medium, in comparison with Mueller-Hinton broth, resulted in an increase in the observed resistance of methicillin-resistant strains to the penicillinase-resistant semisynthetic penicillins.

INTRODUCTION

The antistaphylococcal capability of non-β-lactam antimicrobics is of importance for several reasons. First, methicillin-resistant (MR) staphylococci have been isolated in the United States and Europe in association with hospital- and community-acquired infections (1, 3, 4, 8, 9; M. B. DiCostanzo, T. J. Bird, and H. G. Grieble, Abstr. Annu. Meet. Am. Soc. Microbiol. 1976, A15, p. 3; S. L. Krause, S. A. Pappas, P. R. Bey, R. Dorger, T. J. Bird, and H. G. Grieble, Abstr. Annu. Meet. Am. Soc. Microbiol. 1976, C137, p. 48). Second, allergy to the β-lactam drugs may proscribe their use. Third, in patients with compromised cellular defenses or certain infections, such as endocarditis, enhanced bactericidal action resulting from synergy between two different antimicrobics may be desirable. Therefore, 14 antimicrobics (3 penicillinase-resistant [PR] penicillins, 7 aminocyclitols [5 new], 2 macrolides [1 new], clindamycin, and a new polysaccharide) were tested in vitro for activity against 22 penicillin-susceptible (PS), 51 PR, and 47 MR strains of *Staphylococcus aureus*.

Antimicrobic susceptibility of some bacteria may be influenced by the concentration of divalent cations in the test medium (5, 10, 11). Furthermore, the divalent cation concentration of commercial Mueller-Hinton broth (MHB) may vary by batch and manufacturer (11). A totally defined medium, such as the bacterial synthetic amino acid medium (SAAMB), may be advantageous for antimicrobial susceptibility testing because the concentration of all components is constant and protein and other antagonists of antimicrobial agents are absent (6). Before a defined medium could be considered for routine susceptibility testing, it must be shown to perform well with commonly isolated bacteria in comparison with other media. We have compared the results of susceptibility testing performed in MHB and SAAMB.

MATERIALS AND METHODS

Bacteria. PS and PR strains of *S. aureus* were isolated from specimens submitted to the Clinical Microbiology Laboratory, University of California (Davis)-Sacramento Medical Center. MR strains were collected from the United States and Europe (7). All strains gave a positive reaction for coagulase, catalase, and heat-stable nuclease. Strains giving a zone of inhibition of 9 mm or less when tested on Mueller-Hinton agar against a 5-μg methicillin disk at 35°C using the Bauer-Kirby method (2) were defined as MR strains. A capillary tube penicillinase test was used to distinguish PS from PR strains. For storage, the cultures were suspended in skim milk and lyophilized.

Culture mediums. MHB was purchased from Difco Laboratories, Detroit, Mich. SAAMB, as modified from the formula originally reported (6), was purchased from the Grand Island Biological Co., Grand Island, N.Y. The composition of modified SAAMB is given in Table 1.

Antimicrobics. Nafcillin (obtained from Wyeth

TABLE 1. *Synthetic amino acid medium (SAAM)*[a]

Medium	Ingredients (g/liter)	
SAAM base	L-Arginine	1.05
	L-Lysine	0.58
	L-Histidine	0.31
	L-Tyrosine	0.36
	L-Tryptophane	0.10
	L-Phenylalanine	0.32
	L-Cystine	2.24
	L-Methionine	0.15
	LThreonine	0.48
	L-Leucine	0.52
	L-Isoleucine	0.52
	L-Valine	0.46
	L-Proline	1.00
	Glycine	0.50
	L-Glutamine	2.52
	L-Asparagine	1.00
	D-Glucose	1.00
	Fumaric acid	1.50
	Sodium pyruvate	1.00
	Ammonium acetate	0.50
	$K_2HPO_4 \cdot 3H_2O$	0.50
	MOPS[b]	16.45
	Tris[c]	10.45
	Biotin	0.0005
	Folic acid	0.005
	Choline chloride	0.025
	Nicotinamide	0.005
	D-Calcium pentothenate	0.025
	Pyridoxal-HCl	0.005
	Thiamine-HCl	0.005
	Riboflavin	0.005
	i-inositol	0.025
	$MgCl_2$ anhydrous	0.09535
	$FeCl_3 \cdot 6H_2O$	0.00270
	$ZnSO_4 \cdot 7H_2O$	0.00080
	$MnSO_4 \cdot 4H_2O$	0.00036
	$CaCl_2$ anhydrous	0.00557
	Phenol red	0.0020
SAAMB	SAAM base plus:	
	uracil	0.025
	adenine	0.025
SAAMF	SAAM base plus:	
	glucose	19.0

[a] Available in any one of the three forms from GIBCO, P.O. Box 4385, Madison, WI 53711.

[b] MOPS, Morpholinopropane sulfonic acid.

[c] Tris, Tris(hydroxymethyl)aminomethane.

Laboratories, George Warren), oxacillin, and methicillin (Bristol Laboratories, Paul Jones) were dissolved in sterile distilled water.

Amikacin (Bristol Laboratories, Paul Jones), gentamicin B, gentamicin C_1, C_2, and C_{1a} (hereafter labeled gentamicin as this mixture is the gentamicin in clinical use), sisomicin, verdamicin (Schering Corp., George Arcieri), and tobramycin (Eli Lilly & Co., R. S. Griffiths) were weighed and dissolved in sterile distilled water. Erythromycin (Eli Lilly & Co., R. S. Griffiths), everninomicin, and rosamicin (Schering Corp., George Arcieri) were first dissolved in 10% methanol; subsequent dilutions were made in sterile distilled water. Clindamycin (Upjohn Co., George Whitfield) was dissolved in sterile distilled water. Stock solutions of all antimicrobics were prepared eight times more concentrated than required for the highest test concentration.

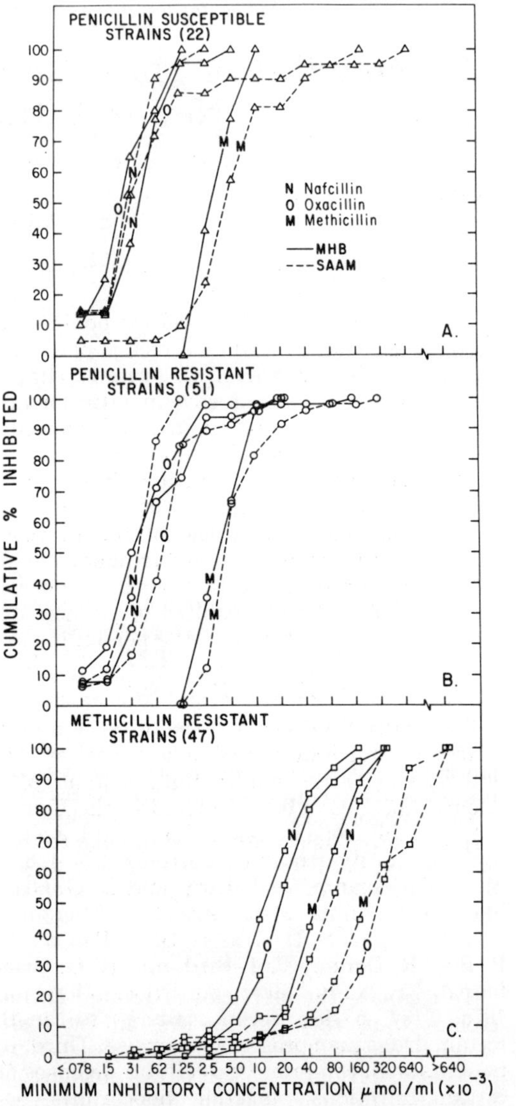

FIG. 1. *Activity of three penicillinase-resistant penicillins against S. aureus. Susceptibility testing was performed in MHB or SAAMB.*

TABLE 2. *Molecular weights and attainable serum concentrations of antimicrobics*

Antimicrobic	Mol wt		Concn attainable in serum	
	Free base or acid	Salt	μg/ml	μmol/ml
Nafcillin	414	436 (Na)	50–100	0.115–0.229
Oxacillin	401	423 (Na)	50–100	0.118–0.236
Methicillin	380	402 (Na)	100–200	0.249–0.498
Amikacin	586	782 ($2^1/_2$ H_2SO_4)	15–25	0.0192–0.0320
Gentamicin B	482	678 (2 H_2SO_4)	3–10	0.00442–0.0147
Gentamicin C_1	478	723 ($2^1/_2$ H_2SO_4)	3–10	0.00415–0.0138
Gentamicin $C_1C_2C_{1a}$	464	709 ($2^1/_2$ H_2SO_4)	3–10	0.00423–0.0141
Sisomicin	448	693 ($2^1/_2$ H_2SO_4)	3–10	0.00433–0.0144
Tobramycin	468	713 ($2^1/_2$ H_2SO_4)	3–10	0.00421–0.0140
Verdamcin	461	702 ($2^1/_2$ H_2SO_4)	3–10	0.00427–0.0142
Erythromycin	734		1–2	0.00136–0.00272
Rosamicin	581		0.5–1	0.000860–0.00172
Clindamycin	441	487 (HCl)	5–20	0.0103–0.0411
Everninomicin	1,553	1,575 (Na)	2–5[a]	0.00127–0.00317[a]

[a] Probably attainable.

Procedure. Twofold dilutions of the antimicrobics were made either in MHB or SAAMB in plastic trays using the Autotiter IV (Canalco, Rockville, N.J.). The loaded trays, containing 0.10 ml/well, were kept at −20°C for 24 to 48 h prior to use.

After overnight growth on sheep blood agar, brain heart infusion broth was inoculated with 10 to 15 colonies. After 5 to 6 h of incubation at 35°C, the cultures were diluted 1:100 in sterile distilled water to provide inocula. One microliter of inoculum (approximately 10^5 bacteria) was added to each well. A row of inoculum controls was included on each plate. After incubation at 35°C for 48 h, the plates were inspected using light transmitted through the base of the plates. The lowest concentration of antimicrobic that resulted in no visible growth was taken as the minimal inhibitory concentration.

RESULTS

To compare the activities of related antimicrobics that vary up to 13% in molecular weight, the results have been expressed as molar concentrations. The salt of the antimicrobic used and the concentration attainable in the serum, expressed in micromoles per milliliter and micrograms per milliliter, are given in Table 2.

Nafcillin and oxacillin were equally active against PS and PR strains (Fig. 1A and B). As previously shown (7), methicillin was the least active. Good agreement was obtained against the three penicillins between the results of testing PS and PR strains, in MHB and SAAMB. In contrast, the three β-lactamase-resistant penicillins were significantly less active against the MR strains in accordance with the disk susceptibility test results (Fig. 1C). The increased resistance of MR strains was more apparent when SAAMB was used as the culture medium.

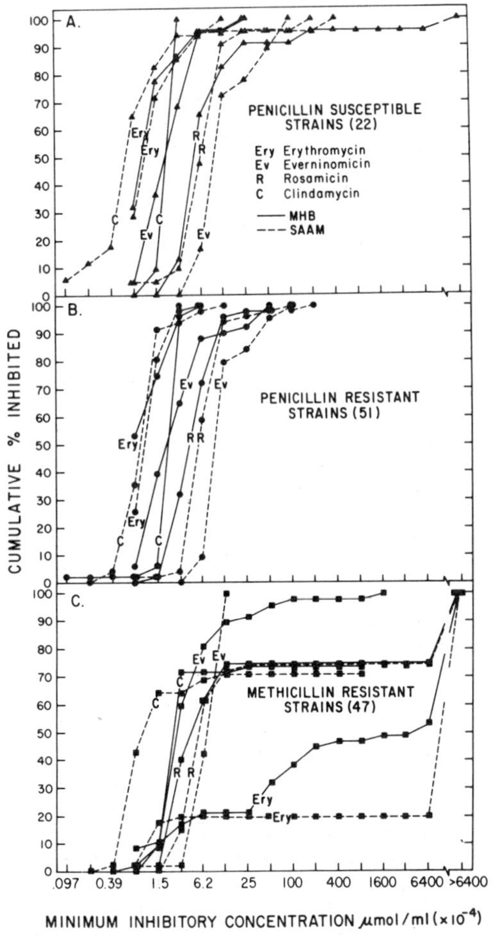

FIG. 2. *Activity of erythromycin, rosamicin, clindamycin, and everninomicin against S. aureus. Susceptibility tests were performed in MHB or SAAMB.*

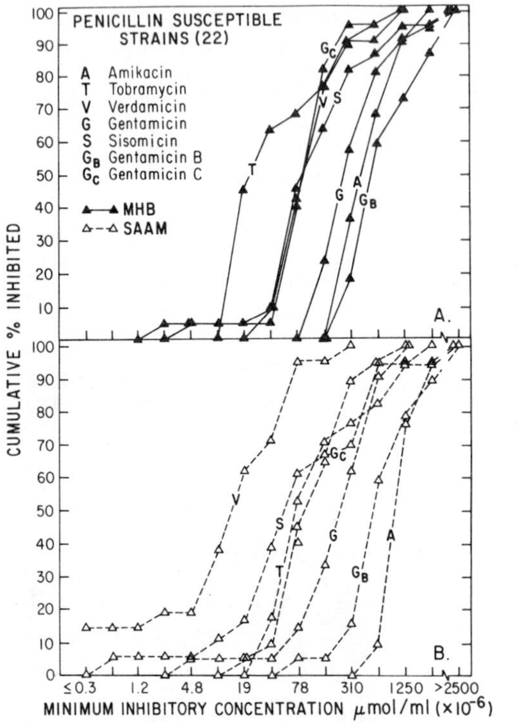

FIG. 3. *Activity of seven aminocyclitols (amikacin, tobramycin, verdamicin, gentamicin, sisomicin, gentamicin B, and gentamicin C) against 22 strains of PS S. aureus. Susceptibility tests were performed in MHB or SAAMB.*

Both PS and PR strains were comparably susceptible to erythromycin, everninomicin, rosamicin, and clindamycin (Fig. 2A and B). MR strains were equally susceptible to everninomicin; however, approximately 25% of MR strains were resistant to rosamicin and clindamycin, whereas 80% were resistant to erythromycin (Fig. 2C). Susceptibility testing in MHB and SAAMB gave similar results for rosamicin and erythromycin, except erythromycin resistance was more sharply defined in SAAMB (Fig. 2). Staphylococci appeared to be more susceptible to clindamycin but less susceptible to everninomicin when tested in SAAMB (Fig. 2).

The aminocyclitols were as active against PR as they were against MR staphylococci (Fig. 3 to 5). In descending order of antistaphylococcal activity on a molar basis they were: verdamicin, tobramycin, sisomicin, gentamicin C, gentamicin, gentamicin B, and amikacin. In MHB, approximately 10% of all staphylococci (Fig. 3 to 5) were resistant to the highest concentration of gentamicin B and amikacin, whereas 20% of MR strains demonstrated resistance to these two antimicrobics when tested in SAAMB (Fig. 5). In comparing the results obtained in MHB and SAAMB, verdamicin susceptibility was increased, whereas susceptibility to amikacin was decreased when tested in SAAMB (Fig. 3 to 5).

DISCUSSION

S. aureus strains that are resistant to the PR penicillins have been observed in several European countries, especially Denmark (8) and Switzerland (9). Such strains have also been encountered in the United States (11). MR staphylococci continue to be observed as causes of serious staphylococcal sepsis, particularly in a hospital environment (4; DiCostanzo et al., Abstr. Annu. Meet. Am. Soc. Microbiol. 1976, A15, p.3; Krause et al., Abstr. Annu. Meet. Am. Soc. Microbiol. 1976, C137, p. 48). The MR strains used in the present study were collected from the United States and Europe and were isolated from blood, cerebrospinal fluid, sputum, and pus from abscesses. Other associated diseases included osteomyelitis, septic arthritis, parotitis, and necrosis of the skin.

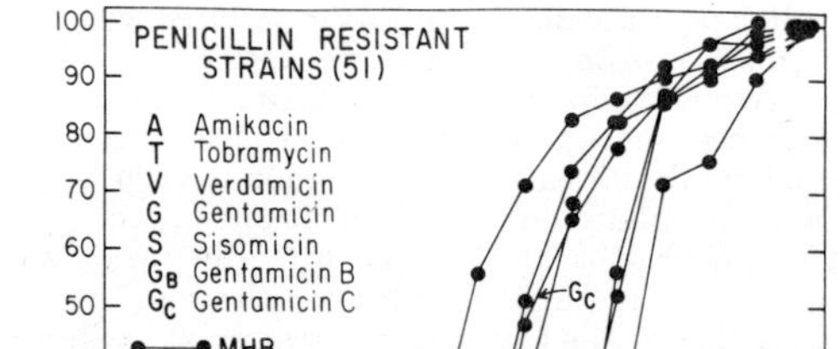

FIG. 4. *Activity of seven aminocyclitols (amikacin, tobramycin, verdamicin, gentamicin, sisomicin, gentamicin B, and gentamicin C) against 51 strains of PR S. aureus. Susceptibility tests were performed in MHB or SAAMB.*

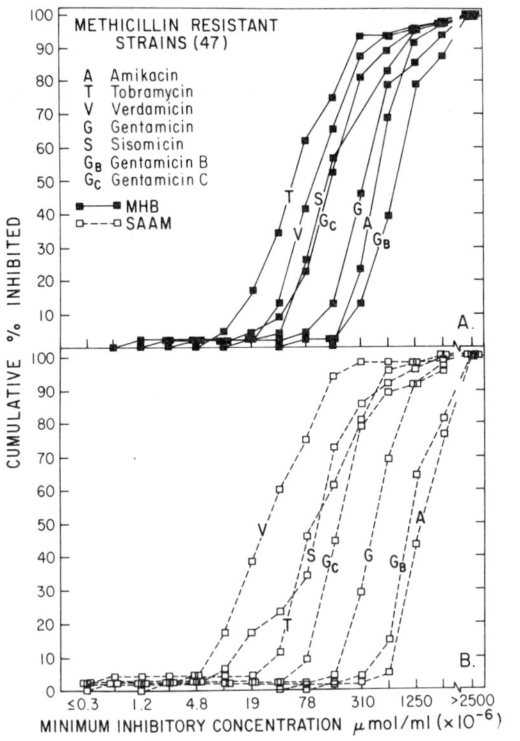

FIG. 5. *Activity of seven aminocyclitols (amikacin, tobramycin, verdamicin, gentamicin, sisomicin, gentamicin B, and gentamicin C) against 47 strains of MR S. aureus. Susceptibility tests were performed in MHB or SAAMB.*

All of the aminocyclitols tested were active against PS, PR, and MR strains of *S. aureus* at concentrations achievable in serum (Table 2). Gentamicin, tobramycin, sisomicin, and verdamicin inhibited almost all strains at concentrations less than 1 μg/ml, an easily attainable and nontoxic concentration. The minimal inhibitory concentrations were virtually the same for the MR strains. A significant number of strains were resistant to amikacin and gentamicin B. The new polysaccharide antimicrobic everninomicin also appeared to be equally active against PS, PR, and MR strains. In contrast, many of the MR strains were resistant to erythromycin, rosamicin, and clindamycin at concentrations attainable in the serum.

The use of the totally defined medium SAAMB may have certain advantages over undefined media. Although the concentration of divalent cations is critically important to the activity of the aminocyclitols against certain gram-negative bacteria (10), antistaphylococcal activity is not known to be similarly affected. The differences in the dose-response curves for verdamicin and amikacin (Fig. 3 to 5) and for clindamycin and everninomycin (Fig. 2), according to the medium of testing, may be the result of differences in the concentration of divalent cations or other components. The use of SAAMB caused an accentuation of the resistance of the MR strains to the PR semisynthetic penicillins (Fig. 1C) and resulted in a sharply defined level of erythromycin resistance (Fig. 2C). The use of SAAMB also avoids the problem of variation between different batches or different suppliers that is inherent in undefined media and does affect the results of susceptibility tests with some bacteria (11).

It appears that the newer aminocyclitols, gentamicin, tobramycin, verdamicin, and sisomycin, and the polysaccharide antimicrobic everninomicin are active against MR strains of *S. aureus* in concentrations relevant to therapeutics. In contrast, from 25 to 80% of MR strains were resistant to erythromycin, rosamicin, and clindamycin, necessitating susceptibility testing before using these antimicrobics against these strains of *S. aureus*.

ACKNOWLEDGMENTS

This research was supported by Public Health Service research grant AI 08955-07 from the National Institute of Allergy and Infectious Diseases and grants-in-aid from Eli Lilly & Co. and Schering Corp.

We are grateful to Lee Effinger for expert technical assistance.

LITERATURE CITED

1. **Barrett, F. F., R. F. McGehee, and M. Finland.** 1968. Methicillin-resistant *Staphylococcus aureus* at Boston City Hospital: bacteriologic and epidemiologic observations. N. Engl. J. Med. **279**:441–448.
2. **Bauer, A. W., W. M. Kirby, J. C. Sherris, and M. Turck.** 1966. Antibiotic susceptibility testing by a standardized single disc method. Am. J. Clin. Pathol. **45**:493–496.
3. **Benner, E. J., and V. Morthland.** 1967. Methicillin-resistant *Staphylococcus aureus*: antimicrobial susceptibility. N. Engl. J. Med. **277**:678–680.
4. **Blackwell, C. C., and D. S. Feingold.** 1975. Frequency and some properties of clinical isolates of methicillin-resistant *Staphylococcus aureus*. Am. J. Clin. Pathol. **64**:372–377.
5. **D'Amato, R. F., C. Thornsberry, C. N. Baker, and L. A. Kirven.** 1975. Effect of calcium and magnesium ions on the susceptibility of *Pseudomonas* species to tetracycline, gentamicin, polymyxin B, and carbenicillin. Antimicrob. Agents Chemother. **7**:596–600.
6. **Hoeprich, P. D., A. L. Barry, and G. D. Fay.** 1971. Synthetic medium for susceptibility testing, p. 494–497. Antimicrob. Agents Chemother. 1970.
7. **Hoeprich, P. D., E. J. Benner, and F. H. Kayser.** 1970. Susceptibility of methicillin-resistant *Staphylococcus aureus* to 12 antimicrobial agents, p. 104–110. Antimicrob. Agents Chemother. 1969.
8. **Jessen, O., K. Rosendal, P. Bulow, V. Faber, and K. R. Eriksen.** 1969. Changing staphylococci and staphylococcal infections. N. Engl. J. Med. **281**:627–635.

9. **Kayser, F. H., and A. Hollinger.** 1968. Methicillin resistente Staphylokokken. Bakteriologie, Klinik, und Epidemiologie. Dtsch. Med. Wochenschr. 93:1933–1937.

10. **Medeiros, A. A., T. F. O'Brien, W. E. C. Wacker, and N. J. Yulug.** 1971. Effect of salt concentration on the apparent *in vitro* susceptibility of *Pseudomonas* and other gram-negative bacilli to gentamicin. J. Infect. Dis. 124(Suppl.):559–564.

11. **Reller, L. B., F. O. Schoenknecht, M. A. Kenny, and J. C. Sherris.** 1974. Antibiotic susceptibility testing of *Pseudomonas aeruginosa*: selection of a control strain and criteria for magnesium and calcium content in media. J. Infect. Dis. 130:454–463.

ANTIMICROBIAL AGENTS AND CHEMOTHERAPY, Jan. 1977, p. 13-20 Vol. 11, No. 1

Temperature-Sensitive R Plasmid Obtained from Naturally Isolated Drug-Resistant *Vibrio cholerae* (Biotype El Tor)

TAKESHI YOKOTA* AND SHOGO KUWAHARA

Department of Bacteriology, School of Medicine, Juntendo University, Tokyo 113, and Department of Microbiology, School of Medicine, Toho University, Tokyo 143, Japan*

Received for publication 13 August 1976

A temperature-sensitive fi^- R plasmid, pJY1, which confers resistance to chloramphenicol, streptomycin, and sulfonamide, was found in a drug-resistant strain of *Vibrio cholerae* (biotype El Tor) isolated in the Philippines in 1973. The R plasmid is temperature sensitive for transferability but not for stability in the hosts. pJY1 is stably maintained either in *V. cholerae* or in *Escherichia coli* at a range of culture temperatures from 27 to 42°C. Compatibility tests with reference R plasmids revealed that pJY1 belongs to the J group. Growth of *V. cholerae* carrying pJY1 is poor on TCBS (thiosulfate-citrate-bile-sucrose) selective plates when the microbe is subcultured in nutrient broth at temperatures higher than 37°C.

It is known that R plasmids can be transferred between various species of gram-negative rods. In 1963, soon after the discovery of a transferable drug resistance factor(1), Goto and Kuwahara (4) reported that R plasmids were successfully transmitted from *Shigella flexneri* to *Vibrio cholerae* (both classical and El Tor biotypes), although most were unstable in the latter microbe. Prescott et al. (12) and Goto and Kuwahara (4) also published papers dealing with the discovery of transferable R plasmids in multiply drug-resistant *V. cholerae* isolated in Calcutta, India, in 1967 and in Manila, Philippines, in 1964–1965, respectively.

Conjugative R plasmids, however, were so unstable even in the natural host vibrios that the original strain, *V. cholerae* D226-R, had lost the drug resistance as early as 1 year after the isolation (4).

Owing to the instability of conjugative R plasmids in vibrios, some confusion occurred in the following years. Yamada et al. (16) failed to confirm tranmission of R plasmids from *Escherichia coli* to *V. cholerae,* and they could not succeed in transfer experiments of drug resistance from nine multiply drug-resistant strains of *V. cholerae,* isolated in Manila in 1969 by Kobari et al. (7), to *E. coli* strains.

We (19) reconfirmed successful transfer of R plasmids from *E. coli* to *V. cholerae* and revealed that a temperature-sensitive kanamycin resistance factor, Rts1(15), could be stably maintained in *V. cholerae* at low temperatures.

This paper deals with a new, temperature-sensitive R plasmid found in a multiply drug-resistant strain of *V. cholerae* (biotype El Tor) isolated in Manila in 1973.

MATERIALS AND METHODS

Bacteria. Sixty strains of *V. cholerae* (biotype El Tor) were isolated in Manila in 1973 from patients with cholera and were provided by H. Kitamura, Kawasaki Quarantine Station, Kawasaki, Japan. Thirty-nine strains of *V. cholerae* were isolated in Calcutta in 1973 by one of the authors and D. B. Chatterjee, School of Tropical Medicine, Calcutta, India. Nine multiply drug-resistant strains of *V cholerae* isolated by Kobari et al. (7) in Manila in 1969 were given by C. Yamada, National Institute of Health, Tokyo, Japan. Derivatives of *E. coli* K-12 used for genetic analysis are listed in Table 1.

Media. L broth(11) was used as the liquid medium. TCBS(thiosulfate-citrate-bile-sucrose) agar (2) (Oxoid Ltd., London, England), sensitivity disk agar (Eiken Chemical Co. Ltd., Tokyo, Japan), Wellcotest sensitivity agar (Wellcome Foundation, London, England), and minimal eosin methylene blue agar (9) containing 1% lactose or glucose as the sole carbon source were used as plating media. For selection of certain auxotrophic *E. coli,* eosin methylene blue agar was supplemented with the appropriate vitamins and amino acids.

Chemicals. Crystalline powdered tetracycline (TC), sulfamethoxazole (SMX), and nalidixic acid (NAL) were gifts from Japan Lederle Co. (Tokyo), Shionogi Pharmaceutical Co. Ltd. (Osaka), and Daiichi Pharmaceutical Co. Ltd. (Tokyo), respectively. Commercially available chloramphenicol (CM; Sankyo Pharmaceutical Co. Ltd., Tokyo), streptomycin sulfate (SM; Meiji Seika Co., Tokyo), kanamycin sulfate (KM; Shionogi), cephaloridine (Shionogi), and aminobenzylpenicillin (ABPC;

Toyama Chemical Co. Ltd., Toyama) were also used.

Method for sensitivity test of *V. cholerae*. All strains of *V. cholerae* were kept as stab cultures in twice-diluted semisolid agar at room temperatures. The microbes were repurified on TCBS agar plates just before the experiment and subcultured in L broth at 37°C, with shaking, overnight. The cultures were diluted 100-fold with sterile saline, and one-loopful portions of the samples were streaked on sensitivity disk agar plates containing serially increasing amounts of antibiotics. The minimal growth inhibitory concentration (MIC) of each antibiotic was determined 24 h after incubation at 37°C. For examination of the MIC of sulfamethoxazole, Wellcotest sensitivity test agar was substituted for sensitivity disk agar.

Method for transfer of conjugative R plasmids. One milliliter of an overnight culture in L broth of a NAL-resistant mutant of *E. coli* CSH2 was mixed with 4 ml of fresh L broth and 0.1 ml of an overnight culture of each of 14 multiply drug-resistant strains of *V. cholerae,* including A27, B27, B28, C21, C22, C24, C28, D11, and H1 (isolated in 1969) and 189, 191, 199, 204, and I-13 (isolated in 1973) (Table 2). The mixed cultures were incubated at 27 and 37°C overnight with shaking, and samples of 0.1 ml were spread, after appropriate dilution, on MacConkey agar plates containing 100 μg of NAL and 10 μg of CM or TC per ml. The plates were incubated at 37°C overnight, and the number of colonies appearing on the plates was scored as the fraction of the NAL-resistant recipient clone inheriting R plasmids. The secondary transfer of R plasmids was performed from *E. coli* CSH2(R^+) to *E. coli* AB1157, using MacConkey agar plates containing 1,000 μg of SM and 10 μg of CM or TC per ml as the selective medium. The influence of culture temperatures and pH on the transfer frequency of R plasmids was investigated by incubation of the mixed cultures at 27, 32, 37, 40, or 42°C in a Monod multishaker(Taiyo Science Industry Co. Ltd., Tokyo), consisting of five water baths which can be adjusted to different temperatures, and using L broths adjusted to pH 6.0, 6.5, 7.0, 7.5, or 8.0.

Method for examination of stability of R plasmids. Strains of *V. cholerae* and *E. coli* bearing R plasmids were cultured in L broth containing antibiotics in concentrations inhibitory to R^- strains, but not to R^+ bacteria, at 27°C overnight. The cells were harvested by centrifugation and resuspended in the same volume of fresh L broth, followed by a 10^6-fold dilution. Samples of 0.1 ml of the diluted culture were inoculated into three tubes, each con-

TABLE 1. *List of E. coli K-12 substrains used for genetical analysis*

Strain	Genotype	Plasmid	Reference
CSH2	*metB*	F^-, R^-	2
CSH2 ($R100^+$)	*metB*	F^-, R100 *tet cat aadA sul tra*$^+$	19
CSH2 ($Rts1^+$)	*metB*	F^-, Rts1 *aphA* (*kan*)	15
CSH2 ($YR5^+$)	*metB*	F^-, YR5 *aphA* (*kan*)	17
CSH2 *nal*	*metB nal*$^+$	F^-, R^-	
AB1157	*thi argE thr leu proC his str ara lac gal mtl xyl*	F^-, R^-	2
20SO	*lac str sul azi*	F^-, R^-	2
HfrR1	*metB*	(F)Hfr	2
J53	*pro met*	F^-, R^+ (reference R plasmids)	5

TABLE 2. *List of V. cholerae strains used for the R plasmid transfer experiment*

Strain	MIC (μg/ml) of:				Isolation	
	CM	TC	SM	SMX	Place	Year
A27	50.0	0.39	1,000	>1,000	Philippines	1969
B27	25.0	0.39	500	500	Philippines	1969
B28	50.0	0.39	1,000	>1,000	Philippines	1969
C21	25.0	12.5	500	>1,000	Philippines	1969
C22	50.0	0.78	500	1,000	Philippines	1969
C24	25.0	25.0	100	500	Philippines	1969
C28	25.0	0.39	500	500	Philippines	1969
D11	25.0	0.2	500	500	Philippines	1969
H1	25.0	0.39	500	500	Philippines	1969
189	6.25	50.0	1,000	>1,000	Philippines	1973
191	3.13	0.78	25	>1,000	Philippines	1973
199	3.13	100.0	100	>1,000	Philippines	1973
204	12.5	0.2	40,000	>1,000	Philippines	1973
I-13	3.13	0.78	250	>1,000	Philippines	1973
E2	0.2	0.1	6.25	1.56	Philippines	1964

taining 5 ml of drug-free L broth, followed by incubation at 27, 37, and 42°C overnight with shaking. After streaking one-loopful samples of the cultures on drug-free MacConkey agar plates, they were again diluted 10^6-fold and inoculated into secondary subcultures. This procedure was repeated for 10 subcultures, and the proportion of the cells retaining R plasmids compared to the total viable number was scored by the replica-plating method (8) at each subculture step and at each culture temperature.

Compatibility test of R plasmids. Strains of *E. coli* J53 carrying reference R plasmids were provided by Y. Terawaki, Department of Bacteriology, School of Medicine, Shinshu University, Matsumoto, Japan, and the plasmids are listed in Table 5. Since *E. coli* J53 is susceptible to NAL, NAL-resistant *E. coli* CSH2 subclones bearing the test R plasmids were used as recipients. A 1-ml overnight culture of the recipient was mixed with a 0.1-ml overnight culture of one of the donors and 4 ml of fresh L broth, followed by incubation at 37°C (27°C for Rtsl) for 4 h with shaking. Samples of 0.1 ml of the mixed cultures were spread on MacConkey agar plates containing 100 μg of NAL and 10 μg of TC per ml, 25 μg of KM per ml, or 50 U of ABPC per ml, according to the donor markers. The plates were incubated at 37°C overnight, and transfer frequencies of reference R plasmids from the same donor were compared to *E. coli* CSH2 with and without test plasmids. Subclones of *E. coli* CSH2, which were assumed to carry both reference and test R plasmids, were purified on the same selective plates and inoculated into drug-free liquid medium. The liquid cultures were incubated at 37°C (27°C for Rtsl) overnight and subcultured successively. The secondary subcultures were streaked on drug-free MacConkey agar plates, and resistance markers of the transconjugants were examined by the replica-plating method. At least 50 colonies were checked for the presence of both plasmids by testing for the presence of their respective drug resistance markers.

When direct transfer of reference R plasmids to *E. coli* CSH2 could not be detected, *E. coli* AB1157 and *E. coli* 20SO carrying the test R plasmid were used as the recipients.

Fertility inhibition test. Test R plasmids were transferred from *E. coli* CSH2 to *E. coli* HfrRl, and F-mediated fertility between this strain and *E. coli* AB1157 was studied. Susceptibility of R^- and R^+ *E. coli* HfrRl to the male-specific phages Qβ, MS2, and Fl was compared by a spot test.

Method for examination of growth behavior of *V. cholerae* carrying R plasmids. *V. cholerae* bearing R plasmids were subcultured in L broth at 27, 37, and 42°C overnight with shaking, and the number of colony-forming units in the subcultures was compared by plating on nutrient agar plates and TCBS agar plates with and without one-fifth the MIC of CM.

RESULTS

Multiply drug-resistant strains of *V. cholerae* isolated in 1973. The average MICs of CM, TC, SM, and SMX to *V. cholerae* isolated in Manila (60 strains) and Calcutta (39 strains) in 1973 were 0.78, 0.2, 25.0, and 3.1 μg/ml, respectively. No multiply drug-resistant strains were found in the isolates from Calcutta; 2 of the 39 strains were moderately resistant to SMX only. However, 5 multiply drug-resistant strains were discovered among the 60 isolates from Manila. There were two CM.TC.SM.SMX-resistant strains (189 and 199), two CM.SM.SMX-resistant strains (204 and I-13), and one CM.SMX-resistant strain (191) (Table 2). *V. cholerae* E2, isolated in Manila in 1964(19) and used as a drug-susceptible (R^-) reference strain, is included in the table.

Transfer of drug resistance from *V. cholerae* to *E. coli*. Transfer of CM resistance from *V. cholerae* 204 (Cm Sm Su) to *E. coli* CSH2 *nal* was determined by mixed culture. Since 100 subclones of *E. coli* CSH2 *nal* that had received CM resistance were found to be simultaneously resistant to SM and SMX, it seemed likely that an R plasmid conferring resistance to CM, SM, and SMX was transferred from *V. cholerae* 204 (Table 3). This plasmid was designated pJY1. Retransfer of pJYl was successfully performed from *E. coli* CSH2(pJYl$^+$) to *E. coli* AB1157(F^-), *E. coli* HfrRl, or *V. cholerae* E2 (Table 3). It may be noteworthy that pJYl confers rather low resistance to CM and high resistance to SM in its host. No drug resistance transfer was found from the 13 other multiply drug-resistant strains of *V. cholerae*.

The results indicate that a conjugative R plasmid occurs only in one out of five multiply drug-resistant strains of *V. cholerae* isolated in

TABLE 3. *Resistance levels of V. cholerae and E. coli carrying and not carrying the pJY1 plasmid*

Species	Strain	Plasmid	MIC (μg/ml) of:					
			CM	TC	SM	SMX	KM	ABPC
V. cholerae	204	pJY1	12.5	0.2	40,000.0	>1,000.0	6.25	6.25
	E2	R^-	0.2	0.1	6.25	1.56	6.25	6.25
	E2	pJY1	25.0	0.1	40,000.0	>1,000.0	6.25	6.25
E. coli	CSH2	R^-	0.78	0.39	0.78	12.5	3.13	3.13
	CSH2	pJY1	100.0	0.39	500.0	>1,000.0	3.13	3.13

Manila in 1973 and in none of those isolated in 1969.

Temperature-sensitive transfer of pJYl. Transfer of pJYl became detectable 1 h after mixing the culture at 37°C and increased gradually thereafter (Fig. 1). Thus, a 4-h mixed culture was used as a standard for the subsequent experiments. The figure also shows pJYl is transferred better at 27 than 37°C.

Figure 2 indicates the influence of culture temperatures on the transfer frequency of pJYl from *V. cholerae* 204(pJYl$^+$) and *E. coli* AB1157(pJYl$^+$) to *E. coli* CSH2 *nal* or a NAL-resistant mutant of *V. cholerae* E2. In this experiment, all donors and recipients were subcultured overnight at 27°C, further incubated at the indicated temperatures after mixing, and tested for transfer frequencies of pJYl by plating on MacConkey agar or L agar containing 100 μg of NAL and 10 μg of CM per ml followed by incubation at 37°C. The highest transfer frequency was observed at 27°C, whereas no transfer at 42°C occurred with any combination of donor and recipient.

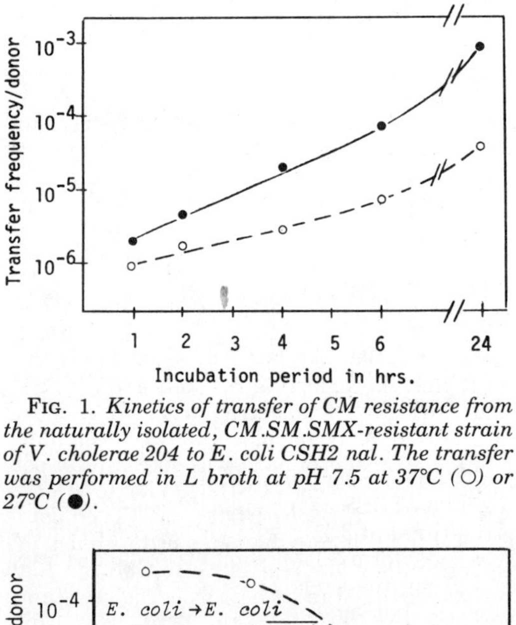

FIG. 1. *Kinetics of transfer of CM resistance from the naturally isolated, CM.SM.SMX-resistant strain of V. cholerae 204 to E. coli CSH2 nal. The transfer was performed in L broth at pH 7.5 at 37°C (○) or 27°C (●).*

The temperature-sensitive transfer of pJYl was compared with that of the known thermosensitive YR5 and non-thermosensitive R100 plasmids (Fig. 3). The optimal temperature for the transfer of ordinary R plasmids was around 40°C, although pJYl was transferred with the highest frequency at 27 to 30°C, as was observed in the case of the thermosensitive YR5 plasmid (17).

Stability of pJYl in *V. cholerae* at various temperatures. It is known that some temperature-sensitive R plasmids are thermosensitive not only in their transferability, but also in their stability in host bacteria (15, 17). Also, almost all R plasmids discovered in species of *Enterobacteriaceae* are unstable in *V. cholerae* regardless of culture temperatures, leading to rapid elimination of drug resistance from the host after several subcultures. Stability of pJYl in *V. cholerae* and *E. coli* was examined by successive subcultures from small inocula, and it was shown that the percentage of progeny containing the plasmid at all temperatures was greater than 99% in either *V. cholerae* or *E. coli*, even after 10 subcultures. Furthermore, pJYl was stably maintained in *V. cholerae* 204 and *E. coli* CSH2 after 3 years of conservation in drug-free semisolid agar.

Influence of pH on the transfer of pJYl. The pJYl plasmid was transferred better at an acidic pH than at an alkaline pH. It is interesting to note that the growth of *V. cholerae* is

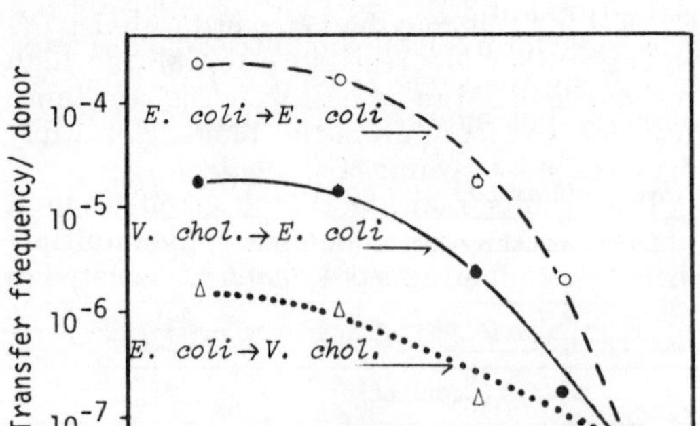

FIG. 2. *Influence of culture temperature on the transfer frequency of pJY1 between V. cholerae and E. coli. Symbols: ○, from E. coli AB1157 to E. coli CSH2 nal; ●, from V. cholerae 204 to E. coli CSH2 nal; △, E. coli AB1157 to V. cholerae E2.*

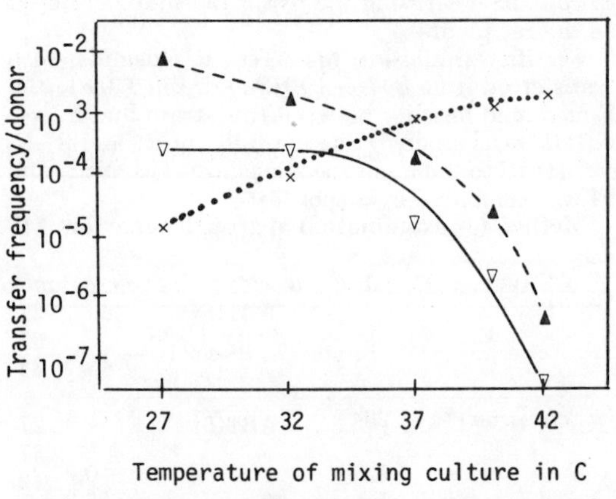

FIG. 3. *Influence of culture temperature on the transfer frequency of pJY1, YR5(ts), and R100(non-ts) plasmids from E. coli AB1157 to E. coli CSH2 nal. Symbols: ▲, YR5; ▽, pJY1; ×, R100.*

better at a slightly alkaline pH, although transfer of the R plasmid from that microbe is more efficient at acidic pH values (Fig. 4).

***fi* type of pJYl.** The frequency of F-mediated chromosomal recombination was identical whether *E. coli* HfrRl carried pJyl or not (Table 4). Furthermore, it was demonstrated that *E. coli* HfrRl carrying pJYl remained as susceptible to F-specific phages Qβ, MS2, and Fl as the R⁻ strain. These results indicate that the pJYl plasmid is of the *fi*⁻ type.

Incompatibility grouping of pJYl. Conjugative transfer of reference R plasmids belonging to FI, FIV, M, Iγ, N, O, and T groups from *E. coli* J53(R⁺) to *E. coli* CSH2 *nal* was suppressed by the presence of pJYl in the recipient strain. A small number of transconjugants, however, stably maintained both pJYl and the reference R plasmid, even after subcultures in drug-free liquid media (Table 5). It is suggested that pJYl does not belong to these groups, even though some entry exclusion was observed with them. Neither entry exclusion nor incompatibility was found between pJYl and reference R plasmids of the A, C, H, Iα, L, P, and S groups.

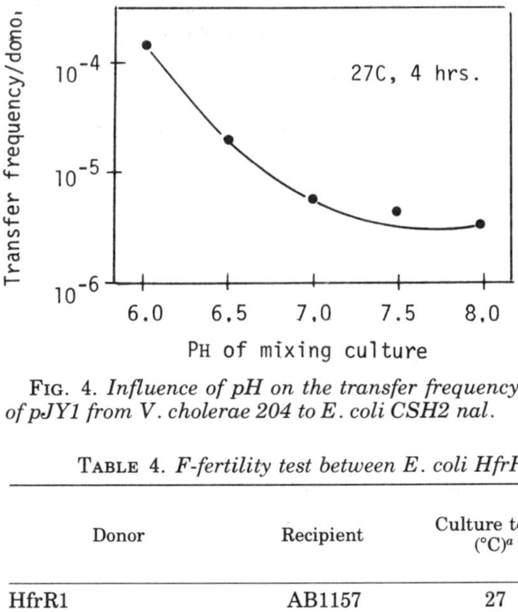

FIG. 4. *Influence of pH on the transfer frequency of pJY1 from V. cholerae 204 to E. coli CSH2 nal.*

Although transfer frequency of group J plasmids was little reduced by the presence of pJYl in the recipient bacteria, transconjugants carrying both plasmids lost either one at a frequency of 36 to 56% (Table 5). It is thus concluded that pJYl belongs to the J group.

Growth behavior of *V. cholerae* bearing pJYl. Since *V. cholerae* 204(pJYl⁺) grew sparsely on TCBS selective plates when it was inoculated from the culture in L broth at 37°C, the growth behavior on different agar plates of *V. cholerae* 204 (original host) or *V. cholerae* E2 (conjugant) carrying pJYl was investigated in detail. The growth of these strains was generally poorer on TCBS agar plates than the comparative R⁻ strains. This difference became more pronounced in the overnight culture in L broth at temperatures higher than 37°C prior to plating. Ninety percent of the cells viable on nutrient agar could form colonies on TCBS agar when *V. cholerae* 204(pJYl⁺) was precultured at 27°C, although only 30% and less than 1% of them were capable of producing colonies on the same selective medium if they were precultured at 37 and 42°C, respectively, overnight (Table 6). Temperatures for incubation of the plates did not affect this phenomenon, and thus all plates were incubated at 37°C.

Table 6 indicates also that a small amount of CM (almost one-fifth of the MIC) reduced the number of colonies not only on TCBS agar plates but also on nutrient agar plates when the microbe was precultured at temperatures higher than 37°C, although the reduction was more prominent on TCBS agar than on nutrient agar. More than two-thirds of the cells were inhibited for colony formation by 2.5 μg of CM per ml on TCBS agar plates if the microbe was precultured at 37°C, whereas about 80% of the cells could form colonies on nutrient agar plates containing the same amount of CM. Since all colonies that appeared on drug-free TCBS or

TABLE 4. *F-fertility test between E. coli HfrR1 with or without pJY1 and E. coli AB1157(F⁻)*

Donor	Recipient	Culture temp (°C)[a]	Chromosomal recombination frequency[b] with selective marker of:	
			proC	*his*
HfrR1	AB1157	27	6.1×10^{-4}	1.3×10^{-5}
		37	3.2×10^{-3}	6.8×10^{-5}
		42	3.0×10^{-4}	1.1×10^{-5}
HfrR1 (pJY1⁺)	AB1157	27	8.6×10^{-4}	1.1×10^{-5}
		37	4.7×10^{-3}	7.2×10^{-5}
		42	2.1×10^{-4}	9.3×10^{-6}

[a] Subculture of the donor strain and mixed culture was performed at indicated temperatures. The recipient strain was subcultured at 37°C.

[b] Nine milliliters of a late logarithmic-phase culture of recipient was mixed with 1 ml of a late logarithmic-phase culture of donors, followed by further incubation for 60 min.

TABLE 5. *Incompatibility test of pJY1 with reference R plasmids*

Reference plasmids[a]			Interrelationships with pJY1					
Group	Name	Selective marker	Transfer frequencies of reference plasmids to: CSH2 (R^-)	Transfer frequencies of reference plasmids to: CSH2 ($pJY1^+$)	Entry exclusion	No. of transconjugants: $pJY1^-$	No. of transconjugants: Reference R^-	Incompatibility
FI	R386	*tet*	3.5×10^{-4}	7.0×10^{-7}	+	0/50	0/50	−
FIV	R124	*tet*	2.0×10^{-5}	2.0×10^{-7}	+	0/50	0/50	−
M	R4466	*tet sul*	1.3×10^{-4}	1.2×10^{-6}	+	0/50	1/50	−
Iγ	R621a	*tet*	2.8×10^{-4}	7.2×10^{-8}	+	0/50	0/50	−
N	N3	*tet str sul*	7.9×10^{-5}	1.1×10^{-8}	+	1/50	0/50	−
O	R16	*tet amp str sul*	3.2×10^{-4}	1.3×10^{-6}	+	0/50	0/50	−
T	Rts1	*kan*	1.5×10^{-3}	1.1×10^{-5}	+	0/50	0/50	−
A	RA1	*tet sul*	2.0×10^{-6}	2.5×10^{-6}	−	0/50	0/50	−
C	R40a	*amp kan sul*	1.7×10^{-5}	1.0×10^{-5}	−	0/50	0/50	−
H	R27	*tet*	6.1×10^{-5}	1.8×10^{-4}	−	1/50	0/50	−
Iα	R144	*tet kan*	3.4×10^{-4}	4.9×10^{-4}	−	0/50	0/50	−
L	R471a	*amp*	6.2×10^{-3}	5.5×10^{-3}	−	0/50	1/50	−
P	RP4	*amp kan*	3.8×10^{-3}	4.1×10^{-3}	−	0/50	0/50	−
S	R477-1	*tet str sul*	1.6×10^{-5}	1.9×10^{-5}	−	0/50	0/50	−
J	R391	*kan*	3.9×10^{-4}	1.0×10^{-4}	±	18/50	28/50	+

[a] The following plasmids were not tested: FII, R1, *cml str sul amp*; K, R387, *cml sul*; W, S-a, *cml str kan sul*.

TABLE 6. *Temperature-sensitive growth behavior of V. cholerae 204[a] carrying pJY1 on TCBS selective plates*

Preculture temp in L broth (°C)	No. of colonies[b] formed on: Nutrient agar containing: No drug	Nutrient agar containing: CM (2.5 μg/ml)	TCBS agar containing: No drug	TCBS agar containing: CM (2.5 μg/ml)
27	2.4×10^{9}	2.0×10^{9}	2.1×10^{9}	8.7×10^{8}
37	3.2×10^{9}	2.4×10^{9}	9.8×10^{8}	2.5×10^{8}
42	1.6×10^{9}	4.3×10^{8}	1.0×10^{7}	$>1.0 \times 10^{7}$

[a] *V. cholerae* 204, which lost pJY1 spontaneously, and *V. cholerae* E2(R^-) could form the same numbers of colonies on either nutrient agar or TCBS agar regardless of the preculture temperature in L broth.

[b] Expressed as number per milliliter of the preculture.

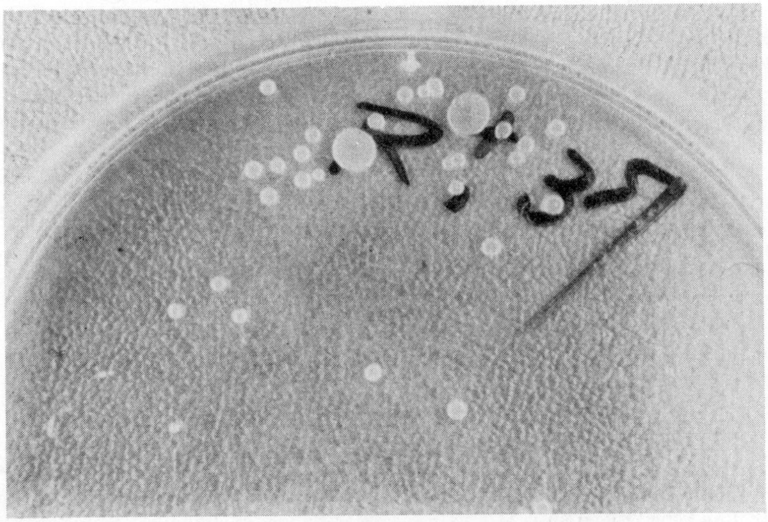

FIG. 5. *Colonies of V. cholerae 204 carrying the pJY1 plasmid, subcultured in L broth at 37°C and plated on TCBS selective agar.*

nutrient agar plates were confirmed to retain pJYl by replica plating, it was suggested that the phenotypic expression of CM resistance specified by pJYl was poor in drug-free L broth incubated at higher temperatures. Similar results were obtained with *V. cholerae* E2 carrying pJYl.

When more than 10^5 cells of *V. cholerae* 204(pJYl$^+$) precultured in L broth at 37 or 42°C overnight were spread on drug-free TCBS agar plates, several large colonies appeared (Fig. 5). It was found that about one-half of the colonies were comprised of entirely drug-susceptible cells(pJYl$^-$), the remaining colonies retaining the pJYl plasmid.

DISCUSSION

In spite of a marked increase of conjugative R plasmids in various gram-negative rods, no reports have appeared of any outbreak of a chemotherapy-tolerant epidemic by *V. cholerae* carrying R plasmids. This fortunate situation may depend partly on the instability of many R plasmids in cholera vibrios (4, 8, 19). Multiply drug-resistant strains of *V. cholerae,* however, were sporadically isolated in some parts of the world. Kobari et al. (7) reported that 11 multiply drug-resistant strains of *V. cholerae* (biotype El Tor) were obtained in Manila in 1969 from 11 out of 1,109 patients with cholera, whereas we found that 5 out of 60 clinical isolates of *V. cholerae* isolated in Manila in 1973 were multiply drug resistant (present results).

Although no conjugative R plasmids were confirmed in nine multiply drug-resistant cholera vibrios isolated in Manila in 1969 (see above), K. Bhaskaran found that CM, TC, SM, and sulfanilamide resistance of one of those strains was capable of simultaneous elimination by nitrosoguanidine treatment (personal communication). Furthermore, Yamada et al. (16) identified CM acetyltransferase in the cell-free extracts of those strains. These results in *V. cholerae* is of plasmid origin rather than of chromosomal origin.

We reported previously that a temperature-sensitive KM-resistant plasmid, Rtsl, was able to remain in *V. cholerae* at low temperatures (19). It may be interesting to note that the newly discovered conjugative R plasmid pJYl is also temperature sensitive, but for transferability only. A distinct difference between the two plasmids Rtsl and pJYl is that the latter plasmid can be retained stably in *V. cholerae* at a high culture temperature and belongs to the J compatibility group, different from the T group in which Rtsl has been classified. On the other hand, group S plasmids were reported to be temperature sensitive for transferability but not for stability in the hosts, although no evidence was demonstrated that they were stably maintained in *V. cholerae* (14).

Rahal et al. (13) and Hedges and Jacob (6) found that a strain of *V. cholerae* isolated in Algeria and southern U.S.S.R., respectively, carried conjugative R plasmids conferring resistance to ABPC, SM, TC, CM, KM, and sulfanilamide and to SM, TC, and CM. Both plasmids were reported to belong to the A–C complex in the system of R. W. Hedges and colleagues (5).

These results suggest that neither temperature sensitivity nor a special incompatibility group is an essential characteristic of R plasmids that can be maintained in *V. cholerae.* Since only one plasmid was isolated by us, by Rathal et al. (13), or by Hedges and Jacob (6), further R plasmids from *V. cholerae* need to be isolated for a better understanding of them.

A distinct finding from study of the *V. cholerae* bearing pJYl was its poor growth on TCBS selective agar, which is widely used for primary isolation of the pathogen. Although the generality of this phenomenon based on the study of one plasmid is uncertain, selective media other than TCBS agar may be preferable for the isolation of *V. cholerae* carrying R plasmids.

The reason why *V. cholerae* carrying pJYl grows poorly on TCBS agar when it is precultured in a liquid medium at temperatures higher than 37°C remains unanswered. However, it can be postulated that pJYl modifies the surface structure of the host vibrios in liquid media at high temperatures and ingredients of TCBS agar such as sodium thiosulfate and bile salts may affect growth strongly. Cells modified in such a way may form colonies on nutrient agar but not on TCBS agar. We reported that deficiency of cyclic adenosine 3′,5′-monophosphate in *V. cholerae* resulted in an abnormal formation of the cell wall at high culture temperatures (20). The poor growth of *V. cholerae* carrying pJYl, however, could not be overcome by the addition of cyclic adenosine 3′,5′-monophosphate to the preculture.

When a large number of *V. cholerae* 204(pJYl$^+$) (about 10^5 cells) was spread on TCBS agar plates, several large colonies, clearly distinguishable from many other tiny colonies, were obtained, and half of them were comprised of entirely pJTl$^-$ cells, the remaining colonies retaining the plasmid. This evidence suggests that the growth of *V. cholerae* strains (204 and E2) carrying pJYl can revert to normal either by losing the plasmid or by an unknown mechanism (presumably mutation of the host vibrio).

A poor phenotypic expression of the CM resistance specified by pJYl is another problem. We found recently that *E. coli* strains carrying pJYl showed inducible CM resistance which was increased two- to fourfold by pretreatment with 1/100 the MIC of CM for 60 min. A paper dealing with the inducible CM resistance conferred by pJYl will appear elsewhere (in preparation).

ACKNOWLEDGMENTS

This work was supported by the Scientific Research Fund of the Ministry of Education of Japan and by the United States Japan Cooperative Medical Science Program Cholera Panel.

We are indebted to H. Kitamura, C. Yamada, and Y Terawaki for supplying bacterial strains, and to W. Watanabe for supplying male-specific phages Qβ, MS2, and Fl.

LITERATURE CITED

1. **Akiba, T., K. Koyama, Y. Isshiki, S. Kimura, and T. Fukushima.** 1960. On the mechanism of the development of multiple drug resistant clones of *Shigella*. Jpn. J. Microbiol. **4**:219–227.
2. **Bachman, B. J.** 1972. Pedigree of some mutant strains of *Escherichia coli* K-12. Bacteriol. Rev. **36**:525–557.
3. **Difco Laboratories.** 1968. Bacto-TCBS agar, p. 388. Difco Supplementary Literature. Difco Laboratories, Detroit.
4. **Goto, S., and S. Kuwahara.** 1970. Transmission of multiple drug resistance between enterobacteria and vibrio through conjugation, p. 419–423. *In* Progress in antimicrobial and anticancer chemotherapy (Proc. 6th Int. Natl. Congr. Chemother.), vol. 1. University of Tokyo Press, Tokyo.
5. **Hedges, R. W.** 1974. R factor from Providence. J. Gen. Microbiol. **81**:171–181.
6. **Hedges, R. W., and A. E. Jacob.** 1975. A 98 megadalton R factor of compatibility group C in a *Vibrio cholerae El Tor* isolated in southern U.S.S.R. J. Gen. Microbiol. **89**:383–386.
7. **Kobari, K., I. Takakura, M. Nakatomi, S. Sogame, and C. Uylangco.** 1970. Antibiotic-resistant strains of *El Tor Vibrio* in the Philippines and the use of furalazine for chemotherapy. Bull. W.H.O. **43**:365–371.
8. **Kuwahara, S., T. Akiba, K. Koyama, and T. Arai.** 1963. Transmission of multiple drug resistance from *Shigella flexneri* to *Vibrio cholerae* through conjugation. Jpn. J. Microbiol. **7**:61–68.
9. **Lederberg, J.** 1949. Aberrant heterozygotes in *Escherichia coli*. Proc. Natl. Acad. Sci. U.S.A. **35**:178–184.
10. **Lederberg, J., and E. M. Lederberg.** 1952. Replica plating and indirect selection of bacterial mutants. J. Bacteriol. **63**:399–406.
11. **Lennox, E. S.** 1955. Transduction of linked genetic characters of the host by bacteriophage Pl. Virology **1**:190–206.
12. **Prescott, L. M., A. Datta, and G. C. Datta.** 1968. R factors in Calcutta strains of *Vibrio cholerae* and members of *Enterobateriaceae*. Bull. W.H.O. **39**:971–973.
13. **Rahal, K., G. R. Gerbaud, and Y. A. Chabbert.** 1973. Characterization d'un facteur de resistance transferable de *Vibrio cholerae* biotype El Tor. Ann. Microbiol.(Inst. Pasteur) **124B**:283–294.
14. **Rodriguez-Lemoine, V., A. E. Jacob, R. W. Hedges, and N. Datta.** 1970. Thermosensitive production of their transfer systems by group S plasmids. J. Gen. Microbiol. **62**:1–4.
15. **Terawaki, Y., H. Takayasu, and T. Akiba.** 1967. Thermosensitive replication of a kanamycin resistance factor. J. Bacteriol. **94**:687–690.
16. **Yamada, C., Y. Suzuki, M. Takao, and H. Shishigu.** 1969. Chloramphenicol acetyltransferase and nontransferable chloramphenicol resistance in multiple drug resistant strains of *Vibrio cholerae*. (In Japanese) Jpn. J. Bacteriol. **24**:144.
17. **Yamamoto, T., A. Fujii, and T. Yokota.** 1975. A multiply temperature sensitive kanamycin resistance factor and its spontaneous mutants relating to temperature sensitivity, p. 125–133. *In* Microbial drug resistance. University of Tokyo Press, Tokyo.
18. **Yokota, T., Y. Kanamaru, R. Mori, and T. Akiba.** 1969. Recombination between a thermosensitive kanamycin resistance factor and a non-thermosensitive multiple drug resistance factor. J. Bacteriol. **98**:863–873.
19. **Yokota, T., T. Kasuga, M. Kaneko, and S. Kuwahara.** 1972. Genetic behavior of R factors in *Vibrio cholerae*. J. Bacteriol. **109**:440–442.
20. **Yokota, T., and S. Kuwahara.** 1974. Adenosine 3′,5′-cyclic monophosphate-deficient mutants of *Vibrio cholerae*. J. Bacteriol. **120**:106–113.

Antimicrobial Agents and Chemotherapy, Jan. 1977, p. 21-25 Vol. 11, No. 1

Therapy of Murine Aspergillosis with Amphotericin B in Combination with Rifampin or 5-Fluorocytosine

JULIO ARROYO, GERALD MEDOFF,* AND GEORGE S. KOBAYASHI

Divisions of Infectious Diseases, Dermatology, and Laboratory Medicine, Department of Medicine, Washington University School of Medicine, St. Louis, Missouri 63110*

Received for publication 19 July 1976

Suboptimal doses of amphotericin B in combination with either rifampin or 5-fluorocytosine were better than single-drug therapy in the treatment of disseminated *Aspergillus fumigatus* infection in mice. Despite the increased effectiveness of combination therapy, none of the therapeutic regimens we used completely eradicated infections in the mice when evaluated by mycological culture, even in long-term survivors.

The combined use of amphotercin B (AmB) plus 5-fluorocytosine (5FC) has been shown to be more effective than either agent alone against *Candida albicans* both in vitro (14, 15) and in vivo (18). Similar results were observed when this combination was tested against *Cryptococcus neoformans* in vitro (15) and when used in the treatment of murine and human cryptococcosis (5, 19).

AmB used together with rifampin has been found to be more effective than either drug alone when tested against *C. albicans* (16) and *Aspergillus* (10) in vitro and against *Histoplasma capsulatum* and *Blastomyces dermatitidis* in vitro (12, 13) and in mice (9).

Based on our observations on the in vitro effectiveness of both of these drug combinations against species of *Aspergillus* (10, 11), we have studied the in vitro efficacy of AmB plus rifampin and AmB plus 5FC in mice infected with a clinical isolate of *A. fumigatus*.

MATERIALS AND METHODS

Animals. AKR female mice weighing 18 to 20 g, obtained from Jackson Laboratories, Bar Harbor, Me., were used in some experiments to determine whether strain differences occurred in response to therapy. In all subsequent experiments, female CD_1 mice weighing 18 to 22 g, purchased from Charles River, Wilmington, Mass., were employed as experimental animals since their responses were equivalent and they were more readily available. All animals were housed in plastic cages in groups of five and received food and water ad libitum.

Organism. *A. fumigatus* no. 1 (10, 11), a clinical isolate and part of our permanent laboratory collection, was maintained at 37°C and transferred weekly on Sabouraud agar slants. Sporulating subcultures of this organism were rinsed with sterile saline to collect the spores. Vigorous shaking of the resulting suspension with small glass beads yielded a uniform suspension consisting mainly of single spores. The spore concentration was determined by hemocytometer counts, and the number of viable spores per milliliter was assessed by colony counts.

Drugs. AmB (Fungizone) was purchased from E. R. Squibb and Sons, Inc., Princeton, N.J. Rifampin (Rifadin) was obtained from Dow Chemical Co., Zionsville, Ind. 5FC (Ancobon) was obtained from Hoffman-LaRoche, Inc., Nutley, N.J.

Treatment groups. All animals were inoculated by the intravenous (i.v.) route with 0.1 ml of a freshly prepared spore suspension. The mice were then randomly distributed into cages in groups of five. In each experiment the inoculating dose of spores varied, but was always greater than the mean lethal dose. The mean lethal dose was 2×10^5 for AKR mice and for CD_1 mice it was 1×10^6; the virulence of the organism remained constant throughout these experiments.

Antifungal treament was started 2 days after inoculation and was continued for 28 days thereafter. All of the drugs were freshly prepared just before use. AmB was dissolved in sterile 5% dextrose in water to a concentration of 0.10 mg/ml. A 10-μg (= 0.5 mg/kg) dose of AmB was injected through a lateral tail vein on Mondays, Wednesdays, and Fridays for 4 weeks. Rifampin (8 mg) was dissolved in 0.5 ml of 50% ethanol and diluted with sterile water to the desired concentrations. Rifampin and 5FC were administered daily by mouth using a curved, round-tip, 20-gauge gavage needle. Treatment groups usually consisted of 10 mice each. Control mice received sterile 5% dextrose in water and/or sterile water without antibiotics i.v. and orally, respectively. In all of the experiments, the efficacy of drug treatment was measured by the number of surviving mice at the cessation of therapy, which was 30 days after infection. In the different experiments the periods of observation after 30 days were variable.

Histology and culture of organs. A number of treated and untreated mice were necropsied, and sections of various organs were cultured on Mycosel agar. Brain and kidney sections were fixed in formalin and stained with hematoxylin and eosin and methanamine silver dyes.

RESULTS

Treatment groups. Figure 1 shows the combined results of two separate experiments with AKR mice. The administration of AmB and rifampin in combination was significantly better than either drug alone in preventing deaths from aspergillosis ($P < 0.05$) (P values calculated by simple chi-square analysis). The infecting dose in these experiments was 5×10^5 spores. AmB, at a dose of 10 μg, was minimally effective in increasing the survival as compared with controls. Rifampin alone, at 50 or 100 μg, had no beneficial effect and actually appeared detrimental in these and other experiments. Since the curves for rifampin, 50 and 100 μg, were similar, only the former concentration is represented in the figures.

A similar experiment using CD_1 mice and an inoculum of 2×10^6 spores is shown in Fig. 2. The combination of AmB plus rifampin, 50 or 100 μg, was more effective against *Aspergillus* infection than either agent alone. The difference between the survival rates of the combination treatment groups and the single ($P < 0.005$)-drug and untreated groups ($P < 0.001$) was highly significant. After stopping treatment, the survivors were observed for 1 month, and six more animals died in the combination groups. The cause of these late deaths was not definitely established, but, on the basis of histopathological evidence, it appeared that continued renal infection resulted in obstructive nephropathy and uremia.

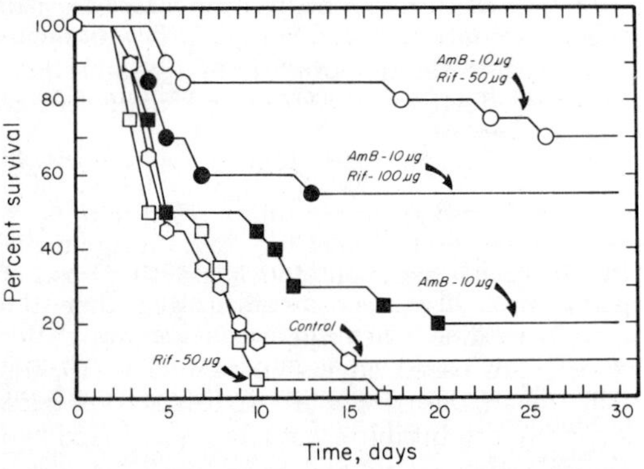

FIG. 1. *AKR mice were infected on day 0 with 5 × 10⁵ spores of A. fumigatus. Treatment was begun on day 2. AmB was given i.v. on Monday, Wednesday, and Friday, and rifampin (Rif) was given orally daily for 28 days. There were 10 mice in each treatment group, and the results are the average of two separate experiments.*

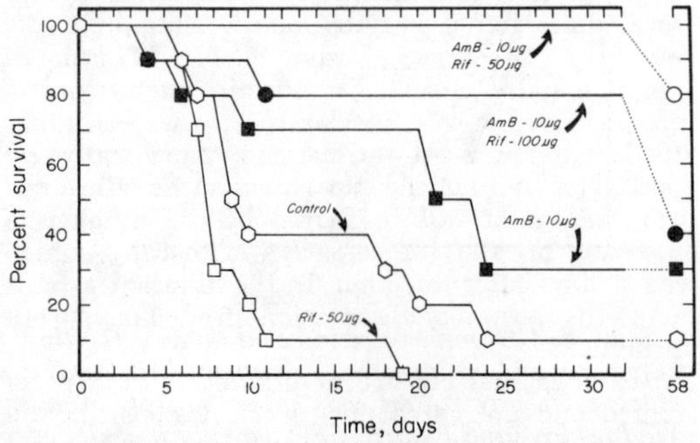

FIG. 2. *Same as in the legend to Fig. 1. CD_1 mice were used and the inoculum was 2×10^6 spores of A. fumigatus.*

When the infectious dose was increased to 5.5 $\times 10^6$ spores (Fig. 3), the effectiveness of the combination therapy was less and was not significant ($P < 0.12$). A one-sided test makes it significant at 0.06.

To determine the maximum infectious dose at which combination drug therapy would still be effective, groups of mice were inoculated with increasing numbers of spores. The salutary effect of combination AmB-rifampin treatment was lost when a dose greater than 1×10^7 spores was given (Fig. 4).

When CD_1 mice received 2×10^6 spores and then were treated with different doses of AmB, we found that a dose of 250 μg of AmB was required to approach the survival rate of the mice treated with the combination of 10 μg of AmB and 50 μg of rifampin (Fig. 4b).

Figure 5 shows the combined results of two separate experiments designed to test the efficacy of 5FC alone and in combination with AmB in the treatment of murine aspergillosis. CD_1 mice were infected with 2×10^6 spores and divided into the treatment groups shown. 5FC was given orally in doses of 5 and 1.25 mg daily, alone or combined with 10 μg of AmB. The difference in survival rate between each of the combination treated groups and the groups receiving the same dose of single-drug therapy was significant ($P < 0.015$). In these experi-

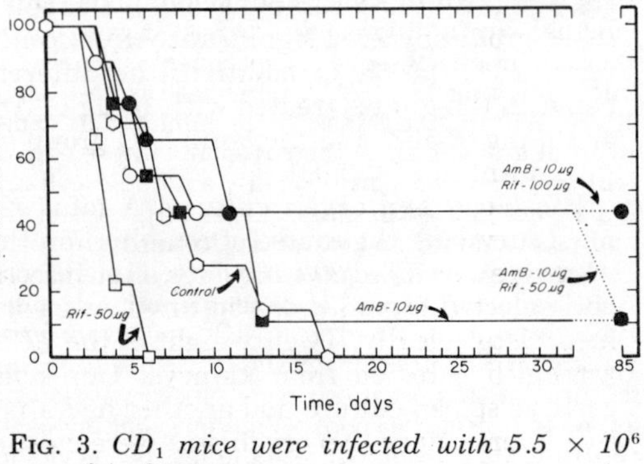

FIG. 3. *CD_1 mice were infected with 5.5×10^6 spores of A. fumigatus.*

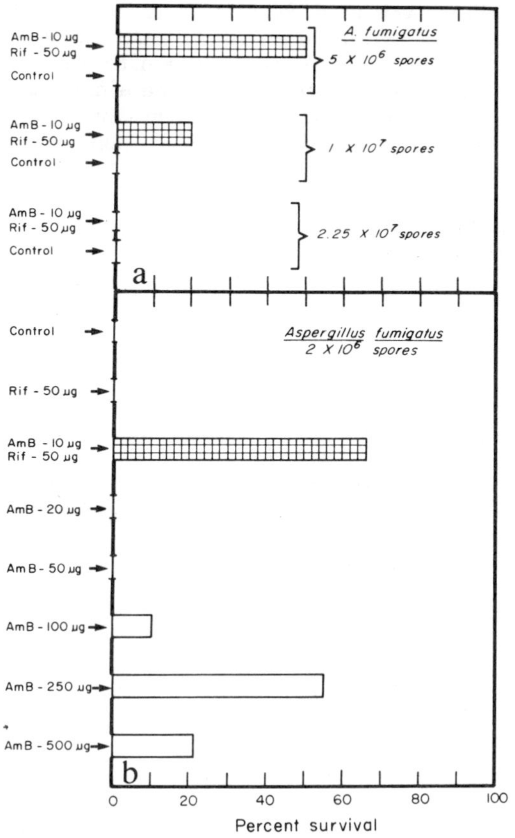

FIG. 4. *(a) Percentage of mice surviving 30 days after infection of groups of 10 CD_1 mice infected with increasing numbers of spores of A. fumigatus and treated with the regimens shown. The groups receiving 10 µg of AmB alone and 50 µg of rifampin alone had no survivors at the end of 30 days (data not shown). (b) Percentage of mice surviving 30 days after infection of groups of 10 CD_1 mice infected with 2×10^6 spores and treated with the regimens shown.*

ments, 5FC alone at a dose of 5 mg was as effective as the lower dose combination group (10 µg of AmB and 1.25 mg of 5FC), and both of these groups differed significantly from control mice ($P < 0.006$). In addition, the difference between the groups treated with 10 µg of AmB and 5 mg of 5FC and the 5-mg 5FC group was significant at $P < 0.001$.

Histology and organ culture. A total of 77 mice surviving the course of combination therapy were sacrificed 30 to 60 days after infection and selected organs were cultured and examined histologically. Twenty-eight of the 77 had aspergilli cultured from kidneys. One had a positive spleen culture and another had a positive liver culture. No organisms were cultured from the brains or the lungs of these long-term survivors. Macroscopically, the kidneys in most of these animals were hydronephrotic, with large pelvic abscesses. Histologically, mycelia were seen in the renal pelvices in the form of fungus balls, without apparent invasion of pelvic tissue. In contrast, untreated animals dying of *Aspergillus* infection had invasive disease of brain, lung, and kidney.

DISCUSSION

Using a model of disseminated *Aspergillus* infection in mice, we have confirmed our in vitro observations that the combination of AmB and rifampin is better than either of these agents alone against a clinical isolate of *A. fumigatus*.

Since rifampin alone had no therapeutic value and AmB at a dose of 10 µg was only marginally active, we believe that the in vivo interaction of these two drugs is synergistic. Whereas 5FC alone at the 5-mg dose was effective against this organism, at equivalent doses the combination of AmB and 5FC was better than either agent alone. These data indicate that the effectiveness of combined drug therapy was synergistic.

In the previous report in which we showed that these same combinations were synergistic in vitro against this strain of *Aspergillus*, the levels of 5FC and rifampin required for synergism were higher than clinically achievable concentrations when measurements of synergism were based on visual turbidity (10, 11). But, when the effects of the drugs were measured by the inhibition of ribonucleic acid synthesis or dry weight increase, much lower concentrations were effective.

The results we report here, which show an

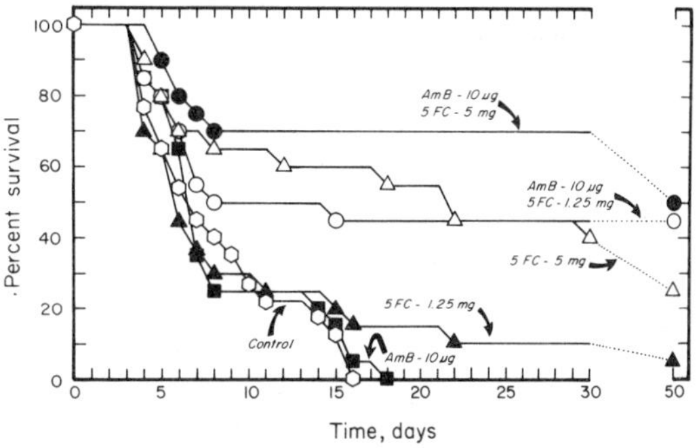

FIG. 5. *CD_1 mice were infected on day 0 with 2×10^6 spores of A. fumigatus. Treatment with AmB was started on day 2 and was given i.v. on Monday, Wednesday, and Friday. 5FC was given orally every day for 28 days. There were 10 mice in each treatment group, and the results shown are the average of two separate experiments.*

enhanced effectiveness of these two drug combinations at clinically achievable blood levels against *Aspergillus* infection in mice, indicate that the use of effects on ribonucleic acid synthesis and dry weight as measures of susceptibility to rifampin and 5FC may be a more accurate determinant of in vivo susceptibility than the usual methods that use growth on agar or turbidity.

The cause of death in the mice dying during therapy was disseminated infection involving many organ systems. This confirms other studies which showed that early in the course of infection aspergilli could be cultured from many different organs. These studies also show that as the animals survived for longer periods aspergilli disappeared, first from the lungs and followed by the spleen, liver, and brain, but the kidneys in these studies usually remained culture positive (17). Our histopathological data for the long-term survivors also confirm these latter observations, and the deaths that occurred several weeks or months after the infection of our animals appeared to be related to the persistence of aspergilli in the kidneys. Because there was no evidence of late dissemination in these mice, we think that obstructive nephropathy and uremia was a major cause of death. Using a similar experimental model, Corbel and Eades (7) also found that mice chronically infected with *Absidia ramosa* suffered moderate to severe uremia.

The reason for the failure of therapy to eradicate kidney infection is unknown, but local conditions in the kidney, such as depressed activity of phagocytic cells (6) or inactivation of complement (3), might account for the persistence of infection.

In regard to drug levels, serum levels of 5FC in our mice (S. A. Garding and H. M. Solomon, Prog. Abstr. Intersci. Conf. Antimicrob. Agents Chemother., 15th, Washington, D.C., Abstr. 416, 1975) were 92 and 43 μg/ml at 1 and 6 h after a single oral dose of 5 mg. These levels are in the high therapeutic range. Rifampin serum levels were not measured, but we feel we used maximum dosages because the 100 μg of rifampin was no better, and was perhaps worse, than the 50-μg dose (2). However, according to serum measurements, the dose of AmB we used in our experiments was suboptimal. AmB serum levels at 1 and 24 h after a 10-μg i.v. dose were 0.2 μg/ml (4, 8, 9). Therefore, it is possible that by using higher doses of AmB together with 5FC or rifampin in the treatment of *Aspergillus* infection, mycological sterility in the kidneys might be achieved.

In summary, AmB in combination with either rifampin or 5FC was better than single-drug therapy in the treatment of disseminated *A. fumigatus* infection in mice. Our observation that 5FC alone at a daily dose of 5 mg (250 mg/kg) was also effective confirms the clinical experience of others (1). Because none of the therapeutic regimens we used completely eradicated infections, even in long-term survivors, higher doses of AmB in the combinations should be tried.

ACKNOWLEDGMENTS

The AmB serum level determinations were performed by John E. Bennet, National Institute of Allergy and Infectious Diseases, Bethesda, Md., and the 5-fluorocytosine levels were performed by Harvey M. Solomon, Johns Hopkins Hospital, Baltimore, Md. We are grateful to Sung C. Choi for furnishing the statistical analysis of our data.

This work was supported by Public Health Service grants AI 10622 and AI 06213 and training grants AI 00459 and AI 07015 from the National Institute of Allergy and Infectious Diseases, grants from John A. Hartford Foundation, Inc., a Brown-Hazen grant, and a special Public Health Service training fellowship, AI 00199, for Julio Arroyo from the National Institute of Allergy and Infectious Diseases.

LITERATURE CITED

1. **Atkinson, G. W., and H. L. Israel.** 1973. 5-Fluorocytosine treatment of meningeal and pulmonary aspergillosis. Am. J. Med. 55:496–505.
2. **Bassi, L., L. DiBerardino, V. Arioli, L. G. Silvestri, and E. L. Cherie-Ligniere.** 1973. Conditions for immunosuppression by rifampicin. J. Infect. Dis. 128:736–744.
3. **Beeson, P. B., and D. Rowley.** The anticomplementary effect of kidney tissue: its association with ammonia production. J. Exp. Med. 110:685.
4. **Bindschadler, D. D., and J. E. Bennett.** 1969. A pharmacologic guide to the clinical use of amphotericin B. J. Infect. Dis. 120:427–436.
5. **Block, E. R., and J. E. Bennett.** 1973. The combined effect of 5-fluorocytosine and amphotericin B in the therapy of murine cryptococcosis. Proc. Soc. Exp. Biol. Med. 142:476–480.
6. **Charnew, I., and A. I. Braude.** 1962. Depression of phagocytosis by solutes in concentrations found in the kidney and urine. J. Clin. Invest. 41:1945.
7. **Corbel, M. J., and S. M. Eades.** 1975. Factors determining the susceptibility of mice to experimental phycomycosis. J. Med. Microbiol. 8:551–574.
8. **Green. W. R., J. E. Bennett, and R. D. Goos.** 1965. Ocular penetration of amphotericin B. Arch. Ophthalmol. 73:769–775.
9. **Kitahara, M., G. S. Kobayashi, and G. Medoff.** 1976. Enhanced efficacy of amphotericin B and rifampicin combined treatment of murine histoplasmosis and blastomycosis. J. Infect. Dis. 133:663–668.
10. **Kitahara, M., V. K. Seth, G. Medoff, and G. S. Kobayashi.** 1976. Activity of amphotericin B, 5-fluorocytosine, and rifampin against six clinical isolates of *Aspergillus*. Antimicrob. Agents Chemother. 9:915–919.
11. **Kitahara, M., V. K. Seth, G. Medoff, and G. S. Kobayashi.** 1976. Antimicrobial susceptibility testing of six clinical isolates of *Aspergillus*. Antimicrob. Agents Chemother. 9:908–914.
12. **Kobayashi, G. S., S. C. Cheung, D. Schlessinger, and G. Medoff.** 1974. Effects of rifamycin derivatives, alone and in combination with amphotericin B, against *Histoplasma capsulatum*. Antimicrob.

Agents Chemother. 5:16–18.

13. **Kobayashi, G. S., G. Medoff, D. Schlessinger, C. N. Kwan, and W. E. Musser.** 1972. Amphotericin B potentiation of rifampin as an antifungal agent against the yeast phase of *Histoplasma capsulatum*. Science 177:709–710.
14. **Kwan, C. N., G. Medoff, G. S. Kobayashi, D. Schlessinger, and H. J. Raskas.** 1972. Potentiation of the antifungal effects of antibiotics by amphotericin B. Antimicrob. Agents Chemother. 2:61–65.
15. **Medoff , G., M. Comfort, and G. S. Kobayashi.** 1971. Synergistic action of amphotericin B and 5-fluorocytosine against yeast-like organisms. Proc. Soc. Exp. Biol. Med. 138:571–574.
16. **Medoff, G., G. S. Kobayashi, C. N. Kwan, D. Schlessinger, and P. Venkov.** 1972. Potentiation of rifampicin and 5-fluorocytosine as antifungal antibiotics by amphotericin B. Proc. Natl. Acad. Sci. U.S.A. 69:196–199.
17. **Smith, G. R.** Experimental aspergillosis in mice: aspects of resistance. J. Hyg. 70:741–754.
18. **Titsworth, E., and E. Grunberg.** 1973. Chemotherapeutic activity of 5-fluorocytosine and amphotericin B against *Candida albicans* in mice. Antimicrob. Agents Chemother. 4:306–308.
19. **Utz, J. P., I. L. Garriques, M. A. Sande, J. F. Warner, G. L. Mandell, R. F. McGehee, R. J. Duma, and S. Shadomy.** 1975. Therapy of cryptococcosis with a combination of fluorocytosine and amphotericin B. J. Infect. Dis. 132:368–373.

ANTIMICROBIAL AGENTS AND CHEMOTHERAPY, Jan. 1977, p. 26-30 Vol. 11, No. 1

Lysis of Enterobacteria by Cefoxitin, Cefuroxime, and Cephalothin

C. S. GOODWIN[1]* AND JOYCE P. HILL

Division of Hospital Infection, Clinical Research Centre, Harrow, Middlesex HA1 3UJ, England

Received for publication 2 June 1976

Cefoxitin, cefuroxime, and cephalothin were added to dense populations of beta-lactamase-producing enterobacteria, and the subsequent turbidity changes were monitored continuously. Viable counts and antibiotic assays were made at intervals after the addition of antibiotic, and the morphological appearances of the organisms were observed. Cephalothin caused lysis of most of the organisms tested, but even at high concentrations, after a few hours the antibiotic was destroyed and the organisms recommenced logarithmic growth. Cefoxitin produced lysis of all the strains of *Escherichia coli* and *Klebsiella* species tested, with supression of regrowth. With cephalothin and cefoxitin the viable counts after the addition of antibiotic correlated with the turbidity measurements. Cefuroxime infrequently caused lysis that suppressed multiplication, and the organisms became long and filamentous while the turbidity readings increased; the viable counts did not correlate with the turbidity measurements. Cefuroxime and cefoxitin were not destroyed by the beta-lactamases of any of the strains of enterobacteria that were studied.

Many enterobacteria produce beta-lactamases, including cephalosporinases; cephaloridine and cephalothin lyse such enterobacteria, but are destroyed after a few hours and the organisms recommence logarithmic growth (3, 6). Cefazolin appears to be more stable to cephalosporinases (3, 5). Cefuroxime is a new semisynthetic cephalosporin that is active against indole-positive *Proteus* species and very active against *Haemophilus influenzae* (9). Cefoxitin is one of the cephamycin antibiotics, which have been shown to be significantly resistant to cephalosporinases (2, 7) and are active against enterobacteria and *Bacteroides* that are normally resistant to cephalothin and cephaloridine (1). Intravenous doses of cefoxitin in humans produce higher serum concentrations than does cephalothin (4). Using continuous turbidimetric monitoring in a biophotometer, we have studied the ability of cefoxitin, cefuroxime, and cephalothin to lyse dense populations of enterobacteria and then suppress the phase of regrowth. Other workers with the biophotometer have related their results to the minimal inhibitory concentrations (MICs) of antibiotics determined with an inoculum of 10^4 organisms/ml (6), but we have related our results to MICs for the denser population of bacteria that we found at the time of addition of the antibiotic. The morphological appearance of organisms after the action of cefoxitin and cefuroxime has been contrasted and correlated with the viable count at intervals after the addition of the antibiotic and with the biophotometer tracings.

[1] Present address: Microbiology Department, Royal Perth Hospital, Box X 2213, GPO Perth, Western Australia 6001.

MATERIALS AND METHODS

Bacterial strains and their beta-lactamase activities. Isolates of *Escherichia coli*, *Klebsiella* spp., and *P. vulgaris* were obtained from clinical specimens at Northwick Park Hospital Harrow, London, England. The strains studied in the biophotometer were selected to cover the range of speed of beta-lactamase production as shown by the chromogenic cephalosporin 87/312 (8). One drop of a solution of 87/312 (500 μg/ml) was added to an overnight broth culture of each organism at 37°C; cleavage of the beta-lactam ring was shown by a color change from yellow to red, and the time taken for this change was noted.

MICs. Serial dilutions of cefoxitin, cefuroxime, and cephalothin were made in Sensitest Agar (Oxoid, London); within 48 h of being poured, plates were inoculated from a multiple inoculator that delivered approximately 0.03 ml of a suspension containing 1×10^5 or 2×10^7 bacteria/ml. After incubation for 18 h the lowest concentration showing no growth was regarded as the MIC.

Growth medium. The medium of Greenwood and O'Grady (6), which has an osmolality of about 325 mosmol/kg, was used.

Turbidimetric system. Cultures were grown from 0.04 ml of an overnight broth culture inoculated into 8 ml of medium to produce a concentration of approximately 3×10^6 bacteria/ml. This inoculum was chosen because it produced a short lag phase but still allowed 100% transmission. Six stirred broth cultures, at 37°C, were continuously monitored in a Jouan (Paris) biophotometer. To one culture antibiotic was not added, and to each of the others a different antibiotic concentration was added at the same point in the logarithmic growth phase; before the antibiotic was added, a sample was taken for a viable count of each culture. The concentrations of antibiotic were usually two, four, and eight times the MIC for the denser population of the organism (see MICs above). In some experiments a viable count was done at hourly intervals after the addition of the antibiotic, wet preparations of the organisms were examined by bright-field microscopy, and their morphological appearance was noted.

Assay of antibiotic in the culture medium. Antibiotic assays were done at intervals after the addition of the antibiotic. Experiments identical to those described above were performed, but for the antibiotic assay all of the broth mixture was removed and centrifuged, and the supernatant was passed through a membrane filter (Millipore; pore size, 0.45 μm) to remove remaining bacteria. The filtrate, undiluted and at suitable dilutions, was placed in wells in agar plates. For the assay of cephalothin, a suspension of *Staphylococcus aureus* (NCTC 6571) was flooded over a plate of Sensitest Agar (Oxoid) and the plate was dried; for the assay of cefoxitin and cefuroxime, a suspension of *Bacillus subtilis* spores was incorporated into a plate of nutrient agar (10). Each plate also included three wells filled with known concentrations of the antibiotic being assayed. After overnight incubation the diameters of the zones of inhibition were measured. A graph was constructed from the results of the standards, and the antibiotic concentration of each test solution was calculated.

Resistance of antibiotics to commercial beta-lactamase. A commercial beta-lactamase preparation (Whatman Biochemicals) made from *B. cereus* 569H contained beta-lactamases I and II. Each vial contained 50 U of beta-lactamase II (cephalosporinase). The contents of the vial were dissolved in 5 ml of distilled water, and 0.1 ml of this solution was used for each test. Solutions containing 20 μg of each antibiotic per ml were prepared in nutrient broth; 0.1 ml of beta-lactamase solution was added to 0.5 ml of antibiotic; the pH of all mixtures was 7. Each was assayed immediately and after 10, 30, 60, and 120 min. All were incubated at 37°C between samplings. The antibiotic solutions, without beta-lactamase, were also assayed. The assays were performed by the method described above.

RESULTS

Beta-lactamase activity. The chromogenic cephalosporin 87/312 (Fig. 1), used to estimate beta-lactamase activity, undergoes a distinct change from yellow to red when it is hydrolyzed by beta-lactamases. The time taken for this to occur depends on the amount of lactamase produced by the strain being tested. Some of the strains we examined and the times taken for the color change to occur were: *E. coli* strains 17, 150, and 103, 5, 5, and 10 min, respectively; *Klebsiella* strains 19 and 21, 30 and 120 min. *P. vulgaris* strains failed to produce a color change, even after overnight incubation.

MICs. The MICs with two different inocula are shown in Table 1; the larger inoculum was the concentration of organisms found at the time of antibiotic addition in the turbidimetric studies. The larger inoculum resulted in a two- to fourfold increase of MIC in most strains.

Turbidimetric studies. A typical example of the changes in turbidity of *E. coli* is shown in Fig. 2. After the addition of cephalothin and cefoxitin to *E. coli* 103, lysis of the organism occurred within 15 to 30 min. With 32 μg of cephalothin per ml, twice the MIC against the larger inoculum, the organism started to regrow at 2.5 h after the addition of antibiotic; with a concentration four times the MIC, regrowth was delayed for 6 h. With cephalothin, similar results were obtained for all of the strains of enterobacteria that produced beta-

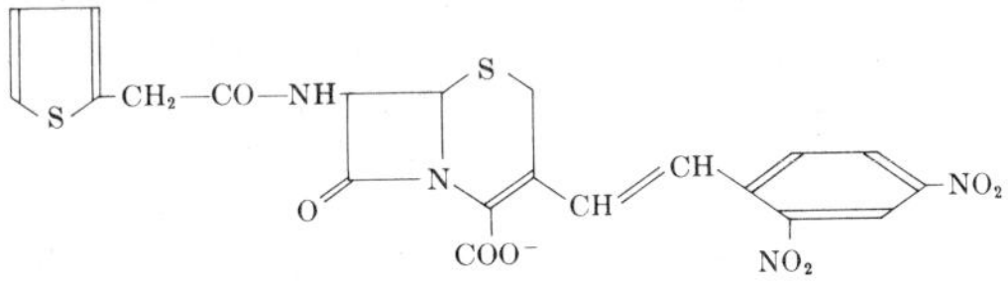

FIG. 1. *Structure of the chromogenic cephalosporin 87/312.*

TABLE 1. *MICs of three cephalosporins against two sizes of inocula*

Species	Strain	MIC (μg/ml) against: 1 × 10^5 organisms/ml			2 × 10^7 organisms/ml		
		Cephalothin	Cefuroxime	Cefoxitin	Cephalothin	Cefuroxime	Cefoxitin
E. coli	17	4	8	4	8	8	4
E. coli	55	8	4	2	12	8	8
E. coli	103	8	4	4	16	8	4
E. coli	150	8	8	4	12	12	8
Klebsiella	19	2	2	2	8	8	8
Klebsiella	21	2	2	2	2	1	4
P. vulgaris	24	4	4	4	8	2	4

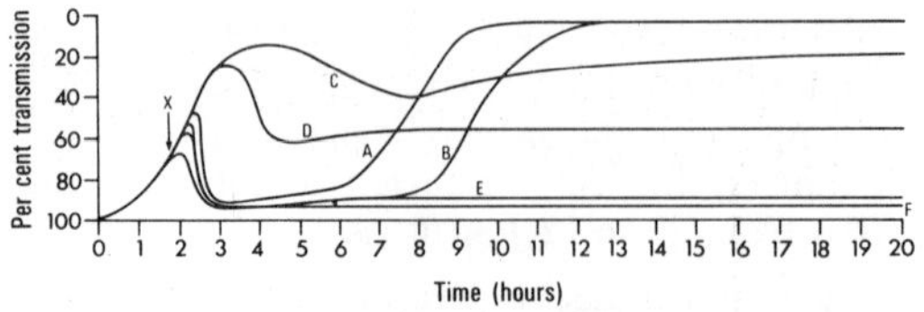

FIG. 2. *Copies of biophotometer tracings of six cultures of E. coli 103, showing the effect of addition, at time x, of: (A) cephalothin, 32 µg/ml, twice the MIC; (B) cephalothin, 64 µg/ml, four times the MIC; (C) cefuroxime, 16 µg/ml, twice the MIC; (D) cefuroxime, 32 µg/ml, four times the MIC; (E) cefoxitin, 8 µg/ml, twice the MIC; and (F) cefoxitin, 16 µg/ml, four times the MIC.*

lactamase: after lysis, regrowth occurred even with concentrations eight times the MIC, up to 128 µg/ml, although with the slowest beta-lactamase producer, *E. coli* 55, regrowth was delayed for up to 12.5 h. Regrowth did not occur after lysis by cefoxitin. After the addition of cefuroxime at 16 and 32 µg/ml, turbidity continued to increase for 2.5 and 1.5 h, respectively. This was followed by partial lysis, and turbidity fell to an intermediate level that was maintained until the end of the experiment.

When each antibiotic, at a concentration twice the MIC for the larger inoculum, was added to *E. coli* 150, cephalothin almost disappeared from the culture medium within 4 h, but cefuroxime and cefoxitin remained in their initial concentrations (Table 2). The disappearance of cephalothin was accompanied by regrowth of the organism, commencing at 3 h after the addition of the antibiotic, when the antibiotic concentration had fallen below the MIC for the smaller inoculum. A similar correlation between the concentration of the antibiotic and regrowth of the organism, as shown by a biophotometer tracing, was found for the other organisms and antibiotics.

The time between the addition of antibiotic and the recommencement of growth after lysis, as shown by turbidity measurements, is illustrated graphically in Fig. 3. After the addition of some concentrations of antibiotic, lysis did not occur; for example, *E. coli* 17 with cephalothin at the lowest concentration. The turbidity measurements suggested that, with a concentration of cefuroxime twice the MIC and *E. coli* 17, multiplication of the organism continued without a decrease in turbidity; however, viable counts during the first few hours after the addition of antibiotic showed that there was a 10-fold decrease in the viable count, with a suppression of regrowth and the formation of very long filamentous forms (see below).

Even at low concentrations of cefoxitin, lysis

TABLE 2. *Antibiotic concentrations remaining at intervals after the addition of cephalothin, cefuroxime, and cefoxitin to E. coli 150*

Antibiotic and concn (µg/ml)	Antibiotic concn (µg/ml) at time (h) after addition of antibiotic:			
	0	1	2.5	4
Cephalothin, 32	32	8	1.5	0.5
Cefuroxime, 25	25	25	25	25
Cefoxitin, 12	12	11	14	12

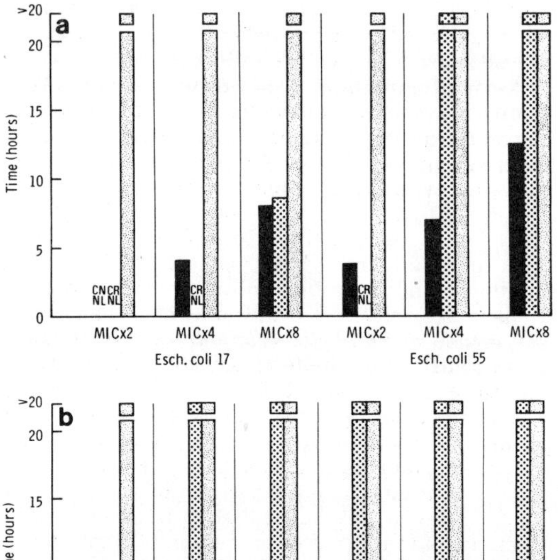

FIG. 3. *Time from addition of antibiotic to recommencement of growth after lysis of: (a) E. coli 17 and E. coli 55; (b) E. coli 103 and E. coli 150; (c) Klebsiella sp. 19 and Klebsiella sp. 21. NL, No lysis. Symbols: ■, cephalothin (CN); ⊠, cefuroxime (CR); □, cefoxitin.*

was followed by a complete suppression of regrowth with all strains of *E. coli* and with *Klebsiella* sp. 21; with *Klebsiella* sp. 19, the recovery was delayed for at least 8 h with the lowest concentration of cefoxitin.

Viable counts and morphological appearances. Cephalothin and cefoxitin caused lysis of the strains of *E. coli* and *Klebsiella* spp., and the surviving organisms morphologically were predominantly spheroplasts with occasional rod forms. With these two antibiotics the turbidity measurements correlated with the viable counts; cultures without antibiotic multiplied, reaching up to 1×10^9 organisms/ml, and lysed cultures resulted in counts of 1×10^4 organisms/ml. With *P. vulgaris* 24 the biophotometer tracing did not show evidence of lysis after the addition of cephalothin and cefoxitin, but the turbidity remained at 60% transmission and viable counts revealed that there was suppression of growth; after 4 h without antibiotic the count was 1×10^9 organisms/ml, and with 8 μg of cefoxitin per ml, twice the MIC, the count was 5×10^7 organisms/ml and morphologically all the organisms were spheroplasts.

After the addition of cefuroxime the viable counts did not correlate with the turbidity measurements. For example, for *E. coli* 17 the viable count at antibiotic addition was 3×10^7 organisms/ml, and after 4 h it had fallen to 2×10^6 organisms/ml, but there was increase in turbidity and the final plateau was only slightly lower than that of the culture without antibiotic. At 2 h after the addition of cefuroxime only long filamentous forms were seen in the wet preparation, and after 4 h even longer filamentous forms were seen. With *E. coli* 55 the turbidity measurements showed a decrease to 50% turbidity, and the viable count decreased by 99% to 1×10^5 organisms/ml; with *E. coli* 150 there was a turbidity decrease to 50%, with a viable count after 4 h of 2×10^4 organisms/ml. Regrowth was suppressed, and the turbidity remained the same. Similar results were found with cefuroxime for all of the other strains studied. When a high concentration of cefuroxime, 32 μg/ml, was added to *E. coli* 17, long filamentous forms were seen without any reduction in turbidity.

Antibiotic assays. In incubated broth without any organism, after 18 h of incubation a solution of cefoxitin decreased from a concentration of 16 to 12 μg/ml and a solution of cefuroxime decreased from 8 to 6 μg/ml.

Resistance of antibiotics to commercial beta-lactamase. In mixtures of beta-lactamase (Whatman Biochemicals) with cephalothin and cefuroxime the antibiotic had disappeared completely after approximately 15 s; i.e., there were no zones on the assay plate. After 2 h of incubation the concentration of cefoxitin had fallen from 20 to 12 μg/ml.

DISCUSSION

Biophotometer tracings are a useful method for continuous monitoring of the interaction between beta-lactam antibiotics and bacteria that produce beta-lactamases. However, the limitations of this method are shown by the viable counts after the addition of an antibiotic, such as cefuroxime, when there may be a 90% reduction of organisms but the tracing shows increasing turbidity and a final turbidity only slightly less than a culture without antibiotic. The morphological response profile of beta-lactam antibiotics has been extensively described by Greenwood and O'Grady (6) and Greenwood et al. (5): these workers used medium with a lower osmolality for *Proteus* than that of the medium for *E. coli* because they found that *Proteus* spheroplasts were protected in the lower osmolality. We preferred to use the same osmolality in all of our experiments, and we found that *P. vulgaris* 24, after the addition of cefoxitin, showed a total absence of rods with a large number of viable spheroplasts, but complete suppression of multiplication.

For strains of *E. coli* and *Klebsiella,* even at an osmolality of 325 mosmol/kg, cefoxitin causes rapid lysis of dense populations of enterobacteria, with complete suppression of regrowth, in contrast to cephalothin which allowed regrowth after a few hours. The resistance of cefoxitin to beta-lactamases is confirmed by its stability in the presence of a commercial beta-lactamase that immediately destroyed cefuroxime and cephalothin.

For clinical use cefoxitin would be expected to be superior to cephalothin, even for strains with a similar MIC, and might allow less frequent administration, for example, twice daily. Cefuroxime has been found to be very similar in action to cephalexin (6), producing long filamentous forms without much lysis in many strains of beta-lactamase-producing *E. coli*. Multiplication of organisms was suppressed and cefuroxime was not destroyed by beta-lactamases, and these features may be sufficient to give a good clinical effect.

ACKNOWLEDGMENTS

We thank R. Blowers for encouragement and advice; Merck, Sharp and Dohme Research Laboratories, West Point, Pa., for the supply of cefoxitin; and Glaxo Laboratories Ltd., Greenford, Middlesex, England, for the supply of cefuroxime and cephalosporin 87/312.

LITERATURE CITED

1. **Brumfitt, W., J. Kosmidis, J. M. T. Hamilton-Miller, and J. N. G. Gilchrist.** 1974. Cefoxitin and cephalothin: antimicrobial activity, human pharmacokinetics, and toxicology. Antimicrob. Agents Chemother. 6:290–299.
2. **Daoust, D. R., H. R. Onishi, H. Wallick, D. Hendlin, and E. O. Stapley.** 1973. Cephamycins, a new family of beta-lactam antibiotics: antibacterial activity and resistance to beta-lactamase degradation. Antimicrob. Agents Chemother. 3:254–261.
3. **Goodwin, C. S., and J. P. Hill.** 1975. Beta-lactamase resistance of cephazolin and other cephalosporins. Scott. Med. J. 20:236–239.
4. **Goodwin, C. S., E. B. Raftery, A. D. Goldberg, H. Skeggs, A. E. Till, and C. M. Martin.** 1974. Effects of rate of infusion and probenecid on serum levels, renal excretion, and tolerance of intravenous doses of cefoxitin in humans: comparison with cephalothin. Antimicrob. Agents Chemother. 6:338–346.
5. **Greenwood, D., C. H. Chan-Teoh, and F. O'Grady.** 1975. Activity of cefazolin against dense populations of enterobacteria. Antimicrob. Agents Chemother. 7:191–195.
6. **Greenwood, D., and F. O'Grady.** 1973. Comparison of the responses of *Escherichia coli* and *Proteus mirabilis* to seven beta-lactam antibiotics. J. Infect. Dis. 128:211–222.
7. **Miller, A. K., E. Celozzi, B. A. Pelak, E. O. Stapley, and D. Hendlin.** 1972. Cephamycins, a new family of β-lactam antibiotics. III. In vitro studies. Antimicrob. Agents Chemother. 2:281–286.
8. **O'Callaghan, C. H., A. Morris, S. M. Kirby, and A. H. Shingler.** 1972. Novel method for detection of beta-lactamases by using a chromogenic cephalosporin substrate. Antimicrob. Agents Chemother. 1:283–288.
9. **O'Callaghan, C. H., R. B. Sykes, A. Griffiths, and J. E. Thornton.** 1976. Cefuroxime, a new cephalosporin antibiotic: activity in vitro. Antimicrob. Agents Chemother. 9:511–519.
10. **O'Callaghan, C. H., R. B. Sykes, D. M. Ryan, R. D. Foord, and P. W. Muggleton.** 1976. Cefuroxime—a new cephalosporin antibiotic. J. Antibiot. 29:29–37.

ANTIMICROBIAL AGENTS AND CHEMOTHERAPY, Jan. 1977, p. 31-33 Vol. 11, No. 1

Bioassay Method for Polyene Antibiotics Based on the Measurement of Rubidium Efflux from Rubidium-Loaded Yeast Cells

R. F. COSGROVE AND J. E. FAIRBROTHER

Squibb International Development Laboratory, Moreton, Wirral, Merseyside L46 IQW, England

Received for publication 9 July 1976

A bioassay method for the polyene antibiotics nystatin and amphotericin B is proposed based on the measurement of the efflux of rubidium ions from a rubidium-loaded yeast culture challenged with the antibiotics. For this purpose a major proportion of the intracellular K^+ ions in a *Saccharomyces cerevisiae* culture has been substituted by Rb^+ ions. The rubidium leakage is measured by atomic absorption spectrophotometry, and a straight-line, dose-response correlation has been obtained for both antibiotics.

It has been recognized since the early 1960s that one of the principal effects of polyene antibiotic action on susceptible microorganisms is the leakage of vital cytoplasmic constituents from the cells (8-11). The work of Sutton et al. (11) and Marini et al. (10) highlighted the leakage of K^+ ions and NH_4^+ ions particularly. Since these early papers, many authors have examined induced potassium efflux from yeast cells by polyenes (4, 5, 7, 12-14).

From some of the literature referred to above a correlation between polyene concentration and potassium efflux can be identified, and the prognosis for a possible rapid bioassay of this class of antibiotics, by measuring ion release from cells, is good.

Smithler et al. (E. A. Smithler, H. S. Commager, and N. J. Kauffman, 31st Int. Cong. Pharm. Sci., Washington, D.C., 1971) measured the efflux of proteins released from yeast cells treated with nystatin. They sought to use this effect as a bioassay for nystatin, quantitating the chromophore (570 nm) produced by reacting the released protein with ninhydrin. Further work along these lines by Williams (personal communication), using cultures of *Candida albicans* and *Saccharomyces cerevisiae*, confirmed the linear relationship between nystatin concentration and absorption at 570 nm but gave variable response slopes from day to day. It was thought that the measurement of efflux of a simple ion would yield less variable results, and attention was directed towards the possible development of a bioassay for nystatin based on K^+ ion leakage. This possibility was examined in depth using a culture of *S. cerevisiae*.

However, in almost every application envisaged for the nystatin bioassay, the level of K^+ ions occurring as natural contaminants in the sample is of a similar order to that released by the yeast cells. This would give an unacceptably high blank value and result in poor assay performance characteristics.

To overcome this problem, an alternative ion, which could be introduced into the yeast cells without affecting their viability or membrane function but which had a very low level of natural occurrence, was sought.

To reproduce as closely as possible the characteristics of K^+ ion leakage across the nystatin-impaired yeast cell membrane, it is necessary to find an ion of like charge and ionic radius. K^+ ions exist in solution in a hydrated form, and the hydrated ionic radii of K^+ (0.232 nm) and Rb^+ (0.228 nm) are very similar, as are the ionic mobilities of these two ions.

Rubidium ions are known to be well tolerated by erythrocytes, and an examination of the literature revealed a number of papers reporting the uptake of Rb^+ ion by the yeast *S. cerevisiae* (1-3). Rubidium can also be determined at low levels with precision by atomic absorption spectrophotometry. It was therefore decided to examine the feasibility of using Rb^+ uptake and subsequent release from yeast cells by the action of the polyene antibiotics nystatin and amphotericin as a bioassay system. The work reported here clearly shows such a system to be feasible in that a linear dose-response relationship can be obtained.

MATERIALS AND METHODS

Yeast culture. *S. cerevisiae* SQ.1600 (from the Squibb Culture Collection) was used throughout.

The culture was maintained on slants of Sabouraud agar and grown at 30°C. A loopful of inoculum from an 18-h slant was transferred to 100 ml of medium of the following composition: yeast extract, 5 g; glucose, 30 g; rubidium chloride, 6.0 g; 0.1 M citric acid solution, 280 ml; 0.1 M sodium citrate, 220 ml; distilled water to 1 liter (pH 4.6; autoclaved at 15 lb/in^2 for 15 min). After incubation in this medium for 17 h at 30°C, cells were harvested by centrifugation and washed eight times with 25-ml amounts of sterile distilled water. (It was found that a minimum of six washes was required to remove extracellular Rb^+.) The cells were finally resuspended in distilled water to a transmission of 30% at 623 nm using a water blank.

Antibiotics. Nystatin and amphotericin B were used in this study. (i) Nystatin stock solutions were prepared in dimethyl formamide (DMF) at a concentration of 8,000 units of activity (U) per ml. Further dilutions were made in DMF to concentrations of 6,000, 4,000, and 2,000 U/ml. (ii) Amphotericin B stock solutions were prepared in DMF at a concentration of 300 μg/ml. Further dilutions were made in DMF to concentrations of 225, 150, and 75 μg/ml.

Rubidium leakage. A 0.01-ml sample of each of the above nystatin or amphotericin B solutions was added to 10 ml of the cell suspension in universal bottles. These were immediately shaken and placed in a 37°C incubator for exactly 30 min. A 10-ml amount of the cell suspension containing 0.01 ml of DMF and 10 ml of the untreated cell suspension were incubated with samples as controls.

After 30 min the suspensions were immediately centrifuged at 5,000 rpm for 5 min, and the supernatant solutions were removed. The supernatant solutions were then examined for Rb^+ ion concentration using a Southern Analytical A3000 atomic absorption spectrophotometer with a conventional rubidium-sensitive hollow-cathode lamp source (784.5 nm) and an air-acetylene flame. The instrument was calibrated with standard rubidium chloride solutions in distilled water before and during each test run.

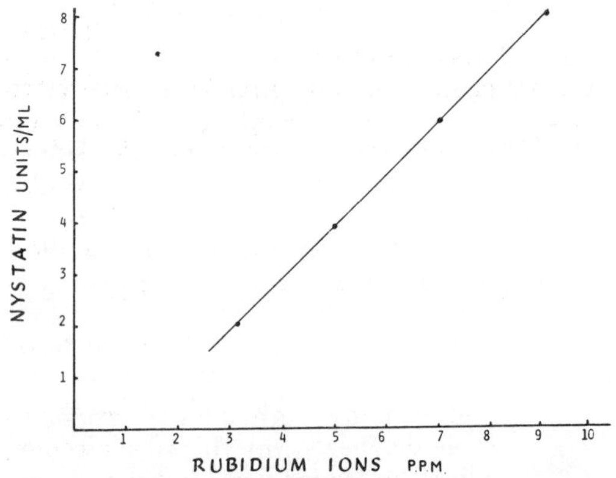

FIG. 1. *Dose-response curve; nystatin concentration versus mean supernatant Rb^+ concentration. Coefficient of linear correlation = 0.999.*

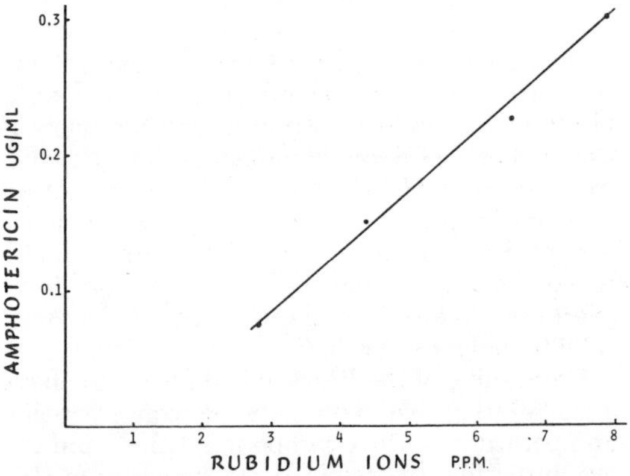

FIG. 2. *Dose-response curve; amphotericin concentration versus mean supernatant Rb^+ concentration. Coefficient of linear correlation = 0.996.*

TABLE 1. *Efflux of Rb^+ ions from S. cerevisiae exposed to standard levels of nystatin*

Nystatin (U/ml)	Supernatant Rb^+ (μg/g)					Mean	Standard deviation
	Day 1	Day 2	Day 3	Day 4	Day 5		
8	9.05	9.15	9.30	9.00	9.25	9.15	0.127
6	7.10	7.00	7.20	7.25	7.00	7.11	0.114
4	5.10	5.10	5.15	5.10	5.00	5.09	0.055
2	3.15	3.00	3.05	3.05	3.20	3.09	0.082
DMF control	0.70	0.70	0.75	0.80	0.85	0.76	0.065
Cell blank	0.70	0.70	0.70	0.80	0.80	0.74	0.055

TABLE 2. *Efflux of Rb^+ ions from S. cerevisiae exposed to standard levels of amphotericin*

Amphotericin (μg/ml)	Supernatant Rb^+ (μg/g)					Mean	Standard deviation
	Day 1	Day 2	Day 3	Day 4	Day 5		
0.300	7.80	7.85	7.85	7.90	7.80	7.84	0.041
0.225	6.45	6.55	6.45	6.40	6.45	6.46	0.055
0.150	4.30	4.30	4.35	4.30	4.30	4.31	0.022
0.075	2.85	2.75	2.75	2.75	2.80	2.78	0.045
DMF control	0.65	0.70	0.80	0.80	0.85	0.76	0.082
Cell blank	0.70	0.70	0.75	0.85	0.85	0.77	0.075

RESULTS AND DISCUSSION

Table 1 records the micrograms of Rb^+ ions per gram of supernatant (p.p.m.) released from yeast cells by nystatin concentrations between 8 and 2 U/ml. Figure 1 shows this to be a linear arithmetic response, and this is confirmed by the coefficient of linear correlation in Fig. 1.

Table 2 records the micrograms of Rb^+ ions per gram of supernatant (p.p.m.) released from yeast cells by amphotericin B concentrations between 0.300 and 0.075 μg/ml. Figure 2 shows this to be a linear arithmetic response, and this again is confirmed by the coefficient of linear correlation in Fig. 2. The reproducibility of the data is apparent from the five sets of figures and the standard deviations quoted.

For an assay to be precise and accurate the dose-response curve is critical, and therefore the factors influencing the curve are most important.

To date, the growth phase of the yeast cells, the temperature of incubation of the cells, the temperature at which the cells are challenged with the nystatin, and the length of time of contact between the cells and the nystatin have been examined. The conditions detailed in Materials and Methods have been found to be most satisfactory for obtaining a linear response.

Stationary-phase cells grown at 30°C have the most suitable susceptibility to nystatin and amphotericin B; log-phase cells and cells grown at 20 or 37°C are unsuitable for a linear response.

It has been found that, once initiated, the release of Rb^+ ions from yeast cells, similarly to K^+ ions, is a continuous process until all Rb^+ or K^+ is depleted. Not only is the release of the ions time dependent, but it is also temperature dependent, and 30 min at 37°C have been found to be the optimum conditions for a satisfactory dose response.

Data produced from rubidium ion leakage measurement has been found to correlate well with that produced with potassium ion leakage measurements in the absence of extracellular K^+ contamination, and therefore the substitution of K^+ ions by Rb^+ ions would appear to be valid.

In summary, the assay of polyene antibiotics by measurement of ion leakage from susceptible cells is feasible. A linear response can be produced with both nystatin and amphotericin B.

LITERATURE CITED

1. **Azoulay, L., and G. W. F. H. Borst-Pauwels.** 1974. Net Rb^+ transport by Rb^+ loaded yeast cells and the electrokinetical formulism. Acta Bot. Neerl. 23:505–512.
2. **Borst-Pauwels, G. W. F. H., P. Schnetkamp, and P. Van Well.** 1973. Activation of Rb^+ and Na^+ uptake into yeast by monovalent cations. Biochim. Biophys. Acta 291:274–279.
3. **Borst-Pauwels, G. W. F. H., G. H. J. Wolters, and J. J. Henricks.** 1971. The interaction of 2,4-dinitrophenol with anaerobic Rb^+ transport across the yeast cell membrane. Biochim. Biophys. Acta 225:269–276.
4. **Clements-Jewery, S.** 1976. Nystatin-induced potassium efflux from *Saccharomyces cerevisiae* measured by flame photometry: a potential bioassay approach. Antimicrob. Agents Chemother. 9:585–586.
5. **Gale, E. F.** 1974. The release of potassium ions from *Candida albicans* in the presence of polyene antibiotics. J. Gen. Microbiol. 80:451–465.
6. **Hammond, S. M., and B. N. Kliger.** 1976. Mode of action of the polyene antibiotic candicidin: binding factors in the wall of *Candida albicans*. Antimicrob. Agents Chemother. 9:561–568.
7. **Hammond, S. M., P. A. Lambert, and B. N. Kliger.** 1974. The mode of action of polyene antibiotics; induced potassium leakage in *Candida albicans*. J. Gen. Microbiol. 81:325–330.
8. **Kinsky, S. C.** 1961. Alterations in the permeability of *Neurospora crassa* due to polyene antibiotics. J. Bacteriol. 82:889–897.
9. **Lampen, J. O., P. M. Arnow, Z. Borowska, and A. I. Laskin.** 1962. Location and role of sterol at nystatin-binding sites. J. Bacteriol. 84:1152–1160.
10. **Marini, F., P. Arnow, and J. O. Lampen,** 1961. The effect of monovalent cations on the inhibition of yeast metabolism by nystatin. J. Gen. Microbiol. 24:51–62.
11. **Sutton, D. D., P. M. Arnow, and J. O. Lampen.** 1961. Effect of high concentrations of nystatin upon glycolysis and cellular permeability in yeast. Proc. Soc. Exp. Biol. Med. 108:170–175.
12. **Venables, P., and A. D. Russell.** 1972. Some effects of nystatin on *Saccharomyces cerevisiae*. Microbios 6:239–246.
13. **Venables, P., and A. D. Russell.** 1975. Nystatin-induced changes in *Saccharomyces cerevisiae*. Antimicrob. Agents Chemother. 7:121–127.
14. **Zygmunt, W. A.** 1966. Intracellular loss of potassium in *Candida albicans* after exposure to polyene antifungal antibiotics. Appl. Microbiol. 14:953–956.

ANTIMICROBIAL AGENTS AND CHEMOTHERAPY, Jan. 1977, p. 34-37 Vol. 11, No. 1

Printed in U.S.A.

Production of Megacins C and Cx: Presumptive Evidence of Extrachromosomal Control

HELEN D. DONOGHUE[1]

Bacteriology Department, The Medical School, Bristol University, Bristol BS8 1TD, England

Received for publication 3 June 1976

Exposure of growing cultures of *Bacillus megaterium* C4A$^-$ to ethidium bromide or an elevated growth temperature was found to eliminate megacin C production. Ethidium bromide resulted in a cure rate of up to 13%. Growth at 43°C gave a cure rate of up to 99%. Megacin C production was lost spontaneously at a rate of 4% or less. There was a greater rate of spontaneous loss of megacin Cx production by *B. megaterium* 337, up to 14%. Growth at 43°C resulted in a cure rate of up to 24% in this organism. Reversion to the Meg$^+$ state by cured clones has never been demonstrated. These observations support the hypothesis that production of megacins C and Cx is plasmid mediated. Meg$^-$ clones adsorbed more megacin than either parent strain and were more susceptible to megacin action.

Megacins are bacteriocins produced by strains of *Bacillus megaterium*. "Megacine" was first described by Ivánovics and Alföldi (16). Later it was realized that the term covered a number of different agents. Megacin C appears to be similar in its effect to certain colicins (22), acting on deoxyribonucleic acid (DNA) synthesis in susceptible organisms (13-15). Megacin Cx, first thought to be similar to megacin C (6, 8), is now known to inhibit protein synthesis in susceptible bacteria (7).

Little is known of the genetic regulation of bacteriocin production by gram-positive organisms, although some staphylococcins are apparently plasmid mediated and can be cured by an elevated growth temperature or by ethidium bromide (3, 4, 17, 24). Kawakami and Landman (18) noted that megacin C production could not be cured by acriflavine treatment, yet Donoghue (5) observed that production of megacins C and Cx could be eliminated by incubating Meg$^+$ cultures at 43°C.

This paper examines the effect of chemical curing agents or an elevated initial incubation temperature on the production of megacin C or Cx by two strains of *B. megaterium*.

(This paper is taken in part from a Ph.D. thesis submitted by H.D.D. to Bristol University.)

MATERIALS AND METHODS

Organisms. *B. megaterium* C4A$^-$ (MegA$^-$C$^+$) was obtained from I. B. Holland, Department of Genetics, University of Leicester, England. *B. megaterium* 337 (MegCx$^+$) was obtained from G. Ivánovics, Institute of Microbiology, University Medical School, Szeged, Hungary. *B. megaterium* 162u is a streptomycin-resistant indicator strain that was originally isolated from soil.

Media. Oxoid blood agar base no. 2 (4%, wt/vol; NA) was used for routine subculture and counts of bacteria. The liquid medium used was peptone-water, which contained 1% (wt/vol) each of peptone and tryptone (Difco) and 0.05% (wt/vol) NaCl. Soft agar used for overlayering plates contained 1.6% (wt/vol) Difco nutrient broth, 0.5% (wt/vol) NaCl, and 0.7% (wt/vol) agar. Peptone-glucose broth (12) was used for megacin production and broth cultures.

Megacin. Megacins C and Cx were produced according to the method described by Donoghue (5). Crude culture supernatants were used as a source of both megacins.

Demonstration of megacin production. Cultures were diluted in saline, and 0.1 ml of appropriate dilutions was spread on NA plates. After overnight incubation at 37°C, plates showing well-distributed colonies were replicated onto NA plates seeded with 162u (0.1 ml of an overnight 162u peptone-water culture per 4 ml of soft agar). The replicated plates were kept at 5°C overnight and then incubated at 37°C for 8 to 12 h. Meg$^-$ colonies were easily identified by the absence of an inhibition zone (Fig. 1).

Elimination by chemical agents. A growing C4A$^-$ culture in peptone-glucose broth was diluted 1:10 and 1:100 in warm broth, and an aqueous acriflavine solution added to give a final concentration of 10.0, 1.0, or 0.1 μg/ml. The organisms were incubated at 37°C overnight, together with control cultures without acriflavine. To examine the effect of culture age, C4A$^-$ was inoculated into peptone-glucose broth and samples were taken at various times after incubation. The optical density of samples was adjusted with warm broth to give a reading of 0.06 to 0.07

[1] Present address: School of Medical Sciences, University of Bradford, Bradford, West Yorkshire BD7 1DP, England.

(Unicam SP600, 610 nm). Volumes (10 ml) of diluted sample were mixed with various concentrations of aqueous acriflavine or ethidium bromide solutions. These and control cultures were incubated overnight at 37°C and then tested for megacin production.

Effect of temperature. Two peptone-water cultures of the test organism, inoculated from the same colony, were set up. One was incubated overnight at 37°C and the other at 43°C. Samples were then tested for megacin production. All subsequent incubation was at 37°C.

Adsorption of megacin and susceptibility to megacin action. The organisms to be used for megacin adsorption were grown as a confluent layer on the surface of a large (304.8 mm² or 12 by 12 inch) NA plate. After overnight incubation, they were scraped off the agar, suspended in saline, and washed twice with saline. A sample from each cell suspension was counted by the Miles and Misra method (21), using triplicate plates. Equal volumes of sterile megacin solution and either undiluted or diluted cell suspension were mixed and left for 1 to 2 h at 5°C to allow adsorption to occur. The bacterial cells were then spun down, resuspended in saline, and counted. The supernatant was assayed for residual megacin by a punch-hole assay (20). The percentage of megacin adsorbed was calculated, and when different strains were compared, the figures were corrected to allow for differences in cell numbers.

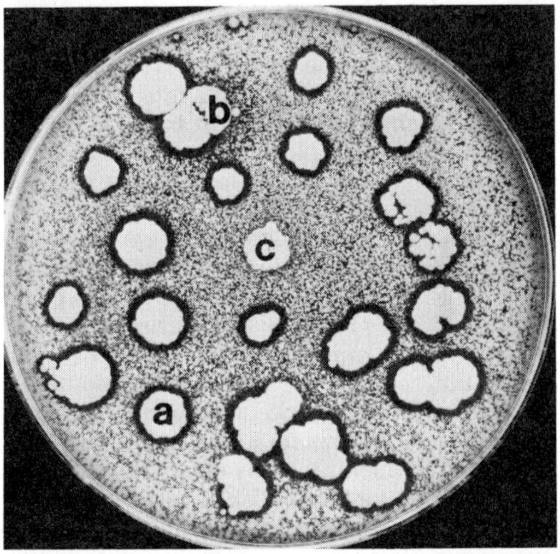

FIG. 1. *Demonstration of megacin production by replica plating on to agar seeded with the indicator strain B. megaterium 162u. (a) Meg⁺ colony; (b) Meg± colony; (c) Meg⁻ colony.*

RESULTS

A summary of the results is shown in Table 1.

Chemical curing agents. Acriflavine, at a concentration of 0.1, 1.0, or 10.0 μg/ml, had little curing effect on C4A⁻ cultures containing 1.3×10^6, 2.5×10^7, or 2.8×10^8 viable organisms per ml. A concentration of 10 μg of acriflavine per ml was bactericidal except in the undiluted C4A⁻ culture. Acriflavine had no curing effect on C4A⁻ cells obtained from 1- to 5-h-old cultures. In a similar experiment, there was an increase in the proportion of Meg⁻ colonies when 1×10^{-5} M ethidium bromide was added to a 3-h (exponential phase) culture of C4A⁻. The cure rate was 13% (15/116), compared with 2% (4/196) in the control.

Effect of high temperature. An initial incubation temperature of 43°C was highly effective in eliminating megacin C production. A maximal cure rate of 99% (110/111) could be obtained by this procedure. Using data from several experiments, an average cure rate of 85% (468/550) was realized after initial growth at 43°C, compared with a rate of 1.7% (17/975) in the controls. Using strain 337, there was a slight increase in cure rate of megacin Cx production. In one experiment a rate of 24% (44/184) was noted, compared with 2% (4/198) in the corresponding control. Average rates, however, were 10.6% (125/1,174) at 43°C and 6.3% (54/854) at 37°C.

Spontaneous loss of megacin Cx production. Because MegCx⁻ clones appeared to arise so readily, individual MegCx⁺ colonies were examined to see whether they too contained

TABLE 1. *Comparison of the effect of various curing agents on megacin production*

Treatment	Megacin C		Megacin Cx	
	No. of colonies cured/ no. tested	Maximum percent cured	No. of colonies cured/ no. tested	Maximum no. percent cured
Ethidium bromide (1×10^{-5} M)	15/116	12.9	NT	NT
Control	4/196	2.0	NT	NT
Acriflavine (1.0 μg/ml)	3/111	2.7	NT	NT
Control	0/89	0	NT	NT
Growth at 43°C	110/111	99.1	44/184	23.9
Control	2/152	1.3	4/196	2.0

[a] NT, Not tested.

MegCx⁻ cells. Both MegCx⁺ colonies and those colonies surrounded by a hazy zone, termed MegCx$^{\pm}$, contained a significant proportion of viable Meg$^-$ cells, 13.5% (8/133) and 9.8% (19/193), respectively.

Reversion from Meg$^-$ to Meg$^+$. No Meg$^-$ clone has yet been shown to have reverted to the Meg$^+$ state. From the data currently available, if reversion does occur it must be at a rate less than 0.22% (0/456) for MegCx and 0.073% (0/1,371) for MegC.

Activity spectrum of Meg$^+$ and Meg$^-$ organisms. Using an overlay technique, both Meg$^+$ strains were apparently nonsusceptible to megacins C and Cx. Meg$^-$ clones were susceptible to both megacins. This was the only difference in activity spectrum observed. In broth cultures, Meg$^+$ strains could be shown to be megacin susceptible when high multiplicities of megacin were used. A typical result as shown in Fig. 2.

Adsorption of megacin. Meg$^-$ cultures adsorbed more megacin than Meg$^+$ cells (Fig. 2). In this example, cells of the indicator organism 162u adsorbed about five times more megacin than did MegCx$^-$ cells of strain 337. The Meg$^-$ cells adsorbed approximately 50 times more megacin Cx than did the MegCx$^+$ cells.

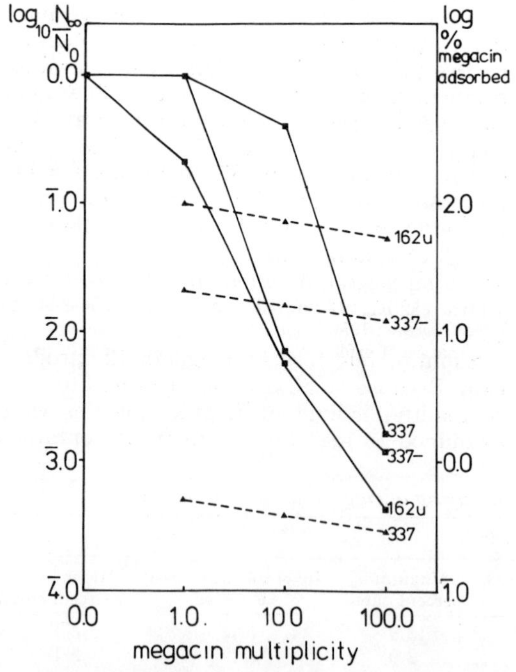

FIG. 2. *Adsorption of megacin Cx to MegCx$^+$ and MegCx$^-$ cells of B. megaterium and their subsequent survival. Symbols: (■) Survival curve after an "infinite" time for megacin adsorption. Log_{10} survivor ratio plotted against megacin multiplicity. (▲) Adsorption curve. Log_{10} percent megacin adsorbed per cell plotted against megacin multiplicity.*

DISCUSSION

An elevated incubation temperature has been shown to eliminate megacin C production highly effectively from *B. megaterium* C4A$^-$. Ethidium bromide has a lesser effect. These observations, when compared with staphylococcal studies (1, 3, 17, 19, 24), strongly suggest that the determinant for megacin C production is situated on a plasmid. Failure to eliminate megacin C production with acriflavine is not unexpected. Curing of plasmids is highly unpredictable, and agents active against one organism may have no effect even on another strain of the same species (3, 10).

Too little is known of the genetics of *B. megaterium* to enable plasmid linkage to be established by the other criteria suggested by Novick (23). It is known that a high proportion of the DNA in *B. megaterium* is in the form of heterogeneous circular DNA segments (2, 11). Although an additional element could not be distinguished in one Meg$^+$ strain examined, the existence of a megacin plasmid has not been disproved.

The megacin Cx determinant is probably also plasmid borne, but since its high rate of spontaneous loss masks the effect of possible curing agents, *B. megaterium* 337 cultures were not tested with chemical curing agents. The demonstration of mixed clones of strain 337 is rather surprising, since it would be expected that a Meg$^-$ cell arising in a Meg$^+$ colony would be killed immediately by the megacin being produced by adjacent cells. Possibly most of this megacin is adsorbed to the cell walls of the producing organisms or rapidly diffuses away into the surrounding agar. If Meg$^-$ organisms are being killed, their proportions as reported in this paper may be underrepresented.

Previous work (5) has demonstrated the presence of megacin on the surface of Meg$^+$ cells. This may explain the low levels of megacin adsorption found in Meg$^+$ cultures. However, the difference in megacin susceptibility between Meg$^+$ and Meg$^-$ cultures of the same bacterial strain suggests that, as with other bacteriocins (9), there may be an immunity substance present in the cytoplasm of Meg$^+$ organisms that can be overwhelmed by high megacin levels.

B. megaterium is a particularly suitable organism for future investigations along these lines since its cell wall can be completely removed by treatment with lysozyme. Kawakami and Landman (18) have already shown that the capacity of $C4A^-$ to produce megacin C is not lost when cultures are converted into protoplasts. The study of megacin production and its action on protoplasts should, therefore, prove most rewarding.

ACKNOWLEDGMENTS

The advice and helpful discussions of the late Anna Mayr-Harting, formerly of this Department, are gratefully acknowledged. Vilma Stanisich is thanked for her constructive criticism of the manuscript. Most of the work was carried out while I was in receipt of an M.R.C. scholarship for training in research methods.

LITERATURE CITED

1. **Bouanchaud, D. H., M. R. Scavizzi, and Y. A. Chabbert.** 1968. Elimination by ethidium bromide of antibiotic resistance in enterobacteria and staphylococci. J. Gen. Microbiol. 54:417–425.
2. **Carlton, B. C., and D. R. Helinski.** 1969. Heterogeneous circular DNA elements in vegetative cultures of *Bacillus megaterium*. Proc. Natl. Acad. Sci. U.S.A. 64:592–599.
3. **Dajani, A. S., and Z. Taube.** 1974. Plasmid-mediated production of staphylococcin in bacteriophage type 71 *Staphylococcus aureus*. Antimicrob. Agents Chemother. 5:594–598.
4. **Dastidar, S. G., S. Mitra, S. N. Sarkar, and A. N. Chakrabarty.** 1974. Transformation with bacteriocin factors in staphylococci. J. Gen. Microbiol. 84:245–252.
5. **Donoghue, H. D.** 1972. Properties and comparative starch-gel electrophoresis of megacins from several *Bacillus megaterium* strains. J. Gen. Microbiol. 72:473–483.
6. **Durner, K.** 1970. Anreicherung, Reinigung und Charakterisierung eines Bacteriocins aus *Bacillus megaterium* 337. Z. Allg. Mikrobiol. 10:93–102.
7. **Durner, K.** 1970. Untersuchungen zur Wirkungsweise von Megacin Cx auf *Bacillus megaterium* KM. Z. Allg. Mikrobiol. 10:373–382.
8. **Durner, K., and F. Mach.** 1966. Physiologische Untersuchungen eines Bacteriocines aus *Bacillus megaterium* 337. Zentralbl. Bakteriol. Parasitenkd. Infektionskr. Hyg. Abt. II Orig. 120:565–575.
9. **Frédéricq, P.** 1958. Colicins and colicinogenic factors. Symp. Soc. Exp. Biol. 12:104–122.
10. **Hale, E. M., and R. D. Hinsdill.** 1975. Biological activity of staphylococcin 462: bacteriocin from *Staphylococcus aureus*. Antimicrob. Agents Chemother. 7:74–81.
11. **Henneberry, R. C., and B. C. Carlton.** 1973. Characterization of the polydisperse closed circular deoxyribonucleic acid molecules of *Bacillus megaterium*. J. Bacteriol. 114:625–631.
12. **Holland, I. B.** 1961. The purification and properties of megacin, a bacteriocin from *Bacillus megaterium*. Biochem. J. 78:641–648.
13. **Holland, I. B.** 1963. Effect of a bacteriocin preparation (Megacin C) on DNA synthesis in *Bacillus megaterium*. Biochem. Biophys. Res. Commun. 13:246–250.
14. **Holland, I. B.** 1965. A bacteriocin specifically affecting DNA synthesis in *Bacillus megaterium*. J. Mol. Biol. 12:429–438.
15. **Holland, I. B., and C. F. Roberts.** 1964. Properties of a new bacteriocin formed by *Bacillus megaterium*. J. Gen. Microbiol. 35:271–285.
16. **Ivánovics, G., and L. Alföldi.** 1954. A new antibacterial principle: megacine. Nature (London) 174:465.
17. **Jetten, A. M., and G. D. Vogels.** 1973. Characterization and extrachromosomal control of bacteriocin production in *Staphylococcus aureus*. Antimicrob. Agents Chemother. 4:49–57.
18. **Kawakami, M., and O. E. Landman.** 1966. Retention of episomes during protoplasting and during propagation in the L state. J. Bacteriol. 92:398–404.
19. **May, J. W., R. H. Houghton, and C. J. Perret.** 1964. The effect of growth at elevated temperatures on some heritable properties of *Staphylococcus aureus*. J. Gen. Microbiol. 37:157–169.
20. **Mayr-Harting, A., A. J. Hedges, and R. C. W. Berkeley.** 1972. Methods for studying bacteriocins, p. 315–422. *In* J. R. Norris and D. W. Ribbons (ed.), Methods in microbiology, vol. 7A. Academic Press Inc., London.
21. **Miles, A. A., and S. S. Misra.** 1938. The estimation of the bactericidal powers of the blood. J. Hyg. 38:732–748.
22. **Nomura, M.** 1967. Colicins and related bacteriocins. Annu. Rev. Microbiol. 21:257–284.
23. **Novick, R. P.** 1969. Extrachromosomal inheritance in bacteria. Bacteriol. Rev. 33:210–263.
24. **Warren, R., M. Rogolsky, B. B. Wiley, and L. A. Glasgow.** 1974. Effect of ethidium bromide on elimination of exfoliative toxin and bacteriocin production in *Staphylococcus aureus*. J. Bacteriol. 118:980–985.

ANTIMICROBIAL AGENTS AND CHEMOTHERAPY, Jan. 1977, p. 38-43 Vol. 11, No. 1

Printed in U.S.A.

Effect of Atebrin on Bacterial Membrane Adenosine Triphosphatases in Relation to the Divalent Cation Used as Substrate and/or Activator

JOSÉ CARREIRA AND EMILIO MUÑOZ*

Consejo Superior Investigaciones Científicas, Membrane Biochemistry Unit, Velázquez, 144, Madrid-6, Spain

Received for publication 2 June 1976

The action of atebrin on purified adenosine triphosphatase (ATPase) from *Micrococcus lysodeikticus* was studied as well as on the membrane-bound and soluble ATPases from *Escherichia coli* and *Bacillus megaterium*. Atebrin inhibited the Ca^{2+}-dependent activity of all these enzymes, and the inhibition was reversed by an excess of Ca^{2+} ions. Kinetic studies carried out with the purified enzyme from *M. lysodeikticus* showed that the inhibition by atebrin was strongly cooperative, suggesting the complex nature of the process. On the other hand, atebrin stimulated the Mg^{2+}ATPase activity of the *M. lysodeikticus* enzyme, displacing its adenosine 5′-triphosphate (ATP)/Mg^{2+} optimum ratios, but inhibited the Mg^{2+}-ATPase activity of *E. coli* provided that ATP was in excess over Mg^{2+}, i.e., that the ATP/Mg^{2+} ratio was higher than its optimum. These results suggest that divalent cations influence the bacterial ATPases in different ways depending on the type of divalent ion and/or enzyme. The effect of atebrin on bacterial ATPases may reflect those differences, and its complex mechanism of action might be related to the existence of more than one site for divalent cations and/or distinct conformational states in these enzymes.

In spite of the considerable structural similarities emerging between adenosine triphosphatases (ATPases) from bacteria (1, 3, 7, 26) and organelles (23, 24), the inhibitors of these energy-transducing ATPases show a certain degree of specificity, suggesting that they act according to specific mechanisms. Some inhibitors, i.e., oligomycin, atebrin, and Dio 9, affected certain types of ATPase (6, 8, 12–14, 16, 17), whereas azide and *N*,*N*′-dicyclohexyl carbodiimide behave as general inhibitors (10, 14, 21, 25). The molecular basis of this specificity is unknown except in a few cases, e.g., oligomycin. The selective action of this drug on mitochondrial ATPase was related to the association of the enzyme into membranal, vesicular complexes and was found to be dependent on a protein of molecular weight 18,000 (6).

Atebrin, an uncoupler of photophosphorylation, stimulated a light-triggered, Mg^{2+}-dependent activity in chloroplasts, but inhibited the Ca^{2+}-ATPase of the soluble coupling factor (8). The effect of atebrin on bacterial ATPases was earlier studied with membrane-bound enzymes (12, 13) or with crude "soluble" preparations (12). In previous work from this laboratory, it was noticed that atebrin stimulated or inhibited the Mg^{2+}-dependent membrane-bound ATPase of *Micrococcus lysodeikticus* depending upon the degree of cation depletion of the membranes and/or the concentration of inhibitor (M. Lastras, Ph.D. thesis, University of Madrid, Madrid, 1974). Furthermore, atebrin at low concentrations stimulated, and at high concentrations inhibited, the Ca^{2+}-ATPase activity of the crude soluble enzyme of *M. lysodeikticus* (C. Muñoz, unpublished observations). These studies did not establish a clear mechanism for the inhibition of ATPases by atebrin. On the other hand, atebrin apparently did not inhibit either the membrane-bound or the soluble ATPase of *Escherichia coli* K-12 using adenosine 5′-triphosphate (ATP)-Mg^{2+} (2:1) as substrate (10). To ascertain whether the specificity of the inhibition by atebrin would reside in its interaction with the protein or with the activating cation, we studied its effect on a highly purified Ca^{2+}-ATPase from *M. lysodeikticus* assayed in the presence of either Ca^{2+} or Mg^{2+} as activating ion. This study suggested that the stimulatory or inhibitory effect of atebrin was in fact related to the cation used with ATP as substrate or activator. An extension of these studies to *E. coli* and *Bacillus megaterium* ATPases confirmed the above suggestion but pointed out that the inhibition of ATPase by atebrin was also selectively dependent on the type of enzyme but independent of its physical state (soluble or membrane-bound).

MATERIALS AND METHODS

Microorganisms and membrane preparation. The growth characteristics and membrane isolation of *M. lysodeikticus* were described elsewhere (21). The conditions for cultivation and isolation of membranes of *E. coli* K-12 (Hfr, Thr$^-$) have been reported previously (9, 11). The conditions of culture and membrane isolation of *B. megaterium* KM were essentially as described by Mirsky (19).

Solubilization of bacterial ATPases. *M. lysodeikticus* ATPase was solubilized by the "shock-wash" procedure applied to divalent cation-depleted membranes (21). The crude shock-wash enzyme was purified by gel filtration on Sephadex G-200 as described (21), but 30 mM tris(hydroxymethyl)aminomethane (Tris)-hydrochloride buffer (pH 8.0) was used as the effluent. Solubilization of *E. coli* ATPase was achieved by treatment of the membranes with 3 mM ethylenediaminetetraacetate at alkaline pH (9.0) as reported by Carreira et al. (9). *B. megaterium* ATPase was solubilized following the procedure of Mirsky et al. (20).

Measurement of ATPase activity and protein concentration. The ATPase activity at pH 7.5 in 30 mM Tris-hydrochloride buffer was measured by the liberation of ^{32}P from [γ-^{32}P]ATP as reported elsewhere (22). Incubations were carried out at 37°C for 3 min (*M. lysodeikticus* ATPase) and 5 min (membrane-bound and soluble ATPases from *E. coli* and *B. megaterium*). The concentrations of ATP and activating divalent cations were varied according to the type of experiment and ATPase used (9, 20, 21, 25). A detailed description of each of the experimental conditions is given under Results.

Protein concentration was estimated by the method of Lowry et al. (18) with bovine serum albumin as standard.

Chemicals. Adenosine triphosphate-disodium salt (Na_2ATP) was purchased from P-L Biochemicals Inc., Milwaukee, Wis. [γ-^{32}P]ATP (2,506 mCi/mmol) was from Amersham, The Radiochemical Center. Atebrin (quinacrine dihydrochloride) and Tris (Trizma base) were products from Sigma Chemical Co., St. Louis, Mo. All other reagents of the highest quality commercially available were from Merck, Darmstadt, West Germany.

RESULTS

Effect of atebrin on the Ca^{2+}-dependent activity of pure *M. lysodeikticus* ATPase. Table 1 shows the inhibition of purified *M. lysodeikticus* at 2 mM substrate concentration using the optimum ATP/Ca^{2+} = 1 ratio previously determined (21) and its reversal by an excess of Ca^{2+} ions. These results suggested that the inhibition by atebrin of the Ca^{2+}-ATPase activity of the enzyme may be dependent on different ATP/Ca^{2+} ratios.

The above suggestion was confirmed by two types of experiments. Figure 1 illustrates the effect of variable concentrations of atebrin at three different ATP/Ca^{2+} ratios. The results showed that the inhibition by atebrin was strongly cooperative and varied with the concentration of Ca^{2+}. Figure 2 shows the results obtained with variable concentrations of ATP at a fixed concentration of Ca^{2+} and increasing concentrations of atebrin. The curve representing no inhibitor confirms the optimum ATP/Ca^{2+} ratio (21), and a K_m, app can be calculated for ATP = 1 mM (see inset of Fig. 2). The pattern of inhibition by atebrin was noncompetitive. However, the inhibition was not directly proportional to the concentration of inhibitor as deduced from Fig. 2. This was further evidenced by plotting the slopes against inhibitor

TABLE 1. *Reversion by Ca^{2+} ions of the inhibition by atebrin of M. lysodeikticus Ca^{2+}-ATPase*

Ca^{2+} (mM)	ATPase activity[a]	
	Sp act (μmol/min per mg of protein)	Inhibition (%)
2 (−atebrin)	14.3	0
2 (+atebrin)	6.4	55.3
3 (+atebrin)	10.8	25.0
4 (+atebrin)	12.8	10.5
5 (+atebrin)	13.9	2.8
6 (+atebrin)	13.9	2.8

[a] The conditions of enzyme assay were as those described in Materials and Methods. Each assay mixture contained (in 500 μl), 2 mM [γ-^{32}P]ATP (specific radioactivity in the assay was 200,000 cpm/μmol), 2 mM $CaCl_2$, and 6 μg of enzyme protein. Where present, the concentration of atebrin was 1 mM.

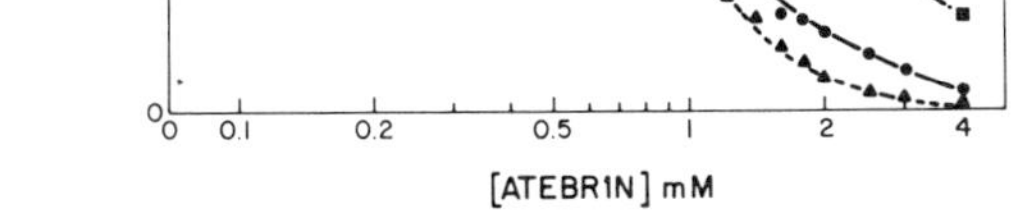

FIG. 1. *Semilogarithmic plot of relative velocity of the purified M. lysodeikticus ATPase versus atebrin concentration at three different ATP/Ca^{2+} ratios. The assay mixtures (500 μl) contained 4 mM [γ-^{32}P]ATP (specific radioactivity 100,000 cpm/μmol), 6 μg of enzyme protein and (- -▲- -), 2 mM $CaCl_2$; (— ●—), 4 mM $CaCl_2$; (· — ■— ·), 8 mM $CaCl_2$. For other details see Materials and Methods.*

concentrations. This plot (not shown) gave a parabolic pattern of inhibition and, therefore, a single K_i value for the inhibitor could not be calculated. All these results suggested that the inhibition by atebrin of *M. lysodeikticus* ATPase is very complex and difficult to analyze by a kinetic approach. This difficulty was even more apparent when the effect of atebrin on *M. lysodeikticus* ATPase was examined as a function of Ca^{2+} concentration at a fixed ATP concentration. The addition of increasing concentrations of atebrin changed the hyperbolic form of the Ca^{2+}-saturation curve (not shown) into a sigmoid form, and the inhibitor affected both the K_m and V_{max} values.

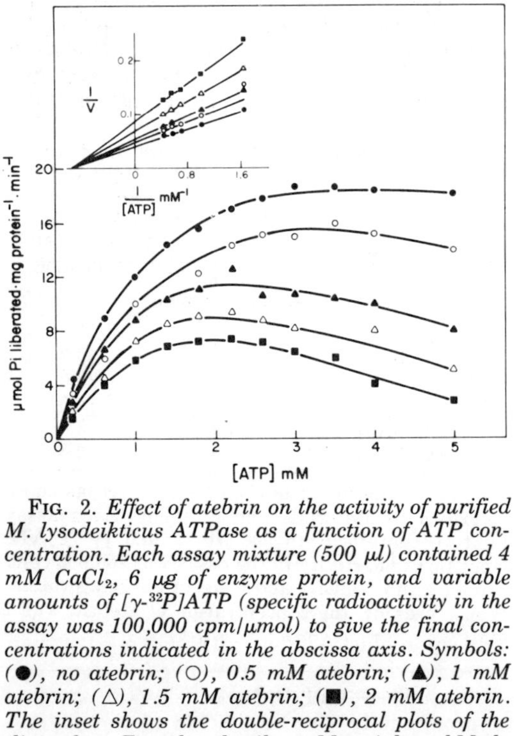

FIG. 2. *Effect of atebrin on the activity of purified M. lysodeikticus ATPase as a function of ATP concentration. Each assay mixture (500 µl) contained 4 mM $CaCl_2$, 6 µg of enzyme protein, and variable amounts of [γ-^{32}P]ATP (specific radioactivity in the assay was 100,000 cpm/µmol) to give the final concentrations indicated in the abscissa axis. Symbols: (●), no atebrin; (○), 0.5 mM atebrin; (▲), 1 mM atebrin; (△), 1.5 mM atebrin; (■), 2 mM atebrin. The inset shows the double-reciprocal plots of the direct data. For other details see Materials and Methods.*

TABLE 2. *Effect of atebrin on the Mg^{2+}-dependent activity of M. lysodeikticus ATPase*

Mg^{2+} (mM)	ATPase activity[a] (µmol/min per mg of protein)		
	No atebrin	Atebrin	
		50 µM	0.5 mM
0.05	3.3	10.5	2.6
1	6.1	8.1	8.7
2	4.1	6.3	10.7
8	4.0	3.8	6.8

[a] The conditions of enzyme assay were as described in Materials and Methods and Table 1, but with Mg^{2+} instead of $CaCl_2$.

Effect of atebrin on the Mg^{2+}-dependent activity of *M. lysodeikticus* ATPase. Table 2 illustrates the effect of atebrin on purified *M. lysodeikticus* ATPase using ATP-Mg^{2+} as substrate. The first column indicates that the optimum activity was reached at an ATP/mg^{2+} ratio of 2, which agrees with previous studies of the crude soluble enzyme (21). Also, Mg^{2+} appeared to be a more effective activator than Ca^{2+} at low concentrations but less effective at the optimum and higher concentrations (21). Unlike with Ca^{2+}-ATPase activity, atebrin stimulated the Mg^{2+}-ATPase activity of the *M. lysodeikticus* enzyme and displaced the optimum ATP/Mg^{2+} ratios depending on the concentrations of inhibitor used in most cases.

Effect of atebrin on membrane-bound and soluble ATPase of *E. coli*. To test whether the antagonistic effect of atebrin on the Ca^{2+}- or Mg^{2+}-ATPase of *M. lysodeikticus* was specific to the protein or not, we examined its effect on the soluble and membrane-bound ATPases from *E. coli* and *B. megaterium* whose specificities for divalent cations are known to differ from that of *M. lysodeikticus* (9, 10, 20, 25). In most cases atebrin inhibited the Mg^{2+}- and Ca^{2+}-dependent activities of *E. coli* ATPase (Table 3). At a given concentration of atebrin, its inhibitory effect was dependent on the type and concentration of the divalent cation used. As found for *M. lysodeikticus* ATPase, the Ca^{2+}-dependent activity of *E. coli* ATPase was more sensitive than the Mg^{2+}-dependent activity. However, unlike in the case of *M. lysodeikticus* ATPase, atebrin did not stimulate the Mg^{2+}-ATPase activity of *E. coli* at low concentrations of the divalent cation. On the other hand, a lack of inhibition or even a slight stimulation by atebrin was observed at the optimum ATP/Mg^{2+} 2 ratio, thus confirming previous results from this laboratory (10). Again, as found for *M. lysodeikticus* ATPase, an excess of Ca^{2+} ions over ATP prevented or markedly reduced the inhibition by atebrin of the Ca^{2+} ATPase of *E. coli*. It is worth noting that the effect of atebrin was virtually independent of the physical state of the protein, soluble or membrane bound.

Effect of atebrin on Ca^{2+}-ATPase of *B. megaterium*. The effect of atebrin on *B. megaterium* ATPase was examined by its Ca^{2+}-dependent activity because the low values were obtained with Mg^{2+} as the activating ion. Table 4 illustrates the inhibition by atebrin of Ca^{2+}-soluble and membrane-bound ATPase, as well as their partial reversion by addition of an ex-

TABLE 3. *Effect of atebrin on the membrane-bound and soluble ATPase of E. coli*

Enzyme prepn	Me^{2+}	ATPase activity[a] (μmol/min per mg of protein)			
		No atebrin	Atebrin (mM)		
			0.5	1	2
Membrane	2 mM $MgCl_2$	0.43	0.34 (21)	0.22 (49)	0.11 (74)
	4 mM $MgCl_2$	0.46	0.47 (0)	0.35 (24)	0.22 (52)
	2 mM $CaCl_2$	0.18	0.11 (39)	0.06 (67)	0.02 (89)
	4 mM $CaCl_2$	0.21	0.15 (28)	0.1 (52)	0.04 (80)
	8 mM $CaCl_2$	0.18	0.19 (0)	0.14 (22)	0.09 (50)
Soluble	2 mM $MgCl_2$	2.37	1.84 (23)	1.58 (33)	1.11 (53)
	4 mM $MgCl_2$	3.3	3.7 (+)	3.88 (+)	3.56 (+)
	2 mM $CaCl_2$	1.33	0.71 (47)	0.54 (59)	0.44 (67)
	4 mM $CaCl_2$	2.65	1.03 (39)	0.83 (69)	0.47 (82)
	8 mM $CaCl_2$	2.7	2.19 (19)	1.36 (50)	0.62 (77)

[a] The assay mixtures (500 μl) contained: 8 mM [γ-^{32}P]ATP (specific radioactivity 100,000 cpm/μmol), the concentrations of $MgCl_2$ or $CaCl_2$ and atebrin as indicated in the table, and 100 μg of membrane protein or 20 μg of soluble protein. Numbers in parentheses indicate the percentage of inhibition with respect to controls (no atebrin); (+) denotes stimulation of the activity.

TABLE 4. *Effect of atebrin on the Ca^{2+}-dependent membrane-bound and soluble ATPase of B. megaterium*

Ca^{2+} (mM)	ATPase activity[a]			
	Membrane bound		Soluble	
	Sp act (μmol/min per mg)	Inhibition (%)	Sp act (μmol/min per mg)	Inhibition (%)
8 (−atebrin)	0.42	0	1.83	0
8 (+atebrin)	0.11	74	0.38	79
12 (+atebrin)	0.18	57	0.51	72
16 (+atebrin)	0.24	43	0.83	55
24 (+atebrin)	0.29	31	1.26	34

[a] The assay mixtures (500 μl) contained: 8 mM [γ-^{32}P]ATP (specific radioactivity 100,000 cpm/μmol), the concentrations of $CaCl_2$ indicated in the table; 1 mM atebrin, and 100 μg of membrane protein or 10 μg of soluble protein.

cess of Ca^{2+} ions, again confirming previous findings. However, a typical result obtained with *B. megaterium* ATPase was the inability of higher concentrations of atebrin to inhibit its activity further. As a matter of fact, 10 mM atebrin inhibited only 85% of the control Ca^{2+}-ATPase.

DISCUSSION

The early reports by Greenawalt et al. (12) on *B. megaterium* ATPase and by Gross and Coles on *Staphylococcus aureus* ATPase (13) are among the few that describe an inhibition of bacterial ATPases by atebrin. Interestingly enough, Greenawalt et al. found differences in the amount of the inhibition depending upon the use of Ca^{2+} or Mg^{2+} as the activating ion (12). More recently, we reported the lack of inhibition by atebrin of *E. coli* ATPase (10). There have been a great number of studies on the inhibition by atebrin of phosphorylation and chloroplast ATPase, although most of them were carried out on unresolved systems (8). Baltscheffsky and Baltscheffsky (5) observed approximately 90% inhibition of the ATPase activity of the photosynthetic bacterium *Rhodospirillum rubrum,* with relatively low concentrations of atebrin. From these studies, it appeared that atebrin mainly affected the coupling factors related to phosphorylating systems that behaved as Ca^{2+}-soluble ATPases. However, none of these studies explored the mechanisms of inhibition by atebrin of these energy-transducing proteins in depth.

This report presents one of the first attempts to analyze the molecular mechanisms underlying this inhibition. The studies carried out with the purified ATPase of *M. lysodeikticus* suggest that atebrin inhibited its activity by a very complex mechanism. It is also worth noting that the inhibitory effect of the drug was greater on the Ca^{2+}-dependent ATPase than on the Mg^{2+}-dependent activity. As a matter of fact, it stimulated in most cases the Mg^{2+}-dependent activity, thus confirming the antagonistic effects of the two cations on *M. lysodeikticus* ATPase (15, 21). The use of a highly purified ATPase ruled out the existence of two different ATPase systems as suggested earlier by Greenwalt et al. (12). Therefore, it seemed reasonable to conclude that atebrin inhibited preferentially the Ca^{2+}-ATPase activity of the purified enzyme from *M. lysodeikticus*. This conclusion was confirmed from the studies with *E. coli* ATPase, which were of particular relevance because Mg^{2+} was a better activator than Ca^{2+} for *E. coli* ATPase. They also provided a basis to justify the result previously obtained by us (10) when the inhibition by atebrin of *E. coli* ATPase was studied.

The simplest explanation to account for the reversal by excess of divalent cations of inhibition by atebrin of bacterial ATPases might be that atebrin and divalent cations interact with each other with different affinities. However, the kinetic studies with *M. lysodeikticus* ATPase did not support it. Moreover, all the attempts to detect the formation of Me^{2+}-atebrin complexes by either fluorimetry or differential spectrophotometry gave negative results. On the other hand, in preliminary experiments we detected the interaction between atebrin and *M. lysodeikticus* ATPase by an enhancement of the intrinsic fluorescence of atebrin (J. Carreira and E. Muñoz, unpublished observations). The interaction was only partially reversed by Ca^{2+} or ATP/Ca^{2+}, suggesting that a mechanism of pure competitive inhibition could not solely account for the inhibition of the enzyme by atebrin. Therefore, it seems reasonable to propose that there are at least two classes of divalent cation sites in bacterial ATPases: one may be involved at the active site where ATP is bound; and a second, less defined, may be related to the general structure or conformation of the enzyme. Atebrin would interact preferentially with this second site. On kinetic grounds, Ahlers et al. (2) proposed that Mg^{2+} plays a complex role on the Mg^{2+}-ATPase of *E. coli* as part of the substrate and as activator and inhibitor. On a similar basis, we (10) proposed the existence of two sites for Mg^{2+} in *E. coli* ATPase. The results presented in this work are also interesting in connection with recent reports on the influence of divalent cations, i.e., Mg^{2+} or Ca^{2+}, on the ATPase or ATP synthase activity of mitochondrial, bacterial, and chloroplast coupling factors (4, 15, 23, 24, 27). It seems possible, therefore, that divalent cations play an important and selective role at the molecular level, perhaps by inducing conformational changes in the energy-transducing proteins, in the processes of conservation of energy. This possibility is currently being explored.

ACKNOWLEDGMENTS

This work was supported in part by a grant from the Fondo Nacional para el Desarrollo de la Investigación Científica. J.C. thanks the Plan de Formación del Personal Investigador for a fellowship. We are indebted to M. Nieto for many discussions, to C. Muñoz for valuable information on the effect of atebrin on the crude ATPase of *M. lysodeikticus*, and to the reviewers for their help in the interpretation of data.

LITERATURE CITED

1. **Abrams, A., and J. B. Smith.** 1974. Bacterial membrane ATPases, p. 395–429. *In* P. D. Boyer (ed.), The enzymes, vol. 10. Academic Press Inc., New York.
2. **Ahlers, J., D. Kabisch, and T. Günther.** 1975. The functional groups of the Mg-Ca ATPase from *Escherichia coli*. Can. J. Biochem. **53**:658–665.
3. **Andreu, J. M., J. A. Albendea, and E. Muñoz.** 1973. Membrane adenosine triphosphatase of *Micrococcus lysodeikticus*. Molecular properties of the purified enzyme unstimulated by trypsin. Eur. J. Biochem. **37**:505–515.
4. **Bakker-Grunwald, T.** 1974. A Ca^{2+}-stimulated incorporation of phosphate into ATP in chloroplasts; the problem of allotopy. Biochim. Biophys. Acta **347**:141–143.
5. **Baltscheffsky, H., and M. Baltscheffsky.** 1958. On light-induced phosphorylation in *Rhodospirillum rubrum*. Acta Chem. Scand. **12**:1333–1335.
6. **Beechey, R. B.** 1974. Structural aspects of the mitochondrial membrane-bound adenosine triphosphatase, p. 41–62. *In* J. R. Bronk (ed.), Membrane adenosine triphosphatases and transport processes. The Biochemical Society, London.
7. **Bragg, P. D., and C. Hou.** 1975. Subunit composition function and spatial arrangement in the Ca^{2+}- and Mg^{2+}-activated adenosine triphosphatases of *Escherichia coli* and *Salmonella typhimurium*. Arch. Biochem. Biophys. **167**:311–321.
8. **Carmeli, C.** 1969. Properties of ATPases in chloroplasts. Biochim. Biophys. Acta **189**:256–266.
9. **Carreira, J., J. A. Leal, M. Rojas, and E. Muñoz.** 1973. Membrane ATPase of *Escherichia coli* K 12. Selective solubilization of the enzyme and its stimulation by trypsin in the soluble and membrane-bound states. Biochim. Biophys. Acta **307**:541–556.
10. **Carreira, J., and E. Muñoz.** 1975. Membrane bound and soluble adenosine triphosphatase of *Escherichia coli* K 12. Kinetic properties of the basal and typsin-stimulated activities. Mol. Cell. Biochem. **9**:85–95.
11. **Corao, M., J. A. Serrano, J. A. Leal, J. Puig, and E. Muñoz.** 1974. Isolation of murein-free spheroplast "ghosts" from a strain of *Escherichia coli* K 12. Microbiol. Esp. **27**:233–298.
12. **Greenawalt, J. W., C. Weibull, and H. Löw.** 1962. The hydrolysis of adenosine triphosphatase by cell fractions of *Bacillus megaterium*. J. Biol. Chem. **237**:853–858.
13. **Gross, R., and N. W. Coles.** 1968. Adenosine triphosphatase in isolated membranes of *Staphylococcus aureus*. J. Bacteriol. **95**:1322–1326.
14. **Harold, F. M.** 1972. Conservation and transformation of energy by bacterial membranes. Bacteriol. Rev. **36**:172–230.
15. **Lastras, M., and E. Muñoz.** 1974. Membrane adenosine triphosphatase of *Micrococcus lysodeikticus:* effect of millimolar Mg^{2+} in modulating the properties of the

membrane-bound enzyme. J. Bacteriol. **119**:593–601.

16. **Löw, H.** 1959. On the participation of flavin in mitochondrial adenosine triphosphatase reactions. Biochim. Biophys. Acta **32**: 1–10.
17. **Löw, H.** 1959. The effects of promazines on mitochondrial adenosine triphosphatase reactions. Biochim. Biophys. Acta **32**: 11–18.
18. **Lowry, O. H., N. J. Rosebrough, A. L. Farr, and R. J. Randall.** 1951. Protein measurements with the Folin phenol reagent. J. Biol. Chem. **193**:265–275.
19. **Mirsky, R.** 1969. Membrane proteins from *Bacillus megaterium* KM. Biochemistry **8**:1164–1169.
20. **Mirsky, R., and V. Barlow.** 1971. Purification and properties of ATPase from the cytoplasmic membrane of *Bacillus megaterium* KM. Biochim. Biophys. Acta **241**:835–845.
21. **Muñoz, E., M. R. J. Salton, M. H. Ng, and M. T. Schor.** 1969. Membrane adenosine triphosphatase of *Micrococcus lysodeikticus*. Purification, properties of the "soluble" enzyme and properties of the membrane-bound enzyme. Eur. J. Biochem. **7**:490–501.
22. **Nieto, M., E. Muñoz, J. Carreira, and J. M. Andreu.** 1975. Conformational and molecular responses to pH variation of the purified membrane adenosine triphosphatase of *Micrococcus lysodeikticus*. Biochim. Biophys. Acta **413**:394–414.
23. **Pedersen, P. L.** 1975. Mitochondrial and chloroplast ATPases, p. 375–394. *In* P. D. Boyer (ed.), The enzymes, vol. 10. Academic Press Inc. New York.
25. **Roisin, M. P., and A. Kepes.** 1972. The membrane ATPase of *Escherichia coli*. I. Ion dependence and ATP-ADP exchange reaction. Biochim. Biophys. Acta **275**:333–346.
26. **Schnebli, H. P., and A. Abrams.** 1970. Membrane adenosine triphosphatase from *Streptococcus faecalis*. Preparation and homogeneity. J. Biol. Chem. **245**:1115–1121.
27. **Sone, N., M. Yoshida, H. Hirata, and Y. Kagawa.** 1975. Purification and properties of a dicyclohexylcarbodiimide-sensitive adenosine triphosphatase from a thermophilic bacterium. J. Biol. Chem. **250**:7917–7923.

ANTHMICROBIAL AGENTS AND CHEMOTHERAPY, Jan. 1977, p. 44-46 Vol. 11, No. 1
 Printed in U.S.A.

Microassay for Amphotericin B

ROBERT M. BANNATYNE,* ROSE CHEUNG, AND HANNA R. DEVLIN

Department of Bacteriology, The Hospital for Sick Children, Toronto, Ontario M5G 1X8, Canada

Received for publication 3 August 1976

Depending on the hematocrit, duplicate or triplicate determinations of serum amphotericin B concentration may be made on as little as 100 μl of capillary blood obtained by finger prick. In an accurate plate diffusion bioassay, using *Paecilomyces varioti* as the indicator organism, levels of the drug in the therapeutic range can be determined fast enough for clinicians to modify their next dose.

Traditional bioassay methods for amphotericin B (1, 2) require quantities of blood which are most conveniently obtained by venipuncture. Since therapy with amphotericin B is often prolonged, repeated venipuncture over a long period for the purpose of following serum levels of the drug is distressing to the patient and inconvenient for the clinician. Also, in the pediatric age group, particularly in neonates, it is often impractical to obtain blood regularly in this way. This report describes a miniaturized amphotericin B bioassay system utilizing only 100 μl of capillary blood collected from the heel or by finger prick and suitable for determining the amount of this drug in serum.

MATERIALS AND METHODS

The assay method of Shadomy et al. (2), with minor modifications, was used.

Media and cultures. *Paecilomyces varioti* (MSSC 5605, National Institute of Allergy and Infectious Diseases) was grown at 37°C on dry slants of unmodified Sabouraud dextrose agar for 2 to 3 days. Mature cultures of *P. varioti* consisting mostly of conidia were harvested by washing with sterile saline, and the spore suspension was adjusted to a light transmission of 30% at 360 nm on a Bausch & Lomb Spectronic 20 spectrophotometer (approximately 5×10^6 spores/ml). This suspension remains stable for 5 days at 4°C.

Sterile, melted agar (nystatin assay agar, Difco) in 150-ml volumes was cooled to 50 to 52°C and inoculated with the adjusted spore suspension of *P. varioti* at a 1% (vol/vol) ratio. The inoculated medium was then well mixed without excess agitation and dispensed in 15-ml volumes with a wide-bore serological pipette into sterile plastic petri dishes (150 by 15 mm; Fisher or Falcon) placed on a special, heated level surface (Bio-Tech Co., Canada). After the plates had set, they were held at 4°C for at least 1 h. Prior to use the cooled plates were dried at 37°C for 10 min to remove excess surface moisture, and 21 wells were cut with a 4.5-mm cork borer in a formation such as to minimize the variation in zone size as a result of unevenness of the agar depth. Before filling the wells any excess moisture in them was removed with a sterile disposable pipette.

Preparation of stock drug solution for use in the dose response curve. Amphotericin B (E. R. Squibb & Sons, Inc.), 50 mg of active drug, was dissolved in 5 ml of 100% dimethyl sulfoxide. This was diluted 1:10 in sterile 60% dimethyl sulfoxide to give a solution containing 100 μg/ml. This stock solution is stable for at least 4 months if stored at −70°C. Further dilutions were prepared freshly for each experiment by diluting the stock solution 1:20 in alkalinized 50% isopropyl alcohol (6 drops of 10% NaOH plus 100 ml of diluted alcohol) to give a solution containing 50 μg/ml. This solution retains its potency for up to 7 days if stored at 4°C.

Dose response curve. The 50-μg/ml amphotericin B solution was diluted in pooled normal human serum (heat inactivated and filtered) and 5 μg/ml. Using fresh pipettes for each transfer, doubling dilutions in serum were made from 2.5 to 0.078 μg/ml. Heparinized capillary tubes (Instrumentation Laboratory) of 100-μl volume were filled with each of the standards and, using a micro-rubber bulb to expel the fluid, the wells were filled in duplicate. Plates were incubated on a level surface at 30°C for 24 h. Zones of inhibition were measured in two diameters against a 1-mm square grid taped to the stage of a Bausch & Lomb plate microscope. The standard curve was obtained by plotting the average zone diameter (in millimeters) against the concentration of the standards (in micrograms per milliliter) on 4-cycle, −70-division semilog graph paper and joining these with the best-fit straight line.

Preparation of biological fluids for assays. Capillary blood obtained from a heel or by finger prick was collected in 100-μl heparizined tubes. The cells were packed by centrifugation at 1,000 rpm for 1 min in a microhematocrit centrifuge (Clay-Adams Inc., New York) and separated from the serum by filing through the capillary tube at the cell-serum interface. A micro-rubber bulb was used to expel the serum from the sawed capillary tube and to fill duplicate wells with approximately 20 μl. Depending on the hematocrit, two or three determinations could easily be made from the 100-μl heparinized capillary samples. Using a 21-well template, it was possible to assay in duplicate seven standards and three patient samples on one plate. Plates were incubated and read as above.

Reproducibility. Assay precision was assessed on 27 specimens by performing the determination twice (i.e., two sets of duplicates) on different plates with the same or different standards. "Within sample" standard deviation (SD) of the paired results was calculated according to the equation SD = $(\sum d^2/2n)^{1/2}$, where d is the difference in micrograms per milliliter between the results of the two assays of the same specimen and n is the number of specimens.

RESULTS

A composite dose response curve derived from the measurements on 124 separate curves is shown in Fig. 1. The curve was linear over the normal range for amphotericin B serum levels at recommended doses. The lower limit of sensitivity was of the order of 0.07 μg/ml. The indicated ranges of the zones of diameter at each of the standard concentrations were within acceptable limits.

The precision of the assay technique is shown in Fig. 2. The closeness of the paired values to the line of identity emphasizes the high degree of reproducibility. The within sample SD of each pair of results was 0.026 μg/ml.

Figure 3 depicts the correlation between daily incremental doses of amphotericin B in a representative case during week 1 of therapy and the serum levels of the drug obtained by this assay method when specimens were withdrawn at 1 to 3 h after the end of each infusion. The almost linear relationship of dose to level and the capacity of the assay to detect low concentrations of amphotericin B after even small doses provide an indication of the accuracy of this method in a clinical setting.

DISCUSSION

The standard agar diffusion assay of Shadomy et al. (2), on which the present miniaturized version is modeled, requires 0.2 ml of serum for duplicate determinations. In the absence of details on the need for special processing of the blood samples from which these quantities of serum are obtained, it is presumed that collection was by the traditional method of venipuncture. Depending on the hematocrit, the assay described here requires only one-fifth as much serum (approximately 40 μl) conveniently collected as heparinized capillary blood. The nature of the standard curve, the high degree of reproducibility of the technique, and the excellent correlation between dose and serum level illustrated in Fig. 1, 2, and 3 attest to the accuracy and sensitivity of this micromethod for amphotericin B assay. With usual doses of amphotericin B, serum levels rarely exceed 2.01 μg/ml (1) and, although the assay as described covers the expected range of serum levels, additional studies not reported here confirm that much higher levels can be measured with equal accuracy.

The microassay method offers advantages in two principal situations. First, repeated, even

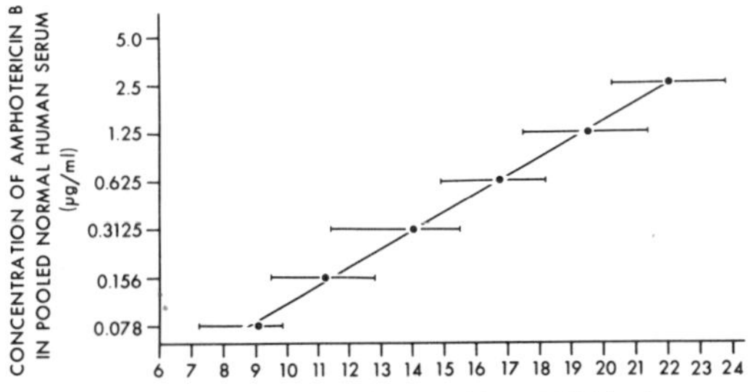

FIG. 1. *Bioassay for amphotericin B. This represents a composite dose response curve, with ranges, derived from mean values for 124 separate dose response curves.*

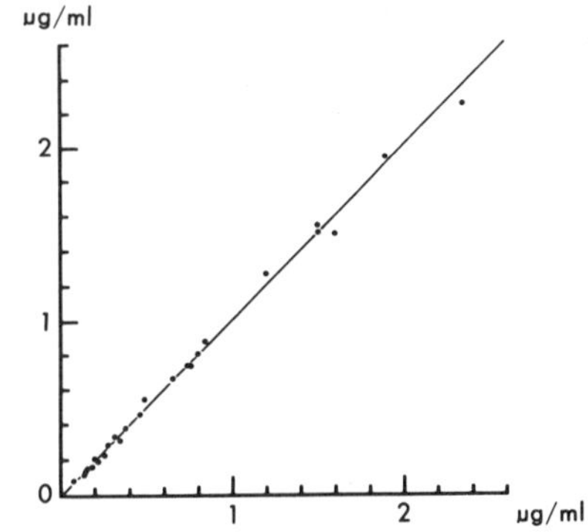

FIG. 2. *Reproducibility of assay results for amphotericin B. Each point represents the results of two separate duplicate assays performed on one serum sample, one value plotted on the ordinate and the other plotted on the abscissa. The line of identity is included for reference.*

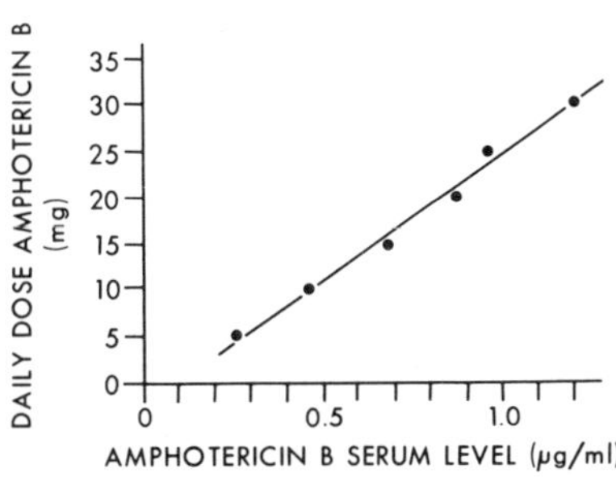

FIG. 3. *Relationship between daily dose of amphotericin B and assayed serum level (patient's weight, 69.3 kg).*

daily, patient sampling throughout the long courses of amphotericin B therapy generally employed now becomes possible. Serum levels can be accurately monitored and correlated with biochemical indexes of altered renal function, and ultimately the determination of a "toxic" amphotericin B level can be achieved. The second major area of attraction is in pediatrics, where economy of blood sampling, particularly in the neonatal age group, is desirable. In addition, from a pharmacokinetic viewpoint a neonate is unique in the way that it handles drugs and, although little is known of the fate of amphotericin B in an adult, its behavior in a neonate is a totally uncharted region. With the provision of a microtechnique for assaying amphotericin B in the above circumstances, perhaps the answers to many of these questions will be forthcoming.

ACKNOWLEDGMENTS

This work was supported by Ontario Provincial Health Research grant PR568.

LITERATURE CITED

1. **Fields, B. T., Jr., J. H. Bates, and R. S. Abernathy.** 1970. Amphotericin B serum concentrations during therapy. Appl. Microbiol. **19**:955–959.
2. **Shadomy, S., J. A. McCay, and S. I. Schwartz.** 1969. Bioassay for hamycin and amphotericin B in serum and other biological fluids. Appl. Microbiol. **17**: 497–503.

Antimicrobial Agents and Chemotherapy, Jan. 1977, p. 47–50 Vol. 11, No. 1

Mechanisms of Gentamicin Resistance in *Staphylococcus aureus*

J. E. DOWDING[1]

Department of Pharmacology, University of Cambridge Medical School, Cambridge CB2 2QD, England

Received for publication 19 July 1976

Three clinical isolates of *Staphylococcus aureus* resistant to gentamicin and other aminoglycosides have been examined for antibiotic modifying enzymes. The strains contain a number of these enzymes, most of them similar to those commonly found in aminoglycoside-resistant gram-negative strains. All three strains (and a transductant derived from one of them) contain two enzymes mediating gentamicin resistance, an aminoglycoside 6′-*N*-acetyltransferase and a novel enzyme, gentamicin phosphotransferase.

There have been a number of recent reports of gentamicin resistance in clinical isolates of *Staphylococcus aureus*. Soussy et al. (6) reported plasmid-coded resistance to gentamicin, kanamycin, and tobramycin and suggested that a single modifying enzyme was responsible. An inactivating enzyme was also implicated in a gentamicin-resistant strain isolated by Porthouse et al. (5). Speller et al. (7) demonstrated the presence of an acetyltransferase and an adenylyltransferase, both inactivating gentamicin, kanamycin, and tobramycin, and a second adenylyltransferase, inactivating streptomycin.

A number of gentamicin-resistant strains of *S. aureus* have recently been isolated in two Cambridge hospitals. The epidemiology of these strains and the transduction of resistance by means of a phage isolated from one of them have been described by Warren (manuscript submitted for publication).

The mechanisms of resistance to gentamicin in these strains are examined here to test further the suggestion that most antibiotic resistance mechanisms will be basically similar in all bacteria (3). There are at present five known aminoglycoside-modifying enzymes that mediate resistance to gentamicin in gram-negative bacteria, namely, aminoglycoside 6′-*N*-acetyltransferase, aminoglycoside 2″-adenylyltransferase, and three distinct aminoglycoside acetyltransferases (4).

In this report the aminoglycoside-modifying enzymes in the Cambridge strains are characterized, and a previously undescribed enzyme (a gentamicin-kanamycin-tobramycin phosphotransferase) is demonstrated.

[1] Present address: Department of Biochemistry, Adrian Building, University of Leicester, Leicester, England.

MATERIALS AND METHODS

Bacterial strains. The bacterial strains used were all clinical isolates of *S. aureus* provided by R. Warren, Department of Bacteriology, New Addenbrooke's Hospital, Cambridge. Aminoglycoside resistances were as follows (abbreviations: Gm, gentamicin; Km, kanamycin; Tm, tobramycin; Sm, streptomycin; Nm, neomycin): strain C1 was Gm^r Km^r Tm^r Sm^r, Nm^r; strains C2 and C4 were Gm^r Km^r Tm^r; and strain T1 was a Gm^r Km^r Tm^r Sm^s Nm^s transductant from strain C1. Strains C1, C2, and C4 were of different phage types (Warren, manuscript submitted for publication).

Preparation of cell-free extracts. Cells were grown by diluting 0.5 ml of an overnight culture into 100 ml of medium (grams per liter: tryptone, 10; yeast extract, 5; and NaCl, 10). Flasks were incubated at 37°C with shaking until the late logarithmic phase of growth. Cells were harvested, washed once in buffer I {0.01 M tris(hydroxymethyl)-aminomethane[Tris]-hydrochloride, pH 7.8, 0.01 M $MgCl_2$, 0.025 M NH_4Cl, 0.001 M dithiothreitol}, and frozen at −20°C. Frozen cell pellets (approximately 0.5 g, wet weight) were ground with alumina, 3 to 4 ml of buffer I was added, and the lysate was spun at a low speed to remove alumina and unbroken cells. The crude extract was spun at 105,000 × *g* for 90 min, and 250-μl portions of the supernatant (S100) were stored at −20°C. Protein concentration in the S100 fraction was normally 1 to 3 mg/ml.

Enzyme assays. Phosphocellulose paper binding assays were performed as described by Haas and Dowding (4). All reaction mixtures consisted of 10 μl of phosphotransferase buffer, 10 μl of radiolabeled substrate, 10 μl of crude enzyme (S100), and 5 μl of antibiotic (1 mg/ml of free base). Assays were incubated at 35°C for 30 min.

Sephadex chromatography. A 4-ml amount of S100 was concentrated approximately 10-fold by dialysis against buffer I containing 20% polyethylene glycol (carbowax 6000), and the sample, containing 4.8 mg of protein, was applied to a 10-ml bed volume column of Sephadex G-100 swollen in buffer I. After elution of the void volume (determined with blue dextran 2000) 2-min fractions (flow rate, 0.1 ml/min) were collected and assayed for enzyme activities.

Polyacrylamide gel electrophoresis. Lower gels (80 by 6 mm) were prepared by mixing 3 parts solution A (Tris, 12.1 g; 1 N HCl, 16 ml; tetramethyleneethylenediamine, 0.18 ml; water to 100 ml), 4 parts solution B (acrylamide, 15 g; methylenebisacrylamide, 0.4 g; water to 100 ml), and 1 part ammonium persulfate (0.56% in water). Stacking gels (12 by 6 mm) were prepared by mixing 2 parts solution C (Tris, 3 g; 1 N HCl, 24 ml; water to 100 ml), 3 parts solution D (acrylamide, 6.67 g; methylenebisacrylamide, 1.67 g; water to 100 ml), 1 part riboflavin (4 mg/100 ml of water), and 2 parts water with the addition of 1 μl of dimethylaminopropionitrile (10% in water) per ml of gel. A total of 200 μl of S100 was layered onto the gel and electrophoresed at 2.5 mA/tube for 2 to 3 h at 4°C. Buffer chambers contained 0.025 M Tris-0.019 M glycine, pH 8.3. After electrophoresis, gels were sliced to give 2-mm fractions; one-half of each fraction was assayed for aminoglycoside 6′-*N*-acetyltransferase and one-half was assayed for gentamicin phosphotransferase.

RESULTS

The three strains examined here all contain a similar aminoglycoside 6′-*N*-acetyltransferase (1). Table 1 shows the efficiencies of a number of aminoglycosides as substrates for this enzyme in vitro (for structures of aminoglycosides, see Fig. 3 and 4). The fact that neomycin B is a substrate but that paromomycin is not suggests that acetylation occurs on the 6-amino group of the purpurosamine ring of gentamicin (ring I, Fig. 4). Furthermore, when a number of purified components of the gentamicin complex were tested as substrates, it was found that increasing substitution at carbon 6 of this ring led to a decreasing ability of the compound to act as a substrate (gentamicin C_{1a}, 100%; gentamicin C_2, 16%; gentamicin C_1, 1%). In addition, 6′-*N*-acetylneomycin is known to retain considerable antibacterial activity, a fact that is compatible with the observation that strains C2 and C4, which both contain the acetyltransferase, are susceptible to neomycin.

In some gram-negative strains a single adenylyltransferase inactivates both streptomycin and spectinomycin (2). In the strains examined here there are two enzymes of narrower substrate specificity. Strain C1 inactivates streptomycin by means of a specific adenylyltransferase that does not modify spectinomycin, and strain C2 inactivates spectinomycin by means

TABLE 1. *Efficiencies of various aminoglycosides as substrates for aminoglycoside 6′-N-acetyltransferase and aminoglycoside 3′-phosphotransferase*[a]

Substrate	Efficiency (%)		
	Strain C1	Strain C2	Strain C4
Aminoglycoside 6′-*N*-acetyltransferase			
Kanamycin B	100	100	100
BBK8 (amikacin)	61	53	46
Gentamicin	45	64	47
Tobramycin	79	82	83
Neomycin B	35	29	18
Butirosin	12	ND[b]	ND
Paromomycin	0	0	0
Lividomycin A	0	ND	ND
Aminoglycoside 3′-phosphotransferase			
Neomycin B	100		
Kanamycin B	581		
Butirosin	220		
Lividomycin A	222		

[a] Results are expressed relative to kanamycin B (100%) and neomycin B (100%), respectively. All figures are averages from duplicate assays.

[b] ND, Not determined.

TABLE 2. *Efficiencies of various aminoglycosides as substrates for gentamicin phosphotransferase*[a]

Substrate	Efficiency (%)		
	Strain C1	Strain C2	Strain C4
Gentamicin	100	100	100
Sisomicin	103	100	ND[b]
Kanamycin B	87	42	40
Tobramycin	52	49	50
BBK8 (amikacin)	33	27	18

[a] Results are expressed relative to gentamicin (100%). All figures are averages from duplicate assays.

[b] ND, Not determined.

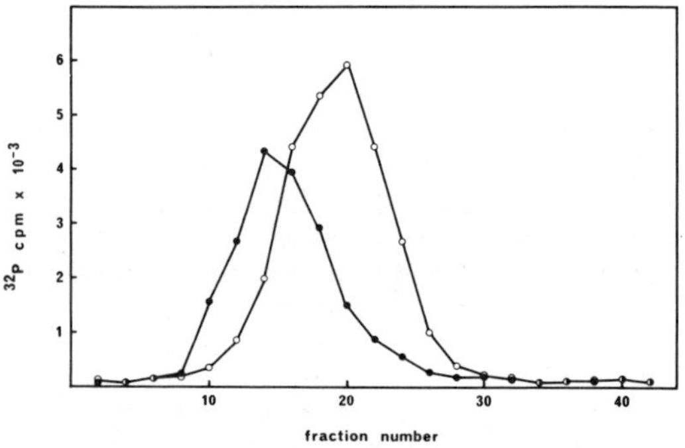

FIG. 1. *Separation of gentamicin phosphotransferase and aminoglycoside 3′-phosphotransferase from strain C1 by Sephadex G-100 chromatography. Symbols:* ●, *phosphorylation of gentamicin;* ○, *phosphorylation of neomycin.*

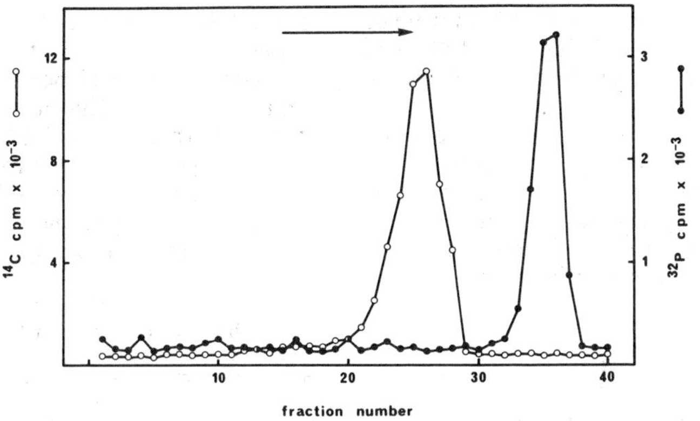

FIG. 2. *Separation of gentamicin phosphotransferase and aminoglycoside 6'-N-acetyltransferase from strain C1 by polyacrylamide gel electrophoresis. Symbols: ●, phosphorylation of gentamicin; ○, acetylation of kanamycin. Electrophoresis was towards the anode in the direction indicated by the arrow.*

of a distinct adenylyltransferase that does not modify streptomycin.

Table 1 shows that strain C1 also contained an aminoglycoside 3'-phosphotransferase. The unusually high level of kanamycin phosphorylation by extracts of this strain prompted the testing of a number of other compounds of the kanamycin-gentamicin group for their ability to act as substrates. These assays revealed (Table 2) that in all three strains there was a phosphotransferase present capable of modifying the gentamicins, kanamycins, tobramycin, and BBK8 (amikacin). The two phosphotransferase activities from strain C1 were shown to be distinct by chromatography on Sephadex G-100 (see Fig. 1). Under these conditions, however, the gentamicin phosphotransferase and the acetyltransferase coeluted. This fact, coupled with the observation that all three strains contained both activities and the finding that they shared many common substrates, raised the possibility that only one enzyme was present, capable of phosphorylating or acetylating a range of substrates, depending on the cofactor available. That two enzymes were, in fact, present was shown by separating the activities on a polyacrylamide gel (Fig. 2).

The aminoglycosides may be divided into two structural groups (Fig. 3 and 4), depending on the positions of the substitutions (4,5- or 4,6-) on the deoxystreptamine moiety. When the gentamicin phosphotransferase from strain C2 was assayed with all available substrates, it was found that all 4,6-substituted compounds tested were phosphorylated (kanamycins A and B, gentamicins C_{1a}, C_2, and C_1, sisomicin, BBK8, and tobramycin), whereas the 4,5-substituted compounds (neomycin B, paromomycin, ribostamycin, butirosin, and lividomycin A) were not. These findings demonstrate that

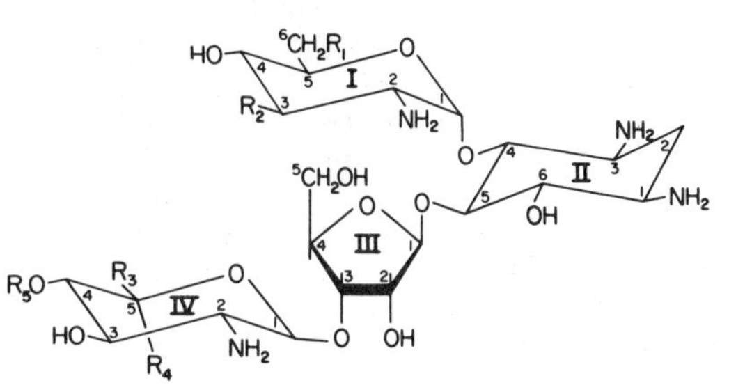

FIG. 3. *Structure of the neomycins*

	R_1	R_2	R_3	R_4	R_5
Neomycin B	NH_2	OH	H	CH_2NH_2	H
Neomycin C	NH_2	OH	CH_2NH_2	H	H
Paromomycin	OH	OH	{H / CH_2NH_2	CH_2NH_2 / H}	H
Lividomycin A	OH	H	H	CH_2NH_2	Mannose
Lividomycin B	OH	H	H	CH_2NH_2	H

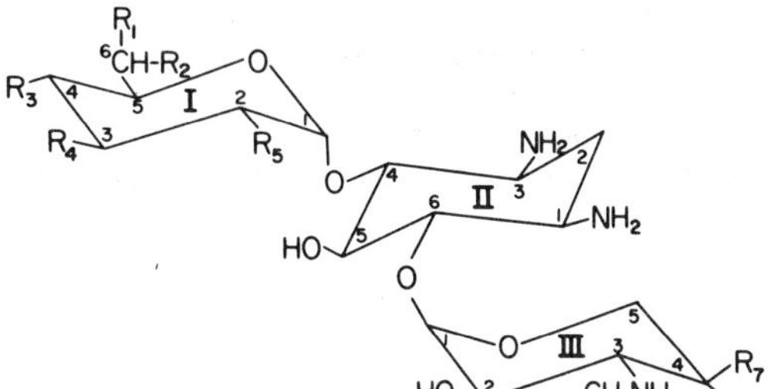

FIG. 4. *Structure of the gentamicins*

	R_1	R_2	R_3	R_4	R_5	R_6	R_7
Gentamicin A	H	OH	OH	OH	NH_2	H	OH
Gentamicin B	H	NH_2	H	OH	OH	OH	CH_3
Gentamicin C_{1a}	H	NH_2	H	H	NH_2	OH	CH_3
Gentamicin C_2	CH_3	NH_2	H	H	NH_2	OH	CH_3
Gentamicin C_1	CH_3	$NHCH_3$	H	H	NH_2	OH	CH_3

modification does not occur on the neosamine or purpurosamine ring (ring I Fig. 3 and 4) as is the case for the aminoglycoside 3′-phosphotransferases.

The four enzymes present in strain C1 appear to be produced constitutively. The addition of streptomycin, kanamycin, or neomycin (all at 10 μg/ml) to the growth medium resulted in no apparent overall increase in enzyme activity or change in the relative activities of any of the enzymes.

DISCUSSION

There has recently been a sudden increase in resistance to gentamicin among clinical isolates of *S. aureus*, and it is becoming apparent that this resistance is mediated by modifying enzymes similar to those found in many gram-negative strains. The strains studied here possess two mechanisms of resistance to gentamicin and related antibiotics. One of these is an enzyme that closely resembles aminoglycoside 6′-*N*-acetyltransferase (1) in that it appears to 6′-*N*-acetylate a similar range of compounds, including BBK8. The second mechanism is one that has not previously been detected in any strain, namely phosphorylation of the gentamicin-kanamycin group of antibiotics. The site at which this enzyme modifies is, as yet, unknown, but substrate studies suggest that it is either on deoxystreptamine or on the garosamine moiety of gentamicin. One possible site of modification is the 2″-hydroxyl of garosamine (ring III, Fig. 4) as this group is known to be available for modification by gentamicin adenylyltransferase (8).

The fact that both enzymes, with their very similar substrate ranges, are present in all three original isolates may be more than coincidence. Selection with gentamicin after transduction from strain C1 produced strain T1, which also harbors both of the gentamicin-modifying enzymes but not the aminoglycoside 3′-phosphotransferase or the aminoglycoside 3″-adenylyltransferase. The resistance phenotypes observed can, in theory, be explained by the possession of either of the enzymes alone, and it is possible that for some as yet unknown reason both are required for resistance. It is thus also possible that a re-examination of oher strains carrying aminoglycoside 6′-*N*-acetyltransferase may reveal that these, too, elaborate a gentamicin phosphotransferase.

ACKNOWLEDGMENTS

I wish to thank Rod Warren for supplying the strains and information about them, Eric Cundliffe for helpful discussions and comments on the manuscript, and Julian Davies for supplying antibiotics.

This work was supported by grants to Eric Cundliffe from the Medical Research Council and the Wellcome Foundation.

LITERATURE CITED

1. **Benveniste, R., and J. E. Davies.** 1971. Enzymatic acetylation of aminoglycoside antibiotics by *Escherichia coli* carrying an R factor. Biochemistry **10**:1787–1796.
2. **Benveniste, R., T. Yamada, and J. E. Davies.** 1970. Enzymatic adenylylation of streptomycin and spectinomycin by R-factor-resistant *Escherichia coli*. Infect. Immun. **1**:109–119.
3. **Dowding, J. E., and J. E. Davies.** 1975. Mechanisms and origins of plasmid-determined antibiotic resistance, p. 179–186. *In* D. Schlessinger (ed.), Microbiology – 1974. American Society for Microbiology, Washington, D.C.
4. **Haas, M. J., and J. E. Dowding.** 1975. Aminoglycoside-modifying enzymes, p. 611–628. *In* J. H. Hash (ed.), Methods in enzymology, vol. XLIII, Antibiotics. Academic Press Inc., New York.
5. **Porthouse, A., D. F. J. Brown, R. Graeme Smith, and T. Rogers.** 1976. Gentamicin resistance in *Staphylococcus aureus*. Lancet **i**:20–21.
6. **Soussy, C. J., D. H. Bouanchaud, J. Fouace, A. Dublanchet, and J. Duval.** 1975. A gentamicin-resistance plasmid in *Staphylococcus aureus*. Ann. Microbiol. (Paris) **126B**:91–94.
7. **Speller, D. C. E., D. Raghunath, M. Stephens, A. C. Viant, D. S. Reeves, P. J. Wilkinson, J. M. Broughall, and H. A. Holt.** 1976. Epidemic infection by a gentamicin-resistant *Staphylococcus aureus* in three hospitals. Lancet **i**:464–466.
8. **Yagisawa, M., H. Naganawa, S. Kondo, M. Hamada, T. Takeuchi, and H. Umezawa.** 1971. Adenylyl-dideoxykanamycin B, a product of the inactivation of dideoxykanamycin B by *Escherichia coli* carrying R factor. J. Antibiot. **24**:911–912.

ANTIMICROBIAL AGENTS AND CHEMOTHERAPY, Jan. 1977, p. 51–63 Vol. 11, No. 1

Laboratory Evaluation of FR10024, a New Cephalosporin Derivative

MINORU NISHIDA, TAKEO MURAKAWA, TOSHIAKI KAMIMURA, NAOHIKO OKADA, SHIGEMI FUKADA, HIROSHI SAKAMOTO, SHOJI NAKAMOTO, YOSHIKO YOKOTA, AND YOKO KONO

Research Laboratories, Fujisawa Pharmaceutical Co., Ltd., Osaka, Japan

Received for publication 20 July 1976

FR10024 is a broad-spectrum antibiotic. The in vitro antibacterial activity of FR10024 against clinical isolates of *Staphylococcus aureus, Escherichia coli, Klebsiella pneumoniae,* and *Proteus mirabilis* is greater than that of any of the cephalosporins developed to date. Indole-positive *Proteus, Enterobacter,* and *Citrobacter* are resistant to FR10024, as is true for the other cephalosporins. However, more than half of the strains of *Enterobacter* and *Citrobacter* tested were susceptible to FR10024 at an inoculum of 10^6 cells/ml. A single subcutaneous injection of FR10024 to mice with peritoneal infections due to *S. aureus* and several species of gram-negative bacilli gave a protective effect inferior to that of cefazolin but appeared to be superior to that of cephalothin. When given in two divided doses, however, the protective effect of FR10024 was enhanced and almost equaled that of cefazolin. The serum levels and rates of urinary recovery of FR10024 varied in different animal species. The mean peak serum level of FR10024 in humans after a single intramuscular injection of 500 mg was two times higher than that of cephalothin. The serum half-life after intramuscular injections of 250 and 500 mg was slightly shorter than that of cephalothin. After receiving 250 mg of FR10024 intramuscularly the urinary recovery rate was 87.7% in healthy volunteers. The biliary excretion rate of FR10024 was particularly high. The 24-h excretion of FR10024 in rats was 63.3%, this being six to seven times higher than that for cefazolin, which has the highest biliary excretion of the other known cephalosporins. When FR10024 was injected intramuscularly (20 mg/kg), it was found that the hepatic levels of FR10024 in rats were the highest of all the cephalosporins, including cefazolin, but the levels of FR10024 in other tissues were not as high as those of cefazolin.

In an effort to develop better cephalosporins, a great number of derivatives have been synthesized and evaluated in the Research Laboratories of Fujisawa Pharmaceutical Co., Ltd., Osaka. Cefazolin (4) and ceftezole (5), both having excellent antibacterial activity and tolerance, were found in this screening program and both are now in clinical use. FR10024, a new cephalosporin derivative [sodium 7-(2-thienyl)acetamido-3-(1-methyltetrazol-5-yl)-thiomethyl-3-cephem-4-carboxylate] recently developed in our Research Laboratories, has proved superior in antibacterial activity to both cefazolin and ceftezole (Fig. 1). In animal experiments with FR10024, it was found that its biliary excretion pattern was unqiue when compared with that of other known cephalosporins (1, 3–5). We report here the results obtained thus far.

MATERIALS AND METHODS

Test antibiotics. FR10024 and cephalosporin C were provided by Fujisawa Research Laboratories; cefazolin by Fujisawa Pharmaceutical Co., Ltd.; cephaloridine, cephalothin, and cephalexin by Eli Lilly & Co.; cephapirin by Bristol Laboratories; and cephacetrile by Ciba Geigy AG.

Subjects. The antibiotics were tested in the following subjects: (i) male ICR strain mice aged 4 weeks, each weighing 21 to 25 g; (ii) male SD strain rats aged 6 weeks, each weighing 190 to 240 g; (iii) male beagle dogs, each weighing 9.5 to 14.5 kg; (iv) male rhesus monkeys, each weighing 6.4 to 9.9 kg; (v) male healthy adult volunteers, each weighing 56 to 65 kg.

In vitro antibacterial activity. The in vitro antibacterial activity of the test antibiotics was determined by the agar dilution method (2). One drop of an overnight broth culture and decimal dilutions thereof were inoculated on heart infusion agar (Difco) containing graded concentrations of the test drugs. The minimum inhibitory concentration (MIC) was determined after incubation at 37°C for 20 h.

Bactericidal activity. (i) MBC. Each heart infusion broth containing graded concentrations of the test antibiotics was inoculated with test organisms to obtain a concentration of about 10^6 cells/ml. After

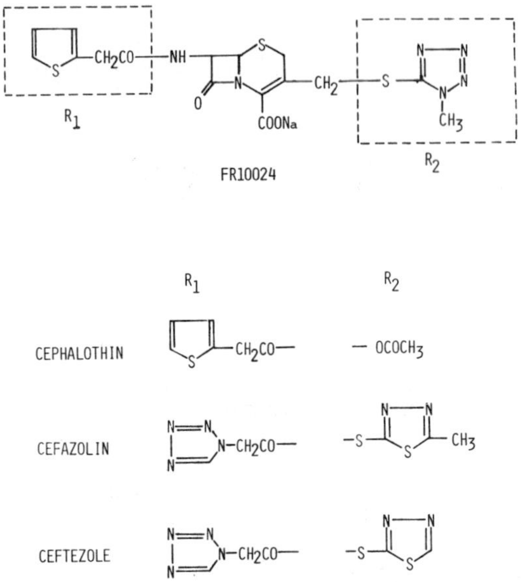

FIG. 1. *Chemical structure of FR10024 and other cephalosporins.*

incubating at 37°C for 20 h, the minimum bactericidal concentration (MBC) was determined as the lowest antibiotic concentration in which viable cell counts were decreased to less than 10^2 cells/ml.

(ii) Initial killing rate. Heart infusion broths containing a concentration of 10 μg of each of the test antibiotics per ml, were inoculated with four strains of *Escherichia coli* or *Klebsiella pneumoniae* (10^6 cells/ml) and were then incubated at 37°C for 60 min. After inactivation with *Citrobacter* β-lactamase, which destroyed the residual antibiotic in 5 min at 37°C, viable cell counts in the culture fluids were measured.

Serum-protein binding. A 0.5-ml portion of the antibiotic solution (300 μg/ml), in 0.067 M phosphate buffer (pH 7.0), was added to 4.5 ml of fresh serum and was then incubated at 37°C for 1 h. This reaction liquid was poured into a Visking tube (size 8/32), suspended in a 15-ml polypropylene tube, and centrifuged at 1,000 × *g* for 30 min (10). The free antibiotic concentration in the ultrafiltrate was determined by the disk method (2).

Protective effect on infections in mice. *Staphylococcus aureus, E. coli, K. pneumoniae, Proteus mirabilis,* and *Citrobacter freundii,* precultured overnight on agar slants at 37°C, were suspended in a mucin solution to obtain specified cell counts of test organisms. Male ICR strain mice aged 4 weeks, each weighing 21 to 25 g, were used, and each group consisted of 10 mice. Mice were inoculated intraperitoneally with 0.5 ml of the suspension and were given a single subcutaneous dose of the test antibiotics 1 h after challenge. In another experiment, mice were given two divided doses of the test antibiotics 1 h and either 2 or 3 h after challenge. The 50% effective dose values were found by the probit method from the number of mice surviving after 2 weeks of observation.

Serum levels. The test antibiotics were injected intramuscularly (i.m.) in animals (20 mg/kg) and in human volunteers (250 and 500 mg). The serial data on rats were obtained on the different groups used at each bleeding, and the serial data in other animals and volunteers were obtained on the same subjects throughout the test period. The antibiotic levels in each serum sample were determined by the disk method, using standard solutions prepared with animal and human sera. The serum half-life was calculated from the linear descending slope of mean antibiotic concentrations in the serum plotted semilogarithmically against time.

Urinary excretion. Urine of rats, monkeys, and healthy volunteers was collected at specified intervals (5) after i.m. injection of the test antibiotics, 20 mg/kg in rats and monkeys and 250 and 500 mg in healthy volunteers. The antibiotic levels in each urine sample were bioassayed by the standard solutions prepared with 0.067 M phosphate buffer, pH 7.0, because there were no significant differences in standard curves between the standard solutions prepared with the buffer and those prepared with urine.

Biliary excretion. Rats and dogs anesthetized intraperitoneally with pentobarbital (25 mg/kg) were fixed in the supine position, and a polyethylene cannula was inserted into the bile duct. Bile samples were collected at 0 to 3, 3 to 6, and 6 to 24 h after i.m. injection of 20 mg of the test drugs per kg. The antibiotic levels in the bile samples were bioassayed with the standard solutions prepared with 0.067 M phosphate buffer, pH 7.0, for the same reason as in the case of urine.

Identification of active antibiotic substances in urine and bile samples. After i.m. injection of FR10024, urine samples were collected from rats, monkeys, and healthy volunteers, and bile samples were collected from rats at specified intervals. Each sample was examined by thin-layer chromatography and bioautography. For thin-layer chromatography, the following solvent was used: *n*-butanol-acetic acid–water (4:1:2). The absorbent was Eastman chromagram sheet no. 6061. For bioautography, sheets developed with the above solvent were dried and set on the agar media, which were inoculated with 0.2% spore suspensions of *Bacillus subtilis* ATCC 6633 (2 × 10^8 spores/ml) for approximately 15 min. After the sheets were removed and the agar plate was incubated at 37°C for 20 h, the bioactive substances were identified.

Tissue distribution. Rats that had received 20 mg of the test antibiotics per kg were bled at set intervals and their organs were removed. After the organs were lightly washed with saline solution, the tissues were homogenized in twice their weight of ethanol with the polytron homogenizer. The antibiotic levels in the supernatant, obtained by centrifuging the homogenate at 10,000 × *g* for 10 min, were bioassayed with a standard solution prepared with 0.067 M phosphate buffer at pH 7.0 containing 66% ethanol, since there were no significant differences in standard curves between the standard solution with 0.067 M phosphate buffer, pH 7.0, containing 66% ethanol and the supernatant obtained from the control tissues in the same manner. The tissue levels of the test drugs were thus calculated.

RESULTS

Antibacterial activity: Antibacterial spectrum. FR10024, like other well-known cephalosporins, is a broad-spectrum antibiotic active against gram-positive and gram-negative organisms. When it was compared with other antibiotics for antibacterial activity against various standard strains, FR10024 was slightly more active against gram-positive bacteria than cefazolin and cephacetrile but less active than cephaloridine. However, the activity of FR10024 against gram-negative bacteria was greater than that of any other cephalosporin tested. FR10024 was less active against *Streptococcus faecalis* 6733 and was inactive against *Proteus vulgaris* IAM-1025 and *Pseudomonas aeruginosa* IAM-1095 (Table 1).

Susceptibility distribution. MICs of FR10024 against 42 strains of *S. aureus* ranged from 0.05 to 0.39 μg/ml for an inoculum of 10^6 cells/ml, and no strains resistant to FR10024 were found (Table 2). The antibacterial activity of FR10024 against *S. aureus* was greater than that of cefazolin.

The MICs of FR10024 against 21 strains of *S.*

TABLE 1. *Antibacterial spectra of FR10024 and other cephalosporins*[a]

Organism	MIC (μg/ml)					
	FR10024	Cefazolin	Cephaloridine	Cephalothin	Cephapirin	Cephacetrile
S. aureus 209P JC-1	0.1	0.39	0.1	0.39	0.1	0.39
S. aureus Newman	0.2	0.78	0.1	0.39	0.1	0.78
S. aureus Smith	0.1	0.39	0.025	0.2	0.1	0.39
B. subtilis ATCC 6633	0.025	0.39	0.05	0.05	0.025	0.2
M. luteus PCI-1001	0.05	0.39	0.025	0.1	0.05	0.39
S. pneumoniae III[b]	0.2	0.39	0.1	0.2	0.2	0.2
S. pyogenes S-23[b]	0.1	0.2	0.05	0.1	0.05	0.39
S. faecalis 6733[b]	25	50	25	25	25	12.5
C. diphtheriae PW-8[b]	0.05	0.1	0.05	1.56	0.05	0.2
E. coli NIHJ JC-2	3.13	3.13	6.25	25	50	12.5
K. pneumoniae NCTC 418	1.56	3.13	12.5	25	6.25	12.5
P. vulgaris IAM-1025	100	>100	100	100	>100	>100
P. aeruginosa IAM-1095	>100	>100	>100	>100	>100	>100
S. typhi T-287	0.2	1.56	3.13	1.56	3.13	6.25
S. paratyphi A 1015	0.1	3.13	3.13	3.13	3.13	12.5
S. schottmuelleri 8006	0.2	3.13	3.13	12.5	6.25	6.25
S. typhimurium 1406	0.2	3.13	3.13	3.13	6.25	12.5
S. enteritidis 1891	0.2	3.13	3.13	3.13	3.13	12.5
S. dysenteriae A1 Shiga	0.78	3.13	6.25	12.5	12.5	12.5
S. flexneri 1a EW-8	0.39	6.25	6.25	6.25	25	12.5
S. sonnei I EW-33	0.78	0.78	1.56	6.25	12.5	6.25

[a] Conditions: Heart infusion streak method, 37°C, 20 h, 10^8 cells/ml.
[b] Supplemented with 10% rabbit blood.

TABLE 2. *Distribution of susceptibilities of clinical isolates to FR10024 and other cephalosporins*[a]

Organism	Antibiotic	No. of strains showing MIC (μg/ml) of:											
		0.05	0.1	0.2	0.39	0.78	1.56	3.13	6.25	12.5	25	50	100
S. aureus (42 strains)	FR10024	1	4	27	10								
	Cefazolin			2	23	16	1						
	Cephaloridine	7	29	6									
	Cephalothin		1	18	22	1							
	Cephapirin		1	25	16								
	Cephacetrile				1	15	24	2					
S. faecalis (21 strains)	FR10024										10	11	
	Cefazolin										8	13	
	Cephaloridine								1	15	5		
	Cephalothin										3	18	
	Cephapirin										20	1	
	Cephacetrile								1	14	6		

[a] Conditions: Heart infusion agar, stamp method, 37°C, 20 h, 10^6 cells/ml.

faecalis ranged from 25 to 50 μg/ml. The activity of FR10024 was almost the same as that of cefazolin and was weaker than that of cephaloridine, cephapirin, and cephacetrile.

Table 3 shows the distribution of susceptibility of each of the 42 strains of *E. coli*, *K. pneumoniae*, and *P. mirabilis* to the antibiotics. For *E. coli*, the MICs of FR10024 ranged from <0.78 to 100 μg/ml. The MIC was <0.78 to 6.25 μg/ml for 34 (81.0%) of the 42 strains and 12.5 to 50 μg/ml for 7 (16.6%) strains and was not more than 100 μg/ml for 1 (2.4%) strain. The antibacterial activity of FR10024 against *E. coli* was considered to be very similar to that of cefazolin. However, the number of strains highly susceptible to FR10024 at a MIC of 0.78 μg/ml or less was greater than that to cefazolin.

When the susceptibility of *K. pneumoniae* to FR10024 was compared with that of the other drugs, the activity of FR10024 appeared to be greater than that of the other cephalosporins, including cefazolin. The MICs of FR10024 against 41 (97.6%) of the 42 strains were 3.13 μg/ml or less. The MIC of the antibiotic against 19 (45.2%) highly susceptible strains was less than 0.78 μg/ml. The MIC against one (2.4%) strain was 50 μg/ml; this strain was moderately resistant. No highly resistant strains were found.

When the susceptibility of *P. mirabilis* to FR10024 was compared with that of other cephalosporins, including cefazolin, the MICs against 28 (66.7%) strains were not more than 6.25 μg/ml, whereas those against 14 (33.3%) strains ranged from 12.5 to 50 μg/ml. No highly resistant strains were observed. FR10024 had the best antibacterial activity of all the cephalosporins tested.

Table 4 shows the distribution of susceptibility of indole-positive *Proteus*, *Enterobacter*, and *Citrobacter* to the test antibiotics. All 20 strains of *P. rettgeri* were susceptible to FR10024. The MICs of FR10024 against 19 (90.5%) of the 21 strains of *P. inconstans* B ranged from 6.25 to 50 μg/ml. The MICs of FR10024 against 43% of *E. cloacae*, 62% of *E. aerogenes*, and 86% of *Citrobacter* were not more than 50 μg/ml.

Influence of various test conditions on antibacterial activity. (i) Test medium. The MIC of FR10024 against three strains was determined using five kinds of conventional agar media. No differences in antibacterial activity of FR10024 against the three strains were noted with any of the five media (Table 5).

(ii) pH. The pH of heart infusion agar ranged from 5.4 to 9.4, and the MIC of FR10024 against the three strains was determined. The MIC of FR10024 did not greatly fluctuate when the pH values changed.

(iii) Inoculum. Generally, the MIC of FR10024 against various test strains became correspondingly smaller when the inoculum size was reduced.

(iv) Serum. Rabbit serum (10, 20, or 50%) was added to each medium, and changes in antibacterial activity of FR10024 against the test strains were studied. The antibacterial ac-

TABLE 3. *Distribution of susceptibilities of clinical isolates to FR10024 and other cephalosporins*[a]

Organism	Antibiotic	No. of strains showing MIC (μg/ml) of:											
		<0.78	0.78	1.56	3.13	6.25	12.5	25	50	100	200	400	>400
E. coli (42 strains)	FR10024	10		12	11	1	2	3	2	1			
	Cefazolin	4		16	12	2	2	4	1		1		
	Cephaloridine	1		14	6	5	9	2	1	2	2		
	Cephalothin			5		10	15	5	1	2		3	1
	Cephapirin	1		2	3	6	15	7	2	2			4
	Cephacetrile				2	20	10	3	4	2	1		
K. pneumoniae (42 strains)	FR10024	19		14	8				1				
	Cefazolin			30	5	4	2	1					
	Cephaloridine				27	11	2	1		1			
	Cephalothin	1		5	28	3	3	1	1				
	Cephapirin			6	21	9	4	1		1			
	Cephacetrile					20	19	2	1				
P. mirabilis (42 strains)	FR10024			2	10	16	10	3	1				
	Cefazolin				9	14	16	3					
	Cephaloridine					7	26	8			1		
	Cephalothin				3	17	18	3	1				
	Cephapirin				1	10	17	11	2	1			
	Cephacetrile						4	32	6				

[a] Conditions: Heart infusion agar, stamp method, 37°C, 20 h, 10^6 cells/ml.

TABLE 4. *Distribution of susceptibilities of clinical isolates to FR10024 and other cephalosporins*[a]

Organism	Antibiotic	No. of strains showing MIC (μg/ml) of:										
		<1.56	1.56	3.13	6.25	12.5	25	50	100	200	400	>400
P. rettgeri (20 strains)	FR10024	2				1	1		3	13		
	Cefazolin	2				2		1	1	1	6	7
	Cephaloridine			1	1		1		1	9	6	1
	Cephalothin				1		1		1	1	1	15
	Cephapirin					2				1	1	16
	Cephacetrile				1	1		2	1	2	13	
P. inconstans B (21 strains)	FR10024				5	4	3	7	2			
	Cefazolin				1	3	2	6	6		2	1
	Cephaloridine							4	3	6	7	1
	Cephalothin						1	4	4	9	3	
	Cephapirin							4	4	5	7	1
	Cephacetrile						3	4	9	5		
E. cloacae (21 strains)	FR10024				1	3	3	2	2	3		7
	Cefazolin						1			1	1	18
	Cephaloridine								1			20
	Cephalothin							1		2	1	17
	Cephapirin								1		2	18
	Cephacetrile								1			20
E. aerogenes (21 strains)	FR10024			2	1	5	3	2	2	1	4	1
	Cefazolin					2	1		5	8	1	4
	Cephaloridine						1	1	1	3	13	2
	Cephalothin					1		1	1		1	17
	Cephapirin								2	1	1	17
	Cephacetrile							2		1	7	11
Citrobacter (21 strains)	FR10024			7	2	7	2			1		2
	Cefazolin							5	4	6	4	2
	Cephaloridine								5	6	8	2
	Cephalothin						1	4	5	5	4	2
	Cephapirin						1	4	3	7	3	3
	Cephacetrile									5	7	9

[a] Conditions: Heart infusion agar, stamp method, 37°C, 20 h, 10^6 cells/ml.

tivity of FR10024 tended to decrease when the serum was present in high concentrations.

Bactericidal activity. (i) Initial killing rate. The killing rate of the specified levels (10 μg/ml) of FR10024 against isolated strains of *E. coli* and *K. pneumoniae* was compared with that of the other cephalosporins. Figure 2A and B gives the mean viable cell counts at 60 min after incubation. No significant differences in the killing rate against the four strains of *E. coli* were noted between FR10024 and cephaloridine. The killing rate of FR10024 was slightly higher than that of cefazolin and was much higher than that of cephalothin and cephalexin. For the four strains of *K. pneumoniae,* a similar pattern was observed; i.e., the killing rate was the highest for cephaloridine, followed in descending order by FR10024, cefazolin, cephalothin, and cephalexin.

(ii) MBC. The MBC and the MIC of FR10024 against 11 strains were compared with those of cefazolin and cephalothin (Table 6).

The ratios of MBC to MIC of FR10024 at an inoculum of 10^6 cells/ml varied with the test organism. The MBCs of FR10024 against three strains of *S. aureus* ranged from 16 to 64 times the MIC. The MBCs of FR10024 against eight strains of gram-negative bacilli were very close to the MIC and ranged from one to eight times the MIC. The MBCs of cefazolin and cephalothin against two of the eight strains of gram-negative bacilli, *K. pneumoniae* no. 11 and *P. mirabilis* no. 1, were 16 and 32 times the MIC. When the MBC of FR10024 was compared with those of cefazolin and cephalothin, it was lower than that of cefazolin against 10 of the 11 test strains and lower than that of cephalothin for all of the strains.

Serum-protein binding. The extent of the binding of FR10024 to serum proteins of different animal species was compared with that of the other antibiotics (Table 7). The binding of FR10024 to rabbit serum protein was 97%, and it was 89% to rat serum protein, which was

TABLE 5. *Influence of various factors on the antimicrobial activity of FR10024*

Factor	MIC (μg/ml)		
	S. aureus 209P JC-1	*E. coli* NIHJ JC-2	*K. pneumoniae* no. 11
Medium[a]			
Nutrient agar (Difco)	0.1	3.13	6.25
Mueller-Hinton agar (Difco)	0.1	3.13	6.25
HI agar (Difco)	0.1	6.25	3.13
BHI agar (Difco)	0.1	6.25	3.13
Trypticase soy agar (BBL)	0.1	3.13	3.13
pH			
5.4	≦0.1	3.13	1.56
6.4	≦0.1	3.13	3.13
7.4	0.1	3.13	3.13
8.4	≦0.1	3.13	3.13
9.4	≦0.1	12.5	3.13
Inoculum size			
10^8	0.1	3.13	3.13
10^7	≦0.1	3.13	1.56
10^6	≦0.1	3.13	1.56
10^5	≦0.1	1.56	0.78
10^4	≦0.1	1.56	0.78
Serum (%)[b]			
0	0.1	3.13	3.13
10	0.1	6.25	3.13
20	0.2	12.5	6.25
50	0.39	25	25

[a] HI, Heart infusion; BHI, brain heart infusion.
[b] Rabbit serum.

similar to that of human serum protein (94%), 46% to dog serum protein, and 60% to horse serum protein.

Protective effect on infections in mice. FR10024 and the other test antibiotics were each given subcutaneously to mice 1 h after intraperitoneal infections experimentally induced by *S. aureus*, *E. coli*, *K. pneumoniae*, and *P. mirabilis*.

The in vitro antibacterial activity of FR10024 against *S. aureus* no. 26 was greater than that of cefazolin, but its therapeutic effect was lower (Table 6); the 50% effective dose value of FR10024 was greater than that of cefazolin (35.5 mg/kg for FR10024 and 11.5 mg/kg for cefazolin). This tendency was also noted in infections with six strains of gram-negative bacilli. The MICs of cefazolin and FR10024 against *K. pneumoniae* no. 1 were both 1.56 μg/ml. The MICs of FR10024 and cefazolin against *P. mirabilis* no. 2 were 3.13 and 12.5 μg/ml, respectively. However, FR10024 was not found to be superior in therapeutic effect when compared with cefazolin. One the other hand, the in vitro antibacterial activity of FR10024 was about eight times greater than that of cefazolin against *E. coli* no. 22 and four times greater against *P. mirabilis* no. 22, and in these instances the therapeutic effect of FR10024 was superior to that of cefazolin.

The therapeutic effect of FR10024 after two subcutaneous injections in mice infected intraperitoneally with *E. coli* or *C. freundii* was compared with that of the other antibiotics. In mice infected with *E. coli* no. 22 or 29, the beneficial effect of a single injection of cephaloridine was most marked (Table 9). The therapeutic effect of cephaloridine did not increase with more than one or with divided doses. However, the effect of FR10024, cefazolin, and cephalothin was greatly enhanced by dividing the dose into two equal injections. The therapeutic effect of FR10024 in divided doses was about the same as that of cefazolin and cephaloridine. FR10024 exhibited the greatest effect in mice infected with *C. freundii* no. 19.

Absorption and excretion: serum levels. (i) Rats. Figure 3 shows the serum levels of FR10024 and of the other cephalosporins in SD strain rats after i.m. injection of 20 mg/kg.

The serum levels of FR10024 peaked at 23.3 μg/ml 15 min after administration and decreased to 0.4 μg/ml at 2 h. The peak levels of FR10024 were nearly the same as those of cephaloridine and were about one-third those of cefazolin. The serum levels of FR10024, however, were generally higher than those of cephalothin (peak level, 14.1 μg/ml) and cephapirin (peak level, 14.6 μg/ml). The serum half-life under these conditions was the longest for cefazolin, followed in descending order by cephaloridine, FR10024, cephacetrile, cephalothin, and cephapirin.

(ii) Monkeys. Figure 4 shows the serum levels of FR10024 and the other antibiotics in monkeys after i.m. injection of 20 mg/kg. The serum levels of FR10024 peaked at 47.6 μg/ml at 30 min. The peak level after i.m. injection was 75.3 μg/ml for cefazolin, 35.7 μg/ml for cephaloridine, and 17.6 μg/ml for cephalothin. The peak level of FR10024 was second only to cefazolin. However, the serum half-life was 33 min for FR10024, 60 min for cefazolin, and 51 min for cephaloridine. Since the half-life of FR10024 was shorter than that of the other antibiotics, the serum levels of FR10024 at 1 and 2 h after administration were commensurately lower than those of cephaloridine.

Thus, it was found that the serum levels of FR10024 after i.m. injection of 20 mg/kg varied according to the species. The serum half-life of FR10024 was short in all of the animals tested.

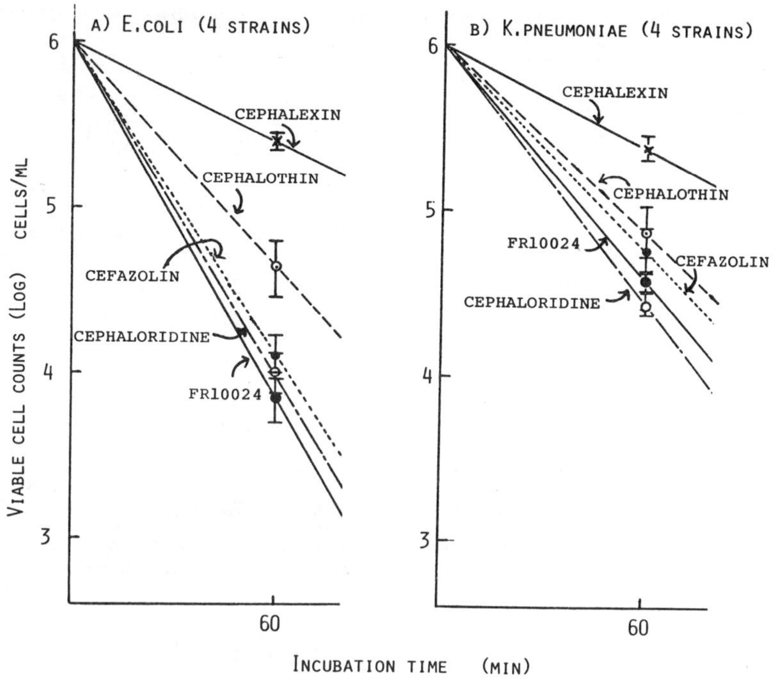

FIG. 2. *Initial bacterial velocity of FR10024 and other cephalosporins against some species of bacteria.*

TABLE 6. *Comparison of MBC and MIC (in micrograms per milliliter)*[a]

Organism	FR10024			Cefazolin			Cephalothin		
	MBC	MIC	MBC/MIC	MBC	MIC	MBC/MIC	MBC	MIC	MBC/MIC
S. aureus 209P JC-1	6.25	0.1	64	12.5	0.2	64	12.5	0.2	64
S. aureus 6	12.5	0.39	32	25	1.56	16	25	0.39	64
S. aureus 31	3.13	0.2	16	6.25	0.39	16	6.25	0.2	32
E. coli NIHJ JC-2	3.13	3.13	1	25	6.25	4	50	25	2
E. coli 19	1.56	≦1.56	≧1	6.25	3.13	2	25	12.5	2
K. pneumoniae 11	6.25	1.56	4	50	3.13	16	100	6.25	16
K. pneumoniae 20	1.56	≦1.56	≧1	12.5	6.25	2	50	6.25	8
P. mirabilis 1	25	3.13	8	200	12.5	16	100	3.13	32
P. mirabilis 18	25	6.25	4	25	12.5	2	50	12.5	4
C. freundii 49	200	50	4	>1,600	1,600	>1	1,600	400	4
E. aerogenes 13	800	200	4	1,600	800	2	1,600	1,600	1

[a] Conditions: Heart infusion broth (Difco), 37°C, 20 h; inoculum size, 10^6 cells/ml. The MBC was determined as the lowest concentration that kills 99.99% of the inoculum.

TABLE 7. *Extent of protein binding of FR10024 and related antibiotics*[a]

Antibiotic	Extent of protein binding (%)[b]				
	Human[c]	Dog	Rabbit	Rat	Horse
FR10024	94	46	97	89	60
Cefazolin	94	40	97	97	54
Cephaloridine	55	22	55	67	17
Cephalothin	86	44	86	87	42
Cloxacillin	96	92	96	94	79

[a] Serum concentration, 90%; drug concentration, 30 μg/ml; method, centrifugal ultrafiltration.
[b] Mean values of three determinations.
[c] Type of serum.

The elimination rate of FR10024 in the serum was similar to that of cephalothin and cephacetrile.

(iii) Healthy volunteers. The serum levels of FR10024 in healthy volunteers after i.m. injection are shown in Fig. 5. The mean serum levels of FR10024 after administration of 250 and 500 mg peaked at 8.6 and 25.0 μg/ml, respectively, at 15 min. At 1 h they were 4.5 and 13.6 μg/ml, and at 4 h they were 0.1 and 0.5 μg/ml. FR10024 was not detectable at 6 h, except in one volunteer who received 500 mg. The serum levels of FR10024 and cephalothin were compared in five healthy volunteers after i.m. in-

TABLE 8. *Protective effect of a single dose of FR10024 and other cephalosporins against experimental infections in mice*[a]

Organism	Challenge size (cells/mouse)	ED$_{50}$ (mg/kg)				MIC (μg/ml)			
		FR10024	Cefazolin	Cephaloridine	Cephalothin	FR 10024	Cefazolin	Cephaloridine	Cephalothin
S. aureus 26	1.3 × 10^7 (5% M)	35.5 (20.0–65.5)[b]	11.5 (6.0–23.5)	6.0 (3.5–11.0)	122 (57.5–298)	0.1	0.78	0.2	0.39
S. aureus 30	6.6 × 10^7 (5% M)	5.0 (2.5–9.5)	2.9 (1.4–5.5)	<1.0	15.0 (6.0–31.5)	0.2	0.39	0.05	0.2
E. coli 22	1.1 × 10^4 (2.5% M)	11 (0.05–2.4)	5.5 (3.0–7.5)	7.0 (5.0–9.5)	25.0 (17.5–34.0)	0.2	1.56	3.13	6.25
E. coli 29	5.7 × 10^4 (2% M)	5.5 (3.0–11.0)	2.2 (1.1–4.8)	ND	55.0 (38.0–79.5)	0.78	0.78	1.56	1.56
K. pneumoniae 1	3.6 × 10^2 (2% M)	31.0 (18.5–54.5)	3.0 (1.0–6.5)	8.0 (2.0–17.0)	79.5 (42.5–153)	1.56	1.56	3.13	3.13
K. pneumoniae 6	5.8 × 10^5 (2% M)	8.5 (7.0–10.5)	1.6 (1.1–2.2)	1.6 (1.1–2.2)	18.5 (12.0–29.0)	1.56	0.78	3.13	3.13
P. mirabilis 2	7.0 × 10^5 (5% M)	53.0 (29.5–98.5)	13.5 (7.0–26.0)	28.0 (21.0–37.5)	146 (58.5–401)	3.13	12.5	12.5	12.5
P. mirabilis 22	1.3 × 10^8 (5% M)	7.0 (3.8–13.0)	10.5 (6.0–18.0)	9.0 (5.0–15.5)	13.5 (6.5–26.0)	0.78	3.13	12.5	1.56

[a] Mice: ICR strain, male, 4 weeks old, 21 to 25 g, 10/group. Infection: Mucin suspension, 0.5 ml/mouse, intraperitoneally. Therapy: 1 h after challenge, subcutaneously. 50% Effective dose (ED$_{50}$): Probit method. Inoculum: 10^6 cells/ml. ND, Not done.

[b] 95% confidence limit.

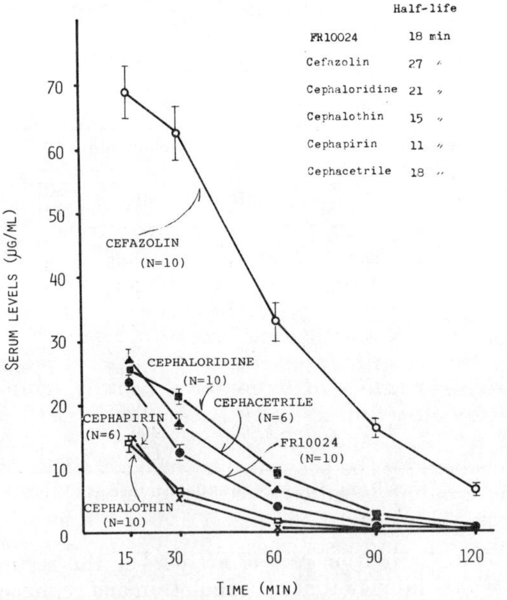

FIG. 3. *Serum levels of FR10024 and other cephalosporins in rats after i.m. injection.*

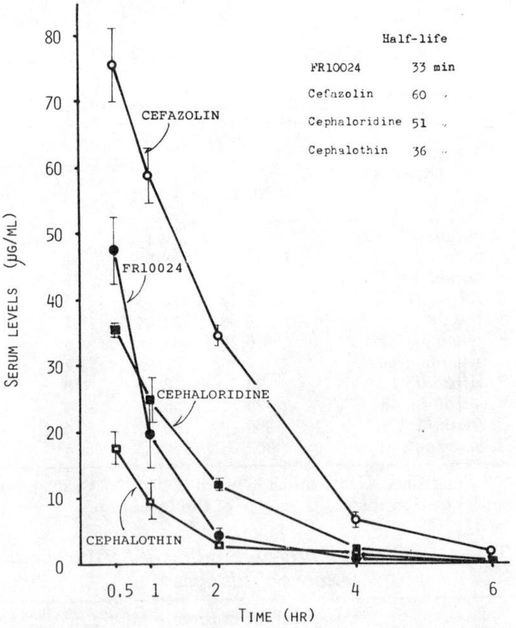

FIG. 4. *Serum levels of FR10024 and other cephalosporins in three monkeys after i.m. injection.*

jection of 500 mg in a crossover study. The peak level of cephalothin was 11.4 μg/ml at 15 min after administration, which was about one-half that of FR10024.

The serum half-life in healthy volunteers after i.m. injection was calculated from the above results to be 39 min for FR10024 and 48 min for cephalothin.

Urinary excretion. (i) Rats. The 24-h urinary recovery rate of FR10024 in SD strain rats after i.m. injection of 20 mg/kg was 28.6% (Table 10). The 24-h urinary recovery rate under the same conditions was about 80% for cefazolin and cephaloridine and about 35% for cephapirin and 42% for cephacetrile. The low urinary re-

TABLE 9. *Protective effect of two divided doses of FR10024 and other cephalosporins against experimental infections in mice*[a]

Organism	Challenge size (cells/mouse)	ED$_{50}$ (mg/kg)							
		Single dose				Two divided doses			
		FR10024	Cefazolin	Cephaloridine	Cephalothin	FR10024	Cefazolin	Cephaloridine	Cephalothin
E. coli 22[b]	7.2×10^3 (2.5% M)	7.0 (3.8–13.0)[c]	3.3 (1.6–6.5)	1.2 (0.05–2.6)	23.0 (12.0–46.0)	2.7 (0.1–6.5)	3.0 (1.2–5.5)	2.5 (1.1–3.5)	23.0 (11.3–51.5)
E. coli 29[b]	8.3×10^4 (2% M)	8.0 (6.5–10.0)	5.5 (3.5–8.0)	2.3 (1.3–4.0)	31.0 (16.0–55.0)	0.95 (0.7–1.5)	3.1 (2.2–4.3)	3.5 (2.6–4.7)	5.0 (3.0–9.0)
C. freundii 19[d]	1.3×10^7 (5% M)	119 (57.4–252)	280 (184–423)	280 (184–423)	>1,000	70.1 (35.9–134)	125 (63.8–245)	148 (78.7–278)	>1,000

[a] Mice: ICR strain, male, 4 weeks old, 21 to 25 g, 10/group. Infection: Mucin suspension, 0.5 ml/mouse, intraperitoneally. 50% Effective dose (ED$_{50}$): Probit method.

[b] Therapy: 1 and 2 h after challenge, subcutaneously.

[c] 95% confidence limit.

[d] Therapy: 1 and 3 h after challenge, subcutaneously.

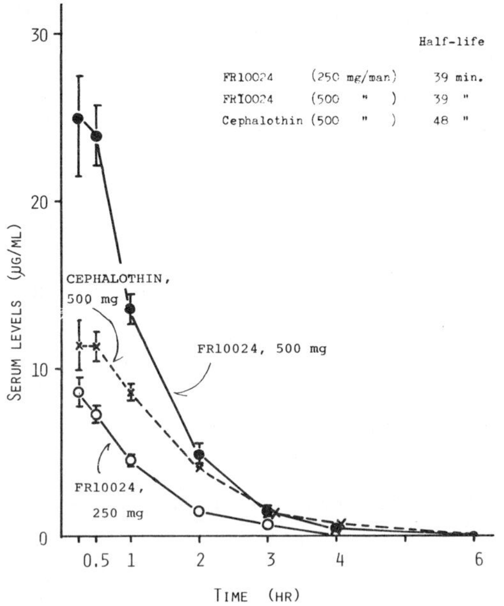

FIG. 5. *Serum levels of FR10024 and cephalothin in five healthy volunteers after i.m. injection.*

covery in rats was due to the high biliary excretion of FR10024, as mentioned below.

(ii) Monkeys. The 24-h urinary recovery rate of FR10024 in monkeys after i.m. injection of 20 mg/kg was compared with that of the other test drugs (Table 11). The recovery rate of FR10024 in monkeys, unlike that in rats, was 76.6%, i.e., almost the same as that of cefazolin (80.3%) and cephaloridine (74.4%). However, the recovery rate of FR10024 varied with the species, as was the case for serum levels.

(iii) Healthy volunteers. The 24-h urinary recovery rate of FR10024 in five healthy volunteers after i.m. injection was as high as 87.7% for 250 mg and as high as 88.5% for 500 mg (Table 12). The peak urinary levels of FR10024 after administration were 694 μg/ml at 0 to 2 h for 250 mg and 1,560 μg/ml at 0 to 2 h for 500 mg, and decreased thereafter. The majority of the 24-h excretion of FR10024 was obtained within 4 h after each i.m. injection of 250 or 500 mg. The 24-h urinary recovery rate of cephalothin in five volunteers after i.m. injection was as high as 51.2% for 500 mg; i.e., it was lower than that of FR10024.

Biliary excretion. (i) Rats. The 24-h biliary excretion rate of FR10024 after i.m. injection of 20 mg/kg was compared with that of the other cephalosporins (Table 13). The biliary excretion of FR10024 was especially high; 63.3% of the administered dose was excreted in the bile within 24 h after administration. The biliary

TABLE 10. *Urinary excretion of FR10024 and other cephalosporins in rats after i.m. injection*[a]

Antibiotic	0–3 h		3–6 h		6–24 h		Total	
	µg/ml	%	µg/ml	%	µg/ml	%	mg	%
FR10024	1,060	26.3	59.2	1.42	8.10	0.92	1.18	28.6
	(214)	(2.0)	(16.9)	(0.31)	(4.88)	(0.53)	(0.07)	(1.9)
Cefazolin	1,580	75.7	171	4.05	4.04	0.44	3.59	80.2
	(195)	(1.9)	(24.7)	(0.50)	(0.90)	(0.09)	(0.06)	(1.7)
Cephaloridine	1,430	79.7	83.6	2.20	2.02	0.31	3.54	82.2
	(125)	(2.1)	(12.6)	(0.30)	(0.35)	(0.05)	(0.12)	(2.2)
Cephalothin	395	21.8	12.2	0.30	0.25	0.02	0.95	22.1
	(60.4)	(1.5)	(3.2)	(0.07)	(0.15)	(0.01)	(0.06)	(1.5)
Cephapirin	570	34.7	20.7	0.39	0.28	0.04	1.52	35.1
	(102)	(2.1)	(8.2)	(0.16)	(0.15)	(0.02)	(0.08)	(2.1)
Cephacetrile	1,030	40.5	51.2	1.16	0.46	0.07	1.86	41.7
	(222)	(1.1)	(16.6)	(0.40)	(0.23)	(0.03)	(0.08)	(1.0)

[a] Dose: 20 mg/kg, i.m. Rats: SD strain, male, 6 weeks old, 190 to 240 g, 5 to 10/group. Numbers in parentheses are standard errors.

TABLE 11. *Urinary excretion of FR10024 and other cephalosporins in monkeys after i.m. injection*[a]

Antibiotic	0–2 h		2–4 h		4–6 h		6–24 h		Total	
	µg/ml	%	µg/ml	%	µg/ml	%	µg/ml	%	mg	%
FR10024	1,420	61.5	839	13.3	153	1.38	9.2	0.43	110	76.6
	(341)	(4.9)	(200)	(2.6)	(48.3)	(0.70)	(5.3)	(0.18)	(4.4)	(4.3)
Cefazolin	1,410	45.0	1,240	28.6	139	4.6	48.6	2.2	120	80.3
	(139)	(8.3)	(441)	(6.8)	(38)	(0.7)	(17.5)	(0.7)	(10)	(0.5)
Cephaloridine	764	58.6	780	15.8	218	2.2	6.3	0.3	115	74.4
	(37)	(2.9)	(234)	(3.2)	(75)	(0.6)	(2.0)	(0.1)	(10)	(1.5)
Cephalothin	602	38.8	405	9.8	25.4	0.83	0.25	0.02	77.2	49.4
	(92)	(4.7)	(63.3)	(4.1)	(9.1)	(0.27)	(0.03)	(0.01)	(8.2)	(2.7)

[a] Dose: 20 mg/kg, i.m. Monkeys: rhesus monkeys, male, 6.4 to 9.9 kg, three/group. Numbers in parentheses are standard errors.

TABLE 12. *Urinary excretion of FR10024 and cephalothin in healthy volunteers after i.m. injection*

Antibiotic	Volunteer (body weight, kg)	0–2 h		2–4 h		4–6 h		6–8 h		8–24 h		Total	
		µg/ml	%	µg/ml	%	µg/ml	%	µg/ml	%	µg/ml	%	mg	%
FR10024 (250 mg/man)	A (63)	749	68.9	294	20.0	42.0	1.5	2.0	0.3	0.4	0.2	228	90.9
	F (62)	255	53.6	202	18.6	42.0	1.7	3.2	0.3	0.5	0.2	186	74.4
	I (64)	794	79.4	97.2	12.6	13.3	1.9	2.3	0.3	0.3	0.1	236	94.3
	H (56)	871	78.0	80.0	7.7	36.6	1.0	5.6	0.2	0.6	0.2	218	87.4
	S (65)	802	77.0	227	12.2	34.5	1.5	6.5	0.3	1.0	0.3	228	91.3
	Mean	694	71.4	180	14.2	33.7	1.5	3.9	0.3	0.6	0.2	219	87.7
	SE[a]	100	4.3	36	2.0	4.7	0.1	0.8	0.02	0.1	0.03	8	3.1
FR10024 (500 mg/man)	A (63)	2,080	85.0	168	8.2	24.7	0.76	3.19	0.12	0.61	0.11	471	94.2
	F (62)	762	57.2	290	11.3	37.3	1.70	8.70	0.40	1.29	0.29	355	70.9
	I (64)	1,210	76.3	253	14.4	17.7	0.83	16.0	0.94	1.80	0.14	462	92.6
	H (56)	1,580	79.2	367	8.2	73.6	1.10	10.5	0.22	0.99	0.13	444	88.9
	S (65)	2,180	77.6	805	15.0	105	2.66	17.0	0.44	0.93	0.15	479	95.9
	Mean	1,560	75.1	377	11.4	51.7	1.41	11.1	0.42	1.12	0.16	442	88.5
	SE	238	4.2	100	1.3	14.7	0.32	2.3	0.13	0.18	0.03	20	4.1
Cephalothin (500 mg/man)	A (63)	842	43.0	420	8.4	45.9	1.1	3.8	0.13	0.12	0.02	263	52.7
	F (62)	1,220	36.6	565	9.0	55.2	1.2	8.7	0.23	0.36	0.04	235	47.1
	I (64)	737	40.6	243	7.3	33.9	0.6	2.7	0.11			243	48.6
	H (56)	1,970	51.2	377	7.9	41.4	0.7	6.7	0.11	0.30	0.04	300	58.6
	S (65)	617	35.8	551	9.9	104	2.4	35.7	0.64	1.90	0.24	245	49.0
	Mean	1,080	41.4	431	8.5	56.1	1.2	11.5	0.24	0.54	0.07	257	51.2
	SE	219	2.5	53	0.4	11.2	0.3	5.5	0.09	0.31	0.04	10	1.8

[a] SE, Standard error.

excretion rate of cefazolin was about 10%. For the other cephalosporins, the biliary excretion rate was 1.6% for cephapirin and less than 1% for cephaloridine, cephalothin, and cephacetrile.

(ii) Dogs. The 24-h biliary excretion rate of FR10024 in beagle dogs after i.m. injection of 20 mg/kg was 9.6% (Fig. 6). In this experiment, the biliary excretion of FR10024 was not compared with that of other antibiotics; however, the biliary excretion of other cephalosporins in dogs is known to be comparatively low. The biliary excretion of FR10024 was approximately three times higher than that reported previously for cefazolin. The biliary levels of FR10024 in dogs were 1,770 μg/ml at 1 h and 215 μg/ml at 6 h after administration.

Antibacterial substances in urine and bile. Using thin-layer chromatography-bioautography, the bioactive substances in the urine and bile of rats, monkeys, and healthy volunteers were investigated after i.m. injection of FR10024 (Fig. 7). Spots of bioactive substances in the urine or bile of each animal and of humans were detected only at the positions corresponding to the standard reference for FR10024.

Tissue distribution. Table 14 shows the tissue levels of FR10024 in rats after i.m. injection of 20 mg/kg. FR10024 was distributed into all the tissues 30 min after administration. In the case of the tissue distribution of FR10024, it was found that hepatic levels were higher than those of the other cephalosporins. At 30 min the hepatic levels were 24.9 μg/g for FR10024, 16.3 μg/g for cefazolin, and 8.6 μg/g for cephaloridine. Renal levels were 70.3 μg/g for cephaloridine, 45.4 μg/g for cefazolin, and 28.4 μg/g for FR10024. Renal levels of the other cephalosporins were all lower than those of FR10024. Other tissue levels, such as of the lungs, heart, and spleen, were the highest for cefazolin, followed by cephaloridine, FR10024, cephacetrile, cephapirin, and cephalothin.

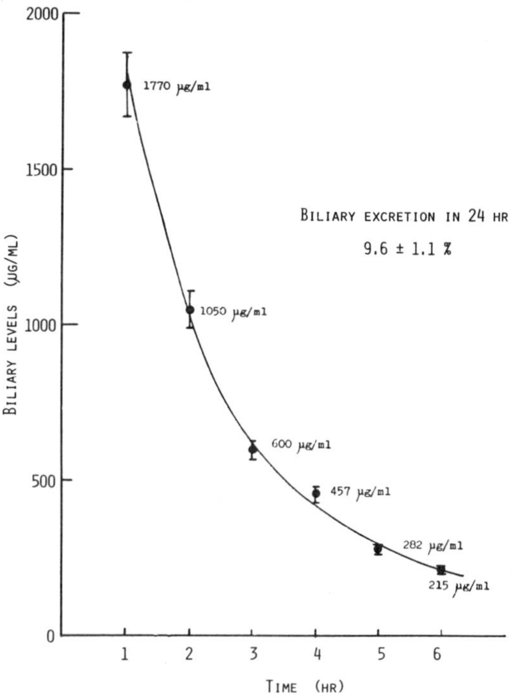

FIG. 6. *Biliary levels of FR10024 in five dogs after i.m. injection.*

DISCUSSION

Although *Citrobacter*, *E. cloacae*, and *E. aerogenes* are generally regarded as bacteria that are resistant to cephalosporins, a significant number are susceptible to FR10024 at an inoculum of 10^6 cells/ml. Clinical studies will be necessary to confirm whether the antibacterial activity of FR10024 against these strains is of

TABLE 13. *Biliary excretion of FR10024 and other cephalosporins in rats after i.m. injection*[a]

Antibiotic	0–3 h		3–6 h		6–24 h		Total	
	μg/ml	%	μg/ml	%	μg/ml	%	mg	%
FR10024	939	61.8	31.0	1.42	0.28	0.06	2.73	63.3
	(104)	(6.7)	(5.2)	(0.24)	(0.04)	(0.01)	(0.29)	(6.7)
Cefazolin	141	9.4	12.3	0.50	0.05	0.01	0.43	9.9
	(17.1)	(1.3)	(1.3)	(0.05)	(0.02)	(0.00)	(0.06)	(1.3)
Cephaloridine	6.0	0.37	1.23	0.05	0.05	0.01	0.017	0.44
	(0.72)	(0.05)	(0.14)	(0.01)	(0.02)	(0.00)	(0.002)	(0.06)
Cephalothin	12.0	0.90	0.05	0.00	0.05	0.01	0.041	0.91
	(1.8)	(0.14)	(0.02)	(0.00)	(0.02)	(0.00)	(0.007)	(0.14)
Cephapirin	22.9	1.59	0.26	0.01	0.10	0.02	0.060	1.62
	(1.3)	(0.13)	(0.07)	(0.00)	(0.00)	(0.00)	(0.005)	(0.13)
Cephacetrile	<0.60	<0.04	<0.60	<0.12	<0.60	<0.05	<0.010	<0.22
	(0.00)	(0.00)	(0.00)	(0.01)	(0.00)	(0.01)	(0.001)	(0.01)

[a] Dose: 20 mg/kg, i.m. Rats: SD strain, male, 6 weeks old, 190 to 240 g, 6 to 10/group. Numbers in parentheses are standard errors.

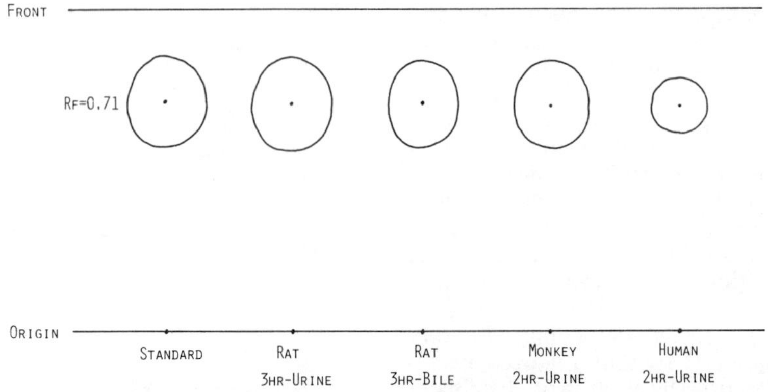

FIG. 7. *Bioautograms of urine and bile samples after i.m. injection of FR10024. Thin-layer chromatography: Eastman chromagram no. 6061; development: n-butanol–acetic acid–water (4:1:2), ascending.*

TABLE 14. *Tissue distribution of FR10024 and other cephalosporins in rats after i.m. injection*[a]

Antibiotic	Time (min)	Tissue levels (μg/g)					Serum (μg/ml)
		Liver	Kidneys	Lungs	Heart	Spleen	
FR10024	30	24.9	28.4	3.6	2.2	0.9	10.3
	60	7.0	8.7	1.0	0.8	0.2	3.8
	90	1.4	0.9				0.4
Cefazolin	30	16.3	45.4	10.9	5.8	2.7	50.0
	60	9.5	33.4	6.6	4.7	1.8	30.8
	90	5.0	13.6	3.5	2.1	1.0	12.5
Cephaloridine	30	8.6	70.3	6.8	3.0	2.1	19.6
	60	6.8	27.9	3.3	1.4	1.1	7.8
	90	4.9	8.7	1.3	0.7	1.0	2.7
Cephalothin	30	2.4	8.5	0.6	0.3		5.5
	60	0.4	1.6	0.1			1.4
	90						0.3
Cephapirin	30	1.1	8.1	0.9	0.5	0.2	6.3
	60	0.6	3.0	0.2	0.04		1.2
	90						
Cephacetrile	30	3.6	15.2	2.5	2.0	0.4	19.3
	60	2.5	3.6	0.9	0.3		6.3
	90						

[a] Dose: 20 mg/kg, i.m. Rats: SD strain, male, 6 weeks old, 180 to 230 g, 9/group.

therapeutic value. Also, it was found that the MBC of FR10024 against the tested strains was lower than that of cefazolin, and the bactericidal activity against the test strains of *E. coli* and *K. pneumoniae* was slightly greater than that of cefazolin.

FR10024 given in two divided doses to mice with experimentally induced infections was as effective as cefazolin and cephaloridine, both of which provide high bactericidal activity. An insufficient therapeutic effect of FR10024 after only a single dose is presumed to be due to rapid excretion of this antibiotic in mice.

Of the commercially available cephalosporins, cefazolin is known to be the drug with the highest biliary excretion (6, 9). In our animal experiments, the 24-h biliary excretion rate after i.m. injection of 20 mg of cefazolin per kg was about 10% in rats and about 3% in dogs (3). In patients, biliary levels of cefazolin were higher than those of cephalothin and cephaloridine (6–9). In the animal experiments, the biliary excretion rate of FR10024 at the same doses averaged 63.3% in rats and 9.6% in dogs, significantly higher than that of cefazolin. These findings suggest that it will be of special interest to evalute the therapeutic effect of FR10024 in patients with biliary tract infections.

LITERATURE CITED

1. **Brogard, J. M., P. Haegele, M. Dorner, and J. Laviliaureix.** 1973. Biliary excretion of a new semisynthetic cephalosporin, cephacetrile. Antimicrob. Agents Chemother. 3:19-23.
2. **Nishida, M., T. Matsubara, T. Murakawa, Y. Mine, and Y. Yokota.** 1970. Cefazolin, a new semisynthetic cephalosporin antibiotic. II. J. Antibiot. 23:137-148.
3. **Nishida, M., T. Matsubara, T. Murakawa, Y. Mine, and Y. Yokota.** 1970. Cefazolin, a new semisynthetic cephalosporin antibiotic. III. J. Antibiot. 23:184-194.
4. **Nishida, M., T. Matsubara, T. Murakawa, Y. Mine, Y. Yokota, S. Kuwahara, and S. Goto.** 1970. In vitro and in vivo evaluation of cefazolin, a new cephalosporin C derivative, p. 236-243. Antimicrob. Agents Chemother. 1969.
5. **Nishida, M., T. Murakawa, T. Kamimura, N. Okada, H. Sakamoto, S. Fukada, S. Nakamoto, Y. Yokota, and K. Miki.** 1976. In vitro and in vivo evaluation of ceftezole, a new cephalosporin derivative. Antimicrob. Agents Chemother. 10:1-13.
6. **Nishida, M., T. Murakawa, T. Matsubara, Y. Kohno, Y. Yokota, T. Yasutomi, and M. Okamoto.** 1976. Characteristics of biliary excretion of cefazolin and other cephalosporins with reference to the relationship between serum levels and administration conditions. Chemotherapy 22:30-36.
7. **Ram, M. D.** 1971. Cephalothin levels in human bile. Clin. Res. 19:401.
8. **Ram, M. D., and S. Watanatittan.** 1973. Levels of cefazolin in human bile. J. Infect. Dis. 128(Suppl.): S361-S363.
9. **Ratzan, K. R., C. Ruiz, and G. L. Irvin III.** 1974. Biliary tract excretion of cefazolin, cephalothin, and cephaloridine in the presence of biliary tract disease. Antimicrob. Agents Chemother. 6:426-431.
10. **Shimizu, T.** 1974. Studies on protein binding of cefazolin and other antibiotics. Jpn. J. Antibiot. 27: 296-301.

ANTIMICROBIAL AGENTS AND CHEMOTHERAPY, Jan. 1977, p. 64-73 Vol. 11, No. 1
 Printed in U.S.A.

In Vitro Studies with Netilmicin Compared with Amikacin, Gentamicin, and Tobramycin

VIJAY DHAWAN, EUGENE MARSO, WILLIAM J. MARTIN, AND LOWELL S. YOUNG*

Department of Medicine, Department of Pathology, and Department of Microbiology and Immunology, UCLA Medical Center, Los Angeles, California 90024*

Received for publication 12 August 1976

Netilmicin, a new semisynthetic aminoglycoside derived by ethylation of the 1-*N* position of the deoxystreptamine ring of sisomicin, was tested in vitro with 4,070 strains of gram-negative bacilli isolated at the UCLA Medical Center during 1975 to 1976, using the agar dilution technique and an inoculum of approximately 10^4 organisms. Results were compared with those simultaneously obtained for amikacin, gentamicin, and tobramycin. Using Mueller-Hinton medium, inhibitory concentrations in broth correlated with those obtained by the agar dilution method except for *Pseudomonas aeruginosa,* where a 2- to 16-fold difference in susceptibility was noted. For most clinically significant *Enterobacteriaceae* and *P. aeruginosa,* the activity of netilmicin in vitro was comparable or superior to that of gentamicin, tobramycin, and amikacin with respect to potency by weight and achievable blood levels. Against gentamicin-resistant strains (MIC > 16 μg/ml), the activity of netilmicin paralleled that of amikacin with the exception of *Providencia stuartii,* which was inhibited by amikacin but not by netilmicin.

Gram-negative bacilli are responsible for an increasing number of the serious infections occurring in hospitalized patients (3). Gentamicin and other aminoglycoside antibiotics have been used successfully to treat many such infections. Nonetheless, the emergence of resistant gram-negative bacilli in certain clinical settings (5, 7, 9, 13, 16) and toxic side effects of these agents present a serious problem. There are increasing reports of bacterial resistance to gentamicin on the basis of either selection of naturally occurring resistant organisms or spread of highly resistant strains that possess resistance transfer factors (2). This changing pattern of antimicrobial susceptibility serves as a constant stimulus for the development of new antimicrobial agents and for structural modification of existing compounds. For these reasons, the evaluation of a new aminoglycoside antibiotic with a broadened anti-gram-negative bacillary spectrum but with increased potency and relatively less toxicity is an important goal of laboratory and clinical research.

Netilmicin (Sch 20569) is a new semisynthetic aminoglycoside antibiotic derived by ethylation of the 1-*N* position of the deoxystreptamine ring of sisomicin. This synthetic modification has resulted in a compound that is resistant to inactivation by gentamicin adenyltransferase 1 and relatively resistant to gentamicin acetyltransferase 1. Netilmicin possesses no active site for kanamycin phosphotransferase inactivation, but the compound is inactivated by kanamycin acetyltransferase and gentamicin acetyltransferase 2. Preliminary reports (12, 15) have indicted that netilmicin has a broad spectrum of activity against most *Enterobacteriaceae* and *Pseudomonas aeruginosa*. In this respect, it resembles the parent compound, sisomicin. Because the biosynthetic reaction that has yielded netilmicin is similar to the process by which amikacin was derived from kanamycin A, we were particularly interested in the comparison of netilmicin with amikacin and specifically its activity against gentamicin-resistant strains. This report focuses on the results of in vitro susceptibility testing of netilmicin against more than 4,000 clinical isolates of gram-negative bacilli, and compares the results to simultaneous in vitro results obtained for amikacin, gentamicin, and tobramycin.

MATERIALS AND METHODS

Agar dilution tests. In vitro susceptibility of 4,070 clinical isolates of gram-negative bacilli to netilmicin, amikacin, gentamicin, and tobramycin was assessed principally by using the agar dilution method. These organisms were isolated from clinical material between October 1975 and January 1976 in the Clinical Microbiology Laboratories of the UCLA Medical Center. Taxonomic identification of members of the family *Enterobacteriaceae* was carried out by use of the API 20 E test system (Analytab Products Inc., Plainview, N.Y.) (18, 20), whereas isolates of *P. aeruginosa* and other gram-negative bacilli were identified by the use of standard criteria (8, 10). Dehydrated Mueller-Hinton medium (control no. 02520, Difco Laboratories, Detroit, Mich.) with 1.7 g of agar per liter was prepared to contain two fold increments of each antibiotic. Gentamicin (lot no. GMC-4-M-6162; potency, 584 μg/mg) and netilmicin (lot no. 75184D/7989-53; potency 592 μg/mg) were obtained in sulfate form from George Arcieri and Sadhna Sathe of the Schering Corp., Bloomfield, N.J. Amikacin (lot no. 74F/339; potency, 911 μg/mg) was obtained from Edward Yevak of Bristol Laboratories, Syracuse, N.Y. Tobramycin base (potency, 1,000 μg/ml) was obtained from William Miller of Eli Lilly and Co., Indianapolis, Ind.

Plastic petri dishes containing serial twofold dilutions of antibiotics in agar ranging from 32 to 0.25 μg/ml were prepared. An inoculum of approximately 10^4 organisms diluted from broth cultures in the logarithmic phase of growth was used. The organisms were delivered to dry agar surfaces using the inoculum replicating device of Steers et al. (18). To insure the purity of each isolate, a loopful of the broth from each well of the Steers replicator was removed after the plates had been inoculated and was streaked to one-half of a blood agar plate. The minimum inhibitory concentration (MIC) was read as the lowest concentration of antibiotic that completely prevented visible growth. A very fine haze of growth of one or two colonies was ignored in determining the MIC. Control plates with no antibiotic were always used to insure that there was adequate growth of each test isolate.

Broth dilution tests. Broth dilution susceptibility tests were performed with Mueller-Hinton broth medium (control no. 598597, Difco). An inoculum of approximately 5×10^5 organisms was used in accordance with the guidelines of the International Collaborative Study sponsored by the World Health Organization (4). Broth MICs were obtained by recording the lowest concentration of antibiotics that yielded a clear tube at 24 h. Aliquots (0.01-ml calibrated loop) from all clear tubes were subcultured onto blood agar, and the minimal bactericidal concentration (MBC) was the concentration that yielded growth of less than five colonies after 24 h of incubation.

The Mg^{2+} content of Mueller-Hinton agar was determined and ranged between 2.4 and 2.6 mg/100 ml by freeze-thaw extraction of the liquid contained in agar, followed by measurement in an atomic absorption spectrophotometer. The Mg^{2+} content of Mueller-Hinton medium in broth by the same method was found to range between 0.4 and 0.6 mg/100 ml.

Standard reference strains of *Escherichia coli* ATCC 25922 and *P. aeruginosa* ATCC/27853 (Boston strain) were tested with agar and broth dilution as an internal control. All MICs and MBCs were in the susceptible range on repetitive testing; these values differed by no more than one dilution.

Additionally, 30 highly gentamicin-resistant (MIC > 32 μg/ml) strains of *P. aeruginosa, Serratia marcescens*, and *Providencia stuartii* isolated at Wadsworth Veterans Administration Hospital, Los Angeles, were obtained through the courtesy of Richard D. Meyer. Some characteristics of these strains have been previously reported (12). None of these gentamicin-resistant isolates is included in data summarized for the agar dilution tests. Other highly gentamicin-resistant strains tested against netilmicin include some that have been previously reported (21).

Criteria for susceptibility. Isolates or organisms were considered susceptible if they were inhibited at or below the peak serum level achieved during administration of the drug to hospitalized patients or normal volunteers. For gentamicin and tobramycin, this was 4 μg/ml at a dose of 1.5 mg/kg; for amikacin it was 16 μg/ml at a dose of 7.5 mg/kg. Data made available from Schering Corp. and our initial clinical experience indicate that peak serum levels achieved after administration of 1.5 mg of netilmicin per kg and 2.5 mg intramuscularly usually exceed 4 and 8 μg/ml, respectively. To relate results of susceptibility tests to achievable blood levels in humans, we have assessed these results by calculating inhibitory indexes, using a technique previously described (20, 21). The inhibitory index refers to the ratio between the mean peak serum levels given above and the MIC for at least two-thirds of each species tested.

RESULTS

Agar dilution susceptibility. As determined by agar and broth dilution methods, MICs and MBCs for the two reference strains are summarized in Table 1. The MBC was usually one dilution higher than the MIC. In vitro susceptibility of organisms assessed by the agar dilution method is summarized in Fig. 1 through 13. Susceptibilities to netilmicin, gentamicin,

TABLE 1. *Comparative activity of four aminoglycosides against standard reference strains*[a]

Organism	Netilmicin			Amikacin			Gentamicin			Tobramycin		
	Agar MIC	Broth		Agar MIC	Broth		Agar MIC	Broth		Agar MIC	Broth	
		MIC	MBC		MIC	MBC		MIC	MBC		MIC	MBC
Escherichia coli ATCC 25922	2	2	2	2	2	4	2	2	2	1	1	2
Pseudomonas aeruginosa ATCC 27853	4	0.5	2	8	2	4	4	0.25	0.5	1	0.25	0.5

[a] All values are expressed as micrograms per milliliter.

and tobramycin closely paralleled each other for most groups of organisms tested, and amikacin was usually inhibitory at two- to fourfold higher concentrations.

Figure 1 summarizes the results of netilmicin alone by the agar dilution method. Ninety-eight percent of *E. coli* (1,687 strains tested), 97% of *K. pneumoniae* (636 strains), 86% of *S. marcescens* (116 strains), 99% of *Enterobacter* sp. (280 strains), 95% of *Proteus mirabilis* (383 strains), and 98% of *P. morganii* (60 strains) were inhibited at 4 μg/ml. Netilmicin was less active at 4 μg/ml against *Acinetobacter calcoaceticus*, since only 73% of 92 organisms were inhibited. Results for *P. vulgaris* (38 strains) and *P. rettgeri* (11 strains) were pooled, and only 71% were inhibited at 4 μg/ml. However, susceptibility results for *P. aeruginosa* were found to be highly medium dependent (see below).

The specific comparative activity of the four aminoglycosides versus gram-negative bacilli is summarized in Fig. 2 through 13. Slightly more than 95% of isolates of *E. coli* were inhibited by all four antibiotics at clinically achievable concentrations (Fig. 2). Similar results were obtained with *K. pneumoniae* (Fig. 3); 97% of *K. pneumoniae* were inhibited by 4 μg of netilmicin, gentamicin, and tobramycin per ml and 8 μg of amikacin per ml. At 4 μg/ml, 95% of *S. marcescens* were inhibited by gentamicin, 86% by netilmicin, 81% by amikacin, but only 73% by tobramycin (Fig. 4). However, amikacin inhibited 95% of *S. marcescens* at 16 μg/ml, which is clearly a clinically attainable blood level. At 4 μg/ml, 95% of isolates of *P. mirabilis* were inhibited by netilmicin, 97% by tobramycin and gentamicin, and 93% by amikacin (Fig. 5). For *P. vulgaris* and *P. rettgeri*, susceptibilities at 4 μg/ml were comparable for netilmicin (71%), gentamicin (82%), tobramycin (81%), and amikacin (79%). However, at 16 μg/ml (Fig. 6), 91% of these *Proteus* strains were inhibited by amikacin. At 4 μg/ml, 80% of isolates of *A. calcoaceticus* were inhibited by gentamicin, 87% by tobramycin, 89% by amikacin, but only 73% by netilmicin (Fig. 7). Better than 95% of isolates of *Enterobacter* sp., *P. morganii*, and *Citrobacter freundii* were inhibited by netilmicin, gentamicin, and tobramycin at 4 μg/ml and amikacin at 8 μg/ml (Fig. 8–11). Against *P. aeruginosa* (632 strains tested), only 18% were inhibited by netilmicin and 96% by tobramycin at 4 μg/ml (Fig. 12), whereas 52% were inhibited by netilmicin, 87% by gentamicin, and 98% by tobramycin at 8 μg/ml. In comparison, only 74% of isolates were inhibited at 8 μg of amikacin per ml and 91% at 16 μg/ml. Against other gram-negative bacilli, netilmicin was highly effective at 4 μg/ml against *Serratia liquefaciens* (100% of seven strains), *Pseudomonas fluorescens* (89% of 9 strains), *Enterobacter hafniae* (94% of 16 strains), *P. stutzeri* (86% of 7 strains), *Salmo-*

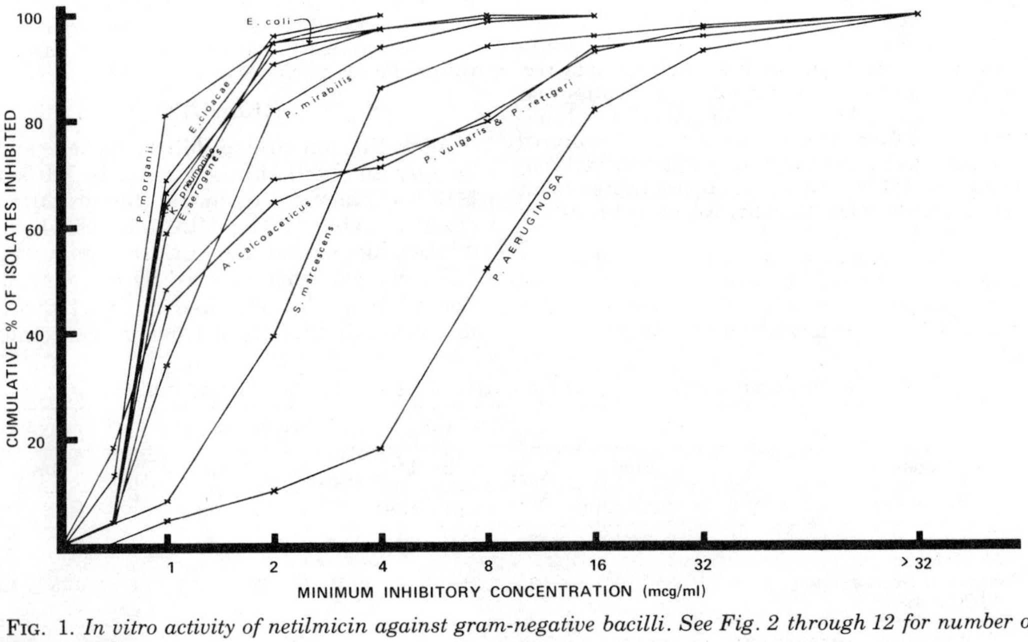

FIG. 1. *In vitro activity of netilmicin against gram-negative bacilli. See Fig. 2 through 12 for number of isolates tested.*

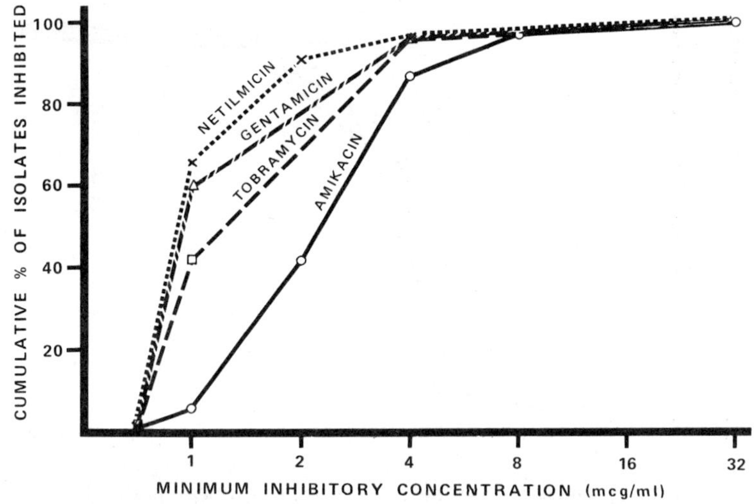

FIG. 2. *Activity of four aminoglycoside antibiotics against Escherichia coli (1687 isolates) by the agar dilution method.*

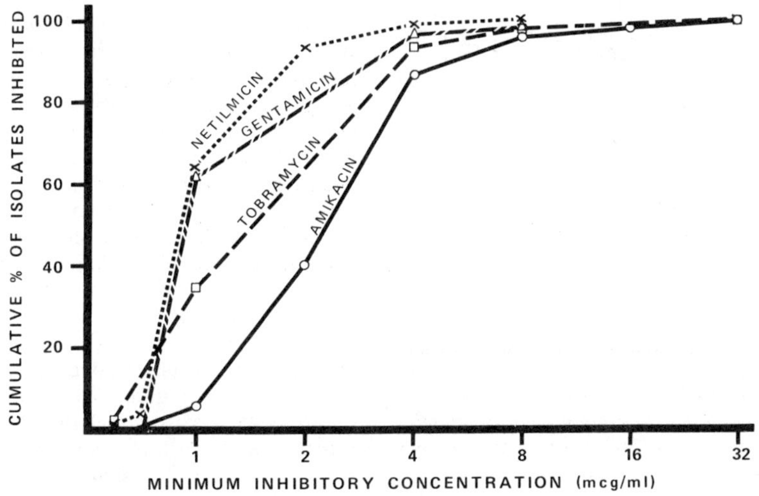

FIG. 3. *Activity of four aminoglycoside antibiotics against Klebsiella pneumoniae (636 isolates) by the agar dilution method.*

nella sp. (100% of 21 strains), *Shigella* sp. (100% of 14 strains), and *Aeromonas* sp. (80% of 5 strains). However, netilmicin showed less activity against *Pseudomonas cepacia* (only one of four strains inhibited) and *Providencia stuartii* (two of six strains inhibited) at 4 μg/ml.

Broth dilution susceptibility. Results using Mueller-Hinton medium in broth dilution correlated with the agar dilution method except for *P. aeruginosa*. It is now widely recognized that results of in vitro susceptibility tests for *P. aeruginosa* markedly differ depending on the divalent cation content of the medium and that Mueller-Hinton agar and broth significantly differ in such cationic content. To assess the apparent resistance of *P. aeruginosa* to various agents, 40 strains of *P. aeruginosa* isolated from clinical material were simultaneously tested by agar and broth dilution methods (Fig. 13). A 2- to 16-fold difference in susceptibility was noted between agar and broth media, since only 46% of isolates of *P. aeruginosa* were inhibited by 8 μg and 78% by 16 μg of netilmicin per ml in agar. In comparison, 65% were inhibited by 8 μg of amikacin per ml and 91% by 16 μg/ml. When these 40 *P. aeruginosa* strains were tested in broth, 94% were inhibited by 4 μg of netilmicin per ml and 100% by 8 μg/ml. the MBC of netilmicin against *P. aeruginosa*

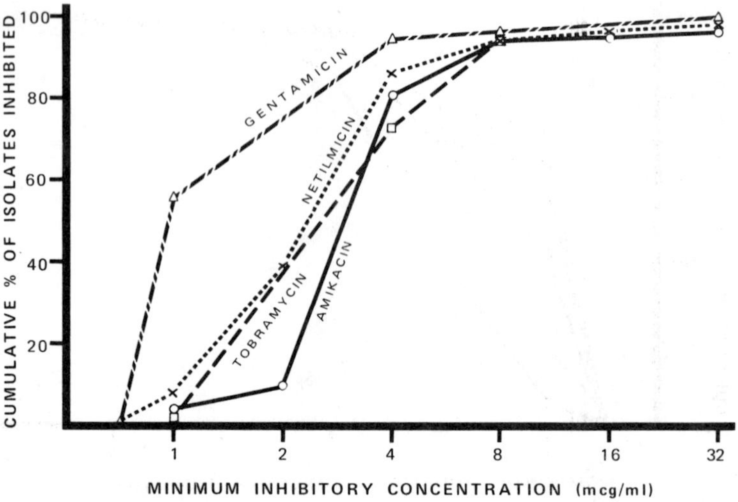

FIG. 4. *Activity of four aminoglycoside antibiotics against Serratia marcescens (116 isolates) by the agar dilution method.*

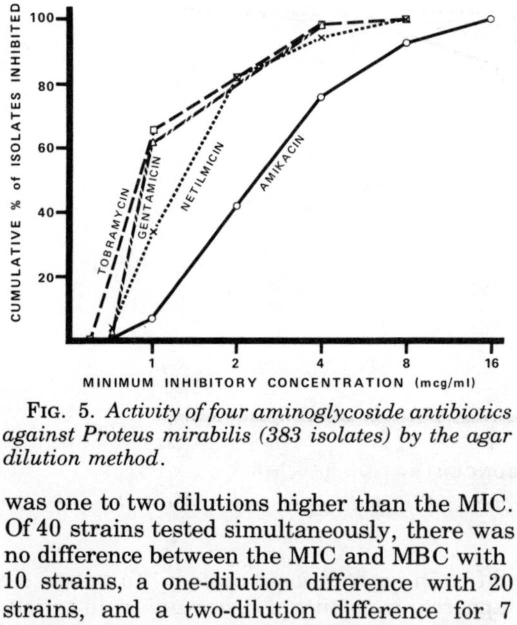

FIG. 5. *Activity of four aminoglycoside antibiotics against Proteus mirabilis (383 isolates) by the agar dilution method.*

was one to two dilutions higher than the MIC. Of 40 strains tested simultaneously, there was no difference between the MIC and MBC with 10 strains, a one-dilution difference with 20 strains, and a two-dilution difference for 7 strains.

Results of studies with highly gentamicin-resistant strains (Table 2). Of 11 strains of *S. marcescens* highly resistant to gentamicin, 9 were inhibited by netilmicin at 4 μg/ml. However, amikacin inhibited 10 of 11 of these organisms, and one strain was resistant to both amikacin and netilmicin. In broth dilution tests, netilmicin inhibited most gentamicin-resistant strains of *P. aeruginosa* at broth concentrations of 4 μg/ml or less. One strain of *P. aeruginosa* with a netilmicin MIC of 8 μg/ml in broth was inhibited by lower concentrations of amikacin, whereas complete cross-resistance was observed for two *P. aeruginosa* isolates that were resistant to all four aminoglycosides. All gentamicin-resistant strains of *P. stuartii* were resistant to netilmicin but were inhibited by amikacin. Tobramycin was not compared because of the close similarity between R-factor-mediated enzymes known to inactivate both tobramycin and gentamicin (1).

Comparison of inhibitory indexes. The activity of weight of an antimicrobial agent may be less meaningful than the relationship between potency by weight and the achievable peak serum levels. For each group of organisms and each aminoglycoside, the ratio between mean peak serum level and MIC required to inhibit two-thirds of each group of organisms (in agar dilution tests) was calculated (Table 3). Thus, higher ratios reflect higher achievable blood levels in relation to most of the MICs for a group of organisms. Results indicate that inhibitory indexes for netilmicin are within the ranges observed for amikacin with a twofold range of *E. coli*, *K. pneumoniae*, *S. marcescens*, *Proteus mirabilis*, *P. morganii*, *P. aeruginosa*, and *Enterobacter* sp. (data pooled for *E. aerogenes* and *E. cloacae*). Against *Proteus vulgaris* and *P. rettgeri*, amikacin showed fourfold greater inhibitory index than did netilmicin.

DISCUSSION

On the basis of this study, in which a very large number of clinical isolates were tested, netilmicin appears to have a wide spectrum of antimicrobial activity against gram-negative

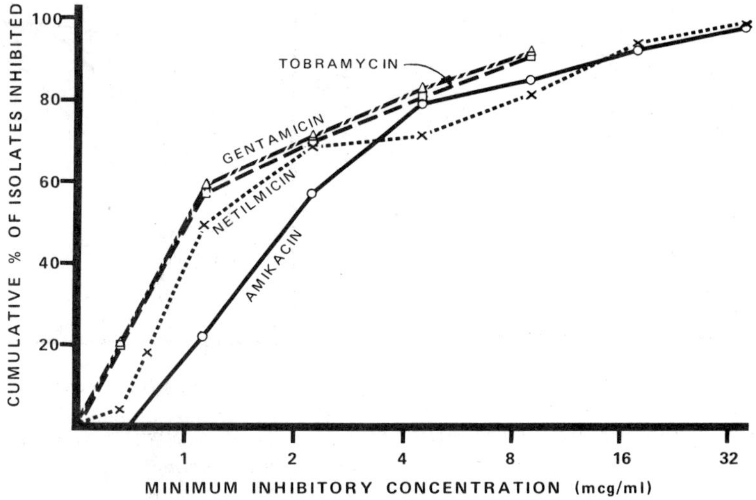

FIG. 6. *Activity of four aminoglycoside antibiotics against Proteus vulgaris (38 isolates) and Proteus rettgeri (11 isolates) by the agar dilution method.*

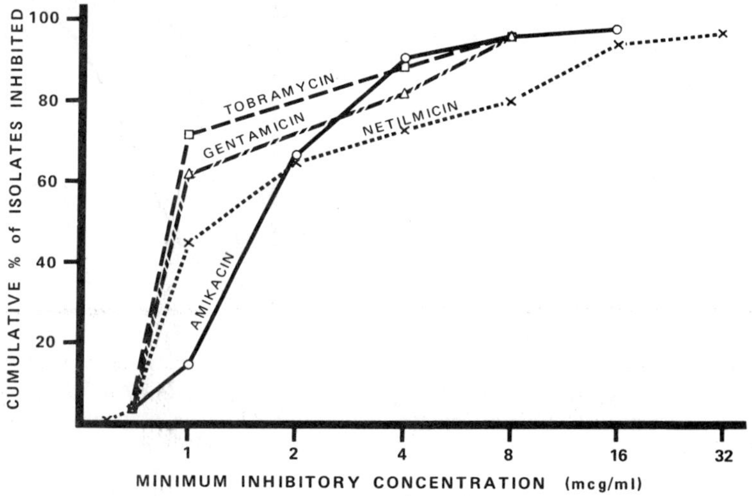

FIG. 7. *Activity of four aminoglycoside antibiotics against Acinetobacter calcoaceticus (92 isolates) by the agar dilution method.*

bacilli. This in vitro activity against most strains of *Enterobacteriaceae* and *P. aeruginosa* is comparable to or superior to that of amikacin, gentamicin, and tobramycin. Few reports have been published (12, 15) that document the in vitro effectiveness of netilmicin against gentamicin-resistant strains of *Enterobacteriaceae* and *P. aeruginosa*. However, any comparison of in vitro data of aminoglycoside activity must be interpreted in light of several factors such as the composition of the medium used, including its divalent cation concentration (6, 11, 22; K. P. Nu and H. C. Neu, Abstr. Annu. Meet. Am. Soc. Microbiol. 1976, A30, p.6) and achievable blood levels in humans. Marked differences in agar-versus-broth MICs of netilmicin against *P. aeruginosa* as reported in a previous report by Meyer et al. (12) were confirmed in our study. We found a 2- to 16-fold difference in agar and broth MICs of netilmicin against *P. aeruginosa* and also that these differences were more marked with netilmicin than with amikacin or gentamicin. Since the relationship between in vitro results and clinical response has not been established, there is a widely recognized need for standardization of the test procedure for susceptibility testing of *P. aeruginosa*. What can be said from our data

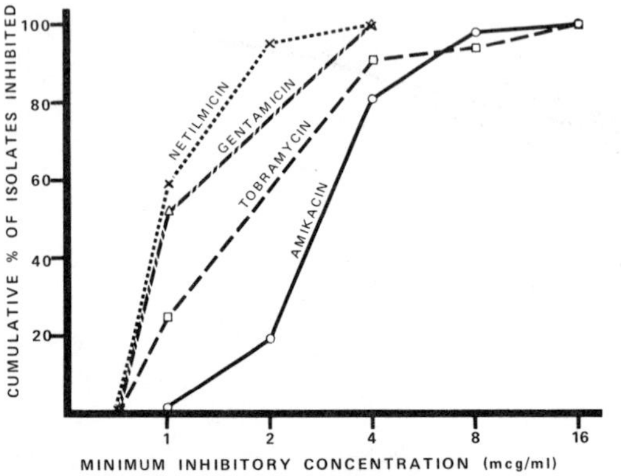

FIG. 8. *Activity of four aminoglycoside antibiotics against Enterobacter aerogenes (86 isolates) by the agar dilution method.*

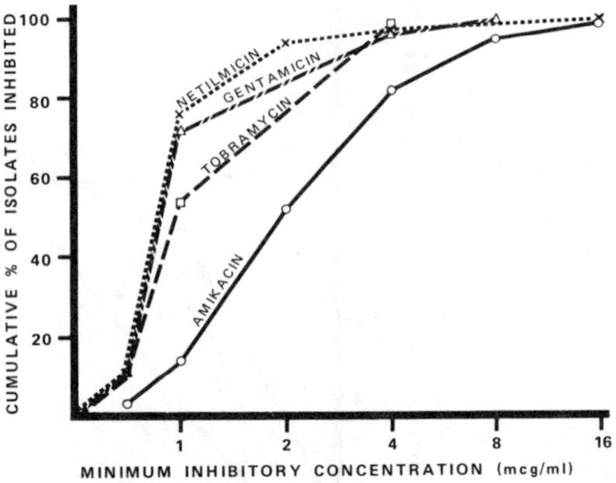

FIG. 10. *Activity of four aminoglycoside antibiotics against Citrobacter freundii (69 isolates) by the agar dilution method.*

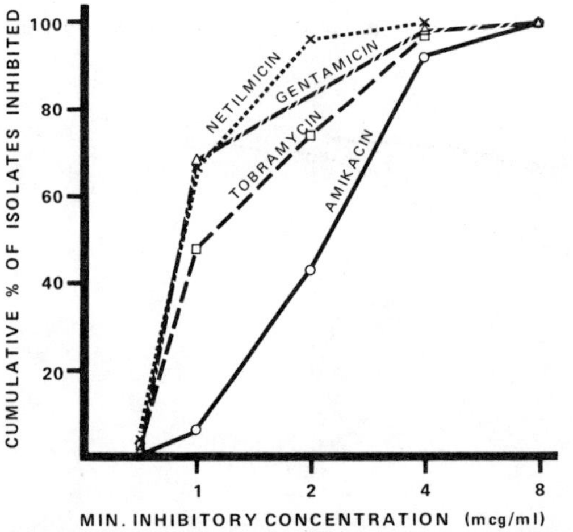

FIG. 9. *Activity of four aminoglycoside antibiotics against Enterobacter cloacae (193 isolates) by the agar dilution method.*

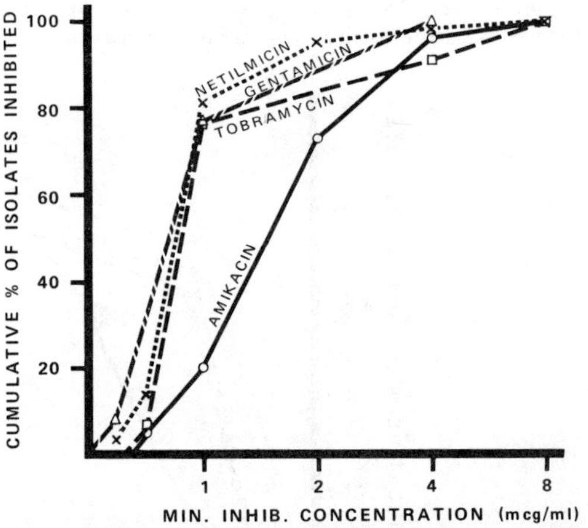

FIG. 11. *Activity of four aminoglycoside antibiotics against Proteus morganii (60 isolates) by the agar dilution method.*

is that for *P. aeruginosa* strains that are susceptible to all four agents, the inhibitory indexes are within a twofold range.

Against gentamicin-resistant strains of *S. marcescens and P. aeruginosa,* our results indicate that the activity of netilmicin parallels that of amikacin. In contrast, netilmicin appears to have little activity against gentamicin-resistant strains of *Providencia stuartii,* whereas all of these organisms were inhibited by amikacin at readily obtainable blood levels. The results with the previous report by Meyer et al. (12), who demonstrated that gentamicin-resistant strains of *Enterobacteriaceae* and *P. aeruginosa* that are susceptible to amikacin are not consistently inhibited by netilmicin. In this respect amikacin appears to have wider range of activity than netilmicin.

Studies in normal volunteers (private communication from G. Arcieri) and our own initial clinical investigations with netilmicin indicate that the blood levels achieved are equal to or greater than those obtained with gentamicin at comparable loading doses. Further, netilmicin can be given safely in individual doses as high as 3 mg per kg of body weight to achieve mean peak serum levels exceeding 10 μg/ml. Comparative assessment of aminoglycoside activity in vitro should, however, take into consideration differences in safe achievable blood levels between various compounds. Thus, we have resorted to calculations of inhibitory indexes to relate potency by weight to anticipated blood levels. The figures for the mean peak serum levels of amikacin and netilmicin used in our calculations are rather conservative, and

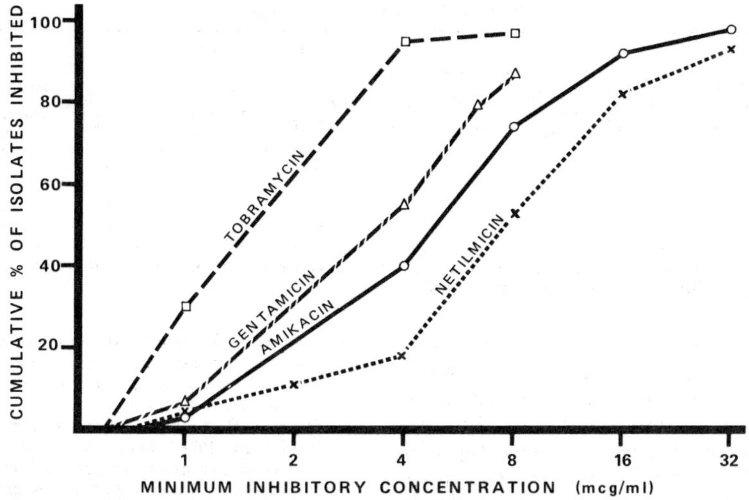

FIG. 12. *Activity of four aminoglycoside antibiotics against Pseudomonas aeruginosa (632 strains) by the agar dilution method.*

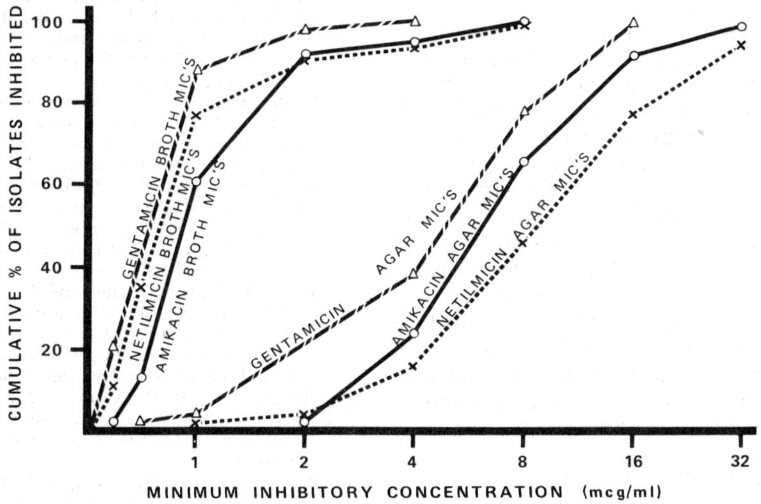

FIG. 13. *Comparison of agar MICs and broth MICs of 40 different clinical isolates of Pseudomonas aeruginosa with netilmicin, gentamicin, and amikacin.*

TABLE 2. *Comparative activity of netilmicin and amikacin against highly gentamicin-resistant strains by the broth dilution method*

Organisms	Total no. of strains tested	No. of strains growing with:		
		Gentamicin (MIC ≥ 16 μg/ml)	Netilmicin (MIC ≥ 16 μg/ml)	Amikacin (MIC ≥ 32 μg/ml)
Serratia marcescens	11	11	2	1
Pseudomonas aeruginosa	10	10	2	2
Providencia stuartii	10	10	10	0

higher blood levels are likely to be achieved in clinical practice. The safe maximal dose for netilmicin has not yet been determined. Though we recognize that these inhibitory indexes are arbitrary and have no established or predictive clinical value, a fourfold or greater variation in inhibitory indexes between various agents may be significant. Our data indicate

TABLE 3. *Inhibitory indexes*[a]

Agent	Mean peak level (μg/ml)	Inhibitory index							
		Escherichia coli	*Klebsiella pneumoniae*	*Serratia marcescens*	*Proteus mirabilis*	*P. vulgaris, P. rettgeri*	*P. morganii*	*Pseudomonas aeruginosa*	*Enterobacter* sp.
Netilmicin	8	4	4	2	4	1	8	0.5	4
Amikacin	16	4	4	4	4	4	4	1	4
Gentamicin	4	2	2	2	2	1	4	0.5	2
Tobramycin	4	1	1	0.5	2	1	4	1	1

[a] Expressed as the ratio of the mean peak serum level to the concentration required to inhibit two-thirds of the isolates (in micrograms per milliliter) in agar dilution susceptibility tests.

that these indexes for netilmicin are comparable to those for gentamicin and amikacin against *E. coli*, *K. pneumoniae*, *S. marcescens*, and *Enterobacter* sp. and superior to those for tobramycin. All antibiotics showed a high index against *P. mirabilis* and *P. morganii*. Against *P. vulgaris* and *P. rettgeri*, amikacin appeared to have a significant advantage over the other antibiotics, which is consistent with a previous report (12).

Aside from considerations of antimicrobial spectrum, pharmakokinetics, and resistance to enzymatic degradation, another important factor in the assessment of aminoglycosides is that of relative toxicity. Our preliminary data indicate that netilmicin may be safely given to patients who have aminoglycoside-associated cochlear and vestibular damage. This parallels animal tests suggesting that netilmicin is less toxic than gentamicin (G. Arcieri, private communication). In view of our in vitro results and results of initial clinical trials, comparative studies in humans now appear indicated to determine whether netilmicin has advantages over other aminoglycosides from the viewpoint of therapeutic efficacy or lessened toxicity.

ACKNOWLEDGMENTS

This study was supported by a grant from the Schering Corp.

We gratefully acknowledge the excellent technical assistance of Qamar Murtaza and Charlotte Findell.

LITERATURE CITED

1. **Benveniste, R., and J. Davies.** 1973. Mechanisms of antibiotic resistance in bacteria. Annu. Rev. Biochem. 42:471.
2. **Bryan, L. E., M. S. Shahrbadi, and H. M. Vanden Elzen.** 1976. Gentamicin resistance in *Pseudomonas aeruginosa:* R-factor-mediated resistance. Antimicrob. Agents Chemother. 6:191–199.
3. **Dupont, H. L., and W. W. Spink.** 1969. Infections due to gram-negative organisms. Medicine 48:307–332.
4. **Ericsson, H. M., and J. C. Sherris.** 1971. Antibiotic sensitivity testing. Report of an international collaborative study. Acta Pathol. Microbiol. Scand. Sec. B, Suppl. 217.
5. **Finland, M.** 1972. Changing patterns of susceptibility of common bacterial pathogens to antimicrobial agents. Ann. Intern. Med. 76:1009–1036.
6. **Garrod, L. P., and P. M. Waterworth.** 1969. Effects of media composition on the apparent sensitivity of *Pseudomonas aeruginosa* to gentamicin. J. Clin. Pathol. 22:537–538.
7. **Holmes, R. K., B. H. Minshew, K. Gould, and J. P. Sanford.** 1974. Resistance to *Pseudomonas aeruginosa* to gentamicin and related aminoglycoside antibiotics. Antimicrob. Agents Chemother. 6:253–262.
8. **Hugh, R.** 1970. *Pseudomonas and Acromonas,* p. 175–190. *In* J. E. Blair, E. H. Lennette, and J. P. Truant (ed.), Manual of clinical microbiology, 1st ed. American Society for Microbiology, Bethesda, Md.
9. **Martin, C. M., N. S. Ikari, V. Zimmerman, and A. V. Waitz.** 1971. A virulent nosocomial *Klebsiella* with a transferable R-factor for gentamicin. J. Infect. Dis. 124(Suppl): S24–S29.
10. **Martin, W. J.** 1970. *Enterobacteriaceae,* p. 151–174. *In* J. E. Blair, E. H. Lennette, and J. P. Truant (ed.), Manual of clinical microbiology, 1st ed. American Society for Microbiology, Bethesda, Md.
11. **Mederios, A. A., T. F. O'Brien, W. E. C. Wache, and N. F. Yulug.** 1971. Effects of salt concentration on the apparent in vitro susceptibility of *Pseudomonas* and other gram-negative bacilli to gentamicin. J. Infect. Dis. 124(Suppl.):S29–S64.
12. **Meyer, R. D., L. L. Kraus, and K. A. Pasiecznik.** 1976. In vitro susceptibility of gentamicin-resistant *Enterobacteriaceae* and *Pseudomonas aeruginosa* to netilmicin and selected aminoglycoside antibiotics. Antimicrob. Agents Chemother. 10:677–681.
13. **Meyer, R. D., R. P. Lewis, J. Halter, and M. White.** 1976. Gentamicin resistant *Pseudomonas aeruginosa* and *Serratia marcescens* in a general hospital. Lancet i:580–583.
14. **Price, K. E., T. A. Pursiano, M. D. DeFuria, and G. E. Wright.** 1974. Activity of BB-K8 (Amikacin) against clinical isolates resistant to one or more aminoglycoside antibiotics. Antimicrob. Agents Chemother. 5:143–152.
15. **Rahal, J. J., Jr., M. S. Simberkoff, K. Kagan, and N. H. Moldover.** 1976. Bactericidal efficacy of Sch 20569 and amikacin against gentamicin-sensitive and -resistant organisms. Antimicrob. Agents Chemother. 9:595–599.
16. **Schulman, J. A., P. M. Terry, and C. E. Hough.** 1971. Colonization with gentamicin resistant *Pseudomonas aeruginosa,* pyocine type S in a burn unit. J. Infect. Dis. 124(Suppl.):S18–S23.
17. **Smith, P. B., K. M. Tomfohrde, D. L. Rhoden, and A. Balows.** 1972. API system: a multitube micromethod for identification of *Enterobacteriaceae*. Appl. Microbiol. 24:449–452.
18. **Steers, E., E. L. Foltz, and B. S. Graves.** 1959. An inoculum replicating apparatus for routine testing of bacterial susceptibility to antibiotics. Antibiot. Chemother. 9:307–311.
19. **Washington, J. A., II, P. K. W. Yu, and W. J. Martin.** 1971. Evaluation of accuracy of multitest micro-

method system for the identification of *Enterobacteriaeceae*. Appl. Microbiol. 22:267–269.
20. **Weinstein, R. J., L. S. Young, and W. L. Hewitt.** 1975. Activity of three aminoglycosides and two penicillins against four species of gram-negative bacilli. Antimicrob. Agents Chemother. 7:172–178.
21. **Young, L. S., and W. L. Hewitt.** 1973. Activity of five aminoglycoside antibiotics in vitro against gram-negative bacilli and *Staphlococcus aureus*. Antimicrob. Agents Chemother. 4:617–625.
22. **Zimelis, V. M., and G. G. Jackson.** 1973. Activity of aminoglycoside antibiotics against *Pseudomonas aeruginosa,* specificity and site of calcium and magnesium antagonism. J. Infect. Dis. 127:663–669.

Antimicrobial Agents and Chemotherapy, Jan. 1977, p. 74-79
Vol. 11, No. 1

Mezlocillin: In Vitro Studies of a New Broad-Spectrum Penicillin

GERALD P. BODEY* AND THERESA PAN

The University of Texas System Cancer Center, M. D. Anderson Hospital and Tumor Institute, Houston, Texas 77030

Received for publication 9 July 1976

Mezlocillin is a new semisynthetic penicillin that inhibited 71% of the isolates of *Serratia marcescens*, 67% of *Escherichia coli*, 50% of *Enterobacter* spp., and 49% of *Klebsiella* spp. at a concentration of 12.5 μg/ml. It is also active against both indole-positive and -negative *Proteus* spp. and gram-positive cocci, except penicillin G-resistant *Staphylococcus aureus*. At a concentration of 100 μg/ml, it inhibited 94% of the isolates of *Pseudomonas aeruginosa*. It is more active than ampicillin, carbenicillin, and cephalothin against some gram-negative bacilli.

Gram-negative bacilli continue to be a major cause of infection in hospitalized patients. This is especially true among patients with malignant diseases and patients receiving immunosuppressive therapy (3, 4). Often these patients do not respond, despite the in vitro susceptibility of the etiological organism to the antibiotic utilized (1). Consequently, there is a continuing need for the development of new antibiotics. The ureido-penicillins are an interesting group of semisynthetic penicillins that have broad-spectrum activity against gram-negative bacilli, including *Pseudomonas aeruginosa* (2). Figure 1 shows the chemical structure of mezlocillin (D-α[2-oxo-3-mesyl-imidazolidinyl)-carbonyl]-aminobenzylpenicillin; BAY 1353), a new ureido-penicillin recently undergoing investigation (H. B. Konig, K. G. Metzger, H. A. Offe, and W. Schrock, Prog. Abstr. Intersci. Conf., Antimicrob. Agents Chemother., 14th, San Francisco, Calif., Abstr. 372, 1974; K. Metzger, Prog. Abstr. Intersci. Conf. Antimicrob. Agents Chemother., 15th, Washington, D.C., 332, 1975). This report presents the results of in vitro studies of mezlocillin, which indicate that it may be a potentially useful antibiotic.

MATERIALS AND METHODS

Susceptibility tests were conducted on 556 clinical isolates of gram-negative bacilli and 88 clinical isolates of gram-positive cocci, using the dilution technique with an automatic microtiter system (Canalco, Autotiter instruction manual). All organisms were inoculated into Mueller-Hinton broth (Difco) and incubated at 37°C for 18 h. For gram-negative bacilli, a 0.05-ml sample of a 10^{-3} dilution of this broth culture (approximately 10^5 colony-forming units [CFU]/ml) was used as the inoculum. For gram-positive cocci, a 0.05-ml sample of a 10^{-2} dilution of this broth culture (approximately 10^6 CFU/ml) was used as the inoculum for susceptibility testing.

All gram-negative bacilli used in this study were cultured from blood specimens obtained from patients between 1967 and 1975. The patients were hospitalized at this institution and had underlying malignant diseases. A total of 100 isolates each of *P. aeruginosa*, *Klebsiella* spp., and *Escherichia coli*, 98 isolates of *Proteus* spp., 69 isolates of *Serratia* spp., and 89 isolates of *Enterobacter* spp. were used. All gram-positive cocci used in this study were cultured from specimens obtained from hospitalized patients, most of whom did not have cancer. A total of 22 isolates of *Streptococcus pyogenes*, 14 isolates of *S. pneumoniae*, and 62 isolates of *Staphylococcus aureus* were used. The susceptibility of isolates of *S. aureus* to penicillin G was determined by the broth dilution method. Isolates inhibited by less than 0.10 μg/ml were selected as penicillin G susceptible, and those isolates resistant to more than 25 μg/ml were selected as penicillin G resistant.

Mezlocillin (BAY 1353) was supplied as a powder by Delbay Pharmaceuticals, Inc., Bloomfield, N.J. Ampicillin and BL-P1654, 6-[D-α-(3-guanylureido)-phenylacetamido] penicillanic acid, were supplied by Bristol Laboratories, Syracuse, N.Y. Carbenicillin and ticarcillin were supplied by Beecham Pharmaceuticals, Bristol, Tenn. Twofold serial dilutions of the antibiotics were made with Mueller-Hinton broth, and the minimal inhibitory concentration (MIC) was determined after incubation at 37°C for 18 h. All wells containing trace growth or no discernible growth were subcultured on sheep blood agar. A calibrated pipette was used to transfer 0.01 ml of the inoculum. The minimum bactericidal concentration (MBC) was determined after incubation at 37°C for 18 h. The MBC was defined as the lowest concentration of drug that yielded less than 50 colonies on subculture (less than 5 colonies/0.001 ml of inoculum). Comparison studies were conducted simultaneously.

RESULTS

The in vitro activity of mezlocillin against gram-positive cocci and gram-negative bacilli is shown in Fig. 2. Although the majority of isolates of *S. pneumoniae* were quite susceptible to mezlocillin, 14% required concentrations of 6.25 to 25 μg/ml to inhibit their growth. Likewise, the majority of penicillin G-susceptible *S. aureus* were inhibited by 0.20 μg or less of mezlocillin per ml, whereas penicillin G-resistant *S. aureus* were also resistant to mezlocillin. Isolates of *S. pyogenes* were quite susceptible to mezlocillin. Over 95% of the isolates of *P. mirabilis* and 70% of the isolates of indole-positive *Proteus* spp. were susceptible to 1.56 μg or less of mezlocillin per ml. A concentration of 12.5 μg/ml inhibited 71% of the isolates of *S. marcescens*, 67% of *E. coli*, 50% of *Enterobacter* spp., and 49% of *Klebsiella* spp., but only 27% of *P. aeruginosa*. However, at a concentration of 100 μg/ml, mezlocillin inhibited 94% of the isolates of *P. aeruginosa*. Generally, the MIC was also the MBC, but this was not true for *P. aeruginosa*. The MBC for most isolates of *P. aeruginosa* was twice as high as the MIC.

The effect of inoculum size on the MIC and MBC was determined for 10 isolates each of *K. pneumoniae*, *E. coli*, and *P. aeruginosa* (Fig. 3). For all isolates of *K. pneumoniae* and most

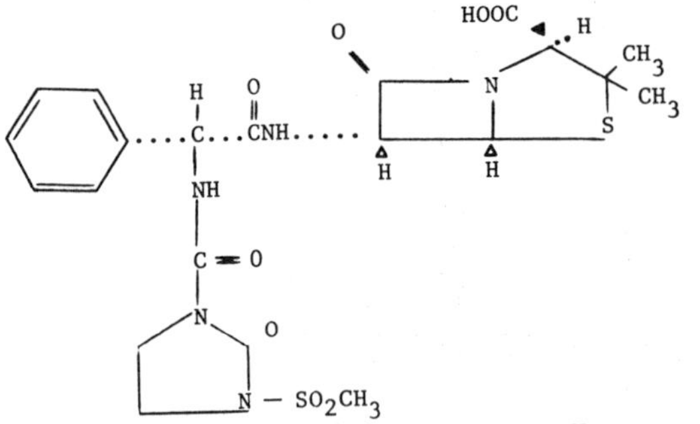

FIG. 1. *Chemical structure of mezlocillin.*

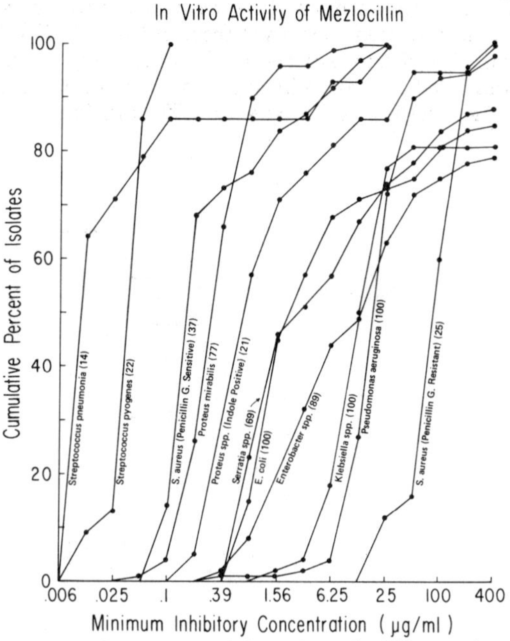

FIG. 2. *In vitro activity of mezlocillin against gram-negative bacilli and gram-positive cocci. Numbers in parentheses indicate the number of isolates tested.*

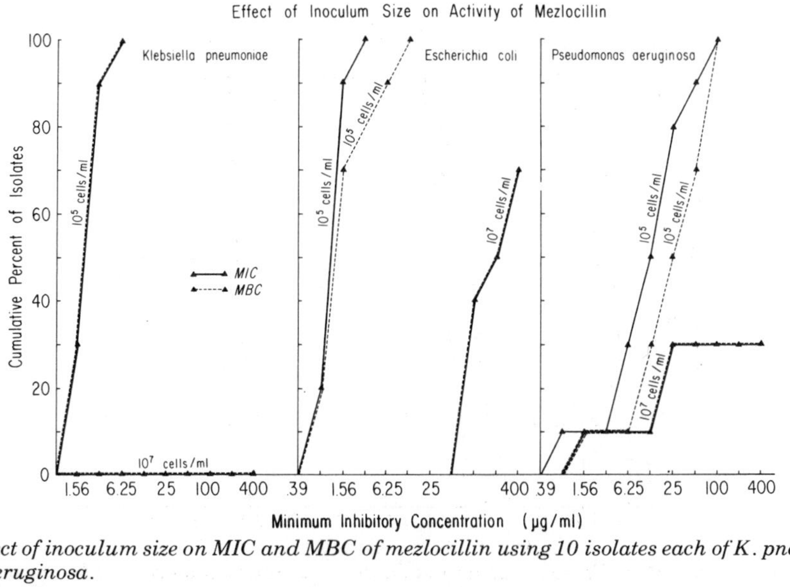

FIG. 3. *Effect of inoculum size on MIC and MBC of mezlocillin using 10 isolates each of K. pneumoniae, E. coli, and P. aeruginosa.*

isolates of *E. coli*, the MIC and MBC were the same. Inoculum size had the greatest effect on the activity of mezlocillin against *K. pneumoniae*. Using an inoculum of 10^5 CFU/ml, all isolates were inhibited at a concentration of 6.25 μg/ml, whereas using an inoculum of 10^7 CFU/ml, none was inhibited at a concentration of 400 μg/ml. The MIC and MBC for isolates of *E. coli* increased sixfold or more when the inoculum size was increased from 10^5 to 10^7 CFU/ml. All of the isolates of *P. aeruginosa* were inhibited by 100 μg or less of mezlocillin per ml when the inoculum was 10^5 CFU/ml, but only 30% were inhibited by 400 μg/ml when the inoculum was 10^7 CFU/ml.

The effect of pH on the susceptibility of 10 isolates each of *E. coli*, *K. pneumoniae*, and *P. aeruginosa* is shown in Fig. 4. The pH was adjusted by the addition of phosphate buffer to Mueller-Hinton broth. The greatest effect was observed against isolates of *E. coli*, which were more susceptible at alkaline pH. The pH had no appreciable effect on the activity of mezlocillin against isolates of *P. aeruginosa*. Media had little effect on the activity of mezlocillin (Fig. 5). However, isolates of *K. pneumoniae*, *E. coli*,

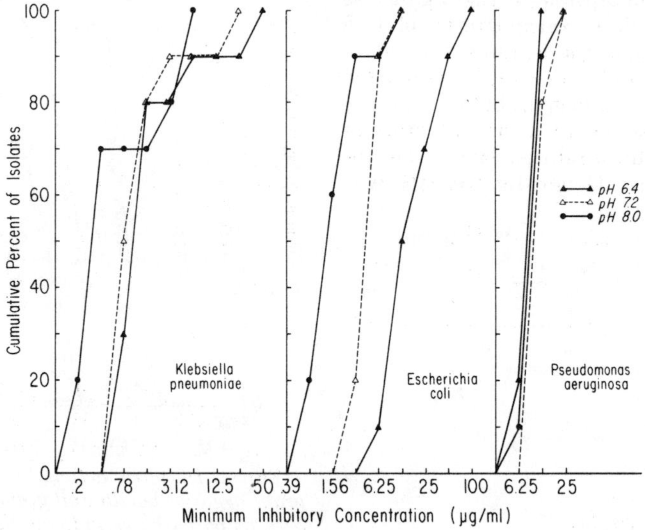

FIG. 4. *Effect of pH on the activity of mezlocillin against K. pneumoniae, E. coli, and P. aeruginosa. Ten isolates of each gram-negative bacillus were tested.*

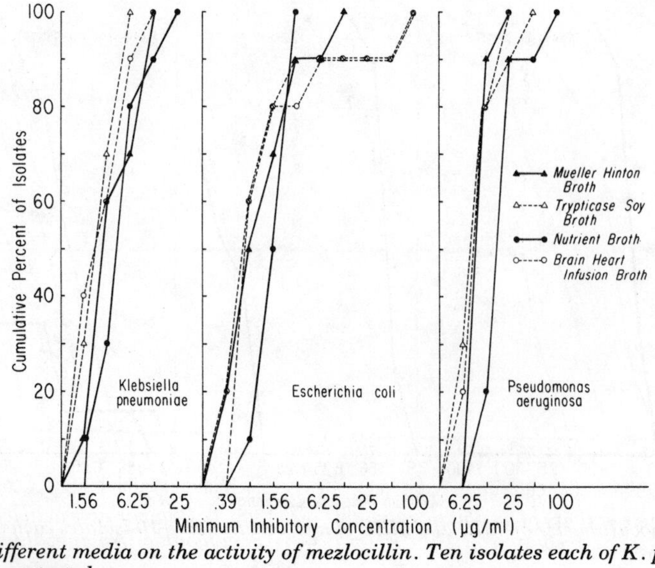

FIG. 5. *Effect of different media on the activity of mezlocillin. Ten isolates each of K. pneumoniae, E. coli, and P. aeruginosa were tested.*

and *P. aeruginosa* were slightly more resistant when tested in nutrient broth, with the exception of one isolate of *E. coli* which was considerably more susceptible to mezlocillin when tested in nutrient broth.

The activity of mezlocillin against 50 isolates each of various gram-negative bacilli was compared with ampicillin, carbenicillin, and cephalothin (Fig. 6 to 10). Figure 10 shows similar data for 21 isolates of indole-positive *Proteus* spp. Mezlocillin was the most active drug against isolates of *E. coli*, although about 30% of the isolates were resistant to 25 μg/ml and some of these isolates were more susceptible to cephalothin. Cephalothin was the most active antibiotic against *K. pneumoniae*, although mezlocillin was the most active penicillin. Mezlocillin was substantially more active than any of the other antibiotics against *S. marcescens*. Cephalothin was virtually inactive, whereas carbenicillin was active against nearly 50% of these isolates. Mezlocillin was the most active antibiotic against *Enterobacter* spp. although 56% of the isolates were resistant to 25 μg/ml. Carbenicillin was the second most active antibiotic, but 74% of the isolates were resistant to 25 μg of this drug per ml. All three penicillins were equally active against *P. mirabilis*. Two isolates that were resistant to ampicillin and cephalothin and one isolate that was relatively resistant to carbenicillin were inhibited by 6.25 μg of mezlocillin per ml. Mezlocillin was also the most active antibiotic against indole-positive *Proteus* spp. and was consistently four times more active than carbenicillin. Ampicillin and cephalothin had minimal activity against these isolates.

The activity of mezlocillin was compared with that of BL-P1654, carbenicillin, and ticarcillin against 50 isolates of *P. aeruginosa* (Fig. 11). The most active antibiotic was BL-P1654 and the least active was carbenicillin. Mezlocillin and ticarcillin had comparable activity.

DISCUSSION

Mezlocillin is a broad-spectrum semisynthetic penicillin with activity against both gram-positive cocci and gram-negative bacilli. It is of particular interest because it is marginally active against *S. marcescens*, *K. pneumoniae*, and *P. aeruginosa*. It is more active in vitro than ampicillin or carbenicillin against *E. coli* and as active as these two penicillins against *P. mirabilis*. It is also more active in vitro than carbenicillin against indole-positive *Proteus* spp. and *Enterobacter* spp. It is as active as cephalothin against 80% of the isolates

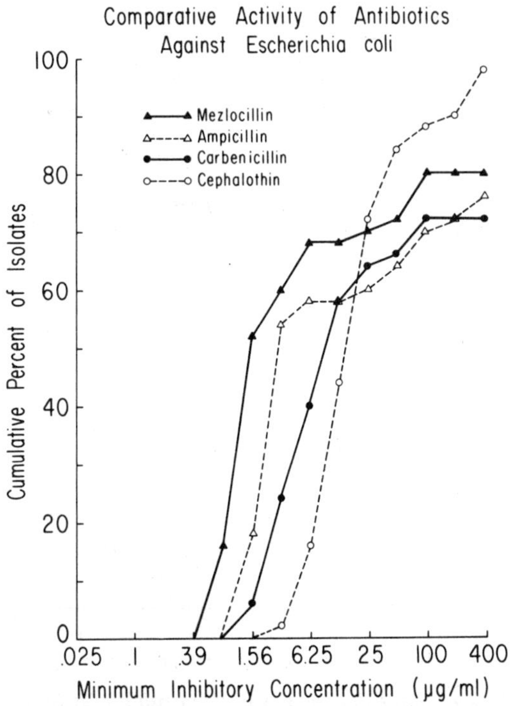

FIG. 6. *Comparative activity of antibiotics against 50 isolates of E. coli. An inoculum of 10^5 CFU/ml was used.*

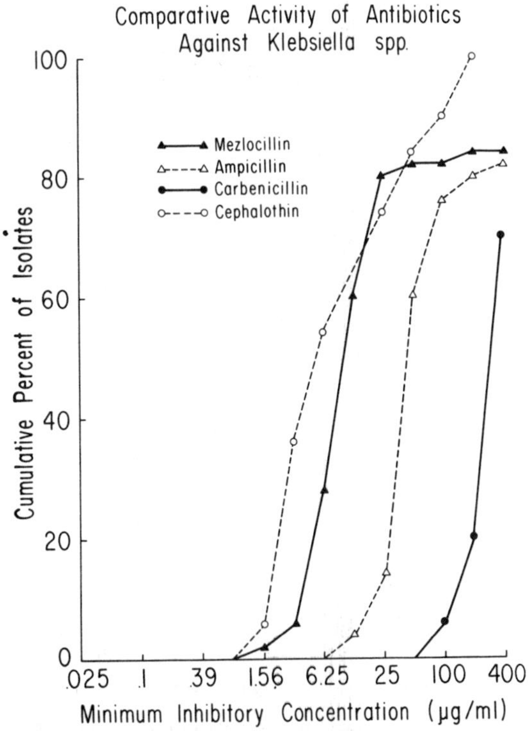

FIG. 7. *Comparative activity of antibiotics against K. pneumoniae. An inoculum of 10^5 CFU/ml was used.*

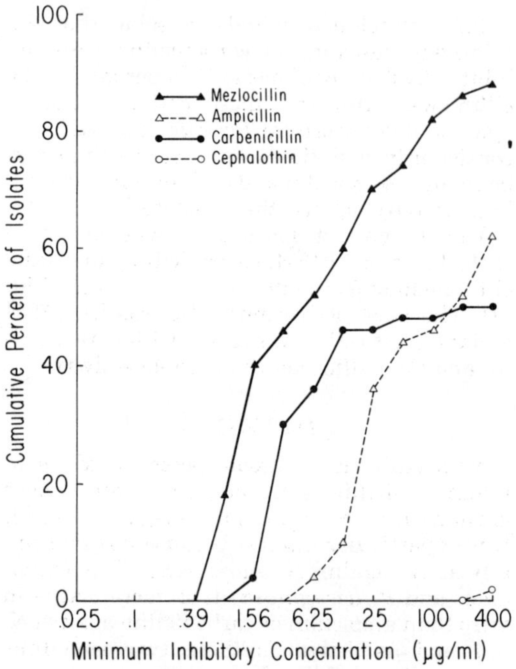

FIG. 8. *Comparative activity of antibiotics against S. marcescens. An inoculum of 10^5 CFU/ml was used.*

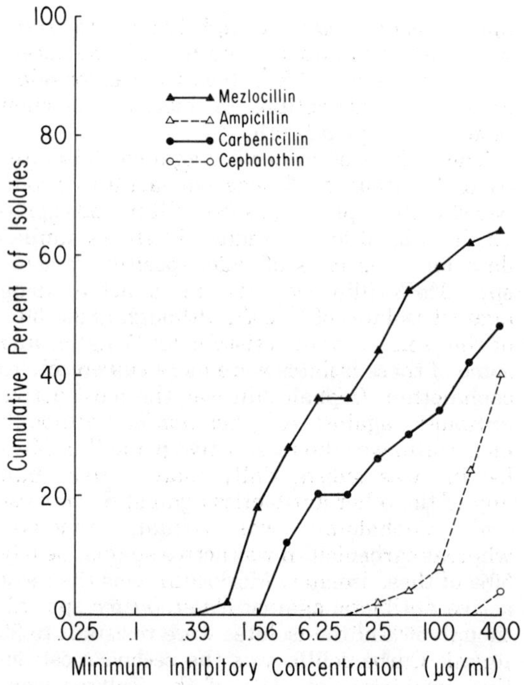

FIG. 9. *Comparative activity of antibiotics against Enterobacter spp. An inoculum of 10^5 CFU/ml was used.*

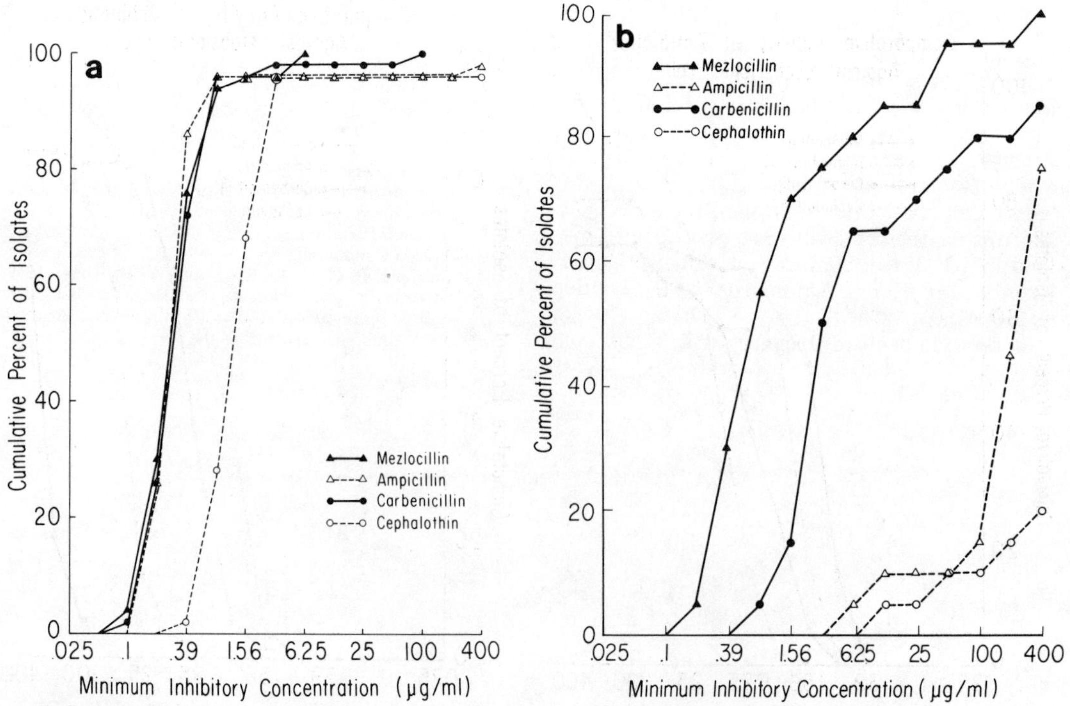

FIG. 10. *Comparative activity of antibiotics against Proteus spp. Fifty isolates of P. mirabilis (a) and 21 isolates of indole-positive Proteus spp (b) were tested. An inoculum of 10^5 CFU/ml was used.*

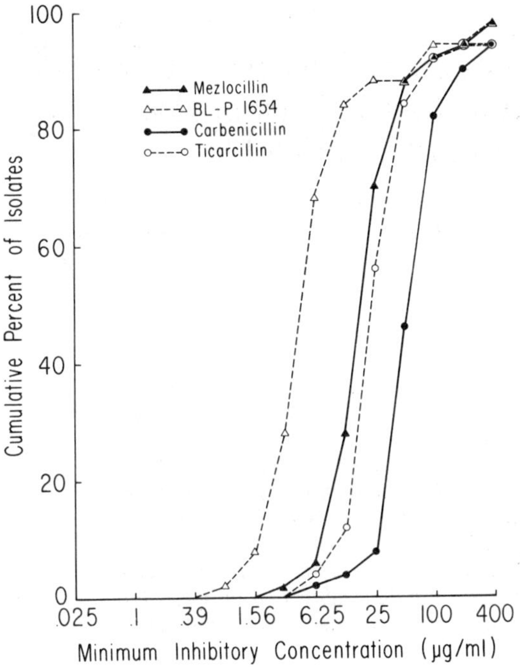

FIG. 11. *Comparative activity of penicillins against 50 isolates of P. aeruginosa. An inoculum of 10^5 CFU/ml was used.*

of *Klebsiella* spp. and is the most active of the four antibiotics against *S. marcescens*. However, another ureido-penicillin, BP-P1654, is more active than mezlocillin in vitro against *P. aeruginosa*. The ureido-penicillins have been shown to be relatively resistant to destruction by the β-lactamase of isolates of *E. coli* and *S. marcescens* resistant to ampicillin, which may account for the better in vitro results with mezlocillin (B. Wiedemann, V. Kremery, and H. Knothe, Int. Kongr. Chemother., 9th, London, Abstr. M366, 1975).

There has been controversy in the past over the bactericidal activity of ureido-penicillins. Generally, mezlocillin was bactericidal at the MIC, but this was not true for isolates of *P. aeruginosa*. Inoculum size had a major effect on the activity of mezlocillin. It was ineffective against all isolates of *K. pneumoniae* and most isolates of *P. aeruginosa* when a large inoculum was used. This suggests that these cells are not uniformly susceptible to mezlocillin, and a large inoculum includes more cells that are inherently resistant to the antibiotic. This adverse effect of inoculum size has been observed with other penicillins (5, 6).

Mezlocillin is an interesting new penicillin because of its broad-spectrum activity. The drug deserves further evaluation because it is potentially more active than ampicillin, carbenicillin, and cephalothin against some gram-negative bacilli.

ACKNOWLEDGMENTS

This work was supported by Public Health Service grant CA-10042 from the National Cancer Institute and a grant-in-aid from Delbay Pharmaceuticals, Inc., Bloomfield, N.J.

LITERATURE CITED

1. **Bodey, G. P., E. Middleman, T. Umsawasdi, and V. Rodriguez.** 1972. Infections in cancer patients—results with gentamicin sulfate therapy. Cancer 29:1697–1701.
2. **Bodey, G. P., and D. Stewart.** 1971. In vitro studies of semisynthetic α-(substituted-ureido) penicillins. Appl. Microbiol. 21:710–717.
3. **Eickhoff, T. C.** 1973. Infectious complications in renal transplant patients. Transplant. Proc. 5:1233–1238.
4. **Inagaki, J., V. Rodriguez, and G. P. Bodey.** 1974. Causes of death in cancer patients. Cancer 33:568–573.
5. **Neu, H. C., and E. B. Winshell.** 1971. In vitro studies of semisynthetic penicillin, 6-[D(-)-α-carboxy-3-thienylacetamido] penicillanic acid (BRL 2288), active against *Pseudomonas*, p. 385–389. Antimicrob. Agents Chemother. 1970.
6. **Standiford, H. C., A. C. Kind, and W. M. Kirby.** 1969. Laboratory and clinical studies of carbenicillin against gram-negative bacilli, p. 286–291. Antimicrob. Agents Chemother. 1968.

ANTIMICROBIAL AGENTS AND CHEMOTHERAPY, Jan. 1977, p. 80-83 Vol. 11, No. 1

Interferon Induction in Cynomolgus and Rhesus Monkeys After Repeated Doses of a Modified Polyriboinosinic-Polyribocytidylic Acid Complex

M. L. SAMMONS, E. L. STEPHEN,* H. B. LEVY, S. BARON, AND D. E. HILMAS

U.S. Army Medical Research Institute of Infectious Diseases, Fort Detrick, Frederick, Maryland 21701, National Institute of Allergy and Infectious Diseases, Bethesda, Maryland 21714, and University of Texas Medical Branch, Galveston, Texas 77550*

Received for publication 19 August 1976

Serum interferon activity was determined in 12 cynomolgus and 12 rhesus monkeys injected intravenously once daily for 10 days with from 0.1 to 6.0 mg of a stabilized polyriboinosinic acid·polyribocytidylic acid complex per kg, composed of polyriboinosinic acid·polyribocytidylic acid, poly-1-lysine, and carboxymethylcellulose [poly(ICLC)]. Interferon activity was detected 2 h after the first injection, with maximum activity occurring 8 h after the second injection. A period of hyporesponsiveness occurred after the third injection of poly(ICLC) in all monkeys and lasted until the sixth injection in the rhesus monkeys, when interferon activity again became more elevated. The delayed rebound was not as apparent in cynomolgus monkeys. Rhesus monkeys injected with 6 mg/kg did not exhibit serious side effects.

Polyriboinosinic acid·polyribocytidylic acid [poly(I)·poly(C)] is effective as an interferon inducer in rodents (3-6, 14), but not in cattle, humans, or subhuman primates (7, 13). Failure of poly(I)·poly(C) to induce interferon in these latter species has been ascribed to the action of a serum nucleolytic enzyme, which inactivates the compound (10, 11). By complexing the poly(I)·poly(C) with poly-1-lysine and carboxymethylcellulose, it was found that interferon could be induced in rhesus monkeys and chimpanzees by intravenous injection of the resulting stabilized compound [poly(ICLC)] (11).

The effectiveness of this stabilized compound for therapy against viral infection has been demonstrated in rhesus monkeys infected with simian hemorrhagic fever virus (11), yellow fever virus (our unpublished observations), or street rabies virus (G. Baer, S. Baron, and H. B. Levy, unpublished data). A possible barrier to antiviral therapy with poly(ICLC) is the period of hyporesponsiveness, manifested by diminished levels of serum interferon activity during the administration of repeated doses of interferon inducers or viral agents which has been reported by others in rodents and cattle (2-5, 8, 13, 14). This study describes the early interferon responses and a period of hyporesponsiveness that occurs after repeated injections with multiple doses of poly(ICLC) in cynomolgus (*Macaca fasicularis*) and rhesus (*Macaca mulatta*) monkeys.

MATERIALS AND METHODS

Drugs. Poly(ICLC), lot 66, prepared at the National Institutes of Health as previously described (11), was diluted with equal volumes of pyrogen-free 0.85% NaCl prior to injections into monkeys. Ketaset (ketamine hydrochloride, Bristol Laboratories, Syracuse, N.Y.), 10 mg/kg, was injected intramuscularly for restraint of the monkeys to facilitate injection of poly(ICLC).

Monkeys. Twelve healthy, young adult, male cynomolgus monkeys, weighing 1.8 to 2.2 kg, and 12 healthy, young adult, male rhesus monkeys, weighing 3 to 4 kg, were housed in individual cages and maintained throughout the experimental period at a constant room temperature (25°C) and a 12-h light cycle. Monkeys were fed four to six commercial monkey chow biscuits per day (Wayne Monkey Diet, Allied Mills, Inc., Chicago, Ill.), and water was available ad libitum. Apples were given each day 3 h after injection of poly(ICLC).

Injection and bleeding schedules. Four groups of three cynomolgus monkeys each were injected intravenously with 0.1, 0.3, 1.0, or 3.0 mg of poly(ICLC)/kg of body weight per day for 10 days. In addition, four groups of three rhesus monkeys each were injected intravenously with 0.3, 1.0, 3.0, or 6.0 mg of poly(ICLC)/kg per day for 10 days. A 3- to 4-ml amount of venous blood was collected twice daily, prior to the time of each injection of poly(ICLC) and again 8 h later. Two serum samples were collected from each monkey before treatment was initiated to determine base line values of interferon activity. A concurrent control group consisted of four monkeys injected daily with saline and bled according to the same schedule as the monkeys that received poly(ICLC). These dose levels were generally well tolerated, except for some anorexia and fever produced by the higher doses. Details of the clinical responses to the daily injections of poly(ICLC) will be published separately.

Interferon assays. One-milliliter aliquots of serum from each sample were stored at −70°C until assayed for interferon activity. Interferon activity was measured by determining the dilution of the sample that would cause a 50% reduction of the cytopathic effect induced by vesicular stomatitis virus in HFS-1 tissue culture cells, as previously described (1). Activity was expressed as interferon units per milliliter of serum normalized to reference units per milliliter of human serum interferon standard (National Institute of Allergy and Infectious Diseases reference reagent catalog no. G023901-527).

Statistics. Geometric mean interferon titers were calculated for each group of monkeys. Samples that showed no detectable interferon activity were arbitrarily assigned a value of 10 interferon units/ml, one-half of the lower limit of the test. Interferon activity at various times was plotted, and the area under the curves, representing total serum interferon activity, was determined with a planimeter for each monkey. Two-way analysis of variance was used for intergroup comparisons of the area.

RESULTS

Interferon activities over the 10-day experimental period are shown in Fig. 1 for cynomolgus monkeys and in Fig. 2 for rhesus monkeys. Serum interferon activity was not detected in samples collected prior to the first injection of poly(ICLC) or in samples from control monkeys. Interferon activity was detected in rhesus monkeys 2 h after the first injection of poly(ICLC). To minimize blood loss in the smaller animals, cynomolgus monkeys were not bled at 2 h. Twenty of the 24 monkeys had serum interferon activity ranging from 25 to 800 interferon units/ml 8 h after the first injection of poly(ICLC). Interferon activity 24 h after the first injection of poly(ICLC) remained above base line in 19 of the 20 monkeys that responded to the first injection. Maximum interferon activity was found in 23 of 24 monkeys 8 h after the second injection of poly(ICLC), with individual monkeys having interferon activity up to 16,000 interferon units/ml.

The area under the interferon curves, representing total interferon activity (Fig. 3 and 4) for the cynomolgus and rhesus monkeys, re-

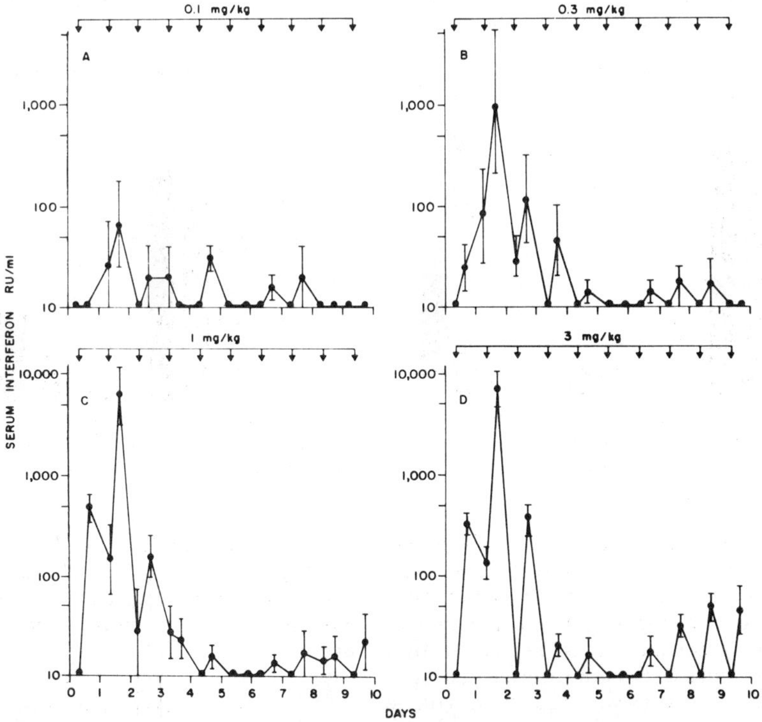

FIG. 1. *Serum interferon response of cynomolgus monkeys to multiple intravenous injections of poly(ICLC) in varying amounts. Monkeys were injected daily (arrows), and serum interferon activity was determined at times indicated by (●). Standard errors of the means are shown.*

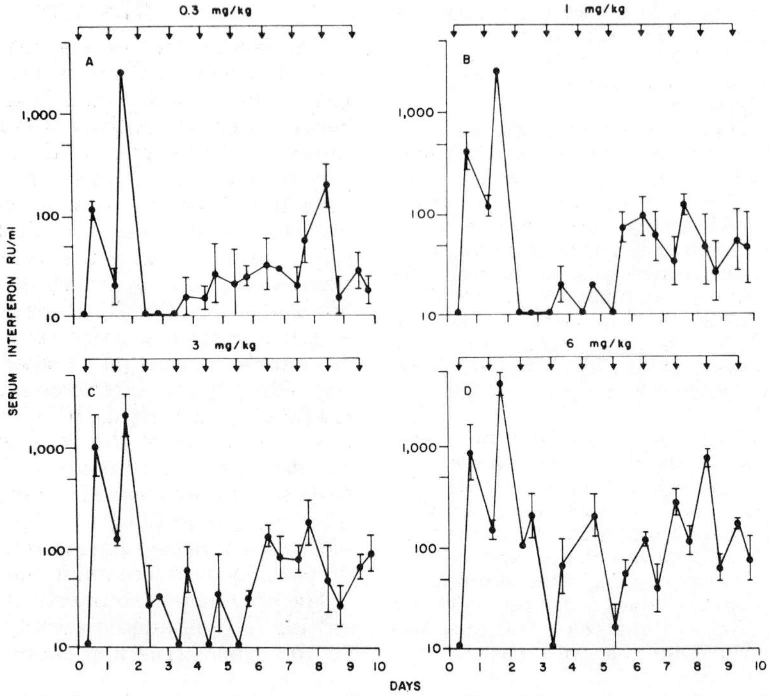

FIG. 2. *Serum interferon response of rhesus monkeys to multiple intravenous injections of poly(ICLC) in varying amounts. Monkeys were injected daily (arrows), and serum interferon activity was determined at times indicated by (●). Standard errors of the means are shown.*

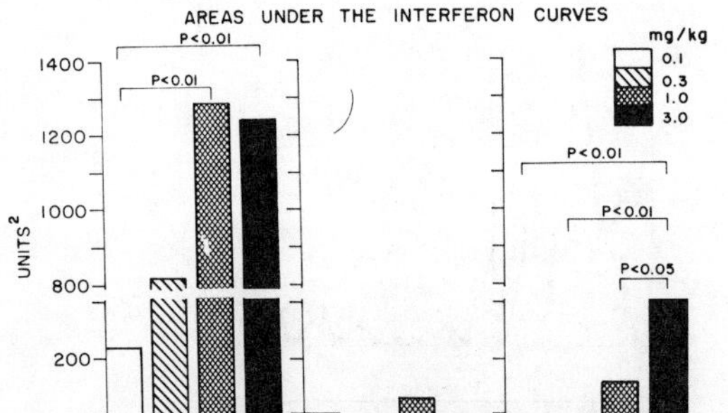

FIG. 3. *Relative total interferon activity of cynomolgus monkeys divided according to similar interferon responses.*

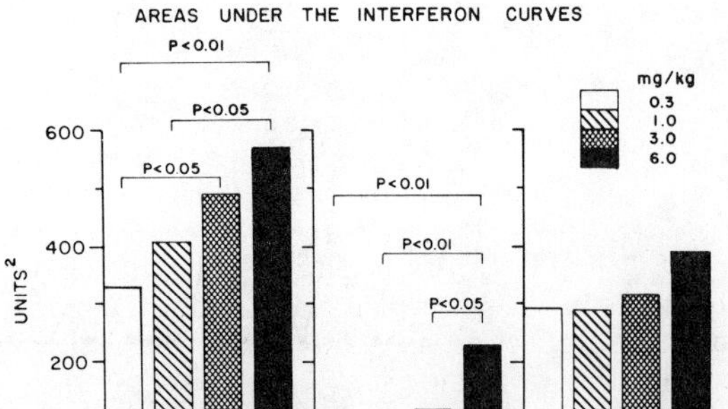

FIG. 4. *Relative total interferon activity of rhesus monkeys divided according to similar interferon responses.*

spectively, showed dose-related increase of interferon response during the first 3 days. Significantly lower interferon activity was noted throughout the remainder of the experiment. This period was considered to represent the hyporesponsive period. Serum interferon activity in the rhesus monkeys was higher from days 7 to 10 than on days 4 to 6. The recovery phase was not as evident in cynomolgus monkeys. The 0.1-mg/kg dose of poly(ICLC) was not an effective interferon inducer in cynomolgus monkeys. The rhesus monkeys injected with 6 mg of poly(ICLC) per kg were anorectic and had a fever after each injection, but no severe clinical signs were observed and deaths did not occur.

DISCUSSION

We found that poly(ICLC) effectively induced serum interferon activity in cynomolgus and rhesus monkeys. Further, the first injection of poly(ICLC) primed the monkey for a potentiated response to the second injection of poly(ICLC). A similar potentiation has been demonstrated in vitro using mouse L cells with moderate concentrations of interferon (12).

The hyporesponsiveness in interferon activity after the third injection of poly(ICLC) is consistent with similar observations in rodents and cattle (2–5, 13, 14) and may be a limiting factor in the potential clinical usefulness of poly(ICLC) as an antiviral compound. However, serum interferon may not be a complete measure of the degree of resistance to virus in animals. The monkeys given 3.0 or 6.0 mg of poly(ICLC) per kg had more interferon activity than the other groups during the hyporesponsive period. One possible explanation for the difference in dose response during the hyporesponsive phase and subsequent increase of interferon activity in the rhesus monkeys is that some population of new cells normally being produced each day in the monkey could be induced to produce interferon by the higher doses of poly(ICLC). Other possible interferon control mechanisms include circulating, refractory repressor products, which, if depleted by repeated injections of interferon inducers, could also result in interferon activity in the higher-dosage groups and in the recovery phase reported in rhesus monkeys (14).

Homan et al. (9) reported that poly (I)·poly(C) was toxic and lethal at 5 mg/kg after four doses in rhesus monkeys. Poly(ICLC) was not lethal when 6.0 mg/kg was given daily for 10 days to these macaques. Our studies indicate that poly(ICLC) is safe for use in monkeys as an interferon inducer. This is supported by the observation that poly(ICLC) induces interferon in rhesus monkeys and chimpanzees and is an effective antiviral compound against simian hemorrhagic fever (11) and yellow fever virus infections in rhesus monkeys.

In view of changing interferon responses after sequential injections of poly(ICLC), the time of initial antiviral therapy and frequency and length of treatment in relation to infection with interferon-sensitive viruses are important potential factors to consider when using poly(ICLC). As might have been predicted from experiments in rodents, the hyporesponsive period cannot be avoided by increasing the dosage of inducer. Higher dosages (3.0 or 6.0 mg/kg) do, however, induce the release of significant amounts of serum interferon during the hyporesponsive period in monkeys. Since the anorexia and fever are more pronounced with higher dosages of poly(ICLC) and 0.3 mg of the complex per kg stimulated the release of significant amounts of serum interferon, a regimen of therapy consisting of two injections at 0.3 mg/kg followed by three injections at 3.0 or 6.0 mg/kg might be expected to induce maximum interferon responses and concomitant antiviral activity.

LITERATURE CITED

1. **Armstrong, J. A.** 1971. Semi-micro, dye-binding assay for rabbit interferon. Appl. Microbiol. **21**:723–725.
2. **Borden, E. C., and F. A. Murphy.** 1971. The interferon refractory state: *in vivo* and *in vitro* studies of its mechanism. J. Immunol. **106**:134–142.
3. **Borden, E. C., E. V. Prochownik, and W. A. Carter.** 1975. The interferon refractory state. II. Biological characterization of a refractoriness-inducing protein. J. Immunol. **114**:752–756.
4. **Buckler, C. E., H. G. DuBuy, M. L. Johnson, and S. Baron.** 1971. Kinetics of serum interferon response in mice after single and multiple injections of polyI·polyC. Proc. Soc. Exp. Biol. Med. **136**:394–398.
5. **DuBuy, H. G., M. L. Johnson, C. E. Buckler, and S. Baron.** 1970. Relationship between dose size and dose interval of polyinosinic-polycytidylic acid and interferon responsiveness in mice. Proc. Soc. Exp. Biol. Med. **135**:340–344.
6. **Field, A. K., A. A. Tytell, G. P. Lampson, and M. R. Hilleman.** 1967. Inducers of interferon and host resistance. II. Multistranded synthetic polynucleotide complexes. Proc. Natl. Acad. Sci. U.S.A. **58**:1004–1010.
7. **Hill, D. A., S. Baron, J. C. Perkins, M. Worthington, J. E. Van Kirk, J. Mills, A. Z. Kapikian, and R. M. Chanock.** 1972. Evaluation of an interferon inducer in viral respiratory disease. J. Am. Med. Assoc. **219**:1179–1184.
8. **Ho, M., Y. Kono, and M. K. Breinig.** 1965. Tolerance to the induction of interferons by endotoxin and virus: role of a humoral factor. Proc. Soc. Exp. Biol. Med. **119**:1227–1232.
9. **Homan, E. R., R. P. Zendzian, L. D. Schott, H. B. Levy, and R. A. Adamson.** 1972. Studies on poly I·C toxicity in experimental animals. Toxicol. Appl. Pharmacol. **23**:579–588.
10. **Nordlund, J. J., S. M. Wolff, and H. B. Levy.** 1970. Inhibition of biologic activity of poly I:poly C by human plasma. Proc. Soc. Exp. Biol. Med. **133**:439–444.
11. **Levy, H. B., G. Baer, S. Baron, C. E. Buckler, C. J. Gibbs, M. J. Iadarola, W. T. London, and J. Rice.** 1975. A modified polyriboinosinic-polycytidylic acid complex that induces interferon in primates. J. Infect. Dis. **132**:434–439.
12. **Margolis, S. A., H. Oie, and H. B. Levy.** 1972. The effect of interferon, interferon inducers or interferon induced virus resistance on subsequent interferon production. J. Gen. Virol. **15**:119–128.
13. **Rosenquist, B. D.** 1971. Polyriboinosinic-polyribocytidylic acid-induced interferon in calves. Am. J. Vet. Res. **32**:35–39.
14. **Stringfellow, D. A., and L. A. Glasgow.** 1972. Hyporeactivity of infection: potential limitation to therapeutic use of interferon-inducing agents. Infect. Immun. **6**:743–747.

ANTIMICROBIAL AGENTS AND CHEMOTHERAPY, Jan. 1977, p. 84-87 Vol. 11, No. 1

Printed in U.S.A.

Cefoxitin Activity Against Multiply Antibiotic-Resistant *Klebsiella pneumoniae* In Vitro

ROGER T. JACKSON,* FRANK E. THOMAS, AND ROBERT H. ALFORD

Medical Service, Veterans Administration Hospital, and Department of Medicine Vanderbilt University School of Medicine, Nashville, Tennessee 37203*

Received for publication 16 August 1976

Due to the emergence of cephalothin- and gentamicin-resistant *Klebsiella pneumoniae* at this institution, we investigated the in vitro activity of two new cephalosporin compounds—cefoxitin and cefamandole. Whereas both drugs were active against cephalothin- and gentamicin-susceptible isolates of *Klebsiella*, only cefoxitin exhibited significant activity against cephalothin- and gentamicin-resistant isolates. Seventeen of 20 (85%) of the cephalothin- and gentamicin-resistant isolates were inhibited by ≤12.5 μg of cefoxitin per ml. The minimum bactericidal concentration in broth of representative isolates equaled the agar dilution minimum inhibitory concentration. Kirby-Bauer disk susceptibility testing correlated well with the agar dilution minimum inhibitory concentration. Cephalothin and cefamandole resistance of isolates could be correlated with antibiotic degradation by β-lactamase. Cephalothin and cefamandole evoked only a transient decrease in viable bacterial cell count with rapid inactivation of antibiotics, and full regrowth of the organisms. Cefoxitin, on the other hand, was quite effective in vitro against multiply resistant *Klebsiella*. No β-lactamase degradation of cefoxitin was detected. Growth curves with antibiotics indicated rapid killing of cephalothin- and gentamicin-resistant isolates by cefoxitin.

Emergence of multiply antibiotic-resistant *Klebsiella pneumoniae* has become a serious therapeutic problem at this institution and at others in recent years (10). The ongoing epidemic of *Klebsiella* infections at this hospital with multidrug resistance, including cephalothin and gentamicin, is due to three serotypes: 2, 21, and 22. Because of the broad resistance of these organisms, we investigated the in vitro activity of two new cephalosporin compounds against these multiply resistant *Klebsiella*.

Cefoxitin, a cephamycin derivative structurally related to the cephalosporins, is active against *Klebsiella* and is resistant to β-lactamase degradation (8). Cefamandole, a new cephalosporin, is reported to show greater activity in vitro against *Klebsiella* than currently available cephalosporins (3). These new antibiotics were compared to cephalothin in vitro to assess their relative effectiveness against cephalothin- and gentamicin-susceptible and -resistant clinical isolates of *Klebsiella*.

MATERIALS AND METHODS

Bacterial isolates. Twenty consecutive *Klebsiella* isolates resistant to both cephalothin and gentamicin by the Bauer-Kirby method (1) and 10 consecutive isolates of *Klebsiella* susceptible to both cephalothin and gentamicin by the same method were collected from clinical laboratory specimens from the Nashville Veterans' Administration Hospital in March 1976. Most of the isolates were recovered from urine, but also from sputum, wound, and blood cultures.

Antibiotics. Cefoxitin was supplied as the sodium salt by Merck Sharp & Dohme Research Laboratories (Rahway, N.J.). Cefamandole was supplied as the lithium salt by Eli Lilly & Co. (Indianapolis, Ind.). The commercial preparation of cephalothin (Keflin, Lilly) was employed.

Disk susceptibility testing. Disks containing 30 μg of cefoxitin, cefamondole, or cephalothin were supplied by the manufacturers. Susceptibility testing was performed by the standard Bauer-Kirby method.

Agar dilution minimum inhibitory concentrations (MICs). Test organisms were allowed to grow overnight at 37°C in Mueller-Hinton broth to final concentrations of approximately 10^9 bacteria per ml. Antibiotics were added to Mueller-Hinton agar by serial twofold dilutions, achieving concentrations from 100 to 1.56 μg/ml. By using a calibrated loop to deliver 0.001 ml, the bacterial inoculum was streaked on the agar surface. After 18 h of incubation at 37°C, plates were examined for growth. The presence of less than five colonies was recorded as indicating growth inhibition >99.9% of the bacterial inoculum.

MBC in broth. Antibiotic concentrations from

100 to 1.56 μg/ml by serial twofold dilutions were prepared in Mueller-Hinton broth. After overnight growth, broth cultures were diluted 10^{-4} in broth, and 0.5 ml was added to each antibiotic dilution. The least concentration of antibiotic resulting in no visible growth after 18 h at 37°C was recorded as representing the tube dilution MIC. The minimum bactericidal concentration (MBC) was determined by subculturing 0.01 ml on antibiotic-free blood agar plates, and the least antibiotic concentration without visible growth after 18 h at 37°C was recorded as the MBC.

β-Lactamase assay. The Rosen (9) acidometric technique for assaying β-lactamase was used with cephalothin, cefamandole, or cefoxitin as a substrate. A 20-mg amount of each antibiotic was added to 10 ml of of distilled water containing 2 ml of 0.5% phenol red indicator. The pH was adjusted to 8.5 with 1 N NaOH added dropwise. *Klebsiella* isolates freshly grown on Mueller-Hinton agar were pressed into the tip of capillary tubes containing the antibiotic-indicator solution to form a plug. The capillary tubes were incubated vertically for 1 h at room temperature, and a change from violet to yellow color was interpreted as indicating a positive result. A group A *Streptococcus pyogenes* isolate and a noninoculated antibiotic indicator solution served as negative controls.

The microbiological method of Kjellander and Myrback as modified by Findell and Sherris (4), in which a β-lactamase-producing organism allows growth of a susceptible indicator organism around an antibiotic disk in a "cloverleaf" pattern, was employed. A swab of an 18-h broth culture of *Sarcina lutea* ATCC 9341 was used to inoculate a Mueller-Hinton agar plate. The *Klebsiella* isolates to be tested for β-lactamase were swabbed in the shape of a cross across the plate from an overnight broth culture. A 30-μg of disk of cephalothin, cefamandole, or cefoxitin was placed in the center of the cross and then incubated overnight at 37° and then at 22°C for another 24 h to allow full growth and yellow color of *S. lutea*. Patterns of *Sarcina* growth were read at 24 and 48 h and tracings were made. The cloverleaf pattern of growth of the susceptible indicator organism next to the *Klebsiella* indicated β-lactamase degradation of the antibiotic diffusing from the disk, whereas a circular zone of inhibition indicated absence of β-lactamase degradation.

Growth curves and antibiotic inactivation. Bacterial growth in the presence of cephalothin, cefamandole, or cefoxitin was determined for representative isolates of each of the three serotypes of cephalothin- and gentamicin-resistant *Klebsiella*. A total of 20 μg of each antibiotic per ml was added to a 10^{-4} broth dilution of an overnight growth of bacteria, and portions were sampled at 3, 6, 12, and 24 h for quantitative viable cell counts by the pour plate technique with appropriate dilutions.

Portions of each sample were membrane filtered (Millipore Corp., Bedford, Mass.; 0.45-μm pore size) and frozen at −70°C until the antibiotic assay. Before the assay, samples and antibiotic standards were heated at 56°C for 30 min to inactivate β-lactamase. A comparison of heated and nonheated samples indicated insignificant degradation (<10%) of any antibiotic. Assay of antibiotics was by the well diffusion method in brain heart infusion agar, with *Staphylococcus aureus* MB2786d (provided by C. Martin, Merck Sharp & Dohme) as the indicator organism.

Gentamicin resistance. For the purpose of this study, resistance to gentamicin was detected by confluent growth to 10-μg gentamicin disks by Bauer-Kirby testing. This was confirmed by growth from 10^4 to 10^8 organisms per ml in Mueller-Hinton broth containing 10 μg of gentamicin per ml, with viability subsequently confirmed by growth on antibiotic-free Mueller-Hinton agar. All isolates had gentamicin MICs >6.25 μg/ml, with the mean MIC to gentamicin of 18.7 μg/ml.

RESULTS

Cefamandole and cefoxitin inhibited the cephalothin- and gentamicin-susceptible isolates as shown in Fig. 1. All strains were inhibited in the agar dilution studies by ≤12.5 μg of each of the three cephalosporin compounds per ml. In Bauer-Kirby susceptibility testing, the zone of inhibition was >18 mm for all isolates with either cephalothin, cefamandole, or cefoxitin disks.

However, cefoxitin was the only antibiotic with significant activity against cephalothin- and gentamicin-resistant isolates (Fig. 2). The agar dilution MIC was ≤50 μg of cefoxitin per ml for all isolates, and 17 of 20 (85%) isolates were inhibited by ≤12.5 μg of cefoxitin per ml. In Bauer-Kirby susceptibility testing, cefoxitin produced zones of inhibition of ≥18 mm against 18 isolates (90%), with an agar dilution MIC ≤25 μg/ml. In contrast, cefamandole and cephalothin inhibited only two isolates (10%) at ≤50 μg/ml, and the other isolates were not inhibited by 100 μg of either drug per ml. In Bauer-Kirby

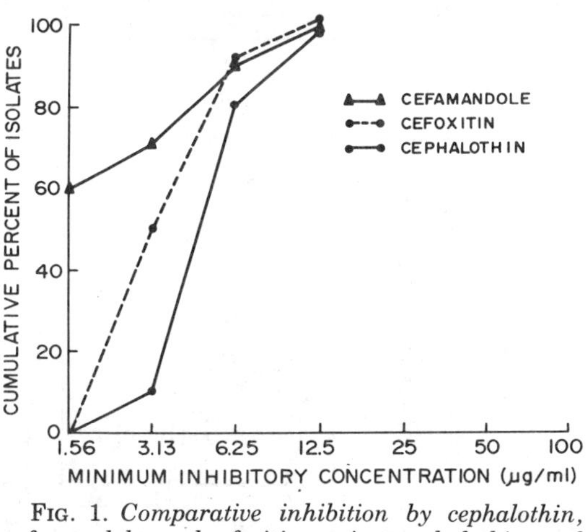

FIG. 1. *Comparative inhibition by cephalothin, cefamandole, and cefoxitin against cephalothin- and gentamicin-susceptible isolates of Klebsiella.*

testing neither cefamandole nor cephalothin produced zones of inhibition greater than 15 mm against any isolate.

Tube dilution MICs and MBCs were determined with cefoxitin for 10 of the isolates including all isolates having agar dilution MICs of >12.5 μg/ml. The tube dilution MIC was one dilution less than the agar dilution MIC in 4 of 10 isolates. In all isolates the MBC equaled the agar dilution MIC.

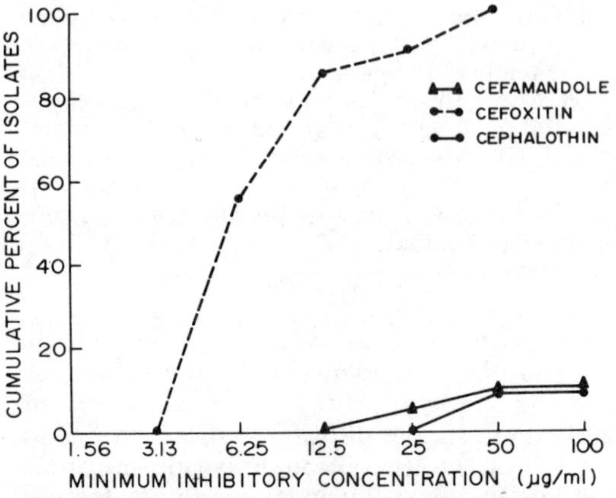

FIG. 2. *Comparative activity of cephalothin, cefamandole, and cefoxitin against cephalothin- and gentamicin-resistant isolates of Klebsiella.*

β-Lactamase assay. By the acidometric assay, none of 10 cephalothin-susceptible isolates or controls gave positive reactions for antibiotic degradation by β-lactamase. In contrast, all 20 cephalothin-resistant isolates gave positive reactions with cephalothin and cefamandole, but not with cefoxitin.

The microbiological assay demonstrated striking cloverleaf patterns with all 20 cephalothin-resistant isolates to cephalothin and cefamandole, but not cefoxitin. Eight of ten cephalothin-susceptible isolates also produced cloverleaf patterns (always to a less pronounced degree than the cephalothin-resistant isolates) with cephalothin and cefamandole. Again, zones around the cefoxitin disks were circular, indicating absence of β-lactamase degradation.

Growth curves and antibiotic inactivation. Cephalothin and cefamandole inhibited bacterial growth only transiently, with the antibiotic rapidly inactivated in the culture (Fig. 3). In

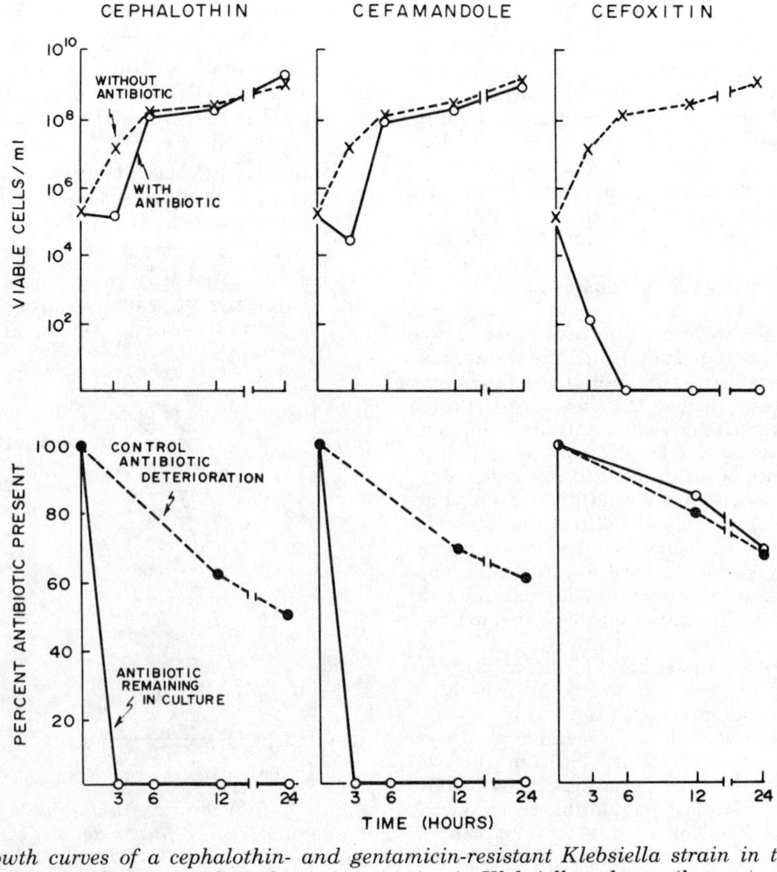

FIG. 3. *Growth curves of a cephalothin- and gentamicin-resistant Klebsiella strain in the presence of caphalosporin compounds (top), and antibiotic inactivation in Klebsiella cultures (bottom).*

contrast, cefoxitin caused a rapid decline in viable cell count with no significant antibiotic inactivation compared with control antibiotic deterioration in broth.

DISCUSSION

Cefoxitin is demonstrably effective in vitro when tested against our cephalothin- and gentamicin-resistant *Klebsiella*. Cefamandole appers to be ineffective in vitro against those same multiply resistant strains. Cefoxitin has previously been reported to be effective in vitro against cephalothin-resistant *Klebsiella* (7). Cefamandole has been reported to show promising in vitro activity against cephalothin-susceptible *Klebsiella,* but is only minimally effective against cephalothin-resistant isolates (7).

The indifference of cefoxitin to β-lactamase degradation appears to be the major factor contributing to the drug's efficacy against our multiply resistant *Klebsiella*. Cefamandole and cephalothin were readily degraded by the β-lactamase of our resistant isolates. In contrast, β-lactamase activity failed to significantly degrade cefoxitin according to the acidometric assay or during growth curves with the antibiotic. No β-lactamase degradation of cefoxitin occurred with the microbiological cloverleaf procedure to Findell and Sherris (4), which offers good conditions for enzyme induction due to exposure of organisms to graduations of the diffusing antibiotic.

Resistance to cefoxitin by *Klebsiella* is readily induced in vitro by exposure to subinhibitory concentrations in an incremental fashion. However, the resistance appears to be intrinsic in nature and not due to inactivation by β-lactamase (6).

Cefoxitin achieves serum and urine levels comparable to those of cephalothin, and toxicity appears minimal (5). If clinical trials in progress here confirm the efficacy of cefoxitin against our multiply antibiotic-resistant *Klebsiella,* cefoxitin will be a welcome new antibiotic for therapy of these troublesome infections.

LITERATURE CITED

1. **Bauer, W. W., W. M. M. Kirby, J. C. Sherris, and M. Turck.** 1966. Antibiotic susceptibility testing by a standardized single disc method. Am. J. Clin. Pathol. 45:493–496.
2. **Bodey, G. P., and S. Weaver.** 1976. In vitro studies of cefamandole. Antimicrob. Agents Chemother. 9:452–457.
3. **Eykyn, S., C. Jenkins, A. King, and I. Phillips.** 1973. Antibacterial activity of cefamandole, a new cephalosporin antibiotic, compared with that of cephloridine, cephalothin, and cephalexin. Antimicrob. Agents Chemother. 3:657–661.
4. **Findell, C. M., and J. C. Sherris.** 1976. Susceptibility of *Enterobacter* to cefamandole: evidence for a high mutation rate to resistance. Antimicrob. Agents Chemother. 9:970–974.
5. **Goodwin, C. S., E. B. Raftery, A. D. Goldberg, H. Skeggs, A. E. Till, and C. M. Martin.** 1974. Effects of rate of infusion and probenecid on serum levels, renal excretion, and tolerance of intravenous doses of cefoxitin in humans: comparison with cephalothin. Antimicrob. Agents Chemother. 6:338–346.
6. **Hoeprich, P. D., and A. C. Huston.** 1976. Induction of resistance in *Staphylococcus aureus* and *Klebsiella pneumoniae* by exposure to cephalothin and cefoxitin. J. Infect. Dis. 133:681–685.
7. **Lewis, R. P., R. D. Meyer, and L. L. Kraus.** 1976. Antibacterial activity of selected beta-lactam and aminoglycoside antibiotics against cephalothin-resistant *Enterobacteriaceae*. Antimicrob. Agents Chemother. 9:780–786.
8. **Onishi, H. R., D. R. Daoust, S. B. Zimmerman, D. Hendlin, and E. O. Stapley.** 1974. Cefoxitin, a semisynthetic cephamycin antibiotic: resistance to beta-lactamase inactivation. Antimicrob. Agents Chemother. 5:38–48.
9. **Rosen, I. G., J. Jacobson, and R. Rudderman.** 1972. Rapid capillary tube method for detecting penicillin resistance in *Staphylococcus aureus*. Appl. Microbiol. 23:649–650.
10. **Schaberg, D. R., R. A. Weinstein, and W. E. Stamm.** 1976. Epidemics of nosocomial urinary tract infection caused by multiply resistant gram-negative bacilli: epidemiology and control. J. Infect. Dis. 133:363–366.

Antimicrobial Agents and Chemotherapy, Jan. 1977, p. 88–91
Vol. 11, No. 1

Comparative In Vitro Activity of Nafcillin, Oxacillin, and Methicillin in Combination with Gentamicin and Tobramycin Against Enterococci

CHATRCHAI WATANAKUNAKORN* and CHERYL GLOTZBECKER

Department of Internal Medicine, University of Cincinnati College of Medicine, Cincinnati, Ohio 45267

Received for publication 7 July 1976

The in vitro activity of nafcillin, oxacillin, and methicillin alone and in combination with gentamicin and tobramycin against 30 strains of enterococci was investigated. The penicillinase-resistant penicillins were less active than penicillin and ampicillin against the enterococci. Nafcillin was more active than oxacillin and methicillin. Sixty-six percent of strains were inhibited by nafcillin at 6.25 μg/ml, but none was inhibited by oxacillin and methicillin at the same concentration. At 12.5 μg/ml, 83, 16, and 0% were inhibited by nafcillin, oxacillin, and methicillin, respectively. By using a variety of criteria and analyses, it was shown that none of the antibiotic combinations studied demonstrated enhanced killing of all strains of enterococci. Nafcillin-gentamicin was the best combination, and enhanced killing was demonstrated against most strains. Oxacillin was more effective than methicillin when combined with gentamicin. Tobramycin was probably less effective than gentamicin in combination with the penicillinase-resistant penicillins against enterococci.

The combination of a penicillinase-resistant penicillin and gentamicin is often used in the empirical antimicrobial therapy of suspected sepsis because of its spectrum against *Staphylococcus aureus, Pseudomonas aeruginosa,* and other gram-negative bacilli. However, neither the penicillinase-resistant penicillins nor the aminoglycosides alone were very effective against enterococci. The adequacy of such a combination in clinical situations where enterococcal infection is a possibility is not certain. It is especially important in a heroin addict who may have endocarditis caused by *S. aureus, P. aeruginosa,* or an enterococcus (1, 10). Although good universal synergism of the combination of penicillin and gentamicin against enterococci has been demonstrated (8, 9, 11, 15, 17), there have been only limited data regarding the synergistic activity of nafcillin, oxacillin, or methicillin in combination with gentamicin against enterococci. Furthermore, conflicting results were obtained (3, 7). Tobramycin, a recently released aminoglycoside with an in vitro antimicrobial spectrum and clinical pharmacology similar to that of gentamicin, is now used instead of gentamicin by some clinicians. There have been no data regarding the effects of the combination of tobramycin with nafcillin, oxacillin, or methicillin against enterococci.

This study was undertaken to determine the bactericidal effects of the three penicillinase-resistant penicillins against enterococci alone and in combination with gentamicin or tobramycin.

MATERIALS AND METHODS

Enterococci. Thirty strains of enterococci were studied, 21 of which were isolated from blood cultures of patients with endocarditis. All strains were gram-positive cocci in chains, grew as nonhemolytic or alpha-hemolytic colonies on sheep blood agar, gave a positive reaction on bile-esculin agar, and grew in 6.5% NaCl brain heart infusion broth.

Antibiotic susceptibility test. The minimal inhibitory concentrations (MICs) of penicillin G, ampicillin, nafcillin, oxacillin, methicillin, gentamicin, and tobramycin were determined by the ICS agar dilution method (2). Mueller-Hinton agar was used. The inoculum was 0.002 ml of a 10^{-2} dilution of an overnight culture (approximately 10^3 to 10^4 organisms) delivered by a Steers replicator (13).

Test for synergism. The time-kill curve method was utilized. The enterococci were grown overnight and diluted with Mueller-Hinton broth to give between 10^6 and 10^7 colony-forming units (CFU) per ml and incubated with different antibiotics in a water bath at 37°C. The final concentrations of antibiotics were as follows: (i) nafcillin, 20 μg/ml; oxacillin, 20 μg/ml; methicillin, 20 μg/ml; (ii) gentamicin, 4 μg/ml; tobramycin, 4 μg/ml; and (iii) combinations of each antibiotic in (i) with each antibiotic in (ii). A culture with no antibiotic was set up as a control. At 6, 24, and 48 h of incubation, viable CFU were enumerated by subculturing on Mueller-Hinton agar.

RESULTS

The MICs of the five penicillins and two aminoglycosides for the 30 strains of enterococci are listed in Table 1. The penicillinase-resistant penicillins were much less active than penicillin and ampicillin against enterococci. Nafcillin was more active than oxacillin and methicillin. As expected, all enterococci were resistant to gentamicin and tobramycin. Tobramycin was much less active than gentamicin.

Figure 1 shows the effects of nafcillin, oxacillin, methicillin, gentamicin, and tobramycin alone in killing enterococci. Among the penicillinase-resistant penicillins tested, nafcillin was the best in comparison with oxacillin and methicillin. In general, gentamicin and tobramycin had negligible effects in killing enterococci; some killing did occur with a few strains.

The effects of the antibiotic combinations in comparison with single antibiotics against the 30 strains of enterococci are shown in Table 2. The data were analyzed according to the magnitude of increase in the killing of enterococci (≥10-fold, ≥100-fold, and ≥1,000-fold) as compared with the most effective antibiotic alone at different time intervals (6, 24, and 48 h). In general, the enhancement of killing became more obvious as the period of incubation increased. No antibiotic combination tested demonstrated enhanced killing of all strains of enterococci tested. There were more strains showing enhanced killing by the combination of oxacillin and gentamicin than by the nafcillin-gen-

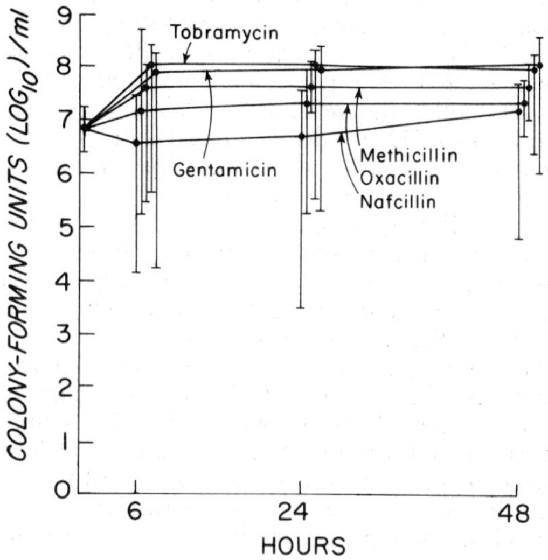

FIG. 1. *Effect of nafcillin (20 μg/ml), oxacillin (20 μg/ml), methicillin (20 μg/ml), gentamicin (4 μg/ml) and tobramycin (4 μg/ml) in killing enterococci. Range (I) and mean (●——●) viable CFU per milliliter for 30 strains are shown.*

TABLE 1. *Antimicrobial susceptibility of 30 strains of enterococci*

Antibiotic	No. of strains with MIC (μg/ml) at:									
	0.78	1.56	3.12	6.25	12.5	25	50	100	200	>200
Ampicillin	15	10	4	1						
Penicillin	1	15	11	3						
Nafcillin			2	18	5	1	2		2	
Oxacillin					5	17	4	2	1	1
Methicillin						7	11	2	8	2
Gentamicin						1	17	12		
Tobramycin						2	9	9	2	8

TABLE 2. *Effect of antibiotic combinations in comparison with that of single antibiotics against 30 strains of enterococci*

Antibiotic combination	Magnitude of increase in killing of enterococci[a]								
	≥10-fold			≥100-fold			≥1,000-fold		
	6 h	24 h	48 h	6 h	24 h	48 h	6 h	24 h	48 h
Nafcillin + gentamicin	8[b]	16	27	1	7	25	0	4	21
Nafcillin + tobramycin	4	6	20	0	1	19	0	1	15
Oxacillin + gentamicin	22	26	24	4	18	20	0	5	8
Oxacillin + tobramycin	14	20	19	1	12	17	0	4	8
Methicillin + gentamicin	8	17	16	0	7	7	0	2	2
Methicillin + tobramycin	5	10	13	1	5	5	0	2	1

[a] As compared with the most effective antibiotic alone at the designated time intervals.
[b] Number of strains.

tamicin and methicillin-gentamicin combinations. However, in the case of the nafcillin-gentamicin combination, the apparent less enhancement of killing by the combination was due partly to the much greater effectiveness of nafcillin than oxacillin alone in killing enterococci (Fig. 1), resulting in less difference in viable CFU when gentamicin was added. It is worth noting that at 48 h a ≥1,000-fold decrease in viable CFU was demonstrated in the largest number of strains when nafcillin-gentamicin and nafcillin-tobramycin were tested.

For all strains tested, none of the culture systems became sterile at the end of 6, 24, or 48 h. Data were then analyzed according to the number of viable CFU at 6, 24, and 48 h. Table 3 shows the number of strains with $<9 \times 10^3$ viable CFU per ml in different antibiotic combinations. If a stricter criterion is used, namely the number of strains with $<9 \times 10^2$ viable CFU per ml, the results are as follows: at 6 h, none; at 24 h, one strain with the nafcillin-gentamicin combination and two strains with the nafcillin-tobramycin combination; at 48 h, eight and ten strains with the nafcillin-gentamicin and nafcillin-tobramycin combinations, respectively, and one strain each with the oxacillin-gentamicin and oxacillin-tobramycin combinations. Thus, nafcillin-gentamicin and nafcillin-tobramycin were the most effective combinations in reducing viable CFU.

Nafcillin was more effective than oxacillin and methicillin in killing enterococci when it was used alone. In combination with gentamicin or tobramycin, nafcillin was also superior to oxacillin and methicillin. Gentamicin was probably more effective than tobramycin when used in combination with methicillin, oxacillin, or methicillin against enterococci.

DISCUSSION

There have been few data regarding the in vitro susceptibility of enterococci to the penicillinase-resistant penicillins, but it is known that the penicillinase-resistant penicillins are less active than penicillin against these organisms (3, 14). In our study, 100% of enterococcal strains tested were inhibited by penicillin and ampicillin at 6.25 μg/ml, whereas only 66% were inhibited by nafcillin and 0% by oxacillin and methicillin at the same concentration. At 12.5 μg/ml, 83, 16, and 0% were inhibited, and at 25 μg/ml, 86, 73, and 23% were inhibited by nafcillin, oxacillin, and methicillin respectively. Our data were comparable with those of two other studies and showed that nafcillin was the most active of the three penicillinase-resistant penicillins against enterococci (3, 4).

It has been shown that penicillin, ampicillin, amoxicillin, carbenicillin, or vancomycin in combination with gentamicin gives enhanced killing of enterococci (4–6, 8, 9, 11, 12, 15–17). However, no uniform results were obtained regarding combinations of a penicillinase-resistant penicillin and gentamicin against enterococci. Glew et al. studied 14 strains of enterococci by the time-kill curve method and reported synergism of the nafcillin-gentamicin combination against 10 of 14 strains, whereas oxacillin-gentamicin and methicillin-gentamicin were synergistic against only three and one strains, respectively (3). By using a different method (checkerboard), Marier et al. reported synergism by the oxacillin-gentamicin combination against 27 of 34 strains of enterococci studied (7). In our studies, by using a variety of criteria and types of analyses similar to those used by Glew et al., it was shown that none of the combinations studied demonstrated enhanced killing of all strains of enterococci. Nafcillin-gentamicin was the best combination; significant enhanced killing was demonstrated against most strains. Oxacillin was more effective than methicillin when combined with gentamicin.

Tobramycin has not been studied extensively against enterococci. One study reported that tobramycin was less active than gentamicin against enterococci, the MIC being >250 μg/ml for about 15% of the strains (9). In this same study it was shown that whereas the penicillin-gentamicin combination was synergistic against all 27 strains of enterococci tested, the penicillin-tobramycin combination was ineffective against 4 strains; all 4 strains were *Streptococcus faecium*. In our study, the MIC of tobramycin for 8 of 30 strains (26%) was >200 μg/ml. It was also shown that tobramycin was probably less effective than gentamicin in combination with the penicillinase-resistant penicillins against enterococci.

TABLE 3. *Effect of antibiotic combinations against 30 strains of enterococci*

Antibiotic combination	No. of strains with viable $<9 \times 10^3$ CFU/ml at:		
	6 h	24 h	48 h
Nafcillin + gentamicin	2	21	25
Nafcillin + tobramycin	3	15	18
Oxacillin + gentamicin	0	6	5
Oxacillin + tobramycin	1	3	5
Methicillin + gentamicin	0	1	2
Methicillin + tobramycin	0	1	0

ACKNOWLEDGMENTS

This investigation was supported by a grant from the Schering Corp., Bloomfield, N.J., and the Morton Hamburger Memorial Fund.

We thank Dexter Balterman for his assistance.

LITERATURE CITED

1. **El-Khatib, M. R., F. M. Wilson, and A. M. Lerner.** 1976. Characteristics of bacterial endocarditis in heroin addicts in Detroit. Am. J. Med. Sci. 271:197-201.
2. **Ericsson, H. M., and J. C. Sherris.** 1971. Antibiotic sensitivity testing: report of an international collaborative study. Acta Pathol. Microbiol. Sect. B 217(Suppl.):1-90.
3. **Glew, R. H., R. C. Moellering, Jr., and C. Wennersten.** 1975. Comparative synergistic activity of nafcillin, oxacillin, and methicillin in combination with gentamicin against enterococci. Antimicrob. Agents Chemother. 7:828-832.
4. **Harwick, H. J., G. M. Kalmanson, and L. B. Guze.** 1973. In vitro activity of ampicillin or vancomycin combined with gentamicin or streptomycin against enterococci. Antimicrob. Agents Chemother. 4:383-387.
5. **Libke, R. D., C. Regamey, J. T. Clarke, and W. M. M. Kirby.** 1973. Synergism of carbenicillin and gentamicin against enterococci. Antimicrob. Agents Chemother. 4:564-568.
6. **McCracken, G. H., Jr., J. D. Nelson, and M. L. Thomas.** 1973. Discrepancy between carbenicillin and ampicillin activities against enterococci and *Listeria*. Antimicrob. Agents Chemother. 3:343-349.
7. **Marier, R. L., N. Joyce, and V. Andriole.** 1975. Synergism of oxacillin and gentamicin against enterococci. Antimicrob. Agents Chemother. 8:571-573.
8. **Moellering, R. C., Jr., C. Wennersten, and A. N. Weinberg.** 1971. Synergy of penicillin and gentamicin against enterococci. J. Infect. Dis. 124:S207-S209.
9. **Moellering, R. C., Jr., C. Wennersten, and A. J. Weinstein.** 1973. Penicillin-tobramycin synergism against enterococci: a comparison with penicillin and gentamicin. Antimicrob. Agents Chemother. 3:526-529.
10. **Reiner, N. E., K. V. Gopolakrishna, and P. I. Lerner.** 1976. Enterococcal endocarditis in heroin addicts. J. Am. Med. Assoc. 235:1861-1863.
11. **Ruhen, R. W., and J. H. Darrell.** 1973. Antibiotic synergism against group D streptococci in the treatment of endocarditis. Med. J. Aust. 2:114-116.
12. **Russell, E. J., and R. Sutherland.** 1973. Activity of amoxycillin against enterococci and synergism with aminoglycoside antibiotics. J. Med. Microbiol. 8:1-10.
13. **Steers, E., E. L. Foltz, and B. S. Graves.** 1959. An inocula replicating apparatus for routine testing of bacterial susceptibility to antibiotics. Antibiot. Chemother. 9:307-311.
14. **Toala, P., A. McDonald, C. Wilcox, and M. Finland.** 1969. Susceptibility of group D streptococcus (enterococcus) to 21 antibiotics in vitro, with special reference to species differences. Am. J. Med. Sci. 258:416-430.
15. **Watanakunakorn, C.** 1971. Penicillin combined with gentamicin or streptomycin: synergism against enterococci. J. Infect. Dis. 124:581-586.
16. **Watanakunakorn, C., and C. Bakie.** 1973. Synergism of vancomycin-gentamicin and vancomycin-streptomycin against enterococci. Antimicrob. Agents Chemother. 4:120-124.
17. **Wilkowske, C. J., R. R. Facklam, J. A. Washington II, and J. E. Geraci.** 1971. Antibiotic synergism: enhanced susceptibility of group D streptococci of certain antibiotic combinations, p. 195-200. Antimicrob. Agents Chemother. 1970.

ANTIMICROBIAL AGENTS AND CHEMOTHERAPY, Jan. 1977, p. 92-97 Vol. 11, No. 1
 Printed in U.S.A.

Evaluation of Various Analogues of Tilorone Hydrochloride Against Venezuelan Equine Encephalitis Virus in Mice

RALPH W. KUEHNE,* WALLACE L. PANNIER, AND EDWARD L. STEPHEN

United States Army Medical Research Institute of Infectious Diseases, Fort Detrick, Frederick, Maryland 21701

Received for publication 25 August 1976

The antiviral activity of tilorone hydrochloride and three of its analogues (11,002, 11,567, and 11,877) was assessed by oral and intraperitoneal (i.p.) administration to Venezuelan equine encephalitis (VEE) virus-infected mice. Significant increases in the percentage of survival ($P < 0.01$) were apparent after oral administration of tilorone and analogue 11,877 at dosages of 250 and 500 mg/kg. Neither tilorone nor 11,877 increased percentage of survival when dosages of 31.25 to 500 mg/kg were given by the i.p. route. Orally administered analogue 11,002 was effective against 100 mouse intracranial median lethal doses ($MICLD_{50}$) of VEE virus at doses at 250 to 1,000 mg/kg; doses of 31.25 to 250 mg/kg given i.p. were effective against 10 $MICLD_{50}$. Oral dosages of 250 to 1,000 mg of analogue 11,567 per kg were active against 100 $MICLD_{50}$ of virus. By the i.p. route, 250 mg of 11,567 per kg protected mice against 1,000 $MICLD_{50}$, and a dose of 125 mg/kg protected against 100 $MICLD_{50}$. Oral treatment of VEE infection with analogue 11,567 24 h after subcutaneous inoculation of VEE virus resulted in no significant increase in the percentage of survivors. All survivors of these studies were susceptible to rechallenge 21 days after the first inoculation of virus.

Numerous substances induce interferon both in vitro and in vivo. Interferon inducers appear to be promising antiviral compounds for protection of humans and animals from viral infections (4, 5, 12). Tilorone hydrochloride, the water-soluble dihydrochloride salt of 2,7-bis[2-(diethylamino)ethoxy]fluorene-9-one, is a low-molecular-weight, broad-spectrum, antiviral agent that presumably acts by inducing endogenous interferon (1, 10). In mice, prophylactic oral administration of tilorone hydrochloride has been shown to be effective against vesicular stomatitis virus (VSV), mengovirus, encephalomyocarditis virus, influenza virus, and herpes simplex virus (8). Intraperitoneal (i.p.) administration of tilorone is protective against the virus designated MM (3), and it is effective against Semliki forest virus when given by the oral, subcutaneous (s.c.), and i.p. routes (9). Consequently, we have studied protection against Venezuelan equine encephalitis (VEE) virus in mice elicited by different prophylactic dosages of tilorone hydrochloride and three of its analogues given by either the oral or i.p. routes. In addition, results are presented of a preliminary therapeutic study with analogue 11,567 given by the oral route.

MATERIALS AND METHODS

Compounds. Tilorone {2,7-bis[2-(diethylamino)-ethoxy]fluorene-9-one dihydrochloride}, analogue 11,002 {2,7-bis[2-(dimethylamino)acetyl]fluorene dihydrochloride}, analogue 11,567 {2,8-bis[2-(dimethylamino)acetyl]-dibenzofuran dihydrochloride}, and analogue 11,877 {2,8-bis[2-(dimethylamino)acetyl]-dibenzothiophene dihydrochloride} were supplied by Merrell-National Laboratories, Cincinnati, Ohio. All compounds were dissolved in pyrogen-free 0.85% NaCl solution prior to use. Dosages ranged from 31.25 to 250 mg/kg by the i.p. route and from 250 to 1,000 mg/kg by the oral route.

Animals. Weanling outbred albino Swiss male mice (CD-1), weighing 14 to 20 g, were obtained from Charles River Mouse Farms, Inc., Wilmington, Mass. The mice were housed 4 to 6 per pan, fed, and given water ad libitum.

Virus. The Trinidad donkey strain of VEE virus was used in these studies (14). The virus was originally isolated in guinea pigs and has been maintained by 13 serial passages in embryonated chicken eggs. This strain of VEE virus produces fatal paralytic disease in mice inoculated s.c. or i.p. Inocula were diluted in modified Hanks balanced salt solution containing 2% fetal calf serum.

Animal techniques. Virus inoculations administered s.c., containing 0, 10, 100 and 1,000 mouse intracranial median lethal doses ($MICLD_{50}$), were administered midventrally. Tilorone and the designated analogues were given by gavage or i.p. on a milligram/kilogram of body weight basis. In the prophylaxis experiments, compounds were given 20 to 24 h prior to inoculation of the virus. Group sizes averaged 10 mice, with a total of 200 to 300 mice receiving each compound by the i.p. route and 80 to 120 receiving the compounds by the oral route. Each study included both infected, untreated mice and uninfected, treated mice as controls. Mice were observed daily for 14 days postchallenge. Increased percentage of survivors 14 days after virus inoculation was the criterion selected for evaluation of antiviral activity. Mean death times were calculated only on animals that died during the 14-day observation period and were thus unaffected by survivors. The experimental design of the oral studies was similar to that used in the i.p. studies, except for the dosages of compounds administered. All survivors were rechallenged at 21 days after first challenge with 1,000 $MICLD_{50}$ of Trinidad VEE virus by the s.c. route.

Statistical analysis of data. Independent comparisons were made for each virus dose by partitioning the overall chi-square for the given virus dose into independent chi-squares with single degrees of freedom (16). For a given comparison among virus dose levels, the proportion surviving a zero dose of drug was compared to the response for the lowest given dose of drug. If no significance was found ($P < 0.01$), the two responses were averaged and compared with the response to the next higher dose. This averaging of responses for comparison to the next higher dose was continued until a significant difference was found in the proportion surviving. Data from replicate experiments for each compound did not differ significantly and were combined. Analysis of variance was used to determine significant differences in mean death time.

RESULTS

The effects of i.p. administration of tilorone hydrochloride or one of its three analogues 24 h prior to s.c. inoculation of mice with Trinidad VEE virus are presented in Table 1. Dosages equal to or greater than 125 mg of tilorone hydrochloride per kg, 250 mg of 11,877 per kg, and 500 mg of 11,002 or 11,567 per kg administered by the i.p. route showed significant ($P <$ 0.01) toxicity to mice and are not included. Dosages lower than 125 mg of tilorone hydrochloride per kg or 250 mg of 11,877 per kg did not significantly increase the percentage of survival when compared with survival of untreated infected mice. Dosages of 31.25 to 250 mg of 11,002 per kg administered prophylactically protected mice against 10 $MICLD_{50}$ of

TABLE 1. *Effect of prophylactic i.p. administration of tilorone hydrochloride, 11,002, 11,567, or 11,877 on the survival of mice inoculated s.c. with VEE virus*

Dose (mg/kg)	% Survival (survivors/total) at 14 days postchallenge			
	0[a]	10	100	1,000
Tilorone				
0	95 (19/20)	20 (4/20)	0 (0/20)	0 (0/20)
31.25	80 (16/20)	40 (8/20)	10 (2/20)	0 (0/20)
62.5	80 (16/20)	45 (9/20)	15 (3/20)	0 (0/20)
11,002				
0	88 (14/16)	13 (2/16)	0 (0/16)	0 (0/16)
31.25	100 (6/6)	100[b] (6/6)	17 (1/6)	0 (0/6)
62.5	83 (5/6)	50[b] (3/6)	33 (2/6)	0 (0/6)
125	94 (15/16)	56[b] (9/16)	38 (6/16)	0 (0/16)
250	100 (16/16)	69[b] (11/16)	19 (3/16)	0 (0/16)
11,567				
0	88 (14/16)	81 (13/16)	0 (0/16)	0 (0/16)
31.25	90 (9/10)	40 (4/10)	10 (1/10)	0 (0/10)
62.5	80 (8/10)	80 (8/10)	10 (2/20)	0 (0/10)
125	100 (16/16)	100 (16/16)	50[b] (8/16)	6 (1/16)
250	94 (15/16)	88 (14/16)	88[b] (14/16)	31[b] (5/16)
11,877				
0	100 (16/16)	38 (6/16)	0 (0/16)	0 (0/16)
31.25	100 (10/10)	60 (6/10)	0 (0/10)	0 (0/10)
62.5	70 (7/10)	30 (3/10)	20 (2/10)	0 (0/10)
125	81 (13/16)	44 (7/16)	25 (4/16)	13 (2/16)

[a] $MICLD_{50}$ of the virus.
[b] $P < 0.01$ compared to untreated, infected mice.

VEE virus but not against 100 or 1,000 $MICLD_{50}$. Significant antiviral activity was found with 125 mg of 11,567 per kg against 100 $MICLD_{50}$ of virus, and a dose of 250 mg/kg was active against 100 and 1,000 $MICLD_{50}$ of virus.

Typical dose-response curves using analogue 11,877 administered by the i.p. route are shown in Fig. 1. Although no significant increase in percentage survival occurred with any of the i.p. dosages of 11,877 (Table 1), a significant ($P < 0.01$) increase in survival time occurred with a dose of 125 mg/kg against a virus dose of 100 $MICLD_{50}$.

The effects of oral administration of the four compounds on the percentage of survival of mice inoculated s.c. with Trinidad VEE virus are given in Table 2. Preliminary trials indicated that all four compounds were less toxic

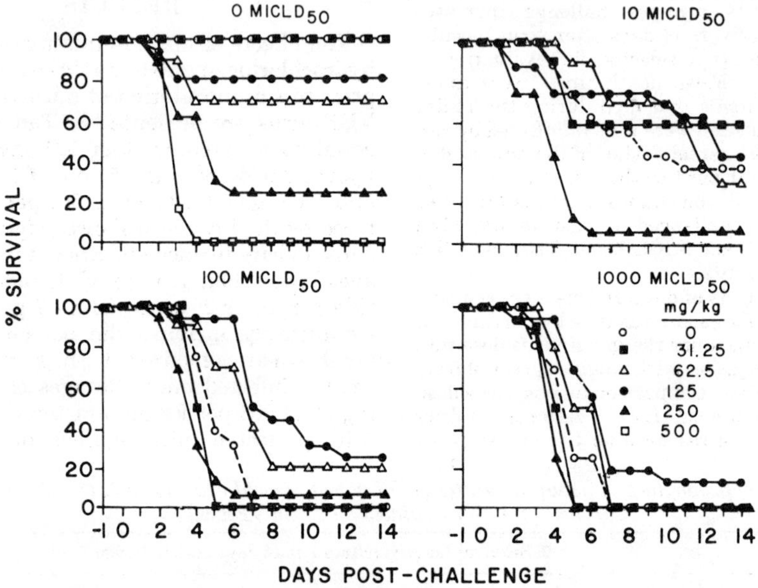

FIG. 1. *Effect of a single i.p. 24-h prophylactic dose of analogue 11,877 on VEE virus infections in mice.*

TABLE 2. *Effect of prophylactic oral administration of tilorone hydrochloride, 11,002, 11,567, or 11,877 on the survival of mice inoculated s.c. with VEE virus*

Dose (mg/kg)	% Survival (survivors/total) at 14 days postchallenge			
	0[a]	10	100	1,000
None	100 (10/10)	20 (2/10)	0 (0/10)	0 (0/10)
Tilorone				
250	90 (9/10)	100[b] (10/10)	70[b] (7/10)	30 (3/10)
500	90 (9/10)	100[b] (10/10)	80[b] (8/10)	23 (2/10)
11,002				
250	100 (10/10)	60[b] (6/10)	50[b] (5/10)	0 (0/10)
500	100 (10/10)	80[b] (8/10)	80[b] (8/10)	30 (3/10)
1,000	100 (10/10)	80[b] (8/10)	90[b] (9/10)	20 (2/10)
11,567				
250	100 (10/10)	80[b] (8/10)	70[b] (7/10)	20 (2/10)
500	100 (10/10)	100[b] (10/10)	60[b] (6/10)	20 (2/10)
1,000	100 (10/10)	100[b] (10/10)	60[b] (6/10)	30 (3/10)
11,877				
250	100 (10/10)	100[b] (10/10)	80[b] (8/10)	10 (1/10)
500	100 (10/10)	100[b] (10/10)	90[b] (9/10)	20 (2/10)
1,000	100 (10/10)	100[b] (10/10)	70[b] (7/10)	50[b] (5/10)

[a] $MICLD_{50}$ of the virus.

[b] $P < 0.01$ compared to untreated, infected mice.

orally than i.p., so higher oral doses could be administered. Only tilorone hydrochloride showed significant toxicity by the oral route at a concentration of 1,000 mg/kg. Lower dosages of tilorone (250 and 500 mg/kg) protected mice against 10 and 100 $MICLD_{50}$ of virus. Oral administration of 250 to 1,000 mg of 11,002, 11,567 or 11,877 per kg protected mice against 10 and 100 $MICLD_{50}$. In addition, 1,000 mg of analogue 11,877 per kg significantly increased the percentage of survival of mice inoculated with 1,000 $MICLD_{50}$ of virus.

Figure 2 depicts typical dose-response curves after oral administration of analogue 11,877 and prior to infection with VEE virus. No significant increases in mean death time were observed in treated mice.

A therapy study was conducted to assess the effect of treatment of VEE virus infection of mice with orally administered analogue 11,567. Groups of mice received 250 or 500 mg of 11,567 per kg 24 h after s.c. inoculation of 0, 10, 100 or 1,000 $MICLD_{50}$ of Trinidad VEE virus. Additional mice were treated with either 250 or 500 mg of 11,567 per kg/day for 3 consecutive days after virus inoculation (Table 3). Neither oral treatment schedule resulted in significant protection against 10, 100 or 1,000 $MICLD_{50}$ of VEE virus. Significant increases in mean death time did not occur as a result of treatment with 11,567 (Fig. 3).

Survivors of all studies were uniformly susceptible to rechallenge with 1,000 $MICLD_{50}$ of Trinidad VEE virus by the s.c. route 21 days after the first administration of virus.

DISCUSSION

Tilorone hydrochloride and three analogues designated 11,002, 11,567 and 11,877 are effective antiviral compounds when given prophy-

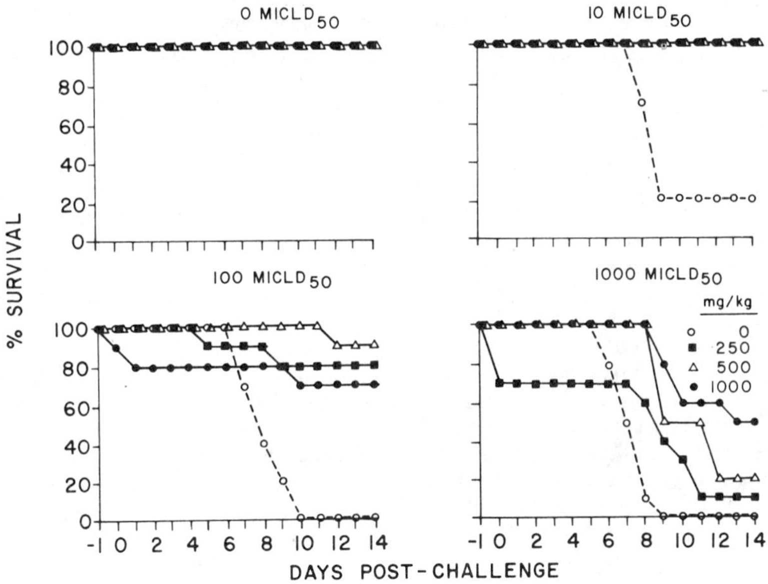

FIG. 2. *Effect of a single oral 24-h prophylactic dose of analogue 11,877 on VEE virus infections in mice.*

TABLE 3. *Effect of therapeutic oral administration of analogue 11,567 on the survival of mice inoculated s.c. with VEE virus*

Dose (mg/kg)	% Survival (survivors/total) at 14 days postchallenge			
	0[a]	10	100	1,000
24 h				
0	100 (10/10)	0 (0/10)	0 (0/10)	0 (0/10)
250	90 (9/10)	10 (1/10)	0 (0/10)	0 (0/10)
500	100 (10/10)	40 (4/10)	0 (0/10)	0 (0/10)
24, 48 and 72 h				
0	100 (10/10)	0 (0/10)	0 (0/10)	0 (0/10)
250	100 (10/10)	30 (3/10)	0 (0/10)	0 (0/10)
500	100 (10/10)	30 (3/10)	0 (0/10)	0 (0/10)

[a] $MICLD_{50}$ of the virus.

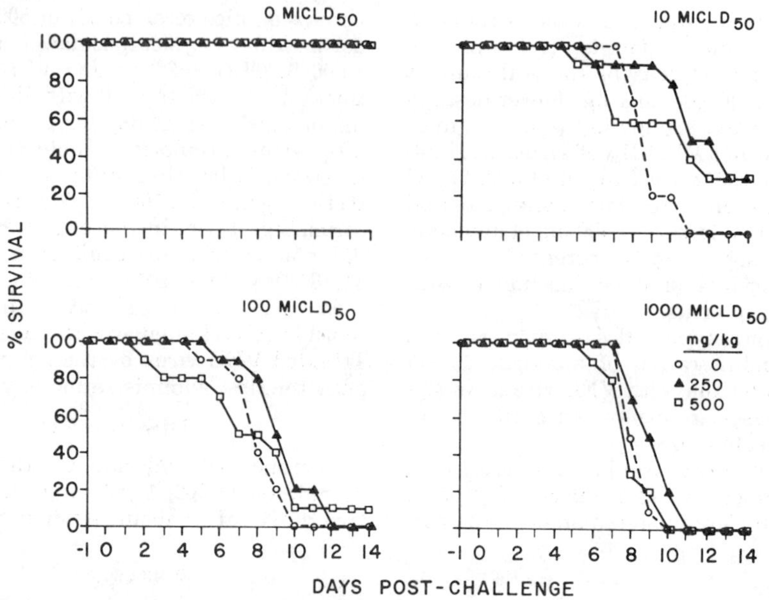

FIG. 3. *Effect of oral treatment of mice with analogue 11,567 at 24, 48, and 72 h post-VEE infection.*

lactically to VEE virus-infected mice. R. W. Krueger and S. Yoshimura (Fed. Proc. 29:635, 1970) reported that a single prophylactic dose of tilorone hydrochloride given 24 h before a lethal s.c. inoculation of Semliki forest virus provided maximal protection. Further, they reported the oral and i.p. mean lethal dose of tilorone to be 959 and 145 mg/kg, respectively. The most uniform increases in the percentage of survivors in the present studies occurred in mice given the compounds orally. When treatment was initiated 24 h after virus inoculation, analogue 11,567 had no significant effect on survival. Consistent with these findings, others have shown that treatment of mice with the optimal oral dose of 250 mg of tilorone hydrochloride per kg 24 to 48 h after a fatal challenge of Semliki forest virus did not significantly change the incidence of mortality (9).

Although the antiviral activity of tilorone hydrochloride has been attributed to induction of interferon (1, 10), exceptions have been reported with several viruses. Giron et al. (3) reported that protection of mice with tilorone hydrochloride against MM virus is apparently not dependent on interferon induction. In their studies, circulating interferon was not detected with i.p. tilorone doses of less than 150 mg/kg. Others have reported that detectable interferon induced by pyran, polyriboinosinic acid · polyribocytidylic acid and bacterial endotoxin does not correlate with the degree of protection obtained by use of these agents against MM virus (13) and mengovirus (11) infections in mice. Giron et al. (3) concluded that determination of circulating interferon concentration is of limited value in assessing antiviral activity, since protection can be demonstrated without the simultaneous detection of interferon. In contrast, others report that protection of mice against intranasal infection with VSV is directly related to the concentrations of interferon induced by different doses of tilorone (1). It appears that MM virus is much more susceptible to the action of tilorone, since lower doses of this compound that do not induce detectable amounts of circulating interferon are effective against MM virus but not against VSV (3).

Virulent Trinidad strain and attenuated TC-83 strain of VEE virus are sensitive to the antiviral activity of interferon (6). Tilorone and structurally related compounds increase serum interferon levels in rodents but not in monkeys or humans (7; H. E. Kaufman and Y. M. Centifanto, J. Clin. Invest. 50:53, 1971). However, antiviral activity has been shown with tilorone hydrochloride against rubella virus in man (G. M. Schiff, C. C. Linnemann, T. Rotte, G. D. Mayer, and S. Trimble, Clin. Res. 21:882, 1973) and with tilorone and its three analogues against the attenuated TC-83 strain of VEE virus in monkeys (G. D. Mayer, A. C. Hagan, and F. Bray, Fed. Proc. 32:704, 1973). The mechanism of this antiviral activity is unclear. Recent in vitro data (W. L. Pannier, unpublished observations) obtained from tilorone-treated, VEE virus-infected Vero cell cultures have shown that 50 μg of tilorone per ml results in 50% virus plaque reduction with no evidence of cytopathic effects in these cell cultures. These data suggest that other mechanisms may be involved, since it is reported that interferon cannot be induced in Vero cells (2, 15). Other possibilities for protection in the absence of detectable interferon are the stimulation of cellular immunity, the production of lymphokines, and insensitivity of the interferon assay techniques employed.

The interaction of challenge doses of virus with administration of potential antiviral compounds and the importance of route of administration of these compounds is emphasized in our studies. In the case of tilorone and analogue 11,877, their effectiveness by the i.p. route is marginal at best but is greatly increased when given orally. The importance of route is also evident when a dosage of 250 mg of analogues 11,002 and 11,567 per kg is compared by the oral and i.p. routes: significant protection against 100 $MICLD_{50}$ of VEE virus is conferred by 250 mg of 11,002 per kg only when given orally, whereas 250 mg of 11,567 per kg is significantly protective against 1,000 $MICLD_{50}$ of VEE virus only when given i.p.

ACKNOWLEDGMENT

We gratefully acknowledge Glen A. Higbee for the statistical analysis of our data.

LITERATURE CITED

1. **De Clercq, E., and T. C. Merigan.** 1971. Bis-DEAE-fluorenone: mechanism of antiviral protection and stimulation of interferon production in the mouse. J. Infect. Dis. 123:190–199.
2. **Desmyter, J., J. L. Melnick, and W. E. Rawls.** 1968. Defectiveness of interferon production and of rubella virus interference in a line of African green monkey kidney cells (Vero). J. Virol. 2:955–961.
3. **Giron, D. J., J. P. Schmidt, and F. F. Pindak.** 1972. Tilorone hydrochloride: lack of correlation between interferon induction and viral protection. Antimicrob. Agents Chemother. 1:78–79.
4. **Hilleman, M. R.** 1970. Prospects for the use of double-stranded ribonucleic acid (poly I:C) inducers in man. J. Infect. Dis. 121:196–211.
5. **Hilleman, M. R.** 1970. Double stranded RNAs (poly I:C) in the prevention of viral infections. Arch. Intern. Med. 126:109–124.
6. **Jordan, G. W.** 1973. Interferon sensitivity of Venezuelan equine encephalomyelitis virus. Infect. Immun. 7:911–917.
7. **Kaufman, H. E., Y. M. Centifanto, E. D. Ellison, and D. C. Brown.** 1971. Tilorone hydrochloride: human toxicity and interferon stimulation. Proc. Soc. Exp. Biol. Med. 137:357–360.
8. **Krueger, R. F., and G. D. Mayer.** 1970. Tilorone hydrochloride: an orally active antiviral agent. Science 169:1213–1214.
9. **Krueger, R. F., G. D. Mayer, S. Yoshimura, and K. A. Ludwig.** 1971. In vivo evaluations of tilorone hydrochloride against Semliki Forest virus, p. 486–490. Antimicrob. Agents Chemother. 1970.
10. **Mayer, G. D., and R. F. Krueger.** 1970. Tilorone hydrochloride: mode of action. Science 169:1214–1215.
11. **Merigan, T. C., E. De Clercq, M. S. Finkelstein, L. Clever, S. Walker, and D. J. Waddell.** 1970. Clinical studies employing interferon inducers in man and animals. Ann. N.Y. Acad. Sci. 173:746–759.
12. **Merigan, T. C., and M. S. Finkelstein.** 1968. Interferon-stimulating and *in vivo* antiviral effects of various synthetic anionic polymers. Virology 35:363–374.
13. **Pindak, F. F., J. P. Schmidt, D. J. Giron, and P. T. Allen.** 1971. Interferon levels and resistance to viral infection associated with selected interferon inducers. Proc. Soc. Exp. Biol. Med. 138:317–321.
14. **Randall, R., and J. W. Mills.** 1944. Fatal encephalitis in man due to the Venezuelan virus of equine encephalomyelitis in Trinidad. Science 99:225–226.
15. **Schafer, T. W., and R. Z. Lockart, Jr.** 1970. Interferon required for viral resistance induced by poly I·poly C. Nature (London) 226:449–450.
16. **Steel, R. G. D., and J. H. Torrie.** 1960. Principles and procedures of statistics. McGraw-Hill Book Co., New York.

ANTIMICROBIAL AGENTS AND CHEMOTHERAPY, Jan. 1977, p. 98-104 Vol. 11, No. 1

Inactivation of Lipid-Containing Viruses by Long-Chain Alcohols

WALLACE SNIPES,* STANLEY PERSON, GREGORY KELLER, WILLIAM TAYLOR, AND ALEC KEITH

Biophysics Laboratory, Department of Biochemistry and Biophysics, The Pennsylvania State University, University Park, Pennsylvania 16802

Received for publication 9 July 1976

This report describes the inactivation of lipid-containing viruses by several long-chain alcohols. A striking peak in antiviral activity was found for saturated alcohols having chain lengths from 10 to 14 carbons. Viruses having different membrane structure showed different susceptibilities to alcohols having different chain lengths and structural features. Decanol, dodecanol, and tetradecanol readily inactivated herpes simplex virus and the enveloped bacterial virus ϕ6. The lipid-containing virus PM2 was susceptible to decanol and dodecanol but comparatively unsusceptible to tetradecanol. The branched-chain alcohol phytol, a naturally occurring component of chlorophyll, was active against ϕ6 and herpes simplex virus but not against PM2. Polyoma virus and the bacteriophage ϕ23-1-a, which do not contain lipids, were not susceptible to inactivation by any of the alcohols tested. Experiments were also carried out to determine the effects of these compounds on cells. At 0.5 mM, decanol lysed human embryonic lung cells, erythrocytes, and the bacterial hosts for ϕ6 and PM2. Dodecanol, tetradecanol, and phytol at this concentration were less damaging to cells. At 0.05 mM, none of the alcohols caused observable cytopathic effects on human embryonic lung cells, although several of the alcohols at this concentration were active against herpes simplex virus. Our findings suggest that dodecanol, tetradecanol, and phytol may warrant further studies as potential antiviral agents, particularly for topical application to virus-infected areas of the skin.

Most antiviral agents being developed for clinical use are designed to interfere with viral nucleic acid metabolism. Many of these are structural analogues to deoxyribonucleic acid and ribonucleic acid precursors, their activity being due to their competitive inhibition of enzymatic reactions (2, 8, 10, 13, 16). There are several properties of this class of compounds that limit their desirability for use as antiviral agents. Some of the more serious ones are: (i) their frequently limited selectivity for inhibiting viral nucleic acid synthesis in comparison to that of the cell; (ii) the development of virus mutants, either spontaneous or induced, that are resistant to the agent; and (iii) the potential mutagenic and teratogenic effects that may occur when dividing cells are exposed to nucleoside analogues, particularly those that become incorporated into nucleic acid polymers. These considerations suggest that additional, alternative approaches to the design of antiviral compounds is a worthy endeavor.

The effective treatment and eventual control of many viral diseases will quite likely rely on the development of drugs that complement each other in their activity, acting at different points in the virus life cycle. In our laboratory we are exploring the possibility that certain viruses, namely, those that are enveloped, can be inactivated by hydrophobic, membrane-perturbing molecules under conditions comparatively harmless to the host cells. This approach was prompted by our discovery that butylated hydroxytoluene (BHT), a commonly used food additive with apparent low toxicity to humans, is nevertheless a potent inactivator of lipid-containing viruses, including herpes simplex virus (HSV) (3, 15, 18). This combination of low toxicity and effectiveness against viruses has generated considerable interest in the potential use of BHT as an antiviral agent, particularly for topical application to virus-infectd areas of the skin. Clinical evaluation of the effectiveness of BHT as an antiviral substance is forthcoming.

The proper design of antiviral agents whose action is due to their perturbation of viral membranes will rely on an understanding of their physical properties and the nature of their interactions with membrane structures. We are currently carrying out experiments to investigate the structural parameters important to the activity of these agents. Compounds that appear to be particularly effective have a hydrophobic component, such as a hydrocarbon chain, to pull the compound into the virus membrane and a polar group to orient the molecule at the membrane-aqueous interface. In the work described in this report, we have investigated the antiviral properties of a series of alcohols varying in chain length from 4 to 18 carbons and the branched-chain alcohol phytol, a naturally occurring component of chlorophyll. A striking peak in activity was observed for alcohols having chain lengths from 10 to 14 carbons, suggesting that a proper balance between the polar and hydrophobic components can lead to maximal perturbation of the viral membrane. For comparative purposes, studies were also carried out to determine the effects of these same compounds on several types of cells, including the host cells in which the virus replicates and erythrocytes. Our findings suggest that some of these compounds, particularly dodecanol, tetradecanol, and phytol, may warrant further studies as potential antiviral agents.

MATERIALS AND METHODS

Viruses and cells. The enveloped bacterial virus ϕ6 was originally isolated by Vidaver et al. (17). The virion contains 25% phospholipid, located in a loose membrane structure similar to that of enveloped animal viruses (17). ϕ6 infects the bacterium *Pseudomonas phaseolicola* strain HB10Y. Our procedures for the routine culture of ϕ6 and HB10Y have been reported (12, 18).

The bacteriophage ϕ23-1-a was obtained from Anne Vidaver. It is insensitive to treatment with organic solvents, such as chloroform and ether, and is presumed to contain no lipid. ϕ23-1-a infects the same host cell as does ϕ6 and is useful in comparative studies for susceptibility to antiviral agents.

The lipid-containing bacterial virus PM2 was isolated by Espejo and Canelo (4). Its structure has been studied extensively by Franklin and co-workers (1, 5, 6). The virion, which contains 13% lipid, has an icosahedral protein coat external to the lipid bilayer (6) and is therefore unlike any known animal viruses. PM2 infects the marine bacterium *Pseudomonas* BAL-31. Procedures for maintaining PM2 and BAL-31 have been described (3, 14).

A syncytia-forming mutant of HSV type 1, designated here HSV-*syn* 20, was used in these experiments. Its isolation and partial characterization have been reported (9). HSV-*syn* 20 was assayed for plaque-forming units on monolayers of human embryonic lung (HEL) cells in plastic petri dishes. The procedures for growth and maintenance of stocks of HSV-*syn* 20 and HEL cells have been published (9).

A wild-type, large-plaque strain of polyoma virus, kindly provided by W. Eckhard was used. The virus was maintained and assayed for plaque-forming units on the mouse embryo cultured cell line 3T3 (A31 clone) obtained from Todaro.

Treatment of virus with alcohols. The longer-chain alcohols having 10 carbons and greater are extremely insoluble in aqueous media. Therefore, the following prcoedure was adopted for treating viruses with these compounds. Stocks of the compounds were prepared in 95% ethanol at 100 times the desired final concentration. A 0.1-ml portion of this stock was added to 5 ml of an appropriate buffered solution, the solution was vortexed, and 30 s later an equal volume of a virus suspension in the same buffered solution was added. After incubation at room temperature for an appropriate time, usually 30 min, the samples were diluted and assayed for plaque-forming units. Minor modifications in volumes, maintaining the same proportions, were used for those viruses available in more limited quantity. None of the viruses are affected by the 1% ethanol present in the culture at the time of treatment. For the longer-chain alcohols at high concentrations, cloudy suspensions formed when the ethanol stocks were added to the aqueous solutions. The concentrations reported, therefore, are those used to form the solution or suspensions and in some cases do not necessarily represent the dissolved concentration of the compound.

Buffer solutions. ϕ6 and ϕ23 were treated in a tris(hydroxymethyl)aminomethane(Tris)-buffered solution containing 6 g of NaCl, 3 g of KCl, 2 g of NH_4Cl, 0.2 g of $MgSO_4 \cdot 7H_2O$, 0.05 g of KH_2PO_4, and 12.1 g of Tris base per liter of distilled water. The pH was adjusted to 7.6 with concentrated HCl. PM2 was treated in a Tris-buffered solution containing 26 g of NaCl, 9.9 g of $MgCl_2 \cdot 6H_2O$, 1.5 g of $CaCl_2 \cdot 2H_2O$, 1.1 g of NH_4Cl, 0.7 g of KCl, 0.025 g of KH_2PO_4, 0.023 g of Na_2SO_4, and 12.1 g of Tris base per liter of distilled water. The pH was adjusted to 7.6 with concentrated HCl. HSV-*syn* 20 was treated in a tricine-buffered solution containing 8 g of NaCl, 0.38 g of KCl, 0.1 g of $MgCl_2 \cdot 6H_2O$, 0.1 g of $CaCl_2 \cdot 2H_2O$, and 4.5 g of tricine per liter of distilled water. The pH was adjusted to 7.3. Polyoma was treated in a phosphate-buffered solution containing 8 g of NaCl, 0.2 g of KCl, 1.15 g of Na_2HPO_4, 0.2 g of KH_2PO_4, 0.133 g of $CaCl_2 \cdot 2H_2O$, and 0.1 g of $MgCl_2 \cdot 6H_2O$ per liter of distilled water. The pH of this solution was 7.2.

RESULTS

Effects of straight-chain alcohols on ϕ6 and ϕ23-1-a. We have found ϕ6 and ϕ23-1-a to be very convenient for initial studies on the antiviral activity of compounds whose mode of action is through membrane perturbations. ϕ6 is especially susceptible to these compounds, and in most cases those agents effective against ϕ6 are also active, usually at higher concentrations, against HSV. ϕ23-1-a, which infects the same host cell as does ϕ6, is generally unsusceptible to compounds that act on membranes and therefore provides a convenient distinction between the classes of compounds in which we are interested and those that may act by some other mechanism.

Extensive data were accumulated on the effects of straight-chain alcohols on ϕ6 at varying concentrations. Striking differences were observed in the effectiveness of alcohols with different chain lengths. Figure 1 shows the percentage of inactivation of $\phi 6$ by alcohols having 8- and 14-carbon chains as a function of concentration of alcohol. The virus was exposed to the compounds for 30 min at room temperature. We have repeatedly observed that the maximum inactivation is reached in less than 15 min, so a 30-min exposure was used for all the experiments reported here. Graphs such as those of Fig. 1 were used to determine, for each alcohol, the concentration required to give 50% inactivation of the virus. The results (Table 1) show that tetradecanol is effective against $\phi 6$ by this assay at lower concentrations than any of the other straight-chain alcohols. Butanol, hexadecanol, and octadecanol gave insignificant inactivation at concentrations up to 1 mM, the highest tested. In comparing the three most active alcohols with data previously reported for BHT (15), it may be noted that dodecanol and tetradecanol are active against $\phi 6$ at lower concentrations than for BHT, whereas about three times more decanol than BHT is required to give 50% inactivation.

$\phi 23$-1-a showed no susceptibility to inactivation by any of the alcohols tested. The highest concentration used was 1 mM.

Inactivation of PM2. In general, PM2 is less susceptible to the straight-chain alcohols than $\phi 6$ but was readily inactivated by several compounds at the higher concentrations. The profile for inactivation as a function of chain length was similar, but not identical, to that for $\phi 6$. Data taken at a concentration of 0.4 mM are displayed in Fig. 2. For PM2, only decanol and dodecanol inactivate more than 50% of the virus at this concentration. This was also found to be the case in another experiment where a concentration of 1 mM was used. No further experiments were carried out with this virus.

HSV-*syn* 20 and polyoma. The effects of the straight-chain alcohols on two mammalian cell viruses, one that is enveloped and one that contains no lipids, were studied. HSV contains approximately 22% lipid (11) located in a membrane envelope that surrounds the nucleocapsid. HSV-*syn* 20 is a plaque morphology mutant of HSV that causes extensive cell fusion when monolayers are infected in vitro (9). The virions of *syn* mutants of HSV are morphologically indistinguishable from wild-type virus, the dif-

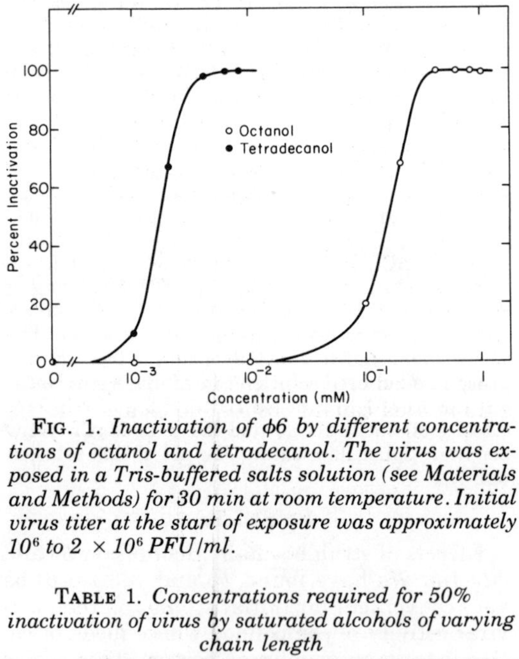

FIG. 1. *Inactivation of $\phi 6$ by different concentrations of octanol and tetradecanol. The virus was exposed in a Tris-buffered salts solution (see Materials and Methods) for 30 min at room temperature. Initial virus titer at the start of exposure was approximately 10^6 to 2×10^6 PFU/ml.*

TABLE 1. *Concentrations required for 50% inactivation of virus by saturated alcohols of varying chain length*

Alcohol chain length	Conc of alcohol required (mM)	
	$\phi 6$	$\phi 23$-1-a
4	>1	>1
6	0.15	>1
8	0.15	>1
10	0.03	>1
12	0.007	>1
14	0.002	>1
16	>1	>1
18	>1	>1

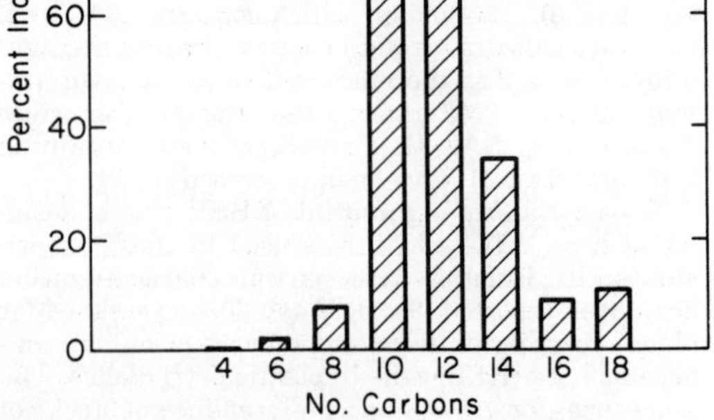

FIG. 2. *Profile for the inactivation of PM2 by saturated alcohols of varying chain length, indicated as the number of carbons on the abscissa. The virus was exposed to 0.4 mM solutions in a Tris-buffered salts solution (see Materials and Methods) with conditions otherwise as stated for Fig. 1.*

ference apparently being due to the patterns of glycosylation of membrane proteins during infection (7). We determined the effects of straight-chain alcohols on HSV-*syn* 20; data for a 30-min exposure to 0.5 mM solutions are shown in Fig. 3. The alcohols that are most active against HSV-*syn* 20, as was the case for ϕ6, are decanol, dodecanol, and tetradecanol. Dodecanol and tetradecanol are also active at lower concentrations (Table 2).

Polyoma is a small deoxyribonucleic acid virus that productively infects mouse cells and transforms hamster cells. It has a diameter of about 45 nm and is non-enveloped. We carried out a limited number of experiments with polyoma and the alcohols phytol and dodecanol. At a concentration of 0.5 mM, polyoma was not inactivated by either compound (data not shown), further substantiating that inactivation by alcohols is due to their effects on virus membranes.

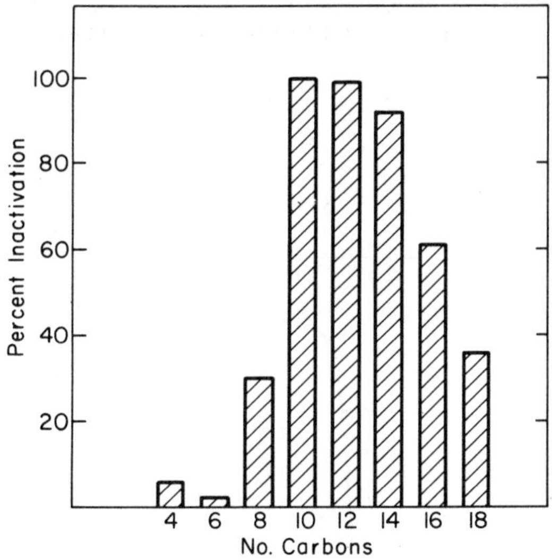

FIG. 3. *Profile for the inactivation of HSV-syn 20 by saturated alcohols of varying chain length. The virus was exposed to 1 mM solutions in a tricine-buffered salts solution (see Materials and Methods) with conditions otherwise as for Fig. 1.*

TABLE 2. *Inactivation of HSV-syn 20 by different concentrations of the most active alcohols*

Alcohol chain length	Conc (mM)	% Inactivation
10	0.5	>99
	0.05	<10
	0.005	<10
12	0.5	>99
	0.05	98
	0.005	<10
14	0.5	91
	0.05	77
	0.005	14

Effects of straight-chain alcohols on host cells. For the bacterial host cells BAL-31 and HB10Y, experiments were carried out to quantify the effects of alcohols on the growth rate of the cells. Cultures growing exponentially were diluted fivefold into medium containing alcohol at 0.5 mM final concentration and further incubated with aeration at 25°C. Growth was monitored by measuring the absorbance at 620 nm using a Bausch and Lomb Spectronic 20 colorimeter. When necessary, corrections were made for the turbidity contributed by the alcohol suspension. A quantitative estimate of growth rate was calculated as the reciprocal of the doubling time for each culture. These data, normalized to that for control cultures, are presented in Table 3. For both BAL-31 and HB10Y, decanol at 0.5 mM caused considerable cell lysis, so no growth rate could be determined. For all the other alcohols the cells grew well, although at reduced rates for octanol and dodecanol. Comparison of these data with those for ϕ6 and PM2 show that the viruses are far more susceptible to dodecanol and tetradecanol than are their host cells.

HEL cells. Monolayers of HEL cells were treated for 2 h with different concentrations of the straight-chain alcohols and then observed for the appearance of any noticeable cytopathic effect. The experiment was performed in such a manner that the samples were scored without knowledge of the conditions of treatment. The results of this experiment are reported in Table 4. At the highest concentration, 0.5 mM, decanol caused cell lysis and both dodecanol and tetradecanol caused observable changes in the monolayer of cells. At 0.05 mM, no cytopathic effect was observed for any of the alcohols. Significant inactivation of HSV-*syn* 20 occurs at 0.05 mM for both dodecanol and tetradecanol,

TABLE 3. *Effect of 0.5 mM saturated alcohols on growth rate of host bacterial cells*

Alcohol chain length	Relative growth rate[a]	
	HB10Y	BAL-31
6	1.0	1.03
8	0.91	0.75
10	Lysed	Lysed
12	0.77	0.43
14	0.93	1.03
Control	1.00	1.00

[a] Calculated as the reciprocal of doubling time for exponentially growing cultures, normalized to the control.

again indicating that the virus is more susceptible than the host cell to these compounds.

Erythrocyte lysis. A more quantitative comparison of the effects of different alcohols on cells of human origin was obtained with erythrocytes. Freshly drawn blood was centrifuged at low speed, and the cells were resuspended in 0.88% NaCl and washed twice in the same saline solution. Samples were treated for 30 min at 37°C with the different alcohols at 0.5 mM final concentration. After removal of unlysed cells by centrifugation and filtering through a 0.22-μm membrane filter (Millipore Corp.), the absorbance of hemoglobin in the filtrate was

TABLE 4. *Cytopathic effect observed for HEL cells treated for 2 h with different concentrations of alcohols*

Chain length	Conc (mM)	Remarks
4	0.5	No effect
6	0.5	No effect
8	0.5	Few vacuoles
10	0.5	Many cells lysed
	0.05	No effect
12	0.5	About half of the cells off glass; remainder rounded
	0.05	No effect
14	0.5	Few vacuoles
	0.05	No effect
16	0.5	Few off glass; remainder normal
18	0.5	No effect

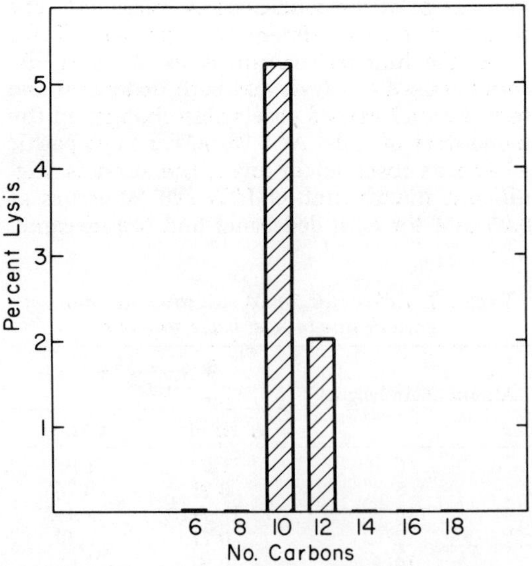

FIG. 4. *Lysis of erythrocytes by saturated alcohols of varying chain length. The cells were exposed to 1 mM solutions in 0.88% NaCl solutions for 30 min at 25°C. Hemoglobin absorbance at 540 nm was measured in the supernatants and compared with that for a control artificially lysed by sonication.*

measured at 540 nm. To express the data as percentage of lysis, a sample was sonicated to cause complete lysis and then processed in the same manner. Figure 4 shows a profile for the effect of the straight-chain alcohols on erythrocytes. Only decanol and dodecanol caused lysis that was significantly greater than untreated controls. These results, along with those for HEL, BAL-31, and HB10Y cultures, clearly indicate that of the alcohols, decanol has the most harsh effect on the cells. Furthermore, these collective data suggest that dodecanol and tetradecanol are the two straight-chain alcohols that show the most promise as potential antiviral agents.

Phytol. In addition to the experiments just described, we investigated the antiviral potential of phytol, a branched-chain alcohol that occurs in nature as a component of chlorophyll. Its structure is shown in Fig. 5. Data for the effects of phytol on the different viruses are given in Fig. 6 and Table 5. φ6 is unusually

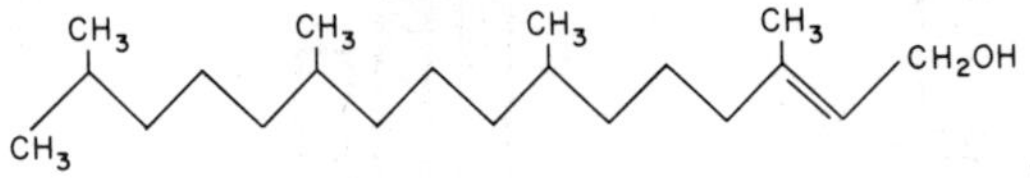

FIG. 5. *Structure of phytol.*

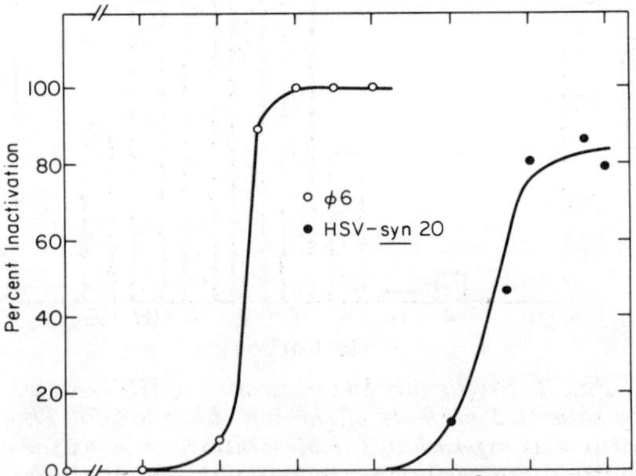

FIG. 6. *Inactivation of φ6 and HSV-syn 20 by different concentrations of phytol. Conditions are as described in Materials and Methods and in the legends for Fig. 1 and 3.*

TABLE 5. *Concentrations of phytol required for 50% inactivation of different viruses*

Virus	Conc required (mM)
φ6	0.00002
φ23-1-a	>1
HSV-*syn* 20	0.035
Polyoma	>1
PM2	>1

susceptible to phytol, HSV-*syn* 20 is inactivated at higher concentrations, and PM2 is not affected by this compound. As expected, ϕ23 and polyoma virus were not susceptible to treatment with phytol.

Phytol gave no reduction in growth rate for BAL-31 and HB10Y cells. HEL cells, when exposed to 0.5 mM phytol for 2 h, contained a few vacuoles but otherwise showed little damage. No effect was observed in HEL cells exposed to 0.05 mM phytol. Due to the abundance of phytol as a natural product, it is expected to have low toxicity to humans and other animals.

DISCUSSION

In considering the design and development of successful antiviral agents, an operational distinction can be made between those compounds that inactivate the virus on contact and those that inhibit the further production of infectious virus particles. For contact inactivation, the agent may be removed after a period of treatment and the virus assayed for infectivity in its absence. For inhibition of virus production, the agent is generally present in the infected culture. In either case, to be useful clinically, the substance must possess antiviral activity at concentrations and under conditions where the organism being treated is comparatively unaffected. The available literature on the selective inhibition of viral functions indicates that the most common approach, by far, has been the search for compounds to inhibit virus production, with very little consideration being given to the contact inactivation of viruses. This may be due, in part, to the fact that many viruses are quite resistant to chemicals that are harmful to cells. Thus, the development of a safe agent that would inactivate all or a large proportion of the pathogenic viruses on contact seems quite unlikely.

As research in antiviral chemotherapy advances, it is becoming apparent that many of the active agents may be effective against only one or a few types of viruses. Nevertheless, the discovery of a drug that would successfully control a single viral disease would constitute a significant advance in the field. The fact that membrane-perturbing antiviral agents, by their very nature, are limited to certain classes of viruses does not appear to detract from their usefulness. Of the viruses that are pathogenic to man and domesticated animals, we estimate that approximately half are encolosed in a lipid-containing membrane structure.

In this report, evidence has been presented that phytol and certain long-chain saturated alcohols are quite effective at inactiviting lipid-containing viruses in vitro. Some of these compounds, notably phytol, dodecanol, and tetradecanol, are active against viruses under conditions that appear to be much less detrimental to the host cells. For the different viruses studied, there exists some degree of specificity with regard to which compounds are most active against which viruses. Phytol, for example, is the most active compound against ϕ6 but is without effect on PM2. Decanol, on the other hand, is more active than tetradecanol against PM2, with the reverse being the case for ϕ6. HSV-*syn-20* appears more susceptible than either ϕ6 or ϕ23 to alcohols having chain lengths greater than 14 carbons. The reasons for and the nature of these specificities are not known at the present time. We anticipate that the structure-function relationships that result in one virus being more susceptible than another to a membrane perturber may also be related to the reasons why a virus may be more susceptible to inactivation than its host cell.

Our findings suggest that dodecanol, tetradecanol, and phytol warrant further studies as potential antiviral agents. It will be of special interest to determine if membrane perturbers that inactivate enveloped viruses on contact do so by inactivating envelope proteins, perturbing lipids, or interrupting lipid-protein interactions. The more thorough our understanding of the similarities and differences between virus and cell membranes, the more rational will be our design and development of this class of antiviral agents.

ACKNOWLEDGMENTS

Financial support for this research was provided by the Energy Resources and Development Administration and the National Institutes of Health. Technical assistance was provided by Lisa Breon, Kathy Kenny, and Vincent Bond.

LITERATURE CITED

1. **Braunstein, S., and R. Franklin.** 1971. Structure and synthesis of a lipid-containing bacteriophage. V. Phospholipids of the host BAL-31 and the bacteriophage PM2. Virology **43**:685–695.
2. **Ch'ien, L. T., F. M. Schabel, Jr., and C. A. Alford, Jr.** 1975. Arabinosyl nucleosides and nucleotides, p. 227–256. *In* W. A. Carter (ed.), Selective inhibitors of viral functions. The Chemical Rubber Co., Cleveland.
3. **Cupp, J., P. Wanda, A. Keith, and W. Snipes.** 1975. Inactivation of the lipid-containing bacteriophage PM2 by butylated hydroxytoluene. Antimicrob. Agents Chemother. **8**:698–706.
4. **Espejo, R., and E. Canelo.** 1968. Properties of PM2: a lipid-containing bacterial virus. Virology **34**:738–747.
5. **Franklin, R.** 1974. Structure and synthesis of bacteriophage PM2 with particular emphasis on the viral lipid bilayer. Curr. Top. Microbiol. Immunol. **68**:107–159.
6. **Harrison, S., D. Caspar, R. Camerini-Otero, and R. Franklin.** 1971. Lipid and protein arrangement in bacteriophage PM2. Nature (London) New Biol. **229**:197–201.

7. **Knowles, R., and S. Person.** 1976. Effects of 2-deoxyglucose, glucosamine, and mannose on cell fusion and the glycoproteins of herpes simplex virus. J. Virol. 18:644–651.
8. **Maugh, T. H., II.** 1976. Chemotherapy: antiviral agents come of age. Science 192:128–132.
9. **Person, S., R. Knowles, G. Read, S. Warner, and V. Bond.** 1976. Kinetics of cell fusion induced by a syncytia-producing mutant of herpes simplex virus type I. J. Virol. 17:183–190.
10. **Prusoff, W. H.** 1972. Viral and host cell interactions with 5-iodo-2′-deoxyuridine (idoxuridine), p. 135–148. *In* D. Shugar (ed.), Virus-cell interactions and viral antimetabolites, 7th FEBS meeting, vol. 22. Academic Press Inc., New York.
11. **Russell, W., D. Watson, and P. Wildy.** 1963. Preliminary chemical studies on Herpes Virus. Biochem. J. 87:26.
12. **Sands, J., J. Cupp, A. Keith, and W. Snipes.** 1974. Temperature sensitivity of the assembly process of the enveloped bacteriophage $\phi 6$. Biochim. Biophys. Acta 373:277–285.
13. **Shugar, D.** 1972. Alkylated pyrimidine nucleosides and (poly)nucleotides as potential anti-viral agents, p. 193–207. *In* D. Shugar (ed.), Virus-cell interactions and viral antimetabolites, 7th FEBS meeting, vol. 22. Academic Press Inc., New York.
14. **Snipes, W., J. Cupp, J. Sands, A. Keith, and A. Davis.** 1974. Calcium requirement for assembly of the lipid-containing bacteriophage PM2. Biochim. Biophys. Acta 339:311–322.
15. **Snipes, W., S. Person, A. Keith, and J. Cupp.** 1975. Butylated hydroxytoluene inactivites lipid-containing viruses. Science 187:64–66.
16. **Sugar, J., and H. E. Kaufman.** 1975. Halogenated pyrimidines in antiviral therapy, p. 295–311. *In* W. A. Carter (ed.), Selective inhibitors of viral functions. The Chemical Rubber Co., Cleveland.
17. **Vidaver, A., R. Koski, and J. Van Etten.** 1973. Bacteriophage $\phi 6$: a lipid-containing virus of *Pseudomonas phaseolicola*. J. Virol. 11:799–805.
18. **Wanda, P., J. Cupp, W. Snipes, A Keith, T. Rucinsky, L. Polish, and J. Sands.** 1976. Inactivation of the enveloped bacteriophage $\phi 6$ by butylated hydroxytoluene and butylated hydroxyanisole. Antimicrob. Agents Chemother. 10:96–105.

ANTIMICROBIAL AGENTS AND CHEMOTHERAPY, Jan. 1977, p. 105-109
Vol. 11, No. 1
Printed in U.S.A.

Rapid Analysis of Cefazolin in Serum by High-Pressure Liquid Chromatography

JOHN S. WOLD

Toxicology Division, Lilly Research Laboratories, Eli Lilly and Company, Greenfield, Indiana 46140

Received for publication 16 August 1976

A high-pressure liquid chromatography (HPLC) method has been developed for the analysis of cefazolin in serum. Serum was deproteinized by the addition of 6% trichloroacetic acid and injected onto a reverse-phase column with a mobile phase of 10 to 15% methanol in 1% aqueous acetic acid. Cefazolin chromatographed without interference from ultraviolet-absorbing components of serum, with a retention time of 3.1 min. Standard curves comparing peak area with concentration prepared from dog or human sera were linear over a range of 1.6 to 200 μg/ml. Results from the HPLC assay were compared with microbiological assays (cylinder plate method) on both standard serum samples and sera from dogs and human subjects receiving intramuscular cefazolin. The HPLC method was somewhat more accurate in comparison with the microbiological assay performed on serum samples of known concentration. The comparison of results from an analysis of serum levels of dogs or human subjects receiving cefazolin indicated that the two methods would lead to identical conclusions concerning pharmacokinetics or the achievement of therapeutic serum levels. The HPLC assay method presents an alternative to conventional microbiological assays, with marked improvement in speed (30 min) and considerable potential for future development.

The antibiotics as a class are unique among drugs or xenobiotics in that the analytical methods used in the routine determination of serum levels have involved bioassay rather than chemical methodology.

Cephalosporins are a widely used group of drugs that have traditionally been assayed in serum by microbiological assays. Sera from patients, clinical pharmacology test subjects, or experimental animals receiving cephalosporings are usually assayed by the disk plate, cylinder plate, or agar well diffusion methods, which depend on the inhibition of growth of *Bacillus subtilis* or *Sarcina lutea*.

The conventional methods routinely used for drug assay in serum, such as gas chromatographic, photometric, or fluorometric methods, have not been applied to the cephalosporins, except to a very limited extent. Tune (5) determined cephaloridine concentrations in serum by a method involving the fluorometric determination of pyridine released by acid hydrolysis. Mullen et al. (3) reported an indirect method for the determination of cephaloridine, involving the gas chromatographic determination of pyridine released by alkaline hydrolysis.

Polarographic methods for the determination of cephaloridine, cephalothin, and cephalexin in an ultrafiltrate of serum have been reported by Benner (1). The chemical methods described above, although satisfactory under the conditions used, do not appear to have widespread utility.

The cephalosporins as a group do not lend themselves to simple gas chromatographic or photometric assays because of their low volatility and poor extraction from serum into organic solvents.

High-pressure liquid chromatography (HPLC) seems to offer the advantages of gas chromatography, such as simultaneous separation and quantitation, in a system that does not necessarily require either extraction or volatilization of the antibiotics.

An HPLC technique for the analysis of tetracycline after extraction from serum has recently been reported by Nilsson-Ehle et al. (4). Cooper et al. (2) reported on the use of HPLC, employing anion exchange chromatography of cephalothin and deacetylcephalothin after ion pair extraction from human serum.

This report describes the development of a method for determining cefazolin in serum by a direct injection of deproteinized serum onto a reverse-phase liquid chromatographic column. The advantages of this approach are simplicity and speed, with accurate determination of serum concentrations available in a properly prepared laboratory within 30 min after the receipt of a serum sample.

MATERIALS AND METHODS

Antibiotics. Cefazolin sodium (Kefzol) was obtained from Eli Lilly & Co., Indianapolis, Inc.

HPLC. Chromatography was carried out on a model ALC 202 liquid chromatograph (Waters Associates, Milford, Mass.). A stainless-steel column (57 cm by 2 mm) was packed with Phenyl Corasil (37 to 50 μm, reverse phase; Waters Associates, Milford, Mass.).

The mobile phase consisted of 10 to 15% methanol in 1% aqueous acetic acid. The concentration of methanol in the mobile phase was adjusted daily for optimum separation and peak shape. The flow rate was maintained at 2.0 ml/min at pressures of 1,500 to 2,000 lb/in. The detector monitored absorption at 254 nm, recorded at 0.02 to 0.04 absorbance units (full scale).

Standard solutions were prepared by dissolving weighed amounts of cefazolin sodium in dog or human sera at various concentrations. The cefazolin sodium standard had been previously assayed by conventional methodology and was shown to contain 815 mg of cefazolin activity per g. Concentrations of cefazolin sodium were obtained from the HPLC analysis by a comparison with standard curves prepared daily, relating the peak area to cefazolin sodium concentrations. The resultant data were then corrected by the above factor to allow comparison with microbiological assay results expressed as cefazolin activity.

Sample preparation. Frozen serum samples obtained from dogs receiving 10 mg of cefazolin sodium per kg intramuscularly or human volunteers receiving a 1-g intramuscular dose were thawed just prior to analysis. A 0.5- to 1-ml portion of serum was removed and an equal volume of cold 6% trichloroacetic acid was added. The samples were kept at 0°C for 5 min and centrifuged at 1,800 rpm for 10 min (model K laboratory centrifuge, International Equipment Co., Needham Heights, Mass.). The supernatant solution was removed and kept at 0°C until a 90-μl portion was injected into the liquid chromatograph. Standards in serum were prepared in an identical manner.

RESULTS

Chromatography. Representative chromatographic tracings resulting from the injection of samples prepared from blank dog serum or from dog serum containing 20 μg of cefazolin sodium per ml are shown in Fig. 1. The chromatographic conditions provided adequate separation of the cefazolin peak from ultraviolet-absorbing components of the serum sample. Control serum contained no interfering ultraviolet-absorbing components. Chromatography of blank and cefazolin-containing samples of human serum was identical to the results described for dog serum.

Standard curves. The reproducibility and linearity of a standard curve generated from dog or human serum containing various amounts of cefazolin sodium are shown in Fig. 2. The standard curve represents triplicate analyses. A standard curve was prepared daily from single analyses at each concentration. When higher serum concentrations were expected, standard curves were prepared over a concentration range of 10 to 200 μg/ml, with a full-scale absorbance at an optical density of 0.04 with similar reproducibility and linearity.

The reproducibility of the analytical method was demonstrated by the analysis of 12 portions of blank human serum containing cefazolin sodium at a concentration of 25 μg/ml assayed against a standard curve prepared from single samples containing 5, 10, 20, 30, and 50 μg of cefazolin sodium per ml. The resultant data gave a mean of 24.3 μg/ml, with a standard deviation of 1.2 and a coefficient of variation of 4.9%. The range of values was from 21.9 to 26.6 μg/ml.

Comparison with microbiological assay. (i) Standards. Two sets of standard solutions were prepared in dog serum. One set was prepared by the HPLC laboratory and the other by the laboratory performing the microbiological as-

FIG. 1. *HPLC tracings of control dog serum and dog serum containing 20 μg of cefazolin sodium per ml. The retention time of the cefazolin peak is 3.1 min (optical density, 0.02, full scale).*

says. Standards were then assayed by both laboratories. The results are shown in Table 1.

The HPLC assay gave results ranging from 85 to 113% (mean, 104%) of the actual cefazolin concentration, and the relative deviation from the actual value was similar over the complete range of concentrations studied (1.6 to 100 μg ml). The microbiological assay gave results that ranged from 72 to 106% of the actual values (mean, 87%). The values determined by the microbiological assay were consistently lower than the actual value, and the deviation became more exaggerated at higher serum concentrations.

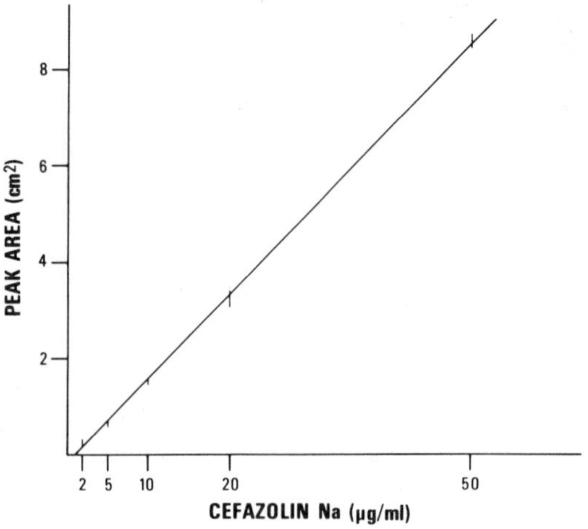

FIG. 2. *Typical standard curve relating the area of the HPLC peak to the standard concentration of cefazolin sodium in dog serum. Vertical bars represent the range of triplicate analyses at each concentration. The line is the least-squares regression line with slope = 0.1743, intercept = 0.2037, correlation coefficient = 0.999.*

(ii) Serum levels. Serum samples from dogs receiving 10 mg of cefazolin per kg intramuscularly and human subjects receiving 1-g intramuscular doses were analyzed by both HPLC and microbiological methods. The resultant serum level-time curves are presented in Fig. 3 and 4.

There is generally good agreement between the two assay methods. The correlation coefficient between the HPLC and microbiological assay in dog and human sera over all time points was 0.96. The HPLC technique gave slightly higher values at most time points although the agreement between the two methods was better at the lower serum levels observed in dogs (Fig. 3).

In cases in which there was a significant discrepancy between the two methods, as shown in Fig. 4 (subject F, 3 h), the HPLC assay appeared to give a more reasonable value since there is no pharmacokinetically logical explanation for a rise in the serum level from 3 to 4 h, as indicated by the microbiological assay.

DISCUSSION

The liquid chromatographic analysis of cefazolin in serum offers an alternative to the conventional microbiological assay. The HPLC method is accurate and reproducible and appears to give results that are at least comparable to or perhaps slightly better than the microbiological assay. The differences between the results obtained by the two methods are not of a great enough magnitude, however, to alter any

TABLE 1. *Comparison of HPLC and microbiological assays of standard cefazolin solutions in dog serum*

Source of standard sera	Actual concn of cefazolin (μg/ml)	HPLC assay[a] concn of cefazolin (μg/ml)	%	Microbiological assay[b] concn of cefazolin (μg/ml)	%
HPLC laboratory	1.6	1.9	119	1.7	106
	4.1	3.5	85	3.9	95
	8.2	8.8	107	6.7	82
	16.3	15.7	96	11.7	72
	40.8	40.8	100	30.9	76
Microbiological assay laboratory	5	5.1	102	4.7	94
	10	9.7	97	8.8	88
	25	26.4	106	21.5	86
	50	55.6	111	46.3	93
	100	113	113	81.7	82
Mean			104		87
Standard error			3.1		3.2
Standard deviation			9.8		10.0

[a] HPLC assay values are the result of single determinations.

[b] Microbiological assay values are the result of one assay (two plates) against *B. subtilis,* using the cylinder plate method.

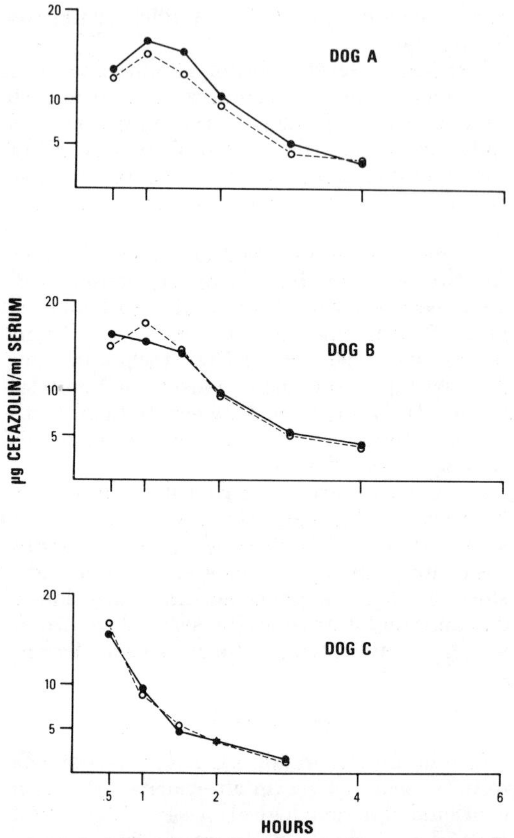

FIG. 3. *Serum levels of cefazolin in dog serum after the administration of 10 mg/kg intramuscularly: comparison of HPLC and microbiological assay. Symbols: ●, single HPLC assay corrected to cefazolin activity; ○, microbiological assay against B. subtilis, using the cylinder plate method (single assay, two plates); *, coincident points.*

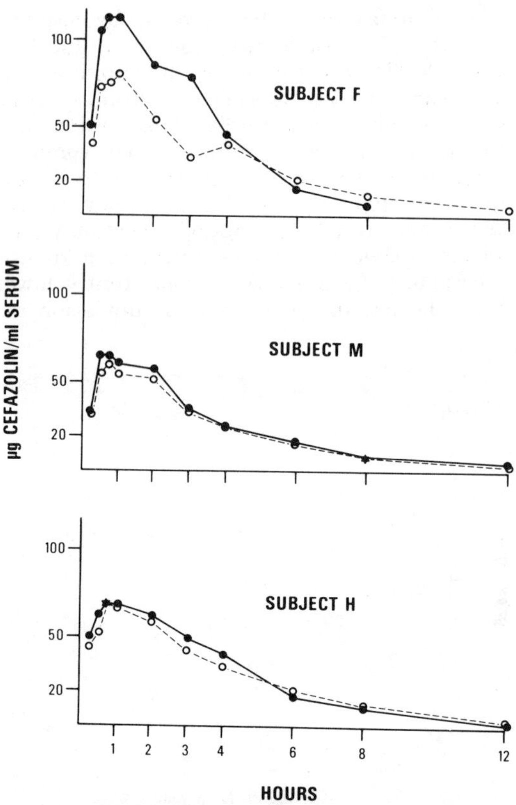

FIG. 4. *Serum levels of cefazolin in human subjects after the administration of 1 g intramuscularly: comparison of HPLC and microbiological assay. Symbols: ●, single HPLC assay corrected to cefazolin activity; ○, microbiological assay against B. subtilis, using the cylinder plate method (single assay, four plates, two zones per plate); *, coincident points.*

conclusions about pharmacokinetics or the attainment of therapeutic serum levels. The most significant advantage of the HPLC method is the speed with which results can be obtained. The concentration of cefazolin in serum can be determined within 30 min of venipuncture through use of the HPLC assay as compared with the 16- to 18-h overnight incubation used in conventional microbiological assays.

With continued importance being placed on the monitoring of antibiotic serum levels in special clinical situations, such as impaired renal function, the advantage of rapid analytical methods will become increasingly important.

This report describes an assay for cefazolin. Similar assays have been developed in this laboratory for cephaloridine and cefamandole, using different mobile phases (unpublished data), and the chromatographic method should be applicable to most cephalosporins.

Another potential advantage of the HPLC assay technique is in the simultaneous determination of two antibiotics in serum resulting from combination therapy. This approach has not yet been investigated.

ACKNOWLEDGMENTS

I wish to acknowledge the excellent technical assistance of Brenda L. Miller. I also wish to thank John W. Lamb and Patricia L. Resener for the microbiological assays.

LITERATURE CITED

1. **Benner, E. J.** 1971. Two-hour assay for content of penicillins and cephalosporins in serum, p. 201–204. Antimicrob. Agents Chemother. 1970.
2. **Cooper, M. J., M. W. Anders, and B. L. Mirkin.** 1973. Ion pair extraction and high speed liquid chromatography of cephalothin and deacetylcephalothin in human serum and urine. Drug Metab. Dispos. 1:659–662.

3. **Mullen, P. W., G. E. Mower, and J. A. Tooth.** 1974. An indirect method for the determination of cephaloridine in serum by gas chromatography. Res. Commun. Chem. Pathol. Pharmacol. 7:85–94.
4. **Nilsson-Ehle, I., T. T. Yoshikawa, M. C. Schotz, and L. B. Guze.** 1976. Quantitation of antibiotics using high-pressure liquid chromatography: tetracycline. Antimicrob. Agents Chemother. 9:754–760.
5. **Tune, B. M.** 1972. Effect of organic acid transport inhibitors on renal cortical uptake and proximal tubular toxicity of cephaloridine. J. Pharmacol. Exp. Ther. 181:250–256.

Antimicrobial Agents and Chemotherapy, Jan. 1977, p. 110–113
Vol. 11, No. 1

Comparative Penetration of Amikacin, Gentamicin, and Penicillin G into Exudate Fluid in Experimental Sterile Peritonitis

ROB ROY MacGREGOR

Infectious Diseases Section, University of Pennsylvania School of Medicine, Philadelphia, Pennsylvania 19174

Received for publication 8 September 1976

Using a rabbit sterile peritonitis model, we compared the penetration of intravenously administered amikacin, gentamicin, and penicillin G into peritoneal exudate. Peritonitis was induced with sterile normal saline, and the peritoneal exudate contained 23,751 ± 3,039 granulocytes 8 h later. Antibiotics were administered intravenously 3 h after initiating peritonitis, and serum and peritoneal fluid concentrations were measured for 5 h. Peritoneal levels of each antibiotic exceeded simultaneous serum levels by 1 h after dose and remained above serum levels thereafter. The maximum peritoneal fluid concentration of amikacin reached 71.2% ± 12.7 of the maximum serum concentration, whereas maximum gentamicin peritoneal concentration achieved 37.1% ± 2.7, and penicillin achieved 23.2% ± 4.5, of their respective maximum serum concentrations.

Our laboratory has developed a rabbit model for sterile peritonitis (8), which offers the opportunity to study the penetration of various antibiotics into peritoneal exudate. Peritonitis can develop after abdominal surgery, spontaneous rupture of a viscus, in alcoholics with cirrhosis, and as a complication of peritoneal dialysis. In all of these clinical settings, gram-negative rod infections are common, and aminoglycoside antibiotics offer the widest spectrum of effectiveness for these organisms. Because Smithivas et al. (12) had reported that "peritoneal gentamicin levels remained in a suboptimal range despite the development of high levels in the serum" in some patients with peritonitis, we measured the kinetics of gentamicin penetration into peritoneal exudate in our experimental model and compared them with the new aminoglycoside, amikacin. This new drug, produced by acetylation of the deoxystreptamine residue of kanamycin A, is more active than kanamycin against most strains of *Pseudomonas* species, including most of those that have inactivating enzymes for gentamicin, tobramycin, and kanamycin (3). Therefore, it might represent a reasonable antibiotic choice in cases of peritonitis if its penetration into the exudate is adequate. To broaden our comparison of relative efficiency of penetration, we also studied penicillin G, because its structure and pharmacology are quite different from the aminoglycosides, and because much already is known regarding its behavior in the peritoneum (4, 10).

MATERIALS AND METHODS

Sterile peritonitis was induced in 2- to 3-kg New Zealand white rabbits by the instillation of 120 ml of sterile normal saline into the peritoneal cavity through a 16-gauge multiply fenistrated intravenous polyethylene catheter (Deseret Pharmaceutical Co., Sandy, Utah) inserted carefully into the peritoneal cavity to avoid the bowel. During the next 8 h, the catheter was held in place with an elastic bandage, and the peritoneal fluid was sampled at 2-h intervals. The animals developed an acute peritonitis, with mean exudate granulocyte counts of 885 ± 309 (standard error) at 2 h, 10,808 ± 2,623 at 4 h, 19,408 ± 3,733 at 6 h, and 23,751 ± 3,039 at 8 h. The catheter was removed after 8 h and, by 24 h after the saline instillation, the animals had neither physical evidence of continued peritoneal reaction nor any apparent aftereffects.

Peritonitis was allowed to develop for 3 h before antibiotic administration, by which time the animals' abdominal musculature was tense and tender to pressure. At that time, blood and peritoneal exudate fluid was taken for "preantibiotic" measurement, and a dose of the antibiotic to be studied was infused through an ear vein over 2 to 3 min. Blood and exudate samples were drawn at 15 min, and then at 1, 3, and 5 h after the end of infusion. Samples were centrifuged for 15 min at 3,000 rpm, and the clear serum or peritoneal fluid was frozen at −70°C until time of antibiotic assay.

The antibiotic dosages for the rabbits were chosen on the basis of normal doses used in humans: amikacin, 7.5 mg/kg; gentamicin, 2 mg/kg; or penicillin G, 200,000 U/kg. The goal was not to compare the peak concentrations achievable with each of the three antibiotics in peritoneal exudate, but rather to determine how close the peak peritoneal fluid concentration of each drug would come to its peak serum concentration, and to study the pharmacokinetics of the drugs between blood and exudate.

The antibiotics were measured with an agar diffusion assay using *Bacillus globigii* as the test organism (13). Wells were filled with the serum or peritoneal samples from the test animals or with freshly prepared antibiotic standards added to normal rabbit serum, which had been shown previously to give no zone of inhibition on the assay plates. The plates were incubated for 6 h at 37°C, and the zones of inhibition of growth of the test organisms were measured to the nearest 0.1 mm. Standard curves were then constructed for each antibiotic using the number of millimeters of clearing around each well of the standards, and the concentrations in the serum and peritoneal fluid samples were read from the standard curve. Each unknown was run in duplicate, and the results were averaged.

RESULTS

The pharmacokinetics of amikacin and gentamicin in rabbits with sterile peritonitis is shown in Fig. 1. Six animals were given each antibiotic, and each isobar represents plus or minus the standard error of the mean. For both antibiotics, the levels in the peritoneal fluid exceeded those in the serum by 1 h, and thereafter remained above simultaneous serum levels. Figure 2 shows that high doses of penicillin are rapidly excreted: by h 3 after injection, most penicillin had been cleared from the serum, whereas the peritoneal fluid concentrations remained high. Figure 3 displays the peritoneal fluid concentration of each antibiotic as a percentage of the peak serum level for that antibiotic. Amikacin proved most effective in entering the peritoneal exudate, with levels reaching 71.2% ± 12.7 (standard error) of peak serum levels; gentamicin reached 37.1% ± 2.7, and penicillin reached 23.2% ± 4.5.

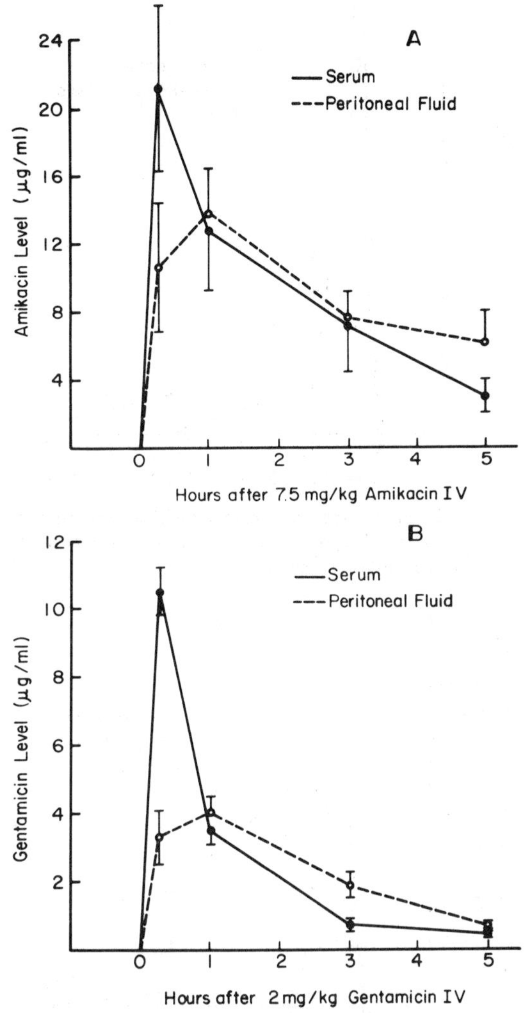

FIG. 1. *Serum and peritoneal fluid concentrations of amikacin and gentamicin after intravenous administration. Each antibiotic was given 3 h after initiation of sterile peritonitis. The points represent mean concentrations in six animals, and the brackets indicate plus or minus standard errors of the means.*

DISCUSSION

The penetration of aminoglycoside and penicillin antibiotics into the peritoneal space has been studied in settings of ascitic fluid accumulation, peritoneal dialysis, and peritonitis. Ascitic fluid was produced by Gerding et al. by constricting the thoracic inferior vena cava in dogs (Prog. Abstr. Intersci. Conf. Antimicrob. Agents Chemother., 15th, Washington, D.C., Abstr. 405, 1975). These investigators reported that both gentamicin and amikacin developed ascites concentrations 17% of those in serum and that the peritoneal levels of the cephalosporins reached 21 to 26% of serum levels. In a different model, Gerding and Hall obtained peritoneal fluid by placing hollow, fenestrated balls in the peritoneal cavity of rabbits and aspirating from them percutaneously thereafter (6). The fluid had the characteristics of ascitic fluid: 1,560 leukocytes/mm^3, 55% neutrophils, and a protein level of 4.1 g/100 ml. Gentamicin and tobramycin peritoneal levels reached only 16.5% of peak serum levels, but amikacin was more effective, reaching 32.4% of peak serum level. Cephalosporins varied from 11.9 to 26.6% of serum levels.

In studies of antibiotic distribution during peritoneal dialysis, Smithivas reported effluent levels 17.4 and 36.4% of simultaneous serum levels in two patients receiving gentamicin intramuscularly during dialysis (12). Gary stud-

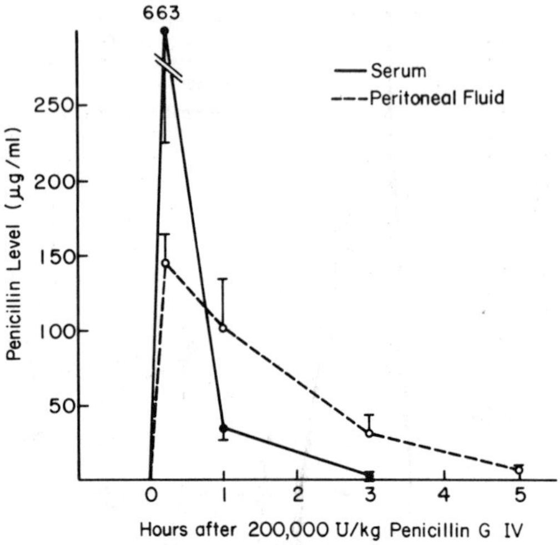

FIG. 2. *Serum and peritoneal fluid concentrations of penicillin G after intravenous administration. Conditions parallel Fig. 1.*

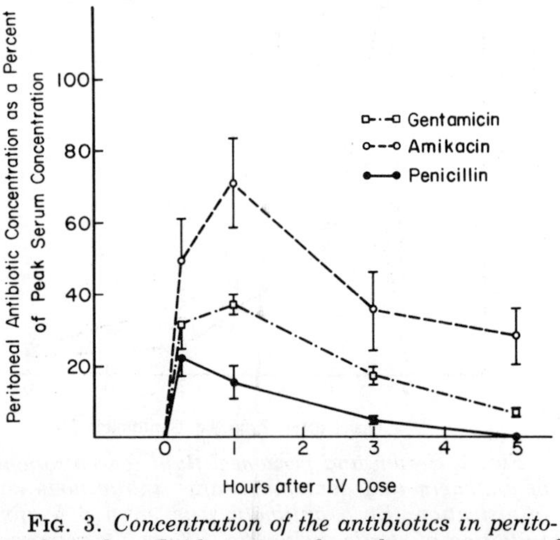

FIG. 3. *Concentration of the antibiotics in peritoneal exudate fluid, expressed as the percentage of peak serum concentration for each antibiotic.*

ied two patients during three episodes of dialysis and found serum gentamicin clearance rates of 2.0 to 19.4 ml/min, removing from 286 to 659 μg of the drug per h (5). In a larger group of patients receiving peritoneal dialysis, Mahon et al. found a mean gentamicin clearance rate of 7.5 ± 1.3 ml/min and a gentamicin plasma half-life of 36 h (compared with 8 h in patients on hemodialysis [9]). Data on peritoneal transfer of kanamycin (included because of the similarity of this drug to amikacin [3]) show that one-third of an injected dose is removed in 24 h of peritoneal dialysis, for a clearance rate of 5.3 to 8.3 ml/min (1, 7). Kanamycin plasma half-life of 70 to 84 h was reduced to 12 h, and recommendations for drug replacement on the day of dialysis suggest either 3.5 mg/kg (1) or a standard dose of 250 mg (7). Madhaven et al. reported that peritoneal dialysis had minimal effect on the serum half-life of amikacin in three patients, and they found levels of 0.7 to 4.98 μg/ml in the dialysis fluid (T. Madhavan, E. Fisher, K. Burch, E. Haas, F. Cox, K. Yaremchuk, N. Levin, and E. L. Quinn, Prog. Abstr. Intersci. Conf. Antimicrob. Agents Chemother., 15th, Washington, D.C., Abstr. 89, 1975). For penicillins, Ruedy reported dialysis fluid levels of oxacillin and ampicillin that were 31.2 and 21.3%, respectively, of their serum levels (10), and Sher et al. reported that methicillin levels in the dialysis effluent were 56 and 32% of maximum serum levels in two patients (11). An authoritative guide to therapy in renal failure states that there is "no significant dialysis of penicillin G with peritoneal dialysis" (2).

In cases of active peritonitis, Smithivas reported that passage of gentamicin from serum to dialysate was quite variable, with a mean peritoneal level 23.8% of serum levels during the first 12 h of treatment (12). Therefore, they recommended addition of gentamicin to the dialysis fluid to assure therapeutic levels in the peritoneal space. Gerding et al. reported much more favorable results in patients with alcoholic cirrhosis and spontaneous peritonitis: gentamicin levels in the peritoneal fluid varied from 54 to 117% of serum levels in six patients, tobramycin exudate concentrations were 14 to 100% of serum concentrations in seven patients, and penicillin and ampicillin proportions were 60 to 100% (D. N. Gerding, W. H. Hall, and E. Schierl, Prog. Abstr. Intersci. Conf. Antimicrob. Agents Chemother., 15th, Washington, D.C., Abstr. 406, 1975).

Our data suggest that both gentamicin and amikacin enter the peritoneal exudate effectively. Therefore, physicians can anticipate therapeutic peritoneal levels when treating peritonitis with either aminoglycoside in doses sufficient to produce high but subtoxic serum levels (e.g., 6 to 10 μg/ml for gentamicin and 20 to 25 μg/ml for amikacin). In clinical situations in which the difference between the antibiotic level required for therapeutic effect and the toxic concentration of that drug is small, amikacin may be preferred because a higher percentage of its serum concentration penetrates into the peritoneum.

ACKNOWLEDGMENTS

This study was supported by a grant from the Bristol Co. Elvira Ventura's handling of the rabbit peritonitis experiments and Mollie Gallagher's measurement of antibiotic levels made the study a success. Kathleen Ludden prepared the manuscript.

LITERATURE CITED

1. **Atkins, R. C., C. Mion, E. Despaux, N. Van-Hai, C. Julien, and H. Mion.** 1973. Peritoneal transfer of kanamycin and its use in peritoneal dialysis. Kidney Int. **3**:391-396.
2. **Bennett, W. M., I. Singer and C. J. Coggins.** 1974. A guide to drug therapy in renal failure. J. Am. Med. Assoc. **230**:1544-1553.
3. **Clarke, J. T., R. D. Libke, C. Regamey, and W. M. M. Kirby.** 1974. Comparative pharmacokinetics of amikacin and kanamycin. Clin. Pharmacol. Ther. **15**: 610-616.
4. **Comber, K. R., C. D. Osborne, and R. Sutherland.** 1975. Comparative effects of amoxycillin and ampicillin in the treatment of experimental mouse infections. Antimicrob. Agents Chemother. **7**:179-185.
5. **Gary, N. E.** 1971. Peirtoneal clearance and removal of gentamicin. J. Infect. Dis. **124**(Suppl.):S96-S97.
6. **Gerding, D. N., and W. H. Hall.** 1975. The penetration of antibiotics into peritoneal fluid. Bull. N.Y. Acad. Med. **51**:1016-1019.
7. **Greenberg, P. A., and J. P. Sanford.** 1967. Removal and absorption of antibiotics in patients with renal failure undergoing peritoneal dialysis. Ann. Intern. Med. **66**:465-479.
8. **Lentnek, A. L., A. D. Schreiber, and R. R. MacGregor.** 1976. The induction of augmented granulocyte adherence by inflammation. J. Clin. Invest. **57**:1098-1103.
9. **Mahon, M. A., J. I. Ezer, S. S. A. Fenton, and D. C. Cattran.** 1973. Studies on gentamicin clearance during peritoneal and hemodialysis. Clin. Res. **21**: 1018.
10. **Ruedy, J.** 1966. The effects of peritoneal dialysis on the physiological disposition of oxacillin, ampicillin, and tetracycline in patients with renal disease. Can. Med. Assoc. J. **94**:257-261.
11. **Sher, L., H. Shinaberger, and K. G. Barry.** 1965. Peritoneal transport of antibiotics in man. N. Engl. J. Med. **272**:666-669.
12. **Smithivas, T., P. J. Hyams, R. Matalon, M. S. Simberkoff, and J. J. Rahal, Jr.** 1971. The use of gentamicin in peritoneal dialysis. I. Pharmacologic results. J. Infect. Dis. **124**(Suppl):S77-S83.
13. **Winters, R. E., K. D. Litwack, and W. L. Hewitt.** 1971. Relation between dose and levels of gentamicin in blood. J. Infect. Dis. **124**(Suppl):S90-S95.

ANTIMICROBIAL AGENTS AND CHEMOTHERAPY, Jan. 1977, p. 114–117 Vol. 11, No. 1

Rapid Method for Determining the Minimum Inhibitory Concentration of Ampicillin for *Haemophilus influenzae*

RAYMOND RYAN AND RICHARD C. TILTON*

University of Connecticut Health Center, Farmington, Connecticut 06032

Received for publication 13 July 1976

A rapid method for determining the minimal inhibiton concentrations (MICs) of ampicillin using *Haemophilus influenzae* as the test organism is described. This semiautomated technique using the Autobac system was compared with the agar dilution MIC method. Fifty-seven isolates of both susceptible and resistant *H. influenzae* were tested. There was exact quantitative agreement with 65% of the isolates, and 91% of the isolates showed no more than a one-dilution-interval difference when MICs were determined by both methods. Total testing time was 3 to 4 h.

Until recently, ampicillin was the drug of choice for the treatment of *Haemophilus*, infection. Several reports (2, 6–8, 11) have documented the resistance of *Haemophilus influenzae* to certain antibiotics. Ampicillin resistance appears to be mediated by the acquisition of a beta-lactamase enzyme (4, 13). Isolates of *H. influenzae* may be rapidly tested for beta-lactamase (9), and minimum inhibitory concentrations (MICs) may then be determined. This communication describes a rapid semiautomated method for determining the MIC of ampicillin using the Autobac system (12). Results can be generated in 3 to 4 h and be essentially available on the same day that organisms are observed on chocolate agar plate.

MATERIALS AND METHODS

Organisms. Fifty-seven isolates of *H. influenzae* type b were used for the study. The organisms were obtained from the Hartford Hospital, Hartford, Conn.; The Center for Disease Control (Clyde Thornsberry), Atlanta, Ga.; Pfizer, Inc., Groton, Conn.; and the clinical laboratories of the University of Connecticut Health Center, Farmington. Isolates were maintained on chocolate agar slants until tested. Before analysis, a subculture was made on a chocolate agar plate (BBL).

Antibiotics. USP reference ampicillin was used throughout the study. Ampicillin disks of varying concentrations were prepared by applying 10 μl of ampicillin diluted in Eugonic broth to a Pfizer blank disk with an Eppendorf 10-μl micropipette. The disks were air-dried in a laminar-flow hood and then stored in a desiccator at −20°C until used. The disks were made as shown in Table 1. There was no apparent disk deterioration during at least 4 weeks.

Ampicillin for agar dilution susceptibility tests was prepared in Trypticase soy broth and added to molten agar. Final concentration of ampicillin in the chocolate agar plates ranged from 80 to 0.15 μg/ml in twofold serial dilutions.

Autobac methodology. Hemin and reduced nicotinamide adenine dinucleotide (X and V factors) were added to Eugonic broth (Pfizer) in one of two modes: (i) addition of XV factor strips (BBL) to the broth before inoculum addition, and (ii) addition of Fildes reagent (BBL) to Eugonic broth. The 10% concentration of Fildes reagent in Eugonic broth was prepared by the addition of 2.0 ml of the reagent to 16.0 ml of Eugonic broth. The *H. influenzae* inoculum was prepared by the addition of growth from a chocolate agar plate to 5 ml of 0.85% saline solution in an Autobac inoculum standardization tube. The concentration of the inoculum was standardized with the Autobac nephelometer to 1.5×10^7 to 3.0×10^7 colony-forming units per ml. Two milliliters of this inoculum was added to 18 ml of the supplemented Eugonic broth. Ampicillin disks were added to the cuvette, and the cuvette was filled as previously described (12) and incubated at 36°C in the Autobac shaker.

Reading of the Autbac test. The MIC was determined by reading the cuvette in "normal mode" on the Autobac. The "normal mode" compares growth in the control well of the cuvette with growth in each of the wells containing decreasing concentrations of ampicillin. The MIC was taken as the lowest concentration of ampicillin in which no growth of the organism occurred. The arbitrary dilution end point for the reaction can be described as follows: light-scattering indexes (LSIs) of 0.0 to 0.50 and 0.50 to 1.00 were interpreted as indicating growth (resistance) and no growth (susceptibility), respectively.

Agar dilution. The agar dilution susceptibility test was prepared according to the method described by Ericsson and Sherris (3). The agar plates were incubated at 36°C in a CO_2 incubator (8% CO_2) for 24 h and read.

RESULTS

Experiments to determine optimal conditions for the Autobac test revealed that (i) the addition of either XV strips or Fildes reagent to Eugonic broth resulted in identical MICs and no prolongation of incubation time; (ii) no growth of *H. influenzae* was observed in Eugonic broth without added cofactors; and (iii) the addition of Fildes reagent did not alter the final test result by increasing the number of nonbiological particles in the medium. However, the high fiber content of the XV strips contributed significantly to background light scattering.

Figure 1 compares the MICs of ampicillin for 57 strains of *H. influenzae* by the Autobac method and by agar dilution. Twenty-eight isolates were resistant to ampicillin by both methods. With 65% of the isolates (37/57), there was precise quantitative agreement between the Autobac method and the agar dilution method. That is, an MIC of 1.0 μg/ml by Autobac was paralleled by an agar dilution MIC of 1.0 μg/ml. With 91% (52/57) of the isolates, there was no more than a one-dilution-interval difference observed between the methods. Exact interpretive agreement was noted between the two methods.

Figure 2 shows the distribution of MICs as determined by the Autobac method. Two definite populations may be observed: one susceptible (MICs ≤ 0.6 μg/ml) and one resistant (MICs ≥ 10 μg/ml). Five isolates exhibited ampicillin MICs ranging from 1.2 to 5.0 μg/ml.

Representative Autobac readouts for a resistant and a susceptible *H. influenzae* isolate are seen in Fig. 3. The arbitrary LSI value of 0.50 is used as an MIC breakpoint. Comparison with parallel agar dilution MICs has justified the 0.50 cutoff. LSIs of 0.50 to 0.60 for an ampicillin dilution, although indicated by the Autobac computer as "indeterminant," are considered to represent susceptibility of the test organism to the stated concentration of ampicillin in the medium.

DISCUSSION

With only a few clinically significant bacteria, clinicians have been able to predict with 100% reliability that a subsequent in vitro assay would confirm the susceptibility of such an organism to an antibiotic. These include *Streptococcus pyogenes* (penicillin), *Streptococcus pneumoniae* (penicillin), and *H. influenzae* (ampicillin). Recently, however, the emerging resistance of *H. influenzae* to ampicillin has been confirmed. Consequently, the American Academy of Pediatrics (1) recommends that initial therapy for severe *Haemophilus* infections be both chloramphenicol and ampicillin until the susceptibility profile of the isolated *Haemophilus* has been determined in the laboratory.

If the disk diffusion test for susceptiblity of *H. influenzae* is used, then the modifications as proposed by Thornsberry and Kirven (13) must be strictly followed. Problems of false resistance may arise from the lack of standardization of the disk diffusion test. The reliability of test results is of extreme importance, as is the rapidity of generating results.

The development of the Autobac MIC method stemmed from its routine use for screening nonfastidious microorganisms for susceptibility to multiple antibiotics. The multiwelled growth

TABLE 1. *Composition of ampicillin disks*

Disk content (μg)	Final concn in cuvette well (μg/ml)
15.0	10.0
7.5	5.0
3.75	2.5
1.88	1.2
0.94	0.62
0.47	0.31
0.24	0.15

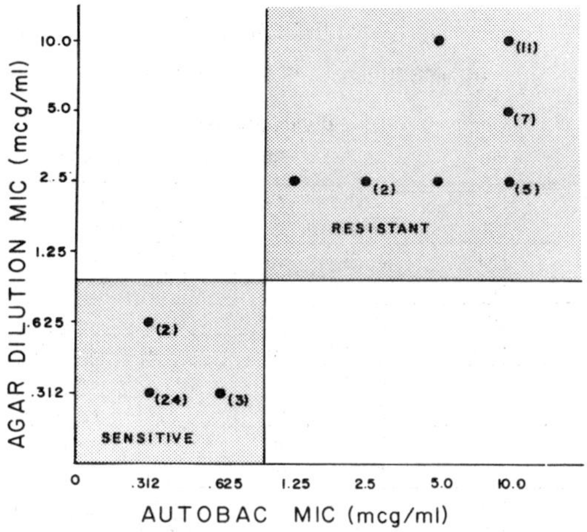

FIG. 1. *Comparison of the ampicillin MICs for Haemophilus influenzae by Autobac and agar dilution.*

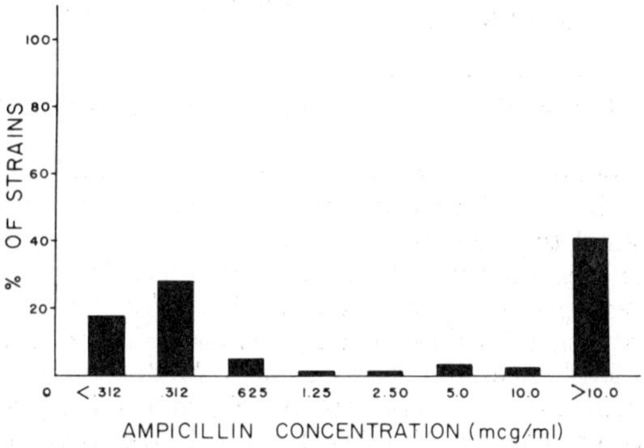

FIG. 2. *Distribution of ampicillin MICs for 57 strains of Haemophilus influenzae.*

autobac 1

ANTIMICROBIAL SUSCEPTIBILITY REPORT

NO.	LSI	INTERPRETATION	ANTIMICROBIAL
12	0.00	R	CONTROL
11	0.00	R	CONTROL
10	0.00	R	CONTROL
09	0.00	R	CONTROL
08	0.04	R	0.156 mcg/ml
07	0.03	R	0.312 mcg/ml
06	0.05	R	0.625 mcg/ml
05	0.04	R	1.25 mcg/ml
04	0.07	R	2.50 mcg/ml
03	0.10	R	5.00 mcg/ml
02	0.15	R	10.00 mcg/ml
01	0.00	R	CONTROL

GRAM NEGATIVE

AMPICILLIN
Concentration

autobac 1

ANTIMICROBIAL SUSCEPTIBILITY REPORT

NO.	LSI	INTERPRETATION	ANTIMICROBIAL
12	0.00	R	CONTROL
11	0.00	R	CONTROL
10	0.00	R	CONTROL
09	0.00	R	CONTROL
08	0.04	R	0.156 mcg/ml
07	0.26	R	0.312 mcg/ml
06	0.57	I	0.625 mcg/ml
05	0.81	S	1.250 mcg/ml
04	0.82	S	2.50 mcg/ml
03	0.88	S	5.00 mcg/ml
02	0.80	S	10.00 mcg/ml
01	0.00	R	CONTROL

GRAM NEGATIVE

AMPICILLIN
Concentration

FIG. 3. *Representative Autobac printouts for resistant and susceptible isolates of Haemophilus influenzae.*

chamber, the antibiotic carrier disk, and the sensitive light-scattering nephelometer provided the technology for a rapid MIC procedure. In the routine use of the Autobac, Eugonic broth is the growth medium. *H. influenzae* will not grow in this medium unless cofactors are added. Supplementation with Fildes reagent promoted detectable growth in 3 to 4 h. Jorgenson and Jones (5) suggested that Fildes reagent caused difficulty in the reading of turbidity. Although such a criticism may be valid for visual scanning of a test, no such difficulty was observed when the test cuvette was read by the nephelometer. Repeated analyses indicated that the particle background of 10% Fildes reagent was minimal, and no interference was observed. This was in contrast to the use of XV disks for nutritional supplementation, which were seen to shed fibers into the medium and cause excessive light scattering.

Early experiments with the Autobac system suggested that there be a provision in the cuvette for use of an increased CO_2 environment. CO_2-generating tablets were added to two empty wells. Subsequently, it was found that the addition of CO_2 prolonged the growth of *H. influenzae,* apparently by increasing the acidity of the medium. Sufficient ambient CO_2 is available in the cuvette to support growth of *H. influenzae* for 5 to 6 h.

Fifty-two of 57 isolates of *H. influenzae* were categorized as either susceptible ($\leq$0.6 μg/ml) or resistant ($\geq$10 μg/ml) by the Autobac MIC method. The remaining five isolates (MICs from 1.2 to 5.0 μg/ml) were arbitrarily classified as resistant to ampicillin. When tested by the agar dilution method, three of these five organisms showed MICs of one to two dilution intervals higher (Fig. 1). The MIC breakpoint for ampicillin between resistant and susceptible populations of *H. influenzae* is unresolved. Smith (10) has stated that the MIC of ampicillin that will inhibit growth ranges from 0.1 to 12.5 μg/ml, whereas resistant organisms require 3 to 500 μg/ml. Such overlap is a function of variability in test methods, particularly inoculum size. As the inoculum is increased, the apparent MIC increases. The Autobac method, as described, uses a final inoculum concentration of 1×10^6 colony-forming units per ml. The use of a larger inoculum might result in fewer isolates with equivocal MICs.

Although the present study used pure cultures of *H. influenzae* growing on chocolate agar plates, the method has been used for the past 6 months on all clinical isolates of *H. influenzae* that require antibiotic susceptibility testing. In practice, the isolates were from cerebrospinal fluid and were observed on chocolate agar after overnight incubation. As with the pure culture isolates, the majority of ampicillin MICs showed exact quantitative agreement with a confirmatory agar dilution test. Because of these results, the Autobac method is being used as the primary method for determining ampicillin MICs.

ACKNOWLEDGMENTS

This study was supported, in part, by a grant from Pfizer Diagnostics, Groton, Conn.

LITERATURE CITED

1. **American Academy of Pediatrics, Committee on Infectious Disease.** 1975. Ampicillin resistant strains of *Haemophilus infleunzae* type b. Pediatrics 55:145–146.
2. **Clymo, A. B., and I. A. Harper.** 1974. Ampicillin resistant *Haemophilus influenzae* meningitis. Lancet i:453–454.
3. **Ericsson, H. M., and J. C. Sherris.** 1971. Antibiotic sensitivity testing. Report of an international collaborative study. Acta Pathol. Microbiol. Scand. Sect. B, Suppl. 217.
4. **Farrar, W. E., and N. M. O'Dell.** 1974. Beta-lactamase activity in ampicillin-resistant *Haemophilus influenzae*. Antimicrob. Agents Chemother. 6:625–629.
5. **Jorgensen, J. H., and P. H. Jones.** 1975. Simplified medium for ampicillin susceptibility testing of *Haemophilus infleunzae*. Antimicrob. Agents Chemother. 7:186–190.
6. **Khan, W., S. Ross, W. Rodriquez, G. Controni, and A. K. Saz.** 1974. *Haemophilus influenzae* type B resistant to ampicillin. A report of two cases. J. Am. Med. Assoc. 229:298–301.
7. **Manten, A., B. van Klingeren, and M. Dessens-Kroon.** 1976. Chloramphenicol resistance in *Haemophilus infleunzae*. Lancet i:702.
8. **Mathies, A. W.** 1972. Penicillins in the treatment of bacterial meningitis. J. R. Coll. Physicians London 6:139–146.
9. **Rubin, F. A., and D. H. Smith.** 1973. Characterization of R-factor beta-lactamases by the acidimetric method. Antimicrob. Agents Chemother. 3:68–73.
10. **Smith, A. L.** 1976. Antibiotics and invasive *Haemophilus infleunzae*. N. Engl. J. Med. 294:1329–1331.
11. **Thomas, W. J., J. W. McReynolds, C. R. Mock, and D. W. Bailey.** 1974. Ampicillin resistant *Haemophilus influenzae* meningitis. Lancet i:313.
12. **Thornsberry, C., T. L. Gavan, J. C. Sherris, A. Balows, J. M. Matsen, L. D. Sabath, F. Schoenknecht, L. D. Thrupp, and J. A. Washington II.** 1975. Laboratory evaluation of a rapid, automated susceptibility testing system: report of a collaborative study. Antimicrob. Agents Chemother. 7:467–480.
13. **Thornsberry, C., and L. A. Kirven.** 1974. Ampicillin resistance in *Haemophilus infleunzae* as determined by a rapid test for beta-lactamase production. Antimicrob. Agents Chemother. 6:653–654.

ANTIMICROBIAL AGENTS AND CHEMOTHERAPY, Jan. 1977, p. 118-121
Copyright © 1977 American Society for Microbiology
Vol. 11, No. 1
Printed in U.S.A.

Antimicrobial Activity In Vitro of Netilmicin and Comparison with Sisomicin, Gentamicin, and Tobramycin

BURT R. MEYERS AND SHALOM Z. HIRSCHMAN*

Divison of Infectious Diseases, Department of Medicine, The Mount Sinai School of Medicine of the City University of New York, New York, New York 10029

Received for publication 13 July 1976

The antimicrobial activity of netilmicin, a new semisynthetic aminoglycosidic aminocyclitol, was determined against 123 recent gram-negative clinical isolates susceptible to gentamicin and 60 isolates resistant to either sisomicin, gentamicin, or tobramycin. The minimal inhibitory concentrations and minimal bactericidal concentrations of netilmicin, sisomicin, gentamicin, and tobramycin against *Pseudomonas, Escherichia coli, Klebsiella, Enterobacter, Proteus mirabilis,* and indole-positive *Proteus* were, in general, quite similar. Gentamicin was the most active against *Serratia*. A total of 54, 67, and 88% of gentamicin-resistant *Pseudomonas, Serratia,* and *Klebsiella,* respectively, were susceptible to netilmicin. Strains of indole-positive *Proteus, Acinetobacter, Providencia,* and *E. coli* resistant to gentamicin were likely to be resistant also to netilmicin.

Netilmicin (Sch 20569) is a new semisynthetic aminoglycosidic aminocyclitol antibiotic similar both in structure and spectrum of antimicrobial activity to gentamicin and sisomicin. Initial work has suggested that netilmicin may be effective against gentamicin-resistant strains of gram-negative bacteria (3) and may have less oto- and nephrotoxicity than gentamicin (Informational material for investigational drug Sch 20569, Schering Corp., Bloomfield, N.J., 1975). We report results of the comparison of the antimicrobial activity in vitro of netilmicin, sisomicin, gentamicin, and tobramycin against recent clinical gram-negative isolates.

MATERIALS AND METHODS

Gram-negative bacterial isolates from recent clinical specimens were obtained from the diagnostic microbiology laboratory of The Mount Sinai Hospital. The isolates included 123 strains susceptible to gentamicin and 60 strains resistant to either gentamicin, sisomicin, or tobramycin. The gentamicin-susceptible strains included 20 *Pseudomonas* sp., 21 *Escherichia coli,* 24 *Klebsiella* sp., 22 *Enterobacter* sp., 9 *Proteus mirabilis,* 9 *Proteus* sp. (indole positive), and 18 *Serratia* sp. The gentamicin-resistant isolates included 13 *Pseudomonas* sp., 2 *Enterobacter* sp., 17 *Klebsiella* sp., 4 indole-positive *Proteus* sp., 13 *Serratia* sp., 2 *Providencia* sp., 6 *E. coli,* and 3 *Acinetobacter* sp. Minimum inhibitory concentrations (MICs) and minimum bactericidal concentrations (MBCs) of netilmicin, sisomicin, gentamicin, and tobramycin for the isolates were determined by the standard twofold tube dilution method in Mueller-Hinton broth as previously described (1, 2). Bacterial isolates inhibited by concentrations ≥6.25 μg/ml of the aminoglycosides were considered to be resistant strains. Netilmicin, sisomicin, and gentamicin were obtained from Schering Corp., Bloomfield, N.J., and tobramycin was obtained from Eli Lilly and Co., Indianapolis, Ind.

RESULTS

The antimicrobial activity in vitro of netilmicin overall was comparable to that of sisomicin, gentamicin, and tobramycin against 123 gram-negative isolates susceptible to gentamicin (Table 1). Neticilin (mean MIC, 0.95 μg/ml) was slightly less active than gentamicin (mean MIC, 0.73 μg/ml) against the 20 strains of gentamicin-susceptible *Pseudomonas* sp. tested; 71% of strains of *Pseudomonas* were inhibited at a concentration of netilmicin of 0.78 μg/ml, whereas 81% were inhibited at the same concentration of gentamicin. Both sisomicin (mean MIC, 0.37 μg/ml) and tobramycin (mean MIC, 0.39 μg/ml) were much more active against these strains. The MICs were only slightly lower than the MBCs.

The mean MIC of netilmicin for 21 strains of *E. coli* tested (0.75 μg/ml) was slightly higher than the mean MIC of gentamicin (0.63 μg/ml), but was lower than the mean MICs of sisomicin (0.85 μg/ml) and tobramycin (0.93 μg/ml) for these strains (Table 1). Eighty-one percent of *E. coli* tested were inhibited by a concentration of 0.78 μg of netilmicin or sisomicin per ml; 90% were inhibited at the same concentration of gentamicin. The mean MICs of the four aminoglycosides were similar against 24 strains of *Klebsiella* sp. tested. Eighty-three percent of *Klebsiella* were inhibited at a concentration of

TABLE 1. *Comparison of in vitro antibacterial activity of netilmicin (N), sisomicin (S), gentamicin (G), and tobramycin (T)*

Microorganism	No. of strains	MIC (μg/ml)				MBC (μg/ml)			
		N	S	G	T	N	S	G	T
Pseudomonas sp.	20	0.95 ± 0.65[a]	0.37 ± 0.16	0.73 ± 0.40	0.39 ± 0.18	1.79 ± 1.45	0.62 ± 0.65	1.18 ± 0.82	0.66 ± 0.61
		(0.39 – 3.12)[b]	(0.2 – 0.78)	(0.2 – 1.56)	(0.2 – 0.78)	(0.39 – 6.25)	(0.2 – 3.12)	(0.2 – 3.12)	(0.2 – 3.12)
Escherichia coli	21	0.75 ± 0.44	0.85 ± 0.38	0.63 ± 0.37	0.93 ± 0.67	1.19 ± 1.32	1.02 ± 0.62	0.97 ± 0.65	1.44 ± 0.92
		(0.2 – 1.56)	(0.39 – 1.56)	(0.2 – 1.56)	(0.2 – 3.12)	(0.2 – 6.25)	(0.39 – 3.12)	(0.2 – 3.12)	(0.9 – 3.12)
Klebsiella sp.	24	0.41 ± 0.20	0.41 ± 0.18	0.45 ± 0.2	0.5 ± 0.22	0.67 ± 0.62	0.58 ± 0.37	0.54 ± 0.36	0.56 ± 0.31
		(0.2 – 0.78)	(0.2 – 0.78)	(0.2 – 0.78)	(0.2 – 0.78)	(0.2 – 3.12)	(0.2 – 1.56)	(0.2 – 1.56)	(0.2 – 0.78)
Enterobacter sp.	22	0.76 ± 0.59	0.67 ± 0.58	0.61 ± 0.59	0.78 ± 0.58	1.04 ± 0.90	0.83 ± 0.79	0.75 ± 0.79	0.9 ± 0.6
		(0.39 – 3.12)	(0.2 – 3.12)	(0.2 – 3.12)	(0.39 – 3.12)	(0.39 – 3.12)	(0.2 – 3.12)	(0.2 – 3.12)	(0.39 – 3.12)
Proteus mirabilis	9	0.95 ± 0.48	0.98 ± 0.56	0.56 ± 0.26	0.67 ± 0.40	1.39 ± 0.78	0.99 ± 0.55	0.87 ± 0.90	1.3 ± 1.09
		(0.39 – 1.56)	(0.39 – 1.56)	(0.2 – 0.78)	(0.2 – 0.78)	(0.78 – 3.12)	(0.39 – 1.56)	(0.02 – 0.78)	(0.2 – 3.12)
Proteus sp. (indole positive)	9	0.56 ± 0.20	0.65 ± 0.19	0.60 ± 0.39	0.73 ± 0.36	1.25 ± 1.11	1.35 ± 1.06	1.12 ± 0.85	1.4 ± 0.72
		(0.39 – 0.78)	(0.39 – 0.78)	(0.39 – 1.56)	(0.39 – 1.56)	(0.39 – 3.12)	(0.39 – 3.12)	(0.39 – 3.12)	(0.78 – 3.12)
Serratia sp.	18	2.73 ± 0.77	1.69 ± 0.72	1.25 ± 0.79	3.91 ± 2.10	3.29 ± 1.5	1.82 ± 0.75	1.47 ± 0.87	4.76 ± 2.53
		(0.78 – 3.12)	(0.78 – 3.12)	(0.39 – 3.12)	(1.56 – 6.25)	(1.56 – 6.25)	(0.78 – 3.12)	(0.78 – 3.12)	(1.56 – 12.5)

[a] Mean ± standard deviation.
[b] Range.

0.39 μg of netilmicin or sisomicin per ml, whereas 75 and 63% were inhibited at the same concentration of gentamicin and tobramycin, respectively. Gentamicin and sisomicin were slightly more active against *Enterobacter* than netilmicin and tobramycin; 95% of strains of *Enterobacter* tested were inhibited by 1.56 μg of netilmicin, sisomicin, gentamicin, and tobramycin per ml. Gentamicin and tobramycin were more active against the strains of *P. mirabilis* tested than were netilmicin and sisomicin. The activities of netilmicin, sisomicin, and gentamicin against nine strains of indole-positive *Proteus* were equivalent. Gentamicin and sisomicin were more active against the 18 strains of *Serratia* tested than were netilmicin and tobramycin. Netilmicin was slightly more active than tobramycin against these strains. Ninety percent of the strains of *Serratia* were inhibited at a concentration of gentamicin of 1.56 μg/ml, whereas 24% of the strains were inhibited at the same concentration of netilmicin; 81% were inhibited by a concentration of 1.56 μg of sisomicin per ml, but only 5% were inhibited at the same concentration of tobramycin.

The antimicorbial activity of netilmicin against 60 gram-negative isolates resistant to either sisomicin, gentamicin, or tobramycin is presented in Fig. 1 and Table 2. Fifty-four percent of gentamicin-resistant strains of *Pseudomonas* were susceptible to netilmicin; 38% of the strains were susceptible to tobramycin, but all were resistant to sisomicin (Fig. 1). Sixty-seven percent of gentamicin-resistant *Serratia* were susceptible to netilmicin (Fig. 1). All the gentamicin-resistant strains of *Serratia* were resistant to sisomicin, whereas 33% were susceptible to tobramycin. Eighty-eight percent of gentamicin-resistant *Klebsiella* were susceptible to netilmicin; all the strains were resistant to sisomicin, whereas only 12% were susceptible to tobramycin (Fig. 1). The two isolates of gentamicin-resistant *Enterobacter* tested were susceptible to netilmicin (Table 2). However, all the gentamicin-resistant strains of indole-positive *Proteus*, *Acinetobacter*, *Providencia*, and *E. coli* were resistant also to netilmicin (Table 2).

DISCUSSION

Our results confirm the data presented recently by Rahal et al. (3) indicating that netilmicin may be an effective antimicrobial agent against gram-negative bacteria and may be especially useful for treatment of infections caused by gentamicin-resistant *Enterobacteriaceae*. All gentamicin-resistant *E. coli* and *Klebsiella* tested by Rahal et al. (3) were susceptible to netilmicin, but these authors did not find netilmicin to be useful against gentamicin-resistant *Pseudomonas*. In contrast, 54% of gentamicin-resistant strains of *Pseudomonas* we tested were susceptible to netilmicin, whereas all our gentamicin-resistant strains of *E. coli* were resistant also to netilmicin. Netilmicin was active against gentamicin-resistant strains of *Serratia, Klebsiella,* and *Enterobacter*. However, gentamicin-resistant strains of indole-positive *Proteus, Acinetobacter,* and *Providencia* appear likely to be resistant also to netilmicin.

Chronic toxicity studies in the rat, dog, and cat suggest that netilmicin may have significantly less oto- and nephrotoxicity than gentamicin. In contrast, acute toxicity studies in these animals revealed netilmicin to have greater toxicity than gentamicin, perhaps due to greater neuromuscular blockade by netilmicin at the higher dose levels. Blood levels of netilmicin in animals are equivalent to those of gentamicin when similar doses are administered (Informational material for the investigational drug Sch 20569, Schering Corp., Bloomfield, N.J., 1975). The effectiveness of netilmi-

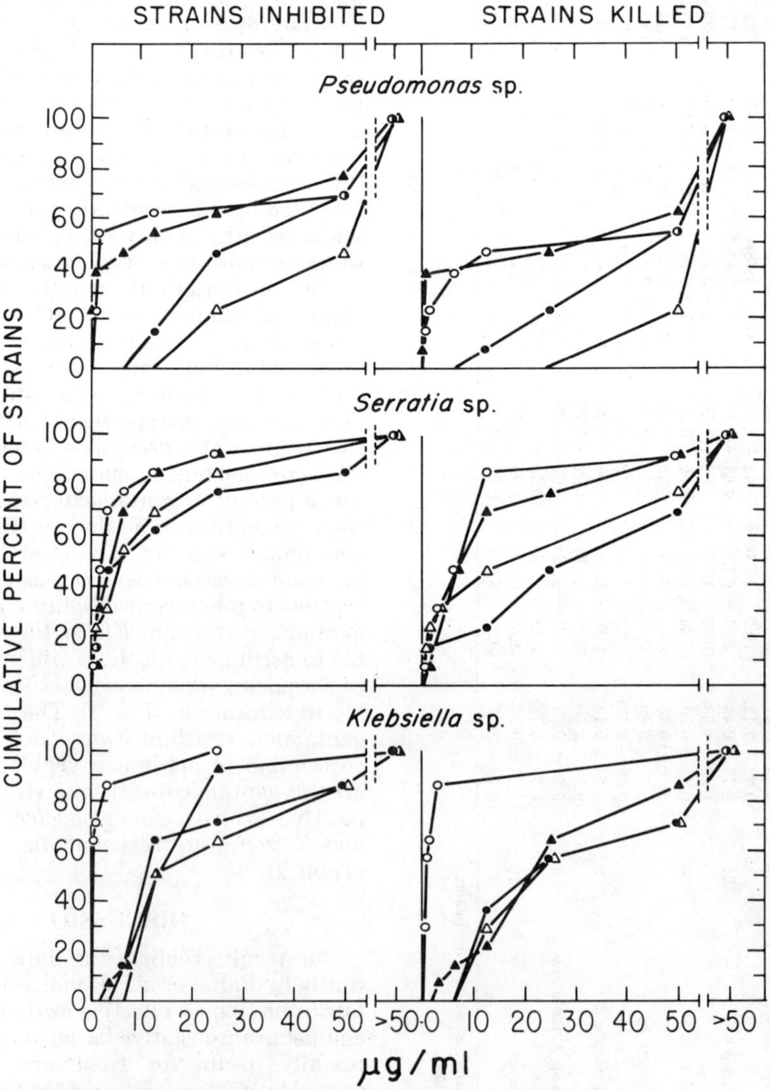

FIG. 1. *Activity of netilmicin against 13 strains each of Pseudomonas sp. and Serratia sp. and 17 strains of Klebsiella sp. resistant to either sisomicin, gentamicin, or tobramycin. Symbols: (○) netilmicin, (●) sisomicin; (△) gentamicin; (▲) tobramycin.*

TABLE 2. *Susceptibility to netilmicin (N) of gram-negative isolates resistant to either sisomicin (S), gentamicin (G), or tobramycin (T)*

Isolate	MIC (μg/ml)				MBC (μg/ml)			
	N	S	G	T	N	S	G	T
Enterobacter sp.	0.78	>12.5	>12.5	1.56	3.12	>12.5	>12.5	6.25
A.A. 676	1.56	>12.5	>12.5	6.25	3.12	>12.5	>12.5	12.5
A.Cl. 314								
Proteus sp. (indole positive)								
101	>50	>50	>50	>50	>50	>50	>50	>50
494	6.25	6.25	6.25	1.56	6.25	6.25	6.25	6.25
168	50	>50	>50	12.5	>50	>50	>50	>50
172	50	>50	>50	12.5	50	>50	>50	12.5
Acinetobacter sp.								
988	>50	25	>50	12.5	>50	25	>50	12.5
163	>50	25	>50	12.5	>50	25	>50	12.5
444	>50	25	>50	6.25	>50	25	>50	12.5
Providencia sp.								
185	50	6.25	50	12.5	50	6.25	50	50
196	>50	>50	>50	>50	>50	>50	>50	50
E. coli								
170	50	>50	>50	25	50	>50	>50	>50
173	25	>50	>50	50	50	>50	>50	50
175	25	>50	>50	50	50	>50	>50	>50
180	3.12	1.56	3.12	6.25	3.12	3.12	3.12	12.5
181	50	>50	>50	>50	>50	>50	>50	>50
193	>50	>50	>50	>50	>50	>50	>50	>50

cin in in vitro studies against gram-negative isolates, especially against gentamicin-resistant bacteria, suggests that this new aminoglycosidic aminocyclitol warrants clinical investigation for the treatment of patients with infections due to gram-negative bacteria, especially those resistant to gentamicin.

ACKNOWLEDGMENTS

We are grateful for the technical assistance of Z. Sadka. This work was supported by a grant from Schering Corp.

LITERATURE CITED

1. **Meyers, B. R., and S. Z. Hirschman.** 1972. Tobramycin: in vitro antibacterial spectrum of a new aminoglycoside. J. Clin. Pharmacol. 12:313–320.
2. **Meyers, B. R., B. Leng, and S. Z. Hirschman.** 1975. Comparison of the antimicrobial activities of sisomicin and gentamicin against gram-negative bacteria. Antimicrob. Agents Chemother. 8:757–758.
3. **Rahal, J. J., Jr., M. S. Simberkoff, K. Kagan, and N. H. Moldover.** 1976. Bactericidal efficacy of Sch 20569 and amikacin against gentamicin-sensitive and -resistant organisms. Antimicrob. Agents Chemother. 9:595–599.

ANTIMICROBIAL AGENTS AND CHEMOTHERAPY, Jan. 1977, p. 122-125
Vol. 11, No. 1

Inhibition of Multiplication of *Mycobacterium leprae* by Polyinosinic-Polycytidylic Acid

LOUIS LEVY AND THOMAS C. MERIGAN*

*Leprosy Research Unit, Public Health Service Hospital, San Francisco, California 94118, and Division of Infectious Diseases, Department of Medicine, Stanford University School of Medicine, Stanford, California 94305**

Received for publication 17 May 1976

Contrary to the results of an earlier study in which polyinosinic-polycytidylic acid [poly(I:C)] administered intraperitoneally to mice had no effect on multiplication of *Mycobacterium leprae* in the mouse footpad, the local administration of poly(I:C) every 12 h for 15 doses during logarithmic multiplication was found both to inhibit bacterial multiplication and to produce high tissue levels of interferon (IF). Local administration of poly(I) alone inhibited multiplication of *M. leprae* to almost as great a degree without at the same time producing a measurable IF titer in the footpad tissues. Mouse IF and "mock" IF both inhibited bacterial multiplication to the same degree, but administration of only the former resulted in a measurable IF titer. Polyadenylic-polyuridylic acid administered locally neither inhibited multiplication nor induced IF; fetal calf serum, administered in the same concentration as found in the preparations of IF and mock IF, was modestly inhibitory, without inducing IF. Thus, the local administration of poly(I:C) appears to have inhibited multiplication of *M. leprae* independently of IF induction.

Polyinosinic-polycytidylic acid [poly(I:C)] is a synthetic double-stranded ribonucleic acid that stimulates production of interferon (IF) both in vivo and in vitro (2). In addition, the compound inhibits multiplication in vivo of a number of bacterial, fungal, and protozoal pathogens, apparently by mechanisms distinct from that of IF induction (reviewed in 6). It was somewhat surprising to find that, in an earlier study (5), poly(I:C) administered intraperitoneally (i.p.) to mice in a dosage of 150 μg three times weekly for 5 months, beginning at the time of inoculation, exhibited no effect on multiplication of *Mycobacterium leprae* in the mouse footpad. The subsequent demonstration that a state of tolerance quickly develops upon repeated administration of poly(I:C) (4) stimulated us to carry out a series of experiments in which the compound was administered locally every 12 h for 1 week during logarithmic multiplication of the organisms. When poly(I:C) was administered in this manner, multiplication of *M. leprae* was inhibited; the mechanism of inhibition appeared to be independent of IF induction.

MATERIALS AND METHODS

Locally bred female BALB/c mice were used in this study, as were *M. leprae* of the strain that had been employed in an earlier study (5). Poly(I:C) was prepared from crystalline poly(C) and poly(I) purchased from Miles Laboratories Inc., Elkhart, Ind. Polyadenylic-polyuridylic acid [poly(A:U)] was prepared from crystalline poly(A) and poly(U), also purchased from Miles Laboratories. IF was prepared as described elsewhere (3) by stimulation with Newcastle disease virus and concentrated 10-fold by pressure dialysis using an Amicon UM-10 membrane. Mock IF was prepared in an identical fashion except that the cells were not infected with Newcastle disease virus. This material, which represents an uninfected tissue culture supernatant, shows no antiviral activity.

Three experiments were carried out. In each experiment, mice were inoculated in both hind footpads with $10^{3.7}$ *M. leprae*. Beginning 70 days later, various treatments were administered every 12 h for 15 doses to groups of 30 mice. Eight mice were exsanguinated 1 h after dose 3, and eight more were exsanguinated after dose 15; serum was separated and stored frozen for later IF assay. At these same intervals, footpad tissues were excised, pooled, homogenized, and stored frozen for IF assay. At about 100 days after inoculation, two mice from each group were sacrificed, and *M. leprae* were harvested from the pooled tissues of four footpads and enumerated by published methods (7, 8). Subsequent harvests of *M. leprae* also from the pooled tissues of four footpads were scheduled by the results of these initial harvests. The results of at least two harvests of *M. leprae* from the footpads of treated and untreated mice were employed to construct bacterial growth curves, to which straight lines were fit by the method of least squares. From each straight line, which represented the logarithmic phase of bacterial multiplication, the time required for multiplication to the level of 10^6 *M. leprae* per footpad was estimated. These estimates of the time elapsed between inoculation and multiplication to 10^6 organisms per footpad were used to calculate the time interval between pairs of growth curves. Based on 129 measurements of the doubling time of this strain of *M. leprae* during logarithmic multiplication in the footpad of the BALB/c mouse (W. M. Krushat, K. E. Schilling, S. A. Edlavitch, and L. Levy, Lepr. Rev., in press), a displacement in the growth curves of 14 days represents a significant delay in multiplication of organisms.

In experiment 1 (m 1-29-74), 0.3 ml of phosphate-buffered saline (PBS) and 150 μg of poly(I:C) were administered i.p. to two groups of mice. Other groups of mice were injected in both hind footpads with 0.05 ml of PBS, 12.5 μg of poly(I:C), and 12.5 μg of poly(I). In experiment 2 (m 4-19-74), 0.05 ml of PBS, 12.5 μg of poly(I:C), 0.05 ml of IF, and 0.05 ml of mock IF were administered in the footpads. To the mice of experiment 3 (m 8-26-75), 0.05 ml of PBS, 12.5 μg of poly(I:C), 12.5 μg of poly(A:U), 0.05 ml of mock IF, and 0.05 ml of a 2% solution of fetal calf serum (FCS) were injected into both hind footpads.

Mouse sera and the homogenates of footpad tissues were assayed for IF by plaque assay using vesicular stomatitis virus and L cell monolayers (3).

RESULTS

The results of harvests of *M. leprae* from footpad tissues and of assays of IF in sera and footpad tissue homogenates are summarized in Table 1. In addition, the effects of treatment of mice with the synthetic polynucleotides are shown in Fig. 1. The i.p. administration of PBS and of poly(I:C) was without effect on multiplication of *M. leprae*. Administration of PBS into the footpads inhibited multiplication to a minor degree in two experiments and not at all in the third. The local administration of poly(I:C) was associated with marked inhibition of multiplication of *M. leprae* in all three experiments. In addition, poly(I) was markedly inhibitory in the first experiment, and poly(A:U) was without effect in the third experiment. The latter two synthetic polynucleotide preparations were used because they are known to exhibit some of the biological activities of poly(I:C) but are not as active in interferon stimulation (1).

In the second experiment, local administration of both IF and mock IF was markedly inhibitory; the effects of the two treatments were virtually identical. In the final experiment, locally administered mock IF was again found to produce marked inhibition of multiplication of *M. leprae,* whereas 2% FCS was only modestly effective.

A high IF titer was measured in the serum after the third i.p. dose of poly(I:C), and a small but significant titer was measured after the last dose; no IF was detected in footpad homogenates after i.p. administration of poly(I:C). Administration of poly(I:C) into the footpads produced measurable levels of IF both in serum and in the injected tissues. The highest titer of

TABLE 1. *Inhibition of multiplication of M. leprae and interferon titers after various treatments of mice*

Treatment	Route[a]	Expt no.	Delay of multiplication of *M. leprae*[b] (days)	Interferon titer 1 h after dose: Serum (U/ml) 3[c]	Serum (U/ml) 15	Homogenate (U/g) 3	Homogenate (U/g) 15
PBS	i.p.	1	0	–[d]	–	<390	–
	f.p.	1	22	–	–	–	<390
		2	17	–	–	–	–
		3	0	<10	<10	<166	<166
Poly(I:C)	i.p.	1	0	>1,000	56	<390	<390
	f.p.	1	93	310	–	2,300	312
		2	67	1,428	–	<390	–
		3	55	233	20	431	580
Poly(I)	f.p.	1	74	<20	–	<390	<390
Poly(A:U)	f.p.	3	0	<10	<10	<166	<166
IF	f.p.	2	54	–	–	2,850	–
Mock IF	f.p.	2	48	–	–	–	–
		3	52	<10	<10	<166	<166
FCS	f.p.	3	28	<20	<10	<166	<166

[a] i.p., Intraperitoneal; f.p., footpad.

[b] The delay is measured as the interval between the growth curve of *M. leprae* in treated mice and that in the appropriate control mice. For PBS treatment, the delay is that compared to multiplication in untreated mice. For all other treatments, the delay is that compared to multiplication in PBS-treated mice. A delay of 14 days or longer is significant.

[c] Dose number.

[d] –, Not measured.

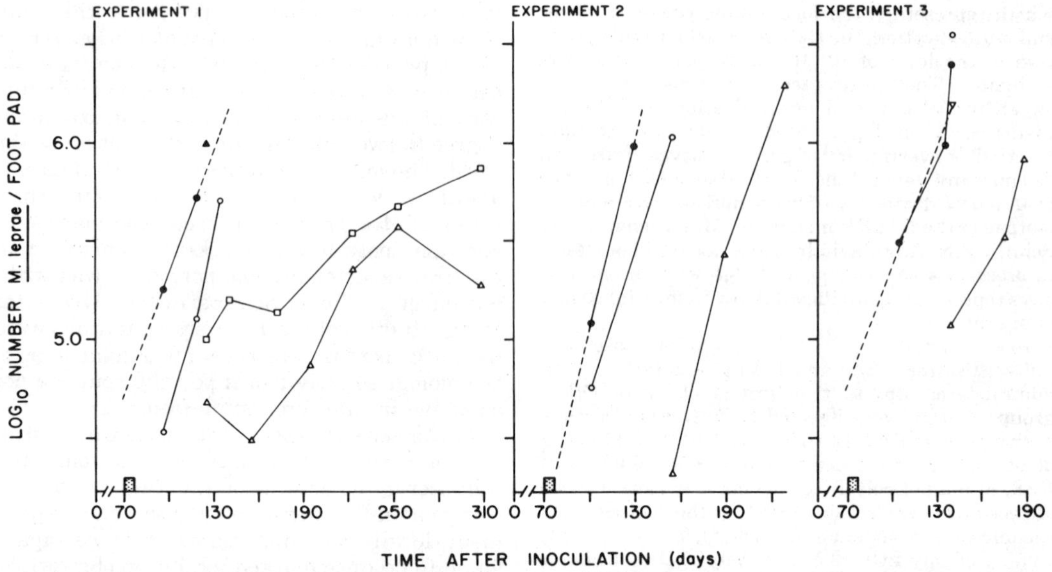

FIG. 1. *Log_{10} number of M. leprae per mouse footpad as a function of time after inoculation. Mice were inoculated with $10^{3.7}$ M. leprae on day zero. Treatments were administered at intervals of 12 h for 15 doses during the interval indicated by the stippled bar on each abscissa. Symbols:* (●) *results of harvests of M. leprae from untreated control mice;* (○) *harvests from saline-injected mice;* (□) *harvests from mice administered poly(I), 12.5 μg/footpad;* (▲) *harvest from mice administered poly(I:C), 50 μg i.p.;* (△) *harvests from mice administered poly(I:C), 12.5 μg/footpad;* (▽) *harvest from mice administered poly(A:U), 12.5 μg/footpad. The broken lines represent logarithmic multiplication of M. leprae in control mice.*

IF (7,200 U/g) was measured in homogenates of footpad tissues excised 10 min after dose 3 of IF in experiment 2; the titer had decayed to an undetectable level by 6 h after the dose. No significant level of IF was detected in serum or in footpad tissue homogenates after footpad administration of mock IF, FCS, poly(I), and poly(A:U).

DISCUSSION

The purpose of this study was twofold. We wished to study the action of poly(I:C) in *M. leprae*-infected mice when the compound was administered locally by a schedule designed to produce high IF titers in the infected footpad tissues. In addition, we wished to learn whether or not an effect of poly(I:C) on multiplication of *M. leprae* could be related to its activity as an inducer of IF.

In our earlier experiment, IF titers in the serum ranged from 10 to 65 U/4 ml during thrice-weekly administration of poly(I:C) over a period of 5 months, beginning with the day mice were inoculated with *M. leprae* (5). If the low titers may be accepted as evidence that the mice had become tolerant to the IF-inducing activity of poly(I:C), then the development of tolerance while the *M. leprae* were still in lag phase could account for the failure of poly(I:C) to inhibit multiplication of the organisms in that experiment. However, this explanation is unlikely because of the lack of effect of i.p. administered poly(I:C), despite a high titer of IF in the serum in our experiment 1. It is perhaps more significant that i.p. administration of poly(I:C) did not produce detectable levels of IF in footpad tissue homogenates.

In the current experiments, the local administration of poly(I:C) produced a considerable effect on multiplication of *M. leprae* concomitant with high IF titers in both the infected tissues and serum. This effect may have been produced by one of four mechanisms: (i) the effect may have been mediated by IF produced in response to the poly(I:C); (ii) the local inflammatory response to repeated needling of the footpad tissues could have been responsible for the effect observed; (iii) poly(I:C) may have nonspecifically enhanced the immune response of the mice to *M. leprae*; (iv) poly(I:C) may have exerted a direct antimicrobial effect on the organisms.

The results of administration of poly(I) and of IF to the footpads appear to exclude the first mechanism. Thus, poly(I) administration inhibited bacterial multiplication without producing high local titers of IF. Furthermore, IF administration resulted in high titers of IF in the footpad tissues and yet inhibited multiplication of *M. leprae* to no greater a degree than did local administration of mock IF. Taken together, these results suggest that poly(I:C) affected multiplication of *M. leprae* independently of its activity as an inducer of IF.

The histopathological examination of footpad tissues obtained from mice of all treatment groups 8 h after the last injections did not distinguish among the treatments. All of the tissues revealed large infiltrates in which large mononuclear cells with vacuolated cytoplasm were the dominant cell type. A few polymorphonuclear leucocytes and even fewer lymphocytes were noted. Although the inconsistent effects of saline injection could perhaps be attributed to the inflammation produced by repeated needling of the tissues, most of the other treatments produced significantly greater effects. Neither mock IF nor FCS could be considered to have acted in a specific fashion. The repeated injection of a foreign protein may well have sensitized the animals and provoked delay-type hypersensitivity, resulting in an inflammatory reaction more intense than that to the repeated injection of saline. It appears also that its content of FCS is only a partial explanation of the activity of mock IF.

The most likely explanation of the activity of poly(I:C) is that of nonspecific enhancement of the immune response of the mice to *M. leprae* or that of a direct antimicrobial effect of the drug. The results of the experiments reported here do not permit a distinction between the two alternatives. However, the great variety of infectious process in which poly(I:C) is active (6) argues against a direct antimicrobial effect on *M. leprae*.

Finally, the nature of the effect of locally administered poly(I:C) on multiplication of *M. leprae* must be considered. The delayed multiplication of *M. leprae* in the footpads of treated mice may represent inhibition of multiplication that endured for a time somewhat longer than the period of treatment. Alternatively, the delay may be attributed to a bactericidal effect of the treatment that falls short of eradication of the infection. In this latter instance, the delay occurs because multiplication resumes from only the surviving fraction of the population of *M. leprae*. The duration of the delay is proportional to the fraction of organisms killed; although the surviving organisms may resume multiplication immediately upon withdrawal of the drug, the first generations result in numbers of acid-fast bacillus too small to be detected. The parallel character of many of the growth curves suggests that the surviving *M. leprae* multiply at the same rate as in untreated mice. This interpretation appears to fit best the data shown in Fig. 1. Particularly in experiment 1, the suggestion that treatment with poly(I:C) was accompanied by bacterial killing is supported by the failure of multiplication of *M. leprae* to increase beyond the level of $10^{5.6}$ organisms per footpad in poly(I:C)-treated mice and by the apparent decrease of the number of *M. leprae* between 253 and 308 days after inoculation. It appears likely that the infection had been eradicated in some of the inoculated footpads and that tissues devoid of *M. leprae* diluted the organisms present in other footpads when the tissues of a number of footpads were pooled for harvesting.

ACKNOWLEDGMENTS

This work was supported by Public Health Service grants AI-05629 and AI-07801, from the National Institute of Allergy and Infectious Diseases.

Michael J. Evans, Stanford Research Institute, Menlo Park, Calif., graciously performed the histopathological examination of the injected footpad tissues.

LITERATURE CITED

1. **Beers, R. F., and W. Braun (ed.).** 1971. Biological effects of polynucleotides. Springer-Verlag, New York.
2. **Field, A. K., A. A. Tytell, G. P. Lampson, and M. R. Hilleman.** 1967. Inducers of interferon and host resistance. II. Multistranded synthetic polynucleotide complexes. Proc. Natl. Acad. Sci. U.S.A. **58:**1004–1010.
3. **Hanna, L., T. C. Merigan, and E. Jawetz.** 1966. Inhibition of TRIC agents by virus-induced interferon. Proc. Soc. Exp. Biol. Med. **122:**417–421.
4. **Ho, M., M. K. Breinig, B. Postic, and J. A. Armstrong.** 1970. The effect of pre-injections on the stimulation of interferon by a complexed polynucleotide, endotoxin, and virus. Ann. N.Y. Acad. Sci. **173:**680–693.
5. **Levy, L., and T. C. Merigan.** 1970. Failure of an interferon inducer to inhibit multiplication of *Mycobacterium leprae*. Proc. Soc. Exp. Biol. Med. **134:**87–89.
6. **Merigan, T. C.** 1973. *In* N. B. Finter (ed.), Interferons and interferon inducers. North-Holland Publishing Co., Amsterdam.
7. **Shepard, C. C.** 1960. The experimental disease that follows the injection of human leprosy bacilli into footpads of mice. J. Exp. Med. **112:**445–454.
8. **Shepard, C. C., and D. H. McRae.** 1968. A method for counting acid-fast bacteria. Int. J. Lepr. **36:**78–82.

Antimicrobial Agents and Chemotherapy, Jan. 1977, p. 126–131
Vol. 11, No. 1

In Vitro Activity of Netilmicin, Gentamicin, and Amikacin

ROBERT J. KANTOR and CARL W. NORDEN*

Department of Medicine, Montefiore Hospital and University of Pittsburgh School of Medicine, Pittsburgh, Pennsylvania 15213

Received for publication 11 August 1976

The in vitro activity of netilmicin (Sch 20569), a new semisynthetic derivative of gentamicin, was compared with that of gentamicin and amikacin. One hundred and ninety-two clinical isolates of *Enterobacteriaceae*, *Pseudomonas aeruginosa*, and *Staphylococcus aureus* were tested using both agar and broth dilution techniques. Netilmicin was comparable to gentamicin, with the following exceptions: (i) for *Serratia marcescens* and *P. aeruginosa*, gentamicin was more active than netilmicin; (ii) all strains of *Escherichia coli*, *Klebsiella*, *Enterobacter*, *Proteus mirabilis*, and *Citrobacter freundii*, which were resistant to gentamicin, were susceptible to netilmicin; (iii) some strains of *S. marcescens*, indole-positive *Proteus*, and *Providencia*, which were resistant to gentamicin, were susceptible to netilmicin. Netilmicin was more active than amikacin for all *Enterobacteriaceae* and *S. aureus* and equal to amikacin in activity against gentamicin-susceptible strains of *P. aeruginosa*. All strains of *P. aeruginosa*, resistant to gentamicin, were also resistant to netilmicin but were susceptible to amikacin. Minimal inhibitory concentrations (MICs) obtained with broth and agar showed no significant differences except for *P. mirabilis*, where broth MICs were twofold greater than agar MICs, and for *P. aeruginosa*, where agar MICs were twofold higher than broth MICs. The minimal bactericidal concentration (MBC) was either identical to or within one twofold dilution of the MIC for the strains tested. A 100-fold increase in inoculum size produced less increase in MIC and MBC with netilmicin than with gentamicin or amikacin.

Although gentamicin has proven to be an effective antibiotic for treatment of serious infections due to gram-negative bacteria, several problems have developed which limit its usefulness. First, administration of the maximum nontoxic doses of gentamicin often results in serum concentrations that are just above the minimal inhibitory concentrations (MICs) for many pathogens. Second, the ratio between therapeutic and toxic levels of gentamicin is narrow and the level obtained after a given dose is not always predictable, thus necessitating frequent monitoring of blood levels. Third, nosocomial infections are being caused with increasing frequency by organisms resistant to gentamicin. Newer antibiotics are being sought and tested in an effort to overcome these problems. One such agent is netilmicin (formerly Sch 20569), a semisynthetic aminoglycoside which is a derivative of sisomycin (4). This report presents the results of in vitro susceptibility testing of netilmicin, amikacin, and gentamicin for 192 clinical isolates. The MICs as determined in broth and agar were compared, the effect of increased inoculum size on MIC and minimal bactericidal concentration (MBC) was determined, and the bactericidal activity of the three antibiotics was measured.

MATERIALS AND METHODS

Antimicrobial agents. Netilmicin and gentamicin were supplied by the Schering Corp., and amikacin was supplied by Bristol Laboratories. The 1,000-μg/ml standards, prepared in 0.1 M phosphate buffer (pH 8.0), were stored at −70°C. Subsequent dilutions were made in 0.1 M phosphate buffer (pH 8.0).

Bacterial isolates. One hundred and eighty-two strains were obtained from isolates from clinical material submitted to the microbiology laboratory at Montefiore Hospital, Pittsburgh, Pa. Additional organisms resistant to gentamicin were obtained from specimens submitted to the microbiology laboratories at Mercy Hospital, Pittsburgh, Pa. (four *Pseudomonas aeruginosa*), Presbyterian University Hospital, Pittsburgh, Pa. (one indole-positive *Proteus*), and the Veteran's Administration Hospital, Pittsburgh, Pa. (two *Escherichia coli*, one *Klebsiella*, one *Enterobacter aerogenes*, and one *Providencia*).

A total of 192 bacterial strains were tested, including: 31 *E. coli*, 28 *Klebsiella*, 22 *Proteus mirabilis*, 16 indole-positive *Proteus*, 48 *P. aeruginosa*, 23 *Staphylococcus aureus*, 11 *Serratia marcescens*, and 13 miscellaneous (7 *Providencia*, 1 *E. aerogenes*, and

5 *Citrobacter freundii*). For analysis, the strains were divided into two groups: 133 that were susceptible to gentamicin (MIC ≤8.0 μg/ml) and 59 (34 *Enterobacteriaceae* and 25 *P. aeruginosa*) that were resistant to gentamicin (MIC >8.0 μg/ml). The 34 *Enterobacteriaceae* that were resistant to gentamicin included: 5 *E. coli*, 3 *Klebsiella*, 1 *E. aerogenes*, 3 *S. marcescens*, 8 indole-positive *Proteus*, 7 *Providencia*, 2 *P. mirabilis*, and 5 *C. freundii*.

Susceptibility testing. MICs for netilmicin, gentamicin, and amikacin were determined by both the agar and broth dilution methods.

(i) Agar dilution method. Square petri dishes were each filled with 20 ml of Mueller-Hinton agar containing twofold dilutions of antibiotic ranging from 0.12 to 256 μg/ml. The bacterial inoculum was prepared by growing individual strains overnight in 1 ml of Mueller-Hinton broth (MHB) and then diluting 1:100 in MHB just prior to inoculation onto drug-containing plates. A Steers replicating device was used which delivered 36 inocula, each containing approximately 0.002 ml, onto the surface of the agar plates. The plates were then incubated at 37°C for 18 h. The MIC was defined as that concentration of antibiotic at which fewer than five colonies grew at the site of inoculation.

(ii) Broth dilution methods. Disposable plastic microtiter U plates with 96 wells were used. Antibiotics were diluted in MHB, and 50 μl was placed in each well. A culture, grown overnight in MHB, was diluted 1:10,000, and 50 μl was then added to each well containing antibiotic. The trays were incubated at 37°C for 18 h. The MIC was defined as that concentration at which there was no visible growth. After determining the MIC, 0.01 ml was removed from each well containing no visible growth, plated on antibiotic-free media, and incubated for 18 h. The MBC was defined as the concentration of antibiotic at which 99.9% of the organisms were killed.

Bactericidal activity. One strain of *Klebsiella* and one strain of *P. aeruginosa* were each grown overnight in MHB. Each suspension was then diluted 1:100 in MHB and added to an equal volume of antibiotic to make a final concentration that was eight times the MIC for that organism. The mixtures were incubated at 37°C, and the number of colony-forming units (CFU) was determined by pour-plate dilutions just after mixing and 3, 6, and 24 h later.

RESULTS

Susceptibility of gentamicin-susceptible organisms to netilmicin and amikacin. The activity of netilmicin, gentamicin, and amikacin was compared for 133 clinical isolates that were susceptible to gentamicin (MIC ≤8 μg/ml). Results of MICs as measured in broth and agar were generally comparable except as noted later. Unless specified otherwise, all results were obtained with the broth dilution method.

Netilmicin showed a wide spectrum of activity against the gram-negative organisms and *S. aureus* (Fig. 1). At a concentration of 1 μg/ml, netilmicin inhibited 100% of *E. coli*, *K. pneumoniae*, and *S. aureus*, 75% of indole-positive *Proteus* and *S. marcescens*, 58% of *P. aeruginosa*, and 30% of *P. mirabilis*. At a concentration of 2 μg/ml, 85% or more of strains of *P. mirabilis*, indole-positive *Proteus*, *S. marcescens*, and *P. aeruginosa* were inhibited. At a concentration of 4 μg/ml, 100% of gentamicin-susceptible strains tested were inhibited by netilmicin except for two isolates of *P. aeruginosa*, which had MICs of 8 and 64 μg/ml; the MICs to gentamicin for these isolates were 2 and 8 μg/ml, respectively.

In general, netilmicin was comparable to gentamicin but more active than amikacin for *Enterobacteriaceae* and *S. aureus* (Table 1; Fig. 2). With *S. marcescens*, however, gentamicin was more active than both netilmicin and amikacin. At 1 μg/ml, 100% of *Serratia* strains were inhibited by gentamicin, with a geometric mean MIC of 0.46 μg/ml. At this same concentration, only 75% of *Serratia* strains were inhibited by netilmicin (geometric mean MIC, 1.09 μg/ml) and 63% by amikacin (geometric mean MIC, 1.68 μg/ml).

Netilmicin was found to be comparable to amikacin but less active than gentamicin against *P. aeruginosa*. At 1 μg/ml, 87% of *Pseudomonas* strains were inhibited by gentamicin (geometric mean MIC, 0.59 μg/ml) compared to 66% by amikacin (geometric mean MIC, 1.22 μg/ml) and 58% by netilmicin (geometric mean MIC, 1.41 μg/ml).

Susceptibility of gentamicin-resistant organisms to netilmicin and amikacin. The activity of netilmicin was compared with that of amikacin for 34 *Enterobacteriaceae* and 25 *P. aeruginosa* that were resistant to gentamicin

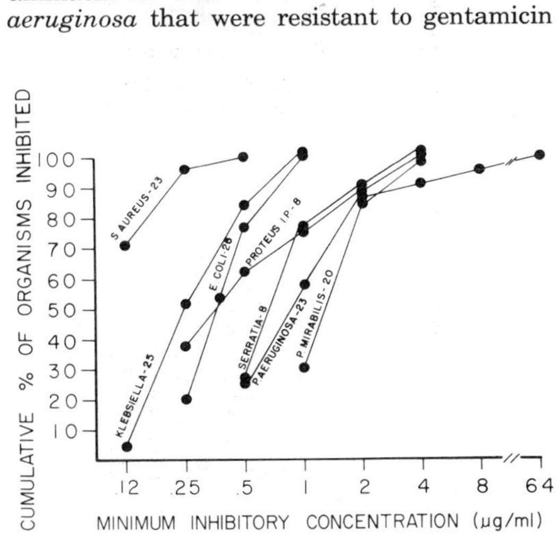

FIG. 1. *Susceptibility of gentamicin-susceptible isolates to netilmicin. The number of strains tested is indicated.*

TABLE 1. *Comparison of in vitro activity in broth and agar for netilmicin, gentamicin, and amikacin against gentamicin-susceptible isolates*

Isolates (no.)	Geometric mean MIC (range)					
	Netilmicin		Gentamicin		Amikacin	
	Broth	Agar	Broth	Agar	Broth	Agar
E. coli (26)	0.51 (0.25–1)	0.51 (0.25–1)	0.57 (0.25–1)	0.50 (0.25–2)	2.20 (1–4)	1.90 (1–8)
K. pneumoniae (25)	0.38 (0.12–1)	0.40 (0.25–1)	0.57 (0.125–8)	0.45 (0.125–8)	1.50 (1–4)	1.28 (0.5–4)
P. mirabilis (20)	1.80 (1–4)	0.81 (0.5–2)	1.27 (0.5–4)	0.66 (0.25–1)	4 (2–8)	2.30 (1–4)
Indole-positive *Proteus* (8)	0.65 (0.25–4)	0.56 (0.12–4)	0.71 (0.125–4)	0.60 (0.25–4)	1.19 (0.25–4)	1.19 (0.25–4)
S. marcescens (8)	1.09 (0.5–4)	1.30 (0.5–4)	0.46 (0.25–1)	0.50 (0.25–1)	1.68 (1–4)	1.83 (1–4)
P. aeruginosa (23)	1.41 (0.5–64)	2.87 (0.5–64)	0.59 (0.125–8)	1.20 (0.5–8)	1.22 (0.5–4)	1.73 (1–4)
S. aureus (23)	0.16 (0.125–0.5)	0.18 (0.125–0.5)	0.15 (0.125–0.25)	0.15 (0.125–0.5)	0.46 (0.25–2)	0.75 (0.125–2)

(MIC >8 μg/ml) (Table 2). At 8 μg/ml, amikacin inhibited 32 (94%) of 34 *Enterobacteriaceae* isolates, compared to 24 (71%) for netilmicin. Five isolates of indole-positive *Proteus* were resistant to netilmicin but susceptible to amikacin, with MICs ranging from 1 to 4 μg/ml. Four isolates of *Providencia* were resistant to netilmicin with MICs ≥64 μg/ml; the MICs to amikacin ranged from 2 to 16 μg/ml. One isolate of *S. marcescens* was resistant to netilmicin, with an MIC of 16 μg/ml; the MIC to amikacin was 4 μg/ml.

All 25 isolates of *P. aeruginosa* were resistant to netilmicin and had comparable MICs to gentamicin. Amikacin inhibited 24 (96%) of 25 isolates at 4 μg/ml and inhibited all isolates at 8 μg/ml.

Comparison of MICs in agar and broth. Comparison of the MICs obtained with MHB and agar showed no significant differences for *Enterobacteriaceae* except for *P. mirabilis* strains, where broth MICs were usually twofold greater than agar MICs (Table 1). The opposite effect was seen for *P. aeruginosa* in that the agar MIC generally averaged twofold greater. Amikacin showed less discrepancy between agar and broth MICs for *Pseudomonas* than did netilmicin or gentamicin. For *S. aureus*, broth and agar MICs were comparable with netilmicin and gentamicin; however, for amikacin, MICs measured by the broth dilution technique were slightly lower than when measured in agar.

Comparison of MBC to MIC. The MBC was determined by the broth dilution technique for eight *Enterobacteriaceae* and three *P. aeruginosa* strains. Inocula of 10^5 and 10^7 CFU/ml were tested. The MBC was identical to or within one tube difference of the MIC for the three aminoglycosides regardless of inoculum size; however, for one strain of *E. coli*, the MBC to amikacin was fourfold greater than the MIC at an inoculum size of 10^7 CFU/ml.

Effect of increasing the inoculum size on MIC and MBC. Twenty-four strains (5 *E. coli*, 5 *Klebsiella*, 5 *P. mirabilis*, 5 *P. aeruginosa*, 2 *S. marcescens*, 2 indole-positive *Proteus*) were tested to determine the effect on the MIC (measured by broth dilution) of increasing the inoculum size 100-fold, i.e., from 10^5 to 10^7 CFU/ml (Table 3). A fourfold increase was seen in four strains with netilmicin, 11 strains with gentamicin, and 14 strains with amikacin.

Eleven strains (2 *E. coli*, 3 *Klebsiella*, 2 *S. marcescens*, 4 *P. aeruginosa*) were tested to determine the effect on the MBC of increasing the inoculum size from 10^5 to 10^7 CFU/ml. A fourfold increase was seen in two strains with netilmicin, five strains with gentamicin, and seven strains with amikacin.

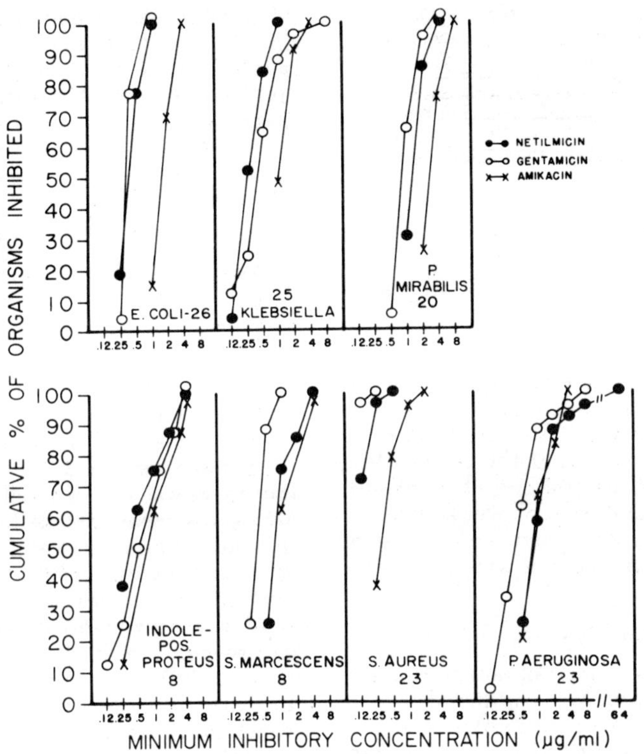

Fig. 2. *Comparison of activity of netilmicin with gentamicin and amikacin against gentamicin-susceptible isolates. The number of strains tested is indicated.*

Table 2. *Comparison of MICs to netilmicin and amikacin for organisms resistant to gentamicin*

Isolates (no.)	Antibiotic[a]	No. of strains with MIC (μg/ml) equal to:									
		0.12	0.25	0.5	1	2	4	8	16	32	64[b]
E. coli (5)	N			2	2		1				
	A					2	3				
Klebsiella (3)	N						2	1			
	A					1		2			
E. aerogenes (1)	N			1							
	A					1					
S. marcescens (3)	N					1		1	1		
	A					1	1	1			
C. freundii (5)	N			1	1	3					
	A			2	2		1				
P. mirabilis (2)	N						1	1			
	A					1	1				
Indole-positive *Proteus* (8)	N						1	2	2		3
	A				3	3	2				
Providencia (7)	N							3			4
	A	1				3		1	2		
P. aeruginosa (25)	N									5	20
	A			4	3	7	10	1			

[a] N, Netilmicin; A, amikacin.
[b] MIC is 64 μg/ml or greater.

TABLE 3. *Effect of a 100-fold increase in inoculum size on the MIC for netilmicin, gentamicin, and amikacin*

Isolates (no.)	No. of isolates with fourfold or greater increase in MIC		
	Netilmicin	Gentamicin	Amikacin
E. coli (5)	1	2	2
Klebsiella (5)	0	1	2
P. mirabilis (5)	0	3	4
Indole-positive *Proteus* (2)	1	2	2
S. marcescens (2)	2	2	2
P. aeruginosa (5)	0	1	2

Results of in vitro killing studies. Bactericidal activity, as a function of time, was similar for the three antibiotics. Rapid killing of *K. pneumoniae* occurred (Fig. 3); there was a 4-log reduction in organisms at 3 h, and no colonies were detected at 6 and 24 h. Slower killing was seen with *P. aeruginosa*; there was a 4-log reduction at 6 h, and no colonies were detected at 24 h (Fig. 3).

DISCUSSION

In this study, the activity of netilmicin, gentamicin, and amikacin was measured against 192 clinical isolates. Our data support and extend the observations of Rahal et al. (4), Kabins et al. (1), and Watanakunakorn (6), who previously reported on the in vitro activity of netilmicin. Netilmicin was comparable to gentamicin in in vitro activity, with the following exceptions: (i) for *S. marcescens*, gentamicin was more active than netilmicin; (ii) for strains of *P. aeruginosa*, which were susceptible to gentamicin, gentamicin was more active than netilmicin; (iii) all strains of *E. coli*, *Klebsiella*, *Enterobacter*, *P. mirabilis*, and *C. freundii* that were resistant to gentamicin were susceptible to netilmicin; (iv) some strains of *Serratia*, indole-positive *Proteus*, and *Providencia*, which were resistant to gentamicin, were susceptible to netilmicin. Netilmicin was more active than amikacin for all *Enterobacteriaceae* and *S. aureus*. For strains of *P. aeruginosa* susceptible to gentamicin, netilmicin and amikacin were equal in activity. All strains of *P. aeruginosa* resistant to gentamicin that were tested in this study were resistant to netilmicin but susceptible to amikacin.

Our studies with netilmicin and *Pseudomonas* show the MICs to be higher when measured by agar dilution than by broth dilution techniques. This discrepancy has previously been reported with aminoglycosides (1, 3, 7) and is presumably due to the different concentrations of calcium and magnesium in broth and agar (3).

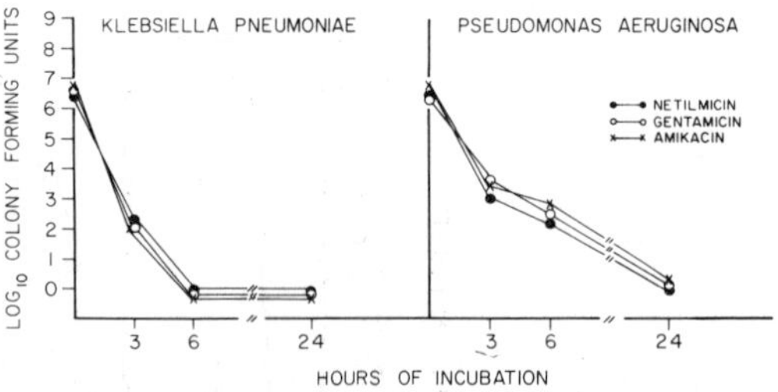

FIG. 3. *Comparison of bactericidal activity as a function of time for netilmicin, gentamicin, and amikacin against one strain each of Klebsiella and P. aeruginosa.*

Several studies have shown the effect of increasing inoculum size on the MICs for amikacin and gentamicin (2, 3, 8). Our study suggests that there was less of an effect on the MICs and MBCs (as measured in broth) for netilmicin than for gentamicin or amikacin when the inoculum was increased 100-fold.

This in vitro study shows that netilmicin has a wide spectrum of activity against clinical pathogens. The frequency with which resistance to different aminoglycosides is reported will vary depending on which inactivating enzymes are present in the bacterial population being investigated (1). Among the isolates we studied, resistance to netilmicin was uncommon with *E. coli*, *Klebsiella*, *Enterobacter*, *Serratia*, *P. mirabilis*, and *C. freundii* but frequent with *P. aeruginosa*, *Providencia*, and indole-positive *Proteus*. Initial studies in animals indicated that the ototoxic and nephrotoxic potential of netilmicin is considerably less than that of gentamicin (5). Because of its broad range of in vitro activity and the possibility of decreased toxicity in clinical use, netilmicin may have advantages over present aminoglycosides and warrants further evaluation.

ACKNOWLEDGMENTS

This study was supported by a grant from the Schering Corp.

We wish to thank Yvonne Korica for identification of the clinical isolates tested, Arnold Brown and Spyros Kominos for providing several clinical isolates, JoAnne Reitz for preparing the manuscript, and Frederick Ruben for critically reviewing the manuscript.

LITERATURE CITED

1. **Kabins, S., C. Nathan, and S. Cohen.** 1976. In vitro comparison of netilmicin, a semisynthetic derivative of sisomicin, and four other aminoglycoside antibiotics. Antimicrob. Agents Chemother. **10:**139–145.
2. **Karney, W., K. Holmes, and M. Turck.** 1973. Comparison of five aminocyclitol antibiotics in vitro against *Enterobacteriaceae* and *Pseudomonas*. Antimicrob. Agents Chemother. **3:**338–342.
3. **Kelly, M., and J. Matsen.** 1976. In vitro activity, synergism, and testing parameters of amikacin, with com-

parisons to other aminoglycoside antibiotics. Antimicrob. Agents Chemother. 9:440–447.
4. **Rahal, J., M. Simberkoff, K. Kagen, and N. Moldover.** 1976. Bactericidal efficacy of Sch 20569 and amikacin against gentamicin-sensitive and -resistant organisms. Antimicrob. Agents Chemother. 9:595–599.
5. **Schering Corporation.** 1976. Informational material for the investigational drug, Sch 20569. Schering Corp., Bloomfield, N.J.
6. **Watanakunakorn, C.** 1976. Comparative in vitro activity of Sch 20656, netilmicin, gentamicin, and tobramycin. Antimicrob. Agents Chemother. 10:382–383.
7. **Young, L., and W. Hewitt.** 1973. Activity of five aminoglycoside antibiotics in vitro against gram-negative bacilli and *Staphylococcus aureus*. Antimicrob. Agents Chemother. 4:617–625.
8. **Yu, P., and J. Washington.** 1973. Comparative in vitro activity of three aminoglycoside antibiotics: BB-K8, kanamycin, and gentamicin. Antimicrob. Agents Chemother. 4:133–139.

ANTIMICROBIAL AGENTS AND CHEMOTHERAPY, Jan. 1977, p. 132-141
Vol. 11, No. 1

Pharmacokinetics of Amoxicillin: Dose Dependence After Intravenous, Oral, and Intramuscular Administration

DANIEL A. SPYKER,* RAYMOND J. RUGLOSKI, ROBERT L. VANN, AND WILLIAM M. O'BRIEN

Department of Internal Medicine, University of Virginia School of Medicine, Charlottesville, Virginia 22901, and Beecham Laboratories, Bristol, Tennessee 37620*

Received for publication 16 September 1976

Amoxicillin was studied in normal subjects after intravenous, oral, and intramuscular administration of 250-, 500-, and 1,000-mg doses. Serum drug levels were analyzed using a two-compartment open model, as well as area under the curve (AUC) and urinary recovery. The variations of these pharmacokinetic parameters were then examined using the three-way analysis of variance and linear regression equations. These results confirmed nearly complete oral absorption: AUC was 93% of intravenous absorption, and urinary recovery was 86%. The intramuscular administration of amoxicillin results in complete and reliable absorption with peak drug levels, AUCs, and urinary recovery equivalent to oral dosage. The absorption of lyophilized amoxicillin after intramuscular injection resulted in an AUC that was 92% of intravenous absorption and urinary recovery of 91%. The peak serum levels, time to peak, and other pharmacokinetic parameters for intramuscular injection were nearly identical to those for oral administration. Kinetics of both intramuscular and oral administration exhibited dose-dependent absorption (absorption rate constant, 1.3/h for 250 mg and 0.7/h for 1,000 mg). This resulted in relatively later and lower peak serum levels for increasing dose. Total absorption, however, showed no dose dependence, as indicated by urinary recovery and AUC, which changed by less than 10%.

Amoxicillin (alpha-amino-*p*-hydroxybenzyl penicillin) is a new semisynthetic penicillin, similar in structure and spectrum of activity to ampicillin (14, 29). Amoxicillin produces higher serum levels than ampicillin with similar absorption and excretion kinetics (10, 21). We report a pharmacokinetic comparison of serum levels and urinary excretion data for amoxicillin administered by mouth (p.o.), intramuscularly (i.m.), and intravenously (i.v.), for three doses in in normal volunteers.

Abbreviations used in this report include the following: ANOVA, analysis of variance; RMS, root mean square; SEM, standard error of the mean; AUC, area under the curve (hours × micrograms per milliliter); alpha, slope of log concentration–early (distribution) phase, per hour; beta, slope of log concentration–late (elimination) phase per hour; V_1, volume of central (plasma) compartment, liters per kilogram; V_2, volume of peripheral (tissue) compartment, liters per kilogram; V_d, total volume of distribution (central+tissue), liters per kilogram; K_{12}, transfer rate constant (central to peripheral), per hour; K_{21}, transfer rate constant (peripheral to central), per hour; K_a, absorption rate constant, per hour; K_e, elimination rate constant, per hour; Do, dose of drug (milligrams); f, fraction of the drug absorbed.

A group of eight subjects was given amoxicillin i.v. in doses of 250, 500, and 1,000 mg and then subsequently received the same doses p.o. In this group, distribution and excretion were characterized using a two-compartment linear model. A second group of 24 subjects, separate from the above group, was given 250-, 500-, and 1,000-mg doses p.o. and also given the same doses via i.m. injection. The administration of three doses permitted the evaluation of a dose effect on drug absorption, distribution, and excretion.

MATERIALS AND METHODS

Description of subjects. Subjects were healthy adult male volunteers ranging in age from 18 to 32, and in weight from 57 to 98 kg. They were selected on the basis of a complete medical history to exclude those having a history of hematological, hepatic, or renal disease, and those with a history of allergic sensitivity to penicillins. A complete blood count, urinalysis, and blood chemistry screen (including levels of total protein, albumin, calcium, inorganic phosphorus, cholestrol, glucose, blood urea nitrogen, uric acid, total bilirubin, alkaline phosphatase, serum glutamic oxalacetic transaminase, serum glutamic pyruvic transaminase, and lactic dehydrogenase) were performed on all subjects before starting the study and repeated at the end of each day on which the drug was administered. Previously screened alternate subjects replaced the few who dropped out during the study.

Administration of amoxicillin. (Drugs were provided by Beecham Laboratories, Bristol, Tenn.)

Eight subjects participated in each of three crossovers, i.v. versus p.o., studies at dosages of 250, 500, and 1,000 mg of sodium amoxicillin. A 1-week washout period was observed between each dosage change, necessitating nearly 6 weeks of involvement. Half the subjects randomly received amoxicillin i.v., whereas the other half received the same dose of the drug p.o.; after a week interval, the routes of administration were crossed over. This was sequentially done through 250-, 500-, and 1,000-mg dosages, so that each subject received all three doses both i.v. and p.o. When administered i.v., amoxicillin was given as a 10-s bolus, and blood samples were drawn beforehand (at zero time) and at 1, 2, 5, 10, 15, 20, 25, 30, 45, 60, 75, and 90 min and 2, 2.5, 3, 4, and 6 h after dosing. From those receiving amoxicillin p.o., blood was drawn at zero time, and at 20, 40, 60, and 90 min and 2, 4, and 6 h after ingestion. Urine was collected over intervals of 0 to 1, 1 to 2, 2 to 3, 3 to 4, and 4 to 6 h.

In the i.m. versus p.o. study 24 volunteers participated. The same general procedures and crossover design as the i.v. versus p.o. study were followed, i.e., each subject received all three doses both i.m. and p.o. The dosages of amoxicillin were 250, 500, and 1,000 mg. (Lyophilized sodium amoxicillin was provided for i.m. injection.) Blood samples were taken immediately before (at zero time) and at 20, 40, 60, and 90 min and at 2, 4, 6, and 8 h after dosing. Urine was collected over intervals of 0 to 4 and 4 to 8 h.

Bioassay. Blood was collected in evacuated glass tubes without anticoagulant, and serum was obtained by centrifugation. All samples were stored in duplicate and deep frozen until assayed. The amoxicillin content of the serum and urine samples was determined by a large plate (13 by 16 inches [33 by 40 cm]) cup assay method using *Bacillus subtilis* (ATCC 6633) as the assay microorganism. As described elsewhere (3), the sensitivity of this assay is 0.5 μg/ml, and the precision is $\pm$5%. Complete standard curves were prepared for each assay using human serum or urine as appropriate; five samples were assayed per each plate (3).

Data handling. Data for each subject were entered via computer terminal and stored directly on disk files. Verification of these master data files was achieved by having a second person enter the data and the computer check for discrepancies. Thereafter, data were manipulated only by pharmacokinetic and statistical programs. Appropriate data files were constructed for each group of subjects at various stages in the analysis as described below. All programs were generalized (as to number of subjects, number of observations, number of parameters, etc.), and subsequent analysis required a minimum number of programs and virtually no operator intervention.

Nonparametric analysis. Nonparametric (model-independent) evaluation of the kinetic data was completed for each subject as an initial step. This included a regression analysis of log of concentration versus time for the following: (i) elimination rate constant from last three data points; (ii) distribution rate constant by exponential peeling (i.v. data); (iii) peak and time to peak from quadratic function fit to three highest drug levels (i.m. or p.o. data); and (iv) absorption delay and rate constant, derived using the method of Wagner and Nelson (30) (i.m. or p.o. data).

AUC was computed using the trapezoid approximation. Correction for the area after the last blood sample was based on the elimination rate constant [as mentioned in (i) above]. An individual plot for each administration trial, along with a summary of derived data, was plotted for each subject (Fig. 1 and Table 1).

Two-compartment linear model. The data were then examined using a two-compartment linear model that has been shown to adequately describe the course of many drugs in humans (24). All absorption and elimination takes place through the central compartment and thus, the absorption rate constant (K_a) and elimination rate constant (K_e) of the drug are characterized as processes involving the central compartment. The parameters K_{12} and K_{21} represent the rate constants of drug transfer between the central and peripheral compartments as summarized in Fig. 2.

General solutions for the two-compartment model have been detailed by Bischoff and Dedrick (4) and recently presented in the clinical context (11, 12). The solution for drug level in the central compartment (C_1) can be written as an exponential equation (Fig. 3).

Experience has shown that the absorption of tablets administered p.o. can usually be well described as a simple first-order, i.e., exponential, process with a time delay (18). The solution equation for central compartment concentration then becomes as shown in Fig. 4.

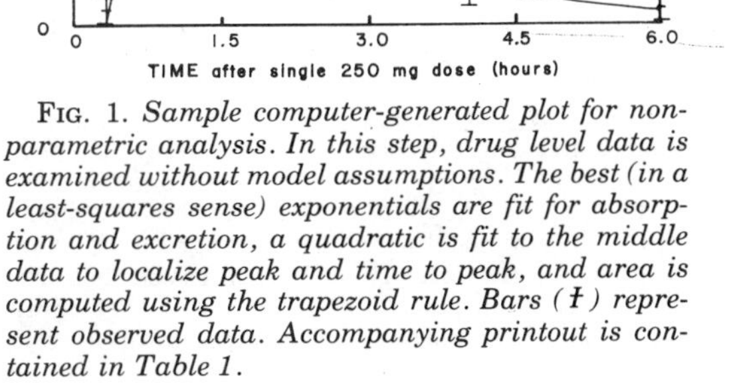

FIG. 1. *Sample computer-generated plot for nonparametric analysis. In this step, drug level data is examined without model assumptions. The best (in a least-squares sense) exponentials are fit for absorption and excretion, a quadratic is fit to the middle data to localize peak and time to peak, and area is computed using the trapezoid rule. Bars (Ɨ) represent observed data. Accompanying printout is contained in Table 1.*

TABLE 1. *Sample of nonparametric analysis. Computer printout of observed data and derived, model-free measures for subject 1 following oral administration of 250 mg of amoxicillin (accompanies Fig. 1)*

Subject No. 1

Weight = 97.73 kg

OBSERVED DATA

Sample Times (min)	Observed Serum Levels (μg/ml)
20	<0.5
40	1.7
60	2.5
90	2.8
120	2.5
240	0.5
360	<0.5

Urinary Recovery = 130.6 mg at 6 h, = 52% of dose

EXPONENTIAL FIT FOR ABSORPTION PHASE

Absorption Delay[a] = 0.33 h

Absorption Rate Constant = 1.57/h, Half Time = 0.44 h

QUADRATIC FIT FOR PEAK

Time to Peak = 1.50 h, Peak = 2.84 μg/ml

EXPONENTIAL FIT FOR EXCRETION PHASE, Last 3 Points

Excretion Rate Constant = 0.58/h, Half Time = 1.20 h

Area Under the Curve[b] (h×μ/ml)–0 to 6 h	=	7.5
>6 h	=	0.4[c]
Total	=	7.9
Percent excreted in the Urine–0 to 6 h	=	52.3
>6 h	=	2.6[c]
Total	=	54.9

[a] Time after administration when absorption process appears to begin.

[b] AUC computed using trapezoid approximation.

[c] Corrections based on extrapolation beyond 6 h using the above computed half-time (1.2 h).

Least-squares fitting. Given the above assumptions on model form and the generalized solutions it only remains to find the parameters K_a, K_e, K_{12}, and K_{21} to fit the observed data for each subject. The starting values for these parameters are obtained from the previously described nonparametric analysis. For example, first approximations to alpha and beta were provided, respectively, by the distribution and elimination rate constants as previously defined. In the case of i.v. data, a parameter space gradient technique is used to find A, B, alpha, and beta, such that the difference between observed and model drug levels is minimized. This program iteratively minimizes the sum of the squares of distance between observed drug levels and model solution values until the best fit is achieved (27) (Table 2 and Fig. 5).

Individual plots of this type are produced for each subject and examined at this point. Subjective examination is important in the overall pharmacokinetic analysis. Levy and Hollister have demonstrated that a model which fits averaged data is not necessarily qualitatively or quantitatively best for drug levels from individual subjects (18). We agree and report only parameter averages after kinetic analysis of each subject.

Statistical analysis. Using the methods outlined, the serum level for each subject in each trial is described in terms of four or more model parameters. A quantitative estimate of the importance of dosage level, route of administration, and intrasubject variation is obtained through the use of ANOVA (5). In the bioavailability study of i.m. amoxicillin, the principle concern was in the demonstration of equivalent or better availability for the i.m. route; thus, a three-way ANOVA (dose × subject × route) was employed. When a significant effect of dosage on a model parameter has been demonstrated by ANOVA, then this "dose effect" can be described and analyzed by means of regression analysis (9). That is, if the percentage absorbed were found to change significantly as a function of dosage administered, then the least-squares linear regression of K_a on dose or log dose is relevant. Since the reliability, i.e., repeatability of absorption, after i.m. administration was of interest, Bartlet's test for homogeneity of variance was applied to the model parameters (26).

The common use of reporting "significant" results as those achieving $P < 0.05$ or even $P < 0.01$ dates from the precomputer era when tables were necessary to arrive at the P value for a given F ratio. A

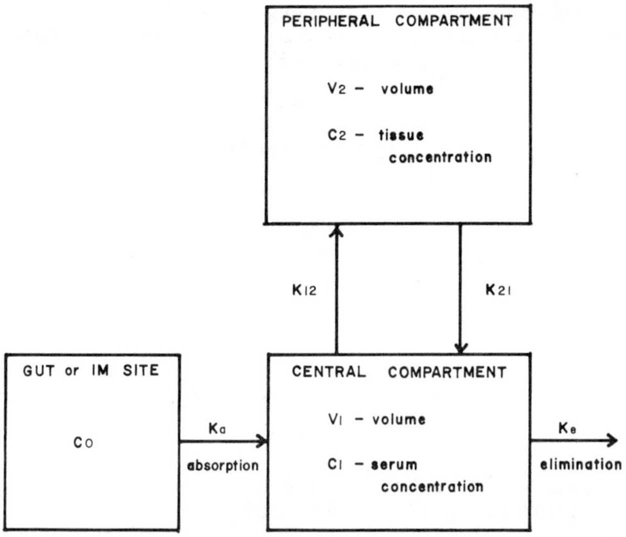

FIG. 2. *Schematic of two-compartment linear pharmacokinetic model. Absorption and elimination are restricted to the central compartment, which is usually considered to represent serum and highly perfused tissue. The peripheral compartment is associated with less well perfused tissue, and thus acts somewhat like a depot for the drug. Each K represents a rate constant of drug transfer and has units of liters per hour. The addition of a third compartment representing the gut (if oral) or injection site (if parenteral) permits description of p.o. or i.m. administration.*

$$C_1(t) = Ae^{-\alpha t} + Be^{-\beta t}$$

Where

$$A = \frac{Do}{V_1} \quad \frac{(K_{21}-\alpha)}{(\beta-\alpha)}$$

$$B = \frac{Do}{V_1} \quad \frac{(K_{21}-\beta)}{(\alpha-\beta)}$$

$$\alpha = \tfrac{1}{2}\left(b + \sqrt{b^2 - 4K_{21}Ke}\right)$$

$$\beta = \tfrac{1}{2}\left(b - \sqrt{b^2 - 4K_{21}Ke}\right)$$

$$b = K_{12} + K_{21} + Ke$$

FIG. 3. *Exponential equation for solution for drug level in the central compartment (C_1).*

few lines of coding in BASIC or FORTRAN are all that is necessary to compute *P* values (1). In this report, computed *P* values are used wherever hypothesis testing is involved.

RESULTS

Intravenous dosage. The results of analysis for the drug levels following i.v. administration

$$C_1(t) = -(P+Q)\,e^{-Ka t} + P\,e^{-\alpha t} + Q\,e^{-\beta t}$$

Where

$$P = \frac{Ka\ f\ Do}{V_1\ (\alpha-\beta)} \quad \frac{(\alpha-K_{21})}{(Ka-\alpha)}$$

$$Q = \frac{Ka\ f\ Do}{V_1\ (\alpha-\beta)} \quad \frac{(K_{21}-\beta)}{(Ka-\beta)}$$

FIG. 4. *First-order equation describing absorption of tablets given p.o.*

are summarized in Table 3. This includes the parameter means for each of the five rate constants, clearance in liters per kilogram per hour, the volume distribution for the central compartment, and the total volume distribution. The means are given for the individual 250-, 500-, and 1,000-mg dosages and finally, the overall average across all doses for total trial observations with the standard deviation and SEM are reported. The urinary recovery is reported as percentage of administered dose.

Analysis of variance for this data (Table 3) revealed no significant intrasubject variation, and only clearance exhibited statistically significant dose effect, though neither K_e nor V_1 showed significant dose effect (clearance $= K_e \times V_1$).

The averaged parameters (K_{12}, K_{21}, K_e, and V_1) were then used in subsequent pharmacokinetic analysis for i.m. and p.o. administration.

TABLE 2. *Sample of two-compartment model analysis. Computer printout of observed levels, predicted levels, and derived model parameters for subject 21 following i.m. administration of 500 mg of amoxicillin (accompanies Fig. 5)*

Subject No. 21

Weight = 81.8 kg

OBSERVED DATA

Sample Times (min)	Observed Serum Levels (μg/ml)	Predicted Serum Levels[d] (μg/ml)
20	8.09	7.72
40	8.80	8.61
60	6.91	7.25
90	5.71	5.18
120	5.18	3.67
240	0.97	0.93
360	<0.50	0.24

Giving weighted RMS error of 0.64 μg/ml

MODEL PARAMETERS[b]

Absorption Delay = 0.94 h, Fraction Absorbed = 1.00
Absorption Rate Constant = 2.00/h, Half Time = 0.35 h
Excretion Rate Constant[c] = 1.98/h, K12,[c] K21[c] = 1.77, 1.91/h

MEASURES BASED ON MODEL

Peak Drug Level = 8.81 μg/ml, Time to Peak = 0.54 h
Area under the curve = 17.3 h$\times\mu$g/ml, versus 17.3 for i.v.

[a] Based on model parameters given below.
[b] Chosen to best fit (minimize RMS error) the observed data.
[c] These parameters are based on the i.v. study.

TABLE 3. *Parameters derived using two-compartment model–i.v. administration. Means for each dose and overall means, standard deviations, and SEMs*

Dose (mg)	Distribution: Alpha (/h)	Distribution: K_{12} (/h)	Distribution: K_{21} (/h)	Elimination: Beta (/h)	Elimination: K_e (/h)	Elimination: Clearance (liters/kg/h)	Volumes: V_1 (liters/kg)	Volumes: V_d (liters/kg)	Urinary Recovery (% dose)
250	5.90	3.05	2.76	2.55	2.65	0.32	0.17	0.29	55.8
500	4.04	1.43	1.64	0.72	1.68	0.32	0.22	0.46	60.0
1000	2.72	0.70	1.22	0.79	1.56	0.34	0.22	0.49	50.9
Across all doses for 20 trial observations									
Means	4.30	1.77	1.91	1.37	1.98	0.32	0.20	0.41	56.4
Standard deviation	4.00	2.27	1.12	2.50	1.20	0.08	0.08	0.18	26.9
SEM	0.90	0.51	0.25	0.56	0.27	0.02	0.02	0.04	6.5

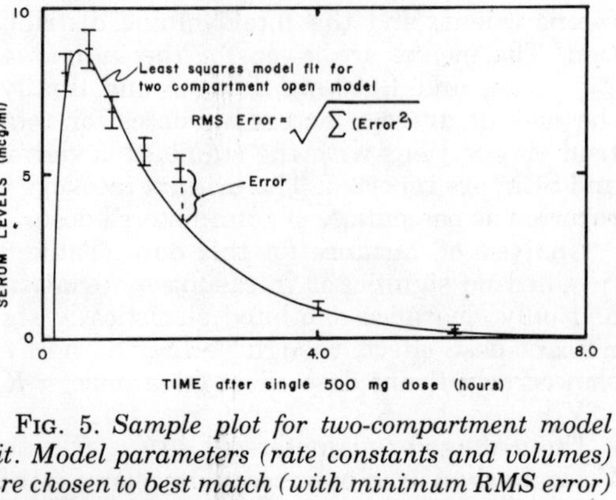

FIG. 5. *Sample plot for two-compartment model fit. Model parameters (rate constants and volumes) are chosen to best match (with minimum RMS error) the observed drug levels. Accompanying printout is contained in Table 2.*

Bioavailability of i.v. injections. A separate group of 24 subjects received amoxicillin by i.m. and p.o. routes. Distribution kinetics are assumed to be those determined in the i.v. study (preceding section). Table 4 shows the results of the i.m. administration for each of the three dosages studied, as well as the overall means. Peak and area values are corrected for 70-kg body weight and 1,000-mg dose to facilitate comparison among doses (i.e., data for 250-mg dose are multiplied by 4; data for 500-mg dose are multiplied by 2).

The results of analysis of variance and least-squares regression for i.m. administration, dose effect, subject effect, and regression are included in Table 4. Table 5 presents the equivalent data for p.o. dosage in the same subjects.

TABLE 4. *Analysis of parameters derived using two-compartment model–i.m. administration. Means for each dose, overall means, standard deviations, analysis of variance for dose and subjects, and linear regression for dose*

Dose (mg)	Absorption		Peak		Area			Urinary recovery (% dose)
	Delay (h)	K_a (/h)	Time (h)	Concn (μg/ml)	i.m. (h·μg/ml)	i.v.	i.m./i.v. (%)	
250	0.15	1.43	0.89	15.4	38.4	40.5	94.8	53.4
500	0.21	0.77	1.28	10.9	38.7	40.5	95.6	48.7
1,000	0.21	0.76	1.33	9.7	34.5	40.5	85.2	51.6
Across all doses for 72 trial observations								
Mean	0.19	0.98	1.16	12.0	37.1	40.5	91.7	51.3
Standard deviation	0.10	0.69	0.51	5.5	4.3	0.0	10.5	15.4
Two-way analysis of variance—subjects versus dose levels								
Dose[a]								
F =	4.54	14.4	12.2	14.3	13.9	0.0	13.9	
P =	0.0160	0.00007	0.00017	0.00007	.00008	1.00	0.00008	
Subjects[b]								
F =	3.25	2.40	3.74	2.87	3.26	0.00	3.26	
P =	0.00055	0.00618	0.00017	0.00149	0.00053	1.00	0.00053	
Least-squares linear regression (for log dose)								
Intercept[c]	−0.066	4.06	−0.796	37.2	51.9	40.5	128	
Slope[c]	0.097	−1.14	0.731	−9.35	−5.43	0.000	−13.4	
F =	4.06	15.4	10.8	16.0	9.61	1.85	9.61	
P =	0.0451	0.00042	0.00197	0.00035	0.00315	0.175	0.00315	

[a] F ratio and corresponding *P* value for main effect of dose, 3 and 45 degrees of freedom.
[b] F ratio for main effect of subjects, 24 and 45 degrees of freedom.
[c] Intercept and slope of the regression line for each parameter versus log of dose.

TABLE 5. *Analysis of parameters derived using two-compartment model—p.o. administration. Means for each dose, overall means, standard deviations, analysis of variance for dose and subjects, and linear regression for dose*

Dose (mg)	Absorption		Peak		Area			Urinary recovery (% dose)
	Delay (h)	K_a (/h)	Time (h)	Concn (μg/ml)	p.o. (h·μg/ml)	i.v.	p.o./i.v. (%)	
250	0.36	1.23	1.07	14.8	39.3	40.4	97.0	49.0
500	0.31	0.90	1.21	11.8	37.6	40.5	93.0	49.5
1,000	0.37	0.66	1.46	9.5	36.2	40.5	89.4	47.2
Across all doses for 71 trial observations								
Mean	0.35	0.93	1.25	12.0	37.7	40.5	93.1	48.5
Standard deviation	0.14	0.49	0.41	4.3	4.1	0.0	10.2	15.1
Two-way analysis of variance—subjects versus dose levels								
Dose								
F =	1.11	13.8	8.5	18.9	3.38	0.00	3.37	
P =	0.338	0.00009	0.0011	0.00001	0.0428	1.000	0.0428	
Subjects								
F =	0.96	2.13	2.21	2.83	1.78	0.00	1.78	
P =	0.528	0.0154	0.0118	0.00179	0.0495	1.000	0.0495	
Least-squares linear regression (for log dose)								
Intercept	0.336	3.42	−0.397	34.8	49.4	40.5	122	
Slope	0.001	−0.92	0.606	−8.43	−4.28	0.000	−10.6	
F =	0.000	19.7	11.5	22.9	5.32	1.76	5.32	
P =	0.982	0.00013	0.00154	0.00006	0.0228	0.186	0.0228	

The statistical comparison of i.m. versus p.o. kinetics is accomplished via three-way ANOVA (subject × dose × route) and Bartlet's test of homogeneity of variance (Table 6).

From these results, it can be seen that the delay is slightly greater ($P = 0.0001$), 0.347 h (p.o.) versus 0.192 h (i.m.), although the time to peak concentration is not statistically different

(P = 0.189). The concentration peak is identical, 12.0 μg/ml, for each. The area under the curve is essentially identical (P = 0.296): for the p.o. route, 37.7 h · μg/ml versus 37.1 h · μg/ml for i.m. Examination for homogeneity of variances shows that the standard deviation of delay is larger for p.o. (0.139 versus 0.104 h). For K_a and peak, i.m. shows more spread, but for the time to peak and area there is no statistical difference. Based on the above results, it is concluded that the i.m. preparation provides equivalent bioavailability and, moreover, is more rapidly available.

DISCUSSION

Comparison with other intravenous studies. The kinetics of amoxicillin after i.v. administration of 250 mg over 33-min infusion in two subjects with four replications has been presented by Zarowny et al. (32). They reported distribution constants (K_{12}, K_{21}, K_e) and volumes (V_1 and V_d) as summarized in Table 7. Within the dosage range studied, a two-compartment linear model does provide a useful description of the distribution and excretion of amoxicillin.

Comparison with other oral studies. Previous studies comparing amoxicillin with ampicillin and/or epicillin have shown that amoxicillin gives higher peak serum concentrations after p.o. doses (6, 7, 10, 21, 23). These results are collected in Table 8 and show reasonable agreement, among the seven studies, in peak levels after p.o. administration. AUC is probably the best single bioavailability parameter. This study found a 93% ratio of p.o. to i.v. AUC as compared with 89% by Zarowny (32). Urinary recovery data provides a useful, separate bioavailability parameter. (Urinary recovery is independent of serum levels or pharmacokinetic models.) We found about 50% recovery, compared with other reports of 60%. This may relate to sensitivity of other assay techniques to metabolites that cannot be measured in our method.

TABLE 6. *Three-way analysis of variance (subject × dose × route). Analysis for i.m. versus p.o. and test for homogeneity of variance*

	Absorption		Peak		Area		
	Delay (h)	K_a (/h)	Time (h)	Concn (μg/ml)	i.m. or p.o. (h · μg/ml)	i.v.	Ratio (%)
Dose							
F =	0.8	23.1	14.8	25.7	13.4	0.0	13.4
P =	0.550	0.00000	0.00002	0.00000	0.00004	1.000	0.00004
Subjects							
F =	1.4	2.7	3.0	2.9	2.1	0.0	2.1
P =	0.145	0.00053	0.00014	0.00020	0.00669	1.000	0.00669
Route							
F =	58.9	0.5	1.7	0.02	1.1	0.00	1.1
P =	0.00000	0.506	0.189	0.893	0.296	1.000	0.296
Bartlet's test of homogeneity of variance							
Route							
Chi-square[a]	5.82	7.87	2.88	4.71	0.12	0.00	0.12
P^b =	0.0153	0.00532	0.0861	0.0284	0.733	0.0000	0.733

[a] Represents a measure of the differences in the observed variation (standard deviation) of each parameter.

[b] P value for the chi-square, 1 degree of freedom. Small value infers a statistical difference in variability of that parameter.

TABLE 7. *Pharmacokinetic studies of amoxicillin–i.v. route*

Source	Parameters from i.v. administration					
	K_{12} (/h)	K_{21} (/h)	K_e (/h)	Clearance (liters/kg/h)	V_1 (liters/kg)	V_d (liters/kg)
Zarowny (32)	1.29	1.94	1.43	0.245	0.187	0.282
This study	1.77	1.91	1.98	0.324	0.199	0.410

TABLE 8. *Pharmacokinetic studies of amoxicillin – p.o. route*

Source	Parameters from p.o. administration				
	Dose (mg)	Peak serum level (μg/ml)	AUC		Urinary recovery (%)
			(h · μg/ml)	% of i.v.	
Neu (21)	250	5.2			58.0
Zarowny (32)	250	3.5	9.2	89	
This study	250	3.8	9.8	97	49.0
Neu (21)	500	7.6			75.2
Croydon (7)	500	10.8			
Gorden (10)	500	7.6			60.0
Philipson (23)	500	6.2			56.8
This study	500	5.9	18.8	93	49.5
This study	1,000	10.2	36.2	89	47.2

Bioavailability after i.m. administration. The i.m. administration of several drugs, most notably diphenylhydantoin (25, 31) and benzodiazepines (2, 13), demonstrates unreliable absorption and resulting unpredictable serum levels. The spectrum and clinical efficacy of p.o. amoxicillin (8, 14–17, 19, 20, 22, 28) have been reasonably well established. If amoxicillin is to provide a complete therapeutic alternative to ampicillin, then demonstration of complete and reliable absorption after i.m. administration is important. In this study the mean AUC, delay, peak, and time to peak are compared in Table 9. Both i.m. and p.o. exhibit intrasubject effects in all parameters except delay in p.o. (Tables 4 and 5). Not only were the mean values similar for i.m. versus p.o., but the amount of scatter for the two preparations was similar, as summarized in Table 6.

Probably the best evidence for completeness of absorption after p.o. and i.m. administration is the similarity in urinary recovery. The averages across all trials were 56% for i.v., 51% for i.m., and 49% for p.o. There was no statistical difference between i.v. and i.m., or i.m. and p.o.

The drug administered i.m. was sodium amoxicillin prepared by lyophilization, an early formulation that has been superceded by a preparation that is obtained by precipitation. Though kinetics of the precipitated drug are still being studied, preliminary results suggest that higher peak serum concentrations are reached than with the lyophilized preparation.

Dose dependence. A statistically significant dose effect in most parameters for both routes was also apparent. After i.m. injection, the 1,000-mg dose resulted in proportionately lower peak serum levels and AUCs (Table 4). This reduction is expressed by the regression equation. For example, the peak serum level expected is given by the slope and intercept (Table 4), viz.: peak concentration = 37.17 − 9.348·log (dose) (in units of μg/ml per 70 kg per 1,000 mg).

TABLE 9. *Summary comparison of i.m. versus p.o. administration. Values are means ±1.0 standard deviation, averaged across all trials, corrected for 1000-mg dose in 70-kg man*

Parameter	Route of administration	
	i.m.	p.o.
AUC (h · μg/ml)	37.1 + 4.2	37.7 + 4.1
Delay to absorption (h)	0.192 + 0.104	0.347 + 0.139
Peak serum level (μg/ml)	12.0 + 5.5	12.0 + 4.3
Time to peak (h)	1.16 + 0.51	1.25 + 0.41

Very similar results occur in these subjects after p.o. dosage. The peak concentration occurs only slightly later than in i.m. (1.25 versus 1.16 h), and the concentration itself falls from 14.8 μg/ml for the 250-mg p.o. dose to 9.54 μg/ml for the 1,000-mg p.o. dose (Table 4). This is largely explained by the reduction in rate of absorption (1.23/h for 250 mg to 0.66/h for 1,000 mg p.o.). Area ratios (p.o.:i.v.) also are reduced, though proportionately much less, from 95 to 85%. These effects, although statistically significant (P = 0.00008) in this study, are probably not clinically significant, since average absorption is still approximately 90% by either route. Figure 6 shows comparison of AUC and delay by dose for i.m. and p.o. administration. As exhibited in Table 6, the only parameter that shows a statistical difference in route is delay, although the time of peak serum levels shows no difference. Figure 7 shows plots of average serum levels for i.v., p.o., and i.m. administration.

Thus, amoxicillin does indeed appear to be rapidly and reliably absorbed after i.m. administration, producing equivalent serum levels, and should prove therapeutically bioequivalent to p.o. amoxicillin or i.m. ampicillin.

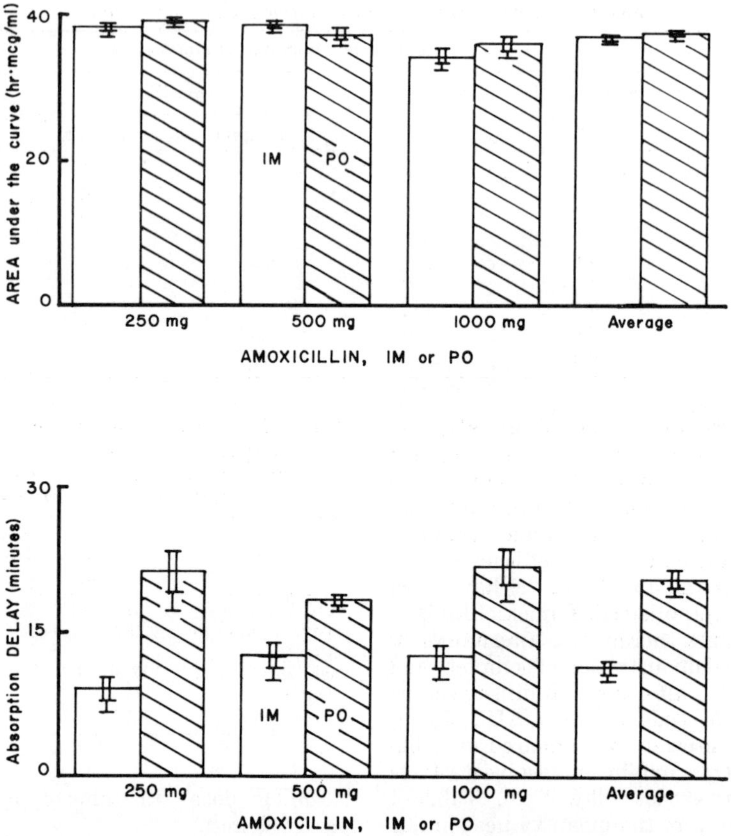

FIG. 6. *Comparison of bioavailability of i.m. and p.o. amoxicillin by dose. Bars indicate the average for all subjects after normalizing to 70-kg body weight and 1,000-mg dose. Double bars (⌶) span ±1.0 SEM for the estimate. Thus, nonoverlapping between two parameters indicates that the parameters are statistically different at the P = 0.05 level. Single bar (I) is −1.96 SEM. If this bar does not reach the base line, then that parameter is statistically nonzero at the P = 0.05 level.*

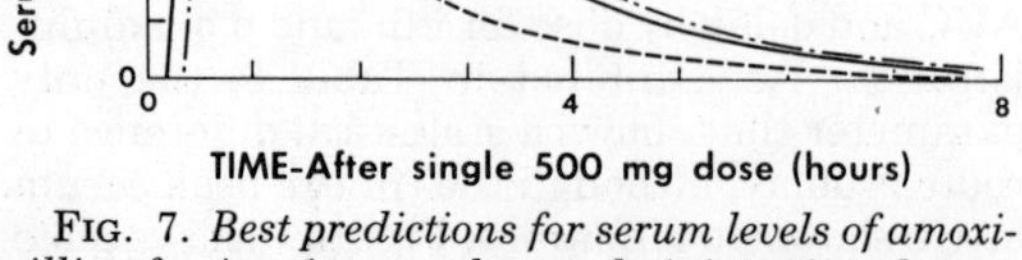

FIG. 7. *Best predictions for serum levels of amoxicillin after i.v., i.m., and p.o. administration. Curves are based on averaged pharmacokinetic parameters assuming a 70-kg patient receiving a single 500-mg dose.*

ACKNOWLEDGMENTS

We are grateful to Fred Barr, Beecham Laboratories, Bristol, Tenn., for performance of bioassays.

LITERATURE CITED

1. **Abramowitz, M., and I. A. Stegnum (ed.).** 1970. Handbook of mathematical functions with formulas, graphs, and mathematical tables. U. S. Government Printing Office, Washington, D. C.
2. **Baird, E. S., and D. M. Hailey.** 1972. Plasma levels of diazepam and its major metabolite following intramuscular administration. Br. J. Anaesth. 45:546–548.
3. **Bennett, J. V., J. L. Brodie, E. J. Benner, and W. M. M. Kirby.** 1966. Simplified accurate method for antibiotic assay of clinical specimens. Appl. Microbiol. 14:170–177.
4. **Bischoff, K., and R. L. Dedrick.** 1970. Generalized solution to linear, two-compartment, open model for drug distribution. J. Theor. Biol. 29:63–68.
5. **Bliss, C. I.** 1967. Statistics in biology. McGraw-Hill Book Co., New York.
6. **Bodey, G. P., and J. Nance.** 1972. Amoxicillin: in vitro and pharmacological studies. Antimicrob. Agents Chemother. 1:358–362.
7. **Croydon, E. A., and R. Sutherland.** 1971. α-Amino-p-hydroxybenzyl penicillin (BRL 2333), a new semisynthetic penicillin: absorption and excretion in man, p. 427–433. Antimicrob. Agents Chemother. 1970.
8. **Croydon, E. A. P.** 1973. Clinical experience of amoxy-

cillin in the United Kingdom. Chemotherapy 18(Suppl.):112–118.
9. **Draper, N. R., and H. Smith.** 1966. Applied regression analysis. John Wiley & Sons, New York.
10. **Gordon, R. C., C. Regamey, and W. M. M. Kirby.** 1972. Comparative clinical pharmacology of amoxicillin and ampicillin administered orally. Antimicrob. Agents Chemother. 1:504–507.
11. **Greenblat, D. J., and J. Koch-Weser.** 1975. Clinical pharmacokinetics (second of two parts). N. Engl. J. Med. 293:964–970.
12. **Greenblatt, D. J., and J. Koch-Weser.** 1975. Clinical pharmacokinetics (first of two parts). N. Engl. J. Med. 293:702–705.
13. **Greenblatt, D. J., and R. I. Shader.** 1974. Benzodiazepines (first of two parts). N. Engl. J. Med. 291:1011–1015.
14. **Handsfield, H. H., H. Clark, J. Wallace, K. K. Holmes, and M. Turck.** 1973. Amoxicillin, a new penicillin antibiotic. Antimicrob. Agents Chemother. 3:262–265.
15. **Harding, J. W., and L. J. Less.** 1972. Trial of a new broadspectrum penicillin (amoxycillin) in general practice. Practitioner 209:363–368.
16. **Holloway, W. J.** 1973. Clinical experience with amoxicillin – a preliminary report. Infect. Dis. Rev. 2:245–251.
17. **Leigh, D. A.** 1972. Diagnosis of urinary tract infections in general practice, and treatment with a new penicillin – amoxycillin. Curr. Med. Res. Opin. 1:10–18.
18. **Levy, G., and L. E. Hollister.** 1964. Inter- and intrasubject variations in drug absorption kinetics. J. Pharm. Sci. 53:1392–1403.
19. **Middleton, F. G., D. M. Poretz, and R. J. Duma.** 1973. Clinical and laboratory evaluation of amoxicillin (BRL 2333) in the treatment of urinary tract infections. Antimicrob. Agents Chemother. 4:25–30.
20. **Neu, H. C., and E. B. Winshell.** 1970. In vitro antimicrobial activity of 6[d(−)a-amino-p-hydroxyphenylacetamido] penicillanic acid, a new semisynthetic penicillin, p. 407–410. Antimicrob. Agents Chemother. 1969.
21. **Neu, H. C., and E. B. Winshell.** 1970. Pharmacological studies of 6[D(-)α-amino-*p*-hydroxyphenylacetamido] penicillanic acid in humans, p. 423–426. Antimicrob. Agents. Chemother. 1969.
22. **Neu, H. C.** Just how good is amoxicillin? Med. Times, February 1975.
23. **Philipson, A., L. D. Sabath, and B. Rosner.** 1975. Sequence effect on ampicillin blood levels noted in an amoxicillin, ampicillin, and epicillin triple crossover study. Antimicrob. Agents Chemother. 8:311–320.
24. **Riegelman, S., J. C. K. Loo, and M. Rowland.** 1968. Shortcomings in pharmacokinetic analysis by conceiving the body to exhibit properties of a single compartment. J. Pharm. Sci. 57:117–123.
25. **Serrano, E. E., D. B. Roye, R. H. Hammer, et al.** 1973. Plasma diphenylhydantoin values after oral and intramuscular administration of diphenylhydantoin. Neurology 23:313–317.
26. **Sokal, R. R., and F. J. Rohlf.** 1969. Biometry – the principles and practice of statistics in biological research. W. H. Freeman, San Francisco.
27. **Spyker, D. A. 1970.** Simulation in the analysis and control of a cardio-circulatory assist device. Simulation 15:196–205.
28. **Stam, J.** 1973. Preliminary clinical study with amoxycillin (brl 2333) in complicated lower respiratory tract infections. Chemotherapy 18(Suppl.):27–33.
29. **Sutherland, R., E. A. P. Croydon, and G. N. Rolinson.** 1972. Amoxycillin: a new semi-synthetic penicillin. Br. Med. J. 3:13–16.
30. **Wagner, J. G., and E. Nelson.** 1963. Per cent absorbed time plots derived from blood level and/or urinary excretion data. J. Pharm. Sci. 52:610–611.
31. **Wilensky, A. J., and J. A. Lowden.** 1973. Inadequate serum levels after intramuscular administration of diphenylhydantoin. Neurology 23:318–324.
32. **Zarowny, D., R. Ogilvie, D. Tamblyn, C. Macleod, and J. Reudy.** 1974. Pharmacokinetics of amoxicillin. Clin. Pharmacol. Ther. 16:1045–1051.

Antimicrobial Agents and Chemotherapy, Jan. 1977, p. 142-146 Vol. 11, No. 1

Beta-Lactamase Activity in Strains of *Bacteroides melaninogenicus* and *Bacteroides oralis*

A. A. SALYERS,* J. WONG, and T. D. WILKINS

Anaerobe Laboratory, Virginia Polytechnic Institute and State University Blacksburg, Virginia 24061

Received for publication 10 August 1976

β-Lactamase from strains of *Bacteroides melaninogenicus* and *Bacteroides oralis* hydrolyzed penicillin more rapidly than ampicillin or carbenicillin. Cephalothin and a chromogenic cephalosporin (87/312) were also hydrolyzed by the enzyme. Activity was found only in β-lactam-resistant strains, but there was considerable variation in activity among strains having the same minimal inhibitory concentrations of antibiotic. β-Lactamase activity was cell bound and appeared to be tightly associated with the cell envelope since detergents were required to elute this activity.

Bacteroides melaninogenicus and *B. oralis* are components of the normal flora of the human upper respiratory tract and are frequently isolated from infections of that area. In the past, these species have been considered to be susceptible to β-lactam antibiotics, with resistance occuring in about 10% of the strains tested (5, 10). However, in a current survey, 40% of all clinical isolates of these species were resistant to penicillin (P. Murray and J. Rosenblatt, private communication).

Hydrolysis of penicillin and ampicillin by a strain of *B. oralis* was first demonstrated by Pinkus et al. (8). Recently, Hackman and Wilkins reported penicillinase activity by penicillin-resistant strains of both *B. melaninogenicus* and *B. oralis* (3). Since these strains are also resistant to other β-lactam antibiotics, we determined the ability of β-lactamases from these organisms to hydrolyze ampicillin, carbenicillin, and cephalothin. We also investigated the cellular location of the enzyme activity.

MATERIALS AND METHODS

Source of bacterial strains. Two strains of *B. melaninogenicus* were obtained from V. L. Sutter, Wadsworth Hospital, Los Angeles, Calif.: WAL 2721 (VPI 9465B) and WAL 2784 (VPI 9466). All other strains were obtained from the culture collection of the Anaerobe Laboratory, Virginia Polytechnic Institute and State University (VPI), Blacksburg, Va. Identifications were made according to previously published procedures (4).

MIC determinations. Except for strains of *B. melaninogenicus* subsp. *asaccharolyticus*, minimal inhibitory concentrations (MICs) were determined by using an agar dilution technique (12) with brucella blood agar plates. All manipulations were carried out in an anaerobic chamber (Coy Manufacturing Co., St. Louis, Mo.), with an atmosphere of 85% nitrogen, 10% hydrogen, and 5% carbon dioxide. Since strains of *B. melaninogenicus* subsp. *asaccharolyticus* did not grow well on the brucella blood agar plates, MICs for these strains were determined by using a broth dilution method (13) with chopped-meat broth (4) substituted for brain heart infusion broth.

Source of antibiotics. Benzylpenicillin, potassium salt, was obtained from Sigma Chemical Co. (St. Louis, Mo.). Carbenicillin and ampicillin were provided by Bristol Laboratories (Syracuse, N.Y.). Cephalothin was obtained from the Eli Lilly & Co. (Indianapolis, Ind.). The chromogenic cephalosporin 87/312 was a gift from C. O'Callaghan (Glaxo Research Inc., Middlesex, England).

Preparation of cells. For determinations of β-lactamase in whole cells, 16-h cultures in 100 ml of Trypticase-yeast extract-glucose (TYG) medium (4) were harvested by centrifugation at 10,800 × *g* for 15 min at 4°C and then washed twice in 0.1 M potassium phosphate buffer (pH 5.9). Cells were resuspended in 10 ml of buffer, and the concentration of cells was determined by measuring optical density and comparing with a standard curve. The standard curve (optical density versus concentration of cells) was obtained using a *B. melaninogenicus* strain. Since standard curves for most *Bacteroides* species have the same slope, this standard curve was used for all strains tested. The final cell suspension had an optical density of approximately 10. Portions (0.1 ml) were assayed for enzyme activity.

Whole cells that had been washed and resuspended in buffer were mechanically disrupted by shaking aerobically with glass beads in a Bronwill cell disintegrator (Bronwill Scientific Inc., Rochester, N.Y.) for 3 min. Glass beads were allowed to settle and the lysed cell suspension was decanted. The lysed cell suspension was then centrifuged at 20,000 × *g* for 30 min at 4°C. The supernatant was saved and the pellet was resuspended in 10 ml of buffer. Both the supernatant and pellet were assayed for enzyme activity.

Adsorption of enzyme to the glass beads used for breaking cells was estimated by adding 2-g glass beads to 5 ml of lysed cell suspension and mixing for 1 to 2 min. Enzyme activity after mixing was compared with enzyme activity before the addition of the glass beads. Approximately 10% of the activity was removed by adsorption to glass beads.

To determine the effect of growth phase on activity, cells growing in TYG medium were harvested at 4-h intervals after inoculation and prepared for assay as described above. Four strains (VPI 7795, VPI 9465B, VPI 9466, and VPI 9611) were tested.

β-Lactamase assays. β-Lactamase activity was determined using the microiodometric method of Sykes and Nordstrom (9) with penicillin, ampicillin, carbenicillin or cephalothin as the substrate. Cephalosporinase activity was also determined by using the chromogenic cephalosporin method of O'Callaghan et al. (7), except that assays were run at 30°C. Enzyme activities were determined by averaging triplicate assays. Activity obtained with washed whole cells was expressed as units per 10^{11} cells. One unit is defined as hydrolysis of 1 μmol of substrate/min.

To determine whether the different rates of hydrolysis obtained using the microiodometric method might be due, in part, to conditions of the iodometric assay (e.g., the presence of iodine), the hydrolysis of penicillin, ampicillin, and carbenicillin was also followed by using the thin-layer chromatographic method of Pinkus et al. (8). Washed whole cells were added to phosphate buffer (pH 7.0) containing 1 mg of antibiotic per ml. At 30-min intervals, 10-μl portions were spotted on silica gel plates and developed in ethanol-water (79:21, vol/vol). Spots were visualized using starch-iodine reagent (8). R_f values were as follows: penicillin, 0.8; penicilloic acid, 0.4; carbenicillin, 0.6; carbenicilloic acid, 0.3; ampicillin, 0.7; ampicilloic acid, 0.3. The amount of time required to hydrolyze 100% of the antibiotic was estimated and compared with that predicted by the rate obtained using the iodometric method.

Spheroplast formation. To determine whether cell-bound activity was in the periplasmic space, spheroplasts were made from washed whole cells using the lysozyme-ethylenediaminetetraacetate technique of Birdsell and Cota-Robles (1), except that cells were incubated 4 h. Spheroplast formation was checked microscopically. Spheroplasts were centrifuged and resuspended in 20% sucrose. β-Lactamase activities in the spheroplast supernatant and in the resuspended spheroplasts were determined by using the chromogenic cephalosporin method. Four strains (VPI 7795, VPI 9465B, VPI 9466, and VPI 9611) were used in these experiments.

Solubilization of β-lactamase activity. To elute β-lactamase activity from the lysed cell pellet, the pellet was resuspended in each of the following: 1 M NaCl in phosphate buffer (pH 7.0), 2% Triton X-100 (vol/vol) in phosphate buffer (pH 7.0), 2% sodium dodecyl sulfate (vol/vol) in tris(hydroxymethyl)aminomethane-hydrochloride buffer (pH 7.0), 10% sodium taurocholate (vol/vol) in phosphate buffer. After 1 h at room temperature, the mixture was centrifuged at 20,000 × g for 30 min (4°C). The supernatant and resuspended pellet were assayed for β-lactamase activity by using the chromogenic cephalosporin method.

Inducibility of β-lactamase activity. To determine whether exposure of strains to antibiotics prior to assay affected activity, four strains (VPI 9331, VPI 7795, VPI 9611, and VPI 9465B) were grown in the presence of 2 μg of penicillin or cephalothin per ml. β-Lactamase activities in these strains were compared with activities in the same strains grown in the absence of antibiotics.

RESULTS

MICs for the strains used in these experiments are given in Table 1. Penicillin-resistant strains were equally resistant to the other three antibiotics. Penicillin-susceptible strains were susceptible to the other antibiotics.

There was no detectable β-lactamase activity in any of the strains that were susceptible to β-lactam antibiotics. β-Lactamase activity was found only in the resistant strains. Activity appeared to be cell bound since no activity was detected in the culture supernatant.

TABLE 1. *MICs of penicillin, carbenicillin, ampicillin, and cephalothin for the Bacterioides strains used in this study*

Bacteroides strain (VPI no.)	MIC value (μg/ml)			
	Penicillin	Carbenicillin	Ampicillin	Cephalothin
B. melaninogenicus subsp. *intermedius*				
8944, 9145	<0.125	<0.125	<0.125	<0.25
9931, 9466	16–32	16–32	8–16	32
B. melaninogenicus subsp. *melaninogenicus*				
4196	<0.125	<0.125	<0.125	<0.125
9465B	32	16	16	64
B. melaninogenicus subsp. *asaccharolyticus*				
8107DP, 8544A	<0.125	<0.125	<0.125	<0.125
7795, 9848	16	16	8–16	32–64
B. oralis				
5933, 6733	<0.125	<0.25	<0.125	<0.25
4533C, 9611	16–32	16–32	8–16	16–32

Although the resistant strains were equally resistant to all four antibiotics, β-lactamase activity varied considerably, depending on the strain and the antibiotic used as substrate (Table 2). Strains of *B. oralis* and the two saccharolytic subspecies of *B. melaninogenicus* (*B. melaninogenicus* subsp. *intermedius* and *B. melaninogenicus* subsp. *melaninogenicus*) hydrolyzed penicillin much more rapidly than carbenicillin or ampicillin. Hydrolysis of cephalothin was less rapid than hydrolysis of penicillin but more rapid than hydrolysis of ampicillin or carbenicillin (Table 2). Strains of *B. melaninogenicus* subsp. *asaccharolyticus* had much lower activity on both penicillin and cephalothin than did strains of *B. oralis* or the other two *B. melaninogenicus* subspecies, but hydrolyzed ampicillin and carbenicillin at the same rate.

The different rates of hydrolysis of penicillin, ampicillin, and carbenicillin obtained by using the iodometric test were confirmed qualitatively by the thin-layer chromatographic method. When hydrolysis of penicillin, carbenicillin, and ampicillin was followed by using chromatography of the hydrolysis products, the conversion of penicillin to penicilloic acid by strains of *B. melaninogenicus* (*B. melaninogenicus* subsp. *intermedius* and *B. melaninogenicus* subsp. *melaninogenicus*) and *B. oralis* was completed in less than one-fourth the time required for the conversion of carbenicillin and ampicillin. Under these conditions, hydrolysis of all three antibiotics by strains of *B. melaninogenicus* subsp. *asaccharolyticus* occurred within the same time period. Since the qualitative results of the thin-layer chromatographic method agreed with the relative rates of hydrolysis obtained by the iodometric method, it appears that differences in activities on different substrates were not due to the special conditions of the iodometric assay, such as the presence of iodine.

Cephalosporinase activity, determined by using the chromogenic cephalosporin method, was at least 10-fold higher than activity obtained using the iodometric method with cephalothin as a substrate (Table 2). However, relative rates of cephalosporin hydrolysis by the different strains were the same with both methods.

Using logarithmically growing cells instead of stationary-phase cells did not affect the level of activity detected. β-Lactamase activity (per 10^{11} cells) of cultures sampled at 4-h intervals remained constant. β-Lactamase activity did not appear to be inducible by penicillin or cephalothin since the same activities were obtained with cells grown in penicillin or cephalothin as with cells grown in the absence of antibiotics.

In some cases, mechanical disruption of the cells increased activity. In Table 3, the percent increase in activity due to lysis is given for those strains in which such a difference occurred. No decrease in activity with lysis was observed in any of the strains tested. When lysed cell suspensions were centrifuged for 30 min at 20,000 × *g*, activity was found only in the pellet (cell envelope fraction). Except in the case of VPI 9465B, in which 3 to 10% of the activity appeared in the supernatant, no activity was detected in the supernatant. Enzyme activity could be extracted from the pellet with 2% Triton X-100 and 10% taurocholate but not with 1 M NaCl. Enzyme activity was lost when sodium dodecyl sulfate was added to the lysed cell suspension.

Treatment of cells with ethylenediaminetetraacetate-lysozyme resulted in the conversion of nearly all of the cells to spheroplasts. Spheroplast formation released 7 to 12% of the enzyme activity into the medium.

TABLE 2. *β-Lactamase activity in resistant strains of B. melaninogenicus and B. oralis*

Bacteroides (VPI no.)	β-Lactamase activity (μmol/min per 10^{11} cells)				
	Iodometric assay				Chromogenic cephalosporin 87/312
	Penicillin	Carbenicillin	Ampicillin	Cephalothin	
B. melaninogenicus subsp. *intermedius*					
9331	0.5	0.1	0.1	0.2	2.4
9466	1.1	0.4	0.2	0.6	10.0
B. melaninogenicus subsp. *melaninogenicus*					
9465B	1.4	0.2	0.1	1.3	12.8
B. melaninogenicus subsp. *asaccharolyticus*					
7795	0.2	0.1	0.1	<0.1	1.0
9848	<0.1	0.1	0.1	<0.1	0.8
B. oralis					
4533C	1.7	0.2	0.1	0.4	8.6
9611	1.8	0.3	0.1	0.6	8.0

TABLE 3. *Percent increase in β-lactamase activity in lysed cells of B. melaninogenicus*

Bacteroides (VPI no.)	β-Lactamase activity[a]			
	Penicillin	Carbenicillin	Ampicillin	Chromogenic cephalosporin 87/312
B. melaninogenicus subsp. *intermedius*				
9331	240	150	100	150
9466	210	110	120	140
B. melaninogenicus subsp. *melaninogenicus*				
9465B	210	110	100	110

[a] Expressed as a percentage of the activity in whole cells of the same strain on the same antibiotic.

DISCUSSION

Strains of *B. melaninogenicus* and *B. oralis* that are resistant to β-lactam antibiotics have enzymes that can hydrolyze both penicillins and cephalosporins. Since β-lactamase activity was found only in resistant strains of these species, it is probable that the production of β-lactamase is involved in the resistance of these organisms to β-lactam antibiotics. However, there was considerable variation in levels of activity found in strains with the same MIC values. The low β-lactamase activity on carbenicillin and ampicillin, as compared with penicillin, was not accompanied by a higher susceptibility to these antibiotics. Thus, production of β-lactamase may not be the only mechanism of resistance in these strains.

Levels of activity and hydrolysis patterns of *B. oralis* were almost identical with those of *B. melaninogenicus* subsp. *intermedius* and *B. melaninogenicus* subsp. *melaninogenicus*. *B. melaninogenicus* subsp. *asaccharolyticus*, which differs from the other *B. melaninogenicus* subspecies in a number of taxonomic characteristics, including deoxyribonucleic acid base composition (14), also differed from these subspecies and *B. oralis* in the level of enzyme activity on penicillin and cephalothin. These results indicate that *B. oralis* and the two saccharolytic *B. melaninogenicus* subspecies may have similar enzymes, whereas the enzyme produced by *B. melaninogenicus* subsp. *asaccharolyticus* may be distinct from these.

In all cases, β-lactamase activity appeared to be associated mainly with the cell envelope and could only be solubilized by detergents. This may be due in part to the method of mechanical disruption. The use of sonification rather than shaking with glass beads to disrupt cells may increase the percentage of soluble enzyme (R. G. Wilkinson, private communication). The fact that lysis of the cells increased activity indicates that there may be a permeability barrier separating the enzyme from the antibiotic. Also, spheroplast formation did not release significant amounts of activity into the medium. Thus, the enzyme may be associated with the inner membrane of the cell.

β-Lactamase activity in *B. melaninogenicus* and *B. oralis* differs from β-lactamase activities reported in other *Bacteroides* species. Whereas the enzymes from *B. melaninogenicus* and *B. oralis* were generally more active against penicillin than ampicillin, carbenicillin, or cephalothin, β-lactamase from *B. fragilis* has been reported to be more active on cephalosporins than on penicillins (2, 11). A β-lactamase from *B. clostridiiformis* was found to be active primarily on penicillin and ampicillin but not on carbenicillin and cephalosporins (11). Moreover, previous exposure to penicillin increased the activity of *B. clostridiiformis*, whereas previous exposure of *B. fragilis, B. melaninogenicus*, and *B. oralis* strains to penicillin did not increase β-lactamase activity.

β-Lactamases have now been found in resistant strains from a number of species of gram-negative bacteria. However, resistance to β-lactam antibiotics is not always correlated with high β-lactamase activities, and there is still some question about the true role of these enzymes (6). In the case of *B. melaninogenicus, B. oralis*, and *B. fragilis*, strains with similar patterns of resistance to β-lactam antibiotics produce β-lactamases that differ considerably in levels of activity and substrate specificity. Further work is needed to determine the significance of β-lactamase and the possible contribution of other mechanisms to penicillin and cephalosporin resistance in these *Bacteroides* species.

ACKNOWLEDGMENTS

This research was supported by Public Health Service grant GM14604 from the National Institute of General Medical Sciences and by a grant from the Upjohn Co.

LITERATURE CITED

1. **Birdsell, D. C., and E. H. Cota-Robles.** 1967. Production and ultrastructure of lysozyme and ethylenediaminetetraacetate-lysozyme spheroplasts of *Esche-*

richia coli. J. Bacteriol. **93**:427–437.
2. **Del Bene, V. E., and W. E. Farrar.** 1973. Cephalosporinase activity in *Bacteroides fragilis*. Antimicrob. Agents Chemother. 3:369–372.
3. **Hackman, A. S., and T. D. Wilkins.** 1976. Influence of penicillinase production by strains of *Bacteroides melaninogenicus* and *Bacteroides oralis* on penicillin therapy of an experimental mixed anaerobic infection in mice. Arch. Oral Biol. **21**:385–389.
4. **Holdeman, L. V., and W. E. C. Moore (ed.).** 1975. Anaerobe laboratory manual, 3rd ed. Virginia Polytechnic Institute and State University, Blacksburg, Va.
5. **Martin, W. J., M. Gardner, and J. A. Washington.** 1972. In vitro antimicrobial susceptibility of anaerobic bacteria isolated from clinical specimens. Antimicrob. Agents Chemother. **1**:148–158.
6. **Neu, H. C.** 1972. The role of β-lactamases in the resistance of gram-negative bacteria to penicillin and cephalosporin derivatives. Infect. Dis. Rev. **3**:133–149.
7. **O'Callaghan, C. H., A. Morris, S. M. Kirby, and A. H. Shingler.** 1972. Novel method for detection of β-lactamases by using a chromogenic cephalosporin substrate. Antimicrob. Agents. Chemother. **1**:283–288.
8. **Pinkus, G., G. Veto, and A. I. Braude.** 1968. Bacteroides penicillinase. J. Bacteriol. **96**:1437–1438.
9. **Sykes, R. B., and K. Nordstrom.** 1972. Microiodometric determination of β-lactamase activity. Antimicrob. Agents Chemother. **1**:94–99.
10. **Thornton, G. F., and J. A. Cramer.** 1971. Antibiotic susceptibility of *Bacteroides* species, p. 509–513. Antimicrob. Agents Chemother. 1970.
11. **Weinrich, A. E., and V. E. Del Bene.** 1976. β-Lactamase activity in anaerobic bacteria. Antimicrob. Agents. Chemother. **10**:106–111.
12. **Wilkins. T. D., and M. D. Appleman.** 1976. Review of methods for antibiotic susceptibility testing of anaerobic bacteria. Lab. Med. **7**:12–15.
13. **Wilkins. T. D., and T. Thiel.** 1973. Modified broth-disk method for testing the antibiotic susceptibility of anaerobic bacteria. Antimicrob. Agents Chemother. **3**:350–356.
14. **Williams, R. A. D., G. H. Bowden, J. M. Hardie, and H. Shah.** 1975. Biochemical properties of *Bacteroides melaninogenicus* subspecies. Int. J. Syst. Bacteriol. **25**:298–300.

ANTIMICROBIAL AGENTS AND CHEMOTHERAPY, Jan. 1977, p. 147-153 Vol. 11, No. 1

Printed in U.S.A.

L-Glyceraldehyde 3-Phosphate, a Bactericidal Agent

CHU-TAY TANG, ROBERT ENGEL, AND BURTON E. TROPP*

Department of Chemistry, Queens College of the City University of New York, Flushing, New York 11367

Received for publication 3 August 1976

At a concentration of 2.5 mM, DL-glyceraldehyde 3-phosphate has a bactericidal effect upon *Escherichia coli*. The glycerol 3-phosphate transport system is required for the entry of the biologically active L-enantiomer. L-Glyceraldehyde must be phosphorylated by the cell to exert its full effect upon growth. The addition of DL-glyceraldehyde 3-phosphate to a culture of *E. coli* caused no preferential inhibition of the accumulation of deoxyribonucleic acid, ribonucleic acid, or phosphoglycerides, although protein accumulation was less affected. Studies with mutant strains ruled out catabolic glycerol 3-phosphate dehydrogenase, anabolic nicotinamide adenine dinucleotide (phosphate):*sn*-glycerol 3-phosphate oxidoreductase, and fructose 1,6-diphosphate aldolase as the primary sites of action. L-Glyceraldehyde 3-phosphate is a competitive inhibitor of *sn*-glycerol 3-phosphate in the reactions catalyzed by acyl coenzyme A:*sn*-glycerol 3-phosphate acyltransferase (K_i of 1.8 mM) and cytidine 5'-diphosphate-diglyceride:*sn*-glycerol 3-phosphate phosphatidyltransferase (K_i of 2.7 mM). A K_m mutant for the former enzyme was susceptible to the inhibitor. L-Glyceraldehyde 3-phosphate does not affect acyl coenzyme A:lysophosphatidate acyltransferase activity. In vivo, phosphatidylethanolamine and phosphatidylglycerol accumulation are inhibited to the same extent by the addition of DL-glyceraldehyde 3-phosphate to a culture of *E. coli*.

Previous studies with 3,4-dihydroxybutyl-1-phosphonate made us aware that analogues of glycerol 3-phosphate can have profound effects upon cellular metabolism (4, 15–17). The hydrated form of L-glyceraldehyde 3-phosphate may be considered to be an analogue of *sn*-glycerol 3-phosphate in which a hydroxyl group replaces a hydrogen at C1. In aqueous solution, glyceraldehyde 3-phosphate exists as an equilibrium mixture of the geminal diol (hydrated form) and free aldehyde in a molar ratio of 29:1 (19). The data in the present report indicate that L-glyceraldehyde 3-phosphate is bactericidal and interferes with two enzymes involved in phosphoglyceride synthesis.

MATERIALS AND METHODS

Chemicals. L-[^{3}H]isoleucine, *sn*-[^{14}C]glycerol 3-phosphate, and carrier-free [^{33}P]phosphate were purchased from the New England Nuclear Corp., Boston, Mass. The following materials were obtained from the Sigma Chemical Co., St. Louis, Mo.: reduced nicotinamide adenine dinucleotide phosphate, type III; dithiothreitol; DL-glyceraldehyde 3-phosphoric acid (diethyl acetal, monobarium salt); *N,N*-bis-(2-hydroxyethyl) glycine, Bicine; 5,5'-dithiobis-(2-nitrobenzoic acid), DTNB; tris(hydroxymethyl)aminomethane; D- and L-glyceraldehyde; and octylphenoxypolyethoxyethanol, the nonionic detergent Triton X-100; and bovine serum albumin. D-Glyceraldehyde 3-phosphoric acid (diethyl acetal, dicyclohexyl ammonium salt) was a product of Boehringer Mannheim Corp., New York, N.Y. Glyceraldehyde 3-phosphoric acid was generated from the corresponding acetals by mixing with an aqueous suspension of Dowex 50, hydrogen ion form, using the procedure recommended by the Sigma Chemical Co.

1-Palmitoyl glycerol 3-phosphate (lysophosphatidic acid) and cytidine diphosphate-dipalmitin (CDP-dipalmitin) were purchased from Serdary Research Laboratories Inc., London Ontario, Canada. Oleoyl coenzyme A and palmitoyl coenzyme A (CoA) were obtained from P-L Biochemicals, Inc., Milwaukee, Wis. The bacterial phospholipid standards phosphatidylethanolamine, phosphatidylglycerol, and cardiolipin were purchased from Supelco Inc., Bellefonte, Pa.

Silica Gel G thin-layer plates were obtained from Analabs, Inc., North Haven, Conn. Eugonagar was a product of Fisher Scientific, Fair Lawn, N.J. 2-Mercaptoethanol was a product of Matheson, Coleman and Bell, Norwood, Ohio. All other chemicals were of reagent grade.

Bacterial strains and culture conditions. The bacterial strains studied are described in Table 1. The glycerol 3-phosphate transport-negative mutants are derivatives of *E. coli* 8. A complete description of their isolation and characterization will be the subject of a future report. Briefly, strain 8 was mutagenized with *N*-methyl-*N'*-nitronitrosoguanidine. Cells resistant to 3,4-dihydroxybutyl-1-phosphonate were selected, and assayed for the glycerol 3-phosphate transport system.

The effect of glyceraldehyde 3-phosphate and related compounds upon growth was determined by monitoring growth turbidimetrically in a Klett-Summerson colorimeter with a 660-nm filter. Cells were cultured in 10 to 25 ml of medium in 250-ml Erlenmeyer flasks fitted with side arms. Incubations were in a New Brunswick Aquatherm G86 or Metabolyte G77 water bath shaker at 200 rpm. In all cases, several generations of exponential growth were allowed for the dilute starting cultures to attain the cell density at which the experiments were initiated. Viability studies were performed by diluting cultures and plating on Eugonagar. All incubations were at 37°C.

Three types of minimal media were employed in growth studies. *E. coli* CY 115 and 7 were cultured in Vogel and Bonner minimal medium (21) containing 0.5% glycerol as the sole carbon source and supplemented with thiamine-hydrochloride, 2 mg/liter; methionine, 50 mg/liter; and tryptophan, 50 mg/liter. *E. coli* strains 8, NP 315, and derivatives of strain 8 defective in the glycerol 3-phosphate transport system were cultured in Garen and Levinthal minimal medium containing 0.6 mM phosphate (8) with 0.5% potassium succinate as the sole carbon source. A Bicine-buffered medium was utilized in experiments involving the effects of glyceraldehyde on the growth of *E. coli* 8 and 9. This medium contained Bicine-hydrochloride, 100 mM (pH 7.4); NaCl, 90 mM; KCl, 40 mM; NH_4Cl, 200 mM; and all the other salts in concentrations required for the Garen and Levinthal synthetic medium (8). Cells used for the preparation of enzyme extracts were cultured in Garen and Levinthal minimal medium as described above and harvested in late-logarithmic phase.

Macromolecular and phospholipid synthesis. Cultures of *E. coli* 8 at a cell density of 15 to 20 Klett units (1 Klett unit is equivalent to approximately 5×10^6 cells/ml) were simultaneously mixed with various concentrations of DL-glyceraldehyde 3-phosphate or water and 1 to 3 μCi of [^{33}P]phosphate per ml. Samples of 1 ml were removed at the indicated times and treated as previously described (16) to measure the synthesis of deoxyribonucleic acid (DNA), ribonucleic acid (RNA), and phosphoglyceride. A portion of the chloroform-soluble material was retained for thin-layer chromatography of the phosphoglycerides (14).

Protein synthesis was followed by measuring the conversion of isolecucine into a trichloroacetic acid-insoluble material. One milliliter of culture medium was simultaneously mixed with 0.45 μCi of L-[^{3}H]isoleucine and 15 μg of L-isoleucine and DL-glyceraldehyde 3-phosphate. Samples of 0.1 ml were removed and assayed as previously described (15).

Assay of acyl CoA:*sn*-glycerol 3-phosphate acyltransferase. Membranes were prepared from *E. coli* 8 or BB26-36 R2 as described previously (4). The activity of acyl CoA:*sn*-glycerol 3-phosphate acyltransferase of the membrane preparation was assayed by determining the incorporation of [^{14}C]glycerol 3-phosphate (12.4 mCi/mmol) into lipid. The assays were performed at 30°C and initiated by the addition of palmitoyl CoA. The specific activity at maximum velocity of the strain 8 preparations was 2.4 nmol/min per mg. In some cases, the activity of acyl CoA:*sn*-glycerol 3-phosphate was also assayed by monitoring the release of CoA by measuring its chemical interaction with DTNB by a modification of the procedure of Cronan et al. (6). The assay mixture (total volume, 1 ml) contained 100 μmol of Bicine-hydrochloride, pH 8.5; 5 μmol of $MgCl_2$; 1 mg of bovine serum albumin; 50 nmol of palmitoyl CoA; 1.0 μmol of DTNB; 60 μg of enzyme; and 0.75 μmol of *sn*-glycerol 3-phosphate. The initial rates were monitored by measuring absorbance at 25°C in a Gilford model 250 spectrophotometer equipped with a multiple-sample absorbance recorder.

Assay of acyl CoA:lysophosphatidate acyltransferase. The preparation of this particulate enzyme was the same as that of acyl CoA:*sn*-glycerol 3-phosphate acyltransferase. The acyl CoA:lysophosphatidate acyltransferase was assayed by a colorimetric procedure that was essentially the same as described above for acyl CoA:glycerol 3-phosphate acyltransferase (6, 20). The reaction mixture (total volume of 1 ml) contained 100 μmol of Bicine-hydrochloride, pH 8.5; 0.5 μmol of $MgCl_2$; 1 mg of bovine

TABLE 1. *Bacterial strains studied*[a]

Strain	Mating type	Genotype	Source and reference
7	HfrC	*glpR*^{c}*2 phoA8 tonA22* T_2^R *rel-1* (λ)	E. C. C. Lin, Harvard Medical School (10)
8	HfrC	Same as 7, *glpD3*	J. Cronan, Jr., Yale University (9)
9	HfrC	Same as 8, *glpK*	E. C. C. Lin, Harvard Medical School (9)
BB26-36 R2	HfrC	Same as 8, *gpsA3*^{FR} *plsB26*	R. Bell, Duke University Medical Center (2)
NP 315 (formerly h8)	Hfr	*tonA22 thi*$^-$ *rel-1* T_2^R *fda*(Ts)	F. C. Neidhardt, University of Michigan (3)
CY 115	F$^-$	*gpsA20 metE70 trpE8 xyl-5 tsx-67 str-109*	J. Cronan, Jr., Yale University (5)

[a] Genetic nomenclature is that of Taylor and Trotter (18). The allele numbers are those of the Coli Genetic Stock Center at Yale University.

serum albumin; 60 nmol of oleoyl CoA; 1.0 μmol of DTNB; 60 μg of enzyme; and 25 nmol of 1-palmitoyl glycerol 3-phosphate.

Assay of CDP-diglyceride:*sn*-glycerol 3-phosphate phosphatidyltransferase. The particulate fraction was prepared from *E. coli* 8 as described previously (4). The activity of CDP-diglyceride:*sn*-glycerol 3-phosphate phosphatidyltransferase was assayed by monitoring the conversion of [^{14}C]glyerol 3-phosphate into chloroform-extractable material as described previously (4). The assay mixture (total volume of 0.25 ml) contained 62.5 μmol of Bicine-hydrochloride, pH 8.0; 20 μmol of CDP-dipalmitin; 2.5 μmol of $MgCl_2$; 1.25 μmol of 2-mercaptoethanol; 0.5 mg of Triton X-100; 55 μg of particulate enzyme; and the indicated concentrations of *sn*-[^{14}C]glycerol 3-phosphate (24.8 mCi/mmol). The enzyme assay was performed at 37°C and initiated by the addition of enzyme preparation.

All enzyme preparations were prepared at 1 to 4°C. Protein concentrations were determined by the method of Lowry et al. (12). The rates of reaction were linearly dependent upon enzyme concentration and time in the range reported.

RESULTS

DL-Glyceraldehyde 3-phosphate is a potent inhibitor of the growth of *E. coli* 8. Figure 1 shows the effects of various concentrations of this compound upon the growth of *E. coli* 8. The data presented in Fig. 2 reveal that 2.5 mM DL-glyceraldehyde 3-phosphate is bactericidal. The L enantiomer of the phosphate, not currently available for study, must account for the inhibition, since D-glyceraldehyde 3-phosphate does not influence cell growth. The *sn*-glycerol 3-phosphate transport system is required for inhibition of cell growth, since several independently isolated transport-negative mutants were resistant to DL-glyceraldehyde 3-phosphate. One such experiment is depicted in Fig. 3.

We examined the question of whether L-glyceraldehyde 3-phosphate or its nonphosphorylated derivative was the true inhibitor. As evident from Fig. 4A, L-glyceraldehyde has some inhibitory effect upon strain 9, a glycerokinase-deficient mutant of strain 8 (9). However, strain 8 was considerably more susceptible to L-glyceraldehyde (Fig. 4B). The ability of glycerokinase to catalyze the phosphorylation of L-glyceraldehyde (10) provides an explanation for the difference in susceptibility observed between the two strains. These results clearly indicate that the phosphorylated derivative is important in the bactericidal effects. The slight inhibition observed in strain 9 may be due to leakiness of the mutation, a second kinase activity, or an effect of the nonphosphorylated aldehyde. We do not have sufficient data to

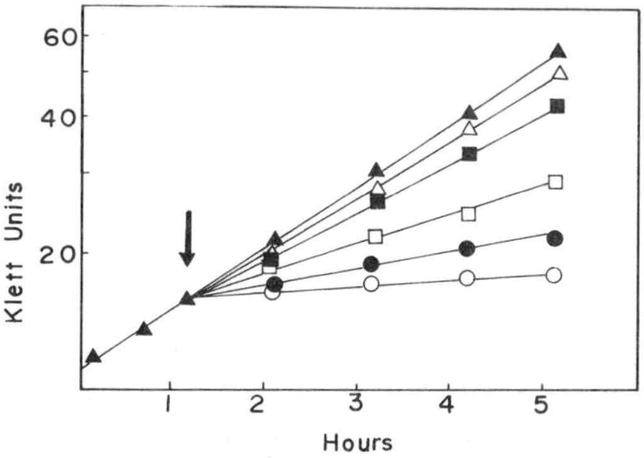

FIG. 1. *Effects of various concentrations of DL-glyceraldehyde 3-phosphate on the growth of E. coli 8 cultured in Garen and Levinthal medium (8) supplemented with 0.5% potassium succinate. At the time indicated by the arrow, the inhibitor was added to the following final concentrations: ○, 2.5 mM; ●, 1.0 mM; □, 0.5 mM; ■, 0.25 mM; △, 0.10 mM; and ▲, untreated.*

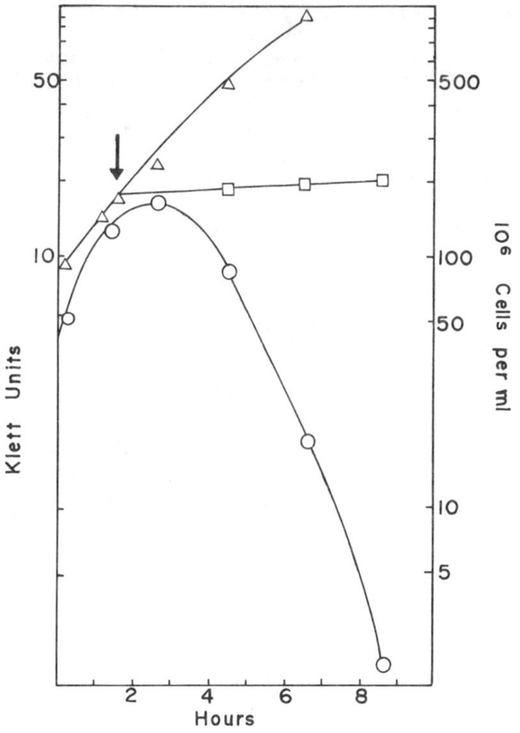

FIG. 2. *Effect of 2.5 mM DL-glyceraldehyde 3-phosphate on the viability of E. coli 8 cultured in Garen and Levinthal medium (8) supplemented with 0.5% potassium succinate. The inhibitor was added at the time indicated by the arrow. Cell viability was determined as described in Materials and Methods. Symbols: △, cell turbidity in Klett units of untreated cultures; □, cell turbidity in Klett units of inhibitor-treated cultures; and ○, viability of inhibitor-treated cultures. The bactericidal effects were also found in Bicine-hydrochloride-buffered medium.*

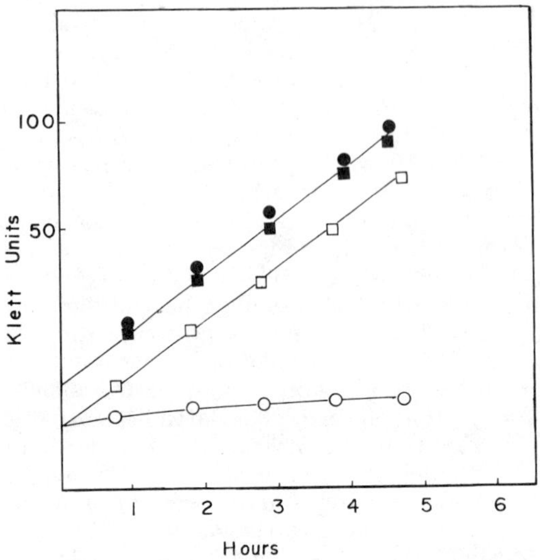

FIG. 3. *Effects of DL-glyceraldehyde 3-phosphate on the growth of E. coli 8 and a glycerol 3-phosphate transport-negative mutant of this strain. Cells were cultured in Garen and Levinthal medium (8) supplemented with 0.5% potassium succinate. DL-Glyceraldehyde was added to early-logarithmic-phase cultures at the start of the experiment. The additions were as follows: strain 8: □, untreated; ○, 2 mM DL-glyceraldehyde 3-phosphate. Glycerol 3-phosphate transport negative-mutant of strain 8: ■, untreated; ●, 2 mM DL-glyceraldehyde 3-phosphate.*

distinguish among the possibilities. D-Glyceraldehyde has an equally slight effect upon strains 8 and 9 (Fig. 4 A and B), which was not studied further.

One method for delineating the site of action of a drug is to examine the effects of various concentrations of the drug on macromolecular and lipid synthesis. This approach has been helpful in studies with another glycerol 3-phosphate analogue, 3,4-dihydroxybutyl-1-phosphonate (16, 17), and with phenethyl alcohol (14). However, as evident from Table 2, this method failed to reveal a single most sensitive site of action for DL-glyceraldehyde 3-phosphate. Experiments similar to those reported in Table 2 for shorter incubation periods and different glyceraldehyde 3-phosphate concentrations also failed to differentiate a site of action. Among the processes examined, protein synthesis appears to be the least affected by glyceraldehyde 3-phosphate. It is therefore unlikely that this agent exerts its primary effect upon amino acid synthesis or energy metabolism.

A second approach to the site of action involves a study of the effects of a drug on various mutants. The lack of catabolic glycerol 3-phosphate dehydrogenase activity in strain 8 is not related to the inhibitory effects observed, since strain 7 and other cells having this activity were quite susceptible to DL-glyceraldehyde 3-

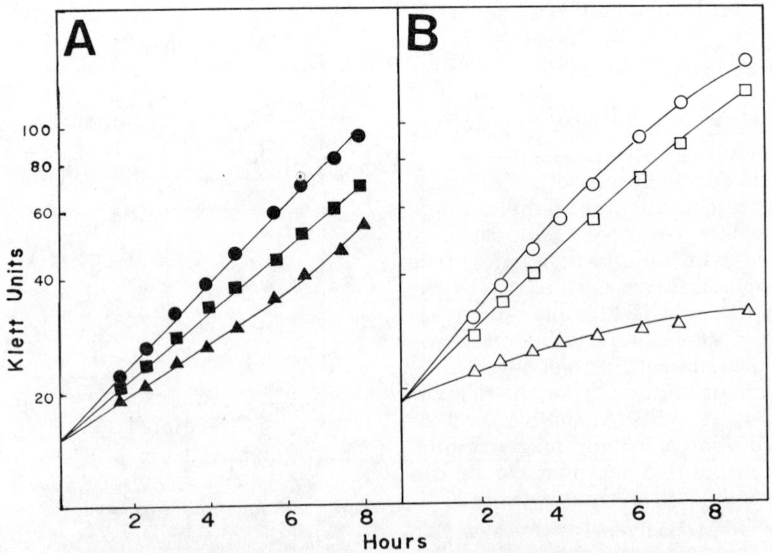

FIG. 4. *Effects of L- and D-glyceraldehyde on the growth of E. coli 8 and 9 in Bicine-buffered medium, as described in Materials and Methods, supplemented with 0.5% potassium succinate. L- or D-Glyceraldehyde was added to a final concentration of 2.5 mM to early-logarithmic-phase cultures at the start of the experiment. Symbols: (A) Strain 9: ●, untreated; ■, D-glyceraldehyde; ▲, L-glyceraldehyde. (B) Strain 8: ○, untreated; □, D-glyceraldehyde; △, L-glyceraldehyde.*

TABLE 2. *Effect of various concentrations of* DL-*glyceraldehyde 3-phosphate on macromolecular and lipid synthesis*[a]

Macromolecular synthesis	DL-Glyceraldehyde 3-phosphate 0.05 M: Total cpm per ml of cells	0.05 M: % of untreated cultures	0.25 M: Total cpm per ml of cells	0.25 M: % of untreated cultures
DNA	2,780	85	1,380	42
RNA	52,800	83	25,200	40
Protein	9,550	101	6,600	69
Phosphoglyceride	28,300	66	15,800	37

[a] DNA, RNA, protein, and phospholipid synthesis by *E. coli* 8 cultured in Garen and Levinthal medium (8) supplemented with 0.5% potassium succinate were monitored as a function of different concentrations of DL-glyceraldehyde 3-phosphate. Labeled precursors of DNA, RNA, and phospholipid, [^{33}P]phosphate, or the precursor of protein, [^{3}H]isoleucine, were added at the same time as the inhibitor and incubated for 60 min. The incorporation studies were performed as described in Materials and Methods.

phosphate. The doubling time of strain 7 increased from 1.8 h to greater than 19 h upon addition of inhibitor.

One possible site of activity for DL-glyceraldehyde 3-phosphate is the anabolic NAD(P):*sn*-glycerol 3-phosphate oxidoreductase (11). This enzyme is inhibited by 3,4-dihydroxybutyl-1-phosphonate (4). This possibility was eliminated by the observation that strain CY 115 (an anabolic dehydrogenase-deficient strain [5], cultured on synthetic medium containing glycerol as the sole carbon source, was quite susceptible to DL-glyceraldehyde 3-phosphate.

L-Glyceraldehyde 3-phosphate might also serve as a substrate of fructose 1,6-diphosphate aldolase. In this case, L-sorbose 1,6-diphosphate would be formed, which might then be the true inhibitor. This possibility was ruled out by the observation that *E. coli* NP 315, a temperature-sensitive fructose 1,6-diphosphate aldolase mutant (3), was quite susceptible to DL-glyceraldehyde 3-phosphate at either 30°C or the nonpermissive temperature, 42°C. At the higher temperature, the addition of 2.5 mM DL-glyceraldehyde 3-phosphate caused an increase in the doubling time from 2 h to greater than 20 h. The other glycolytic enzymes are not likely targets because of their greater sterospecificity for D-glyceraldehyde 3-phosphate.

A third approach to the site of action is to determine whether the drug inhibits a specific enzymatic activity in an in vitro assay. Acyl CoA:*sn*-glycerol 3-phosphate acyltransferase, the first enzyme of the phosphoglyceride biosynthetic pathway, is one of the potential target sites. When assayed by the radioactive assay method as shown in Fig. 5, DL-glyceraldehyde 3-phosphate is a competitive inhibitor of the acyltransferase. D-Glyceraldehyde 3-phosphate does not inhibit the acyltransferase. The apparent K_i for L-glyceraldehyde 3-phosphate is 1.8 mM. The results involving acyltransferase referred to thus far are for palmitoyl CoA as substrate. The incorporation of the oleoyl residue from oleoyl CoA was also inhibited by DL-glyceraldehyde 3-phosphate. The spectrophotometric assay confirmed the glyceraldehyde 3-phosphate inhibition of acyltransferase activity. Furthermore, this assay revealed that DL-glyceraldehyde 3-phosphate does not stimulate the hydrolysis of either palmitoyl CoA or oleoyl CoA and is therefore not a substrate for the acyltransferase.

It appeared possible that K_m mutants for the acyltransferase (2), by virture of an inability to recognize L-glyceraldehyde 3-phosphate, might be resistant to this compound. In agreement with the report of Bell and Cronan (2), we observed that the acyltransferase of BB26-36 R2 had a K_m of 577 μM for *sn*-glycerol 3-phosphate. In the presence of 400 μM *sn*-glycerol 3-phosphate, 7.1 mM DL-glyceraldehyde 3-phosphate inhibited mutant acyltransferase by greater than 60% when assayed at either 25 or 30°C. The acyltransferase of BB26-36 R2 therefore recognizes glyceraldehyde 3-phosphate. The drug is also bactericidal to strain BB26-36 R2. We have not examined other acyltransferase mutants.

Acyl CoA:lysophosphatidate acyltransferase, the second enzyme of phosphoglyceride biosynthesis, was not sensitive to DL-glyceraldehyde

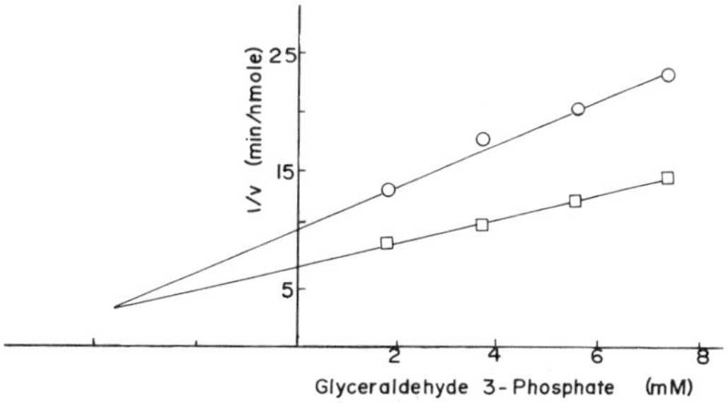

FIG. 5. *Determination of the apparent K_i of* DL-*glyceraldehyde 3-phosphate for acyl CoA:sn-glycerol 3-phosphate acyltransferase by the Dixon method (7). The assay conditions are described in Materials and Methods. The reaction mixtures were* □, *64.6 μM, and* ○, *32.3 μM, in sn-[^{14}C]glycerol 3-phosphate 4 and contained varying concentrations of* DL-*glyceraldehyde 3-phosphate.*

3-phosphate. This is significant, since it indicates that all the sensitivity observed in the *sn*-glycerol 3-phosphate:acyl CoA acyltransferase assay is specific for this enzyme.

DL-Glyceraldehyde 3-phosphate is a competitive inhibitor of CDP-diglyceride:*sn*-glycerol 3-phosphate phosphatidyltransferase (Fig. 6). The D enantiomer was without effect. The apparent K_i for L-glyceraldehyde 3-phosphate is 2.7 mM. The physiological significance of this result was examined by determining the effect of concentrations of DL-glyceraldehyde 3-phosphate to 0.50 mM on the distribution of phosphoglycerides accumulated by *E. coli* 8 for 1 h. At 0.05, 0.10, 0.25, and 0.50 mM DL-glyceraldehyde 3-phosphate, phosphatidylglycerol accumulation was 73, 60, 44, and 25% of untreated cultures, respectively. The percentage of control for phosphatidylethanolamine was 73, 66, 44, and 23%, respectively. Thus, there was no differential effect on the accumulation of these major phospholipids. Cardiolipin accumulation was not noticeably affected by glyceraldehyde 3-phosphate. Although the above results were obtained using [^{33}P]phosphate to monitor phospholipid accumulation, similar results were obtained when [^{14}C]acetate served as the radioactive tracer. These findings are in striking contrast to the effects of 3,4-dihydroxybutyl-1-phosphonate, which preferentially inhibits the accumulation of phosphatidylglycerol (16, 17). The phosphonate analogue also has a lower apparent K_i for the phosphatidyltransferase, 740 μM (4).

DISCUSSION

DL-Glyceraldehyde 3-phosphate, an analogue of glycerol 3-phosphate, enters the cell via the

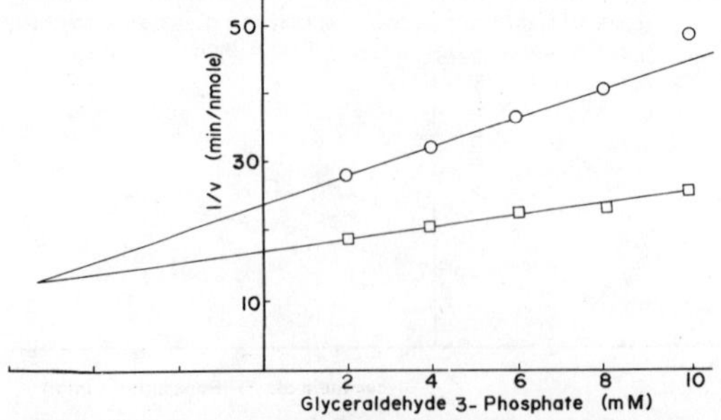

FIG. 6. *Determination of the apparent K_i of DL-glyceraldehyde 3-phosphate for CDP-diglyceride:sn-glycerol 3-phosphate phosphatidyltransferase by the Dixon method (7). The assay conditions are described in Materials and Methods. The reaction mixtures were □, 64.6 μM, and ○, 32.3 μM, in sn-[^{14}C]glycerol 3-phosphate and contained varying amounts of DL-glyceraldehyde 3-phosphate.*

sn-glycerol 3-phosphate transport system (Fig. 3) and is bactericidal (Fig. 2). Several lines of evidence point to L-glyceraldehyde 3-phosphate being the active agent. The D enantiomer is without effect, whereas the racemic mixture is quite active. Hayashi et al. have demonstrated that DL-glyceraldehyde 3-phosphate is an inhibitor of *sn*-glycerol 3-phosphate transport (9). The stereospecificity of this system and its requirement for cell susceptibility strongly suggests that the L form is the active one. Finally, L-glyceraldehyde is quite an effective inhibitor of cell growth in strains capable of phosphorylating this compound. The D form is considerably less active.

Comparison between the inhibitory effects of 3,4-dihydroxybutyl-1-phosphonate and glyceraldehyde 3-phosphate reveals several differences. Among these are the following: (i) 3,4-Dihydroxybutyl-1-phosphonate preferentially inhibits phosphatidylgycerol synthesis (16, 17), whereas the aldehyde does not. (ii) The phosphonate is bacteriostatic (15), whereas glyceraldehyde 3-phosphate is bactericidal (Fig. 2). (iii) L-Glyceraldehyde 3-phosphate is a competitive inhibitor for acyl CoA:*sn*-glycerol 3-phosphate acyltransferase (Fig. 5), whereas the phosphonate is not an inhibitor of this enzyme (4). (iv) Although both analogues are recognized by CDP-diglyceride:*sn*-glycerol 3-phosphate phosphatidyltransferase, the K_i for the phosphonate is 740 μM (4) and the K_i for L-glyceraldehyde 3-phosphate is 2.7 mM (Fig. 6).

The mechanism by which L-glyceraldehyde 3-phosphate kills cells is not known. Studies with mutants (1) and inhibitors (13, 14, 16, 17) indicate that a block in phosphoglyceride synthesis is frequently accompanied by an inhibition of macromolecular synthesis. If, as appears possible, the primary target of L-glyceraldehyde 3-phosphate is at the level of phosphoglyceride biosynthesis, this compound should prove to be an important research tool in the study of phosphoglyceride metabolism. This is particularly so, since the nonphosphorylated derivative should be quite permeable to many cell membranes and, therefore, not require a special transport system. Once inside the cell, glycerokinase can activate the L-glyceraldehyde as shown for *E. coli* (Fig. 4). Preliminary experiments with *Bacillus subtilis* and yeast revealed that the former is quite susceptible to L-glyceraldehyde and DL-glyceraldehyde 3-phosphate, whereas the latter is not (unpublished data of D. Klein, R. Engel, and B. Tropp). Further work is required to determine the primary target. We are currently examining this question.

It is of interest that, although D-glyceraldehyde 3-phosphate and *sn*-glycerol 3-phosphate are ubiquitous metabolic intermediates, L-glyceraldehyde 3-phosphate is not a naturally occurring biological compound. The close structural relationship between glyceraldehyde 3-phosphate and glycerol 3-phosphate may be responsible for the evolution of optically unrelated intermediates for carbohydrate and phosphoglyceride metabolism.

ACKNOWLEDGMENTS

This investigation was supported by Public Health Service grant GM 21400-03 from the National Institute of General Medical Sciences and a grant from the Faculty Research Award Program of City University.

LITERATURE CITED

1. **Bell, R. M.** 1974. Mutants of *Escherichia coli* defective in membrane phospholipid synthesis in an *sn*-glycerol 3-phosphate acyltransferase K_m mutant. J. Bacteriol. 117:1065–1076.
2. **Bell, R. M., and J. E. Cronan, Jr.** 1975. Mutants of *Escherichia coli* defective in membrane phospholipid synthesis: phenotypic suppression of *sn*-glycerol 3-phosphate acyltransferase K_m mutants by loss of feedback inhibition of the biosynthetic *sn*-glycerol 3-phosphate dehydrogenase. J. Biol. Chem. 250:7153–7158.
3. **Bock, A., and F. C. Neidhardt.** 1966. Isolation of a mutant of *Escherichia coli* with a temperature-sensitive fructose 1,6-diphosphate aldolase activity. J. Bacteriol. 92:464–469.
4. **Cheng, P.-J., W. D. Nunn, R. J. Tyhach, S. L. Goldstein, R. Engel, and B. E. Tropp.** 1975. Investigations concerning the mode of action of 3,4-dihydroxybutyl-1-phosphonate on *Escherichia coli*. *In vitro* examination of enzymes involved in glycerol 3-phosphate metabolism. J. Biol. Chem. 250:1633–1639.
5. **Cronan, J. E., Jr., and R. M. Bell.** 1974. Mutants of *Escherichia coli* defective in membrane phospholipid synthesis: mapping of the structural gene for L-glycerol 3-phosphate dehydrogenase. J. Bacteriol. 118:598–605.
6. **Cronan, J. E., Jr., T. K. Ray, and P. R. Vagelos.** 1970. Selection and characterization of an *E. coli* mutant defective in membrane lipid biosynthesis. Proc. Natl. Acad. Sci. U.S.A. 65:737–744.
7. **Dixon, M., and E. C. Webb.** 1964. Enzyme inhibitors, p. 315–359. *In* Enzymes. Academic Press Inc., New York, N.Y.
8. **Garen, A., and C. Levinthal.** 1960. A fine-structure genetic and chemical study of the enzyme alkaline phosphatase of *E. coli*. I. Purification and characterization of alkaline phosphatase. Biochim. Biophys. Acta 38:470–483.
9. **Hayashi, S., J. P. Koch, and E. C. C. Lin.** 1964. Active transport of L-α-glycerophosphate in *Escherichia coli*. J. Biol. Chem. 239:3098–3105.
10. **Hayashi, S., and E. C. C. Lin.** 1967. Purification and properties of glycerol kinase from *Escherichia coli*. J. Biol. Chem. 242:1030–1035.
11. **Kito, M., and L. I. Pizer.** 1969. Purification and regulatory properties of the biosynthetic L-glycerol 3-phosphate dehydrogenase from *Escherichia coli*. J. Biol. Chem. 244:3316–3323.
12. **Lowry, O. H., N. J. Rosebrough, A. L. Parr, and R. J. Randall.** 1951. Protein measurement with the Folin phenol reagent. J. Biol. Chem. 193:265–275.
13. **Nunn, W. D.** 1975. The inhibition of phospholipid synthesis in *Escherichia coli* by phenethyl alcohol. Biochim. Biophys. Acta 380:403–413.
14. **Nunn, W. D., and B. E. Tropp.** 1972. Effects of phenethyl alcohol on phospholipid metabolism in *Escherichia coli*. J. Bacteriol. 109:162–168.
15. **Shopsis, C. S., R. Engel, and B. E. Tropp.** 1972. Effects of phosphonic acid analogues of glycerol 3-phosphate on the growth of *Escherichia coli*. J. Bacteriol. 112:408–412.
16. **Shopsis, C. S., R. Engel, and B. E. Tropp.** 1974. The inhibition of phosphatidylglycerol synthesis in *Escherichia coli* by 3,4-dihydroxybutyl-1-phosphonate. J. Biol. Chem. 249:2473–2477.
17. **Shopsis, C. S., W. D. Nunn, R. Engel, and B. E. Tropp.** 1973. Effects of phosphonic acid analogues of glycerol 3-phosphate on the growth of *Escherichia coli*: phospholipid metabolism. Antimicrob. Agents Chemother. 4:467–473.
18. **Taylor, A. L., and C. D. Trotter.** 1972. Linkage map of *Escherichia coli* K-12. Bacteriol. Rev. 36:504–524.
19. **Trentham, D. R., C. H. McMurray, and C. I. Pogson.** 1969. The active chemical state of D-glyceraldehyde 3-phosphate in its reactions with D-glyceraldehyde 3-phosphate dehydrogenase, aldolase, and triose phosphate isomerase. Biochem. J. 114:19–24.
20. **Van Den Bosch, H., and P. R. Vagelos.** 1970. Fatty acyl CoA and fatty acyl acyl carrier protein as acyl donors in the synthesis of lysophosphatidate and phosphatidate in *Escherichia coli*. Biochim. Biophys. Acta 218:233–248.
21. **Vogel, H. J., and D. M. Bonner.** 1956. Acetyl-ornithinase of *Escherichia coli*: partial purification and some properties. J. Biol. Chem. 218:97–106.

Antimicrobial Agents and Chemotherapy, Jan. 1977, p. 154-160
Vol. 11, No. 1

Printed in U.S.A.

Effects of Amphotericin B on Macrophages and Their Precursor Cells

HSIU-SAN LIN,* GERALD MEDOFF, AND GEORGE S. KOBAYASHI

Section of Cancer Biology, Mallinckrodt Institute of Radiology; and Divisions of Infectious Disease and Dermatology, Department of Internal Medicine and Department of Microbiology and Immunology, Washington University School of Medicine, St. Louis, Missouri 63110*

Received for publication 17 June 1976

The effect of amphotericin B (AmB) treatment on the mononuclear phagocyte system of mice was investigated. Peritoneal macrophages from mice that received AmB treatment showed a higher phagocytic and antibacterial activity than those from normal untreated mice. When the levels of macrophage precursor cells in bone marrow and spleen were followed in mice after AmB treatment, an eightfold increase in the splenic content of limited stem cells for both macrophages and granulocytes (colony-forming units in culture) and a threefold increase in the number of pluripotent hemopoietic stem cells (colony-forming units in spleen) were observed on day 4. These were also accompanied by a slight increase in the colony-forming units in spleen and in culture in femoral marrows. AmB was capable of inducing a large number of peritoneal colony-forming cells in the peritoneum, and caused a significant rise in the serum level of colony-stimulating factor. No significant change in the level of blood monocytes was noted, although a transient increase in the proportion of neutrophils was observed within 24 h after AmB treatment.

We recently demonstrated that amphotericin B (AmB) can increase the survival of mice with a transplantable leukemia (12), delay the occurrence of spontaneous lymphoma in AKR mice (19), and affect the percentage of mice surviving infection with *Listeria monocytogenes* (17). In these cases, one of the hypothesized mechanisms of AmB effect was a nonspecific potentiation of host resistance.

Because of the hypothesized "adjuvant-like" property of AmB, we started to examine its effect on isolated components of the host defense system. Elsewhere we reported on the effect of AmB on T and B lymphocyte function and showed that AmB augments B cell responses to immunization with a hapten-protein complex and also increases certain graft-versus-host reactions (1).

In this paper we describe the effects of AmB on the mononuclear phagocyte system in mice and show that AmB can increase the phagocytic and antibacterial activities of macrophages and the level of various precursor cells of macrophages in hemopoietic organs.

MATERIALS AND METHODS

Mice. The animals used in these experiments were 2- to 3-month-old AKR female mice weighing 20 to 24 g. Some were obtained from the Jackson Laboratories, Bar Harbor, and others were obtained from the Jewish Hospital, St. Louis, Mo. The mice were housed, in cages, in groups of five and fed Wayne Lab Blox F-6 (Allied Mills, Inc., Chicago, Ill.) and water ad lib.

Chemicals. AmB (Fungizone) was purchased from E.R. Squibb & Sons, Princeton, N.J. Fungizone was supplied in vials as a sterile lyophilized powder; each vial contained 50 mg of AmB and 41 mg of sodium deoxycholate with 25.2 mg of sodium phosphate as a buffer. Sodium deoxycholate was obtained from Sigma Chemical Co., St. Louis, Mo. All chemicals were dissolved in sterile, nonpyrogenic 5% glucose in water (Travenol Laboratories, Inc., Deerfield, Ill.) and were not contaminated by endotoxin as determined by the amebocyte-gelation assay and pyrogene test in rabbits (17).

Organism. Our strain of *L. monocytogenes* was originally obtained from a human infection. It was maintained on nutrient agar at 4°C and transferred weekly with periodic passage in animals. Its virulence for mice (mean lethal dose, 2.5×10^4 organisms) has remained constant since its isolation.

Phagocytosis and bactericidal activity. Groups of 10 mice were treated with AmB according to one of two schedules. They were either given one intraperitoneal (i.p.) injection of 0.5 mg of AmB in 0.1 ml of 5% glucose in sterile water or injected intravenously (i.v.) through a tail vein with 20 μg of AmB in 0.1 ml of sterile 5% glucose in water on 3 successive days. Control mice were injected i.p. or i.v. with sterile 5% glucose in water or with sodium deoxycholate (0.5 mg) in sodium phosphate buffer.

Twenty-four hours after the last injection of AmB

or control solutions, peritoneal exudate cells were obtained by irrigation of the peritoneal cavity of the mice with tissue culture medium 199 (Microbiological Associates, Inc., Bethesda, Md.). The cells were then washed with phosphate-buffered saline and suspended in medium 199 with 10% fetal calf serum.

The ability of the peritoneal exudate cells to phagocytize polystyrene beads 0.81 μm in diameter was measured by incubating 10^6 cells per ml in Leighton tubes on flying cover slips with 10^7 beads per ml for 1 h. In some experiments, cells were incubated in the Leighton tubes overnight, and the unattached cells were washed out the next morning with medium before incubation with the beads. This constituted our preparation of "pure macrophages."

After the cells were incubated with the beads for 1 h, the cover slips were removed from the Leighton tubes and then washed and stained with Wright stain. The number of intracellular beads was then determined microscopically by counting the bead content of 200 cells. The counts were done in duplicate by two different observers and the results were averaged.

The ability of the adherent peritoneal exudate cells to limit the growth of *L. monocytogenes* was tested by incubation of 10^7 bacteria with 10^6 cells in 2 ml of medium 199 with 10% fetal calf serum.

In addition, the effects of in vitro exposure of cells to AmB on phagocytic and antibacterial properties were measured by exposing peritoneal exudate cells harvested from unstimulated mice to 1 μg of AmB per ml for 1 h, washing the cells free of AmB, and incubating them in fresh medium with polystyrene beads or bacteria.

The bacterial incubations were carried out in duplicate in plastic tubes (12 by 75 mm; Falcon Plastics, Oxnard, Calif.) in 5% CO_2 at 37°C for the times shown. The tubes were rotated at 6 rpm and samples were taken at the times shown. Cells were sonically treated in a Branson Probe 75 sonifier at setting no. 6, which disrupted the cells without affecting the bacteria. Samples were then streaked on nutrient agar plates to determine bacterial colony counts.

Preparation of cells suspensions for assay. Bone marrow cells from the femurs of drug-treated and untreated mice were flushed out with alpha medium (Flow Laboratories, Inc., Rockville, Md.) (6) supplemented with 10% fetal calf serum. Blood was collected in heparin by cardiac puncture. Spleens were minced with scissors, and the minces were then pushed through a fine stainless-steel screen to make a single-cell suspension.

Assay for precursor cells of macrophages. Pluripotent hemopoietic stem cells, colony-forming units in spleen (CFU-S), were assayed for their ability to produce macroscopic colonies in the spleens of supralethally irradiated recipients in 10 days, as described by Till and McCulloch (18).

The number of hemopoietic colony-forming units in culture (CFU-C), cells considered to be the limited stem cells for both granulocytes and monocytes-macrophages (2, 14), was determined by a single-layer agar technique described previously (9). L cell-conditioned medium was used as the source of colony-stimulating factor (CSF). Cultures were incubated at 37°C in 10% CO_2 in air. These dishes were examined with an inverted microscope 7 days after plating, and any aggregates containing more than 50 cells on day 7 were defined as colonies.

Counting and classification of leukocytes. The leukocyte count of heparinized blood collected by cardiac puncture was done with a hemocytometer. Blood smears were stained with Leishman stain, and the classification of cells was done by two persons.

Induction of PCFC. Three days after one i.p. injection of various doses of AmB, the peritoneal cells were collected and assayed for their content of peritoneal colony-forming cells (PCFC). The culture technique for assaying the number of PCFC was essentially the same as that for CFU-C, except PCFC are defined as cells that do not form colonies before day 7 but that can form aggregates containing more than 50 cells by day 28 (8, 9).

Assay for CSF. The blood obtained by cardiac puncture from three to five mice was mixed and the serum was separated. The sera were sterilized by passage through a membrane filter (Millipore Corp., Bedford, Mass.) and kept frozen until use. Serum from endotoxin-treated mice was obtained by injecting 25 μg of endotoxin (*Salmonella typhosa*, Difco) into a group of AKR mice 3 h before they were bled. All sera were diluted 1:6 with alpha medium before use. The stimulating activity of these sera on the growth of CFU-C was tested by incorporating 0.1 ml from each group into 1 ml of agar medium from which L cell-conditioned medium was omitted. The agar medium contained 5×10^4 nucleated bone marrow cells from normal AKR mice. The data were normalized to the control, which contained 0.1 ml of L cell-conditioned medium and gave 72 ± 19 colonies.

Statistical analysis. Statistical significance was determined by Student's *t* test.

RESULTS

Effect of AmB on the functional capabilities of peritoneal macrophages. The differential counts of the peritoneal exudate cells from AmB-treated mice were not significantly different from control animals. In both cases about 65% of the cells were macrophages; this confirmed previous results (17). Macrophages (adherent cells) in peritoneal cells isolated from mice previously treated i.v. or i.p. with AmB have increased phagocytic function when compared with macrophages from control mice, as determined by the number of polystyrene beads phagocytized (Fig. 1a and b). In both cases the macrophages from AmB-treated animals ingested more beads than the control animals. This increased phagocytic function was also induced in peritoneal cells or pure macrophages from unstimulated mice treated in vitro with 1 μg of AmB per ml for 1 h and then incubated with beads in AmB-free medium (data not shown).

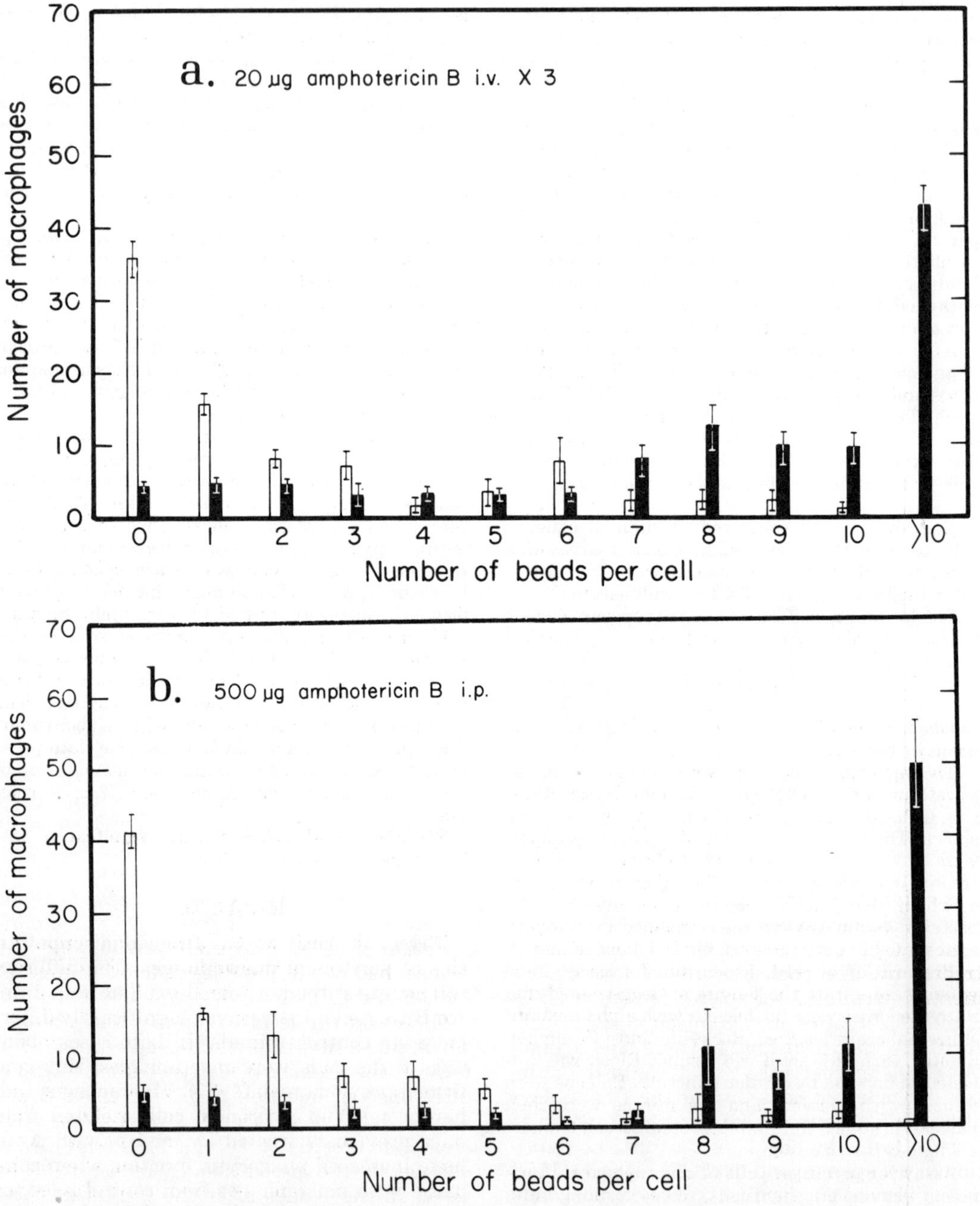

FIG. 1. *Histograms of polystyrene bead count distribution in peritoneal macrophages obtained from (a) mice given 3 injections of 20 μg of AmB i.v. and (b) mice given 500 μg of AmB i.p. Symbols:* □, *controls;* ■, *AmB treated. Experiments were done in duplicate three times. Values represent mean ± standard error of the mean.*

Peritoneal exudate cells or purified macrophages isolated from AmB-treated animals also had a greater inhibitory effect on the growth of *L. monocytogenes* than controls (Fig. 2a and b). Cells from AmB-treated animals had temporarily decreased bacterial counts at 3 h, but the decrease was followed by regrowth of organisms at the same rate as controls. Peritoneal cells treated in vitro for 1 h with AmB were also more active against *L. monocytogenes* than

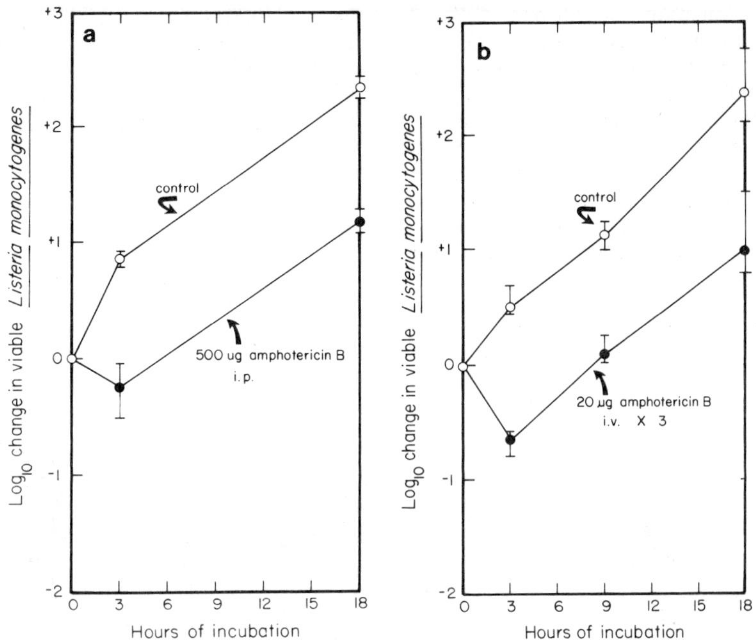

FIG. 2. *Growth inhibition of L. monocytogenes in vitro by peritoneal macrophages obtained from AmB-treated mice; (a) AmB given i.p. and (b) AmB given i.v. The experiments were done in duplicate thre times. Values represent mean ± standard error of the mean.*

controls (Fig. 3), but purified macrophages incubated for 1 h in AmB did not show this enhanced antibacterial activity (data not shown). AmB by itself had no effect in the viability of *L. monocytogenes*. Sodium deoxycholate alone, in the same concentration as that found in the Fungizone used in the individual experiments, had no effect on the functional capabilities of peritoneal macrophages.

Levels of CFU-S and CFU-C after AmB treatment. The pooled results of four experiments determining the splenic content of CFU-S and CFU-C after one i.p. injection of 0.5 mg of AmB are shown in Fig. 4. There was a small but consistent decrease ($P < 0.05$) in the number of nucleated cells during the first 2 days after AmB treatment, followed by a return to normal levels by day 4. In contrast, no reduction in the splenic content of CFU-C and CFU-S was observed in the first 2 days; however, a significant increase of these two classes of cells was noted between 4 and 7 days after the injection. There was, on the average, an eightfold increase in the number of CFU-C by day 4. The magnitude of the increase in the number of CFU-S was smaller than that of CFU-C; the value of CFU-S on day 7 was three times that of controls. No significant change in the splenic content of CFU-C and CFU-S was seen after one injection of 0.5 mg of sodium deoxycholate.

The number of hemopoietic stem cells in femoral bone marrow was also followed serially after AmB treatment (Table 1). The number of CFU-C and CFU-S reached a maximum 4 days after treatment and returned to pretreatment levels by day 7. The change in bone marrow was not as marked as that in spleen since there was no more than a twofold increase of these precursor cells in bone marrow. The i.p. administration of sodiu..n deoxycholate (0.5 mg per mouse) had no effect on the marrow content of CFU-S and CFU-C.

Effect on the level of monocytes in blood. There was a small but significant increase ($P < 0.05$) in the number of leukocytes in blood 3 h after one i.p. injection of 0.5 mg of AmB per mouse, but the number returned to the pretreatment level by 24 h (Table 2). No significant change in the proportion of monocytes was noted in the 7 days after the treatment. The most prominent change after AmB treatment was a transient reversal in the proportion of lymphocytes and neutrophils. The reduced proportion of lymphocytes was observed within 3 h; the level reached its nadir on day 1. The reduction was accompanied by a proportionate increase in the percentage of neutrophils. By day 3, the proportion of lymphocytes and neutrophils had returned to the pretreatment level.

Serum CSF level after AmB treatment.

After one i.p. injection of 0.5 mg of AmB, groups of mice were bled as a function of time, and the level of CSF in their sera was assayed. The pooled results from four experiments are presented in Table 3. A considerable variation in the level of CSF existed from one experiment to another. The serum from normal AKR mice contained very little CSF. Within 3 h after AmB, an increase in CSF level was noted. The level of CSF reached its maximum on day 1, and the activity persisted for at least 5 days. Colonies formed in the presence of sera from AmB-treated mice were generally smaller in diameter than those grown in the presence of L cell-conditioned medium or serum from mice treated with endotoxin. It was quite possible that AmB itself possessed colony-stimulating

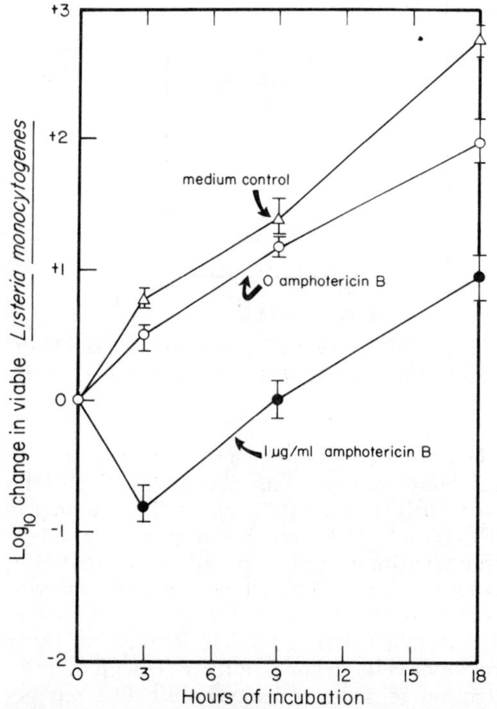

FIG. 3. *Growth inhibition of L. monocytogenes by peritoneal cells preincubated with AmB in vitro. The experiments were done in duplicate three times. The medium control values show colony count changes in medium without peritoneal cells and without AmB. The other two curves show the effects of peritoneal exudates with and without AmB.*

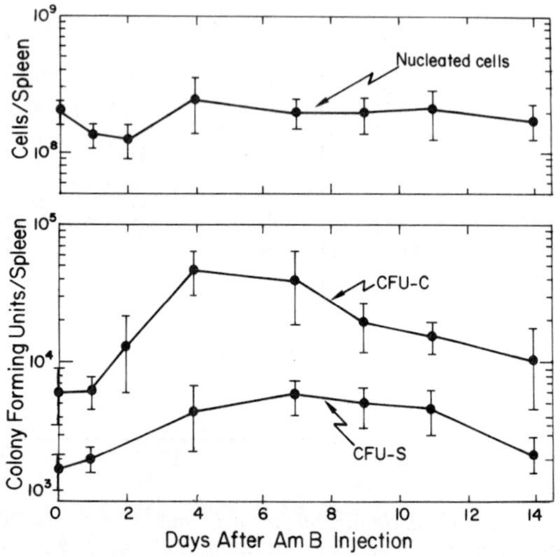

FIG. 4. *Splenic content of nucleated cells, CFU-C, and CFU-S in mice after one i.p. injection of 0.5 mg of AmB. Error bars denote standard deviation.*

TABLE 1. *Effect of AmB treatment on femoral bone marrow*

Time after AmB	Nucleated cells/femur ($\times 10^{-7}$)	CFU-C/ femur ($\times 10^{-4}$)	CFU-S/ femur ($\times 10^{-3}$)[a]
Control (no AmB)	1.73 ± 0.28[b]	2.37 ± 0.31	2.73 ± 0.39
3 h	1.30 ± 0.15	2.51 ± 0.22	2.52 ± 0.19
1 day	1.64 ± 0.34	3.46 ± 0.42	2.68 ± 0.31
2 days	1.69 ± 0.21	3.43 ± 0.39	
3 days	1.75 ± 0.61	3.64 ± 0.31	3.21 ± 0.29
4 days	1.72 ± 0.32	4.86 ± 0.62	4.50 ± 0.58
7 days	1.66 ± 0.20	2.67 ± 0.21	2.54 ± 0.28

[a] No correction was made for cells that did not get into the spleens of recipient mice.
[b] Mean ± standard deviation from four experiments.

TABLE 2. *Effect of AmB on blood leukocytes*

Time after AmB	Total leukocytes/mm^{3}[a] ($\times 10^{-3}$)	Classification (%)				
		Lymphocyte	Neutrophil	Eosinophil	Basophil	Monocyte
Control	6.4 ± 1.8[a]	70.3 ± 5.9	24.0 ± 6.3	2.6 ± 1.0	0.2	2.9 ± 1.6
3 h	8.2 ± 1.6	45.9 ± 6.7	49.6 ± 7.0	1.1 ± 0.5	0.2	3.2 ± 1.1
1 day	6.3 ± 2.2	31.1 ± 9.4	65.4 ± 9.2	0.7 ± 0.7	0.1	2.7 ± 1.3
2 days	6.9 ± 2.3	64.4 ± 7.6	30.5 ± 6.5	1.5 ± 1.2	0.2	3.4 ± 1.5
3 days	5.5 ± 1.3	69.1 ± 4.7	24.5 ± 4.4	1.6 ± 1.0	0.2	4.6 ± 1.4
4 days	6.0 ± 1.6	69.0 ± 7.0	27.3 ± 3.5	1.0 ± 0.9	0.1	2.6 ± 1.4
7 days	5.6 ± 1.8	67.8 ± 4.9	26.7 ± 3.2	1.8 ± 1.1	0.1	3.6 ± 1.0

[a] Mean ± standard deviation.

activity and that the elevation of colony-stimulating activity in the sera of treated animals merely reflected the amount of AmB present in them. To rule out this possibility, varying amounts of AmB were added to the bone marrow cell culture dishes containing serum from normal unstimulated mice in place of L cell-conditioned medium. The addition of AmB, ranging from 0.01 to 100 μg per dish, failed to increase the number of colonies, indicating that AmB does not have colony-stimulating activity.

Induction of PCFC by AmB. A large number of PCFC was detected in the peritoneum of AmB-treated mice; the number of PCFC induced appeared to be dose dependent (Table 4). Since only a slight increase in the number of PCFC was noticed when mice were given sodium deoxycholate, AmB present in Fungizone appeared to be the agent responsible for the induction of PCFC. Three daily i.v. injections of 10 μg of AmB (maximum tolerated single i.v. dose was 20 μg) gave a small but significant increase in the number of PCFC.

TABLE 3. *Serum CSF level after AmB treatment*

Time after AmB treatment (0.5 mg, i.p.)	CSF level[a] (% of control)
L cell-conditioned medium (control)	100
Serum from endotoxin-treated mice	92 (85–120)[b]
No AmB	3 (0–15)
3 h	21 (0–30)
6 h	18 (4–24)
12 h	31 (18–31)
1 day	60 (30–82)
3 days	41 (32–54)
5 days	26 (10–42)

[a] The amount of CSF was determined by the ability of 0.1 ml of serum to stimulate 5×10^4 bone marrow cells to form colonies in vitro. The activity was normalized to that of 0.1 ml of L cell-conditioned medium.

[b] Mean (range).

TABLE 4. *Induction of PCFC by AmB*[a]

Treatment	No. of cells/ peritoneal lavage ($\times 10^{-6}$)	No. of PCFC/10^5 cells
None	1.74 ± 0.34[b]	<1
AmB		
0.01 mg i.p. (day 0)	2.12 ± 0.56	39 ± 8
0.1 mg i.p. (day 0)	5.42 ± 1.20	108 ± 20
0.5 mg i.p. (day 0)	10.24 ± 2.38	514 ± 72
AmB		
0.01 mg i.v. × 3 (days 0, 1, and 2)	1.68 ± 0.29	24 ± 8
Sodium deoxycholate, 0.5 mg i.p. (day 0)	2.24 ± 0.41	5 ± 2

[a] Peritoneal cells were collected and assayed on day 3.

[b] Mean ± standard deviation.

DISCUSSION

Various tissue macrophages and their precursors are now included in one system called the mononuclear phagocyte system (7). Recent studies showed that mononuclear phagocytes originate from precursor cells present in bone marrow and other hemopoietic organs, are transported by way of the bloodstream as monocytes, and eventually become tissue macrophages (4). At least two classes of cells that are capable of differentiating into macrophages have been described. One is the pluripotent hemopoietic stem cells (CFU-S) that are the progenitor cells for all cellular elements in blood (18). Another class of cells is more differentiated than CFU-S and is known to be the progenitor of both granulocytes and monocytes—macrophages (CFU-C) (2, 14). Recently, another class of mononuclear phagocytes, PCFC, which appear in large numbers only when an acute inflammatory response is induced, was described (8, 9). Although the nature of PCFC has not been fully elucidated, they appear to be a subclass of inflammatory exudate macrophages that are capable of extensive proliferation in vitro.

If AmB is to exert its antitumor activity through the mononuclear phagocyte system, there are several possible ways for it to increase the activity of this system. These include "activation" of the preexisting mature tissue macrophages, increasing the supply of macrophages, movement of "active macrophages" to the site of action, or a combination of all of the above.

The present study shows that macrophages from mice treated i.v. or i.p. with AmB had an increased phagocytic and antibacterial function. This is consistent with our previous observations on AmB effects on mouse resistance to tumors and *Listeria* infection. The increase in phagocytic function probably represents a primary effect of AmB on macrophages because it occurs in vitro with purified macrophage preparations. The antibacterial effect may require the presence of lymphocytes and may represent an effect secondary to lymphokines, elaborated by lymphocytes exposed to AmB, because this effect did not occur when macrophages were exposed to AmB in the absence of lymphocytes. This is consistent with other data (1) that showed that AmB stimulates lymphocytes. The mechanism of the stimulating effect of AmB is unknown, but its binding to sterols in the cytoplasmic membrane of eukaryotic cells (6) may be involved.

The present data show that AmB, like other substances possessing adjuvant activity (3, 5, 10, 11), induces a generalized increase in the levels of CFU-S and CFU-C. However, it is not clear at this time whether the marked increase in the splenic content of these two classes of cells is the result of migration of cells from bone marrow of replication of preexisting cells in situ, or the combination of these two mechanisms.

Although the requirement of CSF for the proliferation and differentiation of CFU-C (2, 14) and PCFC (8, 9) in vitro has been well established, the role of this factor in vivo is not yet clear. The present study shows that AmB treatment is capable of increasing the level of CSF in serum although it is not as potent as endotoxin (13) or Freund adjuvant (11).

Like Freund adjuvant and other irritants known to induce a sterile inflammatory reaction (8), AmB, when given i.p., induces PCFC in the peritoneal cavity of mice. Thus, AmB appears to be capable of inducing an acute inflammatory reaction locally, of activating macrophages or attracting active macrophages to the site of inflammation, or both.

Since monocytes, the immediate precursor cells of tissue macrophages, are known to migrate to the site of inflammation, it is not surprising that the blood level of monocytes remained unchanged despite the marked increase in the number of CFU-C in spleen and bone marrow after i.p. AmB treatment. As soon as monocytes are produced in hemopoietic organs and released into the blood, they emigrate to the peritoneal cavity.

In summary, we have shown that AmB stimulates the function and the supply of certain classes of cells that belong to the mononuclear phagocyte system. Whether this is a sufficient explanation for its immunoadjuvant properties will have to be determined by further studies.

ACKNOWLEDGMENTS

We thank Barbara Devaraj, Scott Sauerbrunn, and Mary Comfort Blum for their technical assistance.

This work was supported by Public Health Service grants CA-15665, CB-43872 and CA-13053 from the National Cancer Institute, and grants AI-00459 and AI-10622 from the National Institute of Allergy and Infectious Diseases and a grant from the John A. Hartford Foundation. H. Lin is a recipient of Public Health Service Research Career Development Award CA-70730 from the National Cancer Institute.

LITERATURE CITED

1. **Blanke, T., R. Little, R. Lynch, H. Lin, and G. Medoff.** 1975. Immunostimulant properties of amphotericin B, p. 349. *In* J. Schultz and R. C. Leif (ed.), Critical factors in cancer immunology, vol. 10. Miami Winter Symposia. Academic Press Inc., New York.
2. **Bradley, T. R., and D. Metcalf.** 1966. The growth of mouse bone marrow cells in vitro. Aust. J. Exp. Biol. Med. Sci. 44:287–300.
3. **Dimitrov, N. V., A. Simonne, G. Eliopoulos, and B. Halpern.** 1975. Effect of *Corynebacterium parvum* on bone marrow cell cultures. Proc. Soc. Exp. Biol. Med. 148:440–442.
4. **Gordon, S., and Z. A. Cohn.** 1973. The macrophage. Int. Rev. Cytol. 36:171–214.
5. **Hanks, G. E., and E. J. Ainsworth.** 1964. Endotoxin protection and colony-forming units. Radiat. Res. 32:367–382.
6. **Kinsky, S. C.** 1970. Antibiotic interactions with model membranes. Annu. Rev. Pharmacol. 10:119–142.
7. **Langevoort, H. L., Z. A. Cohn, J. G. Hirsch, J. H. Humphrey, W. G. Spector, and R. van Furth.** 1970. The nomenclature of mononuclear phagocytic cells, p. 1–6. *In* R. van Furth (ed.), Mononuclear phagocytes. F. A. Davis Co., Philadelphia.
8. **Lin, H.** 1974. Peritoneal exudate cells. II. Kinetics of appearence of colony-forming cells. J. Cell. Physiol. 84:159–164.
9. **Lin, H., and C. C. Stewart.** 1974. Peritoneal exudate cells. I. Growth requirement of cells capable of forming colonies in soft agar. J. Cell. Physiol. 83:369–378.
10. **McCulloch, E. A., M. W. Thompson, L. Siminovitch, and J. E. Till.** 1970. Effects of bacterial endotoxin on hemopoietic colony-forming cells in the spleens of normal mice and mice of genotype sl/sl^d. Cell Tissue Kinet. 3:47–54.
11. **McNeil, T. A., W. A. Fleming, S. F. McClure, and M. Killen.** 1973. Granulocyte-macrophage precursor cell responses in mice of different strain, sex and age. Immunology 25:91–101.
12. **Medoff, G., F. Valeriote, R. G. Lynch, D. Schlessinger, and G. Kobayashi.** 1974. Synergistic effect of Amphotericin B and 1,3-bis (2-chloroethyl)-1-nitrosourea against a transplantable AKR leukemia. Cancer Res. 34:974–978.
13. **Metcalf, D.** 1971. Acute antigen-induced elevation of serum colony stimulating factor (CSF) levels. Immunology 21:427–436.
14. **Pluznik, D. H., and L. Sachs.** 1965. The cloning of normal "mast" cells in tissue culture. J. Cell Comp. Physiol. 66:319–324.
15. **Quesenberry, P. J., A. Morley, M. Ryan, D. Howard, and F. Stohlman.** 1973. The effect of endotoxin on murine stem cells. J. Cell. Physiol. 82:239–244.
16. **Stanners, C. P., G. L. Eliceiri, and H. Green.** 1971. Two types of ribosome in mouse-hamster hybrid cells. Nature (London) New Biol. 230:52–54.
17. **Thomas, M. Z., G. Medoff, and G. Kobayashi.** 1973. Changes in murine resistance to *Listeria monocytogenes* infection induced by amphotericin B. J. Infect. Dis. 127:373–377.
18. **Till, J. E., and E. A. McCulloch.** 1961. A direct measurement of the radiation sensitivity of normal mouse bone marrow cells. Radiat. Res. 14:213–222.
19. **Valeriote, F., R. Lynch, G. Medoff, and B. V. Kumar.** 1976. Protective effect of Amphotericin B against spontaneous and transplantable murine tumors. J. Natl. Cancer Inst. 56:557–560.

ANTIMICROBIAL AGENTS AND CHEMOTHERAPY, Jan. 1977, p. 161-166
Vol. 11, No. 1

Comparison of the Binding Properties of Two 6β-Amidinopenicillanic Acid Derivatives That Differ in Their Physiological Effects on *Escherichia coli*

BRIAN G. SPRATT

Department of Genetics, University of Leicester, Leicester LE1 7RH, England

Received for publication 23 July 1976

The 6-β-amidinopenicillanic acid derivative, mecillinam, was highly specific in its action on the growth of *Escherichia coli*. Concentrations from the minimal inhibitory concentration (0.05 μg/ml) up to at least 200 μg/ml resulted in the conversion of *E. coli* rods into osmotically stable spherical cells without significantly inhibiting cell growth or causing cell lysis. A second amidinopenicillanic acid derivative [6-([4-morpholinylmethylene] amino) penicillanic acid] showed identical effects on cell growth at concentrations from its minimal inhibitory concentration (0.2 μg/ml) up to at least 5 μg/ml but, at higher concentrations, increasing amounts of lysis occurred. Neither of these compounds showed the immediate inhibition of cell division that is observed with typical β-lactam antibiotics. We have compared the binding of these two amidinopenicillanic acids to the individual penicillin-binding proteins of *E. coli*. Both compounds showed a high specificity of binding to penicillin-binding protein 2 at low concentrations. At higher concentrations mecillinam still maintained its high specificity for protein 2 and very little binding of mecillinam to any of the other binding proteins was detected with concentrations up to 1 mg/ml. The morpholino compound, however, showed extensive binding to proteins 1 and 4, and slight binding to proteins 5 and 6 at high concentrations. The morpholino compound therefore combined both the physiological properties and the binding properties of mecillinam with some of those of typical penicillins and cephalosporins. Lysis probably occurs at high concentrations of morpholino compound because it binds to penicillin-binding protein 1, since this is believed to be the target with which β-lactams interact to inhibit cell elongation.

The amidinopenicillanic acid derivative, mecillinam (Fig. 1A), is the prototype of a new class of β-lactam antibiotics (6). The replacement of the usual 6-acylamino side chain of normal β-lactams by the 6-amidino linkage in mecillinam results in a compound with properties strikingly different from those of typical penicillins and cephalosporins. Mecillinam (previously called FL1060) is relatively ineffective against gram-positive organisms but is about 100 times more active than other β-lactams against most gram-negative organisms (6, 9, 15). This antibiotic converts *Escherichia coli* cells into large osmotically stable spherical forms (6, 9). Although cell division is eventually inhibited (5) and cell lysis occurs after several hours of growth in the presence of mecillinam (7, 16), these effects are quite different from the rapid lysis and immediate inhibition of division observed with typical β-lactams (4, 11, 14).

The biochemical properties of mecillinam are also unusual. Penicillin-susceptible D-alanine carboxypeptidase 1, peptidoglycan transpeptidase, and endopeptidase activities are only slightly inhibited by this compound at concentrations far above those required to inhibit the growth of *E. coli* (7, 10). Mecillinam was originally reported not to compete for the binding of [^{14}C]benzylpenicillin to membranes of *E. coli* (7), but recently the separation of the individual penicillin-binding proteins (PBPs) of this organism has shown that it competes with high affinity for one of the six proteins in the cytoplasmic membrane that bind [^{14}C]benzylpenicillin (13). [^{14}C]mecillinam was subsequently shown to bind exclusively to this protein (PBP 2), and mutants of *E. coli* have been isolated that fail to bind either [^{14}C]benzylpenicillin or [^{14}C]mecillinam to PBP 2 (12).

Mecillinam clearly exerts its effects on *E. coli* by interacting with PBP 2. The penicillin-susceptible enzyme that presumably corresponds to this binding protein has not been identified.

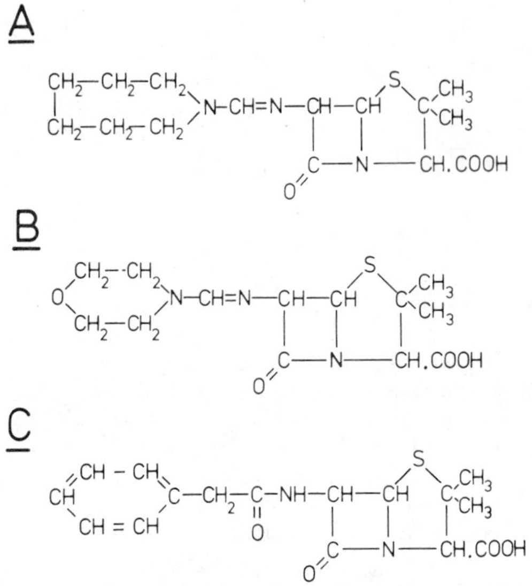

FIG. 1. *Structures of (A) mecillinam, (B) morpholino compound, and (C) benzylpenicillin.*

Typical β-lactams generally show low affinity for PBP 2 but bind with high affinity to other PBPs which are believed to be the targets at which these antibiotics inhibit cell division and cause cell lysis (12).

A new amidinopenicillanic acid derivative, 6-([4-morpholinylmethylene] amino) penicillanic acid (Fig. 1B), (referred to as morpholino compound) which combines the properties of mecillinam with some of those of typical β-lactams has been brought to our notice by F. Lund of Leo Pharmaceutical Laboratories. In this paper we compare the physiological and binding properties of mecillinam with the morpholino compound.

MATERIALS AND METHODS

Bacterial strains and conditions of growth. *E. coli* KN126 F^- *tryE8929* tyr^- ilv^- *sup-126* was used in all experiments and was originally obtained from T. Nagata. Cells were grown in Penassay broth (Difco antibiotic medium number 3) at 37°C with vigorous aeration. Exponentially growing cells were used in all experiments.

Measurement of cell growth. Absorbance of the culture was monitored at 550 nm with a Gilford model 300 automatic sampling spectrophotometer using sterile broth as a blank. Total cell numbers were measured with a Coulter counter model B. Cells were diluted into ice-cold membrane-filtered (Millipore Corp.) 0.9% NaCl containing 0.37% formaldehyde and then counted with a 30-μm probe.

Preparation of membranes. Three-liter batches of exponentially growing cells were cooled on ice, harvested by centrifugation for 6 min at 6,000 × *g* at 4°C, and resuspended in 80 ml of ice-cold 10 mM sodium phosphate buffer, pH 7.0. An 0.8-ml amount of 2-mercaptoethanol was added and the cells were disrupted by three 30-s periods of sonication with intermittent periods of cooling. Cell debris was removed by centrifugation for 20 min at 8,000 × *g*, and the cell membranes were pelleted from the supernatant at 100,000 × *g* for 40 min at 4°C. The membranes were washed twice and finally resuspended in the above buffer at a protein concentration of approximately 40 mg/ml and stored at −80°C. These membrane preparations consist of both inner and outer membranes.

Binding of [^{14}C]mecillinam. Two-hundred-microliter portions of membranes (5 to 10 mg of protein/ml in 50 mM sodium phosphate buffer, pH 7.0) were incubated for 10 min at 30°C with 10 μl of twofold increasing concentrations of [^{14}C]mecillinam (53 mCi/mmol). The binding was terminated by the addition of 5 μl of 40-mg/ml nonradioactive mecillinam and 10 μl of 20% (wt/vol) Sarkosyl NL-97. After 20 min at room temperature, the Sarkosyl-insoluble peptidoglycan and outer membrane were pelleted at 100,000 × *g* for 40 min at 10°C and the Sarkosyl-soluble inner-membrane proteins were removed and fractionated on a 10% sodium dodecyl sulfate-polyacrylamide slab gel as described previously (12, 13). The dried gel was fluorographed by exposure to Kodak RP Royal X-Omat X-ray film at −80°C (12, 13).

Binding of amidinopenicillanic acids by competition for the binding of [^{14}C]benzylpenicillin. Portions (200 μl) of membranes (as above) were preincubated for 10 min at 30°C with 10 μl of increasing concentrations of nonradioactive amidinopenicillanic acids, and the binding proteins remaining accessible were measured by the addition of 20 μl of 50-μCi/ml [^{14}C]benzylpenicillin (54 mCi/mmol) for a further 10 min at 30°C. This concentration of [^{14}C]benzylpenicillin is sufficient to saturate all PBPs under these conditions (B. G. Spratt, manuscript in preparation). The binding was terminated by the addition of 5 μl of 120-mg/ml nonradioactive benzylpenicillin and 10 μl of 20% (wt/vol) Sarkosyl NL-97, and the binding proteins in the Sarkosyl-soluble fraction were detected as described above.

Binding proteins were quantitated by densitometry of their images on the X-ray films with a Joyce-Loebl Mk111c microdensitometer.

Measurement of minimal inhibitory concentrations. The minimal inhibitory concentration (MIC) was defined as the lowest concentration of the antibiotic that produced a clear alteration of the rod morphology of *E. coli* KN126 when added to a culture of 2 × 10^7 organisms/ml growing at 37°C in Penassay broth.

Chemicals. [^{14}C]benzylpenicillin (54 mCi/mmol) was purchased from The Radiochemical Centre, Amersham, England. [^{14}C]mecillinam (53 mCi/mmol), nonradioactive mecillinam (batch GA 32138) and morpholino compound (batch GA 33086) were kindly provided by F. Lund of Leo Pharmaceutical Products, Ballerup, Denmark. Benzypenicillin and cephalexin were kindly provided by Glaxo Laboratories, Greenford, Middlesex, England. Solutions of all β-lactams were freshly prepared immediately before use. Sarkosyl NL-97 was purchased from Geigy Industrial Chemicals, New York.

RESULTS

Comparison of the effects of mecillinam and morpholino compound on the morphology, growth, and division of E. coli KN126. The MICs of mecillinam and morpholino compound were 0.05 μg/ml and 0.2 μg/ml, respectively. Addition of mecillinam at concentrations up to at least 200 μg/ml had little effect on the growth rate during a 90-min period at 37°C. During this period absorbance increased by 10.6-fold in the control and 10.1-fold in the presence of 200 μg of mecillinam per ml (Fig. 2), and the latter culture consisted entirely of large osmotically stable spherical cells. The morpholino compound also produced little inhibition of growth at concentrations up to 5 μg/ml, and the morphology of the cells was indistinguishable from that produced by mecillinam; at higher concentrations increasing amounts of lysis occurred (Fig. 2).

Mecillinam at 200 μg/ml (or 2 μg/ml) had no effect on cell division for 30 min at 37°C, and then division slowed and stopped. Total cell number increased by about 170% after the addition of mecillinam (Fig. 3). The morpholino compound (2 μg/ml) gave an identical increase in cell number and even 200 μg of this compound per ml allowed division to occur at the normal rate for 20 min at which time cell number could no longer be followed because cell lysis took place. At the time lysis began the increase in cell number was 72% and this should be compared with the 10 to 20% residual division that was obtained with 50 μg of cephalexin per ml (a typical β-lactam antibiotic; MIC, 3 μg/ml). Benzylpenicillin (MIC, 6 μg/ml) at concentrations of 25 μg/ml and 50 μg/ml also inhibited cell division within 10 min and only allowed a residual increment in cell number of 21.8% and 19.1% respectively (data not shown).

Binding of [^{14}C]mecillinam. Figure 4 shows the binding of increasing concentrations of [^{14}C]mecillinam to the inner-membrane proteins of *E. coli* KN126. No binding to the Sarkosyl-insoluble outer-membrane proteins has been detected with this, or any other, ^{14}C-labeled β-lactam (12). Binding was observed with high affinity for one inner-membrane protein with an electrophoretic mobility identical to that of [^{14}C]benzylpenicillin-binding protein 2 as previously observed (12). In this experiment 50% saturation of PBP 2 with mecillinam was obtained at 0.023 μg/ml for 10 min at 30°C. A trace of high-affinity binding was also seen to a protein with a mobility slightly faster than PBP 4. This is almost certainly a proteolytic product of PBP 2 since mutants that fail to bind [^{14}C]mecillinam to PBP 2 also fail to show any binding to this minor protein (B. G. Spratt, unpublished observations).

Binding of amidinopenicillanic acids by competition with [^{14}C]benzylpenicillin. Mecillinam at concentrations up to at least 2 μg/ml binds exclusively to PBP 2 (see above and reference 12). Since morpholino compound was not available radioactively labeled, we have studied its binding by competition for [^{14}C]benzylpenicillin binding. Figure 5 shows

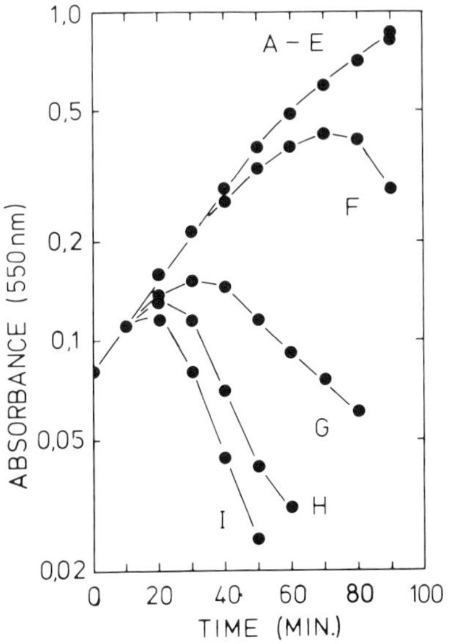

FIG. 2. *Growth of E. coli KN126 in the presence of various concentrations of mecillinam and morpholino compound. Mecillinam: (A) control, (B) 2 μg/ml, and (C) 200 μg/ml. (D) Morpholino compound: 2 μg/ml, (E) 5 μg/ml, (F) 50 μg/ml, (G) 100 μg/ml, (H) 150 μg/ml, and (I) 200 μg/ml.*

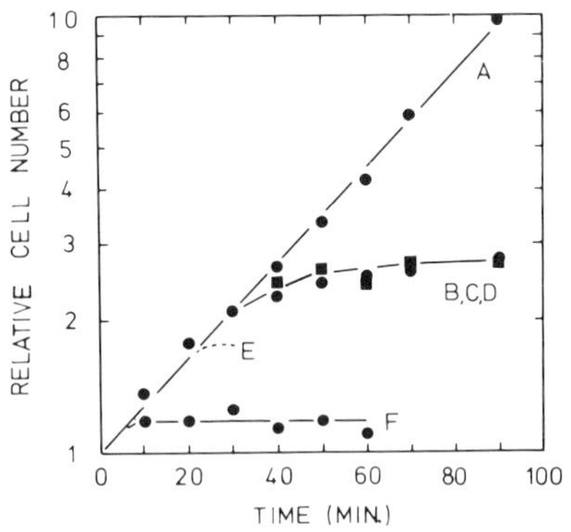

FIG. 3. *Cell division of E. coli KN126 in the presence of mecillinam, morpholino compound, and cephalexin. Mecillinam: (A) control, (B) 2 μg/ml, and (C) 200 μg/ml. Morpholino: (D) 2 μg/ml, and (E) 200 μg/ml. Cephalexin: (F) 50 μg/ml. The cell number at zero time was 8.6 × 10^6 organisms/ml.*

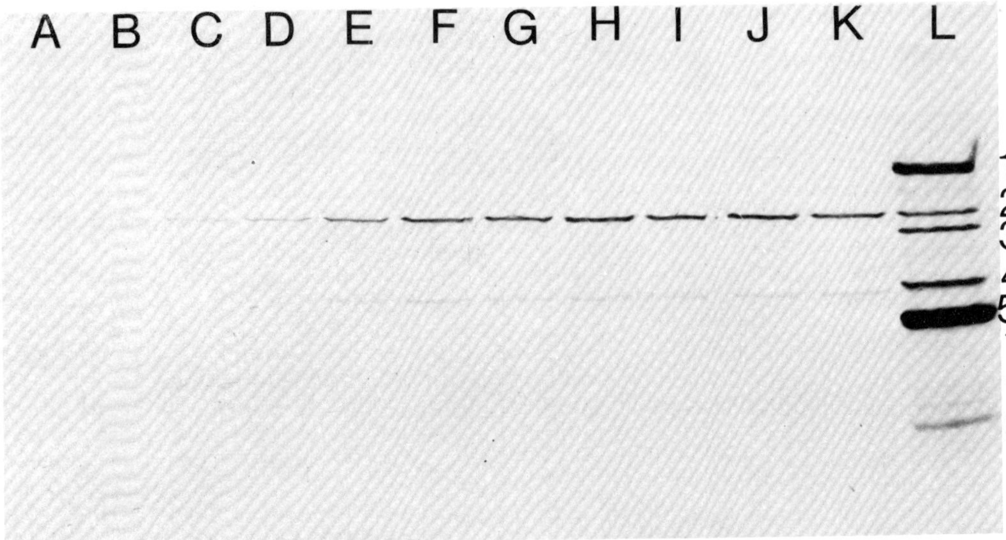

FIG. 4. *Binding of [^{14}C]mecillinam and [^{14}C]benzylpenicillin to membranes of E coli KN126. (A) 0.001 μg/ml and then twofold increasing concentrations up to (K) 1.0 μg of [^{14}C]mecillinam per ml; (L) 31.0 μg of [^{14}C]benzylpenicillin per ml. Electrophoresis was from top to bottom, and the gel was exposed to X-ray film for 92 days. PBPs 5 and 6 have not resolved into two proteins on this gel.*

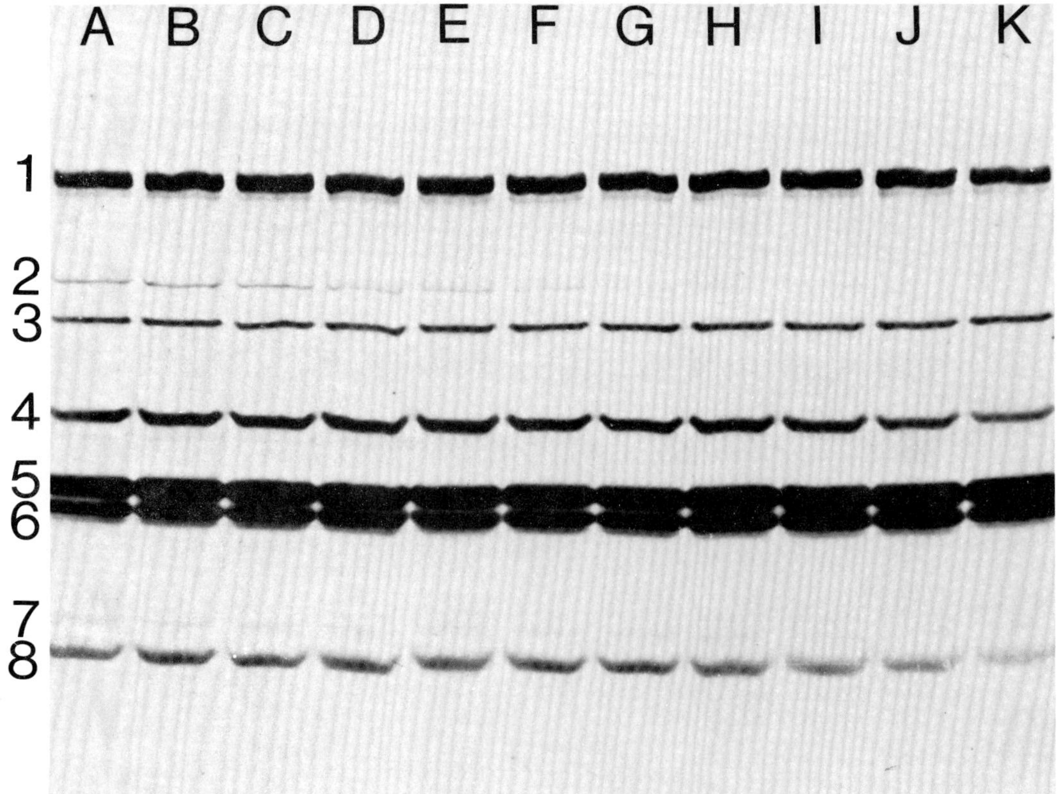

FIG. 5. *The competition of low concentrations of morpholino compound for the binding of [^{14}C]benzylpenicillin to membranes of E. coli KN126. (A) Control, (B) 0.0024 μg/ml and then threefold increasing concentrations up to (K) 47.6 μg of morpholino compound per ml. Morpholino compound was prebound at the above concentrations, and the residual binding of [^{14}C]benzylpenicillin (31.0 μg/ml) was measured. Electrophoresis was from top to bottom and the gel was exposed to X-ray film for 60 days.*

an X-ray film from an experiment in which the competition of a range of concentrations (up to 47.6 μg/ml) of morpholino compound was studied. At these concentrations the morpholino compound showed strong competition for PBP 2 but only very slight competition for any of the other PBPs. The minor protein with a mobility slightly faster than PBP 4 is probably the minor proteolytic product of PBP 2 discussed above. Two other binding proteins of low molecular weight (PBPs 7 and 8) were also seen on this gel. These proteins have been found in several experiments (although in this experiment PBP 8 is unusually prominent) and may also be proteolytic products of other PBPs as they are only detected in some membrane preparations and are highly variable in amount. Fifty percent inhibition of the binding of [^{14}C]benzylpenicillin to PBP 2 was obtained with 0.066 μg of the morpholino compound per ml.

The morpholino compound, in contrast to mecillinam, showed typical penicillin lysis at concentrations of 50 μg/ml and above (Fig. 2), and we therefore compared the competition of high concentrations (up to 1 mg/ml) of these compounds for [^{14}C]benzylpenicillin binding. Figure 6 and Table 1 shows that the morpholino compound competed extensively for the binding of [^{14}C]benzylpenicillin to PBPs 1 and 4 and to a lesser extent to PBPs 5 and 6, whereas mecillinam, even at 1 mg/ml, competed little for any of the PBPs (except PBP 2). Very little competition for PBP 3 was observed with either amidinopenicillanic acid.

DISCUSSION

The morphological and physiological effects of mecillinam and morpholino compound were identical at concentrations up to 5 μg/ml. Neither compound caused cell lysis or significantly inhibited cell mass increase at these concentrations. Cell division was also not inhibited during the first 30 min but then division slowed and finally ceased, and the cells were converted to large osmotically stable spherical forms. Similar effects of mecillinam have been reported by other investigators (2, 5–8).

Mecillinam inhibits the growth of *E. coli* by interacting with PBP 2 (12, 13), and as expected the morpholino compound bound exclusively to this protein at low concentrations. Fifty percent binding of both mecillinam and morpholino compound was attained at concentrations close to the MIC values of these antibiotics.

At concentrations above about 50 μg/ml these two amidinopenicillanic acid derivatives had distinctly different properties. Two hundred micrograms of mecillinam per ml had no more effect on the growth, division, and morphology than did 2 μg/ml, whereas increasing amounts of morpholino compound resulted in cell lysis which occurred earlier and to a greater extent as the concentration was raised further. At 200 μg of morpholino compound per ml lysis resulted within 20 min and was indistinguishable from that produced by typical penicillins and cephalosporins (4, 11). Even at this concentration cell division continued at the same rate as in the control culture until lysis

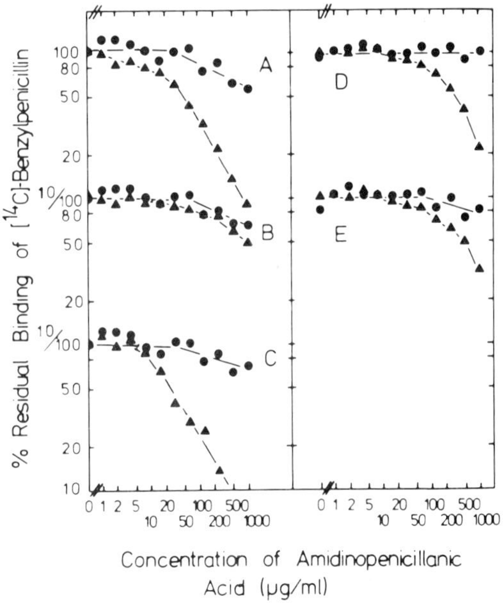

FIG. 6. *The competition of high concentrations of mecillinam (●) and morpholino compound (▲) for the binding of [^{14}C]benzylpenicillin. The experiment was performed as described in the legend to Fig. 5 and the PBPs were quantitated by densitometry. (A) PBP 1; (B) PBP 3; (C) PBP 4; (D) PBP 5; (E) PBP 6.*

TABLE 1. *Concentration of amidinopenicillanic acids required to give 50% binding or competition*

Amidinopenicillanic acid	MIC (μg/ml)	Conc of amidinopenicillanic acids required to give 50% binding or competition (μg/ml)					
		PBP 1	PBP 2	PBP 3	PBP 4	PBP 5	PBP 6
Mecillinam (direct binding)	0.05	ND[a]	0.023	ND	ND	ND	ND
Mecillinam (competition)	0.05	>1,000	0.04	>1,000	>1,000	>1,000	>1,000
Morpholino compound (competition)	0.2	49.0	0.066	956	25.7	324	468

[a] ND, None detected at [^{14}C]mecillinam concentration of 1 μg/ml.

precluded further measurements. The extent of residual division at this time was at least three times that obtained with cephalexin or benzylpenicillin. High concentrations of morpholino compound therefore showed the lysis (4), but not the immediate inhibition of cell division (14), which is typical of other β-lactams. The different responses of *E. coli* to high concentrations of mecillinam and morpholino compound were paralleled by a difference in their binding properties to the PBPs. Mecillinam, at concentrations up to 1 mg/ml, bound virtually exclusively to PBP 2 and showed very little competition for [^{14}C]benzylpenicillin binding to any of the other PBPs. The morpholino compound, however, showed (in addition to its binding to PBP 2) extensive competition for PBPs 1 and 4 at high concentrations.

Morpholino compound clearly functions identically to mecillinam at concentrations up to about 5 μg/ml; at higher concentrations the ability of the former compound to lyse *E. coli* correlates very well with its affinity for PBPs 1 and 4. This result is additional evidence for our suggestion (12) that lysis by β-lactams is caused by their binding to PBP 1. However, the correlation between lysis and binding to PBP 4 is also good and this protein cannot be excluded as the possible target at which β-lactams bind to cause lysis. Hopefully the isolation of a temperature-sensitive cell lysis mutant which has a thermolabile PBP 1 (or PBP 4) will definitively answer this problem. The failure of either amidinopencillanic acid to show typical penicillin inhibition of cell division agrees well with the failure of these compounds to bind to PBP 3 since this protein has been shown to be involved in the inhibition of division by penicillins and cephalosporins (12). The eventual inhibition of division caused by mecillinam is thought to result from the inhibition of an early step in the division cycle of *E. coli* and is not thought to be related to the immediate inhibition of division caused by other β-lactams (5).

The selectivity of binding of mecillinam to PBP 2 is remarkable. Modification of the side chain of this compound though can result in derivatives (e.g., the morpholino compound) which still maintain their mecillinam-like properties but which also have the lytic ability of typical β-lactams. Since mecillinam and typical β-lactams show synergy, both in vivo (3) and in vitro (1, 16), a compound that combines both these types of activity in the same molecule might be of clinical importance.

ACKNOWLEDGMENTS

I am extremely grateful to Frantz Lund of Leo Laboratories for the gifts of radioactive and non-radioactive amidinopenicillanic acids. I would like to thank Vinay Jobanputra for technical assistance and the Medical Research Council of Great Britain for a project grant.

LITERATURE CITED

1. **Baltimore, R. S., J. O. Klein, C. Wilcox, and M. Finland.** 1976. Synergy of mecillinam (FL1060) with penicillins and cephalosporins against *Proteus* and *Klebsiella*, with observations on combinations with other antibiotics and against other bacterial species. Antimicrob. Agents Chemother. **9**:701–705.
2. **Greenwood, D., and F. O'Grady.** 1973. FL1060: a new beta-lactam antibiotic with novel properties. J. Clin. Pathol. **26**:1–6.
3. **Grunberg, E., R. Cleeland, G. Beskid, and W. F. DeLorenzo.** 1976. In vivo synergy between 6β-amidinopenicillanic acid derivatives and other antibiotics. Antimicrob. Agents Chemother. **9**:589–594.
4. **Hahn, F. E., and J. Ciak.** 1957. Penicillin-induced lysis of *Escherichia coli*. Science **125**:119–120.
5. **James, R., J. Y. Haga, and A. B. Pardee.** 1975. Inhibition of an early event in the cell division cycle of *Escherichia coli* by FL1060, an amidinopenicillanic acid. J. Bacteriol. **122**:1283–1292.
6. **Lund, F., and L. Tybring.** 1972. 6β-Amidinopenicillanic acids-a new group of antibiotics. Nature (London) New Biol. **236**:135–137.
7. **Matsuhashi, S., T. Kamiyro, P. M. Blumberg, P. Linnett, E. Willoughby, and J. L. Strominger.** 1974. Mechanism of action and development of resistance to a new amidino penicillin. J. Bacteriol. **117**:578–587.
8. **Melchior, N. H., J. Blom, L. Tybring, and A. Birch-Anderson.** 1973. Light and electron microscopy of the early response of *Escherichia coli* to a 6β-amidinopenicillanic acid (FL1060). Acta Pathol. Microbiol. Scan. Sect. B. **81**:393–407.
9. **Neu, H. C.** 1976. Mecillinam, a novel penicillanic acid derivative with unusual activity against gram-negative bacteria. Antimicrob. Agents Chemother. **9**:793–799.
10. **Park, J. T., and L. Burman.** 1973. FL1060, a new penicillin with a unique mode of action. Biochem. Biophys. Res. Commun. **51**:863–868.
11. **Schwarz, U., A. Asmus, and H. Frank.** 1969. Autolytic enzymes and cell division in *Escherichia coli*. J. Mol. Biol. **41**:419–429.
12. **Spratt, B. G.** 1975. Distinct penicillin-binding proteins involved in the division, elongation, and shape of *Escherichia coli*. Proc. Natl. Acad. Sci. U.S.A. **72**:2999–3003.
13. **Spratt, B. G., and A. B. Pardee.** 1975. Penicillin-binding proteins and cell shape in *E. coli*. Nature (London) **254**:516–517.
14. **Starka, J., and J. Moravova.** 1967. Cellular division of penicillin-induced filaments of *Escherichia coli*. Folia Microbiol. (Prague) **12**:240–247.
15. **Tybring, L.** 1975. Mecillinam (FL1060), a 6β-amidinopenicillanic acid derivative: in vitro evaluation. Antimicrob. Agents Chemother. **8**:266–270.
16. **Tybring, L., and N. H. Melchior.** 1975. Mecillinam (FL 1060), 6β-amidinopenicillanic acid derivative: bactericidal action and synergy in vitro. Antimicrob. Agents Chemother. **8**:271–276.

ANTIMICROBIAL AGENTS AND CHEMOTHERAPY, Jan. 1977, p. 167–170
Vol. 11, No. 1

NOTES

Nalidixic Acid-Induced Protein Alterations in *Escherichia coli*

LEE CHAO

Department of Biochemistry, Medical University of South Carolina, Charleston, South Carolina 29401

Received for publication 15 July 1976

The effect of nalidixic acid on pulse-labeled protein patterns was analyzed by sodium dodecyl sulfate-polyacrylamide slab gel electrophoresis. The drug was found to alter protein patterns in a drug-sensitive strain but not in the isogenic drug-resistant strain of *Escherichia coli*. The drug-induced alteration of protein patterns was demonstrated by the appearance of some and the disappearance of other pulse-labeled peptides elicited by the drug.

Nalidixic acid is an extensively used antibacterial drug whose mode of action is poorly understood. It is known that nalidixic acid specifically inhibits bacterial deoxyribonucleic acid (DNA) synthesis but only partially inhibits the synthesis of ribonucleic acid (RNA) and proteins (2, 12). The primary target of inhibition is the semiconservative DNA replication (21), with a possible effect on the repair synthesis of DNA (10). The inhibition of DNA synthesis is not attributable to any interaction between nalidixic acid and the DNA template (3, 4). It has been shown (18) that the thermal susceptibility of a DNA ligase temperature-sensitive mutant is enhanced by nalidixic acid, but the search for a direct interference of the drug with enzymes involved in DNA metabolism has been so far unsuccessful (4, 19). A recent report by Crumplin and Smith (8) indicates that, in addition to inhibiting DNA synthesis, nalidixic acid may inhibit RNA synthesis as a second target site. However, the inhibition of bacterial RNA synthesis is only partial (12) and may or may not affect bacterial growth significantly, since the rate of bacterial RNA synthesis can also vary widely depending on the growth conditions. Studies have therefore been conducted to investigate the possibility that nalidixic acid may alter the expression of many gene products in a qualitative manner. Results of these studies, reported here, indicate that the protein pattern in bacteria is indeed altered by nalidixic acid treatment. The alteration is quite complex in that the synthesis of certain proteins is depressed whereas that of other proteins is induced by the drug.

The bacterial strains used were *Escherichia coli* KL161 and KL166. These two strains are isogenic except that KL166 is a NalA derivative of KL161 (1). The growth of KL161 is totally inhibited by nalidixic acid at a concentration of 10 μg/ml in minimum medium M9 supplemented with 100 μg of thymine per ml. (5). The growth of KL166 is unaffected by nalidixic acid at 500 μg/ml in the same medium. A direct analysis of the effect of nalidixic acid on the profiles of pulse-labeled RNA is clearly not feasible. An indirect approach of analyzing pulse-labeled proteins on sodium dodecyl sulfate-polyacrylamide gel was used. This approach is based on the assumption that the profile of pulse-labeled proteins reflects that of the RNA and that nalidixic acid does not act on translation (8).

Cells at a density of 3×10^8 per ml in M9 medium plus 100 μg of thymine per ml were treated with nalidixic acid (Sigma Chemical Co.) at 100 μg/ml. Nalidixic acid-treated and untreated samples were then divided and were separately pulse labeled with [^{14}C]thymidine (0.5 μCi/ml), [^{3}H]uridine (1 μCi/ml), and ^{14}C-labeled amino acid mixtures (2 μCi/ml) at predetermined time intervals. All labeled chemicals were purchased from New England Nuclear. [^{14}C]thymidine- and [^{3}H]uridine-labeled samples of 1 ml each were stopped with 10% trichloroacetic acid and counted. Samples (1 ml each) labeled with ^{14}C-labeled amino acids were stopped by adding 2 ml of ice-cold 2% unlabeled amino acid mixture and 10% glycerol. Labeled cells were pelleted and lysed in the extraction buffer (15). Portions of the lysate were precipitated with 5% trichloroacetic acid and counted. Another portion of each sample was used for sodium dodecyl sulfate-polyacrylamide gel electrophoresis according to the standard method (16).

The results of the pulse-labeling experiment are shown in Fig. 1. The rate of protein synthesis in KL161 and KL166 was reduced by nalidixic acid treatment by about 25 and 10%, respectively. The rate of RNA synthesis in these two strains was also reduced proportionately as reported by others (12). Thymidine incorporation was inhibited in KL161 but not in KL166 (data not shown). Thus, the bactericidal action of nalidixic acid does not seem to be related specifically to its action on bacterial RNA or protein synthesis. However, a close examination of individual peptides by sodium dodecyl sulfate-polyacrylamide gel analysis indicates otherwise. Certain major qualitative differences in protein patterns between KL161 and KL166 elicited by nalidixic acid are shown in Fig. 2. The pattern of pulse-labeled proteins was drastically altered by nalidixic acid in KL161 but not in KL166. Furthermore, in KL161 the synthesis of many proteins was depressed whereas that of others was induced by nalidixic acid. The most prominent protein bands whose synthesis was depressed by nalidixic acid were the 165-K (165,000 daltons), 155-K, 95-K and 30-K peptides. Of these peptides, only the 165- and 155-K peptides have been identified. These are the β' and β subunits of RNA polymerase, respectively (17; my unpublished data). The synthesis of these two subunits was depressed by about 10-fold in KL161 but only by about 30% in KL166 by nalidixic acid as revealed by direct scanning of the bands on radioautograms (data not shown). In KL161 the following peptides were induced by nalidixic acid: 135, 110, 90, 59, 55, 52, 40, and 18 K. The 135-K peptide has been identified as β-galactosidase (unpublished data). Shuman and Schwartz have shown (20) that nalidixic acid reduces the level of induced β-galactosidase in *E. coli* strain K-12. Unfortunately, they did not mention the effect of nalidixic acid on the level of β-galactosidase in uninduced cultures. The relationship between the action of nalidixic acid and the induction of β-galactosidase, and possibly the induction of other catabolite-repressible operons, appears to be complex in that β-galactosidase is only poorly induced by isopropyl-β-D-thiogalactoside in KL166 as compared with KL161 even in the absence of nalidixic acid (L. Chao, manuscript in preparation). The other readily identifiable peptide is the 40-K peptide, which corresponds to protein X previously reported by Inouye and Pardee (14). This protein has been implied to function in DNA repair (13). Note that certain peptides, such as the 59- and 52-K peptides, are only induced transiently in KL161 by nalidixic acid. The induction of other peptides in KL161 persists until the viability of the cells begin to drop significantly (data not shown).

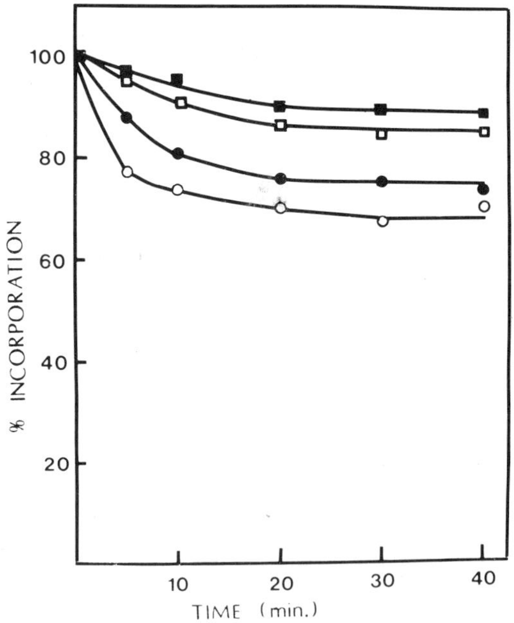

FIG. 1. *Effect of nalidixic acid on the rate of RNA and protein synthesis. E. coli KL161 and KL166 were grown in M9 minimal medium supplemented with 100 µg of thymine per ml at 30°C to 3 × 10^8 cells/ml. Nalidixic acid was added to each culture at zero time to give a final concentration of 100 µg/ml. Samples of 1 ml each were taken at the indicated time and pulse labeled with either [^{3}H]uridine (1 µCi/ml) for 1 min or ^{14}C-labeled amino acid mixture (2 µCi/ml) for 3 min. Labeled RNA and proteins were determined by scintillation counting. Acid-precipitable counts were plotted as the percentage of the control which was pulse labeled before the drug addition. [^{3}H]uridine incorporation: (○) KL161; (□) KL166. ^{14}C-labeled amino acid incorporation: (●) KL161; (■) KL166.*

It is known that nalidixic acid treatment converts cellular DNA into acid-soluble fragments and that this solubilization is antagonized by conditions restricting RNA and protein synthesis (6). In addition, nalidixic acid, like other agents that cause lesions in DNA, induces prophages (7, 11, 22). It is therefore very attractive to implicate nalidixic acid in inducing a DNA lesion or inhibiting DNA repair, or both. The results presented here are very suggestive of such actions by nalidixic acid. First, nalidixic acid drastically alters the pattern of newly syn-

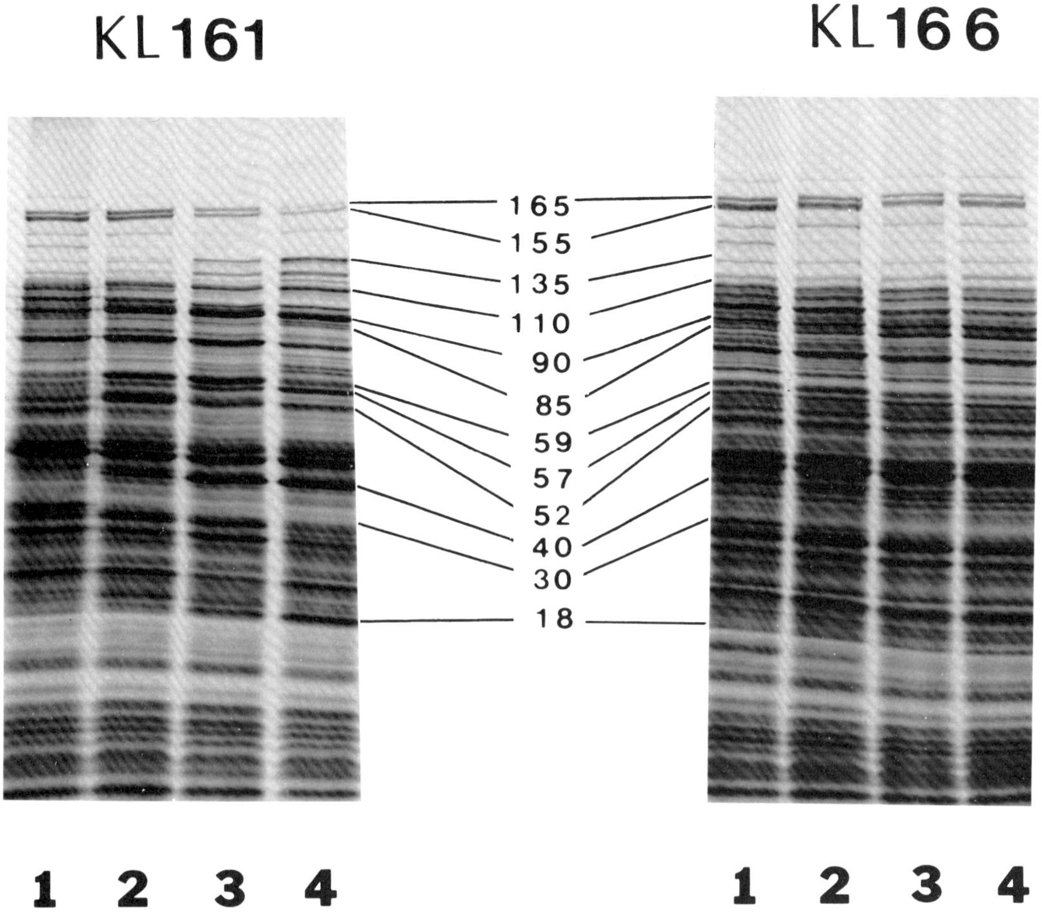

FIG. 2. *Effect of nalidixic acid on pulse-labeled protein patterns. KL161 and KL166 were treated with nalidixic acid and pulse labeled with ^{14}C-labeled amino acid mixture as described in the legend to Fig. 1. Samples corresponding to 5 × 10[7] cells were lysed and analyzed on a 7.5 to 12.5% gradient sodium dodecyl sulfate-polyacrylamide slab gel. Pulse-labeled protein patterns were obtained by autoradiography. The following proteins were electrophoresed on the same gel for molecular weight determination: E. coli RNA polymerase subunits (165, 155, 90 and 39 K), bovine serum albumin (67 K), ovalbumin (45 K), uricase (33 K) and myoglobin (18 K). (1) Control; (2) 10 min, (3) 20 min, and (4) 30 min after drug addition. The molecular weights (in kilodaltons) of relevant peptides are indicated.*

thesized proteins in sensitive but not in resistant strains of bacteria. This alteration is likely due to a direct or indirect effect of nalidixic acid on gene expression at the RNA level and not at the level of translation (8). However, a modification of the translational machinery by the drug cannot be totally excluded at the present time. Second, nalidixic acid elicits different effects on different gene products, as shown by the induction of certain proteins and the depression of others. Some of the induced proteins, such as β-galactosidase, are apparently not related to the bactericidal effect of the drug. Other induced or depressed proteins may play a role in the drug action. One of the possibilities is that some of the drug-depressed proteins may be involved in cellular DNA metabolism in a way similar to DNA repair enzymes or nucleases. Recently Crumplin and Smith reported (9) that the step blocked by nalidixic acid in DNA synthesis is the conversion of 38*S* single-stranded DNA fragments into high-molecular-weight DNA in sensitive cells. The nalidixic acid-induced proteins may therefore directly interfere with the conversion of the 38*S* fragments into full-sized DNA or rapidly degrade the 38*S* intermediate fragments, and thus exert the bactericidal action of the drug. This notion is supported by the observation that competent RNA and protein syntheses are essential prerequisites for both exonuclease action and the bactericidal action of nalidixic acid (6, 8).

I am grateful to J. D. Karam for his generosity in providing equipment and his patience in instructing in the use of slab gel techniques. I also wish to thank J. D. Karam and B. Baggett for their critical reading of the manuscript. The bacterial strains were kindly provided by Barbara Bachman.

This work was supported by Public Health Service General Research Grant RR05420 (from the Division of Research Resources) to the Medical University and by the South Carolina State Appropriation for Biomedical Research.

LITERATURE CITED

1. **Bachman, B. J.** 1972. Pedigrees of some mutant strains of *Escherichia coli*. J. Bacteriol. 36:525–557.
2. **Bauernfeind, A., and G. Grummer.** 1965. Biochemical effects of nalidixic acid on *Escherichia coli*. Chemotherapia 10:95–102.
3. **Bourguignon, G. J., M. Levitt, and R. Sternglanz.** 1973. Studies on the mechanism of action of nalidixic acid. Antimicrob. Agents Chemother. 4:479–486.
4. **Boyle, J. V., T. M. Cook, and W. A. Goss.** 1969. Mechanism of action of nalidixic acid on *Escherichia coli*. VI. Cell-free studies. J. Bacteriol. 97:230–236.
5. **Champe, S. P., and S. Benzer.** 1962. Reversal of mutant phenotypes by 5-fluorouracil: an approach to nucleotide sequences in messenger-RNA. Proc. Natl. Acad. Sci. U.S.A. 48:532–546.
6. **Cook, T. M., W. H. Deitz, and W. A. Gross.** 1966. Mechanism of action of nalidixic acid on *Escherichia coli*. IV. Effect on the stability of cellular constituents. J. Bacteriol. 91:774–779.
7. **Cowlishaw, J., and W. Ginoza.** 1970. Induction of λ prophage by nalidixic acid. Virology 41:244–255.
8. **Crumplin, G. C., and J. T. Smith.** 1975. Nalidixic acid: an antibacterial paradox. Antimicrob. Agents Chemother. 8:251–261.
9. **Crumplin, G. C., and J. T. Smith.** 1976. Nalidixic acid and bacterial chromosome replication. Nature (London) 260:643–645.
10. **Eberle, H., and W. Masker.** 1971. Effect of nalidixic acid on semiconservative replication and repair synthesis after ultraviolet irradiation in *Escherichia coli*. J. Bacteriol. 105:908–912.
11. **Geissler, E.** 1967. Untersuchungen über den Mechanismus der Induktion lysogener Bakterien. XI. Der Einfluss von DNA-Synthesehemmern auf lysogene Bakterien. Biol. Zentralbl. 86(Suppl.):55–67.
12. **Gross, W. A., W. H. Deitz, and T. M. Cook.** 1965. Mechanism of action of nalidixic acid on *Escherichia coli*. II. Inhibition of deoxyribonucleic acid synthesis. J. Bacteriol. 89:1068–1074.
13. **Gudas, L. J., and A. B. Pardee.** 1975. Model for regulation of *Escherichia coli* DNA repair functions. Proc. Natl. Acad. Sci. U.S.A. 72:2330–2334.
14. **Inouye, M. and A. B. Pardee.** 1970. Changes of membrane proteins and their relation to deoxyribonucleic acid synthesis and cell division in *Escherichia coli*. J. Biol. Chem. 245:5813–5819.
15. **Karam, J. D., and M. G. Bowles.** 1974. Mutation to overproduction of bacteriophage T4 gene products. J. Virol. 13:428–438.
16. **Laemmli, U. K.** 1970. Cleavage of structural proteins during assembly of the head bacteriophage T4. Nature (London) 227:680–685.
17. **Matzura, H., S. Molin, and O. Maaløe.** 1971. Sequential biosynthesis of the β and β' subunits of the DNA-dependent RNA polymerase from *Escherichia coli*. J. Mol. Biol. 59:17–25.
18. **Nishida, M., Y. Mishima, J. Kawada, and K. L. Yielding.** 1975. Enhancement by nalidixic acid of the thermal susceptibility of the Ts-7 mutant of *Escherichia coli* TAU-bar. Antimicrob. Agents Chemother. 8:384–386.
19. **Pedrini, A. M., D. Geroldi, A. Siccardi, and A. Falashi.** 1972. Studies on the mode of action of nalidixic acid. Eur. J. Biochem. 25:359–365.
20. **Shuman, H., and M. Schwartz.** 1975. The effect of nalidixic acid on the expression of some genes in *Escherichia coli* K-12. Biochem. Biophys. Res. Commun. 64:204–209.
21. **Simon, T. J., W. E. Masker, and P. C. Hanawalt.** 1974. Selective inhibition of semiconservative DNA synthesis by nalidixic acid in permeabilized bacteria. Biochim. Biophys. Acta 349:271–274.
22. **Taketo, A., and H. Watanbe.** 1967. Effect of nalidixic acid on the growth of bacterial viruses. J. Biochem. 61:520–522.

ANTIMICROBIAL AGENTS AND CHEMOTHERAPY, Jan. 1977, p. 171-173
Vol. 11, No. 1

Printed in U.S.A.

Susceptibility of *Propionibacterium acnes* to Seventeen Antibiotics

WEN LAN LOU WANG,* E. DALE EVERETT,[1] MARCIA JOHNSON, AND EVELYN DEAN

Microbiology Laboratory, Laboratory Service, Veterans Administration Hospital, and Department of Pathology, School of Medicine, University of Colorado, Denver, Colorado 80220*

Received for publication 13 July 1976

The in vitro susceptibility of 96 isolates of *Propionibacterium acnes* to 17 antibiotics was determined by utilizing an agar dilution technique. With the exception of the aminoglycosides, these organisms are susceptible to virtually all of the commonly used antimicrobial agents.

Propionibacterium species are unusual causes of illness, but are known to produce a variety of infections (4, 6). Only a few in vitro antibiotic susceptibility studies against these organisms have been made in which multiple antibiotics and/or large numbers of isolates were used (1, 7, 10).

In the present study, we have examined the in vitro susceptibility of 96 strains of *P. acnes* to 17 antibiotics, including several antimicrobial agents not previously tested against *P. acnes* (1, 7, 10). Of particular interest is the susceptibility of these organisms to cephalosporins and semisynthetic penicillins, because these drugs are frequently used as prophylaxis in procedures such as cerebrospinal fluid shunts and cardiac valvular surgery where *Propionibacterium* infections are prone to occur (4, 6).

The majority of the 96 strains studied were clinical isolates from the microbiology laboratories of the Veterans Administration Hospital, Colorado General Hospital, and St. Joseph Hospital, Denver, Colo. Eleven strains, five with known minimal inhibitory concentration (MIC) values by broth dilution, were supplied by George Lombard of the Center for Disease Control (CDC), Atlanta, Ga. Speciation was done by standard methods (2, 5, 8).

The antibiotics tested are indicated in Table 1. Antimicrobial susceptibility was done by using the agar dilution technique on brain heart infusion agar supplemented with hemin (5 μg/ml) and vitamin K (0.5 μg/ml). Stock solutions of the test drugs were prepared in sterile distilled water; further dilutions were made in brain heart infusion broth supplemented with hemin (5 μg/ml) and vitamin K_1 (1.0 μg/ml) and added to similarly supplemented brain heart infusion agar at 46°C to yield final drug concentrations ranging from 0.1 to 50 μg/ml. The antibiotic-containing plates were stored at 4 to 8°C for not longer than 5 days and were reduced in an anaerobic chamber for 24 h before use.

The inoculum was prepared by diluting a 24-h supplemented brain heart infusion broth culture to provide an inoculum size of approximately 10^4 colony-forming units—a Steers replicator was then used to deliver the diluted inoculum to the surface of the agar (9). After inoculation, all plates were incubated in an anaerobic chamber at 36°C. After 48 h of incubation, the MIC values were read as the lowest concentration permitting no growth, a barely visible fine haze, or not more than one discrete colony (3). A limited number of antibiotic dilutions and inoculating procedures, not requiring more than 30 min, were done at ambient atmosphere. All other steps were done in an anaerobic chamber.

Table 1 shows the cumulative percentages of the strains of *P. acnes* inhibited at various concentrations of 17 antibiotics. Ninety-six strains of *P. acnes* were susceptible to all antibiotics tested, except the aminoglycosides: gentamicin, tobramycin, and amikacin. These results are in general agreement with the published data (1, 7, 10). Penicillin G and erythromycin were the most active, inhibiting all strains at 0.1 μg/ml. The MICs of the semisynthetic penicillins were higher than penicillin, but were within the range of achievable blood levels.

Cephalothin was the most active cephalosporin tested. Clindamycin showed activity comparable to cephalothin. The MICs of chloramphenicol and vancomycin were similar, with 100% inhibition at 1.6 and 0.8 μg/ml, respectively. Gentamicin inhibited 100% of the strains at 50 μg/ml and 76% at 25 μg/ml. Tetracycline inhibited all of the strains at 3.1 μg/ml and 64% at 1.6 μ/ml.

The CDC MICs of seven antibiotics against

[1] Present address: Brooke Army Medical Center, Fort Sam Houston, Texas.

the five strains, by broth dilution, are compared with our results in Table 2. Some of the differences may be more apparent than real, because the lowest test concentration in our method was 0.1 μg/ml, whereas the minimal concentration tested by the CDC method was 0.01 μg/ml. Our MICs for gentamicin and tetracycline are substantially higher than those of the CDC, although our results are similar to those obtained by Martin (7), who also used an agar dilution method. As with certain facultative organisms, the differences in MICs of gentamicin and tetracycline, between the two methods, could possibly be due to the differences in concentrations of divalent ions and pH of the media (3). Nevertheless, these discrepancies between broth and agar dilution methods point out the need for a standardized susceptibility test method for *P. acnes*.

The MIC results from this study indicate that *P. acnes* is susceptible to almost all commonly used antibiotics, including the cephalosporins and semisynthetic penicillins, which are frequently used for prophylaxis in certain neurosurgical and cardiovascular procedures. Our results also indicate that *P. acnes* is not susceptible to some of the commonly used aminoglycosides.

TABLE 1. *Susceptibility of propionibacterium acnes to 17 antibiotics*

Antibiotics	No. of strains tested	Cumulative % of organisms inhibited at various concn (μg/ml)									
		0.1	0.2	0.4	0.8	1.6	3.1	6.2	12.5	25.0	50.0
Penicillins											
Ampicillin	96	65	99	99	100						
Dicloxacillin	90	3	3	19	78	98	100				
Methicillin	96	12	26	47	89	91	99	100			
Nafcillin	96	16	48	83	97	98	100				
Oxacillin	96	43	79	88	100						
Penicillin G	96	100									
Cephalosporins											
Cephalexin	95		1	56	97	99	100				
Cefoxitin	96	51	98	100							
Cephalothin	96	92	99	100							
Aminoglycosides											
Amikacin	96						1		2	58	92
Gentamicin	96				2	2	9	32	64	76	100
Tobramycin	96									2	13
Others											
Chloramphenicol	94	1	5	29	94	100					
Clindamycin	95	94	96	100							
Erythromycin	96	100									
Tetracycline	96			4	23	64	100				
Vancomycin	96			5	100						

TABLE 2. *MICs (μg/ml) of five strains of propionibacterium acnes: agar dilution versus broth dilution method*[a]

Antibiotic	MIC (μg/ml) in strain no.									
	1		3		7		92		95	
	Agar	Broth	Agar	Broth	Agar	Broth	Agar	Broth	Agar	Broth
Cephalothin	≤0.1	0.06	≤0.1	0.06	0.2	0.12	≤0.1	0.5	≤0.1	0.06
Chloramphenicol	0.8	0.5	0.8	0.25	0.8	0.5	0.4	1.0	0.4	0.25
Clindamycin	0.2	0.12	≤0.1	≤0.015	≤0.1	≤0.015	≤0.1	0.03	≤0.1	0.03
Erythromycin	≤0.1	≤0.015	≤0.1	≤0.015	≤0.1	≤0.015	≤0.1	0.01	≤0.1	0.01
Gentamicin	12.5	0.12	12.5	0.5	3.1	0.25	50	16	50	4.0
Penicillin	≤0.1	≤0.015	≤0.1	≤0.015	≤0.1	≤0.015	≤0.1	0.5	≤0.1	0.06
Tetracycline	1.6	≤0.015	3.1	0.06	1.6	0.12	3.1	0.12	3.1	0.12

[a] MICs by the broth dilution method were obtained from the CDC.

We thank George Lombard, the National Communicable Disease Center, for supplying 11 strains of *P. acnes,* and Florence Rogers for assistance in preparation of the manuscript.

LITERATURE CITED

1. **Chow, A. W., V. Pattern, and L. B. Guze.** 1975. Comparative susceptibility of anaerobic bacteria to minocycline, doxycycline, and tetracycline. Antimicrob. Agents Chemother. 7:46–49.
2. **Dowell, V. R., and T. M. Hawkins.** 1974. Laboratory methods in anaerobic bacteriology. *In* Public Health Service, Monogr. no. 74-8272, Washington, D.C.
3. **Ericsson, H. M., and J. C. Sherris.** 1971. Antibiotic sensitivity testings, report of an international collaborative study. Acta Pathol. Microbiol. Scand. Sect. B. Suppl. no. 217, 27–32, 68.
4. **Everett, E. D., T. C. Eickhoff, and R. H. Simon.** 1976. Cerebrospinal fluid shunt infections with anaerobic diphtheroids. J. Neurosurg. 44:580–584.
5. **Holdeman, L. D., and W. E. Moore.** 1975. Anaerobic laboratory manual. Virginia Polytechnic Institute and State University, Blacksburg, Va.
6. **Johnson, W.D., and D. Kaye.** 1970. Serious infections caused by diphtheroids. Ann. N.Y. Acad. Sci. 174:568–576.
7. **Martin, W. J., M. Gardener, and J. A. Washington II.** 1972. In vitro antimicrobial susceptibility of anaerobic bacteria isolated from clinical specimens. Antimicrob. Agents Chemother. 1:148–158.
8. **Moore, H. B., V. L. Sutter, and S. M. Finegold.** 1975. Comparison of three procedures for biochemical testing of anaerobic bacteria. J. Clin. Microbiol. 1:15–24.
9. **Steers, E., E. L. Foltz, B. S. Graves, and J. Riden.** 1959. An inocula replicating apparatus for routine testing of bacterial susceptibility to antibiotics. Antibiot. Chemother. 9:307–311.
10. **Tally, F. P., N. V. Jacobs, J. G. Bartlett, and S. L. Gorbach.** 1975. Susceptibility of anaerobes to cefoxitin and other cephalosporins. Antimicrob. Agents Chemother. 7:128–132.

ANTIMICROBIAL AGENTS AND CHEMOTHERAPY, Jan. 1977, p. 174-175 Vol. 11, No. 1

Stability of Cephalosporins in Horse Serum

M. A. FOGLESONG

The Lilly Research Laboratories, Eli Lilly and Company, Indianapolis, Indiana 46206

Received for publication 30 July 1976

The antibiotic activity of cephalothin, cephaloridine, cephalexin, cephaloglycin, cefazolin, and cefamandole was determined after storage for up to 30 days in horse serum at −10 and 4°C. Cephalothin, cefamandole, cefazolin, and cephalexin were stable for at least 30 days at −10°C, whereas cephaloridine lost 29% of its initial activity and cephaloglycin lost more than 50%. Cefamandole, cefazolin, and cephalexin could only be stored for 3 days at 4°C without significant loss in activity, whereas cephalothin, cephaloridine, and cephaloglycin could be stored for only 1 day. Repeated freezing and thawing had a detrimental effect on the stability of cephaloridine.

Frequently, the nature of antibiotic bioavailability studies is such that prolonged freezing or repeated freezing and thawing of samples is required. Information is available concerning the stability of antibiotics in aqueous and frozen solutions (2, 5–10), but little is known about the stability of antibiotics in serum. Berti and Maccari (1) have recently examined the stability of 11 different antibiotics, including cephaloridine and cephalexin, stored in frozen rat plasma for 8 weeks at −20°C. Under these conditions, cephalexin was shown to be significantly more stable than cephaloridine.

The present study was undertaken to examine the stability of cephalothin, cephaloridine, cephalexin, cephaloglycin, cefazolin, and cefamandole stored in horse serum under the following conditions: (i) frozen in serum at −10°C and the same sample assayed at 1-, 2-, 3-, and 30-day intervals: (ii) frozen in serum at −10°C for 30 days; and (iii) stored in serum at 4°C and assayed at 1-, 2-, 3-, and 30-day intervals.

Using pooled horse serum as a diluent, antibiotic solutions were prepared by volumetric dilutions to the following reference concentrations: cefazolin, 4.0 μg/ml; cephalothin, cephaloridine, and cefamandole, 1.0 μg/ml; cephalexin, 0.4 μg/ml; and cephaloglycin, 0.2 μg/ml. Microbiological activity was determined by a cylinder-plate assay (4). *Sarcina lutea* was used as the test organism for the cephalexin and cephaloglycin plate assays, and *Bacillus subtilis* was used for the remaining cephalosporins. The format used for the assays is outlined in the *Code of Federal Regulations* (3).

Immediately after the initial assay, each antibiotic solution was divided into three portions. One sample was frozen at −10°C and then thawed, refrozen, and assayed at 1-, 2-, 3-, and 30-day intervals. The second sample was frozen at −10°C and assayed after 30 days. This sample functioned as a control for the freeze-thaw portion of the study. The third sample was stored at 4°C and assayed at 1-, 2-, 3-, and 30-day intervals.

The microbiological activity as the precentage of initial activity of the six cephalosporins after storage at −10°C is listed in Table 1. Thawing and refreezing of the samples at 1-, 2-, and 3-day intervals had little effect on the activity of cephalothin, cephaloridine, cephalexin, cefazolin, and cefamandole. These compounds retained at least 94% of their initial antibiotic activity for 3 days. Cephaloglycin, however, retained only 75% of its activity after 1 day and 50% of its activity after 3 days. After 30 days at −10°C, cephalothin, cephalexin, cefazolin, and cefamandole showed no loss in

TABLE 1. *Antibiotic activity as the percentage of initial activity of cephalosporins stored at −10°C in pooled horse serum and assayed at various time intervals*[a]

Antibiotic	Antibiotic activity (%) after storage (days):					Antibiotic activity (%) of freeze-thaw control
	0	1	2	3	30	
Cephalothin	100 (±8)	93 (±4)	92 (±6)	94 (±4)	91 (±8)	93 (±3)
Cephaloridine	100 (±3)	97 (±3)	94 (±5)	94 (±1)	71 (±3)	90 (±8)
Cephalexin	100 (±1)	105 (±7)	NS[b]	95 (±1)	98 (±1)	98 (±1)
Cephaloglycin	100 (±2)	75 (±1)	55 (±1)	<50	<50	<50
Cefazolin	100 (±8)	101 (±6)	94 (±4)	97 (±4)	100 (±2)	101 (±5)
Cefamandole	100 (±3)	100 (±10)	94 (±2)	99 (±8)	100 (±3)	104 (±6)

[a] Average of six determinations ± standard deviation.
[b] NS, Not sampled.

activity. However, under the same conditions, cephaloridine lost 29% of its initial activity. Cephaloglycin possessed less than 50% of its activity when stored for 30 days at −10°C.

Of the cephalosporins tested, only cephaloridine appeared to be affected by repeated freezing and thawing. The cephaloridine control sample, which was thawed only once prior to being assayed, contained 90% of the initial activity after 30 days. The cephaloridine sample that was thawed and refrozen on days 1, 2, 3, and 30 possessed only 71% of its initial activity after 30 days.

Storage at 4°C (Table 2) had a more drastic effect on the stability of the antibiotics than storage at −10°C or repeated thawing and freezing. After 3 days at 4°C, cephalexin, cefazolin, and cefamandole retained greater than 90% of their initial activity, cephalothin and cephaloridine retained approximately 80%, and cephaloglycin possessed less than 50%. After 30 days of storage at 4°C, cefamandole retained 70% of its initial activity, cephalexin retained 56%, and cefazolin retained 42%. Cephalothin, cephaloridine, and cephaloglycin all possessed less than 50% of their initial activity.

TABLE 2. *Antibiotic activity as the percentage of initial activity of cephalosporins stored at 4°C in pooled horse serum and assayed at various time intervals*[a]

Antibiotic	Antibiotic activity (%) after storage (days):				
	0	1	2	3	30
Cephalothin	100 (±8)	94 (±3)	85 (±3)	79 (±3)	<25
Cephaloridine	100 (±3)	102 (±5)	78 (±4)	80 (±2)	<25
Cephalexin	100 (±2)	98 (±5)	NS[b]	95 (±3)	56 (±2)
Cephaloglycin	100 (±10)	65 (±5)	<50	<50	<50
Cefazolin	100 (±8)	100 (±5)	98 (±2)	99 (±7)	42 (±1)
Cefamandole	100 (±6)	95 (±4)	95 (±2)	92 (±5)	70 (±2)

[a] Average of six determinations ± standard deviation.
[b] NS, Not sampled.

The technical assistance of Jack Scott is gratefully acknowledged.

LITERATURE CITED

1. **Berti, M. A., and M. Maccari.** 1975. Stability of frozen rat plasma containing different antibiotics. Antimicrob. Agents Chemother. 8:633–637.
2. **Boylan, J. C., J. L. Simmons, and C. L. Winely.** 1972. Stability of frozen solutions of sodium cephalothin and cephaloridine. Am. J. Hosp. Pharm. **29**:687–689.
3. **Code of federal regulations.** Vol. 39, no. 105, part III, §436.105(a)(b)(c)(d).
4. **Grove, D. C., and W. A. Randall.** 1955. Penicillin section A: microbiologic assay methods for penicillin, p. 7–14. Assay methods of antibiotics. Medical Encyclopedia, Inc., New York.
5. **Hou, J. P., and J. W. Poole.** 1969. Kinetics and mechanism of degradation of ampicillin in solution. J. Pharm. Sci. **58**:447–454.
6. **Kuchinskas, E. J., and G. N. Levy.** 1972. Comparative stabilities of ampicillin and hetacillin in aqueous solution. J. Pharm. Sci. **61**:727–729.
7. **Mann, J. M., D. L. Coleman, and J. C. Boylan.** 1971. Stability of parenteral solutions of sodium cephalothin, cephaloridine, potassium penicillin G (buffered), and vancomycin hydrochloride. Am. J. Hosp. Pharm. **28**:760–763.
8. **Sauello, D. R., and R. F. Shangrau.** 1971. Stability of sodium ampicillin solutions in the frozen and liquid states. Am. J. Hosp. Pharm. **28**:754–759.
9. **Stolar, M. H., H. S. Carlin, and M. I. Blake.** 1968. Effect of freezing on the stability of sodium methicillin injection. Am. J. Hosp. Pharm. **25**:32–35.
10. **Yamana, T., A. Tsuji, K. Kanayama, and O. Nakano.** 1974. Comparative stabilities of cephalosporins in aqueous solutions. J. Antibiot. **27**:1000–1002.

ANTIMICROBIAL AGENTS AND CHEMOTHERAPY, Jan. 1977, p. 176-177
Vol. 11, No. 1

Bactericidal Effects of Combinations of Ampicillin with Anti-R-Plasmid Compounds on *Salmonella typhimurium* R1+

FRED E. HAHN* AND JENNIE CIAK

Department of Molecular Biology, Walter Reed Army Institute of Research, Washington, D.C. 20012

Received for publication 28 June 1976

Salmonella typhimurium R1$^+$, resistant to 2,500 μg of ampicillin per ml, was rapidly killed by combinations of 60 μg of ampicillin per ml with quinacrine (4×10^{-4} M), ethidium bromide (10^{-4} M), tilorone (10^{-4} M), or Nitroakridin 3582 (5×10^{-6} M).

We have shown that deoxyribonucleic acid-intercalating compounds eliminate resistance determinants from R-plasmid R1 carried by *Salmonella typhimurium* LT-2 and, hence, restore antibiotic susceptibility to this bacterium (2). The purpose of this work was to investigate if sensitization of *S. typhimurium* R1$^+$ to antibiotics and the bactericidal actions of such antibiotics can occur concurrently in the same bacterial cultures. Preliminary experiments with combinations of kanamycin and ethidium bromide did not demonstrate any influence of this drug combination on growth and viability of *S. typhimurium* R1$^+$. Other work on the influence of antibiotics on the spontaneous or chemically enforced elimination of their resistance determinants from R plasmids in *Salmonella* has been reviewed recently (1).

The R-plasmid R1 carries a determinant of resistance to ampicillin (2). In serial dilution test tube assays, *S. typhimurium* R1$^+$ incubated overnight was resistant to 2,500 μg of ampicillin per ml.

Figure 1 presents growth curves from plate counts of *S. typhimurium* R1$^+$ growing in Penassay broth (Difco). A drug-free control culture showed rapid exponential growth. A second culture to which 60 μg of ampicillin per ml (1.7×10^{-4} M) was added showed an initial decline in viability. Growth resumed at h 5 and attained a rate identical to that of the drug-free control culture. A third culture was supplied with 10^{-4} M ethidium bromide. This, too, showed an initial decline in viability and resumed growth at h 6 at an accelerating rate, which by h 14 had still not attained that of the drug-free control culture. However, upon further incubation, this culture grew to the same bacterial density as the drug-free control culture. Serial dilution test tube assays of these bacteria showed that their susceptibility to ethidium was unchanged.

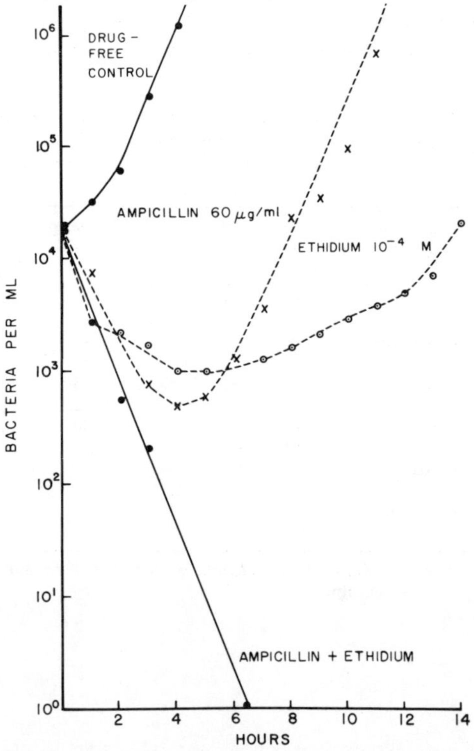

FIG. 1. *Growth or loss of viability of S. typhimurium R1$^+$ exposed to ampicillin, ethidium bromide, or to a combination of both drugs. Penassay broth (Difco) was prepared in 10^{-2} M potassium phosphates buffer, adjusted to pH 8. The bacteria were grown in this aerated medium to early-log phase. The cultures were then standardized to an optical density of 0.01 at 540 nm in a Beckman model 25 spectrophotometer and diluted by a factor of 100 to yield cultures containing 2×10^4 bacteria per ml. After addition of test compounds, these cultures were incubated further, and portions were removed at intervals for serial dilution, plating on meat extract agar, and colony counting after incubation overnight.*

A combination of 1.7×10^{-4} M ampicillin and 10^{-4} M ethidium bromide, however, was rapidly bactericidal from the moment of addition, so that by h 6 only one or no viable bacteria remained per milliliter. Further incubation of such experimental cultures for several days demonstrated that they remained sterile. These results were obtained in the pH range 7.4 to 8.0, to which the medium was buffered with potassium phosphates.

Analogous results were obtained with combinations of ampicillin with quinacrine (4×10^{-4} M), tilorone (10^{-4} M), or Nitroakridin 3582 (5×10^{-6} M), i.e., 2.5 μg/ml. The minimal growth inhibitory concentration of Nitroakridin 3582 for *S. typhimurium* is $>2 \times 10^{-4}$ M (4). Cultures that were exposed to ethidium bromide alone for the first 6 h were rapidly sterilized when ampicillin was added at that point in time. In contrast, cultures that were initially exposed to ampicillin and had resumed growth by 6 h continued to grow when ethidium bromide was added.

Resistance of *S. typhimurium* R1$^+$ to ampicillin was of the "intrinsic" type (3). Assays for ampicillin on the membrane-filtered (Millipore Corp.) growth medium of *S. typhimurium* R1$^+$, using *Staphylococcus aureus* (ATCC 25923) as a highly susceptible test strain, showed that at h 5, when *S. typhimurium* resumed growth, the concentration of ampicillin in the medium was still 30 μg/ml. Only by h 14 had the medium lost all growth-inhibitory activity for *S. aureus*. It is doubtful, therefore, that the ability of *S. typhimurium* R1$^+$ to resist ampicillin resulted from an exhaustive hydrolysis of the antibiotic by β-lactamase(s).

We interpret our results as indications that the deoxyribonucleic-intercalative compounds ethidium bromide, quinacrine, tilorone, and Nitroakridin 3582 acted as template poisons for R-plasmid deoxyribonucleic acid (1, 2) and prevented either the replication of the ampicillin resistance determinant or its phenotypic expression. This enabled ampicillin to exert its bactericidal effect.

LITERATURE CITED

1. **Hahn, F. E.** 1976. Experimental elimination of R factors. Antibiot. Chemother. (Basel) **20**:196–226.
2. **Hahn, F. E., and J. Ciak.** 1976. Elimination of resistance determinants from R-factor R1 by intercalative compounds. Antimicrob. Agents Chemother. **9**:77–80.
3. **Richmond, M. H., and R. B. Sykes.** 1973. The β-lactamases of Gram-negative bacteria and their possible physiological role. Adv. Microbiol. Physiol. **9**:31–88.
4. **Wolfe, A. D., T. M. Cook, and F. E. Hahn.** 1971. Antibacterial nitroacridine, Nitroakridin 3582: effects on bacterial growth and macromolecular biosynthesis in vivo. J. Bacteriol. **108**:320–327.

U.S. POSTAL SERVICE

STATEMENT OF OWNERSHIP, MANAGEMENT AND CIRCULATION

(Required by 39 U.S.C. 3685)

1. TITLE OF PUBLICATION: ANTIMICROBIAL AGENTS AND CHEMOTHERAPY

2. DATE OF FILING: 10/1/76

3. FREQUENCY OF ISSUE: Monthly

A. NO. OF ISSUES PUBLISHED ANNUALLY: 12

B. ANNUAL SUBSCRIPTION PRICE: Mem.$13, N-Mem.$50

4. LOCATION OF KNOWN OFFICE OF PUBLICATION *(Street, City, County, State and ZIP Code) (Not printers)*: 1913 Eye St.,N.W., Washington, D.C. 20006

5. LOCATION OF THE HEADQUARTERS OR GENERAL BUSINESS OFFICES OF THE PUBLISHERS *(Not printers)*: 1913 Eye St., N.W., Washington, D.C. 20006

6. NAMES AND COMPLETE ADDRESSES OF PUBLISHER, EDITOR, AND MANAGING EDITOR

PUBLISHER *(Name and Address)*: AMERICAN SOCIETY FOR MICROBIOLOGY, 1913 Eye St.,N.W.,Washington,DC.20006

EDITOR *(Name and Address)*: Dr. Gladys L. Hobby,Inf. Disease Res. Inst., P.O. Box 495, East Orange, NJ. 07019

MANAGING EDITOR *(Name and Address)*: Robert A. Day, 1913 Eye St., N.W., Washington, D.C. 20006

7. OWNER *(If owned by a corporation, its name and address must be stated and also immediately thereunder the names and addresses of stockholders owning or holding 1 percent or more of total amount of stock. If not owned by a corporation, the names and addresses of the individual owners must be given. If owned by a partnership or other unincorporated firm, its name and address, as well as that of each individual must be given.)*

NAME	ADDRESS
American Society for Microbiology	1913 Eye St., N.W. Washington, D.C. 20006

8. KNOWN BONDHOLDERS, MORTGAGEES, AND OTHER SECURITY HOLDERS OWNING OR HOLDING 1 PERCENT OR MORE OF TOTAL AMOUNT OF BONDS, MORTGAGES OR OTHER SECURITIES *(If there are none, so state)*

NAME	ADDRESS
None	

9. FOR COMPLETION BY NONPROFIT ORGANIZATIONS AUTHORIZED TO MAIL AT SPECIAL RATES *(Section 132.122, PSM)*
The purpose, function, and nonprofit status of this organization and the exempt status for Federal income tax purposes *(Check one)*

[XX] HAVE NOT CHANGED DURING PRECEDING 12 MONTHS [ ] HAVE CHANGED DURING PRECEDING 12 MONTHS *(If changed, publisher must submit explanation of change with this statement.)*

10. EXTENT AND NATURE OF CIRCULATION	AVERAGE NO. COPIES EACH ISSUE DURING PRECEDING 12 MONTHS	ACTUAL NO. COPIES OF SINGLE ISSUE PUBLISHED NEAREST TO FILING DATE
A. TOTAL NO. COPIES PRINTED *(Net Press Run)*	5412	5626
B. PAID CIRCULATION 1. SALES THROUGH DEALERS AND CARRIERS, STREET VENDORS AND COUNTER SALES	None	None
2. MAIL SUBSCRIPTIONS	4193	4908
C. TOTAL PAID CIRCULATION *(Sum of 10B1 and 10B2)*	4193	4908
D. FREE DISTRIBUTION BY MAIL, CARRIER OR OTHER MEANS SAMPLES, COMPLIMENTARY, AND OTHER FREE COPIES	2	3
E. TOTAL DISTRIBUTION *(Sum of C and D)*	4195	4911
F. COPIES NOT DISTRIBUTED 1. OFFICE USE, LEFT OVER, UNACCOUNTED, SPOILED AFTER PRINTING	1217	715
2. RETURNS FROM NEWS AGENTS	None	None
G. TOTAL *(Sum of E, F1 and 2—should equal net press run shown in A)*	5412	5626

11. I certify that the statements made by me above are correct and complete.
SIGNATURE AND TITLE OF EDITOR, PUBLISHER, BUSINESS MANAGER, OR OWNER: Robert A. Day Managing Editor

12. FOR COMPLETION BY PUBLISHERS MAILING AT THE REGULAR RATES *(Section 132.121, Postal Service Manual)*

39 U. S. C. 3626 provides in pertinent part: "No person who would have been entitled to mail matter under former section 4359 of this title shall mail such matter at the rates provided under this subsection unless he files annually with the Postal Service a written request for permission to mail matter at such rates."

In accordance with the provisions of this statute, I hereby request permission to mail the publication named in Item 1 at the phased postage rates presently authorized by 39 U. S. C. 3626.

SIGNATURE AND TITLE OF EDITOR, PUBLISHER, BUSINESS MANAGER, OR OWNER: Robert A. Day Managing Editor

PS Form 3526 *(Page 1)* Apr. 1976 (See instructions on reverse)

ERRATA

New Method for Detecting In Vitro Inactivation of Penicillins by *Haemophilus influenzae* and *Staphylococcus aureus*

WIE-SHING LEE* AND LOUIS KOMARMY
Microbiology Laboratory, Children's Hospital, San Francisco, California 94119

Volume 10, no. 3, p. 565, Table 1, column 6 (no. of penicillinase producers), line 3: "0" should read "21."

Antibiotic Resistance Among Coliform and Fecal Coliform Bacteria Isolated from Sewage, Seawater, and Marine Shellfish

MARYLYN D. COOKE
Cawthron Institute, Nelson, New Zealand

Volume 9, no. 6, p. 883, column 1, line 23: "MNP" should read "MPN." p. 883, column 2, reference 4: "*Hydridella*" should read "*Hyridella.*"

Antibiotic Resistance Among Coliform and Fecal Coliform Bacteria Isolated from the Freshwater Mussel *Hydridella menziesii*

MARYLYN D. COOKE
Cawthron Institute, Nelson, New Zealand

Volume 9, no. 6, p. 885, title, abstract, and column 1, line 21: "*Hydridella*" should read "*Hyridella.*"

Inhibition of *Neisseria gonorrhoeae* by a Bacteriocin from *Pseudomonas aeruginosa*

STEPHEN A. MORSE,* PATRICK VAUGHAN, DEANNE JOHNSON, AND BARBARA H. IGLEWSKI
Department of Microbiology and Immunology, University of Oregon Health Sciences Center, Portland, Oregon 97201

Volume 10, no. 2, p. 355, column 2, line 17 should read: "...0.85% NaCl and 0.1% cysteine-HCl (pH 6.4) and adjusted to a ..."

Antimicrobial Agents and Chemotherapy, Feb. 1977, p. 179–184
Vol. 11, No. 2

Emergence of Gentamicin-Resistant *Klebsiella* in a General Hospital

R. P. RENNIE* and I. B. R. DUNCAN

Department of Medical Microbiology, University of Toronto, and Microbiology Department, Sunnybrook Medical Centre, Toronto, Ontario M4N 3M5, Canada*

Received for publication 5 August 1976

Gentamicin had been in use in a general hospital for over 7 years before any gentamicin-resistant *Klebsiella* were observed. In 1974 and 1975, nine different gentamicin-resistant serobiotypes of *Klebsiella* were isolated from 35 patients. The first strain to appear had R-factor-mediated gentamicin resistance, and it infected 19 patients during a period of almost 2 years, spreading largely by case-to-case infection in patients with urinary catheters. It appeared to lose the capacity to transfer its gentamicin resistance after it had infected five of the patients. We had previously isolated on the same ward a gentamicin-susceptible *Klebsiella* of identical type, and it was found to be capable of acquiring an R-factor for gentamicin resistance. All of the other types of gentamicin-resistant *Klebsiella* infected few patients and did not persist in the hospital; four of them had R-factor-mediated resistance to gentamicin and all four, as did the original strain, cotransferred kanamycin, neomycin, and tobramycin resistance. Every gentamicin-resistant *Klebsiella* was susceptible to amikacin and netilmicin.

The appearance of multiresistant strains of *Klebsiella* in hospitals has been clearly associated with the widespread use of antimicrobial agents (12, 13, 16, 17). Strains of *Klebsiella* isolated from healthy individuals who had no association with hospitals were shown by Davis and Matsen (5) to be resistant only to ampicillin and carbenicillin. By contrast, these workers found that strains carried by hospital patients in the same city were frequently resistant to many other antibiotics and often possessed transmissible R-factors.

Until recently even multiresistant hospital strains of *Klebsiella* have retained their susceptibility to gentamicin. There have been few reports of gentamicin-resistant *Klebsiella* causing outbreaks of nosocomial infection (8, 10). In these cases the gentamicin resistance was transferable from the *Klebsiella* to recipient laboratory strains of *Escherichia coli*. In our own hospital, gentamicin was used for 7 years before the first gentamicin-resistant strains of *Klebsiella* appeared. The present report gives an account of their emergence and spread and describes the main characteristics of the gentamicin-resistant strains.

MATERIALS AND METHODS

Identification and typing of *Klebsiella*. All of the *Klebsiella* studied were clinical isolates from inpatients at Sunnybrook Medical Centre, Toronto, which is a 1,000-bed teaching hospital with almost equal numbers of acute and chronic patients. Isolates were first identified in the diagnostic laboratory as *Klebsiella* species by standard methods (7). The capsular serotypes of gentamicin-resistant isolates were determined by quellung reaction by the method reported by Casewell (3). Typing antisera against the 72 recognized capsular types of *Klebsiella* were prepared by immunizing rabbits and were absorbed to remove cross-reacting antibodies (7). The gentamicin-resistant *Klebsiella* were further subdivided by the numerical biotyping scheme that we described previously (14). The results of the two typing methods were combined as the serobiotype of the strain, and this provided a more discriminating system for differentiating *Klebsiella* than did either typing method used alone.

Antimicrobial susceptibility testing. Routine susceptibility tests were done in the diagnostic laboratory by inoculating isolates with a Steers inocula replicator to Mueller-Hinton agar (BBL) plates containing antimicrobials in the following concentrations: chloramphenicol (Ch), 16 μg/ml; tetracycline (Te), 4 μg/ml; cephalothin (Ce), 16 μg/ml; ampicillin (A), 16 μg/ml; carbenicillin (Ca), 100 μg/ml; colistin (Co), 10 μg/ml; nalidixic acid (Na), 12 μg/ml; nitrofurantoin (Ni), 30 μg/ml; sulfamethoxazole (Su), 10 μg/ml; kanamycin (K), 8 μg/ml; and gentamicin (G), 4 μg/ml. Isolates not inhibited at these concentrations were considered resistant for the purposes of clinical reporting. Isolates not inhibited by 4 μg of gentamicin per ml had full minimal inhibitory concentration (MIC) estimations performed for gentamicin, streptomycin (Str), neomycin (Ne), kanamycin, tobramycin (To), sisomicin (Si), amikacin, and netilmicin (an experimental semisynthetic aminoglycoside developed by Schering Corp. and originally designated Sch 20569). Serial two fold dilutions of the antibiotics were made so that their final concentrations in Mueller-Hinton agar ranged from 0.25 to 128 μg/ml. The inoculum for MIC estimations was an 18-h broth culture diluted in saline to contain 2×10^7 bacteria/ml; the number transferred by the inocula replicator to each plate was approximately 1×10^5 organisms.

Cephalosporinase activity of *Klebsiella* isolates was determined qualitatively by a modification of an iodometric method (9, 11) with cephalothin (2.5 mg/ml) as the substrate. The reaction mixture consisted of 1 ml of cephalothin solution and 1 ml of an overnight broth culture of *Klebsiella*. After 2 h of incubation at 37°C, 0.4 ml of iodine reagent and 0.1 ml of soluble starch (0.4%, wt/vol) were added; the formation of a blue color that disappeared within 1 min was recorded as a positive test. Appropriate positive and negative controls were included in the assay.

Transfer of gentamicin resistance. Conjugation experiments were performed by mixing diluted (1:100) overnight broth cultures of gentamicin-resistant *Klebsiella* with a similarly diluted culture of a mutant strain of *E. coli* K-12 (*lac*$^-$ *hys*$^+$ *cys*$^+$ Hfr) that was resistant only to nalidixic acid (MIC > 1,000 μg/ml) and had a gentamicin MIC of 0.25 μg/ml. This recipient strain was kindly provided by R. B. Grant, Hospital for Sick Children, Toronto. The mating mixtures were made in a 1:5 ratio of donor to recipient. After overnight incubation at 37°C, the mixed cultures were plated on brain heart infusion agar (BBL) and MacConkey agar (Oxoid), each containing 100 μg of nalidixic acid per ml and 4 μg of gentamicin per ml. Neither the donor strains of *Klebsiella* nor the recipient *E. coli* would grow on the selective media, even after 72 h of incubation. Representative colonies from the antibiotic selection plates were picked and purified on antibiotic-free medium. Antimicrobial susceptibility tests and gentamicin MIC estimations were done on transconjugants from these experiments to determine the nature of the resistance determinants that had been transferred by conjugation.

RESULTS

Incidence and epidemiology of gentamicin-resistant *Klebsiella*. Gentamicin was released for general use in Canada in August 1966, and, as shown in Table 1, use of the antibiotic in our hospital has increased steadily since. In the 6-year period from January 1968 to March 1974, gentamicin-resistant *Klebsiella* were not isolated from patients in the hospital. Then, from April 1974 to the end of 1975, 98 gentamicin-resistant *Klebsiella* were found among a total of 2,300 isolates identified as *Klebsiella* species in our laboratory. These resistant strains were isolated from 35 patients on nine different wards. They were found only in urine specimens in 23 of the 35 cases, only in sputum in 4 cases, in wound specimens in 2 cases, and in blood cultures in 2 cases. In the other four patients, the resistant *Klebsiella* were isolated from more than one body site, but both urinary and respiratory tracts were involved in each case.

TABLE 1. *Gentamicin usage and isolations of gentamicin-resistant Klebsiella*

Yr	Amt of gentamicin used[a]	Total no. of *Klebsiella* isolates	No. of gentamicin-resistant *Klebsiella* isolates	No. of patients infected
1968	1,800	1,460	0	0
1969	1,200	1,160	0	0
1970	2,600	990	0	0
1971	4,700	1,270	0	0
1972	5,300	1,070	0	0
1973	6,200	1,190	0	0
1974	7,200	1,240	46	23
1975	9,900	1,440	52	12

[a] Expressed as the number of 80-mg vials.

The gentamicin-resistant *Klebsiella* were subdivided by combined typing into eight distinct serobiotypes (Table 2). The 27 isolates obtained from five patients did not react with any of our 72 monospecific antisera of the international set, but did give positive quellung reactions with an antiserum (labeled SK1) prepared by immunizing rabbits with one of these isolates. Two other strains did not type with the standard antisera or with antiserum SK1. These two strains, NT:4/3/4 and NT:1/1/1, were differentiated from each other by their biotypes and from other isolates by the combination of biotype and failure to react with any of the antisera. Table 2 shows that four of the resistant serobiotyes were isolated from only one patient each and that serobiotypes SK1:1/1/1, NT:4/3/4, and K45:1/1/2 each infected only a very small number of patients over a relatively short period of time. We also found that these strains did not spread from one ward to another.

By contrast, gentamicin-resistant *Klebsiella* of serobiotype K22:1/1/2 have persisted in the hospital for almost 2 years since they were first isolated in April 1974. In all, gentamicin-resistant type 22 *Klebsiella* with indistinguishable biochemical characteristics were isolated from 20 patients on five different wards. One strain of serobiotype K22:1/1/2 differed from the other 19 strains, which were entirely homogeneous in their antibiotic susceptibilities, in having much lower MICs for tetracycline, neomycin, and sulfonamide than the others and a higher amikacin MIC. It also had no detectable cephalosporinase activity, whereas the others all did. It was therefore considered to be distinct from the other type 22 *Klebsiella* and was designated subsequently as K22:1/1/2 (P).

The 19 identical K22:1/1/2 *Klebsiella* were associated with two distinct episodes of cross-

TABLE 2. *Properties of 98 gentamicin-resistant Klebsiella isolates*

Serotype	Biotype	Reistance pattern[a]	No. of strains	No. of isolates	Dates of isolations	No. of wards
K22	1/1/2	K Ne G To Si Str Ch Te A Ca Ni Su Ce	19	33	Apr 1974–Dec 1975	4
K22[b]	1/1/2	K G To Si Str Ch Te A Ca Ni	1	1	Dec 1974	1
NT[c]	4/3/4	K Ne G To Si Str Ch Te A Ca Ni Su	3	5	Sept–Oct 1974	1
SK1	1/1/1	K Ne G To Ch Te A Ca Ni	5	27	Dec 1974–Jan 1975	1
NT[c]	1/1/1	K Ne G To Si Str Ch Te A Ca Ni Su Ce	1	4	Jan 1975	1
K9	1/1/1	K Ne G To Ch A Ca	1	4	Apr 1975	1
K21	7/1/4	K Ne G To Ch Te A Ca Ni Ce	1	1	May 1975	1
K37	3/1/2	K Ne G To Str Ch Te A Ca Ni Su	1	2	July 1975	1
K45	1/1/2	K Ne G To Ch Te A Ca Ni	3	21	Sept–Dec 1975	1

[a] Abbreviations are given in the text.
[b] Strain subsequently designated as K22:1/1/2 (P).
[c] NT, Not typable with any of the international typing antisera.

infection. The first, which is illustrated in Fig. 1, affected 14 patients on three wards between April and December 1974. As indicated in Fig. 1, the spread of these type 22 *Klebsiella* from a chronic care ward to a general medical ward and subsequently to an urology ward occurred when patients were transferred from one ward to another. Between January and July 1975, gentamicin-resistant type 22 *Klebsiella* were not isolated from any specimens sent to the diagnostic laboratory. Then, five patients on an orthopedic ward acquired the strain during the remaining 5 months of the year. There was no evidence of patients on other wards being involved during this second limited series of infections.

Table 3 shows the association of bladder catheterization and the acquisition of gentamicin-resistant *Klebsiella*. Of the 27 patients from whom urinary isolates were obtained, 22 had an indwelling catheter in place when the strain was isolated, 1 had been catheterized shortly before, and 4 were seriously debilitated patients with no history of bladder instrumentation. Both patients with bacteremia had bladder catheters in place when the *Klebsiella* was isolated from blood cultures, and this is a probable route of entry of the organisms. However, urine samples were not submitted at the times that would have been necessary to prove a urinary infection by the organism. Two of the four patients with resistant *Klebsiella* in their sputum were intubated and received frequent bronchial suction, one had recent anesthesia with intubation, and the last had no respiratory manipulations but was in the terminal stage of bronchogenic carcinoma. All except 2 of the 35 patients infected with gentamicin-resistant *Klebsiella* had received antibiotics prior to their acquisition of the strain; only 11 of them had received gentamicin.

Characteristics of the gentamicin resistance. The range of gentamicin MICs found in strains of *Klebsiella* obtained from the 35 patients is shown in Table 4. Although considerable variation was observed in the MICs of strains of the same serobiotype isolated from different patients, the gentamicin MICs of repeat isolates of the same serobiotype recovered from any particular patient remained constant.

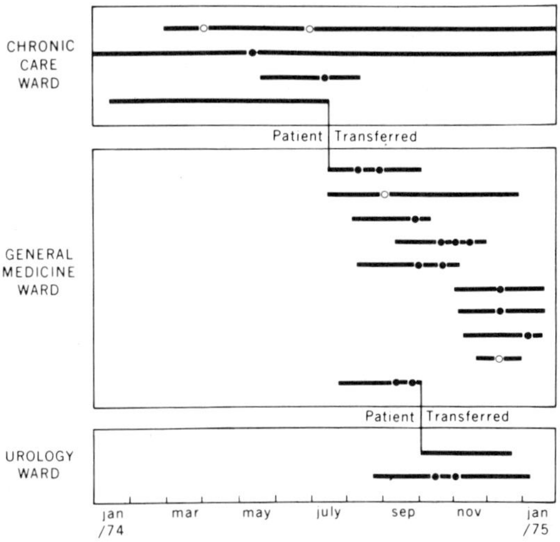

FIG. 1. *Ward location and duration of hospital stay of 14 patients infected with gentamicin-resistant type K22:1/1/2 Klebsiella. Symbols: ●, time of isolation of the strain from a patient's urine; ○, time of its isolation from another body site.*

TABLE 3. *Bladder catheterization and sites yielding the organism in 35 patients acquiring gentamicin-resistant Klebsiella in the hospital*

Site of isolation of *Klebsiella*	No. of patients catheterized in hospital	
	Yes	No
Urine only	19	4
Urine + other	4	0
Blood only	2	0
Sputum only	2	2
Wound only	0	2

TABLE 4. *Gentamicin MICs of 35 resistant strains of Klebsiella*

Strain	No. of patients	No. of strains with gentamicin MIC (μg/ml) of:			
		8	16	32	64
K22:1/1/2	19	1	11	3	4
SK1:1/1/1	5	0	4	1	0
K45:1/1/2	3	0	3	0	0
NT:4/3/4	3	0	1	1	1
Other types[a]	5	1	3	1	0

[a] Includes strain K22:1/1/2 (P).

TABLE 5. *Patterns of resistance transferred to E. coli recipient by gentamicin-resistant Klebsiella*

Donor type	No. of strains transferring	Resistances transferred[a]	Transfer frequency[b]
K37:3/1/2	1	K Ne G To Ch Te	5×10^{-6}
SK1:1/1/1	5	K Ne G To Ch Te A Ca	2×10^{-5}
K45:1/1/2	3	K Ne G To Ch Te A Ca	1×10^{-6}
K9:1/1/1	1	K Ne G To Ch A Ca	5×10^{-6}
K22:1/1/2	1	K Ne G To Ch Te	1×10^{-5}
K22:1/1/2	4	K Ne G To Ch Te A Ca	3×10^{-6}

[a] Abbreviations are given in the text.
[b] Average number of recombinants per number of recipient cells in the mating mixture.

The gentamicin-resistant *Klebsiella* isolated from 15 of the 35 patients transferred their gentamicin resistance to the recipient *E. coli* strain. Table 5 shows that the 10 strains of the four capsular types K37, SK1, K45, and K9 all transferred gentamicin resistance and lists the frequency of transfer and the other antibiotic resistances that were cotransferred in each case. However, only the strains isolated from the first 5 of the total of 19 patients involved in the chain of cross-infection with the type 22 *Klebsiella* transferred their gentamicin resistance. The first strain isolated cotransferred K Ne To Ch Te resistance, those from the next 4 patients infected cotransferred these five plus A Ca, and those from the remaining 14 patients failed to demonstrate any transferable gentamicin resistance. Since we selected only for transferable gentamicin resistance, we do not know whether the strains that did not transfer their gentamicin resistance had any other transferable resistance determinants.

Among all of the *Klebsiella* that were shown to transfer their gentamicin resistance, resistance to kanamycin, tobramycin, and neomycin was cotransferred in each case and resistance to chloramphenicol was also cotransferred. Although a number of the strains were resistant to sisomicin and streptomycin (Table 2), these resistances were never cotransferred.

Origin of gentamicin-resistant *Klebsiella* at Sunnybrook Medical Centre. About a month before the appearance of the first gentamicin-resistant *Klebsiella,* which was of serobiotype K22:1/1/2, a gentamicin-susceptible strain (MIC = 0.5 μg/ml) was isolated from a catheter urine and the amputation wound of another patient on the same chronic care ward. The serobiotype of this strain of *Klebsiella* was also K22:1/1/2; it was resistant to ampicillin, carbenicillin, nitrofurantoin, kanamycin, neomycin, and streptomycin and susceptible to other antimicrobials.

To determine whether the gentamicin-susceptible type 22 *Klebsiella* was capable of acquiring an R-factor, a gentamicin-resistant *E. coli* transconjugant, recovered from the mating of the first resistant type 22 *Klebsiella* with the *E. coli* recipient strain, was used as a donor culture and was mated with the gentamicin-susceptible type 22 *Klebsiella*. "Laboratory-derived" gentamicin-resistant type 22 *Klebsiella,* with cotransferred resistance to chloramphenicol, tetracycline and tobramycin, were recovered after the mixed culture was plated on selective media containing gentamicin (4 μg/ml) and ampicillin (16 μg/ml). This laboratory-derived strain was then found to be capable of transferring its gentamicin resistance to the original *E. coli* recipient.

Activity of other aminoglycosides against gentamicin-resistant *Klebsiella*. All of the strains had kanamycin MICs > 64 μg/ml, and all had neomycin MICs > 128 μg/ml, except for the single strain of K22:1/1/2 (P) which had an MIC of 8 μg/ml. The tobramycin MIC of every strain was consistently the same as its gentamicin MIC. Resistance to streptomycin varied with different serobiotypes. Types SK1, K45, K9, and K21 had streptomycin MICs < 8 μg/ml, whereas the MICs of the other five types were all >128 μg/ml. Sisomicin MICs ranged from 4 to 16 μg/ml with all of the types of *Klebsiella*. All serobiotypes had amikacin MICs of 1 to 2 μg/ml, except for the K22:1/1/2 (P) strain which had an MIC of 16 μg/ml. Netilmicin showed the lowest MICs of all the aminoglycosides tested. All of the gentamicin-resistant *Klebsiella* had netilmicin MICs of 0.25 or 0.5 μg/ml.

DISCUSSION

Despite the increasing use of gentamicin in our hospital since it was first introduced about 8 years ago, gentamicin resistance has been slow to develop in strains of *Klebsiella* isolated in the institution. Other workers (10) have suggested that the incidence of gentamicin-resistant *Klebsiella* may be directly related to the amount of the antibiotic used in a hospital, but we did not find any obvious association between gentamicin usage and the number of resistant *Klebsiella* we isolated (Table 1). Most of the resistant strains failed to spread in the hospital. The small outbreaks of infection that did occur were largely the result of case-to-case spread of urinary tract infections on individual wards, sometimes following the transfer of an infected patient from one ward to another.

It is probable that the emergence of gentamicin-resistant *Klebsiella* in our hospital resulted from the in vivo acquisition of an R-factor by a strain previously susceptible to gentamicin. This strain was of an identical serobiotype (K22:1/1/2) to that of the first gentamicin-resistant *Klebsiella;* it was isolated earlier on the same ward, and it was shown to be capable of acquiring an R-factor mediating gentamicin resistance. Only gentamicin-resistant type 22 *Klebsiella* were isolated from the index case (Fig. 1) and, therefore, the exact sequence of events that led to the R-factor acquisition could not be determined. However, transferable gentamicin resistance has been described in other bacteria found commonly in hospitals (2, 15, 18), and it seems likely that the source of the R-factor for gentamicin resistance in this *Klebsiella* was another enteric bacterium.

Of particular clinical significance was the observation that the resistant type 22 *Klebsiella,* the strain with a known gentamicin-susceptible precursor, was the only strain that persisted for more than a few months. This strain was also one in which the R-factor for gentamicin resistance appeared to lose its conjugative capacity and was not detected either after the strain had cross-infected a number of patients or when it reemerged in a different area of the hospital after a latent period of several months. We did not attempt transfer-enhancing techniques and, therefore, we cannot say with absolute certainty that the R-factor in the later type 22 isolates had become nonconjugative. However, even if the R-factor in these later isolates was conjugative, but at levels too low to detect by our simple methods, these findings still raise the question of the stability and survival advantage of this kind of strain over other strains possessing R-factors that transfer them at higher frequencies. In another study it was shown, even if somewhat artificially, that enterobacteria carrying transferable R-factors survived less readily in the gut than strains which appeared to be R-factor free (1). It may well be that the gentamicin-resistant type 22 *Klebsiella* is peculiar in having a mechanism which assists its ability to survive by suppressing the frequency of R-factor transfer, deletion of an undesirable portion of an R-factor, or stable integration into the chromosome. Further studies will be required to determine whether one of these mechanisms is operating in this strain.

Our resistant *Klebsiella* have not yet been tested for gentamicin-inactivating enzyme activity, and therefore we cannot discount other mechanisms of inactivation of the antibiotic (4). However, an enzymatic mechanism seems the most probable, particularly as kanamycin, tobramycin, and neomycin, but not other aminoglycosides, were cotransferred in every strain that transferred its gentamicin resistance. Since the specificity of an aminoglycoside-3′-transferase has been shown to reside in these substrates (6), it will be necessary to have our strains examined for such an enzymatic mechanism of gentamicin inactivation. The likelihood of finding a single enzyme responsible for R-factor-mediated gentamicin resistance in our *Klebsiella* seems quite high and could have significant epidemiological implications for other enterobacteria in our hospital that are capable of acquiring R-factors.

Of all the aminoglycosides tested, only amikacin and netilmicin inhibited all of the gentamicin-resistant *Klebsiella* at levels that can be achieved in the blood with normal doses. In particular, every strain was highly susceptible to netilmicin. Streptomycin and sisomicin MICs were variable, depending on the strain or serobiotype isolated. All of the gentamicin-resistant strains were susceptible to colistin and nalidixic acid. However, as both of these have definite therapeutic limitations, the efficacy of amikacin and netilmicin against gentamicin-resistant *Klebsiella* is likely to be of real clinical importance in the future.

ACKNOWLEDGMENTS

This investigation was supported by National Health Grant No. 606-1104-28 awarded by Health and Welfare, Canada.

We wish to thank K. Kruschel for her skilled technical assistance and J. J. Iazzetta, Pharmacy Department, Sunnybrook Medical Centre, for providing the data on gentamicin usage.

LITERATURE CITED

1. **Anderson, J. D.** 1974. The effect of R-factor carriage on the survival of *Escherichia coli* in the human intestine. J. Med. Microbiol. **7:**85–90.
2. **Bryan, L. E., M. S. Shahrabadi, and H. M. Van Den Elzen.** 1974. Gentamicin resistance in *Pseudomonas aeruginosa:* R-factor-mediated resistance. Antimicrob. Agents Chemother. **6:**191–199.
3. **Casewell, M. W.** 1972. Experiences in the use of commercial antisera for the capsular typing of *Klebsiella*

species. J. Clin. Pathol. 25:734–737.
4. **Davies, J.** 1971. Bacterial resistance to aminoglycoside antibiotics. J. Infect. Dis. 124(Suppl.):S7–S10.
5. **Davis, T. J., and J. M. Matsen.** 1974. Prevalence and characteristics of *Klebsiella* species: relation to association with a hospital environment. J. Infect. Dis. 130:402–405.
6. **Dowding, J., and J. Davies.** 1975. Mechanisms and origins of plasmid-determined antibiotic resistance, p. 179–186. *In* D. Schlessinger (ed.), Microbiology—1974. American Society for Microbiology, Washington, D.C.
7. **Edwards, P. R., and W. H. Ewing (ed.).** 1972. Identification of *Enterobacteriaceae,* 3rd., p. 290–300. Burgess, Minneapolis.
8. **Martin, C. M., N. S. Ikari, J. Zimmerman, and J. A. Waitz.** 1971. A virulent nosocomial *Klebsiella* with a transferable R-factor for gentamicin: emergence and suppression. J. Infect. Dis. 124(Suppl.):S24–S29.
9. **Medeiros, A. A., and T. F. O'Brien.** 1966. Association of cephalosporinase activity, cephalothin resistance, and episome-mediated drug resistance in *Klebsiella* strains. Antimicrob. Agents Chemother. 6:321–327.
10. **Noriega, E. R., R. E. Leibowitz, A. S. Richmond, E. Rubinstein, S. Schaefler, M. S. Simberkoff, and J. J. Rahal.** 1975. Nosocomial infection caused by gentamicin-resistant streptomycin-sensitive *Klebsiella*. J. Infect. Dis. 131(Suppl.):S45–S50.
11. **Perret, C. J.** 1954. Iodometric assay of penicillinase. Nature (London) 174:1012–1013.
12. **Pollack, M., P. Charache, R. E. Nieman, M. P. Jett, J. A. Reinhardt, and P. H. Hardy.** 1972. Factors influencing colonisation and antibiotic-resistance patterns of Gram-negative bacteria in hospital patients. Lancet ii:668–671.
13. **Price, D. J. E., and J. D. Sleigh.** 1970. Control of infection due to *Klebsiella aerogenes* in a neurosurgical unit by withdrawal of all antibiotics. Lancet ii:1213–1215.
14. **Rennie, R. P., and I. B. R. Duncan.** 1974. Combined biochemical and serological typing of clinical isolates of *Klebsiella*. Appl. Microbiol. 28:534–539.
15. **Richmond, A. S., J. J. Rahal, M. S. Simberkoff, and S. Schaefler.** 1975. R factors in gentamicin-resistant organisms causing hospital infection. Lancet ii:1176–1178.
16. **Rose, H. D., and J. Schreier.** 1968. The effect of hospitalization and antibiotic therapy on the Gram-negative fecal flora. Am. J. Med. Sci. 255:228–236.
17. **Selden, R., S. Lee, W. L. L. Wang, J. V. Bennett, and T. C. Eickhoff.** 1971. Nosocomial klebsiella infections: intestinal colonization as a reservoir. Ann. Intern. Med. 74:657–664.
18. **Shafi, M. S., and N. Datta.** 1975. Infection caused by *Proteus mirabilis* strains with transferable gentamicin-resistance factors. Lancet i:1355–1357.

ANTIMICROBIAL AGENTS AND CHEMOTHERAPY, Feb. 1977, p. 185-190
Vol. 11, No. 2

Pharmacological and Clinical Study of Bacampicillin in Acute Peritonsillitis—a Comparison with Ampicillin

HANS O. HALLANDER,* ANDERS FLODSTRÖM, AND JAN SJÖVALL

Department of Clinical Bacteriology and ENT-Department, Central Hospital S-72189 Västerås, and Astra Pharmaceuticals AB, S-15785, Södertälje, Sweden*

Received for publication 12 July 1976

The pharmacological and clinical properties of bacampicillin in three dosage groups were studied in 66 hospitalized patients with unilateral acute peritonsillitis in a comparison with ampicillin. Bacampicillin is a new semisynthetic aminopenicillin which is rapidly converted to ampicillin but is better absorbed. Both drugs were given orally. The mean individual peak serum levels achieved with 200, 400, and 800 mg of bacampicillin in the first morning dose were 4.9, 6.8, and 11.9 mg/liter, respectively, with an almost linear dose response. The peak level of 800 mg of bacampicillin was significantly higher than the 6.8 mg/liter noted after a nearly equimolar dose of 500 mg of ampicillin. A linear relationship was also seen between dose and area under the serum concentration-time curve. Preliminary antibiotic concentration studies in five patients indicated therapeutic levels in peritonsillar pus. Beta-streptococci alone or in combination with anaerobes were isolated from about half of the abscesses, whereas anaerobes were isolated from the other half. Treatment was supplemented by surgical procedures in the majority of cases. The clinical effect was good in all treatment groups, with only one relapse. All beta-streptococci were eliminated during therapy. The total number of gastrointestinal side effects was significantly lower in patients treated with bacampicillin, although the difference in frequency of diarrhea alone was not significant.

In the continued development of ampicillin, special interest has been paid to certain esters such as bacampicillin (1), pivampicillin (3), and talampicillin (2), which have proved to be better absorbed than ampicillin itself when taken orally. Higher serum concentrations of ampicillin are obtained as a result of rapid hydrolysis in the body, and more complete absorption results in fewer intestinal side effects.

Bacampicillin, which was synthesized by the Astra Läkemedel laboratories in Södertälje, Sweden, is the hydrochloride of 1′-ethoxycarbonyloxyethyl-6-(D-α-aminophenylacetamido) penicillinate. In the present investigation the pharmacological and clinical properties of the drug have been studied in patients with acute peritonsillitis.

In earlier studies (5, 7) betastreptococci were isolated from the abscesses in about 50% of cases with acute peritonsillitis, and one or more anaerobic microorganisms were isolated in the remaining cases. In vitro, some of these anaerobes are substantially more susceptible to ampicillin compared with penicillin V (6), which is often used to treat quinsy.

MATERIALS AND METHODS

Diagnostic criteria. Acute peritonsillitis, the term used synonymously with quinsy, is defined as "an infection of the pharynx mainly or primarily involving the peritonsillar tissues on one or both sides."

Patients. The initial series consisted of 68 hospitalized patients with unilateral acute peritonsillitis treated in the Department of Otolaryngology, Central Hospital, Västerås, during the period February through December 1974.

There were as many men as women in the series. The average age was 27, the youngest patient being 12 and the oldest 77.

Patients with a previously established allergy to penicillin, malignancies, renal disease, or disease of the liver were excluded from the trial, as were children under 12 years of age and pregnant women. Any antibiotic therapy started earlier was discontinued. Twelve patients received antibiotic therapy before inclusion in the study. Most of them received penicillin V for an average of 2 days. In spite of this, the symptoms had progressed. This therapy, evidently insufficient, was considered not to influence the outcome of the forthcoming therapy. For dropouts, see Table 2.

Treatment. All patients entering the trial were randomly allocated to one of the following four groups, with an attempt to have groups of equal size: (i) bacampicillin, 200 mg twice a day; (ii) bacampicillin, 400 mg twice a day; (iii) bacampicillin, 800 mg twice a day; (iv) ampicillin (Doktacillin), 500 mg three times a day. The 12-h dosage interval for bacampicillin was chosen at the suggestion of the manufacturer. The antibiotic was given by mouth for 10 days.

Apart from medication given for other illnesses (Rinomar tablets [cinnarizine and 2-amino-1-phenylpropanol], owing to simultaneous sinusitis, in one case and Plaquenil tablets [hydroxychloroquine sulfate] plus injections of Acton Prolongatum for rheumatoid arthritis in another), no other drug was given during the course of the trial except paracetamol (Alvedon) when an analgesic was needed.

Every patient with an abscess diagnosed by inspection and aspiration was treated by incision and debridement on day 1 of treatment, followed by daily debridement until no more pus was produced. Before the primary incision the patient was anesthetized with Xylocaine dental spray applied topically to the mucous membrane in a dose of 40 to 80 mg of lidocaine. In 55 cases abscess formation was demonstrated. These patients had their antibiotic therapy supplemented by surgery.

Clinical evaluation of therapy. Ambulatory follow-ups were carried out 5 to 8 days after the start of antibiotic therapy and about a fortnight after the termination of therapy, the question of side effects being included in the interviews. The evaluation included the following criteria: (i) satisfactory healing—clinical symptoms subsided in a reasonable length of time with no signs of infection after 10 days of treatment or during follow-up; (ii) satisfactory healing but prolonged course—cases needing debridement for more than 3 days; (iii) unsatisfactory healing—(a) patients requiring surgical or antibiotic treatment for more than 10 days and (b) recurrences within 2 months.

Pharmacological data. The first morning dose was used as a test dose for the study of serum concentrations. At this time the patients had been fasting for at least 9 h. The test dose was given at 9 a.m. with a glass of water. Breakfast was served at 11 a.m., after which time the patients were allowed to take food and drink at will. Blood samples for the serum concentration study were taken before giving the first tablet and then 30 min and 1, 1.5, 2, 4, and 8 h afterwards.

Assay of antibiotics. (i) Sampling procedure. Blood samples were drawn by capillary puncture. At 6 and 8 h a parallel venous puncture was drawn to be used in the cup-plate method if the capillary method did not yield detectable values.

(ii) Culture medium and test strain. Penassay seed agar (antibiotic medium I, Difco) and *Sarcina lutea* ATCC 9341 were used for all determinations.

(iii) Assay procedure. For the determination of ampicillin, the paper disk method as described by Jalling et al. was used (8). Two series of standard disks and two disks for each test sample were always used. The standard series was prepared from ampicillin sodium (Doktacillin; Astra Läkemedel AB) as twofold dilutions in pooled human serum. When concentrations in pus were assayed, the standard solution was diluted in peritonsillar pus aspirated from the same patient before antibiotic therapy. Petri dishes (14 cm) with 60 ml of medium adapted for concentrations between 0.5 and 16 mg/liter, were used for samples taken after 30, 60, and 90 min. For increased sensitivity a petri dish with 25 ml of medium, adapted for concentrations between 0.06 and 2 mg/liter, was added for 120- and 240-min samples, as well as for material collected before the antibiotic was given. When no zone of inhibition could be recorded, an additional assay by the cup method, with a sensitivity of 0.03 to 0.008 mg/liter, was performed.

Bacteriology. Bacteriological specimens were collected before the start of therapy and at both ambulatory follow-ups. On all occasions specimens were taken from the nasopharynx and throat for aerobic culture. In addition, in cases with abscesses, material was aspirated from the abscess for both aerobic and anaerobic culture. The specimens were processed as previously described (7).

Laboratory tests. A series of clinical chemistry laboratory tests was performed before giving the first dose of the antibiotic and at both follow-ups. The following parameters were investigated: erythrocyte sedimentation rate, hematocrit, Hb, erythrocyte count, platelets, leukocyte count, leukocyte differential count, serum bilirubin (conjugated/unconjugated), serum alkaline phosphatase, serum aspartate-aminotransferase, serum alanine, aminotransferase, lactate dehydrogenase, serum creatinine, serum urea, urinary sediment, urinary albumin, and urinary glucose. Any pathological findings were checked until they returned to normal or occasioned further investigation.

Statistical evaluation. The area under the serum concentration-time curve was calculated by the method of overlapping parabolas (4). For statistical evaluation of the pharmacological results, Student's t test for independent observations was used, whereas Fisher's exact probability test was used in the evaluation of side effects.

RESULTS

Serum concentrations. Serum concentration determinations were performed in 64 patients. Two of the original 68 patients were excluded, one owing to inability to swallow the tablets and one because the wrong preparation was given inadvertently. Two patients were excluded because of the presence of measurable concentrations of antibiotic in the pretreatment specimens without a plausible explanation.

The mean individual serum peak levels appeared after 1.06, 1.25, and 1.22 h, respectively, in the 200-, 400-, and 800-mg bacampicillin dosage groups. This was 20 to 25 min earlier than in the ampicillin group, in which the peak level was reached after 1.41 h.

The peak values of the mean serum concentration curves (Fig. 1) were, respectively, 3.9, 4.5, and 9.9 mg of ampicillin per liter in the

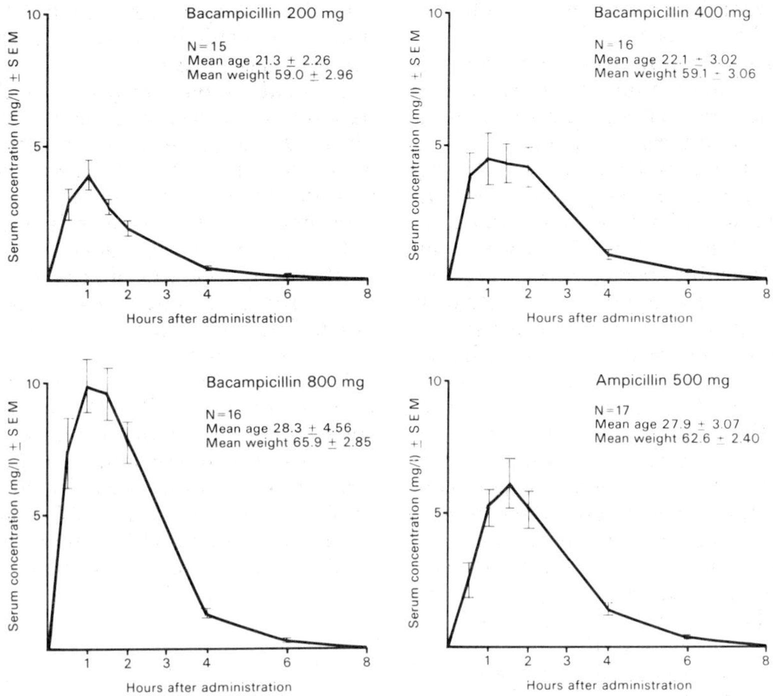

FIG. 1. *Mean serum concentration curves ± standard error of the mean after oral administration of bacampicillin or ampicillin in patients with peritonsillitis (age in years, weight in kilograms).*

bacampicillin groups. After 500 mg of ampicillin the mean peak level was 6.1 mg/liter, as compared to 9.9 mg/liter after 800 mg of bacampicillin, which is equimolar to 556 mg of ampicillin.

However, patients given 400 mg retained serum levels of 4 mg/liter for 2 h, whereas the concentrations in subjects in the 200-mg group (Fig. 1) had fallen to 2 mg/liter. In contrast to the lack of correlation between dose and serum concentrations expressed as peaks of the mean serum curves, there was a nearly linear relationship when the area under the mean serum concentration-time curve was calculated. The area values in the bacampicillin groups were 7.81, 13.73, and 25.73 h × mg/liter, respectively, whereas that of ampicillin was 16.21 h × mg/liter.

The same linear relation between dose and serum concentration was also obtained when mean individual peak serum levels were used instead of mean serum curves (Fig. 2). The peak concentration of 11.9 ± 1.14 (standard error of the mean) mg/liter after 800 mg of bacampicillin differs significantly from the 6.8 ± 0.87 mg/liter noted with 500 mg of ampicillin ($P < 0.01$). The peak values calculated in this manner in the 200- and 400-mg bacampicillin groups were 4.9 and 6.8 mg/liter, respectively.

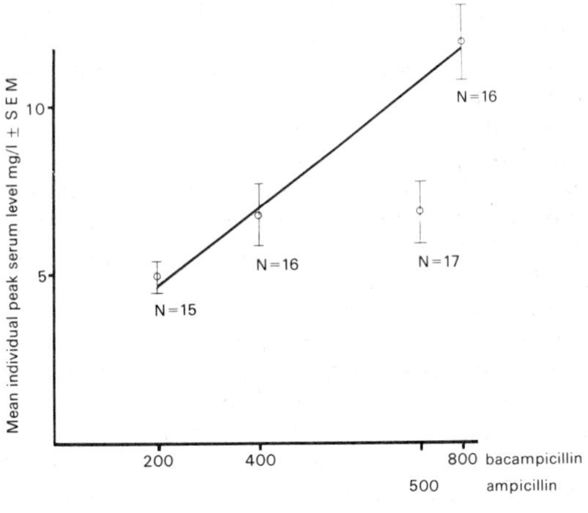

FIG. 2. *Mean individual peak serum levels after oral administration of bacampicillin (200, 400, and 800 mg) or ampicillin (500 mg) in patients with peritonsillitis.*

There were no significant differences between ampicillin and these two dosages of bacampicillin. For the sake of comparison, an equimolar scale has been used in Fig. 2.

An analysis of the relationship between body weights and peak concentrations in each treatment group revealed no significant correlation, as might have been expected.

Pus concentrations. It was not possible to determine the concentrations of pus other than as isolated assays in a small number of cases: three in the ampicillin group, one in the 200-mg bacampicillin group, and one in the 400-mg bacampicillin group. In the patients investigated, values between 0.4 and 1.6 mg/liter were noted after 2 to 4 h. It is not known at what point on the ampicillin abscess curve the specimens were taken; consequently, no conclusions can be drawn as to the relationship between serum and pus concentrations. It seems likely, however, that concentrations are reached in pus that are higher than the minimum inhibitory concentration values for most of the aerobic and anaerobic bacteria in question.

Bacteriology. (i) Tonsils and nasopharynx. In the 62 patients who completed the course of treatment, beta-streptococci were isolated from the nasopharynx and/or tonsils before treatment in 24 cases: 21 in Lancefield group A, two in group C, and one in group G. All streptococci were eliminated during and after therapy, except in three patients with initial findings of beta-streptococci group A. Bacteria of this type were also isolated at the second follow-up visit after not being detectable during the course of treatment. Two of these patients were treated with bacampicillin (200 mg) and one with ampicillin. In one case culture was not done initially, and in seven cases culture was not done at the second follow-up.

(ii) Abscess. Aspiration in the 62 cases produced evidence of abscess formation in 55 patients. All these cases were treated by incision and debridement. The bacteriological findings in 30 of these patients, who had no previous antibiotic treatment, have been studied thoroughly (Table 1). In the remaining 25 cases a full bacteriological analysis was not made either because the diagnosis was made on a Sunday, when full bacteriological service was not available, or because the patient had received antibiotics before aspiration and incision. These antibiotics were usually given before the patient was included in the trial. In a few cases, however, abscess formation could not be demonstrated until the test drug had been given for 12 to 24 h.

The anaerobic flora included peptostreptococci, peptococci, bifidobacteria, *Veillonella*, fusobacteria, and species of *Bacteroides*. According to the "paper disk method," the bacteria isolated from the abscesses were susceptible to ampicillin (minimum inhibitory concentration, ≤1 mg/liter), with the excepion of two strains of *Bacteroides* with reduced susceptibility (minimum inhibitory concentration, 1 to 16 mg/liter) and two penicillinase-producing strains of *Staphylococcus aureus*.

Clinical effect. Sixty-two of the 68 initial patients completed the course of treatment (Table 2). Three patients in the ampicillin group discontinued treatment because of intolerable side effects. In the 800-mg bacampicillin group, treatment was discontinued in a female patient with progressive laryngeal edema necessitating tracheotomy. She was later given antibiotics by the parenteral route. An additional patient dropped out after failing to complete the follow-up examinations.

One relapse occurred 4 days after termination of therapy in the 400-mg bacampicillin (twice a day) group and could not be explained in terms of drug resistance in the bacteria encountered in the abscess, which were mainly fusobacteria and species of *Bacteroides*. After repeated incision and treatment with the same antibiotic for 20 days, the infection was cured without further relapse.

TABLE 1. *Bacteria recovered from peritonsillar abscesses by aspiration in 30 cases*

Bacteria isolated	No. of cases
Beta-hemolytic streptococci, group A	8
Beta-hemolytic streptococci, group A, + anaerobes	5
Beta-hemolytic streptococci, group C, + anaerobes	1
Anaerobes	8
Anaerobes + sparse normal throat flora	8

TABLE 2. *Clinical evaluation*

Treatment	No. of patients receiving: Bacampicillin twice a day			Ampicillin three times a day	Total no. of patients
	200 mg	400 mg	800 mg	(500 mg)	
Patients	17	17	17	17	68
Excluded before trial	2				2
Discontinued treatment			1	3	4
Completed treatment	15	17	16	14	62
Not assessable	1				1
Satisfactorily healed	14	16	16	14	60
Prolonged course	4	1		1	6
Recurrence		1			1

The remaining patients showed satisfactory healing, although in six cases with a delayed course. Four of these were in the group given the lowest dose of bacampicillin, an interesting but not statistically significant difference. The two-dose schedule for bacampicillin does not appear to have had any negative effect on healing compared with ampicillin given in three doses.

Side effects. Two cases of diarrhea were recorded in the ampicillin group (Table 3). In both cases the discomfort was so pronounced that the drug had to be withdrawn. The patients with one or two loose stools continued their treatment without omitting any dose or taking any other measure against the condition, which ceased spontaneously.

A comparison of the total incidence of gastrointestinal side effects (diarrhea plus loose stools) of the preparations revealed a statistically significant difference ($P < 0.05$). The difference in the frequency of diarrhea alone is not significant.

Urticaria occurred in two patients, and this caused withdrawal of the drug in the case occurring in the ampicillin group. The patient with urticaria in the bacampicillin group did not react to the preparation until day 8 of treatment and pursued the entire 10-day course in spite of a very troublesome itch.

The laboratory tests revealed few, and only insignificant, deviations from the values held to be normal, or the deviations were entirely attributable to the infection itself. No changes in hepatic or renal function were noted. A case of slight eosinophilia (13%) during treatment occurred in the bacampicillin group. Ten cases of slight thrombocytosis (350,000 to 500,000) were noted, seven in the bacampicillin group and three in the ampicillin group. One patient on bacampicillin showed thrombocytopenia with a count down to 78,000/mm^3. All the above-mentioned values returned to normal spontaneously. The changes in the platelet count are difficult to explain; it is probably impossible to determine whether they are an effect of the infection itself or of the treatment given.

TABLE 3. *Side effects*

Side effects	No. of patients showing side effects in:	
	Bacampicillin group (n = 47)	Ampicillin group (n = 17)
Urticaria	1 (2%)	1 (6%)
Diarrhea, possibly also abdominal pains	0	2 (12%)
1–2 loose stools	1 (2%)	2 (12%)

DISCUSSION

Studies of healthy subjects have shown that bacampicillin produces 2.5 to 3 times as high peak serum levels as equimolar doses of ampicillin (11, 12). The values noted in the present investigation appear to be slightly lower in the 200- and 400-mg bacampicillin groups and somewhat higher for the 500-mg ampicillin groups, whereas comparable values were noted for 800 mg of bacampicillin. These differences may have been caused by heterogeneity in the series, which might have been eliminated if the study had been of the crossover type, or by the fact that the tests were performed in sick subjects confined to bed.

Calculations of the area under the mean serum concentration-time curve or mean individual peak serum concentrations showed a linear relation between the dose and serum concentrations that was not entirely evident from the peaks of the mean serum curves alone. This is in agreement with the study in healthy volunteers by Magni et al. (11). The discrepancy between the mean serum curves and individual peak values can be explained by the dispersion of the time of individual peak levels, which was particularly large in the 400-mg bacampicillin group, as shown by the broader shape of the curve in Fig. 1. Thus, the mean serum concentration curve does not always give a good description of the actual peak levels achieved.

The small number of pus concentration determinations performed indicated that therapeutic levels are obtained in pus. In a more systematic study Maesen et al. (10) reported fully satisfactory concentrations in the sputum of patients with chronic bronchitis treated with bacampicillin, 400 or 800 mg.

In the cases in which beta-streptococci were isolated initially, these microorganisms disappeared during the course of treatment. However, in three cases showing normal clinical responses, they reappeared after treatment.

With the exception of one recurrence in the 400-mg bacampicillin group, healing was satisfactory in all treatment groups. However, the effect of the antibiotics on healing must be judged in light of the fact that 55 out of 62 patients were treated concurrently by incision and debridement. The 12 patients given antibiotics before the trial consulted the hospital due to progressive symptoms, so this treatment was considered to have a negligible effect on healing.

Traditionally, therapy of quinsy in Sweden

consists of pecicillin V and, if abscesses are present, surgical drainage. After the first incision and debridement daily debridements are generally performed until all suppuration has ceased. Theoretically, however, the in vitro susceptibilities of certain anaerobes, primarily fusobacteria, might suggest that penicillin V is not the drug of choice (6). On the basis of the present findings, it is not possible to say that bacampicillin would be a more suitable antibiotic adjunct in the treatment of peritonsillitis than penicillin V.

The total incidence of gastrointestinal disorders has proved to be significantly lower in patients treated with bacampicillin. Bacampicillin, in contrast to reports on the other ampicillin esters (9, 13), produced no complaints of gastritis in any of the treatment groups. A larger series of ampicillin patients is needed, however, for statistical confirmation of differences between bacampicillin and ampicillin with regard to diarrhea alone.

LITERATURE CITED

1. **Bodin, N.-O., B. Ekström, U. Forsgren, L.-P. Jalar, L. Magni, C. H. Ramsay, and B. Sjöberg.** 1975. Bacampicillin: a new orally well absorbed derivative of ampicillin. Antimicrob. Agents Chemother. 8:518–525.
2. **Clayton, J. P., M. Cole, S. W. Elson, and H. Ferres.** 1974. BRL 8988 (talampicillin), a well-absorbed oral form of ampicillin. Antimicrob. Agents Chemother. 5:670–671.
3. **Daehne, W., E. Fredicksen, E. Gundersen, F. Lun, P. Morck, H. J. Peterson, K. Roholt, L. Tybring, and W. O. Godtfredsen.** 1970. Acyloxymethyl esters of ampicillin. J. Med. Chem. 13:607–612.
4. **Davis, P. J., and P. Rabinowitz.** 1967. Numerical integration, p. 22. Blaisdell Publishing Co., London.
5. **Flödstrom, A., and H. O. Hallander.** 1976. Microbiological aspects on peritonsillar abscesses. Scand. J. Infect. Dis. 8:157–160.
6. **Gorbach, S. L., and J. G. Bartlett.** 1974. Anaerobic infections. N. Engl. J. Med. 290:1289–1294.
7. **Hallander, H. O., A. Flodström, and K. Holmberg.** 1975. Influence of the collection and transport of specimens on the recovery of bacteria from peritonsillar abscesses. J. Clin. Microbiol. 2:504–509.
8. **Jalling, B., A.-S. Malmborg, A. Lindman, and L.-O Boréus.** 1972. Evaluation of a micromethod for determination of antibiotic concentrations in plasma. Eur. J. Clin. Pharmacol. 4:150–157.
9. **Knudsen, E. T., and J. W. Harding.** 1975. A multicentre comparative trial of talampicillin and ampicillin in general practice. Br. J. Clin. Pract. 10:255–264.
10. **Maesen, F. P. V., H. Beeuwkes, B. I. Davies, H. J. Buytendijk, P. J. Brombacher, and J. Wessman.** 1976. Bacampicillin in acute exacerbations of chronic bronchitis—a dose-range study. J. Antimicrob. Chemother. 2:279–285.
11. **Magni, L., B. Sjöberg, J. Sjövall, and J. Wessman.** 1976. Clinical pharmacological studies with bacampicillin, p. 109. *In* J. D. Williams and A. M. Geddes (ed.), Chemotherapy, vol. 5. Penicillins and cephalosporins, Proceedings of the 9th International Congress of Chemotherapy, London, July, 1975. Plenum Press, New York.
12. **Rozencweig, M., M. Staquet, and J. Klastersky.** 1976. Antibacterial activity and pharmacokinetics of bacampicillin and ampicillin. Clin. Pharmacol. Ther. 19:592–597.
13. **Wilcox, J. B., R. N. Brogden, and G. S. Avery.** 1973. Pivampicillin: a preliminary report of its pharmacokinetic properties and therapeutic efficacy. Drugs 6:94–103.

ANTIMICROBIAL AGENTS AND CHEMOTHERAPY, Feb. 1977, p. 191-197

Vol. 11, No. 2
Printed in U.S.A.

Antiviral Activities of Acyl Derivatives of 2,2′-Anhydro-1-β-D-Arabinofuranosylcytosine and 1-β-D-Arabinofuranosylcytosine in Cell Culture[1]

KOSABURO SATO,* AKIO NOMURA, AND JOHN G. MOFFATT

Shionogi Research Laboratory, Shionogi & Co., Ltd., Fukushima-ku, Osaka, 553 Japan, and Institute of Molecular Biology, Syntex Research, Palo Alto, California 94304*

Received for publication 20 May 1976

Antiviral activities of acyl derivatives (3′-*O*-octanoyl and 3′-*O*-decanoyl) of 2,2′-anhydro-1-β-D-arabinofuranosylcytosine (cyclo-C) and 1-β-D-arabinofuranosylcytosine (Ara-C) were compared with other antiviral nucleosides, and some biological characteristics of the antiviral activity were investigated. Among those synthesized acyl derivatives, 3′-*O*-decanoyl ara-C was the most active against deoxyribonucleic acid viruses, with an activity comparable to that of Ara-C. Acyl derivatives of cyclo-C were somewhat less active than their Ara-C counterparts. In the value of therapeutic index, 1-β-D-arabinofuranosyladenine was superior to the others, followed by 5-iodo-2′-deoxyuridine. In comparing the sensitivity of two serotypes of herpes simplex virus it was found that Ara-C and its ester, as well as its cyclo-C counterpart, were more active against the type 2 than the type 1 strain. The activity of 3′-*O*-decanoyl Ara-C, like that of its parent, was diminished by treatment with cytidine deaminase from mouse kidney, but 3′-*O*-decanoyl cyclo-C was resistant to this treatment. In comparative studies of 3′- and 5′-*O*-acyl Ara-C's, antivaccinia virus activity of 3′-*O*-palmitoyl Ara-C was significantly superior to its 5′-counterpart. The inhibitory activity of 5′-*O*-decanoyl Ara-C was markedly reduced by the presence of a threefold molar excess of eserine sulfate, a choline esterase inhibitor, whereas the 3′-acyl Ara-C was not affected by the inhibitor in any combination. This result indicates that enzymatic hydrolysis of the 3′-ester to Ara-C, which is inhibited by eserine sulfate, did not occur in this cell culture.

The pronounced antiviral (3, 5, 15, 16, 28), antileukemic (9, 26, 29), and immunosuppressive (10, 11) activities of 1-β-D-arabinofuranosylcytosine (Ara-C) reported by numerous investigators have stimulated the synthesis of a considerable number of derivatives of the parent compound. Particular attention has been focused upon derivatives with a high biological activity of long duration that are not substrates for cytidine deaminase. These studies covered various 5′-esters of Ara-C prepared by the Upjohn group (8, 31), and a number of 2,2′-anhydro-1-β-D-arabinofuranosylcytosine (cyclo-C) derivatives (7, 24, 27) also were synthesized. We have been engaged in a systematic study on the synthesis of acylated derivatives of Ara-C and cyclo-C and have examined the relationship between antiviral activity as well as antileukemic activity in mice and chemical structure (12–14, 17). From our study on antiviral activity, we concluded that the introduction of short-chain acyl groups results in somewhat diminished activity relative to the parent nucleosides. As the acyl groups increase in size, however, the antiviral activities are enhanced, reaching optimum values in the vicinity of the decanoyl esters. A further increase in the chain length of the acyl groups leads to decreased activities. Detailed studies of the antiviral activity against deoxyribonucleic acid viruses were made for selected acyl derivatives, and the activities were compared with those of other antiviral nucleosides. The results, together with some characteristics of the antiviral activity, are reported in this paper.

[1] Contribution no. 129 from the Institute of Molecular Biology, Syntex Research, Palo Alto, CA 94304.

MATERIALS AND METHODS

Cell culture. The BGM line of African green monkey kidney cells (25), AV_3 cells (human amnion cells), or HeLa cells were grown in Eagle minimal essential medium (MEM) supplemented with 10% bovine serum. Rabbit kidney cells were established in our laboratory and grown in the same medium.

All cell cultures were grown in Falcon flasks (30 ml) and maintained with MEM supplemented with 2% bovine serum, except in the case of adenovirus where 3% fetal calf serum was used instead.

Virus. HF and Oda strains of herpes simplex virus type 1 (HSV-1) and UW-268 and Hata strains of HSV-2 were used. They were kindly provided by S. Nii, Research Institute for Microbial Disease, Osaka University, Suita, Japan. Vaccinia virus (strain IHD) was kindly provided by N. Ishida, Tohoku University, Sendai, Japan. Adenovirus (type 3), was kindly provided by T. Kurimura, Osaka Prefectural Institute of Public Health, Osaka, Japan. IUdR-resistant HSV was isolated by repeated passage of the virus through progressively higher concentrations of IUdR. The viruses were further purified by the technique of single plaque isolation in the presence of 50 μg of IUdR per ml. These stock viruses were prepared from infected BGM cell cultures for HSV-1 and HSV-2 and from AV3 cultures for adenovirus, harvested at the time of about 90% cytopathic effect, treated with three cycles of freezing and thawing, clarified by low-speed centrifugation, and stored at −70°C.

Plaque assay. For the assay of vaccinia virus and the HF strain of HSV, BGM cell monolayers were used. RK cells were used for the Oda strain of HSV-1 and the strains of HSV-2, and 400 μg of diethylaminoethyl-dextran (Pharmacia, Uppsala, Sweden) per ml was added to the overlay medium. In these plaque assays, the second overlay agar containing neutral red (1:20,000) was added on day 4, and the plaques that appeared were counted on day 6. Adenovirus type 3 was titered on an AV_3 cell monolayer in a petri dish (6 mm), with an overlay medium of 0.9% agar (Special Agar-Noble, Difco) in MEM supplemented with 5% fetal calf serum and 70 μg of arginine per ml. Overlay was added on days 5 and 8 with 3 ml of the medium. The final overlay contained neutral red (1:40,000). Plates were incubated for 12 days at 37°C in 5% CO_2 in air and the number of plaques was counted.

Plaque reduction test. A confluent monolayer of BGM cells in a Falcon flask was infected with 100 to 200 plaque-forming units (PFU) and then overlaid with agar medium (1.25% agar in MEM with 2.0% bovine serum) containing different concentrations of the compound to be tested. On day 4, the second overlay was added with the same medium plus neutral red (1:20,000). The flasks were incubated, and the plaques were counted on day 6. The 50% plaque reduction concentration of the compound (ED_{50}) was calculated by the method of Reed and Muench (22) from the dose response curve. ED_{50} was expressed in terms of the micromolar concentration of the test compound in an experiment.

Virus growth inhibition test. BGM cells grown in Falcon flasks were infected with virus at a multiplicity of infection of 1.0. After adsorption of viruses, the infected monolayer was washed twice with Hanks balanced salt solution, treated with maintenance medium containing different concentrations of the compound to be tested, and incubated at 37°C until the maximum virus yield in the one-step growth cycle was reached in an untreated culture. The harvested cultures were frozen and thawed three times and then clarified by low-speed centrifugation at 4°C. Virus titration was performed by the plaque assay mentioned above. Inhibition of virus growth was expressed by a $\log_{10}$ reduction in virus titer.

Deamination with mouse kidney homogenate. The preparation of enzyme from mouse kidney, a rich source of pyrimidine nucleoside deaminase activity, was essentially done by the method of Camiener and Smith (2). After clarification of the homogenate (20%) by high-speed centrifugation at 20,000 rpm for 2 h in a 30 PA rotor of a Hitachi centrifuge, the supernatant obtained was filtered through a membrane filter (Millipore Corp., 0.45 μm) to eliminate contaminating bacteria, and the filtrate was used as soon as possible. The compounds to be tested were dissolved in the filtrate to the desired concentration and incubated at 37°C for 2 h with shaking. The control samples were dissolved in filtrate that had been inactivated by heating in boiling water for 3 min. After the reaction period, samples were heated to terminate the reaction, centrifuged, and assayed for remaining antiviral activity by the plaque assay method.

Chemicals. Ara-C hydrochloride and IUdR were purchased from Sigma Chemical Co., St. Louis, Mo. 1-β-D-Arabinofuranosyladenine (Ara-A) was synthesized by Yoshio Nosaki in our laboratory. The other nucleosides were synthesized at Syntex Research, Palo Alto, Calif. (12–14). Solutions of all chemicals were made in maintenance medium immediately prior to use, except for compounds insoluble in water, which were initially dissolved in methanol.

RESULTS

Comparative antiviral activity of nucleosides. 3′-*O*-decanoyl Ara-C was the most active compound among those synthesized in our systematic study (12–14). The compounds had substantial activity against deoxyribonucleic acid viruses, but were inactive against ribonucleic acid viruses, including measles, Sendai virus, poliovirus, and influenza virus. Vaccinia virus was always somewhat more sensitive than HSV to the test compounds as well as to other antiviral nucleosides (Table 1). In a parallel experiment, the antiviral activities were compared with those of other nucleosides in the plaque reduction test (Table 1). The antiviral activities of 3′-*O*-decanoyl Ara-C against vaccinia virus and herpesvirus were comparable to those of Ara-C, and 3′-*O*-decanoyl cyclo-C was somewhat less active than the Ara-C derivative. The activities of the Ara-C and cyclo-C esters against adenovirus were of a lower order. Comparisons were made with Ara-A and IUdR in our test system. The two nucleosides were less active than Ara-C analogues, and IUdR was the least active of the compounds tested on the basis of the inhibitory effect on the multiplication of the viruses tested. However, the high level of antiviral activity of cyclo-C or Ara-C derivatives was accompanied by a high cytotoxicity toward HeLa cells, but antiviral activities of Ara-A and IUdR were shown to a lesser degree. Based upon a comparison of the therapeutic index (TI) value, Ara-A appeared to be the most effective compound, followed by IUdR. Ara-C analogues showed low TI values.

Cytotoxicity. Additionally, morphological change associated with cytotoxicity was also examined by using BGM cell monolayers. Five-day-old cells were exposed to concentrations of the drugs from 100 to 0.1 μg per ml of maintenance medium for 2 days at 37°C. The cells were fixed and stained with hematoxylin and eosin and observed for morphological changes under a microscope. With concentrations of 10 μg or less per ml, no signs of toxicity were noted in any of the drugs tested. At a concentration of 30 μg of Ara-C and cyclo-C derivatives per ml, enlarged nuclei were observed, although to a small degree. At 100 μg of these drugs per ml, however, considerable cellular damage was observed after 72 h, represented by increased granularity, frequent vacuolization, and abnormal mitotic figures. The mitotic index of Ara-C or cyclo-C derivatives was low when using concentrations of 10 μg per ml or more, but at 1 μg or less per ml no change occurred.

Comparative antiviral activities of Ara-C and cyclo-C acylates and other nucleosides against HSV-1 and HSV-2. Susceptibility of HSV-1 and HSV-2 to the nucleosides (10 μM) was examined in the virus growth inhibition test (Table 2). In the case of Ara-C derivatives, 3′-*O*-octanoyl derivatives of Ara-C and of cyclo-C as well as Ara-C itself were more active against HSV-2 than against HSV-1, using low-passage strains (Oda and Hata strains) in cell culture. Additionally, low-passage strains in both HSV-1 and HSV-2 were more sensitive than high-passage strains, including the HF strain of HSV-1 and the UW-268 strain of HSV-

TABLE 1. *Comparative antiviral activity of nucleosides*

Compound	Concn for ED_{50} (μg/ml)			Cytotoxicity[a] ED_{50} (μg/ml)	TI[b]	
	Vaccinia virus	HSV[c]	Adenovirus type 3		Vaccinia virus	HSV
3′-*O*-decanoyl cyclo-C	0.062	0.43	9.98	0.20[d]	3.22	0.46
3′-*O*-decanoyl Ara-C	0.019	0.09	13.51	0.09[d]	4.73	1.00
Cyclo-C	0.10	0.18	ND[e]	0.05[d]	0.50	0.27
Ara-C	0.017	0.038	5.35	0.05[d]	2.94	1.31
Ara-A	0.36	0.53	>26.72	25.0	69.4	47.16
IUdR	3.39	3.66	27.25	45.0	13.3	12.29

[a] HeLa cells (10^5 cells/ml) were grown in MEM supplemented with 10% bovine serum for 2 days at 37°C. At this time, the medium was replaced with fresh medium containing a serial dilution of the test compound. After 48 h the cells were dispersed with 0.02% trypsin and 0.04% Versene and counted with a model B Coulter counter. ED_{50} values were determined graphically.

[b] TI = ED_{50} in cytotoxicity/ED_{50} in antiviral activity.

[c] HF strain.

[d] These values were presented from the data described previously (12, 14).

[e] ND, Not done.

TABLE 2. *Comparative antiviral activities of acylates and other nucleosides against HSV-1 and HSV-2*[a]

Drug (10 μM)	HF (type 1)		Oda (type 1)		UW-268 (type 2)		Hata (type 2)	
	PFU/ml (log_{10})	Inhibition[b]	PFU/ml (log_{10})	Inhibition[b]	PFU/ml (log_{10})	Inhibition[b]	PFU/ml (log_{10})	Inhibition[b]
3′-*O*-octanoyl Ara-C	4.98	3.03	2.28	4.29	3.82	3.60	0.87	4.93
3′-*O*-octanoyl cyclo-C	6.83	1.18	2.54	4.03	4.50	2.92	1.30	4.50
Ara-C	5.15	2.86	2.38	4.19	3.74	3.68	1.09	4.71
IUdR	5.58	2.43	3.12	3.45	5.20	2.22	3.69	2.11
Ara-A	7.17	0.84	4.66	1.91	5.66	1.76	3.90	1.90
Control	8.01		6.57		7.42		5.80	

[a] BGM cell monolayers were infected with HSV, including type 1 (HF and Oda) and type 2 (UW-268 and Hata), respectively. After adsorption of the viruses, the infected cells were treated with maintenance medium containing a 10 μM concentration of the drugs or without drugs for 30 h at 37°C. Virus titration was made by the plaque assay. Inhibition of virus growth was expressed by a log_{10} reduction in PFU per milliliter. Further details of the method are described in the text.

[b] Log_{10} reduction in virus titer (PFU per milliliter).

2. There was little difference between the inhibitory activity of IUdR and Ara-A against HSV-1 and HSV-2, except that the HF strain was the least sensitive toward Ara-A and IUdR was more active against the Oda strain of HSV-1 than other HSV strains. In general, the HF strain of HSV was the least sensitive one toward the nucleosides.

Antagonism of cyclo-C derivative. The antiviral activity of IUdR is reversed by thymidine (23), whereas that of Ara-C is unaffected and reversed specifically by deoxycytidine (CdR) (4). We found that 3′-*O*-acetyl cyclo-C is also reversed by CdR, one of the nucleoside analogues tested. Thus, the concentration relationship between viral inhibition by 3′-*O*-acetyl cyclo-C and reversal by CdR was compared with that of Ara-C. As shown in Fig. 1, the inhibition of plaque formation caused by various concentrations of 3′-*O*-acetyl cyclo-C (8 to 64 μM) was competitively reversed by equimolar amounts of CdR. Full reversal of the inhibition by Ara-C, however, required a four- to eightfold molar excess of the antagonist. This result may indicate that the mode of action of the cyclo-C derivate also involves the CdR pathway, analogous to that of Ara-C.

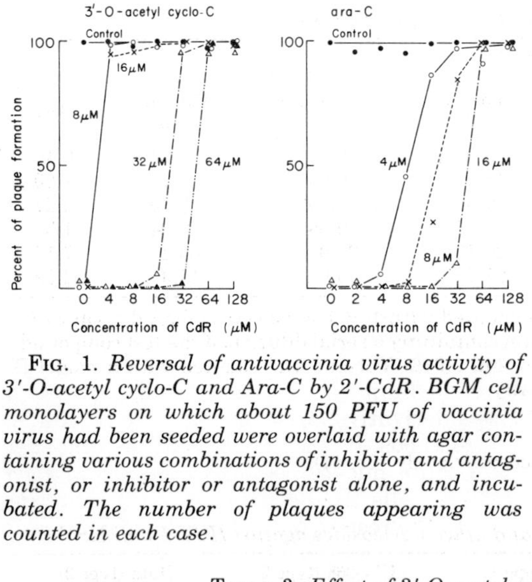

FIG. 1. *Reversal of antivaccinia virus activity of 3′-O-acetyl cyclo-C and Ara-C by 2′-CdR. BGM cell monolayers on which about 150 PFU of vaccinia virus had been seeded were overlaid with agar containing various combinations of inhibitor and antagonist, or inhibitor or antagonist alone, and incubated. The number of plaques appearing was counted in each case.*

Effect of cyclo-C against IUdR-resistant HSV. The sensitivity of IUdR-resistant HSV to 3′-*O*-acetyl cyclo-C and Ara-C was examined by the plaque reduction method. Table 3 shows that the number of plaques of IUdR-resistant HSV was not reduced, even in the presence of 100 μg of IUdR per ml, whereas plaque formation of the parent viruses was suppressed by 95% with a concentration of 3 μg of IUdR per ml. With 3′-*O*-acetyl cyclo-C and Ara-C, on the other hand, sensitivity was shown by IUdR-resistant viruses as well as the parent viruses.

Deamination of 3′-*O*-decanoyl Ara-C and of cyclo-C with homogenate from mouse kidney. Ara-C is rapidly converted to the inactive product uracil arabinoside by cytidine deaminase (1, 2). On the other hand, cyclo-C (21, 30) is resistant to the deaminase, as are 5′-*O*-acyl derivatives of Ara-C (18). Therefore, it is of interest to determine whether 3′-esters of cyclo-C and Ara-C are also inactivated by cytidine deaminase. As shown in Table 4, Ara-C is converted by mouse kidney homogenates to an inactive product, a process that probably involves deamination to form uracil arabinoside. The antiviral activity of 3′-*O*-decanoyl Ara-C also disappeared upon treatment with the mouse kidney homogenate for 2 h. In contrast to this catabolism of the Ara-C derivatives, the antiviral activity of 3′-*O*-decanoyl cyclo-C was not affected by treatment with this system. This result shows that the 3′-ester of cyclo-C was resistant to deamination by cytidine deaminase, an enzyme known to be present in such homogenates.

Comparative antiviral activity between 3′- and 5′-acylates. Antiviral activities of the 3′-

TABLE 3. *Effect of 3′-O-acetyl cyclo-C againt IUdR-resistant HSV*

Concn (μg/ml)[a]	Inhibition of plaque formation (%)					
	IUdR		3′-*O*-acetyl cyclo-C		Ara-C	
	S[b]	R[c]	S	R	S	R
100	100	0	NT[d]	NT	NT	NT
30	100	0	100	100	NT	NT
10	100	NT	100	100	100	100
3	94.6	NT	79.7	73.6	100	100
1	54.1	NT	24.3	17.5	91.8	89.4

[a] Concentrations of drug indicated were added into agar overlay medium.
[b] IUdR-sensitive virus (HVS-1, HF).
[c] IUdR-resistant virus.
[d] NT, Not tested.

TABLE 4. *Deactivation of derivatives of Ara-C and cyclo-C by homogenate of mouse kidney*[a]

Concn (μg/ml)	Inhibition of plaque formation (%)[b]								
	Ara-C			3′-O-decanoyl Ara-C			3′-O-decanoyl cyclo-C		
	A	B	C	A	B	C	A	B	C
1.25	100	100	2.8	70.4	100	0	100	100	100
0.40	100	100	0.9	33.3	86.1	0	100	100	100
0.125	100	100	0.9	2.8	49.1	0	50.0	63.9	65.7

[a] The drugs were dissolved in C to concentrations as indicated in the table and incubated at 37°C for 2 h. The control samples were dissolved in A or B. Samples were then heated to terminate the reaction, and remaining antiviral activities were assayed by the plaque assay method.

[b] A, With phosphate-buffered saline (pH 7.2); B, with inactivated homogenate (100°C for 3 min); C, with homogenate.

and 5′-decanoyl and palmitoyl derivatives of Ara-C were compared with the plaque reduction test. Results based upon average micromolar ED_{50} values from three separate tests are shown in Table 5 and analyzed by means of the eight-point parallel line assay method. Anti-vaccinia virus activity of 3′-O-palmitoyl Ara-C was significantly superior to its 5′-counterpart ($P \leq 0.05$). In the others, however, no significant differences were shown by means of statistical analysis.

Prevention of the antiviral activities of 3′- and 5′-acylates by eserine sulfate. The question was raised as to whether hydrolysis of 3′-O-acyl Ara-C to Ara-C is required for antiviral activity as has been suggested for 5′-O-acyl Ara-C (18). To solve this problem we tested whether the antiviral activity of the compound is inhibited by the addition of eserine sulfate (physostigmine sulfate, Merck), a choline esterase inhibitor, to the assay system. Table 6 shows the comparative effects of eserine sulfate on the antiviral activities of 3′- and 5′-decanoyl Ara-C against HSV in the plaque reduction test. At concentrations of 10 μM, the nucleosides alone inhibited plaque formation of HSV by 99.6 and 74.1%, respectively. Eserine sulfate at the concentrations used (3 to 30 μM) also possessed inhibitory activity (17 to 50.4%). A combination of the 5′-ester and eserine sulfate reduced the activity of the compound itself. Thus, the inhibitory activity of the 5′-ester was reduced from 62.6 to 23.9% when 30 μM eserine sulfate was added. In contrast to this, the antiviral activity of the 3′-ester was not affected with eserine sulfate in any combination.

TABLE 5. *Comparative antiviral activities of 3′- and 5′-O-acyl Ara-C's*[a]

Tested virus	ED_{50} (μM)			
	3′-Decanoyl	5′-Decanoyl	3′-Palmitoyl	5′-Palmitoyl
Vaccinia	0.11	0.18	0.14[b]	0.30[b]
Herpes simplex[c]	0.64	0.86	0.67	1.14

[a] The tests were made by the plaque reduction method in three separate experiments, and the results obtained were analyzed by means of the eight-point parallel line assay method.

[b] Difference with $P \leq 0.05$.

[c] HF strain.

DISCUSSION

The antiviral activities of several 3′-O-acyl Ara-C and 3′-O-acyl cyclo-C derivatives have been examined. It was hoped that the introduction of an acyl group at the 3′-position of the sugar moiety would increase penetration into the host cells, due to the lipophilicity of the ester. In fact, the addition of a 3′-O-acyl group of appropriate chain length (C_6 to C_{12}) to cyclo-C was accompanied by enhanced antiviral activity (Table 1). A further increase in chain length, however, led to reduced activity due to the insolubility of such compounds in the culture medium (12–14, 17). The cytotoxicity of these derivatives was examined by two different methods. It is generally accepted that antimetabolite nucleosides are particularly active against cells in the growing state, affecting cells in the resting state, a confluent cell monolayer, to a lesser degree, probably due to the slower rates of uptake of the chemical and cellular metabolism. In fact, Ara-C derivatives exhibit strong inhibitory activities against the replication of HeLa cells (Table 1), but a morphological change in cell monolayers treated is observed to a lesser degree, even at a high concentration of the drugs (10 μg/ml). In cases of acylates of Ara-C or cyclo-C, as with their parents, a high level of antiviral activity was accompanied with a pronounced cytotoxicity toward the host cell culture. Cyclo-C is resistant to pyrimidine nucleoside deaminase cleavage (21, 30), unless it is first converted to Ara-C by a nonenzymatic process under physiological conditions (30). Our studies confirmed that 3′-

TABLE 6. *Prevention of the antiviral activities of 3'- and 5'-acylates by eserine sulfate*[a]

Concn of eserine sulfate (μM)	Inhibition of plaque formation (%)				
	Eserine sulfate alone	3'-*O*-decanoyl		5'-*O*-decanoyl	
		Eserine sulfate	Calculated[b]	Eserine sulfate	Calculated[b]
0		99.6		74.1	
30	50.4	97.8	95.5	62.6	23.9
10	28.6	100	100	67.0	53.9
3	17.0	98.9	98.7	74.4	69.2

[a] Infected BGM cell monolayers with 150 PFU of HSV-1 (HF) were overlaid with the agar medium containing a combination of various concentrations of eserine sulfate and a 10 μM concentration of the nucleoside. Antiviral activities of eserine sulfate and the nucleoside to be tested alone and the mixtures were examined in the plaque reduction test as described in the text. Inhibition by the combination of eserine sulfate and the nucleoside was calculated by the method of Neil et al. (18).

[b] Calculated percent inhibition due to a 10 μM concentration of the nucleoside in the presence of eserine sulfate = $100\{1 - [Ge + d]/Ge]\}$, where Ge = the number of plaques in the presence of a particular eserine sulfate concentration and $Ge + d$ = the number of plaques in the presence of 10 μM concentration of the nucleoside and a particular eserine sulfate concentration.

O-acyl derivatives of cyclo-C are also resistant to the enzyme (Table 4). Therefore, the acylated cyclo-C derivatives might be able to serve as stable reservoir forms of Ara-C, which is responsible for the antiviral activity of the compounds. In general, the activities of 3'-*O*-acyl cyclo-C compounds were somewhat lower than those of their 3'-*O*-acyl Ara-C counterparts. It seems likely that the activity of the cyclo-C derivative depends upon the rate of cleavage of the 2,2'-anhydro bond. The wide variation in sensitivity of HSV-1 and HSV-2 to antiviral agents has been described (6, 19, 20). The results have shown that these differences in susceptibility depend on the cell culture system, the prior passage history of the virus, and the assay system used. The sensitivity of the serotype of HSV to the nucleosides also varied in our assay system (Table 2). This study has demonstrated that, under certain conditions, the type 2 strain is more sensitive to Ara-C derivatives than the type 1 strain. Our data have also made clear that the difference in sensitivity to the agent can vary depending upon the strain of virus used and the number of passages of the virus in cell culture. A comparison of the antiviral activities of 3'-esters of Ara-C with their 5'-acyl counterparts was interesting, the 3'-esters being somewhat more active. On the other hand, in contrast to the resistance of 5'-esters of Ara-C to pyrimidine nucleoside deaminase, the 3'-esters were metabolized by a mouse kidney homogenate to an inactive product. Neil et al. (18) have reported that inhibition of enzymatic hydrolysis with eserine sulfate, an esterase inhibitor, markedly reduced the cytotoxicity of 1-β-D-arabinofuranosylcytosine 5'-admantoate (Ado-Ara-C) against L1210 cells in culture and concluded that hydrolysis of Ado-Ara-C to Ara-C is required for cytotoxic activity. We also observed the same effect, i.e., the antiviral activity of 5'-*O*-decanoyl Ara-C being markedly reduced by the addition of eserine sulfate. In contrast, the activity of 3'-*O*-decanoyl Ara-C was not affected under comparable conditions. Thus, the esterase that is responsible for cleavage of the 5'-esters and that is inhibited by eserine sulfate does not seem to be responsible for the hydrolytic conversion of 3'-*O*-acyl Ara-C derivatives to Ara-C.

ACKNOWLEDGMENTS

We are particularly grateful to T. Okabayashi and T. Ishigami, who have contributed much to our liaison, and to O. Shiratori and S. Takase for cytotoxicity tests.

LITERATURE CITED

1. **Camiener, G. W.** 1968. Studies of the enzymatic deamination of ara-cytidine. V. Inhibition *in vitro* and *in vivo* by tetrahydrouridine and other reduced pyrimidine nucleosides. Biochem. Pharmacol. **17**:1981–1991.
2. **Camiener, G. W., and C. G. Smith.** 1965. Studies of the enzymatic deamination of cytosine arabinoside. I. Enzyme distribution and species specificity. Biochem. Pharmacol. **14**:1405–1416.
3. **Chow, A. W., A. Ronald, M. Fiala, W. Hryniuk, M. L. Well, J. St. Geme, Jr., and L. B. Guze.** 1973. Cytosine arabinoside therapy for herpes simplex encephalitis—clinical experience with six patients. Antimicrob. Agents Chemother. **3**:412–417.
4. **Chu, M. Y., and G. A. Fischer.** 1962. A proposed mechanism of action of 1-β-D-arabinofuranosylcytosine as an inhibitor of the growth of leukemic cells. Biochem. Pharmacol. **11**:423–430.
5. **Feldman, L. A., and F. Rapp.** 1966. Inhibition of adenovirus replication by 1-β-D-arabinofuranosyl cytosine. Proc. Soc. Exp. Biol. Med. **122**:243–247.
6. **Fiala, M., A. Chow, and L. B. Guze.** 1972. Susceptibility of herpesviruses to cytosine arabinoside: standardization of susceptibility test procedure and relative resistance of herpes simplex type 2 strains. Antimicrob. Agents Chemother. **1**:354–357.

7. **Fox, J. J., E. A. Falco, I. Wempen, D. Pomeroy, M. D. Dowling, and J. H. Burchenal.** 1972. Oral and parenteral activity of 2,2′-anhydro-1-β-D-arabinofuranosyl-5-fluorocytosine against both intraperitoneally and intracerebrally inoculated mouse leukemia. Cancer Res. 32:2269–2272.

8. **Gish, D. T., R. C. Kelly, G. W. Camiener, and W. J. Wechter.** 1971. Nucleic acids. II. Synthesis of 5′-esters of 1-β-D-arabinofuranosyl cytosine possessing antileukemic and immunosuppressive activity. J. Med. Chem. **14**:1159–1166.

9. **Gluckman, E., A. Basch, B. Varet, and B. Dreyfus.** 1973. Combination chemotherapy with cytosine arabinoside and rubidomycin in 30 cases of acute granulocytic leukemia. Cancer **31**:487–491.

10. **Gordon, R. O., M. E. Wada, and M. S. Mitchell.** 1969. The production of tolerance to human erythrocytes in the rat with cytosine arabinoside or cyclophosphamide. J. Immunol. **103**:233–243.

11. **Gray, G. W., F. R. Nichol, M. M. Mickelson, G. W. Camiener, D. T. Gish, R. C. Kelly, W. J. Wechter, T. E. Moxley, and G. L. Neil.** 1972. Immunosuppressive, antiviral and antitumor activities of cytarabine derivatives. Biochem. Pharmacol. 21:465–475.

12. **Hamamura, E. K., M. Prystasz, J. P. H. Verheyden, J. G. Moffatt, K. Yamaguchi, N. Uchida, K. Sato, A. Nomura, O. Shiratori, S. Takase, and K. Katagiri.** 1976. Reactions of 2-acyloxyisobutyryl-halides with nucleosides. 6. Synthesis and biological evaluation of some 3′-acyl derivatives of 2,2′-anhydro-1-(β-D-arabinofuranosyl)cytosine hydrochloride. J. Med. Chem. **19**:654–662.

13. **Hamamura, E. K., M. Prystasz, J. P. H. Verheyden, J. G. Moffatt, K. Yamaguchi, N. Uchida, K. Sato, A. Nomura, O. Shiratori, S. Takase, and K. Katagiri.** 1976. Reactions of 2-acyloxyisobutyryl-halides with nucleosides. 7. Synthesis and biological evaluation of some 2,2′-anhydro-1-(3′,5′-di-*O*-acyl-β-D-arabinofuranosyl)cytosine hydrochlorides. J. Med. Chem. 19:663–667.

14. **Hamamura, E. K., M. Prystasz, J. P. H. Verheyden, J. G. Moffatt, K. Yamaguchi, N. Uchida, K. Sato, A. Nomura, O. Shiratori, S. Takase, and K. Katagiri.** 1976. Reactions of 2-acyloxyisobutyryl-halides with nucleosides. 8. Synthesis and biological evaluation of some 3′-acyl and 3′,5′-diacyl derivatives of 1-β-D-arabinofuranosylcytosine. J. Med. Chem. 19:667–674.

15. **Kaufman, H. E., J. A. Capella, E. D. Maloney, J. E. Robbins, G. M. Cooper, and M. H. Uotila.** 1964. Corneal toxicity of cytosine arabinoside. Arch. Ophthalmol. 72:535–540.

16. **Leuter, C. B., E. J. Bailey, and A. M. Lerner.** 1974. Assessment of cytosine arabinoside as an antiviral agent in humans. Antimicrob. Agents Chemother. 6:598–602.

17. **Moffatt, J. G., E. K. Hamamura, A. F. Russell, M. Prystasz, J. P. H. Verheyden, K. Yamaguchi, N. Uchida, K. Sato, S. Nishiyama, O. Shiratori, and K. Katagiri.** 1974. Synthesis and biologic examination of some derivatives of 2,2′-anhydro-1-(β-D-arabinofuranosyl) cytosine hydrochloride. Cancer Chemother. Rep. 58:451–469.

18. **Neil, G. L., H. H. Buskirk, T. E. Moxley, R. C. Manak, S. L. Kuentzel and B. K. Bhuyan.** 1971. Biochemical and pharmacologic studies with 1-β-D-arabinofuranosyl cytosine 5′-admantoate, a depot form of cytarabine. Biochem. Pharmacol. 20:3295–3308.

19. **Nutter, R. L., and F. Rapp.** 1973. The effect of cytosine arabinoside on virus production in various cells infected with herpes simplex virus types 1 and 2. Cancer Res. 33:166–170.

20. **Person, D. A., P. J. Sheridan, and E. C. Hermann, Jr.** 1970. Sensitivity of types 1 and 2 herpes simplex virus to 5-iodo-2′-deoxyuridine and 9-β-D-arabinofuranosyladenine. Infect. Immun. 2:815–820.

21. **Pizer, L. I., and S. S. Cohen.** 1960. Metabolism of pyrimidine arabinonucleosides and cyclonucleosides in *Escherichia coli*. J. Biol. Chem. 235:2387–2392.

22. **Reed, L. J., and H. Muench.** 1938. A simple method of estimating fifty per cent end points. Am. J. Hyg. 27:493–497.

23. **Roizman, B., L. Aurelian, and P. R. Roane, Jr.** 1963. The multiplication of herpes simplex virus. I. The programming of viral DNA duplication in HEP-2 cells. Virology 21:482–498.

24. **Russell, A. F., M. Prystasz, E. K. Hamamura, J. P. H. Verheyden, and J. G. Moffatt.** 1974. Reaction of 2-acyloxyisobutyryl halides with nucleosides. V. Reactions with cytidine and its derivatives. J. Org. Chem. 39:2182–2186.

25. **Sato, K., F. Righthand, and D. T. Karzon.** 1971. Effect of host cell on distribution of a lysosomal enzyme during virus infection. J. Virol. 7:467–472.

26. **Talley, R. W., R. M. O'Bryan, W. G. Tucker, and R. V. Loo.** 1967. Clinical pharmacology and human antitumor activity of cytosine arabinoside. Cancer 20:809–816.

27. **Tanai, T., M. Ichino, A. Hoshi, F. Kanazawa, and K. Kuretani.** 1974. Pyrimidine nucleosides. 6. Synthesis and anticancer activities of N^4-substituted 2,2′-anhydronucleosides. J. Med. Chem. 17:1076–1078.

28. **Underwood, G. E.** 1962. Activity of 1-β-D-arabinofuranosyl cytosine hydrochloride against herpes simplex keratitis. Proc. Soc. Exp. Biol. Med. 111:660–664.

29. **Vadlamudi, S., and A. Goldin.** 1971. Influence of mitotic cycle inhibitors on the antileukemic activity of cytosine arabinoside in mice bearing leukemia L1210. Cancer Chemother. Rep. 55:547–560.

30. **Wang, M. C., R. A. Sharma, and A. Bloch.** 1973. Studies on the mode of action of 2,2′-anhydro-1-β-D-arabinofuranosylcytosine. Cancer Res. 33:1265–1271.

31. **Wechter, W. J., M. A. Johnson, C. M. Hall, D. T. Warner, A. E. Berger, A. H. Wenzel, D. T. Gish, and G. L. Neil.** 1975. Ara-cytidine acylates. Use of drug design predictors in structure-activity relationship correlation. J. Med. Chem. 18:339–334.

ANTIMICROBIAL AGENTS AND CHEMOTHERAPY, Feb. 1977, p. 198-201

Vol. 11, No. 2
Printed in U.S.A.

Comparative Study of the Antiviral Activity of Acyl Derivatives of 2,2′-Anhydro-1-β-D-Arabinofuranosylcytosine and Other Nucleosides Against Encephalitis in Mice[1]

SHINYA NISHIYAMA, KOSABURO SATO,* TOSHIHIKO YAMANAKA, AND JOHN G. MOFFATT

Shionogi Research Laboratory, Shionogi & Co., Ltd., Fukushima-ku, Osaka, 553 Japan, and Institute of Molecular Biology, Syntex Research, Palo Alto, California 94304

Received for publication 20 May 1976

Anti-deoxyribonucleic acid virus activities of 3′-*O*-acyl derivatives of 2,2′-anhydro-1-β-D-arabinofuranosyl cytosine (cyclo-C) and 1-β-D-arabinofuranosylcytosine (Ara-C) were evaluated by using an in vivo test system in mice. Among the derivatives tested, 3′-*O*-decanoyl cyclo-C hydrochloride was the most effective against herpes simplex virus-induced encephalitis in mice when the drug was administered directly into infected brains of mice (target-organ treatment). A comparative study of the treatment of herpetic encephalitis in mice with 3′-*O*-decanoyl cyclo-C and other nucleosides, including Ara-C, 9-β-D-arabinofuranosyladenine (Ara-A), and 5-iodo-2′-deoxyrudine (IUdR), proved Ara-A to be more efficacious than the other nucleosides, followed by 3′-*O*-decanoyl cyclo-C, which was more active than Ara-C and IUdR. Administration of 3′-*O*-acyl cyclo-C's by intraperitoneal injection, however, failed to demonstrate activity against herpetic encephalitis in mice. The antivaccinial activity of 3′-*O*-decanoyl cyclo-C was also compared with that of other compounds against encephalitis and dermal tail lesions in mice caused by vaccinia virus infection. Interaperitoneally administered 3′-*O*-decanoyl cyclo-C and Ara-C also showed no significant activity against the diseases. Under these test conditions, *N*-methylisatin-β-thiosemicarbazone (Marboran) was the most active compound, followed by Ara-A.

The marked in vitro anti-deoxyribonucleic acid virus activities of 3′-*O*-acyl derivatives of 1-β-D-arabinofuranosylcytosine (Ara-C) and 2,2′-anhydro-1-β-D-arabinofuranosylcytosine (cyclo-C), as have previously been demonstrated (11), prompted a series of investigations to determine whether the drugs were also active in animal systems against the same viruses. Experiments were carried out to demonstrate the effectiveness of the drugs, using different routes of administration, against encephalitis in mice caused by herpes simplex virus (HSV) and vaccina virus (VV) and against VV-induced dermal lesions on the tails of mice. The results obtained, together with a comparison with the activity of other known antiviral substances, are presented in this paper.

MATERIALS AND METHODS

Virus. Strains of HSV used in this study were: HF and Oda strains for type 1 and UW-268 and Hata strains for type 2. The IHD strain of VV was used. Details concerning the history of the stock virus preparations and the plaque assay method used in this study were described in a previous report (11). For HSV employed, titers of viral inocula (mean lethal dose [LD_{50}]) were calculated by the method of Reed and Muench (10) for 14-day mortality of mice inoculated intracerebrally with the viruses.

Mice. Randomly-bred albino JCL:ICR mice (purchased from CLEA, Takatsuki, Osaka, Japan) weighing 14 to 15 g were used. Mouse encephalitis experiments were conducted by two methods described below.

Target-organ treatment. The experiment procedure for target-organ treatment was essentially that of Allen and Sidwell (1), except that 30 LD_{50} of the HF strain of HSV in 0.025 ml of solution containing the drug to be tested was directly inoculated into the brains of mice.

Vaccinial and herpetic encephalitis. Mice were inoculated intraperitoneally (i.p.) with 10 LD_{50} of VV or subcutaneously with 30 LD_{50} of the Oda strain of HSV and treated i.p. with the compound to be tested once daily for 5 days, beginning 24 h before virus inoculation, unless indicated otherwise. The antiviral activity in these experiments was evaluated by the increase in the survival rate among the treated, infected mice. The animals were examined for 14 days, and deaths occurring were recorded daily. In some experiments, mean effective dose (ED_{50}) values based on survival rate and mean sur-

[1] Contribution no. 130 from the Institute of Molecular Biology, Syntex Research, Palo Alto, CA 94304.

vival day (SD_{50}) were calculated (10). Toxicity control mice, which were sham infected, were also included in each test.

Tail lesion method. For the tail lesion method, the mice were inoculated intravenously in the tail with 5×10^3 plaque-forming units of VV per 0.05 ml. Dermal lesions appeared 5 to 7 days after virus inoculation and reached a maximum level in the number of lesions at 9 days. The number of lesions was counted after staining with 0.5% methylene blue (2). The drugs were administered i.p. in the various regimens.

Chemicals. The various 3′-*O*-acyl derivatives of cyclo-C and Ara-C were synthesized at Syntex Research, Palo Alto, Calif. (5, 6, 9). Marboran was kindly provided by N. Ishida, Tohoku University, Sendai, Japan. The other compounds were supplied as mentioned in the accompanying report (11). Drug preparations of all chemicals were made in sterile Hanks balanced salt solution, except for insoluble compounds, which were suspended with 0.5% gum arabic in sterile saline.

RESULTS

In an initial experiment, a series of 3′-*O*-acyl derivatives of cyclo-C and Ara-C was examined for antiherpetic activity against HSV-induced encephalitis in mice by administration directly into the brain (target-organ treatment method; Table 1). As was the case with esters of cyclo-C in cell culture (11), introduction of the C_8 to C_{12} acyl groups at the 3′-*O*-position led to an increase in activity relative to the parent compound (cyclo-C). In the Ara-C series, however, no increase in activity was observed upon introduction of 3′-*O*-acyl groups. Against HSV, maximum effectiveness was shown by 3′-*O*-decanoyl cyclo-C. The antiherpetic activity of the 3′-*O*-decanoyl derivative was compared with other antiviral nucleosides in the same test system. Table 2 shows that, among the compounds tested, 9-β-D-arabinofuranosyladenine (Ara-A) showed the most pronounced activities. The activity of 3′-*O*-decanoyl cyclo-C was higher than that of Ara-C and 5-iodo-2′-deoxyuridine (IUdR), being roughly twice as effective as Ara-C. The activity was also examined by systemic treatment against encephalitis in mice infected subcutaneously with 30 LD_{50} of HSV (Oda strain). In this experiment, the drug was administered i.p. twice a day for 5 days, beginning 24 hr before virus inoculation. No antiherpetic activity appeared in this test system at the dosage used (Table 3). Treatment with 200 mg of 3′-*O*-decanoyl cyclo-C per kg was toxic. Antivaccinial activity of the nucleosides was also evaluated by systemic treatment of the dermal tail lesions (Table 4) and encephalitis (Table 5) in mice caused by VV infection. Various concentrations of the drugs in serial two-

TABLE 1. *Antiherpetic activities of acyl derivatives of cyclo-C and Ara-C by the target-organ treatment method*[a]

Compound	ED_{50} (mg/kg) of 3′-substituted: *O*-2,2′-cyclo-C	ED_{50} (mg/kg) of 3′-substituted: Ara-C
	>12.5	3.4
3′-*O*-acetyl	>12.5	4.3
3′-*O*-octanoyl	4.2	9.0
3′-*O*-decanoyl	1.3	>12.5
3′-*O*-lauroyl	6.25	>12.5
3′-*O*-myristoyl	>12.5	>12.5
3′-*O*-palmitoyl	>12.5	>12.5

[a] Serial dilutions of the drugs were administered (0.025 ml/mouse) directly into the brain of mice with 30 LD_{50} of the HF strain of HSV. Deaths of mice (10 mice/group) were recorded daily for 14 days. The ED_{50} was calculated by the method of Reed and Muench (10), based on the survival rate.

TABLE 2. *Comparative antiherpetic activity of nucleosides by the target-organ treatment method*

Compound	Dose (mg/kg)	No. of survivors/ total no. of mice	Survival rate (%)	SD_{50} (days)
3′-*O*-decanoyl cyclo-C	3.1	10/10	100	>14.0
	1.5	6/10	60	>14.0
	0.7	2/10	20	8.8
	0	O/10	0	4.0
Ara-C	6.2	5/5	100	>14.0
	3.1	3/5	60	>14.0
	1.5	1/5	20	7.5
	0	0/5	0	5.8
IUdR	20	4/5	80	>14.0
	10	2/5	40	9.2
	5	4/5	80	>14.0
	0	0/5	0	7.5
Ara-A	0.6	5/5	100	>14.0
	0.3	4/5	80	>14.0
	0.15	3/5	60	>14.0
	0	0/5	0	7.5

TABLE 3. *Antiviral activity of 3'-O-decanoyl cyclo-C administered i.p. against herpetic encephalitis in mice*[a]

Dose (mg/kg)	No. of survivors/total no. of mice	Survival rate (%)	SD_{50} (days)
100	0/5	0	6.6
50	0/5	0	6.6
25	1/5	20	6.6
0	0/5	0	6.3

[a] Mice were inoculated subcutaneously with 30 LD_{50} of the Oda strain of HSV and were treated i.p. with the drug twice daily for 5 days beginning 24 h before virus inoculation. The animals were examined for 14 days.

fold dilutions were administered i.p. for 5 days, beginning 24 h before virus inoculation. In the two test systems, Marboran was the most active compound against vaccinia virus, followed by Ara-A. 3'-*O*-octanoyl cyclo-C and Ara-C failed to demonstrate antivaccinial activity in this system, even using a dosage regimen of twice a day. Susceptibility of serotypes of HSV towards the nucleosides was examined by the target-organ treatment method, and the results are shown in Table 6. The compounds tested were somewhat more active against type 2 than type 1 HSV in both high- and low-passage strains.

TABLE 4. *Comparative antivaccinial activity of nucleosides and Marboran in tail lesion method*[a]

Compound	Dose (mg/kg)	No. of mice	No. of lesions	Avg no. of lesions	Inhibition (%)
3'-*O*-octanoyl cyclo-C[b]	100	7	8 4 26 12 8 10 16	12.0	26.7
	50	8	11 43 53 55 40 16 11 21	31.3	0
	0	8	18 10 22 12 24 13 24 8	16.4	
Ara-C[b]	50	7	6 23 47 16 16 6 8	17.4	0
	0	8	18 10 22 12 24 13 24 8	16.4	
Ara-A[c]	100	10	12 23 2 24 13 23 8 14 31 8	15.8	41.3
	50	10	7 32 8 40 9 19 21 11 26 25	19.8	26.4
	0	15	31 12 16 36 23 22 41 30 19 25 20 21 19 40 49	26.9	
Marboran[c]	50	5	1 2 12 5 3	4.6	84.1
	25	5	20 21 14 20 30	19.0	34.5
	0	5	32 10 55 28 20	29.0	

[a] The mice were inoculated intravenously in the tail with vaccinia virus (5×10^3 plaque-forming units/0.05 ml). The infected mice were treated with the drugs in the regimens as indicated in the table. The number of lesions was counted at 9 days after inoculation of virus.

[b] Administered i.p. twice daily for 5 days, beginning 24 h before virus inoculation.

[c] Administered i.p. once daily for 5 days, beginning 24 h before virus inoculation.

TABLE 5. *Comparative antivaccinial activity of nucleosides and Marboran against vaccinial encephalitis*[a]

Compound	Dose (mg/kg)	No. of survivors/total no. of mice	Survival rate (%)	SD_{50} (days)
3'-*O*-octanoyl cyclo-C[b]	50	0/5	0	4.1
	25	0/5	0	3.8
	0	0/5	0	5.6
Ara-C[b]	100	0/5	0	5.5
	50	0/5	0	5.6
	25	0/5	0	5.8
	0	0/5	0	5.6
Ara-A[c]	100	3/5	60	>14.0
	50	1/5	20	8.5
	25	0/5	0	7.8
	0	0/5	0	8.8
Marboran[c]	100	3/5	60	>14.0
	50	2/5	40	8.7
	25	0/5	0	5.8
	0	5	0	3.8

[a] Mice were inoculated i.p. with 10 LD_{50} of VV and were treated i.p. with the drugs in the regimens as indicated in the table. Deaths were recorded daily for 14 days.

[b] Administered i.p. twice daily for 5 days, beginning 24 h before virus inoculation.

[c] Administered i.p. once daily for 5 days, beginning 24 h before virus inoculation.

TABLE 6. *Comparison of antiherpetic activities of Ara-C and 3'-O-octanoyl cyclo-C on HSV types 1 and 2 infection in mice*[a]

Compound	Antiherpetic activity (ED_{50}, mg/kg)			
	HSV type 1		HSV type 2	
	HF[a]	ODA[b]	UW-268[a]	HATA[b]
3'-*O*-octanoyl cyclo-C	5.8	3.12	2.6	1.1
Ara-C	2.5	3.2	1.9	1.1

[a] Serial dilutions of drugs were administered (0.025 ml/mouse) directly into the brains of mice with 30 LD_{50} of each strain of HSV. The mice were examined for 14 days. The ED_{50} values based on the survival rate were calculated (10).

[b] High passage strain in tissue culture.

[c] Low passage strain in tissue culture.

DISCUSSION

3'-*O*-acyl derivatives of cyclo-C and Ara-C that have been shown to possess anti-deoxyribonucleic acid virus activity in cell culture systems were tested for in vivo activity, and their activities were compared with those of other antiviral compounds. Examination of structure-activity relationships showed that in the series of 3'-*O*-acyl derivatives of cyclo-C, but not in the comparable Ara-C derivatives, the introduction of an adequately long acyl chain (C_8 to C_{12}) led to an increase in activity relative to that of the parent compound. Maximum activity was found with 3'-*O*-decanoyl cyclo-C hydrochloride. A further increase in the chain length of the acyl group led to reduced activity; the C_{14} and C_{16} esters showed no significant activity. This reduced activity of the higher esters may be related to their low solubilities. The results with the cyclo-C derivatives obtained in this experiment coincided with that from cell culture studies. The test system employed, target-organ treatment, is a sensitive assay method for the evaluation of antineurotropic virus activity. The advantages of this system, particularly in primary antivirus assay, include the small amount of test compound used, the high concentration of drug introduced into the target organ, and an elimination of the alteration of the test chemical by enzymes prior to its reaching the organ (1). Although derivatives of cyclo-C and Ara-C showed marked activity against VV and HSV in cell culture (11) and in an animal test system by topical treatment (K. Sato, S. Nishiyama, T. Yamanaka, J. Hara, and J. G. Moffat, manuscript in preparation), the drugs failed to show antiviral activity when administered systemically by i.p. injection. We assumed that this ineffectiveness of Ara-C may be due to its rapid degradation to the biologically inactive 1-β-D-arabinofuranosyl uracil (Ara-U) by the ubiquitous enzyme cytidine deaminase before it reached the target organ (3, 4). Cyclo-C is known to be readily hydrolyzed, apparently via a nonenzymatic process, to Ara-C (8) and is likely to be further converted to Ara-U, although the cyclo-C derivative itself is resistant to the deaminase (7, 11).

LITERATURE CITED

1. **Allen, L. B., and R. W. Sidwell.** 1972. Target-organ treatment of neurotropic virus diseases: efficacy as a chemotherapy tool and comparison of activity of adenine arabinoside, cytosine arabinoside, idoxuridine, and trifluorothymidine. Antimicrob. Agents Chemother. 2:229–223.
2. **Boyl, J. J., R. F. Haff, and R. C. Stewart.** 1967. Evaluation of antiviral compounds by suppression of tail lesions in vaccinia-infected mice, p. 536–539. Antimicrob. Agents Chemother. 1966.
3. **Camiener, G. W., and C. G. Smith.** 1965. Studies of the enzymatic deamination of cytosine arabinoside. I. Enzyme distribution and species specificity. Biochem. Pharmacol. 14:1405–1416.
4. **Creasey, W. A., R. J. Papac, M. E. Markiw, P. Calabresi, and A. D. Welch.** 1966. Biochemical and pharmacological studies with 1-β-D-arabinofuranosylcytosine in man. Biochem. Pharmacol. 15:1417–1428.
5. **Hamamura, E. K., M. Prystasz, J. P. H. Verheyden, J. G. Moffatt, K. Yamaguchi, N. Uchida, K. Sato, A. Nomura, O. Shiratori, S. Takase, and K. Katagiri.** 1976. Reactions of 2-acyl-oxyisobutyryl halides with nucleosides. 6. Synthesis and biological evaluation of some 3'-acyl derivatives of 2,2'-anhydro-1-(β-D-arabinofuranosyl) cytosine hydrochloride. J. Med. Chem. 19:654–622.
6. **Hamamura, E. K., M. Prystasz, J. P. H. Verheyden, J. G. Moffatt, K. Yamaguchi, N. Uchida, K. Sato, A. Nomura, O. Shiratori, S. Takase, and K. Katagiri.** 1976. Reactions of 2-acyloxyisobutyryl halides with nucleosides. 8. Synthesis and biological evaluation of some 3'-acyl and 3',5'-diacyl derivatives of 1-β-D-arabinofuranosylcytosine. J. Med. Chem. 19:667–674.
7. **Hoshi, A., F. Kanzawa, K. Kuretani, M. Saneyoshi, and Y. Arai.** 1971. 2,2'*O*-Cyclocytidine, an anti-tumor cytidine analog resistant to cytidine deaminase. Gann 62:145–146.
8. **Kessel, D.** 1974. On the characteristics of inhibition of deoxyribonucleic acid synthesis by 2,2'-anhydro-1-β-D-arabinofuranosyl cytosine. Biochem. Pharmacol. 23:2657–2662.
9. **Moffatt, J. G., E. K. Hamamura, A. F. Rusell, M. Prystasz, J. P. H. Verheyden, K. Yamaguchi, N. Uchida, K. Sato, S. Nishiyama, O. Shitatori, and K. Katagiri.** 1974. Synthesis and biologic examination of some derivatives of 2,2'-anhydro-1-(β-D-arabinofuranosyl) cytosine hydrochloride. Cancer Chemother. Rep. 58:451–469.
10. **Reed, L. J., and H. Muench.** 1938. A simple method of estimating fifty percent end points. Am. J. Hyg. 27:493–497.
11. **Sato, K., A. Nomura, and J. G. Moffatt.** Antiviral activities of acyl derivatives of 2,2'-anhydro-1-β-D-arabinofuranosylcytosine and 1-β-D-arabinofuranosylcytosine in cell culture. Antimicrob. Agents Chemother. 11:191–197.

ANTIMICROBIAL AGENTS AND CHEMOTHERAPY, Feb. 1977, p. 202-208
Vol. 11, No. 2

Printed in U.S.A.

Synthesis of Vaccinia Viral Antigens in HeLa Cells in the Presence of Isatin Beta-Thiosemicarbazone

EHUD KATZ* AND HAYA FELIX

The Chanock Centre for Virology, Hebrew University–Hadassah Medical School, Jerusalem, Israel

Received for publication 15 September 1976

Vaccinia virus antigens, in HeLa cells treated with the antipox virus drug isatin β-thiosemicarbazone (IBT), were analyzed by immunoprecipitation, followed by sodium dodecyl sulfate-polyacrylamide gel electrophoresis. The total radioactivity in the immunoprecipitate was decreased to almost 50% in the presence of the drug as compared to its absence. An inhibition also occurred with an IBT-dependent mutant (IBT^D) when growing in the absence of IBT. However, similar levels of radioactivity were observed in the immunoprecipitates from an IBT-resistant mutant (IBT^R) grown in either the absence or presence of the drug. When the antigens within the immunoprecipitates were analyzed by sodium dodecyl sulfate-polyacrylamide gel electrophoresis, it was shown that the inhibition observed in the wild-type-infected cells in the presence of IBT and in the IBT^D-infected cells in the absence of the drug, was quantitative, affecting the amounts of the different polypeptides more or less equally.

Isatin β-thiosemicarbazone (IBT) is an efficient drug active against pox-viruses, which inhibits late stages during virus growth (21). Viral deoxyribonucleic acid (DNA) and early viral proteins are synthesized in the presence of the drug; however, the viral DNA fails to be coated with proteins and remains sensitive to deoxyribonuclease (4, 26). Easterbrook (4), who studied vaccinia virus infection in KB cells in the presence of IBT, did not observe inhibition in viral antigen synthesis, even at the late period after infection, using complement fixation and fluorescent-antibody staining techniques. On the other hand, Appleyard et al. (1) followed rabbit pox infection in HeLa cells by precipitation in agar and found that several late viral antigens were missing in the presence of IBT.

The aim of the present study was to analyze the antigens formed in the absence and presence of the drug, using the combined method of immunoprecipitation followed by sodium dodecyl sulfate (SDS)-polyacrylamide gel electrophoresis. An IBT-resistant mutant (IBT^R), recently isolated by us, served as a control in this study.

MATERIALS AND METHODS

Cells. HeLa S3 and BSCl cells were grown in monolayer cultures with M199 media supplemented with 10% calf serum.

Viruses. Vaccinia WR strain (wild type [WT]), IBT^R, and IBT^D mutants were grown in HeLa S3 cells and purified as previously described (8). Titration of virus infectivity by the plaque assay technique in BSCl cells was performed as described before (10).

Immune serum. Antisera to purified vaccinia virus (WT) were prepared. Rabbits were weekly injected intramuscularly and subcutaneously with 2 ml of a mixture containing approximately 5 mg of purified virus and 1 ml of complete Freund adjuvant (Difco Laboratories, Detroit, Mich.). Seven days after the fourth injection, the rabbits were bled and the serum was separated. The antiserum was heated at 56°C for 30 min before use.

Preparation of soluble antigen fraction. HeLa cells in 60-mm plastic petri dishes (Nunc, Denmark), containing approximately 5×10^6 cells, were infected with purified virus to give an input multiplicity of 10 plaque-forming units/cell. After 30 min at 37°C, 4 ml of Eagle minimal essential medium (MEM) containing 5% of the regular concentration of methionine, supplemented with 2% calf serum, was added. A 50-μCi portion of [^{35}S]methionine was added to each culture at the indicated time. The harvest of the cells was performed by removing the cells with a rubber policeman, after washing them twice with cold phosphate-buffered saline (PBS). The cells were centrifuged at $1,000 \times g$ for 10 min and resuspended in 0.5 ml of PBS containing 0.5% of the nonionic detergent Nonidet P-40. The cell extract was shaken by a Vortex mixer for 30 s and centrifuged in a Sorvall SS-34 rotor at 10,000 rpm for 20 min. The supernatant referred to as soluble antigen fraction was collected and the pellet was suspended in PBS containing 2% SDS. A soluble antigen fraction of uninfected cells was similarly prepared. For tryptophan labeling, the infected cultures were supplied with Eagle MEM containing 10% of the regular concentration of amino acids, supplemented with 2% calf serum. A 50-μCi amount of the isotope per culture was used.

Radioimmune precipitation reactions. Immune

precipitations were performed by incubating 0.5 ml of the radioactively labeled soluble antigen preparation with 0.5 ml of a 1:5 dilution of the rabbit antiserum in a tapered glass tube at 4°C for 15 h. The mixtures were then centrifuged at 1,000 × g for 10 min. The supernatant fluids were removed, and the pellets were rinsed twice with 1 ml of ice-cold PBS. The washed pellets were drained of excess fluid and resuspended in 0.2 ml of PBS.

Polyacrylamide gel electrophoresis. Gel electrophoresis was performed essentially as described previously (22). Gels (10 by 0.6 cm) were prepared of 7.5% acrylamide, 0.2% N',N-methylene bisacrylamide in 0.1 M sodium phosphate (pH 7.1), and 0.1% SDS. Prior to use, excess catalyst was removed from the gels by electrophoresis at 5 mA/gel for 1 h. The samples for electrophoresis (50 μl) were reduced and dissociated with 2% SDS and 1% mercaptoethanol for 1 min at 100°C. Sucrose was added to 10% and 100 μl was applied to each gel. Electrophoresis was carried out at 3.5 mA/gel for 17 h. After electrophoresis, the gels were placed in 10% trichloroacetic acid, stained with 0.1% Coomassie brilliant blue in 10% trichloroacetic acid, and washed in 7.5% acetic acid. The gels were sliced into 1-mm fractions, the slices were dissolved in H_2O_2, and radioactivity was measured.

Isotopes and drugs. [^{35}S]methionine (290 Ci/mmol) and [^{3}H]tryptophan (6 Ci/mmol) were purchased from the Radiochemical Centre, Amersham, England. IBT was obtained from Schwarz/Mann, Orangeburg, N.Y. A stock solution was freshly prepared before use by dissolving 5 mg in 1 ml of acetone, and then 4 ml of 0.25 N NaOH was added. The drug was further diluted to a final concentration of 14 μM in culture media.

RESULTS

The antiserum used in this study was prepared by repeated inoculations of a purified vaccinia virus (WT, strain WR) preparation into rabbits. As a result, active replication of the virus occurred in the rabbits, and a wide spectrum of antibodies, also to nonstructural proteins, was made. If virus replication induces synthesis of proteins coded for by the genome of the cell, it is unlikely that these proteins would be antigenic for rabbits. Thus, the antiserum prepared would be expected to detect only those proteins coded for by the viral genome. However, it will not detect all of these proteins equally, since viral-induced polypeptides differ in their antigenicity and also in the amount at which they are produced.

First we examined the neutralization capability of the antiserum and its specificity for virus-induced antigens, and then the immunoprecipitate and its polypeptide composition were analyzed.

Neutralization of virus infectivity. The capability of antiserum, prepared with the WT strain, to neutralize the infectivity of the virus was examined. Purified WT virus suspension was incubated with the antiserum diluted 1:10 at 37°C. At time intervals, samples were removed, diluted 100-fold, and kept on ice. The samples were then used to infect monolayers of BSC1 cells. The results presented in Fig. 1 show the kinetics of the neutralization of virus infectivity by the antiserum. Amost 90% of the infectivity was neutralized within the first 3 min, and then the rate of neutralization was reduced. Neutralization of virus infectivity by the antiserum was also observed in embryonated eggs. These findings indicate that the antiserum used in this study was efficient in neutralizing the infectivity of virus in both in vitro and in vivo systems.

Specificity of the immunoprecipitation reaction. The characterization of intracellular viral proteins by immunoprecipitation requires adequate serological specificity and conditions that yield maximal precipitation of viral polypeptides. HeLa cells were infected with a purified stock of the WT strain of vaccinia virus at a multiplicity of infection of 10 plaque-forming units/cell. The radioactively labeled methionine was added 2 h after infection, a time when host-cell protein synthesis was greatly inhibited (3, 5, 9, 14, 16, 18, 20). The cells were harvested 7 h after infection. A soluble antigen fraction was prepared from the cell cytoplasm as described in Materials and Methods. After immunoprecipitation, radioactivity in the trichloroacetic acid-precipitable fraction of the immunoprecipitate was determined. Preliminary studies revealed that a 1:5 dilution of the antiserum was very efficient in the immune precipitation reaction, when undiluted soluble antigen fraction was used.

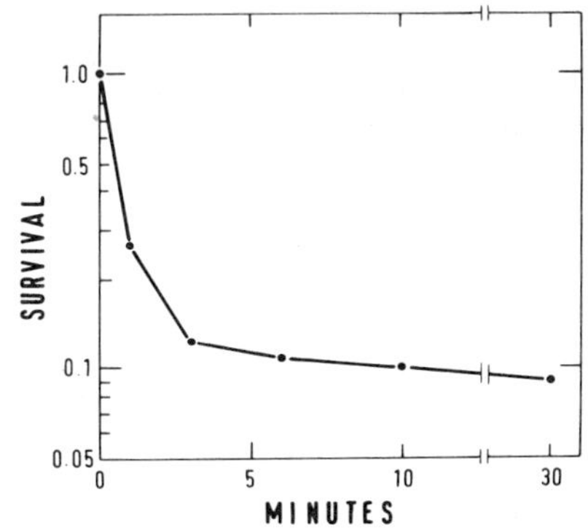

FIG. 1. *Kinetics of neutralization of infectious vaccinia virus. A suspension of purified vaccinia virus (WT strain) was incubated with antiserum at 37°C. At time intervals, samples were removed and virus infectivity was determined by plaque assay in BSC1 cells.*

Since the antiserum was prepared in the rabbits against purified virus grown in HeLa cells, we wished to determine whether formation of antibodies against antigens of uninfected HeLa cells was also induced in the animals. This would also enable antigens of uninfected cells to be precipitated by the antiserum. Another question that was raised was whether rabbit serum, before starting the immunization procedure, was capable of precipitating viral antigens. The results presented in Table 1 show that the immune serum precipitated 100-fold more labeled antigens from infected cells than from uninfected cells and that the serum from the preimmunized rabbit precipitated less than 2% of proteins, as compared with labeled proteins precipitated by the rabbit antiserum.

Identification of viral polypeptides in the immunoprecipitate. The virus-induced polypeptides, which are made in cells after vaccinia virus infection, are divided into two groups (17, 25). The first consists of viral polypeptides, the synthesis of which takes place before initiation of synthesis of the viral DNA. These polypeptides are "early" ones and are made also when DNA synthesis is blocked by inhibitors of DNA synthesis. The second group are the "late" polypeptides, which are produced after synthesis of the viral DNA. Since IBT affects late stages during vaccinia virus growth, we examined the viral antigens formed during this period. Cells were labeled with [^{35}S]methionine between 4 and 7 h after infection with vaccinia virus and then were harvested. The [^{35}S]methionine-labeled polypeptides of the cell cytoplasm were separated by polyacrylamide gel electrophoresis (Fig. 2A). When the soluble antigen fraction of these cells was run in the gels, a similar pattern was obtained (Fig. 2B). However, in the immunoprecipitate (Fig. 2C), mainly three polypeptide peaks were observed, one migrating at 2 cm and the other two located at the gel area between 4 and 5 cm. The first migrates in the gel region, which is characteristic for the polypeptide P4a, a high-molecular-weight precursor of the virion core polypeptide 4a (12, 13, 15). The identification of this polypeptide as P4a can be confirmed by its tryptophan deficiency (12). Infected cells were labeled with [^{3}H]tryptophan. The high-molecular-weight polypeptide was very poorly labeled, as compared with the other polypeptides of the cytoplasmic extract (Fig. 2D), of the soluble antigen fraction (Fig. 2E), and of the immunoprecipitate (Fig. 2F), thus confirming its identification as P4a.

Synthesis of viral antigens in the presence of IBT. Two mutants of vaccinia virus were isolated by us recently: one is resistant to IBT (IBT^{R}) and another requires IBT for growth (IBT dependent, IBT^{D}) (11). The use of the IBT^{R} mutant in the present study was helpful in distinguishing specific effects of IBT on the synthesis of viral antigens of the WT strain from nonspecific effects resulting from toxicity of the drug for the host cell. We also wished to find out whether there are viral antigens of the IBT-dependent mutant that are not formed in the absence of IBT.

Since the total radioactivity of the immunoprecipitate represents almost exclusively viral-induced polypeptides (Table 1), we first studied the values obtained with the three virus strains, WT, IBT^{R}, and IBT^{D}, in the absence and presence of IBT. The results are summarized in Table 2. The amount of the IBT^{R}-labeled antigens in the immunoprecipitate from infected cultures grown in the absence of IBT appeared quite similar to that of cultures treated with IBT. However, the values were quite different for the WT strain, where more than twice the labeled antigens were precipitated when the virus was grown in the absence of the drug than in its presence. On the other hand, the radioactivity of the IBT^{D}-labeled antigens precipitated by the antiserum was more

TABLE 1. *Immunoprecipitation of labeled proteins from uninfected and infected cells*[a]

Cells	Radioactivity: Soluble antigen fraction (cpm)	Immunoprecipitate: Preimmune serum cpm	Preimmune serum %	Immune serum cpm	Immune serum %
Uninfected	3,568,065	1,087	0.03	1,954	0.05
Infected	4,653,565	4,745	0.10	239,323	5.14

[a] HeLa cells were labeled with [^{35}S]methionine (15 μCi/culture) starting at 2 h after infection with the WT strain of vaccinia virus. The cells were harvested at 7 h after infection. Uninfected cells were labeled in parallel. The sera used for the immunoprecipitation were rabbit sera taken before the first injection of the antigen and at the end of the immunization procedure. The radioactivities of the soluble antigen fraction and the immunoprecipitate, after precipitation in cold trichloroacetic acid, were determined and calculated per culture.

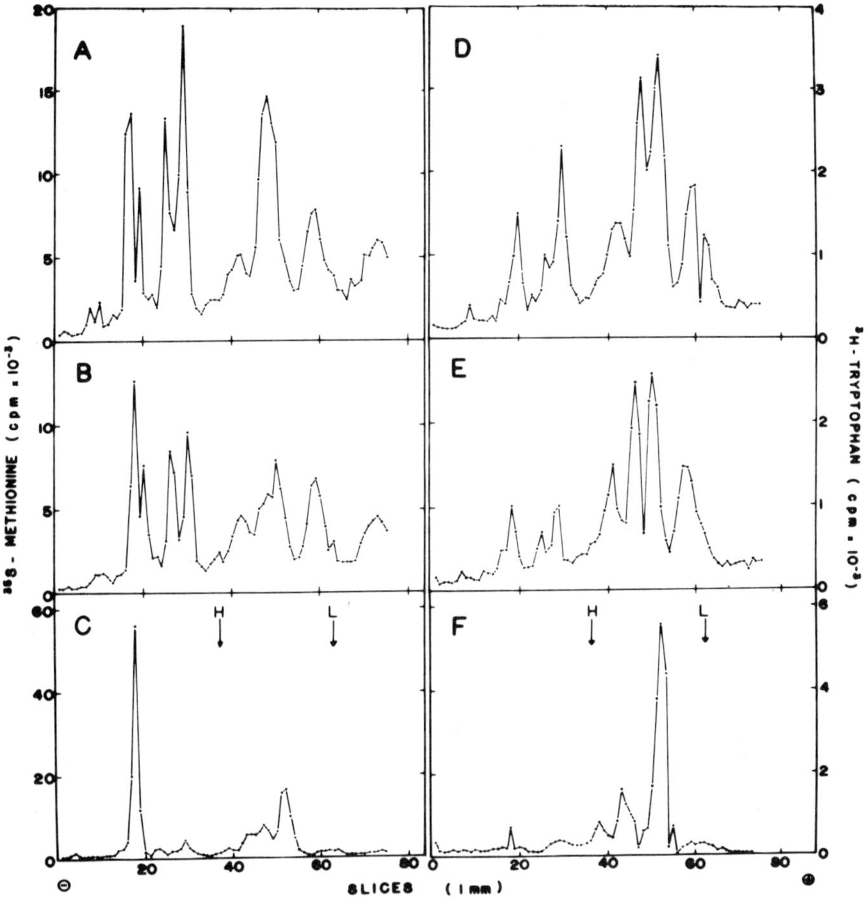

FIG. 2. *Gel electrophoresis of "late" viral polypeptides. Cells were labeled with [^{35}S]methionine or [^{3}H]tryptophan between 4 and 7 h and then harvested. The profiles of the labeled polypeptides (after gel electrophoresis) of the cell cytoplasm (A and D), the soluble antigen fraction (B and E), and the immunoprecipitate (C and F) are presented. The internal polypeptide markers of the immunoprecipitate are the heavy (H) and light (L) chains of rabbit gamma globulin stained with Coomassie brilliant blue.*

TABLE 2. *Immunoprecipitation of "late" proteins from WT-, IBT^{R}-, and IBT^{D}-infected cells synthesized in the absence and presence of IBT*[a]

Virus strain	Radioactivity of the immunoprecipitate		
	cpm		−IBT/+IBT
	−IBT	+IBT	
WT	71,500	33,700	2.12
IBT^{R}	56,500	49,800	1.13
IBT^{D}	21,120	48,740	0.43

[a] Infected cells were labeled with [^{35}S]methionine between 4 and 7 h after infection and then harvested. The soluble antigen fraction was prepared, and the immune precipitation reaction was carried out as described in Materials and Methods. The radioactivity of the immunoprecipitate was determined after precipitation in cold trichloroacetic acid. Each value represents an average of three experiments.

than twice as high when the cultures were grown in the presence of IBT as in its absence. It can be concluded that almost 50% of the viral antigens precipitated by the antiserum are formed under the nonpermissive conditions, either when the WT strain is grown in the presence of IBT or when the IBT^{D} mutant is grown in the absence of the drug.

Next we analyzed the labeled antigens of the immunoprecipitate, to determine whether the decrease in the radioactivity is quantitative rather than qualitative. The immunoprecipitates were dissolved by treatment with SDS and mercaptoethanol at 100°C, and the polypeptides were separated by SDS-polyacrylamide gel electrophoresis. Equal amounts of radioactivity (approximately 100,000 cpm) of each sample were applied to each gel. The results are presented in Fig. 3. In the WT-infected cells, it

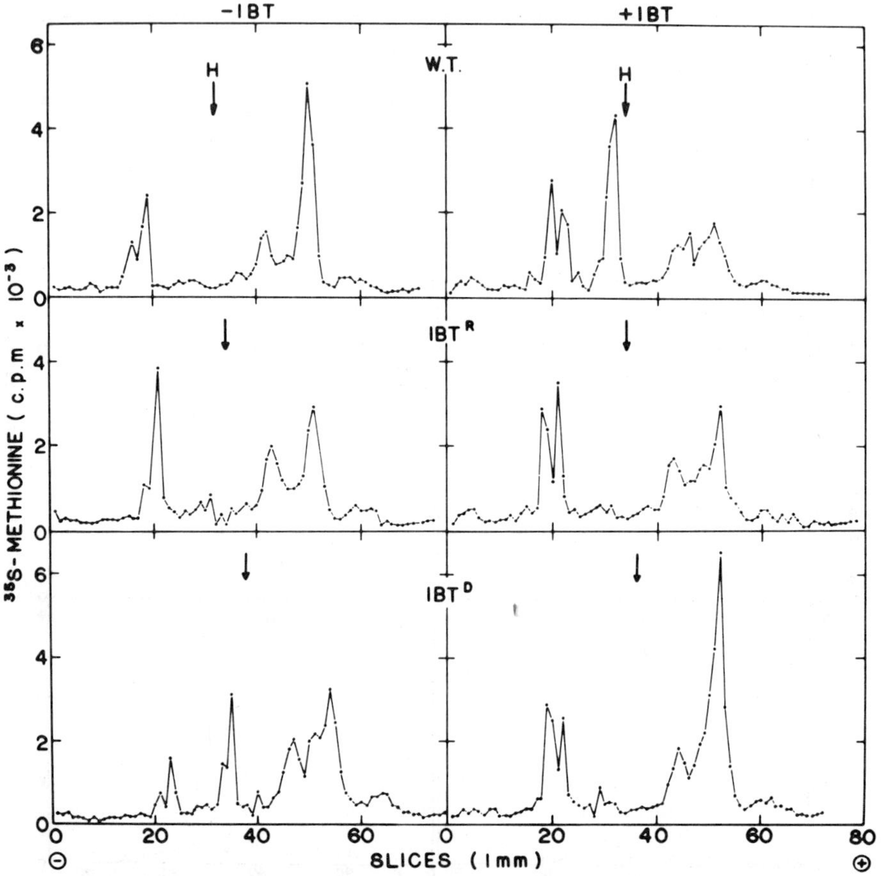

FIG. 3. *Gel electrophoresis of the polypeptides of the immunoprecipitates. Cells were infected with the WT strain of vaccinia virus and with the two mutants, IBT^R and IBT^D, in the absence and presence of IBT (14 μM). The cells were labeled with [^{35}S]methionine from 4 to 7 h after infection. The polypeptides of the immunoprecipitates were separated by polyacrylamide gel electrophoresis.*

is possible to detect all the main viral polypeptides, which are synthesized in the absence of IBT, in the IBT-treated cells. There is one prominent radioactive peak formed in the presence of IBT (at gel slice 32) that appears in significantly smaller amounts in the absence of IBT. This peak is the virus core polypeptide 4b, which is known to be integrated into virus particles during virus maturation (13). Because the block in virus maturation occurred in the presence of IBT, this polypeptide may fail, to a certain extent, to integrate into the forming virus structures and therefore is found in excess in the soluble antigen fraction and in the immunoprecipitate derived from the IBT-treated cells. The immunoprecipitate of the IBT^R mutant, obtained from cultures grown in the absence and presence of IBT, consists of a similar labeled polypeptide profile, except that the high-molecular-weight polypeptide (P4a) appears at a somewhat higher level in the presence of IBT. In the immunoprecipitate of the IBT^D mutant, all the main virus antigens are seen in both the absence and presence of IBT. Polypeptide 4b appears in a higher amount in the absence of IBT, perhaps because of partial failure of its integration into the particulate fraction under the nonpermissive growth conditions (absence of IBT).

It is possible to conclude that the decrease in the radioactivity of the immunoprecipitate of the WT infection in the presence of IBT and of the IBT^D infection in the absence of IBT is quantitative rather than qualitative.

DISCUSSION

The methods previously used to determine whether IBT prevents synthesis of vaccinia viral antigens were complement fixation, fluorescent antibody staining and precipitation in agar. In the last few years, a technique was introduced that enables the analysis and identification of the antigens that comprise the immunoprecipitate by polyacrylamide gel electrophoresis. This method was previously used with adenoviruses (7), influenza virus (2), oncornaviruses (19, 23, 24), and herpes simplex virus (6). Analysis based on this technique enables detection of those virus-induced polypeptides that are efficient antigens, even if they are present in the infected cells in relatively low quantities. It is possible that a virus-induced polypeptide would not be revealed when gel electrophoresis only is used, because its migration is identical to that of another polypeptide. The combined methods of immunoprecipitation and gel electrophoresis can preferably detect a polypeptide when it is a better antigen. The rabbits were injected with infectious purified vaccinia virus grown in HeLa cells. The injected virus caused local infection in the rabbits, so that the antibodies produced were directed against both structural and nonstructural virus-induced polypeptides and not against normal rabbit antigens. Cell extract from uninfected HeLa cells gave very low levels of precipitation with the rabbit antiserum (Table 1). Furthermore, no significant radioactive polypeptide was detected after gel electrophoresis of such an immunoprecipitate (not shown).

By determination of the radioactivity of the immunoprecipitate, it was possible to show that there is approximately a 50% inhibition of viral antigen synthesis between 4 and 7 h after infection as a result of the presence of IBT in WT-infected cells. Similar inhibition was observed in IBT^D-infected cells in the absence of the drug. However, when the immunoprecipitates were analyzed by SDS-polyacrylamide gel electrophoresis, no antigen was missing from the preparation of the WT-infected cells in the presence of the drug or from the IBT^D-infected cells in the absence of the drug. This suggests that the inhibition observed in the total radioactivity of the immunoprecipitate resulted from a slow-down in protein synthesis, due to the block in virus maturation, and not an inhibitory effect on synthesis of a certain polypeptide of the soluble fraction. The failure of Appleyard et al. (1), who followed rabbit pox infection in HeLa cells treated with IBT, to detect few viral antigens by precipitation in agar may be a consequence of the decrease in synthesis of these antigens and the lower sensitivity of the technique of immunoprecipitation in the agar that was used. Although we previously had observed partial inhibition of the cleavage of the polypeptide P4a forming 4a in WT-infected cells in the presence of IBT, and also in IBT^D-infected cells in the absence of the drug, the lower level of 4a was not detected in the present study. The reason for this is that 4a does not appear in the soluble fraction of the cell cytoplasm and its cleavage from P4a is strictly associated with a particulate fraction (13). Only when the total cytoplasmic fraction of the cell is examined, after SDS and mercaptoethanol treatment at 100°C, can the lower amount of 4a be observed.

ACKNOWLEDGMENTS

The continuous interest of N. Goldblum in this work is appreciated. This study was supported by grant no. 690 of the United States-Israel Binational Science Foundation, Jerusalem, Israel.

LITERATURE CITED

1. **Appleyard, G., V. B. M. Hume, and J. C. N. Westwood.** 1965. The effect of thiosemicarbazones on the growth of rabbit pox virus in tissue culture. Ann. N.Y. Acad. Sci. 130:92–104.
2. **Dimmock, N. J., and D. H. Watson.** 1969. Proteins specified by influenza virus in infected cells: analysis by polyacrylamide gel electrophoresis of antigens not present in the virus particle. J. Gen. Virol. 5:499–509.
3. **Dubbs, D. R., and S. Kit.** 1964. Isolation and properties of vaccinia mutants deficient in thymidine kinase inducing activity. Virology 22:214–225.
4. **Easterbrook, K. B.** 1961. Interference with the maturation of vaccinia virus by isatin β thiosemicarbazone. Virology 17:245–251.
5. **Holowczak, J. A., and W. K. Joklik.** 1967. Studies on the structural proteins of vaccinia virus. II. Kinetics of the synthesis of individual groups of structural proteins. Virology 33:726–739.
6. **Honess, R. W., and D. H. Watson.** 1974. Herpes simplex virus specific polypeptides studied by polyacrylamide gel electrophoresis of immune precipitates. J. Gen. Virol. 22:171–185.
7. **Horwitz, M. S., and M. D. Sharff.** 1967. Immunological precipitation of radioactively labeled viral proteins, p. 297–315. *In* K. Habel and N. P. Salzman (ed.), Fundamental techniques in virology. Academic Press Inc., New York.
8. **Joklik, W. K.** 1962. The purification of four strains of poxvirus. Virology 18:9–18.
9. **Joklik, W. K., and T. C. Merigan.** 1966. Concerning the mechanism of action of interferon. Proc. Natl. Acad. Sci. U.S.A. 56:558–565.
10. **Katz, E., E. Margalith, and B. Winer.** 1974. The effect of isatin β thiosemicarbazone (IBT)-related compounds on IBT-resistant and on IBT-dependent mutants of vaccinia virus. J. Gen. Virol. 25:239–244.
11. **Katz, E., E. Margalith, B. Winer, and A. Lazar.** 1973. Characterization and mixed infections of three strains of vaccinia virus: wild type, IBT-resistant and IBT-dependent mutants. J. Gen. Virol. 21:469–475.
12. **Katz, E., and B. Moss.** 1970. Formation of a vaccinia virus structural polypeptide from a higher molecular weight precursor: inhibition by rifampicin. Proc. Natl. Acad. Sci. U.S.A. 66:677–684.
13. **Katz, E., and B. Moss.** 1970. Vaccinia virus structural polypeptide derived from a high molecular weight precursor: formation and integration into virus particles. J. Virol. 6:717–726.
14. **Moss, B.** 1968. Inhibition of HeLa cell protein synthesis by vaccinia virion. J. Virol. 2:1028–1037.
15. **Moss, B., and E. N. Rosenblum.** 1973. Protein cleavage

and poxvirus morphogenesis: tryptic peptide analysis of core precursors accumulated by blocking assembly with rifampicin. J. Mol. Biol. 81:267-269.
16. **Moss, B., and N. P. Salzman.** 1968. Sequential protein synthesis following vaccinia virus infection. J. Virol. 2:1016-1027.
17. **Pennington, T. H.** 1974. Vaccinia virus polypeptide synthesis: sequential appearance and stability of pre and post replicative polypeptides. J. Gen. Virol. 25:433-444.
18. **Salzman, N. P., and E. D. Sebring.** 1967. Sequential formation of vaccinia virus proteins and viral deoxyribonucleic acid replication. J. Virol. 1:16-23.
19. **Shanmugham, G., G. Vecchio, D. Attardi, and M. Green.** 1972. Immunological studies on viral polypeptide synthesis in cells replicating murine sarcoma-leukemia virus. J. Virol. 10:447-455.
20. **Shatkin, A. J.** 1963. The formation of vaccinia virus protein in the presence of 5-fluorodeoxyuridine. Virology 20:292-301.
21. **Sheffield, F. W., D. J. Bauer, and S. Stephenson.** 1960. The protection of tissue cultures by isatin β thiosemicarbazone from the cytopathic effects of certain pox viruses. Br. J. Exp. Pathol 41:638-647.
22. **Summers, D. F., J. V. Maizel, Jr., and J. E. Darnell, Jr.** 1965. Evidence for virus specific non-capsid proteins in poliovirus infected HeLa cells. Proc. Natl. Acad. Sci. U.S.A. 54:505-513.
23. **Van Zaane, D., A. L. J. Gielkens, M. J. A. Dekkens Michielsen, and H. P. J. Bleomers.** 1975. Virus specific precursor polypeptides in cells infected with Rauscher leukemia virus. Virology 67:544-552.
24. **Vogt, V. M., and R. Eisenman.** 1973. Identification of a large polypeptide precursor of avian oncornavirus proteins. Proc. Natl. Acad. Sci. U.S.A. 70:1734-1738.
25. **Woodson, B.** 1968. Recent progress in poxvirus research. Bacteriol. Rev. 32:127-137.
26. **Woodson, B., and W. K. Joklik.** 1965. The inhibition of vaccinia virus multiplication by isatin β thiosemicarbazone. Proc. Natl. Acad. Sci. U.S.A. 54:946-953.

ANTIMICROBIAL AGENTS AND CHEMOTHERAPY, Feb. 1977, p. 209-213 Vol. 11, No. 2

Printed in U.S.A.

Drug Resistance and R Plasmids in *Salmonella typhi* Isolated in Korea

DOKI CHUN,* SUNG YONG SEOL, DONG TAEK CHO, AND RYUNBIN TAK

Department of Bacteriology, Kyungpook National University School of Medicine, Taegu, Korea

Received for publication 17 June 1976

A total of 949 strains of *Salmonella typhi* isolated in Korea from 1968 to 1975 were tested for drug resistance and distribution of R plasmids. Resistance was mostly restricted to streptomycin (SM) and sulfisomidine (SA), singly or in combination, at a low degree. A small number of strains (1.5%) were resistant to four or more drugs: chloramphenicol (CM), tetracycline (TC), SM, SA, ampicillin (AP), and kanamycin (KM). No strain was resistant to nalidixic acid or to a 1:20 mixture of trimethoprim and sulfamethoxazole. Nor was there any strain singly resistant to CM, TC, AP, or KM. Transfer experiments of multiple-drug resistance to *Escherichia coli* ML1410 showed that all the strains resistant to four or more drugs carried R plasmids, whereas those weakly resistant to three or less drugs did not. The quadruply resistant strains carried one R plasmid determining CM, TC, SM, and SA resistance, and sextuply resistant ones carried two plasmids, one determining CM, TC, SM, and SA resistance and the other determining AP and KM resistance. One strain carrying a plasmid determining AP and KM resistance was also found. The transfer frequency of CM, TC, SM, and SA resistance was much higher than that of AP and KM resistance. The resistance of *S. typhi* was more efficiently transferred to *E. coli* at 25°C than at 37°C.

Typhoid fever is prevalent throughout the year in Korea, probably due to unsanitary conditions. The cases reported to the public health authorities amount to approximately 4,000 annually (6), but this represents only a small portion of actual incidences. Since many cases are treated without being reported, the real number of patients would be several times higher than that reported.

The drug resistance of *Salmonella typhi* in Korea has been reported by several workers, with the indication that most strains are susceptible to chloramphenicol (CM), tetracycline (TC), ampicillin (AP), and some other drugs, with only a small number of strains resistant to one or more drugs (2, 5, 6, 8). In contrast to a large number of reports on multiply resistant and R plasmid strains of *Escherichia coli, Shigella,* and *Salmonella* other than *S. typhi,* as reviewed by Mitsuhashi (11), reports on that of *S. typhi* strains are much less frequent (1, 3, 4, 14). This report describes the drug resistance and prevalence of R plasmids in *S. typhi* isolated in Korea during the 8-year period from 1968 to 1975.

MATERIALS AND METHODS

Test strains. A total of 949 strains of *S. typhi* were isolated between 1968 and 1975 in the laboratories of Kyungpook University Hospital, Taegu Presbyterian Hospital, and the National Institute of Health, Korea. They were confirmed biochemically and immunologically, but Vi phage typing was not attempted. The majority of strains were cultured from patients' blood, and a small number were cultured from stools, urine, and other specimens. The strains were maintained in rubber-stoppered, soft nutrient agar stabs, and typical colonies were selected on MacConkey agar plates before use.

Drugs. Freshly prepared solutions of the following drugs were used: CM (Parke, Davis & Co.), TC (Lederle Laboratories), streptomycin (SM; Banyu Seiyaku Co., Japan), sulfisomidine (SA; Daiichi Seiyaku Co., Japan), nalidixic acid (NA; Sterling-Winthrop Laboratories), AP (Beecham Research Laboratories), kanamycin (KM; Banyu Seiyaku Co., Japan), and a 1:20 mixture of trimethoprim (TMP; Burroughs Wellcome Co.) and sulfamethoxazole (SMZ; Roche Co.). TMP was dissolved in 0.1 N lactic acid, SMZ was dissolved in 0.1 N NaOH, and the other drugs were dissolved in appropriate solvents. They were further diluted before use (9, 15).

Test for drug resistance. A plate dilution method was used throughout the study. Brain heart infusion (BHI) (pH 7.2; Difco) agar plates containing serial twofold concentrations of each drug were prepared as described by Williams and Ewing (20). For the test of SA and TMP-SMZ resistance, Mueller-Hinton (pH 7.2; BBL) agar plates containing the drugs were used. The concentration of drugs in the media ranged from 0.2 to 400 μg/ml. Overnight cultures of test strains in BHI broth were diluted 100 times with sterile buffered saline and inoculated in media with a multiple inoculator (17). Results were read after 24 h of incubation at 37°C, and the minimum inhibitory concentration (MIC) was defined as the lowest concentration of drugs that exhibited no growth, except SA and TMP-SMZ, for which the MIC was defined as the lowest concentration of drugs inhibiting confluent growth of large colonies (10). Strains that grew in media containing 12.5 μg of CM, TC, and NA per ml, 25 μg of SM and SA per ml, and 3.1 μg of AP, KM, and TMP-SMZ per ml were considered resistant.

Transfer of drug resistance. The recipient strain used was NA-resistant *E. coli* ML1410, kindly supplied by S. Mitsuhashi, Gunma University School of Medicine, Maebashi, Japan. Single colonies of donor and recipient strains were cultured in BHI broth for 18 h at 37°C. One drop of each culture was inoculated in 5 ml of BHI broth and incubated for 3.5 h with gentle shaking. One milliliter of donor and 4 ml of recipient cultures were mixed and conjugated for 18 h at 37°C and then were spread on BHI or Mueller-Hinton agar plates containing 25 μg of NA per ml and one of the selecting drugs (25 μg of CM, TC, and SM per ml, 100 μg of SA per ml, or 12.5 μg of AP and KM per ml). After incubation for 24 h at 37°C, plates were inspected for colonies of resistant *E. coli*. Ten colonies were picked, purified on MacConkey agar, confirmed to be *E. coli* by biochemical reactions, and tested for the patterns and levels of drug resistance by the plate dilution method. No growth of *S. typhi* on selecting media was confirmed by plating a mixed culture on MacConkey agar containing 25 μg of NA per ml. To count the number of transconjugants, appropriate decimal dilutions of mixed cultures were thoroughly spread on selective media, and colonies were counted after 24 h of incubation. The frequency of resistance transfer was expressed as the number of transconjugants per number of donor cells in mixed cultures at 18 h of incubation (7).

RESULTS

Figure 1 illustrates the antimicrobial spectrum of 949 strains of *S. typhi* tested. Most strains were highly susceptible to AP and, to a lesser degree, to TMP-SMZ, TC, CM, KM, and NA in decreasing order. They were less susceptible to SM and SA, with approximately 10 and 40% resistant strains, respectively. No strain resistant to NA and TMP-SMZ was encountered, but a small number of strains were resistant to AP, TC, CM, and KM. Resistance patterns of *S. typhi* resistant to two or more drugs are shown in Table 1. Thirty-five strains (3.7%) were doubly resistant to SM and SA, followed by 10 (1.1%) strains quadruply resistant to CM, TC, SM, and SA. Three strains (0.3%) were sextuply resistant to CM, TC, SM, SA, AP, and KM, and strains resistant to the other combinations of drugs were very few. No strain singly resistant to CM, TC, AP, and KM was encountered. The resistance level of quadruply resistant strains was fairly high, with an MIC of 100 μg or more per ml to each drug, but the MIC of AP and KM to sextuply resistant strains was low as compared with that of the above four drugs. Strain 73-KH50 was resistant to five drugs but might be considered doubly resistant to AP and KM, since its level of resistance to CM, TC, and SA was very low (Table 2).

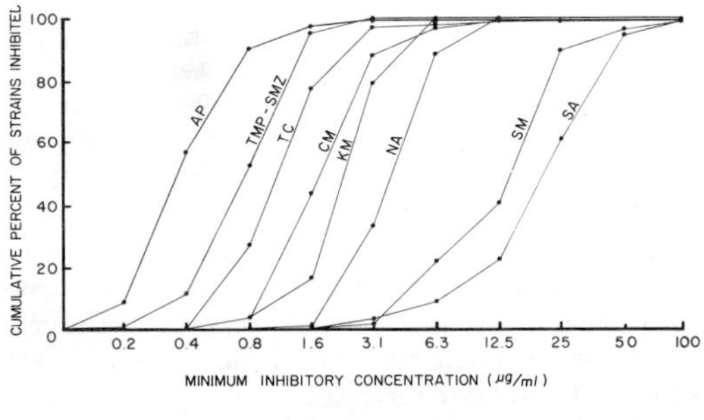

FIG. 1. *Antimicrobial spectrum of S. typhi isolated in Korea. TMP-SMZ, 1:20 mixture.*

TABLE 1. *Multiple drug resistance patterns of S. typhi isolated in Korea from 1968 to 1975*

Multiple drug resistance pattern[a]	No. of strains isolated in: 1968–1970 (119)[b]	1971 (30)	1972 (115)	1973 (113)	1974 (336)	1975 (236)	Total (%) strains isolated (949)
CM, TC, SM, SA, AP, KM	0	0	0	0	3	0	3 (0.3)
CM, TC, SA, AP, KM	0	0	0	1	0	0	1 (0.1)
CM, TC, SM, SA	0	0	1	4	4	1	10 (1.1)
CM, SM, SA	0	0	0	0	1	0	1 (0.1)
TC, SM	0	0	0	0	2	0	2 (0.2)
SM, SA	0	1	2	6	14	12	35 (3.7)
%		0.1	0.3	1.2	2.5	1.4	

[a] Strains that grow in media containing 12.5 μg of CM and TC per ml, 25 μg of SM and SA per ml, and 3.1 μg of AP and KM per ml are considered resistant.

[b] Number of strains tested is given in parentheses.

TABLE 2. *Levels of resistance to drugs of multiply resistant S. typhi*

Strain no.[a]	IC (μg/ml)					
	CM	TC	SM	SA	AP	KM
74-62, 74-D48	200	400	400	>400	25	25
74-KS3	200	100	200	400	100	25
73-KH50	25	25	s[b]	100	50	25
72-45, 73-40	400	200	400	>400	s	s
73-67, 73-KH64	400	200	200	>400	s	s
73-8, 75-131	200	200	400	>400	s	s
74-D12, 74-D18 74-D19, 74-D25	100	200	400	400	s	s
74-D98	25	s	100	100	s	s

[a] Strains resistant to three or more drugs are listed.
[b] s, Susceptible by the criteria described in Table 1.

TABLE 3. *Resistance transfer of multiply resistant strains of S. typhi to E. coli ML1410*

Drug resistance of donor strains	Selecting drugs	Resistance transferred	Strain no.
CM, TC, SM, SA, AP, KM	CM	CM, TC, SM, SA	74-62, 74-D48
(2 strains)	TC	CM, TC, SM, SA	
	SM	CM, TC, SM, SA	
	SA	CM, TC, SM, SA	
	AP	AP, KM	
	KM	AP, KM	
CM, TC, SM, SA	CM	CM, TC, SM, SA	72-45, 73-40
(10 strains)	TC	CM, TC, SM, SA	73-67, 73-KH64
	SM	CM, TC, SM, SA	73-8, 74-D12
	SA	CM, TC, SM, SA	74-D18, 74-D19
			74-D25, 75-131
CM, TC, SM, SA, AP, KM	CM	CM	74-KS3
(1 strain)	TC	–[a]	
	SM	–	
	SA	–	
	AP	AP, KM	
	KM	AP, KM	
CM, TC, SA, AP, KM	CM	–	73-KH50
(1 strain)	TC	–	
	SA	–	
	AP	AP, KM	
	KM	AP, KM	

[a] –, Resistance not transferred.

All the other strains singly, doubly, and triply resistant to drugs were only weakly resistant, with the level of resistance barely exceeding the MIC.

A resistance transfer experiment (Table 3) indicated that all strains quadruply resistant to CM, TC, SM, and SA consistently transferred their complete resistance to the recipient in any case where one of the four drugs was used as the selecting agent. Sextuply resistant strains transferred two different patterns of resistance, CM, TC, SM, and SA resistance and AP and KM resistance, suggesting that these strains were infected with two R plasmids. One strain (74-KS3) transferred CM resistance and AP and KM resistance, and one other (73-KH50), which was resistant to five drugs, transferred AP and KM resistance only. The other strains, resistant to three or fewer drugs, did not transfer the resistance to the recipient even when selected with lower concentrations of drugs. Purified transconjugants obtained by transfer experiment were tested for resistance to drugs, and all of them were found to maintain the same patterns and degrees of resistance as those of the donor strains when 10 randomly selected colonies of transconjugants were tested. To eliminate the possibility of transduction by phages, culture filtrates of donor strains were tested, and all of them were confirmed not to transfer the resistance to the recipient. The transfer frequency of CM, TC, SM, and SA resistance from *S. typhi* to *E. coli* was from $10^{-3.0}$ to $10^{-4.9}$ at 18 h of incubation at 37°C, and that of AP and KM resistance was from $10^{-5.3}$ to $10^{-6.7}$. Each selecting drug produced an almost similar degree of transfer frequency within a single donor strain, and the difference in frequency was marked by donor strains rather than by selecting drugs. With some randomly selected, quadruply resistant *S. typhi,* the transfer frequency was compared at two temperatures (Table 4), and conjugation at 25°C was found to result in a much higher frequency than that at 37°C.

DISCUSSION

Many reports have appeared on the emergence of *S. typhi* resistant to CM, and this resistance was frequently accompanied by resistance to other drugs (1, 3, 4, 12–14, 19). However, in spite of the extensive use of CM for the treatment of typhoid fever for more than 15 years, CM-resistant strains were rare in Korea, as shown in this study and in other works (2, 5, 8). The frequency of *S. typhi* multiply resistant to drugs was very low among our isolates, as compared with results obtained in the United States (16.5%) (3). Our quadruply resistant strains carried exclusively one R plasmid causing CM, TC, SM, and SA resistance, as reported in the United States and Vietnam (3, 4), and sextuply resistant strains carried one more factor causing AP and KM resistance, as noted for strains in Mexico (14). An R plasmid causing TC resistance was noted among strains isolated in Mexico, but none has been noted in Korean strains as yet. The complete patterns of transferable resistance of *S. typhi* will require further studies. Some strains were weakly resistant to three or fewer drugs and were proved not to carry transmissible R plasmids within the limits of our test and with the recipient strains used.

TABLE 4. *Frequency of resistance transfer of S. typhi to E. coli at different temperatures*

Strain no.	Selecting drug	Transfer frequency[a] at conjugation temp of: 25°C	37°C
73-8	CM	$10^{-1.0}$	$10^{-3.7}$
	TC	$10^{-1.0}$	$10^{-3.9}$
	SM	$10^{-1.0}$	$10^{-4.3}$
	SA	$10^{-1.3}$	$10^{-3.8}$
73-40	CM	$10^{-1.3}$	$10^{-4.8}$
	TC	$10^{-1.2}$	$10^{-4.7}$
	SM	$10^{-1.0}$	$10^{-4.9}$
	SA	$10^{-1.2}$	$10^{-4.9}$
74-D12	CM	$10^{-0.7}$	$10^{-3.3}$
	TC	$10^{-1.5}$	$10^{-3.1}$
	SM	$10^{-1.6}$	$10^{-3.0}$
74-D48	CM	$10^{-2.2}$	$10^{-3.7}$
	TC	$10^{-1.6}$	$10^{-3.9}$
	SM	$10^{-2.7}$	$10^{-4.3}$
	SA	$10^{-2.0}$	$10^{-3.8}$

[a] Transfer frequency was calculated as the number of exconjugants per number of donor cells after 18 h of incubation at 37°C.

The multiple-drug resistance of *S. typhi* was transferred more easily at 25°C than at 37°C, as observed in *S. typhimurium* (18), and this result suggests that receipt of multiple resistance by *S. typhi* would be more easily attained in defecated stools during warm seasons, when the ambient temperature is approximately 25°C, than in the intestinal canal. The transfer of multiple resistance to *S. typhi* from *E. coli* of various origins is being studied at different temperatures.

The occurrence of R plasmids in *S. typhi* is a warning to physicians, as well as to public health authorities, especially where the isolation of patients and the supervision of carriers are not well controlled. The presence of these strains also suggests the possibilities of epidemics due to these organisms (14) and of a yearly increase in R plasmid strains (4). Fortunately, the emergence of these strains was very infrequent when compared with that of *E. coli* and *Shigella* (11, 18).

LITERATURE CITED

1. **Anderson, E. S., and H. R. Smith.** 1972. Chloramphenicol resistance in the typhoid bacillus. Br. Med. J. 3:329–331.
2. **Baik, S. H., H. K. Lee, Y. H. Kim, J. M. Park, and J. S. Chun.** 1970. Resistance of *Salmonella typhi* to various antimicrobial agents. (In Korean) Korean J. Mod. Med. 2:155–159.
3. **Bissett, M. L., S. L. Abbott, and R. M. Wood.** 1974. Antimicrobial resistance and R factors in *Salmonella* isolated in California (1971–1972). Antimicrob. Agents Chemother. 5:161–168.
4. **Butler, T., N. N. Linh, K. Arnold, and M. Pollack.** 1973. Chloramphenicol resistant typhoid fever in Vietnam associated with R factor. Lancet ii:983–985.
5. **Chun, D.** 1964. A review of *Salmonella* and *Shigella* in Korea. Endemic Dis. Bull. Nagasaki Univ. (Japan) 6:125–138.
6. **Chun, D., and I. S. Suh.** 1971. *Salmonella* in the Republic of Korea. J. Res. Inst. Med. Sci. (Korea) 3:489–497.
7. **Davey, R. B., and J. Pittard.** 1974. Genetic and biophysical study of R plasmids conferring sulfonamide resistance in *Shigella* strains isolated in 1952 and 1956. J. Bacteriol. 120:1186–1195.

8. **Kong, J. K., D. W. Lee, H. W. Yoon, D. H. Ahn, and H. S. Lee.** 1971. Types of *Salmonella* and *Shigella* isolated from patients in Taegu in 1971. (In Korean) Korean Cent. J. Med. 21:433-436.
9. **MacLowry, J. D., M. J. Jaqua, and S. T. Selepak.** 1970. Detailed methodology and implementation of a semiautomated serial dilution microtechnique for antimicrobial susceptibility testing. Appl. Microbiol. 20:46-53.
10. **Marks, M. I., M. Kazemi, and E. MacKay.** 1973. In vitro sensitivity of *Salmonella* to ten antimicrobial agents including sulfamethoxazole and trimethoprim, alone and in combination. Antimicrob. Agents Chemother. 4:555-559.
11. **Mitsuhashi, S.** 1969. The R factor. J. Infect. Dis. 119:89-100.
12. **Murti, B. R., K. Rajavalakshmi, and C. S. Bhaskaren.** 1962. Resistance of *Salmonella typhi* to chloramphenicol. J. Clin. Pathol. 15:544-554.
13. **Nare, I. J.** 1967. Drug resistance in *Salmonella typhosa*. S. Afr. Med. J. 41:703-704.
14. **Olarte, J., and E. Galindo.** 1973. *Salmonella typhi* resistant to chloramphenicol, ampicillin, and other antimicrobial agents: strains isolated during an extensive typhoid fever epidemic in Mexico. Antimicrob. Agents Chemother. 4:597-601.
15. **Rudoy, R. C., J. D. Nelson, and K. C. Haltalin.** 1974. In vitro susceptibility of *Shigella* strains to trimethoprim and sulfamethoxazole. Antimicrob. Agents Chemother. 5:439-443.
16. **Sato, G., H. Kodama, and N. Terakado.** 1974. Detection of an R factor showing temperature-sensitive transfer in *Salmonella typhimurium* isolated from calves. Antimicrob. Agents Chemother. 5:541-543.
17. **Steers, E., E. L. Flotz, and B. S. Graves.** 1959. Inocula replicating apparatus for routine testing of bacterial susceptibility to antibiotics. Antibiot. Chemother. 9:307-311.
18. **Tanaka, T., K. Ikemura, M. Tsunoda, T. Sasakawa, and S. Mitsuhashi.** 1976. Drug resistance and distribution of R factors in *Salmonella* strains. Antimicrob. Agents Chemother. 9:61-64.
19. **Vasquez, V., E. Calderon, and R. S. Rodriquez.** 1972. Chloramphenicol-resistant strains of *Salmonella typhosa*. N. Engl. J. Med. 286:1220.
20. **Williams, R. B., and W. H. Ewing.** 1964. The susceptibility of *Shigella* and *Escherichia* to antimicrobial agents. Communicable Disease Center, Atlanta.

ANTIMICROBIAL AGENTS AND CHEMOTHERAPY, Feb. 1977, p. 214-218 Vol. 11, No. 2

Pharmacokinetics of Amikacin During Hemodialysis and Peritoneal Dialysis

LISBETH REGEUR, HANNE COLDING,* HERLUF JENSEN, AND JENS P. KAMPMANN

Department of Clinical Bacteriology, Clinical Pharmacology Research Unit, Medical Department P, Division of Nephrology, Rigshospitalet, University of Copenhagen, Copenhagen, Denmark

Received for publication 21 September 1976

The pharmacokinetics of amikacin were examined in six bilaterally nephrectomized patients undergoing hemodialysis and in four patients with a minimal residual renal function undergoing peritoneal dialysis. The mean elimination half-life before the dialysis was 86.5 h in the anephric patients and 44.3 h in the patients with minimal residual kidney function. The results from the anephric patients suggest that some extrarenal elimination of amikacin may occur. The mean volume of distribution was about 25% of the total body weight. This is in accordance with values reported from subjects with normal renal function. During hemodialysis the half-life decreased to less than 10% (5.6 h) of the pretreatment value. The effectiveness of peritoneal dialysis was less as the half-life decreased to only about 30% (17.9 h) of the pretreatment value. During the dialyses a significant correlation between the half-life of amikacin and the decrease in blood urea and serum creatinine was demonstrated. The pharmacokinetic data were used to make dosage regimen recommendations for the treatment of patients undergoing intermittent hemodialysis or peritoneal dialysis.

Amikacin is a new semisynthetic aminoglycoside antibiotic with kinetics and toxicity similar to those of kanamycin (4, 5, 7). The antimicrobial activity differs, however, as amikacin is active against various isolates of gram-negative bacilli resistant to other aminoglycosides including kanamycin, gentamicin, and tobramycin (10, 12, 17).

Severe bacterial infections are common in uremic patients, and treatment with aminoglycosides is often required. Like other aminoglycosides, amikacin is mainly eliminated by glomerular filtration of the unchanged drug, and a correlation between the elimination half-life and the serum creatinine concentration in patients with varying degrees of reduced renal function has recently been demonstrated (13, 15).

The purpose of the present study has been to evaluate the kinetics of amikacin in bilaterally nephrectomized patients undergoing hemodialysis and in patients with minimal residual renal function undergoing peritoneal dialysis. The kinetics have been investigated both before and during the dialyses.

MATERIALS AND METHODS

Patients. Ten patients, five females and five males, were studied. Their ages ranged from 23 to 58 years, and their weights ranged from 41 to 76 kg. All of the patients had terminal renal insufficiency that required regular treatment with dialysis. Six of the patients were nephrectomized bilaterally and treated with intermittent hemodialysis. The other four patients had an endogenous creatinine clearance between 2.8 and 4.9 ml/min and were treated with intermittent peritoneal dialysis. All patients were treated as outpatients, and they were in reasonably good health during the study. The weight varied maximally 4.3% during the dialyses and not more than 2.9% between the dialyses. The patients did not receive any other medication during the study. None of the patients suffered from edema or ascites.

Informed consent was obtained from each patient after an explanation of the risks and inconveniences reasonably to be expected.

Dialysis. The hemodialysis was performed twice weekly over 7 to 10 h. In five cases a plate kidney (type Gambro-Lundia Optima; 17 μm) was used, and in one case (see Table 1, patient no. 2) a capillary kidney (Cordis Dow model 4) was used. The peritoneal dialysis was performed once weekly with a Tenckhoff catheter, using about 60 liters of dialyzing fluid over a period of about 30 h.

Administration of antibiotic. A 125-mg amount of amikacin dissolved in 200 ml of isotonic saline was infused intravenously over a period of 1 h in all patients immediately after dialysis (1.7 to 3.1 mg/kg). Blood samples for the determination of amikacin, creatinine, and urea were drawn 1 h after termination of the infusion and once or twice daily until the next dialysis. During the hemodialysis four blood samples were taken every 2 to 3 h, beginning at the onset of the dialysis. In patients undergoing peritoneal dialysis five samples were drawn every 5 to 6 h.

Antibiotic assay. The serum concentration of amikacin was measured microbiologically with filter paper disks (19). A laboratory strain of *Bacillus subtilis* was used as the test organism. The intra- and interassay variation was below 5%.

Data analysis. The pharmacokinetic parameters were calculated according to an open one-compartment model.

(i) Elimination half-life. Elimination half-life was obtained from the linear part of the curve of log concentration versus time by a least-squares regression.

(ii) Apparent volume of distribution. Apparent volume of distribution was calculated by dividing the dose given with the extrapolated zero concentration obtained in the period before the dialysis.

(iii) Total body clearance of amikacin. Total body clearance of amikacin was calculated from the above data according to the formula: clearance = $(0.693 \cdot V_d)/T_{1/2}$, where V_d is the apparent volume of distribution and $T_{1/2}$ is the elimination half-life. In the model used, both the apparent volume of distribution and clearance are slightly overestimated. The error, however, is minor because of the very rapid tissue distribution of all aminoglycosides.

The data were subjected to statistical evaluation, using Student's *t* test and linear correlation analysis.

RESULTS

The measured and calculated parameters are shown in Table 1. The mean elimination half-life was 86.5 h (range, 56.1 to 150.6 h) in the six anephric patients and 44.3 h (range, 33.5 to 49.9 h) in the four patients with minimal residual renal function. The total body clearance was 1.6 ± 0.5 and 2.5 ± 0.4 ml/min (mean ± standard deviation) in the two groups, respectively. These differences are significant ($P < 0.05$). The mean volumes of distribution expressed as a percentage of the total body weight were 28.1 and 25.8%, respectively. No significant difference was found between these two values ($P > 0.05$).

During dialysis the half-lives decreased and the total body clearances increased significantly ($P < 0.01$) in both groups. In the patients hemodialyzed the half-life decreased to a mean value of 5.6 h (range, 4.1 to 7.3 h), and in the group subjected to peritoneal dialysis it decreased to a mean value of 17.9 h (range, 13.6 to 21.1 h). The increase in serum creatinine and blood urea before the dialyses equaled the decrease resulting from the dialyses ($P > 0.05$).

Figure 1 shows the logarithmic decline of the serum concentrations of amikacin in the individual patients. After an initial phase of distribution the mean serum concentration was 8.1 μg/ml in the group undergoing hemodialysis (mean body weight, 55.2 ± 11.5 kg) and 5.9 μg/ml in the group undergoing peritoneal dialysis (mean body weight, 67.2 ± 6.3 kg). Immediately before the next dialysis the values had decreased to 5.1 and 2.9 μg/ml, respectively. After termination of the dialysis the mean value of amikacin in the patients treated with hemodialysis was 2.0 μg/ml (a decrease of 61%), whereas the patients treated with peritoneal dialysis had a mean value of 0.8 μg/ml (a decrease of 72%).

Figures 2 and 3 show a significant inverse correlation between the half-life of amikacin during the dialysis and the decrease in the concentrations of serum creatinine and blood urea, respectively ($r = -0.88$ and -0.71; $P < 0.05$).

DISCUSSION

The present study shows that amikacin in common with other aminoglycosides has a prolonged half-life in patients with reduced renal function. Although most of the drug is excreted unchanged by the renal route, the decay of the serum concentration in six patients without kidneys shows that some extrarenal elimination may occur. In accordance with this finding, only about 90% of a parenteral dose is recovered in urine (7). A comparison between the anephric patients and the patients with minimal residual renal function shows that even an endogenous creatinine clearance of about 3 ml/min results in a significantly lower half-life of amikacin in the latter group. The average serum concentration of creatinine before dialysis in the four patients on peritoneal dialysis was about 12 mg/100 ml, and the measured average half-life of 44.3 h is in good agreement with the values presented by Levy and Klastersky (13). A volume of distribution of about 0.25 liter/kg is in accordance with the values reported from subjects with normal renal function (4, 5), indicating that the delayed excretion does not influence the distribution of the drug.

The pharmacokinetics of the aminoglycosides during dialysis have been reported in several works (1, 6, 8, 9, 14). It has been shown that the serum concentrations of kanamycin, gentamicin, and tobramycin decreased more than 70% during an 8- to 10-h period of hemodialysis (Kiil dialyzer), and during peritoneal dialysis the serum concentrations of kanamycin and tobramycin have been shown to decrease 32 and 65% during 22 and 12 h of dialysis, respectively (2, 16).

The present study shows that amikacin is also substantially cleared from the body of anephric patients during hemodialysis, with a de-

TABLE 1. *Pharmacokinetic parameters of amikacin before and during hemodialysis and peritoneal dialysis*

Patient no.	V_d[a] (% of total body weight)	Before dialysis				During dialysis			
		Half-life (h)	Clearance of amikacin (ml/min per m²)	Increase in blood urea (mmol/liter)	Increase in serum creatinine (mmol/liter)	Half-life (h)	Clearance of amikacin (ml/min per m²)	Decrease in blood urea (mmol/liter)	Decrease in serum creatinine (mmol/liter)
Hemodialysis									
1	34.3	56.1	2.2	17.5	0.44	4.6	25.9	20.7	0.45
2	29.6	79.0	2.1	27.6	0.63	4.1	27.1	25.6	0.61
3	34.8	150.6	1.6	21.8	0.87	5.3	27.3	22.7	0.94
4	29.9	84.5	2.0	24.9	0.80	6.4	17.6	24.5	0.77
5	15.1	63.0	1.0	11.5	0.41	7.3	15.5	22.0	0.69
6	24.6	85.6	1.2	12.4	0.49	6.0	17.0	14.3	0.47
Mean ± SD[b]	28.1 ±6.7	86.5 ± 30.7	1.6 ± 0.5	19.3 ± 6.0	0.61 ± 0.18	5.6 ± 1.1	21.5 ± 5.1	21.6 ± 3.6	0.66 ± 0.17
Peritoneal dialysis									
7	21.3	49.0	1.9	9.8	0.31	21.1	4.4	8.5	0.20
8	32.1	44.7	3.0	5.5	0.20	16.1	8.4	14.5	0.39
9	27.9	49.9	2.3	8.0	0.28	13.6	8.5	15.7	0.63
10	21.7	33.5	2.9	0.0	0.04	20.9	4.6	9.5	0.30
Mean ± SD	25.8 ± 4.5	44.3 ± 6.5	2.5 ± 0.04	5.8 ± 3.7	0.21 ± 0.10	17.9 ± 3.2	6.4 ± 2.0	12.1 ± 3.6	0.38 ± 0.18

[a] V_d, Apparent volume of distribution.
[b] SD, Standard deviation.

crease in half-life to less than 10% of the pretreatment values, approaching the value of 2 h in humans with normal kidney function (4, 5). The effectiveness of peritoneal dialysis is less as the half-life is decreased to only about 30% of the pretreatment value.

The serum concentration of amikacin prior to dialysis was 3 to 6 μg/ml in most of the patients. The highest concentrations were found in patients on hemodialysis, which is to be expected from the smaller total body weight. After dialysis the concentration decreased to levels less than 2 μg/ml, which is below the minimum inhibitory concentration for various isolates of bacterial strains (11). The toxic peak

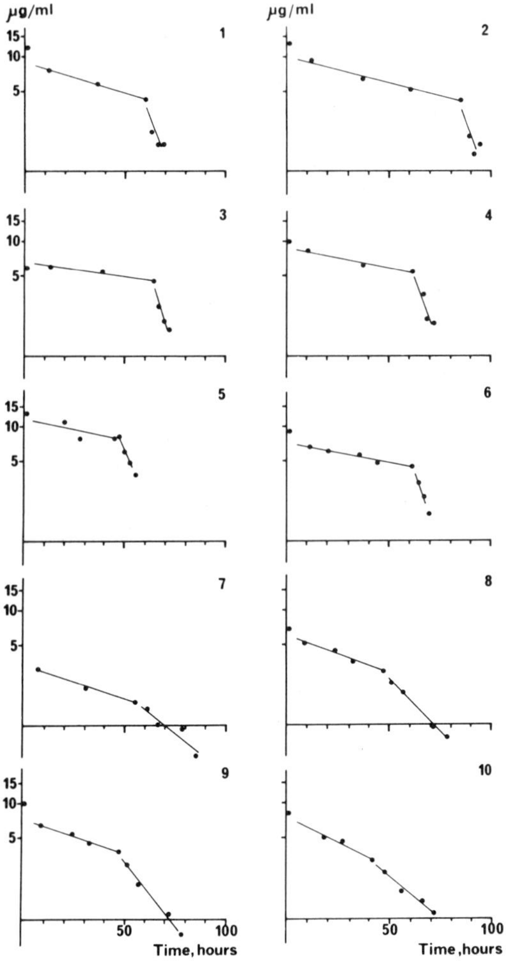

FIG. 1. *Serum concentrations of amikacin before and during dialysis in six patients undergoing hemodialysis (patients 1 to 6) and in four patients undergoing peritoneal dialysis (patients 7 to 10). The regression lines have been calculated by the method of least squares.*

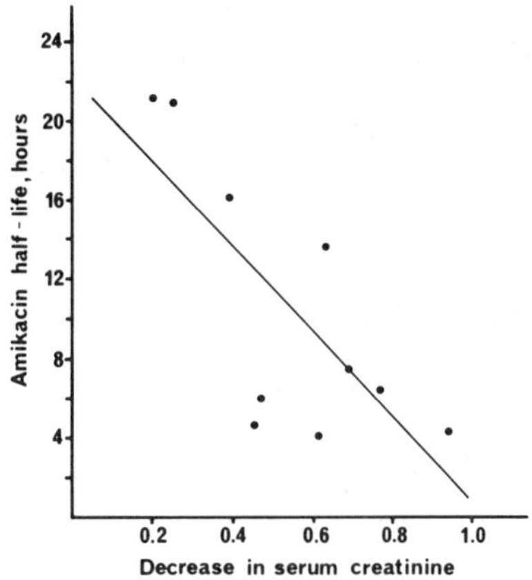

FIG. 2. *Correlation between the half-life of amikacin and the decrease in serum creatinine during hemodialysis and peritoneal dialysis. $r = -0.71$; $P < 0.05$.*

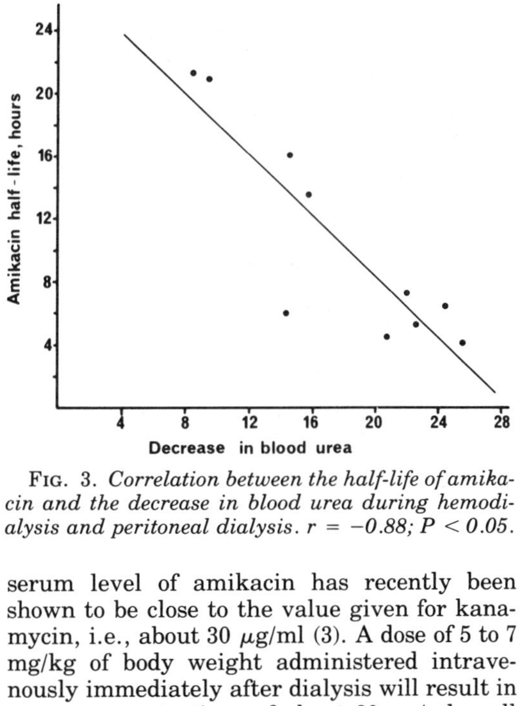

FIG. 3. *Correlation between the half-life of amikacin and the decrease in blood urea during hemodialysis and peritoneal dialysis. $r = -0.88$; $P < 0.05$.*

serum level of amikacin has recently been shown to be close to the value given for kanamycin, i.e., about 30 μg/ml (3). A dose of 5 to 7 mg/kg of body weight administered intravenously immediately after dialysis will result in serum concentrations of about 20 μg/ml, well above the minimum inhibitory concentration, but below the toxic level. With a serum half-life in anephric patients of about 3 days, this dose will suffice until the next dialysis, even if dialysis is performed only once weekly. In patients with minimal residual renal function (i.e., endogenous creatinine clearance between 2 and 5 ml/min) the half-life is about 2 days, and one extra dose after 4 days may well be necessary.

During dialysis a significant correlation between the half-life of amikacin and the decrease in blood urea and serum creatinine was demonstrated. This finding differs from a previous observation concerning gentamicin and kanamycin (9), but is in agreement with Riff and Jackson (18), who demonstrated a significant correlation between the degree of dialysis of creatinine and gentamicin during hemodialysis. However, the studies are not directly comparable as different kinds of artificial kidneys were used.

It is obvious that large individual differences exist regarding the various kinetic parameters of amikacin. The dose schedule suggested is therefore only to be considered as a clinical guideline and should be supplemented with serum concentration measurements whenever possible.

LITERATURE CITED

1. **Altmann, G., B. Bogokowsky, G. Boner, and H. E. Eliahou.** 1970. Blood levels of ampicillin, kanamycin, and gentamycin in the uremic patient. Isr. Med. J. 6:683–690.
2. **Atkins, R. C., C. Mion, E. Despaux, N. Van-Hai, C. Julien, and H. Mion.** 1973. Peritoneal transfer of kanamycin and its use in peritoneal dialysis. Kidney Int. 3:391–396.
3. **Black, R. E., W. K. Lau, R. J. Weinstein, L. S. Young, and W. L. Hewitt.** 1976. Ototoxicity of amikacin. Antimicrob. Agents Chemother. 9:956–961.
4. **Bodey, G. P., M. Valdivieso, R. Feld, and V. Rodriguez.** 1974. Pharmacology of amikacin in humans. Antimicrob. Agents Chemother. 5:508–512.
5. **Cabana, B. E., and J. G. Taggart.** 1973. Comparative pharmacokinetics of BB-K8 and kanamycin in dogs and humans. Antimicrob. Agents Chemother. 3:478–483.
6. **Christopher, T. G., D. Korn, A. D. Blair, A. W. Forrey, M. A. O'Neill, and R. E. Cutler.** 1974. Gentamycin pharmacokinetics during hemodialysis. Kidney Int. 6:38–44.
7. **Clarke, J. T., R. D. Libke, C. Regamey, and W. M. M. Kirby.** 1974. Comparative pharmacokinetics of amikacin and kanamycin. Clin. Pharmacol. Ther. 15:610–616.
8. **Curtis, J. R., S. J. McDonald, and J. H. Weston.** 1967. Parenteral administration of gentamycin in renal failure: patients undergoing intermittent hemodialysis. Br. Med. J. 2:537–539.
9. **Danish, M., R. Schultz, and W. Jusko.** 1974. Pharmacokinetics of gentamicin and kanamycin during hemodialysis. Antimicrob. Agents Chemother. 6:841–847.
10. **Editorial.** 1975. Amikacin. Lancet ii:804–805.
11. **Kelly, M. T., and J. M. Matsen.** 1976. In vitro activity, synergism, and testing parameters of amikacin, with comparison to other aminoglycoside antibiotics. Antimicrob. Agents Chemother. 9:440–447.
12. **Klastersky, J., B. Nyamubeya, and L. Vandenborre.** 1974. Antimicrobial effectiveness of kanamycin, aminosidin, BB-K8, sisomicin, gentamicin and tobramycin combined with carbenicillin or cephalotin against gram-negative rods. J. Med. Microbiol. 7:465–472.
13. **Levy, J., and J. Klastersky.** 1975. Correlation of serum creatinine concentration and amikacin half-life. J. Clin. Pharmacol. 15:705–707.
14. **Lockwood, W. R., and J. D. Bower.** 1973. Tobramycin and gentamicin concentrations in the serum of normal and anephric patients. Antimicrob. Agents Chemother. 3:125–129.
15. **McHenry, M. D., J. G. Wagner, P. M. Hall, D. G. Vidt, and T. L. Gavan.** 1976. Amikacin in renal failure. Clin. Pharmacol. Ther. 19:112.
16. **Malacoff, R. F., F. O. Finkelstein, and V. T. Andriole.** 1975. Effect of peritoneal dialysis on serum levels of tobramycin and clindamycin. Antimicrob. Agents Chemother. 8:574–580.
17. **Reynolds, A. V. J. M. T. Hamilton-Miller, and W. Brumfitt.** 1974. Newer aminoglycosides—amikacin and tobramycin: an in-vitro comparison with kanamycin and gentamycin. Br. Med. J. 3:778–780.
18. **Riff, L. J., and G. G. Jackson.** 1971. Pharmacology of gentamicin in man. J. Infect. Dis. 124(Suppl.):S98–S105.
19. **Rosdahl, V. T., V. Vejlsgaard, N. Rosdahl, and R. Vejlsgaard.** 1969. A micromethod for determination of antibiotics in serum. Dan. Med. Bull. 16:133–139.

ANTIMICROBIAL AGENTS AND CHEMOTHERAPY, Feb. 1977, p. 219-224
Vol. 11, No. 2

Requirements of Glucose and Incubation Under Static Conditions for Optimal Colicin E1 Induction

ATSUSHI NAKAZAWA,* NOBUO SUZUKI, AND TERUMI TAMADA

Department of Biochemistry, Chiba University School of Medicine, Inohana, Chiba, Japan

Received for publication 23 August 1976

A rapid rate and large amounts of colicin E1 synthesis were induced by incubating colicinogenic cells without aeration in the presence of glucose. The decrease in ability of colicin induction by aeration was not due to an ample supply of oxygen, but to the simple agitation of the bacterial suspension. Sugars other than glucose that support colicin synthesis were mannose, fructose, glucose-6-phosphate, and mannitol. The effect of sugars in mutants deficient in enzymes of glucose metabolism suggested that some intermediary metabolites between glucose and pyruvate are closely related to the stimulation of colicin synthesis under these conditions. Analyses of deoxyribonucleic acid replication indicated that the induced replication of the colicin E1 plasmid deoxyribonucleic acid occurred even under conditions in which colicin was not actively synthesized.

Synthesis of an antimicrobial protein, colicin E1 (19), depends on the presence of colicin E1 plasmid deoxyribonucleic acid (DNA) (ColE1) (4.2×10^6 daltons) (2). ColE1 is present in 10 to 20 copies per colicinogenic cell (3), but normally is dormant with regard to active colicin production. Treatment of the cells, however, with agents such as mitomycin C (14) or ultraviolet light (23) results in active colicin synthesis after a certain lag period. Although it has been shown that the DNA molecule of ColE1 is multiplied after mitomycin treatment (5), there was conflicting evidence as to the requirement of ColE1 plasmid replication for induction (6), and little is known about the control mechanisms involved in the overall process of colicin E1 induction.

In the course of studies to clarify the biochemical events of the induction process, we attempted to define the optimal conditions for colicin E1 synthesis. Systematic studies of cultural and induction conditions have apparently been neglected, although such studies would allow some insight into the mechanism of induction. This paper includes data that the presence of glucose and incubation without aeration are required for optimal colicin E1 induction.

MATERIALS AND METHODS

Bacterial strains. The genotypes and sources of *Escherichia coli* strains used in these experiments are listed in Table 1.

Media. M9 Casamino Acids medium used as a basal medium has been described (20). Routinely, the bacteria were grown and induced to synthesize colicin E1 in basal medium supplemented with 0.4% carbohydrate unless stated otherwise. Indicator strains were grown in nutrient broth (Difco) medium.

In experiments with mutants of glucose metabolism, the strains 1100 (ColE1), 1103 (ColE1), 897 (ColE1), and DF1311 (ColE1) were grown and induced in the M9 salt medium supplemented with 0.3% Casamino Acids (vitamin free, Difco). Strain AceE20 (ColE1) was grown and induced in basal medium supplemented with 0.4% glucose and 0.34% $CH_3COONa \cdot 3H_2O$. For the growth of K1.1.2.5[c] (ColE1), thymine (40 μg/ml) was added to the basal medium supplemented with glucose. All of these strains were treated with tris(hydroxymethyl)-aminomethane and ethylenediaminetetraacetate to facilitate and transport of phosphorylated compounds by the method described by Pastan and Perlman (24). The bacteria were grown at 37°C with constant bubbling.

Induction of colicin. When the culture reached an absorbancy of 0.400 at 660 nm, the cells were collected by centrifugation and incubated with fresh basal medium containing various carbon sources together with mitomycin C (2 μg/ml) (Kyowa Hakko, Ltd., Tokyo). This concentration of inducing agent was optimal for colicin E1 induction in most of the strains (22). Routinely, 1 ml of the reaction mixture was incubated in a small test tube (diameter, 1 cm) without aeration at 37°C. When aeration was required, 3 ml of the mixture was bubbled constantly at 37°C (flow rate of air, 80 to 100 ml/min) in a test tube (diameter, 25 mm). Shaking the medium during induction was performed at a frequency of 130 strokes/min in an incubator (model M-IV, Taiyo Co., Ltd., Tokyo).

In ultraviolet induction, the cells suspended in saline buffer at concentrations of 1×10^9 to 2×10^9/ml were irradiated for 15 s in thin layers at 72 cm from a 15-W Toshiba germicidal bulb in dim light. Irradiated cells were incubated in the medium for induction as described above.

Colicin assay. To the incubation mixture (1 ml) was added 2 ml of distilled water and absorbancy was read at 660 nm. The mixture (3 ml) was treated with a sonic oscillator (100 W, 20 kHz; MS Co., Ltd., Osaka) for 90 s to obtain a clear colicin solution. Colicin activity was determined as previously described (20). The amount of colicin E1 produced was expressed as units per an absorbancy of 1.0 at 660 nm of the incubation mixture unless otherwise stated.

ColE1 DNA analysis. Cleared lysates were prepared as previously described (21). Diluted cleared lysates were centrifuged through linear 5-ml 5 to 20% neutral sucrose gradients for 2.5 h at 45,000 rpm and 18°C in an RPS 65TA rotor in a Hitachi 65P ultracentrifuge. Sucrose gradients were prepared in 0.5 M NaCl-0.005 M ethylenediaminetetraacetate-0.03 M tris(hydroxymethyl)aminomethane-hydrochloride, pH 8.0. Fractions (12 drops) were collected directly from the bottom of the tube on 25-mm square papers. The papers were washed successively with cold 5% trichloroacetic acid and ethanol, and the radioactivity was counted in a Beckman LS-100 liquid scintillation counter. Toluene containing 4.0 mg of PPO (2,5-diphenyloxazole) per ml served as a fluor. In all cases the cleared lysates contained more than 90% of the circular plasmid present in the cell as measured by CsCl-ethidium bromide equilibrium centrifugation and velocity sedimentation through sucrose. The pellets obtained after centrifugation for preparing cleared lysates were used for the determination of chromosomal DNA.

TABLE 1. *Bacterial strains* [a]

E. coli K-12 strain	Genetic markers	Source (reference)
Y20	*thi thr leu* ColE1	S. Luria (8)
AB1157	*pro his arg leu thr thi lac str*^{r}	K. Mizobuchi
W3110	Prototroph	K. Mizobuchi
1100	Prototroph	R. Simoni (9)
1103	*ptsI*, derivative of 1100	R. Simoni (9)
879	*pgm3 thi* Hfr-300	S. Adhya (1)
DF1311	*pgi pgl* HfrC	S. Adhya (17)
AceE20	*pdh*	U. Henning (10)
K1.1.2.5 [c]	*ppc pps thy met iclR*	M. Morikawa (16)

[a] ColE1 derivatives were constructed by conjugation with donor strains containing ColE1 (Y20) and F$^+$ (W3110, F$^+$) by the method of Smith et al. (26). The resultant strain containing both ColE1 and F$^+$ was treated with acridine orange to eliminate F$^+$.

RESULTS

Optimal conditions for colicin E1 induction. A colicinogenic strain, Y20 (ColE1), was grown to log phase with various carbon sources. Mitomycin C was then added and the culture was divided into two portions. One portion was aerated through a bubbling pump, while the other portion was incubated without aeration. Among the conditions tested, incubation without aeration in the presence of glucose proved to be the most adequate for a rapid synthesis of colicin E1 (Table 2). In a separate experiment, up to 99% of the cell population became colicin-producing cells in 2 h in the presence of glucose and under conditions without aeration, as judged by the lacunae test (21). In the presence of glycerol, aeration increased the synthesis of colicin, but the rate of synthesis was less than that in the presence of glucose. In the medium

TABLE 2. *Colicin E1 induction under various conditions in Y20 (ColE1) strain*

Culture medium [a]	Aeration [b]	Colicin E1 produced (U/ml of medium)			
		0 [c]	1	6	24
Glucose (20 mM)	−	3 (0.42) [d]	260 (0.50)	330 (0.59)	580 (0.55)
	+		19 (0.53)	81 (0.63)	250 (0.64)
Glycerol (20 mM)	−	12 (0.40)	15 (0.41)	4 (0.31)	3 (0.24)
	+		19 (0.54)	34 (0.58)	180 (0.54)
Succinate (20 mM)	−	7 (0.35)	9 (0.33)	5 (0.28)	5 (0.28)
	+		7 (0.43)	3 (0.49)	15 (0.40)
Lactate (20 mM)	−	5 (0.26)	12 (0.26)	13 (0.20)	10 (0.20)
	+		19 (0.33)	6 (0.35)	33 (0.30)
Casamino Acids (0.5%) [e]	−	9 (0.44)	11 (0.44)	14 (0.37)	14 (0.37)
	+		240 (0.53)	160 (0.40)	410 (0.39)
Nutrient broth (0.8%) [f]	−	5 (0.38)	3 (0.37)	7 (0.31)	16 (0.33)
	+		28 (0.43)	150 (0.22)	120 (0.21)

[a] The basal medium was supplemented with each sugar.
[b] −, Without aeration; +, with aeration.
[c] Time in hours after the addition of mitomycin C.
[d] Numbers in parentheses are absorbance values at 660 nm of the incubation mixture at the indicated time.
[e] The concentration of Casamino Acids was raised to 0.5% in basal medium when they were used as carbon sources.
[f] Nutrient broth medium was used in place of M9 Casamino Acids medium.

containing Casamino Acids or nutrient broth, aeration facilitated colicin production. Inhibition of synthesis by aeration was also observed in the case of other colicins, such as colicin E2, although they were less severely inhibited than was colicin E1 (Table 3). Glucose stimulation was also observed in colicin E3 induction, whereas colicin E2 synthesis was inhibited by glucose, as reported by Lavoie et al. (18) (Table 4). The stimulation by glucose and inhibition by aeration were observed in other colicinogenic strains, such as AB1157 (ColE1), W3110 (ColE1), and 1100 (ColE1, ColIb), and also in the ultraviolet-induced cells of Y20 (ColE1).

Effect of aeration on induction. Not only aeration but also shaking the medium during incubation decreased the synthesis of colicin E1. The aeration or shaking effect on colicin synthesis did not appear to be due to an oversupply of oxygen to the culture. Either bubbling with nitrogen gas or shaking under reduced pressure inhibited colicin synthesis (Fig. 1).

The aeration effect for colicin E1 induction was not simply attributable to an exhaustion of glucose in the medium. After 1 h of aeration in the standard induction medium, glucose still remained at 10 mM. The addition of glucose (10 mM) to the medium after 30 min of incubation did not prevent the inhibition of synthesis by aeration.

The inhibition of colicin synthesis by aeration appeared reversible. The culture was first aerated for 1 h in the presence of mitomycin C and then centrifuged to separate the cells from the supernatant fluid. Fresh medium was added to the cells and incubation was continued without aeration for 2 h. Colicin E1 was synthesized at almost the same rate as in the culture without aeration.

Effect of sugar on colicin induction. Sugars other than glucose that support colicin E1 synthesis under conditions without aeration were mannose, fructose, glucose-6-P, and mannitol (each at 20 mM). Maltose, ribose, sorbitol, gluconate, arabinose, xylitol, and glucuronate showed moderate stimulation, and galactose, xylose, melibiose, glycerol, sorbose, rhamnose, α-methyl glucoside, 2-deoxyglucose, and inositol were not effective at the same concentration. It should be noted that all of the effective compounds for colicin synthesis are sugars that bring about catabolite repression of the synthesis of some inducible enzymes (13).

Colicin induction in mutants of sugar metabolism. In the mutant strain 1103 (ColE1), which can not phosphorylate glucose because of a deficiency in enzyme I of the phosphotransferase system (*ptsI*$^-$), the amounts of colicin E1 synthesized in 2 h in the presence of glucose under static conditions were very low as compared with those in the parent strain 1100 (Table 5). Glucose-6-P, gluconate, and pyruvate, however, supported colicin synthesis. Therefore, glucose must be phosphorylated to support colicin synthesis. Fructose and glycerol did not stimulate the synthesis because of a failure in being phosphorylated in this mutant (9).

TABLE 3. *Induction of colicin synthesis under various conditions* [a]

Strain	Amt of colicin (U) [b]	
	Static [c]	Aerating
W3110 (ColE1)	79	10
W3110 (ColE2)	420	140
W3110 (ColE3)	750	750

[a] Cells were grown and induced for colicin synthesis in basal medium supplemented with 0.4% glucose.
[b] Per absorbancy at 660 nm of the incubation mixture after 1 hr of incubation.
[c] Incubation conditions.

TABLE 4. *Induction of colicin synthesis in the presence of various carbohydrates* [a]

Strain	Amt of colicin (U) [b]		
	Glucose	Glycerol	Lactate
W3110 (ColE1)	80	11	8
W3110 (ColE2)	59	74	180
W3110 (ColE3)	1,870	150	120

[a] Cells were grown and induced in basal medium supplemented with 0.4% of each carbohydrate.
[b] Per absorbancy at 660 nm of the incubation mixture after 1 h of incubation. Incubation for induction was done under static conditions.

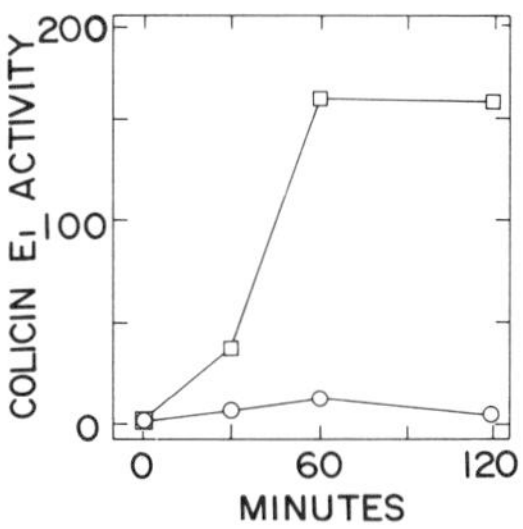

FIG. 1. *Effect of aeration on colicin E1 induction under reduced pressure. Cells of Y20 (ColE1) were grown in basal medium supplemented with 0.4% glucose. The bacterial culture was poured into a Thunberg tube. After evacuation (2 mm of Hg), mitomycin C was added from the side arm and incubated under both aeration (○) and static (□) conditions. Colicin activity was expressed as units per absorbancy at 660 nm of the incubation mixture.*

If reactions such as glucosylation are involved in the colicin induction process, conversion of glucose-6-P to glucose-1-P, the precursor of uridine 5'-diphosphate–glucose, would be necessary. In mutant 897 (ColE1), deficient in phosphoglucomutase activity (*pgm*⁻), however, glucose-6-P was much more effective than glucose-1-P or pyruvate (Table 5). Therefore, it is unlikely that the conversion of glucose-6-P to glucose-1-P is a necessary step for colicin synthesis.

Free glucose-6-P does not seem to have a stimulatory effect because mutant DF1311 (ColE1), which lacks phosphoglucoisomerase and phosphogluconolactonase simultaneously (pgi^- pgl^-), did not require glucose and glucose-6-P for colicin synthesis. In contrast, gluconate and ribose, both of which enter the pentose phosphate pathway after being phosphorylated at the point distal to the mutation step, could support colicin synthesis (Table 5).

In mutant AceE20 (ColE1), deficient in pyruvate dehydrogenase (pdh^-), which is a key enzyme linking the glucose metabolism to the tricarboxylic acid cycle, glucose and pyruvate supported colicin synthesis.

In addition, in mutant K1.1.2.5[c] (ColE1), which lacks both phosphoenolpyruvate (PEP) carboxylase and PEP synthetase (ppc^-, pps^-), PEP was a better substrate than pyruvate (Table 5). In *E. coli*, the conversion of pyruvate to oxalacetate does not occur through the direct carboxylation reaction but through reactions involving PEP synthetase and PEP carboxylase (25). It is therefore hardly conceivable that the conversion of pyruvate to some intermediate of the tricarboxylic acid cycle plays a major role in colicin synthesis. It is suggested that metabolites of glucose between glucose-6-P and PEP have a stimulatory effect in colicin synthesis.

ColE1 DNA replication under conditions in which colicin E1 induction is inhibited. ColE1 plasmid DNA replication occurred in mitomycin C induction in certain cases (5, 6). As judged from the percent radioactivity of plasmid DNA in the total radioactivity incorporated, replication of ColE1 DNA was stimulated upon addition of mitomycin C under bubbling conditions (Table 6). There was essentially no difference in the induced plasmid replication between bubbling and static conditions. Also, the replication was observed independently of carbon sources, although the amounts of colicin E1 synthesized differed significantly. These findings indicate that aeration of the medium and using sugars other than glucose as a carbon source stopped colicin synthesis after the step of ColE1 DNA replication.

DISCUSSION

The time course of induced synthesis of group E colicins varied, depending upon the conditions of incubation. Although stimulation of synthesis in the presence of glucose and inhibition by aeration of the medium were observed in the case of other group E colicins, colicin E1 is the only one that required the presence of glucose and incubation under static conditions for optimal induction. Those effects were observed specifically with colicin E1, even though host strains varied.

The possibility may be raised that colicin E1 is produced actively, but inactivated during aeration. This is hardly conceivable because of the

TABLE 5. *Induction of colicin E1 synthesis in various mutants of glucose metabolism*

Sugar[a]	Amt of colicin (U)[b]					
	1100	1103 ($ptsI^-$)	897 (pgm^-)	DF1311 (pgi^- pgl^-)	AceE20 (pdh^-)	K1.1.2.5[c] (ppc^- pps^-)
Glucose	43	6		4	43	320
Glucose-6-P	37	55	85	5		
Glucose-1-P			50			
Gluconate	12	98		30		71
Fructose	34	11				
Glycerol	12	6			1	
Ribose	11	28		34		58
Arabinose	11	38				
Pyruvate	34	62	47	32	29	92
Lactate					5	
Phosphoenolpyruvate						164
Oxalacetate						16
None	11	10	29	5	1	15

[a] Cells treated with tris(hydroxymethyl)aminomethane and ethylenediaminetetraacetate were incubated with mitomycin C in basal medium supplemented with a 5 mM concentration of each sugar.

[b] Per absorbancy at 660 nm of the incubation mixture after 2 h of incubation under static conditions.

TABLE 6. *ColE1 replication under various conditions* [a]

Strain	Carbon source	Mitomycin C	Aeration	Label ([cpm × 10^3]/3 ml of incubation mixture) incorporated into: ColE1 DNA	Label ([cpm × 10^3]/3 ml of incubation mixture) incorporated into: Chromosomal DNA	Label as ColE1 DNA (%)	Colicin E1 (U/ml)
AB1157 (ColE1)	Glucose	+	+	9.6	930	1.0	5
	Glucose	−	+	15	5,100	0.29	5
Y20 (ColE1)	Glucose	+	+	12	1,400	0.85	5
	Glucose	+	−	2.6	220	1.2	55
	Glucose	+	−	3.7	410	0.9	50
	Glycerol	+	−	4.8	347	1.4	5
	Lactate	+	−	1.7	214	0.79	6

[a] Cells were grown to an absorbancy of 0.4 as described in the text. Incubation was done in 3 ml with deoxyadenosine (250 μg/ml) and [^{3}H]thymine (6.7 μCi/ml) in the presence or absence of mitomycin C (2 μg/ml) for 1 h at 37°C under the condition indicated.

following observations. First, large amounts of colicin E1 were synthesized under aeration conditions upon incubation in Casamino Acids and nutrient broth medium. Second, colicin E1 produced in 1 h under static conditions was not inactivated significantly during further aeration for 1 h. Third, if the cells produced colicin E1 actively and then the protein was inactivated subsequently, a large population of the cells would be dead, since colicin E1 induction is a lethal synthesis (11). However, the majority of the cells remained viable after aeration for 1 h, indicating that colicin E1 synthesis did not occur under these conditions. Finally, there was no evidence that substances which accumulated during aeration destroyed colicin E1 protein. Incubation of the colicin E1 solution (100 U/ml) with the supernatant fluid of the aerated culture medium for 1 h at 37°C did not lead to an inactivation of colicin. Thus, physical agitation of the bacterial suspension is the major factor for an inhibitory effect.

The effect of glucose on colicin E1 induction is difficult to explain at present. A similar observation was reported by Horak in the agar culture system (12). Experiments with mutants that lack enzymes in glucose metabolism suggested that some intermediary metabolites from glucose to pyruvate are closely related to the stimulation effect. Relatively rapid induction with Casamino Acids under aeration conditions could be understood along this line. Amino acids such as alanine, aspartate, and glutamate can be used as target substrates for amphibolic pathways, serving both as the energy source through the tricarboxylic acid cycle and as substrates for biosynthetic pathways such as gluconeogenesis (25).

It is interesting that the stimulatory compounds for colicin induction were sugars, which bring about catabolite repression for synthesis of certain inducible enzymes. In the case of catabolic enzyme systems, glucose repression can be antagonized by cyclic adenosine 5′-monophosphate (AMP). In the colicin E1-synthesizing system, however, cyclic AMP did not act against but rather cooperated with glucose (20). These differences may be related to the difference in incubation conditions, i.e., static versus aerating, or to the distinct mode of action of cyclic AMP in these systems. Cyclic AMP acts at the ColE1 DNA replication step (15, 21), whereas in the inducible enzyme system the nucleotide acts at the transcriptional step (4, 7).

Induction of colicin E1 synthesis has been thought to be accompanied by replication of ColE1 DNA (5). However, there was conflicting evidence on the requirement of plasmid replication for induction (6). Whether this replication is directly linked to transcription and translation upon induction is still unclear. The present result, that even under suboptimal conditions for colicin synthesis induced replication occurred, suggests at least that some host-controlled factors are reponsible for the regulation of transcription and translation of the ColE1 plasmid.

ACKNOWLEDGMENTS

Gratitude is due to M. Tatibana for generous support and encouragement and M. Ohara for her help in preparing the manuscript. We are also grateful to S. Luria, K. Mizobuchi, R. Simoni, S. Adhya, U. Henning, and M. Morikawa for gifts of strains.

This research was supported by the Scientific Research Fund of the Ministry of Education of Japan (CO58008).

LITERATURE CITED

1. **Adhya, S., and M. Schwartz.** 1971. Phosphoglucomutase mutants of *Escherichia coli* K-12. J. Bacteriol. **108**:621–626.

2. **Bazaral, M., and D. R. Helinski.** 1968. Circular DNA forms of colicinogenic factors E_1, E_2 and E_3 from *Escherichia coli*. J. Mol. Biol. **36**:185–194.
3. **Clewell, D. B., and D. R. Helinski.** 1970. Properties of a supercoiled deoxyribonucleic acid-protein relaxation complex and strand specificity of the relaxation event. Biochemistry **22**:4428–4440.
4. **DeCrombrugghe, B., B. Chen, W. Anderson, P. Nissley, M. Gottesman, R. Perlman, and I. Pastan.** 1971. Lac DNA, RNA polymerase, cyclic AMP receptor protein, cyclic AMP, lac repressor and inducer are the essential elements for controlled lac transcription. Nature (London) New Biol. **231**:139–142.
5. **DeWitt, W., and D. R. Helinski.** 1965. Characterization of colicinogenic factor E1 from a non-induced and a mitomycin C-induced *Proteus* strain. J. Mol. Biol. **13**:692–703.
6. **Durkacz, B. W., C. K. Kennedy, and D. J. Sherratt.** 1974. Plasmid replication and the induced synthesis of colicin E1 and E2 in *Escherichia coli*. J. Bacteriol. **117**:940–946.
7. **Eron, L., R. Arditti, G. Zubay, S. Connaway, and J. R. Beckwith.** 1971. An adenosine 3′,5′-cyclic monophosphate-binding protein that acts on the transcription process. Proc. Natl. Acad. Sci. U.S.A. **68**:215–218.
8. **Fields, K. L., and S. E. Luria.** 1969. Effects of colicins E1 and K on transport systems. J. Bacteriol. **97**:57–63.
9. **Fox, C. F., and G. Wilson.** 1968. The role of a phosphoenolpyruvate-dependent kinase system in β-glucoside catabolism in *Escherichia coli*. Proc. Natl. Acad. Sci. U.S.A. **59**:988–995.
10. **Henning, U., W. Busch, G. Deppe, and R. Marek.** 1969. Pyruvate dehydrogenase synthesis in *E. coli* K12, FEBS Symposium, vol. 19, p. 19–28. Academic Press Inc., London.
11. **Herschmann, H. R., and D. R. Helinski.** 1967. Comparative study of the events associated with colicin induction. J. Bacteriol. **94**:691–699.
12. **Horak, V.** 1973. Glucose repression of the synthesis of some colicins. Folia Microbiol. (Prague) **18**:75–76.
13. **Hsie, A. W., and H. V. Rickenberg.** 1967. Catabolite repression in *Escherichia coli*: the role of glucose 6-phosphate. Biochem. Biophys. Res. Commun. **29**:303–310.
14. **Iijima, T.** 1962. Studies on the colicinogenic factor in *Escherichia coli* K12, induction of colicin production by mitomycin C. Biken J. **5**:1–8.
15. **Katz, L., D. T. Kingsbury, and D. R. Helinski.** 1973. Stimulation by cyclic adenosine monophosphate of plasmid deoxyribonucleic acid replication and catabolite repression of the plasmid deoxyribonucleic acid-protein relaxation complex. J. Bacteriol. **114**:577–591.
16. **Kornberg, H. L., and J. Smith.** 1969. Genetic control of hexose phosphate uptake by *Escherichia coli*. Nature (London) **224**:1261–1262.
17. **Kupor, S. R., and D. G. Fraenkel.** 1969. 6-Phosphogluconolactonase mutants of *Escherichia coli* and a maltose blue gene. J. Bacteriol. **100**:1296–1301.
18. **Lavoie, M., L. G. Mathieu, and L. Charron-Alle.** 1974. Inhibition of colicin production by fermentable sugars. Can. J. Microbiol. **20**:269–272.
19. **Luria, S. E.** 1970. Phage, colicins, and macroregulatory phenomena. Science **168**:1166–1170.
20. **Nakazawa, A., and T. Tamada.** 1972. Stimulation of colicin E1 synthesis by cyclic 3′,5′-adenosine monophosphate in mitomycin C-induced *Escherichia coli*. Biochem. Biophys. Res. Commun. **46**:1004–1010.
21. **Nakazawa, A., and T. Tamada.** 1972. Involvement of cyclic 3′,5′-adenosine monophosphate in replication of colicinogenic factor E1 DNA. Biochem. Biophys. Res. Commun. **49**:977–983.
22. **Nakazawa, A., and T. Tamada.** 1974. Induction of colicin E1 synthesis by neocarzinostatin and bleomycin. J. Antibiot. **27**:984–986.
23. **Ozeki, H., B. A. D. Stocker, and H. DeMargerie.** 1959. Production of colicine by single bacteria. Nature (London) **184**:337–339.
24. **Pastan, I., and R. L. Perlman.** 1969. Stimulation of tryptophanase synthesis in *Escherichia coli* by cyclic 3′,5′-adenosine monophosphate. J. Biol. Chem. **244**:2226–2232.
25. **Sanwal, B. D.** 1970. Allosteric controls of amphibolic pathways in bacteria. Bacteriol. Rev. **34**:20–29.
26. **Smith, S., H. Ozeki, and B. A. D. Stocker.** 1963. Transfer of ColE1 and ColE2 during high-frequency transmission of ColI in *Salmonella typhimurium*. J. Gen. Microbiol. **33**:231–242.

ANTIMICROBIAL AGENTS AND CHEMOTHERAPY, Feb. 1977, p. 225–228 Vol. 11, No. 2

Printed in U.S.A.

Microdilution Transfer Plate Technique for Determining In Vitro Synergy of Antimicrobial Agents

PAULA F. DOUGHERTY,[1] DAVID W. YOTTER, AND THOMAS R. MATTHEWS*
Nucleic Acid Research Institute, ICN Pharmaceuticals, Inc., Irvine, California 92715

Received for publication 29 June 1976

A microdilution transfer plate technique for determining in vitro synergy of antimicrobial agents is described. Combinations of gentamicin-nalidixic acid against *Proteus mirabilis* and rifampin-amphotericin B against *Candida albicans* are used as examples to demonstrate the technique. Results correlate with published data obtained by conventional methods. The technique is effective for evaluating the in vitro effects of antimicrobial agent combinations against both bacteria and fungi. The technique enables one to produce a checkerboard gradient in a fast, convenient, and reproducible way; results are easily visualized.

In vitro synergy of antimicrobial agents is traditionally accomplished using a tube broth dilution "checkerboard" in which several concentrations of one drug are each combined with concentrations of a second drug (4, 14). Agar dilution can be applied to this technique (11). Several agar diffusion methods are also described (7, 9, 12).

Microdilution methods have been described for determining synergy (3, 5, 6, 15, 16). Two methods (15, 16) involve dilution of both drugs before pipetting each into the microdilution plate. The method of Kluge et al. (6) requires diluting one drug in the microdilution plate, then adding the second drug (already diluted) to the wells containing the first drug. In two other methods described (3, 5) both drugs are diluted in the same microdilution plate.

This study describes a microdilution technique using the transfer plate (Cooke Engineering Co., Alexandria, Va.). The technique permits one drug dilution sequence to be superimposed upon another. This results in a rapid, reproducible, quantitative determination with simple dilution calculations.

Two known synergistic combinations, gentamicin-nalidixic acid against *Proteus mirabilis* and rifampin-amphotericin B against *Candida albicans* were selected as examples to demonstrate the technique.

MATERIALS AND METHODS

Antimicrobial agents. Rifampin (lot 557303, assay 990 μg/mg) was purchased from Calbiochem. Gentamicin (lot GMC-4M-6231, assay 578 μg/mg) was a gift from Schering Corp. Amphotericin B (lot 3956-001, assay 876 μg/mg) was a gift from E. R. Squibb and Sons, Inc. Nalidixic acid (lot J9463) was a gift from Sterling-Winthrop. All drugs were solubilized in 50% Me_2SO-50% ethanol and diluted in distilled water. Final solvent concentration in the microdilution plate was ≤1.0%.

Cultures and growth media. *P. mirabilis* (ICN 40) was used for the nalidixic acid-gentamicin combination; brain heart infusion (Difco) was the medium used for this example. *C. albicans* (ICN 80) was used for the amphotericin B-rifampin combination; a medium containing a yeast-nitrogen base (Difco), L-asparagine, and dextrose was used (13).

All incubations were for 18 to 24 h at 35°C.

Synergy assay. The test for synergy was performed using a 96-well, flat-bottom microdilution plate (Microtest II, Falcon, Div. of Becton, Dickinson & Co., Oxnard, Calif.) and 50-μl microdiluters (Cooke) to dilute drug I. Drug II was diluted in a transfer plate (Cooke) using 25-μl microdiluters (Cooke). Wells in the transfer plate have a calibrated orifice designed to retain the material in the well by surface tension until contact is made with the fluid in the flat-bottom plate. This contact breaks the surface tension and allows all wells of the transfer plate to drain. The system includes a transfer plate holder and carrier, which were autoclaved before use. Pipetting into plates was accomplished using precision pipettes with sterile, disposable tips (Medical Laboratory Automation Inc., Mt. Vernon, N. Y.).

The flat-bottom plate was prepared by first pipetting 50 μl of growth media into each well. Next, 50 μl of drug I was pipetted into all wells of row B (12 wells across). Twofold serial dilutions were then made from row B through row G using 50-μl microdiluters.

The transfer plate was prepared by first pipetting 25 μl of growth media into each well. Next, 25 μl of drug II was pipetted into all wells of column 2 (8 wells across). Twofold serial dilutions were made from column 2 through column 11 using 25-μl microdiluters.

Before draining drug II from the transfer plate

[1] Present address: Rachelle Laboratories, Inc., Long Beach, CA 90801.

into the flat-bottom plate, the flat-bottom plate was oriented with the highest concentration of drug I at the top. The transfer plate was oriented above the flat-bottom plate with the highest concentration of drug II to the left. Contents of the transfer plate were added to the flat-bottom plate following the manufacturer's instructions. This transfer achieved a concentration gradient (highest in the upper left to lowest in the lower right) of both drugs in the flat-bottom plate (Fig. 1). Each well in the flat-bottom plate was inoculated with 200 μl of growth media containing ~8 10^5 cells/ml. Final well volume was 275 μl.

Plate layout of the assay is given in Fig. 1. The four-corner wells of the plate contained no drug and were used as positive growth controls. The minimum inhibitory concentration (MIC) of drug I alone was determined in columns 1 and 12. The MIC of drug II alone was determined in rows A and H.

After incubation, a lack of growth in wells below the MIC levels of both drugs was an indication of a possible synergistic effect; drug concentrations of these wells were plotted on an isobologram. Definition of synergy was that of Sabath (12).

Minimum lethal concentrations were determined by pipetting 50 μl of the well contents into a tube containing 5.0 ml of broth. No growth after incubation indicated a lethal effect.

The fractional inhibitory concentration (FIC) index and the fractional lethal concentration (FLC) index were calculated as follows (2, 10):

$$\text{FIC index} = \frac{\text{MIC of SMX in combination}}{\text{MIC of SMX alone}} + \frac{\text{MIC of TMP in combination}}{\text{MIC of TMP alone}}$$

(Abbreviations: SMX, sulfamethoxazole; TMP, trimethoprim.) Since rifampin was not inhibitory or lethal by itself, the highest concentration of the drug tested was used to calculate the FIC or FLC index.

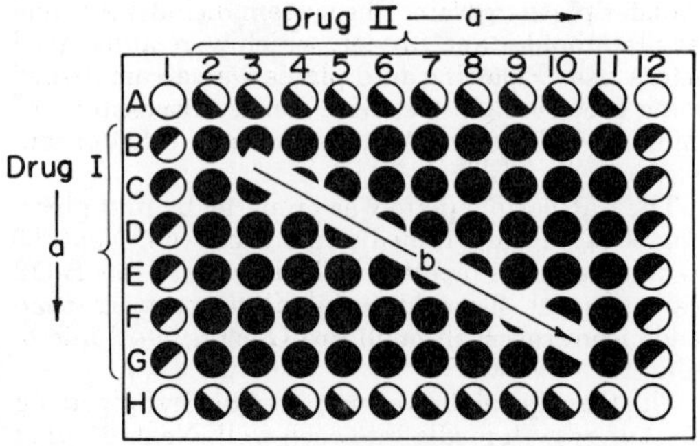

FIG. 1. *Plate layout of microdilution transfer plate synergy assay. a, direction of dilution; b, direction of concentration gradient; ◐, drug I; ◑, drug II; ●, I + II; ○, growth control.*

RESULTS

Nalidixic acid and gentamicin. The results of 10 consecutive tests of the nalidixic acid-gentamicin combination against *P. mirabilis* are given in Tables 1 and 2. Bacteriostatic and bactericidal synergy was produced by this combination. The FIC and FLC indexes were 0.654 ± 0.057 and 0.825 ± 0.038, respectively (tests by P. Dougherty).

Rifampin and amphotericin B. Results of the rifampin-amphotericin B combination against *C. albicans* are given in Tables 3 and 4. Both fungistatic and fungicidal synergies

TABLE 1. *Replicate testing of minimal inhibitory concentrations of gentamicin and nalidixic acid, alone and in combination, against Proteus mirabilis using the microdilution transfer plate technique*

Test	MIC (μg/ml)[a]				FIC index[b]
	Alone Gent	Alone Nal A	Combination		
			Gent	Nal A	
1	1.0	4.0	0.062	2.0	0.56
2	1.0	4.0	0.062	2.0	0.56
3	1.0	4.0	0.062	2.0	0.56
4	1.0	4.0	0.125	2.0	0.62
5	0.5	4.0	0.250	2.0	1.00
6	0.5	4.0	0.250	2.0	1.00
7	1.0	4.0	0.062	2.0	0.56
8	1.0	4.0	0.062	2.0	0.56
9	1.0	4.0	0.062	2.0	0.56
10	1.0	4.0	0.062	2.0	0.56

[a] Gent; Gentamicin; Nal A, nalidixic acid.
[b] Mean of FIC indexes ± standard error: 0.654 ± 0.057.

TABLE 2. *Replicate testing of minimal lethal concentrations of gentamicin and nalidixic acid, alone and in combination, against Proteus mirabilis using the microdilution transfer plate technique*

Test	MLC (μg/ml)[a]				FLC index[b]
	Alone Gent	Alone Nal A	Combination		
			Gent	Nal A	
1	1.0	8.0	0.25	4.0	0.75
2	1.0	8.0	0.50	4.0	1.00
3	1.0	8.0	0.25	4.0	0.75
4	1.0	8.0	0.25	4.0	0.75
5	1.0	8.0	0.50	2.0	0.75
6	0.5	8.0	0.25	4.0	1.00
7	1.0	8.0	0.25	4.0	0.75
8	1.0	8.0	0.50	4.0	1.00
9	1.0	8.0	0.25	4.0	0.75
10	1.0	8.0	0.25	4.0	0.75

[a] Gent, Gentamicin; Nal A, nalidixic acid.
[b] Mean of FLC indexes ± standard error: 0.825 ± 0.038.

TABLE 3. *Replicate testing of minimal inhibitory concentrations of amphotericin B and rifampin, alone and in combination, against Candida albicans using the microdilution transfer plate technique*

Test	MIC (μg/ml)[a]				FIC index[b]
	Alone Am B	Alone Rif	Combination		
			Am B	Rif	
1	1.0	>250	0.06	31.3	0.19
2	1.0	>250	0.06	15.6	0.12
3	1.0	>250	0.06	15.6	0.12
4	1.0	>250	0.06	7.8	0.09
5	1.0	>250	0.03	31.3	0.19
6	1.0	>250	0.06	7.8	0.09

[a] Am B, Amphotericin B; Rif, rifampin.

[b] Mean of FIC indexes ± standard error: 0.133 ± 0.018.

TABLE 4. *Replicate testing of minimal lethal concentrations of amphotericin B and rifampin, alone and in combination, against Candida albicans using the microdilution transfer plate technique*

Test	MCL (μg/ml)[a]				FLC index[b]
	Alone Am B	Alone Rif	Combination		
			Am B	Rif	
1	2.0	>250	0.5	7.8	0.28
2	4.0	>250	0.5	7.8	0.15
3	2.0	>250	0.5	7.8	0.28
4	4.0	>250	0.5	7.8	0.15
5	2.0	>250	0.25	15.6	0.19
6	2.0	>250	0.5	7.8	0.28

[a] Am B, Amphotericin; Rif, rifampin.

[b] Mean of FLC indexes ± standard error: 0.221 ± 0.026.

were observed. The FIC and FLC indexes were 0.133 ± 0.018 and 0.221 ± 0.026, respectively, for six consecutive tests (tests by D. Yotter).

DISCUSSION

The results of this quantitative study confirm the qualitative synergy data reported previously for these combinations. Bactericidal synergy of nalidixic acid and gentamicin against *Enterobacteriaceae* was reported by Michel et al. (9). The potentiation of rifampin by amphotericin B was reported by Beggs et al. (1) and Medoff et al. (8).

We have found the microdilution transfer plate technique useful for evaluating the in vitro effects of antimicrobial agent combinations against both bacteria and fungi. Quantitative inhibitory and lethal synergistic values are reproducible. The FIC and FLC indexes for the nalidixic acid-gentamicin combination, determined by using a single-plate method (3), were 0.625 and 0.75, respectively. These values compare favorably with the FIC and FLC indexes calculated from the microdilution transfer plate data.

The technique provides an efficient and convenient way to produce the desired checkerboard gradient. After the stock drug solutions and inocula are prepared, an experienced worker can set-up, dilute, and inoculate a plate in less than 40 min. Individual well concentrations are easily calculated. Additionally, the layout of the plate permits easy visualization of a possible synergistic effect. Each drug is diluted only once in its respective plate. This reduces the potential variation of diluting both drugs in the same plate.

Occasional problems have been encountered due to inadequate drainage of the transfer plate wells. These have been minimized by following the manufacturer's suggestions for the elimination of static charge.

The transfer plate technique represents a small investment and can be easily applied in any laboratory that uses the microdilution method for susceptibility testing. When preparation time, ease of interpretation, and cost of materials using this technique are compared with many conventional methods, the advantages of this technique are readily apparent.

ACKNOWLEDGMENTS

We wish to thank E. R. Squibb and Sons, Inc. for the amphotericin B, Schering Corp. for the gentamicin, and Sterling-Winthrop Research Institute for the nalidixic acid. *Candida albicans* was provided by Lilly Research Laboratories, and *Proteus mirabilis* was provided by Bristol Laboratories.

LITERATURE CITED

1. **Beggs, W. H., G. A. Sarosi, and F. A. Andrews.** 1974. Synergistic action of amphotericin B and rifampin on *Candida albicans*. Am. Rev. Resp. Dis. **110**:671–673.
2. **Elion, G. B., S. Singer, and G. H. Hitchings.** 1954. Antagonists of nucleic acid derivatives. J. Biol. Chem. **208**:477–488.
3. **Fass, R. J., C. A. Rotilie, and R. B. Prior.** 1974. Interaction of clindamycin and gentamicin in vitro. Antimicrob. Agents Chemother. **6**:582–587.
4. **Garrod, L. P., and P. M. Waterworth.** 1962. Methods of testing combined antibiotic bactericidal action and the significance of the results. J. Clin. Pathol. **15**:328–338.
5. **Kelly, M. T., and J. M. Matsen.** 1976. In vitro activity, synergism, and testing parameters of amikacin, with comparisons to other aminoglycoside antibiotics. Antimicrob. Agents Chemother. **9**:440–447.
6. **Kluge, R. M., H. C. Standiford, B. Tatem, V. M. Young, M. H. Greene, S. C. Schimpff, F. M. Calia and R. Hornick.** 1974. Comparative activity of tobramycin, amikacin, and gentamicin alone and with carbenicillin against *Pseudomonas aeruginosa*. Antimicrob. Agents Chemother. **6**:442–446.
7. **Lee, W. S., and L. Komarmy.** 1975. Simple technique

for the assay of antibiotic synergism against enterococci. Antimicrob. Agents Chemother. 7:82–84.
8. **Medoff, G., G. S. Kobayashi, C. N. Kwan, D. Schlessinger, and P. Veenkov.** 1972. Potentiation of rifampicin and 5-fluorocytosine as antifungal antibiotics by amphotericin B. Proc. Natl. Acad. Sci. U.S.A. 69:196–199.
9. **Michel, J., R. Luboshitzky, and T. Sacks.** 1973. Bactericidal effect of combinations of nalidixic acid and various antibiotics on *Enterobacteriaceae*. Antimicrob. Agents Chemother. 4:201–204.
10. **Phillips, I., and C. Warren.** 1976. Activity of sulfamethoxazole and trimethoprim against *Bacteroides fragilis*. Antimicrob. Agents Chemother. 9:736–740.
11. **Rosenblatt, J. E., and P. R. Stewart.** 1974. Combined activity of sulfamethoxazole, trimethoprim, and polymyxin B against gram-negative bacilli. Antimicrob. Agents Chemother. 6:84–92.
12. **Sabath, L. D.** 1968. Synergy of antibacterial substances by apparently known mechanisms, p. 210–217. Antimicrob. Agents Chemother., 1967.
13. **Shadomy, S.** 1969. In vitro studies with 5-fluorocytosine. Appl. Microbiol. 17:871–877.
14. **Shadomy, S., G. Wagner, A. Espinel-Ingroff, and B. A. Davis.** 1975. In vitro studies with combinations of 5-fluorocytosine and amphotericin B. Antimicrob. Agents Chemother. 8:117–121.
15. **Traub, W. H., and I. Kleber.** 1975. In vitro additive effect of polymyxin B and rifampin against *Serratia marcescens*. Antimicrob. Agents Chemother. 7:874–876.
16. **Zinner, S. H., R. B. Provonchee, K. S. Elias, and G. Peter.** 1976. Effect of clindamycin on the in vitro activity of amikacin and gentamicin against gram-negative bacilli. Antimicrob. Agents Chemother. 9:661–664.

ANTIMICROBIAL AGENTS AND CHEMOTHERAPY, Feb. 1977, p. 229-233
Vol. 11, No. 2

Effects of Purines and Pyrimidines on the Fungistatic Activity of 5-Fluorocytosine in *Aspergillus* Species

GERALD E. WAGNER AND SMITH SHADOMY*

Division of Infectious Diseases, Medical College of Virginia, Virginia Commonwealth University, Richmond, Virginia 23298

Received for publication 17 August 1976

The ability of some exogenously supplied purines, pyrimidines, and their nucleosides to antagonize the in vitro fungistatic activity of 5-fluorocytosine (5-FC) in *Aspergillus* species was examined. All compounds tested except thymidine were capable of altering the minimal inhibitory concentration of 5-FC for seven strains of aspergilli tested. In most instances, there was a reciprocal correlation between the ability of a compound to antagonize the fungistatic activity of 5-FC and the quantity of 5-FC taken up by cells in the presence of the compound over a 72-h period.

5-Fluorocytosine (5-FC, Flucytosine, Ancobon; Roche Laboratories) has been used primarily in the treatment of human candidiasis (4), cryptococcosis (15), and infections due to *Torulopsis glabrata* (2). Occasional reports on the successful use of 5-FC in treating aspergillosis (1) and chromomycosis (7) also have appeared in the medical literature. The observation by Shadomy et al. (13) that in vitro susceptibility testing with 5-FC could be accomplished only in synthetic media that did not contain additional sources of pyrimidines or purines initiated interest in the mode of action of the drug. A number of investigators examined the mode of action of 5-FC in yeastlike organisms (5, 6, 10, 11). It has been concluded that the drug enters the yeast cell via a permease system that recognizes several purines in addition to the natural analogue (9). Once inside the cell, 5-FC is rapidly deaminated to 5-fluorouracil and subsequently incorporated into ribonucleic acid (11). Polak (8) recently demonstrated that the substitution of 5-fluorouracil for uracil in ribonucleic acid produced a direct effect on protein synthesis in *Candida albicans*.

Polak and Scholer (10) examined the capability of pyrimidines, purines, and nucleosides to reverse or antagonize the fungistatic activity of 5-FC against *C. albicans*. These observations, in addition to other data, led to the conclusion that the mode of action of the drug was probably the same in *C. albicans* as described in *Saccharomyces cerevisiae* (6). To date, the mode of action of 5-FC in filamentous fungi has not been studied. The investigation reported here examines the ability of some pyrimidines, purines, and nucleosides to alter the minimal inhibitory concentration (MIC) of 5-FC for several strains of *Aspergillus fumigatus* and *Aspergillus niger*.

MATERIALS AND METHODS

Organisms. Five strains of *A. fumigatus*, two of *A. niger*, and *S. cerevisiae* ATCC 9763 were obtained from the fungus culture collection of the Division of Infectious Diseases, Medical College of Virginia, Virginia Commonwealth University, Richmond. Cultures were maintained on Sabouraud agar (Difco) at room temperature, 20 to 22°C.

Determination of MIC values. MICs of 5-FC were determined by using a modification of the agar dilution technique of Ericsson and Sherris (3). Serial dilutions of 5-FC were prepared in a filter-sterilized 10× concentrate of yeast nitrogen base (YNB, Difco) supplemented with 5% glucose as carbon source. Concentrations of drug ranged from 0.63 to 1,280 μg/ml. The solutions of YNB and drug were then diluted 1:10 with sterile 2% agar and dispensed in 20-ml volumes in square Integrid petri plates (15 by 15 cm, Falcon Plastics). After solidification of the agar, 0.05 ml of inoculum was applied to the surfaces of the medium, using a replica inoculator. Inocula were prepared from 72-h shaking cultures grown in diluted YNB. The cultures were homogenized in a Tenbroek hand tissue grinder (Corning Glass Works), and large pieces of cellular material were allowed to settle out. The resulting suspension of cells was then diluted with sterile physiological saline to an absorbancy of 0.05 at 530 nm. The MIC was defined as the lowest concentration of drug inhibiting visible vegetative growth after 72 h of incubation at 30 ± 1°C.

Reversal studies. The possible reversal or antagonistic effects of pyrimidines, purines, and some of their nucleosides on the fungistatic activity of 5-FC were determined by observing alterations in the MIC values of 5-FC alone and in combination with these compounds. Plates were prepared in the same manner as for the MIC determinations except that a modified 10-fold serial dilution scheme for 5-FC giving final concentrations of drug ranging from 0.04 to 4,000 μg/ml was used. The compounds under study for their potential antagonistic effects were added to the medium at concentrations of 1,000 μg/ml for the aspergilli and 100 μg/ml for the control organism, *S. cerevisiae*. Controls consisted of one plate containing the purported antagonist but no 5-FC and a series of plates for determining the MIC of 5-FC in the absence of antagonist. The alteration in MIC values for each organism was expressed as a power of 10 by comparing the MIC obtained in the presence of the added compound with that of 5-FC alone. The compounds tested included cytosine, cytidine, deoxycytidine, uracil, uridine, thymidine, adenine, adenosine, hypoxanthine, and deoxyguanosine. Each test was repeated six times.

Uptake studies. The quantitative effect of the addition of 1,000 μg of pyrimidines, purines, and their nucleosides per ml on uptake of 5-FC by the aspergilli was determined. Cells were grown with moderate shaking for 72 h at 30°C in YNB in the presence of 0.02 μCi of [2-^{14}C]5-FC per ml (30.87 mCi/mmol) adjusted to 10 μg/ml with unlabeled 5-FC. Cultures were harvested on preweighed membrane filters (1.2-μm pore size; Millipore Corp.), washed once with saline-citrate buffer (14 mM sodium chloride plus 1.5 mM sodium citrate, pH 7.0), air dried, and reweighed. The filters then were placed in liquid scintillation vials with 8.0 ml of scintillation fluid and counted in a Packard Tri-Carb liquid scintillation spectrometer (model 3320) The scintillaton fluid consisted of 4.0 g of 2,5-diphenyloxazole (PPO) and 100 mg of 1,4-bis-[2]-(5-phenyloxazolyl)benzene (POPOP) per liter of toluene. [2-^{14}C]5-FC taken up in the absence of any additional pyrimidines, purines, or nucleosides was designated as 100% uptake for comparative purposes.

Chemicals. [2-^{14}C]5-FC used in these experiments was kindly provided by Hoffmann-La Roche, Inc., Basel, Switzerland; 5-FC (lot 021052) was provided by Hoffman-La Roche, Inc., Nutley, N. J. Pyrimidines, purines, and nucleosides were purchased from Nutritional Biochemicals, Cleveland, Ohio. All other chemicals were of the highest commercial grade available.

RESULTS

MIC determinations. The MIC values for 5-FC measured against the five strains of *A. fumigatus*, two strains of *A. niger*, and *S. cerevisiae* ATCC 9763 used in this study are shown in Table 1. The standardized conditions used for MIC determinations allowed for consistent results, with never more than a one-dilution-step variation in either direction upon repeated trials. Preliminary studies with the aspergilli revealed that the nature of the inoculum, whether strictly spores or strictly hyphae, had no effect on the MIC values. However, control of both inoculum size and temperature of incubation were important in obtaining consistent MIC values.

Effect of exogenous pyrimidines, purines, and nucleosides on 5-FC activity. The effects of the addition of 1,000 μg of various pyrimidines, purines, and some of their nucleosides per ml on the fungistatic activity of 5-FC in solid culture medium are shown in Tables 2 and 3. The numbers indicate the power of 10 by which the MIC was altered when the selected pyrimidine, purine, or nucleoside was added to the culture medium. *S. cerevisiae* ATCC 9763 served as a control, with the compounds being tested at a concentration of 100 μg/ml. The values obtained for the control organism agreed closely with those published by Polak and Scholer (10) from similar experiments with the same organism.

Three patterns of effects emerged among the strains of aspergilli tested. One pattern involved *A. fumigatus* strains 4.6 and 4.28, both of which were resistant to 5-FC (400 μg/ml). The second encompassed the more sensitive *A. fumigatus* strains 4.19, 4.33, and 4.41 (4.0 μg/ml). The third pattern was seen with *A. niger* strains 4.55 and 3884, both of which were sus-

TABLE 1. *Minimal inhibitory concentrations (MIC), minimal sporulation inhibitory concentrations (MSIC), and minimal fungicidal concentrations (MFC) of 5-FC and 5-FU for the aspergilli and S. cerevisiae ATCC 9763*[a]

Organism	5-FC			5-FU		
	MIC	MSIC	MFC	MIC	MSIC	MFC
A. fumigatus						
4.6	>128	0.25	>128	128	8	>128
4.28	>128	0.25	>128	>128	16	>128
4.19	0.5	0.25	>128	128	32	>128
4.33	0.5	0.25	>128	128	8	>128
4.41	0.5	0.25	>128	>128	4	>128
A. niger						
4.55	0.5	0.25	>128	>128	64	>128
3884	0.06	0.06	>128	>128	64	>128
S. cerevisiae						
ATCC 9763	0.06		0.06	0.25		

[a] Values expressed in micrograms per milliliter.

TABLE 2. *Antagonistic effect of pyrimidines and some of their nucleosides on the fungistatic activity of 5-FC*[a]

Organism	MIC (μg/ml)	Cyt	Cyd	dCyd	Ura	Urd	Thyd
S. cerevisiae ATCC 9763	0.04	2[b]	0	0	0	0	0
A. fumigatus							
4.6	400	1	−1	−1	>1	−1	0
4.28	400	1	−1	−1	>1	0	0
4.19	4.0	2	2	2	>3	>3	0
4.33	4.0	3	1	1	3	2	0
4.41	4.0	3	2	1	NG[c]	>3	1
A. niger							
4.55	0.4	>3	>3	>3	>3	1	1
3884	≤0.04	5	>5	5	>5	4	1

[a] Abbreviations: Cyt, Cytosine; Cyd, cytidine; dCyd, deoxycytidine; Ura, uracil; Urd, uridine; Thyd, thymidine.

[b] Power of 10 by which the MIC was altered.

[c] NG, No growth.

TABLE 3. *Antagonistic effect of some purines and their nucleosides on the fungistatic activity of 5-FC*[a]

Organism	MIC (μg/ml)	Ade	Ades	Hypo	dGuas
S. cerevisiae ATCC 9763	≤0.04	2[b]	4	2	4
A. fumigatus					
4.6	400	1	>1	1	>1
4.28	400	1	>1	1	>1
4.19	4.0	>3	>3	3	>3
4.33	4.0	2	>3	3	>3
4.41	4.0	3	>3	3	>3
A. niger					
4.55	0.4	>3	3	>3	3
3884	≤0.04	3	4	3	4

[a] Abbreviations: Ade, Adenine; Ades, adenosine; Hypo, hypoxanthine; dGuas, deoxyguanasine.

[b] Power of 10 by which the MIC was altered.

ceptible to 5-FC although to different degrees (0.4 and 0.04 μg/ml, respectively).

Of the pyrimidines and their nucleosides examined (Table 2), all but thymidine influenced the fungistatic activity of 5-FC against every organism tested. In each case, uracil was the most powerful antagonist. In contrast, cytidine and deoxycytidine decreased by one titer step the MIC of 5-FC for *A. fumigatus* strains 4.6 and 4.28, whereas uridine produced a similar effect on *A. fumigatus* strain 4.6. Thymidine had the least overall antagonistic effect on activity of 5-FC against the aspergilli.

All of the purines and their nucleosides tested antagonized the fungistatic effects of 5-FC (Table 3). The MIC values for the strains more resistant to 5-FC, *A. fumigatus* strains 4.6 and 4.28, were increased to or beyond the limits of detection of 4,000 μg/ml. The MIC values for *A. fumigatus* strains 4.19, 4.33, and 4.41 and *A. niger* strains 4.55 and 3884 were increased by three or four titer steps each.

Uptake of [2-^{14}C]5-FC as influenced by pyrimidines, purines, and nucleosides. The studies on 5-FC taken up as influenced by a number of pyrimidines, purines, and some of their nucleosides were conducted in liquid shaking culture and measured after 72 h of incubation, when cells had reached the stationary phase of growth. On the basis of the alteration of MIC values by pyrimidines, purines, and their nucleosides, *A. fumigatus* strain 4.6, *A. fumigatus* strain 4.19, and *A. niger* strain 4.55 were chosen as representative organisms of the three groups noted above. The percentage of inhibition of radioactivity taken up at the concentration of 10 μg of 5-FC per ml as influenced by 1,000 μg of the various compounds being tested per ml is shown in Table 4. Uptake obtained in the presence of [2-^{14}C]5-FC alone was taken as 100%. Significant decreases of amounts of 5-FC taken up were measured for each pyrimidine, purine, or nucleoside tested except for the following: cytidine in *A. fumigatus* strain 4.6, adenosine in *A. fumigatus* strain 4.19, and cytidine and uridine in *A. niger* strain 4.55.

DISCUSSION

Conflicting reports on the efficacy of 5-FC in treating aspergillosis (14) interested us in in-

TABLE 4. *Percent inhibition of uptake of [2-^{14}C]5-FC (0.02 μCi/ml, 10 μg of 5-FC per ml) when 1,000 μg of various purines, pyrimidines, and nucleosides per ml were added to the growth medium*[a]

Compound	Percent inhibition[b]		
	A. fumigatus 4.6	*A. fumigatus* 4.19	*A. niger* 4.55
Cyt	95	98	94
Cyd	0	80	0
dCyd	88	84	80
Ura	90	97	83
Ade	>99	89	97
Hypo	>99	98	83
Ades	40	0	90
dGuas	91	71	56
Urd	88	51	0
Thyd	58	61	19

[a] Total [2-^{14}C]5-FC taken up in the absence of additional compounds was considered as 100%.

[b] The 5-FC MIC values for the three strains were 400, 4.0, and 4.0 μg/ml for *A. fumigatus* 4.6, *A. fumigatus* 4.19, and *A. niger* 4.55, respectively.

vestigating whether the drug follows a metabolic pathway in *Aspergillus* sp. similar to that described in yeastlike organisms. Our initial step was to examine the ability of exogenous pyrimidines, purines, and some of their nucleosides to inhibit the fungistatic activity of the drug in these organisms.

The basic mechanism by which 5-FC inhibits the growth of yeast cells has been explained (8). In comparing the mode of action of the drug in *C. albicans* with a scheme proposed for *S. cerevisiae* (6), Polak and Scholer (10) examined the capacity of exogenous pyrimidines, purines, and nucleosides to antagonize the fungistatic activity of 5-FC. As expected, they found that cytosine and uridine antagonized the activity of 5-FC in *C. albicans*, but the inability of uracil to produce such an effect seemed paradoxical. This was resolved when it was shown that the uptake of uracil in these organisms was very limited. Also intriguing was the fact that some purines such as adenosine and hypoxanthine were strong antagonists of the fungistatic activity of 5-FC. Further investigations (9) revealed that *S. cerevisiae* as well as *C. albicans* possessed a permease that recognized cytosine, 5-FC, and certain purines. The inability of a compound to inhibit the activity of the drug was correlated with inhibition of uptake of 5-FC in the presence of that compound (10).

In the strains of aspergilli examined, all of the pyrimidines, purines, and nucleosides tested except thymidine consistently produced an alteration of MIC values. Thymidine exhibited antagonism in both strains of *A. niger* used in this study, but this effect was limited to only one strain of *A. fumigatus*. The enhancement of the fungistatic activity of 5-FC by cytidine, deoxycytidine, and uridine in isolated instances remains a paradox at this time. It is interesting to note, however, that this enhancement was limited to the two resistant strains of *A. fumigatus*. In general, a reciprocal correlation existed between the ability of a compound to alter the MIC value and the amount of 5-FC taken up by a strain of the aspergilli. Discrepancies in this correlation may be the result of measuring the amount of [2-^{14}C]5-FC taken up after a 72-h culture time.

From the data obtained in this investigation, no inference as to the mode of action of 5-FC in *Aspergillus* sp. can be made. It is apparent, however, that the aspergilli may possess a common purine and pyrimidine uptake system. Such a common uptake system has been reported for *Neurospora crassa* (12). Further investigations on the mode of action of 5-FC in *Aspergillus* sp. are needed to clarify the mechanisms of uptake and inhibition.

ACKNOWLEDGMENTS

The [2-^{14}C]5-FC used in this study was provided by Hoffman-La Roche, Inc., of Basle, Switzerland.

Funds for this research were provided in part through the Advisory Committee and Board of Directors of the Brown-Hazen Program of Research Corporation of America.

LITERATURE CITED

1. **Atkinson, W., and H. L. Israel.** 1973. 5-Fluorocytosine treatment of meningeal and pulmonary aspergillosis. Am. J. Med. **55:**496–504.
2. **Bennett, J. E.** 1974. Chemotherapy of systemic mycoses. N. Engl. J. Med. **290:**320–323.
3. **Ericsson, H. M., and J. C. Sherris.** 1971. Antibiotic sensitivity testing. Report of an international collaborative study. Acta Pathol. Microbiol. Scand. Sect. B, Suppl. 217.
4. **Fass, R. J., and R. L. Perkins.** 1971. 5-Fluorocytosine in the treatment of cryptococcal and *Candida* mycoses. Ann. Intern. Med. **74:**535–539.
5. **Grenson, M.** 1969. The utilization of exogenous pyrimidines and the recycling of uridine-5-phosphate derivatives in *Saccharomyces cerevisiae*, as studied by means of mutants affected in pyrimidine uptake and metabolism. Eur. J. Biochem. **11:**249–260.
6. **Jund, R., and F. Lacroute.** 1970. Genetic and physiological aspects of resistance to 5-fluoropyrimidines in *Saccharomyces cerevisiae*. J. Bacteriol. **102:**607–615.
7. **Mauceri, A. A., S. I. Cullen, A. G. Vandevelde, and J. E. Johnson III.** 1974. Flucytosine: an oral treatment for chromomycosis. Arch. Dermatol. **109:**873–876.
8. **Polak, A.** 1974. Effects of 5-fluorocytosine on protein synthesis and amino acid pool in *Candida albicans*. Sabouraudia **12:**309–319.
9. **Polak, A., and M. Grenson.** 1973. Evidence for a common transport system for cytosine, adenine and hypoxanthine in *Saccharomyces cerevisiae* and *Candida albicans*. Eur. J. Biochem. **32:**276–282.
10. **Polak, A., and H. J. Scholer.** 1973. Fungistatic activity, uptake and incorporation of 5-fluorocytosine in *Candida albicans*, as influenced by pyrimidines and purines. I. Reversal experiments. Pathol. Microbiol. **39:**148–159.

11. **Polak, A., and H. J. Scholer.** 1973. Fungistatic activity, uptake and incorporation of 5-fluorocytosine in *Candida albicans*, as influenced by pyrimidines and purines. II. Studies on distribution and incorporation. Pathol. Microbiol. 39:334–347.
12. **Schlitz, J. R., and K. D. Terry.** 1970. Nucleoside uptake during the germination of *Neurospora crassa* conidia. Biochim. Biophys. Acta 209:278–288.
13. **Shadomy, S., H. J. Shadomy, J. A. McCay, and J. P. Utz.** 1969. *In vitro* susceptibility of *Cryptococcus neoformans* to amphotericin B, hamycin and 5-fluorocytosine, p. 452–460. Antimicrob. Agents Chemother. 1968.
14. **Steer, P. L., M. I. Marks, P. D. Klite, and T. C. Eickoff.** 1972. 5-Fluorocytosine: an oral antifungal compound. Ann. Intern. Med. 76:15–22.
15. **Utz, J. P., B. S. Tines, H. J. Shadomy, R. J. Duma, M. M. Kannan, and K. N. Mason.** 1969. 5-Fluorocytosine in human cryptococcosis, p. 344–346. Antimicrob. Agents Chemother. 1968.

ANTIMICROBIAL AGENTS AND CHEMOTHERAPY, Feb. 1977, p. 234-239 Vol. 11, No. 2

Printed in U.S.A.

Prevention of 5-Fluorouracil-Caused Growth Inhibition in *Sordaria fimicola*

HOWARD F. SCHOEN[1]* AND JOHN BERECH, JR.

Department of Biology, Queens College of the City University of New York, Flushing, New York 11367, and Graduate School and University Center, City University of New York, New York, New York 10036

Received for publication 1 September 1976

Growth (dry weight accumulation) of *Sordaria fimicola* in standing liquid culture (sucrose-nitrate-salts-vitamins) is inhibited by the presence of 5 μM 5-fluorouracil in the medium. This inhibition is completely prevented by uracil, deoxyuridine, and 5-bromouracil, partly prevented (40 to 90% of growth observed without 5-fluorouracil) by uridine, thymidine, and 5-bromodeoxyuridine, and slightly prevented by trifluorothymine, cytosine, cytidine, deoxycytidine, and 5-methylcytosine (all at 0.5 to 1 mM). Thymidine and thymine riboside were without any apparent effect. Growth is also inhibited by 0.2 mM 6-azauracil, and this inhibition was completely prevented by uracil and uridine, partly prevented by deoxyuridine, 5-bromouracil, cytidine, and 5-methylcytosine, and slightly prevented by thymine, thymidine, 5-bromodeoxyuridine, cytosine, and deoxycytidine. The data suggest that the observed inhibition of growth by 5-fluorouracil is due to inhibition of both ribonucleic acid and deoxyribonucleic acid synthesis. The data also allow inferences concerning pyrimidine interconversions in *S. fimicola;* i.e., thymine can be anabolized to thymidylic acid without first being demethylated, although demethylation appears to occur also.

There is much practical importance in knowing the pathways of nucleic acid precursor interconversions for the design of selective anticancer and antimicrobial drugs. The invention of the anticancer drug 5-fluorouracil (FU) followed the recognition that cancer cells use uracil for nucleic acid biosynthesis to a greater extent than normal cells (5). The success of the antimycotic drug 5-fluorocytosine appears to depend on the ability of fungi to deaminate the drug to FU and the inability of mammalian cells to do so (10).

In our laboratory we have been attempting to elucidate the modes of action of FU in the inhibition of growth and perithecial formation in *Sordaria fimicola*. One of the procedures employed has been to investigate the ability of various pyrimidines and pyrimidine derivatives to prevent FU inhibition. On the basis of these data we also have been able to propose a scheme for the interconversions of some pyrimidine metabolites in this fungus.

(This paper is based on a portion of the Ph.D. thesis of H. F. Schoen [City University of New York, 1975].)

MATERIALS AND METHODS

Organism. A wild-type strain of *S. fimicola* (rob.) Ces. et de Not. was obtained from the American Type Culture Collection (culture 14517) and was maintained on slants of basal medium solidified with 2% agar. Transfers were allowed to grow and develop at room temperature (20 to 28°C) until mature perithecia were present, about 6 days, and then stored at 4 to 6°C.

Medium. A sucrose-nitrate medium, with thiamine and biotin added, modified slightly from that of Bretzloff (1), was the basal medium used in all experiments. It contained (in 1.00 liter of glass-distilled water): sucrose, 20.0 g; KNO_3, 1.0 g KH_2PO_4, 1.0 g; $MgSO_4 \cdot 7H_2O$, 0.5 g; $CaCl \cdot 2H_2O$, 0.12 g; $FeCl_3$, 0.1 mg; $MnSO_4 \cdot 4H_2O$, 0.4 mg; $CuSO_4 \cdot 5H_2O$, 0.4 mg; $Zn(NO_3)_2 \cdot 6H_2O$, 0.9 mg; thiamine-hydrochloride, 0.5 mg; and biotin, 12.5 μg. The pH of the medium is 4.6 before autoclaving and was not adjusted except for experiments in which additions to the medium altered the pH, in which cases it was readjusted to 4.6 with HCl.

The medium was autoclaved at 121°C for 15 min. Additions to the basal medium were incorporated into the medium before autoclaving, except for trifluorothymine solutions, which were filter sterilized separately and then added to the cooled, autoclaved medium.

Inoculum and incubation conditions. The inoculum was prepared by transferring scrapings from a stock slant to a 250-ml Erlenmeyer flask containing 50 ml of basal medium, allowing this to grow without shaking for 5 to 6 days, and then blending in a Virtis homogenizer.

Experimental cultures contained 40 ml of medium in a 250-ml Erlenmeyer flask and were inoculated with 0.4 ml of the blended inoculum. The flasks were

[1] Department of Ophthalmology, Mount Sinai School of Medicine, New York NY 10029.

incubated without shaking at 24 ± 2°C in constant fluorescent white light (Sylvania Powertube, Cool White, FA8T12-CW-VHO).

Dry weight determination. The mycelium was collected on a tared filter paper circle in a Büchner funnel, washed twice with water, dried overnight in an oven at 90°C, and weighed.

RESULTS

Table 1 gives the results of a series of experiments on the prevention of FU inhibition of growth by various pyrimidines and derivatives. Uracil and deoxyuridine were the most effective compounds; at 0.50 mM they completely prevented the growth (dry weight accumulation) inhibition by 5.0 μM FU. Uridine was less effective. Thymine was also quite effective but, at 5.0 μM FU, the effect reached a plateau at 0.50 mM at less than complete restoration of growth. In the presence of 10 μM FU, thymine was more effective at 1.0 mM than at 0.50 mM, but the response was still less than complete. The thymine nucleosides were apparently without any effect.

Some analogues of thymine also were tried as preventives. 5-Bromouracil (bromouracil) was even more effective than thymine, and 5-bromodeoxyuridine (bromodeoxyuridine) was quite effective even though thymidine was not.

Finally, cytosine, its nucleosides, and 5-methylcytosine showed a slight preventive effect.

Dry weights were determined also in older cultures (15 to 25 days old) (data not shown). The overall pattern of results was similar to that seen in the 5-day-old cultures. The percentage of inhibition by FU alone was less. Where the growth as a percentage of control for a preventive was high (as, for example, with 0.50 mM thymine), there was in general no

TABLE 1. *Prevention of FU inhibition by pyrimidines and pyrimidine nucleosides*

FU concn (μM)	Base series	Base series concn (mM)	Growth (%)[a]		
			Free base	Ribonucleoside	Deoxyribonucleoside
5.0	None		10.6 ± 6.7		
	Uracil	0.0010	15.3 ± 1.8	–[b]	–
		0.0050	24.7 ± 1.0	13	19
		0.050	76.5	21	47
		0.50	113 ± 33.2	28.8 ± 8.0	90.6 ± 28.9
		1.0	87	51.3 ± 32.9	109
	Thymine	0.0050	0	–	–
		0.050	26.3 ± 0.4	–	–
		0.50	65.1 ± 14.4	–	–
		1.0	68.0 ± 5.3	5.5	19 ± 9.9
	Bromouracil	0.0050	20	–	5.0
		0.050	39	–	9.5
		0.50	95.0	–	51.0
		1.0	87.0 ± 16.3	–	82.5
	Azathymine	1.0	14.3 ± 0.4	–	–
	Trifluorothymine	0.75	28	–	–
		1.0	32.8 ± 3.2	–	–
	Cytosine	0.50	26	27	22
		1.0	38	–	–
	5-Methylcytosine	0.50	28	–	–
10	None		6.5 ± 3.1		
	Thymine	0.050	12	–	–
		0.10	17 ± 1.4	–	–
		0.50	37	–	–
		1.0	58.5 ± 16.3	–	–

[a] Dry weight after 5 days, as percentage of control without FU, plus or minus the standard deviation of the mean of two replicates where experiment was repeated.

[b] –, Data not avilable.

further increase, relative to the control, in older cultures. Where the degree of reversal was smaller (as with 0.0050 mM uracil), there was an increase in the percentage dry weight in older cultures. However, since the culture with FU alone also increased in percentage dry weight, there was no increase in the relative degree of prevention (in fact, there was usually a decrease).

There was, however, one exception to this pattern. The growth, as percentage of control, with deoxyuridine typically decreased in older cultures (for 0.50 mM deoxyuridine, the average in cultures aged 15 to 25 days was 72%, and for 1.0 mM it was 76%).

In general, the degree of perithecial development was correlated with the degree of restoration of growth. Even in cases where growth restoration was complete, however, there were usually noticeable differences in overall appearance between the control and the cultures with additions. The only preventive restoring the appearance of the culture to one identical to the control was uracil at 0.50 mM and above; 1.0 mM uridine gave almost normal perithecial development, but the overall appearance of the culture was still noticeably different from the control. Thymine and uridine together also gave an appearance like that of the control (see below).

Two additional types of experiments were performed to check on the specificity of the preventive effect. In one, the ability of purines and a purine ribonucleoside (inosine) at 100 times the molarity to prevent inhibition by 5 μM FU was tested. They were totally without effect. In the other, several pyrimidine compounds at 0.50 mM were tested in the absence of FU for their effect on growth. Uracil, uridine, deoxyuridine, and bromouracil were slightly stimulatory (ca. 20% more growth after 5 days than with no additions), and thymine and bromodeoxyuridine were without effect. At 18 days no effects were seen on growth, but bromouracil and bromodeoxyuridine inhibited perithecial development somewhat. (Cytosine compounds were not tested in this manner.)

To account for the effects of uptake and usage peculiarities in *S. fimicola* of these compounds, the ability of the above compounds to prevent the inhibitory effects of the inhibitor of pyrimidine anabolism 6-azauracil (azauracil) was tested. Azauracil inhibits the de novo synthesis of pyrimidines (14). The ability of a compound to prevent the inhibition would indicate: (i) that the compound was taken up and anabolized to the extent that it could replace the needed components that were not being made de novo because of the inhibitor, or (ii) that it interferes with the transport of the inhibitor itself and exerts its preventive effect that way. The procedure is not foolproof, as intermediate steps involved in the interconversions are not known for *S. fimicola*.

The results of the experiment with azauracil are given in Table 2. Surprisingly, all the pyrimidines tested gave some stimulation of growth compared to azauracil alone. Uracil and uridine completely prevented inhibition; deoxyuridine was less effective. Thymine gave relatively less growth here than in the FU experiments; bromouracil, as in the FU experiments, was more effective than thymine, but bromodeoxyuridine was much less effective than in the FU experiments.

One additional experiment was performed to try to determine whether the effects of thymine and deoxyuridine on FU inhibition are separable from the effects of uridine. That is, do thymine and deoxyuridine stimulate growth by a different mechanism (presumably by providing an increased endogenous supply of thymidylic acid) than uridine (presumably by increasing the endogenous supply of uridylic acid)? The experiment consisted of testing the effects of combinations of thymine, uridine, and deoxyuridine. The results are shown in Table 3. The effects of thymine plus deoxyuridine were intermediate between those of thymine alone and deoxyuridine alone. Thymine plus uridine and uridine plus deoxyuridine had a greater effect than either alone. Of the combinations, only thymine plus uridine was like the control in perithecial development and overall appearance. Although these results seem to indicate that thymine and uridine do act in different ways in preventing inhibition by FU, the differ-

TABLE 2. *Prevention of azauracil inhibition by pyrimidines and pyrimidine nucleosides*[a]

Preventive[b]	Growth (%)[c]
None	1
Uracil	117
Uridine	112.5
Deoxyuridine	78.5
Thymine	21
Thymidine	14
Bromouracil	47.5
Bromodeoxyuridine	27.5
Cytosine	29.5
Cytidine	76.5
Deoxycytidine	28
5-Methylcytosine	47

[a] Azauracil at 0.20 mM.

[b] Preventives at 0.50 mM each.

[c] Dry weight after 5 days, as percentage of control without azauracil. Average of two replicates.

TABLE 3. *Prevention of FU inhibition by thymine, uridine, and deoxyuridine, separately and in combinations*[a]

Preventive	Concn (mM)	Growth (%)[b]	
		5 days	15 days
None		14	27
Thymine	0.50	57.5	67
Deoxyuridine	0.50	100.5	56.5
Uridine	0.50	23	81
Thymine + deoxyuridine	0.25 0.25	86	70
Thymine + uridine	0.25 0.25	73.5	94
Deoxyuridine + uridine	0.25 0.25	128	100.5

[a] FU at 5.0 μM.

[b] Dry weight as percentage of control without FU. Average of two replicates.

ences are not necessarily those presumed above (see Discussion).

DISCUSSION

The following mechanisms of the prevention of FU inhibition have been reported (6, 11, 12): (i) inhibition of uptake, (ii) inhibition of anabolism to the active derivative, (iii) inhibition of incorporation of the active derivative into ribonucleic acid (RNA), and (iv) bypass of the block in thymidylic acid synthesis by supplying the cell with an alternate source of thymidylic acid, usually thymine or thymidine (4, 5, 13, 15). Since FU is incorporated into RNA only as 5-fluorouridylic acid residues (5, 12), presumably only those compounds that are ultimately converted to uridine triphosphate or an analogue thereof can prevent FU inhibition by method (iii).

The greater preventive effects of uracil and uridine, compared with cytosine and cytidine, could be due to the action of the former two compounds by all three mechanisms, the action of the latter two being restricted to methods (ii) and/or (iii), presumably after being deaminated to uracil or a uracil derivative.

The situation with regard to deoxyuridine and deoxycytidine is less clear. They may act by somehow reversing the block in thymidylic acid synthesis, possibly by raising the endogenous levels of deoxyuridylic acid. However, the block in thymidylic acid synthesis would by itself be expected to cause the endogenous level of deoxyuridylic acid to rise, and it is questionable whether any exogenously added compound would raise this level further. We feel, therefore, that deoxyuridine and deoxycytidine act by being ultimately converted to uracil or uridylic acid, rather than deoxyuridylic acid, and act through method (ii) or (iii).

Thymine would, at first thought, be expected to act by method (iv). Similarly, bromouracil, which in some organisms is incorporated into deoxyribonucleic acid (DNA) in place of thymine without severe effects on DNA function (2), might also, along with bromodeoxyuridine, be expected to act this way. In *Neurospora crassa*, however, there are no known enzymes for thymine anabolism (3, 10). Thymine and thymidine are, however, converted in vivo to uracil (3, 9, 10). If this were the case in *S. fimicola*, then thymine could not act by method (iv) and would presumably act by method (ii) or (iii). Bromouracil and bromodeoxyuridine could presumably also act this way if they were debrominated (2). But if thymine, bromouracil, and bromodeoxyuridine can be converted to uracil, then one would expect them to prevent inhibition caused by azauracil also. As shown in Table 2, however, these compounds are much less effective in preventing azauracil inhibition than FU inhibition (Table 1). We conclude, therefore, that the enzymes for thymine anabolism are present in *S. fimicola* and that at least part of the preventive effects of these compounds with FU is due to the bypassing of the block in thymidylic acid synthesis (method iv). (If the enzymes for thymine anabolism are indeed present, it is surprising that the analogues trifluorothymine and 6-azathymine have been reported not to inhibit growth or perithecial production in *S. fimicola* [8; H. F. Schoen, Ph.D. thesis, City University of New York, 1975]. On the other hand, if 6-azathymine is converted to azauracil, it should also have an inhibitory effect. Trifluorothymine did have a slight preventive effect with FU [Table 1].) Additional possibilities for the preventive effect of thymine, bromouracil, and bromodeoxyuridine are: antagonism of the uptake or anabolism of FU (and more effective than that of azauracil) and inhibition of catabolism of FU to the tricarboxylic acid cycle inhibitor fluoroacetic acid (7)—inhibition by thymine of FU catabolism has been reported (2).

In the experiment shown in Table 3, where pairs of preventives were used, it was noted that some pairs gave better prevention than the individual preventives, viz., at 5 days, thymine plus uridine, and, at 15 days, thymine plus uridine and deoxyuridine plus uridine. This suggests that the inhibition of both RNA and DNA synthesis is involved in the inhibition of growth by FU. It may, however, indicate only that the conversion of the members of each pair to uridine triphosphate occurs via different pathways, and that the ultimate endogenous level of uridine triphosphate achieved is greater when both pathways are utilized. (We have already mentioned that deoxyuridine and uridine likely act by the same method.)

In summary, we believe that the inhibition of growth by 5 μM FU involves inhibition of DNA synthesis and possibly also normal RNA synthesis. Whether this is also the case at lower FU concentrations, where inhibition of branch density and perithecia formation has been reported (8), is not known.

We can now attempt a synthesis of what the data may tell us about pyrimidine interconversions in *S. fimicola*, in spite of the fact that conclusions from this type of data can be only tentative without supporting enzyme and genetic data and experiments with labeled precursors.

From the experiment on preventives of azauracil-caused growth inhibition (Table 2) it can be seen that all the preventives tried were successful to some degree in preventing growth inhibition. Since azauracil is believed to act by inhibiting de novo pyrimidine synthesis, this implies that either all these compounds are capable of ultimately being converted to a uracil ribonucleotide, at least to some degree, or that they interfere with the uptake or anabolism of azauracil itself. On the basis of our data there is no way of clearly distinguishing between these two possibilities.

Since azauracil inhibits by blocking the de novo synthesis of pyrimidines, those compounds that are converted to a uracil compound past the block (e.g., uridylic acid) to only a very slight degree may nevertheless have a marked effect on allowing growth to proceed. On the other hand, FU is converted to 5-fluorouridine triphosphate and is subsequently incorporated into RNA. Uridine triphosphate formed from potential preventives will thus have to compete with the 5-fluorouridine triphosphate for incorporation, and we therefore can expect that relatively high levels will be required for the competition to be successful. In addition, uridine ribonucleotides presumably continue to be made de novo in the presence of FU, and hence additions to this pool resulting from transformation of exogenous pyrimidines may not have a great effect. Thus, we assume that prevention of FU inhibition is indicative of a major conversion of the preventive to a uridine ribonucleotide. Complications in this interpretation are the possible relief of the thymidylic acid block by certain preventives and the inhibition of the uptake and anabolism of FU by the preventive. One should also bear in mind that differences in the effectiveness of the preventives may be due to differences in the rate of uptake of the preventives themselves.

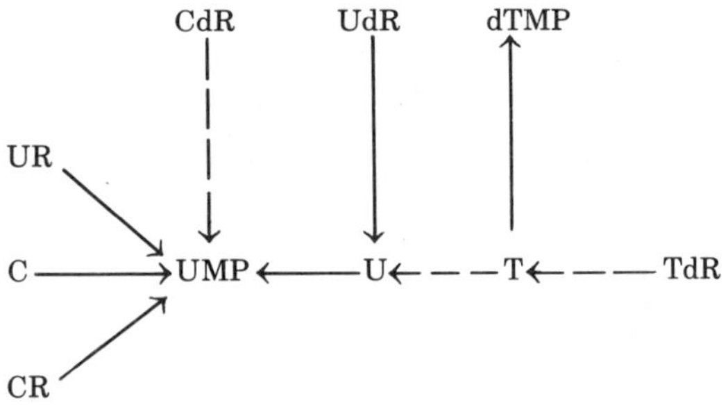

FIG. 1. *Proposed scheme of pyrimidine interconversions in S. fimicola, as determined by studies of prevention of FU and azauracil inhibition by various pyrimidines and pyrimidine derivatives. Dashed lines indicate that the proposed reaction occurs only slightly. Arrows connect only those intermediates that are implicated directly by the data; they do not necessarily show the pathways involved. Abbreviations: U, uracil; UR, uridine; UdR, deoxyuridine; UMP, uracil ribonucleotide, presumably uridylic acid when derived from U or UR; T, thymine; TdR, thymidine; dTMP, thymidylic acid; C, cytosine; CR, cytidine; CdR, deoxycytidine.*

The hypothesized interconversions are summarized in Fig. 1.

LITERATURE CITED

1. **Bretzloff, C. W., Jr.** 1954. The growth and fruiting of *Sordaria fimicola*. Am. J. Bot. 41:58–67.
2. **Brockman, R. W., and E. P. Anderson.** 1963. Pyrimidine analogues, p. 239–285. *In* R. M. Hochster and J. H. Quastel (ed.), Metabolic inhibitors: a comprehensive treatise, vol. 1. Academic Press Inc., New York.
3. **Fink, R. M., and K. Fink.** 1962. Relative retention of H^3 and C^{14} labels of nucleosides incorporated into nucleic acids of *Neurospora*. J. Biol. Chem. 237:2889–2891.
4. **Hahn, G. A., and H. G. Mandel.** 1971. Effects of fluorouracil on RNA synthesis in *Bacillus cereus*. Biochem. Pharmacol. 20:1973–1990.
5. **Heidelberger, C.** 1965. Fluorinated pyrimidines. Prog. Nucleic Acid Res. Mol. Biol. 4:1–50.
6. **Kempner, E. S.** 1961. The selection and utilization of metabolic analogs for nucleic acid synthesis. Biochim. Biophys. Acta 53:111–122.
7. **Koenig, H., and A. Patel.** 1970. Biochemical basis for fluorouracil neurotoxicity. The role of Krebs cycle inhibition by fluoroacetate. Arch. Neurol. 23:155–160.
8. **Lindenmayer, A., and H. F. Schoen.** 1967. Selective effects of purine and pyrimidine analogues and of respiratory inhibitors on perithecial development and branching in *Sordaria*. Plant Physiol. 42:1059–1070.
9. **Liu, C.-K., C. Hsu, and M. T. Abbott.** 1973. Catalysis of three sequential dioxygenase reactions by thymine 7-hydroxylase. Arch. Biochem. Biophys. 159:180–187.
10. **O'Donovan, G. A., and J. Neuhard.** 1970. Pyrimidine metabolism in microorganisms. Bacteriol. Rev. 34:278–343.
11. **Polak, A., and M. Grenson.** 1973. Evidence for a common transport system for cytosine, adenine and hypoxanthine in *Saccharomyces cerevisiae* and *Candida albicans*. Eur. J. Biochem. 32:276–282.
12. **Polak, A., and H. J. Scholer.** 1973. Fungistatic activity, uptake and incorporation of 5-fluorocytosine in *Candida albicans*, as influenced by pyrimidines and pu-

rines II. Studies on distribution and incorporation. Pathol. Microbiol. 39:334–347.
13. **Reich, M., and H. G. Mandel.** 1966. Dissociation of cellular functions in *Bacillus cereus* by 5-fluorouracil. J. Bacteriol. 91:517–523.
14. **Škoda, J.** 1963. Mechanism of action and application of azapyrimidines. Prog. Nucleic Acid Res. 2:196–219.
15. **Ullman, J., J. Krekule, and L. Teltscherová.** 1972. Action of inhibition by fluorodeoxyuridine and its reversal by thymidine o the nucleic acid fractions of the overground parts of photoperiodically induced *Chenopodium rubrum* plants. Biol. Plant. 14:350–355.

Antimicrobial Agents and Chemotherapy, Feb. 1977, p. 240–243 Vol. 11, No. 2

Antimicrobial Prophylaxis for Catheter-Associated Bacteriuria

MICHAEL R. BRITT,* RICHARD A. GARIBALDI, WILLIAM A. MILLER, RICHARD M. HEBERTSON, and JOHN P. BURKE

Departments of Medicine (Infectious Diseases), Medical Biophysics and Computing, and Obstetrics and Gynecology, University of Utah College of Medicine and LDS Hospital, Salt Lake City, Utah 84143

Received for publication 29 June 1976

We evaluated short-term systemic antimicrobial prophylaxis for catheter-associated bacteriuria in women undergoing elective gynecological operations in a prospective, controlled, double-masked study. Nine of 100 placebo-treated patients acquired bacteriuria during catheterization compared with 3 of 96 of the drug-treated group. However, at the time of hospital discharge, clean-voided urine specimens were positive as frequently in the drug-treated group (8 of 82 patients cultured) as in the placebo group (8 of 75 patients cultured). No difference in febrile morbidity due to bacteriuria was noted between the prophylaxis and placebo groups. The incidence of catheter-associated bacteriuria may be reduced by antimicrobial prophylaxis. However, because the protective effect is transient and is associated with the selection of resistant organisms, prophylaxis is not indicated for patients at low risk for acquired bacteriuria and in whom the sequelae of catheter-associated infections are infrequent.

In a prospective survey of patients with indwelling urethral catheters, we observed a lower rate of acquired bacteriuria in patients who were receiving systemic antimicrobials than in untreated patients (3). The apparent protective effect of antimicrobial treatment was noted during each of the first 4 days of catheterization, and was evident for both female and male, old and young, and critically ill and noncritically ill patients. Overall, the average daily incidences of acquiring bacteriuria were 4.1% for patients who received antimicrobials and 12.2% for patients who did not. However, microbial species associated with increased antibiotic resistance were cultured more often from treated patients than from the untreated comparison group. We undertook the present study to evaluate, in a prospective, double-masked trial, the effects of short-term use of an antimicrobial on the rate of acquired bacteriuria.

MATERIALS AND METHODS

From April 1974 to February 1975, data were collected from patients admitted to a 23-bed gynecological division of the LDS Hospital. Patients were included in the study if they gave informed consent, underwent a gynecological operation, received an indwelling urethral or suprapubic urinary catheter, and did not have a rapidly or ultimately fatal disease, an active clinical infection, or allergy to penicillins or cephalosporins. Patients with positive urine cultures at the time of insertion of the catheter were analyzed separately. The study patients received either antimicrobial or placebo provided through the hospital pharmacy by a randomization schedule. Neither the attending physicians, study personnel, nor nursing personnel were aware of the treatment regimen assigned by the pharmacy. If a complication occurred which required release of this information, a note was made in the study record. The first dose of the antimicrobial (cefazolin sodium [Kefzol], 500 mg) was given at the time of operation, and each subsequent dose was given at 8-h intervals, intravenously or intramuscularly, for a total of nine doses.

A clean-voided urine specimen for culture was collected preoperatively upon entry to the study. Additional specimens were collected at the time of catheter insertion and daily during indwelling catheterization by aseptic needle puncture of the catheter tubing. A clean-voided specimen was also collected on the day of discharge from the hospital. All urine specimens were refrigerated within 1 h of collection and 0.1- and 0.01-ml samples were streaked on blood and MacConkey agar plates, respectively. We considered gram-negative bacilli and/or enterococci with colony counts of 10^5 or more per ml from clean-voided specimens and 10^2 or more per ml from catheter specimens indicative of colonization of bladder urine. Colony counts of this magnitude were reproducible by our culture method and were not considered to reflect bacterial contamination during specimen collection or processing. Bacterial identification was performed by standard methods.

The indwelling urinary catheters were inserted by physicians at the time of operation. Povidone-iodine solution was used for meatal cleansing before catheter insertion. The same commercially available closed-drainage bag system was used throughout the study. Nursing personnel were instructed in, and closely monitored, regarding the techniques of closed sterile drainage. A member of the study team visited each patient daily to monitor the quality of catheter care and to collect clinical data and urine specimens. Blood cultures were obtained according to study protocol from patients who had fever greater than 38.3°C orally. Febrile morbidity was defined as an oral temperature of 38.0°C or greater for at least 2 consecutive days, excluding the first 24 h after operation.

RESULTS

Patient population. A total of 215 patients were entered into the study; 14 patients were subsequently excluded because the first clean-voided or catheterized specimen was positive, and five patients were excluded because they were catheterized for less than 1 day. The final study population included 100 in the placebo group and 96 in the active-drug group. The two treatment groups were similar in age (40.6 years in the prophylaxis group versus 38.3 years in the placebo), type of surgery (Table 1), quality of catheter care, and type of catheterization (6 suprapubic catheters in the prophylaxis group versus 12 in the placebo group).

Acquired bacteriuria. Overall, 24 patients acquired bacteriuria; 12 patients became colonized during their period of catheterization and 12 additional patients had more than 10^5 colonies per ml in clean-voided specimens at time of hospital discharge (Table 1). Four patients who acquired bacteriuria during catheterization also had more than 10^5 colonies per ml in clean-voided specimens at the time of hospital discharge. Of those patients who acquired bacteriuria during indwelling catheterization, three had received antimicrobial prophylaxis and nine had received placebo. Only one of the patients in the active-drug group acquired bacteriuria during the period of drug administration. The other two patients acquired bacteriuria while still catheterized but were colonized 2 and 5 days after the prophylaxis has been discontinued. All nine patients in the placebo group who acquired bacteriuria were colonized during the first 3 days of catheterization. The average daily rate of acquired bacteriuria was 1.7% for the prophylaxis group compared with 3.8% for the placebo group. Enterococcus (two) and indole-negative *Proteus* (one) were cultured from the three antimicrobial-treated patients who were colonized during their period of catheterization. The nine placebo-treated patients who acquired bacteriuria were colonized with *Escherichia coli* (eight) and *Enterobacter* (one). No significant differences in rates of bacteriuria were observed between patients who had undergone vaginal versus abdominal hysterectomies. None of the patients who had received suprapubic catheters became bacteriuric.

At the time of hospital discharge, the rates of positive cultures of clean-voided specimens were similar for the prophylaxis and placebo groups (Table 1). The bacterial isolates from patients who received prophylaxis included *E. coli* (three), *Enterobacter* (three), *Pseudomonas* (one), and both *E. coli* and enterococcus (one). Patients who had received placebo were colonized with *E. coli* (six) and enterococci (two).

TABLE 1. *Effect of antimicrobial prophylaxis on acquired bacteriuria*

Acquired bacteriuria	Prophylaxis group ($N = 96$)		Placebo group ($N = 100$)	
	Abdominal hysterectomy ($N = 82$)	Vaginal hysterectomy ($N = 14$)	Abdominal hysterectomy ($N = 82$)	Vaginal hysterectomy ($N = 18$)
During catheterization				
Day 1–3 of catheterization[a]				
10^2–10^4 colonies/ml	1	0	6	0
$\geq 10^5$ colonies/ml	0	0	2	1
Day ≥4 of catheterization				
10^2–10^4 colonies/ml	0	0	0	0
$\geq 10^5$ colonies/ml	2	0	0	0
Positive clean-voided specimen at discharge	0	0	4[b]	0
After catheterization[c]	6[d]	2[d]	4[b]	0

[a] $P < 0.01$ by Fisher exact test for difference between prophylaxis and placebo groups.

[b] Eight positive cultures of 63 clean-voided specimens collected at time of discharge from patients who had not received nonprotocol antimicrobial therapy.

[c] First positive culture was obtained at time of discharge.

[d] Eight positive cultures of 72 clean-voided specimens collected at time of discharge from patients who had not received nonprotocol antimicrobial therapy.

Morbidity. No reduction in febrile morbidity occurred among the abdominal hysterectomy patients who received antimicrobial prophylaxis (Table 2). However, among patients with vaginal hysterectomies, postoperative fever occurred less often in those who received prophylaxis. In addition, significantly fewer of the patients who had received prophylaxis required subsequent therapy with nonprotocol antimicrobial drugs. The average duration of indwelling catheterization was less in vaginal hysterectomy patients who received prophylaxis than in those who received placebo. The prolonged period of catheterization in the placebo group, however, was not associated with an increased risk of acquired bacteriuria. The single instance of acquired bacteriuria in the vaginal hysterectomy group receiving placebo occurred during day 1 of catheterization.

Only 1 of the 29 febrile patients had concurrent bacteriuria, suggesting that urinary tract colonization or infection was not a major cause of fever in these patients. Attending physicians, often without obtaining additional bacterial cultures, diagnosed pelvic, respiratory, urine, or wound infections, or infection at an unknown site, as causes of the febrile episodes. No instance of fever was attributed to drug sensitivity or drug-associated phlebitis. All protocol blood cultures were negative.

We also evaluated the effect of the randomly assigned antimicrobial prophylaxis on the hospital course of the 14 patients found to have positive cultures from their first clean-voided or catheterized specimens. Bacterial isolates included *E. coli* (seven), *Klebsiella* (three), enterococcus (three), and *Enterobacter* (one). Seven patients received cefazolin and seven received placebo. Mean ages, severity of underlying diseases, and types of operations were similar for the two groups. All seven of the patients treated with the antimicrobial were cleared of their bacteriuria within 24 h after drug administration. Only one of the seven had a subsequent febrile episode, and this occurred after the catheter had been removed. Additional antimicrobials were not required, and none of six specimens obtained at time of discharge was positive.

On the other hand, four of the seven patients who received placebo, including two who had fever above 38.9°C orally for 2 or more consecutive days, required subsequent nonprotocol antimicrobial treatment. The other three had persistent bacteriuria at time of discharge. The mean duration of hospitalization was 5.6 days for the seven patients who received cefazolin versus 6.7 days for the seven who received placebo.

DISCUSSION

The results suggest that a brief course of prophylactic antimicrobial may reduce the incidence of catheter-associated bacteriuria. We observed that the group which received antimicrobial prophylaxis had a lower overall rate, as well as a lower average daily incidence, of acquired bacteriuria. This apparent efficacy of antimicrobials for the prevention of catheter-associated bacteriuria has been noted in several studies (1, 3, 4, 6, 7, 10, 12). Allen et al. (1), in a controlled prospective study, demonstrated beneficial effects of prophylaxis against urinary tract infections in gynecological surgery patients who were not studied with daily urine cultures. Their rates of clinical urinary tract infection in placebo and prophylaxis groups (11 and 0%, respectively) are similar to our observed rates of acquired bacteriuria (12 and 3%, respectively).

Quantitative criteria for bacteriuria during constant bladder drainage with an indwelling catheter have not been determined. In a previous study (3), we found that, among patients

TABLE 2. *Effect of antimicrobial prophylaxis on morbidity*

Determination	Prophylaxis group: Abdominal hysterectomy ($N = 82$)	Prophylaxis group: Vaginal hysterectomy ($N = 14$)	Placebo group: Abdominal hysterectomy ($N = 82$)	Placebo group: Vaginal hysterectomy ($N = 18$)
No. with febrile morbidity	11	1	12	5
No. treated with nonprotocol antimicrobial	10	2	10	12[a]
Avg duration of catheterization (days)	1.8	2.4	1.7	5.0
Avg daily incidence of acquired bacteriuria (%)	2.1	0	5.5	1.1
Avg duration of hospitalization (days)	6.0	6.1	5.6	7.6

[a] $P < 0.01$ by Fisher exact test.

who showed colony counts between 10^2 and 10^5 organisms per ml, the first positive culture was noted on the last day of catheterization (so that subsequent cultures were not obtained) or systemic antimicrobials were being used in those with low colony counts on 2 or more days. In the present study, a higher proportion of patients had low colony counts because of the brief duration of catheterization in this population and the frequent occurrence of positive cultures on the last day of catheterization.

The indwelling urinary catheter has been cited as a prime causal factor for nosocomial urinary tract infection and resultant bacteremia. Obviously, certain efforts should be extended to minimize the frequency of these complications. However, our enthusiasm for using antimicrobial prophylaxis for catheter-associated bacteriuria in gynecological surgery patients is dampened by other results of our study. These include: (i) the low incidence of acquired bacteriuria in this population, (ii) the lack of relation between febrile morbidity and acquired bacteriuria, (iii) the failure of prophylaxis to reduce the prevalence of positive urine cultures at the time of discharge, and (iv) the lack of effect of prophylaxis in reducing febrile morbidity or duration of hospitalization of the abdominal hysterectomy patients. However, we noted a trend toward less febrile morbidity and shorter hospital stays for the vaginal hysterectomy patients who received prophylaxis, a finding consistent with a number of previous reports (2, 5, 8, 9, 11).

In our previous report, we noted that the major morbidity and mortality of indwelling urinary catheterization are related to the patients' age, sex, and severity of underlying disease. The patient selection criteria for this study excluded higher-risk patients, thus explaining the low incidence of acquired bacteriuria.

We have no explanation for the high prevalence of bacteriuria at time of discharge in patients who had negative cultures during indwelling catheterization. It seems likely that these patients acquired bacteriuria after subsequent ("straight") catheterizations for urinary retention after their period of constant bladder drainage. However, this aspect of care was not monitored.

The efficacy of antimicrobials was more apparent in patients who had a positive urine culture at time of insertion of the catheter. In these patients, antimicrobial therapy probably reduced subsequent catheter-associated morbidity. On the basis of these observations, we recommend that a urine specimen for culture be submitted from all patients either before or at the time or urethral catheterization. Bacteriuric patients should be treated with a specific antimicrobial as soon as possible. Antimicrobial prophylaxis is not indicated for patients with noncritical underlying diseases undergoing short-term urinary catheterization. Additional study is needed to determine the possible efficacy and potential benefits of prophylaxis in higher-risk patient populations.

ACKNOWLEDGMENTS

This study was supported in part by Public Health Service grant AI-11950 from the National Institute of Allergy and Infectious Diseases, and by a grant from the Eli Lilly & Co., Indianapolis, Ind. We thank Margaret Whelan and Patricia Steinmuller, who performed the bacteriological procedures, Elaine Warner and Steven Chappel, who assisted in monitoring the care of these patients, Tannys M. Last, and the gynecology staff whose cooperation made this study possible, and Charles B. Smith, who reviewed the manuscript.

LITERATURE CITED

1. **Allen, J. L., J. F. Rampone, and C. R. Wheeless.** 1972. Use of a prophylactic antibiotic in elective major *gynecologiic operations. Obstet. Gynecol.* **39**:218–224.
2. **Bolling, D. R., Jr., and G. D. Plunkett.** 1973. Prophylactic antibiotics for vaginal hysterectomies. Obstet. Gynecol. **41**:689–692.
3. **Garibaldi, R. A., J. P. Burke, M. L. Dickman, and C. B. Smith.** 1974. Factors predisposing to bacteriuria during indwelling urethral catheterization. N. Engl. J. Med. **291**:215–219.
4. **Gillespie, W. A., K. B. Linton, A. Miller, and N. Slade.** 1960. The diagnosis, epidemiology, and control of urinary infection in urology and gynecology. J. Clin. Pathol. **13**:187–194.
5. **Goosenberg, J., J. P. Emich, and R. H. Schwarz.** 1969. Prophylactic antibiotics in vaginal hysterectomy. Am. J. Obstet. Gynecol. **105**:503–506.
6. **Kunin, C. M., and R. C. McCormack.** 1966. Prevention of catheter-induced urinary-tract infections by sterile closed drainage. N. Engl. J. Med. **274**:1155–1161.
7. **Lacy, S. S., G. W. Drach, and C. E. Cox.** 1971. Incidence of infection after prostatectomy and efficacy of cephaloridine prophylaxis. J. Urol. **105**:836–839.
8. **Ledger, W. J., C. Gee, and W. P. Lewis.** 1975. Guidelines for antibiotic prophylaxis in gynecology. Am. J. Obstet. Gynecol. **121**:1038–1045.
9. **Ledger, W. J., R. L. Sweet, and J. T.Headington.** 1973. Prophylactic cephaloridine in the prevention of postoperative pelvic infections in premenopausal women undergoing vaginal hysterectomy. Am. J. Obstet. Gynecol. **115**:766–774.
10. **Plorde, J. J., R. P. Kennedy, H. H. Bourne, J. S. Ansell, and R. G. Petersdorf.** 1965. Course and prognosis of prostatectomy. With a note on the incidence of bacteremia and effectiveness of chemoprophylaxis. N. Engl. J. Med. **272**:269–277.
11. **Scott, J. R.** 1973. Pelvic infections following vaginal hysterectomy. Hosp. Pract. **8**:101–110.
12. **Shapiro, S. R., A. Santamarina, and J. H. Harrison.** 1974. Catheter-associated urinary tract infections: incidence and a new approach to prevention. J. Urol. **112**:659–663.

Antimicrobial Agents and Chemotherapy, Feb. 1977, p. 244–247 Vol. 11, No. 2

Bone Marrow Toxicity Associated with 5-Fluorocytosine Therapy

CAROL A. KAUFFMAN,* and PETER T. FRAME

*Department of Internal Medicine, University of Cincinnati Medical Center, and Cincinnati Veterans Administration Hospital, Cincinnati, Ohio 45220**

Received for publication 23 August 1976

Bone marrow toxicity occurred in 4 of 15 patients treated with 5-fluorocytosine (5-FC) for serious fungal infections. The development of marrow toxicity appeared to be related to serum 5-FC levels of 125 μg/ml or greater. In three patients, accumulation of toxic levels of 5-FC was related to diminished renal function. One patient with acute renal failure and prolonged high levels of 5-FC developed marrow aplasia and died of bacterial sepsis. Three patients experienced leukopenia, which was readily reversed when the dosage of 5-FC was decreased and the serum concentration was lowered. With careful monitoring of serum 5-FC concentration and renal function, the dose-related toxic effects of 5-FC on the marrow can be avoided.

Several authors have suggested that bone marrow depression may be associated with the use of 5-fluorocytosine (5-FC) for the treatment of serious fungal infections (2, 7, 10, 11, 15). Leukopenia (2, 15), thrombocytopenia (15), and pancytopenia (7, 10, 11) have been reported. Although the toxic effect on the marrow has been felt to be dose related, serum levels of 5-FC at the time of marrow depression have only infrequently been recorded (7). We have encountered significant marrow toxicity during 5-FC therapy and have related this toxicity to serum concentrations of the drug. This report describes the clinical and laboratory studies in four patients who exhibited bone marrow depression during 5-FC therapy.

PATIENTS AND METHODS

Fifteen patients with serious fungal infections were treated with 5-FC at the University of Cincinnati Medical Center from June 1972 to June 1975. The fungal infections treated were: cryptococcal meningitis (eight patients), disseminated candidiasis (two patients), candida endocarditis (one patient), and *Torulopsis glabrata* septicemia (four patients). From June 1972 to December 1972, five patients received 5-FC alone as initial therapy or after failure of amphotericin B therapy, using a dose of 150 mg/kg per day. Ten patients treated since January 1973 received a combination of 5-FC (150 mg/kg per day) and amphotericin B (1 mg/kg three times a week). Patients were followed with regard to the following parameters: renal function (creatinine, blood urea nitrogen, creatinine clearance), hepatic function (bilirubin, alkaline phosphatase, transaminases), hematologic function (total leukocyte and differential leukocyte count, platelet count, hemoglobulin, and hematocrit).

The minimal inhibitory concentration of 5-FC for each organism was determined by the method of Shadomy (13). All fungi isolated from these 15 patients were inhibited by ≤ 1.9 μg of 5-FC per ml.

Serum levels of 5-FC were measured by a modification of the disk diffusion method of Kaspar and Drutz (5), as previously described (6).

RESULTS

Four of the 15 patients developed marrow toxicity while receiving 5-FC (Table 1). All were receiving 5-FC on a daily dosage schedule of 150 mg/kg. Patient 1 was treated with 5-FC alone; patient 3 received 5-FC alone 6 days after amphotericin B had been stopped (185 mg of amphotericin B had been administered over 7 days); and patients 2 and 4 were treated with 5-FC and amphotericin B concomitantly. All four patients had peak serum 5-FC levels of 125 μg/ml or greater immediately preceding and during the initial period of marrow depression. The serum concentration of 5-FC remained elevated above 125 μg/ml for 2 to 14 days in three patients.

Renal insufficiency appeared to be a very significant factor in the accumulation of excessive amounts of 5-FC in three of the four patients. Patient 1, with fungal pyelonephritis and sepsis, initially had a blood urea nitrogen of 20 mg/100 ml and a creatinine of 2.2 mg/100 ml (Fig. 1). However, renal insufficiency quickly ensued when she developed ureteral obstruction and oliguria secondary to the fungal infection. 5-FC levels increased rapidly and remained at very high levels in spite of discontinuance of the drug. Aplasia of all marrow precursors was documented by bone marrow

TABLE 1. *Leukopenia associated with 5-FC therapy*

Patient	Age/sex	Underlying disease	Other medications	Fungal infection	Renal insufficiency	5-FC serum level[a] (μg/ml)	Days of 5-FC level >125 μg/ml	Leukocyte count[b] (no./mm³)	Neutrophils[b] (%)	Other marrow toxicity
1	63/F	Diabetes mellitus	Gentamicin	*T. glabrata* sepsis	Yes	500	14	300	0	Pancytopenia
2	39/F	Systemic lupus erythematosus	Amphotericin B prednisone	*C. albicans* sepsis	Yes	200	8	2,400	75	None
3	83/F	None	Amphotericin B[c]	*C. neoformans* meningitis	No	125	Not known	2,700	51	None
4	23/M	None	Amphotericin B	*C. neoformans* meningitis	Yes	160	2	3,900	59	None

[a] Maximum serum level immediately preceding development of leukopenia. Levels were obtained 2 h after 5-FC administration in patients 2 through 4.
[b] Lowest leukocyte count and percentage of neutrophils recorded.
[c] A total of 185 mg had been given; the last dose was administered 6 days before 5-FC was begun.

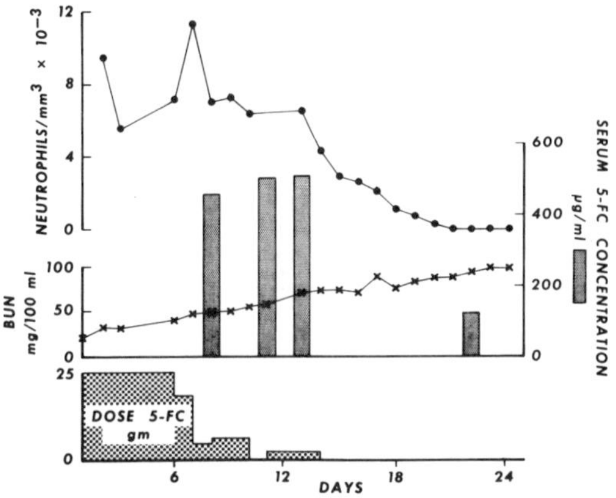

FIG. 1. *Graphic representation of renal function, as shown by the blood urea nitrogen (BUN), 5-FC serum concentration, and the number of circulating neutrophils in patient 1, who developed marrow aplasia during 5-FC therapy.*

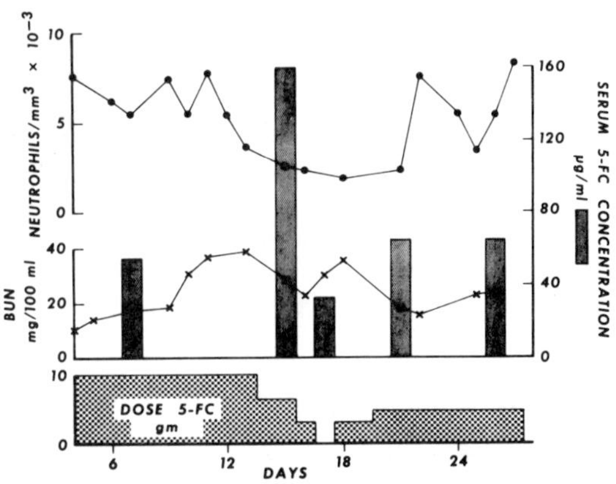

FIG. 2. *Graphic representation of renal function, as shown by blood urea nitrogen (BUN), 5-FC serum concentration, and the number of circulating neutrophils in patient 4, who had reversible neutropenia during the course of therapy with 5-FC.*

aspiration on day 22, and the patient died of *Pseudomonas* sepsis on day 24.

Patient 2 had mild lupus nephritis with a base line creatinine of 1.5 mg/100 ml. In this patient and patient 4, who initially had normal renal function, treatment with amphotericin B led to gradually rising creatinine and blood urea nitrogen. This was accompanied by an increased concentration of 5-FC in the serum. Figure 2 shows the relationships among the blood urea nitrogen level, the 5-FC serum concentration, and the absolute neutrophil count in the blood for patient 4. In this patient, as well as in patients 2 and 3, leukopenia was readily reversed when the dosage of 5-FC was adjusted for the degree of renal insufficiency.

Only one other patient of the 15 treated with 5-FC reached a serum level of 5-FC of 125 μg/ml on one occasion. Unfortunately, this patient was discharged from the hospital the next day, and a leukocyte count was not obtained at that time. The dosage of 5-FC was subsequently reduced, and follow-up leukocyte counts were normal.

Isolated thrombocytopenia was not found in any of our patients; likewise, anemia did not occur other than that normally found during the course of amphotericin B therapy in those patients on both drugs. Hepatic enzymes and serum bilirubin values remained normal throughout the course of treatment with 5-FC in all 15 patients.

DISCUSSION

These studies indicate that the bone marrow suppression associated with 5-FC therapy appears to be dose related. Levels of 125 μg/ml or greater were associated with reversible leukopenia. Very high levels (500 μg/ml) for a prolonged period of time in one patient were probably responsible for marrow aplasia. Whether this was a reversible lesion is unknown, since the patient succumbed to gram-negative bacterial sepsis during the period of aplasia. Record et al. described irreversible marrow failure in one patient treated with 5-FC (10), and Schlegel et al. reported the development of aplasia in a patient with chronic mucocutaneous candidiasis treated for 17 days with 5-FC (11). 5-FC levels were not available in either of these patients at the time of marrow toxicity.

The total amount of drug given during the course of therapy did not seem to be related to the development of marrow toxicity. Leukopenia was reversed by decreasing the dose of 5-FC, and therapy was continued at a lower dosage schedule in three of our patients. No further marrow suppression was found throughout the course of therapy in these patients.

The mechanism of this marrow suppression is not known. Cytosine and its fluorinated analogue 5-FC are not metabolized by mammalian cells. Although in rats a small amount of orally administered 5-FC is converted to 5-fluorouracil by the resident bacteria in the colon, there is no direct evidence for this conversion in humans (8).

It is possible that amphotericin B, through its effects on the membranes of mammalian cells (4), allows enhanced uptake of 5-FC by these cells and, subsequently, greater toxicity (9). This mechanism could be postulated in two of our patients only. The other two patients, as well as others previously reported, received 5-FC alone (2, 10, 11).

Isolated thrombocytopenia was not observed in our patients but did occur in three patients reported by Utz et al. (15). 5-FC levels were not reported in those patients.

Hepatotoxicity was not observed in our patients treated with 5-FC alone or in combination with amphotericin B, although this side effect has been associated with both drugs (3, 10). Record's patient had concomitant marrow and liver toxicity (10), but other patients with probable marrow toxicity due to 5-FC have not demonstrated hepatotoxicity (2, 11).

Renal function assumes a very important role in determining serum levels and subsequent toxicity of 5-FC since this drug is excreted almost wholly by the kidneys (16). In the face of rapidly progressive renal failure, as in patient 1, very high serum levels of 5-FC can occur and persist for several days even though the drug has been discontinued. It is noteworthy that the patient with the most severe degree of marrow toxicity had very high levels of 5-FC for 14 days. 5-FC is readily dialyzable (1), and this procedure should be used in similar situations to remove toxic accumulations of this drug.

Since amphotericin B administration almost invariably leads to diminished renal function (14), combined therapy with amphotericin B and 5-FC is especially likely to result in high serum levels of 5-FC. To avoid toxicity during combined therapy, 5-FC serum concentration and serum creatinine should be monitored closely and the dosage of 5-FC adjusted accordingly. Several methods of adjusting the dosage of 5-FC on the basis of creatinine clearance have been proposed (12, 16). Use of such formulas combined with determination of 5-FC serum concentrations should obviate the problem of 5-FC-related marrow toxicity.

ACKNOWLEDGMENTS

This work was supported by Veterans Administration research grant 4834-01 and by the Morton Hamburger Memorial Research Fund.

LITERATURE CITED

1. **Block, E. R., J. E. Bennett, L. G. Livoti, W. J. Klein, R. R. MacGregor, and L. Henderson.** 1974. Flucytosine and amphotericin B: hemodialysis effects on the plasma concentration and clearance. Studies in man. Ann. Intern. Med. 80:613–617.
2. **Davies, R. R., and D. S. Reeves.** 1971. 5-Fluorocytosine and urinary candidiasis. Br. Med. J. 1:577–579.
3. **Gordon, M. A., and D. K. Vedder.** 1966. Serologic tests in diagnosis and prognosis of cryptococcosis. J. Am. Med. Assoc. 197:961–967.
4. **Hamilton-Miller, J. M. T.** 1973. Chemistry and biology of the polyene macrolide antibiotics. Bacteriol. Rev. 37:166–196.
5. **Kaspar, R. L., and D. J. Drutz.** 1975. Rapid simple bioassay for 5-fluorocytosine in the presence of amphotericin B. Antimicrob. Agents Chemother. 7:462–465.
6. **Kauffman, C. A., J. A. Carleton, and P. T. Frame.** 1976. Simple assay for 5-fluorocytosine in the presence of amphotericin B. Antimicrob. Agents Chemother. 9:381–383.
7. **Kauffman, C. A., and J. S. Tan.** 1974. *Torulopsis glabrata* renal infection. Am. J. Med. 57:217–224.
8. **Koechlin, B. A., F. Rubio, S. Palmer, T. Gabriel, and R. Duschinsky.** 1966. The metabolism of 5-fluorocytosine-2-^{14}C and of cytosine-^{14}C in the rat and the disposition of 5-fluorocytosine-2-^{14}C in man. Biochem. Pharmacol. 15:435–446.
9. **Medoff, G., and G. S. Kobayashi.** 1975. Amphotericin B: old drug, new therapy. J. Am. Med. Assoc. 232:619–620.
10. **Record, C. O., J. M. Skinner, P. Sleight, and D. C. E. Speller.** 1971. Candida endocarditis treated with 5-fluorocytosine. Br. Med. J. 1:262–264.
11. **Schlegel, R. J., G. M. Bernier, J. A. Bellanti, D. A. Maybee, G. B. Osborne, J. L. Stewart, D. J. Pearlman, J. Ouelette, and F. C. Biehausen.** 1970. Severe candidiasis associated with thymic dysplasia, IgA deficiency, and plasma antilymphocyte effects. Pediatrics 45:926–936.
12. **Schonebeck, J., A. Polak, M. Fernex, and H. J. Scholer.** 1973. Pharmacokinetic studies on the oral

anti-mycotic agent 5-fluorocytosine in individuals with normal and impaired kidney function. Chemotherapy 18:321–336.
13. **Shadomy, S.** 1969. In vitro studies with 5-fluorocytosine. Appl. Microbiol. 17:871–877.
14. **Utz, J. P., J. E. Bennett, M. W. Brandriss, W. T. Butler, and G. J. Hill.** 1964. Amphotericin B toxicity. Ann. Intern. Med. 61:334–354.
15. **Utz, J. P., I. L. Garriques, M. A. Sande, J. F. Warner, G. L. Mandell, R. F. McGehee, R. J. Duma, and S. Shadomy.** 1975. Therapy of cryptococcosis with a combination of flucytosine and amphotericin B. J. Infect. Dis. 132:368–373.
16. **Wade, D. N., and G. Sudlow.** 1972. The kinetics of 5-fluorocytosine elimination in man. Aust. N.Z. J. Med. 2:153–158.

Antimicrobial Agents and Chemotherapy, Feb. 1977, p. 248-250
Vol. 11, No. 2

Pharmacokinetics of Cefamandole in Patients with Renal Failure

BURT R. MEYERS and SHALOM Z. HIRSCHMAN*

Department of Medicine, The Mount Sinai School of Medicine of the City University of New York, New York, New York 10029

Received for publication 11 August 1976

The pharmacokinetics of cefamandole were studied in four patients with stable renal failure, two patients undergoing peritoneal dialysis, and four patients undergoing hemodialysis. Peak concentrations of cefamandole in serum were achieved 1 to 2 h after intramuscular injection in the patients with stable renal impairment, and the concentrations declined slowly, with half-life values of 12.3 to 18 h. Cefamandole was removed only very slowly by peritoneal dialysis. Hemodialysis was more efficient in removing cefamandole, with serum half-life values ranging from 3.8 to 7.9 h. The mean apparent volume of distribution of cefamandole in these 10 patients was 21.92 liters, or 31% of the body weight.

Cefamandole, a new cephalosporin derivative, has a broad spectrum of antimicrobial activity against gram-positive and gram-negative bacteria, including *Haemophilus influenzae* (3, 9, 11). Pharmacokinetic studies in healthy human volunteers have shown that excellent concentrations of cefamandole in serum are achieved after both intramuscular and intravenous injections (10). Recent clinical studies have demonstrated that cefamandole is an effective agent for the treatment of seriously ill hospitalized patients with a variety of infections due to gram-positive and gram-negative bacteria (B. R. Meyers, P. Nicholas, and S. Z. Hirschman, manuscript in preparation). In this report we present results of pharmacokinetic studies with cefamandole in patients with stable renal failure and in patients undergoing peritoneal dialysis and hemodialysis.

MATERIALS AND METHODS

Four patients with stable renal failure, two patients undergoing peritoneal dialysis, and four patients requiring hemodialysis were the subjects of this study. Each patient received 1 g of cefamandole intramuscularly. Serum samples were collected from the patients with stable renal failure before injection and at timed intervals postinjection. Dialysate samples were collected from patients undergoing dialysis. Peritoneal dialysis with a solution containing sodium chloride, calcium chloride, magnesium chloride, sodium lactate, and dextrose (Inpersol) was begun 1 h after the injection of cefamandole. All dialysis runs lasted 45 to 60 min, and each patient was treated for 36 exchanges. Patients undergoing hemodialysis were placed on a Travenol coil hemodialysis machine for 6 h at 1 h after the intramuscular administration of cefamandole.

Serum, urine, and dialysate samples were stored at $-70°C$. The concentration of cefamandole in the various specimens was determined by the cup-plate method, using *Bacillus subtilis* as the test organism as previously described (10). The regression lines of the logs of the concentrations of cefamandole in serum versus time and their correlation coefficients (r) were calculated by the method of least squares, using a standard computer program to obtain the half-life ($t_{1/2}$) of the drug in each patient. These calculations were based on a one-compartment model for the pharmacokinetics of the drug (4). The apparent volume of distribution (AVD) of cefamandole was calculated from the formula $AVD = I/C_0$, where I is the intramuscular dose in milligrams and C_0 is the expected serum concentration at the time of injection, assuming rapid equilibration (2). The C_0 was obtained by extrapolation of the regression lines of the log concentration of cefamandole in serum versus time (2).

All patients signed certificates of informed consent for the studies according to institutional policy.

RESULTS

Four patients with stable renal impairment and serum creatinine concentrations ranging from 5 to 9 mg/100 ml were studied (Table 1). Peak concentrations of cefamandole in serum were achieved between 1 and 2 h after intramuscular injection. The serum concentration declined slowly, and drug levels still could be measured at 72 h. The serum $t_{1/2}$ of cefamandole ranged from 12.3 to 18 h and was greater in patients with higher serum creatinine concentrations (Table 1). In this group of patients the

TABLE 1. *Pharmacokinetics of cefamandole in patients with stable renal failure*

Patient	Serum creatinine (mg/100 ml)	Serum concn of cefamandole (μg/ml) at time (h) postinjection:															$t_{1/2}$ (h)	Correlation coefficient (r)
		1	2	4	8	12	13	18	20	22	24	28	36	46	48	72		
1	9	28	46	40		28							12.8	12.5	4.8		18	−0.94
2	7.7	30		27	14											1.3	16.8	−0.99
3	5	23		23	17		12.3		8	4.8		5			1.8	0.45	12.3	−0.99
4	5.9	32	50					28			22				6.1	1.3	13.1	−0.99

TABLE 2. *Pharmacokinetics of cefamandole in patients undergoing peritoneal dialysis*

Patient	Serum creatinine (mg/100 ml)	Serum concn of cefamandole (μg/ml) at time (h) postinjection:												$t_{1/2}$ (h)	Correlation coefficient (r)
		1	2	3	4	6	8	12	16	18	24	30	36		
R.H.	17.2	40	42	36	36					16	11	10.2		13.2	−0.99
E.H.	14.8	56	66		56	50	48	31	18.8		12.4	10	7.2	10.3	−0.99

relationship between $t_{1/2}$ and serum creatinine could be expressed by the equation log $t_{1/2}$ = 0.0443 Cr + 0.8661 (r = 0.99), where Cr is serum creatinine.

Two patients were studied while undergoing peritoneal dialysis. Peak levels of cefamandole in serum were observed during the first 2 h after injection and declined slowly over the next 48 h (Table 2). Both patients still had a concentration of 10 μg of cefamandole per ml in their serum at 30 h. The average serum $t_{1/2}$ during peritoneal dialysis was 11.8 h. The mean dialysate concentration of cefamandole was 4.82 μg/ml; a peak concentration of 19 μg/ml was obtained 2 h after injection.

Four patients were given cefamandole before hemodialysis. The serum creatinine in these four patients ranged from 7.1 to 14.8 mg/100 ml (Table 3). Cefamandole was removed to a greater extent during hemodialysis than during peritoneal dialysis; the serum $t_{1/2}$ values ranged from 3.8 to 7.9 h during the 6-h dialysis period (Table 3).

The mean AVD for the 10 patients in this study was 21.92 ± 10.27 (standard deviation) liters, or 31% of the body weight.

TABLE 3. *Pharmacokinetics of cefamandole in patients undergoing hemodialysis*

Patient	Serum creatinine (mg/100 ml)	Serum concn of cefamandole (μg/ml) at time (h) postinjection:				$t_{1/2}$ (h)	Correlation coefficient (r)
		1	2	4	6		
W.S.	7.1	50	44	37	32	7.9	−0.99
H.H.	14.8	53	60	44	42	7.8	−0.92
J.M.	13.5	57	56	32	27	3.8	−0.96
W.R.	13.4	27	40	30.4	23.2	5.1	−0.99

DISCUSSION

In patients with normal renal function cefamandole is excreted primarily by the kidneys (10). The serum $t_{1/2}$ after intramuscular administration of cefamandole to human volunteers with normal renal function was 1.17 h, and the AVD was 17.11 liters, or 24% of the body weight (10). The serum $t_{1/2}$ of cefamandole in patients with stable renal impairment and serum creatinine values ≥5 mg/100 ml was approximately 10 to 15 times greater than that obtained in volunteers with normal renal function. The $t_{1/2}$ was greater in patients with higher serum creatinine values as has been observed with other cephalosporin derivatives (1, 8). The mean AVD of 21.92 liters in the group of 10 patients with renal failure was higher than that of 17.11 liters found in healthy volunteers. However, the range of values in the ten patients (13.2 to 41 liters) was great and may reflect a poor absorption of the drug after intramuscular injection in the sicker patients, such as those with severe congestive heart failure.

Peritoneal dialysis removed cefamandole at a very slow rate. The serum $t_{1/2}$ in the two patients studied was still markedly prolonged. The average dialysate concentration of cefamandole of 4.8 μg/ml was above the minimum inhibitory concentrations of the drug for suceptible gram-positive bacteria and also for many susceptible gram-negative bacteria (9). Hemodialysis was more efficient in removing cefamandole than was peritoneal dialysis, yet the serum $t_{1/2}$ values were still much greater than those observed in patients with normal renal function.

The effects of peritoneal dialysis and hemodialysis on the removal of other cephalosporins have been studied and can be compared with the results reported here for cefamandole. Perkins et al. (12) found a 24% reduction of mean peak concentrations of both cephalothin and cephaloridine in serum during peritoneal dialysis below those observed in a base line study. The serum $t_{1/2}$ values of the drugs during peritoneal dialysis were about 10 to 12 h. After 1-g intramuscular doses serum cephalothin concentrations fell to 0 at 48 h with peritoneal dialysis, but cephaloridine was still detectable at 72 h. Cephaloridine is significantly removed from blood by hemodialysis (10). Hemodialysis of patients with creatinine clearances ≤ 5 ml/min lowered the serum $t_{1/2}$ of cefazolin, a cephalosporin derivative highly bound to protein, from 56.6 to 8.8 h; peritoneal dialysis had little effect on the $t_{1/2}$ (6). McCloskey et al. (8) reported that hemodialysis removed 23% of an administered dose of cephapirin during a 6-h dialysis period. Linquist et al. (7) showed that the $t_{1/2}$ of cephalexin, an orally administered cephalosporin, was decreased from 30.8 to 6.3 h in patients with renal failure undergoing hemodialysis. Thus, cefamandole is similar to other cephalosporin derivatives in the marked prolongation of serum $t_{1/2}$ in patients with renal failure, the very slow removal of drug during peritoneal dialysis, and the more efficient removal during hemodialysis. As suggested for other cephalosporins in patients with renal failure (6), it would appear that a loading dose of cefamandole followed by one-third to one-half of the loading dose every $t_{1/2}$ would be sufficient dosage. This dosage would also apply to patients undergoing peritoneal dialysis. In patients undergoing hemodialysis, an additional one-third to one-half of the loading dose should be administered at the end of the dialysis. When possible, levels of cefamandole in serum should be measured, at least initially, to correctly adjust the dosage.

ACKNOWLEDGMENTS

We appreciate the technical assistance of Z. Sadka.

This work was supported by a grant from Eli Lilly Laboratories.

LITERATURE CITED

1. **Butcher, R. H., J. K. Dawborn, and G. Pattison.** 1972. Blood and urine levels of cephalexin in patients with impaired renal function. Med. J. Aust. **2**:1282–1284.
2. **Dost, F. H.** 1968. Grundlagen der Pharmakokinetic, p. 36, 238, 275, 311. Georg Thieme Verlag, Stuttgart.
3. **Eykeyn, S., C. Jenkins, and A. King.** 1973. Antibacterial activity of cefamandole, a new cephalosporin antibiotic, compared with that of cephaloridine, cephalothin, and cephalexin. Antimicrob. Agents Chemother. **3**:657–661.
4. **Greenblatt, D. J., and J. Koch-Weser.** 1975. Clinical pharmacokinetics. N. Engl. J. Med. **293**:702–705.
5. **Kunin, C. M., and N. Atuk.** 1966. Excretion of cephaloridine and cephalothin in patients with renal impairment. N. Engl. J. Med. **274**:654–656.
6. **Levison, M. E., S. P. Levison, K. Ries, and D. Kaye.** 1973. Pharmacology of cefazolin in patients with normal and abnormal renal function. J. Infect. Dis. **128**(Suppl.):354–357.
7. **Linquist, J. A., J. Y. Siddiqui, and I. M. Smith.** 1970. Cephalexin in patients with renal disease. N. Engl. J. Med. **283**:720–723.
8. **McCloskey, R. V., E. E. Terry, A. W. McCracken, M. J. Sweeney, and M. F. Forland.** 1972. Effect of hemodialysis and renal failure on serum and urine concentrations of cephapirin sodium. Antimicrob. Agents Chemother. **1**:90–93.
9. **Meyers, B. R., B. Leng, and S. Z. Hirschman.** 1975. Cefamandole: antimicrobial activity in vitro of a new cephalosporin. Antimicrob. Agents Chemother. **8**:737–741.
10. **Meyers, B. R., B. Ribner, S. Yancovitz, and S. Z. Hirschman.** 1976. Pharmacological studies with cefamandole in human volunteers. Antimicrob. Agents Chemother. **9**:140–144.
11. **Neu, H. C.** 1974. Cefamandole, a cephalosporin antibiotic with an unusually wide spectrum of activity. Antimicrob. Agents Chemother. **6**:177–182.
12. **Perkins, R. L., E. J. Smith, and S. Saslaw.** 1969. Cephalothin and cephaloridine: comparative pharmacodynamics in chronic uremia. Am. J. Med. Sci. **257**:116–124.

ANTIMICROBIAL AGENTS AND Chemotherapy, Feb. 1977, p. 251-257 Vol. 11, No. 12

Printed in U.S.A.

Changes in Superhelical Density of Closed Circular Deoxyribonucleic Acid by Intercalation of Anti-R-Plasmid Drugs and Primaquine

RICHARD G. ALLISON AND FRED E. HAHN*

Department of Molecular Biology, Walter Reed Army Institute of Research, Washington, D.C. 20012

Received for publication 1 July 1976

The following compounds, which possess anti-R-plasmid activity (Hahn and Ciak, 1976) in decreasing order, were shown by viscometric titration to change systematically the superhelical density of closed circular PM2 deoxyribonucleic acid in the manner of intercalators: ethidium bromide, quinacrine, acridine orange, quinine, chlorpromazine, chloroquine, and methylene blue. The same effect was caused by the antimalarial drug primaquine, which has not been tested for antiplasmid activity.

It was originally proposed in this laboratory (11) that substances that bind to deoxyribonucleic acid (DNA) by intercalation possess the group property of being able to eliminate bacterial plasmids. Preliminary tests of this hypothesis (11; J. Ciak, S. Wormley, and F. E. Hahn, Bacteriol. Proc., GP154, p. 67, 1969) supported it, but remained less than conclusive. A confirmation of the hypothesis by more rigorous tests with the R-plasmid R1 carried by *Salmonella typhimurium* has recently been published (12), using 15 intercalative compounds.

Although biophysical indications of intercalation binding exist for these 15 anti-R-plasmid drugs, conclusive tests of this type of binding by measuring resulting hydrodynamic changes and, hence, changes in the superhelical density of closed circular DNA, had not been carried out for all of them. Waring proved intercalation binding with the sedimentation method for daunomycin, proflavine, ethidium bromide, hycanthone (a miracil D congener), propidium iodide, and chloroquine (37); his results with chlorpromazine suggested that this drug was not intercalated into the ϕX174 replicative form of DNA (37). By viscometric titration of PM2 DNA, Saucier et al. (32) showed intercalation of proflavine, ethidium bromide, daunomycin, and quinacrine. With the same method (29), we have tested for intercalation binding of ethidium bromide, quinacrine, acridine orange, quinine, chlorpromazine, chloroquine, and methylene blue and report here that all of these anti-R-plasmid substances changes the superhelical density of PM2 DNA in the manner of intercalators. A preliminary report of some of these findings has been published (R. G. Allison and F. E. Hahn, Fed. Proc. 32:700, 1973).

The antimalarial drug primaquine acts as a preferential inhibitor of protein biosynthesis in vivo (28) by causing a rapid breakdown of ribosomes (27). The same effect has been demonstrated for chloroquine in *Bacillus megaterium* (6) and in *Plasmodium knowlesi* (36). At 6×10^{-4} M, primaquine inhibits protein synthesis completely in *B. megaterium* but has only minor effects on the biosyntheses of DNA and ribonucleic acid (28). Evidently, the drug has merely marginal, if any, activity as a DNA template poison.

Holbrook et al. reported (17) that DNA caused a hypochromic shift in the absorption spectrum of primaquine, but the drug did not shift the thermal strand separation profile of DNA to higher temperatures and failed to increase the viscosity of calf thymus DNA; this last observation argued against intercalation binding of primaquine.

Whereas the pK_1 of the terminal nitrogen in the identical side chains of chloroquine and primaquine is approximately 10, the pK_2 for chloroquine is 7.8, but that for primaquine is 3.1. The 8-aminoquinoline, hence, exists at physiological pH values as a monoprotonated cation (17) and cannot bridge the minor groove of DNA in the manner of 4-aminoquinolines (15). The nature of the primaquine-DNA complex has remained unknown. We report here that at low ionic strength, primaquine changed the superhelical density of PM2 DNA in the manner of intercalators.

MATERIALS AND METHODS

Quinacrine HCl, chloroquine diphosphate, primaquine diphosphate, and chlorpromazine HCl were supplied by the Division of Medicinal Chemistry of our Institute. Acridine orange, propidium diiodide, and ethidium bromide were obtained from Calbiochem. Quinine 2HCl was a preparation of Vitarine Co. Inc., and methylene blue was furnished by Mallinkrodt Chemical Works.

Bacteriophage PM2 and its host organism, a marine bacterium, *Pseudomonas* BAL31, were kindly furnished by William R. Bauer. Isolation of PM2 from the infected bacteria was carried out with minor modifications of published methods (7, 31). CsCl was removed from virus suspensions by dialysis against a solution of NaCl (1 M) in tris)hydroxymethyl)aminomethane(Tris)-hydrochloride buffer (0.02 M, at pH 8.1). The virus coats were removed by incubating these suspensions for 30 min with 0.05% Sarkosyl at 37°C. Addition of propidium diiodide (100 μg/ml) to the lytic mixture prior to its incubation increased the final yield of supercoiled DNA. The liberated PM2 DNA was collected by centrifugation overnight in a Beckman 60 rotor at 35,000 rpm and 4°C. The DNA seediment was resuspended in a solution of CsCl (1.55 g/ml) in Tris-hydrochloride buffer (0.02 M), pH 7.4, containing 300 μg of propidium diiodide per ml (18). Isopycnic centrifugation (18) produced one band consisting of supercoiled DNA. This material was stored frozen in liquid nitrogen and reisolated by isopycnic centrifugation prior to its use. Propidium diiodide was removed with Bio-Rad cation exchange resin AG 50W-X8 in a batch operation, and the DNA was immediately dialyzed against a solution containing 0.2 M NaCl, 0.02 M Tris-hydrochloride, and 1 mM ethylenediaminetetraacetic acid at pH 7.35.

The theory of viscometric titration of supercoiled DNA with intercalators has been developed and exemplified with ethidium bromide by Révet et al. (29). Such titrations were carried out by us in a Cannon semimicro dilution viscometer (model K 100), whose associated electronics have been described elsewhere (21). The titrant was added from a Gilmont 0.25-ml micrometer syringe equipped with a glass capillary, which was placed firmly to extend approximately 1 mm below the surface of the DNA test solution. In the regions of the viscosity maxima, the titration curves were fitted to the measured times by computer to a third-degree polynomial (29).

RESULTS

Quinacrine. Intercalation of this drug was originally inferred from classical optical studies (22), and Saucier et al. (32) carried out a viscometric titration of PM2 DNA with quinacrine, which provided hydrodynamic evidence of intercalation binding. We have reproduced these results and obtained a viscometric titration curve (not shown), which shows the typical increase in viscosity (i.e., flow time) when supercoils are removed, an equivalence point (maximum) at which no supercoils are present in PM2 DNA, and a decrease in viscosity when supercoils are reintroduced.

Saucier et al. had estimated that the unwinding angle for quinacrine was 75% of that for ethidium bromide (32). This was based upon an estimate of the extent of intercalation binding of quinacrine from viscometry of fragmented linear DNA. We have reinvestigated the unwinding angle for quinacrine and found that it equaled that of ethidium bromide under our experimental conditions.

Titrations of five different DNA concentrations with quinacrine and of four different DNA concentrations with ethidium bromide were carried out. When ν' is the critical binding ratio at which viscosity becomes maximal, i.e., all supercoils have been removed, c'_T is the total drug concentration added, N_T is the total DNA concentration, and c' is the free drug concentration at equilibrium, the following correlation among these parameters exists (29):

$$c'_T = \nu' N_T + c' \qquad (1)$$

This is an equation for a straight line of which the slope is the critical binding ratio, ν', and the intercept, c', is the free drug concentration. Figure 1 shows these correlations for the titrations of PM2 DNA with quinacrine and ethidium. From these data, the intrinsic association constants under our ionic conditions were calculated to be 2.9×10^4 M^{-1} for quinacrine and 10^6 M^{-1} for ethidium.

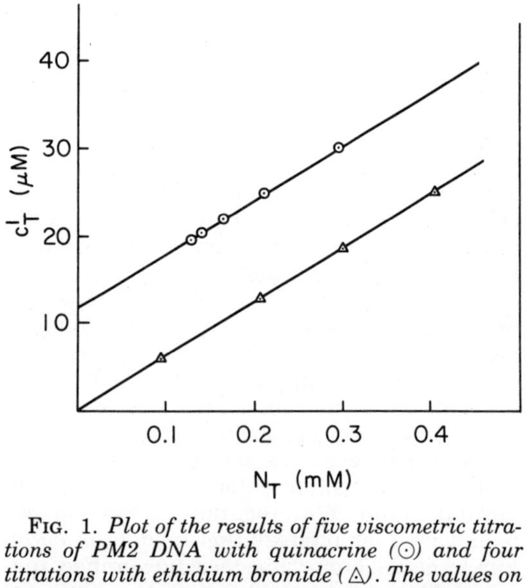

FIG. 1. *Plot of the results of five viscometric titrations of PM2 DNA with quinacrine (⊙) and four titrations with ethidium bromide (△). The values on the ordinate (total drug concentrations added) were obtained by a computer fit of the regions of the principal maxima to a third-degree polynomial. The dimension on the abscissa is the DNA concentration expressed for constituent nucleotides. Solvent was 0.02 M Tris-hydrochloride, containing 0.01 M ethylenediaminetetraacetic acid and 0.2 M NaCl at pH 7.4. The temperature was 20°C.*

The critical binding ratio, ν', at which the superhelical turns disappear entirely is related to the initial superhelix density (in the absence of intercalators), σ_0, and to the unwinding angle of an intercalator, ρ, by equation 2:

$$-\nu' = \frac{\pi}{10\phi}\sigma_0 \quad (2)$$

Assuming the classical unwinding angle for ethidium of 12°, i.e., $\pi/15$ radians (37), the superhelical density of PM2 DNA, σ_0, was calculated to be -4.2×10^{-2}, a value in good agreement with -4.3×10^{-2} reported by Smit and Borst (33) from viscometric experiments under similar ionic conditions. From the identity of the slopes of the two lines in Fig. 1, it follows that the unwinding angles for ethidium bromide and quinacrine were identical at the present ionic concentrations, which minimized nonintercalative binding to DNA.

It is possible that the values for the initial superhelical density and for the unwinding angle of quinacrine will have to be proportionally adjusted, because the unwinding angle for ethidium bromide has recently been revised upward to 26°C (35). For the purpose of our present investigation, this is not of critical importance.

Acridine orange. As concerns its interaction with DNA, acridine orange has been one of the most frequently studied aminoacridines, but we are not aware of published hydrodynamic studies of acridine orange/DNA complexes. Figure 2 shows the results of our viscometric titration of PM2 DNA with acridine orange. Since no data exist for the stoichiometry of binding (number of dye molecules per unit of DNA), the critical binding ratio, ν', was not calculated. However, the shape of the viscometric titration curve (Fig. 2) is typical for a situation in which supercoils are removed, an equivalence point is attained, and supercoils are reintroduced. We conclude that acridine orange was intercalated into PM2 DNA under our experimental conditions.

Chloroquine and quinine. These 4-substituted quinoline derivatives satisfy structural requirements for intercalation binding by possessing a minimal size of their planar heterocyclic systems of 38 Å^2, necessary for antimicrobial activity (1). This requirement has been subsequently recognized to be among those for intercalation into DNA (10). Titrations of PM2 DNA with both compounds were carried out in 1 mM NaCl to forestall inorganic cationic competition with the binding of the substances to DNA. Waring (37) reported that at his standard concentration of 0.05 M Tris-hydrochloride, the interaction of chloroquine with closed circular DNA was "much weaker" than that of other drugs he studied, and we had found (8) that NaCl had marked activity of reversing the hypochromic effects of linear DNA on the absorption spectrum of quinine. Despite an asymmetry of the two titration curves (Fig. 3 and 4), they are qualitatively consistent with intercalation binding.

Chlorpromazine and methylene blue. Intercalation binding of the two phenothiazine derivatives chlorpromazine and methylene blue has remained controversial. Waring (37) found no hydrodynamic evidence that chlorpromazine was intercalated, and hydrodynamic tests have not been carried out on methylene blue/DNA complexes.

In this laboratory, earlier studies on the interaction of methylene blue with DNA (13) were hampered by the tendency of the dye to precipitate DNA, and similar occurrences with chlorpromazine rendered DNA-binding studies in our hands nonfeasible. Others (19) who have reported such experiments have commented on the "precipitation or aggregation" of DNA by chlorpromazine. Precipitability by phenothiazines appears to be a group property of polyphosphates (16).

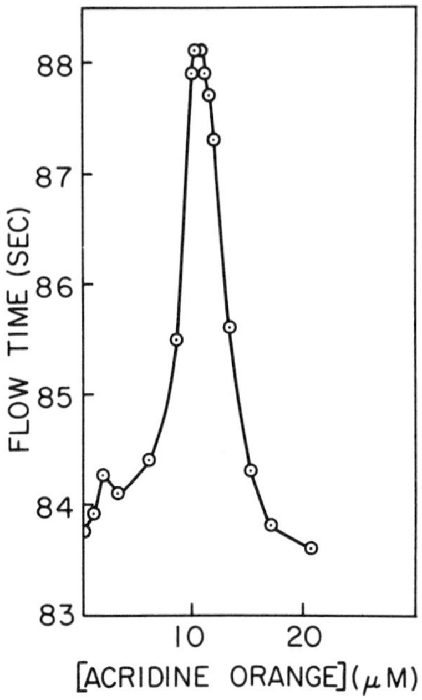

FIG. 2. *Viscometric titration of PM2 DNA with acridine orange. DNA, 2.3 × 10^{-4} M constituent nucleotides, dissolved in mM NaCl at pH 6.0. Acridine orange solution was 3.7 × 10^{-4} M.*

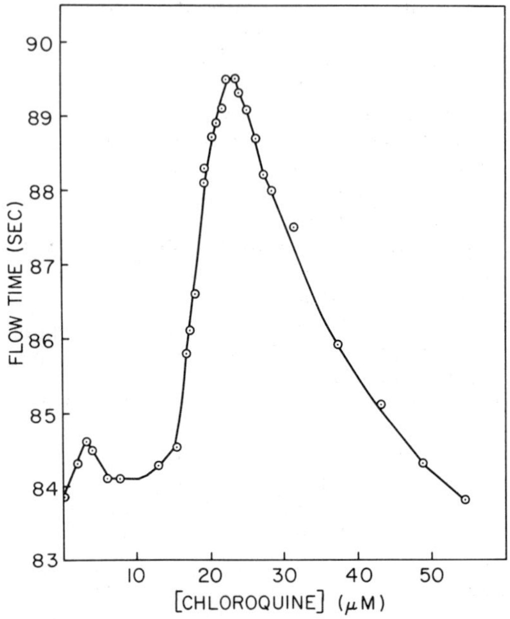

FIG. 3. *Viscometric titration of PM2 DNA with chloroquine in 1 mM NaCl at pH 6.3. Chloroquine solution was 6.6 × 10^{-4} M. DNA concentration was 2.3 × 10^{-4} M constituent nucleotides.*

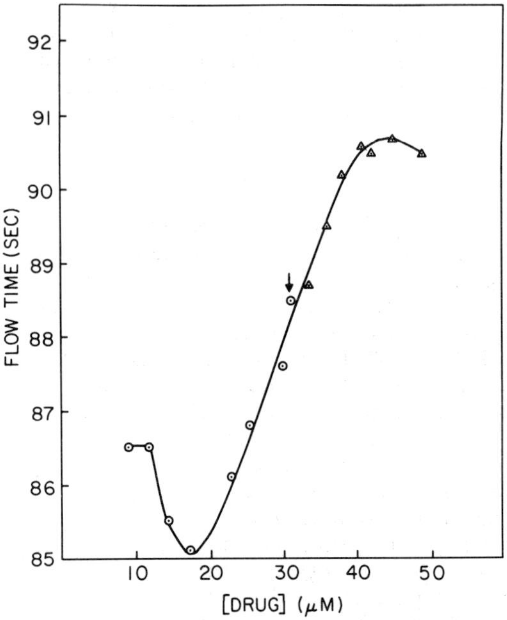

FIG. 5. *Sequential viscometric titration of PM2 DNA with methylene blue (⊙), 5.4 × 10^{-4} M, followed by quinacrine (△), 3.1 × 10^{-4} M. DNA concentration was 4.2 × 10^{-4} M constituent nucleotides. Solvent system was as in Fig. 1.*

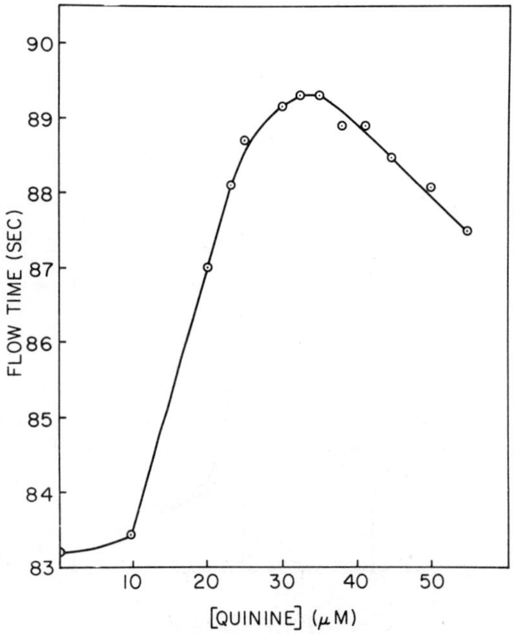

FIG. 4. *Viscometric titration of PM2 DNA with quinine at pH 6.75. The quinine solution was 0.01 M. All other solutions as in Fig. 3.*

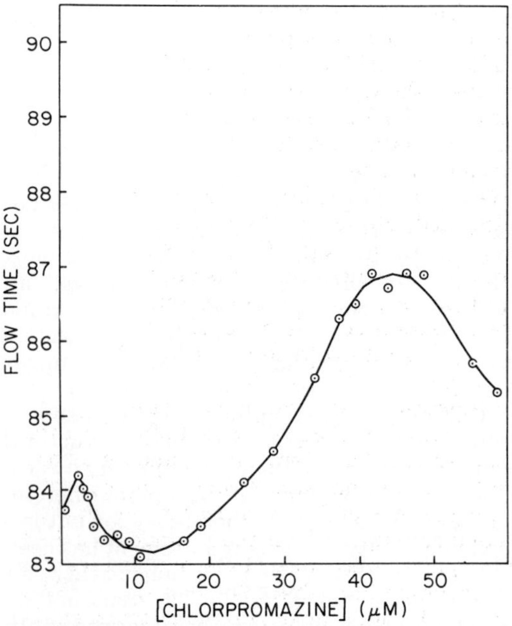

FIG. 6. *Viscometric titration of PM2 DNA with chlorpromazine, 8.4 × 10^{-4} M. DNA concentration was 2.3 × 10^{-4} M constituent nucleotides in 1 mM NaCl, pH 7.2.*

To avoid experimental complications from precipitation of DNA by methylene blue, we carried out a sequential titration (Fig. 5), which was started with methylene blue to a point indicated by the arrow at which the removal of supercoils was apparent, and then we completed the titration with quinacrine. Methylene blue contributed to the systematic change in viscosity of PM2 DNA, as would be expected from an intercalating compound.

A viscometric titration of PM2 DNA with chlorpromazine is shown in Fig. 6. When the addition of chlorpromazine was increased above 60 μM, the viscosity dropped precipitously (not shown), suggesting that DNA was precipitated. Therefore, we carried out, again, a sequential titration, starting with ethidium bromide to the point indicated by the arrow (Fig. 7) and followed by chlorpromazine, which produced a systematic decrease in viscosity, consistent with the systematic reintroduction of supercoils into PM2 DNA.

In previous sequential viscometric titrations of distamycin A and ethidium bromide (20), we have shown that the antibiotic did not contribute to the viscosity changes produced by ethidium bromide and, hence, was not intercalated. Sequential viscometric titration is a method by which intercalation models of DNA-complexing drugs can be studied for substances that precipitate DNA.

Primaquine. This antimalarial drug has no significant effects on nucleic acid biosyntheses (28), and DNA-binding studies have not given indications of intercalation (17). However, the size of the 8-aminoquinoline ring system suggests that intercalation binding should be possible. We tested this by viscometric titration of PM2 DNA, using a low ionic concentration of NaCl of 1 mM. The titration curve (Fig. 8) is consistent with the interpretation that under the present experimental conditions primaquine was, indeed, intercalated into DNA.

DISCUSSION

The present viscometric studies have proved for the first time that acridine orange, quinine, chlorpromazine, methylene blue, and primaquine are intercalated into DNA; they have confirmed intercalation binding of ethidium bromide (29), quinacrine (32), and chloroquine (37). The viscometric method has been used previously to prove intercalation of proflavine, actinomycin D, daunomycin (32), methoxy-9-ellepticine (9, 32), and amikhellin (30); on the other hand, it has shown that distamcyin A binds to DNA without intercalation (20).

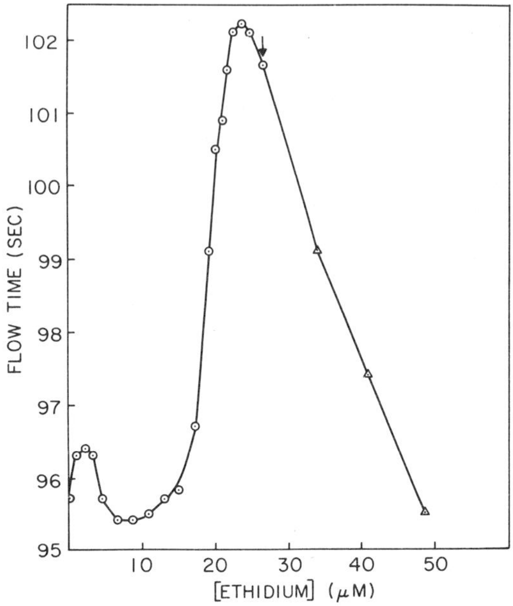

FIG. 7. *Sequential viscometric titration of PM2 DNA with ethidium bromide (⊙), 2.3 × 10^{-4} M, followed by chlorpromazine (△), 8.40 × 10^{-4} M. DNA concentration was 4.4 × 10^{-4} M constituent nucleotides. Solvent was 1 mM NaCl at pH 7.2.*

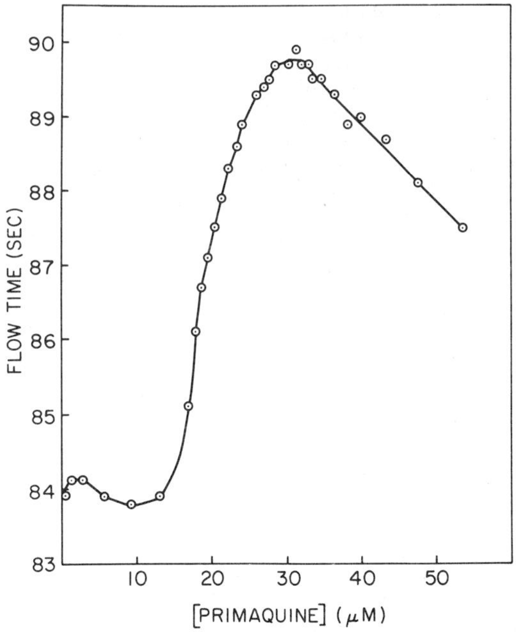

FIG. 8. *Viscometric titration of PM2 DNA with primaquine. Solvent was 1 mM NaCl at pH 6.35. DNA concentration was 2.3 × 10^{-4} M constituent nucleotides; primaquine solution was 9.3 × 10^{-4} M.*

Of acridine orange it was initially believed that the compound was bound to DNA by "stacking" alongside the periphery of the double helix (4), but already in that early work reference was made to two types of complexes, the formation of which was dependent upon the dye/DNA binding ratio (4). Subsequently, it became conventional to consider aminoacridine/DNA complexes of low dye/DNA ratios to be intercalation complexes (3). On the basis of optical studies, intercalation binding of acridine orange has been discussed or inferred by several authors (34, 39).

Intercalation binding of chloroquine was first postulated on the basis of hydrodynamic experiments with linear DNA (25) and has subsequently been proved by Waring (37) in sedimentation studies with closed circular DNA. Intercalation binding of quinine was also inferred from hydrodynamic experiments with linear DNA (8, 14), but a low stoichiometry of 1 drug molecule per 40 base pairs and a numerical value for the apparent association constant were estimated at low quinine/DNA ratios, because at higher concentrations quinine precipitated DNA. Some uncertainty persists, therefore, that these data expressed the binding parameters of the alkaloid at equilibrium.

In the phenothiazine ring, the bond angles and distances of the C—S—C moiety of the ring system cause a localized departure from overall planarity (23), arguing against the possibility of complete intercalation binding. Binding of methylene blue to DNA in equilibrium dialysis revealed an extreme specificity for guanine-plus-cytosine-rich DNA (24). In that work, methylene blue was classified as an intercalator (24), but no tests of this hypothesis are reported in the literature. Electron-spin resonance studies of the binding of the positive radical of chlorpromazine to DNA have suggested intercalation binding (26), but Waring found no hydrodynamic evidence that the drug was intercalated (37). Quenching of the fluorescence of the intercalation complex of acridine orange with DNA by methylene blue and chlorpromazine led Yamabe to the inference that the two phenothiazines were intercalated (40).

Viscometry (32) has confirmed Waring's estimates of the unwinding angles of proflavine and daunomycin to be approximately 66 or 33% of that of ethidium bromide (37). A discrepancy exists, however, between an estimate of the unwinding angle of quinacrine, which Saucier et al. reported to be 75% of that of ethidium bromide (32), and our finding that it was identical to that of ethidium bromide (Fig. 1). Those workers (32) based their estimate of the unwinding angle of quinacrine on determinations of the extent of intercalation binding of quinacrine by viscometry of fragmented linear DNA, whereas our determination is based upon titrations of a series of closed circular DNA concentrations with the drug and determinations of the critical binding parameters from the linear plot of Fig. 1, using the original methodology of Révet et al. (29). Another difference between the work of Saucier et al. (32) and our studies involves ionic concentrations in the viscometric titrations. They used a solvent of an ionic strength of 0.05 M, whereas in the present work a higher ionic strength was selected (see legend to Fig. 1) to minimize electrostatic binding of quinacrine to the periphery of the double helix.

Our present work and studies of others (32, 37) bring to 11 the number of anti-R-plasmid drugs in a set of 15 that have been tested for their ability to eliminate the R-plasmid R1 (12). Intercalation binding has been proved for these 11 compounds. Among the remaining four, intercalation of berberine (14) and tilorone (5) is strongly suggested by hydrodynamic studies of their complexes with linear DNA. Intercalation of Nitroakridin 3582 and of nitroacridine II can be reasonably assumed by analogy to other acridine derivatives. A spectrophotometric titration of Nitroakridin 3582 with DNA from *Escherichia coli* has yielded a biphasic Scatchard plot, with a stoichiometry of 1 drug molecule per ~2 base pairs for the stronger process (38). This number is suggestive of intercalation binding. Intercalation binding of primaquine under non-physiological hypotonic conditions does not appear to result in biochemical effects in vivo (28) in isotonic media.

Our microbiological results (11, 12) and the present biophysical findings, as well as those of others (32, 37), jointly confirm the hypothesis that intercalative compounds have the group property of eliminating bacterial plasmids. This hypothesis now suggests that superior anti-R-plasmid drugs might be discovered by a systematic study of additional intercalative compounds.

LITERATURE CITED

1. **Albert, A., S. D. Rubbo, and M. I. Burvill.** 1949. The influence of chemical constitution on antibacterial activity. Part IV. A survey of heterocyclic bases with special reference to benzquinolines, phenanthridines, benzacridines, quinolines and pyridines. Br. J. Exp. Pathol. 30:159–175.
2. **Bauer, W., and J. Vinograd.** 1968. The interaction of closed circular DNA with intercalative dyes. I. The superhelix density of SV40 DNA in the presence and

absence of dye. J. Mol. Biol. 33:141-171.

3. **Blake, A., and A. R. Peacocke.** 1968. The interaction of aminoacridines with nucleic acids. Biopolymers 6:1225-1253.
4. **Bradley, D. F., and M. K. Wolf.** 1959. Aggregation of dyes bound to polyanions. Proc. Natl. Acad. Sci. U.S.A. 45:944-952.
5. **Chandra, P., F. Zunino, V. P. Gaur, A. Zaccara, M. Woltersdorf, G. Luoni, and A. Götz.** 1972. Mode of tilorone hydrochloride interaction to DNA and polydeoxyribonucleotides. FEBS Lett. 28:5-9.
6. **Ciak, J., and F. E. Hahn.** 1966. Chloroquine: mode of action. Science 151:347-349.
7. **Espejo, R. T., E. S. Canelo, and R. L. Sinsheimer.** 1969. DNA of bacteriophage PM2: a closed circular double-stranded molecule. Proc. Natl. Acad. Sci. U.S.A. 63:1164-1168.
8. **Estensen, R. D., A. K. Krey, and F. E. Hahn.** 1969. Studies on a deoxyribonucleic acid-quinine complex. Mol. Pharmacol. 5:532-541.
9. **Festy, B., J. Poisson, and C. Paoletti.** 1971. A new DNA intercalating drug: methoxy-9-ellipticine. FEBS Lett. 17:321-323.
10. **Hahn, F. E.** 1975. Strategy and tactics of chemotherapeutic drug development. Naturwissenschaften 62:449-458.
11. **Hahn, F. E., and J. Ciak.** 1971. Elimination of bacterial episomes by DNA-complexing compounds. Ann. N.Y. Acad. Sci. 182:295-304.
12. **Hahn, F. E., and J. Ciak.** 1976. Elimination of resistance determinants from R-factor R1 by intercalating compounds. Antimicrob. Agents Chemother. 9:77-80.
13. **Hahn, F. E., and A. K. Krey.** 1969. Deoxyribonucleic acid-induced anomalous optical rotatory dispersion of antimalarial drugs and dyes, p. 15-20. Antimicrob. Agents Chemother. 1968.
14. **Hahn, F. E., and A. K. Krey.** 1971. Interactions of alkaloids with DNA. Prog. Mol. Subcell. Biol. 2:134-151.
15. **Hahn, F. E., R. L. O'Brien, J. Ciak, J. L. Allison, and J. G. Olenick.** 1966. Studies on modes of action of chloroquine, quinacrine and quinine and on chloroquine resistance. Mil. Med. 131:1071-1089.
16. **Hele, P.** 1963. The interaction of phenothiazine derivatives and imipramine with polyphosphates of biological interest. Biochim. Biophys. Acta 76:647-649.
17. **Holbrook, D. J., L. P. Whichard, C. R. Morris, and L. A. White.** 1971. Interaction of antimalarial aminoquinolines (primaquine, pentaquine and chloroquine) with nucleic acids and effects on various enzymatic reactions *in vitro*. Prog. Mol. Subcell. Biol. 2:113-125.
18. **Hudson, B., W. B. Upholt, J. Devinny, and J. Vinograd.** 1969. The use of an ethidium analogue in the dye-buoyant density procedure for the isolation of closed circular DNA: the variation of the superhelix density of mitochondrial DNA. Proc. Natl. Acad. Sci. U.S.A. 62:813-820.
19. **Kantesaria, P., and P. Marfey.** 1975. The effect of chlorpromazine on some properties of DNA in solution. Physiol. Chem. Phys. 7:53-67.
20. **Krey, A. K., R. G. Allison, and F. E. Hahn.** 1973. Interactions of the antibiotic distamycin A, with negative DNA and with synthetic duplex polydeoxyribonucleotides. FEBS Lett. 29:58-62.
21. **Krey, A. K., and F. E. Hahn.** 1975. Studies on the methyl green-DNA complex and its dissociation by drugs. Biochemistry 14:5061-5067.
22. **Lerman, L. S.** 1963. The structure of the DNA-acridine complex. Proc. Natl. Acad. Sci. U.S.A. 49:94-102.
23. **McDowell, J. J. H.** 1973. The molecular structure of phenothiazine derivatives, p. 33-54. *In* I. S. Forrest et al. (ed.), Phenothiazines and structurally related drugs. Raven Press, New York.
24. **Müller, W., and D. M. Crothers.** 1975. Interactions of heteroaromatic compounds with nucleic acids. 1. The influence of heteroatoms and polarizability on the base specificity of intercalating ligands. Eur. J. Biochem. 54:267-277.
25. **O'Brien, R. L., J. L. Allison, and F. E. Hahn.** 1966. Evidence for intercalation of chloroquine into DNA. Biochim. Biophys. Acta 129:622-624.
26. **Ohnishi, S., and H. M. McConnell.** 1965. Interaction of the radical ion of chlorpromazine with deoxyribonucleic acid. J. Am. Chem. Soc. 87:2293.
27. **Olenick, J. G.** 1975. Antibacterial action of primaquine: effects in vitro on polypeptide synthesis and in vivo on ribosomes and ribosomal ribonucleic acid. Antimicrob. Agents Chemother. 8:754-756.
28. **Olenick, J. G., and F. E. Hahn.** 1972. Mode of action of primaquine: preferential inhibition of protein biosynthesis in *Bacillus megaterium*. Antimicrob. Agents Chemother. 1:259-262.
29. **Révet, B. M. J., M. Schmir, and J. Vinograd.** 1971. Direct determination of the superhelix density of closed circular DNA by viscometric titration. Nature (London) New Biol. 229:10-13.
30. **Rucheton, M., and P. Janteur.** 1973. Studies on amikhellin. I. Intercalative binding of double-stranded DNA. Biochimie 55:1415-1420.
31. **Salditt, M., S. N. Braunstein, R. D. Camerini-Otero, and R. M. Franklin.** 1972. Structure and synthesis of a lipid-containing bacteriophage. X. Improved techniques for the purification of bacteriophage PM2. Virology 48:259-262.
32. **Saucier, J. M., B. Festy, and J. B. Le Pecq.** 1971. Change of the torsion of the DNA helix caused by intercalation. II. Measurements of the relative change of torsion induced by various intercalating drugs. Biochimie 53:973-980.
33. **Smit, E. M., and P. Borst.** 1971. The superhelix density of PM2 DNA, determined by a viscometric method. FEBS Lett. 14:125-129.
34. **Takesada, H., E. Saito, H. Fujita, K. Suzuki, and A. Wada.** 1970. Study on the binding nature of acridine orange to DNA by means of flow dichroism. Bull. Chem. Soc. Jpn. 43:181-187.
35. **Wang, J. C.** 1974. The degree of unwinding of the DNA helix by ethidium. I. Titration of twisted PM2 DNA molecules in alkaline cesium chloride density gradients. J. Mol. Biol. 89:783-801.
36. **Warhurst, D. C., and J. Williamson.** 1970. Ribonucleic acid from *Plasmodium knowlesi* before and after chloroquine treatment. Chem. Biol. Interact. 2:89-106.
37. **Waring, M.** 1970. Variation of the supercoils in closed circular DNA by binding of antibiotics and drugs: evidence for molecular models involving intercalation. J. Mol. Biol. 54:247-279.
38. **Wolfe, A. D., T. M. Cook, and F. E. Hahn.** 1971. Antibacterial nitroacridine, Nitroakridin 3582: binding to nucleic acids in vitro and effects on selected cell-free model systems of macromolecular biosynthesis. J. Bacteriol. 108:1026-1033.
39. **Yamabe, S.** 1969. A fluorospectrophotometric study on the binding of acridine orange with DNA and its bases. Arch. Biochem. Biophys. 130:148-155.
40. **Yamabe, S.** 1973. Further fluorospectrophotometric studies on the binding of acridine orange with DNA. Effects of thermal denaturation of DNA and additions of spermine, kanamycin, dihydrostreptomycin, methylene blue and chlorpromazine. Arch. Biochem. Biophys. 154:19-27.

ANTIMICROBIAL AGENTS AND CHEMOTHERAPY, Feb. 1977, p. 258-261 Vol. 11, No. 2

In Vitro Activity of Ticarcillin Against Anaerobic Bacteria Compared with That of Carbenicillin and Penicillin

IRA ROY, VINH BACH, AND HARAGOPAL THADEPALLI*

Division of Infectious Diseases and Department of Internal Medicine, Martin Luther King, Jr. General Hospital; Charles R. Drew Postgraduate Medical School; and University of Southern California School of Medicine, Los Angeles, California 90059*

Received for publication 8 September 1976

A total of 334 clinical anaerobic isolates were tested in an anaerobic glove box by the agar dilution technique for susceptibility to clinically achievable levels of ticarcillin, carbenicillin, and penicillin. Thirty-two micrograms or less of penicillin per milliliter inhibited 91% of all strains, whereas 100 μg of carbenicillin and ticarcillin per ml inhibited 95 and 98%, respectively. A total of 82% (85 strains) of *Bacteroides* were inhibited by penicillin, and 93 and 96% were inhibited by carbenicillin and ticarcillin, respectively. Thirteen (24%) of 55 strains of *Bacteroides fragilis* tested were resistant to 32 μg of penicillin per ml, and 6 (11%) and 3 (5%) were resistant to 100 μg of carbenicillin and ticarcillin per ml, respectively. Within the therapeutic range, ticarcillin was the most effective of the three penicillins tested against *B. fragilis* subsp. *fragilis*.

Ticarcillin, a new semisynthetic penicillin, resembles carbenicillin in structure and in in vitro antimicrobial activity against aerobic bacteria including *Pseudomonas* species. Its effect against anaerobic bacteria is not established. We examined the efficacy of ticarcillin against 334 clinical anaerobic isolates (234 of them were derived from the female genital tract) in comparison with the effect of penicillin and carbenicillin in vitro.

(This work was presented in part at the 76th Annual Meeting of the American Society for Microbiology, Atlantic City, N.J., 2-7 May 1976.)

MATERIALS AND METHODS

Identification of all isolates was done as described in the anaerobic laboratory manual of the Virginia Polytechnic Institute (1). All 334 were human isolates identified in our laboratory between August 1975 and July 1976. Two-thirds of these (i.e., 234) were isolated from healthy cervices or from female genital tract infections, and the remaining were from infections of the lung or abdomen. The inocula were overnight brain heart infusion broth cultures diluted to McFarland standard I delivered with a Steers replicator to deposit 10^5 colony-forming units. Solutions containing concentrations of drug were prepared by dissolving the standard powders of penicillin G (Eli Lilly & Co., Indianapolis, Ind.), sodium carbenicillin (Roerig), and disodium ticarcillin (Beecham Products Inc., Clifton, N.J.) in distilled water. The antibiotic solutions were freshly prepared and added to brain heart infusion agar (Clinical Standard, Torrance, Calif.) and supplemented with defibrinated sheep blood (5%), 10 μg of vitamin K per ml, and hemin (Scott Laboratories, Fiskeville, R. I.). The inocula were planted with a Steers replicator (6), and the plates were incubated in an anaerobic glove box filled with a gas mixture of 85% nitrogen, 5% carbon dioxide, and 10% hydrogen and incubated at 37°C for 48 h. The minimal inhibitory concentration (MIC) was read as the least amount of antibiotic that permitted no growth. A set of aerobic and anaerobic plates without antibiotics was included as a control with each set of tests.

RESULTS

Tables 1, 2, and 3 depict the MIC of penicillin, carbenicillin, and ticarcillin for inhibition of 334 anaerobic isolates. All three penicillins inhibited more than 90% of the anaerobes tested. As expected, 25% of the *B. fragilis* subsp. *fragilis* was resistant to 32 μg of penicillin per ml; correspondingly, 18 and 7% were also resistant to carbenicillin and ticarcillin, respectively. Three of 28 (11%) strains resistant to both penicillin and carbenicillin, but susceptible to ticarcillin, accounted for this difference. Two strains (7%) of *B. fragilis* subsp. *fragilis* were resistant to all three penicillins. *B. fragilis,* other than subsp. *fragilis,* were inhibited by both carbenicillin and ticarcillin alike, but 22% of them were resistant to penicillin. Strains of the *Bacteroides* group, except *B. fragilis,* were highly susceptible to carbenicillin (100%) and ticarcillin (97%). In general, 18% of all strains of *Bacteroides* were resistant to peni-

TABLE 1. *Penicillin concentration and cumulative percentage of susceptible strains*

Organisms	No. of strains	% Susceptible at MIC (μg/ml) of:					
		2	4	8	16	32	64
Gram-negative rods							
Bacteroides (B) *fragilis* subsp. *fragilis*	28	32	36		54	75	96
B. fragilis other than *B. fragilis* subsp. *fragilis*	27	26	41	52	59	78	100
Bacteroides except *B. fragilis*	30	77	80	83	93		97
Bacteroides (all strains)	(85)	46	53	54	69	82	97
Fusobacterium	10	60			70		80
Selanomonas	1	100					
Clostridia (all)	44	52	55	86	95	100	
Nonsporeforming gram-positive rods							
Eubacterium	36	67	72	75	89	92	95
Lactobacilli	16	88		94			94
Propionibacteria	8	75					75
Bifidobacteria	3	100					
Actinomyces	7	100					
Cocci							
Peptococci	75	77	85	88	93		93
Peptostreptococci	43	49	86	88	93	95	95
Veillonella	4		50			100	
Megasphera elsdenii	2		100				
Total (avg)	334	(60)	(70)	(77)	(84)	(91)	(96)

TABLE 2. *Carbenicillin concentration and cumulative percentage of susceptible strains*

Organisms	No. of strains	% Susceptible at MIC (μg/ml) of:					
		5	10	25	50	100	200
Gram-negative rods							
Bacteroides (B) *fragilis* subsp. *fragilis*	28	36	54	68	71	82	100
B. fragilis other than *B. fragilis* subsp. *fragilis*	27	56		67	89	96	100
Bacteroides except *B. fragilis*	30	93	100				
Bacteroides (all above strains)	(85)	62	71	79	87	93	100
Fusobacteria	10	90					90
Selanomonas	1	100					
Clostridia (all)	44	52	55	91	95	97	97
Nonsporeforming gram-positive rods							
Eubacteria	36	83	86	89	97	100	
Lactobacilli	16	87			100		
Propionibacteria	8	75					75
Bifidobacteria	3	100					
Actinomyces	7	71		100			
Cocci							
Peptococci	75	89		94			97
Peptostreptococci	43	86	100				
Veillonella	4	25			100		
Megasphera elsdenii	2	100					
Total (avg)	334	(75)	(77)	(85)	(91)	(96)	(98)

TABLE 3. *Ticarcillin concentration and cumulative percentage of susceptible strains*

Organisms	No. of strains	% Susceptible at MIC (μg/ml) of:					
		5	10	25	50	100	200
Gram-negative rods							
Bacteroides (B) *fragilis* subsp. *fragilis*	28	39	46	50	71	93	100
B. fragilis other than *B. fragilis* subsp. *fragilis*	27	67		70	93	96	100
Bacteroides except *B. fragilis*	30	93	97		100		
Bacteroides (all above strains)	(85)	67	71	73	88	96	100
Fusobacteria	10	80				100	
Selanomonas	1	100					
Clostridia (all)	44	59	66	86	93	100	
Nonsporeforming gram-positive rods							
Eubacteria	36	94	97		100		
Lactobacilli	16	88			100		
Propionibacteria	8	75					75
Bifidobacteria	3	100					
Actinomyces	7	71	100				
Cocci							
Peptococci	75	60	98				99
Peptostreptococci	43	88	93	98			
Veillonella	4	100					
Megasphera elsdenii	2	100					
Total (avg)	334	(77)	(84)	(88)	(94)	(98)	(99)

cillin, and 7 and 4% were resistant to carbenicillin and ticarcillin, respectively.

Forty-four strains of ten different species of clostridia were susceptible to all three penicillins. Twenty-five (57%) of these strains were of species *C. ramosum*. *Actinomyces* (seven strains), including four strains of *A. israellii* and 3 strains of *A. naeslundii,* were susceptible to all three penicillins. Most gram-positive cocci with occasional exceptions were also susceptible to all three penicillins.

DISCUSSION

Ticarcillin, like carbenicillin (also a semisynthetic penicillin), was found to be effective against aerobic bacteria such as *Pseudomonas aeruginosa* both in vitro and in vivo (2–5, 8). It was reported that ticarcillin might even have a greater spectrum of activity and might achieve relatively higher drug concentrations in serum than carbenicillin (5, 8). Its effect on anaerobes in vitro is not well known. The in vivo efficacy of this drug is now being tested. We chose 100 μg/ml as a cutoff point for ticarcillin because the reported concentrations of this drug in serum 0.5 to 1.0 h after a 5-g intravenous injection were found to be from 200 μg (4) to as high as 740 ± 56 μg/ml (5). Nearly two-thirds of the strains reported here were from the female genital tract, which suggests that ticarcillin may find a place in the treatment of postsurgical infections of the female genital tract.

Although all three penicillins exhibited more than 90% efficacy against 334 anaerobic strains, there were important differences in their effectiveness against the *Bacteroides* group of organisms. Both carbenicillin and ticarcillin inhibited 93 to 96% of all strains of *Bacteroides,* including *B. fragilis* other than *B. fragilis* subsp. *fragilis*. Thirty-two micrograms of penicillin per ml was ineffective against 18% of these strains. *B. fragilis* subsp. *fragilis,* however, were the most resistant of all *Bacteroides*. It is difficult to treat a deep-seated infection with penicillin G when the MICs of the infecting organisms are higher than 25 μg/ml (7). Hence, the cutoff point chosen for penicillin was 32 μg/ml. Even at this concentration, nearly 25% of the strains of *B. fragilis* subsp. *fragilis* were resistant to penicillin. Both carbenicillin and ticarcillin inhibited 82 and 93% of these strains, respectively.

The relative resistance of some of the isolates to carbenicillin while susceptible to ticarcillin may be real or may be a spurious reflection of the increased usage of carbenicillin in our hospital in recent years. This remains to be verified.

LITERATURE CITED

1. **Holdeman, L. V., and W. E. C. Moore (ed.).** 1975. Anaerobe laboratory manual. Virginia Polytechnic In-

stitute Anaerobe Laboratory, Virginia Polytechnic Institute and State University, Blacksburg.
2. **Neu, H. C., and G. J. Garvey.** 1975. Comparative in vitro activity and clinical pharmacology of ticarcillin and carbenicillin. Antimicrob. Agents Chemother. **8**:457–462.
3. **Pines, A., G. Khaja, H. Raafat, and K. S. Shreedharan.** 1974. Preliminary clinical experience with Ticarcillin (BRL2288) in 101 patients treated for severe respiratory infections. Chemotherapy **20**:39–44.
4. **Rodriguez, V., G. P. Bodey, N. Horikoshi, J. Inagaki, and K. B. McCredie.** 1973. Ticarcillin therapy of infections. Antimicrob. Agents Chemother. **4**:427–431.
5. **Simon, C., M. Leuth, and V. Malerczyk.** 1974. Ticarcillin. Deutsch. Med. Woschenschr. **99**:2460–2464.
6. **Steers, E., E. L. Foltz, and B. S. Graves.** 1959. An inocula replicating apparatus for routine testing of bacterial susceptibility to antibiotics. Antibiot. Chemother. **9**:307–311.
7. **Sutter, V. L., and S. M. Finegold.** 1975. Susceptibility of anaerobic bacteria to carbenicillin, cefoxitin and related drugs. J. Infect. Dis. **131**:417–422.
8. **Wise, R., and D. S. Reeves.** 1974. Clinical and laboratory investigations on Ticarcillin and anti-pseudomonal antibiotic. Chemotherapy **20**:45–51.

Antimicrobial Agents and Chemotherapy, Feb. 1977, p. 262-266
Vol. 11, No. 2

Pharmacokinetics of Cefamandole in Patients with Normal and Impaired Renal Function

HANS-EBERHARD MELLIN, PETER G. WELLING, AND PAUL O. MADSEN*

Urology Section, Veterans Administration Hospital, Madison, Wisconsin 53705, and Department of Surgery, School of Medicine and School of Pharmacy, University of Wisconsin, Madison, Wisconsin 53706*

Received for publication 16 August 1976

The pharmacokinetics of cefamandole, a new cephalosporin, were investigated in 23 patients with urinary tract infections and normal or varying degrees of impairment of renal function. A daily dose of 1.5 to 3.0 g administered intramuscularly was tolerated well and resulted in very high urine concentrations. The pharmacokinetics of the antibiotic were compared with isotopically labeled [^{131}I]hippurate and [^{125}I]iothalamate, which were used for determination of effective renal plasma flow and glomerular filtration rate, respectively. It was shown that cefamandole was excreted by glomerular filtration as well as by active tubular secretion. Probenecid inhibited the tubular secretion of cefamandole. The serum half-life of cefamandole in patients with normal renal function was approximately 1.5 h and increased in patients along with increasing impairment of renal function. Our studies indicate that a dosage regimen of 1 g of cefamandole every 8 h in patients with normal renal function results in urine concentrations sufficiently high for treatment of most common urinary tract infections. In patients with impaired renal function, the dosage interval should be increased or the dosage lowered according to the serum creatinine values.

Cefamandole, a new cephalosporin antibiotic, is presently being clinically evaluated in the treatment of bacterial infections. It has several advantages over presently available cephalosporins. From in vitro laboratory studies, cefamandole appears to be active against a significant number of gram-negative bacteria, especially indole-positive *Proteus* strains that are resistant to other cephalosporins (2, 6, 11). Generally, the minimum inhibitory concentration values against susceptible gram-positive organisms are lower (0.03 to 1.0 μg/ml) than those for gram-negative strains (1 to 2 μg/ml). The drug has no effect against *Pseudomonas aeruginosa* minimum inhibitory concentrations > 128 μg/ml. However, cefamandole seems to be inferior to cephaloridine and cefazolin in the inhibition of α-hemolytic streptococci, pneumococci, and almost all strains of β-hemolytic streptococci (6, 8, 11).

The effectiveness of this drug is based on interference with the cell wall biosynthesis. Thus, it is only effective against proliferating cells. Similar to other cephalosporins, cefamandole is resistant to many penicillin-hydrolyzing β-lactamases produced by gram-positive as well as gram-negative bacteria (11). Cefamandole appears to have less renal toxic effects than cephaloridine and cefazolin (6).

The present study was designed to evaluate the pharmacokinetics of cefamandole in patients with normal and varying degrees of renal function impairment and urinary tract infection. Other clinical pharmacokinetic studies have also recently been published (3, 7).

MATERIALS AND METHODS

Twenty-three male patients from 32 to 88 years of age (average, 66 years) on a urological ward were treated for urinary tract infections with 1.5 to 3.0 g of cefamandole intramuscularly daily for 5 to 6 days. In five patients, the drug was administered prophylactically before and after instrumentation of the urinary tract. The drug was given at 8-h intervals to all but two patients who had severely impaired renal function. Fourteen patients had normal renal function (serum creatinine ≤ 1.5 mg/100 ml), and nine patients had impaired renal function (serum creatinine ≥ 1.6 mg/100 ml). After intramuscular injection on day 1 of treatment, blood samples were drawn for bioassay at 30, 60, 90, 120, 360 and 450 min. Urine was collected after the injection from 0 to 2, 2 to 4, and 4 to 7.5 h. In thirteen patients, this regimen was repeated on the last day of treatment. In eight of these patients, 1 g of probenecid was given orally every 2 h starting 0.5 h before the last injection on the last day of treatment. In eight patients with normal renal function, approximately 20 μCi of [^{125}I]iothalamate and 40 μCi of *o*-[^{131}I]iodohippurate were injected intramuscularly along with cefamandole. The same blood and urine samples used for bioassays were also used for counting radioactivity in a Gamma well counter. Iothalamate is excreted by the kidneys only by glomerular filtration and iothalamate clearance therefore represents the glomerular filtration rate (1), whereas hippurate is excreted by additional tubular secretion: the hippurate clearance thus represents the effective renal plasma flow (10). These two radioactive drugs, which conveniently can be counted simultaneously, served as additional evaluation of the renal function and as a standard to which the cefamandole could be compared. Creatinine clearances were also carried out in all patients.

Bioassays for determination of plasma and urine concentrations of cefamandole were carried out by a cup plate microbiological assay method using *Bacillus subtilis* (Difco 0453) as test organism on Penassay seed agar (Difco B263) and streptomycin assay agar (Difco 0277). Dilution of serum samples was carried out with pooled normal human serum, and the urine samples were diluted with phosphate buffer at pH 6. All standard curves were made up by diluting the standard antibiotic powder with human serum for the serum readings and with phosphate buffer for the urine readings and were made up simultaneously with the biological samples. No differences were found between standard curves obtained by dilution with urine and dilution with buffer. When equilibration had been reached after about 1 h after injection, a linear decrease could be seen when the serum concentrations were plotted against time on semilogarithmic paper. From this part of the curve, the linear regression line for the serum concentrations against time was determined by the method of the least squares. Half-life, plasma clearance, and renal clearance were calculated by well-established methods (4, 9). The renal clearances were based on the 2- to 4-h and 4- to 7.5-h urine values, and midpoint plasma concentrations were obtained by interpolation.

We determined protein binding in 30 serum samples from patients with normal and varying degrees of impaired renal function using equilibration dialysis for 36 h. After 36 h, antibiotic concentrations inside and outside the dialyzing cellophane bag were measured by the bioassay method, and protein binding was calculated (5).

Determinations of hemoglobin, leukocytes, serum creatinine, serum glutamic oxalacetic transaminase, alkaline phosphates, and serum bilirubin were carried out before drug treatment and after the study to determine whether cefamandole had toxic effects on the hematopoetic system, the liver, or the kidneys.

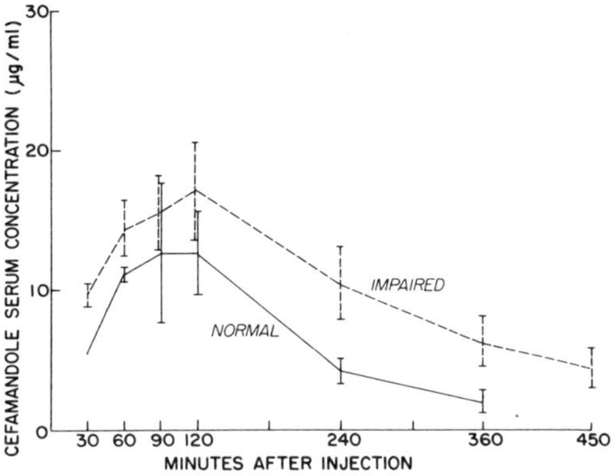

FIG. 1. *Cefamandole serum concentrations after intramuscular injection of 0.5 g of cefamandole in patients with normal (n = 4) and impaired (n = 6) renal function.*

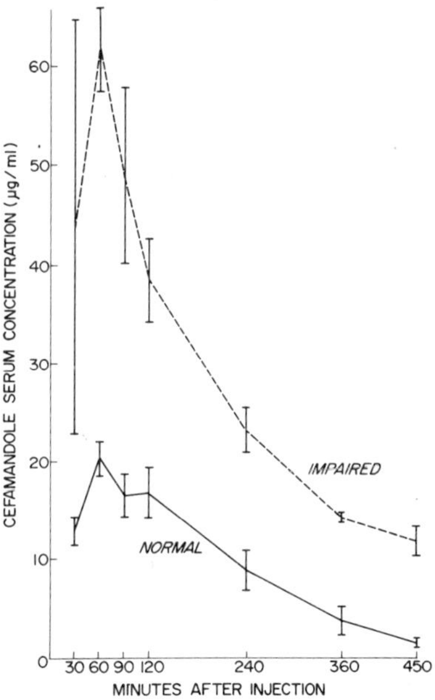

FIG. 2. *Cefamandole serum concentrations after intramuscular injection of 1 g of cefamandole in patients with normal (n = 10) and impaired (n = 3) renal function.*

RESULTS AND DISCUSSION

Figures 1 and 2 show the serum levels of cefamandole after intramuscular injection of 0.5 and 1 g on day 1 of treatment. Cefamandole levels were higher in patients with impaired renal function during the first 6 h after injection, although the differences between these data and those obtained in normals were not statistically significant. This may be due to the small number of patients in this group. After 450 min, the patients with normal function had no measurable serum levels. After administration of 1 g of cefamandole, however, we found a statistically significant difference in serum levels between patients with normal and impaired renal function. The dosage intervals in two patients with severely impaired renal function and receiving 1 g of cefamandole were increased to 12 h, and we did not find accumulation of the drug in any patient after multiple injections. There was no significant difference in serum levels in the two groups of patients 60 min after intramuscular injection of 1 g on the first and the last day of treatment (21 ± 4 versus 18 ± 3 μg/ml and 62 ± 10 versus 52 ± 22 μg/ml, respectively, in patients with normal and impaired renal function). Our dosage regimen for all patients, therefore, appeared to be correct since no accumulation of cefamandole occurred. Table 1 shows urinary excretion of cefamandole after 0.5 and 1 g on day 1 of treatment in patients with normal and impaired renal function. The excretion over a period of 7.5 h was significantly lowered in patients with impaired renal function.

Table 2 shows that the renal clearances of cefamandole significantly exceeded the creatinine clearances in patients with normal as well as impaired renal function. The ratios are significantly different from 1, suggesting active tubular secretion of cefamandole. Table 2 also shows the excretion and renal handling of cefamandole and iothalamate after intramuscular injection. The plasma and renal clearances for cefamandole were significantly higher in patients with normal renal function than in patients with impaired renal function. In all cases, the values for iothalamate were lower than those for the antibiotic. The ratios between the plasma and renal clearances for cefa-

TABLE 1. *Urinary excretion of cefamandole after intramuscular injection*

Dosage (g)	Patient group	Time (h)	% Excretion (range)	Concn range (μg/ml)
0.5	Normal renal function (n = 4)	0–4	61 ± 13[a] (34–93)	450–2,950
		4–7.5	10± 2.5 (6–17)	110–520
0.5	Impaired renal function (n = 6)	0–4	29 ± 5.9 (10–42)	430–3,110
		4–7.5	22 ± 2.5 (12–27)	470–1,220
1.0	Normal renal function (n = 10)	0–4	47 ± 7.6 (15–97)	600–5,150
		4–7.5	18 ± 2.7 (4–29)	270–1,470
1.0	Impaired renal function (n = 3)	0–4	27 ± 9.3 (9–41)	390–3,450
		4–7.5	13 ± 3.7 (8–20)	480–1,660

[a] Mean ± standard error.

TABLE 2. *Cefamandole serum half-life and clearance data of cefamandole, creatinine, and iothalamate*[a]

Patient group	Cefamandole half-life (h)	Cefamandole		Iothalamate		Creatinine clearance (ml/min/1.72 m²)	Ratio: plasma/renal clearancee of cefamandole	Ratio: plasma/renal clearance of iothalamate	Ratio: cefamandole/creatinine renal clearance
		Plasma clearance	Renal clearance	Plasma clearance	Renal clearance				
Normal renal function (n = 14)	1.7 ± 0.1 (0.8–2.6) (n = 14)	303 ± 46 (128–701) (n = 14)	234 ± 41 (77–527) (n = 10)	90 ± 21 (21–170) (n = 8)	94 ± 14 (35–154) (n = 8)	82 ± 7 (36–157) (n = 14)	1.6 ± 0.2 (0.6–3.0) (n = 10)	1.0 ± 0.2 (0.5–2.1) (n = 8)	3.1 ± 0.6[b] (0.9–8.5) (n = 10)
Impaired renal function (n = 9)	3.0 ± 0.3 (1.5–4.1) (n = 9)	98 ± 21 (44–239) (n = 9)	76 ± 13 (30–168) (n = 9)			33 ± 3.5 (10–47) (n = 9)	1.3 ± 0.1 (0.7–1.9) (n = 9)		2.0 ± 0.3[b] (1.1–3.5) (n = 9)

[a] Mean ± standard error (range).
[b] Values are significantly different from 1 (Student's t test).

TABLE 3. *Clearance of cefamandole, hippurate, and iothalamate in eight patients with normal renal function before and after administration of probenecid*[a]

Time	Cefamandole renal clearance (ml/min/ 1.72 m^2)	Iothalamate renal clearance (ml/min/ 1.72 m^2)	Ratio: cefamandole/iothalamate renal clearance	Hippurate renal clearance (ml/min/1.72 m^2)
Before probenecid	302 ± 60	89 ± 14	3.4 ± 0.6[b]	308 ± 44
	(77–527)	(35–154)	(2.2–7.1)	(166–467)
After probenecid	80 ± 14	71 ± 8	1.1 ± 0.1	202 ± 22
	(26–157)	(33–102)	(0.8–1.6)	(132–296)

[a] Mean ± standard error (range).
[b] Value significantly different from 1 (Student's *t* test).

mandole and iothalamate were never significantly different from 1, indicating that both drugs are excreted exclusively by the kidneys. By comparing the renal clearances of cefamandole and iothalamate, we obtained an indicator of the renal handling of the antibiotic. The fact that the ratio of the renal clearances of cefamandole and iothalamate was significantly higher than 1 indicates that cefamandole, in addition to being excreted by glomerular filtration, is also secreted by the renal tubules. This is strongly supported by the inhibiting effect of the probenecid administration.

Table 3 shows that cefamandole and hippurate clearances were significantly lowered after probenecid administration. In addition, although the ratio of cefamandole to iothalamate renal clearances without probenecid was significantly higher than 1, the ratio decreased to 1.1 after probenecid treatment.

Since cefamandole is excreted almost exclusively by the kidneys, the dosage must be adjusted according to renal function. Figure 3 shows the correlation between serum creatinine and half-life of cefamandole after intramuscular injection in 22 patients. The half-life of the drug (Y) at a certain serum creatinine (X) can be calculated simply from the formula for the correlation of X and Y, which is $Y = 0.85 + 0.91X$. For clinical purposes it can be simplified to $Y = 1 + X$. Since the drug should be given about every third half-life, the dosage interval would be $3 \times (1 + X)$. This means that for a patient with a creatinine of 1 mg/100 ml (or less) the dosage interval should be $3 \times 2 = 6$ h, the individual dose being 1 g. For a patient with a serum creatinine of, for example, 3 mg/100 ml, the dosage interval should be $3 \times 4 = 12$ h. If one wants to avoid the wide variations of serum levels following such a dosage regimen, this may be done by giving one-third of the usual dosage every half-life. In both groups of patients we gave 0.5 as well as 1 g of cefamandole with a dosage interval of 8 h, except in two patients with severely impaired renal function,

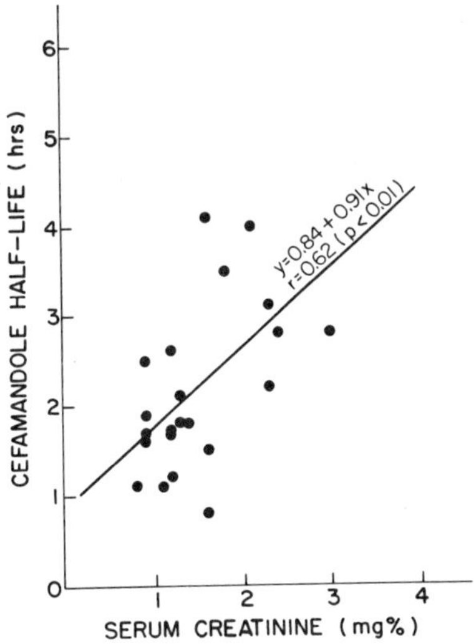

FIG. 3. *Illustration of the correlation between serum creatinine and cefamandole half-life after intramuscular injection in 22 patients.*

who received an injection every 12 h. The dosage regimen of 0.5 g of cefamandole every 8 h appears to be too low for patients with normal renal function, since we found very low serum concentrations after 6 and 8 h after the intramuscular administration. Therefore, we recommend a dose of 1 g every 6 h in patients with normal renal function and adjustment of the dosage according to the renal function in patients with renal failure (Fig. 3).

In 8 patients we found that cefamandole had a protein binding in serum of 32 ± 11% (mean ± standard error) (range, 17 to 58%). There was no significant difference in this respect between patients with normal and impaired renal function. In addition, the protein binding did not depend on the concentration of antibiotic (between 5 and 40 μg/ml.

We did not find toxic effects of cefamandole on the hematopoietic system, liver, or kidneys based on the tests evaluated.

LITERATURE CITED

1. **Elwood, C. M., and E. M. Sigman.** 1967. The measurement of glomerular filtration rate and effective renal plasma flow in man by iothalamate ^{125}I and iodopyracet ^{131}I. Circulation **36**:441–448.
2. **Eykyn, S., C. Jenkins, A. King, and I. Phillips.** 1973. Antibacterial activity of cefamandole, a new cephalosporin antibiotic, compared with that of cephaloridine, cephalothine, and cephalexin. Antimicrob. Agents Chemother. **3**:657–661.
3. **Fong, I. W., E. D. Ralph, E. R. Engelking, and W. M. M. Kirby** 1976. Clinical pharmacology of cefamandole as compared with cephalothin. Antimicrob. Agents Chemother. **9**:65–69.
4. **Goldstein, A., L. Aronow, and S. Kalman.** 1968. Drug elimination: the major routes, p. 194–197. *In* Principles of Drug Action. Harper and Row, New York.
5. **Kunin, C. M.** 1961. Serum binding, distribution and excretion of four penicillin analogues following intravenous injection in man. Proc. Soc. Exp. Biol. Med. **107**:337–341.
6. **Lilly Research Laboratories.** 1974. Cefamandole nafate. Clinical investigation manual. Lilly Research Laboratories, Indianapolis, Ind.
7. **Miyers, B. R., B. Ribner, S. Yancovitz, and S. Z. Hirschman.** 1976. Pharmacological studies with cefamandole in human volunteers. Antimicrob. Agents Chemother. **9**:140–144.
8. **Neu, H. C.** 1974. Cefamandole, a cephalosporin antibiotic with an unusually wide spectrum of activity. Antimicrob. Agents Chemother. **6**:177–182.
9. **Sapirstein, L. A., M. R. Herrold, M. Janakis, and E. Ogden.** 1952. Validity of values for glomerular filtration rate and extracellular fluid obtained from plasma concentration time decay curves after single injections of mannitol in the dog. Am. J. Physiol. **171**:487–491.
10. **Wagoner, R. D., W. N. Tauxe, F. T. Maher, and J. C. Hunt.** 1964. Measurement of effective renal plasma flow with sodium iodohippurate-^{131}I. J. Am. Med. Assoc. **187**:811–813.
11. **Wick, W. E., and D. A. Preston.** 1972. Biological properties of three 3-heterocylic-thiomethyl cephalosporin antibiotics. Antimicrob. Agents Chemother. **1**:221–234.

Antimicrobial Agents and Chemotherapy, Feb. 1977, p. 267-270
Vol. 11, No. 2

Simple, Direct Broth-Disk Method for Antibiotic Susceptibility Testing of *Ureaplasma urealyticum*

MONIEK S. SPAEPEN and RUTH B. KUNDSIN*
Department of Surgery, Peter Bent Brigham Hospital, Boston, Massachusetts 02115

Received for publication 20 August 1976

A simple, direct broth-disk test, utilizing urine sediment as the inoculum and impregnated paper disks as the source of antibiotic, was developed and used to test the susceptibility of 54 isolates of *Ureaplasma urealyticum* (T-strain mycoplasmas) to minocycline, doxycycline, demeclocycline, tetracycline, and erythromycin. The concentration of each antibiotic was calculated to approximate the attainable blood level. Resistance or susceptibility to each antibiotic was determined by growth, indicated by a color change of the medium in each tube, comparable to that of a control culture without antibiotic. Of the 54 T-mycoplasmas tested, 46 (85.2%) were inhibited by 1 μg of minocycline per ml, 45 (83.3%) were inhibited by 1 μg of doxycycline per ml, 38 (72.2%) were inhibited by 1 μg of demeclocycline per ml, 18 (33.3%) were inhibited by 1 μg of tetracycline per ml, and only 2 (3.7%) were inhibited by 3 μg of erythromycin per ml. Seven (13%) of the 54 T-mycoplasmas tested were resistant to all five antibiotics. There was good correlation between results obtained by this direct broth-disk method and minimal inhibitory concentrations obtained by the direct broth dilution method.

With the recent reports of tetracycline-resistant T-mycoplasmas (6, 7, 11), tetracycline can no longer be recommended as the antibiotic of choice for T-mycoplasma infections, unless the specific infecting organisms have been determined to be susceptible in vitro. It has been shown that minocycline and doxycycline are considerably more active than the parent compound against T-mycoplasmas, but resistance to all tetracyclines and erythromycin has been documented. The increasing awareness by physicians of the existence of resistant T-mycoplasmas has resulted in many requests for susceptibility tests.

The indirect broth dilution method described by Braun et al. (3), in which the T-mycoplasmas must be isolated and subcultured, and the direct broth dilution method proposed by Spaepen et al. (11) are both lengthy and time-consuming procedures and, therefore, are not practical for routine susceptibility testing of T-mycoplasmas.

In 1973, Wilkins and Thiel (12) published a simple method for determining the susceptibility of anaerobic bacteria to antibiotics, based on the original idea of Schneierson (10). A concentration of antibiotic approximately equal to that attainable in blood is put into a tube of broth medium. Commercial filter paper disks are the carrier for the antibiotic. Growth of the microorganism at that concentration is considered to constitute resistance.

The present study describes a simple system for testing the antibiotic susceptibility of T-mycoplasmas based on the combination of the Wilkins-Thiel method and the Spaepen direct broth dilution method. The results of the direct broth-disk method are compared with the results of the minimal inhibitory concentration (MIC) determinations obtained by the direct broth dilution technique.

MATERIALS AND METHODS

Fifty-four urine sediments from 54 patients found positive for T-mycoplasmas, in the Surgical Bacteriology Laboratory, Peter Bent Brigham Hospital, Boston, Mass., were used in this study. The patients had a history of reproductive failure. Their specimens (urine and vaginal/cervical or urethral) were sent to the laboratory by private gynecologists and infertility clinics. The study was conducted over a 6-month period (January 1976 to July 1976). The T-mycoplasmas were identified by the simultaneous use of liquid and solid media as described by Kundsin (8). Only urine sediments from which T-mycoplasmas were visualized on agar medium were included in this study.

Susceptibility testing methods. The T-mycoplasmas were tested for susceptibility to minocycline, doxycycline, demeclocycline, tetracycline, and erythromycin. The first three antibiotics were used in both methods, whereas tetracycline and erythromycin were only tested with the broth-disk method. The two methods used were as follows.

(i) **Direct broth dilution method.** The initial and final MICs of the 54 isolates were determined by the direct broth dilution technique (11). The initial MIC was the lowest concentration of antibiotic inhibiting color change at the time the control tube containing the same strain showed a color change. The lowest concentration of antibiotic that completely inhibited color change after 6 days was defined as the final MIC.

(ii) **Direct broth-disk method.** The direct broth-disk method was based on the use of a combination of the Wilkins-Thiel modified broth-disk method for anaerobic bacteria (12) and the direct broth dilution technique for T-mycoplasmas proposed by Spaepen et al. (11).

Sterile, clear plastic screw-cap tubes (Falcon Plastics, Oxnard, Calif.) were filled with 5 ml of Ford medium (5). The appropriate number of standard antibiotic disks was added to each tube with flamed forceps. Per tube of medium, an inoculum of 0.05 ml of urine sediment positive for T-mycoplasmas was added immediately after the addition of the antibiotic disks. A control tube, containing no antibiotic disk, was also inoculated. Tubes were incubated at 36°C for 6 days. They were observed daily for color change of the media and graded from 0 to 4+. Isolates were recorded as "susceptible" when there was no color change (equal to the color of plain Ford medium, 0), as "resistant" when there was complete color change from yellow to deep pink (equal to the color of the control, 4+), and as "exhibiting partial resistance" when the color change was not fully expressed at 6 days (1+ to 3+).

Opinions of various investigators differ as to the concentration of each antibiotic to which an organism must be resistant in order to be termed "clinically resistant." Listed in Table 3 are the test concentrations we chose for the direct broth-disk method. They are based on our findings obtained by correlating the post-treatment urine culture results and the final MIC of the antibiotic used for treatment. A final MIC of ≤ 1 μg of the tetracyclines per ml resulted in a negative post-treatment urine culture (11). Since we had no such data for erythromycin, the most commonly used concentration was chosen.

The minocycline disks were prepared in the laboratory; the four others were purchased from BBL (BBL, Division of BioQuest, Cockeysville, Md.). The minocycline disks were prepared by impregnating sterile blank concentration disks (Difco Laboratories, Detroit, Mich.) with 0.025 ml of a 200-μg/ml minocycline solution. The disks were allowd to dry for 2 h at 36°C, followed by drying for 3 days at 4°C in a desiccator. Dried disks were stored at 4°C in sterile glass vials resembling typical commercial desiccated disk vials.

Comparison of the two methods. The direct broth-disk and the direct broth dilution methods were considered to be in agreement if the final MIC was equal to or less than the concentration in the broth-disk procedure giving a susceptible result, or if the final MIC was greater than the concentration in the broth-disk method giving a resistant result.

Titration of the urine specimens. The titer of each urine sediment was determined by 10-fold serial dilutions up to 10^{-7} in Ford medium and expressed as color-changing units as described previously (11).

RESULTS

The distribution of the titers of the 54 specimens tested and the distribution of the seven resistant strains according to their titer are presented in Table 1. Most urine specimens had a titer of 10^3 color-changing units or greater. The titer of the T-mycoplasmas did not influence resistance or susceptibility. Resistant and susceptible strains were equally distributed throughout.

The T-mycoplasmas were not isolated from their original environment (urine) prior to testing. Table 2 shows the relative occurrence of other microorganisms present in the 54 urine specimens used in this study. Thirty-eight (70%) of the urine specimens contained only T-mycoplasmas.

Table 3 summarizes the susceptibility results of the 54 T-mycoplasmas obtained by the direct broth-disk method. Minocycline was the most active antibiotic in vitro, inhibiting 46 (85.2%) strains in a concentration of 1 μg/ml, followed respectively by doxycycline inhibiting 45 (83.3%) strains in a concentration of 1 μg/ml, demeclocycline inhibiting 38 (72.2%) in a concentration of 1 μg/ml, and tetracycline inhibiting 18 (33.3%) in a concentration of 1 μg/ml.

TABLE 1. *Total number of T-mycoplasma strains and number of resistant strains distributed according to urine titer*

Titer (CCU)[a]	No. of strains[b]	No. resistant
10^2	4 (7.4)	1 (25.0)
10^3	9 (16.7)	2 (22.2)
10^4	19 (35.1)	0 (0)
10^5	13 (24.0)	2 (15.4)
10^6	6 (11.1)	2 (33.3)
$\geq 10^7$	3 (5.5)	0 (0)

[a] CCU, Color-changing units.
[b] Numbers in parentheses are percentages.

TABLE 2. *Occurrence of microorganisms in the 54 urine cultures*

Organism[a]	No. of urine cultures[b]
T-mycoplasmas	38 (70.3)
T-mycoplasmas and *Mycoplasma hominis*	6 (11.1)
T-mycoplasmas and yeast	5 (9.2)
T-mycoplasmas and *Proteus mirabilis*	2 (3.7)
T-mycoplasmas, *M. hominis,* and *Escherichia coli*	2 (3.7)
T-mycoplasmas, *M. hominis,* and yeast	1 (1.8)

[a] Presence of a few gram-positive cocci and/or lactobacilli possible.
[b] Numbers in parentheses are percentages.

TABLE 3. *Broth-disk susceptibility results of 54 T-mycoplasmas in urine*

Antibiotic disk (μg)	Test concn (μg/ml)	No. susceptible	No. intermediate	No. resistant
Minocycline, 5	1	46	0	8
Doxycycline, 5	1	45	2	7
Demeclocycline, 5	1	38	4	12
Tetracycline, 5	1	18	10	26
Erythromycin, 15	3	2	3	39

Erythromycin was considerably less active than the tetracyclines. Only two (3.7%) strains were inhibited by 3 μg/ml. Seven (13%) of the 54 patients had T-mycoplasmas in urine that were resistant to the indicated test concentration of all five antibiotics.

The median values for the initial MIC and final MIC of minocycline, doxycycline, and demeclocycline obtained by the direct broth dilution test are presented in Table 4. Minocycline was the most active antibiotic, with the lowest median values for both the initial MIC and the final MIC.

The results of the direct broth-disk method were in good agreement with the final MICs of minocycline, doxycycline, and demeclocycline. When the final MIC was equal to or less than 1 μg of antibiotic per ml, a color change was never observed with the broth-disk method. When the final MIC was equal to or greater than 4 μg of antibiotic per ml, a color change always occurred with the broth-disk method. When the final MIC was equal to 2 μg/ml, occasionally no color change was observed with the broth-disk method.

DISCUSSION

The main objective of this study was to develop a simple method for antibiotic susceptibility testing of T-mycoplasmas which could be used with ease and yet would give reliable results. Our previous (11) and current experiences with the direct broth dilution method indicated that it is a reliable method for determining the antibiotic susceptibility of T-mycoplasmas. Certain procedures and materials make it relatively simple and convenient, and therefore have been incorporated into the direct broth-disk method. Both methods use the same type of inoculum and medium, and the reading of the results is based on the same color change. The main difference between the two tests is the form in which the antibiotic is added. In the broth-disk method only one concentration is used; therefore, it does not distinguish between the degrees of resistance or susceptibility. The broth dilution method, however, is less feasible for performing large numbers of susceptibility tests. The direct broth-disk method has the following advantages: (i) it is a simple method, easy and quick to perform; (ii) the antibiotic disks are readily available; and (iii) it requires no extra technician to perform a test and is less expensive in time and media.

The results of this study indicate that minocycline is the most active antibiotic in vitro, and are in excellent agreement with our previously published data (11). The median MICs of minocycline and doxycycline were the same. The median initial MIC of demeclocycline was higher, but the median final MIC was the same.

The occasional disagreement between the two methods is most likely due to the inherent error of plus or minus one dilution in the broth dilution method. Many more manipulations are involved with the broth dilution method, and each dilution introduces an opportunity for error. If this factor is taken into account, the disk method may be more precise. One possible source of error in the broth-disk method is the possible deviation from the stated content of antibiotic in the disks. Although it is not possible to check the very disk used in the test, quality control of the method is feasible by checking disks from each cartridge for appropriate zone sizes by the method of Bauer et al. (1), using the American Type Culture Collection control strains of *Escherichia coli* and *Staphylococcus aureus* (2, 9). Since the Food and Drug Administration has enforced standards on antibiotic disk production in the United States (4), the concentration of commercial disks is probably close to the labeled value. Furthermore, no difference was found during the course of this investigation between results from different disk batches or between the commercial disks and the ones prepared in the laboratory.

The direct broth-disk method appears to be an acceptable and simple technique for determining the antibiotic susceptibility of T-mycoplasmas in a clinical laboratory with the facilities for culturing these organisms. The source of antibiotics in readily available disks allows one to perform a one-concentration broth dilu-

TABLE 4. *Broth dilution susceptibility results of 54 T-mycoplasmas in urine*

Antibiotic	No. of strains tested	Median (μg/ml)	
		Initial MIC	Final MIC
Minocycline	54	0.03	0.5
Doxycycline	54	0.06	1.0
Demeclocycline	54	0.125	1.0

tion test without the need to prepare and maintain antibiotic solutions. Furthermore, with this method it becomes feasible to rapidly screen the resistant T-mycoplasmas with antibiotics other than those commonly prescribed for this infection.

LITERATURE CITED

1. **Bauer, A. W., W. M. M. Kirby, J. C. Sherris, and M. Turek.** 1966. Antibiotic susceptibility testing by a single disc method. Am. J. Clin. Pathol. **45**:493–496.
2. **Blazevic, D. J., M. H. Koepecke, and J. M. Matsen.** 1972. Quality control testing with disk antibiotic susceptibility test of Bauer-Kirby-Sherris-Turek. Am. J. Clin. Pathol. **57**:592–597.
3. **Braun, P., J. O. Klein, and E. H. Kass.** 1970. Susceptibility of genital mycoplasmas to antimicrobial agents. Appl. Microbiol. **19**:62–70.
4. **Food and Drug Administration.** 1972. Code of federal regulations, vol. 21, part 460.6. Food and Drug Administration, Washington, D. C.
5. **Ford, D. K., and J. MacDonald.** 1967. Influence of urea on the growth of T-strain mycoplasmas. J. Bacteriol. **93**:1509–1512.
6. **Ford, D. K., and J. R. Smith.** 1974. Non-specific urethritis associated with a tetracycline-resistant T-mycoplasma. Br. J. Vener. Dis. **50**:373–374.
7. **Hofstetter, A., H. Blenk, and R. Rangoonwala.** 1976. Tetrazykline zur Behandlung der Mycoplasmen-Prostato-Urethritis. Muench. Med. Wochenschr. **118**:49–50.
8. **Kundsin, R. B.** 1976. Mycoplasmas in humans. Significance of *Ureaplasma urealyticum*. Health Lab. Sci. **13**:144–151.
9. **Matsen, J. M., and A. L. Barry.** 1974. Susceptibility testing: diffusion test procedures, p. 418–427. *In* E. H. Lennette, E. H. Spaulding, and J. P. Truant (ed.), Manual of clinical microbiology, 2nd ed. American Society for Microbiology, Washington, D.C.
10 **Schneierson, S. S.** 1954. A simple rapid disc-tube method for determination of bacterial sensitivity to antibiotics. Antibiot. Chemother. **4**:125–132.
11. **Spaepen, M. S., R. B. Kundsin, and H. W. Horne.** 1976. Tetracycline-resistant T-mycoplasmas (*Ureaplasma urealyticum*) from patients with a history of reproductive failure. Antimicrob. Agents Chemother. **9**:1012–1018.
12. **Wilkins, T. D., and T. Thiel.** 1973. Modified broth-disk method for testing the antibiotic susceptibility of anaerobic bacteria. Antimicrob. Agents Chemother. **3**:350–356.

ANTIMICROBIAL AGENTS AND CHEMOTHERAPY, Feb. 1977, p. 271-276 Vol. 11, No. 2

Evaluation of the Performance Parameters of a Prediluted, Quantitative Antibiotic Susceptibility Test Device

RICHARD C. TILTON* AND HENRY D. ISENBERG

University of Connecticut School of Medicine, Farmington, Connecticut 06032, and Long Island Jewish-Hillside Medical Center, New Hyde Park, New York 11040*

Received for publication 13 July 1976

A multiwelled plastic strip containing prediluted antibiotics was tested. Antibiotics available at the time of testing included ampicillin, penicillin, methicillin, erythromycin, clindamycin, tetracycline, and minocycline. The effects of inoculum size, inoculum volume, temperature, and time of incubation were determined. A limited clinical evaluation using laboratory strains of selected bacteria proved this product to be a rapid, economical, and reliable method for the determination of the minimal inhibitory concentration of antibiotics.

There is a continuing need for quantitative antibiotic susceptibility methods that do not require the purchase of expensive equipment or hours of a technologist's time for processing.

The antibiotic susceptibility test (AST; Lederle Laboratories, Pearl River, N.Y.) device is a multiwelled plastic strip containing prediluted concentrations of an antibiotic. Inoculation and incubation of these strips results in the determination of the minimum inhibitory concentration (MIC) of the antibiotic to be tested. The MIC of antibiotics may be determined by a number of methods, including agar dilution (2), broth dilution (6), and microdilution (7, 8). No universally recognized reference methods exist for these procedures, although investigators have examined variables and proposed procedures. The present joint study evaluates the performance parameters of the AST strip.

MATERIALS AND METHODS

Antibiotics. The AST is an injection-molded polystyrene multiwelled chamber (Fig. 1). The 10 individual wells hold a maximum fluid volume of 400 μl and are covered by a removable snap-type flexible plastic cover. Each strip contains serial decreasing amounts of an antibiotic in a dried state. Well no. 1 contains 12.5 μg of antibiotic, well no. 2 contains 6.25 μg, etc. Well no. 10 contains no antibiotic. Antibiotics available at the time of testing included ampicillin, penicillin, methicillin, erythromycin, clindamycin, tetracycline, and minocycline. (Information from Lederle Laboratories indicated that these antibiotics were stable at room temperature for a minimum of 6 months.) The strips were stored at room temperature in their packages prior to use. Antibiotics used in the microdilution and agar dilution procedures were obtained as USP reference powders and stored at -20°C until used.

Control organisms. The following reference strains for the stated antibiotics were employed in the evaluation of test conditions for the AST: *Staphylococcus aureus* ATCC 25923, *Escherichia coli* ATCC 25922, *Sarcina lutea* ATCC 9341, *E. coli* WHO-5 (ampicillin, clindamycin); *S. aureus* WHO-4 (penicillin); *S. aureus* 2834 (methicillin); *S. aureus* WHO-6 (erythromycin) and *E. coli* WHO-16 (tetracycline, minocycline).

The limited clinical phase of the study evaluated bacterial strains routinely isolated from the clinical microbiology laboratories of the University of Connecticut Health Center and the Long Island Jewish-Hillside Medical Center. All cultures were either tested immediately after isolation or maintained on Trypticase soy agar slants. *S. aureus* 25923 and *E. coli* 25922 served as the quality control organisms included with each series of tests performed.

AST procedure. An AST strip was removed from its package, unwrapped, and placed on a level table. The cover was removed, and 200 μl of inoculated growth medium was added by pipette to each of the nine antibiotic-containing wells. These wells contained an absolute amount of antibiotic. The volume of the inoculum, therefore, affected the actual MIC value. Thus, the use of 0.2 ml as inoculum approached the usual $\log_2$ dilution of the antibiotics most closely. Two hundred microliters of inoculum was added to well no. 10, the growth control. The cover was replaced, and the strip was incubated at 35°C for the stated time.

Disk diffusion susceptibility test. The standardized disk test was performed in exact accordance with the method of Bauer et al. (1). All diffusion tests were accompanied by plates inoculated with *E. coli* ATCC 25922 and *S. aureus* ATCC 25923.

Agar dilution susceptibility test. The procedure was performed according to the recommendations of Ericsson and Sherris (2).

Microdilution antibiotic susceptibility test. The method of Tilton et al. (8) was followed.

Determination of optimal inoculum concentration for the AST test. Inocula of reference cultures in Mueller-Hinton (M-H) broth for each of the antibiotics to be tested were adjusted by nephelometry (Tilton et al. [8]) to 10^4, 10^5, 10^6, and 10^7 colony-

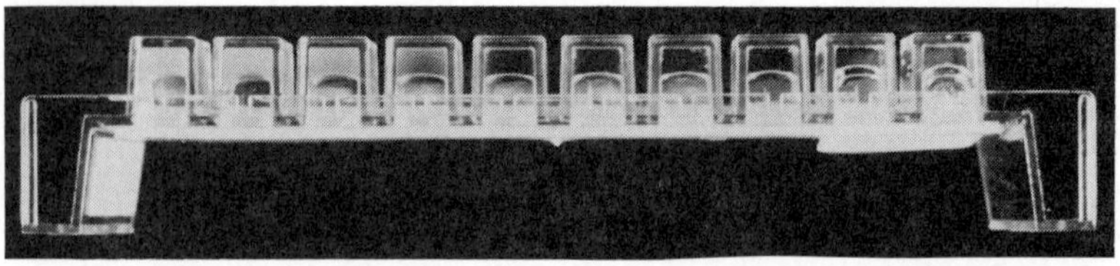

FIG. 1. *The AST, an injection-molded polystyrene device for determining the MIC of antibiotics.*

forming units (CFU) per ml. The AST strips were inoculated in quadruplicate, and incubated for 18 h at 35°C, and the MICs were determined as a function of each inoculum concentration.

Effects of growth on the AST test. Quadruplicate AST strips were inoculated with the reference strains at a concentration of 10^5 CFU per ml in four nutrient media: Trypticase soy broth (Difco), Eugon broth (Difco), M-H broth (BBL), and brain heart infusion broth (Difco). The strips were incubated at 35°C for 18 h and read.

Effects of inoculum volume on the AST test. AST strips were inoculated in quadruplicate with 200, 300, and 400 μl of a 10^5 bacterial inoculum. The strips were incubated for 18 h and the MICs were determined.

Time of incubation. AST strips were inoculated with 200 μl of a 10^5-CFU/ml inoculum and incubated at 35°C. Strips were removed at 2, 4, 6, 8, 18, 24, 40, and 48 h. The MICs on two strips were determined visually, and the MICs of the other two strips were read by the addition of 50 μl of iodonitrotetrazolium to each well. If growth was apparent, the tetrazolium was reduced to a red, insoluble formazan compound.

Limited clinical evaluation. Representative isolates from the clinical laboratories as well as control strains of *E. coli* 25922, *S. aureus* 25923, and *S. lutea* were tested by AST, disk diffusion, agar dilution, and microdilution.

The AST protocol was as follows: inoculum concentration, 10^5 CFU/ml; inoculum size, 200 μl per well; growth medium, M-H broth; incubation temperature, 35°C; incubation time, 6 h; reading of end point, visually in reflected light.

Limited clinical evaluation of fastidious organisms. Selected isolates of *Haemophilus influenzae, Neisseria gonorrhoeae, Neisseria meningitidis, Fusobacterium* sp., and *Bacteroides fragilis* were tested with ampicillin, clindamycin, tetracycline, and penicillin. The M-H medium for growth of the *Haemophilus* and *Neisseria* isolates was supplemented with either supplement C (Difco), yeast extract (1%) and hemoglobin (1%), or 10% Fildes reagent (Difco). The anaerobic gram-negative rods were incubated in a GasPak (BBL) for 24 h prior to reading. All inocula were standardized to 10^5 CFU per ml. The reference method employed was macrotube broth dilution (6) using identical media and environmental conditions.

RESULTS

The first phase of evaluation of the AST focused on the establishment of test conditions. The volume of inoculum added to the wells did not alter the MIC when the concentration of antibiotic per milliliter was adjusted for dilution. In most cases, the MICs were similar regardless of volume and no greater than a 1-dilution interval (d.i.) difference was observed. It was noted, however, that addition of 400 μl of inoculum to a well caused overflow and resultant contamination of the plate. An inoculum of 200 μl was employed for subsequent tests.

Three brands of manual pipettors with disposable tips were used to add a 200-μl inoculum to the wells: Oxford, Clay-Adams, and Pierce (Pierce Chemical Co.). Thirty repetitive tests on each pipette with a methicillin AST strip and *S. aureus* 2834 indicated no change in MIC as a function of pipette type. The Clay-Adams pipettor was used for the remainder of the study because of rapid uptake and release of the inoculum and ease of operation.

Figure 2 shows the effect of inoculum concentration on the AST MICs. Penicillin demonstrated a significant inoculum effect due to the production of penicillinase by *S. aureus*. Inoculum concentrations of 10^6 CFU or greater per ml increased the apparent resistance of the test organism to penicillin. A similar effect was observed when *E. coli* was tested with clindamycin. The lack of inoculum effect with ampicillin, and the presence of one with clindamycin, is unexplained. Inocula of 10^6 to 10^7 CFU per ml caused sufficient turbidity in the medium so as to make visual reading of the MIC difficult. Lesser inocula resulted in extended periods of inoculation.

Figure 3 shows the effect of the growth medium on AST MICs. No marked differences in MIC were seen as a function of nutrient medium except that microorganisms appeared to be more susceptible to some antibiotics when growing in M-H broth. M-H broth was chosen for the remainder of the study for the sake of uniformity with other susceptibility test methods.

Experiments indicated that the AST could be used as a 1-day test of quantitative antimicrobial susceptibility. MICs of all antibiotics for the control cultures, *S. aureus* and *E. coli,* could be determined after incubation for 6 h. Differences of greater than 1 d.i. were not observed when the strips were read at intervals of 6 to 48 h. Occasionally, extended incubation (12 to 18 h) was necessary when testing enterococci and some pseudomonads. It is critical that the strips be read in reflected light through the transparent side of the wells. This procedure allows the reader to shake the bacterial suspension in the well and observe growth. When the

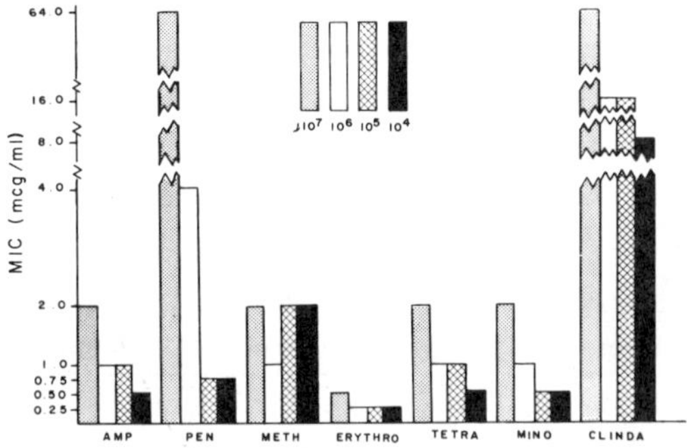

FIG. 2. *Effect of inoculum concentration on AST MICs. Control organisms: E. coli WHO-5 (ampicillin, clindamycin); S. aureus WHO-4 (penicillin); S. aureus 2834 (methicillin); S. aureus WHO-6 (erythromycin); E. coli WHO-16 (tetracycline, minocycline).*

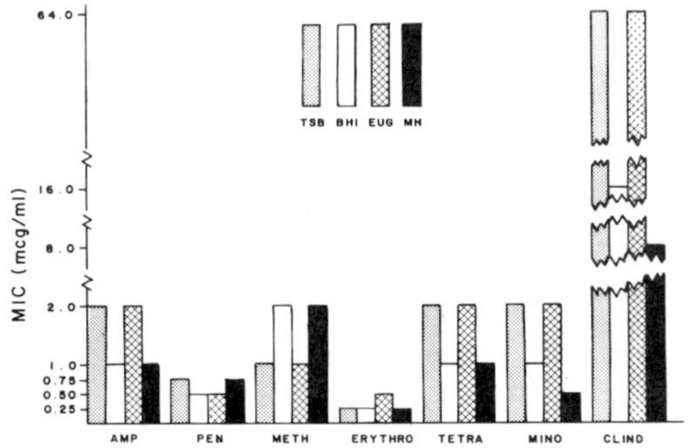

FIG. 3. *Effect of growth medium on AST MICs. Control organisms: E. coli WHO-5 (ampicillin, clindamycin); S. aureus WHO-4 (penicillin); S. aureus 2834 (methicillin); S. aureus WHO-6 (erythromycin); E. coli WHO-16 (tetracycline, minocycline).*

test was read by looking down through the top of the well, turbidity changes could not be observed in 6 h. One of the authors (R.C.T.) added tetrazolium to the wells at 6 h to facilitate the reading of the MIC end point. Results after tetrazolium addition were identical to those in which turbidity alone was assessed. The time necessary to generate a reliable MIC was not shortened by a 2-h preincubation of the inoculum.

Table 1 shows 10 replicate MIC determinations for each of the antibiotics listed. In no case was there a replicate MIC greater than 1 d.i. from the mean of the 10 determinations. MICs, expressed as well numbers, of erythromycin, tetracycline, and minocycline were identical for the 10 replicates.

Table 2 summarizes comparative data between agar dilution, microdilution, broth dilution, disk diffusion, and the AST method using reference strains and the parameters determined to be optimal. In most instances, there was excellent agreement with the macrotube dilution result. In no instance was there interpretative disagreement between the disk diffusion test and any one or more of the dilution tests.

Table 3 is a compilation of data on the limited clinical evaluation of the AST. Gram-negative rods, exclusive of *H. influenzae*, *Fusobacterium* sp., and *B. fragilis*, were tested with ampicillin, tetracycline, and minocycline. Gram-positive bacteria were tested with ampicillin, clindamycin, erythromycin, methicillin, and penicillin. In some instances, isolates were tested by six methods: agar dilution, microdilution, broth dilution, disk diffusion, Autobac, and AST. Other isolates were tested only by AST and broth dilution. The presentation in Table 3 assumes that there is no significant discrepancy in results when there was a 1 d.i. or less difference in MIC as a function of method. Of five strains of *Streptococcus pneumoniae* tested, one isolate showed >1 d.i. difference when tested with penicillin. With either TD or AST, however, the isolate would

TABLE 1. *Variation in replicate AST MICs*

Antibiotic	Control organism[a]	Mean MIC	Range[b]	Standard deviation
Ampicillin	*E. coli* WHO-5	0.85	0.5 (3)–1.0 (7)	0.23
Penicillin	*S. aureus* WHO-4	0.48	0.25 (1)–0.5 (9)	0.07
Methicillin	*S. aureus* 2834	1.70	1.0 (3)–2.0 (7)	0.45
Erythromycin	*S. aureus* WHO-6	0.25	0.25 (10)	0.00
Tetracycline	*E. coli* WHO-16	1.0	1.0 (10)	0.00
Minocycline	*E. coli* WHO-16	1.0	1.0 (10)	0.00
Clindamycin	*E. coli* WHO-5	17.6	16.0 (9)–32 (1)	4.2

[a] Inoculum, 10^5 CFU per ml. Incubation was for 6 h at 35°C.
[b] Parentheses indicate number of replicates with the designated MIC end point.

TABLE 2. *Comparison of AST, broth dilution, agar dilution, microdilution, and agar diffusion methods for antimicrobial susceptibility*

Quality control strain	MIC (μg/ml)[a]					
	Amp	Pen	Meth	Eryth	Clind	Tetra
S. aureus 25923						
AST	<0.25	<0.25	1.0	<0.25	<0.25	0.50
Broth dilution	<0.25	<0.25	1.0	0.5	0.50	0.25
Agar dilution	<0.25	<0.25	0.50	<0.25	<0.25	<0.25
Microdilution	<0.25	<0.25	0.50	<0.25	<0.25	<0.25
Disk diffusion	40 mm	42 mm	36 mm	25 mm	22 mm	29 mm
E. coli 25922						
AST	8	>64	>64	>64	>64	4
Broth dilution	4	>64	>64	>64	>64	4
Agar dilution	4	32	>64	>64	>64	2
Microdilution	4	32	>64	>64	>64	2
Disk diffusion	16 mm	6 mm	6 mm	16 mm	6 mm	20 mm

[a] Amp, Ampicillin; pen, penicillin; meth, methicillin; eryth, erythromycin; clind, clindamycin; tetra, tetracycline.

TABLE 3. *Summary of isolates tested and discrepancies in AST results observed in a limited clinical trial*

Organism	No. of isolates	Method[a]	Discrepancies[b]
Staphylococcus aureus	15	AD, MD, TD, AST, DD, AB	2 (Amp, MD); 2 (Meth, MD); 1 (Meth, AD); 1 (Pen, AD)
Klebsiella pneumoniae	15	Same	1 (Tetra, DD)
Escherichia coli	15	Same	None
Pseudomonas aeruginosa	8	Same	7 (Tetra, AD); 7 (Mino, AD)
Pseudomonas sp.	6	Same	None
Streptococcus faecalis	15	Same	1 (Erythro, AD); 2 (Tetra, AD and MD); 2 (Meth, MD); 7 (Pen, all methods)
Staphylococcus epidermidis	5	AST, TD	None
S. pneumoniae	5	Same	1 (Pen, TD)
S. pyogenes (A)	5	Same	None
S. mitior	5	Same	None
S. agalactae (B)	5	Same	None
Listeria monocytogenes	5	Same	None
Providencia stuartii	5	Same	None
Proteus mirabilis	5	Same	2 (Amp, TD)
Serratia marcescens	5	Same	None
S. liquefaciens	5	Same	None
Enterobacter agglomerans	5	Same	None
E. aerogenes	5	Same	None
Enterobacter hafniae	5	Same	None
Shigella sp.	5	Same	None
Salmonella sp.	5	Same	None
Enterobacter cloacae	5	Same	None

[a] AD, Agar dilution; MD, microdilution; TD, tube dilution; AB, Autobac; AST, Lederle; other abbreviations as in Footnote *a*, Table 2.
[b] Instances in which AST MIC was >1 d.i. from indicated MIC.

have been interpreted as susceptible to penicillin.

S. aureus showed two discrepancies each for ampicillin and penicillin when AST was compared with microdilution and one each for methicillin and penicillin when compared with agar dilution.

Problems of agreement were observed with the enterococci (*Streptococcus faecalis*). Of the discrepancies noted in Table 3, the most numerous were seen with penicillin when AST was compared with microdilution (seven discrepancies) and agar dilution (six discrepancies). Similarly, seven discrepancies were seen when *P. aeruginosa* was tested with tetracycline and minocycline.

Table 4 presents preliminary data that test the versatility of the AST strip. Fastidious organisms such as *H. influenzae*, pathogenic *Neisseria*, and gram-negative anaerobic rods were tested with the modifications of media and incubation conditions as indicated. In all cases, the AST results were within 1 d.i. of the broth dilution results.

DISCUSSION

The continuing use of toxic antimicrobial agents, the appearance of bizarre opportunistic protista, and the increasingly sophisticated therapeutic modalities in infectious disease have dictated the need for a rapid, economical, and accurate MIC. The product known as the AST appears to fulfill these specifications. The AST, a multiwelled tray containing diluted antibiotics, is not a new concept in antimicrobial susceptibility testing. Rather, it is a hybridization of the cumbersome broth dilution test and the microdilution MIC test. The uniqueness of the system is that the significant labor-draining steps of an MIC determination have been circumvented; that is, the preparation of an antibiotic solution and its subsequent dilution in tubes, wells, or agar plates. To determine an MIC, the technologist only standardizes the bacterial inoculum in fresh broth and adds it to the multiwelled chamber before incubation.

The joint study to evaluate this device initially focused on the biological parameters associated with the performance of the test. Once defined, these parameters were incorporated as a routine procedure to test the AST with a limited number of microorganisms commonly encountered in the clinical laboratory.

The test conditions, although predictable from previous investigations (3–5, 7, 8), revealed that the AST was susceptible to inoculum effect as well as the vagaries of the growth medium. It was observed that accurate MICs could be read visually as early as 5 to 6 h after inoculation. This may be a function of the ability to pick up the strip, shake it, and observe turbidity through the side of the chambers. Examining the wells directly through the top with transmitted light did not permit visualization of the turbid end points, as is the case with the microdilution MIC procedure after overnight incubation.

The limited clinical trial of the AST suggested that there was satisfactory interpretive agreement between the AST and other accepted susceptibility test methods. (However, when variation occurred, the AST MIC was usually of a higher value, that is, more resistant than the other methods.) When numerous major discrepancies were observed, such as with penicillin and *S. faecalis*, it was assumed that there were errors in the manufacture of the product. In some cases, the pellet of dried antibiotic adhered to the cover, and a portion of it was lost when the cover was removed. A more extensive clinical trial will quantitate the methodological agreement.

The versatility of the AST for fastidious microorganisms was assessed. *H. influenzae* MICs could be read in 18 h if the nutrient medium was supplemented with supplement C (Difco), yeast extract, or 10% Fildes reagent. The MICs generated showed no significant variation when compared with broth dilution techniques.

The pathogenic *Neisseria* species could be tested similarly. The MICs of some fast-growing isolates of *N. meningitidis* could be read in 6 h. *N. gonorrhoeae* required 18 h of incubation for the assessment of results.

Two genera of anaerobic gram-negative rods were tested. Preliminary data on seven strains

TABLE 4. *Summary of limited clinical testing of the AST method with fastidious bacteria*

Organism	No. of isolates	Method[a]	Environmental/nutritional supplementation	Discrepancies
Haemophilus influenzae	10	BD, AST	Capneic incubation, yeast extract (1%), and hemoglobin (1%) added to M-H broth	None
Neisseria gonorrhoeae	5	BD, AST	Same	None
N. meningitidis	5	BD, AST	Same	None
Fusobacterium sp.	3	BD, AST	Anaerobic incubation (GasPak), thioglycolate broth (hemin-menadione supplement)	None
Bacteroides fragilis	4	BD, AST	Same	None

[a] BD, Broth dilution.

tested against tetracycline, ampicillin, penicillin, and clindamycin indicated that if a thioglycolate broth inoculum was added to the strip and the cover was left loose, then MIC results determined after anaerobic incubation in a GasPak jar consistently agreed with the tube dilution results.

Several features of the AST make it a desirable addition to the clinical microbiology laboratory. They are as follows.

(i) Rapidity of processing and reading. An AST MIC can be set up in less than 5 min. A 6-h reading is possible with the fast-growing organisms.

(ii) Accuracy and reproducibility. The AST showed excellent interpretative agreement with the commonly used dilution tests. Repetitive MICs on replicate AST strips indicated that the test results were reproducible.

(iii) Widespread applicability. The AST test provides the capability for any laboratory, regardless of size or sophistication, to perform MICs. No storage of antibiotic reference powder, no critical weighing of antibiotics, and no serial dilution procedures are necessary.

(iv) Versatility. Preliminary experiments show that with minor modifications of nutrient and/or incubation environment, MICs may be performed on fastidious microorganisms such as the anaerobic bacteria, *Haemophilus*, and *Neisseria*.

LITERATURE CITED

1. **Bauer, A. W., W. M. M. Kirby, J. C. Sherris, and M. Turck.** 1966. Antibiotic susceptibility testing by a standardized single disc method. Am. J. Clin. Pathol. **45:**493–496.
2. **Ericsson, H. M., and J. C. Sherris.** 1971. Antibiotic sensitivity testing: report of an international collaborative study. Acta Pathol. Microbiol. Scand. Sect. B. **217:**(Suppl.):1–90.
3. **Gavan, T. L., and D. Butler.** 1974. Automated microdilution method for antimicrobial susceptibility testing, p. 88–93. *In* Current techniques for antibiotic susceptibility testing. Charles C Thomas Publisher, Springfield, Ill.
4. **Gavan, T. L., and M. A. Town.** 1970. A microdilution method for antibiotic susceptibility testing. Am. J. Clin. Pathol. **53:**880–885.
5. **Gerlach, E. H.** 1974. Microdilution. I. A comparative study, p. 63–76. *In* Current techniques for antibiotic susceptibility testing. Charles C Thomas Publisher, Springfield, Ill.
6. **Lennette, E. H., E. H. Spaulding, and J. R. Truant.** 1974. Manual of clinical microbiology, 2nd ed. American Society for Microbiology, Washington, D.C.
7. **MacLowry, J. D., and H. H. Marsh.** 1968. Semiautomatic microtechnique for serial dilution antibiotic sensitivity testing in the clinical laboratory. J. Lab. Clin. Med. **72:**685–687.
8. **Tilton, R. C., L. Leiberman, and E. H. Gerlach.** 1973. Microdilution antibiotic susceptibility test: examination of certain variables. Appl. Microbiol. **26:**658–665.

Antimicrobial Agents and Chemotherapy, Feb. 1977, p. 277-280 Vol. 11, No. 2
 Printed in U.S.A.

Amphotericin B Susceptibility Testing of Yeasts with a Bactec Radiometric System

ROY L. HOPFER* AND DIETER GRÖSCHEL

Department of Laboratory Medicine, The University of Texas System Cancer Center, M. D. Anderson Hospital and Tumor Institute, Houston, Texas 77030

Received for publication 7 October 1976

The effect of amphotericin B on CO_2 production was studied using a Bactec 225. A radiometric procedure for yeast susceptibility testing that requires 3 h of incubation was developed. A total of 48 yeast isolates was tested in this system and the results were correlated to tube dilution studies. The drug concentration causing at least a 44% decrease in CO_2 production correlated to the tube dilution minimal inhibitory concentration in 85% of isolates tested and was within one tube dilution of the minimal inhibitory concentration in over 95% of yeasts tested.

Amphotericin B suscetibility tests are often requested for yeasts isolated from compromised hosts. Because of the side effects of amphotericin B, knowledge about the susceptibility of a yeast allows the design of a drug regimen that will provide adequate serum levels using the lowest dosage possible. Tube dilution methods are currently used to determine the minimal inhibitory concentration (MIC) of a drug for yeasts (4). Considerable time is required to set up the tests, and results are not available for 24 to 48 h.

Benitez et al. (1) have recently reported a radiometric method that greatly reduces the time needed to determine the effect of antimicrobial agents on mycobacteria and slow-growing fungi. The decrease in the amount of [^{3}H]uracil and [^{3}H]guanine incorporated into ribonucleic acid in the presence of the antibiotics was correlated to traditional susceptibility tests. DeBlanc et al. (2) and DeLand (3) have described a radiometric method for bacteria that provides rapid quantitative measurement of the inhibitory effects of antibiotics. Inhibition of the metabolism of labeled [^{14}C]glucose is measured by the decrease in CO_2 production. A constant relationship was shown between the radiometric results and conventional tube dilution techniques for antibacterial susceptibilities. In this study we determined the usefulness of the $^{14}CO_2$ (Bactec) method for yeast susceptibility testing.

MATERIALS AND METHODS

Yeast strains. Forty-seven fresh isolates were obtained from the Mycology Laboratory at M. D. Anderson Hospital and Tumor Institute. The amphotericin B-resistant strain, *Candida tropicalis* ATCC 28707, was purchased from the American Type Culture Collection, Rockville, Md. All isolates were maintained on Sabouraud dextrose agar slants before testing.

Inoculum preparation. Ehrlenmeyer flasks containing 50 ml of Trypticase soy broth (Bioquest, Cockeysville, Md.) were inoculated from Sabouraud dextrose agar slants and incubated at 37°C for 17 h on a rotary shaker set at 150 rpm. The culture was centrifuged at 800 × g for 10 min, and the resulting pellet was used to prepare a 2% cell suspension in sterile saline. One milliliter of the suspension was used to inject a Bactec 6A bottle (Johnston Laboratories, Inc. Cockeysville, Md.) containing tryptic soy broth (TSB) and ^{14}C-labeled substrates.

Amphotericin B assay. Amphotericin B (Fungizone, E. R. Squibb and Sons, Inc., Princeton, N. J.) was suspended in unlabeled TSB to give a final concentration of 50 μg/ml. Six serial twofold dilutions were prepared in TSB, and 1 ml of each dilution was added to each Bactec 6A bottle, resulting in final drug concentrations of 1.6, 0.8, 0.4, 0.2, 0.1, and 0.05 μg/ml, respectively. One bottle without drug served as the growth reference. After inoculation, the bottles were placed on a rotary shaker incubator (37°C, 150 rpm) for 3 h and then tested on a Bactec 225 automated bacterial detection system (Johnston Laboratories).

Tube dilution procedure. Tube dilutions were performed as described by Shadomy (4). Since no difference in MIC was observed using antibiotic medium 20 or TSB, all tube dilution values were obtained using TSB.

Calculation of the effect of amphotericin B on CO_2 production. Since the growth index values of the Bactec 225 are directly proportional to the amount of radioactive CO_2 produced, the change in CO_2 production ($\triangle$ CO_2) was determined from the growth index (GI) values. Reference values were taken from the drug-free bottles. Percent changes in CO_2 ($\triangle$ CO_2) were calculated by the formula: $\triangle$ CO_2 (%) = GI control − GI test/GI control × 100.

RESULTS

Initial studies indicated that preincubation of the inoculum in TSB reduced the lag period before exponential growth from 12 to 1 h or less. In addition, it was found that an inoculum using actively growing cells (17 h for *Candida* species) provided more rapid CO_2 production after being introduced into the Bactec culture bottles.

Initially, yeast inocula comparable to those used in tube dilution assays were used in the radiometric procedure. With these inocula, amphotericin B concentrations corresponding to the MIC (as determined by tube dilution) prevented detectable CO_2 production; in the drug-free control cultures, 15 to 18 h of incubation were necessary for growth and CO_2 production. Therefore, the inoculum size was steadily increased to reduce the time necessary for CO_2 production in the drug-free bottles. One milliliter of a 2% cell suspension was found to produce adequate levels of CO_2 after 3 h of incubation.

The variation in the number of yeasts in the 2% cell suspension inoculated into each test bottle was determined by performing plate counts immediately after inoculation of six Bactec bottles and after the 3-h incubation period. The plate count varied not more than 3%. The variation in CO_2 production after 3 h of incubation was less than 2%. Deliberate changes (±0.05 ml) in inoculum size caused less than 2% variation in the growth index after 3 h of incubation. The effect of the drug on growth and viability of one strain of *C. albicans* is shown in Fig. 1. Increasing drug concentrations cause a decrease in CO_2 production and in the number of colony-forming units. This particular strain had a tube dilution MIC of 0.2 and a minimal fungicidal concentration (MFC) of 0.8 μg of amphotericin B per ml. In the radiometric procedure, 0.2 μg of amphotericin B per ml caused a 54% decrease in colony-forming units and decreased the CO_2 production by 52%; 0.8 μg of amphotericin B per ml (MFC) decreased colony-forming units by 95% and decreased CO_2 production by 72%.

Table 1 lists all yeast strains tested. The tube dilution MIC ranges from 0.05 to 0.8 μg of amphotericin B per ml, and the range is comparable to published values (4). The tube dilution MIC level caused at least a 44% decrease in CO_2 production in 40 of the 47 susceptible isolates tested. The CO_2 production of five additional isolates was inhibited by at least 44% in the presence of amphotericin B at a level within one dilution of the tube dilution MIC.

The effect of amphotericin B on CO_2 production of 46 isolates tested is shown in Fig. 2. The shaded area represents a composite of 45 susceptible isolates. Considerable variation exists between drug level and CO_2 production, depending on the isolate. For example, the decrease in CO_2 production caused by 0.4 μg of amphotericin B per ml varies from less than 45% for the most resistant strains to near 90% for the most sensitive strains. Also shown are the results obtained when *C. tropicalis* ATCC 28707, a strain resistant to more than 50 μg of amphotericin B per ml, was tested in this system. When values are plotted, the resultant curve is clearly out of the range of the susceptible isolates.

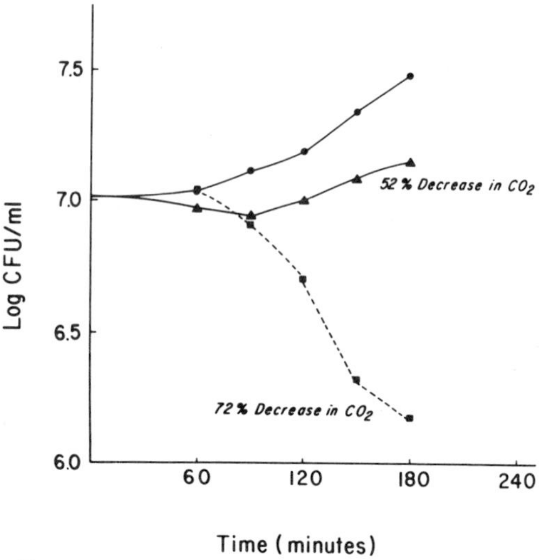

FIG. 1. *Effect of amphotericin B on viability and CO_2 production of Candida albicans strain 701. One milliliter of a 2% cell suspension was inoculated into each Bactec culture bottle. Each point on the graph represents the average colony-forming unit (CFU) per milliliter of two experiments run in duplicate. Amphotericin B concentrations were as follows: none (●); 0.2 μg/ml (▲); and 0.8 μg/ml (■).*

The CO_2 production assay did not correlate to MIC values in two instances. Bactec analysis of both isolates indicated that the strains were resistant to amphotericin B; however, subsequent tube dilution studies showed both isolates to be susceptible to clinically achievable blood levels of the drug. Repeat testing with the Bactec procedure and tube dilution studies failed to resolve these differences.

DISCUSSION

The reduction in CO_2 production by amphotericin B is a more rapid indicator of inhibition than is tube dilution or plate count techniques. Therefore, the measurement of the reduction in

TABLE 1. *Correlation of radiometric results with tube dilution minimal inhibitory concentrations of amphotericin B*

Strain[a]	MIC[b]	No. of strains tested	No. of strains showing 44% reduction in CO_2: At MIC level[c]	No. of strains showing 44% reduction in CO_2: Within range of ±1 dilution[d]
Candida albicans (29)	0.05	2	2	2
	0.10	11	9	11
	0.20	12	10	11
	0.40	3	2	2
	0.80	1	1	1
C. tropicalis (6)	0.20	5	4	5
	0.40	1	1	1
C. parapsilosis (3)	0.10	1	1	1
	0.20	2	1	2
C. pseudotropicalis (2)	0.20	1	1	1
	0.40	1	1	1
C. krusei (2)	0.80	2	2	2
C. guilliermondii (1)	0.20	1	1	1
Cryptococcus neoformans (2)	0.05	2	2	2
Torulopsis glabrata (2)	0.10	1	1	1
	0.40	1	1	1
		47	40 (85.1)	45 (95.7)
C. tropicalis ATCC 28707	>50	1		

[a] Number in parentheses indicates total number of strains tested.
[b] MIC was determined by tube dilution methods.
[c] Number of strains tested in which the amphotericin B concentration causing a 44% decrease in CO_2 production was the same as tube dilution MIC.
[d] Total number of strains tested in which the drug concentration causing 44% decrease in CO_2 production was within one dilution of the tube dilution MIC.

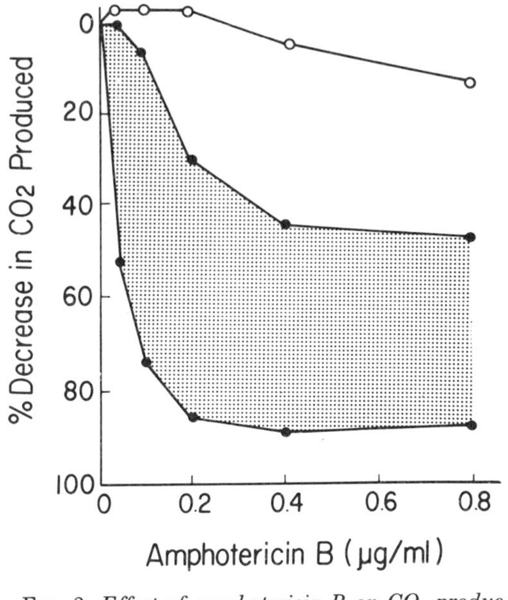

FIG. 2. *Effect of amphotericin B on CO_2 production of 46 yeast strains. Range in CO_2 production of 45 susceptible isolates (shaded area); Candida tropicalis* ATCC 28707 (○).

CO_2 production in a radiometric assay system may provide useful information concerning susceptibility or resistance of a yeast to an antifungal agent.

Comparing MIC values obtained by tube dilution with the radiometric procedure has led to the following observations. The lowest level of drug causing at least a 44% decrease in CO_2 production corresponded to the tube dilution MIC value in 40 of 47 strains and was within one dilution of the MIC value in 5 additional strains. This level of variation is comparable to the variation found with the tube dilution method and does not influence the validity of the Bactec assay.

Two isolates produced results indicating resistance to amphotericin B by the radiometric method, whereas tube dilution studies indicated susceptibility to the drug. These two isolates, upon repeat testing in the Bactec system, consistently produced less than a 30% reduction in CO_2 production at all drug levels tested. Both isolates were killed (as determined by subculturing samples from tube dilution assays) at drug levels fourfold higher than tube dilution MIC. Therefore, all strains determined to be resistant by Bactec assay must be tested by tube dilution methods.

Our study has shown that the radiometric method is capable of determining the susceptibility of yeasts to amphotericin B within 3 h. The degree of inhibition correlates well to MIC values determined by tube dilution. At the present time, other antifungal agents are being tested in the system. In addition to single drug susceptibilities, this method may provide rapid information on synergistic/antagonistic effects of various drug combinations.

ACKNOWLEDGMENTS

This study was supported in part by an American Cancer Society Institutional Research grant ACS-IN-43-0.

LITERATURE CITED

1. **Benitez, P., G. Medoff, and G. S. Kobayashi.** 1974. Rapid radiometric method of testing susceptibility of mycobacteria and slow-growing fungi to antimicrobial agents. Antimicrob. Agents Chemother. 6:29–33.
2. **DeBlanc, Jr., H. J., P. Charache, and H. N. Wagner, Jr.** 1972. Automatic radiometric measurement of antibiotic effect on bacterial growth. Antimicrob. Agents Chemother. 2:361–366.
3. **DeLand, F. H.** 1972. Metabolic inhibition as an index of bacterial susceptibility to drugs. Antimicrob. Agents Chemother. 2:405–412.
4. **Shadomy, S., and A. Espinel-Ingroff.** 1974. Susceptibility testing of antifungal agents, p 569–574. *In* E. H. Lennette, E. H. Spaulding, and J. P. Truant (ed), Manual of clinical microbiology, 2nd ed. American Society for Microbiology, Washington, D. C.

ANTIMICROBIAL AGENTS AND CHEMOTHERAPY, Feb. 1977, p. 281-290 Vol. 11, No. 2

Development of a Chemically Defined Medium for the Synthesis of Actinomycin D by *Streptomyces parvulus*

W. KENNETH WILLIAMS AND EDWARD KATZ*

Department of Microbiology, Georgetown University Schools of Medicine and Dentistry, Washington, D. C. 20007

Received for publication 13 October 1976

A chemically defined medium, consisting of D-fructose, L-glutamic acid, L-histidine, K_2HPO_4, $MgSO_4 \cdot 7H_2O$, $ZnSO_4 \cdot 7H_2O$, $CaCl_2 \cdot 2H_2O$, $FeSO_4 \cdot 7H_2O$, $CoCl_2 \cdot 6H_2O$, and deionized water, was developed for synthesis of high yields (500 to 600 μg/ml) of actinomycin D by *Streptomyces parvulus*. Under these nutritional conditions, growth and actinomycin formation did not follow a typical trophophase-idiophase pattern. The amino acids appeared to have a sparing action on the utilization of D-fructose which was slowly and incompletely metabolized during mycelium development and antibiotic production. A significant repression of actinomycin synthesis by *S. parvulus* was observed when D-glucose (0.01 to 0.25%) was added to the culture medium. The repression was not due to a decline in the pH of the medium during glucose catabolism.

Because of our continued interest in the mechanism of directed biosynthesis (30), we have turned our attention to the metabolic activities of *Streptomyces parvulus* which synthesizes virtually the single antibiotic component, actinomycin D (40). Although the medium described previously (16, 32) proved satisfactory for the production of actinomycin mixtures by *Streptomyces antibioticus*, the synthesis of actinomycin D by *S. parvulus*, under the same conditions, was rather poor and extremely variable. Studies were, therefore, initiated to establish the nutritional factors that would support growth and consistently high yields of the antibiotic by this organism. This report describes a series of experiments that have culminated in the development of a chemically defined medium in which production of high titers of actinomycin D was achieved.

MATERIALS AND METHODS

Organism and conditions of cultivation. *S. parvulus* (ATCC 12434) was maintained on slants of glucose-yeast extract-malt extract agar medium (26). Incubation was carried out for 3 to 5 days at 30°C until gray spores had developed; slants were then kept at 4°C for further use.

For preparation of vegetative inoculum, spores were scraped gently from the surface of a slant(s) with 2.5 ml of NZ-Amine medium (31), and 2-ml quantities of the spore suspension were inoculated into a 250-ml Erlenmeyer flask containing 100-ml amounts of NZ-Amine medium. After incubation on a gyratory shaking incubator (New Brunswick Scientific Co., Inc., New Brunswick, N.J.) for 48 h at 30°C, the mycelium was harvested by centrifugation (30 min at 9,000 rev/min), washed twice with and then suspended in 100 ml of saline as described previously (31, 34). Aliquots (3 ml) of the suspension served as inoculum for each 250-ml Erlenmeyer flask containing 100 ml of chemically defined medium.

Basal medium for nutritional studies. The medium (D-galactose, 10 g; D-glucose, 1.0 g; L-glutamic acid·HCl, 2.5 g; $MgSO_4 \cdot 7H_2O$, 25 mg; $ZnSO_4 \cdot 7H_2O$, 25 mg; $CaCl_2 \cdot 2H_2O$, 25 mg; $FeSO_4 \cdot 7H_2O$, 25 mg; deionized water, 1,000 ml; pH 7.1) routinely utilized for actinomycin production with *S. antibioticus* and *Streptomyces chrysomallus* (16, 33, 34, 60) was employed initially for the studies with *S. parvulus*.

Carbon sources (e.g., sugars, organic acids) generally were sterilized separately and added at appropriate concentrations just prior to inoculation. All other additions were made before sterilization of media. Incubations were carried out in duplicate on a gyratory shaking incubator at 250 rev/min for 6 days at 30°C.

Analytical methods. Growth of the culture was followed by measurement of mycelial dry weight (35). The actinomycin titer per milliliter of culture filtrate was determined spectrophotometrically at 443 nm (34) on samples taken after 2, 4, and 6 days of incubation. The data reported in most experiments represent the yield of actinomycin (in micrograms per milliliter) after 6 days of cultivation.

Residual D-fructose was measured enzymatically as outlined by Bernt and Bergmeyer (5). The culture filtrate (5 ml) was shaken for 20 min with Amberlite MB-3 resin (200 mg, 20 to 50 mesh) in a ground glass-stoppered test tube and then centrifuged for 10 min at 2,000 rev/min. Determination of fructose concentration was then performed in triplicate on aliquots of the supernatant. Examination of the fructose preparation for glucose was performed with the Glucostat reagent (16); these analyses revealed that fructose was essentially free of glucose (<0.01%).

Disappearance of L-glutamic acid and L-histidine from the medium was followed by the paper chromatographic procedure of Naftalin (41) and by means of the automatic analytical Beckman Spinco amino acid analyzer (model 120C) (58, 59). An aliquot of the culture filtrate (5 ml, adjusted to pH 2.5 to 3.0) was passed through a Dowex 50W column (1 by 6 cm, H^+ form, 200 to 400 mesh), and the amino acids were eluted with 2 N NH_4OH (34). The solution was evaporated to dryness and then employed for the Naftalin and amino acid analyzer procedures.

Chromatography and high-voltage electrophoresis. Aliquots of each sample in water were examined by the Naftalin method (41), employing ascending paper chromatography (Whatman no. 1) and the solvent system: *1*-butanol:acetic acid:water (12:3:5); the R_f values for L-glutamic acid and L-histidine were 0.29 and 0.11, respectively. For the analytical determinations with the Beckman analyzer, samples were diluted in 0.2 N sodium citrate buffer, pH 2.2, and developed in 0.2 M sodium citrate buffer, pH 3.05, for L-glutamic acid, or 0.35 M sodium citrate, pH 5.25, for L-histidine (basic column). The flow rate of buffer for L-glutamic acid was 68 ml/h and for L-histidine it was 34 ml/h; the flow rate for ninhydrin throughout was 34 ml/h. Retention time for L-glutamic acid was 90 min and for L-histidine it was 43 min.

D-Fructose (R_f = 0.49) was examined by descending paper chromatography overnight with Whatman no. 1 paper, employing the solvent system ethyl acetate:pyridine:water (3.6:1:1.15). Detection was effected with a silver nitrate reagent (52); the chromatographic study revealed that the fructose preparation was homogeneous.

The actinomycin produced by *S. parvulus* was routinely monitored by means of circular paper chromatography as described in earlier publications (31–33). The solvent systems employed were (i) 10% aqueous sodium-*o*-cresotinate:dibutyl ether:*sym*, tetrachloroethane (4:3:1); (ii) 10% aqueous sodium-*o*-cresotinate: isopropyl ether:chloroform (6:5:1) and (5:3:2); and (iii) 5% aqueous sodium-*o*-cresotinate:amyl acetate, unequilibrated.

Amino acid hydrolysates (34) of actinomycin preparations were examined by a two-dimensional technique (59) employing high-voltage electrophoresis in one direction and paper chromatography (methanol, water, pyridine [20:5:1]) in the second direction. Amino acids were visualized with 0.2% ninhydrin/acetone; imino acids also were detected with 0.2% isatin/acetone.

L-Histidine, D-fructose, and hexokinase (EC 2.7.1.1) were purchased from Calbiochem (San Diego, Calif.). Adenosine-5′-triphosphate, nicotinamide adenine dinucleotide phosphate, glucose-6-phosphate dehydrogenase (EC 1.1.1.49), and phosphoglucose isomerase (EC 5.3.1.9) were obtained from Sigma Chemical Co. (St. Louis, Mo.). L-Glutamic acid·HCl was purchased from Mann Research Lab. (New York, N.Y.); D-glucose was from Fisher Scientific Co. (Pittsburgh, Pa.); and the Glucostat reagent kit was from Worthington Biochemical Corp. (Freehold, N.J.). The Dowex 50W resin (H^+ form, 200 to 400 mesh) was procured from BioRad Lab (Richmond, Calif.) and the Amberlite MB-3 monobed resin was obtained from Mallinckrodt Chemical Works (St. Louis, Mo.). All other compounds used were purchased from commercial sources.

RESULTS

Nature of actinomycin produced by *S. parvulus*. The qualitative nature of the actinomycin (predominantly actinomycin D, >95%) elaborated by *S. parvulus* during the period of medium development did not change significantly from that normally elaborated by the organism as monitored by circular paper chromatography, spectrophotometry, and analyses of the amino acid composition of acid hydrolysates of actinomycin preparations.

Sources of carbohydrates. A number of carbohydrates were investigated as carbon sources for actinomycin production in the glutamic acid-basal mineral salts medium. As control, the same medium was employed with galactose (1%) and glucose (0.1%) as carbohydrate sources. Preliminary experiments revealed that, of a large number of compounds tested, D-fructose (191 μg/ml), D-galactose (128 μg/ml), dextrin (127 μg/ml), and D-glucose (104 μg/ml) singly supported increased yields of actinomycin in comparison with the control medium (87 μg/ml). These four carbohydrates were then retested at a concentration of 0.5 and 1.0%. It can be seen (Fig. 1) that the level of the carbon compound employed had a striking influence on actinomycin production; D-fructose was far superior to the other carbohydrates tested at either concentration. In contrast to our preliminary experiments, actinomycin titers were extremely low when D-glucose served as the sole carbohydrate source.

Effect of different amino acids. With D-fructose (1%) present, various amino acids (5 mM) were examined in lieu of L-glutamic acid for antibiotic production. Several amino acids (e.g., valine, histidine, ornithine, glutamine, asparagine, and leucine) appeared suitable for the biosynthesis of actinomycin D (Table 1). L-Glutamic acid, at 5 mM, was rather ineffective as a nitrogen source; however, at a level of 15 mM, it proved to be an excellent nitrogen source for antibiotic formation (160 μg/ml).

These results prompted an experiment to determine the optimal concentration of selected amino acids (L-valine, L-ornithine, L-glutamic acid, L-histidine, L-proline, and L-glutamine) as sole nitrogen source for actinomycin synthesis. The amino acids were used within the concen-

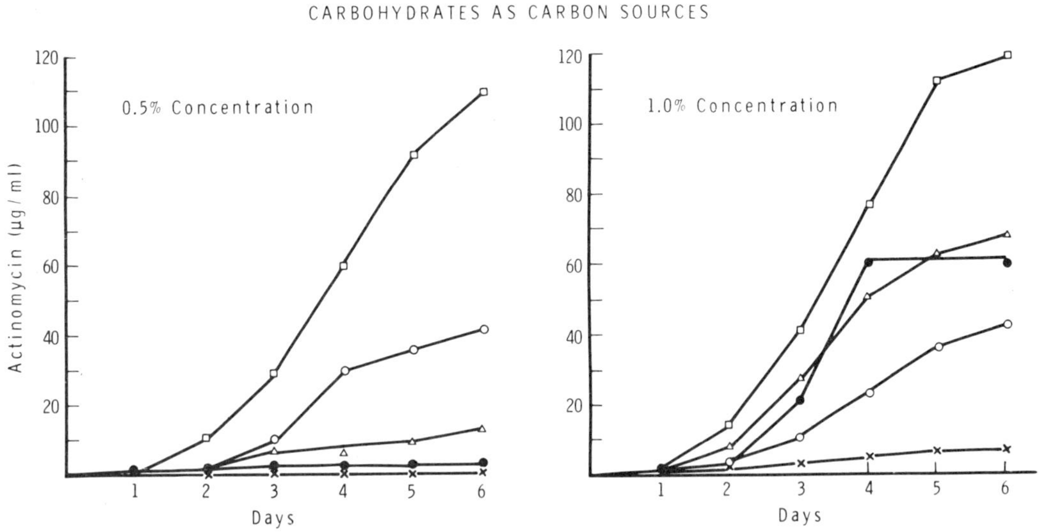

FIG. 1. *Influence of various carbohydrates upon actinomycin synthesis by Streptomyces parvulus in L-glutamic acid-basal mineral salts medium (16). Carbohydrates were employed at the 0.5 and 1% level, except for the control medium. Symbols:* □, *D-Fructose;* △, *D-galactose;* ●, *dextrin;* ×, *D-glucose;* ○, *control (D-galactose, 1.0%; and D-glucose, 0.1%).*

tration range of 3 to 30 mM with D-fructose (1%) and the basal mineral salts; the results are presented in Fig. 2 as a histogram. As seen, histidine (5 mM), ornithine (10 mM), valine (10 mM), glutamic acid (15 mM), glutamine (10 mM), and proline (15 mM) provided the optimum level of each amino acid for actinomycin production. Of interest is the fact that higher concentrations of these amino acids were less effective for antibiotic synthesis. We then compared the effect of L-valine, L-proline, L-ornithine, and L-histidine on actinomycin production when used in combination with L-glutamic acid (15 mM) in the chemically defined medium. The data (Table 2) reveal that antibiotic formation was enhanced if the amino acid in question was combined with glutamic acid as nitrogen source. In particular, valine (3 to 5 mM) and histidine (3 to 5 mM) were the most suitable ancillary amino acids for synthesis of actinomycin.

Influence of fructose concentration upon actinomycin formation. The influence of D-fructose concentration on actinomycin formation was next explored in a medium containing the basal mineral salts, glutamic acid (15 mM) and varying levels of valine or histidine. As shown in Fig. 3, (i) actinomycin synthesis increased as a function of the fructose concentration supplied in the medium, and (ii) the combination of histidine and glutamic acid was somewhat superior to a similar mixture of valine and glutamate for antibiotic production.

Effect of inorganic nitrogen sources. Inorganic nitrates, nitrite, and several ammonium salts were also investigated as sole nitrogen sources for the formation of actinomycin D. The concentrations employed ranged from approximately one-fourth to twice the amount of nitrogen contained in the glutamic acid-histidine medium. At the levels employed, however, none of these compounds were as effective as the combination of glutamic acid and histidine; the maximal titers of actinomycin D attained were one-third that produced with the amino acids present.

Role of organic acids in the production of actinomycin. Although some investigations have shown that organic acids are poor sources of carbon for production of antibiotics when used singly (12, 13), other studies have revealed that the combination of a sugar and the sodium salt of an organic acid produced antibiotic titers higher than those elaborated with these carbon sources used singly (1, 18, 24, 27, 28). Since D-fructose proved to be an excellent carbohydrate for antibiotic production, we examined the role of organic acids (0.1 to 0.5%) as supplemental carbon sources for actinomycin synthesis. Generally, most of the organic acids tested at levels above 0.1% were inhibitory to actinomycin formation.

Effect of carbon-nitrogen ratio on actinomycin formation. To further explore the influence of the organic nutrients upon actinomycin synthesis, the concentration of D-fructose (4%)

TABLE 1. *Effect of various amino acids on actinomycin production by Streptomyces parvulus* [a]

Amino acid	Actinomycin (μg/ml)
L-Glutamic acid·HCl (control) [b]	160
L-Valine	153
L-Histidine	132
L-Ornithine·HCl	124
L-Glutamine	109
L-Asparagine·HCl	105
L-Leucine	104
L-Proline	95
L-Serine	91
L-Alanine	90
β-Alanine	89
L-Threonine	87
L-Aspartic acid	79
L-Citrulline	79
L-Phenylalanine	69
L-Glutamic acid·HCl	65
L-Tyrosine	63
L-Isoleucine	58
L-Lysine·HCl	49
Glycine	47
L-Methionine	37
L-Tryptophan	28
L-Cysteine·HCl	28
L-Cystine	23
L-Arginine·HCl	23

[a] *S. parvulus* was grown in a 1% D-fructose-basal mineral salts medium for 144 h at 30°C.

[b] L-Glutamic acid·HCl was supplied at 15 mM (control); all other amino acids were employed at 5 mM.

was held constant, while the amount of L-glutamic acid and L-histidine was varied to provide different C/N ratios in the medium. The results of these experiments are depicted in Fig. 4. Maximum formation of actinomycin (455 μg/ml) was achieved at a C/N ratio of 41.7. This ratio corresponded to 4% D-fructose, 15 mM L-glutamic acid, and 5 mM L-histidine.

Mineral requirements. Several laboratories have noted that various cations, such as Mg^{2+}, Fe^{2+}, Zn^{2+}, Cu^{2+}, Mn^{2+}, and Co^{2+} are stimulatory to antibiotic production (55). In some instances rigorous methods of purification (e.g., chelation or adsorption) have been employed to free medium constituents from trace metal contamination (1, 4, 8, 39). In other cases no special precautions have been made; the effects of exogenously provided trace elements have been examined over and above that present as contaminants on glassware, chemicals, etc. (9, 18, 47).

Role of trace metals. The relative requirement of several individual microelements for actinomycin production was studied in the medium consisting of: D-fructose, 40.0 g; L-glutamic acid, 15 mM; L-histidine, 5 mM; K_2HPO_4, 1.0 g; $MgSO_4 \cdot 7H_2O$, 25 mg; $ZnSO_4 \cdot 7H_2O$, 25 mg; $CaCl_2 \cdot 2H_2O$, 25 mg; $FeSO_4 \cdot 7H_2O$, 25 mg; and deionized water, 1,000 ml with a pH 7.1. The trace metal under test was added to the basal medium at different concentrations in separate flasks. In the subsequent experiments, the composition of the medium was modified to include this amount of the trace element. Figures 5 to 8 reveal that the optimal concentrations of the various cations tested were 4.88 ppm of Mg^{2+}, 8 to 10 ppm of Fe^{2+}, 7.5 to 14.6 ppm of Ca^{2+}, and 4.6 to 13.7 ppm of Zn^{2+}. The optimal range appeared somewhat broader for Ca^{2+} and Zn^{2+}.

Fosfomycin biosynthesis by *Streptomyces fradiae* (47), gentamicin formation by *Micromonospora* species (R. T. Testa, personal communication), as well as the production of certain other antibiotics by streptomycetes have been found to be stimulated or influenced by the addition of Co^{2+} to the production medium (9, 45). An experiment was carried out to determine whether Co^{2+} would exert a similar effect on actinomycin synthesis by *S. parvulus*. The results of two experiments suggest that Co^{2+} may stimulate antibiotic production (10 to 25%), particularly at a concentration of $CoCl_2 \cdot 6H_2O$ of 1×10^{-7} M to 5×10^{-8} M.

Influence of K_2HPO_4 concentration. The concentration of K_2HPO_4 found optimal for actinomycin production in the chemically defined medium was 0.1% (565 μg/ml), although the level of the inorganic compound that could be employed for excellent synthesis ranged from 0.05 to 0.4%. Even at a concentration of 1.0%, production was still three-fourths that observed at the optimal concentration of K_2HPO_4. Acti-

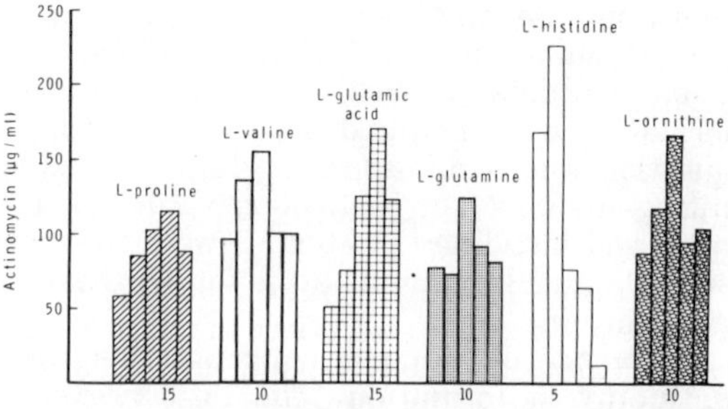

FIG. 2. *Histogram depicting the influence of the concentration of different amino acids upon actinomycin formation in a medium containing 1% D-fructose and basal mineral salts. Concentration of each amino acid (L-proline, L-valine, L-glutamic acid, L-glutamine, L-histidine, and L-ornithine), reading from left to right, was 3, 5, 10, 15, and 30 mM. Incubation was at 30°C for 144 h. The numerical values shown represent the optimal concentration of each amino acid for actinomycin production.*

TABLE 2. *Effect of* L*-amino acids provided singly or in combination with* L*-glutamic acid for actinomycin synthesis by S. parvulus* [a]

L-Glutamic acid (mM)	L-Valine (mM)	L-Ornithine (mM)	L-Histidine (mM)	L-Proline (mM)	Actinomycin (μg/ml)	% of control
15	0	0	0	0	170	1.00
0	3	0	0	0	75	0.44
15	3	0	0	0	190	1.12
0	5	0	0	0	115	0.68
15	5	0	0	0	215	1.26
0	10	0	0	0	126	0.74
15	10	0	0	0	165	0.97
0	0	3	0	0	75	0.44
15	0	3	0	0	160	0.94
0	0	5	0	0	105	0.62
15	0	5	0	0	177	1.04
0	0	10	0	0	85	0.50
15	0	10	0	0	165	0.97
0	0	0	3	0	155	0.91
15	0	0	3	0	215	1.26
0	0	0	5	0	140	0.82
15	0	0	5	0	210	1.24
0	0	0	10	0	55	0.32
15	0	0	10	0	195	1.15
0	0	0	0	3	90	0.53
15	0	0	0	3	155	0.91
0	0	0	0	5	140	0.82
15	0	0	0	5	140	0.82
0	0	0	0	10	110	0.65
15	0	0	0	10	140	0.82

[a] Conditions were the same as in Table 1, except incubation was for 135 h at 30°C. Media contained D-fructose (1%).

nomycin synthesis appears to be far less sensitive to the inorganic phosphate concentration in the medium than the corresponding fermentations of prodigiosin, monamycin, pyocyanine, or vancomycin (57). By contrast, Haavik (21) reported that optimal synthesis of bacitracin was observed at levels of inorganic phosphate in excess of 100 mM, which represents a 20-fold greater amount than required for maximal actinomycin formation.

Repression of actinomycin synthesis by D-glucose. The repressive effect of glucose and related compounds on enzyme synthesis and secondary metabolite formation has been discussed in several reviews (10, 36, 42) and the mechanism of catabolite repression has been critically examined (46). In the case of *S. antibioticus*, glucose markedly repressed synthesis of actinomycin as well as phenoxazinone synthase, a key enzyme required for the formation of the actinomycin chromophore, actinocin (16). It was postulated that the repression of antibiotic synthesis observed with glucose may be due primarily to a repression of the formation of phenoxazinone synthase and other key enzymes required for antibiotic biosynthesis.

Glucose was a poor carbon source when employed as the sole carbohydrate for synthesis of actinomycin (Fig. 1). It significantly repressed antibiotic formation in the fructose-glutamic acid-histidine-mineral salts medium (Fig. 9). Acidity was not responsible for the reduced synthesis of antibiotic since the pH of the media containing glucose (0.01 to 0.25%) was similar to that of the control culture. These data also contrast with the findings of Haavik (20, 22). Formation of bacitracin was not considered to be under catabolite repression control by glucose; the inhibitory nature of the sugar was believed to be due to the low pH created during the first few hours of incubation.

Biochemical analyses of substrate utilization during growth and antibiotic production. A study of the dynamics of the fermentation process was carried out to determine the extent to which the organic substrates were consumed during growth and production of actinomycin by the organism. As shown in Fig. 10, disap-

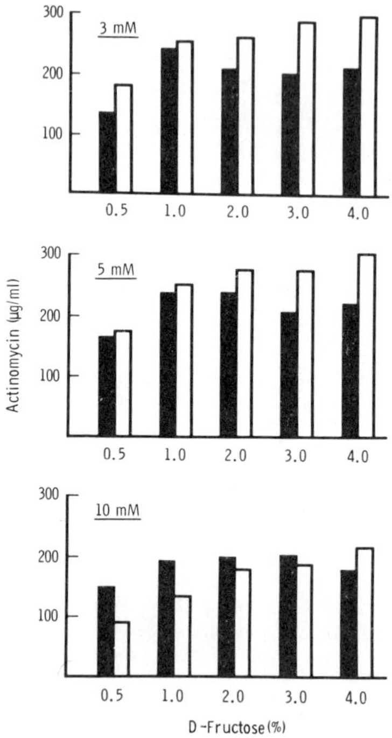

FIG. 3. *Effect of D-fructose concentration upon actinomycin formation in a medium containing basal mineral salts and L-glutamic acid (15 mM) in combination with L-valine or L-histidine employed at 3, 5, or 10 mM. Incubation was for 144 h at 30°C. Solid bars represent L-valine and open bars represent L-histidine.*

pearance of the amino acid substrates was extremely rapid with 50% of histidine and glutamic acid taken up by the cells within 12 h; the amino acids were removed (>99%) by 18 to 20 h, i.e., shortly before the onset of actinomycin production. By contrast, the utilization of fructose was a much slower process. Enzyme assays (5) indicated that there was an initial lag of approximately 8 h before it was taken up by the organism; however, even after 140 h, only 30% of the sugar supplied initially had been utilized.

Growth of the culture and production of the antibiotic did not appear to follow the typical pattern of a trophophase-idiophase fermentation (7, 10, 56). After an initial 3-h lag, there was a rapid increase of mycelium until 48 h; during the ensuing incubation, however, the organism continued to grow slowly until the experiment was terminated. Actinomycin was detected in the culture medium after 24 h; subsequently, its formation and growth of the culture remained parallel for the duration of the experiment.

DISCUSSION

The major purpose of this investigation was to design a chemically defined medium suitable for the growth and for the production of high titers of actinomycin by *S. parvulus*. The data described herein do reveal that yields of 500 to 600 μg of actinomycin D per ml can be consistently obtained by the organism in a glutamic acid-histidine-fructose-mineral salts medium.

Examination of a variety of carbohydrate sources for antibiotic production has revealed that D-fructose is far more effective than any of the other substances examined. Experimentally, we observed that a concentration of 4% was optimal for actinomycin production; however, the analytical results (Fig. 10) reveal that the utilization of the hexose occurred slowly and that only 30% (1.2 g) was consumed by 140 h, i.e., at the termination of the experiment. Similar conclusions were reported by Parit-

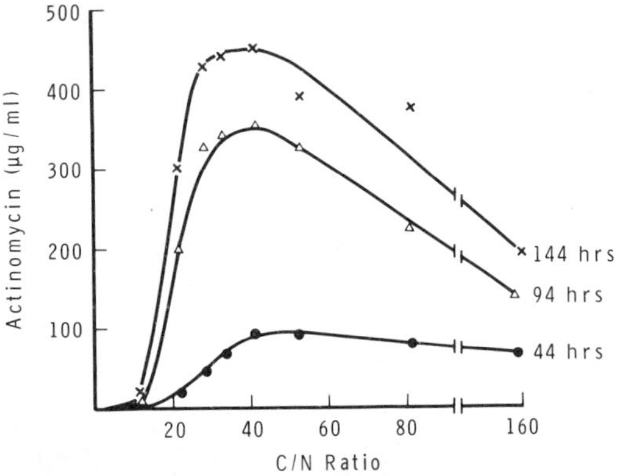

FIG. 4. *Influence of carbon-nitrogen ratio on actinomycin synthesis. S. parvulus was grown in media containing basal mineral salts with 4% D-fructose and varying amounts of L-glutamic acid and L-histidine as shown below:*

L-Glutamic acid (mM)	L-Histidine (mM)	D-Fructose (%)	C/N
3.75	1.25	4	155.3
7.5	2.5	4	79.2
11.25	3.75	4	53.8
15.0	5.0	4	41.7
18.6	6.25	4	33.5
22.5	7.5	4	28.4
30.0	10.0	4	22.0
60.0	20.0	4	12.5

The carbon-nitrogen ratio is based on the following calculations:

Determination	C(%)	N(%)
D-Fructose	40	
L-Glutamic acid	40.8	9.5
L-Histidine	46.4	27.1

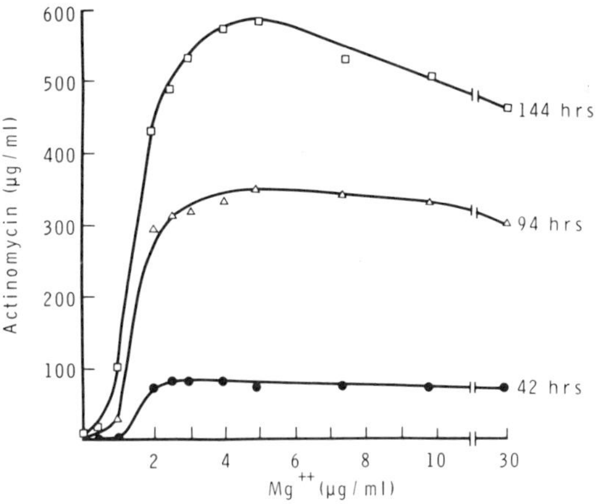

FIG. 5. *Influence of Mg^{2+} ion upon actinomycin production after 42, 94, and 144 h of incubation.*

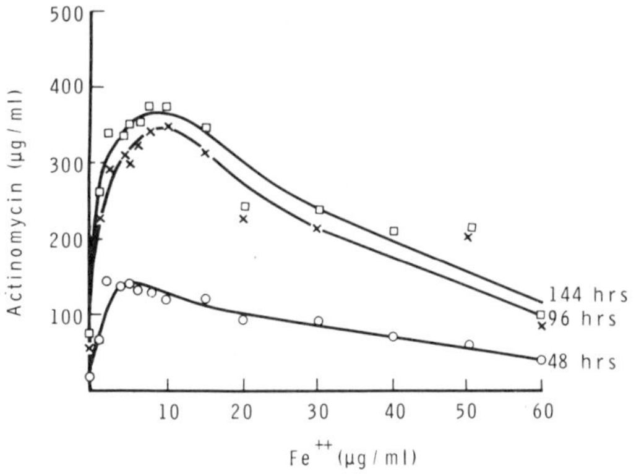

FIG. 6. *Influence of Fe^{2+} ion upon actinomycin production after 48, 96, and 144 h of incubation.*

skaya et al. (43) who examined the growth of *Actinomyces roseoflavus* in a fructose-containing medium. They noted that not more than 10 to 15% of the fructose present in the medium was oxidized irrespective of the initial concentration supplied; addition of mannitol to the fructose-containing medium improved the utilization of fructose to some extent (22 to 27%) (14). The slow utilization of D-fructose by *S. parvulus* throughout the fermentation ensures that a carbon and energy source was available during the period of antibiotic production. It should be pointed out that fructose is also an excellent source of carbon for gramicidin S formation (53).

Although a number of L-amino acids were favorable sources of nitrogen (and carbon) for actinomycin synthesis, when used singly, the combination of L-histidine (5 mM) and L-glutamic acid (15 mM) in the D-fructose-containing medium yielded the highest actinomycin titers. The uptake of these two amino acids by *S. parvulus* was found to occur quite rapidly, with 50% of the histidine and glutamic acid taken up within 12 h and essentially both amino acids (>99%) being removed by 18 to 20 h. The data in Fig. 10 suggest that the amino acids are preferentially employed initially for cell growth and that they exert a sparing effect on the utilization of the hexose. Moreover, the enzymes involved in the transport (44, 54) as well as the subsequent metabolism of fructose (e.g., fructokinase) (49, 50) may be inducible and require time for synthesis before the sugar can be metabolized.

The metabolic fate of glutamic acid and histidine, once they are taken up intracellularly, has not been investigated as yet. L-Glutamic acid has been shown to be a highly favorable source of nitrogen and carbon for growth of *Streptomyces* (12, 17, 48) and for the production of several chemically different antibiotics (24, 38, 39, 47). It also serves as a precursor of L-proline (2), which is an important constituent of

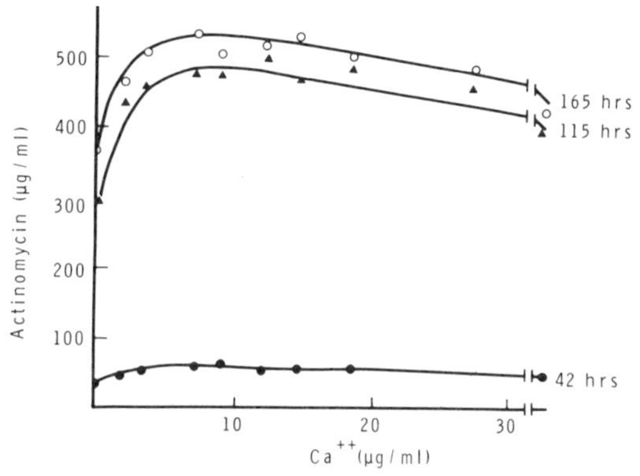

FIG. 7. *Effect of Ca^{2+} ion upon actinomycin synthesis after 42, 115, and 165 h of incubation.*

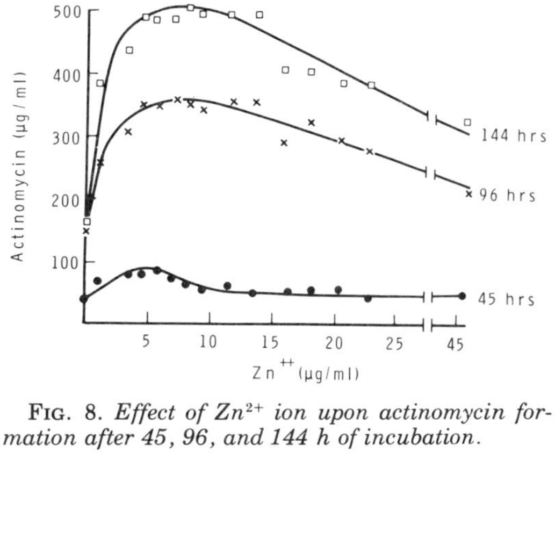

FIG. 8. *Effect of Zn^{2+} ion upon actinomycin formation after 45, 96, and 144 h of incubation.*

the actinomycin pentapeptides (40). L-Histidine has been reported to serve as a source of nitrogen for candicidin production (1). Moreover, it has proved useful in combination with valine and arginine for the formation of streptomycin; Eiser and McFarlane (15) observed that there was a direct correlation between the histidine

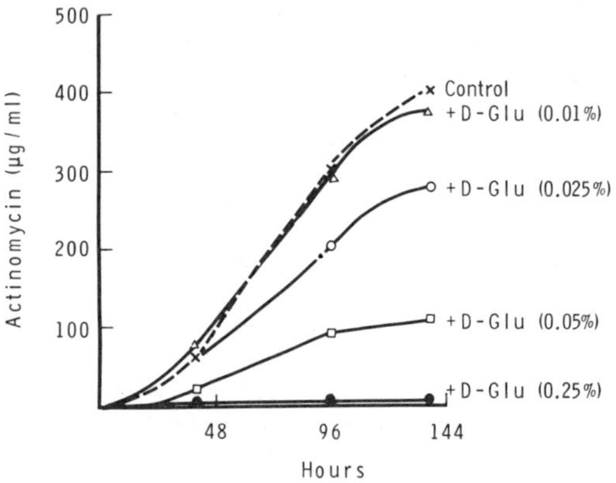

FIG. 9. *Repression of actinomycin formation by D-glucose. D-Glucose, at varying concentrations, was added at zero time to the 4% D-fructose-L-glutamic acid (15 mM)-L-histidine (5 mM)-basal mineral salts medium. Incubation was carried out for 137 h at 30°C. Symbols: ×, control; D-glucose: △, 0.01%; ○, 0.025%; □, 0.05%; ●, 0.25%.*

concentration in the medium and streptomycin production. With regard to *S. parvulus*, the effectiveness of L-histidine may be due in part to its ability to serve as (i) a buffer, (ii) a chelating agent, (iii) a direct source of the amino acid for protein synthesis, and (iv) an indirect source of L-proline through its catabolism to glutamic acid (19, 37).

As the data in Fig. 10 further reveal, growth of *S. parvulus* and production of the antibiotic do not follow the typical pattern of a trophophase-idiophase fermentation (7, 10, 55, 56). After a short lag (3 h), growth of the organism increased rapidly, initially at the expense of the amino acid substrates in the medium. Antibiotic synthesis was observed after 24 h of incubation; however, further growth of the organism and production of the antibiotic continued more or less in parallel throughout the remainder of the incubation. Presumably, D-fructose was then utilized as the chief carbon and energy source, and the intracellular pool provided the nitrogen for cell growth and antibiotic synthesis. Secondary metabolite formation by microorganisms has frequently been reported to occur principally during the stationary phase (idiophase), and numerous examples of this phenomenon are described in the literature (55, 56). However, it is also evident that the synthesis of such compounds may parallel the growth

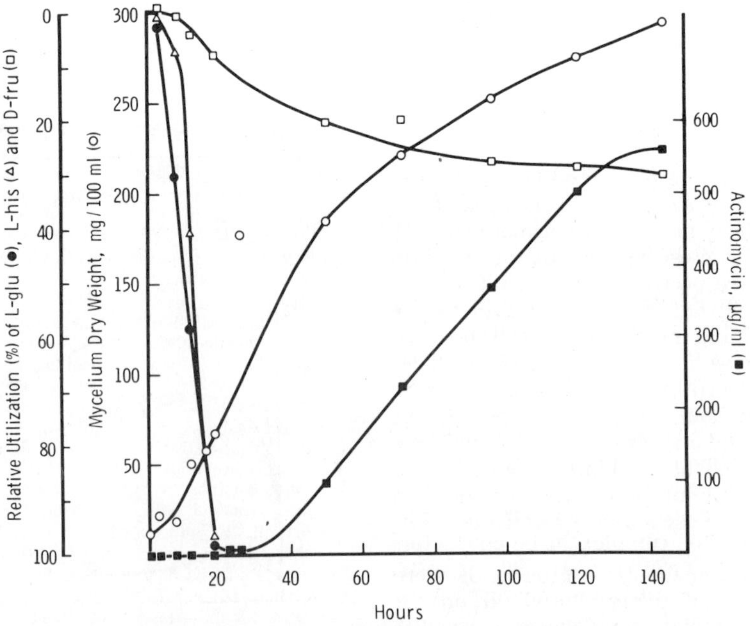

FIG. 10. *Dynamics of actinomycin fermentation: biochemical analyses of organic substrate utilization during growth and antibiotic synthesis by S. parvulus. The organism was cultivated in 4% D-fructose-L-glutamic acid (15 mM)-L-histidine (5 mM)-mineral salts medium for 144 h. Symbols: ●, L-Glutamic acid; △, L-histidine; □, D-fructose; ○, mycelium dry weight; ■, actinomycin.*

of the producing organism (3, 24), or that they may be formed during continuous cultivation of an organism (6, 23). As pointed out by Haavik (20, 22), the production of an antibiotic, after active growth of a culture, may depend on the particular nutritional conditions employed, or could arise as a consequence of the metabolic activities of the producing organism (e.g., formation of organic acids). Antibiotic synthesis may take place simultaneously with the cell's growth and may exert its effects throughout the growth cycle (23, 25, 29).

The repression of antibiotic formation by glucose in *S. parvulus* is similar to our previous experience with *S. antibioticus* (16). As the pH of the control and glucose-containing media increased from 7.1 to 8.0, the reduced antibiotic titer did not appear to be due to the lowering of pH through the production of organic acids (20, 22). The effect of glucose upon actinomycin production noted here may represent a repression of "actinomycin synthetase" formation (16).

Cations have been found to be important factors in the biosynthesis of antibiotics and other metabolic products by microorganisms (55). While we have not examined the role of the microelements systematically, in relation to the cell's growth and antibiotic production, nor rigorously purified the medium constituents, certain tentative conclusions can be drawn from the trace metal experiments (Fig. 5 to 8). The optimal yields of actinomycin were obtained in media containing Mg^{2+}, 4.88 μg/ml; Fe^{2+}, 8 to 10 μg/ml; Zn^{2+}, 4.6 to 13.7 μg/ml; Ca^{2+}, 7.5 to 14.6 μg/ml; and Co^{2+}, 0.003 to 0.006 μg/ml. Poor production was clearly observed if Fe^{2+} and Mg^{2+} (and Zn^{2+}) were omitted from the medium; however, such effects may be secondary to an initial influence on the growth of the producing culture. Additional studies are clearly required to provide insight into these relationships.

S. parvulus produces actinomycin D almost exclusively during antibiotic formation. The use of *S. parvulus* in contrast to *S. antibioticus* or *S. chrysomallus* for directed biosynthetic studies has certain advantages as the latter organisms normally produce five and three actinomycin components, respectively (29, 40). When an amino acid analogue is supplied to either of these cultures, the actinomycin mixtures formed are too complex to be characterized adequately. By contrast, a recent investigation with *S. parvulus,* employing *cis-* or *trans*-4-methyl-DL-proline, revealed that only two novel actinomycins (in major amounts) were synthesized in addition to actinomycin D (unpublished data).

ACKNOWLEDGMENTS

This work was supported by Public Health Service research grant CA-06926 and a contract (NOI-CM-43732) from the National Cancer Institute and a training grant from the National Institute of Allergy and Infectious Diseases (AI-298). We wish to thank Kaarin Mason for her assistance and discussions with regard to the use of the Beckman-Spinco amino acid analyzer.

LITERATURE CITED

1. **Acker, R. F., and H. Lechevalier.** 1954. Some nutritional requirements of *Streptomyces griseus* for growth and candicidin production. Appl. Microbiol. 2:152–157.
2. **Adams, E.** 1970. Metabolism of proline and of hydroxyproline. Int. Rev. Connect. Tissue Res. 5:1–91.
3. **Audhya, T. K., and D. W. Russell.** 1975. Enniatin production by *Fusarium sambucinum*; primary, secondary and unitary metabolism. J. Gen. Microbiol. 86:327–331.
4. **Basek, K., and S. K. Majumdar.** 1975. Mineral nutrition of *Streptomyces kanamyceticus* for kanamycin formation. Antimicrob. Agents Chemother. 8:391–395.
5. **Bernt, E., and H. U. Bergmeyer.** 1974. D-Fructose, p. 1304–1307. *In* H. U. Bergmeyer (ed.), Methods of enzymatic analysis, vol. 3. Academic Press Inc., New York.
6. **Blanch, H. W., and P. L. Rogers.** 1971. Production of gramicidin S in batch and continuous culture. Biotechnol. Bioeng. 13:843–864.
7. **Bu'Lock, J. D.** 1961. Intermediary metabolism and antibiotic synthesis. Adv. Appl. Microbiol. 3:293–342.
8. **Chesters, C. G. C., and G. N. Rolinson.** 1951. Trace elements and streptomycin production. J. Gen. Microbiol. 5:559–565.
9. **Claridge, C. A., V. Z. Rossomano, N. S. Buono, A. Gourevitch, and J. Lein.** 1966. Influence of cobalt on fermentative methylation. Appl. Microbiol. 14:280–283.
10. **Demain, A. L.** 1968. Regulatory mechanisms and the industrial production of microbial metabolites. Lloydia 31:395–418.
11. **Dulaney, E. L.** 1948. Observations on *Streptomyces griseus*. II. Nitrogen sources for growth and streptomycin production. J. Bacteriol. 56:305–313.
12. **Dulaney, E. L.** 1949. Observations on *Streptomyces griseus*. III. Carbon sources for growth and streptomycin production. Mycologia 41:1–10.
13. **Dulmage, H. T.** 1953. The production of neomycin by *Streptomyces fradiae* in synthetic media. Appl. Microbiol. 1:103–106.
14. **Eagon, R. G., and P. V. Phibbs, Jr.** 1971. Kinetics of transport of glucose, fructose and mannitol by *Pseudomonas aeruginosa*. Can. J. Biochem. 49:1031–1041.
15. **Eiser, H. M., and W. C. McFarlane.** 1948. Studies on the metabolism of *Streptomyces griseus* in relation to the production of streptomycin. Can. J. Res. 26:164–173.
16. **Gallo, M., and E. Katz.** 1972. Regulation of secondary metabolite biosynthesis: catabolite repression of phenoxazinone synthase and actinomycin formation by glucose. J. Bacteriol. 109:659–667.
17. **Gottlieb, D., and O. Ciferri.** 1956. Deamination and degradation of amino acids by *Streptomycetes*. Mycologia 48:253–263.
18. **Gottlieb, D., and L. Diamond.** 1951. A synthetic medium for chloromycetin. Bull. Torrey Bot. Club 78:56–60.
19. **Greenstein, J. P., and M. Winitz (ed.).** 1961. Histidine, p. 1971–1995. *In* Chemistry of the amino acids, vol. 3. John Wiley and Sons, New York.

20. **Haavik, H. I.** 1974. Studies on the formation of bacitracin by *Bacillus licheniformis*: effect of glucose. J. Gen. Microbiol. 81:383–390.
21. **Haavik, H. I.** 1974. Studies on the formation of bacitracin by *Bacillus licheniformis*: effect of inorganic phosphate. J. Gen. Microbiol. 84:226–230.
22. **Haavik, H. I.** 1974. Studies on the formation of bacitracin by *Bacillus licheniformis*: role of catabolite repression and organic acids. J. Gen. Microbiol. 84:321–326.
23. **Haavik, H. I., and Ø. Froyshov.** 1975. Function of peptide antibiotics in producer organisms. Nature (London) 254:79–82.
24. **Hendlin, D.** 1949. The nutritional requirements of a bacitracin producing strain of *Bacillus subtilis*. Arch. Biochem. 24:435–446.
25. **Hodgson, B.** 1970. Possible roles for antibiotics and other biologically active peptides at specific stages during sporulation of *Bacillaceae*. J. Theor. Biol. 30:111–119.
26. **Hook, D. J., and L. C. Vining.** 1973. Biosynthetic precursors of etamycin, a peptidolactone antibiotic from *Streptomyces griseoviridus*. Can. J. Biochem. 51:1630–1637.
27. **Hubbard, C. V., and H. H. Thornberry.** 1950. Utilization of some organic acids by *Streptomyces griseus* for streptomycin production and growth. Trans. Ill. State Acad. Sci. 43:61–74.
28. **Jarvis, F. G., and M. J. Johnson.** 1947. The role of the constituents of synthetic media for penicillin production. J. Am. Chem. Soc. 69:3010–3017.
29. **Katz, E.** 1967. Biogenesis of the actinomycins, p. 276–341. *In* D. Gottlieb and P. D. Shaw (ed.), Antibiotics. II. Biosynthesis. Springer-Verlag, Berlin.
30. **Katz, E.** 1974. Controlled biosynthesis of actinomycins. Cancer Chemother. Rep. 58:83–91.
31. **Katz, E., and W. A. Goss.** 1959. Controlled biosynthesis of actinomycin with sarcosine. Biochem. J. 73:458–465.
32. **Katz, E., P. Pienta, and A. Sivak.** 1958. The role of nutrition in the synthesis of actinomycin. Appl. Microbiol. 6:236–241.
33. **Katz, E., C. R. Waldron, and M. L. Meloni.** 1961. Role of valine and isoleucine as regulators of actinomycin peptide formation by *Streptomyces chrysomallus*. J. Bacteriol. 82:600–608.
34. **Katz, E., and H. Weissbach.** 1963. Incorporation of ^{14}C-labeled amino acids into actinomycin and protein by *Streptomyces antibioticus*. J. Biol. Chem. 238:666–675.
35. **Katz, E., M. Wise, and H. Weissbach.** 1965. Actinomycin biosynthesis. Differential effect of chloramphenicol on protein and peptide antibiotic synthesis. J. Biol. Chem. 240:3071–3078.
36. **Magasanik, B.** 1961. Catabolite repression. Cold Spring Harbor Symp. Quant. Biol. 26:249–256.
37. **Mahler, H. R., and E. H. Cordes.** 1966. Biological chemistry. Harper and Row, New York.
38. **Majumdar, S. K., and S. K. Bose.** 1960. Trace element requirements for *Bacillus subtilis* for mycobacillin formation. J. Bacteriol. 79:564–565.
39. **Majumdar, M. K., and S. K. Majumdar.** 1965. Effects of minerals on neomycin production by *Streptomyces fradiae*. Appl. Microbiol. 13:190–193.
40. **Meienhofer, J., and E. Atherton.** 1973. Structure-activity relationships in the actinomycins. Adv. Appl. Microbiol. 16:203–300.
41. **Naftalin, L.** 1948. Quantitative chromatographic estimation of α-amino acids. Nature (London) 161:763.
42. **Paigen, K., and B. Williams.** 1970. Catabolite repression and other control mechanisms in carbohydrate utilization. Adv. Microb. Physiol. 4:251–324.
43. **Paritskaya, N. S., E. T. Nikitina, and L. V. Kalakoutskii.** 1974. Growth features of *Actinomyces roseoflavus* var. roseofungini on synthetic medium with D-fructose. Mikrobiologia 43:686–690.
44. **Phibbs, P. V., Jr., and R. G. Eagon.** 1970. Transport and phosphorylation of glucose, fructose and mannitol by *Pseudomonas aeruginosa*. Arch. Biochem. Biophys. 138:470–482.
45. **Principe, P. A., and H. H. Thornberry.** 1952. Effect of cobalt on production of streptomycin and vitamin B-12 by *Streptomyces griseus*. Phytopathology 42:123–126.
46. **Rickenberg, H. V.** 1974. Cyclic AMP in prokaryotes. Annu. Rev. Microbiol. 28:353–369.
47. **Rogers, T. O., and J. Birnbaum.** 1974. Biosynthesis of fosfomycin by *Streptomyces fradiae*. Antimicrob. Agents Chemother. 5:121–132.
48. **Romano, A. H., and W. J. Nickerson.** 1958. Utilization of amino acids as carbon sources by *Streptomyces fradiae*. J. Bacteriol. 75:161–166.
49. **Sabater, B., J. Sebastian, and C. Asensio.** 1972. Identification and properties of an inducible mannokinase from *Streptomyces violaceoruber*. Biochim. Biophys. Acta 284:406–413.
50. **Sabater, B., J. Sebastian, and C. Asensio.** 1972. Identification and properties of an inducible and highly specific fructokinase from *Streptomyces violaceoruber*. Biochim. Biophys. Acta 284:414–420.
51. **Sivak, A., M. L. Meloni, F. Nobili, and E. Katz.** 1962. Biosynthesis of the actinomycin chromophore. Studies with DL-7α-^{14}C-tryptophan and L-Me-^{14}C-methionine. Biochim. Biophys. Acta 57:283–289.
52. **Smith, I. (ed.).** 1960. Sugars, p. 246–260. *In* Chromatographic and electrophoretic techniques, vol. 1. W. Heinemann Medical Books Ltd., London.
53. **Vandamme, E. J., and A. L. Demain.** 1976. Nutritional Requirements of the gramicidin S fermentation. Prog. Ind. Microbiol. 17:51–60.
54. **Vincente, M., M. A. dePedro, G. deTorrontegui, R. Diaz, and J. L. Canovas.** 1975. Uptake of fructose by *Pseudomonas putida*. Arch. Microbiol. 102:163–166.
55. **Weinberg, E. D.** 1970. Biosynthesis of secondary metabolites; roles of trace metals. Adv. Microb. Physiol. 4:1–44.
56. **Weinberg, E. D.** 1971. Secondary metabolism: raison d'etre. Perspect. Biol. Med. 14:565–577.
57. **Weinberg, E. D.** 1974. Secondary metabolism: control by temperature and inorganic phosphate. Dev. Ind. Microbiol. 15:70–81.
58. **Yajima, T., M. A. Grigg, and E. Katz.** 1972. Biosynthesis of antibiotic peptides with isoleucine stereoisomers. Arch. Biochem. Biophys. 151:565–575.
59. **Yajima, T., K. T. Mason, and E. Katz.** 1975. Branched-chain amino acid substitutions in the biosynthesis of the antibiotic actinomycin. Antimicrob. Agents Chemother. 7:773–780.
60. **Yajima, T., K. T. Mason, and E. Katz.** 1976. Biogenetic origin of the D-isoleucine and *N*-methyl-L-alloisoleucine residues in the actinomycins. Antimicrob. Agents Chemother. 9:224–232.

ANTIMICROBIAL AGENTS AND CHEMOTHERAPY, Feb. 1977, p. 291-298
Vol. 11, No. 2

Relationship Between the Physicochemical Nature of Human Interferon, the Cell Induced, and the Inducing Agent

THOMAS C. CESARIO,[1]* PATRICIA J. SCHRYER, AND JEREMIAH G. TILLES
Department of Medicine, California College of Medicine, University of California, Irvine, California 92664

Received for publication 15 August 1976

To determine the basis for differences in interferons previously noted by others, we prepared five types of human interferon, namely interferon induced in muscle skin fibroblasts using complexed polyinosinic:polycytidylic acid (IC) and Newcastle disease virus (NDV), and interferon induced in leukocytes using IC, NDV, and phytohemagglutinin. We determined the molecular weight, isoelectric point, inactivation rate at 56°C and structural activity relationships for each interferon. Significant differences between these interferons were found, many of which seem related to the cell induced rather than the inducer. We believe these findings have important pharmacological implications for the use of interferon in man.

Recent investigations have established that human fibroblast interferon induced by complexed polyinosinic:polycytidylic acid (IC) is different from human leukocyte interferon induced by viruses (6, 9, 18, 20). Dissimilarities between these two interferons have been found in their antigenicity (9), in the circumstances under which they will renature (18), and in their sensitivity to guanidine (6) and heat (20). Although many issues remain unsolved, particularly pressing questions which are still unanswered include the following: which factors dictate when a given interferon will be elaborated; is there a molecular basis for the observed dissimilarities; and how many human interferons can be expected to exist? The answers to these questions may have particular relevance for identifying a human interferon species which will be pharmacologically superior for clinical application.

We addressed these questions by preparing five varieties of human interferon: interferon prepared in human fibroblasts (muscle skin fibroblast [MSF] cells) using IC and Newcastle disease virus (NDV) as inducers and interferon prepared in leukocytes using IC, NDV, and phytohemagglutinin (PHA) as inducers. We compared these interferons in the crude state with regards to physical properties and sensitivities to chemical reagents known to attack specific bonds and groups. However, because the data presented here were determined on crude interferon, they cannot be considered absolute and could be updated when studies on purified preparations are possible. Nevertheless, since each of the interferons was studied under identical circumstances, the resulting data are clearly valid for comparing interferons and offer insight into the occasional differences among crude interferons that have been observed previously. Additionally, this information will be of value in deciding on purification schemes and ultimately in determining what alteration in native crude interferon (i.e., as it exists in its native state) are caused by a particular purification sequence.

Indeed it has been possible to determine that the cell induced exerts an important influence on the properties of the interferon secreted, that the circumstances of the induction may alter at least some of these properties, and that the observed differences appear to be associated with structural dissimilarities within the interferon molecule.

MATERIALS AND METHODS

Preparation of virus-, IC-, and PHA-induced human interferon in WBCs (WBC-NDV, WBC-IC, and WBC-PHA). After separation by low-speed centrifugation from blood acidified with ammonium chloride for 10 min, human white blood cells (WBCs) were washed twice with Leibovitz medium (L-15). The cells were subsequently suspended at a density of 10 million/ml in L-15 supplemented with 5% fetal calf serum (FCS) and rolled in test tubes for 18 h at 37°C in the presence of NDV (multiplicity of 100 median egg infectious dose [EID_{50}] per cell) for preparation of WBC-NDV interferon. The interferon-containing medium was separated by pelleting the cells at low-speed centrifugation and then sequentially dialyzed against 0.1 M citric acid at pH 2.7 for 5 days and phosphate-buffered saline (PBS) at pH 7.4 for 24 h.

[1] Present address: University of California Irvine Medical Center, 101 City Drive South, Orange, CA 92668.

After centrifugation at 25,000 rpm for 90 min in a Beckman SW27 rotor, 2-ml aliquots of the pooled interferon-containing supernatant were frozen at −80°C. For WBC-IC, the cells, at a similar concentration, were suspended in a solution of IC (10 μg/ml) and diethylaminoethyl dextran (DEAE-D) (100 μg/ml) in PBS, rolled at 4°C for 1 h, washed three times with supplemented L-15, and rolled at 37°C for a further 18 h. The interferon-containing medium was then separated from the cells by low-speed centrifugation, aliquoted, and stored as noted above.

For WBC-PHA, fresh human leukocytes as described above were incubated with a 1:400 dilution of phytohemagglutinin P (Difco) as 2.0-ml aliquots in tissue culture tubes rolled for 18 h at 37°C. After centrifugation at 1,000 rpm for 10 min, the pooled supernatants were dialyzed in PBS (pH 7.4) for 24 h before freezing and storing at −80°C in 2.0-ml aliquots. Separate preparations of WBC-PHA were acid-dialyzed at pH 2.7 as noted above for WBC-NDV. Acid-dialyzed WBC-PHA was found to react identically to PBS-dialyzed WBC-PHA in the heat inactivation and chemical stability experiments, and was not used in the molecular weight and isoelectric focusing studies.

Preparation of IC-induced human interferon in MSF cells (MSF-IC). MSF were exposed to 10 μg of poly IC per ml and 100 μg of DEAE-D (molecular weight 2,000,000) per ml for 3 h, washed three times, and incubated overnight in L-15 supplemented with 5% FCS. The interferon-containing medium was then harvested and stored at −80°C in 2.0-ml aliquots.

Preparation of virus-induced interferon in MSF cells (MSF-NDV). Confluent MSF cells were inoculated with NDV (multiplicity of 30 EID_{50} per cell) and allowed to incubate overnight. The next morning the interferon-containing tissue culture medium was harvested and processed identically to the WBC interferons described above with sequential dialysis versus 0.1 M citric acid and PBS before centrifugation at 25,000 rpm for 90 min. Aliquots (2 ml) of the pooled interferon-containing supernatant were frozen at −80°C.

Preparation of virus-induced chicken interferon. Monolayers of primary chicken embryo fibroblasts (CEF) were exposed to Sindbis virus at a multiplicity of 1 plaque-forming unit per cell for 1 h at 37°C. Further incubation at 37°C in Geys balanced salt solution (BSS), supplemented with 5% calf serum, was carried out for 48 h. The interferon-containing medium was then sequentially dialyzed against 0.1 M citric acid at pH 2.7 for 24 h and Geys BSS at pH 7.4 for 24 h. The dialysate was distributed into 10-ml aliquots and stored at 4°C.

Interferon assays. Human interferon was assayed on MSF using vesicular stomatitis virus (VSV) as the challenge virus. The plaque reduction and microtiter techniques utilized were described previously (4, 19). In such assays, interferon-treated cell monolayers are washed free of test samples prior to virus challenge. Chicken interferon assays were performed on CEF by plaque reduction with VSV as the challenge virus (19).

Heat inactivation. Aliquots of each interferon, containing 1,000 to 2,000 interferon units per ml, were placed in a 56°C water bath. At indicated intervals (10, 20, 30, 60, and 120 min), samples were withdrawn, placed in an ice bath, and titered immediately. Comparisons of differences in the rate of heat inactivation between the fibroblast and leukocyte interferon were performed twice.

Electrofocusing. Electrofocusing was performed by the technique of Wrigley (21). Samples containing 10,000 to 80,000 interferon units were exhaustively dialyzed for 24 h against 0.05 M PBS at 4°C and then mixed with appropriate amounts of catalyst solution, acrylamide solution, and carrier ampholytes. Each interferon was focused either in both the pH 5 to 8 and 3 to 10 ampholyte ranges or twice in the pH 3 to 10 range. A current of 1 mA per tube was applied in a Buchler disc electrophoresis apparatus. The voltage was maintained constant and the amperage was allowed to diminish. Electrofocusing was performed at 4°C for periods ranging from 5 to 25 h. The gels were subsequently sliced into 12 to 15 equal segments, each of which wes homogenized in 0.5 ml of distilled water. After a measurement of pH and an overnight incubation at 4°C, 0.2 ml of a solution containing antibiotics and 4% FCS was added to each fraction prior to assay for interferon activity. Linear pH gradients were established in all experiments.

Molecular weight determinations. Estimations of molecular weight were performed on a column of Sephadex G-200 superfine, which was extensively washed with 0.05 M PBS. The void volume was marked with dextran blue, and the column was calibrated with proteins of known molecular weight. Interferon samples containing 15,000 to 40,000 interferon units in 0.8 ml were applied to the column through a flow adaptor. The specimens were eluted using inverse flow of 0.05 M PBS at pH 7.0 in general; fractions of 0.5 ml were collected at a flow rate of 0.5 ml/h. At the completion of the run, each fraction was passed through a 300-nm membrane filter (Millipore Corp.) and titered immediately. Molecular weight estimates were made by the method of Andrews (1). Each interferon was chromatographed at least twice on Sephadex G-200 superfine. MSF-IC and WBC-NDV were also run on Sepharose 6B.

Additionally, both MSF-IC and WBC-IC interferons were acidified and chromatographed at pH 2.7 using a 0.05 M citric acid eluant on both G-200 and G-75 superfine columns.

Chemical reagents. Solutions were prepared immediately prior to use with reagent-grade chemicals. The diluent for dithiothreitol and urea was PBS containing 250 μg of streptomycin per ml and 150 μg of potassium penicillin G per ml; for iodoacetamide and sodium periodate the diluent was distilled water. Solutions of urea and iodoacetamide were sterilized by membrane filtration (Millipore Corp.). The preparation of acetic anhydride solution occurred in two steps: first, saturated sodium acetate was added to an equal volume of PBS containing the interferon to be exposed; second, acetic anhydride was added with vigorous shaking until its desired final concentration was achieved.

Some preparations of 6 M urea (marked with footnote *c* in Table 3) were either rendered free of extraneous ions through passage on columns of Amberlite MB-3 or purchased "free of cyanide" contamination from Schwarz-Mann.

Exposure of interferon to reagents. One-half milliliter of each interferon was mixed with a like volume of dithiothreitol, allowed to incubate under the conditions defined in Table 1, and then diluted to the appropriate volume in L-15 medium supplemented with FCS (20 ml/100 ml), glutamine (30 μg/ml), arginine (90 μg/ml), glucose (1 μg/ml), potassium penicillin G (150 μg/ml), and streptomycin (250 μg/ml). With all other reagents, interferon was added in 0.2- to 2.0-ml quantities to the reagent solution to make the final volume of 8 ml. When the tests were performed in microtiter, the proportions of the interferon reagent solutions were maintained as above, but the final volume was only 2 ml.

As a control for each test, interferon was also exposed, in the same concentration and under the same conditions, to an identical solution which lacked the test reagents. It was deemed appropriate to make an exception for the interferon control of the iodoacetamide test. Here, to simulate the molarity of the iodoacetamide test solution, 10 mM dextrose was added to the water diluent of the interferon control. Table 1 lists the conditions under which interferon was exposed to the various reagents.

To avert cytotoxicity by test reagents upon exposure to cell culture, test and control solutions were routinely dialyzed against 250 volumes of Geys BSS for 24 h prior to assay for interferon. Dialysis was found to be unnecessary in the case of dithiothreitol and was therefore omitted. The results reported are based on interferon assays which, in every case, were devoid of cytopathic effect due to the test reagent.

To determine if observed differences between human and chicken interferons were artifactual, mixtures containing interferon from both species were also exposed to reagent and control solutions. At the completion of such a test, interferon was assayed both on chicken and human cells.

RESULTS

Thermal sensivitity. Figure 1 demonstrates the decay in biological activity of each interferon upon exposure to heat. Although every type of human interferon tested was inactivated at 56°C, WBC-NDV and WBC-IC interferons were the least susceptible, both by being slowly inactivated initially and by retaining significant activity at 2 h (Table 2). WBC-PHA was more heat labile than were the other two WBC interferons in that it resembled the fibroblast interferons in the first 30 min of exposure but differed from the latter at 2 h time by retaining a small amount of activity (whereas the fibroblast interferons were devoid of all biological activity). Repeat testing gave similar results.

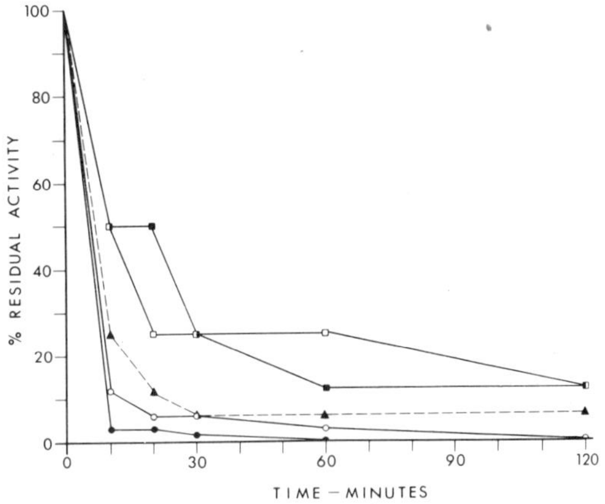

FIG. 1. *Inactivation of human interferon at 56°C. Symbols:* ●, *MSF-NDV;* ○, *MSF-IC;* ■, *WBC-NDV;* □, *WBC-IC;* ▲, *WBC-PHA.*

TABLE 1. *Conditions for exposure of interferon to reagents*

Reagent	Concn (mM)	Temp (°C)	Duration of exposure prior to dialysis at 4°C (min)	pH
Dithiothreitol	5	25	30	7
Urea	6 or 8 M	25	75	7
Iodoacetamide	10	25	24 h	7
Acetic anhydride	100	4	60	5.8
Periodate	33	4	180	6.8

Isoelectric points. The isoelectric points (pIs) determined by peaks of interferon activity after electrofocusing can be seen in Table 2, whereas Fig. 2 demonstrates the pattern of activity after this procedure for MSF-IC and WBC-NDV. Human MSF-IC had a single peak of activity with pI very close to pH 5. MSF-NDV activity resembled the MSF-IC activity, in that the majority of activity resided in a peak found close to pH 5. On the other hand, interferons derived from leukocytes had a much broader range of activity with peaks observed at both ends of the activity range. The more acid peak of the leukocyte-derived interferons induced by NDV and by IC appeared to be close to pH 5.3, whereas the more basic peak was at pH 6.9. WBC-PHA also focused over a broad pH range, with two peaks at slightly more acidic pH values than observed from the other WBC interferons. When fraction pools of WBC-NDV interferon containing the pH ranges of 6.5 to 7.0 or 5.3 to 5.7 were re-electrofocused, single peaks were then identified with pIs identical to those of the initial interferon fractions. Recovery rates for interferons during the electrofo-

TABLE 2. *Physical properties of crude human interferons*

Interferon	Stability at 56°C heat		Mol wt	pIs
	Half-life (min)	Residual activity after 2 h (%)		
Fibroblast (MSF)				
IC	3	0	300,000[a], 14,000[b]	5.1
NDV	2	0	25,000[a]	4.8
Leukocyte (WBC)				
IC	10	12	12,000[a]	5.5, 6.9
NDV	10	12	25,000[a]	5.3, 6.9
PHA	5	6	12,000[a]	4.9, 6.5

[a] As determined by chromatography at pH 7.0.
[b] As determined by chromatography at pH 2.7.

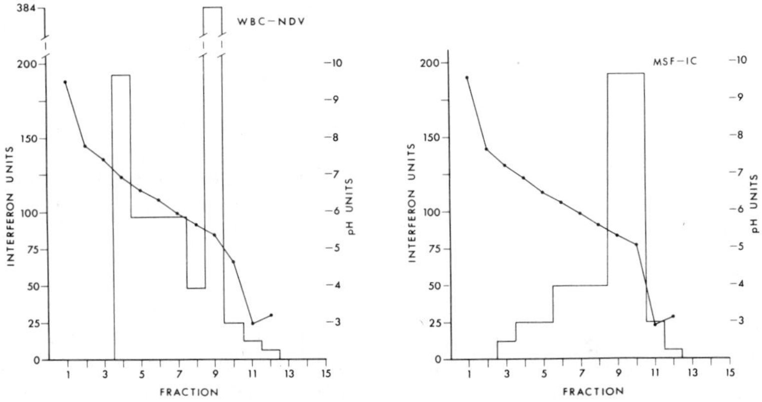

FIG. 2. *Representative patterns of interferon activity after electrofocusing. MSF-IC interferon electrofocused on pH 3 to 10 ampholytes, 9,600 units electrofocused, 38% recovery. WBC-NDV electrofocused on pH 5 to 8 ampholytes, 19,200 units applied, 100% recovery.*

cusing procedure ranged from 10 to 100%, with a mean of 46%.

Molecular weight determination. When chromatography was carried out at pH 7.0, MSF-IC interferon had an estimated molecular weight of 300,000 and MSF-NDV interferon had a molecular weight of 25,000 (Table 2). Leukocyte interferon also had a molecular weight of 25,000 when induced by NDV, but only 12,000 when induced by either IC or PHA. Both fibroblast and leukocyte interferons induced by IC were acidified to pH 2.7 and chromatographed at these lower pH ranges. Acid chromatography of MSF-IC interferon resulted in the absence of a peak at 300,000 molecular weight and in the appearance of a peak antiviral activity at 14,000 molecular weight. Occasionally under these circumstances a second activity peak, representing up to 50% of the recovered biological activity, was detected at 25,000 molecular weight. In contrast, no change occurred in the estimated molecular weight for WBC-IC interferon when chromatographed at acid pH. Molecular weight estimations performed at pH 7 for MSF-IC and WBC-NDV and at pH 2.7 for MSF-IC are shown in Fig. 3. Repeat runs of each of the interferons tested always gave identical results. Recovery rates following chromatography ranged from 5 to 30%, with a mean of 16%.

Chemical sensitivity. All five human interferons tested differed from chicken interferon in two major regards (Table 3): (i) each was considerably more resistant to disulfide bond reduction with dithiothreitol, and (ii) each was more sensitive to disruption of hydrogen bonds by urea. Among the human interferons, those derived from leukocytes were relatively less sensitive to urea than those derived from fibroblasts. Furthermore, whereas the three leukocyte interferons resembled chicken interferon in being completely resistant to attack on sulfhydryl groups by iodoacetamide, both fibroblast interferons were partially inactivated by the reagent. These differences between human leukocyte and human fibroblast interferons are

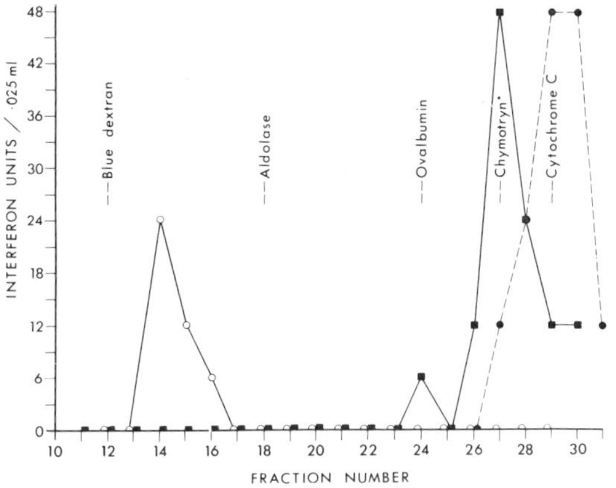

FIG. 3. *Representative molecular weight estimates confirmed from multiple determinations on G-200 superfine column (1.6 by 20 cm) at 6 to 12°C. Chromatography performed at pH 7 for WBC-NDV and at pH 7.0 and 2.7 as noted below for MSF-IC. Column calibrated with dextran blue, aldolase, ovalbumin, chymotrypsinogen, and cytochrome c. Peak fractions of the molecular weight markers were eluted and measured at 280-μm optical density. Fractions containing the peak concentrations of each marker are designated above. Symbols: ○, MSF-IC interferon at pH 7.0, 15,600 units applied to column, 21% recovered; ■, WBC-NDV at pH 7.0, 30,200 units applied, 27% recovered; ●, MSF-IC interferon at pH 2.7, 32,000 units applied to column, 30% recovery.*

both highly significant ($P > 0.01$, Student's t test). Like chicken interferon, all five human interferons were inactivated by acetic anhydride and sodium periodate.

DISCUSSION

The above observations permit both a comparison of interferons induced by different classes of inducer in the same cell type and a comparison of interferons induced by a single kind of inducer in cells of different types. Thus, it is possible to decide the relative role of cell and inducer in determining the nature of the interferon produced. With the exception of WBC-PHA interferon (as noted below), it is apparent that interferons derived from a given cell type tend to resemble each other in pattern of activity after electrofocusing, in heat stability at 56°C, and in chemical reactivity. Such interferons differ only in molecular weights. In contrast, interferons induced by a given inducer in cells of different type resemble each other primarily in molecular weight. Our data, thus, indicate that interferons derived from a given cell by different inducers are very similar whereas interferons stimulated by the same inducer in different cells are substantially different. These findings are not unexpected as isoenzymes have long been noted to have differing properties depending on the cell in which they are produced (5). In view of the fact that differences between interferons from different cell types involve charge, heat stability, and chemical stability (all properties dependent on molecular characteristics), we conclude that there are undoubtedly structural differences between interferons from different cells. Our hypothesis is strengthened by the recent demonstration by Havell et al. (9) of antigenic differences between fibroblast IC- and leukocyte virus-induced interferons. Nevertheless, it does appear that the inducer may exert some influence on at least one physical property, mainly molecular weight, although further investigation may show this property to be only a manifestation of dissimilar packaging. In discussing the effects of the inducer, it is important to point out that virus-induced interferons require acid dialysis to eliminate infectious particles; thus, it is necessary to ask what influence this process may have on the physicochemical properties we have reported. In considering the effects of acid dialysis on the interferon species studied here, it is important to compare the properties of the interferons induced in each cell type by viruses and by IC. In the case of virus, acid treatment was undertaken to eliminate the infectivity of the residual inducer, whereas in the case of the IC, which has no infectivity, acid treatment was unnecessary. Although differing with respect to acid treatment, interferons induced by the two inducers in a single cell strain (either leukocytes or fibroblasts) have identical electrofocusing properties, rates of heat inactivation, and chemical stabilities. If the acid had affected these properties, the interferons induced in the same cell by different inducers might well have been dissimilar rather than similar as was observed here. The reverse argument also holds; i.e., the two acid-treated interferons (i.e., WBC-NDV and MSF-NDV) are dissimilar as are the two nonacid interferons (i.e., WBC-IC and MSF-IC). If the acid treatment was responsible for all the differences observed here, these acid-dialyzed interferons should have been identical as should the nonacid-dialyzed species. In the case of molecular weights, where differences exist between interferons induced in the same cell type, acid treatment could be responsible. However, if acid artifactually creates a difference where one does not exist, it would only strengthen our thesis that the cell induced is the important determinant of the properties of native interferons.

TABLE 3. *Interferon activity after exposure to reagents*

Test	Reagent	Target	Interferon activity (%)					
			Fibroblast			Leukocyte (human)		
			Chicken virus	Human		Virus	IC	PHA
				Virus	IC			
1	Dithiothreitol	S—S	0[a]	50	100	50	50	100
2					67	70		100
3[b]			0		50			
4[b]			0		100			
5[b]			0		87			
1	Urea	H—H	72	3[c]	0[c]	24[c]	14[c]	25[c]
2				6[c]	0[c]	20[c]		50[c]
3				12	0	10		
4					1	18		
5					5			
6[b]			53		0			
1	Iodoacetamide	S—H	100	25	20	50	100	100
2				25	24	100	100	100
3					54	100		
4					35	100		
5					50	100		
6[b]			100		25			
7					50			
1	Acetic Anhydride	NH_2	0	12	6	0	6	3
2			0		1	0		
3[b]			6		6			
1	Periodate	—C(OH)—C(OH)—	0	6		0	6	3
2						0		
3[b]			0		0			
4[b]			0		0			

[a] Expressed as percentage of the activity of the same interferon stock treated simultaneously with the respective control solution.
[b] Test in which a mixture of human and chicken interferon was exposed to the treatment solutions.
[c] Test using deionized 6 M urea.

In addition to the interferons discussed above, human leukocytes may produce a really different interferon during transformation. Thus WBC-PHA, although being identical to other leukocyte interferons in most of the parameters studied here, is significantly more sensitive to thermal inactivation than either WBC-NDV or WBC-IC interferon. We interpret this difference to indicate there are probable structural dissimilarities between WBC-PHA interferon and the other two leukocyte interferons. Considering the unique role leukocytes play in the immune system, and the large number of lymphokines already described, it would not be surprising if immune interferon were structurally different from interferon induced by leukocytes in stationary phase.

It should be noted that our estimated molecular weight of 300,000 for MSF-IC interferon is larger than a previous estimate of 96,000 for the molecular weight of fibroblast IC interferon made by Carter et al. (Bacteriol. Proc., p. 213, 1971). However, in both cases it would appear likely that the large size indicates that the interferon is complexed to another protein molecule. Thus acidification and chromatography at pH 2.7 does result in a drop of molecular weight to 14,000. This lower molecular weight estimate is in close agreement with an earlier observation also made by Carter et al. (3) who reported a 12,000-molecular-weight form of IC-induced fibroblast interferon. However, they made these observations after low-salt dialysis, while we found acid chromatography was necessary to reveal the smaller form. More recently, Reynolds and Pitha (16) reported MSF-IC interferon to have a molecular weight of 25,000 when estimates were performed after sodium dodecyl sulfate electrophoresis under reducing circumstances. We find that IC-induced leukocyte interferon has no large-molecular-weight form; thus, the ability of MSF-IC but not WBC-IC interferon to complex (or less likely to aggregate) can be considered a manifestation of another dissimilarity in physical properties between the two IC-induced interferons.

Our molecular weight estimates for virus-induced interferons both in fibroblasts and in leukocytes are in agreement with those reported by others. Thus, Merigan et al. (12) estimated molecular weights of fibroblast virus-induced interferons at 26,000, whereas Falcoff et al. (7) determined the molecular weight of virus-induced leukocyte interferons to also be 26,000. We are currently exploring the reasons for the differences in molecular weights between the virus-induced interferons and the other interferons.

The pIs for fibroblast interferons are in agreement with those of Stancek et al. (17) and Carter (2), who used IC and NDV, respectively, as the inducer. However, Stancek et al. found different results for virus-induced fibroblast interferon. They used interferon induced by ultraviolet-irradiated NDV (NDV-UV) in human foreskin cells and found a pattern of interferon activity that appeared to have several major activity peaks focusing over a range which began at pH 4.5 and extended to a pH at or above 8. For virus-induced leukocyte interferon using NDV-UV; this group of investigators found the same two peaks we have identified as well as a third peak with a pI at or above 9.

Our findings regarding thermal stability of fibroblast interferon are in keeping with the results of Marshall et al. (11) who found a half-life of 5 to 7 min at 56°C for interferons induced by either IC or virus. For leukocyte interferon induced by virus, our results are consistent with those of Mogensen and Cantell (15), who found the concentrated crude preparation lost 1 log of activity in 12 h, and Valle et al. (20), who reported fibroblast interferon to be more sensitive to 56°C than virus-induced leukocyte interferons after 1 h at 56°C. The finding of the latter authors that PHA-induced leukocyte interferon is more sensitive to 56°C than fibroblast interferon is at variance with our results.

Our results on the stability of chicken interferon to the chemical reagents tested are in complete accord with those published by Fantes and O'Neill (8) and others. Although there have been no comparable studies of human interferon, our findings that human interferon differs from chicken interferon in its resistance to disulfide bond reduction and sensitivity to attack on hydrogen bonds could have been anticipated from work that has been carried out on other mammalian species. Thus, Ke and Ho have found rabbit interferon to be resistant to disulfide bond reduction with 2-mercaptoethanol (10). Merigan et al., on the other hand, have demonstrated that mouse interferon is sensitive to disruption of hydrogen bonds with 8 M urea (13). Thus, the unexpected differences between human and chicken interferon reported here do have analogies in certain other mammalian species. Although Mogensen and Cantell (15) have reported human leukocyte interferon to be susceptible to the effects of mercaptoethanol, another disulfide bond-reducing agent, their conditions were more harsh than those used here and hence are not comparable to ours. We find certain differences in stability between leukocyte and fibroblast interferons. Thus, all three leukocyte-derived interferons are more resistant to hydrogen bond attack and to sulfhydryl oxidation than the fibroblast interferon.

It is clear from the information reported here that different forms of human interferon exist. Furthermore, as we have noted above, the cell type appears to be more significant than the inducing agent in determining the characteristics of the interferon produced. It is important to add that interferons derived from cells other than fibroblasts or leukocytes may be found to differ from those already described. Since human interferons do differ in size, charge, and stability, it is very likely that they will be found to differ in absorption, distribution, metabolism, and elimination in man. Furthermore, the procedures for purification and the relative yield of biologically active products will also necessarily vary. Finally, it is entirely possible that there may be found differences in biological function among these interferons. It is likely that efforts to provide a therapeutic preparation of interferon will be most productive if these differences among the interferons are clearly recognized.

ACKNOWLEDGMENTS

This work was supported, in part, by grant no. 05-041-012 from the National Aeronautics and Space Administration and by Public Health Service grant TO1 AI00466 from the National Institute of Allergy and Infectious Diseases.

LITERATURE CITED

1. **Andrews, P.** 1964. Estimation of the molecular weight of proteins by Sephadex gel-filtration. Biochem. J. 91:222–223.

2. **Carter, W. A.** 1970. Interferon: evidence for subunit structure. Proc. Natl. Acad. Sci. U.S.A. **67**:620–628.
3. **Carter, W. A., and P. M. Pitha.** 1971. Structural requirements of ribopolymers for induction of human interferon: evidence for interferon subunits, p. 89–105. *In* R. F. Beers, Jr., and W. Brann (ed.), Biological effects of polynucleotides. Springer-Verlag, New York.
4. **Cesario, T. C., and J. G. Tilles.** 1973. Inactivation of human interferon by urine. J. Infect. Dis. **127**:311–314.
5. **Dixon, M., and E. Webb.** 1964. Isoenzymes, p. 656–659. *In* enzymes, p. 656–659. Academic Press Inc., New York.
6. **Edy, V. G., A. Billiau, M. Joniau, and P. DeSomer.** 1974. Stabilization of mouse and human interferons by acid pH against inactivation due to shaking and guanidine hydrochloride. Proc. Soc. Exp. Biol. Med. **146**:249–253.
7. **Falcoff, E., F. Fournier, and C. Chany.** 1966. Etude comparative des poids molecularres de deux interferons humans produits in vitro. Ann. Inst. Pasteur (Paris) 111:242–248.
8. **Fantes, K. H., and C. F. O'Neill.** 1964. Some similarities between a viral inhibitor of plant origin and chick interferon. Nature (London) **203**:1048–1050.
9. **Havell, E. A., B. Berman, C. A. Ogburn, K. Berg, K. Paucker, and J. Vilcek.** 1975. Two antigenically distinct species of human interferon. Proc. Natl. Acad. Sci. U.S.A. **72**:2185–2187.
10. **Ke, Y., and M. Ho.** 1968. Studies of the physico-chemical inactivation of rabbit interferon. Proc. Soc. Exp. Biol. Med. **129**:433–438.
11. **Marshall, L. W., P. M. Pitha, and W. A. Carter.** 1972. Inactivation of interferon: the effects of protonation. Virology **48**:607–611.
12. **Merigan, T. C., D. F. Gregory, and J. K. Petralli.** 1966. Physical properties of human interferon prepared in vitro and in vivo. Virology **29**:515–522.
13. **Merigan, T. C., C. A. Winget, and C. B. Dixon.** 1975. Purification and characterization of vertebrate interferon. J. Mol. Biol. **13**:679–691.
14. **Mogensen, K. E., and K. Cantell.** 1973. Stability of human leukocyte interferon toward heat. Acta Pathol. Microbiol. Scand. Sec. B **80**:382.
15. **Mogensen, K. E., and K. Cantell.** 1974. Human leukocyte interferon: a role for disulphide bonds. J. Gen. Virol. **22**:95–103.
16. **Reynolds, F., and P. M. Pitha.** 1975. Molecular weight study of human fibroblast interferon. Biochem. Biophys. Res. Commun. **65**:107–112.
17. **Stancek, D., M. Gressnerove, and K. Paucker.** 1970. Isoelectric components of mouse, human and rabbit interferons. Virology **41**:740–750.
18. **Stewart, W. E., P. DeSomer, V. Edy, K. Paucker, K. Berg, and C. Ogburn.** 1975. Distinct molecular species of human interferons: requirements for stabilization and reactivation of human leukocytes and fibroblast interferons. J. Gen. Virol. **26**:327–331.
19. **Tilles, J. G., and M. Finland.** 1968. Microassay for human and chick cell interferons. Appl. Microbiol. **16**:1706–1707.
20. **Valle, M., G. Jordan, S. Haahr, and T. Merigan.** 1975. Characteristics of immune interferon produced in human lymphocyte cultures compared to other human interferons. J. Immunol. **115**:230–233.
21. **Wrigley, C.** 1968. Gel electrofocusing—a technique for analyzing multiple protein samples by isoelectric focusing. Sci. Tools **15**:18–32.

Antimicrobial Agents and Chemotherapy, Feb. 1977, p. 299–306
Vol. 11, No. 2

Combined Antiviral Effects of Interferon, Adenine Arabinoside, Hypoxanthine Arabinoside, and Adenine Arabinoside-5′-Monophosphate in Human Fibroblast Cultures

YVONNE J. BRYSON[1] AND L. H. KRONENBERG*

Department of Pediatrics, School of Medicine, University of California at San Diego, La Jolla, California 92093

Received for publication 24 September 1976

Adenine arabinoside and human interferon are currently being evaluated in clinical trials against herpes- and poxvirus infections. Interferon production is also a normal antiviral response. It is therefore important to examine the combined actions of interferon and antiviral arabinosides for possible synergy or antagonism. We have examined the antiviral activities of human fibroblast interferon, adenine arabinoside, hypoxanthine arabinoside, and adenine arabinoside 5′-monophosphate individually, using plaque inhibition of vaccinia and herpes simplex type 2 viruses in human skin fibroblast cultures. By combining doses of interferon and arabinosides that, acting alone, give intermediate degrees of plaque inhibition, we were able to compare the combined antiviral activity with that calculated from the activity of each inhibitor alone, assuming that the activities are statistically independent. Our results show that the plaque-inhibitory activities of interferon and the arabinosides tested are statistically independent. The results also show that the arabinosides do not destabilize the antiviral state previously induced by interferon, and that interferon pretreatment does not interfere with subsequent arabinoside action in infected cells. We have also found that arabinosides do not affect the induction of interferon synthesis by either Newcastle disease virus or double-stranded ribonucleic acid, and are not themselves interferon inducers.

Adenine arabinoside (9-β-D-arabinofuranosyladenine, Ara-A) and human interferon are currently being evaluated in clinical trials for therapeutic use against several deoxyribonucleic acid virus infections, including herpes simplex types 1 and 2 (HSV-1 and -2), varicella-zoster, cytomegalovirus, and vaccinia (2 to 9, 14). Hypoxanthine arabinoside (Ara-Hx) is produced in vivo and in vitro by deamination of Ara-A, catalyzed by the enzyme adenosine deaminase; it has significantly lower antiviral activity than the parent compound (4, 5, 11). Ara-AMP, the 5′-monophosphate of Ara-A, also has inhibitory activity against the large deoxyribonucleic acid viruses and is presently in phase I clinical trials. For brevity, we refer to all three of these compounds as "arabinosides."

The interferon system is an important component of the vertebrate host's natural antiviral defenses (3). Therefore, it seemed desirable to examine the effects of any potential chemotherapeutic agent on both the production and the antiviral activity of interferon. We have done so using human diploid foreskin fibroblasts (HSF) infected with either HSV-2 or vaccinia virus. Our results show that the arabinosides tested (Ara-A, Ara-Hx, and Ara-AMP) neither antagonize nor enhance the antiviral activity of HSF interferon; that is, the antiviral activities of the arabinosides and interferon are statistically independent. Our results show that the arabinosides do not interfere with the establishment of the antiviral state induced by interferon, do not destabilize the antiviral state induced by previous exposure of cells to interferon, and do not interfere with the induction of interferon synthesis by either virus or synthetic double-stranded ribonucleic acid.

(A preliminary report of these results has been presented [Y. Bryson, J. D. Connor, and L. H. Kronenberg, Abstr. Annu. Meet. Am. Soc. Microbiol. 1976, p. 239, S211].)

MATERIALS AND METHODS

Cell cultures. The *Bas* strain of HSF was obtained from the Genetics Center, School of Medicine, University of California, San Diego. The cells were

[1] Present address: Department of Pediatrics, School of Medicine, University of California at Los Angeles, Los Angeles, CA 90024.

propagated as monolayers with weekly passage in Eagle minimal essential medium (MEM) containing 10% fetal bovine serum (FBS). For plaque assays, 10^5 cells in 1.0 ml were seeded in each well of 24-well culture trays (Falcon no. 3008) and incubated for 3 to 5 days at 37°C under 5% CO_2 until confluent. Maintenance medium for experiments refers to MEM containing 2% FBS.

Viruses. A clinical isolate of HSV-2 was kindly provided by A. Nahmias. Virus stocks were prepared by passage in HSF and were stored at −70°C. Vaccinia virus was obtained from Wyeth as Dryvax calf lymph vaccine. The lyophilized virus was reconstituted in MEM containing 10% skim milk and stored at −70°C. Newcastle disease virus (NDV, L-Kansas strain) was originally obtained from J. J. Holland and was propagated in 10-day embryonated chicken eggs as previously described (13). Virus-containing allantoic fluids were titrated in primary chicken embryo fibroblast cultures and were stored at −20°C. A wild-type strain of encephalomyocarditis (EMC) virus, also obtained from J. J. Holland, was used for the isolation of small- and large-plaque clones by four serial plaque purifications in mouse CCL-1 cells. The virus stocks used herein were obtained by passage in CCL-1 cells and were stored at −20°C.

All virus plaque assays were carried out as follows: confluent 16-mm HSF cultures were washed once with 1 ml of tris(hydroxymethyl)aminomethane (Tris) buffer, pH 7.4 (18), and infected in 0.06 ml of Tris buffer containing virus diluted to give 50 to 60 plaque-forming units (PFU)/culture. The inoculum was adsorbed for 60 min at room temperature and was redistributed at 15-min intervals. After adsorption, the cultures were drained and replenished with 0.6 ml of maintenance medium containing antiviral substances as described below. For EMC plaques, the medium postinfection also contained 0.6% agarose (Calbiochem), which was removed by aspiration before the cells were fixed. Cultures were incubated at 37°C under 5% CO_2 for 36 h after infection with EMC or for 48 h after infection with HSV-2 or vaccina virus, then washed with 1 ml of Tris buffer, fixed in 100% methanol, and stained with 1% aqueous crystal violet. Plaques were counted using a dissecting microscope at ×10 to 15 magnification.

Interferon. A single interferon preparation was used for all experiments in which arabinosides and interferon were used together. This preparation was produced by inducing diploid human fetal fibroblasts with polyinosinic-polycytidylic acid [poly (I:C)] (18) and was previously characterized as nondialyzable, nonsedimentable (3 h at 100,000 × *g*), stable at pH 2.2, trypsin sensitive but ribonuclease and deoxyribonuclease insensitive, and active against a variety of virus types in human and monkey cells but not in chicken, rabbit, mouse, or cat cells.

For experiments in which interferon was induced in combination with arabinosides (Table 1), confluent 35-mm HSF cultures in Linbro FB-6 dishes were induced as follows: for NDV, the cultures were washed once with 2 ml of Tris buffer and infected at approximately 300 PFU/cell in 0.2 ml of NDV-containing allantoic fluids for 90 min at room temperature. After adsorption, the cultures were washed twice with 2 ml of Tris buffer and refed 2 ml of maintenance medium. For poly(I:C), confluent 35-mm cultures were washed once with 2 ml of MEM and refed 1 ml of MEM, 1% FBS, 100 μg of diethylaminoethyldextran (Pharmacia) per ml, and 10 μg of poly(I:C) (P-L Biochemicals) per ml. After incubation for 3 h at 37°C, the cultures were washed three times with 2 ml of MEM and refed 2 ml of maintenance medium. Twenty-four hours after the beginning of induction, culture fluids were removed, pooled for duplicates, and dialyzed at pH 2.2 and pH 7.4 as described (18). The media were then clarified by centrifugation and stored at −20°C. Interferon yields were measured by a modification of the micro dye-uptake method previously described (1): confluent HSF monolayers in Falcon microtest II plates were incubated overnight in 0.1 ml of maintenance medium per well containing serial threefold dilutions of interferons. The cultures were then washed with Tris buffer, infected with 10 PFU of large-plaque EMC virus per cell and refed 0.12 ml of maintenance medium per well. After 24 h at 37°C, the cultures were fixed in methanol and stained with 1% aqueous crystal violet. Interferon titers given in Table 1 are the reciprocal of the dilution giving approximately 50% protection of the microtest cultures from destruction by EMC virus.

Arabinosyl compounds. Ara-A, Ara-Hx, Ara-AMP, and adenosine deaminase inhibitor (ADAI) (24) were obtained from Parke-Davis and were the kind gifts of James D. Connor. The Ara-Hx was further purified by high-pressure liquid chromatog-

TABLE 1. *Effect of Ara-A and Ara-AMP on interferon production by human skin fibroblasts*

Inducer	Arabinoside	Log_{10} interferon titer[a]
Poly(I:C)	None	3.6
	ADAI	3.6
	Ara-A	3.6
	Ara-A + ADAI	3.6
	Ara-AMP	3.6
	Ara-AMP + ADAI	3.6
NDV	None	3.1
	ADAI	3.1
	Ara-A	2.6
	Ara-A + ADAI	2.6
	Ara-AMP	2.6
	Ara-AMP + ADAI	3.1
None	None	<0
	ADAI	<0
	Ara-A	<0
	Ara-A + ADAI	<0
	Ara-AMP	<0
	Ara-AMP + ADAI	<0

[a] 0.5 log_{10} is approximately the limit of reliability in the assay used.

raphy as previously described (5). Stock solutions were stored at −20°C. ADAI was used at a concentration of 0.83 μg/ml in all experiments with Ara-A and Ara-AMP to prevent deamination, as previously described (5). This concentration of ADAI has no intrinsic antiviral activity in the systems used here. ADAI was not used in experiments with Ara-Hx.

RESULTS

Antiviral activity of arabinosides against vaccinia virus and HSV-2. Initially the antiviral activities of Ara-A, Ara-Hx, and Ara-AMP were measured individually, using plaque inhibition against vaccinia virus or HSV-2. These experiments were similar to those reported previously (5, 10) for Ara-A and Ara-Hx, except that plaque assays were carried out in multiwell tissue culture dishes containing 24 cultures 16 mm in diameter. Confluent HSF monolayers were infected with approximately 60 PFU of either vaccinia virus or HSV-2 per culture as described in Materials and Methods and then refed maintenance medium containing serial twofold dilutions of the arabinosides. At 48 h postinfection, the plaques were scored and expressed as percentage of plaque number in drug-free controls. Points representing intermediate degrees of plaque inhibition were fitted to a least-squares line, and from this line concentrations of inhibitors giving 50% plaque inhibition were calculated. For vaccinia virus (Fig. 1) the median inhibitory doses were: 0.038 μg of Ara-A per ml (0.14 μM); 0.077 μg of Ara-AMP per ml (0.22 μM); and 0.45 μg of Ara-Hx per ml (1.7 μM). For HSV-2 (Fig. 2) the median inhibitory doses were: 0.18 μg of Ara-A per ml (0.67 μM); 0.41 μg of Ara-AMP per ml (1.2 μM); and 15.4 μg of Ara-Hx per ml (57 μM). Expressed in terms of median inhibitory doses, vaccinia plaque development was approximately five times as sensitive to Ara-A, and approximately 34 times as sensitive to Ara-Hx, as was HSV-2 plaque development.

These activity curves (Figs. 1 and 2) were used as a reference for choosing drug doses appropriate to give approximately 25% plaque inhibition for the combined experiments that follow.

Combined antiviral activities of arabinosides and interferon. The strategy of these experiments was as follows: confluent HSF monolayers were incubated overnight in maintenance medium containing serial threefold dilutions of human fibroblast interferon. The cultures were then washed, infected with 60 PFU of either vaccinia virus or HSV-2 per culture, and replenished with maintenance medium containing doses of arabinosides chosen from the data in Fig. 1 and 2 to give approximately 25% plaque inhibition. "Drug controls" refers to cultures pretreated with interferon-free medium and maintained postinfection in medium containing the individual arabinosides. "Interferon controls" refers to cultures pretreated with interferon dilutions but maintained postinfection in drug-free medium. "Virus controls" refers to cultures pretreated with interferon-free medium and maintained postinfection in drug-free medium. At 48 h postinfection, the plaques were scored and expressed as percentage of virus controls. Results representative of the experiments with vaccinia virus are shown in Fig. 3. Panel A shows the interferon controls,

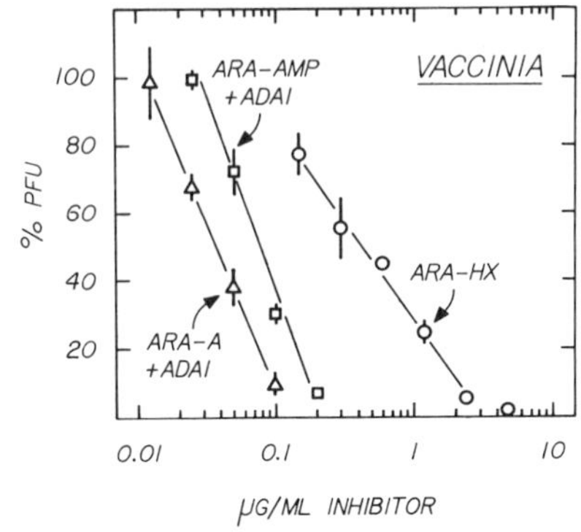

FIG. 1. *Inhibition of vaccinia plaque development (as percentage of control plaque number) by Ara-A, Ara-Hx, and Ara-AMP. Confluent HSF monolayers were infected with 50 to 60 PFU of vaccinia virus and incubated postinfection in maintenance medium containing serial dilutions of arabinosides, and plaques were scored at 48 h postinfection as described in the text. ADAI (0.83 μg/ml) was included with Ara-A and Ara-AMP. Symbols: (△) Ara-A; (□) Ara-AMP; (○) Ara-Hx. Vertical bars represent standard deviation in plaque count for triplicate samples. Linear regression lines calculated from the points are indicated.*

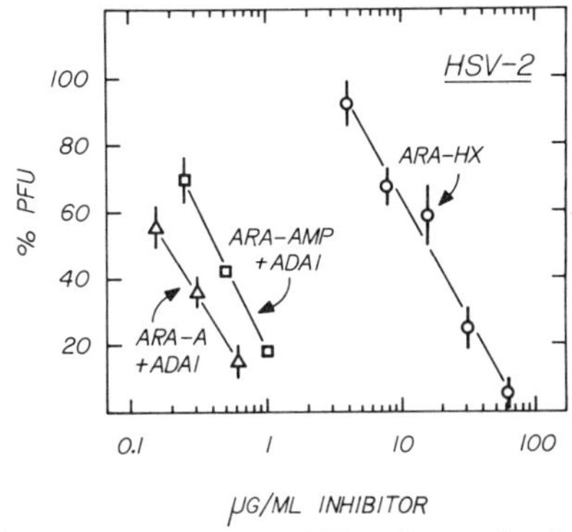

FIG. 2. *Inhibition of HSV-2 plaque development by Ara-A (△), Ara-AMP (□), and Ara-Hx (○). Other details as in Fig. 1.*

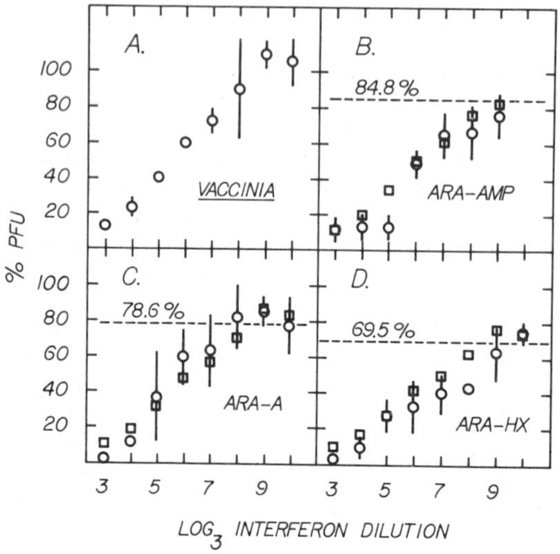

FIG. 3. *Inhibition of vaccinia plaque development by interferon pretreatment alone (A) or in combination with arabinosides postinfection (B, C, D). See text for experimental details. Vertical bars represent standard deviation in plaque counts for triplicate samples. Plaque inhibition due to arabinosides alone (drug controls) is indicated in B, C, and D by horizontal dotted lines. Symbols: (○) observed plaque development expressed as percentage of virus controls; (□) results calculated from the data in panel A and from the arabinoside controls, assuming statistical independence. (A) Interferon pretreatment, drug-free medium postinfection. (B) Interferon pretreatment, 0.04 μg of Ara-AMP per ml (0.11 μM) postinfection. (C) Interferon pretreatment, 0.025 μg of Ara-A per ml (0.094 μM) postinfection. (D) Interferon pretreatment, 1.0 μg of Ara-Hx per ml (3.7 μM) postinfection.*

i.e., cultures pretreated with interferon dilutions and post-treated in drug-free medium. The results are equivalent to a plaque-inhibition assay of our interferon preparation, using vaccinia virus for challenge. In panels B, C, and D the drug controls are shown by the horizontal dotted line. Thus the dose of Ara-AMP used (0.04 μg/ml) produced approximately 15% inhibition of plaque development, Ara-A (0.025 μg/ml) produced approximately 21% plaque inhibition, and Ara-Hx (1.0 μg/ml) produced approximately 30% plaque inhibition. In panels B through D, circles indicate the observed results for cultures pretreated with interferon dilutions (shown on the abscissa) and post-treated with these doses of arabinosides.

Our criterion for antagonism or synergy between the antiviral actions of arabinosides and interferon is as follows: if P_1 is the fraction of control plaques observed in the presence of a given amount of interferon and P_2 is the fraction of control plaques observed in the presence of a given amount of arabinoside, then the fraction of control plaque number observed in the presence of both substances is the product $(P_1)(P_2)$ if the inhibitory activities are statistically independent. We use antagonism to denote plaque survival in excess of that calculated assuming statistical independence, and we use synergy to denote plaque survival less than that calculated assuming statistical independence. Thus the expected results (shown in Fig. 3 by squares) are calculated by multiplying the fraction of control plaque number observed at a given dose of interferon and the fraction of control plaque number observed at the dose of arabinoside used. In Fig. 3 it is evident that the expected and observed results coincide quite closely. Hence we conclude that the antiviral activities of interferon and each of the arabinosides tested are statistically independent.

Identical experiments were performed using HSV-2. Comparison of the abscissae in Fig. 3A and 4A shows that the median inhibitory dose of interferon was approximately eightfold higher for HSV-2 than for vaccinia virus. In Fig. 4, the inhibition due to arabinosides alone (drug controls) is again indicated by horizontal dotted lines. In this case, the dose of Ara-A (0.1 μg/ml) produced approximately 11% plaque inhibition, Ara-AMP (0.2 μg/ml) produced approximately 23% plaque inhibition, and Ara-Hx (6.0 μg/ml) produced approximately 23% plaque inhibition. In each case, the experiments with combined inhibitors (Fig. 4B to D) gave observed results that were experimentally indistinguishable from the expected results calculated assuming statistical independence of the inhibitory activities. For both vaccinia virus and HSV-2, results identical to those obtained for the interferon controls (panel A) were given by cells treated only with ADAI postinfection. We conclude, insofar as HSV-2 and vaccinia virus are concerned, that the plaque-inhibitory activities of human fibroblast interferon and these arabinosides are statistically independent and show no evidence of antagonism or synergy in their actions.

Two further conclusions can be drawn from the results given in Fig. 3 and 4. In these experiments the cells were pretreated overnight with interferon dilutions, infected, and then maintained postinfection in interferon-free medium containing arabinosides. Since the observed results for combined inhibitors were virtually identical with the results calculated on the basis of statistical independence, it follows that neither the arabinosides nor ADAI acts to destabilize the antiviral state induced in the cells by previous exposure to interferon; otherwise, the results would indicate antago-

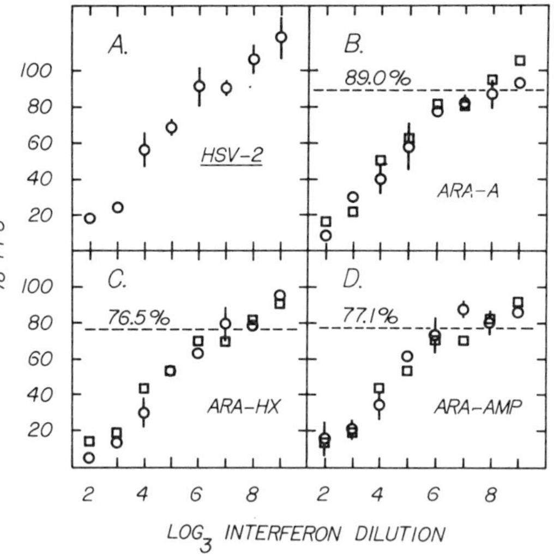

FIG. 4. *Inhibition of HSV-2 plaque development by interferon pretreatment alone (A) or in combination with arabinosides postinfection (B to D). Vertical bars represent standard deviation in plaque counts for triplicate samples. Plaque inhibition due to arabinosides alone (drug controls) is shown by horizontal dotted lines. Symbols: (○) Observed plaque development expressed as percentage of virus controls; (□) results calculated from the data in panel A and from arabinoside controls, assuming statistical independence. (A) Interferon pretreatment, drug-free medium postinfection. (B) Interferon pretreatment, 0.1 μg of Ara-A per ml (0.37 μM) postinfection. (C) Interferon pretreatment, 6.0 μg of Ara-Hx per ml (22 μM) postinfection. (D) Interferon pretreatment, 0.2 μg of Ara-AMP per ml (0.58 μM) postinfection.*

nism between the inhibitory actions of interferon and arabinosides. Conversely, prior exposure of cells to interferon does not interfere with the antiviral action of subsequent doses of arabinosides.

Effect of arabinosides on establishment of the antiviral state induced by interferon. The preceding experiments (Fig. 3 and 4) tested the plaque-inhibitory activities of arabinosides in cells in which an antiviral state was already established by previous exposure of the cells to interferon. The results show that the antiviral arabinosides do not destabilize the antiviral state induced by interferon, but do not rule out the possibility that concomitant exposure of cells to interferon and arabinosides can interfere with establishment of the antiviral state induced by interferon. To test this possibility, confluent HSF monolayers were pretreated overnight with maintenance medium containing interferon dilutions plus relatively high doses of arabinosides (5 μg of Ara-A, 8 μg of Ara-AMP, or 10 μg of Ara-Hx per ml). Controls contained interferon dilutions without arabinosides, with and without ADAI. The cultures were then washed, infected with 60 PFU of small-plaque EMC virus per culture, and scored at 36 h postinfection. Since the arabinosides were washed out of the cultures before infection, and since EMC is ribonucleic acid virus insensitive to the inhibitory activities of these arabinosides (not inhibited in cells even when treated concurrently with arabinosides; our unpublished data), any inhibition of EMC plaque formation in this experiment must be attributed to the antiviral state established in the cells before infection, in response to interferon. The results are shown in Fig. 5. The inhibition curves were identical whether the cells were pretreated with interferon alone or in the presence of Ara-A, Ara-AMP, or Ara-Hx. The results were unchanged for cells treated with interferon and ADAI (data not shown). Hence, neither ADAI nor high concentrations of arabinosides inhibited the establishment of the antiviral state induced by interferon.

Effect of arabinosides on induction of interferon synthesis. A final set of experiments was designed to test whether ADAI or arabinosides interfere with the induction of interferon synthesis by virus or poly(I:C), or might themselves be interferon inducers. Confluent HSF monolayers were induced by NDV or poly(I:C) as described in Materials and Methods and

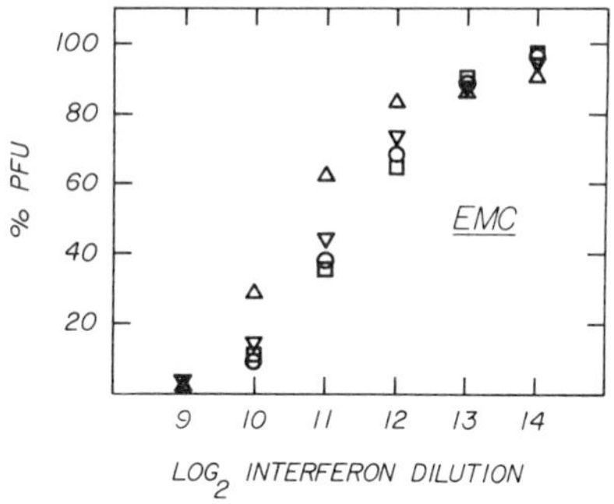

FIG. 5. *EMC plaque development in cultures pretreated with interferon alone or in combination with arabinosides. Cultures were pretreated overnight with serial twofold dilutions of interferon, infected, and maintained postinfection in interferon-free, arabinoside-free medium. The plaque numbers at 36 h postinfection were expressed as percentage of virus controls. Symbols: (○) Pretreatment with interferon alone; (▽) pretreatment with interferon and 8 μg of Ara-AMP per ml (23 μM); (△) pretreatment with interferon and 5 μg of Ara-A per ml (19 μM); (□) pretreatment with interferon and 10 μg of Ara-Hx per ml (37 μM). ADAI (0.83 μg/ml) was included with Ara-A and Ara-AMP.*

refed maintenance medium containing Ara-A (5 μg/ml) or Ara-AMP (8 μg/ml), each with and without ADAI (0.83 μg/ml). Ara-Hx was not tested in these experiments, but was produced by deamination of Ara-A in cultures not containing ADAI. Controls contained no additions. At 24 h postinduction, the extracellular media were removed and the interferon activity was quantitated as described in Materials and Methods (Table 1). Neither arabinosides nor ADAI alone or in combination caused synthesis of any detectable interferon. Control NDV-induced cultures produced 1,200 U of interferon, and neither arabinosides nor ADAI markedly affected this yield. Control poly(I:C)-induced cultures produced about 4,000 U of interferon, and this also was not significantly affected by arabinosides or ADAI. Thus arabinosides and/or ADAI do not impair the production of interferon by human fibroblasts in response to virus or poly(I:C).

DISCUSSION

The experiments reported herein were designed to test whether the antiviral arabinosides Ara-A, Ara-Hx, and Ara-AMP demonstrate antagonistic or synergistic effects upon the production and antiviral activity of human interferon. Interferon production and action are important components of the early antiviral response in vivo (3), and there is increasing evidence that interferon production also serves a regulatory purpose in both cell-mediated and humoral immunity (12, 15–17, 20–22). Therefore it seems desirable to examine the effects of any potential antiviral chemotherapeutic agent on both aspects of the interferon response. Our experiments provide a model by which the combined activities of interferon and antiviral drugs can be examined in vitro. Such information may prove to be important in the chemotherapy of viral diseases since a rational approach to antiviral chemotherapy would require that drugs do not impair the endogenous interferon response. In addition, combined therapy with antiviral drugs and exogenous interferon may provide increased clinical efficacy, provided that the activities are not antagonistic.

We chose HSV-2 and vaccinia viruses as representatives of the herpes- and poxvirus groups. It would also be of interest to examine other herpesviruses such as varicella-zoster and cytomegalovirus. Our experiments measured the antiviral activities of interferon and arabinosides alone and in combination; by combining doses of each that, acting alone, would give intermediate degrees of plaque inhibition, we were able to compare the combined antiviral effects with those calculated from the activity of each inhibitor alone, assuming that the activities are statistically independent. Our results are indistinguishable from those calculated on this basis and lead to the conclusion that the plaque-inhibitory activities of interferon and each arabinoside tested are statistically independent. It should be noted that in these experiments cell cultures were first treated with interferon to establish an antiviral state; the interferon was removed at the time of infection, and infected cultures were then maintained in interferon-free medium containing arabinosides. Therefore, the results also allow us to conclude that treatment with arabinosides postinfection does not destabilize the antiviral state previously induced by interferon, and also that interferon pretreatment does not interfere with the subsequent action of these arabinosides in infected cells.

Our results show that at doses of arabinosides giving intermediate plaque inhibition, there is no synergy at any dose of interferon tested. These results do not preclude possible synergy or antagonism between interferon and higher doses of arabinosides. However, the doses of arabinosides used in our experiments are comparable with serum levels of Ara-A and Ara-Hx achieved after intravenous administration of Ara-A in clinical trials (Y. Bryson and J. D. Connor, in preparation).

In addition, measurement of plaque inhibition is equivalent to measurement of inhibition of viral infectivity, but does not address the yield of progeny virus per infected cell. Hence, our data do not rule out the possibility of synergy between the effects of arabinosides and interferon on virus yields.

Lerner and Bailey (19) reported that the plaque-inhibitory effects of human leukocyte interferon and Ara-A were synergistic in a system using Vero cells infected with HSV-1. Our results do not corroborate this report, and we presume that the discrepancy may arise from the following facts. (i) Lerner and Bailey used a definition of synergy that is not meaningful in the absence of more complete dose-response information and depends, in particular, on the slope of the dose-response curves. When their data (19, Table 2) are recalculated according to our criterion of synergy (statistical independence), some of the data do not, in fact, support the conclusion of synergy. (ii) Lerner and Bailey used Vero cells in their study, whereas we have used human diploid foreskin fibroblasts. (iii) ADAI was not used in their study, necessitating the use of much higher concentrations of Ara-A than were used in the experiments reported here. Hence the plaque inhibition observed by Lerner and Bailey may have been due, in part, to nonspecific cytotoxicity. The doses of inhibitors used in our study are not cytotoxic according to the criteria of trypan blue staining and efficiency of plating of the cells upon subculture (Y. J. Bryson, unpublished data). Also, as demonstrated in Fig. 5 and Table 1, even the highest doses of inhibitors used here were not cytotoxic as measured by the ability of cultures to support virus replication and interferon synthesis, which are the indexes of cytotoxicity most pertinent to our conclusions. (iv) Lerner and Bailey applied interferon at the same time as Ara-A, i.e., immediately after infection of the cultures. Hence the observed antiviral activities must depend on the ability of interferon to establish resistance in cells treated simultaneously with Ara-A and virus, and on the relative kinetics of virus maturation and the development of resistance. Our results show that the arabinosides do not interfere with the establishment of the antiviral state induced by interferon in uninfected cells, but the situation in infected cells may be more complex.

In summary, our results indicate that for vaccinia virus and HSV-2 in HSF, the plaque-inhibitory activities of arabinosides and interferon are statistically independent, with no evidence for synergy or antagonism. Arabinosides do not destabilize the antiviral state induced by previous exposure to interferon, and previous exposure to interferon does not antagonize the subsequent activity of the arabinosides. In addition, neither ADAI nor the arabinosides affect the induction of interferon synthesis by either virus (NDV) or poly(I:C), and are not themselves interferon inducers.

ACKNOWLEDGMENTS

We thank Parke-Davis and Co. and Public Health Service grant GM17702, from the National Institute of General Medical Sciences, for partial support.

Special thanks are due to J. D. Connor and T. Friedmann for their generous support.

LITERATURE CITED

1. **Armstrong, J. A.** 1970. Semi-micro, dye-binding assay for rabbit interferon. Appl. Microbiol., 21:723–725.
2. **Arvin, A. M., A. S. Yeager, and T. C. Merigan.** 1976. Effect of leukocyte interferon on urinary excretion of cytomegalovirus by infants. J. Infect. Dis. 133(Suppl.):205–210.
3. **Baron, S.** 1973. The defensive and biological roles of the interferon system, p. 267–294. *In* N. B. Finter (ed.), Interferons and interferon inducers. American Elsevier, New York.
4. **Bryson, Y., and J. D. Connor.** 1976. The in vitro susceptibility of varicella zoster virus to adenine arabinoside and hypoxanthine arabinoside. Antimicrob. Agents Chemother. 9:540–543.
5. **Bryson, H., J. D. Connor, L. Sweetman, S. Carey, M. A. Stuckey, and R. Buchanan.** 1974. Determination of plaque inhibitory activity of adenine arabinoside (9-β-D-arabinofuranosyladenine) for herpesviruses using an adenosine deaminase inhibitor. Antimicrob. Agents Chemother. 6:98–101.
6. **Ch'ien, L. T., N. J. Cannon, L. J. Charamella, W. E. Dismukes, R. J. Whitley, R. A. Buchanan, and C. A. Alford, Jr.** 1973. Effect of adenine arabinoside on severe herpesvirus hominis infections in man. J. Infect. Dis. 128:658–663.
7. **Ch'ien, L. T., M. H. Cannon, R. J. Whitley, A. G. Diethelm, W. E. Dismukes, C. W. Scott, R. A. Buchanan, and C. A. Alford, Jr.** 1974. Effect of adenine arabinoside on cytomegalovirus infections. J. Infect. Dis. 130:32–39.
8. **Ch'ien, L. T., R. J. Whitley, C. A. Alford, Jr., G. J. Galasso, and the Collaborative Study Group.** 1976. Adenine arabinoside for therapy of herpes zoster in immunosuppressed patients: preliminary results of a collaborative study. J. Infect. Dis. 13(Suppl.):184–191.
9. **Ch'ien, L. T., R. J. Whitley, A. Nahmias, E. Lewis, C. Linnemann, L. Frenkel, J. Bellanti, R. Buchanan, and C. A. Alford, Jr.** 1975. Antiviral chemotherapy and neonatal herpes simplex virus infection. A pilot study—experience with adenine arabinoside. Pediatrics 55:678–685.
10. **Connor, J. D., L. Sweetman, S. Carey, M. A. Stuckey, and R. Buchanan.** 1974. Effect of adenosine deaminase upon the antiviral activity in vitro of adenine arabinoside for vaccinia virus. Antimicrob. Agents Chemother. 6:630–636.
11. **Connor, J. D., L. Sweetman, S. Carey, M. A. Stuckey, and R. Buchanan.** 1975. Susceptibility in vitro of several large DNA viruses to the antiviral activity of adenine arabinoside and its metabolite, hypoxanthine arabinoside: relation to human pharmacology, p. 177–196. *In* D. Pavan-Langston, R. A. Buchanan, and C. A. Alford, Jr. (ed.), Adenine arabinoside: an antiviral agent. Raven Press, New York.
12. **De Maeyer-Guignard, J., A. Cachard, and E. De Maeyer.** 1975. Delayed-type hypersensitivity to sheep red blood cells: inhibition of sensitization by interferon. Science 190:574–576.
13. **Duesberg, P. H., and W. S. Robinson.** 1965. Isolation of the nucleic acid of Newcastle disease virus. Proc. Natl. Acad. Sci. U.S.A. 54:794–800.
14. **Emodi, G., R. O'Reilly, A. Muller, L. K. Everson, U. Biswanger, and M. Just.** 1976. Effect of human exogenous leukocyte interferon in cytomegalovirus infections. J. Infect. Dis. 133(Suppl.):199–204.
15. **Geraldes, A. (ed.).** 1975. Effects of interferon on cells, viruses and the immune system. Proceedings of a meeting held at Oeiras, Portugal, September, 1973. Academic Press, New York.
16. **Gisler, R. H., P. Lindahl, and I. Gresser.** 1974. Effects of interferon on antibody synthesis in vitro. J. Immunol. 113:438–444.
17. **Johnson, H., and S. Baron.** 1975. Interferon, interferon inducers, and the in vitro immune response. J. Immunol. 114:403–413.
18. **Kronenberg, L. H., and T. Friedmann.** 1975. Relative quantitative assay of the biological activity of interferon messenger ribonucleic acid. J. Gen. Virol. 27:225–238.
19. **Lerner, A. M., and E. J. Bailey.** 1974. Synergy of 9-β-D-arabinofuranosyladenine and human interferon against herpes simplex virus, type 1. J. Infect. Dis. 130:549–552.
20. **Lindahl, P., I. Gresser, P. Leary, and M. Tovey.** 1976. Interferon treatment of mice: enhanced expression of histocompatibility antigens on lymphoid cells. Proc.

Natl. Acad. Sci. U.S.A. **73**:1284–1287.

21. **Lindahl, P., P. Leary, and I. Gresser.** 1972. Enhancement by interferon of the specific cytotoxicity of sensitized lymphocytes. Proc. Natl. Acad. Sci. U.S.A. **69**:721–725.
22. **Merigan, T. C. (ed.).** 1976. Antivirals with clinical potential. A symposium held at Stanford University, August, 1975. J. Infect. Dis. **133**(Suppl.).
23. **Sweetman, L., J. D. Connor, R. Seshamani, M. A. Stuckey, S. Carey, and R. A. Buchanan.** 1975. Deamination of adenine arabinoside in cell cultures used in in vitro viral inhibition studies, p. 135–144. *In* D. Pavan-Langston, R. A. Buchanan, and C. A. Alford, Jr. (ed.), Adenine arabinoside: an antiviral agent. Raven Press, New York.
24. **Woo, P. W. K., H. W. Dion, S. M. Lange, L. F. Dahl, and L. J. Durham.** 1974. A novel adenosine and Ara-A deaminase inhibitor. (R)-3-(2-deoxy-β-D-erythro-pentofuranosyl)-3, 6, 7, 8-tetrahydroimidazo (4, 5-D), (1, 3) diazepin-8-ol. J. Heterocycl. Chem. **11**:641–643.

ANTIMICROBIAL AGENTS AND CHEMOTHERAPY, Feb. 1977, p. 307-311
Vol. 11, No. 2

Printed in U.S.A.

Experimental Herpes Simplex Virus Type 1 Encephalitis: Treatment with 5-Trifluoromethyl-2′-Deoxyuridine

D. W. CLOUGH* AND J. RODNEY PARKHURST

The Medical College of Wisconsin, Department of Microbiology, and The Midwest Childhood Cancer Center, Milwaukee, Wisconsin 53233*

Received for publication 30 August 1976

5-Trifluoromethyl-2′-deoxyuridine (F_3dThd) was evaluated for its neurotoxicity and for its ability to increase the life span of mice injected intracerebrally with herpes simplex virus type 1 (HSV-1) and F_3dThd simultaneously. F_3dThd showed no neurotoxicity at the highest concentration tested (100 mg/kg). Mice injected intracerebrally with HSV-1 died within 5 days postinfection. However, all mice injected concurrently with HSV-1 and 100 mg of F_3dThd per kg lived through the termination of the experiment (60 days). Protection of mice from HSV-1 encephalitis by F_3dThd has been shown to be dose dependent, with 100, 75, 50, and 25 mg of F_3dThd per kg yielding a survival rate of 100, 90, 50, and 10%, respectively. HSV-1 titers in mouse brains receiving HSV-1 and 100 mg of F_3dThd per kg concurrently were 100- to 1,000-fold lower at 2 to 4 days postinfection than control mice receiving HSV-1 alone. F_3dThd was shown not to stimulate interferon production. Encephalitis caused by a ribonucleic acid virus, encephalomyocarditis virus, was not modified by F_3dThd treatment.

5-Trifluoromethyl-2′-deoxyuridine (F_3dThd) was first synthesized in 1964 as a thymidine analogue for the treatment of neoplasias (8). Until recently, it had met with limited success in vivo (L. Helson, A. Yagoda, M. McCarthy, M. L. Murphy, and I. H. Krakoff, Proc. Am. Assoc. Cancer Res. **11**:136, 1970) (3). However, more recent evaluations in the treatment of childhood neuroblastoma have shown it to be effective in combination therapy with cyclophosphamide, vincristine, and papaverine (L. Helson, Proc. 67th Annu. Meet. Am. Assoc. Cancer Res. **17**:236, 1976). It inhibits the growth of various mammalian cells in culture (16, 21) and some tumors in mice (7). F_3dThd is also active against herpes simplex and vaccinia viral keratitis in rabbits (11, 12). It has been shown to be highly effective in the treatment of human ocular herpetic keratitis (22).

In vitro studies have demonstrated that deoxythymidine kinase is inhibited by F_3dThd (4) and thymidylate synthetase is inhibited by the nucleotide F_3dThd-5′-P (19). Studies with deoxyribonucleic acid (DNA) polymerase from HeLa cells and from vaccinia-infected HeLa cells indicate that F_3dThd-5′-PPP exhibits competitive inhibition with dThd-5′-PPP and is incorporated into DNA (20).

A major problem encountered when using nucleoside analogues as antiviral agents is the problem of toxicity due to inhibition of host cell DNA biosynthetic functions. Since DNA in neurons of the cerebral cortex replicates at very low levels after birth (14), viral infections of the brain are logical candidates for target-directed antiviral chemotherapy. To effect this target-directed approach, intracerebral (IC) inoculation was used. This technique eliminated any effects mediated by the blood-brain barrier and delivered a high concentration of F_3dThd in close proximity to infected cells. This communication describes the results of an investigation into the effects of simultaneous administration of F_3dThd and herpes simplex virus type 1 (HSV-1) on the course and outcome of experimentally induced HSV-1 encephalitis in mice.

MATERIALS AND METHODS

Animals. Male Swiss albino HA/ICR mice (ARS/Sprague-Dawley, Madison, Wis.) weighing 18 to 22 g were used throughout this study.

Cell culture. Eagle minimum essential medium (GIBCO) supplemented with 10% heat-inactivated calf serum (GIBCO), 50 U of penicillin per ml, and 50 μg of streptomycin per ml was used for growth of HEp-2 monolayer cultures, L_{929} cultures, and virus propagation. Eagle minimum essential medium for Spinner culture (GIBCO) supplemented with 10% heat-inactivated calf serum (GIBCO), 50 U of penicillin per ml, 50 μg of streptomycin per ml, and 0.1% Pluronic F68 (BASF Wyandotte, Wyandotte, Mich.) was used for growth of stock HEp-2 cultures.

Virus. The MacIntyre strain of HSV-1 (ATCC VR-539) was propagated in HEp-2 cells. Confluent HEp-2 monolayers were used to assay infectious HSV-1 (9).

Drug. F_3dThd was generously supplied by Charles Heidelberger of the McArdle Laboratory for

Cancer Research, University of Wisconsin, Madison, Wis.

Virus and drug administration. Mice were injected IC (1) with 30 μl of one of the following preparations: 26 plaque-forming units (PFU) of HSV-1; 26 PFU of HSV-1 with 100, 75, 50, 25, or 0 mg of F_3dThd per kg; drug alone at 100, 75, 50, or 25 mg of F_3dThd per kg; 1.0×10^2 freeze-thawed HEp-2 cells; or saline. Mice were observed for 30 to 70 days, and deaths were recorded daily.

Lethal effects of HSV-1. Various dilutions of HSV-1 in saline were injected IC into mice. Mice were observed for symptoms of encephalitis and length of time until death. It was determined that 26 PFU of HSV-1 was sufficient to kill 100% of the mice injected within 5 days. This inoculum was used throughout this study.

Brain titers of HSV-1. Groups of 20 mice were inoculated with 26 PFU of HSV-1, 26 PFU of HSV-1 with various drug concentrations, or saline. Three mice from each group were sacrificed at 0, 24, 48, 72, and 96 h and 70 days after injection. Three untreated mice were similarly sacrificed for controls. Brains were aseptically removed, disrupted in a Dounce homogenizer, centrifuged at 1,500 rpm for 15 min to remove cellular debris, freeze-thawed once, and assayed for PFU on confluent HEp-2 monolayers.

Inactivation of HSV-1 in the presence and absence of F_3dThd. Dilutions of HSV-1 were made into sterile saline or into F_3dThd. These incubation mixtures contained 1.0×10^7 PFU of HSV-1 per ml and 2.5×10^{-3} M F_3dThd. The samples were incubated at 4°C. Aliquots were removed hourly for dilution and plaque assay. Plaque assays were performed on confluent HEp-2 monolayers (9).

Induction of interferon by F_3dThd. HEp-2 cells were grown to near confluency in 10-ounce (300 ml) bottles. Cells were exposed to 5.0×10^{-6} M, 5.0×10^{-7} M, or 5.0×10^{-8} M F_3dThd. An aliquot of the supernatant was removed at 8, 25, and 49 h after exposure to drug and assayed for interferon by the encephalomyocarditis (EMC) hemagglutinin yield reduction assay method of Grossberg (6). L_{929} cells were grown to near confluency in culture tubes and exposed to 5.0×10^{-6} M, 5.0×10^{-7} M, and 5.0×10^{-8} M F_3dThd for 24 h. The supernatant was removed and assayed for interferon by the GDVII hemagglutinin yield reduction assay (15). Drug toxicity to L_{929} cells was investigated by determining the hemagglutination yield of GDVII virus. Cells were treated with the same concentrations of F_3dThd as was used in the interferon assays and compared with untreated controls (15).

RESULTS

IC toxicity of F_3dThd. To determine the mean lethal dose of F_3dThd in mice, animals were injected IC with either 100, 75, 50, 25, or 0 mg of F_3dThd per kg in a volume of 30 μl and observed for 30 days. No deaths occurred in any of the drug-treated or control mice. Therefore, F_3dThd is not neurotoxic at the highest concentration of drug tested. Concentrations of F_3dThd greater than 0.225 M (drug concentration required to give 100 mg/kg in 0.03 ml) formed precipitates at room temperature; therefore, injections were limited to 100 mg of F_3dThd per kg.

Inactivation of HSV-1 in the presence and absence of F_3dThd. To rule out the possibility that HSV-1 may be inactivated by F_3dThd before IC injection, the following experiment was performed. Duplicate dilutions of HSV-1 were made into sterile saline or into F_3dThd. These incubation mixtures contained 1.0×10^7 PFU of HSV-1 per ml and 2.5×10^{-3} M F_3dThd or saline. The samples were incubated at 4°C. Aliquots were removed hourly for dilution and plaque assay. Figure 1 indicates that the rate of virus inactivation was very similar for both samples. Therefore, preincubation of HSV-1 with F_3dThd does not result in inactivation of the virus beyond that observed in the saline control. This established that mice receiving F_3dThd with HSV-1 in fact receive the same number of PFU of HSV-1 and that these preparations are equally infective. This experiment was repeated at 25 and 37°C with similar results.

Demonstration of a dose-response effect with F_3dThd. To determine the drug concentration necessary to protect mice from fatal encephalitis, the following experiments were conducted. HSV-1 was prepared for injection by

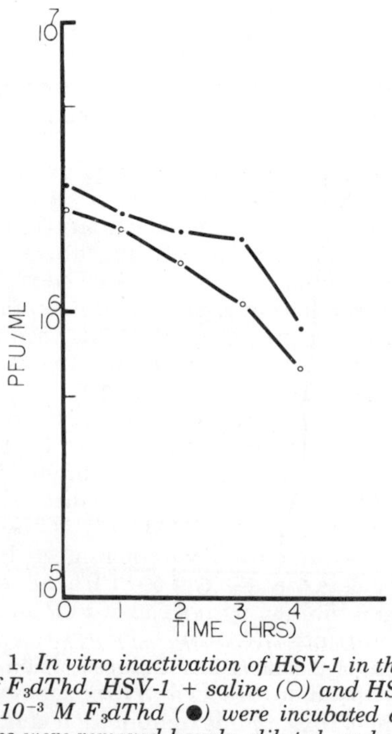

FIG. 1. *In vitro inactivation of HSV-1 in the presence of F_3dThd. HSV-1 + saline (○) and HSV-1 + 2.5×10^{-3} M F_3dThd (●) were incubated at 4°C. Samples were removed hourly, diluted, and assayed for PFU on confluent HEp-2 monolayers.*

dilution into saline or into F$_3$dThd. One group of mice also received freeze-thawed HEp-2 cells as controls. A dose-response effect was observed when either 100, 75, 50, or 25 mg of F$_3$dThd per kg was administered concurrently with HSV-1, resulting in a survival rate of 100, 90, 50, and 10%, respectively (Fig. 2). This experiment was performed in duplicate with 10 mice in each group. These results indicate that F$_3$dThd does in fact modify the course of HSV-1 encephalitis and that this response is dose dependent.

HSV-1 titers in mouse brains after administration of F$_3$dThd. For an antiviral agent to be effective, it must be capable of inhibiting the replication of the virus in the target tissue (2). In these experiments, we evaluated the effectiveness of F$_3$dThd in inhibiting the replication of HSV-1 in mouse brains. Mice were injected with either HSV-1 alone or with HSV-1 and 100 mg of F$_3$dThd per kg concurrently. Three mice each from control and drug-treated groups were sacrificed at 0, 1, 2, 3, 4, and 70 days postinfection. Brains were aseptically removed, disrupted with a Dounce homogenizer, and centrifuged, and the supernatant was assayed for PFU on confluent HEp-2 monolayers. Figure 3 shows the data obtained. Mice receiving 100 mg of F$_3$dThd per kg had brain titers of HSV-1 that were 100- to 1,000-fold lower at 2 to 4 days postinfection than control mice receiving HSV-1 alone. At 70 days postinfection, no virus was detected using the plaque assay, indicating that productive infection had ceased in these brains.

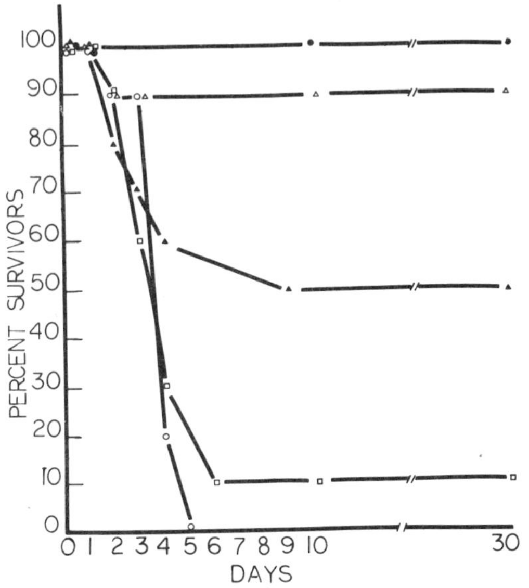

FIG. 2. *Dose-response effect of F$_3$dThd on the outcome of HSV-1 encephalitis. Groups of 10 mice each were infected IC with 26 PFU of HSV-1 alone (○) or concurrently with 100 (●), 75 (△), 50 (▲) or 25 (□) mg of F$_3$dThd per kg and observed for 30 days or until death. Mortalities were recorded daily.*

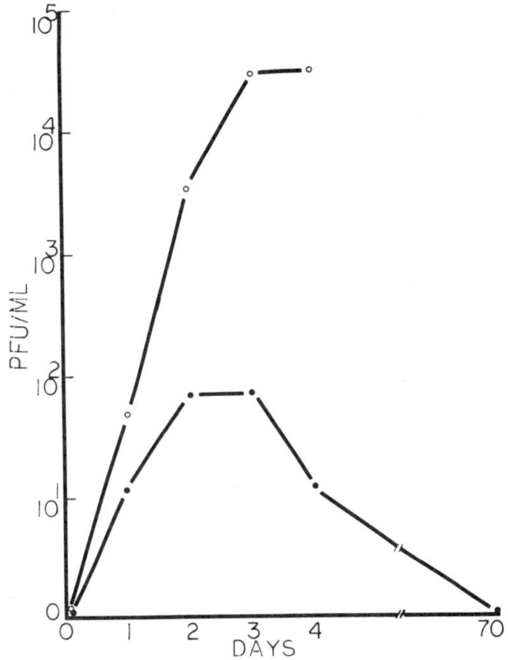

FIG. 3. *Brain titers of HSV-1 in mice at various times postinfection. Groups of mice received 26 PFU of HSV-1 alone (○) or 26 PFU of HSV-1 concurrently with 100 mg of F$_3$dThd (●) per kg. Three mice from each group were sacrificed daily, and brains were aseptically removed, pooled, disrupted with a Dounce homogenizer, and centrifuged at 1500 × g for 15 min. The supernatant fluid was assayed for PFU on confluent HEp-2 monolayers.*

Interferon induction by F$_3$dThd. HEp-2 cells were exposed to 5.0×10^{-6} M, 5.0×10^{-7} M, and 5.0×10^{-8} M F$_3$dThd for 8, 25, or 49 h, and the supernatant was assayed for interferon by the method of Grossberg et al. (6). There was no stimulation of interferon by F$_3$dThd as compared with untreated control cells. Supernatant fluid from L$_{929}$ cells exposed to the same concentrations of F$_3$dThd as above was assayed after 24 h for interferon. This system also showed no stimulation of interferon production as compared with control cells (15). Yield of GDVII virus from cells treated with the same concentrations of F$_3$dThd also showed no difference in hemagglutination yield as compared with untreated controls.

Effect of F$_3$dThd on EMC-induced encephalitis. To eliminate the possibility that the antiviral activity of F$_3$dThd is nonspecific, EMC virus, a ribonucleic acid virus, was used to induce fatal encephalitis in mice. F$_3$dThd, whose mechanism of action involves the inhibition of DNA synthesis, should not affect the outcome of this disease. Groups of 10 mice received 300 PFU of EMC virus in saline or 300 PFU of EMC virus concurrently with 100 mg of F_3dThd per kg. Both groups of mice died within 3 days postinjection, indicating that F_3dThd did not modify the outcome of EMC virus-caused encephalitis.

DISCUSSION

HSV encephalitis is one of the most common causes of sporadic fatal encephalitis in the United States (5). The characteristic presentations of this disease range from a subacute meningitis-like disease to a severe, necrotizing, fatal encephalitis. The majority of the severe cases result in death or permanent neurological sequelae including hemiparesis, aphasia, and memory deficit (13). Untreated cases of this disease have shown a mortality rate of 50 to 60%.

A few antiviral agents that have shown promise in the treatment of other viral diseases have also been evaluated for their effectiveness in the management of HSV-1 encephalitis. The three compounds most thoroughly studied have been 5-iodo-2′-deoxyuridine (IdUrd), 1-β-D-arabinofuranosylcytosine (ara-C), and 9-β-D-arabinofuranosyladenine (ara-A). IdUrd has been shown to be ineffective in the management of human HSV-1 encephalitis, with a high percentage of treatment failures and marked toxicity to the compound (18). Based on the recent clinical trials using IdUrd in the treatment of HSV-1 encephalitis, any further use of this drug in the management of this disease should be seriously questioned (18). Ara-C is not as toxic as IdUrd; however, current reports indicate that this drug is less than satisfactory in the management of herpes encephalitis (5). Ara-A has recently shown promise in the treatment of herpes encephalitis in animal model systems. One study of ara-A treatment of HSV-1 encephalitis has shown that 1,000 mg of ara-A per kg given intraperitoneally gives a 21-day survivor percentage of 50%, while increasing the mean survival time from 5.6 to 8.1 days (17). Experiments of this nature, however, have little bearing on the comparative effectiveness of F_3dThd to ara-A in the treatment of this disease. For completeness, both drugs should be simultaneously tested in identical model systems to clearly establish their comparative effectiveness. Ara-A and F_3dThd have been tested side by side in clinical trials for the treatment of herpetic keratitis. These studies show F_3dThd to be superior in terms of shorter healing time, fewer treatment failures, and the ability to heal more extensively involved disease, at lower drug concentrations, with no significant toxicity (17).

Studies with F_3dThd indicate that in a mouse model system of HSV-1 encephalitis, this antiviral agent is effective by two criteria. First, at doses of 100 mg/kg there is 100% protection against fatal encephalitis. Second, mice treated with 100 mg of F_3dThd per kg have brain titers of HSV-1 that are 100- to 1,000-fold lower than untreated mice between 2 and 4 days postinfection (all control mice succumb to HSV-1 encephalitis by 5 days postinfection). Drug-treated mice brain titers return to zero shortly thereafter. When F_3dThd was tested for neurotoxicity, there was no indication of toxicity at the highest concentration tested, 100 mg/kg. Evidence indicates that HSV-1 is not inactivated by incubation with F_3dThd before injection. Attempts to demonstrate induction of interferon activity by F_3dThd have been unsuccessful. A nonspecific antiviral effect has been eliminated by the failure of F_3dThd to protect mice from EMC-caused encephalitis. Thus, F_3dThd appears to be capable of fulfilling several important criteria of an effective antiviral agent: increased survival time and potent antiviral activity at a nontoxic concentration.

Considering the demonstrated toxicity of F_3dThd to bone marrow and to the gastrointestinal tract (7), a route of administration that bypasses the systemic circulation would be of considerable benefit in the management of HSV-1-caused encephalitis. For instance, administration of F_3dThd into the cerebrospinal fluid could be from one of several anatomical viewpoints: intrathecal, intraventricular, or intracisternal. Current evidence in the treatment of bacterial meningitis indicates that intracisternal and intraventricular routes of administration are beneficial in the management of this disease (10). Further studies into the effectiveness of these routes of administration of F_3dThd may prove to be valuable.

These data have provided sufficient evidence to warrant further investigation of F_3dThd as a potential agent in the treatment of HSV-1 encephalitis.

ACKNOWLEDGMENTS

The technical assistance of Remedios Eudela is gratefully acknowledged. We would also like to thank J. J. Sedmak and Christine Schoenherr for performing the interferon assays.

This investigation was supported by grants from the Regional American Cancer Society, General Research Support Fund (Public Health Service) 5-SO1-RR5434-14, and aided by a Basil O'Connor Starter Research Grant from The National Foundation March of Dimes.

LITERATURE CITED

1. **Ackerfeldt, S., G. Westen, and T. Jansson.** 1971. Aromatic sulfonic acids as viral inhibitors. Structure-activity study using rhino, adeno 3, and influenza viruses. J. Med. Chem. **14**:596–600.
2. **Allen, L. B., and R. W. Sidwell.** 1972. Target organ treatment of neurotropic virus diseases: efficacy as a chemotherapy tool and comparison of adenine arabinoside, cytosine arabinoside, idoxuridine, and triflurothymidine. Antimicrob. Agents Chemother. **2**:229–233.
3. **Ansfield, F. G., and G. Ramirez.** 1971. A phase I-II study of 5-trifluoromethyl-2′-deoxyuridine. Cancer Chemother. Rep. 55:205–208.
4. **Bresnick, E., and S. S. Williams.** 1967. Effects of 5-trifluoromethyl deoxyuridine upon deoxythymidine kinase. Biochem. Pharmacol. **16**:503–507.
5. **Gilbert, D. N., M. T. Johnson, J. P. Luby, and J. P. Sanford.** 1973. Herpesvirus hominis type 1 encephalitis treated with cytarabine, an unresolved problem in encephalitis. Medicine 52:331–338.
6. **Grossberg, S. E., P. Jameson, and J. J. Sedmak.** 1973. Interferon bioassay methods and the development of standard procedures. A critique and analysis of current observations, *In Vitro* Monogr. no. 3, p. 26. The Tissue Culture Association, Rockville, Md.
7. **Heidelberger, C., and S. W. Anderson.** 1964. Fluorinated pyrimidines. XXI. The tumor-inhibitory activity of 5-trifluoromethyl-2′-deoxyuridine. Cancer Res. **24**:1979–1985.
8. **Heidelberger, C., D. Parsons, and D. Remy.** 1964. Syntheses of 5-trifluoromethyluracil and 5-trifluoromethyl-2′-dexoyuridine. J. Med. Chem. **7**:1–5.
9. **Huffman, J. H., R. W. Sidwell, G. P. Khare, J. T. Witkowski, L. B. Allen, and R. K. Robins.** 1973. In vitro effects of 1-β-D-ribofuranosyl-1, 2, 4,-triazole-3-carboxamide (virazole, ICN 1229) on deoxyribonucleic acid and ribonucleic acid viruses. Antimicrob. Agents Chemother. **3**:235–241.
10. **Kaiser, A. B., and Z. A. McGee.** 1975. Aminoglycoside therapy of gram negative bacillary meningitis. N. Engl. J. Med. **293**:1215–1220.
11. **Kaufman, H. E.** 1965. In vivo studies with antiviral agents. Ann. N.Y. Acad. Sci. **130**:168–180.
12. **Kaufman, H. E., and C. Heidelberger.** 1964. Therapeutic antiviral action of 5-trifluoromethyl-2′-deoxyuridine in herpes simplex keratitis. Science **145**:585–586.
13. **Leider, W., R. L. Magoffin, E. H. Lenette, and L. N. R. Leonards.** 1965. Herpes-simplex-virus encephalitis. Its possible association with reactivated latent infection. N. Engl. J. Med. **273**:341–347.
14. **McIlwain, H., and Bacelard, H. S. (ed.).** 1971. Biochemistry and the central nervous system, p. 141. The Williams & Wilkins Co., Baltimore.
15. **Oie, H. K., C. E. Buckler, C. P. Uhlendorf, D. A. Hill, and S. Baron.** 1972. Improved assays for a variety of interferons. Proc. Soc. Exp. Biol. Med. **140**:1178–1181.
16. **Parkhurst, J. R., P. V. Danenberg, and C. Heidelberger.** 1976. Growth inhibition of cells in culture and of vaccinia virus infected HeLa cells by derivatives of trifluorothymidine. Chemotherapy 22:221–232.
17. **Pavan-Langston, D., R. A. Buchanan, and C. A. Alford, Jr. (ed.).** 1975. Adenine arabinoside: an antiviral agent. Raven Press, New York.
18. **Plummer, G., and A. P. Ingerson.** 1974. Iododeoxyuridine and herpes viral encephalitis: lack of inhibitory action against low grade viral replication. Antimicrob. Agents Chemother. 5:672–673.
19. **Reyes, P., and C. Heidelberger.** 1965. Fluorinated pyrimidines. XXVI. Mammalian thymidylate synthetase: its mechanism of action and inhibition by fluorinated nucleotides. Mol. Pharmacol. **1**:14–30.
20. **Tone, H., and C. Heidelberger.** 1973. Fluorinated pyrimidines. XLIV. Interaction of 5-trifluoromethyl-2′-deoxyuridine 5′-triphosphate with deoxyribonucleic acid polymerases. Mol. Pharmacol. **9**:783–791.
21. **Umeda, M., and C. Heidelberger.** 1968. Comparative studies of fluorinated pyrimidines with various cell lines. Cancer Res. 28:2529–2538.
22. **Wellings, P. C., P. N. Audry, F. H. Bors, B. R. Jones, D. C. Brown, and H. E. Kaufman.** 1972. Clinical evaluation of trifluorothymidine in the treatment of herpes simplex corneal ulcers. Am. J. Opthalmol. **73**:932–942.

ANTIMICROBIAL AGENTS AND CHEMOTHERAPY, Feb. 1977, p. 312-317

Vol. 11, No. 2
Printed in U.S.A.

Lethal and Mutagenic Effects of 5-Iodouracil on Bacteriophage T4*td*8*r*II

DANIEL M. BYRD[1]* AND WILLIAM H. PRUSOFF
Department of Pharmacology, Yale University, New Haven, Connecticut 06510

Received for publication 2 September 1976

Evidence was obtained which indicates that the lethal effect of 5-iodouracil (IUra) on bacteriophage T4 is not due to a mutagenic process. T4*td*8*r*II (thymine requiring, rapid lysis) double mutants were constructed. Reversion of T4*td*8*r*II to r^+ was measured. First, reversion by growth in the presence of the structural analogues chlorouracil (ClUra) and bromouracil (BrUra) did not correlate with their relative lethal effects (for mutagenesis: IUra $\leq$ ClUra $\leq$ BrUra; for lethality: ClUra $<$ BrUra $<$ IUra). Second, reversion frequencies of T4*td*8*r*II in infected cells increased linearly with time of growth in the presence of IUra, whereas the frequency of lethality was constant with time. Third, reversion frequencies increased markedly at low levels of IUra substitution, whereas lethal effects were apparent only with extensive IUra substitution. Fourth, the reversion frequency of the nonviable fraction of IUra-substituted T4*td*8*r*II (as examined by multiplicity reactivation) did not differ significantly from that of the viable IUra-substituted T4*td*8 fraction. If mutagenesis caused lethality, then the nonviable T4*td*8*r*II fraction should accumulate mutations and have a higher reversion frequency.

Selective uptake of the antiviral agent 5-iodo-2′-deoxyuridine(IdUrd) explains much of its therapeutic index against herpes simplex virus. Phosphorylated metabolites of IdUrd accumulate in the virus-infected cell because of the induction of virus-specified thymidine kinase (17). However, inhibition of intermediary enzymatic process by IdUrd metabolites does not explain the ability of IdUrd to kill (20). IdUrd is incorporated into viral deoxyribonucleic acid (DNA) in place of thymidine, and malfunction of the resulting iodo-DNA provides an alternative explanation for the lethal effect of IdUrd (9).

We have chosen bacteriophage T4 as a model system to investigate the mechanism(s) of the lethal effect of IdUrd. For the thymine-requiring system of T4*td*8 grown on *Escherichia coli* BT⁻, the lethal effect of 5-iodouracil (IUra) is equivalent to that of IdUrd (6). A monotonic, increasing relationship exists between the concentration of IUra in the medium, the percentage of IUra substitution in DNA, and the extent of the lethal effect (6). Two mechanisms that are qualitatively different account for the lethal effect: (i) sensitivity to incident radiation, particularly near-visible light, or (ii) incorporation of IUra per se (4). Inhibition of DNA replication does not account for the lethal effect in the absence of light (6). Normal yields of progeny particles occur, which absorb and inject competently, and which can be reactivated in several ways, although the particles are IUra substituted and nonviable (5, 13). (By nonviable, we mean that the particle is unable to replicate such that a plaque is formed under standard plating conditions.) IUra is a mutagen for T4 (19). Therefore, we reasoned that the IUra-substituted particles might be killed by accumulation of mutations formed during the DNA incorporation process.

In this paper we investigate the possibility of a mutagenic mechanism of lethality by examining reversion events with a well-characterized system, the *r*II locus of T4 (3). The results are not consistent with a mutagenic mechanism for the lethal effect of IUra.

[1] Present address: Department of Pharmacology, University of Oklahoma Health Sciences Center, Oklahoma City, OK 73190.

MATERIALS AND METHODS

Organisms. W. D. Rupp provided *E. coli* BT⁻. E. B. Freese supplied *E. coli* strains BA, BB, and K(λ). (λ). I. Tessman provided *E. coli* OK 305. E. B. Freese, G. Stent, and S. Champe supplied the T4*r*II C. K. Mathews provided T4*td*8.

Methods. Preparation and purification of substituted T4 stocks, measurement of viability by optical cross section, tris(hydroxymethyl)aminomethane-salts medium, protection from near-visible light, and determination of percentage substitution by CsCl isopycnic centrifugation have been described

(4, 6, 13). Standard plating techniques were used for T4 and to detect the *r*II phenotype (2, 3). The *td* phenotype was determined by the white halo technique of Hall and co-workers (15). Mutation frequency (reversion frequency) was calculated as the ratio of plaque-forming units (PFU) on *E. coli* K(λ) to PFU on *E. coli* BA (K/B) (12). Multiplicity reactivation of IUra-substituted T4 has been described (5). T4*td*8 was recombined with T4*r*II by mixedly infecting *E. coli* BA with both phage types, each at input multiplicities of 4 phage per cell. After one round of growth, progeny were plated on *E. coli* OK 305, and plaques with *td* phenotypes (white halos) were picked. Plaques that did not lyse *E. coli* K(λ) lawns were regrown on *E. coli* BB as described by Fleming and Bessman (10). Stocks derived in this way were retested for *td* and *r*II phenotypes and were used only if recombinant viability, spontaneous reversion frequency, and frequency of white halo phenotype were consistent with those of the appropriate parental stocks. Functional survival of IUra-substituted T4*td*8 was examined with *E. coli* K(λ) grown to 2×10^8 cells per ml in C medium (modified to contain 0.5% glucose instead of maltose [8]) and resuspended in adsorption buffer (supplemented with 0.025% gelatin and 100 μM L-tryptophan [16]) at approximately 2×10^9 cells per ml. One-milliliter portions of cells were mixed with (i) 6×10^9 PFU of T4*td*8*r*II (AP72) (K/B ratio, 0.14×10^{-5}), (ii) 8×10^6 PFU of IUra-substituted T4*td*8 (optical cross section, 17×10^{-11} cm²/PFU), or (iii) (i) and (ii) together. After 10 min at 37° C, unadsorbed phage were removed by centrifuging infected cells, and appropriate dilutions of the pellet were plated on either *E. coli* BA or *E. coli* K(λ) lawns. The "found/expected" ratio is the PFU per milliliter obtained when both phage types are present divided by the sum of the PFU per milliliter obtained with each individual phage type.

RESULTS

Construction and characteristics of double mutants. We studied an *r*II mutant, AP72, that reverts strongly in the presence of bromouracil (BrUra) (12). T4*r*II(AP72) was recombined with T4*td*8 to produce a T4*td*8*r*II(AP72) genotype.

Three tests were performed to demonstrate that T4*td*8*r*II(AP72) did have the same properties attributed to T4*r*II(AP72) and that IdUrd did produce the same effect as bromodeoxyuridine (BrdUrd). First, the ability of both T4*r*II(AP72) and T4*td*8*r*II(AP72) to form plaques on *E. coli* K(λ) lawns increased after growth on either *E. coli* BB in the presence of BrdUrd, or on *E. coli* BT⁻ in the presence of IdUrd. Second, IdUrd-induced reversion was genotypic instead of phenotypic. Stocks grown in the presence of IdUrd were plated, and individual plaques were picked from *E. coli* K(λ) lawns. Stocks were grown from each plaque on *E. coli* BB and tested for *r*II⁺ by plating on *E. coli* BA and *E. coli* K(λ). Nine out of nine plaques picked after IdUrd treatment of T4*r*II(AP72) plated equivalently on either *E. coli* BA or *E. coli* K(λ). Thirty out of thirty-one plaques picked after IdUrd treatment of T4*td*8*r*II(AP72) plated equivalently on *E. coli* BA and *E. coli* K(λ). The remaining plaque yielded progeny that plated less well on *E. coli* BA than on *E. coli* K(λ). All 31 plaques picked retained the *td* genotype. Third, progeny phage obtained after growth in the presence of IdUrd on *E. coli* BT⁻ were regrown on the same host at a low multiplicity of infection in the absence of IdUrd and presence of deoxythymidine. The reversion frequencies of both T4*r*II(AP72) and T4*td*8*r*II(AP72) were not altered appreciably by this second round of growth, demonstrating that the *r*II⁺ revertants resulted from errors of incorporation.

Structure-activity relationships. To examine structure-activity relationships, we studied the closely related halouracils, chlorouracil (ClUra), BrUra, and IUra. During a single, synchronous growth cycle in the absence of light, under conditions where approximately 70% substitution by halouracils occurs, full complements of physically intact phage particles were produced that were normal in their DNA content and ability to absorb to and kill bacteria, but were reduced in viability. Quantitatively, ClUra is less effective than BrUra, which is less effective than IUra with respect to lethality (6). Under the same conditions, the mutagenicity of the three analogues showed a different quantitative relationship (Table 1).

Kinetic relationships. The induction of lethality might increase with growth of intracellular progeny, if the intracellular thymine pool (created from host cell DNA breakdown) were preferentially incorporated into intracellular progeny early during the growth cycle. Previous experiments showed the transfer of *E. coli* BT⁻ DNA-thymine to T4*td*8 progeny DNA to be equivalent with either thymine or IUra present in the growth media (6). Therefore, we examined the viability of intracellular T4*td*8 progeny accumulating in infected *E. coli* BT⁻ cells at different times after growth in the presence of thymine or IUra. The appearance of

TABLE 1. *Comparison of the lethal effect and mutagenicity of ClUra, BrUra, or IUra for T4td8rII(AP72)*

Growth in the presence of:	Burst size (% control)	Reversion frequency (K/B × 10⁴)
Thymine	100	0.004
ClUra	38	1.9
BrUra	25	4.4
IUra	13	1.3

viable intracellular progeny is impaired by IUra to the same extent at earlier times as at the time of spontaneous cell lysis (Fig. 1).

Another possibility was that IUra impaired the synthesis of full complements of virus particles but gave rise to fully viable progeny at early times in the synthesis of intracellular progeny. We eliminated this possibility from consideration in a companion experiment. Infected cells were lysed after 15 min of growth in the presence of IUra, and the optical cross section of the progeny particles obtained after purification was compared with the optical cross section obtained after a complete growth cycle. They were approximately the same (19×10^{-11} cm^2/PFU and 14×10^{-11} cm^2/PFU, respectively).

Since a linear increase with respect to time in the reversion frequency of T4 intracellular progeny in the presence of BrdUrd was obtained by Susman and co-workers, we studied the kinetic correlation of IUra-induced reversion frequency to IUra-induced lethality in T4*td*8*r*II-infected *E. coli* BT⁻ (22). The reversion frequency increased linearly with time from the value of the control to the value found for the progeny after lysis, whereas, as stated previously, lethality is constant at any time during the growth cycle (Fig. 2).

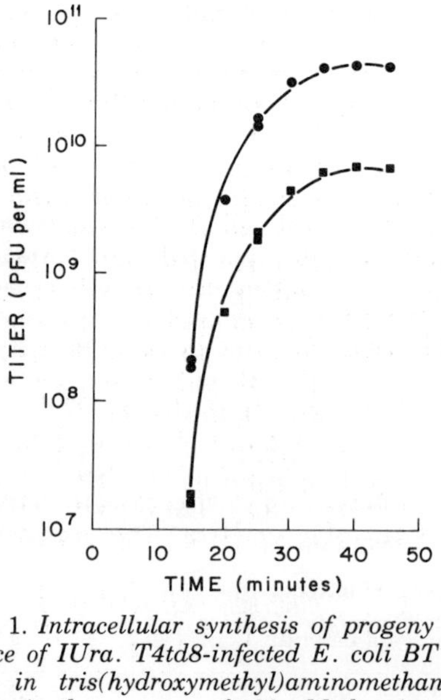

FIG. 1. *Intracellular synthesis of progeny in the presence of IUra. T4td8-infected E. coli BT⁻ were grown in tris(hydroxymethyl)aminomethane-salts medium in the presence of 100 μM thymine (●) or 100 μM IUra (■). At the indicated times, 1-ml samples were mixed with 3 drops of* $CHCl_3$ *and chilled on ice. Portions of each sample were diluted and plated on E. coli BA. The concentration of infected cells in each flask was* 4×10^8 *infected cells per ml, and the burst size was approximately 110 phage per cell.*

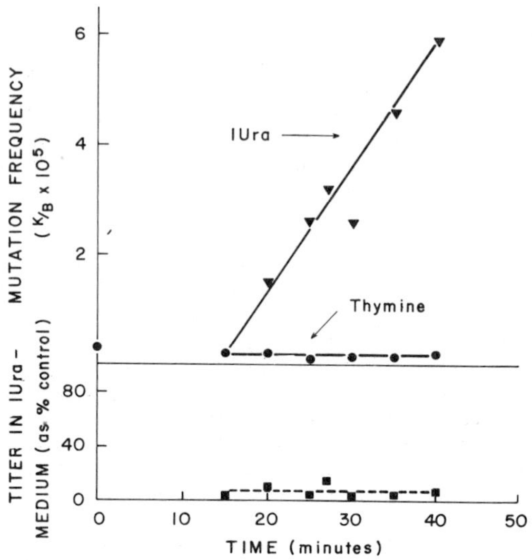

FIG. 2. *Kinetics of lethality and mutagenicity of IUra for T4td8rII(AP72). T4td8rII(AP72) was grown on E. coli BT⁻ in tris(hydroxymethyl)aminomethane-salts medium with 250 μM thymine or IUra. The cells were infected at a multiplicity of 2 phage per cell, and the density of infected cells in the phage growth flasks was* 6×10^9 *cells per ml. At the indicated times, 2-ml portions from each of the flasks were mixed with 8 drops of* $CHCl_3$ *and chilled on ice. Each portion was diluted in adsorption buffer and plated on E. coli BA or E. coli K(λ). The solid lines indicate the K/B ratios that were obtained at different times in the presence of IUra or thymine. The dashed line shows the ratio of PFU on E. coli BA in the presence of IUra to PFU on E. coli BA in the presence of thymine.*

Dose-response relationships. A correlation between IUra-induced mutagenesis and lethal effects was obtained in dose-response studies. As the percentage of substitution of IUra for DNA-thymine increased, both reversion frequency and lethality of T4*td*8*r*II increased (Fig. 3). Percentage substitution varies with the ratio of IUra to thymine in the growth medium (6). However, reversion frequency increased most markedly at lower ratios of IUra to thymine in the medium, whereas the lethal effect is apparent only at higher ratios.

Marker rescue of *r*II. Since IUra substitution impairs the function of some T4 genes (14), we examined the effect of IUra substitution on *r*II⁺. T4*td*8 has equal viability when plated on either *E. coli* BA or *E. coli* K(λ). We infected *E. coli* K(λ) with IUra-substituted T4*td*8 and T4*td*8*r*II together, to see whether IUra-substituted T4*td*8 would supply the *r*II function not expressed by T4*td*8*r*II. As described by Krieg (18), when the mixedly infected *E. coli* K(λ) was plated on *E. coli* K(λ) lawns, where *r*II

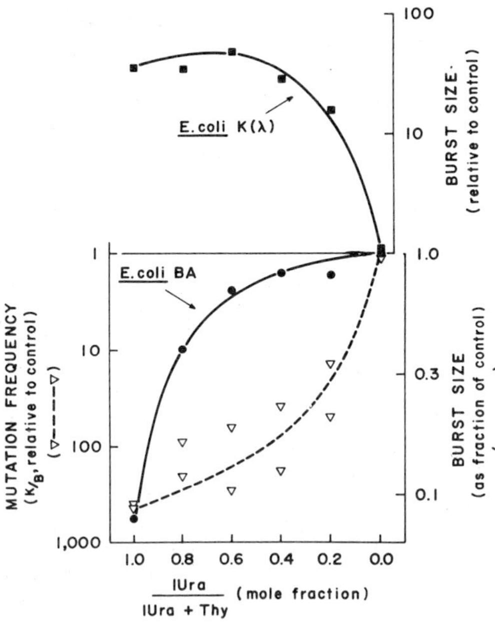

FIG. 3. *Dose-response study of the lethality and mutagenicity of IUra for T4td8rII(AP72). T4td8rII(AP72) was grown on E. coli BT⁻ in tris(hydroxymethyl)aminomethane-salts media in the presence of the indicated mole fractions (of IUra to IUra plus thymine) such that the total concentration of IUra plus thymine was 250 μM. The cells were infected at a multiplicity of 1 phage per cell at a density of 3 × 10⁸ infected cells per ml. $CHCl_3$ was added after 45 min. Duplicate portions from each flask were diluted in adsorption buffer and plated on E. coli BA or E. coli K(λ) lawns. The solid lines show the titer of each flask relative to the titer obtained with no IUra present on either E. coli BA or E. coli K(λ). The dashed line indicates the K/B ratio of progeny from each flask relative to the K/B ratio obtained with no IUra present.*

phage do not survive, genotypic rescue occurs. When plated on *E. coli* BA lawns, where *r*II phage form plaques, phenotypic rescue occurs. IUra-substituted T4*td*8 can both phenotypically and genotypically rescue T4*td*8*r*II (Table 2).

Mutation frequency of nonviable IUra-substituted T4*td*8*r*II. Since T4*td*8*r*II extensively substituted with IUra differs either from T4*td*8*r*II substituted with other halouracils or from T4*td*8*r*II slightly substituted with IUra, in a high degree of lethality relative to mutation frequency, we reasoned that mutations might accumulate in the nonviable fraction of the IUra-substituted T4*r*II*td*8 population. Since nonviable, IUra-substituted T4 reactivates itself at high multiplicities of infection, we could test this hypothesis (5).

Spontaneously arising revertants cannot be detected when highly mutagenized phage stocks are plated, because the number of newly arising revertants is small compared with the number of revertants already present. The burst size of IUra-substituted, multiplicity-reactivated T4*td*8*r*II (AP72) is not known. If it is small, then the reversion frequency of progeny will be about the same as that of the viable parental phage, because the number of r^+ phage reactivated will be small. For this reason, we plated infected cells before lysis. Under these conditions, each cell in which multiplicity reactivation of nonviable phage takes place counts the same as each cell infected with a viable phage. The reversion frequency of multiplicity-reactivated phage in cells infected with substituted T4*td*8*r*II does not differ significantly from the reversion frequency of nonreactivated T4*td*8*r*II surviving the lethal effects of IUra substitution (Table 3).

DISCUSSION

We undertook these experiments to define the lethal effect of IUra in the absence of light. IUra, apparently, does not kill bacteriophage T4 by a mutagenic effect. The absence of a correlation between the structure-activity relationship for lethal effects compared with the

TABLE 2. *Functional survival of IUra-substituted T4td8*

Phage prepn	Phenotypic rescue (*E. coli* BA)	Genotypic rescue (*E. coli* Kλ)
T4*td*8*r*II (PFU/ml)	1.63 × 10⁷	<2.5 × 10⁴
IUra-substituted T4*td*8 (PFU/ml)	0.91 × 10⁷	0.76 × 10⁷
IUra-substituted T4*td*8 plus T4*td*8*r*II (PFU/ml)	5.3 × 10⁷	1.3 × 10⁷
Found/expected (ratio)	2.1	1.7

TABLE 3. *Multiplicity reactivation of IUra-substituted T4td8rII (AP72)*

Determination	Unsubstituted	IUra-substituted
Multiplicity of infection (particles/cell)	0.7	0.6
Multiplicity of infection (PFU/cell)	0.7	0.06
Infected cells expected (PFU/ml ×10⁻⁹)	3.3	0.5
Infected cells found (PFU/ml ×10⁻⁹)	3.6	1.5
Mutation frequency of progeny (K/B ×10⁴)	0.004	1.3
Mutation frequency of infected cells (K/B ×10⁴)	0.04	0.7

relationship for mutagenesis indicates that the lethality and mutagenicity of IUra are unrelated. Further, no kinetic correlation exists between the mutagenicity and the lethality of IUra for T4. Since the reversion frequency of survivors is the same as the reversion frequency of the nonviable fraction of the IUra-substituted population, the relationship between mutagenicity and lethality with respect to percentage of substitution (dose of IUra), if any, cannot be one to one. Finally, reversions do not accumulate in the nonviable fraction, as might be expected if the nonviable fraction experienced more mutational hits.

That extensive mutagenesis does not causally result in extensive lethality is not surprising. For example, Tessman discovered conditions under which hydroxylamine rarely produces lethal hits but is a potent mutagen (24). IdUrd-substituted T4*td*8 induces lower levels of several phage-coded enzymes, including deoxycytidylate deaminase (13). Goz and Aamodt showed IdUrd-substituted T4*td*8-induced deoxycytidylate deaminase to be immunologically equivalent to unsubstituted T4*td*8-induced deoxycytidylate deaminase (1), whereas, if IdUrd-induced mutagenesis caused the lower level of deoxycytidylate deaminase, cross-reacting but enzymatically inactive material would be expected.

In this paper, comparisons of reversion at a single genetic site induced by IUra with the lethal effect of IUra indicate that the mutagenic and lethal effects of IUra are unrelated. This finding applies to reversion at several other sites within the *r*II gene. Studies with T4*td*8*r*II recombinants at other *r*II sites (AP129, DAP-56, *uv-181*, and AP275) do not contradict the results with T4*td*8*r*II(AP72) (D. M. Byrd and W. H. Prusoff, unpublished data). All of the mutants listed revert while incorporating BrdUrd (7, 12). The possibility exists that IUra induces other mutagenic processes within the *r*II gene. However, the predominant evidence indicates that BrUra-induced mutations are errors of incorporation (11). Errors of replication, postulated by Terzaghi and coworkers (23), would not explain the inability of IUra-substituted T4 to induce normal enzyme levels.

Generalization of the present results to all T4 genes warrants some caution. The best evidence that *r*II behaves like other T4 genes with respect to IUra substitution is that *r*II resembles some other T4 genes in undergoing marker rescue. Because AP72 is a point mutant of *r*II, the gene product of AP72 can interfere with the rII^+ phenotypic function. Therefore, the present rescue studies yield a minimal estimate of marker rescue and are subject to an ambiguity not found in previous marker rescue studies of IUra-substituted T4, which utilized *amber* mutants (14).

Impairment of different T4 genes by IdUrd substitution is not constant; some genes are relatively sensitive, whereas others are relatively resistant (14). The present results argue that this distribution is not caused by different "hot spots" for IUra-induced mutagenesis within the genes. Comparison of marker rescue studies with multiplicity reactivation data for IUra-substituted, nonviable T4, led us to reject mechanisms that involve either a few "critical sites" in the genome for lethal damage or characteristic deletions of T4 (5). Instead, we postulated a model in which T4 replication is not perfectly efficient with respect to gene products. In this model, different T4 genes vary in susceptibility to IUra substitution due to variance in either specific susceptibility (length of gene, base sequence, etc.) or the catalytic versus stoichiometric nature of the gene product (21). Although the present results reject mutagenesis as an explanation for impairment of gene product synthesis, we believe that the model remains valid as a working hypothesis for the mechanism of IUra-induced lethal effects.

ACKNOWLEDGMENTS

We thank S. Champe, E. B. Freese, W. D. Rupp, G. Stent, and I. Tessman for the phage and bacterial strains. B. Goz, I. Rubenstein, and I. Tessman provided helpful advice.

This work was supported by Public Health Service grants CA-05262 and CA-1074A from the National Cancer Institute, and by GM-59 from the National Institute of General Medical Sciences.

LITERATURE CITED

1. **Aamodt, L., and B. Goz.** 1970. An immunological study of an enzyme made by phage containing 5-iodo-2′-deoxyuridine-substituted deoxyribonucleic acid. Biochem. Pharmacol. 19:2400–2403.
2. **Adams, M. H.** 1959. Appendix, p. 443–552. *In* Bacteriophages. John Wiley & Sons, Inc., New York.
3. **Benzer, S.** 1955. Fine structure of a genetic region in bacteriophage. Proc. Natl. Acad. Sci. U.S.A. 41:344–354.
4. **Byrd, D. M., B. Goz, and W. H. Prusoff.** 1975. Comparison of the lethal effect of 5-iodouracil incorporated into bacteriophage T4 in the presence and absence of near-visible light. Photochem. Photobiol. 21:407–412.
5. **Byrd, D. M., and W. H. Prusoff.** 1975. Multiplicity reactivation of 5-iodouracil-substituted, nonviable bacteriophage T4*td*8. Antimicrob. Agents Chemother. 8:558–563.
6. **Byrd, D. M., and W. H. Prusoff.** 1976. The effect of 5-iodouracil on the growth and biosynthetic processes of bacteriophage T4*td*8 in the absence of light. Chem. Biol. Interact. 12:197–210.
7. **Champe, S. P., and S. Benzer.** 1962. Reversal of mutant phenotypes by 5-fluorouracil: an approach to nucleotide sequences in messenger-RNA. Proc. Natl. Acad. Sci. U.S.A. 48:532–546.

8. **Cowie, D. B., G. N. Cohen, E. T. Bolton, and H. DeRobichon-Szulmajster.** 1959. Amino acid analogue incorporation into bacterial protein. Biochim. Biophys. Acta 34:39–46.
9. **Dunn, D. B., and J. D. Smith.** 1957. Effects of 5-halogenated uracils on the growth of *Escherichia coli* and their incorporation in deoxyribonucleic acids. Biochem. J. 67:494–506.
10. **Fleming, W. H., and M. J. Bessman.** 1967. The enzymology of virus-infected bacteria. IX. Purification and properties of the deoxycytidylate deaminase of T6-infected *E. coli*. J. Biol. Chem. 242:363–371.
11. **Freese, E.** 1959. The difference between spontaneous and base-analogue induced mutations of phage T4. Proc. Natl. Acad. Sci. U.S.A. 45:622–633.
12. **Freese, E. B., and E. Freese.** 1967. On the specificity of DNA polymerase. Proc. Natl. Acad. Sci. U.S.A. 57:650–657.
13. **Goz, B., and W. H. Prusoff.** 1968. The ability of phage containing 5-iodo-2′-deoxyuridine-substituted deoxyribonucleic acid to induce enzymes. J. Biol. Chem. 243:4750–4756.
14. **Goz, B., and W. H. Prusoff.** 1970. The relation of antiviral activity of IUdR to gene function in phage. Ann. N.Y. Acad. Sci. 173:379–389.
15. **Hall, D. H., I. Tessman, and O. Karlström.** 1967. Linkage of T4 genes controlling a series of steps in pyrimidine biosynthesis. Virology 31:442–448.
16. **Hershey, A. D., and M. Chase.** 1952. Independent functions of viral protein and nucleic acid in growth of bacteriophage. J. Gen. Physiol. 36:39–56.
17. **Kit, S., and D. R. Dubbs.** 1963. Acquisition of thymidine kinase activity by herpes simplex infected mouse fibroblast cells. Biochem. Biophys. Res. Commun. 11:55–59.
18. **Krieg, D. R.** 1959. A study of gene action in ultraviolet-irradiated bacteriophage T4. Virology 8:80–98.
19. **Litman, R. M., and A. B. Pardee.** 1956. Production of bacteriophage mutants by a disturbance of deoxyribonucleic acid metabolism. Nature (London) 178:529–531.
20. **Prusoff, W. H., and B. Goz.** 1975. Halogenated pyrimidine deoxyribonucleosides p. 272–347. *In* A. C. Sartorelli and D. G. Johns (ed.), Antineoplastic and immunosuppressive agents, vol. 2. Springer Verlag, New York.
21. **Snustadt, D. P.** 1968. Dominant interactions in *E. coli* cells mixedly infected with bacteriophage T4 wild-type and amber mutants and their possible implications as to type of gene-product function: catalytic vs. stoichiometric. Virology 35:550–563.
22. **Susman, M., M. M. Piechowski, and D. A. Ritchie.** 1965. Studies on phage development. I. An acridine-sensitive clock. Virology 26:163–174.
23. **Terzaghi, B. E., G. Streisinger, and F. W. Stahl.** 1962. The mechanism of 5-bromouracil mutagenesis in the bacteriophage T4. Proc. Natl. Acad. Sci. U. S. A. 48:1519–1524.
24. **Tessman, I.** 1968. Mutagenic treatment of double- and single-stranded DNA phages T4 and S13 with hydroxylamine. Virology 35:330–333.

Antimicrobial Agents and Chemotherapy, Feb. 1977, p. 318–323 Vol. 11, No. 2
 Printed in U.S.A.

Tetracycline Inhibits Propagation of Deoxyribonucleic Acid Replication and Alters Membrane Properties

MARTIN L. PATO

Division of Molecular and Cellular Biology, National Jewish Hospital and Research Center, and Department of Microbiology, University of Colorado Medical Center, Denver, Colorado 80206

Received for publication 8 November 1976

Tetracycline, at concentrations greater than required for inhibition of protein synthesis, rapidly and completely inhibits replication of deoxyribonucleic acid (DNA) in *Escherichia coli* and *Bacillus subtilis*. At these concentrations of tetracycline, synthesis of ribonucleic acid is not appreciably altered. In addition to inhibiting DNA replication, tetracycline causes alterations of the cytoplasmic membrane resulting in leakage of intracellular pools of nucleotides, amino acids, and the non-metabolizable sugar analogue, thiomethylgalactoside. As DNA is synthesized at a site on the membrane, alterations of membrane structure by tetracycline may be responsible for the observed inhibition of DNA replication.

The tetracyclines (TC) are broad-spectrum antibiotics which were once thought to cause a "bewildering variety of apparently unrelated effects" (5, 9). In the early 1960s some authors despaired of finding a single, unifying mode of action for TC, and suggested that consideration should be given to the order and conditions under which various mechanisms might apply. Though TC may indeed have more than a single mode of action, more recent work has carefully delineated its primary action as an inhibitor of protein synthesis; TC prevents the binding of aminoacyl-transfer ribonucleic acid (RNA) to the postulated "A site" on the ribosome (see reference 5 for review).

As a secondary consequence of inhibition of protein synthesis, initiation of new rounds of deoxyribonucleic acid (DNA) synthesis should be inhibited leading to cessation of replication after nascent molecules have proceeded to completion. That is, propagation of DNA synthesis normally continues after inhibition of protein synthesis, though the rate of movement of replication forks may be decreased (14, 18). This expectation is not the observed effect; instead, as this communication demonstrates, TC rapidly and completely inhibits the propagation of DNA synthesis. Alteration of membrane structure, manifested as changes in cellular permeability, may be responsible for the observed inhibition of DNA replication.

MATERIALS AND METHODS

Bacterial strains and growth conditions. The strains of *Escherichia coli* used were AS19 (an *E. coli* B originally selected for increased sensitivity to actinomycin), B/r *thy*$^-$, and 15 TAU bar. The organisms were grown at 37°C in a phosphate-buffered minimal medium (3) or tris(hydroxymethyl)-aminomethane(Tris)-buffered minimal medium with 0.2% glucose or glycerol as carbon source. Required amino acids were supplied at 50 μg/ml. A combination of 4 μg of thymidine/ml and 100 μg of uridine/ml were used to supply thymine and uracil requirements. The gram-positive *Bacillus subtilis* 168 was grown in *T56T* medium (12).

Measurement of macromolecular syntheses. To monitor macromolecular syntheses, cultures were labeled with [^{3}H]thymidine (4 μg/ml, 10 μCi/ml), uridine (10 μg/ml, 10 μCi/ml), or leucine (10 μg/ml, 2 μCi/ml). Samples of 100 μl were removed from labeled cultures into chilled 5% trichloroacetic acid, collected on membrane filters, and washed with cold 5% trichloroacetic acid and then with hot water. Radioactivity on dried filters was determined in a toluene-based scintillation mixture. Chemical determinations of DNA were performed using the diphenylamine method of Burton (2).

Nucleoside triphosphate pool measurements. Nucleoside triphosphate pools were labeled by growth in Tris medium in the presence of [^{32}P]orthophosphate (300 μCi/μmol) for one cell doubling. The [^{32}P]orthophosphate was purified immediately before use by adsorption to a Dowex-1-Cl column and elution with 0.1 N HCl.

Samples of 2 ml from ^{32}P-labeled cultures were rapidly filtered and suspended in 1 ml of 0.3 M perchloric acid. After 20 min on ice, the extracts were brought to a pH of 5.0 to 5.5, and a 50-μl portion of each extract was spotted on a PEI-cellulose thin-layer chromatography plate. The plates were developed in two dimensions, using procedures similar to those of Neuhard et al. (11). The solvent in the first dimension was 1.25 N LiCl-1 N acetic acid, and the solvent in the second dimension was 0.75 M LiCl-7.5% boric acid. Radioactive spots were located by autoradiography, cut out, and analyzed by counting in a toluene-based scintillation mixture.

CsCl gradient centrifugation. Samples of covalently closed circular PM2 DNA (generously supplied by John Carlson) were added to tubes containing 5.1 g of CsCl, 5.2 ml of TES buffer (0.03 M Tris, pH 8.0, 0.005 M ethylenediaminetetraacetate, 0.05 M NaCl), and either no additional supplement, 400 μg of ethidium bromide/ml or 400 μg of TC/ml. Sedimentation was for 60 h at 44,000 rpm in a Spinco 50Ti rotor at 15°C. Drops were collected from the bottom of the tubes onto squares of Whatman 3MM paper; the squares were washed sequentially in 5% trichloroacetic acid, 95% enthanol, and ether and counted in a toluene-based scintillation mixture.

Leakage of intracellular pools. Leakage of nucleotides was examined by labeling cells with [^{3}H]guanosine (4 μg/ml, 80 μCi/ml) or [^{3}H]uridine (2 μg/ml, 20 μCi/ml) for 20 min before addition of TC. Samples were filtered, and both cells and supernatant were brought to 0.4 M HCOOH. The samples were analyzed by thin-layer chromatography in one dimension using LiCl as the solvent as described by Randerath and Randerath (17). Plates were cut into 1.0-cm strips which were extracted with 0.1 ml 4 N NH_4OH for 20 min before counting in 5 ml of Aquasol (New England Nuclear).

To measure the leakage of radioactively labeled sugars and amino acids from intracellular pools, cells were "loaded" with [^{14}C]thiomethyl-β-D-galactopyranoside (TMG) or radioactive amino acids under appropriate conditions. At intervals before and after addition of TC, 200-μl samples were rapidly filtered on 0.45-μm pore size membrane filters (Millipore Corp.) and washed with 1 ml of nonradioactive medium. Label retained by the cells was then measured. Cells were loaded with [^{14}C]-TMG by inducing a culture of AS19 with isopropyl-β-D-thiogalactopyranoside (5×10^{-4} M) for one generation of growth, removing the isopropyl-β-D-thiogalactopyranoside by filtration, and adding [^{14}C]TMG (10 μg/ml, 0.5 μCi/ml) 10 min before addition of TC. Radioactive amino acids were added 5 min after inhibition of protein synthesis with chloramphenicol (150 μg/ml) and 10 min before addition of TC.

RESULTS

Inhibition of macromolecular synthesis. The incorporation of thymidine, uridine, and leucine by cultures of *E. coli* AS19 in the absence and presence of various concentrations of TC is shown in Fig. 1. TC at 50 to 100 μg/ml rapidly and completely inhibited DNA replication as measured by thymidine uptake. At these concentrations of the antibiotic, RNA synthesis as measured by uridine uptake was not appreciably altered; at later times and/or higher concentrations the uptake of uridine was also affected. Inhibition of protein synthesis in AS19 required only 1 to 10 μg of TC/ml. Complete inhibition of DNA synthesis was observed with thymidine incorporation and with chemical measurements using the diphenylamine assay.

The concentration of TC required to inhibit DNA replication is dependent on the bacterial strain: 50 to 100 μg/ml is sufficient for *E. coli* AS19, whereas 100 to 150 μg/ml is required when using *E. coli* B/r *thy*$^-$, and concentrations of 250 μg/ml are required for *E. coli* TAU bar and the gram-positive organism *B. subtilis* 168. As with strain AS19, these levels of the antibiotic do not appreciably affect the rate of RNA synthesis for at least 20 min after addition.

The results of various attempts to reverse the inhibition of DNA replication are shown in Fig. 2. Removal of TC by filtration restored replication only after a lag of approximately 30 min. As replication in some of the known thermosensitive DNA mutants is restored at the nonpermissive temperature by increasing the osmolarity of the medium (6), the effects of 10% glucose

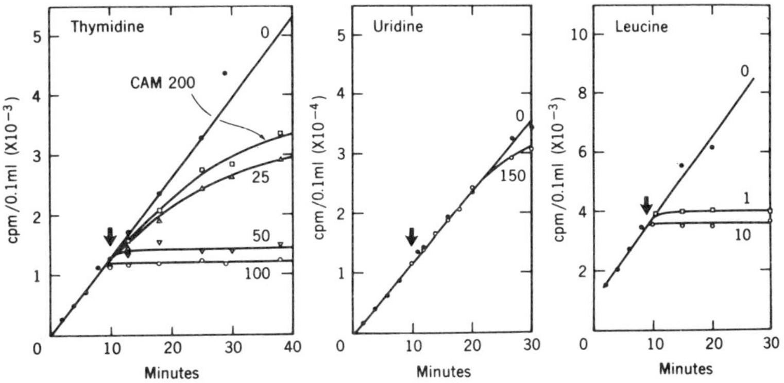

FIG. 1. *Incorporation of [^{3}H]thymidine, -uridine, and -leucine with E. coli AS19 in the presence and absence of TC added 10 min after the labeled precursors. Numbers refer to TC concentration in micrograms per milliliter. Thymidine incorporation in the presence of 200 μg of chloramphenicol/ml is also shown.*

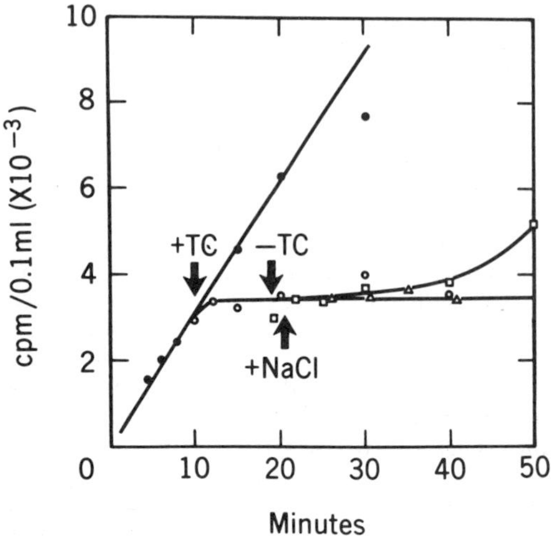

FIG. 2. *Attempts to reverse the effect of addition of 100 μg of TC/ml on thymidine incorporation in E. coli AS19. TC was added (○) 10 min after addition of [^{3}H]thymidine. TC was removed from one portion of the culture (□) by filtration 9 min later, and NaCl (2% final concentration) was added to another portion (△) 10 min after TC addition.*

and 2% NaCl were examined; no reversal of the inhibition was observed.

As TC can chelate divalent cations, the effects of a large molar excess of Mg^{2+}, Mn^{2+}, and Ca^{2+} were examined. Addition of a 5- to 10-fold molar excess of each of these cations after TC addition did not reverse the observed inhibition of DNA synthesis, nor did their prior addition prevent the inhibition (data not shown).

Binding of TC to DNA. Many of the inhibitors of nucleic acid synthesis exert their effect via intercalation into the DNA helix, e.g., proflavine and ethidium (see reference 5 for discussion). The planar structure of the TC molecule suggested that it too might be an intercalating agent. A routine test for intercalation using the density shift of a covalently closed circular DNA molecule in the presence of an intercalating agent is shown in Fig. 3. The intercalating agent ethidium bromide yielded the expected density shift, whereas TC caused no measurable change in density. Other tests designed to measure extensive binding of drugs to DNA were also negative, including the failure to observe bathochromic or hypochromic shifts of the absorption spectra of TC upon the addition of DNA as observed for other drugs which do bind to DNA (19). These results are consistent with earlier experiments which demonstrated only very low levels of binding of TC to DNA (7). It is, of course, difficult to exclude the possibility that very low levels of TC binding may be involved in the observed inhibition of replication.

Effect of TC on nucleoside pools. To investigate the effect of TC on cellular nucleoside triphosphate pools, samples were analyzed by thin-layer chromatography, and the results obtained using AS19 and 15 TAU bar are shown in Table 1. With AS19, no dramatic changes were observed in the presence of 100 μg of TC/ml, a concentration sufficient for rapid inhibition of DNA replication. The general pattern was an initial increase in the size of the pools followed by a decline at later times. It is clear that in the time required for inhibition of replication, generally less than 2 min, no significant decreases were observed. Higher concentrations of TC are required to inhibit replication in 15 TAU bar, and the effects of nucleoside triphosphate pools in 15 TAU bar at these concentrations, 400 μg/ml in this experiment, are strikingly different from those observed with AS19 in the presence of 100 μg of TC/ml. In particular, a rapid and severe shrinking of the deoxyguanosine 5′-triphosphate pool was observed; at later times, all the ribo- and deoxyribonucleoside triphosphate pools decreased in size. However, when this very high level of TC was used with AS19, a similar, extremely rapid shrinking of the deoxyguanosine 5′-triphos-

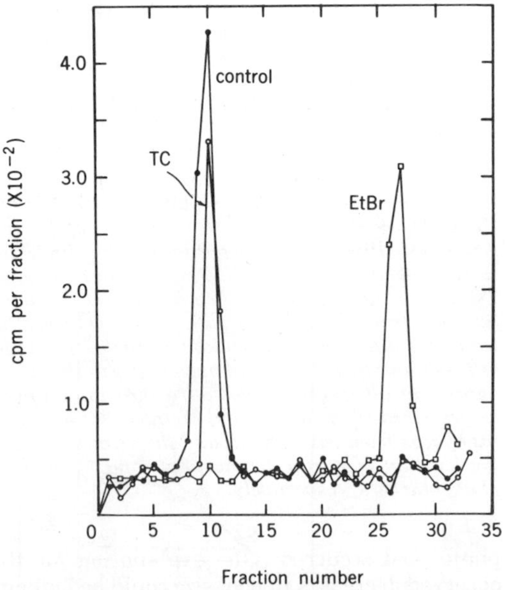

FIG. 3. *CsCl gradient centrifugation of ^{3}H-labeled PM2 DNA. ^{3}H-labeled PM2 DNA was sedimented in CsCl with either no supplements (●), 400 μg of ethidium bromide/ml (□), or 400 μg of TC/ml (○) as described in Materials and Methods.*

TABLE 1. *Intracellular levels of nucleoside triphosphate after TC addition*

Nucleoside triphosphate[b]	Intracellular levels of nucleoside triphosphate after TC addition[a]									
	AS19 (100 μg of TC/ml)			AS19 (400 μg of TC/ml)			15 TAU bar (400 μg of TC/ml)			
	5[c]	15	30	5	15	30	4	10	20	30
G	1.38	0.96	0.48	0.11	0.08	0.08	0.57	0.37	0.28	0.21
U	0.86	0.45	0.14	0.02	0.02	0.02	0.65	0.36	0.21	0.11
A + C	1.25	0.96	0.32	0.15	0.15	0.10	0.89	0.51	0.29	0.20
dG	1.11	0.72	0.36	0.16	0.16	0.11	0.53	0.12	0.06	0.06
T	0.90		0.50			0.26	0.94	0.97	0.59	0.37
dA	1.30	1.20	0.56	0.33	0.62	0.66	1.05	1.05	0.85	0.68
dC	1.12		0.42				1.14	0.92	0.49	0.24

[a] Numbers represent levels relative to those at time of addition of TC.
[b] Abbreviations: G, Guanine; U, uracil; A + C, adenine plus cytidine; dG, deoxyribosylguanine; T, thymine; dA, deoxyribosyladenine; dC, deoxyribosylcytidine.
[c] Minutes after TC addition.

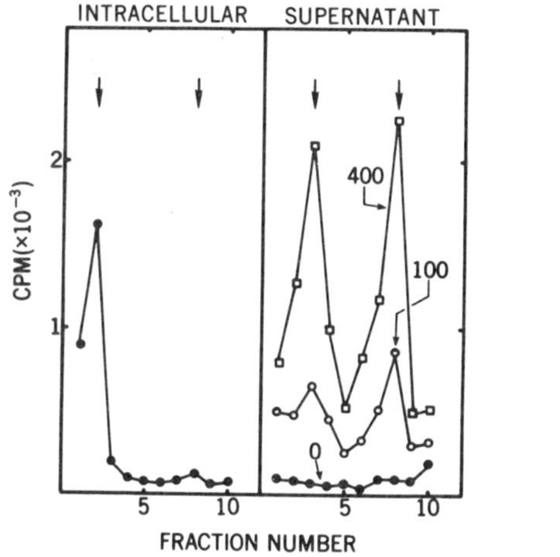

FIG. 4. *Thin-layer chromatography of intracellular and extracellular purine nucleotides. [^{3}H]guanosine was added to a culture of E. coli AS19, and after 20 min one portion of the culture was filtered (●) while 100 μg of TC/ml (○) and 400 μg of TC/ml (□) were added to two additional portions. Samples from the cultures with added TC were filtered 30 min later. Nucleotides extracted from the cells without added TC, and nucleotides in the supernatants of all three samples were chromatographed as described in Materials and Methods. Chromatography was from left to right, and the arrows indicate the location of purine triphosphate and monophosphate markers, respectively.*

phate pool occurred. One explanation for the observed decreases in pool size could be leakage of intracellular material induced by TC. This possibility was therefore examined.

Leakage of intracellular nucleotides. A culture of AS19 was labeled with [^{3}H]guanosine as described in Materials and Methods, and samples were collected before TC addition and 30 min after addition of 100 μg of TC/ml and 400 μg of TC/ml. Cells were filtered rapidly, and the labeled nucleotides present in the supernatant before and after 30 min in TC, as well as the labeled nucleotides in the intracellular pool before TC addition, are shown in Fig. 4. Large amounts of labeled purine triphosphates and monophosphates, and possibly small amounts of purine diphosphates, were found in the supernatant after TC treatment, whereas none was observed in control cultures without added TC. More complete resolution of the nucleotides (data not shown) demonstrated that label was distributed approximately equally between adenine and guanine nucleotides. A similar experiment using [^{3}H]uridine showed leakage of pyrimidine pools; nucleotides in the supernatant were almost exclusively monophosphates.

Leakage of sugar analogues and amino acids. To determine whether the observed leakage is specific for nucleotides or is a more general phenomenon, the effect of TC on intracellular pools of the non-metabolizable lactose analogue TMG was examined. Cells were loaded with [^{14}C]TMG as described in Materials and Methods before TC was added. Intracellular [^{14}C]TMG was measured by filtering the cells and rapidly washing with unlabeled medium. Figure 5 shows that TC addition results in rapid loss of intracellular TMG, higher concentrations of TC leading to more rapid loss of the TMG pool than lower concentrations. The addition of 10^{-5} M carbonyl cyanide *m*-chlorophenyl hydrazone (CCCP), a compound that conducts protons across membranes, thus collapsing the proton-motive force required for transport of TMG (16), also resulted in the loss of the intracellularly accumulated TMG. Gross damage to the cell membrane or lysis of the cells is apparently not occurring, as no β-galactosidase was released into the cytoplasm (data not shown).

The effect of TC addition on loss of amino acid pools was also examined. Two amino acids, histidine and proline, were chosen as representatives of two classes of amino acid transport systems: those requiring proton circulation and those requiring cellular adenosine 5′-triphosphate (ATP) (1). Addition of CCCP should cause release of the pools of amino acids transported via the proton-motive force (proline, in this experiment) but not those whose transport is linked to ATP metabolism (histidine, in this experiment). The data in Fig. 6 show that the expected specificity was seen with CCCP, but TC addition resulted in leakage of both amino acids. These data suggest that the addition of TC results in a membrane alteration causing nonspecific leakage of intracellular pool material.

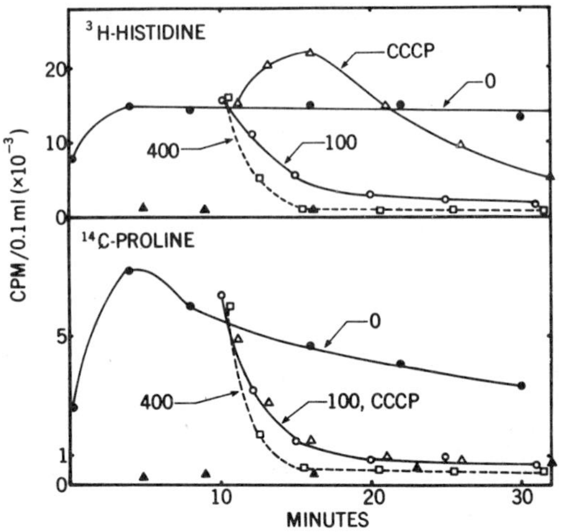

FIG. 6. *Leakage of intracellular amino acids. E. coli AS19 was treated with 150 μg of chloramphenicol/ml for 5 min before addition of [^{3}H]histidine and [^{14}C]proline (t = 0). After 10 min, portions of the culture received either no further addition (●), 100 μg of TC/ml (○), 400 μg of TC/ml (□), or 10^{-5} M CCCP (△). Samples were taken at intervals, and intracellular levels of each labeled amino acid were determined as described in Materials and Methods. Samples were also taken from the portion without added TC and were filtered and washed several times with cold 5% trichloroacetic acid to release total intracellular soluble pools (▲).*

DISCUSSION

TC, at concentrations greater than required for inhibition of protein synthesis, rapidly and completely inhibits replication of DNA. At these elevated levels of the antibiotic, which may be affecting several aspects of cell growth, the synthesis of RNA is not appreciably altered. The observed inhibition is not directly related to the inhibition of protein synthesis, as this primarily affects only the initiation step of DNA synthesis. A decrease in the rate of propagation of DNA synthesis has been described with chloramphenicol addition or amino acid starvation (14, 18), and some degree of premature termination of rounds of DNA replication has been reported (8, 10). However, the complete inhibition of replication demonstrated here with TC has not been observed with other inhibitors of protein synthesis.

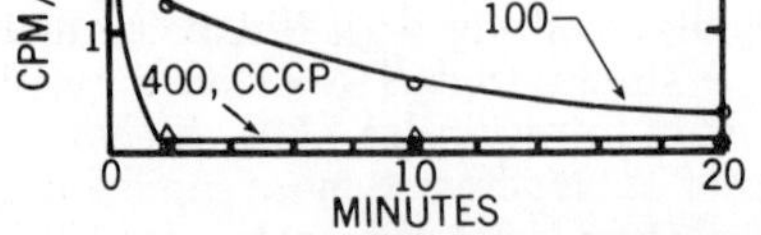

FIG. 5. *Leakage of intracellular [^{14}C]TMG. E. coli AS19 was induced with IPTG for one generation before addition of [^{14}C]TMG. After 10 min (t = 0) portions of the culture received either no further addition (●), 100 μg of TC/ml (○), 400 μg of TC/ml (□), or 10^{-5} M CCCP (△). Samples were collected at intervals, and intracellular [^{14}C]TMG was determined as described in Materials and Methods.*

Some possible explanations for the inhibition of replication by TC have been excluded. Intercalation into the DNA helix or binding of large amounts of TC to DNA does not occur. Though the sizes of nucleoside triphosphate pools do change after TC addition, the kinetics of the changes are too slow to explain, in any simple manner, the inhibition of replication. The marked decreases in ribonucleoside triphosphate levels at late times after TC addition or at high TC concentrations could readily explain the observed inhibition of RNA synthesis under these conditions. It is difficult to exclude a possible involvement of chelation of divalent cations. The observed specificity with regard to RNA synthesis and the failure to prevent or reverse inhibition of replication with excess Mg^{2+}, Mn^{2+}, or Ca^{2+} argues against, but does not exclude, this explanation.

The most likely explanation is an alteration of the cytoplasmic membrane, which, in turn, leads to inhibition of replication. The data presented here show that the membrane properties are altered sufficiently to allow the leakage of nucleotides and of compounds normally accumulated against a concentration gradient. The transport of compounds that utilizes the proton-motive force as well as transport requiring intracellular ATP is affected. However, whatever alteration of membrane structure is occurring is not severe enough to result in leakage of intracellular β-galactosidase.

Replication of chromosomal DNA is believed to take place on the cell membrane (13, 15, 19), perhaps in association with a complex of required enzymes (4), whereas RNA synthesis presumably takes place predominantly in the cytoplasm. Therefore, disruption of membrane structure could affect DNA replication without affecting the synthesis of RNA, and the results reported here can be taken as further evidence for the involvement of the cell membrane in DNA replication. We are presently investigating this possibility and examining the effects of TC on the replication of other DNA elements in *E. coli*.

ACKNOWLEDGMENTS

This research was supported by United States Public Health service grant AI 11075, from the National Institute of Allergy and Infectious Diseases.

I wish to thank Jayna Karpinski for her skillful technical assistance.

LITERATURE CITED

1. **Berger, E. A.** 1973. Different mechanisms of energy coupling for the active transport of proline and glutamine in *Escherichia coli*. Proc. Natl. Acad. Sci. U.S.A. **70**:1514–1518.
2. **Burton, K.** 1968. Determination of DNA concentration with diphenylamine, p. 163–166. *In* L. Grossman and K. Moldave (ed.), Methods in enzymology, vol. 12. Academic Press Inc., New York.
3. **Clark, D. J., and O. Maaløe.** 1967. DNA replication and the division cycle in *Escherichia coli*. J. Mol. Biol. **23**:99–112.
4. **Firshein, W.** 1973. In situ activity of enzymes on polyacrylamide gels of a deoxyribonucleic acid-membrane fraction extracted from pneumococci. J. Bacteriol. **118**:1101–1110.
5. **Gale, E. F., E. Cundliffe, P. E. Reynolds, M. H. Richmond, and M. J. Waring.** 1972. The molecular basis of antibiotic action. J. Wiley and Sons, London.
6. **Gross, J.** 1972. DNA replication in bacteria. Curr. Top. Microbiol. Immunol. **57**:39–74.
7. **Kohn, K. W.** 1961. Mediation of divalent metal ions in the binding of tetracycline to macromolecules. Nature (London) **191**:1156–1158.
8. **Lark, K. G.** 1973. Initiation and termination of bacterial deoxyribonucleic acid replication in low concentrations of chloramphenicol. J. Bacteriol. **113**:1066–1069.
9. **Laskin, A. I.** 1967. *In* D. Gottlieb and P. D. Shaw (ed.), Antibiotics, vol. 1, p. 331. Springer-Verlag, New York.
10. **Marunouchi, T., and W. Messer.** 1973. Replication of a specific terminal chromosome segment in *Escherichia coli* which is required for cell division. J. Mol. Biol. **78**:211–228.
11. **Neuhard, J., E. Randerath, and K. Randerath.** 1965. Ion-exchange thin layer chromatography. XIII. Resolution of complex nucleoside triphosphate mixtures. Anal. Biochem. **13**:211–222.
12. **Pace, N. R., M. L. Pato, J. McKibbin, and C. W. Radcliffe.** 1973. Precursors of 5S ribosomal RNA in *Bacillus subtilis*. J. Mol. Biol. **75**:619–631.
13. **Parker, D. L., and D. A. Glaser.** 1974. Chromosomal sites of DNA-membrane attachment in *Escherichia coli*. J. Mol. Biol. **87**:153–168.
14. **Pato, M. L.** 1975. Alterations of the rate of movement of deoxyribonucleic acid replication forks. J. Bacteriol. **123**:272–277.
15. **Pato, M. L.** 1972. Regulation of chromosome replication and the bacterial cell cycle. Annu. Rev. Microbiol. **26**:347–368.
16. **Pavlasova, E., and F. M. Harold.** 1969. Energy coupling in the transport of β-galactosides by *Escherichia coli:* effect of proton conductors. J. Bacteriol. **98**:198–204.
17. **Randerath, E., and K. Randerath.** 1964. Resolution of complex nucleotide mixtures by two-dimensional anion-exchange thin-layer chromatography. J. Chromatogr. **16**:126–129.
18. **Rodriques, R. L., and C. I. Davern.** 1976. Direction of deoxyribonucleic acid replication in *Escherichia coli* under various conditions of cell growth. J. Bacteriol. **125**:346–352.
19. **Siegal, P. J., and M. Schaechter.** 1973. The role of the host cell membrane in the replication and morphogenesis of bacteriophages. Annu. Rev. Microbiol. **27**:261–282.
20. **Ward, D. C., E. Reich, and I. H. Goldberg.** 1965. Base specificity in the interaction of polynucleotides with antibiotic drugs. Science **149**:1259–1263.

ANTIMICROBIAL AGENTS AND CHEMOTHERAPY, Feb. 1977, p. 324–330
Vol. 11, No. 2

Cefadroxil, a New Broad-Spectrum Cephalosporin

R. E. BUCK[1]* AND K. E. PRICE

Department of Microbiological Research, Bristol-Myers Co., Inc., New York, New York 10022

Received for publication 29 June 1976

Cefadroxil is a new semisynthetic cephalosporin with a broad antibacterial spectrum and a high chemotherapeutic potential when administered orally. The inhibitory activity of this compound was similar to that of cephalexin and cephradine when tested against 602 clinical isolates on Mueller-Hinton medium. In the oral treatment of experimental infections of mice, cefadroxil was more effective than cephalexin against *Streptococcus pyogenes*, and comparably effective against *Streptococcus pneumoniae, Staphylococcus aureus,* and several gram-negative species. Administered orally to mice, at doses ranging from 25 to 100 mg/kg, cefadroxil attained peak concentrations in the blood similar to those of cephalexin. At a dose of 200 mg/kg, however, higher peak levels were noted with cefadroxil than with cephalexin. In regard to other properties which were investigated, the behavior of cefadroxil compared favorably to that of cephalexin.

Two cephalosporins, cephalexin and cephradine, due to their therapeutic efficacy when administered orally, have gained widespread usage in the treatment of a variety of infectious diseases. In this paper we report on laboratory investigations of a new semisynthetic cephalosporin, cefadroxil (Fig. 1), which has been found effective against a variety of gram-positive and gram-negative organisms in vitro and in vivo after oral administration. For comparison, cephalexin and cephradine were included in all studies designed to determine the antibacterial spectrum of cefadroxil. While investigating other antimicrobial and pharmacological properties, cephalexin alone was used as a reference compound.

MATERIALS AND METHODS

Antibiotics. Cefadroxil, 7-[D-(-)-α-amino-α-(4-hydroxyphenyl)-acetamido]-3-methyl-3-cephem-4-carboxylic acid, is a white, crystalline, water-soluble solid with a molecular weight of 363.4. Cephalexin monohydrate is a product of Eli Lilly and Co. and cephradine is a product of E. R. Squibb & Sons, Inc.

(i) Properties in vitro: antibiotic spectrum. The inhibitory activity of cefadroxil, cephalexin, and cephradine was determined for 157 gram-positive and 445 gram-negative organisms, predominantly of clinical origin. The assays were performed by a serial twofold agar dilution technique, the bacterial inoculum being added by the multiple inoculator of Steers et al. (7).

Mueller-Hinton medium (Difco) was used in these assays for all organisms except strains of *Neisseria* and *Haemophilus*. For other fastidious organisms (*Streptococcus, Listeria, Vibrio, Pasteurella,* and *Bordetella*), the medium was supplemented with 4% defibrinated sheep blood. The antibiotic susceptibility of *Haemophilus* and *Neisseria* was determined on GC medium base (BBL) supplemented with 1% hemoglobin (BBL) and 1% Isovitalex (BBL).

An overnight broth culture or an exponentially growing culture (*Neisseria*) served as the source of inoculum. A volume of approximately 0.003 ml of an undiluted or diluted culture was applied to the surface of the antibiotic-containing agar plates. Cultures of *Neisseria, Streptococcus pneumoniae,* and *Streptococcus pyogenes* were used without dilution, whereas all others were diluted 100-fold. Before dilution, however, *Haemophilus* cultures were initially standardized on a Spectronic 20 colorimeter (Bausch and Lomb) to an optical density (OD) of 0.3 at 560 nm, using 11.5-by 100-mm test tubes. All culture plates were incubated at 37°C either overnight (18 h) or for 24 h (*Haemophilus*). Incubation of *Neisseria, Haemophilus,* and all other fastidious organisms was carried out in candle jars in a 5 to 10% CO_2 atmosphere.

After incubation, plates were examined for colony development, and the minimal inhibitory concentration (MIC), i.e., the lowest concentration of antibiotic causing virtually complete inhibition of growth, was recorded. In interpreting these results, inhibition was considered to have occurred if the plates contained only a film of growth or five or less colonies.

Effect of inoculum size. The influence of inoculum size on the inhibitory activity of cefadroxil and cephalexin was determined on solid Mueller-Hinton medium in a manner similar to that described above. The inoculum, however, consisted of three dilutions (10^0, 10^{-2}, and 10^{-4}) of overnight cultures which were first standardized to an OD of 0.45 at 540 nm on a Coleman Jr. II spectrophotometer in 13.5-

[1] Address reprint requests to: P.O. Box 657, Syracuse, NY 13201.

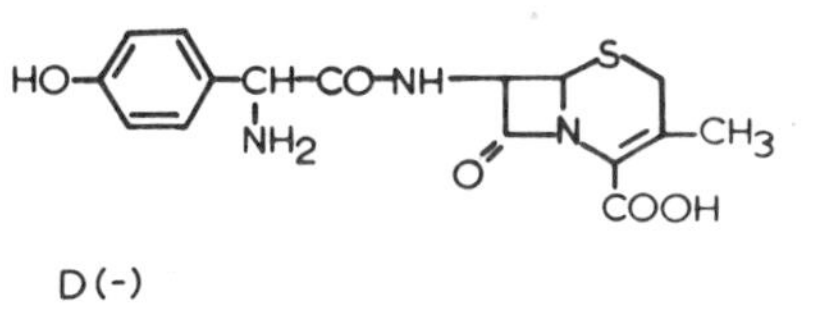

FIG. 1. *Structure of cefadroxil.*

by 150-mm test tubes. The standardized cultures were estimated to contain about 5 × 10^8 cells/ml before dilution.

Bactericidal activity. The bactericidal activity of cefadroxil and cephalexin was determined by exposing various organisms to a twofold series of antibiotic concentrations in Mueller-Hinton broth. The inoculum was an overnight culture diluted so as to yield an initial cell concentration of 10^4 to 10^5 cells/ml. At the termination of a 20- to 24-h incubation period at 37°C, readings were made for MIC determinations and the cultures were then chilled in ice. After this, 0.1-ml samples from each turbidity-free tube were plated on solid medium. Mueller-Hinton medium was used for most organisms but, to minimize spreading, strains of *Proteus* were plated on nutrient agar (Difco). After incubation of plates, colonies were counted to determine the number of viable cells (colony-forming units) in the original MIC tubes. The minimal bactericidal concentration (MBC) was considered to be the lowest concentration yielding a count of <100 cells/ml.

Susceptibility to β-lactamase. Cell-free extracts containing β-lactamases were employed to determine the rates at which the cephalosporins were hydrolyzed by these enzymes. Hydrolytic activity was measured by the iodometric assay of Perret (3) with the following two modifications: (i) gelatin was omitted, and (ii) the buffer was adjusted to pH 7.0. Extracts from gram-negative organisms were obtained by sonic disruption of cell suspensions, followed by removal of cell debris by centrifugation. The preparations were maintained at −20°C for extended periods of time without significant loss of enzyme activity. The extract from *Staphylococcus aureus* was obtained by acetone and ether treatment of a culture grown in the presence of methicillin. The resulting preparation was stored at 4°C.

Binding to serum proteins. The extent to which cefadroxil and cephalexin are bound to human serum proteins was determined by an ultrafiltration method. Samples containing 10 and 25 μg of the compounds per ml in fresh pooled human serum were incubated at 37°C for 15 min. They were then transferred to CF-50A Centriflo filter cones (Amicon Corp.) and centrifuged for 25 min at 900 × *g* at 4°C. The resulting ultrafiltrates were assayed on base agar (BBL) plates seeded with *Sarcina lutea* ATCC 9341. Antibiotic concentrations in the filtrates were then determined from reference standard lines which relate the diameter of the inhibition zone to drug concentration. These lines were constructed on the basis of results obtained from the assay of known concentrations of antibiotic in pH 6.0 phosphate buffer (1%). Adequate controls, consisting of antibiotics added to deproteinized serum, were treated identically to ascertain that any decrease in antibiotic activity was due solely to protein binding.

Stability in solution. In determining the stability of cefadroxil and cephalexin at pH 2.0, a 2 mg/ml solution of each antibiotic was prepared in citric acid-HCl buffer (0.002 M) and incubated at 37°C. Aliquots were removed periodically over a 24-h period, neutralized, and assayed on base agar plates seeded with *Bacillus subtilis* ATCC 6633. Residual antibiotic activity was determined with the aid of standard curves obtained by assaying known concentrations of the drugs in phosphate buffer (0.005 M). The length of exposure (in hours) resulting in a 50% decrease in antimicrobial activity (half-life) was then calculated. Stability at pH 7.4 was determined in a similar manner, except that solutions were prepared and incubated in sodium barbital buffer (0.005 M).

(ii) Properties in vivo: antibiotic concentration in blood. Cefadroxil and cephalexin were administered orally to mice to determine the extent of absorption of these antibiotics into the blood stream. Normal male Swiss-Webster mice weighing 20 (±2) g were used in these experiments, in which blood samples were collected for assay at various intervals over a 3.5-h period. The techniques for blood collection and bioassay were similar to those previously described by Price et al. (5) except that *S. lutea* ATCC 9341 and *B. subtilis* ATCC 6633 were the assay organisms and the animals were fasted for only 4 h pretreatment. A minimum of three tests was carried out in this manner, with eight mice being used per dose level in each experiment.

Recovery in urine. Male Sprague-Dawley rats, weighing 200 (±20) g, were employed to determine the fraction of the orally administered antibiotic that is excreted in the urine. For each drug, a dose of 50 mg/kg in 4 ml of Tween-CMC (carboxymethyl cellulose) was administered by gavage to five rats that were fasted for 18 h pretreatment. Animals were housed individually in metabolism cages and urine specimens were collected over dry ice during intervals of 0 to 6 h and 6 to 24 h postadministration. Aliquots (0.03 ml) of appropriate dilutions of the collected urine were transferred to paper disks (6.35-mm diameter), and antibiotic activity was assayed by the agar diffusion technique on seeded agar plates inoculated with *S. lutea* ATCC 9341. Concentrations of the antibiotic in the urine were calculated from reference standard lines which relate the diameter of the inhibition zone to drug concentration. These lines were constructed from assay data involving known concentrations of the antibiotic added to urine collected from untreated control animals.

To determine the presence of active metabolites, the urine samples were subjected to descending paper chromatography in an *n*-butanol-ethanol-water (80:20:100) system. The paper strips were subsequently assayed in base agar seeded with *B. subtilis* ATCC 6633.

Treatment of experimental infections. Male Swiss-Webster mice weighing 20 (±2) g were challenged intraperitoneally with 0.5 ml of a bacterial suspension containing sufficient organisms to kill

TABLE 1. *Growth inhibitory activity of cefadroxil, cephalexin, and cephradine against miscellaneous bacterial species*

Organism	No. of strains	MIC (μg/ml)[a]		
		Cefadroxil	Cephalexin	Cephradine
Streptococcus faecalis	14	57	84	57
Listeria monocytogenes	7	39	63	39
Bacillus anthracis	1	1	2	1
Edwardsiella tarda	2	4	2	2.8
Arizona hinshawii	2	8	4	8
Citrobacter sp.	5	>72	37	48
Hafnia alvei	2	32	16	32
	1	125	125	125
Serratia marcescens	5	>125	>125	>125
Proteus rettgeri	2	5.7	5.7	8
	1	>125	125	125
Proteus morganii	12	>125	>125	>125
Vibrio cholerae	1	2	2	2
Pasteurella multocida	2	4	2	4
Pseudomonas aeruginosa	3	>125	>125	>125
Alcaligenes sp.	7	7.2	4.4	11
	6	>99	>89	>99
Bordetella bronchiseptica	1	63	125	>125

[a] Geometric mean when applicable.

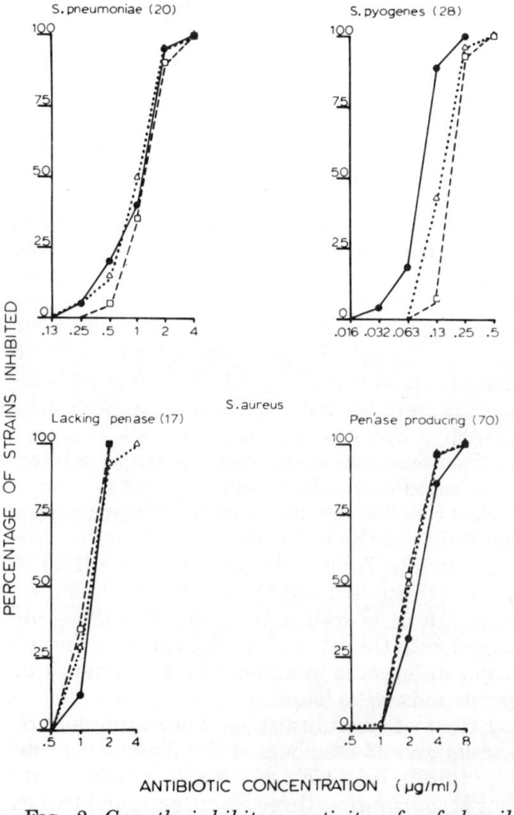

FIG. 2. *Growth inhibitory activity of cefadroxil (●), cephalexin (□), and cephradine (△) against various gram-positive organisms. The number in parentheses indicates the number of strains.*

untreated animals within 72 h. The challenge medium was brain heart infusion broth (Difco) for *Klebsiella pneumoniae* and all streptococci, a suspension of 2% hog gastric mucin (type 1701W, Wilson Laboratories, Inc., Park Forest South, Ill.) for *S. aureus* A9606, and 4% mucin for the remaining organisms. Various concentrations of the antibiotics in a Tween-CMC mixture were administered orally to five mice for each dose level. The animals were treated twice in this manner, in accordance with the treatment schedule shown in Table 4. The number of mice surviving the challenge for 3 or 5 days (depending on the test organism) was recorded and the PD_{50} (dose in milligrams per kilogram required to protect half the infected animals from death) was then estimated by a log probit plot.

RESULTS

(i) Properties in vitro: antibiotic spectrum. Cefadroxil, cephalexin, and cephradine very effectively inhibited a broad spectrum of gram-positive and gram-negative organisms. This is evident upon examination of the susceptibility data shown in Table 1 and Fig. 2 to 5.

Although the three cephalosporins were about equally effective in inhibiting the growth of *S. pneumoniae* and *S. aureus*, cefadroxil was twice as active as cephalexin and slightly more active than cephradine against *S. pyogenes* (Fig. 2). None of the antibiotics displayed any appreciable inhibitory effect for *Streptococcus faecalis* and *Listeria monocytogenes* (Table 1).

In tests involving gram-negative organisms, cefadroxil, cephalexin, and cephradine were comparably active against *Escherichia coli* and

Proteus mirabilis. However, against *K. pneumoniae* (Fig. 3), *Proteus vulgaris* (Fig. 4), and *Salmonella* sp. (Fig. 5), cefadroxil and cephradine were approximately twofold less active then cephalexin. When tested against *Shigella* sp., *Haemophilus influenzae*, and *Neisseria gonorrhoeae*, cefadroxil was again about two-

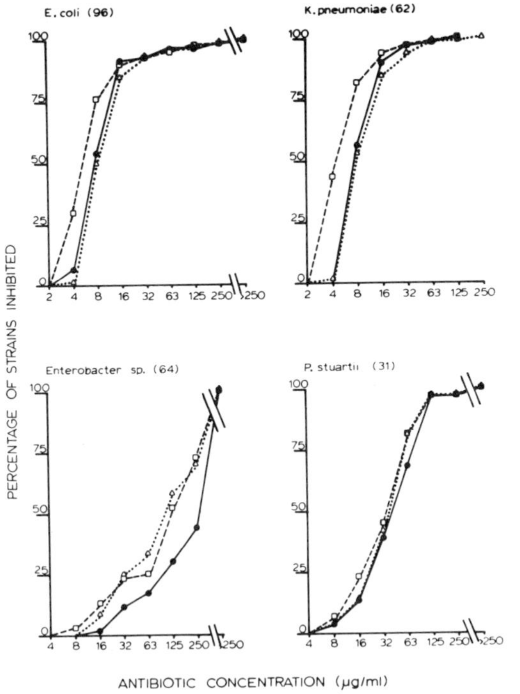

FIG. 3. *Growth inhibitory activity of cefadroxil (●), cephalexin (□), and cephradine (△) against various Enterobacteriaceae. The number in parentheses indicates the number of strains.*

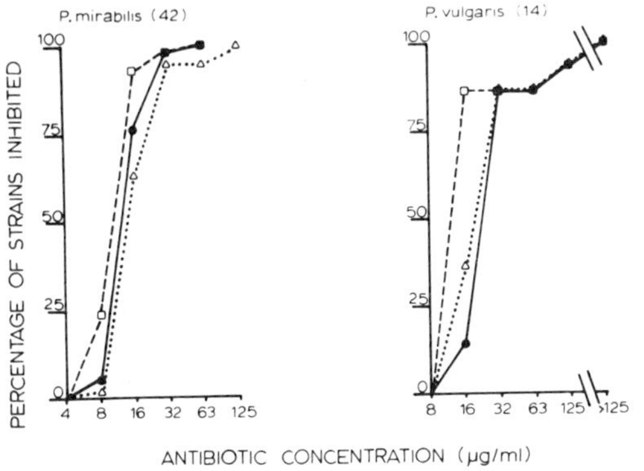

FIG. 4. *Growth inhibitory activity of cefadroxil (●), cephalexin (□), and cephradine (△) against strains of Proteus mirabilis and Proteus vulgaris. The number in parentheses indicates the number of strains.*

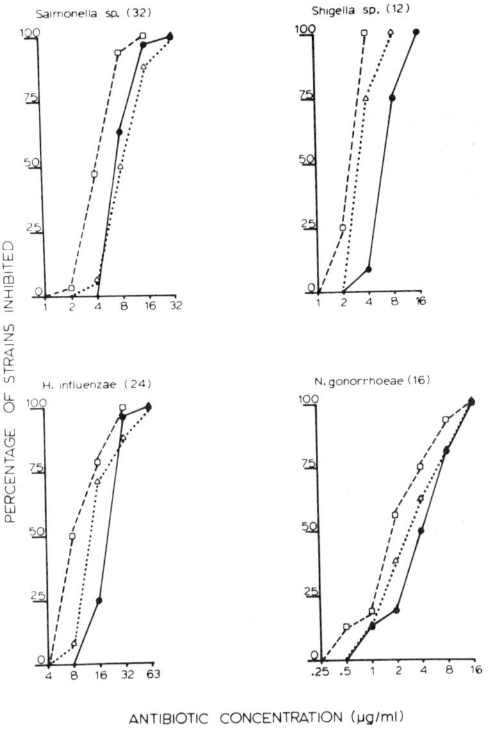

FIG. 5. *Growth inhibitory activity of cefadroxil (●), cephalexin (□), and cephradine (△) against various gram-negative organisms. The number in parentheses indicates the number of strains.*

fold less active than cephalexin, whereas the activity of cephradine was intermediate. On the basis of geometric mean MIC values, cephalexin was more than twice as active as cephradine against sensitive *Alcaligenes* strains, whereas the activity of cefadroxil was closer to that of cephalexin (Table 1). The three cephalosporins were virtually ineffective in inhibiting growth of *Enterobacter* sp., *Providencia stuartii*, *Pseudomonas aeruginosa*, *Serratia marcescens*, and *Proteus morganii*.

Few conclusions can be drawn about the susceptibility of the remaining miscellaneous species listed in Table 1 because of the small number of strains studied. Nevertheless, these results are in overall agreement with those obtained with the other clinical isolates in that no major differences in activity between the three compounds were found.

Effect of inoculum size. Four strains of *S. aureus* and 23 members of the *Enterobacteriaceae* family (eight *E. coli*, six *K. pneumoniae*, four *P. mirabillis*, three *P. rettgeri*, and two *P. vulgaris*) were employed to determine the influence of inoculum size on the activity of cefadroxil and cephalexin. In these studies, the pattern of response to cefadroxil was similar to that of cephalexin in that for about two-thirds of the organisms, the size of the inoculum had relatively little or no effect on antibiotic activity. However, increases in cell concentrations of the remaining strains resulted in a substantial reduction (eightfold or more) in the activity of both antibiotics. Although the greatest inoculum effect on the activity of the two cephalosporins occurred with *Proteus,* a considerable decrease in their inhibitory action was also noted with high inocula of two strains of *E. coli* and one of *K. pneumoniae*.

Bactericidal activity. Bactericidal activity was determined on the basis of antibiotic effectiveness in killing cells of 17 strains of *Enterobacteriaceae* (six each of *E. coli* and *K. pneumoniae,* two of *P. mirabilis,* and three of *P. vulgaris*). Once again, the behavior of the two antibiotics was similar. Both had excellent bactericidal activity since, in every instance, killing concentrations were either equal to or no more than twofold higher than inhibitory concentrations.

Susceptibility to β-lactamase. The relative susceptibility of cefadroxil and cephalexin to hydrolysis by β-lactamases present in cell-free extracts was determined. For comparison, rates of hydrolysis of two other commercially available cephalosporins, cefazolin and cephaloridine, are also presented in Table 2.

Results indicate that cefadroxil and cephalexin are about equally stable to the seven β-lactamases investigated. Both appear to be poor substrates for enzyme types IIa, IIIa, IVa, and the staphylococcal β-lactamase, and are relatively resistant to type IVb. Although cefadroxil, like cephalexin, is hydrolyzed at a significant rate by types Ia and Ib, it is considerably less susceptible to these enzymes than are cefazolin and cephaloridine.

Serum binding. As determined by an ultrafiltration method, cefadroxil and cephalexin are bound to human serum proteins to a similar extent—20 and 17%, respectively. Results obtained with cephalexin are in agreement with those of Kind et al. (2) who reported 13 to 19% binding at a concentration of 10 μg/ml.

Stability in solution. At 37°C, cefadroxil and cephalexin are stable in solution at both pH 2.0 and 7.4, the half-life in all cases being in excess of 24 h.

(ii) Properties in vivo: antibiotic concentration in blood. Concentrations of cefadroxil and

TABLE 2. *Relative susceptibility of several cephalosporins to hydrolysis by β-lactamases in cell-free extracts*

Enzyme[a]		Organism (source of enzyme)	Relative rate of hydrolysis (benzylpenicillin = 100)			
Class	Type		Cefadroxil	Cephalexin	Cefazolin	Cephaloridine
I	a	*Enterobacter cloacae* 214	595	900	10,000	7,900
	b	*Escherichia coli* 719	48	55	760	370
II	a	*Proteus mirabilis* 1266	<1	<1	<1	2
III	a	*Escherichia coli* TEM	<1	<1	12	93
IV	a	*Klebsiella pneumoniae* 53	<1	<1	12	100
	b	*Klebsiella pneumoniae* 1169	2	4	31	50
		Staphylococcus areus A9606	<1	<1	<1	<1

[a] Enzyme classification according to Richmond and Sykes (6).

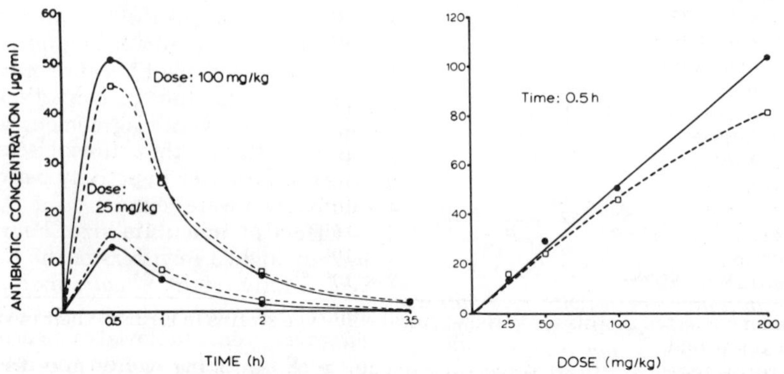

FIG. 6. *Antibiotic concentration in blood after oral administration to mice. Symbols: cefadroxil (●), cephalexin (□).*

cephalexin attained in the blood of mice after oral administration can be seen in Fig. 6. When dosed at 25 and 100 mg/kg, the levels of cefadroxil in blood were virtually identical to those of cephalexin (Fig. 6, left). The highest detectable concentrations of both were found 30 min after administration. Drug levels then declined at similar rates for the two antibiotics. Maximum concentrations (in micrograms per milliliter) observed for cefadroxil and cephalexin were, respectively, 13.7 and 15.1 for a 25 mg/kg dose, as compared to 50.8 and 45.8 when the dose was 100 mg/kg.

Concentrations of the two compounds found at 30 min after administration are plotted as a function of dose (Fig. 6, right). Up to a dose of 100 mg/kg, values for the two cephalosporins were similar, with concentrations being proportional to dose. However, a linear relationship was maintained for cefadroxil, but not for cephalexin, up through a dose of 200 mg/kg.

TABLE 3. *Urinary recovery of cefadroxil and cephalexin after oral administration to rats*

Compound	Urinary recovery as % of administered dose		
	0–6[a]	6–24[a]	0–24[a]
Cefadroxil[b]	63	5	68
Cephalexin	65	3	68

[a] Hours after administration.

[b] The compounds, prepared in Tween-CMC, were administered to five male rats each at a dose of 50 mg/kg body weight.

Urinary excretion. The extent to which cefadroxil and cephalexin were recovered from the urine of rats after a 50 mg/kg dose can be seen in Table 3. A total of 68% of the administered dose of both cephalosporins was found in the urine during the first 24 h postadministration. No bioactive metabolites of either cefadroxil or cephalexin were detected in the urine.

Treatment of experimental infections. The comparative therapeutic effectiveness of cefadroxil and cephalexin in treating mice experimentally infected with various gram-positive and gram-negative bacteria is indicated in Table 4. In vivo, just as in vitro, cefadroxil was more effective than cephalexin against *S. pyogenes*. Against the three infecting strains of this organism, the activity of cefadroxil was three- to sixfold greater than that of cephalexin. In the treatment of mice infected with *S. pneumoniae,* the two compounds were about equally effective. This was also true for the *S. aureus* infections, regardless of ability of the organism to produce penicillinase.

Both compounds were very effective in treating systemic infections caused by *K. pneumoniae, E. coli,* and *P. mirabilis,* although PD_{50} values of cephalexin were somewhat lower (generally less than twofold) than those of cefadroxil.

DISCUSSION

Results reported in this paper for cephalexin and cephradine are consistent with those noted by other workers in the field. Stewart and Bodey (8) showed similarities in antibacterial

TABLE 4. *Therapeutic efficacy of orally administered cefadroxil and cephalexin in experimental infections of mice*

Organism[a]	Challenge (no. of organisms)	PD_{50}/treatment (mg/kg)[b]	
		Cefadroxil	Cephalexin
Streptococcus pyogenes A9604	6×10^4	2.4	6.8
S. pyogenes A15041	7×10^4	0.7	3.5
S. pyogenes A20202	2×10^7	0.6	3.4
S. pneumoniae A20759	1×10^4	18	16
S. pneumoniae A9585	3×10^5	24	38
S. pneumoniae A20769	3×10^4	24	41
Staphylococcus aureus A9537[c]	2×10^5	0.3	0.18
S. aureus A9497[c]	3×10^8	5.1	3.4
S. aureus A20405	4×10^6	8	6
S. aureus A9606	2×10^9	29	24
Klebsiella pneumoniae A9977	4×10^4	85	41
Escherichia coli A15119	2×10^4	12	8
E. coli A9675	1×10^5	18	12
Proteus mirabilis A9900	3×10^6	64	38

[a] The organisms selected for this study were typical wild-type strains in terms of their in vitro susceptibility to the test compounds.

[b] Results are averages of two or three experiments, each consisting of five mice for each dose per experiment. Animals infected with *S. aureus* strains A9497, A20405, and A9606 were treated 0 and 2 h after infection; all others were treated 1 and 3.5 h after infection.

[c] Lack penicillinase. Other strains of *S. aureus* are penicillinase producers.

activity between the two compounds against a series of gram-positive and gram-negative organisms. Clark and Turck (1) also reported on the inhibitory and bactericidal activity of cephalexin and commented on the fact that its activity is reduced in the presence of high inocula of certain strains, particularly *P. mirabilis*. Wick (9), in addition to providing evidence for the bacteriostatic and bactericidal effectiveness of cephalexin, demonstrated good oral absorption in mice and excellent efficacy in treating experimental mouse infections after oral dosage.

It is not surprising that cefadroxil, because of its similarity in structure, possesses many of the same characteristics as cephalexin and cephradine. The most apparent advantages of cefadroxil over the reference compounds, however, lie in its pharmacokinetic properties. In a companion paper (4), cefadroxil has been shown to have a longer serum half-life after oral dosage to humans, a slower urinary excretion rate, and a greater area under the serum level vs. time curve than either cephalexin or cephradine. In addition, it was also noted that the apparent volume of distribution of cefadroxil is greater than that of cephalexin.

Because of cefadroxil's broad range of antimicrobial activity and its favorable pharmacokinetic profile in man, clinical trials with this antibiotic are currently under way.

ACKNOWLEDGMENTS

We would like to acknowledge the excellent technical assistance of M. Christine Arnold, Eileen W. Chaplinsky, Kenneth L. Den Bleyker, Kathlyn F. Frenette, Richard A. Goodhines, Thomas B. Hallett, Angela M. Hill, Thomas Ingram, Antoinette C. Nutting, Christian E. Thater, Martha C. Thiesing, Jacqueline A. Randolph, Erwin B. Williams, and Ellen M. Yastrib. We are also grateful to Terry M. Stickle and Thomas V. Washo for preparing the cultures, and to Evelyn Barenholtz and Maxine C. Postle for their skillful clerical assistance.

LITERATURE CITED

1. **Clark, H., and M. Turck.** 1969. *In vitro* and *in vivo* evaluation of cephalexin, p. 296–301. Antimicrob. Agents Chemother. 1968.
2. **Kind, A. C., D. G. Kestle, H. C. Standiford, and W. M. M. Kirby.** 1969. Laboratory and clinical experience with cephalexin, p. 361–365. Antimicrob. Agents Chemother. 1968.
3. **Perret, C. J.** 1954. Iodometric assay of penicillinase. Nature (London) **174**:1012–1013.
4. **Pfeffer, M., A. Jackson, J. Ximenes, and J. P. de Menezes.** 1976. Comparative human oral clinical pharmacology of cefadroxil, cephalexin, and cephradine **11**:331–338.
5. **Price, K. E., J. A. Bach, D. R. Chisholm, M. Misiek, and A. Gourevitch.** 1969. Preliminary microbiological and pharmacological evaluation of 6-(R-α-amino-3-thienylacetamido)penicillanic acid (BL-P875). J. Antibiot. (Tokyo) **22**:1–11.
6. **Richmond, M. H., and R. B. Sykes.** 1973. The β-lactamases of gram-negative bacteria and their possible physiological role. Adv. Microb. Physiol. **9**:31–88.
7. **Steers, E., E. L. Foltz, and B. S. Graves.** 1959. An inocula replicating apparatus for routine testing of bacterial susceptibility to antibiotics. Antibiot. Chemother. **9**:307–311.
8. **Stewart, D., and G. P. Bodey.** 1976. Comparative *in vitro* activity of cephalosporins. J. Antibiot. **29**:181–186.
9. **Wick, W. E.** 1967. Cephalexin, a new orally absorbed cephalosporin antibiotic. Appl. Microbiol. **15**:765–769.

ANTIMICROBIAL AGENTS AND CHEMOTHERAPY, Feb. 1977, p. 331-338 Vol. 11, No. 2
 Printed in U.S.A.

Comparative Human Oral Clinical Pharmacology of Cefadroxil, Cephalexin, and Cephradine

MORRIS PFEFFER[1]*, ANDRE JACKSON, JOSE XIMENES, AND JAIRO PERCHE DE MENEZES

Bristol-Myers Co., Inc., New York, New York 10022

Received for publication 28 July 1976

At equivalent oral doses, cefadroxil has a longer serum half-life, slower urinary excretion rate, greater area under the serum level versus time curve than cephalexin or cephradine, and peak serum concentrations that are 75 to 80% those of cephalexin. The calculated, apparent in vivo volume of distribution of cefadroxil is greater than that of cephalexin. These properties infer greater persistence of cefadroxil in serum and urine and more prolonged in vivo bacterial exposure to cefadroxil than to cephalexin or cephradine. Neither cefadroxil nor cephalexin demonstrates drug accumulation on repeated administration. The serum levels achieved by cefadroxil are unaffected by food. The pharmacokinetic properties of cefadroxil are supportive of the development of clinical efficacy data which could indicate that cefadroxil could be administered at 12-h intervals.

The studies reported here were undertaken to compare the pharmacokinetic properties in humans of the orally administered cephalosporin antibiotics cefadroxil, cephalexin, and cephradine (structures presented in Fig. 1) and to determine the factors which control their disposition in vivo. A companion paper presents data on the antibacterial activity of cefadroxil (1). The inhibitory activity of cefadroxil on clinical isolates was similar to that of cephalexin and cephradine. Cefadroxil was more effective than cephalexin against *Streptococcus pyogenes* and comparably as effective as cephalexin against *Streptococcus pneumoniae*, *Staphylococcus aureus*, and several gram-negative species in oral treatment of experimental infections in mice.

MATERIALS AND METHODS

Bioassays for antibiotic activity in serum and urine were carried out by standard cup plate assay methodology (4) using *Sarcina lutea* ATCC 9341 as the bioassay organism versus analytical standards of each of the cephalosporin antibiotics employed. All antibiotic doses administered are reported in terms of antibiotic content as established by bioassay.

In all three studies all subjects gave informed consent to their participation. All subjects were between the ages of 23 and 59 years and weighed between 51 and 83 kg. Additional criteria for entrance into the studies included lack of penicillin allergy or sensitivity, a normal routine physical examination, and determinations of hemoglobin, hematocrit, white blood cell and differential count, blood area nitrogen, serum glutamic pyruvic transaminase, bilirubin, urinalysis (including protein test, sugar and microscopy for casts and cells), and stool parasitological examination. Subjects with abnormal values or findings were not admitted into these studies. None of the subjects were to have taken any medication for 3 weeks prior to the study in which they participated.

All subjects were fasted overnight before each study. Oral doses of drugs were always administered at 8:00 a.m. with 250 ml of water, and a further 250 ml of water was ingested every succeeding 2 h for the duration of the study. Except for portions of a study on the effect of food on drug bioavailability, the subjects maintained their fast for 2 h after drug administration.

All studies were designed as balanced, randomized complete crossovers. There was a 6-day washout period between crossover legs.

Study HL-74-41. The first study was a three-period crossover pharmacokinetic and bioavailability comparison between cephalexin and the monohydrate and trihydrate of cefadroxil. The drugs administered were: cefadroxil monohydrate capsules, 300 mg; cefadroxil trihydrate capsules, 300 mg; and commercial cephalexin monohydrate capsules, 250 mg. There were 16 volunteers (13 males, 3 females). Blood samples for the preparation of serum were taken at zero time (before dosage) and at 0.5, 1, 1.5, 3, 6, and 8 h after dosing. Total urine collections were made during the 0- to 4- and 4- to 8-h intervals after dosing.

Study HL-75-47. Study HL-75-47 was a three-period crossover comparison between cefadroxil monohydrate capsules, commercial cephalexin monohydrate capsules, and commercial cephradine capsules. The doses of all three antibiotics were a constant 500 mg. There were 12 volunteers (11 males and 1 female). Blood samples were collected at zero time and at 0.5, 1, 1.5, 2, 4, 6, 8, and 12 h after

[1] Address reprint requests to: P.O. Box 657, Syracuse, NY 13201.

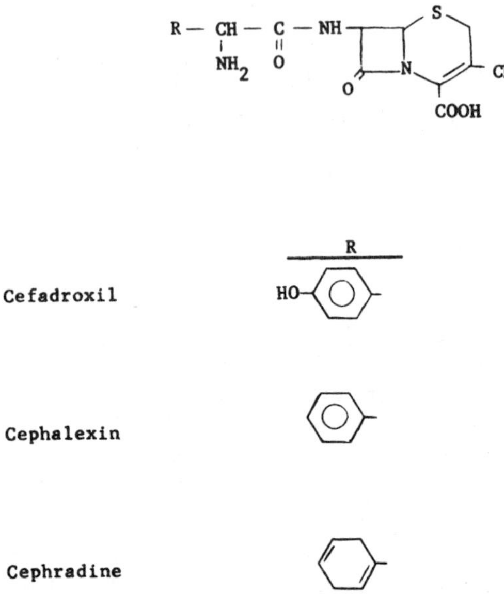

FIG. 1. *Structures.*

dosing. Total urine collections were made over the 0- to 3-, 3- to 6-, and 6- to 12-h intervals after dosing.

Study HL-75-51. Study HL-75-51 was a four-period crossover comparison directed toward the effect of food on the bioavailabilities of cephalexin monohydrate and cefadroxil monohydrate. Cefadroxil monohydrate capsules, 500 mg, and commercial cephalexin monohydrate capsules, 500 mg, were administered. Sixteen volunteers (10 male and 6 female) were employed. Each volunteer received three consecutive doses of each drug with and without food. There were 24-h intervals between the successive doses. All volunteers took both cefadroxil and cephalexin with and without food. On the test days when drug was administered with food, the volunteers ingested 50 g of bacon, one fried egg, one slice of bread, and one cup of coffee with the drug.

On test day 1, blood samples were taken at zero time and at 0.5, 1, 1.5, 3, 6 and 8 h after dosing. On test days 2 and 3, blood samples were taken at 2 and 8 h after dosing. The 8-h blood collections were omitted when the test drug was cephalexin. Total urine collections were made over the 0- to 4- and 4- to 8-h intervals after dosing.

Pharmacokinetic bioavailability and statistical analyses. Serum concentration versus time data for each individual subject were fitted to the following biexponential equation:

$$C = -A_1 \exp(-K_a t) + B_1 \exp(K_{el} t) \quad (1)$$

which describes an open, one-compartment model of drug disposition when drug absorption from the gastrointestinal tract into the systemic circulation occurs by passive diffusion (7). A_1 and B_1 are coefficients; K_a is a first-order rate constant for drug absorption, and K_{el} is a rate constant for drug elimination by first-order processes. The fitting was performed via nonlinear regression analysis using the digital computer program NLIN which employs Marquardt's algorithm (5).

The lag time between drug administration and the onset of absorption, t_o, was found by setting equation 1 equal to zero and rearranging it:

$$t_0 = \ln(A_1/B_1)/(K_a - K_{el}) \quad (2)$$

The time at which peak serum level occurs, $t_{\max}$, was calculated by setting the differential of equation 1 equal to zero and solving for $t_{\max}$:

$$t_{\max} = \ln(A_1K_a/B_1K_{el})/(K_a - K_{el}) \quad (3)$$

$C_{\max}$, the peak serum level, was calculated by substituting $t_{\max}$ into equation 1. The area under the serum concentration versus time curve (AUC) from $t = 0$ to infinity was calculated by integrating equation 1 between these time limits:

$$AUC = -A_1/K_a + B_1/K_{el} \quad (4)$$

The renal clearances (Cl_r) of the drugs were found by plotting the renal excretion rates of the drug ($\Delta M_u/\Delta t$) versus serum concentrations at the midpoint times of the urine collection intervals (9). The total amount of drug in milligrams, M_u, excreted in any given time interval in hours, t_1 to t_2, was divided by the length of the interval to get the renal excretion rate in milligrams per hour:

$$\Delta M_u/\Delta t = M_u/(t_2 - t_1) \quad (5)$$

This was plotted versus serum concentration at time $(t_1 + t_2)/2$. If the serum concentration at a given time had not been experimentally determined, it was estimated by interpolation from a semilogarithmic plot of serum concentration versus time data.

This paper reports the mean results by drug and subject groups rather than the results for each subject. In these three studies there were 44 subjects and 12 different treatments for a total of 528 sets of serum-urine data.

The goodness of fit between the estimates of serum concentration ($\hat{C}_i$) provided by equation 1 and the measured serum concentrations (C_i) was evaluated by F, the sums of squares of the deviations:

$$F = \sum_{i=1}^{n} (C_i - \hat{C}_i)^2 \quad (6)$$

and r^2:

$$r^2 = \left[\sum_{i=1}^{n} C^2_i - \frac{\left(\sum_{i=1}^{n} C_i\right)^2}{n} - F\right] \Bigg/ \left[\sum_{i=1}^{n} C^2_i - \frac{\left(\sum_{i=1}^{n} C_i\right)^2}{n}\right] \quad (7)$$

The serum concentration and urinary excretion data for each subject in each of the studies presented here were each evaluated, using the method presented above, separately. This paper reports the mean data by drug and subject groups, but the results reported for the bioavailability analyses are from the individual subject analyses.

Cefadroxil, cephalexin, and cephradine are each distinctive chemical entities, and it could not be assumed that their in vivo dispositions were identical. For that reason it was inappropriate to consistently test statistical hypotheses regarding bioavailability within each study by a single multiway analysis of variance (ANOVA). Such an ANOVA was appropriate when testing "treatment" affects on bioavailability for a given antibiotic within a single study. Thus, when comparing cefadroxil monohydrate and trihydrate in study HL-74-41 and the effect of food and fasting on cefadroxil monohydrate or cephalexin monohydrate in study HL-75-51, such an ANOVA could be used. A two-period crossover design ANOVA (3) served in these cases. When comparing different antibiotics in a single study or performing interstudy comparisons, the more appropriate one-way ANOVA (6) was used. All hypotheses were tested at the $P = 0.05$ level of significance.

Bioavailability comparisons on a given antibiotic were performed using K_a, t_{max} and C_{max} to characterize rate of availability and AUC to characterize total extent of availability once statistical equivalence of K_{el} values in the crossover had been established (10).

The urine concentrations of the antibiotics have been calculated and compared at their modes (the concentration values corresponding to the greatest concentration frequencies) rather than their means, since the distributions of urine concentrations were skewed and apparently not normal distributions.

RESULTS AND DISCUSSION

Serum concentrations. Tables 1 and 2, 3 and 4, and 5 and 6 contain the mean serum concentrations and pharmacokinetic parameters ± standard error (SE) for studies HL-74-41, HL-75-47, and HL-75-51, respectively. Up to concentrations of 25 μg/ml, the serum protein bindings of cefadroxil and cephalexin were very similar: cefadroxil was 20% bound, and cephalexin was 17% bound (1).

The monohydrate and trihydrate of cefadroxil are fully equivalent to each other. Statistical analyses indicated no significant differences between their rate or total extent of bioavailability.

The data from all three studies indicate that cephalexin is more rapidly absorbed than cefadroxil: K_a for cephalexin was always greater than K_a for cefadroxil. This led to the later t_{max} for cefadroxil than for cephalexin. This later t_{max} for cefadroxil was not due to delayed absorption of the drug; the overall absorption lag times for the two drugs were almost identical at 24 min for cefadroxil and 20 min for cephalexin. At doses of 500 mg, the mean C_{max} for cefadroxil (16 μg/ml) was about 80% of that for cephalexin (21 μg/ml). The overall mean half-life of cefadroxil (1.2 h) was twofold greater than the overall mean half-life of cephalexin (0.6 h); the AUC for cefadroxil (47.4 μgh/ml) was 1.6-fold greater than the AUC for cephalexin (29.0 μgh/ml), indicating that although the peak serum level of cefadroxil is lower than that of cephalexin, cefadroxil persists in the body an appreciably longer time than does cephalexin. At equivalent doses the cefadroxil serum level was higher than the cephalexin serum level by 1.5 h after dose and remained consistently higher thereafter. At the 500-mg dose, cephalexin concentration dropped to 1 μg/ml at about 4 h, and

TABLE 1. *Mean serum antibiotic concentrations for study HL-74-41*

Time (h)	Mean serum antibiotic concn (μg/ml ± SE)		
	Cefadroxil monohydrate (300 mg)	Cefadroxil trihydrate (300 mg)	Cephalexin monohydrate (250 mg)
0	0	0	0
0.5	2.52 ± 0.8	3.38 ± 0.65	4.28 ± 0.79
1	9.19 ± 0.38	9.59 ± 0.55	8.58 ± 0.65
1.5	9.43 ± 0.36	9.29 ± 0.41	5.19 ± 0.39
3	4.13 ± 0.23	3.90 ± 0.19	1.20 ± 0.09
6	0.74 ± 0.06	0.67 ± 0.04	<0.04
8	0.34 ± 0.04	0.28 ± 0.03	<0.04

TABLE 2. *Pharmacokinetic parameters for study HL-74-41*

Parameter	Value ± SE		
	Cefadroxil monohydrate (300 mg)	Cefadroxil trihydrate (300 mg)	Cephalexin monohydrate (250 mg)
AUC (μgh per ml)	26.8 ± 0.8	26.3 ± 0.8	14.0 ± 0.6
K_a (h^{-1})	2.82 ± 0.36	2.97 ± 0.40	4.28 ± 0.42
K_{el} (h^{-1})	0.659 ± 0.028	0.666 ± 0.029	1.35 ± 0.10
t_{max} (h)	1.19 ± 0.05	1.12 ± 0.05	0.86 ± 0.05
C_{max} (μg/ml)	9.82 ± 0.31	10.3 ± 0.5	9.93 ± 0.76
$t_{1/2}$ (h)	1.05 ± 0.05	1.04 ± 0.05	0.51 ± 0.04
t_o (min)	26 ± 0.8	23 ± 2	24 ± 1
F	0.193	0.494	1.365
r^2	0.998	0.994	0.951

cefadroxil concentration dropped to 1 μg/ml at about 7 h.

Figures 2 and 3 contain plots of AUC and C_{max} versus dose for all three studies. Linear regression analysis of AUC and C_{max} versus dose for cefadroxil and cephalexin was performed using individual subject data (each analysis had 42 degrees of freedom). In each case the slope of the curve was significantly greater than zero ($P < 0.005$ for all four analyses) and the y axis intercept was never significantly greater than zero ($P > 0.4$ for all four analyses). The linearity of these plots indicates essential pharmacokinetic linearity for serum level data for cefadroxil and cephalexin up to a 500-mg oral dose. The linearity of cefadroxil and cephalexin indicates that we can calculate serum levels for these antibiotics, at any unknown dose over this range, from serum levels at a known dose by multiplying the known serum levels by the ratio of unknown to known dose (7). We can then calculate the mean serum levels and AUC which would be yielded by a 250-mg dose of cefadroxil. A 250-mg dose of

TABLE 3. *Mean serum antibiotic concentrations for study HL-75-47*

Time (h)	Mean serum antibiotic concn (μg/ml ± SE)		
	Cefadroxil monohydrate (500 mg)	Cephalexin monohydrate (500 mg)	Cephradine (500 mg)
0	0	0	0
0.5	5.61 ± 0.78	14.0 ± 2.2	11.3 ± 2.1
1	14.9 ± 1.7	17.9 ± 1.3	15.2 ± 1.3
1.5	15.0 ± 1.1	10.7 ± 1.1	10.6 ± 1.0
2	12.5 ± 0.8	6.02 ± 0.66	6.33 ± 0.77
4	4.63 ± 0.33	1.05 ± 0.16	0.96 ± 0.13
6	1.84 ± 0.14	0.10 ± 0.04	0.13 ± 0.04
8	0.65 ± 0.07	<0.04	<0.04
12	0.11 ± 0.03	<0.04	<0.04

TABLE 4. *Pharmacokinetic parameters for study HL-75-47*

Parameter	Value ± SE		
	Cefadroxil monohydrate (500 mg)	Cephalexin monohydrate (500 mg)	Cephradine (500 mg)
AUC (μgh per ml)	47.4 ± 2.1	29.0 ± 2.5	27.5 ± 2.2
K_a (h^{-1})	2.44 ± 0.38	4.78 ± 0.59	3.73 ± 0.33
K_{el} (h^{-1})	0.545 ± 0.034	1.21 ± 0.11	1.14 ± 0.09
t_{max} (h)	1.29 ± 0.09	0.71 ± 0.06	0.80 ± 0.08
C_{max} (μg/ml)	16.2 ± 1.4	20.7 ± 1.5	17.7 ± 1.2
$t_{1/2}$ (h)	1.27 ± 0.08	0.57 ± 0.05	0.61 ± 0.05
t_o (min)	22 ± 2	18 ± 4	18 ± 4
F	1.135	5.497	1.430
r^2	0.996	0.978	0.992

TABLE 5. *Mean serum antibiotic concentrations for study HL-75-51*[a]

Drug	Time (h)	Mean serum antibiotic concn (μg/ml ± SE)					
		With food			Without food		
		Day 1	Day 2	Day 3	Day 1	Day 2	Day 3
Cefadroxil monohydrate	0	0	0	0	0	0	0
	0.5	7.31 ± 1.16	ND[b]	ND	6.03 ± 0.69	ND	ND
	1	15.5 ± 1.5	ND	ND	14.3 ± 1.2	ND	ND
	1.5	14.4 ± 1.2	ND	ND	14.7 ± 0.7	ND	ND
	2	ND	13.1 ± 0.7	13.9 ± 0.8	ND	14.4 ± 0.7	14.6 ± 1.2
	3	6.84 ± 0.61	ND	ND	7.68 ± 0.54	ND	ND
	6	1.57 ± 0.16	ND	ND	1.58 ± 0.17	ND	ND
	8	0.50 ± 0.05	0.51 ± 0.06	0.64 ± 0.05	0.55 ± 1.01	0.58 ± 0.08	0.57 ± 0.07
Cephalexin monohydrate	0	0	0	0	0	0	0
	0.5	11.5 ± 1.7	ND	ND	14.0 ± 1.7	ND	ND
	1	15.5 ± 1.2	ND	ND	20.7 ± 1.6	ND	ND
	1.5	12.2 ± 0.9	ND	ND	12.7 ± 0.8	ND	ND
	2	ND	8.17 ± 0.77	8.76 ± 1.00	ND	8.51 ± 0.84	7.90 ± 0.73
	3	3.09 ± 0.33	ND	ND	2.92 ± 0.25	ND	ND
	6	0.25 ± 0.05	ND	ND	0.12 ± 0.05	ND	ND

[a] All doses 500 mg.
[b] ND, Not determined.

TABLE 6. *Pharmacokinetic parameters for study HL-75-51*[a]

Parameter	Value ± SE			
	Cefadroxil monohydrate		Cephalexin monohydrate	
	With food	Without food	With food	Without food
AUC (μgh per ml)	45.1 ± 2.4	43.3 ± 2.4	31.3 ± 1.8	32.8 ± 1.8
K_a (h^{-1})	3.21 ± 0.48	2.47 ± 0.32	5.31 ± 1.67	6.92 ± 2.23
K_{el} (h^{-1})	0.550 ± 0.052	0.546 ± 0.017	0.867 ± 0.085	0.960 ± 0.049
t_{max} (h)	1.17 ± 0.10	1.20 ± 0.06	0.82 ± 0.08	0.74 ± 0.22
C_{max} (μg/ml)	16.3 ± 0.8	14.7 ± 0.8	18.5 ± 1.9	21.4 ± 1.5
$t_{1/2}$ (h)	1.26 ± 0.12	1.27 ± 0.04	0.80 ± 0.08	0.72 ± 0.04
t_o (min)	24 ± 3	20 ± 2	17 ± 3	18 ± 2
F	0.169	2.230	0.666	1.440
r^2	0.999	0.988	0.996	0.995

[a] All doses 500 mg.

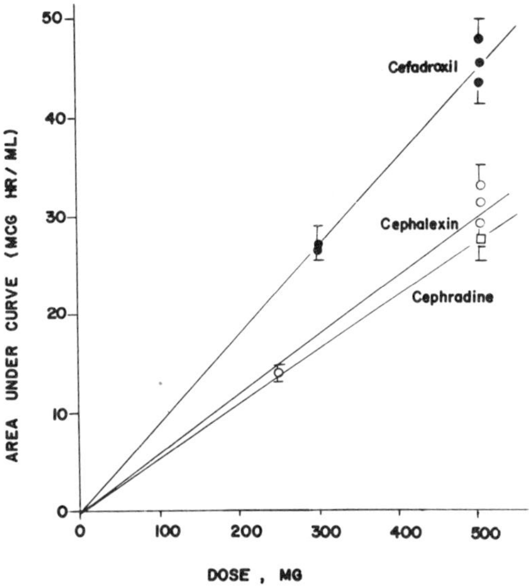

FIG. 2. *Area under curve as a function of dose.*

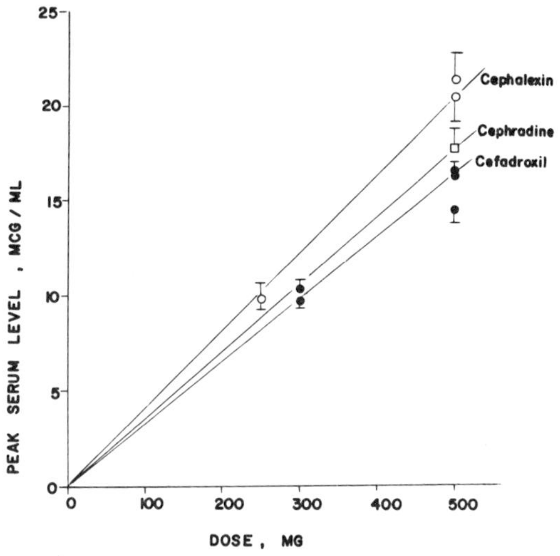

FIG. 3. *Peak serum levels as a function of dose.*

cefadroxil would yield a C_{max} 80% as great and an AUC 1.6-fold greater than those produced by the 250-mg dose of cephalexin.

The pharmacokinetic parameters found for cefadroxil and cephalexin show no more than normal variation between studies. C_{max}, t_{max}, K_a, and AUC values under fasting conditions are very consistent. Cefadroxil half-life varied between 1.05 h in study HL-74-41 and 1.27 h in studies HL-75-47 and HL-75-51. Cephalexin half-life varied between 0.51 and 0.57 h in studies HL-74-41 and HL-75-47 and 0.8 h in study HL-75-51. These half-lives remain in the range of expectable biological variability. Cephalexin half-lives ranging from 0.6 to 1.2 h have been reported in the literature (8). In this series of three studies, cefadroxil consistently had a longer half-life than cephalexin in each of the 44 subjects. We might expect to continue to see consistently longer half-lives for cefadroxil than for cephalexin in humans.

Cephalexin is normally administered every 6 h. At approximately 45 min after dosing, a 250-mg dose of cephalexin yields a mean C_{max} of 10 μg/ml, and at a 500-mg dose it yields a mean C_{max} of 20 μg/ml. By 6 h, at 250 mg, there is no detectable cephalexin present in serum. At a 500-mg dose, the mean 6-h serum level is 0.13 μg/ml. Cefadroxil is more persistent. At a dose of 250 mg it will achieve a mean peak serum level of 8 μg/ml at approximately 70 min and the mean serum concentration will be 0.33 μg/ml at 8 h and 0.06 μg/ml at 12 h. At a dose of 500 mg, cefadroxil has a mean peak serum level of 16 μg/ml at approximately 70 min and the mean serum concentrations will be 0.65 μg/ml at 8 h and 0.11 μg/ml at 12 h. Cefadroxil would have analogous persistence in urine at these doses. It would seem reasonable to develop clinical efficacy data which, supported by these pharmacokinetic properties, could indicate a 12-h dosing interval for cefadroxil.

The disposition of cephradine seems very similar to that of cephalexin. Their serum level curves and the values for their pharmacokinetic parameters are very similar (see Tables 3 and 4).

Concurrent ingestion of food with either cefadroxil or cephalexin on study day 1 (study HL-75-51, Tables 5 and 6) had no statistically significant effect on their bioavailability relative to fasting conditions. Neither rates of availability nor total availability were affected. Continued concurrent administration of food did not markedly affect cefadroxil or cephalexin bioavailability.

The predose, zero-time serum samples on days 2 or 3 did not contain detectable levels of antibiotics. Neither cefadroxil nor cephalexin demonstrated either accumulation of drug or induction of elimination on repeated administration.

Urinary excretion. Plotting $\Delta M_u/\Delta t$ versus serum concentrations for cefadroxil and cephalexin gave the results shown in Fig. 4. These data came from all three studies. Cephradine was excluded for lack of sufficient data. Linear regression analysis indicated that the apparent

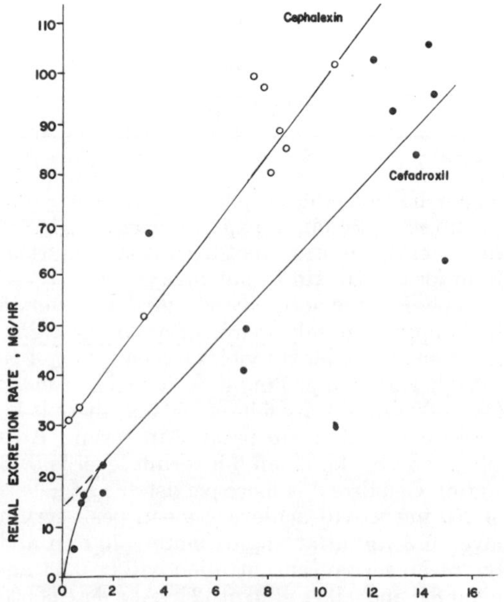

FIG. 4. *Renal excretion rates as a function of serum concentration.*

straight-line portions of these plots were significantly linear. These results enable assignment of specific renal excretion phenomena to glomerular filtration and tubular secretion.

Net renal excretion of antibiotic can be represented as renal excretion rate = glomerular filtration rate + tubular secretion rate, i.e.:

$$dM_u/dt = VK_uC + TmC/(K_m + C) \quad (8)$$

$\Delta M_u/\Delta t$ is the numerical approximation to dM_u/dt; V is the apparent volume of distribution of drug in the body; K_u is the net first-order rate constant for glomerular filtration; C is the serum concentration of drug; Tm is the maximum transport rate for tubular secretion, and K_m is the Michaelis constant. The term $T_mC/(K_m + C)$ describes the capacity-limited process and is exactly analogous to the Michaelis-Menten equation for enzyme activity. When $C \gg K_m$ this reduces to T_m and equation 5 becomes:

$$dM_u/dt = VK_uC + T_m \quad (9)$$

Equation 9 is the best overall description of the curves seen in Fig. 4. At relatively low serum concentrations, less than 0.3 μg/ml for cephalexin and at about 1 μg/ml for cefadroxil, the tubular secretion mechanism has become saturated (i.e., $C \gg K_m$) and tubular secretion proceeds at its maximum rate, T_m. This constant rate is about 30 mg/h for cephalexin and 15 mg/h for cefadroxil. It appears that cephalexin has a greater affinity for the tubular secretion mechanism than does cefadroxil; cephalexin has a higher T_m and a smaller K_m. This is the primary reason for the shorter half-life of cephalexin—it is more readily excreted in the urine.

The slopes of the linear portions of the plots in Fig. 4 are equivalent to the term VK_m, which is the renal clearance rate due to glomerular filtration. This rate is 112 ml/min for cephalexin and 90.1 ml/min for cefadroxil. These rates are statistically equivalent to the commonly accepted value for creatinine clearance rate (gomerular filtration rate) in humans, 95.5 ml/min (2).

Human renal excretion of these two cephalosporin antibiotics does not proceed by a completely linear, first-order process. As cefadroxil or cephalexin dose increases, it would take a longer time to excrete any given percentage of the dose. Since the tubular secretion rate for cefadroxil is less than the tubular secretion rate for cephalexin, the urinary excretion of cefadroxil is of longer duration. Cefadroxil yields initially lower urine concentrations than an equal dose of cephalexin, but cefadroxil maintains higher urine concentrations at the later times (see Tables 7 and 8). Within each given experiment the ranges and means of urine volumes remain reasonably constant. The 0- to 3- or 0- to 4-h modal urine concentrations of cefadroxil are lower than the 0- to 3- or 0- to 4-h modal urine concentrations of cephalexin or cephradine. At the 4- to 8- and 3- to 6- or 6- to 12-h intervals, cefadroxil maintains the highest modal urine levels. In study HL-75-47, urine concentrations of cefadroxil were maintained at a relative constant modal level through 0 to 3 and 3 to 6 h and remained at least twice as high as cephalexin and cephradine modal concentrations from 3 through 12 h.

Figure 5 contains cumulative urinary excretion plots drawn from the three studies being reported here. The total cumulative urinary excretion of active cefadroxil and cephalexin are statistically equivalent with an overall mean of approximately 88% of dose. They are almost completely absorbed; there may be small components of their elimination by biliary excretion or metabolism. All of a dose of cephradine appears to be excreted in the urine; presumably, cephradine is completely absorbed and eliminated completely by renal excretion. The total assayed cumulative urinary excretion of antibiotic in some subjects was greater than 100% of the dose, but the range of these recoveries did not exceed the 10 to 15% variability normally expected from cup-plate assays.

Since cefadroxil is eliminated more slowly than cephalexin or cephradine, it has a longer residence time in the body, time in which it could distribute more extensively. The range of the apparent volumes of distribution can be estimated from the relationship, creatinine clearance rate = G.F.R. = VK_u. Elimination rate constants may be described as $K_{el} = K_u + K_{nr}$ where K_{nr} is a first-order rate constant for drug elimination via nonrenal routes.

If renal excretion is the only elimination route, then $K_{nr} = 0$ and $K_u = K_{el}$. This presumes that the active antibiotic excreted in

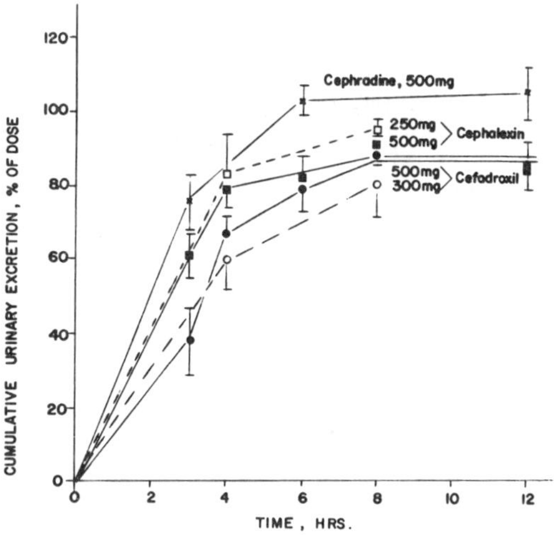

FIG. 5. *Cumulative urinary excretion.*

TABLE 7. *Time course of antibiotic concentrations in urine for studies HL-74-41, HL-75-51*

Drug	Dose (mg)	0–4 h				4–8 h			
		Urine vol (ml)		Urine concn (μg/ml)		Urine vol (ml)		Urine concn (μg/ml)	
		Range	Mean	Range	Mode	Range	Mean	Range	Mode
Cefadroxil	300	100–900	396	203–1,960	497	90–560	262	84–450	243
	500	80–800	348	308–3,500	1,003	100–560	298	84–1,099	293
Cephalexin	250	130–770	361	332–1,697	573	180–470	277	38–270	108
	500	110–950	374	326–3,350	1,140	120–700	327	37–745	201

TABLE 8. *Time course of antibiotic concentration in urine for study HL-75-47*[a]

Drug	0–3 h				3–6 h				6–12 h			
	Urine vol (ml)		Urine concn (μg/ml)		Urine vol (ml)		Urine concn (μg/ml)		Urine vol (ml)		Urine concn (μg/ml)	
	Range	Mean	Range	Mode	Range	Mean	Range	Mode	Range	Mean	Range	Mode
Cefadroxil	70–320	156	730–2360	1211	65–420	184	368–3110	1113	100–320	203	83–263	167
Cephalexin	65–420	172	830–5720	1783	20–430	165	264–1360	607	90–380	210	31–287	78
Cephradine	85–400	170	1068–3805	2136	35–780	231	281–1339	582	85–360	179	9–202	61

[a] All doses 500 mg.

urine represents all of the drug absorbed. If the drug was completely bioavailable, then the difference between the total dose and the cumulative fraction excreted in the urine (F_e) represents the amount eliminated by nonrenal routes and:

$$K_u = K_{el} - K_{nr} = F_e K_{el} \quad (10)$$

since $K_{nr} = (1 - F_e)K_{el}$. Thus, the value of K_u must lie between K_{el} and $F_e K_{el}$. Applying these limits to the relationship V = G.F.R./K_u we can calculate that the possible range of apparent volumes of distribution for cefadroxil is 9.7 to 11.6 liters (i.e., 14 to 17% of body weight) and for cephalexin it is 5.2 to 5.8 liters (i.e., 7.4 to 8.3% of body weight). The longer duration and more extensive distribution of cefadroxil in vito are interrelated factors.

LITERATURE CITED

1. **Buck, R. E., and K. E. Price.** 1976. Cefadroxil, a new broad-spectrum cephalosporin. Antimicrob. Agents Chemother. 11:324–330.
2. **Diem, K.** 1962. Documenta giegy, 6th ed., p. 545. Giegy Pharmaceuticals, Ardsley, N.Y.
3. **Grizzle, J. E.** 1965. The two-period change-over design and its use in clinical trials. Biometrics 21:467–480.
4. **Grove, D. C., and W. A. Randall.** 1953. Assay methods of antibiotics. A laboratory manual. Medical Encyclopedia Inc., N.Y.
5. **Marquardt, D. W.** 1963. An algorithm for least-squares estimation of non-linear parameters. J. Soc. Ind. Appl. Math. 11:431–441.
6. **Snedecor, G. W., and W. G. Cochran.** 1973. Statistical methods, 6th ed., p. 258–298. Iowa State University Press, Ames, Iowa.
7. **Teorell, T.** 1937. Kinetics of distribution of substances administered to the body. I. The extravascular modes of administration. Arch. Int. Pharmacodyn. 57:205–225.
8. **Thrupp, L. D.** 1974. Newer cephalosporins and "expanded-spectrum" penicillins. Annu. Rev. Pharmacol. 14:435–467.
9. **Wagner, J. G.** 1971. Biopharmaceutics and relevant pharmacokinetics, p. 247–248. Drug Intelligence Publishers, Hamilton, Ill.
10. **Wagner, J. G.** 1972. An overview of the analysis and interpretation of bioavailability studies in man. Pharmacology 8:102–117.

ANTIMICROBIAL AGENTS AND CHEMOTHERAPY, Feb. 1977, p. 339-344
Vol. 11, No. 2
Printed in U.S.A.

Transfer of a Plasmid-Specified Beta-Lactamase Gene from *Haemophilus influenzae*

J. R. SAUNDERS[1]* AND R. B. SYKES

Department of Bacteriology, Medical School, Bristol BS8 1TD, and Glaxo Research Limited, Greenford, Middlesex, U.K.

Received for publication 28 June 1976

A number of ampicillin-resistant strains of *Haemophilus influenzae* could donate a gene specifying the type IIIa (TEM) β-lactamase to *Haemophilus parainfluenzae*, *Escherichia coli*, and *Pseudomonas aeruginosa*. Donor strains rapidly lost their ability to transfer ampicillin resistance on storage or subculture. Such strains also apparently contained a single species of covalently closed circular deoxyribonucleic acid of contour length 1.2 μm, equivalent to about 2.5 $\times 10^6$ daltons. No species of plasmid deoxyribonucleic acid large enough to encode sex factor activity was detected. Despite this, transfer occurred to several bacterial genera in the presence of deoxyribonuclease, suggesting that transmissibility was by conjugation. The β-lactamase gene was generally unstable after transfer and was lost in the absence of selection. Where stable transcipients were found, this was evidently by insertion of the β-lactamase gene into the host chromosome. In *P. aeruginosa* insertion was always accompanied by induction of auxotrophy for adenine, suggesting insertion at a specific site. It is believed that insertion also occurred at one site on the chromosome of *Escherichia coli*. Crypticity measurements for β-lactamase activity showed that there was little or no penetration barrier to β-lactam drugs in *Haemophilus*. This may explain the long delay in the acquisition of ampicillin resistance by this organism.

Ampicillin-resistant strains of *Haemophilus influenzae* have become increasingly common in recent years, thus contradicting the previously held assumption that the *H. influenzae* population was uniformly susceptible to this antibiotic. Resistance in all cases so far examined (8, 9, 15, 18, 25, 27) is due to the acquisition by *H. influenzae* of a gene specifying the TEM or type IIIa β-lactamase (22). This gene can form part of the translocatable genetic element transposon A (TnA) (11, 12), which is borne on a range of physically and genetically distinct plasmids found in a variety of bacterial species (13).

Transferable kanamycin resistance has been reported in *H. influenzae* (6). Furthermore, transfer of ampicillin resistance between strains of this organism, but not to *Escherichia coli*, has also been described by Thorne and Farrar (26). We report the transfer of a gene specifying the type IIIa β-lactamase from ampicillin-resistant strains of *H. influenzae* to *H. parainfluenzae*, *E. coli*, and *Pseudomonas aeruginosa*. The behavior and expression of this gene in these bacterial species is described together with possible implications for the spread of drug resistance to previously susceptible strains of *Haemophilus*.

MATERIALS AND METHODS

[2-^{3}H]adenine was obtained from the Radiochemical Centre, Amersham; pancreatic deoxyribonuclease (DNAse) I was from Sigma Chemical Co., London. All other materials have been described previously (3, 10, 25).

Bacterial strains used. See Table 1.

Growth and storage of bacteria. All organisms were grown in brain heart infusion (Difco), supplemented with 5% (vol/vol) Fildes peptic digest (Oxoid) for the growth of *Haemophilus* organisms (BHF). Stock cultures were subcultured in BHF immediately on receipt and stored at −70°C. Where required, liquid medium was solidified by the incorporation of 1.2% (wt/vol) agar (Difco). *Haemophilus* strains were generally grown in an atmosphere supplemented with 5 to 10% CO_2. Where required, antibiotics were incorporated at the following concentrations: ampicillin, 20 μg/ml; carbenicillin, 500 μg/ml; rifampin, 100 μg/ml; streptomycin, 500 μg/ml; and tetracycline, 100 μg/ml.

Detection of β-lactamase. β-Lactamase-producing strains of *E. coli* and *P. aeruginosa* were detected by spotting the chromogenic cephalosporin 87/312 on colonies growing on solid media. Formation of a red color indicated the presence of a β-lactamase.

Suspensions of *H. influenzae* were prepared by

[1] Present address: Department of Microbiology, University of Liverpool, P.O. Box 147, Liverpool L69 3BX, U.K.

TABLE 1. *Bacterial strains used*[a]

Species	Designation	Genetic markers	Origin
Haemophilus influenzae	23142	amp^r	C. Thornsberry
	2486	amp^r	P. Cavanagh
H. parainfluenzae	28366		P. Cavanagh
Escherichia coli	W3110		Ref. 10
	W3110 (R2486)	W3110 × 2486	This paper
	UB1139 (pUB306)	thy^- leu^- met^- nal^r	Ref. 3 and 5
		RP1 – ampicillin susceptible	P. M. Bennett
	J5-3 (pUB307)	pro^- met^- nal^r	
		RP1 – TnA deleted	
Pseudomonas aeruginosa	Ps18	rif^r	Ref. 10
	PAO8	str^r met^- ilv^-	V. Stanisich
	Ps18 (R23142)	rif^r amp^r (Ps18 × 23142)	This paper

[a] Abbreviations: amp^r, nal^r, rif^r, str^r, resistance to ampicillin, nalidixic acid, rifampcin, and streptomycin, respectively. RP1 specifies resistance to ampicillin, tetracycline, and neomycin/kanamycin.

picking several colonies of the test organism from a fresh overnight culture and emulsifying in physiological saline (0.5 ml). Samples (50 μl) of the cell suspensions were distributed into the wells of a Cooke microtiter plate that contained 50 μl of an aqueous solution of 87/312 (500 μg/ml in 0.1 M phosphate buffer, pH 7.0). A color change from yellow to red indicated the presence of β-lactamase.

Preparation of enzymes. Enzymes were prepared as described in reference 25.

β-Lactamase assays. All assays were performed iodometrically by the method of Perret (20) as modified by Novick (19). Ampicillin was used as substrate at a concentration of 6 mM, and assays were performed at pH 7.0 and 37°C. Enzyme units are defined as micromoles of substrate hydrolyzed per minute.

Crypticity measurements. These were determined by incubation of ampicillin with washed cells of the relevant organism (i) intact and (ii) sonicated (for 3 min at 37°C). Estimation of the amount of substrate destroyed in each instance gives a measure of the available β-lactamase activity. Crypticity = (specific enzyme activity of broken cells)/(specific enzyme activity of whole cells).

Genetic transfer. Exponential-phase cultures of donor strains were mixed 1:10 with recipient strains, and incubation continued at 37°C without shaking for 4 h. In some cases, pancreatic DNase I was included in the mating mixture at a concentration of 20 μg/ml. Mating mixtures were Vortex-mixed at the end of the mating period, and dilutions were plated on appropriately supplemented agar.

Elimination of drug resistance. Organisms were grown in the presence of ethidium bromide (2 μg/ml) for 18 h at 37°C. Dilutions of the culture were then plated on drug-free BHF medium and incubated for 18 h at 37°C. Suitable plates were then replicated onto similar medium containing ampicillin.

Isolation of plasmid deoxyribonucleic acid (DNA). *P. aeruginosa* Psa18 (R23142) was labeled with [^{3}H]adenine (5 μCi/ml; 5 μg/ml). All other bacteria were labeled with [^{3}H]thymidine, lysed, and analyzed by ethidium bromide-CsCl gradient centrifugation as described previously (10).

TABLE 2. *Transfer of type IIIa β-lactamase gene from Haemophilus influenzae*

Donor	Recipient	Transfer frequency[a]: In absence of DNase	Transfer frequency[a]: In presence of DNase
H. influenzae 23142	*H. parainfluenzae*	1×10^{-6}	3×10^{-6}
	E. coli W3110	8×10^{-5}	7×10^{-5}
	P. aeruginosa Ps18	3×10^{-5}	2×10^{-5}

[a] Transfer frequencies were determined by dividing the number of ampicillin-resistant recipients present at the end of the mating by the number of donor cells present at the beginning of mating.

Electron microscopy of DNA. Preparations of plasmid DNA were examined by electron microscopy as described in reference 3.

RESULTS

Transferability of ampicillin resistance from *H. influenzae*. All ampicillin-resistant strains of *H. influenzae* examined here contain a type IIIa β-lactamase (25). Because the gene specifying this enzyme is commonly found on R factors (22), attempts were made to transfer ampicillin resistance to other bacteria. The strains used could indeed transfer resistance to a variety of organisms (Table 2). Donor ability, but not resistance, declined rapidly on storage or subculture. However, strains that had apparently lost their ability to transfer directly to *E. coli* could do so indirectly if an intermediate *H. influenzae* donor strain was used in a triparental cross. To eliminate the possibility of gene transfer by transformation, matings were repeated in the presence of DNase (Table 2). No appreciable difference in transfer rate could be determined in the presence or absence of DNase.

The β-lactamase gene was highly unstable when transferred to *H. parainfluenzae*. The presence of the gene could, however, be detected readily in unstable recipient strains by the analytical isoelectric-focusing technique as previously described (25). Direct transfers from *H. influenzae* to *E. coli* were again characterized by instability of the β-lactamase gene. However, transfers either directly to *P. aeruginosa* or by triparental matings to *E. coli* always resulted in stable transcipients. In all cases, furthermore, the β-lactamase gene was not further transferable from such stable transcipients to other strains.

Properties of extrachromosomal DNA in strains carrying the β-lactamase gene. All strains of *H. influenzae* used that were capable of acting as donors of the β-lactamase gene contained covalently closed circular DNA amounting to about 2% of the chromosomal DNA as judged by ethidium bromide-CsCl gradient centrifugation (Fig. 1). Donor strains of *H. influenzae* could be cured of ampicillin resistance by growth in medium containing ethidium bromide (Table 3). Cured strains contained no extrachromosomal DNA (e.g., Fig. 1). Concomitant loss of this DNA and resistance

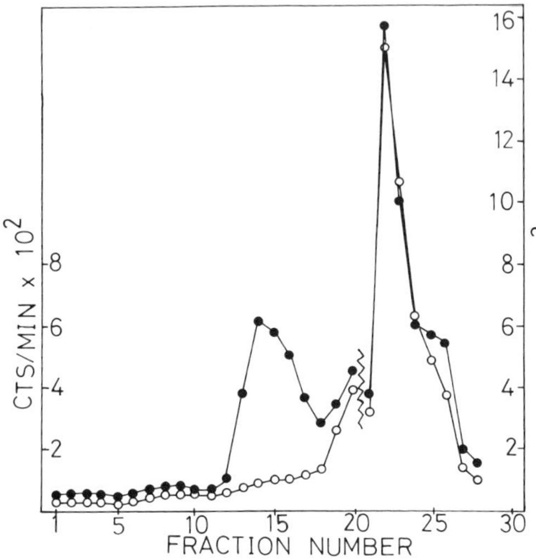

FIG. 1. *Ethidium bromide-CsCl density gradient centrifugation of DNA from strains of H. influenzae. Radioactive cultures were lysed and analyzed separately on ethidium bromide-cell gradients. Symbols:* (●) *DNA from strain 2486 (ampicillin resistant);* (○) *DNA from strain UB 2824 (ampicillin-susceptible variant of 2486). Note the change of scale between fractions 20 and 21 in each case.*

shows that the β-lactamase gene is plasmid linked. Circular DNA in donor strains had a contour length of about 1.2 ± 0.02 μm, equivalent to a molecular weight of about 2.5 Mdal (17) (Fig. 2). No larger plasmid DNA molecules were detected in any donor strain. In addition, transcipients from crosses either to *E. coli* or *P. aeruginosa* that had received the β-lactamase gene contained no detectable extrachromosomal DNA.

Properties of strains of *E. coli* and *P. aeruginosa* receiving the β-lactamase gene. All strains of *P. aeruginosa* tested (30 clones from three separate matings) that had received the β-lactamase gene from *H. influenzae* were found to have become auxotrophic for adenine. Since these strains contain no extrachromosomal DNA (see above), this is probably due to insertion of the β-lactamase gene into the chromosomes of *P. aeruginosa*, causing disruption of one of the two loci known for adenine production in this organism (14). Detailed mapping of the site of insertion was precluded because the strains of *P. aeruginosa* used would not receive the *Pseudomonas* sex factor FP2 (J. R. Saunders, unpublished data).

No equivalent induction of auxotrophic mutations was observed in *E. coli* strains that had received the β-lactamase gene from *H. influenzae*. However, preliminary mapping experiments place the site of insertion of the β-lactamase gene close to *trp* on the chromosome of *E. coli* (J. R. Saunders, unpublished data).

Attempts were made to mobilize the TEM β-lactamase gene from the insertion site in the chromosomes of these two organisms. This was done by infecting such strains with derivatives of the R factor RP1 that no longer specify β-lactamase. These were pUB 306, a derivative of RP1 that contains point mutations both in the type IIIa β-lactamase gene and in the gene specifying intrinsic resistance to penicillins (5; N. Curtis, personal communication), and pUB 307, a variant of RP1 in which the whole of TnA, and hence the β-lactamase gene, has been deleted (23). Strains of *P. aeruginosa* and *E. coli* were maintained for about 20 generations in the absence of drug selection and then tested for transfer ability. Neither R factor was able to mobilize the inserted β-lactamase gene (Table

TABLE 3. *Curing of ampicillin resistance from Haemophilus influenzae*

Strain	Total colonies tested	Ampicillin-susceptible colonies
23142	690	5
2486	403	4

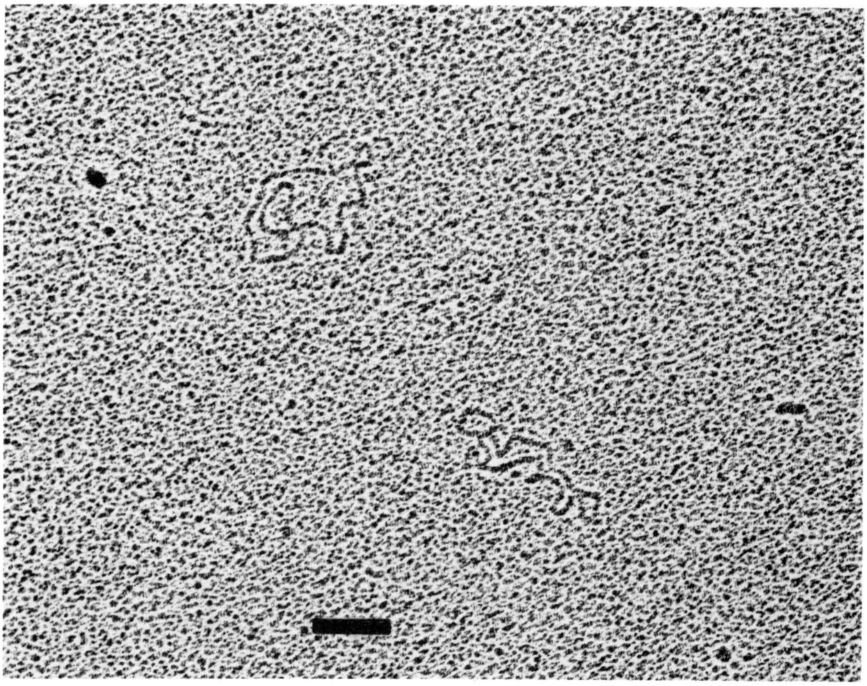

FIG. 2. *Electron micrograph of extrachromosomal DNA from H. influenzae 2486. Bar represents 0.1 μm.*

4) in either species, although the R factors were evidently capable of transferring themselves. Furthermore, the presence of either R factor did not promote the reversion of *P. aeruginosa* to adenine prototrophy.

β-Lactamase production and crypticity values. Both donor and transcipient strains produced similar levels of cell-free β-lactamase (Table 5), as did ampicillin-resistant strains that had lost transfer ability (data not shown). However, hydrolysis of ampicillin by whole-cell preparations varied markedly. Whole-cell cultures of the *Haemophilus* strains hydrolyzed ampicillin at a similar rate to the cell-free extracts. In the case of the *E. coli* and *Pseudomonas* transcipients, whole-cell cultures were much less efficient at hydrolyzing the substrate than their corresponding cell-free enzyme preparations (Table 5).

DISCUSSION

We have demonstrated that the ampicillin resistance found in the *H. influenzae* strains studied here is plasmid linked. Resistance is due to the type IIIa β-lactamase and is specified by an extrachromosomal element of about 2.5 Mdal. We proposed to call this plasmid pUB702. Assuming that the amount of covalently closed circular DNA present in resistant strains (about 2% of the chromosomal DNA) represents

TABLE 4. *Transfer of inserted β-lactamase gene by derivatives of RP1* [a]

Plasmid	Selection on:	Transfer frequency [a]	
		From *P. aeruginosa* Ps18 R23142	From *E. coli* W3110 (2486)
pUB306	Tetracycline (100 μg/ml)	3×10^{-4}	5×10^{-4}
	Carbenicillin (500 μg/ml)	$<10^{-10}$	$<10^{-10}$
pUB307	Tetracycline (100 μg/ml)	1×10^{-4}	3×10^{-4}
	Carbenicillin (500 μg/ml)	$<10^{-10}$	$<5 \times 10^{-9}$

[a] The recipient in all cases was *P. aeruginosa* PAO8, and counterselection was by streptomycin (500 μg/ml).

TABLE 5. *β-Lactamase activity of cell-free preparations and crypticity values*

Organism	Enzyme units/mg of protein	Crypticity value
Haemophilus influenzae 2486	0.03	1
Escherichia coli W3110 (R2486)	0.035	30
H. influenzae 23142	0.03	1
Pseudomonas aeruginosa (R23142)	0.03	40

the lower limit of plasmid DNA and that the molecular weight of the *H. influenzae* chromosome is 1.7×10^9 (7), then this plasmid is present at about 14 copies per chromosome equivalent. The molecular properties of pUB702 are closely similar to those of the smaller (3 Mdal) of two plasmid species, named RSF0885, isolated by Falkow and co-workers (7, 8) from a series of ampicillin-resistant *H. influenzae*. Our strains were capable of donating the TEM β-lactamase gene to other bacteria even in the presence of DNase, thus eliminating transformation as the mechanism of transfer. The ability to transfer to such widely differing organisms as *H. parainfluenzae*, *E. coli*, and *P. aeruginosa* tends also to rule out transduction. It seems more likely that transfer was by conjugation. It is therefore surprising that no plasmid species large enough to encode sex factor activity were found. This may be because such strains contained a sex factor not detected by the methods used, or alternatively lost from the cells relatively rapidly. Support for the latter explanation comes from the observation that donor ability but not β-lactamase production was lost rapidly. Transfer of resistance could therefore have occurred via a plasmid coaggregate (4) or class II transfer system (1), involving an unstable sex factor. An alternative explanation that we cannot rule out is that the donor strains originally contained pUB702 plus another unstable self-transmissible plasmid carrying an identical β-lactamase gene.

Although the TEM β-lactamase gene could be easily transferred to other bacterial species, it was generally unstable in *H. parainfluenzae* and *E. coli*. Similarly, Elwell et al. (8) found that RSF 0885 was unstable when transformed into *E. coli*. Despite this general instability, we could find stable transcipients especially in *P. aeruginosa*, where all such strains were highly stable. Stability was evidently due to insertion at specific sites in the chromosomes of *P. aeruginosa* and *E. coli*. This is in line with the transposable nature of the gene specifying the TEM β-lactamase (3, 11, 12). Generally, transposons can be repeatedly translocated to other genomes (11, 12). This was not the case with the inserted β-lactamase gene studied here, which could not be mobilized by R factors known to accept TnA. De Graaff et al. (7) have shown that the RSF 0885 contains only about one-third of the base sequences found in TnA. Assuming that pUB702 and RSF 0885 are closely similar, insertion of the β-lactamase gene into the genomes of these two bacterial species may therefore have been by normal recombination with pUB702 rather than by transposition per se.

The induction of auxotrophic mutations in *P. aeruginosa* by insertion of the β-lactamase gene from *Haemophilus* is nevertheless consistent with the ability of transposons to cause insertion mutations (12, 16). It is perhaps surprising that there is apparently one (possibly two) site for insertion of the gene in *P. aeruginosa* at *ade*. This suggests relatively limited homology between the gene and the host chromosome. Similarly, in *E. coli* the gene has apparently inserted near *trp*, close to the site reported for TnA in *E. coli* (3, 21). TnC, which specifies linked resistance to streptomycin and trimethoprim, also apparently integrates at a single site on the chromosome of *E. coli* (2).

The ability of the gene specifying TEM β-lactamase to migrate between DNA molecules is well known. This has many implications for the spread of resistance to β-lactam antibiotics to different bacterial species. Because ampicillin resistance has only recently emerged in the population of *H. influenzae*, it seems likely that this species has acquired the TEM β-lactamase by contact with members of the *Enterobacteriaceae*. The molecular properties of R plasmids specifying either ampicillin or tetracycline resistance in *Haemophilus* sp. do not, however, coincide in gross terms with those of any known plasmids found in enteric organisms (7, 8; J. R. Saunders, M. H. Richmond, L. P. Elwell, and S. Falkow, manuscript in preparation). It is possible that the TEM β-lactamase, and other resistance genes, have been deposited in *H. influenzae* by transient passage of an R factor itself incapable of survival in this species. Transposition of the resistance genes to existing replicons in *Haemophilus* has therefore probably resulted in stable acquisition of these genes but not their initial vectors. The reverse of this process, that is, transfer of the β-lactamase gene from *H. influenzae* to *E. coli* and *P. aeruginosa* without concomitant retention of transfer ability, is shown in this paper.

The TEM β-lactamase confers low levels of resistance to ampicillin in *H. influenzae* relative to other bacteria. Moreover, crypticity values for β-lactam antibiotics are extremely low in this organism (18; this paper). It is known in gram-negative bacteria that resistance to these antibiotics depends not only on the possession of a β-lactamase, but also on the penetration barrier afforded by the outer membrane (22, 24). The virtual absence of such a barrier in *H. influenzae* would reduce the effectiveness of the TEM β-lactamase in protecting the organism. Hence the relatively long delay in acquisition of ampicillin resistance could be due both to the likelihood of successful transfer after contact with a resistant enteric organism and to the poor selective advantage conferred by the enzyme in *Haemophilus*.

ACKNOWLEDGMENTS

We are grateful to P. M. Bennett for assistance with electron microscopy and to P. Attfield for technical assistance.

Part of this work was supported by a grant to M. H. Richmond from the Medical Research Council for Molecular and Epidemiological Studies on R-Factors and Other Plasmids.

LITERATURE CITED

1. **Anderson, E. S.** 1965. A rapid screening test for transfer factors in drug sensitive *Enterobacteriaceae*. Nature (London) **208**:1016–1017.
2. **Barth, P. T., N. Datta, R. W. Hedges, and N. J. Grinter.** 1976. Transposition of a deoxyribonucleic acid sequence encoding trimethoprim and streptomycin resistances from R483 to other replicons. J. Bacteriol. **125**:800–810.
3. **Bennett, P. M., and M. H. Richmond.** 1976. Translocation of a discrete piece of deoxyribonucleic acid carrying an *amp* gene between replicons in *Escherichia coli*. J. Bacteriol. **126**:1–6.
4. **Clowes, R. C.** 1972. Molecular structure of bacterial plasmids. Bacteriol. Rev. **36**:361–505.
5. **Curtis, N. A. C., and M. H. Richmond.** 1974. Effect of R-factor mediated genes on some surface properties of *Escherichia coli*. Antimicrob. Agents Chemother. **6**:666–671.
6. **Dang Van, A., F. Goldstein, J. F. Acar, and D. H. Bouanchaud.** 1976. A transferable kanamycin resistance plasmid isolated from *Haemophilus influenzae*. Ann. Inst. Pasteur (Paris) **126A**:397–399.
7. **De Graaff, J., L. P. Elwell, and S. Falkow. 1976.** Molecular nature of two beta-lactamase-specifying plasmids isolated from *Haemophilus influenzae* type b. J. Bacteriol. **126**:439–446.
8. **Elwell, L. P., J. De Graaff, D. Seibert, and S. Falkow.** 1975. Plasmid-linked ampicillin resistance in *Haemophilus influenzae* type b. Infect. Immun. **12**:404–410.
9. **Farrar, W. E., and N. M. O'Dell.** 1974. Beta-lactamase activity in ampicillin-resistant *Haemophilus influenzae*. Antimicrob. Agents Chemother. **6**:625–629.
10. **Grinsted, J., J. R. Saunders, L. C. Ingram, R. B. Sykes, and M. H. Richmond.** 1972. Properties of an R-factor which originated in *Pseudomonas aeruginosa* 1822. J. Bacteriol. **110**:529–537.
11. **Hedges, R. W., and A. Jacob.** 1974. Transposition of ampicillin-resistance from RP4 to other replicons. Mol. Gen. Genet. **132**:31–40.
12. **Heffron, F., C. Rubens, and S. Falkow.** 1975. Translocation of a plasmid DNA sequence which mediates ampicillin resistance: molecular nature and specificity of insertion. Proc. Natl. Acad. Sci. U.S.A. **72**:3623–3627.
13. **Heffron, F., R. Sublett, R. W. Hedges, A. Jacob, and S. Falkow.** 1975. Origin of the TEM beta-lactamase gene found on plasmids. J. Bacteriol. **122**:250–256.
14. **Holloway, B. W.** 1975. Genetic organisation of Pseudomonas, p. 133–161. *In* P. H. Clarke and M. H. Richmond (ed.), Genetics and biochemistry of Pseudomonas. Wiley, London.
15. **Khan, W., S. Ross, W. Rodriguez, G. Controni, and A. K. Saz.** 1974. *Haemophilus influenzae* type b resistant to ampicillin. J. Am. Med. Assoc. **229**:298–301.
16. **Kleckner, N., R. K. Chan, B. K. Tye, and D. Botstein.** 1975. Mutagenesis by insertion of a drug-resistance element carrying an inverted repetition. J. Mol. Biol. **97**:561–575.
17. **Lang, D.** 1970. Molecular weights of coliphages and coliphage DNA. III. Contour length and molecular weight of DNA from bacteriophages T4, T5 and T7, and from bovine papilloma virus. J. Mol. Biol. **54**:557–565.
18. **Medeiros, A. A., and T. F. O'Brien.** 1975. Ampicillin resistant *Haemophilus influenzae* type b possessing a TEM type beta-lactamase but little permeability barrier to ampicillin. Lancet **i**:716–718.
19. **Novick, R. P.** 1952. Staphylococcal penicillinase and the new penicillins. Biochem. J. **83**:229–235.
20. **Perret, C. J.** 1954. Iodometric assay of penicillinase. Nature (London) **174**:1012–1013.
21. **Richmond, M. H., and R. B. Sykes.** 1972. The chromosomal integration of a β-lactamase gene derived from the P-type R-factor RP1 in *Escherichia coli*. Genet. Res. **20**:231–237.
22. **Richmond, M. H., and R. B. Sykes.** 1973. The β-lactamases of gram-negative bacteria and their possible physiological role. Adv. Microb. Physiol. **9**:31–85.
23. **Robinson, M. K., P. M. Bennett, and M. H. Richmond.** 1977. Inhibition of TnA translocation by TnA. J. Bacteriol. **129**:407–414.
24. **Sykes, R. B., and M. Matthew.** 1976. The β-lactamases of gram-negative bacteria and their role in resistance to β-lactam antibiotics. J. Antimicrob. Chemother. **2**:115–157.
25. **Sykes, R. B., M. Matthew, and C. H. O'Callaghan.** 1975. R-factor mediated β-lactamase production by strains of *Haemophilus influenzae*. J. Med. Microbiol. **8**:437–441.
26. **Thorne, G. M., and W. E. Farrar.** 1975. Transfer of ampicillin resistance between strains of *H. influenzae* type b. J. Infect. Dis. **132**:276–281.
27. **Vega, R., H. L. Sadoff, and M. H. Patterson.** 1976. Mechanisms of ampicillin resistance in *Haemophilus influenzae* type b. Antimicrob. Agents Chemother. **9**:164–168.

Antimicrobial Agents and Chemotherapy, Feb. 1977, p. 345–358
Vol. 11, No. 2

Comparison of Colicins B-K260 and D-CA23: Purification and Characterization of the Colicins and Examination of Colicin Immunity in the Producing Strains

ANTHONY P. PUGSLEY* and PETER REEVES

Department of Microbiology and Immunology, The University of Adelaide, Adelaide 5000, South Australia

Received for publication 23 July 1976

Colicins B-K260 and D-CA23 were purified by ammonium sulfate precipitation, gel filtration, and ion-exchange chromatography and were compared with respect to a number of physical and chemical properties. Both colicins were shown to be proteins and were found to have similar molecular weights, isoelectric points and amino acid compositions. The two colicins also have substantial antigenic similarities but are distinguished by the presence of non-cross-reacting antigens and by differences in stability and in sensitivity to heat and reducing conditions. In addition, strains of *Escherichia coli* K-12 producing colicins B-K260 and D-CA23 are not cross-immune. The similarities noted between the two colicins are compatible with their use of a common cell surface receptor while having different modes of action.

Bacteriocins are a diverse group of antibiotic-like proteins produced by many species of bacteria. Colicins are bacteriocins produced by *Escherichia coli* and by related species of bacteria. The production of colicins is controlled by plasmids (col factors; 34), and their activity is limited to *E. coli* and to related organisms (for reviews, see references 13, 16, 34).

Colicins range in size from 18,000 (colicin M-K260; 2) to 92,000 (colicin D-CA23; daltons 42). Several colicins have been purified and characterized, and comparisons of their physical and chemical properties demonstrate the structural diversity of this group of bacteriocins (13, 16, 19). This diversity also extends to the mode of action of colicins on sensitive cells (13). Various studies have shown that colicins with similar modes of action do not necessarily have similar structures, and vice versa (19, 42).

The original classification of the colicins into the various types was based on activity spectra against bacterial isolates and against colicin-resistant mutants of *E. coli* (6, 7). Further differentiation of closely related colicins was based on cross-immunity between the producing strains; bacteria producing a colicin are generally immune (resistant) to that colicin but not to unrelated colicins (9). Recent evidence from our laboratory has indicated that the original identification of colicins B and D as different colicin types may have been in error. We have been unable to isolate mutants of *E. coli* K-12 that are resistant to only one of the two colicin types (3), and both colicins use the same cell surface receptor and are strongly inhibited by the siderophore (iron chelator) enterochelin (31, 32). The colicin B- and D-producing strains originally used by Fredericq in the classification of these colicins (7) have subsequently been shown to produce other colicins in addition to B or D (10, 43). However, strains of *E. coli* that produce only colicins B or D are now available (3, 42), and it is thus possible to compare the two colicins in greater detail. In this paper we compare the physical and chemical properties of purified colicin B-K260 with those of purified colicin D-CA23 and with those determined for the latter colicin by Timmis (42). We find that colicins B-K260 and D-CA23 are indeed very similar but are distinguished from each other by differences in stability and antigenicity. In addition, strains producing colicins B-K260 and D-CA23 are not cross-immune.

MATERIALS AND METHODS

Bacterial strains. Strains of *E. coli* K-12 and colicinogenic bacteria carrying col B or col D factors are listed in Table 1. Other colicinogenic bacteria were as described previously (4).

Culture media. Nutrient broth, nutrient agar, soft nutrient agar, and minimal salts media were as described previously (33).

Transfer of col factors. Transfers of col factors to strain P1684 were performed in nutrient broth buffered to pH 7.8 with Na_2HPO_4 and containing 5 mg of trypsin per ml. Donor and recipient cells in the logarithmic phase of growth were mixed in the ratio 1:5 (final concentration, approximately 10^8 cells/ml) and incubated for 1 to 3 h at 37°C. The

TABLE 1. *Strains of E. coli K-12 and colicinogenic bacteria used in this study*

Strain	Relevant genetic markers	Colicin resistance	Original source of plasmid	Colicins produced[a]	Source/reference
AB1133	*thr leu pro his argE str supE*	–[b]	–	–	A. L. Taylor
P1552	as AB1133, but *aroE spc*	–	–	–	(33)
P1687	as AB1133, but *bfe cir*	A, E1, E2, E3, 1a, S1, V	–	–	This laboratory
P1693	as AB1133, but *tonA cir*	1a, 1b, M, S1, V	–	–	This laboratory
P1684	*trp spc*	–	–	–	Derivatives of JC6256
JC6256 (R64-11)	*trp*	–	–	–	N. Willets
JC6256 (R136 fi⁻)	*trp*	–	–	–	N. Willets
AG097	–	–	K260	B	B. Stocker
T20	–	–	K260	B	This paper
K89	–	–	K89	B, M	P. Fredericq
CA18	–	–	CA18	B, M	P. Fredericq
K252	–	–	K252	B, I, V	P. Fredericq
AG084	–	–	K77	B, M	B. Stocker
K44	–	–	K44	B, I, V	P. Fredericq
UB1082	–	–	CA23	D	K. Timmis (42)
II	–	–	II	D, E1, I, Q	J. Smarda (40)

[a] According to records in this laboratory.
[b] –, No data available.

mixtures were then diluted in nutrient broth and plated onto nutrient agar containing 100 μg of spectinomycin per ml for counter-selection. In the case of self-transferring col factors, selection for col⁺ recipients was by immunity to a crude colicin preparation (2 to 5 arbitrary units/ml of agar) obtained from the donor strain (see below). In the case of R136 fi⁻ or R64-mediated transfer of col factors, donor cells were first mated with bacteria (JC6256) carrying the appropriate R factor (Table 1). Mating mixtures were diluted in glucose minimal salts medium and plated onto glucose minimal agar; counter-selection was for ability to grow in the absence of tryptophan and selection for R⁺ recipients was with 20 μg of tetracycline per ml. Col and R factors were then cotransferred to strain P1684 as above, with selection for R⁺ recipients with or without selection for colicin immunity. All recipient colonies were screened for colicin production, spectinomycin resistance, and tryptophan requirement, and recipients carrying representatives of each col plasmid type were selected for further study.

Isolation of a strain producing increased amounts of colicin B-K260. Strain AG097 was treated with *N*-methyl-*N'*-nitro-*N*-nitrosoguanidine (24), plated directly onto nutrient agar, and incubated for 24 h at 37°C. Single colonies were transferred to two sets of fresh nutrient agar plates and incubated for 24 h at 37°C. Growth on one set of plates was then killed with chloroform vapor, overlayed with 10^6 cells of strain P1552 in 3 ml of soft agar, and reincubated. Isolates showing substantially increased colicin production (increased size of killing zone) were streaked for purity, and single colonies were retested for colicin production. One isolate, named T20, was retained.

Preparation of colicins. The preparation and purification of colicins B-K260 and D-CA23 are described in the text. Partially purified colicins H-CA58, E3-CA38, Ib-P9, K-K235, M-K260, and S1-P1 were as used previously (31). Other colicins used in this study were prepared by growing the producing strains in well-aerated nutrient broth cultures to an optical density (at 660 nm) of 0.60. Mitomycin C (0.4 μg/ml, Sigma) was then added, and incubation was continued for a further 240 min or less if cell lysis occurred. Cells and cell debris were removed from the culture supernatant (crude colicin) by centrifugation (10 min at 4,600 × *g*) and membrane filtration (0.45-μm mean filter pore diameter).

Assay of colicins and detection of colicin activity in polyacrylamide gels. Colicins were assayed by the arbitrary units method as previously described (35), using doubling dilutions of the colicin preparation. Indicator strains P1687 and P1693 were used to detect only colicins B and D of those produced by multicolicinogenic bacteria (see Table 1). Colicins B-K260 and D-CA23 were assayed throughout using strain P1552 as indicator. Colicin activity in polyacrylamide gels (see below) was detected either by embedding the gel in soft nutrient agar containing 10^6 indicator cells/ml or by slicing the gels and placing each section (0.3 mm) onto the surface of soft nutrient agar containing the indicator cells. Both test systems were incubated at 37°C for 24 h, and the diameters of the inhibition zones obtained by the latter procedure were used to compare the colicin activities recovered from the gels.

Colicin resistance patterns and colicin activity spectra. Plate tests for testing colicin resistance/sensitivity were as described previously (4).

Ion-exchange chromatography and gel filtration. Whatman diethylaminoethyl-cellulose (DE52) was used for all ion-exchange column chromatography. Ion-exchange and gel filtration columns were equilibrated with the appropriate buffer before use. Samples for each gel stage of filtration were concentrated to less than 10% of the column liquid volume (less than 1% for high-resolution gel filtration) by dialysis against Aquacide II (Calbiochem) or by Diaflo membrane filtration (Amicon), both at 4°C, or by freeze-drying and resuspending in a reduced volume of solvent (colicin D-CA23 only). All samples were extensively dialyzed against the appropriate buffer at 4°C before being loaded onto columns. All other procedures for gel filtration and column chromatography were as recommended by the manufacturers of the filtration or chromatography media. Fractions from the columns were collected and examined for colicin activity, for optical density at 280 nm, and, where appropriate, for phosphate molarity measured as conductivity. The phosphate buffer (PB) was Na^+ buffer at pH 7.1.

PAGE. Polyacrylamide gel electrophoresis (PAGE) in the presence of sodium dodecyl sulfate (SDS) was performed using the continuous Maizel gel system (23) with 7.5% acrylamide gels in tubes and with the samples solubilized in the phosphate buffer (Na^+, pH 7.3, 0.1 M) containing 1% SDS and 0.1% β-mercaptoethanol. PAGE in the absence of SDS was performed by the method of MacGreggor et al. (22). Gels were fixed, stained, and examined as described previously (31).

Isoelectric focusing. Isoelectric focusing was carried out in acrylamide disc gels containing ampholytes (LKB: wide range, pH 3 to 10). The gels contained 4.8% acrylamide (Eastman), 0.2% bisacrylamide (Eastman), 0.085% *N,N,N',N'*-tetramethylethyldiamine, 2% ampholytes, and 0.034% ammonium persulfate (added as a 2% solution) in distilled water. The mixture was degassed before the addition of the persulfate. Gels were run in the electrolyte bath normally used for PAGE, with 0.01 M phosphoric acid and 0.02 M NaOH as acidic and basic electrolyte solutions, respectively. Excess persulfate was discharged from the gels by prerunning for 30 min at 1 mA/gel. Protein (5 to 50 μg/gel in 10% sucrose) was then loaded, and the gels were run for 20 h at 4°C. An initial voltage of 50 V was applied (1 mA/gel), rising to 400 V for the final 4 h to complete the focusing. Gels were fixed, stained, and scanned in the normal way (31), with extensive dialysis against distilled water between the fixing and staining stages to remove the ampholytes. The pH gradient along the gels was determined by slicing unfixed gels, resuspending the sections in 1 ml of distilled deionized water for 1 h at 20°C, and measuring the pH.

Preparation and assay of antisera. Antisera were prepared in rabbits using multisite intramuscular vaccination with 1 mg of purified colicin B-K260 or D-CA23 in complete Freund adjuvant. The rabbits were vaccinated at 0 and 50 days and bled at 70 days. Colicin neutralization titers of the antisera were determined by mixing 0.1 ml of doubling dilutions of the antisera with an equal volume of nutrient broth containing 1 arbitrary unit of the appropriate colicin per ml. The mixture was incubated for 30 min at 37°C and assayed for residual colicin as above. Neutralization titers were determined from the last dilution of antiserum giving complete inactivation of the colicin.

Immunochemical analyses. Immunodiffusion and immunoelectrophoresis experiments were performed using 1% agarose (Calbiochem) in veronal buffer (pH 8.6; 41) unless otherwise stated. Immunodiffusion tests were performed as described by Ouchterlony and Nilsson (27). Rocket immunoelectrophoresis and cross-immunoelectrophoresis were as described by Weeke (46, 47). Agarose gels were then rinsed extensively in saline and then distilled water and fixed and stained with Coomassie blue as for acrylamide gels (31). PAGE and isoelectric focusing gels loaded with 5 to 50 μg of protein and run as described above were sometimes used in place of the normal agarose first dimension in cross-immunoelectrophoresis by slicing the acrylamide gels longitudinally, dialyzing against veronal buffer for 30 min, and embedding one-half of the acrylamide gel at the edge of the antibody-containing agarose gel. Antisera were used at final concentrations of 5 $\mu l/cm^2$ of agarose gel in each case.

An Ouchterlony-type immunodiffusion test was linked to a colicin activity test in a procedure similar to that described by Ozaki et al. (28). The assay was performed in soft nutrient agar containing 100 μg of streptomycin and 10^6 cells of strain P1552 per ml. Antibody (100 μl) and antigens (100 μg) were incubated at 4°C until clear precipitin lines formed (usually 3 days) and then at 37°C for 8 h to permit growth of the indicator cells.

Chemical analyses. Protein was determined by the method of Schacterle and Pollack (38) using bovine serum albumin as standard. Hexoses were determined by the phenol sulfuric acid method (18) using glucose as standard, and 2-keto-3-deoxyoctonic acid was determined by the method of Warandehar and Shaw (45). Amino acid analyses were performed in a Beckman model 120C amino acid analyzer modified with Chromatronix type LC9MA columns and using Durrum DC1A resin and Durrum pico buffer system III. Samples were hydrolyzed under nitrogen at 110°C for 24 h in 1 ml of 6 N HCl containing 0.1% phenol.

RESULTS

Purification of colicin D-CA23. The method used to purify colicin D-CA23 was essentially that of Timmis (42). Colicin D was extracted from sonicated cells of strain UB1082 as described previously (31; 10-liter nutrient broth culture induced with 0.4 μg of mitomycin C per ml) and purified by sequential steps of ammonium sulfate precipitation (31), gel filtration on Sephadex G200, exchange chromatography on Whatman DE52 cellulose, gel filtration on

Sephadex G200, exchange chromatography on Whatman DE52 cellulose, and high-resolution gel filtration on Sephadex G100. The final four stages of purification are illustrated in Fig. 1. The active material eluted from the Sephadex G100 column (stage 7) was free of detectable hexose and 2-keto-3-deoxyoctonic acid. This material was dialyzed extensively against distilled water at 4°C and lyophilized, and is referred to throughout as purified colicin D-CA23.

Purification of colicin B-K260. An attempt was made to purify colicin B-K260 from strain AG097 using the procedure described above for colicin D-CA23. This attempt failed for several reasons: strain AG097 produced considerably less colicin than strain UB1082, and yields were therefore very low; sedimentation of the crude colicin occurred on standing; and considerable loss of activity occurred during the final stages of purification and during slow freezing and thawing. The latter problems were overcome to some extent by using higher molarity PB to solubilize the colicin and by flash freezing the colicin in ethanol-dry ice mixtures at −20°C. To overcome the problem of low yields of colicin B-K260, we treated a suspension of strain AG097 with *N*-methyl-*N'*-nitro-*N*-nitrosoguanidine (Materials and Methods) and isolated a derivative (T20) that produced increased amounts of colicin in plate tests. Strain T20 was shown to produce only colicin B by its activity spectrum against 18 different classes of colicin-resistant mutants (see references 3, 4).

Strains T20, AG097, and UB1082 were examined for colicin production in nutrient broth after induction with mitomycin C. Twenty-milliliter volumes of broth were inoculated with 2 ml of a standing 16-h broth culture (optical density, 1.0 to 1.2) of each of the three strains and incubated with good aeration at 37°C until the optical density (at 660 nm) reached 0.60. Mitomycin C was then added at final concentrations of 0.2 and 0.4 μg/ml, and incubation was continued for a further 150 min before the cells were harvested by centrifugation. Control cultures (no mitomycin C) were also harvested at this time. The cells were resuspended in 100 mM PB and sonicated for 10 min at 4°C, and cell debris was removed by centrifugation at 46,000 × *g* for 60 min at 4°C. The culture supernatants and cell sonicates were then assayed for colicin activity using strain P1552 on nutrient agar containing 100 μg of streptomycin per ml (Table 2). The production of both colicins B and D was shown to be strongly induced by mitomycin C, as reported previously (12, 42), and strain T20 clearly produced more colicin activity than strain AG097.

For the large-scale production of colicin B-K260, 6 liters of a well-aerated 16-h nutrient broth culture (optical density, 1.1) of strain T20 was used to inoculate 60 liters of nutrient broth in a fermentor. The broth was incubated with good aeration until the optical density (at 660 nm) reached 0.60, at which stage mitomycin C (0.2 μg/ml) was added. Incubation was continued for a further 150 min, and the cells were harvested by centrifugation. The cells (86 g, wet weight) were resuspended in 1 liter of PB (100 mM) at 4°C and disrupted in a French

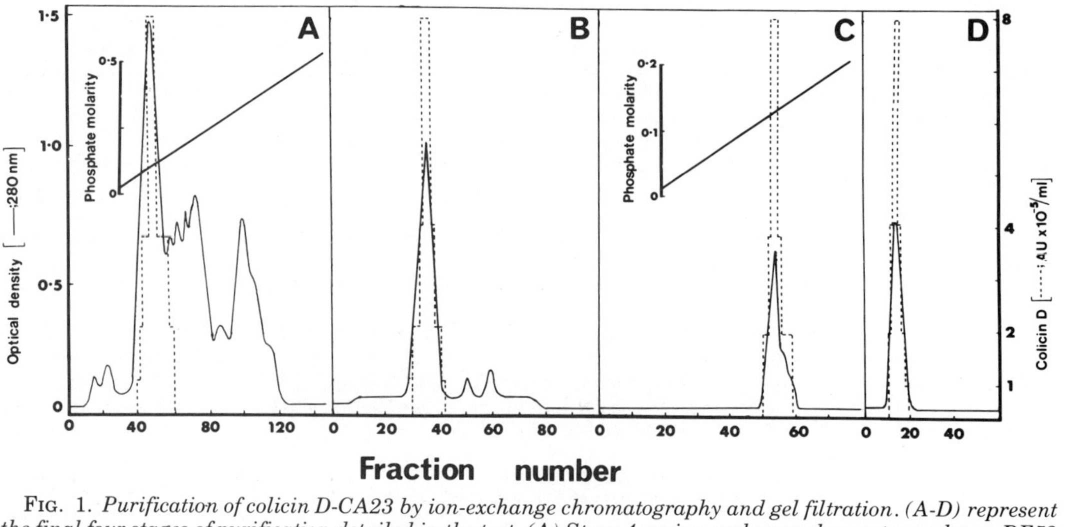

FIG. 1. *Purification of colicin D-CA23 by ion-exchange chromatography and gel filtration. (A-D) represent the final four stages of purification detailed in the text. (A) Stage 4, anion-exchange chromatography on DE52 cellulose; (B) stage 5, gel filtration on Sephadex G200; (C) stage 6, anion-exchange chromatography on DE52 cellulose; (D) stage 7, gel filtration on Sephadex G100.*

pressure cell (Aminco). Cell debris was removed by centrifugation at 46,000 × *g* for 90 min at 4°C. The colicin B-K260 in the supernatant was further purified as detailed in Table 3. Considerable amounts of high- and low-molecular-weight material were removed by gel filtration on Sephadex G200 (stage 3). The final four stages of purification are illustrated in Fig. 2. Samples of the colicin at various stages of purification were assayed for colicin activity and for protein, hexose, and 2-keto-3-deoxyoctonic acid content (Table 4). The colicin eluted from the Sephadex G100 column (stage 7), which was free of detectable hexose and 2-keto-3-deoxyoctonic acid, and was divided into two parts. One part was divided into small aliquots and frozen at −20°C, and the other was dialyzed against distilled water and lyophilized. Both samples are referred to throughout as purified colicin B-K260. Unless otherwise stated, the purified colicin B-K260 frozen in PB, which retained colicin activity, was used in the experiments described in this paper. The final yield of purified colicin B-K260 obtained by this method from strain 720 was 36-fold greater than that obtained from cells of strain AG097 under identical conditions. This indicates that the increased colicin activity obtained from strain T20 was due to increased colicin production and not to altered immunity factor.

Immunochemical analysis of purified colicins B-K260 and D-CA23. Antisera prepared against purified colicins B-K260 and D-CA23 strongly inhibited killing by all colicins of types B and D tested. Each of these colicins was produced by apparently independently isolated strains of bacteria (Table 1), and identical amounts of each colicin (as killing units) were inactivated by the same titers of the antisera (1:1,056 of anticolicin B-K260 and 1:2,122 of anticolicin D-CA23). Neither of the two antisera had any effect on killing by colicins H-CA58, K-K235, M-K260, Ib-P9, S1-P1, and E3-CA38, and normal rabbit serum had no effect on killing by any of the colicins tested.

Purified colicins B-K260 and D-CA23 were examined by the Ouchterlony immunodiffusion technique using homologous and heterologous antisera. Both colicins produced strong single precipitin lines against homologous and heter-

TABLE 2. *Titration of colicins produced by strains AG097, T20, and UB1082 after induction with mitomycin C*

Strain	Colicin produced	Mitomycin C (μg/ml)	Colicin in culture supernatant (AU/ml)[a]	Colicin in cell sonicate (AU/mg of protein)
AG097	B-K260		<1	<1
		0.2	1	1.15×10^2
		0.4	1	1.35×10^2
T20	B-K260		4	23.5
		0.2	1.28×10^3	1.62×10^4
		0.4	1.28×10^3	2.05×10^4
UB1082	D-CA23		4	25.6
		0.2	2×10^3	4.63×10^3
		0.4	1.6×10^4	2.21×10^4

[a] AU, Arbitrary unit.

TABLE 3. *Purification scheme for colicin B-K260*

Stage of purification	Purification procedure
1	Precipitation of cell extract with 30 to 50% saturated $(NH_4)_2SO_4$ at 4°C; precipitate redissolved in 60 ml of 50 mM PB
2	Low-resolution gel filtration on Bio-Gel P100 (50 to 100 mesh, 70 by 2.5 cm) in 50 mM PB at 4°C
3	Divided into two lots for low-resolution gel filtration on Sephadex G200 (70 by 2.5 cm) in 50 mM PB at 4°C
4 (Fig. 2A)	Anion-exchange chromatography on Whatman DE52 cellulose (55 by 2.5 cm); colicin eluted with steps of 50 mM PB (600 ml), 150 mM PB (600 ml), and 500 mM PB (600 ml) at 20°C; active material eluted from this column was concentrated before proceeding to stage 5
5 (Fig. 2B)	Anion-exchange chromatography on Whatman DE52 cellulose (50 by 2.5 cm); colicin eluted with 300 ml of 50 mM PB followed by 1,000-ml linear gradient of 50 to 200 mM PB at 20°C
6 (Fig. 2C)	High-resolution gel filtration on Sephadex G200 (80 by 2.5 cm) in 50 mM PB at 4°C
7 (Fig. 2D)	High-resolution gel filtration on Sephadex G100 (100 by 2.5 cm) in 50 mM PB at 4°C

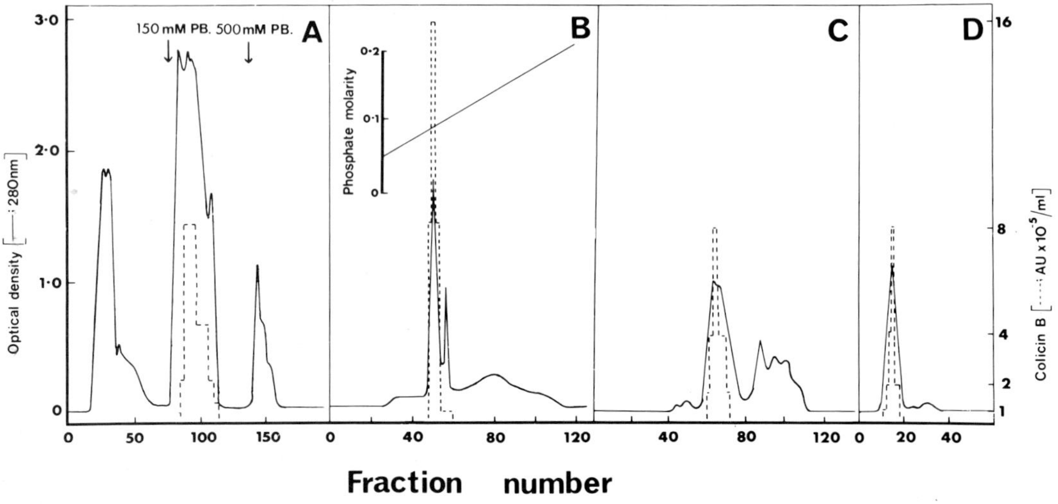

FIG. 2. *Purification of colicin B-K260 by ion-exchange chromatography and gel filtration. (A-D) represent the final four stages of purification detailed in Table 3. (A) Stage 4, anion-exchange chromatography on DE52 cellulose; (B) stage 5, anion-exchange chromatography on DE52 cellulose; (C) stage 6, gel filtration on Sephadex G200; (D) stage 7, gel filtration on Sephadex G100.*

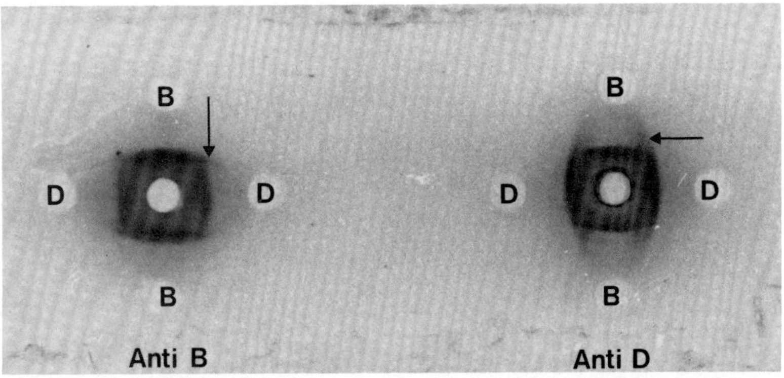

FIG. 3. *Examination of purified colicins B-K260 (B) and D-CA23 (D) by the Ouchterlony immunodiffusion test against homologous and heterologous antisera (anti-B and anti-D). The antibody (10 μl) and antigens (10 μg) were allowed to diffuse for 24 h at 20°C before fixing and staining. Note particularly the spurring reactions present only in reactions with homologous antisera (indicated by arrows).*

TABLE 4. *Colicin activity and chemical analysis of colicin B-K260 at different stages of purification*

	Stage of purification	% Recovery of colicin activity	Sp act (AU/mg of protein)	Protein (mg)	Hexose (μg)	KDO (μg)[a]
	Crude colicin	100	2.8×10^4	5,856	4.9×10^4	2.5×10^3
1	$(NH_4)_2SO_4$ precipitate	78	3.6×10^4	3,325	4.7×10^3	603
2	Bio-Gel P100	56	5.1×10^4	2,916	583	599
3	Sephadex G200	48	8.4×10^4	874	37	0
4	DE52 cellulose	36	2.1×10^5	262	0	0
5	DE52 cellulose	23	5.9×10^5	61	0	0
6	Sephadex G200	17	7.2×10^5	36	0	0
7	Sephadex G100	7.5	7.8×10^5	12	0[b]	0

[a] KDO, 2-Keto-3-deoxyoctonic acid.

[b] No detectable hexose in 1 mg of material.

ologous antisera, with reactions of antigenic identity between the two colicins indicated by merging of the precipitin lines (Fig. 3). Spurring of the precipitin lines (Fig. 3) indicates the presence on both colicin molecules of non-cross-reacting determinants. In addition, we occasionally noted the appearance of a second antigenic species, detected as a very faint precipitin line outside the major line, in samples of the purified colicin B-K260 that had been lyophilized. This second precipitin line was formed only in reactions with homologous antiserum and was only detected in unstained preparations. We suggest that this antigen is a non-cross-reacting component, which is split from the colicin B-K260 molecule in distilled water or by lyophilization (colicin B-K260 is inactivated by dialysis against distilled water).

To confirm that the major precipitin lines formed in the Ouchterlony test resulted from the inactivation of colicin by antiserum and were not due to the presence of contaminating material, we coupled the Ouchterlony test to a colicin activity test (Materials and Methods). The precipitin lines marked the boundary of colicin activity in each case (Fig. 4A). Purified colicin B-K260, which had been partially inactivated by dialysis against distilled water, was used to demonstrate that the spurring of the colicin D-CA23 precipitin line noted above was due to precipitation (and inactivation) of the colicin and not to the presence of contaminating antigens (Fig. 4B). The distortion of the colicin D-CA23 killing zone shown in Fig. 4B is due to competition between colicins B-K260 and D-CA23 for common receptor sites on the indicator cells (31).

Further examination of the purified colicins B-K260 and D-CA23 by rocket immunoelectrophoresis confirmed the presence of strong cross-reactions between the colicins and again indicated the presence of a colicin-specific antigen in the lyophilized colicin B-K260, which was identified on a second precipitin line in Fig. 5 (indicated by arrow). Similar reactions were also indicated by cross-immunoelectrophoresis, in which agarose gels were used for the first electrophoretic dimension (data not shown). Further resolution of the antigenic components of the purified colicins was obtained by using PAGE or isoelectric focusing for the first electrophoretic dimension in the cross-immunoelectrophoreses (Fig. 6 and 7). Figure 8 shows a typical result obtained by these procedures. Both colicins were resolved into three components by these procedures, but only one of these components in each case had colicin activity (Fig. 6 and 7). In the case of purified colicin D-CA23, one or both of the remaining components may be inactive colicin with electrophoretic mobilities (Fig. 6) and isoelectric points (Fig. 7) different from those of the active colicin. In the case of the purified colicin B-K260, however, one or both of the inactive components may be breakdown products derived from the active colicin, since less than 10% of the colicin B-

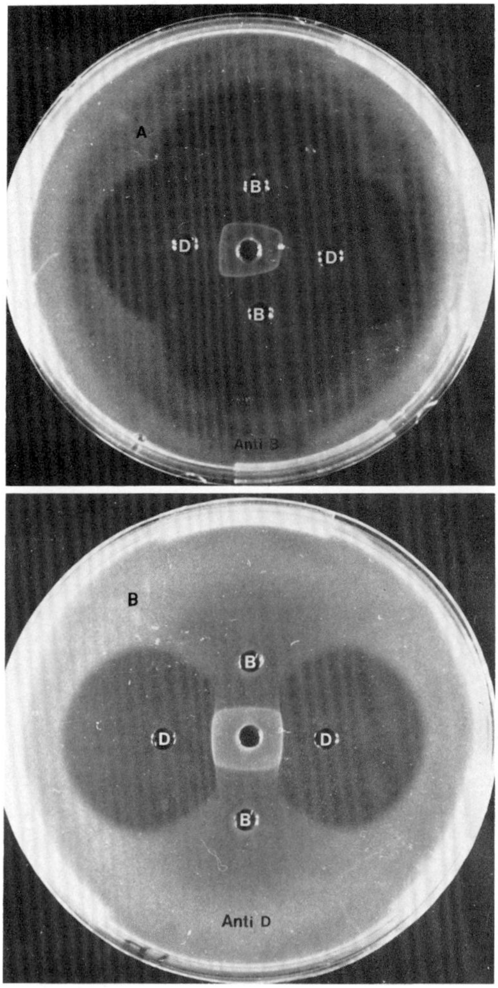

FIG. 4. *Examination of purified colicins B-K260 and D-CA23 by a coupled colicin activity-Ouchterlony immunodiffusion test. (A) shows the reactions between the two colicins (B and D) and antiserum prepared against purified colicin B-K260 (anti-B). An identical pattern was obtained with antiserum against the purified colicin D-CA23. (B) shows a similar reaction between active colicin D-CA23 (D), lyophilized (partially inactivated) colicin B-K260 (B'), and antiserum against purified colicin D-CA23 (anti-D, 50 µl). The clear zone in each case indicates the area of colicin killing of the indicator strain incorporated into the agar.*

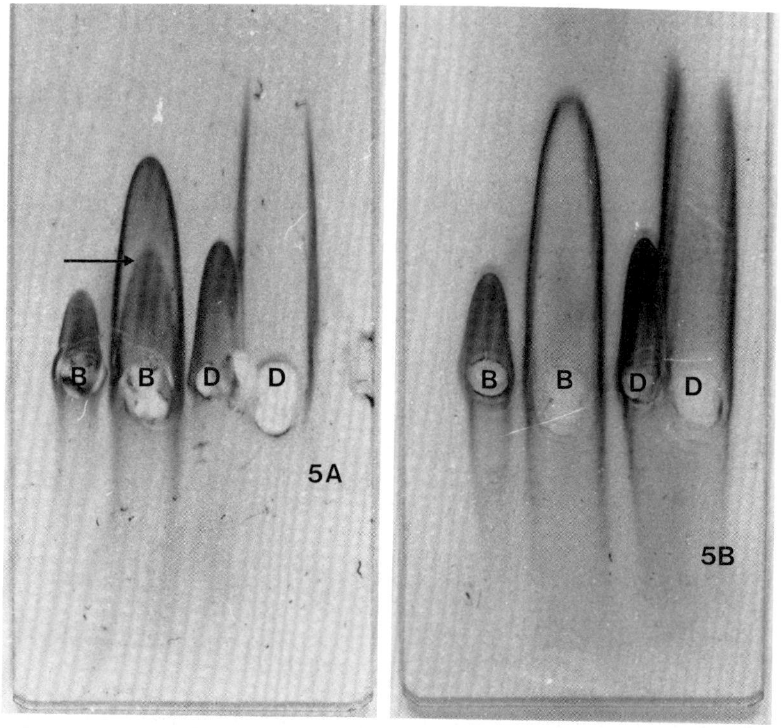

FIG. 5. *Examinaton of purified lyophilized colicins B-K260 (B) and D-CA23 (D) by rocket immunoelectrophoresis against homologous and heterologous antisera. The antigen wells contained 2.5 μg (left) and 15 μg (right) of the appropriate colicins, and the gels were run for 20 h at 80 V/gel slab. (A) shows the reactions between the two colicins and antiserum against purified colicin B-K260. (B) shows the reaction between the two colicins and antiserum against purified colicin D-CA23.*

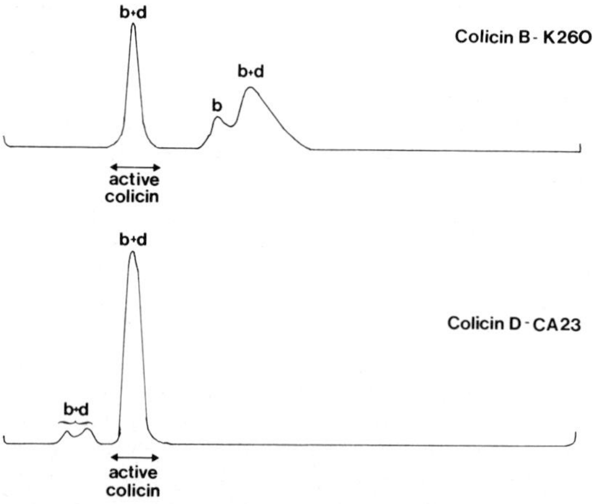

FIG. 6. *Densitometry scans of purified colicins B-K260 and D-CA23 examined by PAGE in the absence of detergent. The figure also shows the location of colicin activity in the gels and identifies the protein peaks that gave precipitin lines with antisera prepared against the purified colicin B-K260 (b) or D-CA23 (d) when the gels were examined by the cross-immunoelectrophoretic technique. The direction of electrophoresis was from left to right.*

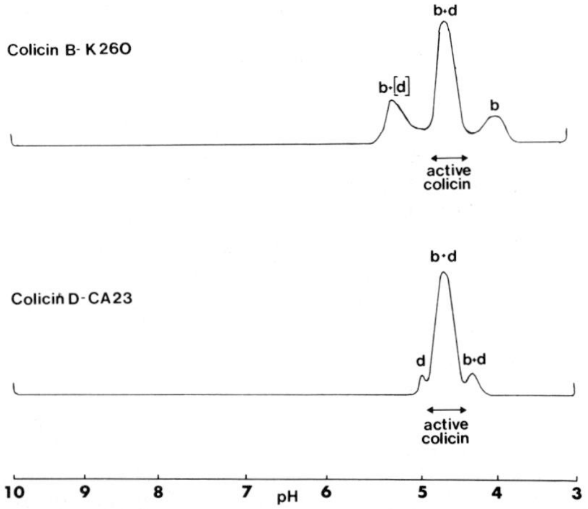

FIG. 7. *Densitometry scans of purified colicins B-K260 and D-CA23 examined by isoelectric focusing in polyacrylamide-ampholyte gels. The figure also shows the location of colicin activity in the gels and identifies the protein peaks that gave precipitin lines with antisera prepared against the purified colicin B-K260 (b) or D-CA23 (d). The scale shows the pH gradient along the length of the gel.*

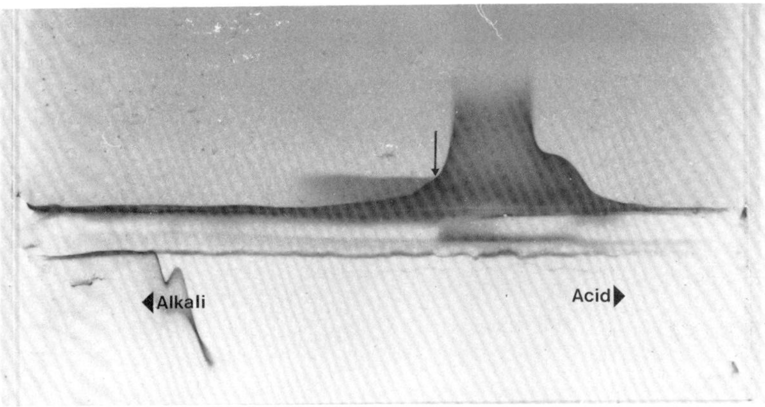

FIG. 8. *Examination of purified colicin D-CA23 by a coupled isoelectric focusing–cross-immunoelectrophoresis technique using homologous antiserum. The acrylamide-ampholyte gel was loaded with 50 μg of protein and subjected to electrophoresis as described in Materials and Methods (first dimension). The second dimension of electrophoresis was at 80 V for 18 h at 20°C. The alkaline end of the acrylamide-ampholyte gel was removed for convenience.*

K260 activity was recovered from the gels compared with the recovery of colicin D-CA23 under the same conditions. Isoelectric focusing revealed the presence of a serologically non-cross-reacting component in both purified colicins (Fig. 7). That present in the colicin B-K260 may be the same component identified in the Ouchterlony test as the additional precipitin line obtained with lyophilized colicin, but the colicin D-CA23 component may be a contaminating protein not detected previously (Fig. 8).

Physical and chemical analysis of purified colicins B-K260 and D-CA23. Purified colicins B-K260 and D-CA23 were compared with respect to a number of physical and chemical properties (Table 5). Although the two colicins had several features in common, there were some notable differences relating to the stability of colicin activity. We have already noted that colicin B-K260 was rapidly inactivated by dialysis against distilled water and by repeated slow freezing and thawing. The results in Table 5 also show that this colicin is unstable at room temperature and is more sensitive than colicin D-CA23 to heat and to the detergent SDS, particularly in the presence of the reducing agent β-mercaptoethanol. The instability of purified colicin B-K260 at room temperature can be reduced to a certain extent by the addition of bovine serum albumin (protein ratio, 1:50), as has been reported previously for colicin E2 (25).

Examination of the purified colicin B-K260 by PAGE in the presence of SDS revealed the presence of two components (labeled I and II in Fig. 8 and 9) whose combined molecular weights were equal to the molecular weight of active colicin B-K260, as determined by gel filtration on Sephadex G200 (Fig. 10). This suggests that treatment with SDS and β-mercaptoethanol results in the breakdown of colicin B-K260 into two components, with a resulting loss of colicin activity. It may be that these two components are identical to the inactive proteins found by PAGE in the absence of SDS and by isoelectric focusing (Fig. 6 and 7). We do not consider that the difference in molecular weights of colicins B-K260 and D-CA23 as demonstrated by gel filtration (Fig. 10, 11) is necessarily significant, as it is probably within experimental error.

Amino acid analyses of purified colicins B-K260 and D-CA23. Table 6 shows the results of amino acid analyses of purified colicins B-K260 and D-CA23. The amino acid composition determined for colicin D-CA23 is very similar to that determined for colicin B-K260 and also to that obtained by Timmis (42) for his preparation of purified colicin D-CA23. However, there is one notable difference between our results and those obtained by Timmis, namely, the absence of cysteine in either of our purified colicins. Control checks with added cysteine on the sensitivity of our amino acid analysis procedure demonstrated that the levels of half-cysteine found by Timmis in his preparation of purified colicin D-CA23 would have been detected by our technique.

Activity spectra of colicins B-K260 and D-CA23. Strains T20 and UB1082 were used to screen a large number of different gram-negative bacterial isolates for sensitivity to the two colicins B-K260 and D-CA23. The two colicinogenic strains produced similar inhibition zones in the agar plate test. In no case did we detect

TABLE 5. *Comparison of chemical and physical properties of purified colicins B-K260 and D-CA23*

Property	Determination for:	
	B-K260	D-CA23
Nonprotein components[a]	Nil	Nil
Sensitivity to proteases[b] – half-life (min) at 37°C in:		
100 μg of Pronase per ml	<1	<1
100 μg of trypsin per ml	5	10
Sensitivity to heat		
Half-life at 56°C (min)	3	35
Half-life at 80°C (min)	<1	3
Half-life at 37°C (days)	8	Stable
Sensitivity to repeated freezing and thawing	Sensitive	Stable
Sensitivity to detergents[c] – relative colicin titer after 30 min at 37°C in:		
0.5% SDS	0.25	1
0.5% Sarkosyl	0.25	0.25
0.5% Nonidet	1	1
0.5% Triton X-100	1	1
0.5% cholic acid	1	1
1% SDS + 0.1% β-mercaptoethanol	0.125	1
Molecular weight		
SDS PAGE[d]	58,000 + 34,500	92,000
Sephadex G200[e]	92,000	96,500
Isoelectric point[f]	4.6	4.7
Maximum adsorption wavelength (nm)	279	279

[a] See Table.
[b] Sensitivity to proteases, heat, and detergents was measured at a final concentration of 100 μg of colicin per ml in 50 mM PB.
[c] Sensitivity to detergents compared with control incubated in 50 mM PB.
[d] PAGE in the presence of SDS; see Fig. 8 and 9.
[e] Gel filtration on Sephadex G200; see Fig. 10.
[f] Isoelectric point of the protein band having colicin activity; see Fig. 7.

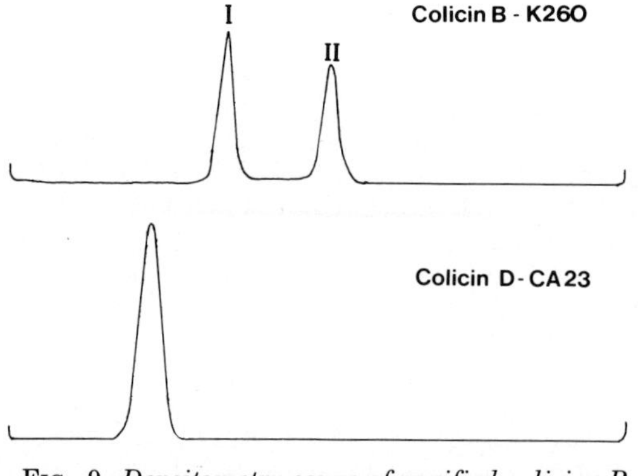

FIG. 9. *Densitometry scans of purified colicins B-K260 and D-CA23 examined by PAGE in the presence of SDS. The direction of electrophoresis was from left to right.*

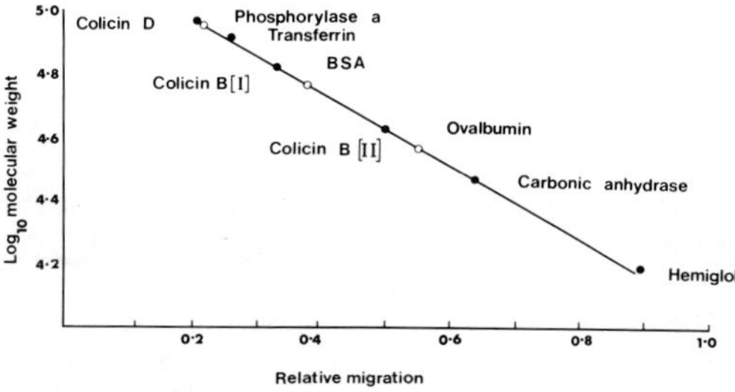

FIG. 10. *Determination of molecular weights of purified colicins B-K260 and D-CA23 by PAGE in the presence of SDS. Gels were loaded with mixtures of 10 μg each of the standard proteins (●) or the two colicins (○) in various combinations, and the migration of each protein relative to the electrophoresis front was determined after electrophoresis. The two components of purified colicin B-K260 revealed by this test are labeled I and II (see Fig. 9). BSA, Bovine serum albumin.*

any difference in the activity of the two colicins. Only *E. coli* (11 of 90 O antigen types tested) and *Shigella sonnei* (6 of 7 strains tested) were found to be sensitive to the two colicins. Strains of *Salmonella* (22, including several deep rough strains), *Serratia* (34), *Enterobacter* (11), *Klebsiella* (9), *Pseudomonas*, (2), *Aeromonas* (13), *Vibrio* (19), *Proteus* (2), *Yersinia* (2), and *Shigella boydii* (4) were resistant to both colicins. Fredericq (7, 8) and Papavasillous (29) have previously reported that both colicins have wider activity spectra against gram-negative

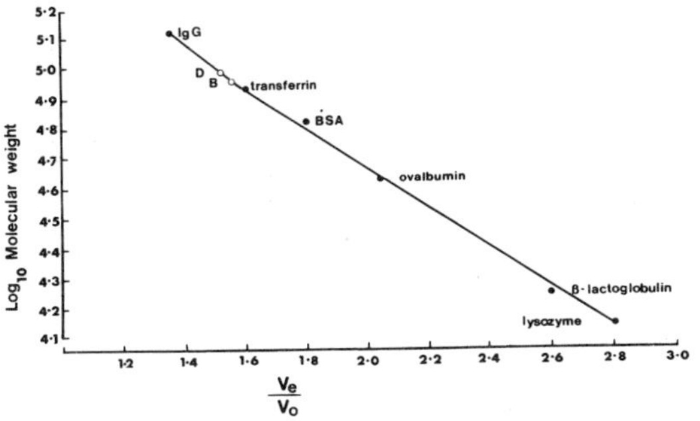

FIG. 11. *Determination of the molecular weights of purified colicins B-K260 and D-CA23 by gel filtration on Sephadex G200. The column (80 by 2.5 cm, equilibrated with 50 mM PB) was loaded with mixtures of 7 to 15 mg each of the various standard proteins (●) and 2 mg of active purified colicin B-K260 or D-CA23 (○) in various combinations. Fractions (1.2 ml) were eluted from the column with 50 mM PB and examined for colicin activity, for protein content (optical density at 280 nm), and, where appropriate, for colicin activity. Blue dextran was included in each run to permit determination of the column void volume (V_o). V_e is the volume at which each component was eluted from the column. BSA, Bovine serum albumin.*

TABLE 6. *Amino acid compositions of purified colicins B-K260 and D-CA23*

Amino acid	% of total amino acid content (M)	
	B-K260	D-CA23
Aspartic acid	12.40	11.10
Threonine	4.04	4.54
Serine	8.62	7.68
Glutamic acid	12.01	10.57
Proline	6.03	6.55
Glycine	9.02	9.37
Alanine	8.48	8.53
Valine	9.15	9.19
Methionine	1.25	2.04
Isoleucine	5.08	5.09
Leucine	8.12	8.47
Tyrosine	2.59	2.20
Phenylalanine	2.24	2.38
Tryptophan[a]	1.82	1.63
Lysine	4.18	5.05
Histidine	0.60	0.96
Arginine	4.23	4.63
Cysteic acid	0	0
Half-cystine	0	0

[a] Derived from tyrosine value and alkaline adsorption spectra (5).

bacteria than found here. This may be due to the production of other colicins by the colicinogenic bacteria in use at that time. In particular, the extremely wide activity spectrum reported for colicin D (7, 8) is probably due to the production by *E. coli* strain CA23 of colicin X, which belongs to a different group of colicins than D-CA23 (3, 42).

Previously, we were unable to isolate mutants of *E. coli* K-12 resistant to only one of the colicins B and D (3). We have now extended this observation with over 300 independently isolated colicin B-K260- or D-CA23-resistant mutants of strains AB1133 and P1552. Mutants were isolated under various conditions of iron deprivation or supplementation and in the presence or absence of enterochelin synthesis to exclude the possibility that interactions between iron uptake systems and colicin killing were preventing the isolation of some mutant classes (31). All mutant classes were of the previously described types (*cbt, cbr, exbC, exbB*, and *tonB;* see references 3, 31), except two representatives of a new phenotypic class of colicin B- and D-resistant mutants (*exbD;* excretion of inhibitor of colicin B, phenotype D). These mutants were isolated as colicin D-CA23-resistant derivatives of strain AB1133 (able to produce enterochelin) and were resistant (tolerant in the triple-layer plate test) to colicins B-K260, D-CA23, G-CA46, H-CA58, Ia-CA53, Ib-P9, S1-P1, and V-CA7 only. The mutants also hypersecreted enterochelin (see reference 33) and became fully sensitive to all colicins upon insertion of the *aroE* marker, which blocks enterochelin biosynthesis (31). We conclude that hypersecretion of enterochelin in this strain blocks killing by colicins B and D in a manner similar to that reported previously for colicin G, H, Ia, Ib, S1, and V action on *exbC* and *exbB* mutants (31).

Cross-immunity between colicin B- and D-producing strains. To study the colicin immunity of *E. coli* carrying col B or col D factors, we transferred col factors of each type to strain P1684. The factors K252, K89, K77, K260, and II were self-transferred at frequencies ranging from 0.01 to 0.1% of potential recipients. Col factor CA18 was not self-transferred at detectable frequencies, but transfer of this col factor could be mediated by R factors R64 and R136 fi^- at rates of 0.6 to 0.9% of potential recipients (70 to 80% cotransfer of col factor and R factors). Col factor CA23 was transferred only in conjunction with the I-like R factor R64 (0.01% of potential recipients, 15% cotransfer of R64 and CA23). Col factor K44 could not be mobilized.

Derivatives of strain P1684 carrying each of the above col factors were tested for colicin production and for immunity to colicins produced by each other and by other strains producing colicins in groups A and B (Davies and Reeves classification; see references 3, 4). Only strains P1684 (K260) and P1684 (CA23) produced single colicins (Table 7); P1684 carrying other col B or col D factors produced colicins of types similar to those produced by the donor strains (Table 1). The tests used to detect colicin production by the P1684 derivatives would, however, only detect colicins secreted in relatively high concentrations. It is evident that colicins D-CA23 and B-K260 do not show cross-immunity and that colicin D-CA23 differs from all of the colicins of type B tested. Thus, although by the usual criterion of resistance colicin D-CA23 would be classed as a colicin of type B, it is nonetheless distinctive in its immunity. This result was also confirmed by titrating the activity of purified colicins B-K260 and D-CA23 against the col^+ derivatives of strain P1684. It is also evident that all the col B factors confer immunity to at least two other colicins in addition to B (Table 7). Indeed, plasmid CA18 conferred immunity to all colicins in group B except D (colicin Q not tested). In addition, we note that P1684 (II) was immune to colicins of type B but not to colicin D-CA23. We conclude that this plasmid codes for the production of colicin B and not colicin D (40). R factors R64 and R136 fi^- did not confer any colicin immunity.

DISCUSSION

The results presented in this paper indicate that considerable purification of colicins B-K260 and D-CA23 was achieved by the techniques used. Although some of the data are compatible with the possible presence of contaminating proteins in our preparations, we believe that a more likely explanation is that some inactive colicin was present in both samples, and in particular in the lyophilized colicin B-K260. In most cases in which cross-immunoelectrophoresis experiments revealed the presence of two antigenic components, of which only one had colicin activity (Fig. 6 and 7), we noted that merging of the precipitin lines occurred (for example, see Fig. 8), indicating antigenic homology between the active colicin and the inactive component. Only in the case of a minor protein present in purified colicin D-CA23 was this merging not demonstrated (Fig. 8), and we concede that this protein could be a contaminant.

The finding that colicins B-K260 and D-CA23 are very similar in many respects is of considerable importance to our understanding of several reported findings with colicins of types B and D. The substantial similarity between the amino acid compositions of the two colicins may account for their similar antigenic determinants; these antigenic determinants presumably have very similar amino acid sequences and tertiary structures. A similar situation may also apply to the receptor-recognition regions of the two colicins, since both use the same cell surface receptor in *E. coli* K-12 (32).

Colicins of types B and D have been reported to have quite distinct modes of action. Colicin D-CA23 specifically inhibits protein synthesis without affecting deoxyribonucleic acid or ribonucleic acid synthesis (44), whereas colicin B-K77 inhibits protein, ribonucleic acid, and deoxyribonucleic acid synthesis (11) and may

TABLE 7. *Colicin production and colicin immunity of strain P1684 carrying various col B and col D factors as determined by the cross-streak plate test*

Plasmid carried	Colicins produced[a]	Immunity/sensitivity to colicins produced by col B and col D factors[b]								Immunity to other colicins[c]
		K260	CA23	CA18	K77	K89	K252	II	K44	
K260	B	I	S	S	S	S	S	S	S	1b-P9, 1a-CA53 (S1-P1)
CA23	D	S	I	S	S	S	S	S	S	
CA18	B, M	I	S	I	I	I	I	S	S	(G-CA46), H-CA58, 1a-CA53, 1b-P9, M-K260, S1-P1, V-CA7
K77	B, M	I	S	I	I	I	I	S	S	1b-P9, M-K260
K89	B, M	I	S	I	I	I	I	I	S	1b-P9, M-K260
K252	B, M	I	S	I	I	I	I	I	S	M-K260, V-CA7
II	B,[d] E1, I-S1, V-Q[e]	I	S	I	I	I	I	I	I	E1-K53, 1a-CA53, 1b-P9, M-K260, (S1-P1), V-CA7

[a] Determined using mutants of known colicin resistance (3, 4; Table 1). Resistance to one of the colicins produced by multicolicinogenic strains was indicated by the appearance of a narrower inhibition zone.
[b] All col factors in strain P1684 except K44. I, Immune (scores as resistant); S, sensitive.
[c] Parentheses indicate partial tolerance (hazy or narrow inhibition zone).
[d] Originally called colicin D.
[e] We are unable to distinguish between colicins 1a, 1b, and S1 and V and Q in these tests.

therefore be similar to colicin K, which affects energy metabolism (21). Although colicin B-K77 may not be identical to the colicin B-K260 studied here, there is substantial antigenic similarity between the two colicins, and *E. coli* producing colicin B-K77 is immune to colicin B-K260. Furthermore, recent results in our laboratory indicate that colicin B-K260 inhibits amino acid uptake, a characteristic of colicins that affect energy metabolism, whereas colicin D-CA23 does not (unpublished data). We therefore suggest that the differences in antigenic structure, and in sensitivity to heat and to reducing agents, and minor differences in amino acid composition are consistent with the differences in modes of action of the two colicins B and D. Colicins E2 and E3 also use a common receptor site on the cell surface of *E. coli* K-12 (37, 39), but have quite distinct modes of action (1, 36) and are only partially cross-immune (17). These colicins also have very similar amino acid compositions, but colicin E2 is sensitive to reducing conditions whereas colicin E3 is not (15), and colicins E2 and E3 each have non-cross-reacting as well as common antigenic specifities (19). This raises the possibility that the common antigenic determinants in colicins B and D and in colicins E2 and E3 are part of the receptor-recognition regions of these colicins, whereas the non-cross-reacting antigens are parts of the "active" regions of the colicin molecules. Colicins Ia and Ib, which are distinguished chiefly by the lack of cross-immunity between the producing strains (20), may also have non-cross-reacting antigens (19). An alternative hypothesis may therefore be that the non-cross-reacting antigens of colicins B and D, E2 and E3, and Ia and Ib are part of the immunity-recognition regions of these colicins. It should be noted, however, that in no case has a range of independently isolated colicins of the two types been compared, and some of the antigenic differences could even be unimportant.

Colicins are generally regarded as secreted proteins, although large amounts of the colicin often remain cell bound (Table 2) even in the absence of the homologous colicin receptors on the producing cells (42). The mechanisms by which colicins are secreted by colicinogenic bacteria remain largely unknown. However, most of the colicins studied in detail have been shown to contain very little or no cysteine (19) and thus conform to the generally accepted view that proteins secreted by bacteria contain very little of this amino acid (30). The only report of a colicin containing appreciable amounts of cysteine is that of Timmis (42) for colicin D-CA23. However, we find that our preparations of colicin D-CA23 and the closely related colicin B-K260 contain no detectable cysteine.

The finding that colicins B and D are very similar also raises some questions relating to the apparent differences between plasmids coding for the production of these colicins. We have previously shown that both colicins are part of a larger subdivision of colicins, which we call group B. Mutants of *E. coli* K-12 resistant to colicins in group B (B, D, G, H, Ia, Ib, M, Q, S1, and V) show no cross-resistance to colicins in group A (A, E1, E2, E3, K, L, N, S4, and X) and vice versa (3, 4). This division into two major groups in general parallels a similar division of col factors into self-transferring and non-self-transferring types (13, 14). Colicins in group B in our classification are generally produced by large self-transferring col factors. The only exception to this observation is colicin D-CA23, which we classify as a group B colicin but which is produced by a small, non-self-transferring col factor. The col factor CA23 is clearly a simple plasmid, coding only for the production of one colicin, and is therefore different from col B factors, which are self-transferring (with the possible exception of K44) and code for the production of at least one additional colicin and produce immunity to at least two other colicins (Table 7). The plasmid K260 used here apparently carries that part of a col I factor coding for immunity, although not producing colicin I. The col factor CA23 is considerably smaller than plasmids coding for production of and immunity to the B colicins (13, 43), and it is possible that this plasmid has been formed by the fragmentation of a larger plasmid with resulting loss of sex factor activity. On the other hand, we note that the complex col B factors also carry col I or col V factor activity (Table 7), and col I and col V factors themselves are known to have sex factor activity (26).

ACKNOWLEDGMENTS

We thank G. Whitfield (Upjohn Ltd.) for a gift of spectinomycin and Stephen Attridge, Max Atkinson, and Irene Pankiweicz for supplying various bacterial strains. We also thank Peter Ey for assistance with the immunochemical analyses, Michael Calder for performing the amino acid analyses, and Antony Richardson for assistance with the polyacrylamide electrophoresis systems.

LITERATURE CITED

1. **Boon, T.** 1972. Inactivation of ribosomes in *vitro* by colicin E3 and its mechanism of action. Proc. Natl. Acad. Sci. U.S.A. **69**:549–552.
2. **Braun, V., K. Schaller, and M. R. Wabl.** 1974. Isolation, characterization, and action of colicin M. Antimicrob. Agents Chemother. **5**:520–533.
3. **Davies, J. K., and P. Reeves.** 1975. Genetics of resistance to colicins in *Escherichia coli* K-12: cross-resistance among colicins of group B. J. Bacteriol. **123**:96–101.
4. **Davies, J. K., and P. Reeves.** 1975. Genetics of resist-

ance to colicins in *Escherichia coli* K-12: cross-resistance among colicins of group A. J. Bacteriol. 123:102-117.
5. **Fraenkel-Conrat, H.** 1957. Methods for investigating the essential groups for enzyme activity, p. 247-269. *In* S. P. Colowick and N. O. Kaplan (ed.), Methods in enzymology, vol. 4. Academic Press Inc., New York.
6. **Fredericq, P.** 1946. Sur la pluralite des recepteurs d' antibiose de *E. coli*. C. R. Soc. Biol. 140:1189-1190.
7. **Fredericq, P.** 1948. Actions antibiotiques reciproques chez les Enterobacteriaceae. Rev. Belge Pathol. Med. Exp. 19(Suppl. 4):1-107.
8. **Fredericq, P.** 1953. Recherches sur les caracteres et la distribution des souches prodactrices de diverses colicines dans les selles normales et pathologiques. Bull. Acad. R. Med. Belg. 18:126-139.
9. **Fredericq, P.** 1956. Recherches sur la frequence des souches transductrices des proprietes colicinogenes. C. R. Soc. Biol. 150:1036-1039.
10. **Fredericq, P., and J. Smarda.** 1970. Complexite du facteur colicinogene B. Ann. Inst. Pasteur Paris 118:767-774.
11. **Guterman, S. K.** 1973. Colicin B: mode of action and inhibition by enterochelin. J. Bacteriol. 114:1225-1230.
12. **Haasmann, C., and R. C. Clowes.** 1971. Mitomycin C and temperature induction of colicin B in the absence of deoxyribonucleic acid synthesis. J. Bacteriol. 107:633-635.
13. **Hardy, K. G.** 1975. Colicinogeny and related phenomena. Bacteriol. Rev. 39:464-515.
14. **Hardy, K. G., G. G. Meynell, and J. E. Dowman.** 1973. Two major groups of colicin factors: their evolutionary significance. Mol. Gen. Genet. 125:217-230.
15. **Herschman, H. R., and D. R. Helinski.** 1967. Purification and characterisation of colicin E2 and colicin E3. J. Biol. Chem. 242:5360-5368.
16. **Holland, I. B.** 1975. Physiology of colicin action, p. 56-133. *In* A. H. Rose and D. W. Tempest (ed.), Advances in microbial physiology, vol. 12. Academic Press Inc., London.
17. **Inselberg, J.** 1974. Incompatability exhibited by colicin plasmids E1, E2, and E3 in *Escherichia coli*. J. Bacteriol. 119:478-483.
18. **Kelchi, G., and W. H. Lederer.** 1974. Handbook of micromethods for the biological sciences. Von Nostrand Reinhold Co., New York.
19. **Konisky, J.** 1973. Chemistry of colicins, p. 41-58. *In* L. P. Hager (ed.), Chemistry and functions of colicins. Academic Press Inc., New York.
20. **Levisohn, R., J. Konisky, and M. Nomara.** 1967. Interaction of colicins with bacterial cells. IV. Immunity breakdown studied with colicins la and lb. J. Bacteriol. 96:811-821.
21. **Luria, S. E., J. Lusk, and C. A. Plate.** Colicins, p. 1-14. *In* L. P. Hager (ed.), Chemistry and functions of colicins. Academic Press Inc., New York.
22. **MacGreggor, C. H., C. A. Schnaitman, D. E. Normansell, and M. G. Hodgins.** 1974. Purification and properties of nitrate reductase from *Escherichia coli* K-12. J. Biol. Chem. 249:5321-5327.
23. **Maizel, J. V., Jr.** 1966. Acrylamide gel electrophoresis by mechanical fractionation: radioactive adenovirus proteins. Science 151:988-990.
24. **Miller, J. H.** 1972. Experiments in molecular genetics. Cold Spring Harbor Laboratory, Cold Spring Harbor, N.Y.
25. **Mitusi, E., and D. Mizuno.** 1969. Stabilization of colicin E2 by bovine serum albumin. J. Bacteriol. 100:1136-1137.
26. **Novick, P. R.** 1974. Bacterial plasmids, p. 537-586. *In* A. I. Laskin and H. A. Lechevalier (ed.), Handbook of microbiology, vol. IV. C. R. C. Press, Cleveland.
27. **Ouchterlony, O., and L. A. Nilsson.** 1973. *In* D. M. Weir (ed.), Handbook of experimental immunology, p. 19.1-19.39. Blackwell, Oxford.
28. **Ozaki, M., Y. Higashi, H. Saito, T. An, and T. Amano.** 1966. Identity of megacin A with phospholipase A. Biken J. 9:201-213.
29. **Papavasillou, J.** 1965. Sensitivity of *Salmonella* to colicines. Isr. J. Med. Sci. 1:627-629.
30. **Pollack, M. R., and M. H. Richmond.** 1972. Low cyst(e)ine content of bacterial extracellular proteins: its possible physiological significance. Nature (London) 194:446-449.
31. **Pugsley, A. P., and P. Reeves.** 1976. Characterization of group B colicin-resistant mutants of *Escherichia coli* K-12: colicin resistance and the role of enterochelin. J. Bacteriol. 127:218-228.
32. **Pugsley, A. P., and P. Reeves.** 1976. Increased production of the outer membrane receptors for colicins B, D and M by *Escherichia coli* under iron starvation. Biochem. Biophys. Res. Commun. 70:846-855.
33. **Pugsley, A. P., and P. Reeves.** 1976. Iron uptake in colicin B-resistant mutants of *Escherichia coli* K-12. J. Bacteriol. 126:1052-1061.
34. **Reeves, P.** 1972. The bacteriocins. Springer-Verlag, Berlin.
35. **Reynolds, B. L., and P. Reeves.** 1969. Kinetics of adsorption of colicin CA42-E2 and reversal of its bactericidal activity. J. Bacteriol. 100:301-309.
36. **Ringrose, P. S.** 1973. Effects of colicin E2 on DNA and the bacterial membrane *in vivo*. Biochim. Biophys. Acta 312:656-666.
37. **Sabet, S., and C. A. Schnaitman.** 1973. Purification and properties of the colicin E3 receptor of *Escherichia coli*. J. Biol. Chem. 248:1797-1806.
38. **Schacterle, G. R., and R. L. Pollack.** 1973. A simplified method for the quantitative assay of small amounts of protein in biologic material. Anal. Biochem. 51:654-655.
39. **Smarda, J., and J. Adler.** 1971. A contribution to the problem of a common receptor of the E-group colicins. Antonie van Leeuwenhoek J. Microbiol. Serol. 37:507-515.
40. **Smarda, J., and V. Obdrzalek.** 1966. Colicine Q. Zentralbl. Bakteriol. Parasitenkd. Infektionskr. Hyg. Abt. 1 Orig. 200:493-497.
41. **Svedson, P. J., and N. H. Axelsen.** 1972. A modified antigen-antibody crossed electrophoresis characterising the specificity and titre of human precipitins against *Candida albicans*. J. Immunol. Methods 1:169-176.
42. **Timmis, K.** 1972. Purification and characterization of colicin D. J. Bacteriol. 109:12-30.
43. **Timmis, K., F. Cabello, and S. N. Cohen.** 1974. Utilization of two distinct modes of replication by a hydrid plasmid constructed *in vitro* from separate replicons. Proc. Natl. Acad. Sci. U.S.A. 71:4556-4560.
44. **Timmis, K., and A. J. Hedges.** 1972. The killing of sensitive cells by colicin D. Biochim. Biophys. Acta 262:200-207.
45. **Warandeher, V. S., and L. D. Shaw.** 1959. A sensitive colorimetric method for the estimation of 2-deoxy sugars with the malonaldehyde-thiobarbituric acid reaction. J. Biol. Chem. 234:1945-1950.
46. **Weeke, B.** 1973. Rocket immunoelectrophoresis, p. 37-47. *In* N. H. Axelsen, J. Krøll, and B. Weeke (ed.), A manual of quantitative electrophoresis. Universitetsforlaget, Oslo.
47. **Weeke, B.** 1973. Crossed immunoelectrophoresis, p. 47-57. *In* N. H. Axelsen, J. Krøll, and B. Weeke (ed.), A manual of quantitative immunoelectrophoresis. Universitetsforlaget, Oslo.

ANTIMICROBIAL AGENTS AND CHEMOTHERAPY, Feb. 1977, p. 359-361
Vol. 11, No. 2

NOTES

Hemagglutination Inhibition Assay for Gentamicin

W. A. MAHON*, RHODA I. FELDMAN, AND GEORGE H. SCHERR

Department of Medicine, Toronto General Hospital, Toronto, Ontario, Canada; Technam, Inc., Park Forest South, Illinois 60466; and Governors State University, Park Forest South, Illinois 60466

Received for publication 4 August 1976

A rapid and simple hemagglutination inhibition test for measuring gentamicin concentrations in serum has been developed. Correlation coefficients for this assay with the radioimmunoassay and microbiological assay were r = 710 and r = 0.864, respectively. Measurements of gentamicin levels in serum by the three methods showed no statistically significant differences. The hemagglutination inhibition assay is fast, reliable, and relatively inexpensive, and should prove valuable for laboratory use.

Gentamicin has an established place in the management of a variety of infections due to gram-negative bacilli. The aminoglycoside is also important in the initial management of serious infections before the results of microbiological cultures are available. The drug is eliminated by the kidney and may accumulate in the plasma in the presence of impaired renal function; such accumulation has been associated with an increased frequency of toxicity (6). A variety of authors and authorities have stated that nephrotoxicity and ototoxicity have been encountered most frequently in patients whose peak serum concentration is in excess of 12 to 15 μg/ml (3, 4). In contrast, concentrations below 4 μg/ml may be ineffective in eradicating infection, particularly that due to *Pseudomonas* (7, 9). Monitoring gentamicin concentrations is required for safe and optimal therapeutic use of the antibiotic (5).

A variety of methods have been devised for monitoring gentamicin concentrations. The most common assays at the present time are the microbiological assay, radioimmunoassay, and enzymatic assay. The relative values of these three assays have been examined (11), and it has been stated that the individual laboratory must ultimately weigh the factors of patient volume, turn-around time, facilities, and costs to determine the method best suited for its needs. There is an obvious need for a rapid and simple assay whose cost approaches that of the microbiological assay and whose specificity approaches that of the radioimmunoassay. In this paper we report such an assay; a rapid and simple hemagglutination inhibition test has been devised for measuring gentamicin concentrations in serum, and the method has been compared with a standard microbiological assay and a radioimmunoassay (9).

MATERIALS AND METHODS

Microbiological assay. The microbiological assay was performed by using a routine cup plate assay with antibiotic medium no. 11 (Difco) at pH 7.9 against a strain of *Enterobacter*. Incubation was for 24 h at 35°C. The microbiological assay used in our clinical laboratory did not allow for the reporting of concentrations of gentamicin less than 0.2 μg/ml.

Radioimmunoassay. The radioimmunoassay techniques for determining gentamicin concentration in serum were performed as previously described (10).

Hemagglutination inhibition assay. The methods of preparation and standardization of antisera and gentamicin-sensitized cells were essentially those described by Adler and Liu for detecting drugs of abuse (1, 2, 9; F. L. Adler and C.-T. Liu, Fed. Proc. 31:807, 1972), except that the gentamicin-bovine serum albumin antigen was covalently attached to the sheep erythrocytes. The cells were then fixed with formaldehyde to yield a preparation that is stable for at least 8 months under refrigeration.

Hemagglutination inhibition tests were done in Linbro microtiter trays (with V wells). Essentially the test involved combining 1 drop of previously diluted patient's serum with 1 drop of gentamicin-specific antiserum, incubating for 5 min at room temperature, and then adding 1 drop of gentamicin-sensitized cells, followed by incubation at room temperature. After 60 to 90 min, the plates were examined for the formation of cell pellets. If the serum samples after dilution contained more than 10 ng/ml, agglutination of the erythrocytes occurred and no pellet was visible. Usually seven dilutions were run for each patient sample. The last dilution giving a pellet was determined by inspection of the plate, and the concentration of gentamicin in the serum sample was then read from a table that had been previously calculated for the dilutions used. Table 1 shows sample table. The drop size was 50 μl.

Using microtiter-type trays and calibrated pipettes, 1 drop (50 μl) of tube no. 1 is added to each of two wells, 1 drop of tube no. 2 is added into each of the second two wells, etc., through to tube no. 7. To well no. 8 is added 50 μl of gentamicin standard containing 10 ng/ml. This will be a control to demonstrate that the antiserum used is, in fact, inhibited by this quantity of gentamicin. Into well no. 9 is added 2 drops of reagent diluent, and this well will be a control to insure that the antibody appropriately reacts with the cells to prevent settling.

A 50-μl amount of reconstituted antiserum is added to all the wells except no. 9, and the tray contents are then mixed by gentle rotation on the bench surface. After 5 to 10 min the reconstituted cells are added in a quantity of 50 μl to all the wells. The tray is again shaken on the tabletop. The reaction tray does not have to be incubated since it works at a very wide range of ambient temperature. After approximately 1 h, the reactions and the end point are read. The well showing a pellet of cells equal to that of the control in tube no. 8 is the end point, and the micrograms of gentamicin per milliliter of sample can be read in the column above opposite the tube number.

Controls were also run to insure that the antiserum and cells were agglutinating properly in the absence of gentamicin (1 drop of reagent diluent, 1 drop of antiserum, and 1 drop of cells) and that the limit of sensitivity for the system was 10 ng/ml (by running a test series of dilutions with a gentamicin standard).

RESULTS

Forty-three samples coming to the microbiological laboratory for assay provided the serum. The mean and standard deviation of results are shown in Table 2. There were no statistically significant differences in the mean values of 4.27 μg/ml for the radioimmunoassay, 4.12 μg/ml for the hemagglutination inhibition assay, and 4.80 μg/ml for the microbiological assay. The mean of the microbiological assay calculates values reported as less than 2.0 μg/ml as 2.0 μg/ml, which may be the reason for the higher mean value.

Figure 1 shows the correlation between the various assays. At the top is a comparison of the radioimmunoassay with the microbiological assay, which reveals a correlation coefficient of $r = 0.707$. In the middle is a comparison between the hemagglutination inhibition assay and the microbiological assay ($r = 0.710$), and at the bottom is a comparison between the ra-

TABLE 1. *Dilutions to be used in calculating gentamicin levels in serum*

Tube no.	Dilution[a]	Gentamicin (μg/ml)
1	0.1 ml of serum + 3.0	0.31
2	12 + 3.0	1.86
3	7 + 3.0	2.97
4	4 + 3.0	4.96
5	3 + 3.0	6.51
6	2 + 3.0	9.61
7	1 + 3.0	18.9

[a] First number indicates drops of stock dilution; second number indicates milliliters of reagent diluent.

TABLE 2. *Results of three assay measurements gentamicin in 43 consecutive samples*

Assay[a]	Mean ± SD[b] (μg/ml)
RIA	4.27 ± 3.40
HIA	4.12 ± 2.79
MA	4.80 ± 2.68

[a] Abbreviations: RIA, Radioimmunoassay; HIA, hemagglutination inhibiton assay; MA, microbiological assay.

[b] SD, Standard deviation. All results were statistically not significant.

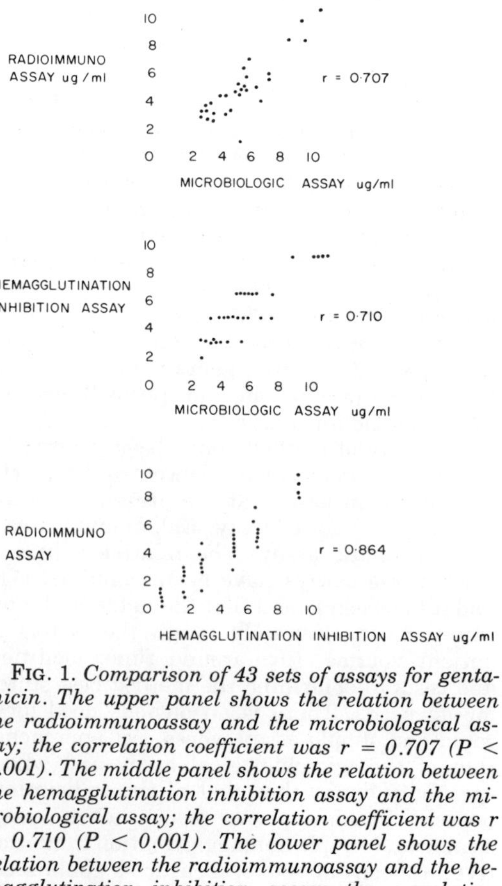

FIG. 1. *Comparison of 43 sets of assays for gentamicin. The upper panel shows the relation between the radioimmunoassay and the microbiological assay; the correlation coefficient was $r = 0.707$ ($P < 0.001$). The middle panel shows the relation between the hemagglutination inhibition assay and the microbiological assay; the correlation coefficient was $r = 0.710$ ($P < 0.001$). The lower panel shows the relation between the radioimmunoassay and the hemagglutination inhibition assay; the correlation coefficient was $r = 0.864$ ($P < 0.001$).*

dioimmunoassay and the hemagglutination inhibition assay ($r = 0.864$). The poorer correlation where the microbiological assay is involved may well be contributed to by the lack of integer values at concentrations less than 2.0 μg/ml, since these figures were not included in the calculation of r. All the correlation coefficients were highly statistically significantly related ($P < 0.001$).

Despite the fact that the hemagglutination inhibition assay method outlined here results in discontinuous values as contrasted with the radioimmunoassay and microbiological assay, the correlation was excellent among all three assay methods. Because of its speed, reliability, low cost per assay, and lack of initial setup cost, the hemmagglutination inhibition test for gentamicin should prove valuable to the clinical laboratory.

The antiserum is lyophilized and is stable for 1 year. Once reconstituted, it is stable at refrigeration temperature for approximately 5 days. Aliquots may be frozen and used as needed over an extended period of time without any decline in activity. The preserved cells are stable for approximately 9 months, and other reagents are stable for at least 6 months.

The specificity of the assay is that of the anti-gentamicin antibody, which does not interact with other aminoglycoside antibiotics or with penicillin, cephalosporins, and tetracyclines (9). The cost of similar assays in kit form for detection of drugs of abuse is $60.00 for a kit to perform 100 to 125 tests, and similar costs are likely with the gentamicin assay. This compares very favorably with the costs estimated for other assays (11).

We wish to thank J. Rennie and Simon Leung for technical assistance in carrying out the various assays, and T. Shaeff, Department of Microbiology, University of Toronto, for advice and assistance.

LITERATURE CITED

1. **Adler, F. L. and C.-T. Liu.** 1971. Detection of morphine by hemagglutination-inhibition. J. Immunol. 106:1684–1685.
2. **Adler, F. L., C.-T. Liu, and D. H. Catlin.** 1972. Immunological studies of heroin addiction. 1. Methodology and application of hemagglutination-inhibition test for detection of morphine. Clin. Immunol. Immunopathol. 1:53–68.
3. A. M. A. Drug Evaluation. 1973. 2nd ed., p. 569–570. Publishing Science Group, Inc., Boston.
4. **Garrod, L. P., H. P. Lambert, and F. O'Grady.** 1973. Antibiotic and chemotherapy, 4th ed., p. 127. Churchill Livingstone, Edinburgh.
5. Handbook of Antimicrobial Therapy, revised. 1976. The Medical Letter, New Rochelle, N. Y.
6. **Jackson, G. G., and G. Arcieri.** 1971. Ototoxicity of gentamicin in man: a survey and controlled analysis of clinical experience in the United States. J. Infect. Dis. 124(Suppl):S130–137.
7. **Jackson, G. G., and L. J. Riff.** 1971. Pseudomonas bacteremia: pharmacologic and other bases for failure of treatment with gentamicin. J. Infect. Dis. 124:S185–191.
8. **Liu, C.-T., and F. L. Adler.** 1973. Immunologic studies on drug addiction. 1. Antibodies reactive with methadone and their use for detection of the drug. J. Immunol. 111:472–477.
9. **Mahon, W. A., J. Ezer, and T. W. Wilson.** 1973. Radioimmunoassay for measurement of gentamicin in blood. Antimicrob. Agents Chemother. 3:585–589.
10. **Noone, P., T. M. C. Parsons, J. R. Pattison, R. C. B. Slack, D. Garfield-Davies, and K. Hughes.** 1974. Experience in monitoring gentamicin therapy during treatment of serious gram-negative sepsis. Br. Med. J. 1:477–481.
11. **Stevens, P., L. S. Young, and W. L. Hewitt.** 1975. Radioimmunoassay, acetylating radio-enzymatic assay and microbioassay of gentamicin: a comparative study J. Lab. Clin. Med. 86:349–359.

ANTIMICROBIAL AGENTS AND CHEMOTHERAPY, Feb. 1977, p. 362-364 Vol. 11, No. 2

Printed in U.S.A.

In Vitro Activity of Netilmicin

J. A. SMITH,* J. R. MORGAN, AND M. MOGYOROS

Division of Microbiology, Mount Sinai Hospital, and Departments of Medical Microbiology and Medicine, University of Toronto, Toronto, Ontario, Canada*

Received for publication 27 September 1976

The activity of netilmicin against a variety of bacteria was similar to that of gentamicin, sisomicin, and tobramycin, but it was less active than these three drugs against *Pseudomonas aeruginosa*. Synergy with penicillin G against enterococci was demonstrated.

Netilmicin is a derivative of sisomicin by the addition of an ethyl radical at the 1-N position on the deoxystreptamine moiety. Preliminary animal studies by the manufacturer (Schering Corp.) suggest that threshold toxicity to kidney and vestibular apparatus occurs at a serum concentration up to five times that of gentamicin. Comparative studies of the in vitro antimicrobial activities of aminoglycosides have suggested that the parent compound sisomicin is equal in activity to, or more active than, gentamicin (1–3). This study evaluates the in vitro activity of netilmicin against 337 strains of aerobic gram-negative rods, including *Pseudomonas aeruginosa* (117 strains, of which 41 were resistant to 8 μg/ml), *Escherichia coli* (73 strains), *Klebsiella* spp. (73 strains), *Enterobacter* spp. (20 strains), *Citrobacter* spp. (10 strains), and *Proteus mirabilis* (40 strains). In addition, the drug was tested against *Staphylococcus aureus* (30 strains) and enterococcus (29 strains).

All strains were tested against netilmicin, sisomicin, tobramycin, amikacin, and gentamicin. Minimum inhibitory concentrations were determined on Mueller-Hinton agar using the Steers multiple inoculator (6) and a broth inoculum containing 10^8 colony-forming units/ml. The antibiotic concentrations used were 0.2, 0.4, 0.8, 1.6, 3.0, 5.0, 8.0, 10.0, 15.0, and 20.0 μg/ml. Cumulative percentages of susceptibility to the various antibiotic concentrations were plotted for each strain, and from these graphs were calculated the concentrations required to inhibit 50 and 90% of the strains.

Against *E. coli*, all five aminoglycosides exhibited almost identical activity with the exception of amikacin, which was slightly less active (Table 1). Netilmicin and sisomicin equalled the activity of gentamicin against 50% of strains of *Klebsiella* spp. (Table 1). However, 98% of the *Klebsiella* strains tested were inhibited by 0.8 μg of sisomicin per ml as compared to 1.6 μg each of netilmicin and gentamicin per ml.

Although the total number of strains of *Enterobacter* spp. and *Citrobacter* spp. (Table 1) was small, the results suggest that netilmicin and sisomicin were more active than the other antibiotics tested. There seemed little apparent difference between the activity of all five aminoglycosides against *P. mirabilis* (Table 1), which is at variance with the findings of Levison and Kaye (2), who ascribed greater activity to gentamicin and sisomicin than to tobramycin and amikacin.

Netilmicin displayed significantly less activity than the other antibiotics against *P. aeruginosa* (Table 2).

All strains of *S. aureus* tested were inhibited by 0.2 μg of each antibiotic per ml, except amikacin, which required 3 μg/ml to inhibit 100% of *S. aureus* strains. Netilmicin, sisomicin, and gentamicin showed activity against enterococcus (Table 1). In particular, at 10 μg/ml, 49% of strains were inhibited by netilmicin, whereas only 7% were inhibited by gentamicin; the other aminoglycosides were ineffective. This prompted an investigation of the synergistic activity of gentamicin (5 μg/ml) and netilmicin (5 μg/ml), respectively, in combination with penicillin (20 μg/ml) against 15 strains of *Streptococcus faecalis* and 1 strain of *Streptococcus faecium*. The method used was that of timed killing curves as described by Moellering et al. (4, 5).

Synergy was demonstrated with both drug combinations against 14 of 15 strains of *S. faecalis*; the remaining strain was completely killed by gentamicin alone at 24 h. Synergy was demonstrated between penicillin and netilmicin against all strains of *S. faecalis* and against the single strain of *S. faecium*. One strain of *S. faecalis* was particularly susceptible to genta-

TABLE 1. *Concentrations of antibiotics at which 50 and 90% of strains tested were inhibited*

Organism	No. of strains	Concn (μg/ml) of antibiotic for inhibition of:									
		50% of strains					90% of strains				
		Gentamicin	Tobramycin	Amikacin	Sisomicin	Netilmicin	Gentamicin	Tobramycin	Amikacin	Sisomicin	Netilmicin
P. aeruginosa	117	2.1	1.6	4.75	1.45	6.75	>20	>20	>20	>20	>20
E. coli	73	0.55	0.6	0.65	0.6	0.7	1.4	1.45	3.8	1.6	1.6
Klebsiella	73	0.35	0.7	0.95	0.35	0.35	1.2	1.5	1.55	0.7	1.1
Proteus mirabilis	44	2.0	1.4	2.3	0.6	1.2	2.85	2.75	2.95	2.5	2.0
Citrobacter spp.	10	1.3	1.8	1.6	0.4	0.4	3.0	3.0	2.0	0.8	1.6
Enterobacter	20	0.4	0.7	1.1	0.5	0.3	1.3	2.3	2.7	0.7	0.8
Enterococcus	29	12.1	>20	>20	11.9	10	14.2	>20	>20	15	15
S. aureus	30	<0.2	<0.2	1.8	<0.2	<0.2	<0.2	0.3	2.8	<0.2	<0.2

TABLE 2. *Cumulative percentages of susceptibility of 117 strains of P. aeruginosa to five aminoglycosides*

Aminoglycoside	% Susceptibility at antibiotic concn (μg/ml) of:									
	0.2	0.4	0.8	1.6	3	5	8	10	15	20
Gentamicin	0.85	4.2	30.7	47.0	56.4	60.6	64.9	67.5	79.4	82.0
Tobramycin	1.7	25.6	46.1	50.4	64.9	66.6	71.7	73.5	74.3	76.9
Amikacin	0.85	1.7	17.0	33.3	35.8	52.1	60.0	67.5	75.2	82.9
Sisomicin	1.7	17.9	34.1	54.7	64.1	67.5	68.3	70.0	74.3	74.3
Netilmicin	0	2.5	7.6	18.8	24.7	42.7	55.5	60.6	64.9	67.5

micin, so that synergy as defined (4, 5) could not be demonstrated at 24 h, but there was a 3-log difference in the number of surviving bacteria at 4 h when either combination was compared with the best single drug.

As previously reported (1–3), the activities of gentamicin, tobramycin, and sisomicin do not differ greatly from each other and netilmicin appears to follow a similar pattern of activity against aerobic gram-negative rods, but with the important difference that netilmicin is significantly less active against *P. aeruginosa*.

We would like to acknowledge the technical assistance of L. Tiosejo, R. Kapun, and J. Campbell and the financial support of Schering Corp. (Canada).

LITERATURE CITED

1. **Klastersky, S., C. Hensgers, M. Gerard, and D. Daneau.** 1975. Comparison of sisomicin and gentamicin in bacteriuric patients with underlying disease of the urinary tract. Antimicrob. Agents Chemother. 7:742–747.
2. **Levison, M. E., and D. Kaye.** 1974. In vitro comparison of four aminoglycoside antibiotics: sisomicin, gentamicin, tobramycin, and BB-K8. Antimicrob. Agents Chemother. 5:667–669.
3. **Meyers, B. R., B. Leng, and S. L. Hirschman.** 1975. Comparison of the antibacterial activities of sisomicin and gentamicin against gram-negative bacteria. Antimicrob. Agents Chemother. 8:757–758.
4. **Moellering, R. C., Jr., C. Wennerstein, and A. N. Weinberg.** 1971. Studies on antibiotic synergism against enterococci. J. Lab. Clin. Med. 77:821–828.
5. **Moellering, R. C., Jr., C. Wennerstein, and A. J. Weinstein.** 1975. Penicillin-tobramycin synergism against enterococci: a comparison with penicillin and gentamicin. Antimicrob. Agents Chemother. 3:526–529.
6. **Steers, E., E. L. Foltz, and B. S. Graves.** 1959. An inocula replicating apparatus for routine testing of bacterial susceptibility to antibiotics. Antimicrob. Agents Chemother. 9:307–311.
7. **Washington, J. A.** 1971. The agar dilution method, p. 127–141. *In* T. L. Gavan, E. L. Cheattle, H. W. McFadden, Jr. (ed.), Antimicrobial susceptibility testing. American Society of Clinical Pathologists, Inc., Chicago.

ANTIMICROBIAL AGENTS AND CHEMOTHERAPY, Feb. 1977, p. 365-368
Vol. 11, No. 2
Printed in U.S.A.

Bioassay for Miconazole

ANA ESPINEL-INGROFF, S. SHADOMY,[1]* AND JOHN F. FISHER

Department of Medicine, Medical College of Virginia, Virginia Commonwealth University, Richmond, Virginia 23298

Received for publication 8 September 1976

A radial diffusion bioassay for miconazole, which employs *Candida stellatoidea* as the indicator organism, is described. Results from three patients treated with the drug are presented.

First described in 1972, miconazole is a β-substituted 1-phenethyl imidazole with broad-spectrum antifungal activity (1, 7). Chemically, it is a white, crystalline substance only sparingly soluble in water (0.03%) and slightly soluble in organic solvents. In vitro it is active against most medically important fungi at concentrations from 0.1 to 10 μg/ml (2, 3, 5, 7). In vivo it has been shown to be protective against *Coccidioides immitis* (3) and curative against *Candida albicans* (7).

Clinical applications of miconazole include topical therapy of dermatophytic infections and vaginal candidosis and oral treatment of gastrointestinal and systemic mycoses (4). The intravenous use of the drug, still in the experimental stage, has been shown to be effective in *Candida* infections and of some potential benefit in other systemic mycoses (6). This report stems from our investigations with the intravenous form of the drug.

The bioassays were performed using a highly susceptible isolate of *Candida stellatoidea* (minimal inhibitory concentration, 0.05 μg/ml) as the indicator organism. Because of the poor solubility of the drug in water, the pharmaceutical preparation of miconazole for intravenous administration was used as standard material rather than pure substance. This preparation consisted of 10 mg of miconazole per ml in a vehicle containing 0.115 mg of polyethoxylated castor oil per ml, 0.5 mg of sodium bisulfate per ml, 1.62 mg of methylparaben per ml, 0.18 mg of propylparaben per ml, and sufficient acetic acid and sodium acetate to adjust the pH to 4.0 ± 0.5 (Janssen R&D, Inc., New Brunswick, N.J.; lot 74LO4/457). A placebo preparation consisting of the vehicle only was shown to be noninhibitory for the indicator organism when tested in a manner identical to that employed in the bioassay procedure. The medium was Sabouraud agar (Difco). Large, rigid plastic plates (23 by 23 cm) were used.

The intravenous preparation of miconazole was first diluted 1:2 with alcohol and then diluted in pooled, normal human serum that previously had been shown to be noninhibitory for the indicator organism. The final concentration in serum was 16 μg/ml. This solution was then serially diluted in the same serum to give concentrations of 8, 4, 2, 1, and 0.5 μg/ml for the standard curve. *C. stellatoidea* MCV 52.10 was harvested from slants of Sabouraud agar and suspended in saline; the density was adjusted to 70% as measured at 570 nm. A 1-ml amount of the suspension was added to 100 ml of molten agar; the seeded agar was mixed and immediately poured into a plate (23 by 23 cm) placed upon a leveling device. Plates were allowed to harden while on the device. A total of 12 stainless-steel antibiotic assay cylinders were placed on each plate in four rows of three cylinders each. Each cylinder received 0.1 ml of diluted drug or of a clinical specimen. Each drug concentration or specimen was tested in duplicate. Controls included a pooled, normal human serum control from the same lot as used for the preparation of the standard curve and pretreatment samples from patients when available. The standard curve and specimen plates were allowed to prediffuse overnight at 4°C before overnight incubation at 30°C. After incubation, zones of inhibition were measured to the nearest 0.1 mm with a dial vernier caliper. Each zone was measured in triplicate, and the average was taken for use in subsequent statistical analyses. Regression analysis was used to derive statistics for the dose response curves, and the estimating equation was used to calculate specimen concentrations of miconazole.

Bioassays for miconazole were performed on five occasions with sera and cerebrospinal fluid specimens from three different patients. These included a case of articular sporotrichosis treated for 30 days, a case of disseminated as-

[1] Address reprint requests to: Dr. S. Shadomy, Box 85, MCV Station, Richmond, VA 23298.

TABLE 1. *Five replicate standard dose response curves for miconazole prepared in pooled, normal human serum*

Assay no.	Diam (mm) of zone of inhibition at drug concn (μg/ml; $\log_2$) of: 16 (4)	8 (3)	4 (2)	2 (1)	1 (0)	0.5 (−1)	r	β	α	Y_c (16 μg/ml)	Y_c (1 μg/ml)
1	20.8	19.2	17.7	16.5	14.5	12.8	0.998	1.58	14.55	20.87	14.55
2	23.0	20.5	18.33	16.0	13.16	11.5	0.999	2.34	13.57	22.93	13.57
3	23.84	22.17	20.84	19.0	17.0	14.84	0.997	1.78	16.94	24.07	16.94
4	19.83	17.0	16.6	14.67	12.5	10.5	0.989	1.77	12.52	19.62	12.52
5	20.0	18.67	17.16	15.5	13.16	12.33	0.995	1.62	13.71	20.18	13.71
Mean, SD[a]	21.49 ± 1.63	19.51 ± 1.74	18.13 ± 1.47	16.33 ± 1.47	14.06 ± 1.61	12.39 ± 1.45	0.998	1.82	14.26	21.53	14.26

[a] SD, Standard deviation.

pergillosis treated for 4 weeks, and a case of cryptococcosis in a renal transplant recipient treated for 5 weeks. The first two patients were treated intravenously with 10 mg of miconazole per kg every 8 h; the third patient received both intravenous and intraventricular drug. All specimens were stored at −20°C prior to bioassay; sera had been removed from blood specimens prior to storage.

Excellent linearity and correlation were demonstrated between the concentrations of drug and the corresponding diameters of the resulting zones of inhibition (Table 1). In four bioassays r, or the coefficient of correlation, was 0.995 ($P < 0.001$) or better; the lowest value for r was 0.989. Calculated regression lines for the standard dose response curves were essentially parallel in four of the five bioassays (Fig. 1). Statistics for these four lines were similar, with values for β, the regression coefficient or slope, ranging from 1.58 to 1.78. Values for α, or intercept (Y_c when $X = 0$), ranged from 12.52 to 14.55 mm in the same four curves. The one nonparallel curve also demonstrated excellent linearity and correlation ($r = 0.999$); however,

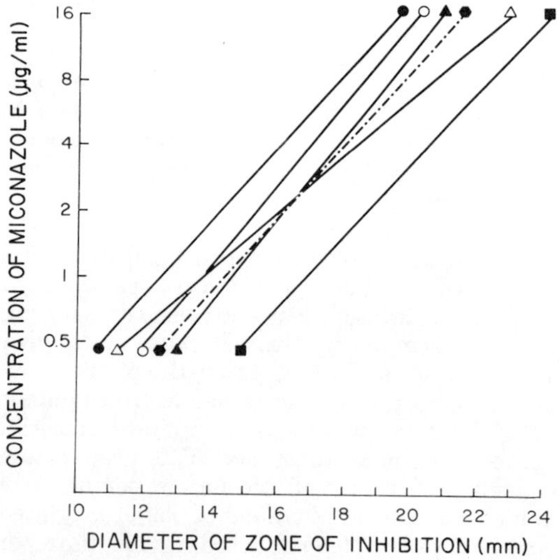

FIG. 1. *Dose response or standard curves obtained for five separate bioassays for miconazole in clinical specimens. The dose response curves were prepared by using an intravenous preparation of the drug diluted in pooled, normal human serum. A highly susceptible isolate of C. stellatoidea was used as the indicator organism. Curves were plotted by using statistics derived by regression analysis. Symbols:* ▲, *assay no. 1;* △, *assay no. 2;* ■, *assay no. 3;* ●, *assay no. 4;* ○, *assay no. 5;* ⬢, *composite standard curve based on averaged zone size values from all five bioassays.*

the slope of this curve, 2.34, differed from the other four, but not significantly ($t = 0.1219$, $P > 0.05$). Excellent correlation was also demonstrated ($r = 0.998$) when a composite regression line based upon mean zone size values of all five curves was derived.

A total of 27 specimens were assayed: sera, 12; cerebrospinal fluids, 6; and ventricular fluids, 9. Eight sera were from the patient with articular sporotrichosis; measurable concentrations of miconazole ranged from 1.41 to 4.35 μg/ml (Table 2). The pretreatment serum was devoid of antifungal activity, and one serum had only a trace amount of less than 0.5 μg/ml. Fourteen specimens from the patient with cryptococcosis were assayed (Table 2). Only three of these contained detectable drug. These included one serum which contained 2.54 μg of drug per ml and two samples of ventricular fluid, obtained immediately after intraventricular administration of 15 mg of miconazole, which contained greater than 120 μg/ml. The results from these two specimens are not to be considered representative of attainable spinal fluid levels. Three sera, including a pretreatment specimen from the patient with disseminated aspergillosis, were assayed; less than 0.5 μg of miconazole per ml was detected in these specimens, including one drawn 30 min after infusion.

Miconazole has been reported to be effective in the treatment of patients with infection due to *C. immitis* (6). In addition, several patients with cryptococcal meningitis are said to have responded to parenteral therapy with this agent (R. Legendre, Janssen R&D, Inc., personal communication). Because of these results and because of its in vitro activity against most fungal pathogens, miconazole may become important clinically. Thus, a reliable bioassay is needed to monitor body fluid levels in terms of bioavailability, therapeutic effectiveness, and potential toxicity. Such a procedure has been described here.

The data presented here have one very important clinical implication. All three fungal isolates from the patients in this study were found to be susceptible to miconazole, being inhibited by 1.56 μg or less of the drug per ml in vitro, yet all three patients failed to respond

TABLE 2. *Results of bioassays for miconazole in 24 clinical specimens from two patients receiving intravenous or intraventricular medication*

Patient	Last miconazole dosage and route[a]	Lapsed time since last dose (h)	Miconazole level (μg/ml) from specimen source: Serum	CSF[b]	Ventricular fluid
Articular sporotrichosis	None	Pretreatment	None		
	10 mg/kg, i.v.	2	4.35	None	
		6.5	1.41	None	
	10 mg/kg, i.v.	7	1.70		
	10 mg/kg, i.v.	9.5	2.00		
	20 mg/kg, p.o.	1	1.70		
		2	1.48		
		8.5	Trace[c]		
Cryptococcal meningitis	10 mg/kg, i.v.	2		None	
	10 mg/kg, i.v.	6.5		None	
	10 mg/kg, i.v.	2	2.54		
	10 mg/kg, i.v.	1.5		None	
	10 mg/kg, i.v.	2			None
	10 mg/kg, i.v.	8			None
	10 mg/kg, i.v.	4.5			None
	10 mg/kg, i.v.	7.5			None
	10 mg/kg, i.v.	3.5		None	None
	10 mg/kg, i.v.	1			None
	15 mg, intraventricularly	5 min			121.8
	10 mg/kg, i.v.	7			None
	15 mg, intraventricularly	5 min			250.3

[a] i.v., Intravenous; p.o., oral.
[b] CSF, Cerebrospinal fluid.
[c] Trace, Less than 0.5 μg/ml, low point of standard curve.

favorably to the drug. These failures may be explained, in part, by our inability to measure significant serum and cerebrospinal fluid levels after apparently adequate dosages in two of the three patients. In the patient with articular sporotrichosis, serum levels, although apparently adequate in terms of the in vitro minimal inhibitory concentration, may have failed to reflect actual drug concentrations at the site of infection. Thus, it is apparent that further data are required regarding distribution, metabolism, and bioavailability of this new antifungal agent.

LITERATURE CITED

1. **Brugmans, J., J. Van Cutsem, J. Heykants, V. Schuermans, and D. Thienpont.** 1972. Systemic antifungal potential, safety, biotransport and transformation of miconazole nitrate. Eur. J. Clin. Pharmacol. 5:93–99.
2. **Holt, R. J.** 1974. Recent developments in antimycotic chemotherapy. Infection 2:95–107.
3. **Levine, H. B., D. A. Stevens, J. M. Cobb, and A. E. Gebhardt.** 1975. Miconazole in coccidioidomycosis. I. Assays of activity in mice and *in vitro*. J. Infect. Dis. 132:407–414.
4. **Sawyer, P. R., R. N. Brogden, R. M. Pinder, T. M. Speight, and G. S. Avery.** 1975. Miconazole: a review of its antifungal activity and therapeutic efficacy. Drugs 9:406–423.
5. **Shadomy, S., and L. Paxton.** 1976. Miconazole and miconazole nitrate, p. 171–178. *In* J. D. Williams and A. M. Geddes (ed.), Chemotherapy 6, Parasites, fungi and viruses. Plenum Press, London.
6. **Stevens, D. A., H. B. Levine, and S. C. Deresinski.** 1976. Miconazole in coccidioidomycosis. II. Therapeutic and pharmacologic studies in man. Am. J. Med. 60:191–202.
7. **Van Cutsem, J. M., and D. Thienpont.** 1972. Miconazole, a broad-spectrum antimycotic agent and antibacterial activity. Chemotherapy 17:392–404.

ANTIMICROBIAL AGENTS AND CHEMOTHERAPY, Feb. 1977, p. 369-371 Vol. 11, No. 2

Antimicrobial Activity of Cefamandole Against *Salmonella typhi*

SHALOM Z. HIRSCHMAN,* BURT R. MEYERS, AND ALBERT MILLER

Division of Infectious Diseases and Division of Pulmonary Diseases, Department of Medicine, Mount Sinai School of Medicine of the City University of New York, New York, 10029*

Received for publication 18 August 1976

A patient with *Salmonella typhi* bacteremia was sucessfully treated with cefamandole, a new cephalosporin derivative. Infection has not recurred during 6 months of follow-up observation. Minimum inhibitory concentrations and minimum bactericidal concentrations of cefamandole, cephalothin, ampicillin, and chloramphenicol were compared against 26 strains of *S. typhi*. All the strains were susceptible to cefamandole in vitro. Seven of the strains were resistant to chloramphenicol, and another seven were resistant to both chloramphenicol and ampicillin. Cefamandole appears to warrant further clinical trial for the treatment of typhoid fever.

Cefamandole, 7-D-mandelamido-3-3 {[(1-methyl-1H-tetrazol-5-yl)-thio] methyl-3-cephem-4 carboxylic acid, is a new semisynthetic cephalosporin derivative with a broad spectrum of antimicrobial activity including strains of *Haemophilus influenzae* (5). Hitherto, the effective agents for therapy of *Salmonella typhi* infections have been chloramphenicol (4) and ampicillin (4, 8). The similarity of cefamandole to ampicillin in the exquisite susceptibility of strains of *H. influenzae* to this new cephalosporin prompted us to consider cefamandole therapy in patients with typhoid fever. We report on the susceptibility in vitro of *S. typhi* to cefamandole, including strains resistant to ampicillin, and the successful therapy of a typhoid fever patient with this new antimicrobial agent.

S. typhi were isolated and identified in the diagnostic microbiology laboratory of The Mount Sinai Hospital by standard methods. The minimum inhibitory concentrations (MIC) and minimum bactericidal concentrations (MBC) of cefamandole, cephalothin, ampicillin, and chloramphenicol for 26 strains of *S. typhi*, initially tested for purity by standard techniques, were determined by the twofold tube dilution method in heart infusion broth (Difco) as described previously (5). Seven of the strains carried an R factor mediating resistance to chloramphenicol (2), and seven others carried an R factor conferring resistance to both ampicillin and chloramphenicol (7).

Case report. D. L., a 34-year-old black male, entered The Mount Sinai Hospital with complaints of fever and malaise. Illness began 17 days before admission, with pain and tenderness (without swelling) of the right ankle. Frontal headaches, myalgia, and malaise soon followed. Two weeks before admission, the patient was admitted to another hospital where red spots were noted on his tongue. Blood, stool, and urine cultures were negative. The patient left against medical advice after 4 days. Three days later, the patient developed fever to 104°F (40°C) orally, generalized arthralgia and myalgia, severe headache, and shortness of breath. These symptoms were followed by 2 days of watery stools and abdominal pain. The patient had lost 15 pounds (ca. 6.8 kg) of weight since onset of the illness. One week before the patient became ill, a friend was admitted to another hospital and treated for "salmonellosis." The patient had been hospitalized with hepatitis in 1964; review of systems was otherwise negative. Physical examination showed a lethargic young man with warm, dry skin. Blood pressure was 140/70 mm of Hg; pulse, 92/min and regular; respirations, 28/min; and rectal temperature, 101°F (38.3°C). The tongue was erythematous, with red spots observed along the lateral anterior borders; the neck was supple. Examination of the lungs and heart was negative. There was no hepatosplenomegaly and no abdominal tenderness. Neurological and rectal exams were normal.

Laboratory data on admission included a hemoglobin of 13.7 g/dl and a leukocyte count of 3,500/mm^3, with a differential count of 25 neutrophils, 29 band forms, 32 lymphocytes, 6 monocytes, and 8 atypical lymphocytes. Urinalysis showed a pH of 5; specific gravity, 1.026; 1+ protein; and 3 to 5 leukocytes per high-power field. Arterial blood gases were normal. The erythrocyte sedimentation rate was 23 mm/h (Westergren). The blood urea nitrogen was 18 mg/dl, and fasting blood sugar was 115 mg/dl. The serum amylase was 136 units; phosphorus, 2.7 mg/dl; cholesterol 123 mg/dl (lower limit of normal, 140 mg/dl); total bilirubin, 0.8 mg/dl; alkaline phosphatase, 62 IμU/ml; glutamic pyruvic transaminase, 50 IμU/ml; oxaloacetic transaminase, 98 IμU/ml (upper limit of normal, 50 IμU/ml); albumin, 4 g/dl; globulin, 4 g/dl; creatine phosphokinase, 419 IμU/ml (upper limit of normal, 145 IμU/ml); and creatinine, 1.4 g/dl. Urinary urobilinogen was positive at a 1:20 dilution. The prothrombin time was 15.4 s, with a control value of 12 s. The slide test for infectious mononucleosis was negative. Stool examination for ova and parasites was negative. The VDRL test for syphilis and the intermediate-strength purified protein derivative skin test were negative. *S. typhi* O and H agglutinins were 1:160 and 1:200, respectively. Electrocardiogram, chest X-ray, and oral cholangiography were normal. Liver-spleen scintigraphy showed patchy hepatic uptake.

Blood cultures taken on admission grew *S. typhi* susceptible to ampicillin, chloramphenicol, gentamicin, tobramycin, kanamycin, and cefamandole by tube dilution test. Stool and urine culture were negative for *S. typhi*. The patient was treated with cefamandole, 2 g intravenously every 6 h for 14 days. The MIC and MBC of cefamandole for the isolate were 0.78 and 1.56 μg/ml, respectively. Defervescence occurred with 24 h after beginning therapy, and within 48 h the patient reported return of his sense of well-being. Blood cultures taken 24 h after beginning therapy were negative for *S. typhi*, and blood cultures remained negative during the hospital stay. One week after therapy was initiated, laboratory data included a hemoglobin of 12.5 g/dl and leukocyte count of 4,600 mm^3, with a differential count of 48 neutrophils, 3 band forms, 36 lymphocytes, 10 monocytes, 2 eosinophils, and 1 basophil. Serum chemistries showed an alkaline phosphatase of 99 IμU/ml; total bilirubin, 0.2 mg/dl; glutamic pyruvic transaminase, 47 IμU/ml; oxaloacetic transaminase, 47 IμU/ml; creatinine phosphokinase, 177 IμU/ml; albumin, 3.9 gm/dl; and globulin, 4.4 g/dl. The patient felt well upon discharge 18 days after admission. Stool cultures have remained negative for *S. typhi* during the 6 months after discharge.

RESULTS

All 19 strains of *S. typhi* tested that were susceptible to ampicillin were very suceptible to cefamandole (Table 1), with 63.2 and 100% of strains inhibited by concentrations of cefamandole of 1.56 and 2.5 μg/ml, respectively. The MBCs were only slightly higher than the MICs; all the strains were killed at a concentration of 5 μg/ml. These strains were inhibited and killed by concentrations of cephalothin and ampicillin of 12.5 and 6.25 μg/ml, respectively (Table 1); seven of the strains tested were resistant to choramphenicol (MIC > 25 μg/ml).

During an epidemic of *S. typhi* infection in Mexico with strains carrying an R factor mediating resistance to chloramphenicol, tetracycline, streptomycin, and sulfonamides, Olarte and Galindo (7) encountered seven strains additionally resistant to ampicillin. The MIC and MBC of cefamandole for these ampicillin- and chloramphenicol-resistant strains are shown in

TABLE 1. *Cumulative percentage of 19 strains of S. typhi inhibited (I) and killed (K) by cefamandole, cephalothin, ampicillin, and chloramphenicol*

Concn (μg/ml)	% Strains inhibited and killed by:							
	Cefamandole		Cephalothin		Ampicillin		Chloramphenicol	
	I	K	I	K	I	K	I	K
0.39	10.5	0	0	0	0			
0.78	36.9	31.6	15.8	5.3	10.5	0		
1.25	52.6	42.1						
1.56	63.2	52.6	36.8	31.6	36.8	15.8		
2.50	100	73.7					0	
3.12		79	57.9	52.6	84.2	73.7	57.9	
5.00		100						
6.25			94.7	84.2	100	100	63.2	0
12.5			100	100				5.3
25								36.8
50								
(>50)[a]							(100)[a]	(100)[a]

[a] Chloramphenicol-resistant strains of *S. typhi*.

TABLE 2. *Susceptibility to cefamandole in vitro of seven strains of S. typhi resistant to both ampicillin and chloramphenicol*

Strain	Cefamandole (μg/ml)		Cephalothin (μg/ml)	
	MIC	MBC	MIC	MBC
P-12	25	25	50	>50
JRR	12.5	12.5	50	50
JM	3.12	3.12	6.25	6.25
H-185	25	25	50	50
LA	25	25	50	>50
LAR I	12.5	25	50	50
LAR II	25	25	50	50

Table 2. The seven ampicillin-resistant strains of *S. typhi* were less susceptible to cefamandole than the 19 ampicillin-susceptible strains, but still were inhibited by concentrations of cefamandole ≤25 μg/ml. The ampicillin-resistant strains were less susceptible to cephalothin (Table 2) and were highly resistant to both ampicillin and chloramphenicol (MICs ≫50 μg/ml).

The patient's clinical response to cefamandole therapy was prompt and complete after almost 3 weeks of continued illness. Defervescence occurred in 24 h and the patient was out of bed within 48 h. Blood cultures became negative within 24 h, and the patient has remained well during 6 months of follow-up observation.

Outbreaks of *S. typhi* infection with organisms resistant to chloramphenicol (1, 2) or to both chloramphenicol and ampicillin (7) have occurred. Although recent reports of the use of the combination of trimethoprim and sulfamethoxazole for the treatment of infections due to chloramphenicol-resistant *S. typhi* are encouraging (3), alternative effective parenteral therapy has hitherto not been available, especially in patients hypersensitive to ampicillin. Cephalothin has not proved clinically reliable despite the susceptibility of *S. typhi* to this antimicrobial agent in vitro (4). Cefamandole appears to be extremely effective against *S. typhi* in vitro and, furthermore, shares a property of ampicillin in its effectiveness in vitro against strains of *H. influenzae*. It is interesting to note that the ampicillin-resistant strains of *S. typhi* isolated by Olarte and Galindo (7) in Mexico were susceptible to cefamandole. Although the MICs of cefamandole for the ampicillin-resistant strains (≤25 μg/ml) were higher than those for the ampicillin-susceptible strains, the required inhibitory and bactericidal concentrations are easily achieved in serum with intravenous cefamandole therapy (6).

Some patients with typhoid fever do recover spontaneously. However, the patient reported here had been ill for almost 3 weeks before admission, and the response to therapy was prompt and marked. Furthermore, illness did not recur after therapy. It would appear that cefamandole warrants clinical trial for the therapy of *S. typhi* infections in areas where this organism is more prevalent.

We thank G. Brier of Eli Lilly and Co. for providing strains of ampicillin-susceptible *S. typhi*, G. T. Keusch and S. Formal for chloramphenicol-resistant organisms, and J. Olarte for his kindness in providing ampicillin-chloramphenicol-resistant strains. The technical assistance of Z. Sadka is appreciated.

LITERATURE CITED

1. **Anderson, S., and H. R. Smith.** 1972. Chloramphenicol resistance in the typhoid bacillus. Br. Med. J. 3:329–331.
2. **Datta, N., and J. Olarte.** 1974. R factors in strains of *Salmonella typhi* and *Shigella dysenteriae 1* isolated during epidemics in Mexico: classification by compatibility. Antimicrob. Agents Chemother. 5:310–317.
3. **Gilman, R. H., M. Terminel, M. Levine, P. Hernandez-Mendosa, E. Calderone, E. Vasquez, E. Martinez, M. J. Snyder, and R. B. Hornick.** 1975. Comparison of trimethoprim-sulfamethoxazole and amoxicillin in therapy of chloramphenicol resistant and chloramphenicol sensitive typhoid fever. J. Infect. Dis. 132:630–635.
4. **Hook, E. W., and W. D. Thompson.** 1972. Typhoid fever, p. 593–601. *In* P. D. Hoeprich, (ed.), Infectious diseases. Harper and Row, New York.
5. **Meyers, B. R., B. Leng, and S. Z. Hirschman.** 1975. Cefamandole: antimicrobial activity in vitro of a new cephalosporin. Antimicrob. Agents Chemother. 8:734–741.
6. **Meyers, B. R., B. Ribner, S. Yancovitz, and S. Z. Hirschman.** 1976. Pharmacological studies with cefamandole in humans volunteers. Antimicrob. Agents Chemother. 9:140–144.
7. **Olarte, J., and E. Galindo.** 1973. *Salmonella typhi* resistant to chloramphenicol, ampicillin, and other antimicrobial agents: strains isolated during an extensive typhoid fever epidemic in Mexico. Antimicrob. Agents Chemother. 44:597–601.
8. **Simon, J. J., and R. C. Miller.** 1966. Ampicillin in the treatment of chronic typhoid carriers. N. Engl. J. Med. 274:807–815.

ERRATA

Laboratory Evaluation of BL-S786, a Cephalosporin with Broad-Spectrum Antibacterial Activity

F. LEITNER,* M. MISIEK, T. A. PURSIANO, R. E. BUCK, D. R. CHISHOLM, R. G. DeREGIS, Y. H. TSAI, AND K. E. PRICE

Department of Microbiological Research, Bristol Laboratories, Syracuse, New York 13201

Volume 10, no. 3, p. 427, column 2, Results, lines 17–21 should read: " . . . ml. At the same concentration, cefazolin inhibited 23% and 44% of the strains, respectively, whereas the percentage of strains inhibited by cephalothin and cephaloridine was negligible for both species. Against *Enterobac-* . . .

Effect of Long-Term Therapies with Penicillin and Sulfadiazine on *Streptococcus mutans* and Lactobacilli in Dental Plaque

H. G. WELD AND H. J. SANDHAM*

Department of Preventive Dentistry, Faculty of Dentistry, University of Toronto, Toronto, Ontario M5G 1G6, Canada

Volume 10, no. 2, p. 202, column 2, last line of Discussion: " . . . that benzathine penicillin has an effect on the . . . " should read " . . . that benzathine penicillin has no effect on the . . ."

R Plasmids in *Streptococcus agalactiae* (Group B)

THEA HORODNICEANU,* D. H. BOUANCHAUD, G. BIETH, AND Y. A. CHABBERT

Service de Bactériologie Médicale, Institut Pasteur, 75015 Paris, France

Volume 10, no. 5, p. 798, column 1, lines 8 and 13, and Table 3, p. 799, column heading 4: "nm" should read "μm."

Antimicrobial Susceptibility Testing of Yeasts: A Turbidimetric Technique Independent of Inoculum Size

JOHN N. GALGIANI* AND DAVID A. STEVENS

Department of Medicine, Santa Clara Valley Medical Center, San Jose, California, Department of Medicine, Stanford, California 94305*

Volume 10, no. 4, byline address: the words "Stanford University" should be inserted before "Stanford, California 94305."

Page 722, column 1, Materials and Methods, line 15: the symbol "%" was substituted after the parentheses; it should have been "×."

ANTIMICROBIAL AGENTS AND CHEMOTHERAPY, Mar. 1977, p. 373–375 Vol. 11, No. 3

Cairomycin B, a New Antibiotic

IBRAHIM R. SHIMI,* NADIA ABEDALLAH, AND SHADIA FATHY
Biochemistry Department, Faculty of Science, Ain Shams University, Cairo, Egypt Arab Republic

Received for publication 28 September 1976

Cairomycin B is a new cyclic peptide antibiotic that was isolated from *Streptomyces* As-C-19 obtained from the soil of Cairo. The antibiotic had the following empirical formula: $C_{10}H_{15}N_3O_3$; on acid hydrolysis, it yielded aspartic acid and lysine. Spectral analysis and its chemical characteristics indicated that it was a cyclic peptide. The antibiotic melted at 120 to 121°C and was freely soluble in chloroform, ethyl acetate, and acetone, slightly soluble in alcohols, and rather insoluble in water and petroleum ether. Cairomycin B was mainly active against gram-positive bacteria, with high toxicity to experimental animals and weak serum-binding properties.

During our screening program to evaluate members of *Streptomyces* from the soil of the Middle East area as producers of antimicrobial substances, an isolate, no. 19, obtained from the soil of Cairo, exerted interesting antimicrobial potentialities. It secretes, in its culture filtrate, several antimicrobial agents; among these, cairomycin B was isolated and its chemical structure was identified.

This paper describes the culture conditions and isolation of the antibiotic, for which the chemical, physical, and biological properties

TABLE 1. *Mass spectrum fragments of cairomycin B*

m/e	% Abundance	Fragment
41	77	$(\overset{O}{\overset{\|}{C}}\text{—}CH)^+$
43	94	$(\overset{H\cdots O}{\overset{\|}{C}}\text{—}CH_2)^+$
55	84	$(\overset{O}{\overset{\|}{C}}\text{—}CH\text{—}CH)^+$
56	34	$(\overset{H\cdots O}{\overset{\|}{C}}\text{—}CH_2\text{—}CH)^+$
57	100	$(CH_2\text{—}NH\text{—}\overset{O}{\overset{\|}{C}})^+$
83	55	$(\overset{O}{\overset{\|}{C}}\text{—}CH\text{—}CH_2\text{—}\overset{O}{\overset{\|}{C}})^+$
85	48	$(\overset{H\text{—}O}{\overset{\|}{C}}\text{—}CH\text{——}CH_2\text{—}\overset{O\text{—}H}{\overset{\|}{C}})^+$
97	36	$(N\text{—}CH_2\text{—}(CH_2)_3\text{—}CH\text{—}NH)^+$
99	23	$(HN\text{—}CH\text{—}(CH_2)_3\text{—}CH\text{—}NH)^+$
225	M	$(C_{10}H_{15}N_3O_3)$
226	10(*m* + 1)	$(C_{10}H_{16}N_3O_3)$

were determined. Finally, a suggested chemical structure was derived from the collected spectroscopic findings.

MATERIALS AND METHODS

Production, isolation and purification of cairomycin B. Microscopic examination of the cairomycin B-producing organism revealed narrow hyphae and straight chains of cylindrical spores, indicating that the organism is a streptomycete, designated as species AS-C-19.

Streptomyces AS-C-19 thrived at 28°C in shake flasks (220 rpm). The medium used for the production of cairomycin B contained the following ingredients (g/100 ml): glucose, 2.5; KNO_3, 0.1; K_2HPO_4, 0.1; $MgSO_4 \cdot 7H_2O$, 0.05; and KCl, 0.05.

The pH of the medium was adjusted to 7.0 before sterilization. The antibiotic contents reached a maximum (7.25 mg/liter) after 5 days of incubation, and the broth was filtered and extracted with a mixture of ethyl acetate and chloroform (vol/vol, 1:1) at pH 7.0. The extract was evaporated in vacuum to dryness, and the residue was dissolved in a minute amount of dry choloroform to which petroleum ether (boiling point, 40 to 60°C) was then added till turbidity appeared. The mixture was left for complete precipitation in a refrigerator and was subsequently separated by centrifugation as a light-brown powder.

The use of thin-layer Silica Gel G F254 and Whatman no. 1 cellulose strips revealed that the crude preparation was composed of three active principles, A, B, and C, contaminated with some inactive materials. For purification, a 200-mg portion of crude preparation was chromatographed on a cellulose CF11 column and eluted with a mixture of chloroform-petroleum ether (vol/vol, 1:1). Three colored, active substances were separated; fraction A (the fastest) was yellowish (1 mg), fraction B, which eluted next was greenish brown (70 mg), and fraction C, which eluted last, was reddish brown (15.4 mg). Fraction B was further purified with preparative Silica Gel G plates using a chloroform-petroleum ether mixture (vol/vol, 1:1) as a developing solvent. Twenty-three milligrams of pure cairomycin B was obtained.

RESULTS AND DISCUSSION

Physical properties. The pure antibiotic melts at 120 to 121°C. It is readily soluble in chloroform, ethyl acetate, and acetone but in-

TABLE 2. *Antibacterial spectrum of cairomycin B using serial agar dilution method*[a]

Test organism[b]	Resistance to other antimicrobials[c]	MIC (μg/ml) after 24 h
Staphylococcus aureus		0.78
S. aureus 209.P		0.78
S. aureus (Terashima's strain)		0.78
S. aureus (Smith's strain)		0.78
S. aureus 252 R	PC, SM, TC, EM, LM, SPM	0.78
S. aureus 199 R	SM, KM, TC, EM, LM	0.78
S. aureus 644 R	EM, SPM	0.78
S. epidermidis 10131	TC, KM, CP, STH, SM	0.78
S. epidermidis (Kawamura's strain)		0.78
Streptococcus faecalis		0.78
S. faecalis (Urayama's strain)	TC, STH, SM, KM, LM, LIM	0.78
Sarcina lutea PCI-1001		0.78
Bacillus subtilis PCI-219		0.78
Escherichia coli NIHJ		100
E. coli K-12		100
E. coli 33-R	PC, SM, KM, TC, CP	100
Salmonella typhimurium		100
Klebsiella pneumoniae PCF602		100
K. pneumoniae R	PC, SM, KM, TC, CP, CI, PL	100
Pseudomonas aeruginosa A3		50
P. aeruginosa 35P	PC, CET, CER, SM, KM, CP	100
Proteus mirabilis 1698		100
Mycobacterium tuberculosis H37RV		50 (14 days)

[a] Medium for all species but *Mycobacterium* was heart infusion agar; *Mycobacterium* was grown in Kirchner medium.

[b] Test organisms were kindly supplied by Tomohoru Okuda, Director of Microbial Chemistry Research Laboratory, Tanabe Seiyaku Co. Ltd., Japan.

[c] EM, Erythromycin; LM, leucomycin; LIM, lincomycin; SPM, spiramycin; CP, chloramphenicol; TC, tetracycline; PC, penicillin; SM, streptomycin; KM, kanamycin; STH, streptothricin; CET, cephalothin; CER, cephaloridine; CI, colistin; PL, polymixin.

TABLE 3. *Antifungal spectrum of cairomycin B using serial agar dilution method*

Fungus[a]	MIC (μg/ml) after 5 days
Trichophyton asteroides	50
T. granulasis	50
T. violaceum	50
T. concentricum	50
Mucor canis	50
Aspergillus fumigatus	50
Candida albicans	50 (2 days)

[a] Fungi were grown in Sabouraud agar. Test organisms were kindly supplied by Tomhoru Okuda, Tanabe Seiyaku Co. Ltd., Japan.

soluble in petroleum and water. The antibiotic has a molar extinction coefficient of 228 at 290 nm. The infrared spectrum of cairomycin B showed absorption at wavelengths of 760, 850, 1,060, 1,243, 1,280, 1,385, 1,435, 1,475, 1,502, 1,625, and 1,695 nm.

Cairomycin B did not migrate on cellulose thin-layer chromatography when developed with methanol, petroleum ether, distilled water, acidified water, and ethyl acetate, whereas it did move with the solvent front of chloroform, ethyl acetate, and acetone. Chloroform-petroleum ether (vol/vol, 1:1) and water saturated with ethyl acetate move the spot of the antibiotic to R_f values of 0.5 and 0.49, respectively. Location of the zones occupied by the antibiotic was determined visually and bioautographically using *Staphylococcus aureus* as the test organism. One definite inhibition zone was always observed.

Chemical properties. Elemental analysis yielded the following data, which correspond to the empirical formula $C_{10}H_{15}N_3O_3$: calculated, $C_{53.33}$, $H_{6.67}$, $N_{18.67}$, and $O_{21.33}$; found, $C_{53.26}$, $H_{6.70}$, $N_{18.72}$, and $O_{21.32}$. Cairomycin B showed a negative response to the following chemical tests: Molisch, Fehling, Biuret, Millons, Sakaguchi, Tollens, and nitration. Also, it did not react with alkaline permanganate, ninhydrin reagent, ferric chloride, and iodine solutions and was reduced with cold acidic permanganate.

After hydrolysis of the pure antibiotic with 6 N HCl at 105°C for 24 h, aspartic acid and lysine were the only products that could be detected. The abundant peaks in mass spectrum analysis of the pure antibiotic are shown in Table 1.

In light of the elemental analysis, acid hydrolysis of the antibiotic and data collected from mass, ultraviolet, and infrared spectra, the following structural formula is suggested.

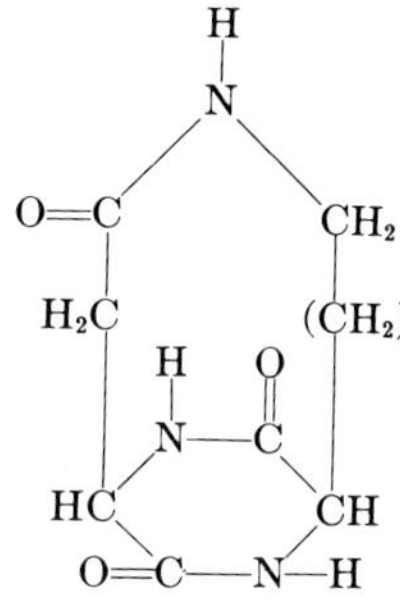

Biological properties. The minimal inhibitory concentrations (MICs) of cairomycin B for a variety of microorganisms are given in Tables 2 and 3. Determination of the MIC was carried out using the following medium (g/100 ml): yeast extract, 0.15; beef extract, 0.15; peptone, 0.5; glucose, 0.1; K_2HPO_4, 0.13; and NaCl, 0.35; the pH was adjusted to 7.0 before sterilization. The test organisms were kindly supplied by Tomohoru Okuda. The results shown in Tables 2 and 3 demonstrate that cairomycin B is mainly active against gram-positive bacteria, whereas very limited activities were exerted against a few of the gram-negative bacteria and fungi.

In vivo tests were then carried out using male Swiss mice, 4 weeks of age. The antibiotic was administered intraperitoneally, and the mice were observed for 7 days, when a delayed toxicity was noticed. The mean lethal dose was 12.5 mg/kg of body weight. The mean protective dose of cairomycin B was 3 mg/kg of body weight using the Swiss mice and *S. aureus*; the challenge inoculum was 2.2×10^4 cells per mouse. The infected animals were kept under observation for 10 days.

Cairomycin B is unique among other antibiotics of a similar nature in its structure, amino acid content, and biological properties. Although amphomycin (1) and aspartocin (2) contain, in their acid hydrolysates, aspartic acid and lysine, among other hydrolytic products, these antibiotics are still distinctly different from cairomycin B in other properties.

LITERATURE CITED

1. **Heinemann, B., and M. A. Kaplan.** 1953. Amphomycin, a new antibiotic. Antibiot. Chemother. 3:1239–1242.
2. **Shay, A. J., and J. Adam.** 1960. Aspartocin. I. Production, isolation and characteristics. Antibiot. Annu., p. 194.

ANTIMICROBIAL AGENTS AND CHEMOTHERAPY, Mar. 1977, p. 376-382 Vol. 11, No. 3

Bacteriostatic and Bactericidal Activities of Selected Beta-Lactam Antibiotics Studied on Agar Plates

GOHTA MASUDA,* SUSUMU TOMIOKA, HIROSHI UCHIDA, AND MITSUTO HASEGAWA

Department of Medicine, School of Medicine, Keio University, and Section of Microbiology, Central Laboratory Department, Keio University Hospital, Shinanomachi, Shinjuku-ku, Tokyo, Japan*

Received for publication 3 September 1976

A novel and time-saving method for assessing bactericidal activities of β-lactam antibiotics on agar plates is described. Minimal inhibitory concentrations (MICs) were determined by the agar dilution method. A potent β-lactamase solution was sprayed onto the plates to inactivate the antibiotic. After further incubation at 37°C overnight, the minimal concentration at which no visible growth occurred on the plates was defined as minimal bactericidal concentration (MBC). With undiluted culture as the inoculum, strains of *Staphylococcus aureus, Escherichia coli,* and *Klebsiella pneumoniae* showed a marked increase in MBC values compared with the values of MIC. There was a marked decrease in both the MICs and MBCs with diminution of inoculum size. The two concentrations were almost the same when the inoculum size was decreased to a 10^{-4} dilution. In contrast, MIC and MBC for enterococci showed no marked decrease with decrease in inoculum size. Although the present study was performed with β-lactamase-unstable penicillins and cephalosporins, the method can be applicable with any β-lactam antibiotic if optimal and potent enzymes are available.

In some special clinical situations, minimal bactericidal concentrations (MBCs) should be determined rather than minimal inhibitory concentrations (MICs) of the antibiotic to be used. At present, MBC can be determined by a loop transfer method following the broth dilution MIC determination; however, the whole procedure is time-consuming.

In the present paper, a simple method is described to assess bactericidal activities of selected β-lactam antibiotics on agar plates.

(This paper was presented in part at the 15th Interscience Conference on Antimicrobial Agents and Chemotherapy, Washington, D.C., 24-26 September 1975.)

MATERIALS AND METHODS

Bacterial strains. All clinical strains were isolated recently at the Keio University Hospital, Tokyo. They were identified as *Staphylococcus aureus* (18 strains), enterococcus (20 strains), *Escherichia coli* (18 strains), and *Klebsiella pneumoniae* (25 strains). The standard strain of *S. aureus* 209P was also used.

Antibiotics. Each of the laboratory standards was supplied by the pharmaceutical company listed in parentheses after the antibiotic: benzylpenicillin (Takeda Chemical Co., Ltd., Osaka), ampicillin (Fujisawa Pharmaceutical Co., Ltd., Osaka), amoxicillin (Fujisawa Pharmaceutical Co., Ltd., Osaka), cephalexin (Shionogi Pharmaceutical Co., Ltd., Osaka), cephaloridine (Shionogi Pharmaceutical Co., Ltd., Osaka), cephalothin (Shionogi Pharmaceutical Co., Ltd., Osaka), and cefazolin (Fujisawa Pharmaceutical Co., Ltd., Osaka). A phosphate buffer solution (pH adjusted to 7.2) was used for the dilution of antibiotics and specimens throughout the experiments.

Media. Heart infusion agar (Difco) and heart infusion broth (Difco) were used.

β-Lactamases. A commercial preparation of penicillinase (Penase, Difco; 50,000 U/ml) was used to inactivate the penicillins. One milliliter of the enzyme solution inactivated up to 5,000,000 μg of each benzylpenicillin, ampicillin and amoxicillin in liquid medium, as assayed by the method described elsewhere (6). A crude enzyme solution obtained by filtering the broth culture of a strain of *Enterobacter cloacae,* known to be a potent β-lactamase producer, was used to inactivate the cephalosporins. One milliliter of the solution was capable of inactivating 350,000 μg of cephaloridine, 300,000 μg of cephalothin or cefazolin, and 200,000 μg of cephalexin, respectively, in liquid medium. This solution was kept at −20°C in a deep freezer until used.

Determination of MIC and MBC in agar. Heart infusion agar plates (10 ml) with serial twofold dilutions of each β-lactam antibiotic were prepared in 90-mm petri dishes. Inoculum sizes were undiluted (10^8 to 10^9 cells/ml), and overnight cultures were diluted to a 10^{-2} dilution (10^6 to 10^7 cells/ml) and a 10^{-4} dilution (10^4 to 10^5 cells/ml). Each of these inocula was inoculated on the agar plates by the use of inocula-replicating apparatus and transferred by a

0.001-ml calibrated loop. These plates were incubated at 37°C overnight. The MIC was defined as the minimal antibiotic concentration that yielded complete inhibition of the bacteria on the plates. β-Lactamase solution was then sprayed uniformly onto the plates by using a perfume atomizer. The amount of the enzyme solution added was about 0.1 ml per plate. These plates were incubated again at 37°C overnight. The minimal antibiotic concentration at which no visible growth occurred on the plates after incubation was arbitrarily defined as MBC. MIC and MBC values were studied in relation to inoculum size.

Confirmative study of antibiotic inactivation on the agar plates. A control study was also carried out simultaneously using the same agar plates that were being used for the determination of MBC values. The strain most susceptible to the antibiotic, the MIC of which was being determined by the study, was selected as the control organism. A loopful (0.001 ml) of a 10^{-4} culture (the greatest dilution used in the study) of the control strain was additionally inoculated on the agar plates that had already undergone β-lactamase treatment. After further incubation at 37°C overnight, the plates showing visible growth of the control bacteria were considered to be optimal for determining MBC values.

Diffusion of β-lactamase into the agar layer. Five milliliters of heart infusion agar containing 1,600 μg of ampicillin per ml of medium was poured into a 90-mm petri dish. After drying, four stainless-steel cylinders (8 mm in diameter) were placed on the agar plate. Additionally, 5 ml of heart infusion agar containing 1,600 μg of ampicillin and cells of *S. aureus* 209P in the concentration of about 10^7 viable cells per ml of medium were poured onto the plate. After solidification, the cylinders were removed, resulting in holes in the plate. A 0.025-ml sample of undiluted and 10-fold, 100-fold, and 1,000-fold diluted penicillinase solutions (Penase, 50,000 U/ml) was introduced in each of the holes on the plate. This plate was allowed to stand in a freezer at 4°C up to 3 h. The plate was then incubated at 37°C overnight (Fig. 1).

Demonstration of inactivation of ampicillin by the application of β-lactamase. A heart infusion agar plate containing 1,600 μg of ampicillin per ml of medium was prepared. A 0.1-ml sample of the penicillinase solution was sprayed onto the agar plate. After drying, each of the undiluted and 10^{-1},

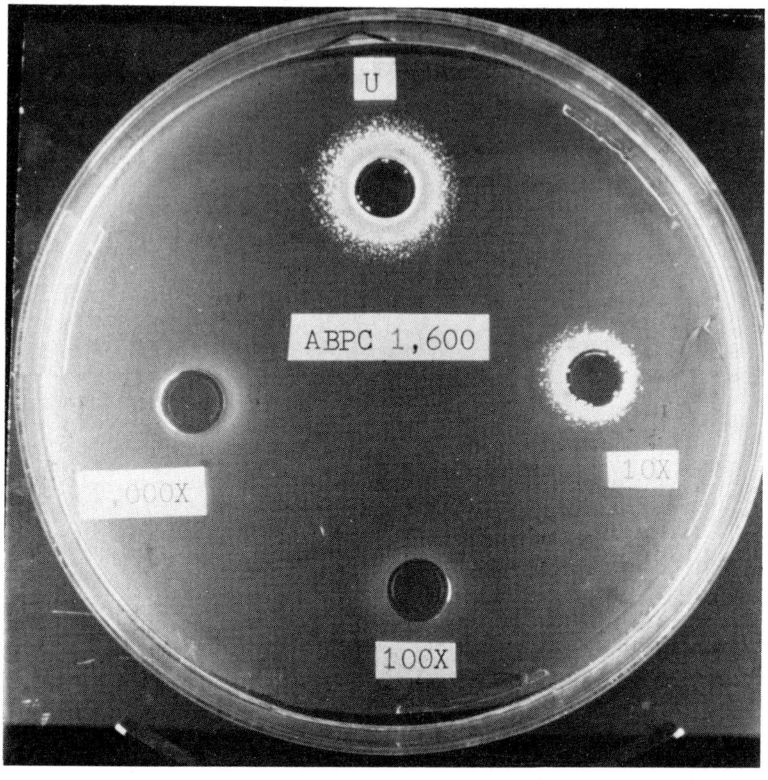

FIG. 1. *Diffusion of β-lactamase into the agar layer of a plate prepared with 1,600 μg of ampicillin (ABPC) and S. aureus 209P at the concentratin of about 10^7 cells per ml of medium. A 0.025-ml sample of variously diluted penicillinase solution had been introduced into each hole on the plate. Around the two holes containing undiluted (U) and 10-fold-diluted (10×) penicillinase solution, growth of S. aureus 209P is apparent. Around the two holes with high dilutions (100× and 1,000×) of the enzyme solution, no growth is visible.*

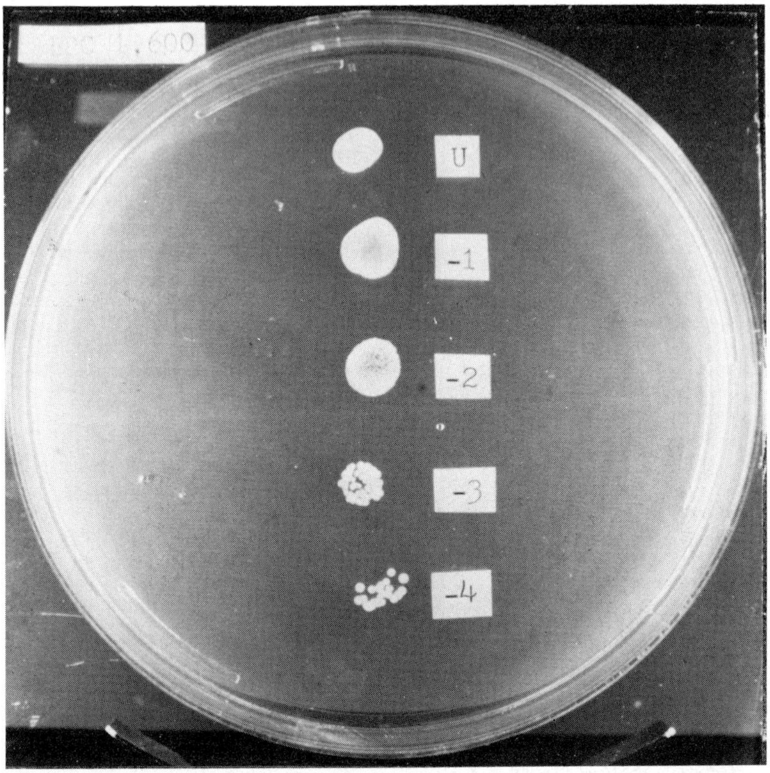

FIG. 2. *Inactivation of ampicillin on an agar plate. The surface of an agar plate containing 1,600 μg of ampicillin per ml of medium was treated with β-lactamase spray. After incubation at 37°C overnight, each of the diluted (U) and 10^{-1} (expressed as −1), 10^{-2} (−2), 10^{-3} (−3), and 10^{-4} diluted overnight cultures of S. aureus 209P formed colonies on the plate.*

10^{-2}, 10^{-3}, and 10^{-4} dilutions of overnight cultures of the standard strain of *S. aureus* 209P, a strain susceptible to ampicillin, was inoculated onto the agar plate. The plate was then incubated at 37°C overnight (Fig. 2).

RESULTS

MIC and MBC values. Figure 3 represents the cumulative percentage of 18 strains of *S. aureus* inhibited (MIC) and/or killed (MBC) by benzylpenicillin, ampicillin, and amoxicillin. With undiluted culture as the inoculum, almost 50% of the strains were inhibited by 25 μg of either of these antibiotics per ml, whereas concentrations as high as 1,600 μg of these drugs per ml killed only 40 to 50% of the strains. The MIC and MBC values markedly decreased in accordance with diminution of inoculum size. The two values almost agreed when the 10^{-4} dilution was used as the inoculum. A concentration of 1.56 μg of these drugs per ml was bacteriostatic or bactericidal for 80 to 90% of these strains. With this dilution, 12.5 μg of these drugs per ml achieved bacteriostatic and bactericidal effect for all the strains tested.

Figure 4 depicts the result obtained with enterococci and the three penicillin antibiotics. With undiluted culture as the inoculum, 6.25 μg of benzylpenicillin, 3.13 μg of ampicillin, or 0.78 μg of amoxicillin per ml each completely inhibited the growth of the test strains, whereas an excess of 1,600 μg of each of these drugs per ml was needed to kill all of the strains tested. In contrast to the *S. aureus*, the inoculum effect of enterococci on MIC and MBC values was smaller. At the 10^{-4} dilution, MIC values of the three penicillins decreased about twofold more than those obtained with the undiluted culture. Likewise, MBC values did not show a marked decrease with decrease in inoculum size.

The result with *E. coli* and the two penicillins and cephalosporins is presented in Fig. 5. With undiluted culture as the inoculum, cefazolin showed the most potent bacteriostatic activity to all of the *E. coli* strains. Cephalothin was less potent bacteriostatically than ampicillin and amoxicillin for almost one-half of the strains, whereas the remaining half were resistant to 1,600 μg of ampicillin and amoxicillin per ml. Such resistant strains also showed high MIC and MBC values at the inoculum size of 10^{-4} dilution.

Figure 6 represents the result using 25 strains of *K. pneumoniae* with cephalexin, cephaloridine, cephalothin, and cefazolin. With undiluted culture, 25 μg of any of these cephalosporin antibiotics per ml was bacteriostatic for 70 to 85% of the *Klebsiella* stains. In contrast, 1,600 μg of these drugs per ml was bactericidal for less than 50% of the strains of *K. pneumoniae*. A marked decrease in MIC and

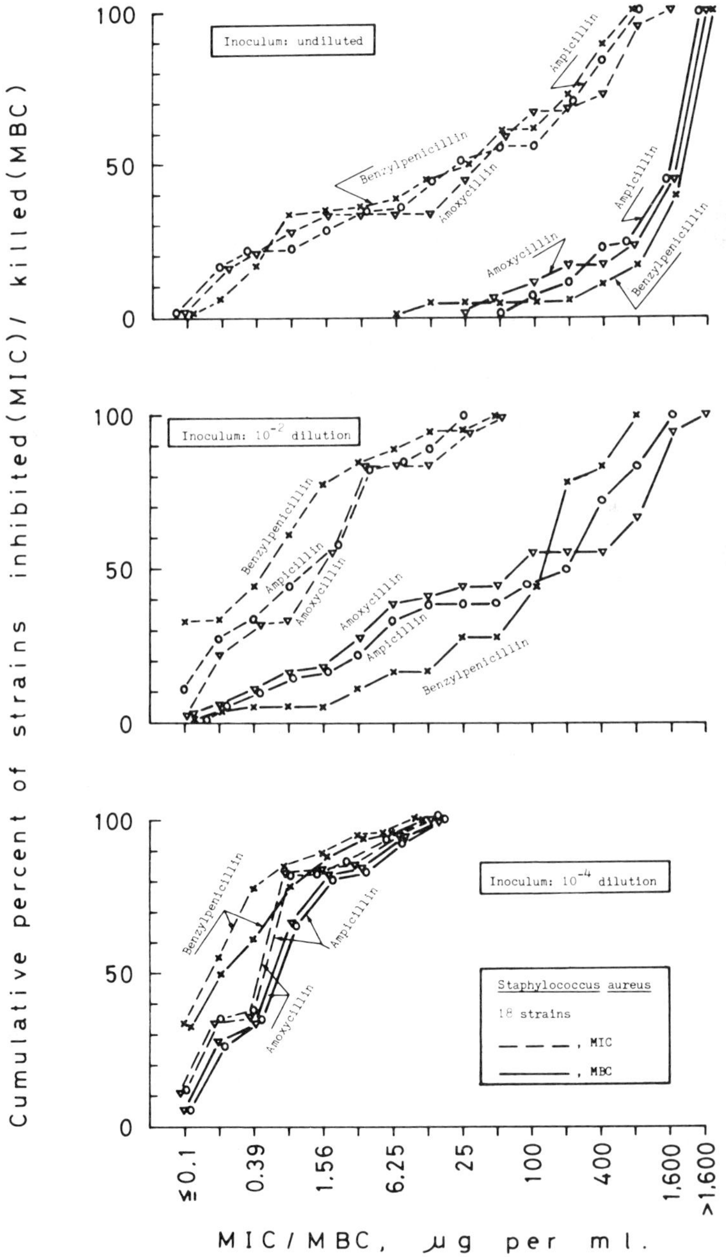

Fig. 3. *Bacteriostatic (MIC) and/or bactericidal activities (MBC) of three penicillins against 18 strains of S. aureus. Symbols:* ×, *benzylpenicillin;* ○, *ampicillin;* ∇, *amoxicillin;* -----, *MIC;* ——, *MBC.*

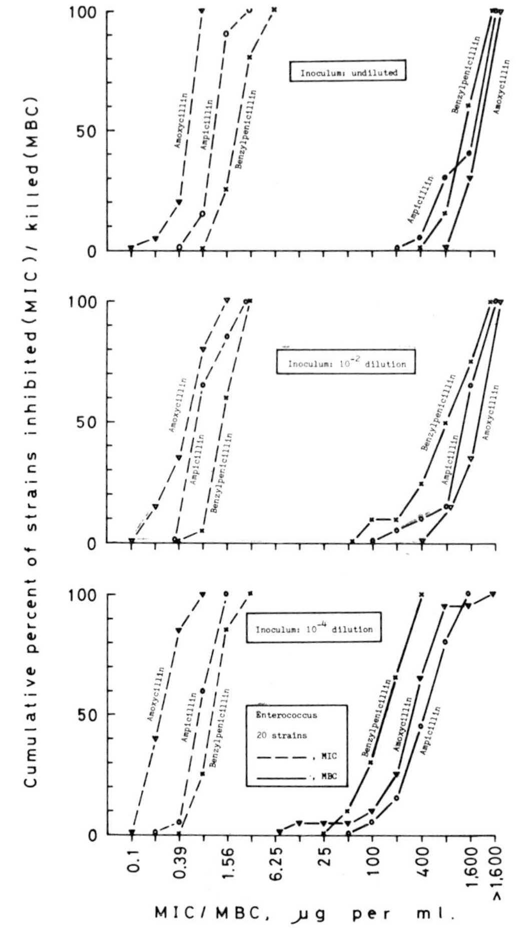

FIG. 4. *Bacteriostatic (MIC) and/or bactericidal activities (MBC) of three penicillins against 20 strains of enterococcus. Symbols: ×, benzylpenicillin; ○, ampicillin; ∇, amoxicillin; -----, MIC; ———, MBC.*

MBC values was obtained in accordance with the decrease in inoculum size. At the 10^{-4} dilution, as high as 6.25 μg of any of these four cephalosporins per ml showed the activity of inhibiting and/or killing to about 80 to 90% of the strains. With this light inoculum, the concentration of 12.5 μg of cephalexin or cefazolin per ml and 25 μg of cephalothin or cephaloridine per ml was enough to inhibit or kill all the strains of *K. pneumoniae* used in the study.

Diffusion of β-lactamase into the agar layer. Growth of *S. aureus* 209P became visible in and on the agar plate to a significant extent surrounding the holes that contained high concentrations of penicillinase solution (Fig. 1). The growth demonstrates the inactivation of ampicillin by the potent penicillinase used. The result suggests that the β-lactam antibiotic significantly loses its activity in the presence of a potent enzyme.

Demonstration of inactivation of ampicillin on an agar plate. Cells of *S. aureus* 209P formed colonies on the agar plate (Fig. 2). The colonies indicated by the position "−4" originated from the inoculum of a 10^{-4} dilution (10 to 10^2 viable cells). This inoculum was the most susceptible to ampicillin among the variously diluted inocula used to study inoculum effect. Such growth demonstrates that ampicillin has significantly lost its potency on the agar surface due to the action of β-lactamase.

DISCUSSION

In this paper we report on comparative studies on bacteriostatic and bactericidal activities of β-lactam antibiotics performed by use of a novel method which had been developed in our laboratory.

The MICs of selected β-lactam antibiotics for several common bacteria were similar to those from other studies. Inoculum effect on MICs was also studied. It is generally accepted that inoculum has a considerable effect on MIC with the β-lactam antibiotics (3, 4). In our study, a marked inoculum effect on MICs was also demonstrated with *S. aureus, E. coli,* and *K. pneumoniae*. Here, almost half the strains of *E. coli* were highly resistant to ampicillin and amoxicillin, which showed no obvious inoculum effect within the range of drug concentrations studied. Presumably, this high drug resistance may be attributable to the intrinsic resistance of the bacteria. With the enterococci, the inoculum effect was smaller.

The MBCs measured were high when the inoculum size was large, whereas these values also decreased in accordance with the decrease in inoculum size. At the 10^{-4} dilution, MICs and MBCs for *S. aureus, E. coli,* and *K. pneumoniae* were almost identical. The MBCs for gram-negative bacteria reported from other institutions were almost the same or slightly higher than the values obtained in the present study (2, 8). A preliminary report from our laboratory with a small number of bacterial strains indicated that the MBC with a light inoculum was almost equal or larger in broth than in agar (5). A discrepancy was observed with the enterococci, however, between the MBCs obtained by the two different methods. With a light inoculum, the MBC for enterococcus strains obtained by the conventional procedure (1, 7) was considerably lower than that obtained by the agar plate method used here.

The β-lactamase solution diffused into the

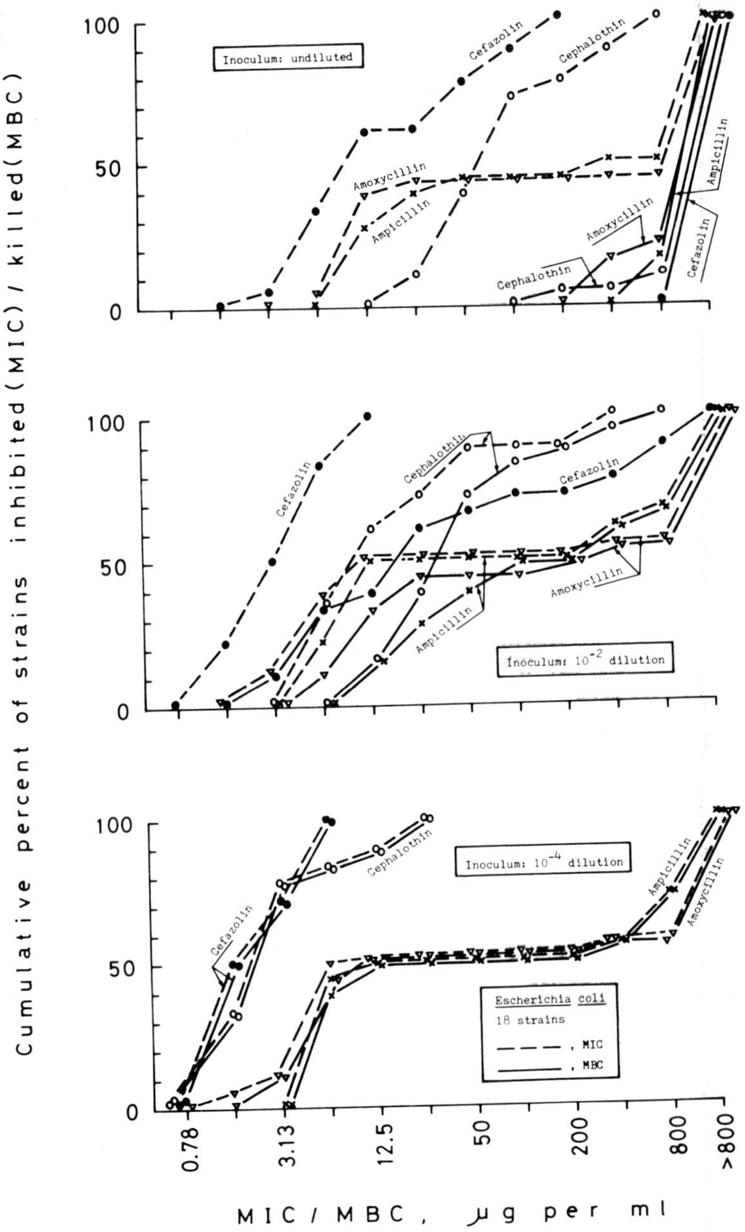

FIG. 5. *Bacteriostatic (MIC) and/or bactericidal activities (MBC) of two penicillins and cephalosporins against 18 strains of E. coli. Symbols: ×, ampicillin; ∇, amoxicillin; ○, cephalothin; ●, cefazolin; -----, MIC; ———, MBC.*

agar layer that produces inactivation of high concentrations of the β-lactam antibiotics adjacent to the enzyme solution. The result indicates that the antibiotic inactivation occurs on the agar surface by the β-lactamase sprayed onto the agar plate. The growth of the ampicillin-susceptible strain on the β-lactamase-treated agar plate also demonstrated that the drug concentration on the agar plate is almost negligible (Fig. 2). However, the possibility still remains that, in some instances, the small amounts of antibiotic activity remaining on the agar surface will influence the MBC values obtained by the method presented. Hence, the

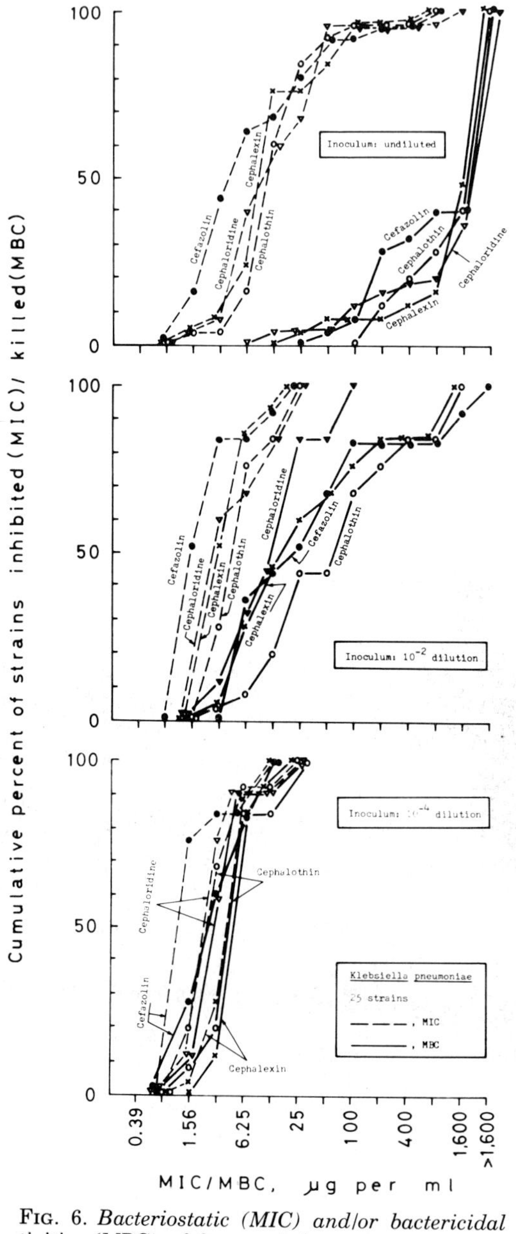

FIG. 6. *Bacteriostatic (MIC) and/or bactericidal activities (MBC) of four cephalosporins against 25 strains of K. pneumoniae. Symbols: ×, cephalexin; ▽, cephaloridine; ○, cephalothin; ●, cefazolin, ------, MIC; ———, MBC.*

use of the 10^{-4} dilution of the most susceptible strain in the experiment, as the indicator, may tentatively be acceptable in the method for determining MBC values.

If one wants to determine quantitative bactericidal activities of the antibiotics, i.e., the concentrations producing a 99.9% kill (arbitrarily defined as minimal lethal concentration) by the agar plate method, a 10^{-2} dilution of overnight cultures (each containing 10^6 to 10^7 cells per ml) plated by a 0.001-ml calibrated loop (10^3 to 10^4 inoculated cells) is recommended. The minimal lethal concentrations could be determined as the lowest concentrations that yield no more than a few colonies at the time of MBC determination. In some instances, however, the inoculum size could be replaced by a 10^{-3} dilution with a 0.01-ml calibrated loop which also produces 10^3 to 10^4 viable cells at the time of inoculation.

Although the present study was performed only with β-lactamase-unstable penicillins and cephalosporins, the method can be applicable to any antibiotic where optimal and potent enzymes are available. The method presented is simple and time-saving for assessing bacteriostatic and bactericidal activities of β-lactam antibiotics against a number of bacterial strains. The method can be useful in the comparison of antibacterial activities of β-lactam antibiotics in the laboratory.

ACKNOWLEDGMENTS

This work was supported by a grant from the Japanese Ministry of Education.

LITERATURE CITED

1. **Beaty, H. N., M. Turck, and R. G. Petersdorf.** 1967. Activity of broad-spectrum antibiotics against enterococci and their efficacy in enterococcal endocarditis. Ann. N. Y. Acad. Sci. **145**:464–472.
2. **Bergeron, M. G., J. L. Brusch, M. Barza, and L. Weinstein.** 1973. Bactericidal activity and pharmacology of cefazolin. Antimicrob. Agents Chemother. **4**:396–401.
3. **Ericsson, H. M., and J. C. Sherris.** 1971. Antibiotic sensitivity testing. Report of an international collaborative study. Acta Pathol. Microbiol. Scand. Sect. B. **217**(Suppl.):1–90.
4. **Hamilton-Miller, J. M. T., J. T. Smith, and R. Knox.** 1964. Effect of penicillinase on the activity of penicillins. Nature (London) **201**:867–868.
5. **Masuda, G.** 1976. Studies on bactericidal activities of β-lactam antibiotics on agar plates: the correlation with the antibacterial activities determined by the conventional methods. J. Antibiot. (Tokyo) **29**:1237–1240.
6. **Masuda, G., S. Tomioka, and M. Hasegawa.** 1976. Detection of β-lactamase production by gram-negative bacteria. J. Antibiot. (Tokyo) **29**:662–664.
7. **Simon, H. J.** 1967. Antimicrobial susceptibility of group D hemolytic streptococci (enterococci). Am. J. Med. Sci. **253**:14–18.
8. **Turck, M., R. A. Clark, H. N. Beaty, K. K. Holmes, W. W. Karney, and L. B. Reller.** 1973. Cefazolin in the treatment of bacterial pneumonia. J. Infect. Dis. **128**(Suppl.):S382–385.

ANTIMICROBIAL AGENTS AND CHEMOTHERAPY, Mar. 1977, p. 383-387 Vol. 11, No. 3

Plasmid-Mediated Chloramphenicol Resistance in *Haemophilus influenzae*

B. VAN KLINGEREN,* J. D. A. VAN EMBDEN, AND M. DESSENS-KROON

Laboratory for Chemotherapy and Laboratory for Bacteriology, National Institute of Public Health, Bilthoven, The Netherlands

Received for publication 20 September 1976

A clinical isolate of *Haemophilus influenzae* HC234 was found to be resistant to chloramphenicol and tetracycline. It was shown that both resistance markers are tranferable as one unit to other *Haemophilus influenzae* strains and also to *Escherichia coli*. Data are presented which indicate that conjugation is the most likely mechanism of resistance transfer. HC234 was shown to carry a single plasmid species with a molecular weight of 38×10^6.

Recent investigations have shown the existence of plasmid-mediated drug resistance in *Haemophilus influenzae* (2, 3, 5, 17). Transfer of resistance, probably by conjugation, was demonstrated for resistance to ampicillin (13, 15) and for resistance to kanamycin (3). Recently, we reported on a chloramphenicol (Cm)-resistant strain of *H. influenzae* isolated from the pharynx of a patient with lymphatic leukemia (10). The resistance to Cm appeared to be due to the production of an enzyme, presumably an acetyltransferase, inactivating this antibiotic. The strain was also resistant to tetracycline (Tc).

This report describes experiments on the transfer of the resistance determinants to susceptible strains of *H. influenzae* and to a strain of *Escherichia coli*. Also, the isolation and characterization of plasmid deoxyribonucleic acid (DNA) from the resistant strain are reported.

MATERIALS AND METHODS

Bacterial strains. The strains used in this study are listed in Table 1. The rifampin- and streptomycin-resistant mutant strains HC215-1, HC217-1, and HC218-1 were obtained by selection on plates containing these antibiotics. All strains of *H. influenzae* investigated in this study were untypable according to Pittman's agglutination method (12). The strain of *E. coli* K-12 (SC181) was kindly provided by E. Lederberg (Stanford University).

Media. Nutrient broth was prepared in this institute from fresh meat and contained in addition 0.5% NaCl, 1% peptone (Difco) and 0.069% Na_2CO_3; the pH was 7.5. Nutrient agar contained, in addition, 2% agar (BBL).

NXV broth was nutrient broth, supplemented with 4% X factor and 4% V factor. X and V factors were freshly prepared from lysed horse blood and lysed yeast cells, respectively. NXV agar was prepared by adding 2% agar to NSV broth.

Stock cultures of *H. influenzae* were maintained and transferred every 2 weeks in semisolid NXV medium containing 1% agar (BBL).

Susceptibility tests were usually carried out on NXV agar. Wellcotest agar, supplemented with X and V factors was used for establishing the susceptibility to cotrimoxazole.

Determination of MICs. The minimum inhibitory concentrations (MICs) were determined by agar dilution, using a Steers replicator. As inocula, undiluted overnight cultures (10^8 to 10^9 colony-forming units/ml) and also the dilutions 10^{-1}, 10^{-2}, and 10^{-3} were used. The antibiotics used were: Cm (Globenicol, Mycofarm), Tc (Tifaco), ampicillin sodium (Amfipen, Mycofarm), erythromycin (Erythrocin, Ab-

TABLE 1. *Bacterial strains used*

Strain	Relevant properties[a]
HC234	Clinical isolate of *H. influenzae*; resistant to Cm and Tc (10)
HC215	Clinical isolate of *H. influenzae*; susceptible to Cm and Tc
HC217	Clinical isolate of *H. influenzae*; susceptible to Cm and Tc
HC218	Clinical isolate of *H. influenzae*; susceptible to Cm and Tc
HC215-1	Mutant of HC215; resistant to rifampin and streptomycin
HC217-1	Mutant of HC217; resistant to rifampin and streptomycin
HC218-1	Mutant of HC218; resistant to rifampin and streptomycin
HC25	Clinical isolate of *H. influenzae*; resistant to ampicillin
SC181	*E. coli* K-12, F$^-$, *leu thi lac sup-44 tonA21 thr chl hsrB*

[a] The nomenclature employed here conforms to the recommendations of Demerec et al. (4), Taylor and Trotter (14), and Novick et al. (11).

bott), kanamycin (Kanymex, Mycofarm), gentamicin (Garamycin, Schering), trimethoprim (Hoffmann-La Roche), and sulfamethoxazole (Hoffmann-La Roche).

Transfer of drug resistance. Matings in liquid medium were carried out by mixing equal volumes of overnight cultures of the donor and the recipient strain, followed by overnight incubation at 37°C. Matings on filters were performed as follows. One-milliliter portions of 1:1 mixtures of overnight cultures of the donor and the recipient were filtered through 13-mm cellulose nitrate filters (Sartorius; pore size, 0.45 μm). The filters were incubated at 37°C during variable times on the surface of NXV agar plates. The filters then were shaken vigorously in 1 ml of NXV broth. Dilutions were plated on NXV agar, supplemented with the appropriate antibiotics (Cm, 2 μg/ml; Tc, 4 μg/ml; and rifampin, 10 μg/ml). To confirm that suspected transcipient colonies were derivatives of the recipient, and not rifampicin-resistant mutants of the donor, replica plating was carried out on plates supplemented with streptomycin (100 μg/ml).

In transfer experiments using *E. coli* as the recipient, dilutions of the mixture of donor and recipient cells were plated on nutrient agar supplemented with Cm (32 μg/ml) or Tc (32 μg/ml).

Isolation and characterization of plasmid DNA. Plasmid DNA was isolated from *H. influenzae* as covalently closed circular DNA (ccc DNA). Cells were lysed by Triton X-100 and, after sedimenting the bulk chromosomal DNA, ccc DNA was separated and purified by equilibrium centrifugation in cesium chloride in the presence of ethidium bromide, as described by Elwell et al. (5). To convert ccc DNA to the open circular form, preparations of ccc DNA were irradiated with ^{60}Co gamma rays for a dose of 2,000 rads (dose rate, 20,000 rads/h).

Electron microscopy of irradiated plasmid DNA preparations and contour length measurements of the molecules have been described previously (16).

RESULTS

MICs. The results of the MIC determinations against the *H. influenzae* strains are listed in Table 2. Strain HC234 appears to be resistant to both Cm and Tc. In comparison with susceptible strains of *H. Influenzae*, a 32- to 64-fold increase in the resistance to these antibiotics was observed. The MICs of both Cm and Tc were influenced very little by the size of the inoculum. HC234 was found to be susceptible to the other drugs tested.

Stability of drug resistance in strain HC234. To see whether there was any spontaneous loss of Cm and Tc resistance, daily transfers (dilution, 1:10^4) were carried out in drug-free NXV broth. After 6 weeks of repeated transfers, no drug-susceptible variants of HC234 were found among any of the approximately 3,000 colonies tested. An attempt was undertaken to cure the cells of the resistance markers by daily transfers for 3 weeks in NXV broth supplemented with 4 μg of ethidium bromide per ml, the highest concentration permitting growth. No loss of resistance was found in any of the approximately 1,000 colonies tested. Overnight incubations in NXV broth supplemented with 32 μg of acridine orange per ml, however, yielded 1% of cells "cured" of their resistance to Cm and Tc.

Transferability and kinetics of transfer of Cm and Tc resistance. To learn whether the Cm and Tc resistance determinants of strain HC234 were transferable, mixtures of cultures of this strain and each of the susceptible recipient strains HC215-1, HC217-1, and HC218-1 were incubated overnight in liquid medium and on filters. The results are shown in Table 3.

No transfer to HC215-1 was detectable, either in liquid medium or on filters. The frequency of transfer of resistance markers to HC217-1 and HC218-1 in liquid medium was low. However, incubation on filters resulted in higher transfer rates of both Cm and Tc resistance determinants. As strain HC217-1 proved to be the best recipient, it was used in further experiments.

The kinetics of the transfer of both the drug resistance markers from HC234 to HC217-1 was studied by incubation of mixed cultures on filters for different periods of time. The results are shown graphically in Fig. 1. As shown in this figure, it takes about 3 h of mixed culturing to reach the maximum frequency of transfer,

TABLE 2. *Susceptibility of H. influenzae to several antibiotic drugs*

Strain	MIC (μg/ml; inoculum about 10^6 cells/ml)[a]						
	Ap	Cm	Tc	Em	Km	Gm	Cotrim
HC234	0.5	16	32	4	4	2	0.03[b]
HC215-1	0.25	0.5	0.5	2	4	2	0.03
HC217-1	0.25	0.5	0.5	2	2	1	0.03
HC218-1	0.25	0.25	0.5	2	4	2	0.03

[a] Ap, Ampicillin; Cm, chloramphenicol; Tc, tetracycline; Em, erythromycin; Km, kanamycin; Gm, gentamicin; cotrim (cotrimoxazole), sulfamethoxazole + trimethoprim in a ratio of 20:1.

[b] For Cotrim, 0.03 = 0.03 μg of TMP per ml + 0.6 μg of SMZ per ml.

TABLE 3. *Transfer frequencies of Cm and Tc resistance of strain HC234 to various recipient strains of H. influenzae*[a]

Recipient	Matings in liquid medium	Matings on filter
HC215-1	$<10^{-8}$	$<10^{-8}$
HC217-1	10^{-7}	10^{-3}–10^{-4}
HC218-1	10^{-8}	10^{-6}

[a] Matings were carried out overnight as described in Materials and Methods. Transfer frequencies are expressed as the number of drug-resistant transcipient cells per total number of donor cells.

i.e., 10^{-3} to 10^{-4} per donor cell. No drug-resistant transcipients were found at time zero and after 30 min of mixed incubation.

In all experiments, the Cm and Tc resistance of HC234 behaved virtually as a single unit of transfer. Replica plating of transcipient colonies, selected for Cm resistance, showed that only 6 out of 2,912 colonies were susceptible to Tc. No Cm-susceptible colonies were found among approximately 10^4 transcipient colonies selected on plates supplemented with Tc.

Once transferred to HC217-1, the aquired Cm and Tc resistance determinants were found to be retransferable to an ampicillin-resistant clinical isolate of *H. influenzae* (HC25) as well as to *E. coli* SC181.

Mechanism of resistance transfer. To find out whether or not transformation was the mechanism of drug resistance transfer, filter matings of HC234 × HC217-1 were performed in the presence of 100 μg of deoxyribonuclease I per ml and 0.01 M $MgCl_2$. These substances were added to the donor and recipient cultures 5 min before mixing and also to the agar plates, which were used for incubation of the filters.

The frequency of transfer of Cm and Tc resistance markers in this mating was not influenced by the presence of deoxyribonuclease I. Consequently, transformation seems not to be the mechanism of transfer.

Also, transduction does not seem to be a mechanism of transfer, as was demonstrated as follows. Transfer experiments were carried out under the conditions of the filter matings, except that cell-free filtrates of the donor were used instead of cultures of the donor. No Tc- or Cm-resistant recipient colonies could be found. Also, dilutions of cell-free filtrates of the donor strain, spotted on NXV agar plates 20 min after these plates had been inoculated with a confluent layer of a logarithmically growing culture of the recipient strain HC217-1, did not reveal any plaques.

Since these experiments suggest that neither transformation nor transduction is a mechanism of resistance transfer in strain HC234, it follows that resistance to Cm and Tc is probably transferred by conjugation.

Transfer to *E. coli*. After unsuccessful trials to transfer Cm and Tc resistance from HC234 to *E. coli* SC181 in liquid medium, positive results were obtained with overnight matings on filters. In these experiments, a transfer frequency was observed that ranged from 10^{-6} to 10^{-7} per donor cell. Twenty-nine transcipient colonies selected on Tc-containing medium were found to be also resistant to Cm. However, 25 of 44 transcipient colonies selected for Cm resistance appeared to be susceptible to Tc (2 μg/ml). The MICs of both antibiotics toward resistant transcipients were $\geq$128 μg/ml, whereas the MICs of Cm and Tc towards the recipient strains SC181 were 8 and 2 μg/ml, respectively.

Presence and characterization of plasmid DNA in HC234. After equilibrium centrifugation (in cesium chloride plus ethidium bromide) of cleared lysates of strain HC234, two DNA bands were found, indicating the presence of ccc DNA. Electron photomicrographs of gamma-ray-irradiated preparations of plasmid DNA revealed the presence of only one species of DNA molecules. Twenty molecules were measured,

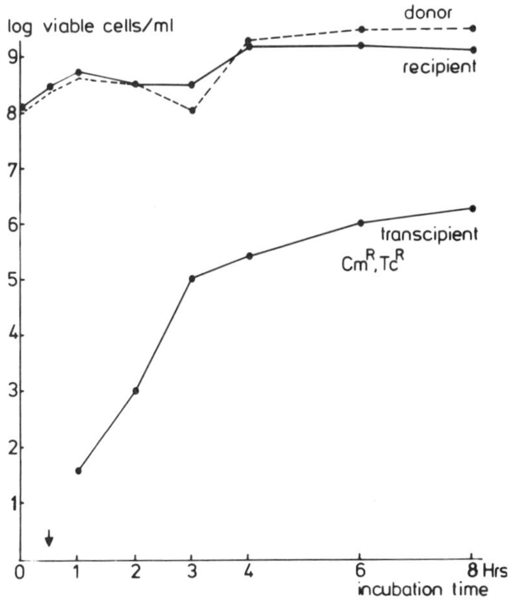

FIG. 1. *Kinetics of transfer of Cm and Tc resistance from H. influenzae HC234 to strain HC217-1 during mixed incubation on membrane filters. At time zero and 30 min, the transfer frequency was below the detection level (arrow).*

and the mean length was found to be 18.4 ± 0.6 μm. This size corresponds to a molecular weight of about 38 × 10^6. This plasmid will be designated as pRI234.

No ccc DNA could be detected in the recipient strain HC217-1. However, in a transcipient (HC217-2), carrying the Cm and Tc resistance markers from HC234, circular DNA was found. The mean contour length of 21 circular molecules was 18.9 ± 0.7 μm.

DISCUSSION

The data presented suggest that the resistance to Cm and Tc in *H. influenzae* HC234 is mediated by a single plasmid. (i) Acridine orange treatment of HC234 results in simultaneous loss of resistance to Cm and Tc. (ii) The drug resistance markers of HC234 are transferred to other *H. influenzae* strains as one single unit of transfer, although occasionally the Tc resistance determinant was lost as a consequence of transfer to the recipient. Furthermore, the acquired resistance of the *H. influenzae* transcipients was retransferable. (iii) Strain HC234 harbors one single plasmid, pRI234, with a molecular weight of 38 × 10^6. A plasmid species of this size was also found in the transcipient HC217-2.

Curing of the resistance markers in HC234 was obtained with acridine orange but not with ethidium bromide. This finding is in accordance with the observations of other investigators, who found that the ampicillin resistance in *H. influenzae* could be cured with acridine orange, but not with ethidium bromide (6, 17).

The most likely mechanism of drug resistance transfer of HC234 is conjugation, since deoxyribonuclease I in the mating mixture did not influence the transfer frequency significantly, and no evidence could be obtained for transduction. Conjugal transfer of ampicillin resistance between *Haemophilus* strains was demonstrated by Thorne and Farrar (15, and cited in reference 8). Conjugation might be the mechanism of transfer of ampicillin resistance as well as was observed by Sykes et al. (13) and in our laboratory (van Klingeren, unpublished observations). The resistance markers of strain HC234 were transferable to *E. coli* K-12, as was found also for a kanamycin resistance plasmid by Dang Van et al. (3). This is in contrast to the findings of de Graaff et al. (8), who attempted unsuccessfully to transfer the conjugative ampicillin resistance plasmid RSF007 to *E. coli* K-12.

Unlike Dang Van et al. (3), we were not able to retransfer the required resistance markers of HC234 once transferred to *E. coli*. Moreover, no ccc DNA could be demonstrated in Cm- and Tc-resistant *E. coli* transconjugants (unpublished observations). Therefore, the resistance determinants of pRI234 are likely to be integrated into the *E. coli* chromosome. A similar phenomenon was observed by Saunders (personal communication), who showed that the ampicillin resistance determinant of *H. influenzae* is integrated into the chromosome of *Pseudomonas aeruginosa* or *E. coli* after conjugal transfer.

The plasmid pRI234 does not seem to be maintained stably in *E. coli* as a plasmid. However, its transferability to an unrelated species like *E. coli* might point to a broad host range like that of the plasmids belonging to compatibility group P (N. Datta, *In Microbiology—1974,* p. 9–15, American Society for Microbiology, Washington D.C., 1974). Therefore, one might speculate that pRI234 is derived from a P-like plasmid. If so, *H. influenzae* HC234 might have acquired its drug resistance by conjugal transfer of such a plasmid from an unrelated organism like *Pseudomonas* or *E. coli,* which are known to carry conjugative plasmids mediating resistance to Cm and Tc. Alternatively, the origin of the drug resistance in HC234 might be similar to that proposed by Falkow and co-workers (5, 8) for the recently observed ampicillin resistance in *H. influenzae:* a conjugative plasmid, indigenous to *H. influenzae,* might have been hooked up with the translocatable sequence TnA, which codes for the widespread TEM-like β-lactamase (9). In analogy, such a plasmid might have acquired a translocatable sequence coding for Cm and Tc resistance. The existance of such translocatable sequences has been demonstrated in some R factors from *Enterobacteriaceae* (1, 7). Further investigations will be carried out to elucidate the origin of the R factor in HC234 and its relatedness to other *Haemophilus* plasmids.

ACKNOWLEDGMENTS

We wish to express our gratitude to M.M.M. van Nesselrooy for her technical assistance.

LITERATURE CITED

1. **Berg, D. E., J. Davies, B. Allet, and J. D. Rochaix.** 1975. Transposition of R factor genes to bacteriophage λ Proc. Natl. Acad. Sci. U.S.A. 72:3628–3632.
2. **Dang Van, A., G. Bieth, and D. H. Bouanchaud.** 1975. Résistance plasmidique à la tétracycline chez *Haemophilus influenzae*. C. R. Acad. Sci. Paris 280:1321–1323.
3. **Dang Van, A., F. Goldstein, J. F. Acar, and D. H. Bouanchaud.** 1975. A transferable kanamycin resistance plasmid isolated from *Haemophilus influenzae*. Ann. Microbiol. Inst. Pasteur Ser. A 126:397–399.
4. **Demerec, M. E., A. Adelberg, A. J. Clark, and P. E.**

Hartman. 1966. A proposal for an uniform nomenclature in bacterial genetics. Genetics 54:61–76.
5. **Elwell, L. P., J. de Graaff, D. Seibert, and S. Falkow.** 1975. Plasmid-linked ampicillin resistance in *Haemophilus influenzae* type *b*. Infect. Immun. 12:404–410.
6. **Farrar, W. E., Jr., and N. M. O'Dell.** 1974. Beta-lactamase activity in ampicillin-resistant *Haemophilus influenzae*. Antimicrob. Agents Chemother. 6:625–629.
7. **Gottesman, M. M., and J. L. Rosner.** 1975. Acquisition of a determinant for chloramphenicol resistance by coliphage lambda. Proc. Natl. Acad. Sci. U.S.A. 72:5041–5045.
8. **Graaff, J. de, L. P. Elwell, and S. Falkow.** 1976. Molecular nature of two beta-lactamase-specifying plasmids isolated from *Haemophilus influenzae* type *b*. J. Bacteriol. 126:439–446.
9. **Heffron, F., R. Sublett, R. W. Hedges, A. Jacob, and S. Falkow.** 1975. Origin of the TEM beta-lactamase gene found on plasmids. J. Bacteriol. *122:*250–256.
10. **Manten, A., B. van Klingeren, and M. Dessens-Kroon.** 1976. Chloramphenicol resistance in *Haemophilus influenzae*. Lancet 1:702.
11. **Novick, R. P., R. C. Clowes, S. N. Cohen, R. Curtiss III, N. Datta, and S. N. Falkow.** 1976. Uniform nomenclature for bacterial plasmids: a proposal. Bacteriol. Rev. 40:168–189.
12. **Pittman, M.** 1931. Variation and type specificity in the bacterial species *Haemophilus influenzae*. J. Exp. Med. 53:471–492.
13. **Sykes, R. B., M. Matthew, and C. H. O'Callaghan.** 1975. R-factor mediated β-lactamase production by *Haemophilus influenzae*. J. Med. Microbiol. 8:437–441.
14. **Taylor, A. L., and C. D. Trotter.** 1972. Linkage map of *Escherichia coli* strain K-12. J. Bacteriol. 90:911–920.
15. **Thorne, G. M., and W. E. Farrar, Jr.** 1975. Transfer of ampicillin resistance between strains of *Haemophilus influenzae* type B. J. Infect. Dis. 132:276–281.
16. **van Embden, J. D. A., and S. N. Cohen** 1973. Molecular and genetic studies of an R factor system consisting of independent transfer and drug resistance plasmids. J. Bacteriol. 116:699–709.
17. **Vega, R., H. L. Sadoff, and M. J. Patterson.** 1976. Mechanisms of ampicillin resistance in *Haemophilus influenzae* type B. Antimicrob. Agents. Chemother. 9:164–168.

ANTIMICROBIAL AGENTS AND CHEMOTHERAPY, Mar 1977, p. 388-391 Vol. 11, No. 3

Changing Patterns of Plasmid-Mediated Drug Resistance During Tetracycline Therapy

J. K. MØLLER,* A. LETH BAK, A. STENDERUP, H. ZACHARIAE, AND H. AFZELIUS

Institute of Medical Microbiology, Bartholin Building, University of Aarhus, Dk-8000 Aarhus C, Denmark, and Department of Dermatology, Marselisborg Hospital, Aarhus, Denmark*

Received for publication 30 August 1976

The patterns of drug resistance and the frequency of conjugative R plasmids in intestinal *Escherichia coli* from 88 patients treated for a skin disease (*acne vulgaris*) with low oral doses of tetracycline are reported. The proportion of patients with resistant bacteria was progressively greater in patients who received tetracycline for 1 week, 4 weeks, or longer (from 50 to 88%). No multiply drug-resistant bacteria were detected before treatment or after 1 week of treatment. After more than 4 weeks of treatment, multiply drug-resistant *E. coli* were isolated from about 50% of the patients. The origin and selection of R plasmid-determined multiple drug resistance are discussed.

The problems related to the increasing prevalence of infectious multiple-drug resistance presently have serious implications on human health all over the world (9). The infectious multiple-drug resistance is mediated by conjugative R (resistance) plasmids, which are extrachromosomal deoxyribonucleic acid molecules possessing genes generally determining the production of enzymes that are able to inactivate the effect of the antibiotics. The pathogenic enteric bacteria, which may become multiply resistant include the organisms that cause bacillary dysentery, typhoid fever, cholera, and plaque. R plasmids are particularly common in *Shigella* and *Salmonella* with frequencies of about 50% as reported from many countries (7, 9, 14, 21, 25). The frequencies of R plasmids in the common enteric bacteria such as *Escherichia coli, Proteus* and *Klebsiella* presently seem to be at least 10 to 20% in populations at large (4, 9, 17, 24) and at least 20 to 30% in hospitals (1, 9, 17).

Extrachromosomal-determined antibiotic resistance is also well known in *Staphylococcus* (18) and is currently reported in species within the genera *Streptococcus* (5, 16), *Haemophilus* (11), *Mycobacterium* (13), *Clostridium* (19), and *Bordetella* (23).

The R plasmid-mediated resistance is often, and presumably with increasing frequency, multiple, which means that the R plasmid-carrying bacteria are resistant to 3 to 5 or even more antibiotics. There are also some indications of an increasing frequency of multiple resistance in especially virulent strains (E. S. Anderson, E. J. Threfall, J. M. Carr, and J. A. Frost, Proc. Soc. Gen. Microbiol., no. 1, p. 3, 1974) of different bacteria and in bacteria that produce plasmid-determined pathogenicity factors (9, 10, 26).

Certain antibiotics, notably tetracycline, have a great potential for selection of bacteria with R plasmid-determined drug resistance (8). Such bacteria may also be resistant to other drugs than the one used for selection of the R plasmids (8). The treatment of severe cases of *acne vulgaris* with low doses of tetracycline for long periods is widely used and generally accepted to be without serious side effects (20). In this paper, we report on the drug resistance patterns and the frequency of R plasmids in *E. coli* isolated from a group of otherwise healthy people that had been treated for different periods with low oral doses of tetracycline for a skin disease (*acne vulgaris*).

MATERIALS AND METHODS

Patients. All patients (88) were seen in the outpatient clinic at the Department of Dermatology, Marselisborg Hospital, Aarhus, for treatment with tetracycline of *acne vulgaris* or *rosacea*. Apart from this treatment, none of the patients had been treated with antbiotics or had been admitted to a hospital for the last 6 months.

The treatment consisted of a single oral dose of tetracycline (250 to 500 mg/day) for the first 2 weeks. Thereafter, the dose generally was 250 mg/day. The patients were divided into four groups. One group consisted of patients (18) not yet treated. A second group (13 patients) had been treated for 7 days, and a third group (16 patients) had been treated for 1 month. The patients in the fourth group (41) had been treated for more than 1 month, some of them even for several years.

Fecal culture. Specimens of feces were collected

from the patients at the outpatient clinic on charcoal-imbibed cottonwool swabs. The swabs were sent to our laboratory in Stuart medium and inoculated on a bromothymol blue agar plate with 1% lactose and on a blood agar plate without peptones and incubated overnight at 37°C. On the blood agar plate were placed nine different paper disks containing antibiotics, and bacteria showing inhibition zones corresponding to a minimal concentration (per ml of agar) of trimethoprim, 10 μg, streptomycin, kanamycin, gentamicin, or tetracycline, 15 μg, chloramsulfonamide, 100 μg, were considered resistant. A secondary susceptibility test was performed on a colony of *E. coli* from the lactose plate. The results of the primary and secondary susceptibility tests were compared with the purpose of excluding loss of resistance in the bacterial strain purified for further examination and were always identical. The lactose plates were examined, and the colonies with the colonial appearance of *E. coli* were streaked separately on a lactose plate with 15 μg of tetracycline per ml of agar. The proportion of the ten colonies able to grow on the plates were scored. Identical results for the ten colonies were obtained in all cases but one. All swabs were inoculated in a tube with 5 ml of brain heart infusion broth (Difco Laboratories) containing 15 μg of tetracycline per ml. If growth appeared in the tubes but not on the plates containing tetracycline, bacteria from the tubes were examined following the procedure described above. This happened in four instances.

Identifications of strains were performed by means of standard bacteriological methods.

Resistance transfer. All resistant strains of *E. coli* were tested for transfer of resistance to the *E. coli* K-12 strain J53-1 according to methods described previously (17). All the J53-1 strains were able to transfer their acquired resistance pattern to another recipient *E. coli* K-12 strain J 62-2. This was done separately for each marker of the resistance pattern.

RESULTS

The 88 patients were divided into four groups as described in Materials and Methods. The results are given in Tables 1, 2, and 3. It is seen that the proportion of patients with resistant *E. coli* increases from 50% before treatment to 69% after 1 week of treatment, to 75% after 4 weeks, and to 88% in the group treated for more than 4 weeks. The figures for the frequencies of R plasmids in the resistant bacteria in the four groups were 63, 67, 75, and 83%. No multiple-resistant *E. coli* (resistant to 3 or more antibiotics) was found in patients before or after 1 week of treatment. However, in the course of the treatment multiple-resistant *E. coli* could be isolated with increasing frequency (from 38% of the patients treated for 4 weeks and from 49% in the group treated for more than 4 weeks). Resistance against gentamicin and nalidixic acid did not occur among the strains investigated. The resistance patterns of these multiply drug-resistant bacteria were partially or completely transferable in 83 and 85% of the cases, respectively. The patterns of resistance transferred are shown in Table 3.

A few points for explanation of the results are needed. It is known that some resistance plasmids are not self-transmissible. Because of that and limitations in the method for determination of transfer, the figures for the fraction of resistant bacteria containing R plasmids are minimum values.

Although only semiquantitative methods are used, it seems safe to conclude that in patients treated for a few weeks or longer, the majority of the population of *E. coli* had the resistance pattern stated in Table 2.

The rather unexpected finding of only susceptible *E. coli* in some of the patients treated for 4 weeks or longer needs an explanation. One would certainly have expected these bacteria to be resistant to tetracycline. It appeared however, that the majority of bacteria isolated in these cases were either mono- or multiple-resistant *Proteus mirabilis* or *Streptococcus faecalis,* while *E. coli* accounted for only a minor

TABLE 1. *Frequency of drug resistance and occurrence of R plasmids in E. coli from patients with acne vulgaris treated with tetracycline*

Duration of treatment	No. of patients	No. (%) of:			
		Resistant[a] strains	R plasmids[b] in resistant strains	Multiply[c, d] resistant strains	R plasmids in multiply resistant strains
Before treatment	18	9 out of 18 (50)	5 out of 9 (63)	0 out of 18 (0)	
1 week	13	9 out of 13 (69)	6 out of 9 (67)	0 out of 13 (0)	
4 weeks	16	12 out of 16 (75)	9 out of 12 (75)	6 out of 16 (38)	5 out of 6 (83)
More than 4 weeks	41	36 out of 41 (88)	30 out of 36 (83)	20 out of 41 (49)	17 out of 20 (85)

[a] t (Rank test) = 2.85, 2p = 0.44%.
[b] t (Rank test) = 1.64, 2p = 10.1%.
[c] t (Rank test) = 4.02, 2p $<$ 0.01%.
[d] Strains resistant to 3 or more of the following drugs: tetracycline, sulfonamide, streptomycin, trimethoprim, chloramphenicol, kanamycin, nalidixic acid, ampicillin, and gentamicin.

TABLE 2. *Patterns of resistance in E. coli from patients before and after treatment with tetracycline*

Before treatment	Treatment for:		
	1 week	4 weeks	More than 4 weeks
Sensitive (9)[a]	Sensitive (4)	Sensitive (4)	Senstitive (5)
Su[b] (1)	Su (1)	Tc (4)	Tc (9)
Tc (6)	Tc (6)	Tc-Su (1)	Tc-Su (2)
Tc-Su (1)	Tc-Ap (2)	Tc-Sm (1)	Tc-Ap (3)
Su-Sm (1)		Tc-Su-Sm (4)	Tc-Sm (3)
		Tc-Su-Sm-Ap (1)	Tc-Su-Sm (10)
		Tc-Su-Sm-Cm-Ap (1)	Tc-Su-Sm-Ap (2)
			Tc-Su-Cm-Ap (1)
			Tc-Su-Sm-Cm-Ap (3)
			Tc-Su-Tp-Sm-Ap (1)
			Tc-Su-Tp-Sm-Cm-Km (1)
			Tc-Su-Sm-Cm-Km-Ap (1)

[a] Number in parentheses is number of patients.
[b] Tc = tetracycline, Su = sulfonamide, Tp = trimethoprim, Sm = streptomycin, Cm = chloramphenicol, Km = kanamycin, Ap = ampicillin, Nx = nalidixic acid, Gm = gentamicin.

TABLE 3. *Patterns of resistance transferred from the drug resistant E. coli strains*

Before treatment	Treatment for:		
	1 week	4 weeks	More than 4 weeks
Su (1)[a]	Tc (5)	Tc (4)	Tc (13)
Tc (4)[b]	Tc-Ap (1)	Tc-Sm (2)	Tc-Su (1)
		Tc-Ap (1)	Tc-Sm (6)
		Tc-Su-Sm (2)	Tc-Ap (1)
			Tc-Su-Sm (4)
			Tc-Su-Sm-Cm (1)
			Tc-Su-Sm-Km-Ap (1)
			Tc-Su-Sm-Cm-Ap (2)
			Tc-Su-Cm-Tp-Km (1)

[a] Number in parentheses is number of patients.
[b] Tc = tetracycline, Su = sulfonamide, Tp = trimethoprim, Sm = streptomycin, Cm = chloramphenicol, Km = kanamycin, Ap = ampicillin, Nx = nalidixic acid, Gm = gentamicin.

fraction of the aerobic organisms in the intestines of these patients.

DISCUSSION

The results clearly illustrate that long-term tetracycline treatment has two main effects on the drug resistance of *E. coli* in the intestinal flora. One is the occurrence of an increasing frequency of R plasmid-determined resistance and the other is the progressive tendency for this resistance to be multiple.

It is known that tetracycline very effectively selects for R plasmid-determined resistance from studies of R plasmids in enteric bacteria from animals given tetracycline in their feed (9) and from patients treated for a shorter time (10 days) with tetracycline (2, 8, 12). It is important to realize that the R plasmid-carrying bacteria, once selected to constitute the majority of the aerobic intestinal flora, disappear slowly only after withdrawal of the antibiotic treatment (2, 6). It is also known that R plasmid-carrying bacteria are, to a great extent, disseminated to other people in the patient's environment (6).

Although it has been reported that treatment with certain antibiotics such as tetracycline, may sometimes select for bacteria that are multiply resistant (8), there is no obvious explanation why this should happen with the frequency and apparent regularity that was seen in this study. The fact implies that the additional resistance genes or other factors somehow make these bacteria more fit in an environment containing tetracycline than are bacteria with R plasmid-determined tetracycline resistance only. It must be remembered that multiply drug-resistant bacteria were not demonstrated at all in patients before or after 1 week of treatment, whereas bacteria with R plasmid-determined tetracycline resistance were detected fairly often in these groups. Therefore, the question is not only why the multiply drug-resistant bacteria came to dominate, but also where they came from.

It is known that R plasmid-carrying bacteria are transferred to humans, either from food contaminated with animal bacteria (3), from other human beings directly (6), or via contaminated food or water (15, 25). Before treatment, the patients may already harbor multiply drug-resistant bacteria at a concentration below the detectability of the methods used, or they may acquire them during the treatment. A third possibility that might play a role in the development of the resistance patterns could be the transfer of drug resistance from the anaerobic bacteria that constitute the majority of the enteric bacteria in the bowel flora.

Finally, we wish to emphasize the need for an intensified research of the factors responsible for the increasing frequency of bacteria that are multiply drug resistant. It is possible that only certain antbiotics, as shown here for tetracycline, have the ability for a preferential selection of multiple resistance. If this is true, a limitation in the use of these drugs should be recommended.

ACKNOWLEDGMENTS

We thank Naomi Datta, London, for the recipient strains J 53-1 and J 62-2.

This work was supported by grants from F.L. Schmidths Jubilaeumsfond, Fonden til Laegevidenskabens Fremme and The Danish Research Council.

LITERATURE CITED

1. **Anderson, F. M., N. Datta, and E. J. Shaw.** 1972. R. factors in hospital infection. Br. Med. 3:82–85.
2. **Anderson, J. D., W. A. Gillespie, and M. H. Richmond.** 1973. Chemotherapy and antibiotic-resistance transfer between enterobacteria in the human gastrointestinal tract. J. Med. Microbiol. 6:461–473.
3. **Babock, G. F., D. L. Berryhill, and D. H. Marsh.** 1973. R-factors of *Escherichia coli* from dressed beef and humans. Appl. Microbiol. 25:21–23.
4. **Baroyan, O. V., V. S. Zueva, V. N. Rybakov, S. P. Mogilskaya, Yu. G. Linevich, L. I. Korobov, A. K. Kashirova, and B. I. Savchenko,** 1973. Natural occurrence of drug-resistant enterobacteria. Antibiotiki (Kiev) 18:1080–1084.
5. **Clewell, D. B., and A. E. Franke.** 1974. Characterization of a plasmid determining resistance to erythromycin, lincomycin, and vernamycin B_α in a strain of *Streptococcus pyogenes*. Antimicrob. Agents Chemother. 5:534–537.
6. **Damato, J. J., D. V. Eitzman, and H. Baer.** 1974. Persistence and dissemination in the community of R-factors of nosocomial origin. J. Infect. Dis. 129:205–209.
7. **Datta, N., and J. Olarte.** 1974. R factors in strains of *Salmonella typhi* and *Shigella dysenteriae* 1 isolated during epidemics in Mexico: classification by compatibility. Antimicrob. Agents Chemother. 5:310–317.
8. **Datta, N., M. C. Faiers, D. S. Reeves, W. Brumfitt, F. Ørskov, and I. Ørskov.** 1971. R factors in *Escherichia coli* in faeces after oral chemotherapy in general practice. Lancet 1:312–315.
9. **Falkow, S.** 1975. Infectious multiple drug resistance. Pion Limited, London.
10. **Gangarose, E. J., J. V. Bennett, C. Wyatt, P. E. Pierce, J. Olarte, P. M. Hernades, V. Vázquez, and D. Bessudo.** 1972. An epidemic-associated episome? J. Infect. Dis. 126:215–218.
11. **Graaff, J. De., L. P. Elwell, and S. Falkow.** 1976. Molecular nature of two Beta-lactamase-specifying plasmids isolated from *haemophilus influenzae* type b. J. Bacteriol. 126:439–446.
12. **Hirsh, D. C., G. C. Burton, and D. C. Blenden.** 1973. Effect of oral tetracycline on the occurrence of tetracycline-resistant strains of *Escherichia coli* in the intestinal tract of humans. Antimicrob. Agents Chemother. 4:69–71.
13. **Jones, W. D., and H. L. David.** 1972. Preliminary observations of the occurrence of a streptomycin R-factor in *Mycobacterium smegmatis* ATCC 607. Tubercle 53:35–42.
14. **Jonsson, M., L. Rutberg, and G. Tunevall.** 1972. Transferable resistance to antibiotics in gram-negative bacteria isolated in a hsopital for infectious diseases. II. Frequency of R factors and their transmission between patients and personnel in a salmonella-shigella ward. Scand. J. Infect. Dis. 4:209–219.
15. **Linton, K. B., M. H. Richmond, R. Bevan, and W. A. Gillespie.** 1974. Antibiotic resistance and R factors in coli-form bacilli isolated from hospital and domestic sewage. J. Med. Microbiol. 7:91–103.
16. **Marder, H. P., and F. H. Kayser.** 1974. Epidemiological and genetic studies of antibiotic resistance in enterococci. Pathol Microbiol. 41:131–132.
17. **Møller, J. K., A. L. Bak, P. Bülow, C. Christiansen, G. Christiansen, and A. Stenderup.** 1976. Transferable and non-transferable drug resistance in enteric bacteria from hospital and from general practice. Scand. J. Infect. Dis. 8:112–116.
18. **Novick, R. P., and D. Bouanchaud.** 1971 Extrachromosomal nature of drug resistance in staphylococcus aureus. Ann. N.Y. Acad. Sci. 182:279–294.
19. **Sebald, M., D. Douanchaud, G. Bieth, and C. R. Hebd.** 1975. Plasmid-linked resistance to four antibiotics in *C. perfringens* type A strain 659. Séances Acad. Sci. Paris. Sér. D. 280:2401–2404.
20. **Sneddon, J. B.** 1966. A clinical trial of tetracycline in rosacea. Br. J. Dermatol. 78:649–652.
21. **Tanaka, T., M. Tsunoda, and S. Mitsuhashi.** 1973. Distribution of R factors among Shigella strains isolated in Japan (II). Jpn. J. Microbiol. 17:291–295.
22. **Tanaka, T., K. Ikemura, M. Tsunoda, I. Sasagawa, and S. Mitsuhashi.** 1976. Drug resistance and distribution of R factors in *Salmonella* strains. Antimicrob. Agents Chemother. 9:61–64.
23. **Terakado, N., and S. Mitsuhashi,** 1974. Properties of R factors from *Bordetella bronchiseptica*. Antimicrob. Agents Chemother. 6:836–840.
24. **Tschäpe, H., H. Kühn, and H. Rische.** 1973. R plasmids of floral *Escherichia coli* of healthy children in one area of the DDR. J. Hyg. Epidemiol. Microbiol. Immunol. 17:208–215.
25. **Tschäpe, H., H. Rische, and J. Stempel.** 1973. R-plasmids in Enterobacteriaceae from river, drinking and waste-water. Zentrabl. Gesamte Hyg. Ihre Grenzgeb. 19:826–829.
26. **Williams Smith, H.** 1974. A search for transmissible pathogenic characters in invasive strains of Escherichia coli: the discovery of a plasmid-controlled toxin and a plasmid-controlled lethal character closely associated or identical with colicine V. J. Gen. Microbiol. 83:95–111.

ANTIMICROBIAL AGENTS AND CHEMOTHERAPY, Mar. 1977, p. 392-395 Vol. 11, No. 3

Printed in U.S.A.

Effect of Penicillin on Streptomycin Production by *Streptomyces griseus*

GY. BARABÁS* AND G. SZABÓ

Institute of Biology, University of Medicine, H-4012, Debrecen, Hungary

Received for publication 11 November 1976

The correlation between the biosynthesis of the cell wall and the formation of streptomycin (SM) in *Streptomyces griseus*, influenced by a specific inhibitor of cell wall synthesis, was investigated. Penicillin, in subinhibitory concentrations (1 to 5 μg/ml), was added to cultures of *S. griseus* in different stages of its life cycle. The inhibitor decreased SM production, when young cultures were treated; however, there was an increase in SM formation when penicillin was added to older cultures. The explanation for these findings is discussed in detail.

The physiological role of streptomycin (SM) in the life of *Streptomyces griseus* has been investigated. We proved that streptidine (SD), a component of the SM molecule, is a constituent of the cell wall (2, 10). This indicates that SM or its SD component plays a role in building up the cell wall network (1, 8–10). These findings prompted us to search for correlations between cell wall synthesis and SM production in *S. griseus*. Use of specific inhibitors of cell wall synthesis in bacteria, such as penicillin, bacitracin, etc., seemed promising as an approach to the problem (Gy. Barabas, Folia Microbiol. 18:266, 1973). Since SD is a component of cell walls, one might expect that the inhibition of cell wall synthesis would change SM production.

In this paper, we describe the effects on SM production by *S. griseus* cultures when penicillin is added at different stages in the *S. griseus* life cycle.

MATERIALS AND METHODS

Strains and cultivation. *S. griseus* LS-1 (code no. 52-1) strain was used. Its cultural and physiological characteristics, as well as the composition of the filtered soybean medium employed throughout the experiments, were previously described (8). Cultivation was carried out on a rotary shaker (250 rpm, 50-mm stroke distance) at 27°C.

Antibiotic assay. SM content of the fermentation liquid was determined by the agar-hole diffusion method against *Bacillus subtilis* ATCC 6633. The fermentation liquid was spun down, and the cell-free supernatants were diluted with 0.067 M phosphate buffer (pH 7.5) containing penicillinase (Neutrapen Riker Laboratories, Loughborough, England, in a final concentration of 100 μg/ml). The samples were incubated at 37°C for 1 h to inactivate penicillin. Then, four to seven replicates were pipetted in the holes of agar plates from every sample, and their mean was used for the calculation. The agar medium for antibiotic assay was prepared as follows: 5 g of meat extract, 1 g of Na_2HPO_4, 0.1 g of KH_2PO_4, and 0.5 g of peptone were dissolved in 100 ml of distilled water and boiled for 2 min. After filtration, 900 ml of distilled water was added, as well as 20 g of agar. The pH of the medium was adjusted to 7.0 after it had melted, and it was finally sterilized by autoclaving. The melted medium was inoculated with *B. subtilis*, poured into petri plates, and incubated at 37°C for 1 h. Samples were then pipetted into the holes. The inhibition zone of the antibiotic was measured after 20 h of incubation at 37°C. Control experiments showed that penicillinase itself did not have any antibiotic activity in the concentration used in our study, nor did it potentiate SM activity. Five hundred-milliliter Erlenmeyer flasks containing 100 ml of medium were employed. In every experiment, three parallel flasks were used for a given penicillin concentration, and the same number of flasks were employed for the control.

Determination of growth rate. Two-milliliter samples of fermentation liquid containing the mycelia were taken. They were spun down, and 0.5 ml of 1 N NaOH was pipetted into the sediment. The preparation was allowed to rest overnight at room temperature, 4.5 ml of distilled water was added, and the protein content was determined (7, 11). The results were expressed as the mycelial protein content of 1 ml of fermentation liquid, and this was taken as the measure of growth.

Chemicals. Penicillin (penicillin G potassium) was a gift of the Biogal Pharmaceutical Factory, Debrecen. One microgram corresponds to 1 IU.

Calculations. For Fig. 1 to 3, calculations were made as follows: $(Pt \times 100/c) - 100$ = percentage (increase or decrease) of SM production, where Pt is penicillin-treated cultures, c is control cultures, and both are expressed as micrograms of SM per milligram of mycelial protein.

RESULTS

The effect of penicillin on bacteria is well known (5). It affects streptomycetes as well (5,

6), although *S. griseus* has not been extensively investigated in this respect. In preliminary experiments, the subinhibitory concentration of penicillin for our strain at different ages was determined. This was found to be in the range of 1 to 5 μg/ml. Penicillin, in subinhibitory concentrations, was added to 24-, 36-, and 48-h cultures of *S. griseus*.

Figure 1 shows that penicillin inhibited SM production, if it was added to a young culture (24 h old) of *S. griseus*. After 24 h of incubation with penicillin at 3 and 5 μg/ml, there was a decrease in antibiotic production. At 1 μg/ml, production was stimulated. After 48 h of incubation, with all concentrations of penicillin, there was a slight increase in SM production.

Penicillin increased SM production, if added to older cultures (36 h) of *S. griseus* (Fig. 2).

The most dramatic effect of penicillin was observed when 48-h cultures of *S. griseus* were treated with the antibiotic (Fig. 3). After 24 h of incubation with penicillin, SM production increased considerably (Fig. 3). However, no correlation existed between the concentration of penicillin employed and the amount of SM produced. This effect continued after 48 h of incubation with the inhibitor. The strain used in the experiment was a "low producer," since the SM production under our conditions was approximately 10, 40, 100, and 120 μg/ml, corresponding to 24-, 48-, 72-, and 96-h incubation times.

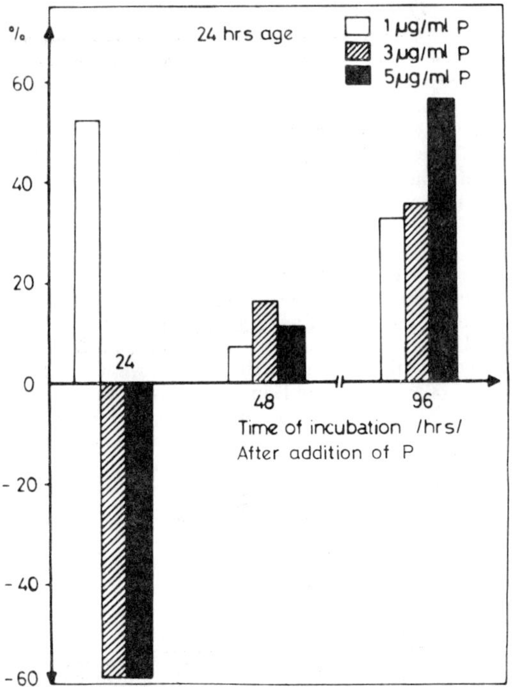

FIG. 1. *Effect of penicillin on SM production of 24-h cultures. The inhibitor was added to 24-h-old strains in submerged cultures in soybean medium. The antibiotic activity was expressed in micrograms per milliliter of mycelial protein, and the values are given as the percentage of the control (untreated) culture. For the details, see Materials and Methods. Time of incubation represents the incubation with penicillin (P).*

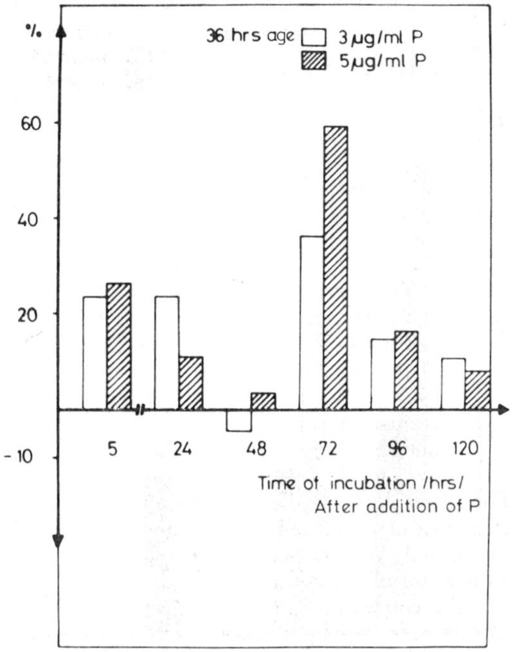

FIG. 2. *Effect of penicillin on SM production of 36-h cultures. Experimental conditions and calculations are the same as described in the legend to Fig. 1, except for the age of the cultures.*

As Fig. 4a-c shows, penicillin did not have a severe inhibitory effect on the growth of *S. griseus*. In this case, the protein content of mycelia was taken as a measure of the growth rate (see Materials and Methods). It is to be noted that, in our soybean medium, the growth curves show a plateau, or slight decrease, between 48 and 96 h of incubation.

DISCUSSION

Our previous findings, which proved that SD is a component of the cell wall of *S. griseus* (2, 10), prompted us to investigate the effect of penicillin on SM production. According to our observations, the effect of this cell wall inhibitor depends on the age of the *S. griseus* culture. The growth curve of our strain was previously

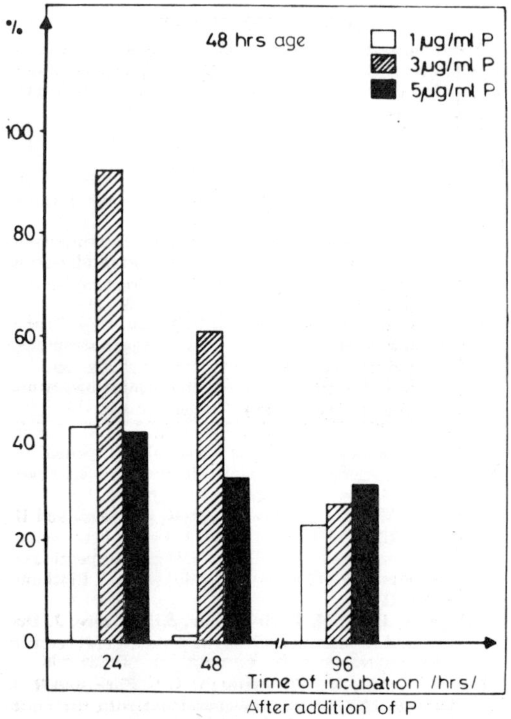

FIG. 3. *Effect of penicillin on SM production of 48-h cultures. Experimental conditions and calculations are the same as described in the legend to Fig. 1, except for the age of culture.*

studied (8). When it was treated in the early stage of life cycle (24-h culture), the production of SM decreased (though in Fig. 1 the effect of 1 µg of penicillin per ml after 24 h of incubation is not yet clarified). The results obtained after prolonged (48-h) incubation with penicillin are hardly attributable directly to the inhibitor, since secondary effects could also occur after incubation for more than 24 h at 27°C. When penicillin was incubated in cell-free soybean medium, the antibiotic activity partly remained after 46 h of incubation. Under similar conditions, but in the presence of 24-h-old cultures of *S. griseus*, penicillin was not detectable in the supernatant of culture liquid after 2 h of incubation (by measuring its activity against SM-resistant, penicillin-susceptible *B. subtilis*). This is probably the effect of irreversible binding of penicillin to the receptor sites that are known to be present in some *Streptomyces* spp. (6). If penicillin was added to cells in a later stage of the life cycle (36- and 48-h cultures), an increase of SM production was observed; this effect was more marked with 48-h cultures. The increased amount of antibiotic was attributable solely to SM, since the antibiotic activity was not measurable with SM-resistant *B. subtilis* in control experiments.

One could raise the question: What is the possible explanation of this phenomenon, since 36- and 48-h cultures are in the stationary phase of their life cycle when cell wall synthesis has presumably ended? Of several possible hypotheses, the following theory seems preferable.

We have observed that cross wall formation occurs in the later stages of the life cycle of *S. griseus*, so that this type of cell wall could be

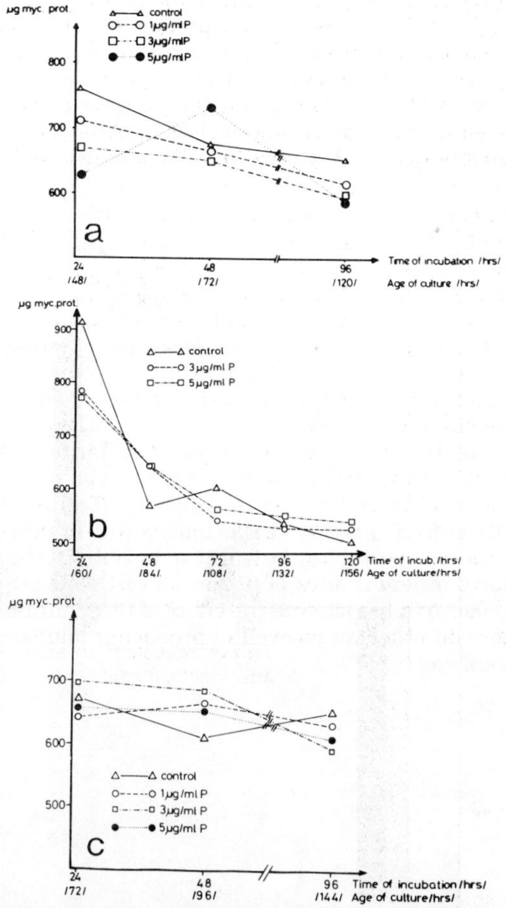

FIG. 4. *Effect of penicillin on the growth of S. griseus. The sediments of samples from cultures of different ages, used for estimating SM production (see Fig. 1–3), were taken for protein determinations. The growth curve was determined as given in Materials and Methods. Time of incubation, on the abscissa, indicates the incubation time after the addition of penicillin (P) to (a) 24-h cultures, (b) 36-h cultures, and (c) 48-h cultures.*

synthesized in the case of 36- and 48-h-old cultures, too. Since SM production begins, under our experimental conditions, in *S. griseus* cultures that are 20 to 24 h old, and the bulk of the antibiotic is formed at 36 to 48 h, it may be possible that the biosynthesis of SM has some correlation with a certain type of cell wall (e.g., cross walls), the biosynthesis of which is inhibited by penicillin, whereby SM production is increased.

It is known of bacteria that elongated, snake-like forms are produced without cross walls as a consequence of penicillin effects. Previous observations showed that there are certain fragments of the hyphae that are more active in SM production than others (3). It is, however, still obscure as to what portion of the cell is responsible for biosynthesis of SM within these hyphae.

It must be mentioned that some component(s) of soybean medium may play a role in the increase in SM production by penicillin that we observed. In a synthetic medium, containing glycerol and sodium asparate as sole carbon and nitrogen sources, respectively, penicillin, in concentrations ranging from 1 to 5 μg/ml, did not alter SM production. In this case, however, the production of SM is very low (under 10 μg/ml). We would like to raise the question. whether in other aminocyclitol antibiotics (neomycin, kanamycin, paramomycin, gentamycin, etc.), in which the structure of the deoxystreptamine component is very similar to that of SD, deoxystreptamine may also be an ingredient in the cell wall of the producer strains, as SD is in *S. griseus*. Experiments are in progress to investigate the effect of inhibitors that have different sites of action on cell wall synthesis and to examine the effect of these inhibitors on other aminocyclitol-producing microorganisms.

ACKNOWLEDGMENTS

We are indebted to D. J. Kushner, University of Ottawa, Department of Biology, for his help in revising the manuscript. We wish to thank A. Ottenberger for excellent technical assistance.

LITERATURE CITED

1. **Barabás, Gy., and G. Szabó.** 1965. Comparison of cell wall composition of *Streptomyces griseus* strains. Arch. Mikrobiol. **50**:156–183.
2. **Barabás, Gy., and G. Szabó.** 1968. Role of streptomycin in the life of *Streptomyces griseus*: streptidine-containing fraction in the cell walls of *Streptomyces griseus* strains. Can. J. Microbiol. **14**:1325–1331.
3. **Barabás, Gy., F. Szeszák, and G. Szabó.** 1974. Transamidinase activity of hyphal fractions of a streptomycin-producing *Streptomyces griseus* strain and enhancement of enzyme activity in a nonproducing mutant. Antimicrob. Agents Chemother. **6**:11–15.
4. **Blumberg, P. M., and J. L. Strominger.** 1974. Interaction of penicillin with the bacterial cell: penicillin-binding proteins and penicillin-sensitive enzymes. Bacteriol. Rev. **38**:291–335.
5. **Frére, J.-M., M. Leyh-Bouille, J.-M. Ghuysen, and H. R. Perkins.** 1974. Interaction between beta-lactam antibiotics and exocellular DD-carboxypeptidase-transpeptidase of *Streptomyces* R61. Eur. J. Biochem. **50**:203–214.
6. **Ghuysen, J.-M., M. Leyh-Bouille, J.-M. Frére, J. Dusart, and A. Marquet.** 1974. The penicillin receptor in *Streptomyces*. Ann. N. Y. Acad. Sci. **235**:236–268.
7. **Lowry, O. H., N. J. Rosebrough, A. L. Farr, and R. J. Randall.** 1951. Protein measurement with the Folin phenol reagent. J. Biol. Chem. **193**:265–275.
8. **Szabó, G., G. Barabás, and R. Ványi-Nagy.** 1961. Comparison of Str. griseus strains which produce streptomycin and those which do not. Arch. Mikrobiol. **40**:261–274.
9. **Szabó, G., Gy. Barabás, and T. Vályi-Nagy.** 1962. Comparison of the carbohydrate composition of the cell walls of strains of *Streptomyces griseus*. J. Bacteriol. **84**:1342–1343.
10. **Szabó, G., Gy. Barabás, T. Vályi-Nagy, and Zs. Magyar.** 1965. A new component from the cell wall of Streptomyces griseus. I. The role of streptomycin in the life of Streptomyces griseus. Acta Microbiol. Acad. Sci. Hung. **12**:109–113.
11. **Szeszák, F., and G. Szabó.** 1967. Application of the Lowry's protein determination method for the mycelium of *Streptomyces griseus* strain no. 52–1. J. Antibiot. Ser. A **20**:295–296.

ANTIMICROBIAL AGENTS AND CHEMOTHERAPY, Mar. 1977, p. 396-401 Vol. 11, No. 3
Printed in U.S.A.

Gardimycin, a New Antibiotic Inhibiting Peptidoglycan Synthesis

SERGIO SOMMA,* WILMA MERATI, AND FRANCESCO PARENTI
Research Laboratories, Lepetit S.p.A., Milano, Italy

Received for publication 12 April 1976

Gardimycin, a new antibiotic, at 100 μg/ml, specifically inhibited cell wall synthesis and induced accumulation of uridine 5'-diphosphate-*N*-acetylmuramylpentapeptide in whole cells of *Bacillus subtilis*. The antibiotic was active in a particulate enzyme preparation from *Bacillus stearothermophilus:* 60 μg/ml caused 50%, and 200μg/ml caused 100%, inhibition of peptidoglycan synthesis. Suppression of peptidoglycan synthesis was accompanied by parallel accumulation of the lipid intermediate. This mechanism of action is discussed in comparison with those of other antibiotics that are known to inhibit bacterial cell wall biosynthesis.

Gardimycin is a new sulfur-containing peptide antibiotic recently isolated from the fermentation broth of *Actinoplanes garbadinensis* sp. nov. (9). It is active against gram-positive bacteria and has very low toxicity. Its chemical characteristics (3) and biological properties (2) have been reported elsewhere. Preliminary experiments indicated that gardimycin interferes with bacterial cell wall biosynthesis. In fact, the drug is inactive on cell wall-lacking bacteria such as *Mycoplasma* and on the L-form of susceptible *Staphylococcus aureus*.

In this paper, a more detailed analysis of its mechanism of action is reported, which confirms the effect of gardimycin on cell wall biosynthesis and indicates that its primary site of action is on the transfer of the disaccharidic pentapeptide unit from the lipid carrier to the acceptor site of the cell wall.

MATERIALS AND METHODS

Bacterial strains. The effects of gardimycin on living cells were studied in *Bacillus subtilis* SB25 (*try*⁻ *his*⁻) and PB 556/1 (*thy*⁻). *Bacillus stearothermophilus* (*calidolactis*) ATCC 10149 was used as the source of particulate enzyme for the studies of in vitro peptidoglycan synthesis.

Bacterial growth. *B. subtilis* was usually grown in flasks at 37°C, with reciprocal shaking, and *B. stearothermophilus* was grown at 55°, in fermenters with forced aeration.

Radiochemicals. [5-^{3}H]uracil, 24.2 Ci/mmol; [2-^{14}C]thymidine, 61 mCi/mmol; [U-^{14}C]phenylalanine, 225 mCi/mmol; L-[U-^{14}C]alanine, 173 mCi/mmol; [1-^{3}H]*N*-acetylglucosamine (GlcNAc), 4 Ci/mmol; and [1-^{14}C]GlcNAc, 58 mCi/mmol; were all obtained from Radiochemical Centre, Amersham, England.

Incorporation of labeled compounds into cell wall and protein fraction. Exponentially growing *B. subtilis* was transferred to Davis minimal medium supplemented with 0.5% glucose, 50 μg of tryptophan per ml, 50 μg of histidine per ml, and the appropriate labeled compound and incubated for 20 min at 37°C. Cells were harvested, washed with buffer [0.1 M tris(hydroxymethyl)aminomethane (Tris)-hydrochloride, pH 7.4], heated for 5 min, and sonicated for 10 min. Unbroken cells were removed by centrifugation at 6,000 × *g* for 10 min. Total incorporated radioactivity was determined at this stage by precipitating a sample of the sonicated cell suspension with cold 10% (wt/vol) trichloroacetic acid; acid-insoluble material was collected on glass-fiber filters (Whatman GF/C) and washed with ethanol and diethyl ether; dried filters were counted for radioactivity. The radioactivity incorporated in the cell wall or the protein fraction of the cells was determined after fractionation as follows. A sample of sonicated cells was treated with pancreatic ribonuclease and deoxyribonuclease I for 30 min, with trypsin for 2 h, and finally with pepsin at pH 2 for 2 h. Trichloroacetic acid-insoluble material, which consists of cell walls, was collected and the radioactivity was determined.

A different sample of sonicated cells was incubated with lysozyme in the presence of 0.05% (wt/vol) sodium dodecyl sulfate for 1 h and then with ribonuclease and deoxyribonuclease for 30 min, and the radioactivity of the trichoroacetic acid-insoluble material, which represents "cellular protein," was determined. All the enzymes were used at a concentration of 1 mg/ml, and the incubation temperature was 37°C.

The specificity of the fractionation procedure was checked as in previous experiments by determining the origin of the radioactivity found in the two fractions obtained from cells grown in the presence of [^{14}C]phenylalanine and [^{3}H]GlcNAc as protein and cell wall precursors, respectively.

Extraction and determination of uridine nucleotide in cells. Cell wall precursors were extracted from exponentially growing *B. subtilis* SB25 incubated in Pennassay (PY) broth (Difco) as described by Garret (4). *N*-acetylhexosamine was determined by the procedure of Reissig et al. (10).

Identification of the accumulated cell wall precursors. To an exponentially growing culture of *B. subtilis* SB25 in PY medium containing 22% (wt/vol) sucrose, 0.4 μCi of [^{3}H]GlcNAc per ml and gardimycin at 200 μg/ml were added. After a further 40-min incubation, the cells were harvested and washed with 22% sucrose in 0.1 M Tris-hydrochloride, pH 7.9. Then, nucleotides were extracted and separated by descending chromatography on Whatman no. 1 filter paper, with a mixture of 95% ethanol and 1 M ammonium acetate, pH 7 (7.5:3), for 16 h. After drying, the paper strip was cut into 0.5-cm segments, and the radioactivity on each segment was counted.

Preparation of uridine 5'-diphosphate *N*-acetyl[^{14}C]muramylpentapeptide (UDP-MurNAc-pentapeptide). Cells of *B. subtilis* SB 25 were treated as described above, except that 0.1 μCi of [^{14}C]GlcNAc per ml and 100 μg of vancomycin per ml were used. The pooled nucleotides were applied to a Dowex 1 column (Cl^- form), 100 to 200 mesh, and eluted with a linear gradient of NaCl (from 0.05 to 0.3 M) in 0.01 N HCl. A main peak absorbing at 260 nm and containing most of the radioactivity was obtained. The fractions making up this peak were pooled and lyophilized. The product thus obtained was homogeneous by paper chromatography and had a specific activity of 104,000 cpm/μmol.

Preparation of particulate enzyme. Cells of *B. stearothermophilus* were grown at 55°C in a medium containing 1% (wt/vol) tryptone, 0.5% (wt/vol) yeast extract, 0.25% (wt/vol) K_2HPO_4, and 0.1% (wt/vol) glucose, harvested in the middle of the exponential phase, washed, suspended in buffer (0.05 M Tris-hydrochloride, pH 7.9, and 0.01 M Mg acetate), and frozen. The frozen-cell paste was ground in a homogenizer with an equal volume of Superbrite (Minnesota Mining & Manufacturing) for three periods of 5 min while being cooled in ice. The Superbrite was removed by filtering on a sintered-glass funnel. The cell suspension was centrifuged twice at 6000 × *g* for 10 min, and the supernatant was centrifuged at 38,000 *g* for 20 min. Then, the pellet was washed twice and resuspended in buffer. The suspension was stored under liquid nitrogen.

In vitro synthesis of peptidoglycan. The reaction mixtures contained 100 mM Tris-hydrochloride, pH 7.9, 25 mM $MgCl_2$, 0.5 mM UDP-GlcNAc, 0.5 mM [^{14}C]UDP-MurNAc-pentapeptide and the particulate enzyme at a concentration of 8 mg of protein per ml (determined with the Folin-Ciocalteau reagent). Final volume was 100 μl. After 40 min of incubation at 30°C, the entire reaction mixture was spread on a 3-cm line at the origin of a strip of Whatman no. 1 chromatographic paper and dried with hot air. Chromatograms were developed in a descending direction with a mixture of isobutyric acid-1 M NH_4OH (5:3). According to Strominger et al. (13), the synthesized peptidoglycan remains at the point of origin, while the substrate and intermediate move down.

Radioactivity measurement. Filter disks and paper segments were counted in a Philips liquid scintillation analyzer with Instagel (Packard) as scintillation fluid; chromatograms were analyzed by a Packard chromatography scanner, and the distribution of radioactivity was determined from the peak areas.

RESULTS

Effect on growth and viability. The minimal inhibitory concentration of gardimycin against *B. subtilis* SB25 is 100 μg/ml. Addition of the antibiotic at this concentration to a growing culture causes an immediate decrease in absorbance, indicating cell lysis (Fig. 1). The effect of gardimycin on cell viability is shown in Fig. 2. When the antibiotic is added at 200 μg/ml to a growing culture, an irreversible loss of viability takes place. At a lower concentration (50 μg/ml), however, there is a resumption of growth after 1 h of incubation. A similar effect of subinhibitory concentrations has already been reported for other antibiotics that interfere with cell wall biosynthesis (5). Addition of gardimycin (200 μg/ml) to resting cells deprived of a carbon source, however, does not affect cell viability.

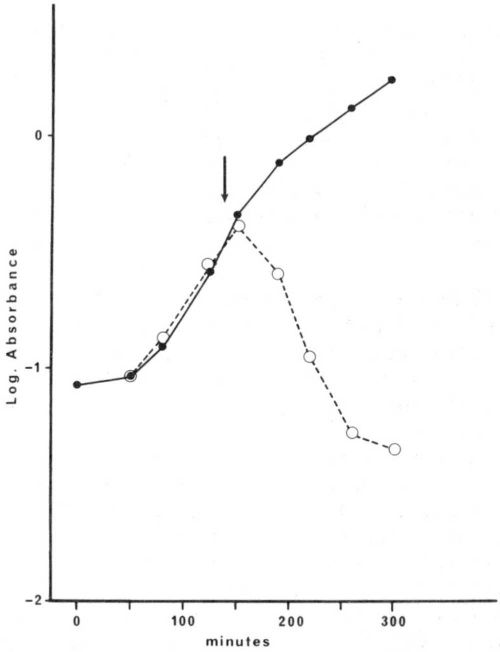

FIG. 1. *Effect of gardimycin on growth. Two cultures of B. subtilis were incubated in PY medium, and the growth was determined by absorbance at 595 nm. At the time indicated by the arrow, gardimycin was added to one of the cultures to a final concentration of 100 µg/ml. Symbols: (●) Control, (○) gardimycin.*

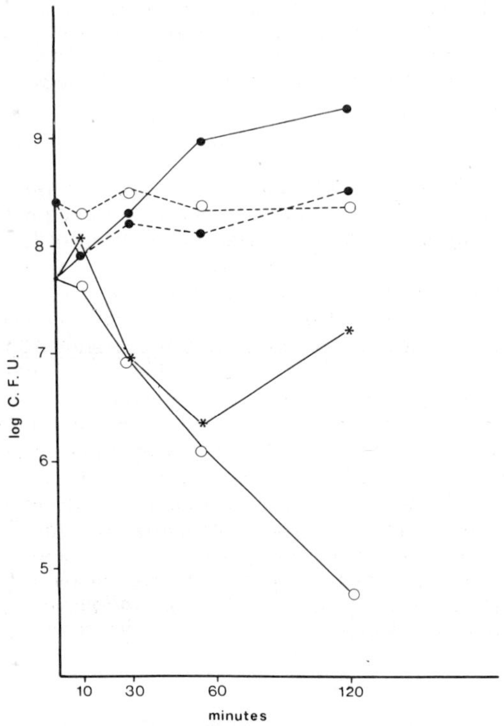

FIG. 2. *Effect of gardimycin on cell viability. The solid line indicates the number of colonies grown on an agar plate after suitable dilution of a culture of B. subtilis growing in PY medium. The dashed line indicates the number of colonies formed after cell washing and incubation in buffer containing 0.15 M NaCl, 0.1 M Tris-hydrochloride (pH 7.9), and 0.01 M $MgCl_2$. Symbols: (●) Control; (*) gardimycin, 50 μg/ml; (○) gardimycin, 200 μg/ml.*

Effect on macromolecular synthesis in vivo. To identify the cellular macromolecular synthesis primarily affected by gardimycin, the rate of incorporation of radioactive precursors was measured in the presence or absence of the antibiotic.

As shown in Fig. 3, the addition of gardimycin (200 μg/ml) to a growing culture immediately suppressed the incorporation of GlcNAc, a specific precursor of peptidoglycan. The syntheses of deoxyribonucleic acid, ribonucleic acid, and protein, measured as incorporation of thymine, uracil, and phenylalanine, respectively, were only slightly affected for the first 20 min, thus suggesting that cell wall synthesis is the primary target of the drug. To ascertain that the target of gardimycin is peptidoglycan synthesis and not merely GlcNAc uptake or utilization, the distribution of labeled alanine, a component of both peptidoglycan and protein, between the cell wall and the protein fractions of bacteria grown in the presence or absence of gardimycin was determined. As a control, the same distribution was also determined in bacteria grown in the presence of the protein synthesis inhibitor, tetracycline. The results of such an experiment are shown in Fig. 4.

Gardimycin did not reduce the amount of alanine incorporated into the protein fraction as compared with the control culture, whereas it strongly decreased its incorporation into the cell wall. As expected, tetracycline inhibited alanine incorporation into the protein fraction, but not into the cell wall fraction.

Accumulation of cell wall precursors. Most antibiotics interfering with peptidoglycan synthesis cause an endocellular accumulation of UDP nucleotides linked to *N*-acetylaminohexoses.

As shown in Fig. 5, such accumulation also occurs in a growing bacterial culture treated with 50 μg of gardimycin per ml. Figure 6 shows the relationship between the antibiotic concentration and the amount of *N*-acetylaminohexose accumulated over a 30-min period of incubation. To identify the accumulated precursors, the nucleotides extracted from cells grown in the presence of [^{3}H]GlcNAc plus 200 μg of gardimycin per ml were co-chromatographed with UDP-NAc[^{14}C]Mur-pentapeptide, obtained from cells treated with vancomycin. Only one main peak of tritium radioactivity was found, with an R_f identical to that of the ^{14}C radioactivity peak, thus indicating that UDP-NAcMur-pentapeptide was the main cell wall precursor accumulated in the presence of gardimycin. The target of the antibiotic is, therefore, the peptidoglycan polymerization process.

Effect on in vitro synthesis of peptidoglycan. The effect of gardimycin on peptidoglycan biosynthesis was studied with a particulate enzyme preparation from *B. stearothermophilus*, capable of synthesizing cross-linked peptidoglycan (11). Gardimycin inhibits the incorporation of labeled MurNAc-pentapeptide into cross-linked peptidoglycan, while causing an accumulation of a phospholipid intermediate (Fig. 7). The same results were obtained when labeled UDP-GlcNAc was used, thus suggesting that the accumulated phospholipid intermediate contains the disaccharide unit GlcNAc-MurNAc-pentapeptide. The effect of gardimycin was compared, in the same experiment, with that of the known peptidoglycan synthesis inhibitors vancomycin and bacitracin. All three antibiotics inhibited precursor utilization. Although vancomycin caused a reduction of pepti-

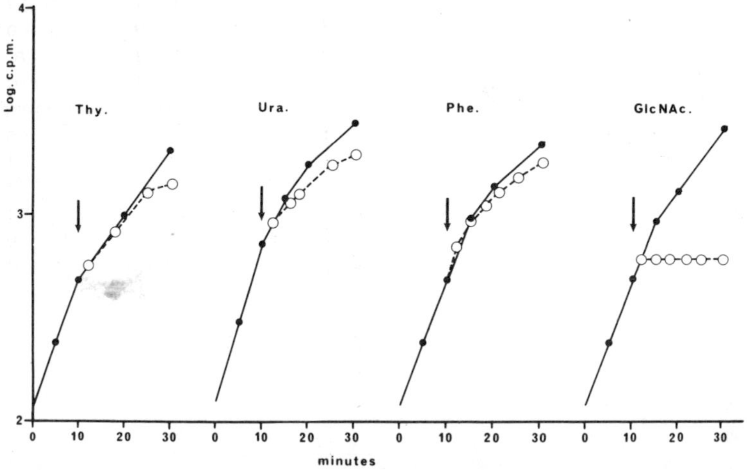

FIG. 3. *Effect of gardimycin on the incorporation of macromolecule precursors into whole cells of B. subtilis 556/1. Cells were grown in Davis minimal medium supplemented with 0.2% Casamino Acids (Difco), 0.5% glucose, and 10 μg of cold thymine per ml in the presence of either [¹⁴C]thymine (0.025 μCi/ml), [¹⁴C]phenylalanine (0.025 μCi/ml), [³H]uracil (0.05 μCi/ml), or [³H]GlcNAc (0.05 μCi/ml). At intervals, aliquots were transferred to cold 5% trichloroacetic acid, and the acid-insoluble material was collected on membrane filters (Millipore Corp.), washed with cold 2% trichloracetic acid, dried, and counted for radioactivity. The arrows indicate the time of antibiotic addition. Symbols: (●) Control; (○) gardimycin, 200 μg/ml.*

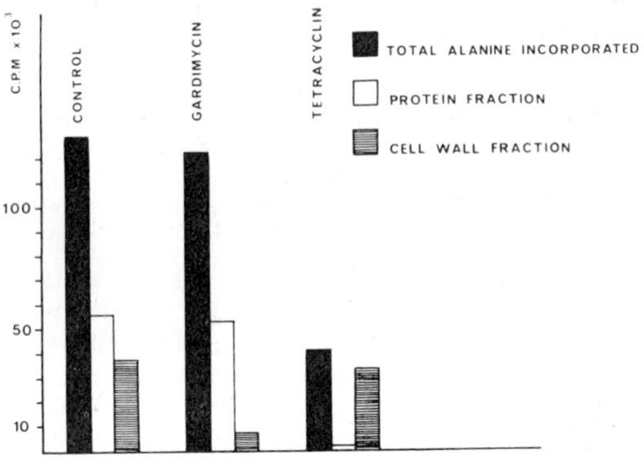

FIG. 4. *Effect of gardimycin and tetracycline on the distribution of [¹⁴C]alanine in the cell wall and in the protein fraction of B. subtilis. Exponentially growing cells were incubated for 20 min in Davis minimal medium supplemented with 0.5% glucose, 50 μg of tryptophan per ml, 50 μg of histidine per ml and 0.8 μCi of [¹⁴C]alanine per ml. Total radioactivity incorporated and the radioactivity incorporated into cell wall and protein fraction were determined as described in Materials and Methods. Three 10-ml cultures were run: the first was kept as a control, 500 μg of gardimycin per ml was added to the second, and 20 μg of tetracycline per ml was added to the third.*

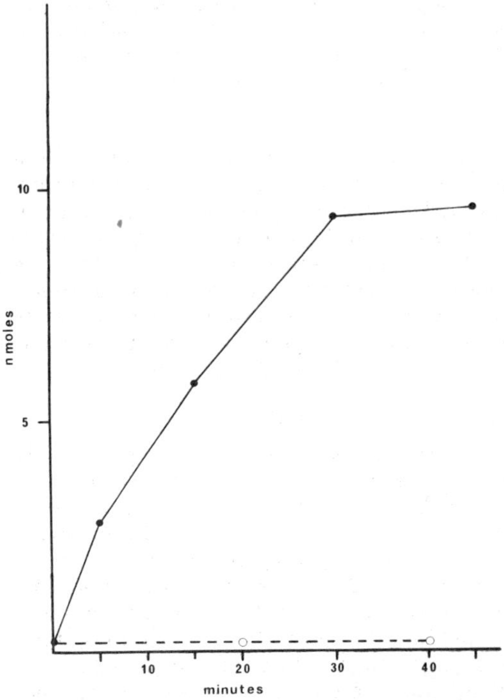

FIG. 5. *Time course of accumulation of cell wall precursors. The amount of N-acetylaminohexoses is expressed as nanomoles per milliliter of culture. Symbols: (○) Control; (●) gardimycin, 50 μg/ml.*

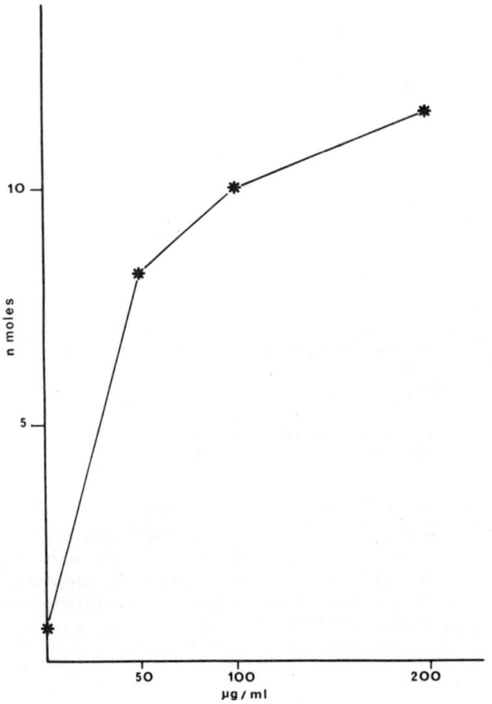

FIG. 6. *Effect of gardimycin concentration on cell wall precursor accumulation. On the ordinate are nanomoles of N-acetylaminohexoses per milliliter of culture, whereas the abscissa shows antibiotic concentrations. Incubation was for 30 min.*

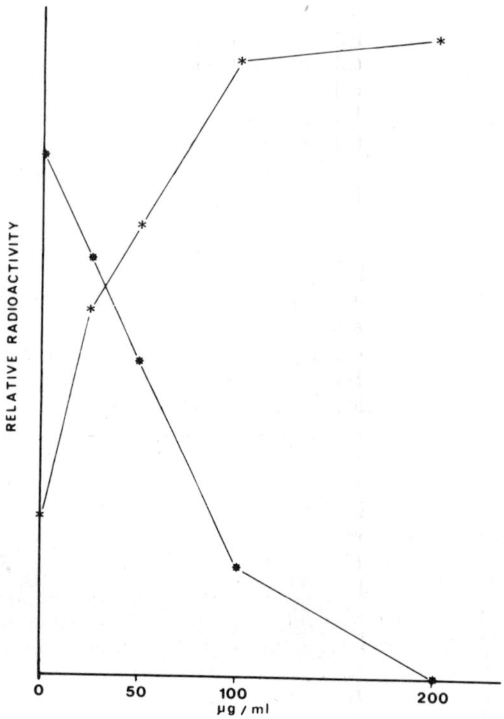

FIG. 7. *Effect of gardimycin on in vitro synthesis of peptidoglycan, catalyzed by a particulate enzyme preparation from B. stearothermophilus. The radioactivity incorporated into the peptidoglycan (●) and into the lipid intermediate (*) is plotted against gardimycin concentration.*

doglycan synthesis with a concomitant accumulation of phospholipid intermediate, bacitracin inhibited the formation of the latter, while allowing some synthesis of peptidoglycan (Table 1). These effects were to be expected from the known mechanism of action of the two antibiotics. Gardimycin behaved in this system exactly like vancomycin, suggesting that its target is the same or similar to that of vancomycin.

DISCUSSION

The results reported in this paper clearly indicate that gardimycin inhibits growth of *B. subtilis* by inhibiting cell wall biosynthesis. This conclusion is supported by the following evidence. First, gardimycin inhibits the incorporation of GlcNAc, a specific precursor, into the cell wall; also, it inhibits incorporation of alanine into the cell wall but not into protein. Second, it induces accumulation of cell wall precursors in growing cells, suggesting that their further utilization is inhibited. Third, the drug has a bactericidal effect on growing cells, but not on resting cells, a phenomenon characteristic of, although not exclusive for, many cell

TABLE 1. *Comparison of effects of gardimycin, vancomycin, and bacitracin on in vitro synthesis of peptidoglycan*[a]

Antibiotic	% of radioactivity added		
	UDP-MurNAc-pentapeptide	Lipid intermediate	Peptidoglycan
None	0	29.0	71.0
Bacitracin	56.0	21.5	22.5
Vancomycin	51.5	48.5	0
Gardimycin	45.5	54.5	0

[a] Antibiotics were present at a concentration of 240 µg/ml.

wall inhibitors. As already mentioned, cell wall-lacking bacteria, such as *Mycoplasma* and L-forms of *S. aureus*, are unsusceptible to high concentrations of the drug.

The synthesis of cell wall peptidoglycan may be conveniently divided into four stages, namely: (i) the syntheis of uridino-diphospho-

N-acetylmuramic acid; (ii) the sequential attachment onto it of a pentapeptide side chain; (iii) the synthesis of a disaccharidic pentapeptide unit and its transfer to the growing polysaccharide chains; and (iv) their cross-linking.

Treatment with gardimycin elicits the accumulation of UDP-MurNAc-pentapeptide, indicating that the drug interferes with reactions at stage (iii) or stage (iv) of cell wall biosynthesis. Stage (iii) consists of several discrete reactions: the binding through a pyrophosphate linkage of UDP-MurNAc-pentapeptide to an isoprenyl phosphate carrier called C_{55}, which is associated with cell membrane. UDP-NAc is then attached to this intermediate, with formation of a disaccharidic pentapeptide unit, which is transferred to a cell wall acceptor, with release of C_{55}-pyrophosphate, which is then dephosphorylated and starts a new reaction cycle.

Gardimycin, added to a cell-free system that is able to carry out all these reactions, results in accumulation of disaccharide-C_{55} intermediate, thus indicating that it is active at the site of the further reaction, namely, its transfer to the cell wall acceptor. In fact, gardimycin behaves like vancomycin, a known inhibitor of such a transfer reaction (1, 14).

Ristocetin (1, 5), macarbomycin (14), diumycin (6, 7), enduracidin (6), meonomycin, prasinomycin, 11.837 RP (8), janemycin, and subtilin (6) have also been reported to interfere with this reaction. The mechanism of action of gardimycin differs from that of bacitracin (12), which prevents the dephosphorylation of C_{55}-pyrophosphate, from that of nisin (6), which does not induce accumulation of the phospholipid intermediate, and from that of the penicillins and cephalosporins, which interfere with transpeptidase and carboxypeptidase activity involved in the cross-linking (5).

LITERATURE CITED

1. **Anderson J. S., M. Matsuhashi, M. A. Naskin, and J. L. Strominger.** 1967. Biosynthesis of the peptidoglycan of bacterial cell wall. II. Phospholipid carrier in the reaction sequence. J. Biol. Chem. 242:3180–3190.
2. **Arioli, V., M. Berti, and L. G. Silvestri.** 1976. Gardimycin, a new antibiotic from Actinoplanes. III. Biological properties. J. Antibiot. 39:511–515.
3. **Coronelli, C., G. Tamoni, and G. C. Lancini.** 1976. Gardimycin, a new antibiotic from Actinoplanes. II. Isolation and preliminary characterization. J. Antibiot. 39:507–510.
4. **Garret, A. J.** 1969. The effect of magnesium ion deprivation on the synthesis of mucopeptide and its precursors in *Bacillus subtilis*. Biochem. J. 115:419–430.
5. **Izaki K., M. Matsuhashi, and J. L. Strominger.** 1968. Biosynthesis of peptidoglycan of bacterial cell walls. XIII. Peptidoglycan transpeptidase and D-alanine carboxypeptidase: penicillin-sensitive enzymatic reactions in strains of *Escherichia coli*. J. Biol. Chem. 243:3180–3192.
6. **Linnet, P. E., and J. L. Strominger.** 1973. Additional antibiotic inhibitors of peptidoglycan synthesis. Antimicrob. Agents Chemother. 4:231–236.
7. **Lugtenberg E. J. J., J. A. Hellings, and G. J. Van De Berg.** 1972. Inhibition of peptidoglycan synthesis by the antibiotic diumycin A. Antimicrob. Agents Chemother. 2:485–491.
8. **Lugtenberg E. J. J., A. van Schijndel-van Dam, and T. M. H. van Bellegem.** 1971. In vivo and in vitro action of new antibiotics interfering with the utilization of *N*-acetyl-glucosamine-*N*-acetyl-muramyl-pentapeptide. J. Bacteriol. 108:20–29.
9. **Parenti, F., H. Pagani, and G. Beretta.** 1976. Gardimycin, a new antibiotic from Actinoplanes. I. Description of the producer strain and fermentation studies. J. Antibiot. 39:501–506.
10. **Reissig, J. L., J. L. Strominger, and F. Leloir.** 1955. A modified colorimetric method for the extimation of N-acetyl-amino sugars. J. Biol. Chem. 217:959–966.
11. **Reynolds, P. E. 1971.** Peptidoglycan synthesis in Bacilli. I. Effect of temperature on the in vitro system from *Bacillus megaterium* and *Bacillus stearothermophilus*. Biochim. Biophys. Acta 237:239–254.
12. **Siewert, G., and J. L. Strominger.** 1967. Bacitracin, an inhibitor of the dephosphorylation of lipidpyrophosphate, an intermediate in biosynthesis of the peptidoglycan of bacterial cell walls. Proc. Natl. Acad. Sci. U.S.A. 57:767–773.
13. **Strominger, J. L., M. Matsuhashi, J. S. Anderson, C. P. Dietrich, G. M. Sievert, and J. M. Gilbert.** 1966. Glycopeptide synthesis in *Staphylococcus aureus* and *Micrococcus lysodeikticus*, p. 473–486. *In* E. N. Neufeld and V. Ginsbury (ed.), Methods in enzymology, vol. 8. Academic Press Inc., New York.
14. **Suzuki J., M. Hori, T. Saeki, and H. Umezawa.** 1972. Macarbomycin, an inhibitor of peptidoglycan synthesis. J. Antibiot. 25:94–104.

ANTIMICROBIAL AGENTS AND CHEMOTHERAPY, Mar. 1977, p. 402–406 Vol. 11, No. 3

Antibacterial Activity of Netilmicin, a New Aminoglycoside Antibiotic, Compared with That of Gentamicin

IAN PHILLIPS,* ANNE SMITH, AND KEVIN SHANNON

Department of Microbiology, St. Thomas's Hospital Medical School, London SE1 7EH, England

Received for publication 13 October 1976

The antibacterial activity of netilmicin (Sch 20569), a new semisynthetic aminoglycoside, was compared with that of gentamicin against a variety of gram-negative bacteria, staphylococci, and streptococci. Both antibiotics had similar activity against most organisms, but netilmicin had appreciably greater activity against gram-negative organisms that were resistant to gentamicin because these species synthesized aminoglycoside 3-*N*-acetyltransferase I or aminoglycoside 2''-*O*-nucleotidyltransferase. Netilmicin was also more active than gentamicin against gentamicin-resistant strains of *Staphylococcus aureus* that produced two enzymes—aminoglycoside-2''-*O*-phosphotransferase and aminoglycoside-6'-*N*-acetyltransferase.

Netilmicin (Sch 20569) (Fig. 1), a new semisynthetic aminoglycoside antibiotic, is a derivative of sisomicin, which itself is a derivative of gentamicin C_{1A}. Although gentamicin and sisomicin have similar activity against most organisms (4, 5), there is evidence that netilmicin is more effective than either gentamicin or sisomicin against certain gentamicin-resistant organisms (6, 9, 11; informational material for SCH 20569, Schering Corp., Bloomfield, N.J., 1975). The purpose of this study was to compare the antibacterial activity of netilmicin with that of gentamicin against a variety of gentamicin-susceptible and gentamicin-resistant bacteria.

MATERIALS AND METHODS

Bacterial strains. The collection consisted of *Acinetobacter anitratus* (7), *A. lwoffi* (9), *Bacteroides fragilis* (19), *Citrobacter freundii* (38), *C. koserii* (30), *Enterobacter aerogenes* (20), *E. cloacae* (29), *Escherichia coli* (41), *Haemophilus influenzae* (16), *Neisseria gonorrhoeae* (39), *Klebsiella aerogenes* (51), *K. ozaenae* (20), *Proteus mirabilis* (31), *P. morganii* (20), *P. rettgeri* (17), *P. vulgaris* (20), *Providencia alkalifaciens* (9), *P. stuartii* (28), *Pseudomonas aeruginosa* (48), *Pseudomonas* spp. (62; *P. acidovorans*, 15; *P. cepacia*, 10; *P. fluorescens*, 3; *P. maltophilia*, 11; *P. pseudoalkaligenes*, 11; *P. putida*, 3; *P. stutzeri*, 7; *P. thomasii*, 5), *Serratia marcescens* (5), *Staphylococcus albus* (41), *S. aureus* (120), *Streptococcus faecalis* (38), *S. pneumoniae* (14), and beta-hemolytic streptococci (56). Most of the strains were isolates from patients in St. Thomas's Hospital, but the collection included the following strains from the National Collection of Type Cultures: *E. aerogenes* (3), *K. ozaenae* (12), *P. rettgeri* (7), *P. Alkalifaciens* (9), *P. Stuartii* (3), *P. Fluorescens* (1), *P. maltophila* (1), *P. pseudoalkaligenes* (1), *P. Stutzeri* (3), and *S. marcescens* (5). Gentamicin-resistant strains from other sources, mostly in Great Britain, were: *E. cloacae* (1), *E. coli* (1), *K. aerogenes* (1), *P. rettgeri* (1), *P. stuartii* (13), *P. aeruginosa* (14), *P. stutzeri* (3), *S. aureus* (6).

Determination of minimum inhibitory concentrations (MICs). Organisms were grown in nutrient broth (Southern Group Laboratories) at 37°C for 18 h. The medium was supplemented with 10% lysed horse blood for *H. influenzae* and *N. gonorrhoeae* and with 10% horse serum for *S. pneumoniae*. The inoculum of *B. fragilis* was prepared by scraping cells off blood agar and suspending them in nutrient broth. Cultures were suitably diluted and 10^3 to 10^4 colony-forming units inoculated on serial doubling dilutions of the antibiotics in Diagnostic Sensitivity Test agar (Oxoid CM 261). For *B. fragilis*, *N. gonorrhoeae*, and *S. pneumoniae*, 6 to 10% lysed horse blood was added. For *H. influenzae*, Columbia agar base (Oxoid CM 331) supplemented with factor V (2%) and factor X (1%) was used. Incubation was at 37°C aerobically (with 10% CO_2 for *N. gonorrhoeae* and *S. pneumoniae*), except for *B. fragilis*, which was incubated in an atmosphere of 10% H_2, 10% CO_2, and 80% N_2. The MIC was the lowest concentration of antibiotic that resulted in complete suppression of growth after overnight incubation. Linear regression of MICs of gentamicin and netilmicin was performed by the method of least squares after transformation of MICs to $\log_2$ of MICs.

Demonstration of enzyme activity. For investigations of aminoglycoside-modifying enzymes, use was made of the cellulose phosphate paper binding system (2). Suspensions, concentrated 10- to 20-fold, of cells grown at 37°C in Oxoid nutrient broth no. 2 (CM 67) were broken with an ultrasonic disintegrator (MSE Mark II). The resulting preparations were tested for their ability to bind radioactivity from acetyl-coenzyme A or adenosine-5'-triphosphate to aminoglycosides.

For acetylation, each tube contained, in a total

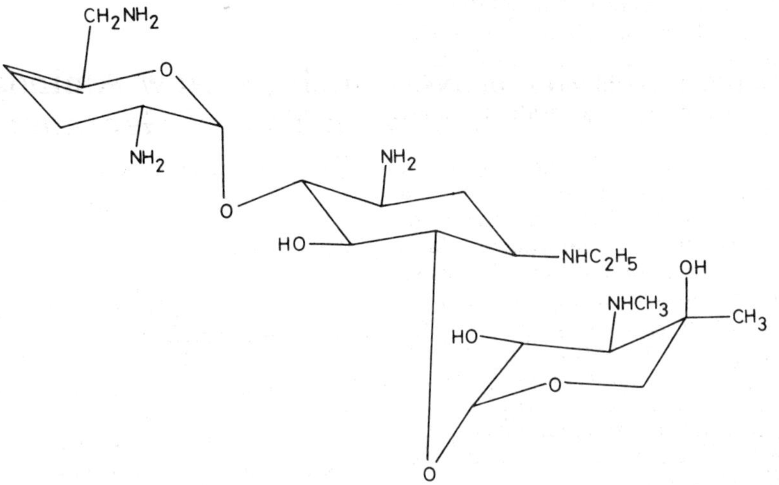

FIG. 1. *Structure of netilmicin.*

volume of 55 μl: 360 ng of aminoglycoside, 1.4 nmol of [1-^{14}C]acetyl-coenzyme A (specific activity, 4.65 Ci/mol), 3 mmol of tris(hydroxymethyl)aminomethane (Tris)-hydrochloride buffer, pH 7.6, 480 nmol of $MgCl_2$, 150 nmol of dithiothreitol, and 15 μl of cell sonicate. For phosphorylation, each tube contained, in a total volume of 55 μl: 360 ng of aminoglycoside, 7 nmol of [γ-^{32}P]adenosine 5′-triphosphate (1.35 Ci/mol), 3 mmol of Tris-hydrochloride buffer, pH 7.6, 480 nmol of $MgCl_2$, 150 nmol of dithiothreitol, and 15 μl of cell sonicate. For adenylylation, each tube contained, in a total volume of 60 μl: 130 ng of aminoglycoside, 2 nmol of [8-^{14}C]adenosine 5′-triphosphate (4 Ci/mol), 4 mmol of Tris-hydrochloride buffer, pH 8.1, 640 nmol of $MgCl_2$, 285 nmol of dithiothreitol, and 28.5 μl of cell sonicate.

After incubation at 37°C for 20 to 60 min, 50-μl amounts of the mixture were pipetted onto squares (20 by 20 mm) of Whatman P81 cellulose phosphate paper. The papers were washed in water, dried, and placed in vials containing scintillation fluid which consisted of toluene containing 2,5-diphenyloxazole (6 g/liter) and 1,4-di-[2]-(5-phenyloxazolyl) benzene (100 mg/liter). Radioactivity was measured in a Beckman liquid scintillation spectrometer. Radioactive materials were obtained from the Radiochemical Centre, Amersham, Bucks, England. Chemicals for scintillation counting were obtained from Koch-Light Laboratories, Colnbrook, Bucks, England.

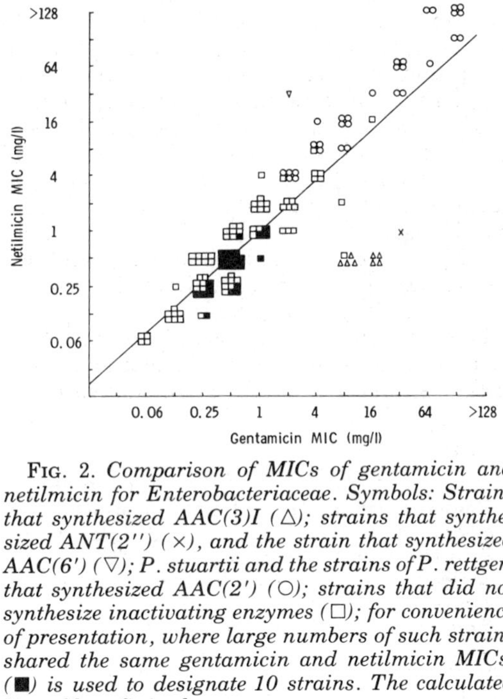

FIG. 2. *Comparison of MICs of gentamicin and netilmicin for Enterobacteriaceae. Symbols: Strains that synthesized AAC(3)I (△); strains that synthesized ANT(2″) (×), and the strain that synthesized AAC(6′) (▽); P. stuartii and the strains of P. rettgeri that synthesized AAC(2′) (○); strains that did not synthesize inactivating enzymes (□); for convenience of presentation, where large numbers of such strains shared the same gentamicin and netilmicin MICs, (■) is used to designate 10 strains. The calculated line of best fit is shown.*

RESULTS

Figure 2 shows MICs of gentamicin versus MICs of netilmicin for the *Enterobacteriaceae*. Of the 332 strains of species other than *P. stuartii*, 95% were susceptible to both gentamicin and netilmicin (MICs, 4 μg/ml). No resistant strains were encountered among isolates of *C. freundii*, *C. koserii*, *E. aerogenes*, *K. ozaenae*, *P. morganii*, *P. vulgaris*, and *P. alkalifaciens*. Strains known to produce enzymes that inactivate aminoglycosides (I. Phillips, King, and K. Shannon, manuscript in preparation) were allocated distinguishing symbols. Seven strains of *K. aerogenes* and one of *E. cloacae* that produced aminoglycoside 3-*N*-acetyltransferase I [AAC(3)I] were resistant to gentamicin but susceptible to netilmicin, as was the strain of *K. aerogenes* that produced aminoglycoside 2″-*O*-nucleotidyltransferase [ANT(2″)]. One strain of *S. marcescens* that produced aminoglycoside 6′-*N*-acetyltransferase [AAC(6′)] was susceptible to gentamicin but resistant to netilmicin. All 28 strains of *P. stuartii* produced aminoglycoside 2′-*N*-acetyltransferase [AAC(2′)], as did three strains of *P. rettgeri*. These strains were generally resistant to both agents.

Results for the genus *Pseudomonas* are shown in Fig. 3. Of the 48 strains of *P. aeruginosa*, 58% were susceptible to gentamicin and 56% were susceptible to netilmicin. Most strains resistant to gentamicin were also resistant to netilmicin, but a few that produced aminoglycoside-inactivating enzymes were susceptible to netilmicin. Fewer strains of *Pseudomonas* spp. (40% of 62 strains) than of *P. aeruginosa* were susceptible to either agent. Only one strain was resistant to gentamicin but susceptible to netilmicin; this strain, of *P. pseudoalkaligenes*, produced AAC(3)I.

Netilmicin was less effective than gentamicin against the genus *Acinetobacter* in which a number of strains produced AAC(6′). All 16 strains were inhibited by gentamicin at a concentration of 2 μg/ml, but five strains were resistant to this concentration of netilmicin.

H. influenzae had similar susceptibilities to both agents; MICs of 0.5 to 2 μg/ml were found for all strains. *N. gonorrhoeae* was more susceptible to netilmicin (MICs, 2 to 8 μg/ml; geometric mean MIC, 3.3 μg/ml) than to gentamicin (MICs, 4 to 16 μg/ml; geometric mean MIC, 5.6 μg/ml). Neither drug had activity against *B. fragilis* (MICs, 128 μg/ml).

More than 90% of strains of *S. aureus* were susceptible to both agents. The gentamicin-resistant strains were often more susceptible to netilmicin (Fig. 4). Most of these strains were found to produce two enzymes: AAC(6′), which does not produce resistance to gentamicin (1), and an enzyme that phosphorylates gentamicin, tobramycin, and kanamycin but not neomycin or amikacin, and so is probably aminoglycoside 2″-*O*-phosphotransferase [APT(2″)] (10). A similar enzyme was found in the first gentamicin-resistant strain of *S. aureus* reported in Great Britain (3, 7).

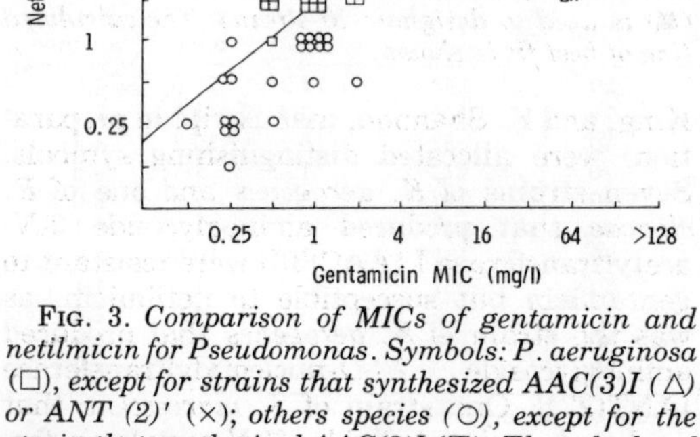

FIG. 3. *Comparison of MICs of gentamicin and netilmicin for Pseudomonas. Symbols: P. aeruginosa (□), except for strains that synthesized AAC(3)I (△) or ANT (2)′ (×); others species (○), except for the strain that synthesized AAC(3)I (▽). The calculated line of best fit is shown.*

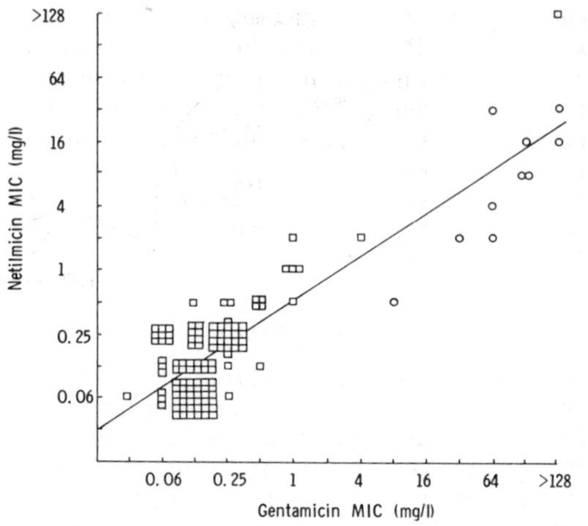

FIG. 4. *Comparison of MICs of gentamicin and netilmicin for S. aureus. Symbols: Strains that synthesized APT(2″) and AAC(6′) (○); other strains (□). The calculated line of best fit is shown.*

S. albus was very susceptible to both drugs, with more than 90% of strains inhibited by 0.25 μg of gentamicin or netilmicin per ml. One strain was resistant to gentamicin but susceptible to netilmicin; it produced the same enzymes as the gentamicin-resistant strains of *S. aureus*.

Most strains of *S. faecalis* were resistant to both agents (MICs, 8 to 32 μg/ml), although 4 of the 38 strains had netilmicin MICs of 4 μg/ml. *S. pneumoniae* was resistant to both agents (MICs, 32 to 64 μg/ml). For beta-hemolytic streptococci, MICs ranged from 0.5 to 32 μg/ml. At a concentration of 4 μg/ml, 70% of strains were inhibited by gentamicin, and 68% were inhibited by netilmicin.

Table 1 shows in vitro modification of gentamicin, sisomicin, and netilmicin by extracts of representative strains that produce aminoglycoside-inactivating enzymes. Netilmicin was a poorer substrate than gentamicin and sisomicin for AAC(3)I and ANT(2″). Sisomicin was a better substrate than gentamicin for AAC(6′), because this enzyme does not acetylate gentamicin C_1 (1). Netilmicin was acetylated by AAC(6′) less well than was sisomicin. For AAC(6′) from *S. aureus* netilmicin was a poorer substrate than gentamicin. There were two types of APT(2″). For the first type, which was more common, sisomicin was a poorer substrate than gentamicin, and netilmicin was phosphorylated only to a small extent. Gentamicin and sisomicin were equally good substrates of the second type and, although it was a poorer substrate, netilmicin was extensively phosphorylated.

DISCUSSION

Despite the general similarity in activity of gentamicin and netilmicin, there was a number of strains against which netilmicin was more active than gentamicin or sisomicin. These strains were mostly ones found to produce enzymes that inactivated gentamicin but for which netilmicin was a poor substrate, although no evidence of inactivating enzymes was detected in one such strain of *E. coli*. Thus, in netilmicin, substitution of an ethyl group on the C1 amino group results in partial protection of the C3 amino and C2″ hydroxyl groups from attack by AAC(3)I, ANT(2″), and APT(2″). This protection usually seems to be sufficient to render producers of AAC(3)I and ANT(2″) fully susceptible to netilmicin. Protection of netilmicin from attack by ANT(2″) has been reported before (6, 11), but for AAC(3)I previous work was contradictory. Soussy and Duval (11) found a strain of *E. coli* that produced AAC(3)I to be susceptible to netilmicin, whereas Kabins et al. (6) found a strain of *P. aeruginosa* to be resistant. Of the organisms that produced this enzyme, we found *Enterobacteriaceae* always to be susceptible to netilmicin; the strain of *P. pseudoalkaligenes* and one of the two strains of *P. aeruginosa* were susceptible and, although the other strain of *P. aeruginosa* was resistant (MIC, 16 μg/ml), it was more susceptible to netilmicin than to gentamicin (MIC, >128 μg/ml). We find producers of AAC(3)I and ANT(2″) generally to be susceptible to amikacin (Phillips et al., manuscript in preparation) in agreement with the suggestion that the L-γ-amino-α-hydroxybutyryl group substituted on the C1 amino group in amikacin has a similar role to the ethyl group of netilmicin (8).

The staphylococci that produced APT(2″) always produced AAC(6′) as well. One cannot separate the individual contributions of these enzymes to resistance, but the strains were generally more susceptible to netilmicin than to gentamicin. They were, however, sufficiently resistant to netilmicin to rule out treatment with this agent. In this finding, we agree with previous work (11).

The C2′ amino group of netilmicin is not protected, since AAC(2′) acetylated the drug. Strains of *P. stuartii* and *P. rettgeri* that produced this enzyme tended to be more resistant to netilmicin than to gentamicin, as was found before (6, 11).

Although acetylated less than sisomicin, netilmicin was a good substrate of AAC(6′) from gram-negative organisms. The strains that produced this enzyme, mostly *Acinetobacter* spp., were the only ones resistant to netilmicin and sisomicin but susceptible to gentamicin. Netilmicin was a poor substrate of AAC(6′) from staphylococci, as is amikacin (3, 10).

For the *Klebsiella-Enterobacter-Serratia* group, in which gentamicin resistance was enzyme mediated, correlation between MICs of gentamicin and netilmicin was poor (correlation coefficient, $r = 0.57$). *P. aeruginosa*, some gentamicin-resistant strains of which produced inactivating enzymes, also had a low correlation coefficient ($r = 0.61$). In contrast, for groups in which there was a sufficiently wide range of MICs there were good correlation coef-

TABLE 1. *In vitro modification of gentamicin, sisomicin, and netilmicin by inactivating enzymes*

Organism	Enzyme	MIC (μg/ml)			Incubation time (min)	Background radioactivity (cpm)[a]	Binding of radioactivity to aminoglycosides[b]		
		Gentamicin	Sisomicin	Netilmicin			Gentamicin	Sisomicin	Netilmicin
K. aerogenes	AAC(3)I	8	16	0.5	20	184	14.9	27.0	4.0
P. aeruginosa	AAC(3)I	128	128	16	20	359	3.4	2.0	1.2
P. stuartii	AAC(2′)	64	128	128	20	552	6.9	10.2	8.3
S. marcescens	AAC(6′)	2	8	32	20	312	1.7	1.7	1.8
A. lwoffi	AAC(6′)	2	32	64	60	167	1.6	2.9	2.0
K. aerogenes	ANT(2″)	32	16	1	60	257	1.3	1.2	1.1
P. aeruginosa	ANT(2″)	128	128	8	30	141	7.3	10.0	1.9
S. aureus	APT(2″) type 1	64	64	2	30	1537	1.8	1.2	1.1
	AAC(6′)	64	64	2	30	202	3.4	4.9	1.6
S. aureus	APT(2″) type 2	128	NT[c]	128	30	384	7.3	7.3	4.2
	AAC(6′)	128	NT	128	30	165	6.6	15.2	4.3

[a] Binding of radioactivity to cellulose phosphate paper in the absence of aminoglycosides.

[b] Shown as multiples of radioactivity bound to cellulose phosphate paper in the absence of aminoglycosides.

[c] NT, Not tested.

ficients. This was true both for groups such as *P. stuartii* (r = 0.96) and *S. aureus* (r = 0.88), in which both gentamicin and netilmicin were substrates of inactivating enzymes and for groups such as *Pseudomonas* spp. (r = 0.97) and beta-hemolytic streptococci (r = 0.94), in which resistance was not the result of inactivation but occurred more or less equally to both drugs.

Our studies suggest that, like sisomicin (4, 5), netilmicin does not have appreciably better antibacterial activity than gentamicin against most organisms, but this it is superior against gram-negative organisms whose gentamicin resistance is the result of synthesis of AAC(3)I or ANT(2'') and against staphylococci whose gentamicin resistance is due to the production of APT(2'') and AAC(6').

ACKNOWLEDGMENTS

We are grateful to Schering Corp. (U.S.A.) for financial support and for providing netilmicin and sisomicin, and to British Schering Limited for providing gentamicin. We also wish to thank N. Datta, P. Noone, A. Percival, D. S. Reeves, R. Sutherland, P. Waterworth, R. E. Warren and J. D. Williams who provided gentamicin-resistant organisms.

LITERATURE CITED

1. **Benveniste, R., and J. Davies.** 1971. Enzymatic acetylation of aminoglycoside antibiotics by *Escherichia coli* carrying an R. factor. Biochemistry 10:1787–1796.
2. **Benveniste, R., and J. Davies.** 1973. Mechanism of antibiotic resistance in bacteria. Annu. Rev. Biochem. 42:471–506.
3. **Brown, D. F. J., F. H. Kayser, and J. Biber.** 1976. Gentamicin resistance in *Staphylococcus aureus*. Lancet 2:419.
4. **Crowe, C. C., and E. Sanders.** 1973. Sisomicin: evaluation in vitro and comparison with gentamicin and tobramycin. Antimicrob. Agents Chemother. 3:24–28.
5. **Hyams, P. J., M. S. Simberkoff, and J. J. Rahal.** 1973. In vitro bactericidal effectiveness of four aminoglycoside antibiotics. Antimicrob. Agents Chemother. 3:87–94.
6. **Kabins, S. A., C. Nathan, and S. Cohen.** 1976. In vitro comparison of netilmicin, a semisynthetic derivative of sisomicin, and four other aminoglycoside antibiotics. Antimicrob. Agents Chemother. 10:139–145.
7. **Porthouse, A., D. F. J. Brown, R. Graeme Smith, and T. Rogers.** 1976. Gentamicin resistance in *Staphylococcus aureus*. Lancet 1:20–21.
8. **Price, K. E., J. C. Godfrey, and H. Kawaguchi.** 1974. Effect of structural modifications on the biological properties of aminoglycoside antibiotics containing 2-deoxystreptamine. Adv. Appl. Microbiol. 18:191–307.
9. **Rahal, J. J., M. S. Simberkoff, K. Kagan, and N. H. Moldover.** 1976. Bactericidal efficacy of Sch 20569 and amikacin against gentamicin-sensitive and -resistant organisms. Antimicrob. Agents Chemother. 9:595–599.
10. **Shannon, K. P., and I. Phillips.** 1976. Gentamicin-resistant *Staphylococcus aureus*. Lancet 2:580–581.
11. **Soussy, C. J., and J. Duval.** 1976. Activité antibactérienne comparée de sept aminosides. Méd Mal. Infect. 6:211–218.

ANTIMICROBIAL AGENTS AND CHEMOTHERAPY, Mar. 1977, p. 407-410 Vol. 11, No. 3
 Printed in U.S.A.

In Vivo Effects of Josamycin, Erythromycin, and Placebo Therapy on Nasal Carriage of *Staphylococcus aureus*

SAMUEL Z. WILSON,* R. RUSSELL MARTIN, AND MARGARET PUTMAN

Departments of Microbiology and Immunology, and Medicine, Baylor College of Medicine, Houston, Texas 77030

Received for publication 27 September 1976

Healthy nasal carriers of *Staphylococcus aureus* were randomly assigned to one of three treatment regimens: josamycin (1.5 g/day), erythromycin stearate (1.0 g/day), or placebo, each administered orally for 7 days. Quantitative nasal cultures were obtained from each subject at intervals before, during, and after treatment. All 25 placebo-treated subjects had positive nasal cultures for *S. aureus* at all culture intervals. Both josamycin and erythromycin were equally effective in reducing the carrier rates and in decreasing the total numbers of *S. aureus* isolated from subjects with positive cultures during treatment. No increase in in vitro antibiotic resistance was detected in isolates obtained after therapy. Both antibiotics were well tolerated, and toxicity was not encountered with either drug.

Josamycin is a new macrolide antibiotic produced by *Streptomyces narboneosis* var. *josamyceticus*. Although josamycin is still an investigational preparation in the United States, it has been used clinically in Japan since 1967 (4). Macrolide antibiotics, especially erythromycin, have been useful as an alternative to semisynthetic penicillins in the treatment of infections caused by *Staphylococcus aureus*. As new macrolide antibiotics are introduced, it is important to determine their relative antistaphylococcal activity, in addition to evaluating toxicity and the incidence of side effects (2).

This study compared the effects of oral therapy with josamycin, erythromycin stearate, and a placebo on *S. aureus* cultured from the nose of healthy carriers. Serial quantitative nasal cultures were obtained to evaluate the effects of therapy on carrier rates and on the number of organisms isolated. In vitro susceptibility of isolates obtained before and after therapy was compared to determine whether resistance was induced by in vivo exposure to either of the antibiotics.

MATERIALS AND METHODS

Subjects for this study were healthy students and staff at the Baylor College of Medicine. Single quantitative nasal cultures were performed on 414 subjects, of which 103 contained *S. aureus*. From this group, a total of 75 *S. aureus* nasal carriers volunteered for the experimental portion of the study after two additional pretreatment nasal cultures obtained 1 week apart had verified the continued presence of pigmented, coagulase-positive staphylococci. The design of the study was explained to each subject and, before the subject was enrolled, written informed consent was obtained on a form approved by the Baylor Institutional Review Board for Human Research.

In selecting an antibiotic dose, preliminary information was available from Endo Laboratories, Inc., Garden City, N.Y., indicating that comparable blood levels were obtained with divided total daily doses of 1.5 g of josamycin and 1.0 g of erythromycin stearate. Consequently, the dose of josamycin chosen for therapy was higher than that of erythromycin stearate, in an attempt to maintain bioequivalence.

Volunteers were randomly assigned to one of three treatment regimens: 1.5 g of josamycin per day, 1.0 g of erythromycin stearate per day, or placebo. All therapy was administered orally in four divided doses for 7 days. Josamycin was supplied by Yamanouchi Pharmaceutical Company, Tokyo, Japan, as a round, orange, film-coated tablet containing 250 mg of josamycin. Erythromycin stearate was obtained from Abbot Laboratories as a round, pink, film-coated tablet bearing the Abbott Co. logo and containing 250 mg of erythromycin stearate. The placebo was identical in appearance to the josamycin tablet and contained microcrystalline cellulose. Because the two antibiotics were not identical in appearance, and because of the higher dose of josamycin than erythromycin, subjects treated with josamycin received alternating doses of two josamycin tablets or one josamycin tablet and one josamycin placebo, to provide a total daily dose of 1.5 g. Subjects treated with placebo received two josamycin placebo tablets every 6 h. Subjects treated with erythromycin stearate received one erythromycin stearate tablet and one josamycin placebo every 6 h. Medication was prepackaged and coded by Endo Laboratories, and supplied in individual-dose packages. The code was unknown to the investigators but was accessible in case identification of the treatment regimen of a particular volunteer was required.

Before enrollment in the study, a preliminary history and physical examination was performed, and all subjects were found to be healthy and free of significant acute or chronic medical problems. Blood and urine samples were obtained twice before and 1 day after completion of therapy, to monitor clinical laboratory tests appropriate to detect possible adverse effects of the drug on hepatic, renal, or hematological function. Standard 12-lead electrocardiograms were obtained before therapy and on day 7 of therapy on all subjects.

A diary of side effects and complaints was maintained by each subject during the 7 days of medication and for 2 weeks after completion of therapy. A diary of drug administration was recorded in relation to meals and other activities during the 7 days of therapy.

Serial quantitative nasal cultures included at least two pretreatment cultures, two cultures during therapy, and three post-treatment cultures, which spanned the interval from 1 day to 4 weeks after completion of therapy. Of the planned cultures, 100% were obtained. *S. aureus* nasal carriers were defined as those subjects whose pretreatment nasal cultures consistently yielded pigmented, coagulase-positive staphylococci. Normal rabbit plasma (Difco) was employed in the coagulase tube test.

Three colonies of coagulase-positive staphylococci were selected and stored from the immediate pretreatment cultures from each subject. From post-treatment cultures of subjects who reacquired staphylococci, or who continued to have staphylococci cultured from the nose, three colonies were also obtained for in vitro testing. Pretreatment and post-treatment *S. aureus* isolates were tested for antibiotic susceptibility by the Kirby-Bauer disk susceptibility method, using antibiotic disks purchased from Baltimore Biological Laboratory (BBL). Strains were considered susceptible to erythromycin if a zone diameter of 18 mm or greater was measured around the 15-μg disk. Three different potencies of josamycin disks were employed (2- 15-, and 30-μg/disk). Strains were considered susceptible if the zone around the 15-μg josamycin disk was 18 mm or greater.

Phage typing of selected strains was performed by the State Public Health Laboratory in Austin, Tex.

Quantitative nasal cultures were performed as previously reported (8), using serial 10-fold dilutions of materials swabbed from the anterior part of the nose diluted in Trypticase soy broth (BBL). In addition to plating the cultures on Trypticase soy agar (where *S. aureus* was recognized by pigment production), aliquots were plated on Vogel and Johnson agar (BBL), on which coagulase-positive staphylococci formed characteristic black colonies. The use of Vogel and Johnson medium allowed quantitation of staphylococci when other organisms overgrew the Trypticase soy agar plates and provided more certainty in collecting isolates when this occurred.

Of the 75 volunteers originally enrolled in the study, 1 withdrew before therapy, and 3 were dropped from the study due to clinical illness or abnormal laboratory values detected before medication. Complete data was obtained from 73 treatment courses in 71 volunteers. Two volunteers were treated twice in courses 6 months apart because of incomplete or questionably abnormal clinical laboratory data from the initial course of therapy. One subject (treated with erythromycin) had base-line serum glutamic oxalacetic transaminase values of 21 units on two separate pretreatment tests, whereas a higher value of 37 units (normal range: <40 units) was obtained after 1 week of therapy. The other subject had a moderate decrease in hemoglobin level (16.3 to 14.6 g/100 ml), hematocrit (46.5 to 41.9%), and erythrocyte count (5.2×10^6 to $4.7 \times 10^6/mm^3$) after 7 days of josamycin therapy. It is doubtful that these alterations represented adverse reactions to either erythromycin or josamycin. However, to be certain, both subjects were retreated, and neither subject had any abnormality after another 7-day course of therapy with the same drug.

RESULTS

Of the 25 subjects treated with placebo, *S. aureus* was isolated from every nasal culture obtained during pretreatment screening and during the 36 days encompassing therapy and post-treatment follow-up (Fig. 1). This documents that the criteria employed in defining *S. aureus* nasal carriers were effective in identifying a true carrier state. Both josamycin (used to treat 22 subjects) and erythromycin (used in 26 subjects) were equally effective in reducing the incidence of positive nasal cultures for *S. aureus* obtained during therapy. When carrier rates for *S. aureus* were compared 1 day or 1 week after completion of therapy, rates were not significantly different for josamycin- or erythromycin-treated subjects. However, from cultures taken 4 weeks after completion of therapy, 24 of 26 erythromycin-treated subjects

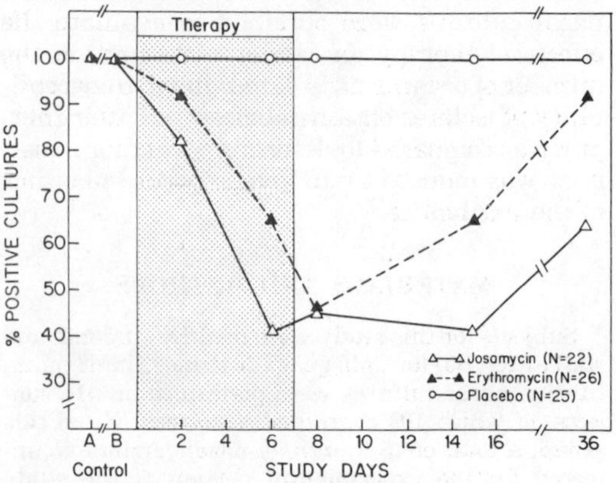

FIG. 1. *Incidence of positive cultures for S. aureus before, during, and after treatment with josamycin, erythromycin, and placebo.*

were once again carriers of *S. aureus* in the nose, whereas only 14 of 22 josamycin-treated subjects were nasal carriers (χ^2, $P < 0.05$).

The mean numbers of *S. aureus* isolated from pretreatment quantitative nasal cultures were very similar from subjects treated with placebo or with erythromycin. The 22 josamycin-treated subjects had slightly lower pretreatment numbers of *S. aureus*, a difference attributable to the presence in the other two groups of several individuals with very high colony counts (Fig. 2). Reproducibility of the quantitative nasal culture method is illustrated by the consistency of the mean numbers obtained from the placebo-treated group, which remained throughout within 0.5 log of the control quantities. In cultures from subjects treated with either of the active antibiotics, over 99% reduction occurred in the numbers of *S. aureus* isolated from cultures that remained positive, and post-therapy numbers of bacteria were similar.

In addition to quantitation of *S. aureus* isolates, the total numbers of all other aerobic bacteria swabbed from the nose were also determined. Colony counts for these organisms were combined, without differentiation as to genera and species. During the 7 days of therapy, and for the 4 weeks after therapy, the total counts of aerobic bacteria isolated from subjects in each of the three treatment regimens ranged within 0.5 log of the control counts for each group. This is in contrast to previous observations of the effects of broad-spectrum, topical therapy with gentamicin in which suppression of the total aerobic nasal flora paralleled the decrease in staphylococci (8).

These pretreatment *S. aureus* colonies from each subject were tested for susceptibility to erythromycin and to josamycin. Post-treatment isolates from all subjects who reacquired or continued to carry *S. aureus* were also tested for susceptibility to both antibiotics. Few of the strains isolated from this group of young, healthy, ambulatory nasal carriers were resistant to either antibiotic. Of the more than 200 pretreatment isolates tested, no josamycin-resistant strains were found, and only three subjects (approximately 4% of the individuals tested) carried erythromycin-resistant strains. None of these three subjects was treated with erythromycin. One subject was treated with placebo, and the same strain (resistant to erythromycin, phage type 85) was consistently isolated. The other two subjects were treated with josamycin. One of these carried phage type 94, 96 before and after therapy. The other (subject no. 160) was a nasal carrier of phage type 52, 52A, 80, 81 on pretreatment culture. Cultures obtained on days 6, 8, and 15 of the study were negative for *S. aureus*. On day 36 (the final day of culture), a new strain of *S. aureus* (phage type 6) was isolated that was susceptible to erythromycin.

No course of therapy was discontinued because of side effects or toxicities. No laboratory abnormalities definitely attributable to therapy with either antibiotic were documented during these studies. Electrocardiograms done on day 7 of therapy showed no changes. After analysis of the symptom diaries, the incidence of diarrhea, loose stools, or increased number of stools was not significantly greater with josamycin (7 of 22) or erythromycin (9 of 26) than with placebo (5 of 25).

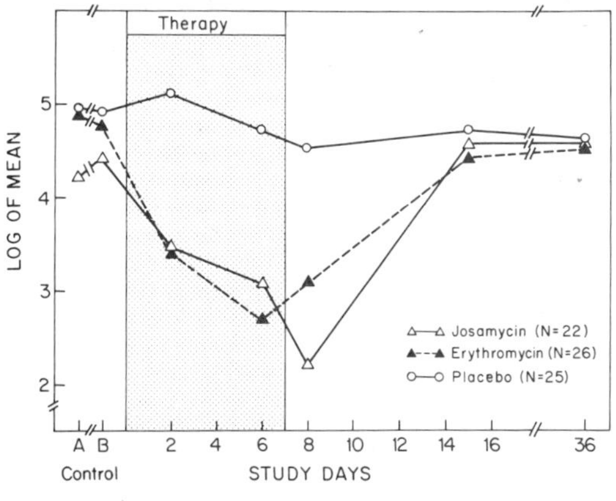

FIG. 2. *Log of mean of colony counts of S. aureus in experiment described in Fig. 1.*

DISCUSSION

Previous studies employing quantitative nasal cultures have shown that antibiotics modify the nasal flora and that results of quantitative nasal cultures provide a reliable indication of in vivo efficacy of an antistaphylococcal compound (2, 3, 9). When staphylococci are suppressed in the nose by therapy, this effect typically persists only as long as the antimicrobial agent is administered or until an antibiotic-resistant strain colonizes the nose. Usually, when the antistaphylococcal agent is discontinued, the carrier state reappears within a short time (2, 8). Thus, it is not usually rewarding to try to eradicate the nasal carrier state for staphylococci by topical or systemic therapy, even of fairly long duration. Temporary suppression of *S. aureus* in the nose may, however, be of clinical benefit by reducing the reservoir from which these organisms seed the skin and cause clinical disease (1, 8).

The present study was designed to determine whether josamycin is effective against *S. au-*

reus in the nose and to compare the in vivo activity of this investigational antibiotic to that of a similar clinically established antibiotic, erythromycin. The results indicate that josamycin and erythromycin are comparable both in reducing nasal carrier rates and in decreasing the numbers of staphylococci cultured during therapy from subjects who remain nasal carriers.

The question of biological equivalence of josamycin and erythromycin is difficult to establish from the present data, since a higher daily dose of josamycin than of erythromycin was selected for treating the staphylococcal carriers. When the study was designed, the decision to use a higher dose of josamycin than erythromycin was based on preliminary bioequivalence information, which indicated that similar blood levels were obtained from oral administration of 1.5 g of josamycin and 1.0 g of erythromycin stearate daily. Subsequently, it has been documented that higher josamycin levels may be obtained after multiple doses, and that these antibiotics may be biologically equivalent (6). Consequently, the amount of antistaphylococcal activity achieved by josamycin may have been higher than that obtained by the dose of erythromycin.

Studies of the acquisition of antibiotic resistance by staphylococci after in vitro exposure to antibiotics have suggested that josamycin is less likely to induce resistance than erythromycin (4). Testing of pre- and post-therapy isolates in the current study failed to identify the development of resistance to either antibiotic after the 7 days of oral therapy. The low incidence of resistance in pretreatment cultures (0% to josamycin and 4% to erythromycin) are similar to reports from other laboratories in the United States in which staphylococci have been tested for in vitro susceptibility (5, 7).

The percentage of carriers who reacquired staphylococci after 1 week of oral therapy was similar for josamycin- or erythromycin-treated subjects until the final culture, 36 days after initiation of therapy, when carrier rates for the josamycin-treated group were significantly lower. The reason for this difference is not readily apparent, since it is difficult to relate the effects of the 1 week of therapy to changes in the carrier rates 4 weeks later.

From subjects whose cultures were positive for *S. aureus*, lower numbers of staphylococci were isolated 1 day after completion of therapy from josamycin-treated subjects than from those who received erythromycin. This may reflect lower initial staphylococcal counts in the subjects treated with josamycin. Alternatively, the effectiveness of josamycin in the nose may have been greater than that of erythromycin 24 h after therapy. In a small group of subjects, josamycin has been documented to be present in saliva and in lacrimal secretions in a concentration higher than those usually obtained with erythromycin (6).

In this study, josamycin was found to have low toxicity, few side effects, and good in vivo effectiveness against nasal *S. aureus*.

ACKNOWLEDGMENTS

R. Martin is the recipient of Public Health Service Research Career Development Award AI 70335 from the National Institute of Allergy and Infectious Diseases. This research was supported by a grant from the E.I. duPont de Nemours Co. and an infectious diseases training grant AI-00446-04 from the National Institute of Allergy and Infectious Diseases.

LITERATURE CITED

1. **Ehrenkranz, N. J.** 1964. Person-to-person transmission of *Staphylococcus aureus*. N. Eng. J. Med. **271**:225–230.
2. **Martin, R. R., and A. White.** 1971. Quantitative nasal culture: a tool in antibiotic research. Appl. Microbiol. **22**:397–400.
3. **Martin, R. R., and A. White.** 1967. The selective activity of lysostaphin in vivo. J. Lab. Clin. Med. **70**:1–8.
4. **Osono, T., and H. Umezawa.** 1971. Macrolide antibodies and lincomycin, p. 41–114. *In* S. Mitsuhasi (ed.), Drug action and resistance. University of Tokyo Press, Tokyo, Japan.
5. **Strausbaugh, L. J., J. A. Dilworth, J. M. Gwaltney Jr., and M. A. Sande.** 1976. In vitro susceptibility studies with josamycin and erythromycin. Antimicrob. Agents Chemother. **9**:546–548.
6. **Strausbaugh, L. J., W. K. Bolton, J. A. Dilworth, R. L. Guerrant, and M. A. Sande.** 1976. Comparative pharmacology of josamycin and erythromycin stearate. Antimicrob. Agents Chemother. **10**:450–456.
7. **Westerman, E. L., T. N. Williams, Jr., and N. Moreland.** 1976. In vitro activity of josamycin against aerobic gram-positive cocci and anaerobes. Antimicrob. Agents Chemother. **9**:988–993.
8. **White, A.** 1964. The use of gentamicin as a nasal ointment. Am. J. Med. Sci. **248**:86–90.
9. **White, A., T. Hemmerly, M. P. Martin, and V. Knight.** 1959. Studies on the origin of drug resistant staphylococci in a mental hospital. Am. J. Med. **27**:26–39.

ANTIMICROBIAL AGENTS AND CHEMOTHERAPY, Mar. 1977, p. 411-414 Vol. 11, No. 3

Antibiotic Metabolites from a Marine Pseudomonad

STEPHEN J. WRATTEN, MARGARET S. WOLFE, RAYMOND J. ANDERSEN, AND D. JOHN FAULKNER*

Scripps Institution of Oceanography, La Jolla, California 92093

Received for publication 29 November 1976

An antibiotic-producing pseudomonad was isolated from a seawater sample from a La Jolla, Calif., tidepool. The pseudomonad produces two novel antibacterial compounds, 2-*n*-pentyl-4-quinolinol and 2-*n*-heptyl-4-quinolinol. It also synthesizes indole-3-carboxaldehyde, 6-bromoindole-3-carboxaldehyde, and the known antibiotic *p*-hydroxybenzaldehyde. Each of these compounds was identified by analysis of spectral data, and the structures were confirmed by synthesis or comparison with authentic samples.

Although the production of antibiotics by marine bacteria is well documented (3, 4), there have been few chemical studies of this phenomenon. In a pioneering chemical study, Burkholder et al. (5) isolated a highly brominated antibiotic I (Fig. 1) from an organism they designated *Pseudomonas bromoutilis*. We have subsequently isolated the same antibiotic, together with tetrabromopyrrole (II) and hexabromo-2,2'-bipyrrole (III) (Fig. 1) from an autotoxic marine bacterium of the genus *Chromobacterium* (1). We could demonstrate that antibiotics I and II were responsible for autotoxicity. In this study we have elucidated the structures of two novel antibiotics and three other interesting metabolites from a marine pseudomonad.

MATERIALS AND METHODS

Isolation, description, and culturing of the bacteria. The marine pseudomonad (designated 102-3) was isolated from a seawater sample taken from a mid-intertidal pool at La Jolla, Calif., on 4 March 1974. The bacterium showed antibiotic activity on the original agar plate spread with the water sample, as demonstrated by the formation of zones of inhibition around individual colonies. Zone-producing colonies were isolated, dilution streaked, and maintained in pure culture.

102-3 is a short (<1 μm), gram-negative, motile rod with no apparent storage granules. Optimum growth occurs in a medium that is 80 to 100% the sodium chloride concentration found in seawater. Potassium chloride will not replace sodium chloride as a required salt. This bacterium will not grow on a minimal medium (i.e., glycerol as the only carbon source) and grows only at temperatures between 9 and 24°C.

The culture medium consisted of peptone (5 g/liter), yeast extract (1 g/liter), and agar (10 g/liter) in filtered seawater. Marine strains used as test organisms were *Vibrio anguillarum* M5900, obtained from W. Fenical of Scripps Institution of Oceanography, and *Vibrio harveyi*, obtained from K. Nealson, also of Scripps Institution of Oceanography. These were grown on the same medium as was 102-3. *Staphylococcus aureus* ATCC 6538P, *Escherichia coli* ATCC 11775, and *Candida albicans* ATCC 10231, obtained from Abbott Laboratories, were cultured on tryptic soy agar. Antibiotic activity was assayed using the agar diffusion method.

Procedures for the indole, methyl red, Voges-Proskauer, nitrate reduction, sucrose, mannitol, catalase, and oxidase tests were those listed by Collins (6).

Large-scale culture and extraction procedures. Large-scale cultures of 102-3 were grown on trays (60 by 30 by 2 cm) of nutrient agar (see above). After 4 days of incubation at room temperature, the cells were gently removed from the agar surface, using a paint scraper. The cells were homogenized in ethyl acetate (100 ml/g of wet cells), the resulting suspension was filtered, and the ethyl acetate extract was dried over anhydrous sodium sulfate. The cellular material was reextracted three times, and the combined extracts were evaporated in vacuo to obtain an oil (~100 mg/tray).

The spent agar medium was sectioned into squares (5 by 5 cm) and covered with ethyl acetate (2:1, solvent:medium). After 48 h, the solvent was decanted; the process was repeated three times. The combined extracts were dried over anhydrous sodium sulfate and the solvent was removed in vacuo to obtain a viscous oil (~200 mg/tray).

Chemical studies: general information. Unless otherwise specified, AR-grade solvents and chemicals were used without further purification. Infrared spectra were recorded on a Perkin-Elmer 700 spectrophotometer, and nuclear magnetic resonance (NMR) spectra were recorded on a Varian HR-220 spectrometer using TMS (δ = 0) as internal standard. Low-resolution mass spectra were recorded at 50 eV on a Hewlett-Packard 5930A mass spectrometer. High-resolution mass measurements were supplied by the Chemistry Department at UCLA. Gas-chromatographic analyses were performed on a Hewlett-Packard 402 instrument, using a column (6 ft [ca. 88 cm] by 2 mm) of 3% SP2250 on Supelco-

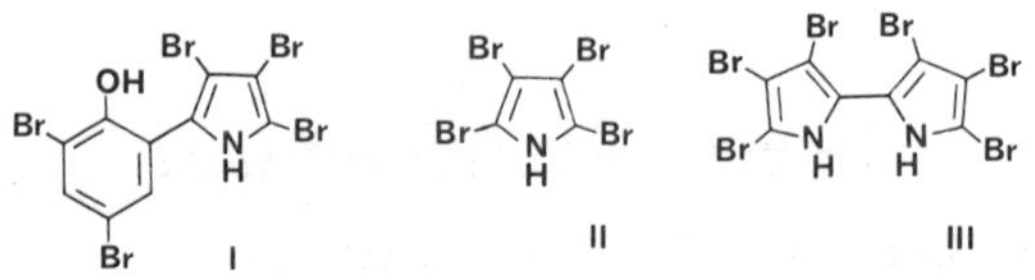

FIG. 1. *Metabolites isolated from Chromobacterium sp.*

port. Melting points were measured on a Fischer-Johns apparatus and are uncorrected.

Chromatography of "agar" extracts. The crude extract (1.3 g) was adsorbed onto florisil (3 g) and the adsorbant was added to the top of a florisil column (30 by 4 cm; 45 g). The components were eluted with solvents of increasing polarity from benzene to 20% methanol in ethyl acetate. Fractions of 125 ml were collected. Fractions 3 and 4 (eluent:benzene) contained a white crystalline solid, melting point (mp), 115 to 116°C, identical in all respects to *p*-hydroxybenzaldehyde; the yield was 68 mg (5% of extract).

Fractions 5 to 7 (eluent: 25% ether in benzene) contained a solid material (49 mg, 3%) which consisted of a 9:1 mixture of two components as revealed by gas chromatographic analysis. The mixture was separated by thin-layer chromatography on silica gel, using 10% acetonitrile in benzene as eluent. The major component, mp, 193 to 195°C, was identical in all respects to authentic indole-3-carboxaldehyde. The minor component, which crystallized from aqueous methanol as fine needles, mp, 200 to 202°C, was shown to be 6-bromoindole-3-carboxaldehyde, identical in all respects to a synthetic sample.

Fractions 11 to 14 (eluent:ether) showed strong activity against *V. anguillarum*. Careful chromatography on silica gel plates, using 15% acetonitrile in chloroform as eluent, allowed separation of two similar compounds. The major component, 2-*n*-pentyl-4-quinolinol (120 mg, 9%) crystallized from benzene:hexane (1:1), mp, 141 to 142°C. NMR ($CDCl_3$) δ 0.80 (t, 3H), 1.23 (m, 4H), 1.72 (m, 2H) 2.70 (t, 1H), 6.26 (s, 1H), 7.34 (t, 1H), 7.59 (t, 1H), 7.85 (d, 1H), 8.38 (d, 1H); ultraviolet (MeOH) λ_{max} 235, 315, 326 nm; infrared ($CHCl_3$) 3300, 1645, 1590, 1550/cm$-^1$. Mass spectrum (*m/e*) 215 (21%), 172 (23%), 159 (100%), 130 (33%), 77 (25%). High-resolution mass measurement: found 215.1309; $C_{14}H_{17}NO$ requires 215.1310. These data were identical to those of a synthetic sample.

The minor component, 2-*n*-heptyl-4-quinolinol (54 mg, 4%), mp, 146 to 147°C, was identical in all respects to authentic material (11).

Synthesis of 6-bromoindole-3-carboxaldehyde (7). A solution of bromine (1.60 g, 10 mmol) in acetic acid (10 ml) was added dropwise to a stirred solution of indole-3-carboxaldehyde (1.45 g, 10 mmol) in acetic acid (60 ml). Stirring was continued for 10 min after the addition was completed, and the resulting mixture was cautiously poured into aqueous sodium bicarbonate solution (100 g in 800 ml of water). The organic material was extracted with ethyl acetate (3 × 100 ml), and the combined extracts were dried over sodium sulfate. Evaporation of the solvent in vacuo gave a dark-red semisolid (2.1 g), which contained mainly unreacted starting material together with two brominated derivatives, 5-bromoindole-3-carboxaldehyde and 6-bromoindole-3-carboxaldehyde. Thick-layer chromatography of the mixture on silica gel, using 10% acetonitrile in benzene, followed by crystallization from aqueous methanol, gave 6-bromoindole-3-carboxaldehyde, mp, 200 to 202°C (reference 7, mp, 203 to 204°C). NMR ($CDCl_3$) δ 7.36 (d, 1H), 7.73 (s, 1H), 8.14 (d, 1H), 8.20 (s, 1H), 10.00 (s, 1H).

Synthesis of 2-*n*-pentyl-4-quinolinol (10). A mixture of ethyl 3-oxo-octanoate (2.2 g, 12 mmol), prepared by the method of Rathke and Deitch (9), aniline (1.11 g, 12 mmol), and 3 N hydrochloric acid (4 drops) was stirred overnight. The mixture was dried over anhydrous sodium sulfate and added to refluxing diphenyl ether under nitrogen. After 30 min at reflux, the solution was cooled and diluted with diethyl ether, and the basic material was extracted with 3 N hydrochloric acid. The combined extracts were basified to pH >10 and extracted with ethyl acetate. The extracts were dried, the solvent evaporated, and the residue was recrystallized from aqueous ethanol to obtain 2-*n*-pentyl-4-quinolinol, mp, 141 to 142°C.

RESULTS AND DISCUSSION

A yellow pseudomonad (designated 102-3) was isolated from a La Jolla tidepool and demonstrated antibiotic activity against *V. anguillarum*, *S. aureus*, *C. albicans*, and *V. harveyi*. 102-3 will not ferment glucose or mannitol, does not reduce nitrate, and gives negative results in the methyl red and Voges-Proskauer tests. It produces indole and is positive in tests for the presence of both oxidase and catalase. After large-scale culturing and the subsequent extraction of the active material, three compounds were isolated and found to be responsible for antibiosis (see Table 1).

By separating the bacterial cells from the spent agar, we were able to investigate both intracellular and extracellular metabolites. The cells and spent agar were extracted separately with ethyl acetate. The spent agar extract contained approximately twice the quantity of material obtained from the cells. The cell extract showed very slight antibiotic activity against *V. anguillarum* and *V. harveyi*. The major constituents of the cell extracts were a mixture of $C_{16:1}$ and $C_{18:1}$ fatty acids. This extract was not investigated further.

The spent agar extracts exhibited strong activity against *V. anguillarum* and *V. harveyi*. Chromatography of the extracts gave three interesting fractions, as judged by thin-layer chromatography, two of which showed antibiotic activity. The first antibiotic fraction contained *p*-hydroxybenzaldehyde (IV) (Fig. 2), which had also been found in *Chromobacter*. A second fraction, which did not show antibiotic

TABLE 1. *Antibiotic activity of 102-3 metabolites*

Compounds tested[a]	Test organisms[b]				
	Staphylococcus aureus	*Escherichia coli*	*Candida albicans*	*Vibrio harveyi*	*Vibrio anguillarum*
4-Hydroxybenzaldehyde (IV) (5 mg/disk)	+	−	+	+	NT
4-Hydroxybenzaldehyde (IV) (50 μg/disk)	−	−	−	−	−
2-*n*-Heptyl-4-quinolinol (VII) (50 μg/disk)	+	−	NT	+	+
2-*n*-Pentyl-4-quinolinol (VIII) (50 μg/disk)	++	−	NT	+	+
Tetracycline (30 μg/disk)	++	NT	NT	NT	NT

[a] Disks used in the antibiotic assays were one-half inch in diameter.
[b] Symbols: ++, >6 mm of inhibition; +, 1 to 6 mm of inhibition; −, no activity. NT, Not tested.

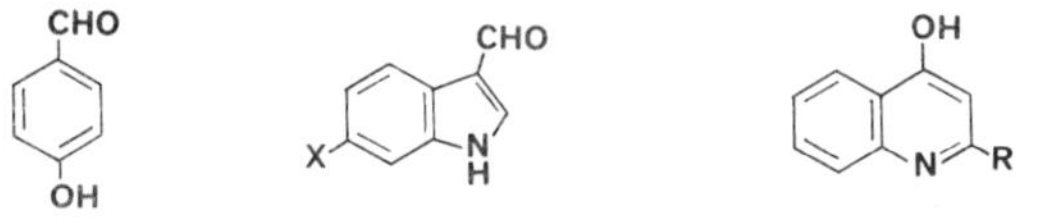

IV V X = H VI X = Br VII R = C_7H_{15} VIII R = C_5H_{11}

FIG. 2. *Metabolites isolated from 102-3. Compounds IV, VII, and VIII displayed antibiotic activity.*

activity, contained a 9:1 mixture of indole-3-carboxaldehyde (V) and 6-bromoindole-3-carboxaldehyde (VI) (Fig. 2). The aldehydes were separated on preparative silica gel plates, and the indole-3-carboxaldehyde (V) was shown to be identical to an authentic sample. The 220-MHz proton magnetic resonance spectrum of the brominated indole aldehyde contained signals that could be interpreted as indicating either a 5- or 6-substituted indole. Comparison of the spectral data with those of authentic 5-bromoindole-3-carboxaldehyde eliminated that possibility. Bromination of indole-3-carboxaldehyde in glacial acetic acid gave a mixture of 5- and 6-bromoindole-3-carboxaldehyde, which was separated on silica gel plates. The synthetic 6-bromoindole-3-carboxaldehyde (VI) was identical in all respects to the natural material.

6-Bromoindoles have been found in other marine organisms. The tyrian purple dye from *Murex* sp. is a dimeric molecule based on 6-bromoindole (2). The acorn worm, *Ptychodera flava laysanica*, contains 6-bromo-3-chloroindole, together with 3-chloro- and 3-bromoindole (8).

The third fraction, which showed the strongest antibacterial activity, contained a mixture of two closely related compounds, which were separated on preparative silica gel plates. The mass spectra of the two compounds contained the same base peak at *m/e* 159, but the molecular weights, 215 and 243, differed by 28. The NMR spectra of the two compounds were identical in the aromatic region, but the minor component contained an additional four protons in the methylene region of the spectrum. The spectral data of the minor component was identical to the reported data for 2-*n*-heptyl-4-quinolinol (VII), a known antibiotic from the terrestrial bacterium *Pseudomonas aeruginosa*. We concluded that the major antibiotic was 2-*n*-pentyl-4-quinolinol (VIII) and synthesized the molecule by the method of Wells et al. (11). The synthetic material was identical in all respects to the natural product.

All three antibiotic-producing marine bacteria which were studied contain brominated material, although, in this case, the brominated metabolite 6-bromoindole-3-carboxaldehyde (VI) was not responsible for the antibiotic activity. The major antibiotic component is a lower homologue of a known antibiotic from *P. aeruginosa*. This result emphasizes the similar biosynthetic capabilities of marine and terrestrial pseudomonads.

ACKNOWLEDGMENTS

We wish to thank K. Nealson for advice and assistance in the area of microbiology. This research was supported by Public Health Service grant AI-11969 from the National Institute of Allergy and Infectious Diseases. Fellowships from the National Science Foundation (to S.J.W.) and the National Research Council of Canada (to R.J.A.) are gratefully acknowledged.

LITERATURE CITED

1. **Andersen, R. J., M. S. Wolfe, and D. J. Faulkner.** 1974. Autotoxic antibiotic production by a marine *Chromobacterium*. Mar. Biol. 27:281–285.
2. **Baker, J. T., and M. D. Sutherland.** 1968. Pigments of marine animals. VIII. Precursors of 6,6′-dibromoindigotin (Tyrian Purple) from the mollusc *Dicathais orbita* gmelin. Tetrahedron Lett., p. 43–46.
3. **Baslow, M. H.** 1969. Schizophyta and eumycophyta, p. 17–29. *In* Marine pharmacology. Williams and Wilkins, Baltimore.
4. **Burkholder, P. R.** 1973. The ecology of marine antibiosis and coral reefs, p. 117–176. *In* O. A. Endean (ed.), Biology and geology of coral reefs, vol. 11, Biology I. Academic Press Inc., New York.
5. **Burkholder, P. R., R. M. Pfister, and R. M. Leitz.** 1966. Production of a pyrrole antibiotic by a marine bacterium. Appl. Microbiol. 14:649–653.

6. **Collins, C. H.** 1967. Microbial methods, p. 164–169. Plenum Press, New York.
7. **Da Settimo, A., M. F. Saettone, E. Nannipieri, and P. Bariti.** 1967. La bromourazione di alcuni derivati indolici. Gazz. Chim. Ital. **97**:1304–1317.
8. **Higa, T., and P. J. Scheuer.** 1975. 3-Chloroindole, principal odorous constituents of the hemichordate *Ptychodera flava laysanica*. Naturwissenschaften **62**:395–396.
9. **Rathke, M. W., and J. Deitch.** 1971. The reaction of lithium ester enolates with acid chlorides. A convenient procedure for the preparation of β-keto esters. Tetrahedron Lett., p. 2953–2956.
10. **Wells, I. C.** 1952. Antibiotic substances produced by *Pseudomonas aeruginosa*. Syntheses of PYO Ib, PYO Ic, and PYO III. J. Biol. Chem. **196**:321–330.
11. **Wells, I. C., W. H. Elliott, S. A. Thayer, and E. A. Doisy.** 1952. Ozonization of some antibiotic substances produced by *Pseudomonas aeruginosa*. J. Biol. Chem. **196**:331–339.

Antimicrobial Agents and Chemotherapy, Mar. 1977, p. 415–419
Vol. 11, No. 3

Chemically Defined Antimicrobial Susceptibility Test Medium for *Pseudomonas aeruginosa*

J. H. JORGENSEN,* J. C. LEE, and P. M. JONES

Departments of Pathology and Microbiology, The University of Texas Health Science Center and the Bexar County Hospitals, San Antonio, Texas 78284*

Received for publication 13 September 1976

A chemically defined growth medium containing physiological concentrations of magnesium and calcium ions was utilized in a microdilution procedure for antimicrobial drug susceptibility testing of *Pseudomonas aeruginosa*. Determinations of growth end points were simplified by use of sodium citrate as a sole carbon source and bromothymol blue as a pH indicator. Growth of the test organisms was detectable by a change in the indicator color from green to blue after alkalinization of the medium due to citrate utilization. Minimal inhibitory concentrations of amikacin, carbenicillin, gentamicin, and tobramycin were determined on 100 recent clinical isolates of *Pseudomonas*. Parallel determinations using the microdilution procedure and a conventional tube-broth dilution technique incorporating Mueller-Hinton broth with identical magnesium and calcium content generally agreed within one twofold dilution. Modal minimal inhibitory concentrations for susceptible strains using the microdilution method were: amikacin, 6 μg/ml; carbenicillin, 50 μg/ml; gentamicin, 1.5 μg/ml; tobramycin, 1.5 μg/ml. This modified microdilution technique allowed rapid, definitive minimal inhibitory concentration determinations, using growth end points defined by a color indicator change.

The magnesium and calcium ion content of antibiotic test media greatly influences the susceptibility of *Pseudomonas aeruginosa* to aminoglycosides, polymyxins, and perhaps carbenicillin (2,3,5,6,10). This phenomenon has not been demonstrated conclusively with other microorganisms tested with these drugs. This effect seems to be a unique property of *P. aeruginosa* mediated by divalent cation stabilization of the cell wall or cell membrane, which assists in preventing antibiotic-induced lysis (15).

For proper use of these potentially toxic antibiotics, clinically relevant susceptibility test results must be readily obtainable. Recently it has been proposed that broth dilution susceptibility testing of *Pseudomonas* with these drugs be performed using Mueller-Hinton (M-H) medium supplemented with physiological concentrations of calcium and magnesium (2, 6, 10). However, it is not yet known if simple adjustment of the concentrations of these cations in M-H medium produced by different manufacturers will yield uniform results. In large part, this is because the composition of M-H is not totally defined nor easily controlled. In an effort to circumvent this problem, a reference *Pseudomonas* strain known to be affected by variations in the ionic content of media has been proposed for development of performance standards applicable to evaluation of various batches of M-H media.

Microdilution techniques were first adapted for antimicrobial susceptibility determinations by Harwick et al. (7). Whereas this technique appeared promising as a simple, rapid method of broth dilution testing, the determination of bacterial growth end points was frequently difficult due to the color of the growth medium and the difficulty of examining individual wells of the plastic microtiter plates. The addition of pH indicators and glucose to the growth medium to clarify growth end points was later proposed for testing organisms such as *Enterobacteriaceae* and staphylococci, which rapidly ferment glucose (13). However, *P. aeruginosa* does not ferment glucose and therefore cannot be successfully tested in this manner. A similar modification of the microdilution technique has not previously been described for use with *Pseudomonas*.

A characteristic of *P. aeruginosa* that would seem useful as an indicator of growth end points is its ability to utilize sodium citrate as a sole carbon source for growth. Therefore, a chemically defined medium that includes sodium citrate as a carbon source and bromothymol blue as a pH indicator was evaluated for drug susceptibility determinations on clinical isolates of *Pseudomonas*, using the microdilution technique.

MATERIALS AND METHODS

Antibiotics. Diagnostic reference standards of gentamicin (Schering Corp.), tobramycin (Eli Lilly & Co.), amikacin (Bristol Laboratories), and carbenicillin (Roerig Division of Pfizer, Inc.) were used to prepare stock solutions for susceptibility tests.

Pseudomonas test strains. One hundred recent clinical isolates of *P. aeruginosa* from the Bexar County Hospital Microbial Pathology Laboratory were used in this evaluation. *Pseudomonas* isolates were grown for 4 to 6 h at 35°C in Trypticase soy broth for preparation of inoculum suspensions. The cell density was then adjusted by dilution in sterile 0.9% NaCl to obtain a turbidity equivalent to that of the one-half no. 1 McFarland standard.

Tube-broth dilution test procedure. As a standard for comparison, tube-broth dilution susceptibility tests were performed on the same day by using the same inoculum suspensions used for the microdilution determinations. M-H broth (Difco) was prepared and sterilized in the usual manner. Samples of filter-sterilized stock solutions of $MgCl_2 \cdot 6H_2O$ and $CaCl_2 \cdot 2H_2O$ were then added aseptically to the M-H broth so as to yield a final ionic content of 25 mg of Mg^{2+} and 75 mg of Ca^{2+} per liter. The actual concentrations of these ions were then verified by atomic absorption spectrophotometry (Perkin-Elmer model 403 spectrophotometer). Serial twofold dilutions of the four antibiotics were prepared in the supplemented M-H broth in disposable glass test tubes (10 by 75 mm). Final test concentrations of gentamicin, amikacin, and tobramycin included dilutions from 12 to 0.38 μg/ml; carbenicillin concentrations ranged from 400 to 12.5 μg/ml. Each tube, plus a positive control tube with antibiotic omitted, was inoculated with a 1:100 dilution of the standardized organism suspension, so as to yield a final inoculum density of 10^5 organisms/ml. After incubation at 35°C for 24 h, the minimal inhibitory concentration (MIC) was defined as the lowest concentration of the antibiotic that inhibited visible turbidity.

Microdilution test procedure. For microdilution tests, a chemically defined test medium was prepared to contain the following: KH_2PO_4, 1.00 g; $NaNH_4HPO_4 \cdot 4H_2O$, 1.50 g; sodium citrate, 3.00 g; $MgCl_2 \cdot 6H_2O$, 0.212 g; $CaCl_2 \cdot 2H_2O$, 0.276 g; bromothymol blue, 0.08 g; distilled water, 1,000 ml; final pH 6.8. In practice the medium was prepared double strength, since the addition of the inoculum suspension diluted the contents of each microtiter well 1:2. After filter sterilization, the actual final concentration of Mg^{2+} and Ca^{2+} was determined as described above. Fifty-microliter aliquots of the 2×-concentrated medium were added to seven rows (labeled B through H) of sterile, disposable, flat-bottom microtiter plates (Falcon). One-hundred microliters of double-strength test medium containing the initial drug concentrations (gentamicin, 24 μg/ml; amikacin, 24 μg/ml; tobramycin, 24 μg/ml; carbenicillin, 800 μg/ml) was added to wells of row A of the microtiter plate. Twofold serial dilutions of the antibiotics were made from rows A through F with flame-sterilized 50-μl microdiluters. Rows G and H were left free of drugs to serve as positive and negative controls. Fifty-microliter aliquots of the 1:500 dilutions of the standardized inoculum suspensions in saline were added to rows A through G to yield a final inoculum density of 10^5 organisms/ml in each test well. The addition of this inoculum to the double-strength citrate medium yielded the appropriate final medium and antibiotic concentrations in each well. Final test concentrations of the four drugs were then identical to those used in the tube-broth dilution procedure. The addition of only citrate medium and inoculum to wells in row G constituted a positive control well for each organism-drug combination, whereas the wells in row H became negative controls after the addition of 50 μl of sterile saline to the citrate medium. Completed microtiter test plates were incubated at 35°C for 24 h and examined for a color change of the indicator from green to blue, indicative of growth by citrate utilization. The MIC was defined as the lowest concentration dilution of the particular drug inhibiting visible growth, i.e., the last green well.

RESULTS

When a chemically defined growth medium containing sodium citrate as a carbon source and bromothymol blue as a pH indicator was used in microtiter plates for drug susceptibility determinations, growth end points were clearly defined and easily interpreted. The change in the indicator from green to blue indicated growth of the organisms at the expense of sodium citrate and a consequent rise in pH of the medium. No change in the color of the medium indicated inhibition of growth of the organisms, as evidenced by no utilization of the citrate. Therefore, the MIC could be easily defined as the lowest drug concentration whose well remained green after incubation.

Table 1 shows the results of paired susceptibility tests on 100 *Pseudomonas* isolates using the microdilution technique with the chemically defined medium and a traditional broth tube dilution procedure with supplemented M-H broth. Results of tests with the four antimicrobials indicated that the two test methods agreed within one twofold dilution in 398 of 400 instances. However, individual MIC values of gentamicin and tobramycin routinely differed by one twofold dilution, depending on the test method used (Table 2).

Gentamicin MICs were frequently one dilution lower with the microdilution method (modal MIC, 1.5 μg/ml) than with the conventional tube-broth dilution procedure (modal MIC, 3 μg/ml). The opposite occurred with tobramycin; i.e., MICs were often higher with the microdilution procedure (modal MIC, 1.5 μg/

TABLE 1. *MICs of 100 P. aeruginosa isolates*

Antimicrobial agent	Method[a]	No. and % of isolates with MIC (μg/ml) of:															
		0.19	0.38	0.75	1.5	3	6	12	25	50	100	200	400	800	1,600	3,200	6,400
Gentamicin	Tube-broth dilution				7	52[b]	23	9	5	1					3[c]		
	Micro-dilution		1	4	41[b]	32	11	4	4						3[c]		
Tobramycin	Tube-broth dilution	1	1	53[b]	23	13	6					3[d]					
	Micro-dilution		2	33	44[b]	13	5					3[d]					
Amikacin	Tube-broth dilution		1		1	30	42[b]	15	7	4							
	Micro-dilution	1			3	25	45[b]	14	7	5							
Carbenicillin	Tube-broth dilution								12	44[b]	17	15	4	2	4	1	1
	Micro-dilution								8	52[b]	19	13	1	2	4		1

[a] With tube-broth dilution, tests were performed using M-H broth with added magnesium and calcium, as described in the text. With microdilution, tests were performed using chemically defined medium.
[b] Indicates modal MIC value.
[c] Gentamicin MIC, >1,500 μg/ml.
[d] Tobramycin MIC, >200 μg/ml.

TABLE 2. *Occurrence of discrepant test results based on the susceptibility test method used*

Drug	Microdilution MIC > tube MIC		Microdilution MIC = tube MIC	Microdilution MIC < tube MIC	
	Two dilutions	One dilution		One dilution	Two dilutions
Gentamicin	0	5	24	70	1
Tobramycin	0	34	51	15	0
Amikacin	1	19	61	19	0
Carbenicillin	0	13	61	26	0

ml, as opposed to 0.75 μg/ml with the tube-broth technique). Table 2 also shows that MICs of amikacin and carbenicillin agreed closely and did not routinely differ based on the test method used.

DISCUSSION

The increased number and severity of infections due to *P. aeruginosa* (1), as well as the inherently limited antimicrobial susceptibility spectrum of this organism (4, 9), have emphasized the importance of appropriate selection of antimicrobial agents for therapy. The relative toxicity of certain drugs used for anti-*Pseudomonas* therapy, such as the aminogycosides, further stresses the importance of knowing accurate MIC values of potential therapeutic agents (1a, 8). The marked effect of medium composition on MICs of aminoglycosides and polymyxins has been recently emphasized by several authors (2, 6, 10, 15). The control of the absolute cation content of test media such as MH broth may help to control these problems. However, the advent of a standardized, readily reproducible, chemically defined medium for susceptibility testing of *P. aeruginosa* would seem to be a more universally acceptable solution.

The results of susceptibility tests with the four antimicrobial agents tested in this study, using cation-supplemented M-H broth, agree closely with previous studies (9, 11, 14) with respect to relative MIC values, i.e., tobramycin MICs < gentamicin MICs < amikacin MICs < carbenicillin MICs. However, the identical modal gentamicin and tobramycin MICs, as determined using the chemically defined medium, suggest instead a similar activity of the two drugs. The most likely explanation for this discrepancy between results obtained using M-H broth and the chemically defined medium is that the starting pH of M-H broth is slightly higher (pH 7.2) than that of the latter (pH 6.8). Thus, it would appear that the slightly more alkaline condition of the M-H broth potentiates the action of gentamicin but not of tobramycin. The starting pH of the chemically defined medium cannot be raised without causing an unacceptable change of the pH indicator to a bluish-green coloration.

The results of this study indicate that a microdilution technique may be easily adapted for susceptibility testing of *Pseudomonas* by use of a chemically defined growth medium incorporating sodium citrate and a pH indicator. The growth of *Pseudomonas* in the medium is easily detected by a pH-induced color change after approximately a 2-log growth of organisms in the medium. Therefore, turbidity is not required for growth to be demonstrated in this system. This modification of the microdilution technique is analogous to the procedure described previously by Tippett et al. for organisms that rapidly ferment glucose (13).

Microtiter plates including growth medium and dilutions of various antibiotics may be prepared and stored at −20°C for at least 1 month prior to use. Automated equipment now available for rapid mechanized pipetting and diluting of fluids allows this type of susceptibility testing to be performed in approximately the same amount of time as is required with the widely used Bauer-Kirby disk diffusion procedure.

In conclusion, a chemically defined growth medium has been used in a microdilution system for rapid, quantitative antimicrobial susceptibility testing of *P. aeruginosa*. This method greatly simplifies the reading of growth end points in the microdilution system when testing the activity of various antimicrobial agents against *Pseudomonas*, and it allows precise control of medium constituents that may potentially alter susceptibility test results.

LITERATURE CITED

1. **Artenstein, M. S., and J. P. Sanford (ed.).** 1974. Symposium on *Pseudomonas aeruginosa*. Session I. The problem: hospital acquired infections and the altered host. J. Infect. Dis. **130** (Suppl.):54–532.

1a. **Atuk, N., A. Mosca, and C. Kunin.** 1964. The use of potentially nephrotoxic antibiotics in the treatment of gram-negative infections in uremic patients. Ann. Intern Med. **60**:28–38.

2. **D'Amato, R. F., C. Thornesberry, C. N. Baker, and L. A. Kirven.** 1975. Effect of calcium and magnesium ions on the susceptibility of *Pseudomonas* species of tetracycline, gentamicin, polymyxin B, and carbenicillin. Antimicrob. Agents Chemother. **7**:596–600.

3. **Davis, S. D., and A. Iannetta.** 1972. Influence of serum and calcium on the bactericidal activity of gentamicin and carbenicillin on *Pseudomonas aeruginosa*. Appl. Microbiol. **23**:775–779.

4. **Duncan, I. B. R.** 1974. Susceptibility of 1500 isolates of *Pseudomonas aeruginosa* to gentamicin, carbenicil-

lin, colistin, and polymyxin B. Antimicrob. Agents Chemother. 5:9–15.

5. **Garrod, L. P., and P. M. Waterworth.** 1969. Effect of medium composition on the apparent sensitivity of *Pseudomonas aeruginosa*. J. Clin. Pathol. 22:534–538.
6. **Gilbert, D. N., E. Kutscher, P. Ireland, J. A. Barnett, and J. P. Sanford.** 1971. Effect of the concentrations of magnesium and calcium on the *in-vitro* susceptibility of *Pseudomonas aeruginosa* to gentamicin. J. Infect. Dis. 124:537–545.
7. **Harwick, H. J., P. Weiss, and F. R. Fekety, Jr.** 1968. Application of microtitration techniques to bacteriostatic and bactericidal antibiotic susceptibility testing. J. Lab. Clin. Med. 72:511–516.
8. **Kunin, C. M.** 1967. A guide to use of antibiotics in patients with renal disease. Ann. Intern. Med. 67:151–158.
9. **Lockwood, W. R., and L. A. Lawson.** 1973. Studies on the susceptibility of 150 consecutive clinical isolates of *Pseudomonas aeruginosa* to tobramycin, gentamicin, colistin, carbenicillin, and five other antimicrobials. Antimicrob. Agents Chemother. 4:281–284.
10. **Reller, L. B., F. D. Schoenknecht, M. A. Kenny, and J. C. Sherris.** 1974. Antibiotic susceptibility testing of *Pseudomonas aeruginosa*; selection of a control strain and criteria for magnesium and calcium content in media. J. Infect. Dis. 130:454–463.
11. **Reynolds, A. V., J. M. T. Hamilton-Miller, and W. Brumfitt.** 1974. Newer aminoglycosides—amikacin and tobramycin: an *in-vitro* comparison with kanamycin and gentamicin. Br. Med. J. 3:778–780.
13. **Tippett, L. O., L. D. Zeleznick, and C. A. Robb.** 1970. Modifications of the microtiter technique for antimicrobial drug susceptibility testing by incorporation of indicators. Appl. Microbiol. 20:342–345.
14. **Waterworth, P. M.** 1972. The *in-vitro* activity of tobramycin compared with that of other aminoglycosides. J. Clin. Pathol. 25:979–983.
15. **Zimelis, V. M., and G. G. Jackson.** 1973. Activity of aminoglycoside and antibiotics against *Pseudomonas aeruginosa*: specificity and site of calcium and magnesium antagonism. J. Infect. Dis. 127:663–669.

ANTIMICROBIAL AGENTS AND CHEMOTHERAPY, Mar. 1977, p. 420-426 Vol. 11, No. 3

Comparative Trial of Carbenicillin and Ampicillin Therapy for Purulent Meningitis

G. D. OVERTURF,* E. A. STEINBERG, A. E. UNDERMAN, J. WILKINS, J. M. LEEDOM, A. W. MATHIES, JR., AND P. F. WEHRLE

Department of Pediatrics and Internal Medicine, and the Hastings Infectious Disease Laboratory, Los Angeles County-University of Southern California Medical Center, Los Angeles, California 90033*

Received for publication 1 September 1976

A randomized therapeutic trial of carbenicillin (CB) or ampicillin (AMP) in purulent meningitis was performed in 86 pediatric and adult patients (41 *Haemophilus influenzae,* 22 *Streptococcus pneumoniae,* 13 *Neisseria meningitidis,* and 10 of unknown etiology). All isolates, incuding *H. influenzae*, were susceptible to CB and AMP. Median cerebrospinal fluid (CSF) antibiotic concentrations were 0.85 and 1.60 μg/ml for CB and AMP, respectively, during administration of daily doses of 400 mg/kg and 0.65 and 0.45 μg/ml, respectively, on daily doses of 200 mg/kg. Higher CSF concentrations, up to a median concentration of 4.5 μg/ml, were observed in patients with CSF protein concentrations ≥75 mg/100 ml. Clinical responses were equivalent on either antibiotic regimen. Among AMP patients (45), 8 had significant residua and 3 died; among CB patients (41), 5 had residua and none died. However, 38% of *H. influenzae* patients treated with CB had positive CSF cultures on day 1 follow-up lumbar punctures, compared with only 5.8% of AMP patients with *H. influenzae*. The significance of a delay of CSF sterilization among CB-treated patients is unknown, since there was no correlation between persistence of hemophilus organisms and the frequency of adverse outcome. AMP and CB are equivalent for the treatment of bacterial meningitis due to susceptible organisms.

Ampicillin (AMP) has received wide acceptance as a single-antibiotic regimen in the treatment of purulent meningitis (20). Early studies demonstrated that AMP had good in vitro activity against strains of *Haemophilus influenzae* type B and activity equivalent to benzylpenicillin G against strains of *Neisseria meningitidis* and *Streptococcus pneumoniae* (4, 5). Subsequent investigations demonstrated adequate cerebrospinal fluid (CSF) levels after administration of AMP and clinical efficacy comparable to standard antibiotic regimens.

However, since the recent isolation of strains of *H. influenzae* type B resistant to AMP, concern has been expressed over the continued use of AMP for treatment of meningitis in children (6, 14). Resistance to penicillins in hemophilus strains is due in part to the presence of a beta-lactamase with marked activity against benzylpenicillin G and AMP; other semisynthetic penicillins and cephalosporins are hydrolyzed less effectively (2, 7). Chloramphenicol, alone or in combination with a penicillin, has been recommended to treat infections suspected to be due to AMP-resistant strains of *H. influenzae* (1). However, the concern of possible antagonism during the use of antibiotic combinations and the potential for severe toxicity after chloramphenicol administration has prompted an evaluation of alternate antimicrobial regimens.

Other investigators have demonstrated that carbenicillin (CB) is less rapidly destroyed by hemophilus beta-lactamases; minimal inhibitory concentrations (MICs) range from 0.8 to 25 μg of CB per ml (2, 10). Because of pharmacological similarities of CB and AMP, as well as the greater in vitro activity of CB against AMP-resistant strains of *H. influenzae,* a pilot study was performed among meningitis patients alternately treated with either AMP or CB.

(This study was presented, in part, to the 16th Interscience Conference on Antimicrobial Agents and Chemotherapy, October 1976).

METHODS

Patient selection. Patients older than 2 months of age, with acute purulent meningitis, admitted from 15 March 1975 through 14 March 1976 to the Communicable Disease Service, Los Angeles County-University of Southern California Medical Center, were eligible for study. Informed written consent was obtained from all patients or their designated guardian. Patients were excluded from study if (i) the etiology of meningitis was confirmed or suspected not to be due to *S. pneumoniae, H. influenzae,* or *N. meningitidis*, (ii) there was a clinical indication for use of a second antimicrobial agent, or (iii) a significant history of penicillin allergy was obtained. The diagnosis of meningitis was confirmed by a positive CSF or blood culture in association with a consistent clinical presentation and CSF changes. Ten patients were included who had negative blood or CSF cultures or Gram stains (i.e., "purulent, unknown"). These patients satisfied two or more of the following criteria: (i) a predominate polymorphonuclear leukocyte pleocytosis (≥500 cells/mm^3) (ii) a protein level of ≥100 mg/100 ml, or (iii) a glucose level of ≥50% of a simultaneously obtained serum glucose value. All patients were assigned a severity classification from 1 to 4 at the time of admission as follows: 4, coma, semicoma, or severe hypotension; 3, convulsions without coma or shock; 2, temperature, ≥105°F (41°C), symptoms for 5 days, or the presence of a complicating disease or marked lethargy; or 1, none of the above.

Treatment regimens. All eligible patients were randomized (nonblinded) by hospital number to receive either CB or AMP. The first 20 patients received either AMP or CB (10 in each treatment group) in a daily dose of 200 mg/kg administered intravenously in six divided doses following an initial loading dose of 65 mg/kg. All subsequent patients received either antibiotic in a daily dose of 400 mg/kg intravenously in six divided doses after the same loading dose; this regimen was selected to evaluate the effect of higher dosage on obtainable CSF antibiotic concentrations. Further, at the lower dose, it was noted that patients with *H. influenzae* more frequently had positive cultures from CSF samples on day 1 if they were receiving CB (five of seven patients) as compared with AMP (one of three patients). Each patient's clinical response was recorded, and attempts were made to obtain CSF on days 1 (12 to 24 h after initiation of treatment), 3, 7, 10, 14, and 21 after the initiation of teatment. Therapy was terminated when the following criteria were met: (i) CSF glucose level was ≥50% of a simultaneously obtained blood sugar value, (ii) CSF protein was ≤75 mg/100 ml, (iii) CSF leukocyte cell count was ≤30/mm^3 with ≤20% polymorphonuclear leukocytes, and (iv) the patient was afebrile for 5 days. If the above criteria were not met at 28 days, therapy was arbitrarily terminated, unless other clinical indications were present to continue therapy (i.e., subdural effusion, pyarthrosis, etc.).

Bacteriology. MICs and minimal bactericidal concentrations (MBCs) of chloramphenicol, AMP, and CB were determined against all available isolates. Susceptibility studies against *H. influenzae* strains were done in modified Levinthal broth as previously described (8), whereas Mueller-Hinton broth (BBL) with 1% supplement B (Difco) and Trypticase soy broth (BBL) were utilized in susceptibility studies against *N. meningitidis* and *S. pneumoniae*, respectively. Beta-lactamase assays were done against all *H. influenzae* isolates by the method of Thornsberry et al. (10).

Microbiological assay. All CSF samples were submitted for microbiological assay for CB or AMP. Whenever possible, a simultaneous serum sample was also obtained. Specimens were immediately refrigerated at 4°C and submitted to assay within 96 h of collection; preliminary observations noted <10% loss in antibiotic activity when samples were held for 5 days at this temperature.

A modification of the standard microbiological assay of Simon and Yin was utilized (9). Assays were performed identically for both antibiotics, except that a temperature of 30°C was utilized for AMP assays, and 25°C was used for CB. Nutrient agar (Difco; pH 6.8) was utilized in both assays; test plates were inoculated with 1.6 ml of a *Bacillus subtilus* spore suspension (Difco) prepared by the addition of one vial of spores to 50 ml of 0.1 phosphate buffer (pH 7.4). Standard curves, appropriately diluted in CSF or serum, were obtained simultaneously by the inclusion of three control wells (0.8, 6.24, and 40 μg/ml).

RESULTS

Patient population. During the study period, 99 patients with purulent meningitis were admitted; 86 were eligible for randomized treatment with CB or AMP and 13 were excluded from study. Eight patients were excluded from randomization to AMP treatment; three patients died before initiation of treatment (one each with infection due to *H. influenzae, N. meningitis,* and *Escherichia coli*), three patients had meningitis due to organisms other than those included for study, and two patients received an inappropriate dosage of AMP. Five patients were excluded from treatment with CB; two patients were allergic to penicillin, and three patients had meningitis due to organisms other than those included for study.

The age and, therefore, the bacterial etiology of each treatment group varied considerably (Table 1). Seventy-three percent of CB-treated patients were in the first decade of life, compared with 55% of AMP-treated patients. Male-female ratios were equal among groups, and there were no significant differences as to racial or ethnic groups; 21% of patients in the total study population were black, which is consistent with the base population served by the hospital.

Despite the differences in age and etiology, each treatment group was equivalent in terms of defined admission severity status. Twenty-seven percent and 22% of the patients were in the most severely affected category for CB and AMP treatment groups, respectively. The median number of days ill before admission was the same in both groups (2.0 days). Antibiotic therapy (oral or parenteral penicillins) had been administered before therapy for at least 12 h in 30% of CB and 35% of AMP patients. Forty percent of blood cultures were positive among

TABLE 1. *Comparison of treatment groups by age and etiology*

Etiology	Age of patient					
	11 months	1–10 years	10–19 years	20–39 years	40–59 years	60 years
CB						
H. influenzae	12	12				
S. pneumoniae	3			2	3	
N. meningitidis			3	2		
Unknown	1	1			1	
AMP						
H. influenzae	10	6				1
S. pneumoniae	4	2	2	3	1	2
N. meningitidis	2	1	1	2	2	
Unknown			2	3		2

CB-treated patients, and 52% were positive among AMP-treated patients. Patients with pneumococcal and meningococcal disease had positive blood cultures more often (71 and 53%, respectively) than patients with meningitis due to *H. influenzae* (45%).

There were no significant differences among treatment groups in regard to the presence of associated purulent conditions; otitis media was present at the time of admission in 27% of patients, and 6% of patients had associated suppurative mastoiditis or sinusitis. No significant differences in the median values for admission hemoglobin (corrected for age), leukocyte count, or serum sodium were noted. Fifty-five percent of the children had anemia on admission (as defined by a hemoglobin value of 9.9 g/100 ml, whereas only 16% of adults had anemia as defined by a hemoglobin value of 10.9 g/100 ml).

Response to treatment. There were no apparent differences in clinical response due to the different dosage regimens and, therefore, the groups were analyzed together. The median duration of antibiotic therapy for each treatment group was 13.5 days. Similarly, the duration of hospitalization was the same for CB (17.1 days) and AMP (16.5 days) patients, and there were no differences according to etiology. One patient, with meningitis due to a CB-susceptible *H. influenzae* organism, required 36 days of treatment with CB because of a relapse confirmed by a positive CSF culture 72 h after discontinuing therapy at 16 days; subsequent evaluation failed to reveal a persistent focus of infection. Prolonged AMP treatment was necessary in two infants because of poor clinical responses; one patient with *H. influenzae* required 32 days of therapy because of an associated pyarthrosis (positive joint cultures, day 6 of therapy), and another child required 37 days of treatment because of subdural effusion, although routine CSF cultures were negative on day 1 taps on both children.

The duration of fever after initiation of antibiotic therapy was the same in both treatment groups (3.5 and 4.0 days for CB and AMP, respectively). Prolonged fever due to a probable drug reaction occurred in a child treated with CB for *H. influenzae* meningitis. There were no significant differences among treatment groups in the number of days required to meet the defined CSF criteria. CSF sugar level was generally normal on day 3 (range 0 to 14 days), whereas a return to normal protein concentrations usually required 3 to 7 days.

Of those patients with culture-proven meningitis, the CSF Gram stain or culture was positive in 65 of 77 (84%) at the time of admission. However, on day 1 (12 to 24 h), the CSF Gram stain or culture or both was positive more frequently in CB-treated patients, compared with those treated with AMP (Table 2). Nine of twenty-four CB-treated patients (38%) with infections due to *H. influenzae* had positive CSF cultures on day 1; none of these patients had positive CSF cultures or Gram stains by day 2 or 3. Persistence of organisms on culture did not correlate with an adverse clinical outcome or a more frequent persistent focus of infection among CB-treated patients. However, persistently positive Gram stains or cultures occurred in two AMP-treated patients with *H. influenzae* infections; one had a bilateral otitis media, and the other had a subdural effusion and subsequently died of his infection. Although the latter patient had a positive CSF culture on day 1, a culture obtained on day 3 was negative. Persistently positive CSF cultures or Gram stains or both on day 1 in patients with infections due to *S. pneumoniae* or *N. meningitidis* had no correlation with subsequent clinical course, despite the treatment regimen.

Adverse effects occurred among 27% of CB-treated patients. Eosinophilia (10%) on differential count (four patients), fever (three patients), and rash (three patients) were the most frequent; diarrhea occurred in a single patient. The occurrence of a rash on day 5 of therapy in a CB-treated patient signaled an apparent hypersensitivity to penicillin and necessitated its discontinuance; therapy was completed with chloramphenicol. Also, one child with a third episode of meningitis (the episodes were due to *H. influenzae*, *S. pneumoniae*, and *S. pneumoniae*, respectively) was not retreated with CB; chloramphenicol was substituted because of the appearance of marked eosinophilia and fever near the termination of therapy with CB during her second episode of meningitis. Adverse effects among AMP-treated patients were less frequent (17.5%) and included eosinophilia (three patients), fever (two patients), rash (two patients), and diarrhea (one patient). No adverse effects necessitated the discontinuance of AMP therapy.

Morbidity and mortality. Three deaths occurred among 86 patients (3.5%) entered into randomization (Table 3); all deaths occurred among AMP-treated patients. Two deaths, due to *H. influenzae*, occurred in children with severe disease due to susceptible organisms. Deaths in these children occurred on days 6 and 9 of disease and followed early clinical courses characterized by the rapid onset of severe neurological complications. A third death occurred in a young adult with meningitis due to *S. pneumoniae* on day 10 of treatment after complications at surgery to drain a middle ear abscess.

Residua were observed with equal frequency among treatment groups: 12% and 17% of CB- and AMP-treated patients, respectively, had significant residua at the time of discharge. Residua involved systems other than the central nervous system in three patients (i.e., one patient with distal extremity gangrene and two patients with mild decrease in joint range of motion after a pyarthrosis). The remainder of residua reflected mild to severe involvement of the central nervous system, including developmental retardation (six patients), mild monoparesis (one patient), and spastic quadraplegia (two patients). Severe residua occurred more frequently in patients with pneumococcal disease.

Relapses occurred in two patients, one in each treatment group. An infant with pneumococcal meningitis had a recurrence of CSF pleocytosis and fever 48 h after completion of a 10-day course of AMP; although the child was retreated with AMP, no organism was isolated during the second episode. Another infant with *H. influenzae* meningitis relapsed 72 h after completing 10 days of CB therapy, and this organism was again isolated from CSF; this child required retreatment with 14 days of CB.

Microbiology. All organisms isolated were susceptible to the antibiotics utilized (Table 4), and differences in susceptibility to CB or AMP among infecting organisms were not significant. Chloramphenicol was less active, on a weight basis, against all organisms, compared with CB or AMP. All *H. influenzae* isolates were confirmed to be type B and none produced beta-lactamase.

Pharmacology. CSF antibiotic concentrations ranged from 0 to 71 μg/ml. Higher CSF antibiotic concentrations were observed in CSF with high protein concentrations (Table 5). Similarly, higher antibiotic concentrations and CSF/serum ratios were attained in CSF obtained during the first 5 days of therapy (Table 6) in contrast to the later days of therapy.

DISCUSSION

Clinical responses after treatment with either CB or AMP were essentially equivalent.

TABLE 3. *Residua and deaths by etiology and treatment group*

Etiology	CB		AMP	
	Residua	Death	Residua	Death
H. influenzae[a]	3	0	2	2
S. pneumoniae[b]	1	0	5	1
N. meningitidis[c]	1	0	0	0
Unknown	0	0	1	0

[a] Residua included residual joint disease (two) and developmental retardation (three).

[b] Residua included severe neurological impairment (three) and developmental retardation (three).

[c] Residua included gangrene with amputation (one).

[d] Residua included mild monoparesis.

TABLE 2. *Incidence of positive CSF stain and culture on day 1 of treatment by treatment group and etiology*

Etiology	% Positive on day 1 with: CB		AMP	
	Gram stain	Culture	Gram stain	Culture
H. influenzae	38 (9/24)	38	11.7 (2/17)	5.8
S. pneumoniae	0 (0/7)	0	21.0 (3/14)	7.1
N. meningitidis	40 (2/5)	0	28.0 (2/7)	0

There were no significant differences between treatment groups in mortality or morbidity. Median CSF concentrations of both antibiotics attained during therapy were similar and exceeded the respective MIC of all isolated organisms. No *H. influenzae* isolates were resistant to AMP and none produced beta-lactamase.

During CB treatment of meningitis due to *H. influenzae*, 38% of the patients had positive CSF cultures on day 1. Despite this, persistently positive Gram stains did not correlate with a subsequent adverse clinical outcome. Wilson and Haltalin noted that 23% of patients with *H. influenzae* meningitis treated with AMP had positive CSF cultures obtained at a mean time of 26 h after the initiation of treatment (18). These investigators noted that persistently positive CSF cultures were more frequent when Levinthal medium was used and suggested that these persistent organisms may represent L-forms due to their unusual "fried-egg" appearance. All our CSF cultures were cultured on chocolate agar, and an atypical colony morphology was not observed.

The performance of a lumbar puncture before completion of 24 h of therapy may explain persistently positive cultures in this study. All day 1 CSF cultures were obtained betweeen 12 and 24 h after initiation of therapy, and CB and AMP patients were comparable in respect to the times of CSF collection. All patients, regardless of treatment or etiology, had negative CSF cultures and Gram stain if obtained at greater than 24 h after the initiation of therapy.

Evaluation of therapy with repeat CSF cultures is required, particularly if the possibility of strains of AMP-resistant *H. influenzae* is considered. However, the first CSF collection should await completion of at least 24 h of therapy; persistently positive cultures, in the face of clinical improvement and improvement of other CSF indexes, may not be an indication to change antibiotic therapy. However, a reevaluation with a subsequent CSF culture at a 24-h interval is advised because continued positive cultures of susceptible organisms beyond 24 h of treatment may signal the presence of a persistent focus of infection or an antibiotic-resistant organism.

Median CSF concentrations of CB and AMP on day 1 exceeded the median MIC of all organisms by 8- to 16-fold. However, measured CSF concentrations did not always exceed the determined MIC of an infecting organism in individ-

TABLE 4. *Antibiotic susceptibilities to bacterial isolates*

Organism	No.	Antibiotic	MIC		MBC	
			Median	Range	Median	Range
H. influenzae	42	CB	0.20	0.1–0.40	0.20	0.1–0.40
		AMP	0.20	0.1–0.40	0.20	0.1–0.80
		CM[a]	0.80	0.4–0.80	1.60	0.8–3.13
S. pneumoniae	14	CB	0.05	0.05–0.20	0.10	0.1–0.20
		AMP	0.05	0.05–0.20	0.10	0.1–0.20
		CM	3.13	0.8–6.25	6.25	1.6–6.25
N. meningitidis	8	CB	0.025	0.025–0.05	0.025	0.025–0.05
		AMP	0.035	0.025–0.050	0.050	0.05
		CM	1.60		3.13	

[a] CM, Chloramphenicol.

TABLE 5. *Relationship of CSF antibiotic concentrations (micrograms of antibiotic per milliliter) to dose and CSF protein concentration (milligrams per 100 ml)*

Drug regimen (mg/kg per 24 h)	Drug concn								
	CSF protein concn ≤74 mg/100 ml			CSF protein concn ≥75 mg/100 ml			CSF protein concn ≥200 mg/100 ml		
	Median	Range	No. of specimens	Median	Range	No. of specimens	Median	Range	No. of specimens
CB (200)	0.65	0–2.2	18	1.30	0.22–41	21	9.10	0.33–41	9
AMP (200)	0.45	0.1–2.3	15	2.20	0.37–30	14	13.80	0.37–30	8
CB (400)	0.85	0–71	41	4.50	0–60	24	8.5	3.2–13.5	2
AMP (400)	1.60	0–11.5	44	4.50	0–50	47	26.0	0–50	12

TABLE 6. *Relationship of CSF antibiotic concentrations and ratios (CSF/serum) versus day of treatment*

Drug regimen[a]	Index	Drug concn/ratio			
		Days 1–5	No. of specimens	Day 6	No. of specimens
CB (200)	Concentration[b]	1.2 (0.02–19)	29	0.42 (0–4.2)	26
	Ratio (%) median[c]	14.5%	20	5.8%	21
AMP (200)	Concentration	0.90 (0.1–14)	14	0.062 (0.1–30)	17
	Ratio (%) median	23.0%	13	4.2%	17
CB (400)	Concentration	1.5 (0–71)	34	1.20 (0–60)	37
	Ratio (%) median	8.3%	17	6.3%	26
AMP (400)	Concentration	3.4 (0–50)	47	1.85 (0–40)	46
	Ratio (%) median	14%		9.5%	36

[a] Daily dose in milligrams per kilogram.
[b] Concentration in micrograms per 100 ml.
[d] CSF/serum antibiotic concentration ratio.

ual cases. The median CSF concentrations of AMP reported in this study are comparable to those previously observed by other investigators (13,18). Further, Thrupp and co-workers noted increased CSF antibiotic concentrations during severe inflammation (13). The higher CSF antibiotic concentrations correlated with the higher levels of CSF protein, earlier days of therapy, and high CSF cell counts. The highest CSF concentrations were observed in patients with severe disease involvement, particularly adults with pneumococcal disease. Median CSF antibiotic concentrations increased with administration of increased doses.

CB has been suggested as a possible alternative to chloramphenicol for meningitis due to AMP-resistant *H. influenzae* (10). The attainable CSF concentration of CB, the in vitro susceptibility of hemophilus strains, and the clinical response documented in this study suggest that CB is adequate for AMP-susceptible *H. influenzae* infections, as well as those due to *N. meningitidis* and *S. pneumoniae*. However, lower cost, as well as the exquisite susceptibility of the meningococcus and pneumococcus to benzylpenicillin, make it the drug of choice for infections due to these organisms.

The susceptibiliy of strains of AMP-resistant *H. influenzae* to beta-lactam antibiotics has been shown to depend on inoculum size (15). When smaller inocula (i.e., 10^5 organisms/ml) of AMP-resistant organisms are utilized in susceptibility studies, apparent in vitro susceptibility to CB may be demonstrated. However, apparent in vitro susceptibility may not adequately predict clinical success. Feldman (3) has demonstrated concentrations of bacteria as high as 3.0×10^8 organisms/ml in the CSF of children with *H. influenzae* meningitis. Despite these high concentrations of bacteria, antibiotic therapy was usually effective; persistently positive cultures were observed only in children with an initial concentration of $\geq 10^7$ organisms/ml. Clinically, it remains undetermined whether CB can effectively treat infections due to AMP-resistant *H. influenzae*. Despite a theoretical advantage of this antibiotic against AMP-resistant *H. influenzae*, meningitis due to an AMP-resistant strain has, as yet, not been treated with CB. Chloramphenicol remains the drug of choice for these infections, and further clinical trials will be required to define the role of CB.

ACKNOWLEDGMENTS

We would like to thank Heather Wren, Paul Marengo, and Ronald Ressler for their assistance in performance of technical studies and Arlene Silva for the manuscript preparation.

This study was supported by a grant from Roerig-Pfizer, New York, and The Hastings Foundation Fund.

LITERATURE CITED

1. **Committee on Infectious Diseases.** 1976. Current status of ampicillin-resistant Hemophilus influenzae type B. Pediatrics 57:417.
2. **Farrar, E. W., and N. M. Odell.** 1974. Beta-lactamase activity in ampicillin-resistant *Haemophilus influenzae*. Antimicrob. Agents Chemother. 6:625–629.
3. **Feldman, W. E.** 1976. Concentrations of bacteria in cerebrospinal fluid of patients with bacterial meningitus. J. Pediatr. 88:549–552.
4. **Hirsh, H., and M. Finland.** 1960. Susceptibility of *Hemophilus influenzae* to 21 antibiotics in vitro. Am. J. Med. Sci. 23:33–39.
5. **Ivler, D., L. D. Thrupp, J. M. Leedom, P. F. Wehrle, and B. Portnoy.** 1964. Ampicillin treatment for bacterial meningitis, p. 335–345. Antimicrob. Agents Chemother. 1963.
6. **Kahn, W., S. Ross W. Rodriguez, G. Controni, and A. K. Saz.** 1974. *Haemophilus influenzae* type B resistant to ampicillin. J. Am. Med. Assoc. 229:298–301.
7. **Medeiros, A. A., and T. F. O'Brien.** 1975. Ampicillin-resistant *Haemophilus influenzae* type B possessing a TEM type beta-lactamase but little permeability barrier to ampicillin. Lancet 1:716–719.
8. **Overturf, G. D., J. Wilkins, J. M. Leedom, D. Ivler, and A. W. Mathies.** 1975. Susceptibility of *Haemophilus influenzae* type B to ampicillin after ten years of use. J. Pediatr. 87:297–300.

9. **Simon, H., and E. J. Yin.** 1970. Microbioassay of antimicrobial agents. Appl. Microbiol. **19**:573–579.
10. **Thornsberry, C., C. N. Baker, L. A. Kirven, and J. M. Swenson.** 1976. Susceptibility of ampicillin-resistant *Haemophilus influenzae* to seven penicillins. Antimicrob. Agents Chemother. **9**:70–73.
11. **Thornsberry, C., and L. A. Kirven.** 1974. Ampicillin resistance in *Haemophilus influenzae* as determined by a rapid test for beta-lactamase production. Antimicrob. Agents Chemother. **6**:653–655.
12. **Thrupp, L. D., J. M. Leedom, D. Ivler, P. F. Wehrle, J. F. Brown, A. W. Mathies, and B. Portnoy.** 1964. *H. influenzae* meningitis: a controlled study of treatment with ampicillin. *In* Proceedings of the Conference of Apothecaries Hall, London.
13. **Thrupp, L. D., J. M. Leedom, D. Ivler, P. F. Wehrle, B. Portnoy, and A. W. Mathies.** 1966. Ampicillin levels in the cerebrospinal fluid during treatment of bacterial meningitis, p. 206–213. Antimicrob. Agents Chemother. 1965.
14. **Tomeh, O. M., S. S. Starr, J. E. McGowan, Jr., P. M. Terry, and A. J. Nahmias.** 1974. Ampicillin-resistant *Haemophilus influenzae* type B. J. Am. Med. Assoc. **229**:295–297.
15. **Vega, R., H. L. Sadoff, and M. J. Patterson.** 1976. Mechanisms of ampicillin resistance in *Haemophilus influenzae* type B. Antimicrob. Agents Chemother. **9**:146–149.
16. **Wehrle, P. F., A. W. Mathies, and J. M. Leedom.** 1967. Management of bacterial meningitis. Clin. Neurosurg. **14**:72–85.
17. **Williams, J. D., and J. Andres.** 1975. Sensitivity of *Haemophilus influenzae* to antibiotics. Br. Med. J. **1**:134–138.
18. **Wilson, J. D., and K. C. Haltalin.** 1975. Ampicillin in *H. influenzae* meningitis. Am. J. Dis. Child. **129**:208–215.
19. **Wilson, F. M., and A. M. Lerner.** 1964. Etiology and treatment of purulent meningitis at the Detroit Receiving Hospital. N. Engl. J. Med. **271**:1235–1238.
20. **Yow, M. D.** 1969. Ampicillin the treatment of meningitis due to *Haemophilus influenzae*: an appraisal after 6 years of experience. J. Pediatr. **74**:848–852.

ANTIMICROBIAL AGENTS AND CHEMOTHERAPY, Mar. 1977, p. 427-434 Vol. 11, No. 3

Printed in U.S.A.

Cefoxitin: Clinical Evaluation in Thirty-Eight Patients

PETER N. R. HESELTINE,* DAVID F. BUSCH, RICHARD D. MEYER, AND SYDNEY M. FINEGOLD

Infectious Disease Section, Medical Service, Wadsworth Hospital Center, Veterans Administration, Los Angeles, California 90073, and Department of Medicine, UCLA School of Medicine, Los Angeles, California 90024

Received for publication 30 September 1976

Clinical and bacteriological efficacy, patient tolerance, and toxicity of cefoxitin, a beta-lactamase-resistant cephamycin, were evaluated in 38 patients; 13 had soft tissue infection, 12 had pneumonia, 3 had urinary tract infection, 2 had peritonitis, and 4 had miscellaneous infections. In five patients, infection was clinically evident, though not bacteriologically proven. The latter patients were evaluated with regard to tolerance and toxicity only. Among the 34 infections in 33 patients, 71% were considered clinically cured; 86% of those patients who could be recultured were bacteriologically cured. Phlebitis was noted in 32% of the total group, and eosinophilia was observed in 16%. Unexplained deterioration in renal function occurred in two patients. Mean peak cefoxitin levels in serum were 72 μg/ml 30 min after a 2-g infusion and 32 μg/ml 30 min after a 1-g infusion. Cefoxitin was more active against facultatively and obligately anaerobic gram-negative organisms isolated from these patients than was cephalothin.

The search for cephalosporin derivatives that are resistant to cephalosporinases and nontoxic to humans has led to the development of cefoxitin, a new beta-lactamase-resistant cephamycin (16, 12). The present study was undertaken to determine the clinical efficacy, patient tolerance, and safety of cefoxitin in the therapy of infections caused by susceptible organisms.

(Presented, in part, at the Western Society for Clinical Research Carmel, Calif., Clin. Res. **23**:113A, 1976.)

MATERIALS AND METHODS

Patients. Patients studied were hospitalized at the Wadsworth Veterans Administration Hospital. In each case, clinical findings and either prior culture or Gram-stained material suggested infection with bacteria likely to be susceptible to the cephalosporins or shown to be susceptible to cefoxitin itself. Informed written consent was obtained from the patients or their relatives.

Cefoxitin was administered via scalp vein infusion set or short catheter as 1 or 2 g, diluted in 100 ml of either normal saline or 5% dextrose in water, given over 20 to 40 min. Doses were administered either every 4 or 6 h. Infusion sites were changed at least every 72 h or at the first sign of inflammation.

Possible toxicity was monitored by daily examination of patients; determinations of complete blood cell count, Coombs test, urinalysis, serum glutamic oxalacetic and glutamic pyruvic transminases, bilirubin, alkaline phosphatase, electrolytes, glucose, creatinine, and blood urea nitrogen determinations were performed at frequent intervals. Appropriate cultures were obtained from all patients before and, when possible, during and after termination of therapy. In all but three suspected cases of pneumonia, transtracheal aspiration was performed to obtain specimens free of oropharyngeal flora.

Efficacy of therapy was evaluated in two principal ways: clinical outcome and bacteriological outcome. Follow-up cultures were not feasible in patients with soft tissue infections who showed resolution, and patients with pneumonia were not subjected to repeat transtracheal aspiration. Clinical cure was defined as recovery from infection achieved either by cefoxitin therapy alone or by local measures, including surgery, in addition to cefoxitin. Eradication of the susceptible initially isolated pathogens without ingrowth of clinically significant organisms on subsequent culture was regarded as evidence of bacteriological cure.

Cefoxitin assays. Blood specimens were collected, and the serum was separated aseptically and frozen for subsequent assay. Assays were performed on the sera of 19 of the 38 patients reported here and from an additional 11 patients subsequently treated. Specimens were obtained immediately at the end of infusion, at 30, 60, and 90 min, and at 2, 4, and 6 h after the end of infusion. Eighty-three serum specimens, three ascitic fluid samples, and two cerebrospinal fluid samples were assayed. Assays were performed by the Infectious Disease Department, UCLA Center for the Health Sciences, Los Angeles, Calif., using a modification of the cup-plate technique of Goodwin et al. (6) with *Micrococcus lysodeikticus* as the test organism. Forty duplicate specimens were assayed by Merck, Sharp & Dohme, West Point, Penn., with comparable results.

Susceptibility testing. Testing of susceptibility to cefoxitin and to cephalothin was performed on 67

clinical isolates by agar or broth dilution technique (5, 15).

RESULTS

Thirty-eight patients (one female, the others male) were treated with cefoxitin between June 1975 and January 1976. The age range was from 21 to 79 years, with a median of 52. Duration of therapy ranged from 2 to 31 days with a median of 8 days. Thirty-three patients received either 4 or 6 g per day. Another 11, considered here for pharmacological evaluation, received 8 to 12 g per day.

Twelve patients had pneumonia, 13 had soft tissue infection, 2 had urinary tract infection, 2 had peritonitis (one with a concurrent urinary tract infection), and 4 had miscellaneous infections. Seven patients were bacteremic. No pathogenic organisms were cultured in five patients despite clinical signs of infection. Bacteriological and clinical outcomes are summarized in Table 1.

Pneumonia. Bacterial isolates from the 12 patients with pneumonia are listed in Table 2.

Of the 12 patients, 10 were clinically cured. Two patients died during therapy. Patient 2, admitted because of pneumonia and alcohol withdrawal, became acutely oliguric 6 h after initiation of therapy; urine output resumed after fluid challenge, and cefoxitin treatment was continued at reduced dosage. The patient suffered a cardiorespiratory arrest 30 h later. At autopsy no organisms were cultured, and the bronchopneumonia, though present, was resolving. Patient 18, with metastatic bronchogenic carcinoma and aspiration pneumonia, had become afebrile and appeared improved after 2 days of therapy. On day 3 of therapy, he had a sudden cardiorespiratory arrest and died.

Follow-up sputum cultures were obtained in seven patients, and, in five, susceptible organisms were eradicated. Despite clinical resolution, *S. pneumoniae* was recultured from the sputum of one, patient 24, on day 6 of therapy, and reemergence of *S. aureus* and *K. pneumoniae* occurred after termination of therapy in the second, patient 16. There was, however, no recurrence of clinical symptoms.

Soft tissue infection. Of 13 patients with soft tissue infection, 11 were considered clinically cured. Nine required drainage of abscesses, two had diagnostic needle aspiration, and another had drainage of an abscess followed by amputation. Bacterial isolates are listed in Table 3. One of the two treatment failures, patient 29, who had an extensive iliofemoral abscess, showed some resolution of the primary process but died of noninfective pulmonary complications after termination of therapy. The second, patient 26, who had a femoral abscess, had eradication of susceptible organisms but showed only moderate clinical improvement.

Follow-up cultures available from seven patients showed six to be bacteriologically cured. In the seventh, patient 25, the initial culture had been sterile, although pus cells and many gram-positive cocci in chains had been seen on initial Gram stain. Reaspiration of the cellulitis after 2 days of therapy yielded moderate growth of group A streptococci. The Gram stain showed a decrease in the number of pus cells and organisms, and this patient progressed to complete clinical resolution on therapy.

Urinary tract infection. All three patients with urinary tract infection (one with concomitant bacterial peritonitis) were clinically and bacteriologically cured (Table 4). *Serratia marcescens,* resistant to cephalothin, was recovered from patient 7 while he was receiving cephalothin. Urine cultures immediately and 5 months after therapy were sterile in this patient; at 6 weeks after therapy, urine cultures were sterile in the other two.

Peritonitis. Two patients with chronic liver disease and ascites had bacterial peritonitis (Table 4). Patient 15 was clinically cured and both patients were bacteriologically cured. Patient 14 required a subsequent course of ampicillin to eradicate persistent *Streptococcus faecalis,* resistant to cefoxitin, from the peritoneal fluid.

Miscellaneous infections. An infected aortofemoral graft, cervical osteomyelitis with associated epidural abscess, necrotizing pharyngitis, and postoperative cholangitis were diagnosed in one patient each (Table 4).

Two patients were clinically cured. One, patient 4, required removal of an infected vascular graft. The second, patient 34, from whom *Staphylococcus aureus* was cultured and anaerobes were clinically implicated by Gram stain and odor, improved markedly on therapy.

In contrast, patient 36 had *Enterobacter aerogenes,* resistant to cefoxitin, recovered repeatedly from biliary drainage and manifested clinical signs of infection, necessitating aminoglycoside therapy. The last, patient 21, had *S. aureus* bacteremia and a spinal epidural abscess demonstrated by radiological and neurological findings. When cerebrospinal fluid pleocytosis was noted, therapy was changed to high-dose oxacillin. However, cerebrospinal fluid and blood cultures obtained during cefoxitin therapy yielded no growth. Granulation tissue obtained at surgery after 24 h of oxacillin therapy also was sterile.

TABLE 1. *Outcome of 34 infections in 33 patients*

Diagnosis	No. of patients	Bacteriological			Clinical	
		Cure	Failure	Unevaluable	Cure	Failure
Pneumonia	12	5	2	5	10	2
Soft tissue infection	13	6	1	6	11	2
Urinary tract infection[a]	3	3			3	
Peritonitis	2	2			1	1
Miscellaneous	4	3		1	2	2

[a] Includes one patient with simultaneous peritonitis.

TABLE 2. *Pneumonias*

Patient no.	Age	Underlying disease	Organisms isolated	Days of treatment	Results	
					Bacteriological	Clinical
2	49	Alcoholism	*Haemophilus influenzae* (S)[a]	3	N/A[b]	Died
3	24	Hypogammaglobulinemia	*H. influenzae* (T)[c] *Neisseria catarrhalis* (T) *Veillonella parvula* (T)	6	Cure	Cure
12	33	Narcotic abuse	*V. alcalescens* (T) *Neisseria* species (T) Diptheroids (T) α-Hemolytic streptococci (T) *H. parainfluenzae* (T)	6	N/A	Cure
16	56	Systemic lupus erythematosis	*Klebsiella pneumoniae* (B)[d] *Staphylococcus aureus* (S)	9	Failure	Cure
18	69	Bronchogenic carcinoma	*H. influenzae* (T) *Eikenella corrodens* (T) α-Hemolytic streptococci (T) *Neisseria* species (T) *Fusobacterium nucleatum* (T) *Bacteroides melaninogenicus* (T) *V. parvula* (T)	4	N/A	Died
19	51	Alcoholism	*H. influenzae* (T) *Streptococcus pneumoniae* (T)	8	Cure	Cure
23	41	Seizure disorder	α-Hemolytic streptococci (T) *Peptostreptococcus micros* (T) *V. parvula* (T)	14	N/A	Cure
24	66	COPD[e]	*S. pneumoniae* (S) *Escherichia coli* (S)	11	Failure	Cure
27	48	Narcotic abuse; COPD	*S. pneumoniae* (T) (B) *H. influenzae* (T) *B. ruminicola* (T) *B. melaninogenicus* (T) *B. oralis* (T)	5	Cure	Cure
28	55	None	*S. pneumoniae* (T) (B) α-Hemolytic streptococci (T) *Corynebacterium* sp. (T) α-Hemolytic streptococci (T) *V. parvula* (T) *Lactobacillus* sp. (T) *B. melaninogenicus* (T) *Eubacterium* sp. (T)	11	Cure	Cure
31	57	Bronchogenic carcinoma–radiation treatment	*S. pneumoniae* (T) Group A streptococci (T) *H. influenzae* (T) α-Hemolytic streptococci (T) *Bacillus* species (T)	11	Cure	Cure
35	53	Squamous cell carcinoma, mouth–resected	*S. pneumoniae* (T) *N. meningitidis* (T) *H. influenzae* (T)	13	N/A	Cure

[a] S, Sputum.
[b] N/A, Not available.
[c] T, Transtracheal aspirate.
[d] B, Blood.
[e] COPD, Chronic obstructive pulmonary disease.

TABLE 3. *Soft tissue infections*

Patient no.	Age	Underlying disease	Organisms isolated	Surgery	Days of therapy	Results	
						Bacteriological	Clinical
6	44	Alcoholism	Group A streptococci	I&D[a]	5	Cure	Cure
8	53	DM[b]	*Staphylococcus aureus* (B)[c]	I&D	31	Cure	Cure
9	59	Laennec cirrhosis	*S. aureus* Group A streptococci *Peptostreptococcus micros*	I&D	8	N/A[d]	Cure
10	42	Narcotic abuse	*Clostridium perfringens*	Needle aspiration	6	N/A	Cure
17	58	DM	*S. aureus* *Peptostreptococcus variabilis*	I&D and subsequent amputation	16	N/A	Cure
22	25	None	*S. aureus*	I&D	6	N/A	Cure
25	27	None	Group A streptococci	Needle aspiration	10	Fail	Cure
26	58	DM, peripheral vascular disease	*Pseudomonas aeruginosa* *Serratia marcesens* *Enterobacter cloacae* *Escherichia coli* Enterococci *S. aureus*	I&D	28	Cure	Fail
29	67	Laennec cirrhosis	*S. aureus*	I&D	19	Cure	Died
30	21	Malabsorption, corticosteroids	*S. aureus*	None	14	N/A	Cure
33	60	Trauma	Group A streptococci α-Hemolytic streptococci *E. aerogenes* (B) *S. aureus*	I&D	14	Cure	Cure
37	32	Narcotic abuse	*S. aureus* α-Hemolytic streptococci *Peptostreptococcus parvulus*	I&D	10	Cure	Cure
38	54	DM	*Propionibacterium acnes*	I&D	20	N/A	Cure

[a] I&D, Incision and drainage.
[b] DM, Diabetes mellitus.
[c] B, Blood.
[d] N/A, Not available.

TABLE 4. *Urinary tract, peritonitis, and miscellaneous infections*

Patient no.	Age	Location	Organism isolated	Surgery	Days of therapy	Results	
						Bacteriological	Clinical
1	59	UTI[a]	*Escherichia coli* (B)[b] (U)[c]	No	5	Cure	Cure
7	47	UTI	*Serratia marcescens*	No	8	Cure	Cure
15	60	UTI	*E. coli*	No	11	Cure	Cure
15	60	Peritonitis	*E. coli* *Bacteroides* species α-Hemolytic streptococci	No	11	Cure	Cure
14	58	Peritonitis	*Staphylococcus aureus* *Klebsiella pneumoniae* *Streptococcus faecalis*	No	16	Cure	Cure
4	53	Infected aortofemoral graft	*S. aureus*	I&D	28	Cure	Cure
21	51	Osteomyelitis-epidural abscess	*S. aureus* (B)	I&D[d]	5	Cure	Fail
34	45	Necrotizing pharyngitis	*S. aureus*[e]	No	5	N/A[f]	Cure
36	79	Cholangitis	*E. coli* (C) *Enterobacter aerogenes*	Biliary drainage	8	Cure	Fail

[a] UTI, Urinary tract infection.
[b] B, Blood.
[c] U, Urine.
[d] I&D, Incision and drainage.
[e] Anaerobes clinically implicated as well.
[f] N/A, Not available.

Bacteremia. Bacteremia occurred in seven of the above patients (Tables 2–4), and follow-up blood cultures were negative after 14 days of incubation in all.

Adverse effects. Four patients showed deterioration of renal function while receiving cefoxitin. In patient 2, oliguria developed 6 h after therapy had begun. After fluid challenge, urine output resumed and remained adequate despite resumption of cefoxitin. The patient died on hospital day 3; postmortem examination of the kidneys showed minimal cortical scarring, minimal thickening of middle-sized arteries, and hyalinization of arterioles. In patient 11, with ascites and cirrhosis of the liver, renal failure, which was present before therapy, progressed and was a contributory cause of death; postmortem examination showed severe alcoholic liver disease and microscopically unremarkable kidneys. There was a very low urine sodium value and it was believed that the patient had hepatorenal syndrome. Two other patients who had no evidence of antecedent renal disease experienced transient elevations of blood urea nitrogen and serum creatinine. Patient 1, who received cefoxitin for a bacteremic urinary tract infection, also had cirrhosis of the liver with ascites. This patient's creatinine level rose to 3.7 μg/ml and returned to 2.1 μg/ml after discontinuation of the drug. Patient 14 had peritonitis that was also associated with ascites cirrhosis of the liver, and an elevated creatinine level (0.8 to 1.4 μg/ml), which returned to normal after therapy was stopped. No specific cause for the azotemia could be documented in either case.

Eosinophilia greater than 6% of the total leukocyte count was noted in six patients during or after the termination of therapy but, of these, only two, patients 8 and 24, had eosinophil counts in excess of 10%. Two patients had conversion of their direct Coombs tests from negative to trace positive during therapy. This was associated with an average decline in hemoglobin level of 1 g/100 ml. Another patient, who initially had a trace positive Coombs test, was negative on subsequent testing.

Patient tolerance. Burning on infusion of cefoxitin, noted by two patients, was not accompanied by phlebitis and did not require discontinuation of the drug. Phlebitis occurred in 12 of the 38 patients. Phlebitis, when it occurred, tended to appear within the first few days of therapy and was persistent, despite changes of infusion site. Degree of involvement was mild in six patients, moderate in four, severe enough to cause discontinuation of therapy in one, and would have resulted in discontinuation in a second had the course not been completed. All responded within 3 days to local measures. Needle aspiration and culture of one severe case, patient 36, yielded no growth.

Drug levels. As shown in Fig. 1, mean serum levels in patients with normal renal function (serum creatinine, ≤1.2 μg/100 ml) after a 1-g infusion ranged from 32 μg/ml 30 min after the end of infusion to <3 μg/ml (lower limit of assay) at 6 h. After a 2-g infusion, levels ranged from a mean of 72 μg/ml at 30 min to 10.4 μg/ml at 4 h (Fig. 2).

Ascitic fluid levels were measured in three patients, 11, 14, and 15, of whom two had abnormal renal function. In all three, ascitic fluid levels of cefoxitin were slightly in excess of simultaneous serum levels 2 h after a 1-g infusion.

Cerebrospinal fluid levels were measured in two patients; one had no meningeal inflammation, the other had mild pleocytosis. At 75 and 180 min after intravenous infusion, respectively, no drug was detected.

Susceptibility results. Susceptibility of gram-negative aerobes was one or more twofold dilutions lower with cefoxitin than with cephalothin; cefoxitin was essentially inactive against *Pseudomonas aeruginosa* and *Enterobacter* species. Gram-negative anaerobic organisms were also more susceptible to cefoxitin than to cephalothin, but gram-positive anaerobic and aerobic organisms were less so (Table 5).

DISCUSSION

Cefoxitin is characterized by a methoxyl group at the 7-position of the cephalosporanic acid nucleus (16). This confers a high degree of resistance to destruction by cephalosporinases (12), notably those produced by indole-positive *Proteus*, certain *S. marcescens* and *B. fragilis* (4, 17), and many cephalosporin-resistant strains of *Escherichia coli, Klebsiella,* indole-negative *Proteus, Providencia, Salmonella,* and *Shigella* (7, 8, 11, 14, 16, 17). It is also active against gram-positive and gram-negative organisms susceptible to currently available cephalosporins (17). Cefoxitin is es-

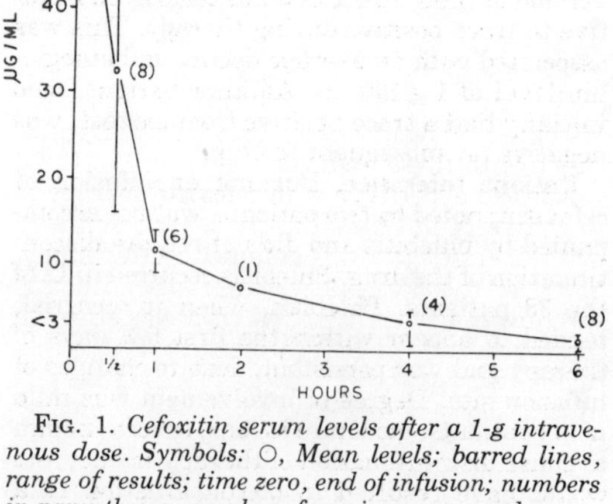

FIG. 1. *Cefoxitin serum levels after a 1-g intravenous dose. Symbols: ○, Mean levels; barred lines, range of results; time zero, end of infusion; numbers in parentheses, number of specimens assayed.*

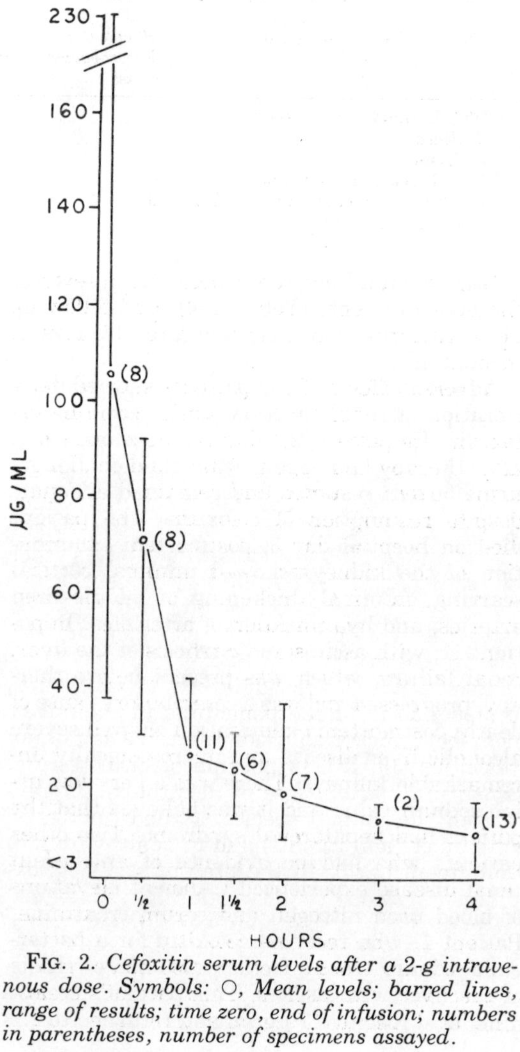

FIG. 2. *Cefoxitin serum levels after a 2-g intravenous dose. Symbols: ○, Mean levels; barred lines, range of results; time zero, end of infusion; numbers in parentheses, number of specimens assayed.*

TABLE 5. *Susceptibilities of isolates to cefoxitin and cephalothin*

Organism	No. of isolates	Minimal inhibitory concentration (μg/ml)			
		Cefoxitin		Cephalothin	
		Median	Range	Median	Range
Staphylococcus aureus	13	2	(≤1 to 4)	≤1	(≤1 to 1)
Streptococcus					
pneumoniae	5	≤1	(≤1 to 2)	≤1 (All)	
Group A	4	2	(≤1 to 8)	≤1 (All)	
Group D	5	>128 (All)		64	(32 to 128)
Escherichia coli	4	4	(≤1 to 16)	32	(≤1 to 64)
Klebsiella pneumoniae	3	32	(16 to 32)	64	(32 to 128)
Enterobacter species	4	>128		>128	
Serratia marcescens	2		(64, 128)		(128 and >128)
Pseudomonas aeruginosa	1	>128		>128	
Haemophilus influenzae	4	32	(8 to 32)	16	(8 to 16)
Bacteroides fragilis	2		(8, 32)		(64, 64)
Bacteroides species (non-*fragilis*)	7	1	(0.25 to 16)	8	(≤0.062 to 256)
Peptostreptococcus micros	2		(0.5, 2)		(0.125, 0.25)
Peptostreptococcus parvulus	1	2		0.5	
Peptococcus variabilis	1	0.25		0.5	
Propionibacterium acnes	1	0.25		0.125	
Clostridium perfringens	1	2		2	
Fusobacterium nucleatum	1	1		≤0.062	
Lactobacillus species	1	1		0.5	
Veillonella alcalescens	1	4		4	
Veillonella parvula	4	0.5	(0.5 to 2)	0.25	(0.25 to 2)

sentially inactive against *P. aeruginosa* and enterococci (11, 16).

Susceptibility testing of clinical isolates from our patients supports the finding that cefoxitin has enhanced activity against cephalothin-susceptible gram-negative organisms and good activity against gram-negative anaerobic organisms (4, 8, 11, 13, 14); this occurs, however, at the expense of some decrease in activity against gram-positive organisms (16, 17). It is of concern that serum levels might not always reach the reported minimal inhibitory concentrations for *B. fragilis*. Certain isolates of *B. fragilis* have been inhibited only by 64 μg of cefoxitin per ml (13, 14).

Except for cephaloridine, the cephalosporin compounds rival the penicillins in their freedom from undesirable side reactions and organ toxicities (10, 18). In pharmacological testing, cefoxitin appeared free of nephrotoxic properties in the animal species studied (monkeys, rats, mice, and rabbits) and in healthy human volunteers (2, 7). In the present study, unexplained transient deterioration in renal function of two patients, 1 and 14, was noted. Since, in each case, other factors (hepatic failure, bacteremia) may have contributed to the renal dysfunction, the possible toxicity of cefoxitin must await further study.

In pharmacological trials, the half-life of intravenous cefoxitin was significantly longer than that of cephalothin (2, 7). It appears that levels of cefoxitin in serum in our patients were somewhat prolonged as compared with those reported for cephalothin. Patients receiving the 2-g doses did have appreciable serum levels at 4 h. Hepatic function did not affect serum levels in the absence of associated renal dysfunction.

Cefoxitin caused phlebitis in approximately one-third of our patients; the incidence was unrelated to the dosage regimen. Phlebitis caused by cephalosporins has been reported with approximately this incidence (1, 3). Transient eosinophilia and Coombs positive reactions have also been described with cephalosporins (10). We observed no adverse clinical reactions associated with these findings.

A broad experience with cefoxitin therapy in a variety of infections commonly encountered in clinical practice was obtained in this study. Many of the patients were seriously ill, and seven were bacteremic. Cefoxitin was effective in eradicating infection in the majority of patients and appeared relatively nontoxic. Although dosages and frequency of administration were increased because of our findings of low serum levels after a 1-g dose, no patient had a clinical failure or developed resistant organisms, even on the lower dosage. Our overall clinical results are comparable to those reported with cephalothin and cefazolin (9).

Further study is required to evaluate the efficacy of cefoxitin in infections. It may prove of specific advantage in the management of intra-abdominal sepsis, where broad-spectrum activity against gram-negative facultative and obligate anaerobes is required.

ACKNOWLEDGMENT

This work was supported by a grant from Merck, Sharp & Dohme, West Point, Penn.

LITERATURE CITED

1. **Berger, S., E. C. Ernst, and M. Barza.** 1976. Comparative incidence of phlebitis due to buffered cephalothin, cephapirin, and cefamandole. Antimicrob. Agents Chemother, 9:575–579.
2. **Brumfitt, W., J. Kosimidis, J. M. T. Hamilton-Miller, and J. N. G. Gilchrist.** 1974. Cefoxitin and cephalothin: antimicrobial activity, human pharmacokinetics, and toxicology. Antimicrob. Agents Chemother. 6:290–299.
3. **Cross, A. S., and E. C. Tramont.** 1976. Comparison of phlebitis produced by cephapirin and cephalothin. Antimicrob. Agents Chemother. 9:722–724.
4. **Del Bene V. E., and W. E. Farrar.** 1973. Cephalosporinase activity in *Bacteroides fragilis*. Antimicrob. Agents Chemother. 3:369–372.
5. **Ericsson, H. M., and J. C. Sherris.** 1971. Antibiotic sensitivity testing: report of an international collaborative study. Acta. Pathol. Microbiol. Scand. Sect. B 217(Suppl.): 67–68.
6. **Goodwin, S. C., E. B. Raftery, A. D. Goldberg, H. Skeggs, A. E. Till, and C. M. Martin.** 1974. Effects of rate of infusion and probenicid on serum levels, renal excretion, and tolerance of intravenous doses of cefoxitin in humans: comparison with cephalothin. Antimicrob. Agents Chemother. 6:338–346.
7. **Kosimidis, J., J. M. T. Hamilton-Miller, J. N. G. Gilchrist, D. W. Kerry, and W. Brumfitt.** 1973. Cefoxitin, a new semi-synthetic cephamycin: an *in vitro* and *in vivo* comparison with cephalothin. Br. Med. J. 4:653–655.
8. **Lewis, R. P., R. D. Meyer, and L. L. Kraus.** 1976. Antibacterial activity of selected beta-lactam and aminoglycoside antibiotics against cephalothin-resistant *Enterobacteriaceae*. Antimicrob. Agents Chemother. 9:780–786.
9. **Madhavan, T., E. L. Quinn, E. Freimer, E. J. Fisher, F. Cox, K. Burch, and D. Pohlod.** 1973. Clinical studies of cefazolin and comparison with other cephalosporins. Antimicrob. Agents Chemother. 4:525–531.
10. **Moellering, R. C., Jr, and M. N. Swartz.** 1976. The newer cephalosporins. N. Engl. J. Med. 294:224–228.
11. **Neu, H. C.** 1974. Cefoxitin, a semisynthetic cephamycin antibiotic: antibacterial spectrum and resistance to hydrolysis by gram-negative beta-lactamases. Antimicrob. Agents Chemother. 6:170–176.
12. **Onishi, H. R., D. R. Daoust, S. B. Zimmerman, D. Hendlin, and E. D. Stapley.** 1974. Cefoxitin, a semisynthetic cephamycin antibiotic. III. Resistance to beta-lactamase inactivation. Antimicrob. Agents Chemother. 5:38–48.
13. **Sutter, V. L., and S. M. Finegold.** 1975. Susceptibility of anaerobic bacteria to carbenicillin, cefoxitin, and related drugs. J. Infect. Dis. 131:417–422.
14. **Tally, F. P., N. V. Jacobus, and J. G. Bartlett.** 1975. Susceptibility of anaerobes to cefoxitin and other cephalosporins. Antimicrob. Agents Chemother. 7:128–132.
15. **Sutter, V. L., V. L. Vargo, and S. M. Finegold.** 1975. Wadsworth anaerobic bacteriology manual, 2nd ed. University of California, Los Angeles Extension Division, Los Angeles.
16. **Wallack, H., and D. Hendlin.** 1974. Cefoxitin, a semisynthetic cephamycin antibiotic. I. Susceptibility studies. Antimicrob. Agents Chemother. 5:25–32.
17. **Washington, J. A.** 1976. The *in vitro* spectrum of the cephalosporins. Mayo Clin. Proc. 51:237–250.
18. **Weinstein, L., and K. Kaplan.** 1970. The cephalosporins: microbiological, chemical and pharmacological properties of use in chemotherapy of infection. Ann. Intern. Med. 72:729–739.

ANTIMICROBIAL AGENTS AND CHEMOTHERAPY, Mar. 1977, p. 435-440 Vol. 11, No. 3
Printed in U.S.A.

Chemotherapy of an Experimental *Bacteroides fragilis* Infection in Mice

CLAY B. WALKER,* DORRIT NITZAN, AND TRACY D. WILKINS

Anaerobe Laboratory, Virginia Polytechnic Institute and State University, Blacksburg, Virginia 24061

Received for publication 24 September 1976

The efficacies of five common antimicrobial agents were determined for a pure *Bacteroides fragilis* infection in mice. Therapy was begun 4 h after bacterial injection and given every 8 h thereafter for 5 days. Blood levels were determined over an 8-h period for each concentration of antibiotic tested. Clindamycin and tetracycline were the most effective in preventing the formation of abscesses. Chloramphenicol, penicillin G, and cephalothin were not effective in protecting the mice from infection.

Bacteroides fragilis is an anaerobic, gram-negative, nonsporeforming bacillus frequently encountered in human clinical specimens. Although the in vitro susceptibility of this organism has been determined to many antimicrobial agents, the lack of a suitable experimental animal model has prohibited the testing of the efficacies of these agents in vivo.

We have recently described the production of a pure *B. fragilis* infection in mice that results in an easily visible subcutaneous abscess (12). This model provides the first opportunity for the testing of antimicrobial agents against a pure *B. fragilis* infection in an experimental animal. Using this model, we have tested the efficacies of five common antimicrobial agents: clindamycin, chloramphenicol, tetracycline, penicillin G, and cephalothin.

MATERIALS AND METHODS

Source of organisms. *B. fragilis* VPI 9032 was originally isolated from a human clinical specimen.

Bacterial inoculum. Before this series of experiments, a chopped-meat broth culture of *B. fragilis* VPI 9032 was lyophilized in a number of ampoules. One ampoule was opened for each experiment into chopped-meat broth. The culture was grown overnight (18 to 20 h), and 0.1 ml was inoculated into 10-ml volumes of chopped-meat–carbohydrate semisolid medium (12). The chopped-meat–carbohydrate semisolid culture was incubated for 18 to 20 h and then injected into mice.

Injection of bacteria. One-half milliliter of the chopped-meat–carbohydrate semisolid culture was injected subcutaneously under the loose skin of the groin on the left side of the mouse as previously described (12).

Source of antibiotics. The antibiotics used and the sources were: penicillin G, potassium salt (1,595 U/mg), and tetracycline-hydrochloride, Sigma Chemical Co., St. Louis, Mo.; chloramphenicol-sodium succinate, and chloramphenicol-hydrochloride, Parke-Davis, Detroit, Mich.; cephalothin, Eli Lilly and Co., Indianapolis, Ind.; clindamycin phosphate and clindamycin-hydrochloride, The Upjohn Co., Kalamazoo, Mich.

Injection of antibiotics. All antibiotics were dissolved in sterile distilled water and given in 0.1-ml volumes. All solutions were made up fresh daily and stored at 4°C with the exception of tetracycline-hydrochloride, which was made up fresh for each injection time. The antibiotics were given intraperitoneally (i.p.) on the animal's right side. Tetracycline-hydrochloride was also given by oral gavage. Two groups of approximately 25 mice each were tested with each concentration of antibiotic. For each experiment, at least 25 mice were used as a control group. The mice received the bacterial injection before being randomly selected for treatment or as controls; the latter received 0.1 ml of sterile distilled water in place of the antibiotic.

Schedule of injections. Antibiotic therapy was begun 4 h after the bacterial injection and then given every 8 h thereafter for a period of 5 days.

Determination of MICs. Minimal inhibitory concentrations (MICs) were determined by the agar dilution procedure (13) with the medium of Wilkins and Chalgren (14). Chloramphenicol-hydrochloride and clindamycin-hydrochloride were used for determinating of MICs to chloramphenicol and clindamycin.

Determination of antibiotic blood levels. The amount of antibiotic present in the blood was determined by the method described by Sabath and Toftegaard (11). For each concentration of antibiotic tested, blood levels were determined in two separate groups of five mice each. Blood was collected from each mouse by tail bleeding at 0.5, 1, 2, 3, 4.5, 6, and 8 h after the last injection of the antibiotic. Ten microliters of blood from each mouse was placed on a 6.35-mm paper disk (Schleicher and Schuell, no. 740-E). The disks were placed on the assay medium (11) and incubated in an anaerobic chamber similar to that described by Aranki and Freter (2). The assay plates were incubated at 37°C for 3 to 5 h until hemolysis of the blood had occurred. The assay medium was made 1 day before use and stored at 4°C. The levels of antibiotics in the blood were determined by comparison with standard curves constructed by exponential regression with a computer. Clindamycin-hydrochloride and chloramphenicol-hydrochloride were used to construct the standard curves for clindamycin and chloramphenicol. Standard curves were constructed by dissolving known amounts of antibiotic in whole sheep blood. Whole sheep blood was used routinely for the standard curves because preliminary trials indicated that no significant differences were detectable between the quantitation of the antibiotics in sheep blood and in mouse blood.

Assay organisms. The strains of *Clostridium perfringens* used as assay organisms for the different antibiotics are given in Table 1.

Anaerobic techniques and media. The media for the cultivation of *B. fragilis* were prepared prereduced (5), and all culture manipulations were performed as described in the *VPI Anaerobe Laboratory Manual* (5).

Mice. Swiss white mice, ICR strain, 18 to 20 g (Flow Laboratories, Dublin, Va.), were used for all experiments. The mice were caged in groups of 25 with a light-dark cycle of 12 h and were allowed to stabilize for at least 48 h before being used in any experiment.

Determination of effects of therapy. The mice were examined daily beginning on the 4th day after bacterial injection and continuing through the 14th day for the presence of a localized subcutaneous abscess. Maximum abscess formation was found to occur by the 7th to the 10th day (11). The mice were not kept past the 14th day.

RESULTS

MICs. The MICs for the five antibiotics tested are given in Table 1. *B. fragilis* VPI 9032 was susceptible to clindamycin, tetracycline, and chloramphenicol and relatively resistant to both penicillin G and cephalothin in vitro.

Blood levels. The antibiotic concentrations in the blood are given in Table 2 for an 8-h period after the final injection of the antibiotic. For all of the antibiotics tested except tetracycline, the peak blood level occurred within the first 0.5 h after injection.

Clindamycin. Intraperitoneal injections of 37.5, 75, 150, or 300 mg of clindamycin per kg were given every 8 h for 5 days. Table 3 gives the percentage of mice protected from infection by each dosage and the peak blood levels obtained. Peak blood levels for clindamycin in humans are generally considered to fall within a range of 3 to 14 μg/ml (7). To obtain comparable blood levels in mice, we found it necessary to give 75 to 150 mg/kg. These dosages gave peak blood levels of 3 and 11 μg/ml and protected 69 and 74% of the mice, respectively. Increasing the dosage to 300 mg/kg yielded peak blood levels of 32 μg/ml and protected 84% of the mice. Although the lowest dosage tested, 37.5 mg/kg, gave a peak blood level of only 0.44 μg/ml, it protected 45% of the mice. This result is not surprising since the MIC for the test organism was only 0.015 μg/ml.

Chloramphenicol. Intraperitoneal injections of 75, 150, or 300 mg of chloramphenicol per kg were given as described for clindamycin. The 150-mg/kg dosage gave peak blood levels of 25 μg/ml, which were comparable to blood levels of 22 μg/ml usually achieved in humans (6). The test organism had an MIC of 4 μg/ml. This dosage protected 43% of the mice that were examined on the 7th day after bacterial injection. By the 10th day, however, the number of mice protected had dropped to 23%. Similar results showing an increase in the number of visible abscesses after cessation of therapy were also observed with dosages of 75 and 300 mg/kg (Table 3).

Penicillin. High dosages of penicillin have been reported by some workers to be effective against *B. fragilis* infections (E. J. Benner, Prog. Abstr. Intersci. Conf. Antimicrob. Agents Chemother, 17th, San Francisco, Calif., Abstr. 396, 1974). We tested the efficacy of very high dosages of penicillin by injecting 500 and 1,000 mg/kg i.p. every 8 h for 5 days. These doses corresponded to 797,500 and 1,595,000 U/kg. The MIC for the test organism was 32 μg/ml. At 500 mg/kg, 84 to 86% of the mice developed abscesses (Table 3), which was not significantly

TABLE 1. *Susceptibilities of various strains of C. perfringens and B. fragilis (VPI 9032) to diverse antimicrobial drugs*

Organism and strain	MIC (μg/ml)				
	Clindamycin	Chloramphenicol	Cephalothin	Tetracycline	Penicillin G
C. perfringens					
ATCC 13124	0.015				
SAL 249[a]		4–8			
VPI 8050A			0.25		
SAL 19				0.125–0.25	0.125
B. fragilis VPI 9032	0.015	4	64	0.5	32

[a] SAL strains were obtained from F. Tally, Tufts Medical Center, Boston, Mass.

TABLE 2. *Concentrations of various antimicrobial agents in whole blood of normal mice after administration of doses used in treating infected mice*

Drug administered	Route	Concn (mg/kg)	μg of drug/ml of whole blood ± SD[b]						
			0.5[c]	1	2	3	4.5	6	8
Clindamycin	i.p.	37.5	0.44 ± 0.17	0.40 ± 0.16	0.16 ± 0.08	0.13 ± 0.1	<0.1	<0.1	<0.1
		75.0	2.9 ± 1.1	0.8 ± 0.2	0.2 ± 0.07	0.1 ± 0.03	<0.1	0.15 ± 0.02	<0.1
		150.0	11.0 ± 7.0	3.0 ± 0.5	0.6 ± 0.03	0.5 ± 0.3	<0.1	0.16 ± 0.1	<0.1
		300.0	32.0 ± 6.0	11.0 ± 3.0	2.9 ± 0.9	2.7 ± 1.0	2.0 ± 1.0	0.5 ± 0.4	0.3 ± 0.3
Chloramphenicol	i.p.	75.0	12 ± 6	9 ± 6	4 ± 2	3 ± 1	ND[d]	ND	ND
		150.0	25 ± 8	18 ± 8	14 ± 12	5 ± 3	<3	ND	ND
		300.0	48 ± 34	34 ± 24	15 ± 11	7 ± 4	<3	<3	<3
Penicillin G	i.p.	500.0	114 ± 40	44 ± 18	1.3 ± 0.25	0.3 ± 0.09	0.2 ± 0.05	0.4 ± 0.2	ND
		1,000.0	228 ± 64	543 ± 104	10 ± 4	0.5 ± 0.1	0.3 ± 0.1	0.3 ± 0.2	0.6 ± 0.8
Cephalothin	i.p.	1,000.0	170 ± 73	70 ± 42	18 ± 16	6 ± 4	4 ± 3	<3	ND
Tetracycline	i.p.	62.5	34 ± 28	35 ± 26	9 ± 9	6 ± 5	1.3 ± 0.9	0.7 ± 0.5	0.5 ± 0.2
		125.0	90 ± 41	92 ± 20	41 ± 13	55 ± 20	28 ± 11	28 ± 13	43 ± 26
	o.p.	125.0	1.6 ± 1.1	1.8 ± 0.6	0.9 ± 0.7	0.5 ± 0.3	<0.2	ND	ND
		250.0	2.1 ± 0.6	2.3 ± 1.1	1.0 ± 0.5	0.7 ± 0.3	0.3 ± 0.05	<0.2	1.2 ± 0.9
		500.0	3.3 ± 1.7	6.6 ± 0.8	4.1 ± 2.3	3.3 ± 2.2	1.0 ± 0.5	1.2 ± 0.9	0.3 ± 0.07

[a] i.p., Intraperitoneal; o.p., oral gavage.
[b] SD, Standard deviation.
[c] Time in hours after drug administration.
[d] ND, None detected.

TABLE 3. *Correlation of protection achieved by administration of various antimicrobial agents with peak concentrations of the agents in whole blood*

	Route[a]	Concn (mg/kg)	Percent of mice protected		μg of drug/ml of whole blood ± SD[b] (peak blood level)
			Day 7	Day 10	
Clindamycin	i.p.	37.5	45	45	0.4 ± 0.2
		75.0	69	69	3.0 ± 1.0
		150.0	74	74	11.0 ± 7.0
		300.0	84	84	32.0 ± 6.0
Chloramphenicol	i.p.	75.0	33	17	12.0 ± 6.0
		150.0	43	23	25.0 ± 8.0
		300.0	51	36	48.0 ± 34.0
Penicillin G	i.p.	500.0	14	16	114.0 ± 40.0
		1,000.0	37	18	543.0 ± 104.0
Cephalothin	i.p.	1,000.0	26	24	170.0 ± 73.0
Tetracycline	i.p.	62.5	45	45	34.0 ± 28.0
	o.p.	125.0	55	55	1.8 ± 0.6
	o.p.	250.0	64	64	2.3 ± 1.1
	o.p.	500.0	77	77	6.6 ± 0.8

[a, b] See Table 2.

different from an 88% incidence of infection in the respective control group. The 1,000-mg/kg dosage conferred limited protection through the 7th day after bacterial injection; however, by the 10th day, 82% of these mice had developed abscesses (Table 3); this finding also was not significantly different from that in the control group.

Cephalothin. Cephalothin had an MIC of 64 μg/ml for the test organism and was tested in vivo at a very high dosage of 1,000 mg/kg i.p. every 8 h for 5 days. This antibiotic conferred only limited protection, protecting approximately one-fourth of the mice from infection (Table 3). This protection, unlike that of penicillin G, remained consistent, without the increase in the incidence of abscesses that occurred from the 7th to the 10th day with penicillin.

Tetracycline. We attempted to inject this antibiotic i.p. as we had with the previous antibiotics. Because of the toxicity of the larger dosages, however, we also gave the drug by oral gavage. The mice injected i.p. received either 62.5 or 125 mg/kg every 8 h for 5 days, and the mice treated by oral gavage received 125, 250, or 500 mg/kg. As expected, the dosages given i.p. produced much higher blood levels due to greater absorption of the drug (Table 3). The 125-mg/kg i.p. dosage killed all of the mice by the 6th day after bacterial injection. The 62.5-mg/kg i.p. dosage caused the mice some discomfort but did not result in death. These mice recovered rapidly after cessation of drug therapy on the 5th day. This dosage protected 45 to 50% of the mice. Of the oral injections, only the 500-mg/kg dosage produced any notable toxicity. These mice, like those that received 62.5 mg/kg i.p., recovered as soon as treatment was terminated. Even though the blood levels achieved with the oral dosages were much lower than those found with the 62.5-mg/kg i.p. dosage, all three of the antibiotic concentrations given by oral injection conferred a higher degree of protection than did the 62.5-mg/kg i.p. dosage. The degree of protection in the oral treatment groups ranged from 55% for the 125-mg/kg dosage to 77% for the 500-mg/kg dosage.

DISCUSSION

In the series of experiments reported here, clindamycin had the highest efficacy of the antimicrobial agents tested. The efficacy observed may be correlated, in part, with the retention of the antibiotic in the blood in concentrations exceeding the MIC of the test organism. We found that all four dosages of clindamycin tested were sufficient to maintain blood levels well above the MIC for most strains of *B. fragilis* for at least 8 h. Our results showed, however, that the larger dosage protected more mice from infection. This increase in protection cannot be explained entirely by increased blood levels since the lowest dosage (37.5 mg/kg) tested gave blood levels seven to eight times higher than the MIC as late as 8 h after administration of the drug. A twofold increase in the dosage to 75 mg/kg gave a dramatic increase in the number of mice protected. The only significant difference in the blood levels produced by these two dosages, however, occurred within 1 to 2 h after injection of the drug. One possible explanation of this observation is that higher blood levels during the 1st or 2nd hour may influence the quantity of the antibiotic that enters the abscess.

For many years tetracycline was the drug of choice for the treatment of anaerobic bacterial infections. Lately its use has decreased because of an increase in the number of anaerobes found to be resistant to it, in particular clinical isolates of *B. fragilis* (7). The *B. fragilis* strain used in these experiments was susceptible to tetracycline. The dosages of tetracycline sufficient to give peak blood levels equivalent to those usually obtained in humans protected the mice from infection almost as well as did clindamycin. On a weight-to-weight basis, however, higher dosages were required for tetracycline than for clindamycin. This finding resulted from the need to use the oral route of administration for tetracycline and from the limited absorption of this drug from the gastrointestinal tract (9). The differences in the amount of protection conferred by oral dosages of tetracycline correlated with the length of time that blood levels of the antibiotic were kept above the MIC. The highest oral dosage tested, 500 mg/kg, was sufficient to maintain blood levels above the MIC for up to 7 h. The lowest oral dosage, 125 mg/kg, only gave blood levels above or equal to the MIC for 4 h. The failure of the i.p. dosage of 67.5 mg/kg to give protection comparable to that of the oral dosages cannot be explained by failure to maintain adequate blood levels. This dosage gave a peak blood level of 34 μg/ml within the first 30 min and the blood level was still equal to or slightly above the MIC of the drug for the test organism 8 h later. Although toxicity was noted in these animals, it was not grossly different from the toxicity observed in the group that was given 500 mg/kg orally. It is possible that differences existed that were not noted.

Most strains of *B. fragilis* are susceptible to chloramphenicol in vitro. The strain that we used had an MIC of 4 μg/ml, which is in the range found for most strains of *B. fragilis* (15). Treatment with this antibiotic, even at levels that gave peak blood levels approximately double that seen in humans, was not very effective against the infection. This result may have been due to the fact that even the highest dosage that we tested gave blood levels that were just equal to or slightly less than the MIC within 3 to 4 h after administration of the drug. The MIC for most anaerobes is only slightly below achievable blood levels, and the antibiotic level is difficult to maintain above the MIC. In addition, the concentration achieved in the abscess may be less than the blood level. The bacteriostatic nature of this antibiotic also appeared to be reflected in the results with all three concentrations tested. Approximately 15 to 20% of the abscesses were not grossly evident during the treatment period or for up to 2 days after cessation of therapy. Previously undetected abscesses were observed as early as 3 days after termination of therapy and rapidly increased in size, so that no differences existed between the sizes of the abscesses present in the control group and in the treatment groups by the 10th day after the bacterial injection. It appeared that chloramphenicol, although present, was somewhat bacteriostatic for the test organisms; but, once therapy was terminated, the organisms were able to continue normal growth.

Penicillin G and cephalothin are both β-lactam antibiotics to which strains of *B. fragilis* are relatively resistant in vitro. Although both these antibiotics were tested at very high dosages, little efficacy was found with either. This agrees with our earlier finding that mixed infections containing *B. fragilis* could not be treated successfully with penicillin or cephalothin (3, 4). Whether this resistance of *B. fragilis* is due to production of β-lactamase or to the rapid clearance from the blood is not known. Several investigators have reported the presence of β-lactamase in *B. fragilis*; however, the levels of the enzyme detected were very low (1, 8, 10). Both these antibiotics initially gave relatively high peak blood levels; however, by the end of 1 to 2 h, blood levels of each had dropped well below the MICs of penicillin G and cephalothin. Although we initially found a higher incidence of protection with the 1,000-mg/kg dosage of penicillin during the period of therapy, there was no significant difference between the 1,000-mg/kg dosage and the 500-mg/kg dosage of penicillin a few days after termination of therapy. In this instance, it appears that the high dosage of penicillin did have a very limited effect on the infection as long as therapy was maintained.

Although caution must be exercised in the extrapolation of data obtained from experimental animals to humans, the results obtained from these experiments reflected very well the clinical findings with these antibiotics against infections in humans with *B. fragilis*. This model may be useful, therefore, for the evaluation of new antimicrobial agents by providing a means for the rapid and economical determination of their efficacies. The model infection provides a method for the testing of antibiotics against *B. fragilis* that may be more relevant to the clinical use of the drugs than the routine testing of in vitro susceptibility.

ACKNOWLEDGMENTS

This research was supported by a grant from The Upjohn Co.

LITERATURE CITED

1. **Anderson, J. D., and R. B. Sykes.** 1973. Characterization of a β-lactamase obtained from a strain of *Bacteroides fragilis* resistant to β-lactamase antibiotics. J. Med. Microbiol. 6:201–206.
2. **Aranki, A., and R. Freter.** 1972. Use of anaerobic glove boxes for the cultivation of strictly anaerobic bacteria. Am. J. Clin. Nutr. 25:1329–1334.
3. **Hackman, A. S., and T. D. Wilkins.** 1975. Comparison of cefoxitin and cephalothin therapy of a mixed *Bacteroides fragilis* and *Fusobacterium necrophorum* infection in mice. Antimicrob. Agents Chemother. 8:224–225.
4. **Hackman, A. S., and T. D. Wilkins.** 1975. In vivo protection of *Fusobacterium necrophorum* from penicillin by *Bacteroides fragilis*. Antimicrob. Agents Chemother. 7:698–703.
5. **Holdeman, L. V., and W. E. C. Moore (ed.).** 1975. Anaerobe laboratory manual, 3rd ed. Virginia Polytechnic Institute and State University, Blacksburg.
6. **Kucers, A., and N. McK. Bennett (ed.).** 1975. The use of antibiotics, p. 244–270, 284–302. Wm. Heinemann Medical Books Ltd., London.
7. **Martin, W. L., M. Gardner, and J. A. Washington.** 1972. *In vitro* antimicrobial susceptibility of anaerobic bacteria isolated from clinical specimens. Antimicrob. Agents Chemother. 1:148–158.
8. **Olsson, B., C-E. Nord, and T. Wadström.** 1976. Formation of β-lactamase in *Bacteroides fragilis*: cell-bound and extracellular activity. Antimicrob. Agents Chemother. 9:727–735.
9. **Pindell, M. H., K. M. Cull, K. M. Doran, and H. L. Dickison.** 1959. Absorption and excretion studies on tetracycline. J. Pharmacol. Exp. Ther. 125:287–294.
10. **Pinkus, G., G. Veto, and A. I. Braude.** 1968. *Bacteriodes* penicillinase. J. Bacteriol. 96:1437–1438.
11. **Sabath, L. D., and I. Toftegaard.** 1974. Rapid microassays for clindamycin and gentamicin when present together and the effect of pH and of each on the antibacterial activity of the other. Antimicrob. Agents Chemother. 6:54–59.
12. **Walker, C. B., and T. D. Wilkins.** 1976. The use of semisolid agar for initiation of pure *Bacteroides fragilis* infection in mice. Infect. Immun. 14:721–725.
13. **Wilkins, T. D., and M. D. Appleman.** 1976. Review of methods for antibiotic susceptibility testing of anaerobic bacteria. Lab. Med. 7:12–15.
14. **Wilkins, T. D., and S. L. Chalgren.** 1976. Medium for use in antibiotic susceptibility testing of anaerobic bacteria. Antimicrob. Agents Chemother. 10:926–928.
15. **Zabransky, R. J., J. A. Johnson, and K. J. Hauser.** 1973. Bacteriostatic and bactericidal activities of various antibiotics against *Bacteroides fragilis*. Antimicrob. Agents Chemother. 3:152–156.

ANTIMICROBIAL AGENTS AND CHEMOTHERAPY, Mar. 1977, p. 441-448 Vol. 11, No. 3

Printed in U.S.A.

Pirbenicillin: Comparison with Carbenicillin and BL-P1654, Alone and with Gentamicin, Against *Pseudomonas aeruginosa*

CARLOS E. LOPEZ, HAROLD C. STANDIFORD,* BEVERLY A. TATEM, FRANK M. CALIA, STEPHEN C. SCHIMPFF, MERRILL J. SNYDER, AND RICHARD B. HORNICK

Department of Medicine, Veterans Administration Hospital, University of Maryland School of Medicine, and Baltimore Cancer Research Center, Baltimore, Maryland 21218*

Received for publication 23 June 1976

Minimum inhibitory concentrations (MIC) of pirbenicillin against 135 clinical isolates of *Pseudomonas aeruginosa* were one-fourth of those required for carbenicillin but two times higher than those for BL-P1654. Increasing the inoculum size produced an adverse effect on the bactericidal activity for all three antibiotics. This was more apparent for pirbenicillin than for carbenicillin, but less than the effect on BL-P1654. When concentrations of antibiotics likely to be achieved clinically were used, gentamicin increased the inhibitory and bactericidal effects of all three semisynthetic penicillins for the majority of isolates. Strains highly resistant to the aminoglycoside antibiotic, however, were inhibited no more by the penicillin-gentamicin combinations than by the most effective of the antibiotics alone.

Pirbenicillin, previously known as CP-33,994-2, is a new semisynthetic penicillin with a spectrum of antibacterial activity similar to that of carbenicillin. It is reported to have greater potency against *Pseudomonas aeruginosa*, *Streptococcus faecalis*, and *Haemophilus influenzae* than carbenicillin but is less active against *Proteus* species (3, 22). The present study compares the in vitro activity of this new penicillin with that of carbenicillin and BL-P1654 against *P. aeruginosa*. BL-P1654 is also a penicillin with activity against *P. aeruginosa* (14, 20, 21, 24, 28, 29) and has been found to have good inhibitory but poor bactericidal activity against these organisms. It was included in this study because it has a chemical structure somewhat similar to that of pirbenicillin (Fig. 1).

MATERIALS AND METHODS

One hundred and thirty-five clinical isolates of *P. aeruginosa* were obtained from the Baltimore Veterans Administration Hospital, Baltimore Cancer Research Center (National Cancer Institute), and the University of Maryland Hospital. Some of the organisms were selected because they were resistant to carbenicillin or gentamicin by routine Kirby-Bauer disk susceptibility testing. Cultures were maintained on Trypticase soy agar (BBL, Cockeysville, Md.) at −70°C until studied, passed twice in Trypticase soy broth prior to testing to produce a luxuriant growth, and plated onto blood agar to insure purity. All comparative studies were performed in parallel in Trypticase soy broth at a pH of approximately 7.3.

The antibiotics, in concentrations of 25,000 μg/ml for pirbenicillin and carbenicillin and 1,000 μg/ml for BL-P1654 and gentamicin, were freshly prepared once a week in Trypticase soy broth and frozen until used. Pirbenicillin and carbenicillin were kindly furnished by Pfizer Laboratories; BL-P1654 and gentamicin were from Bristol Laboratories and the Schering Corp., respectively.

Antibiotic susceptibility studies. The minimum inhibitory concentrations (MIC) of the three penicillins alone and in combination with gentamicin were determined by a microtiter modification of the checkerboard technique, as previously described by this laboratory (12). Utilizing this method, minimum inhibitory concentrations were obtained using twofold dilutions of each penicillin alone, twofold dilutions of gentamicin alone, and each penicillin in combination with gentamicin at every dilution. The inoculum was 0.1 ml of a 10^{-3} dilution of an overnight culture added to 0.1 ml of broth containing the antibiotics. The MIC was the lowest concentration that prevented grossly detectable growth after 18 h of incubation at 37°C. Previous studies have indicated that the MIC obtained by this method is almost identicial to that obtained by the conventional macrotube technique (12).

Minimum bactericidal concentrations (MBC) were determined for 58 carbenicillin-susceptible strains. These strains were selected at random from a pool of strains with an MIC of carbenicillin of less than, or equal to, 100 μg/ml. Because of the difficulty in subculturing from microtiter wells, the bactericidal studies were determined by the conventional macrotube technique, using an inoculum of 0.5 ml of a 10^{-3} dilution of an overnight culture, added to the same volume of broth containing twofold dilutions of the antibiotics. After 18 h of incuba-

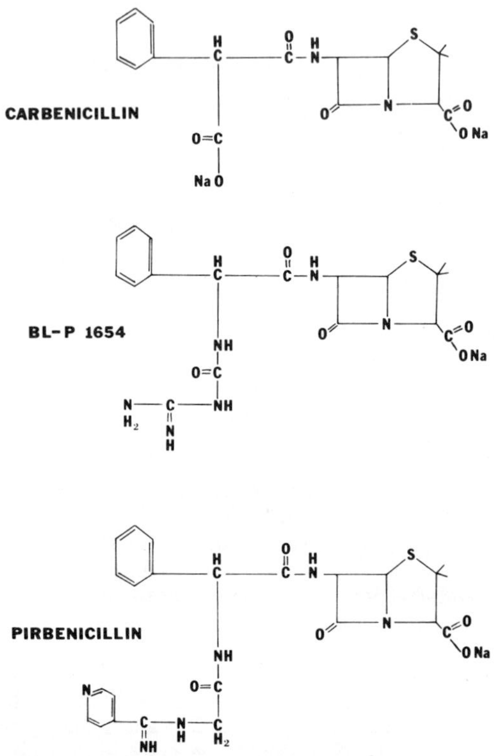

FIG. 1. *Chemical structure of pirbenicillin, carbenicillin, and BL-P1654.*

tion, the inhibitory end points were determined, and the tubes without visible growth were subcultured onto blood agar plates with a 0.01-ml calibrated loop. The MBC was defined as the lowest concentration that resulted in growth of less than 10 colonies (approximately 99.9% killing of the inoculum).

The influence of the inoculum size on the inhibitory and bactericidal end points was determined in a similar manner. The inocula were 0.5 ml of 10^{-2}, 10^{-4}, and 10^{-5} dilutions of an overnight culture and 0.5 ml of the standard 10^{-3} dilution.

The bactericidal effect of adding gentamicin to the three penicillins was determined in a total volume of 2 ml, which contained twofold dilutions of a penicillin, a final subbactericidal concentration of 1.2 μg of gentamicin per ml, and 1 ml of the standard inoculum. Subculturing for bactericidal end points was performed as described above from tubes containing the penicillin-gentamicin combination as well as each antibiotic alone.

The rates of killing of seven carbenicillin-susceptible strains of *P. aeruginosa* (chosen at random from strains with MICs of carbenicillin of less than or equal to 100 μg/ml) by 200 μg of the three penicillins per ml were determined in parallel. The MICs of carbenicillin for six of the seven strains tested were 50 μg/ml, and one strain was inhibited by 100 μg/ml. For pirbenicillin, three strains had an MIC of 25 μg/ml and four were inhibited by 12.5 μg/ml. BL-P1654 inhibited three strains at 12.5 μg/ml and four at a concentration of 6.25 μg/ml. The inoculum was 2 ml of a 10^{-2} dilution of an overnight culture in a total volume of 20 ml. Colony counts were obtained by sampling 0.1 ml at 0, 4, 8, and 24 h, diluting appropriately in buffered saline, and subculturing into melted Trypticase soy agar. The number of colonies representing viable bacteria was counted after 18 h of incubation at 37°C. After the broth was filtered to remove the surviving bacteria, the residual antibiotic in the tubes was assayed by a modified agar well diffusion method, previously described (1), using *P. aeruginosa* NTCC 10701 as the assay organism. Residual antibiotic was also measured in control tubes containing antibiotic and broth, but no organisms, which were incubated in an identical fashion.

RESULTS

MICs. The MICs of each of the three penicillins alone for all 135 isolates of *P. aeruginosa* are shown in Fig. 2. The MICs of pirbenicillin were one-fourth the inhibitory concentrations of carbenicillin but two times higher than those of BL-P1654. Approximately 80% of the strains could be inhibited by 12.5 μg of BL-P1654, 25 μg of pirbenicillin, and 100 μg of carbenicillin per ml. The cross-susceptibility between pirbenicillin and carbenicillin is seen in Table 1. Strains susceptible or moderately resistant to carbenicillin (MIC $\leq$ 200 μg/ml) were susceptible to pirbenicillin, all but two being inhibited by 100 μg or less of this antibiotic per ml. However, all but one of the isolates with MICs of carbenicillin of 400 μg/ml or greater were also resistant to 100 μg of pirbenicillin per ml. On the other hand, strains resistant to 100 μg of pirbenicillin per ml were also resistant to this concentration of carbenicillin. Similar results were obtained when comparing the cross-susceptibility of BL-P1654 and carbenicillin (Table 1).

MBCs. The MBCs and MICs of the three penicillins as performed by the conventional tube dilution technique against 58 carbenicillin-susceptible isolates of *P. aeruginosa* are expressed in Fig. 3. The strains studied were selected at random from strains with MICs of carbenicillin of 100 μg/ml or less. In spite of the greater inhibitory activity of both pirbenicillin and BL-P1654 as compared to that of carbenicillin, the concentrations of these two drugs required to achieve killing were higher; 70% of strains required more than 400 μg/ml. Determinations of pH at the time of subculture from all clear tubes ranged from 7.3 to 7.4 for five of the six strains tested, and therefore a pH change of the medium did not accompany the diminished bactericidal effect.

Inoculum effect. The effect of the inoculum on the MIC and MBC for 10 carbenicillin-susceptible strains is seen in Fig. 4 and 5, respec-

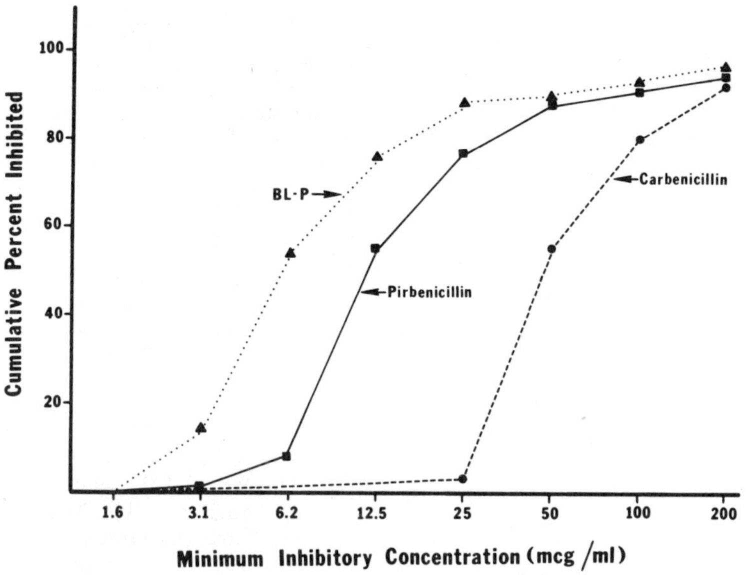

FIG. 2. *MICs of the three semisynthetic penicillins against 135 isolates of P. aeruginosa.*

TABLE 1. *Cross-resistance between carbenicillin, pirbenicillin, and BL-P1654 for 135 isolates of P. aeruginosa*

Carbenicillin MIC	No. of isolates tested	No. of isolates inhibited by: Pirbenicillin MIC (μg/ml) of:					BL-P1654 MIC (μg/ml) of:				
		≤25	50	100	200	≥400	≤25	50	100	200	≥400
≤100	108	100	6	2	0	0	104	2	2	0	0
200	17	4	9	2	2	0	14	1	2	0	0
≥400	10	0	0	1	1	8	0	1	0	3	6

tively. The marked effect of the inoculum on the inhibitory activity of all three antibiotics is apparent. When the inoculum was 10^6 bacteria/ml (our standard inoculum), pirbenicillin and BL-P1654 had greater inhibitory activity than carbenicillin. However, at 10^7 bacteria/ml, the MIC of all three antibiotics was generally greater than 400 μg/ml. The adverse inoculum effect was more apparent for the bactericidal concentrations of the three drugs. With an inoculum of 10^4 bacteria/ml, all three penicillins appeared bactericidal, and both pirbenicillin and BL-P1654 were somewhat superior to carbenicillin. At an inoculum of 10^5 bacteria/ml, a standard inoculum in some laboratories, pirbenicillin was more bactericidal than carbenicillin, but BL-P1654 showed inferior killing against 6 of the 10 isolates. At 10^6 bacteria/ml, pirbenicillin and BL-P1654 were less bactericidal when compared to carbenicillin. The bactericidal activity of pirbenicillin was, therefore, adversely affected more than carbenicillin, but less than BL-P1654, by changes in the inoculum size.

Bactericidal rates. The comparative rates of killing of *P. aeruginosa* by 200 μg of carbenicillin, pirbenicillin, and BL-P1654 per ml were determined in parallel for seven strains. During the first 8 h, the rates of killing of these strains were almost identical for the three antibiotics. By 24 h, however (Table 2), carbenicillin appeared slightly more cidal than the other two penicillins. Colony counts were less than 100 bacteria/ml for all of the strains exposed to carbenicillin but for only four of the seven strains in contact with pirbenicillin. BL-P1654 was the least cidal, with four of the seven strains having greater than 10^4 bacteria/ml at this time.

The percentage of antibiotic deterioration for all three antibiotics during the 24 h of incubation is seen in Table 3. Deterioration was slightly greater when bacteria were present as compared to the antibiotics in broth without bacteria (controls). Twenty percent of the initial concentration of pirbenicillin incubated with the bacteria and 16% of carbenicillin deteriorated over a 24-h period. Fifty-four percent of

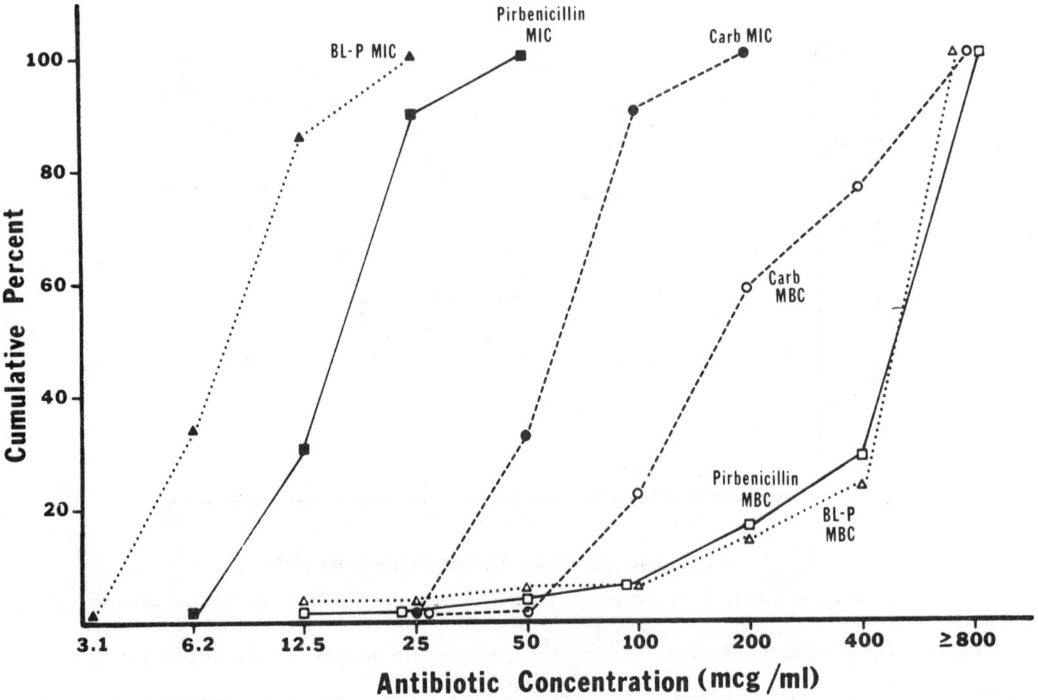

FIG. 3. *Comparative MICs and MBCs of the three penicillins for 58 carbenicillin-susceptible isolates of P. aeruginosa.*

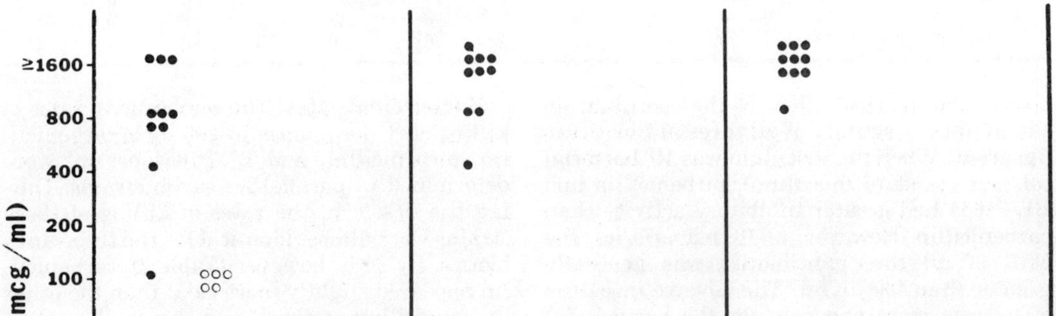

FIG. 4. *Effect of inoculum size (expressed as colony-forming units per milliliter) on the MIC of the three penicillins against 10 isolates of P. aeruginosa.*

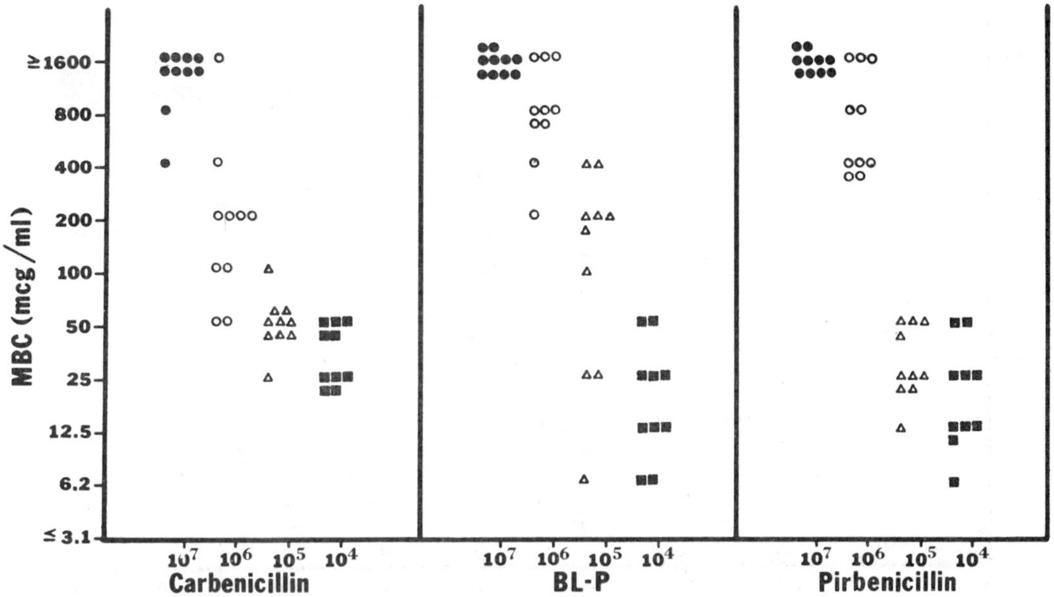

FIG. 5. *Effect of inoculum size (expressed as colony-forming units per milliliter) on the MBC of the three penicillins against 10 isolates of P. aeruginosa.*

TABLE 2. *Comparative killing of seven strains of P. aeruginosa by 200 μg of the three penicillins per ml at 24 h of incubation*

Antibiotic	No. of strains with colony counts per ml at 24 h of:					
	0	1–10	11–100	101–1,000	1,001–10,000	>10,000
Carbenicillin	0	4	3	0	0	0
Pirbenicillin	0	0	4	1	2	0
BL-P1654	0	0	1	2	0	4

TABLE 3. *Comparative percentage of antibiotic deterioration after 24 h of incubation at 37°C with and without (control) bacteria*

Antibiotic	Antibiotic deterioration (%) in 24 h	
	With bacteria[a]	Control[b]
Carbenicillin	16 (10–18)	8
Pirbenicillin	20 (17–24)	12
BL-P1654	54 (52–59)	39

[a] Average (range) for seven determinations.
[b] One determination.

BL-P1654 deteriorated in the same time interval.

Although there was more deterioration of pirbenicillin and BL-P1654 compared to carbenicillin, the ratio of residual antibiotic at 24 h to the MIC for the strains tested was greater for pirbenicillin and BL-P1654. This residual antibiotic-to-MIC ratio was always greater than 6 for pirbenicillin and BL-P1654, whereas it was less than 4 for carbenicillin. It is, therefore, unlikely that antibiotic deterioration alone is responsible for the differences in bactericidal activity among the three antibiotics.

Adding gentamicin to the penicillins. The activity of all three penicillins was enhanced by the addition of gentamicin. This is illustrated in Fig. 6, which compares the inhibitory concentrations of each of the penicillins alone and in combination with a subinhibitory concentration of 0.6 μg of gentamicin per ml. The combination resulted in a greater inhibition (illustrated by a leftward shift of the MIC curves) by each of the penicillins as compared to each of the three drugs alone. In combination with gentamicin, the inhibitory activity of pirbenicillin remained superior to that of carbenicillin but inferior to that of BL-P1654. The addition of gentamicin likewise increased the bactericidal activity of the three penicillins (Fig. 7). The bactericidal effect produced by adding 1.2 μg of gentamicin per ml (not bactericidal for the

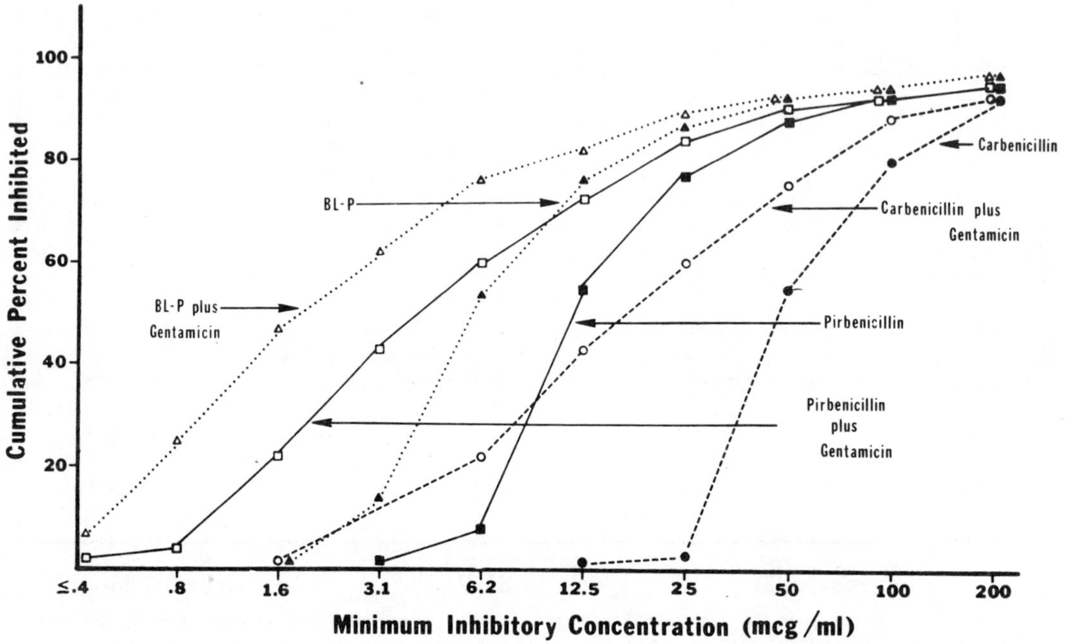

FIG. 6. *Comparison of the MICs of the three penicillins alone and in combination with a subinhibitory concentration of 0.6 μg of gentamicin per ml against 135 isolates of P. aeruginosa.*

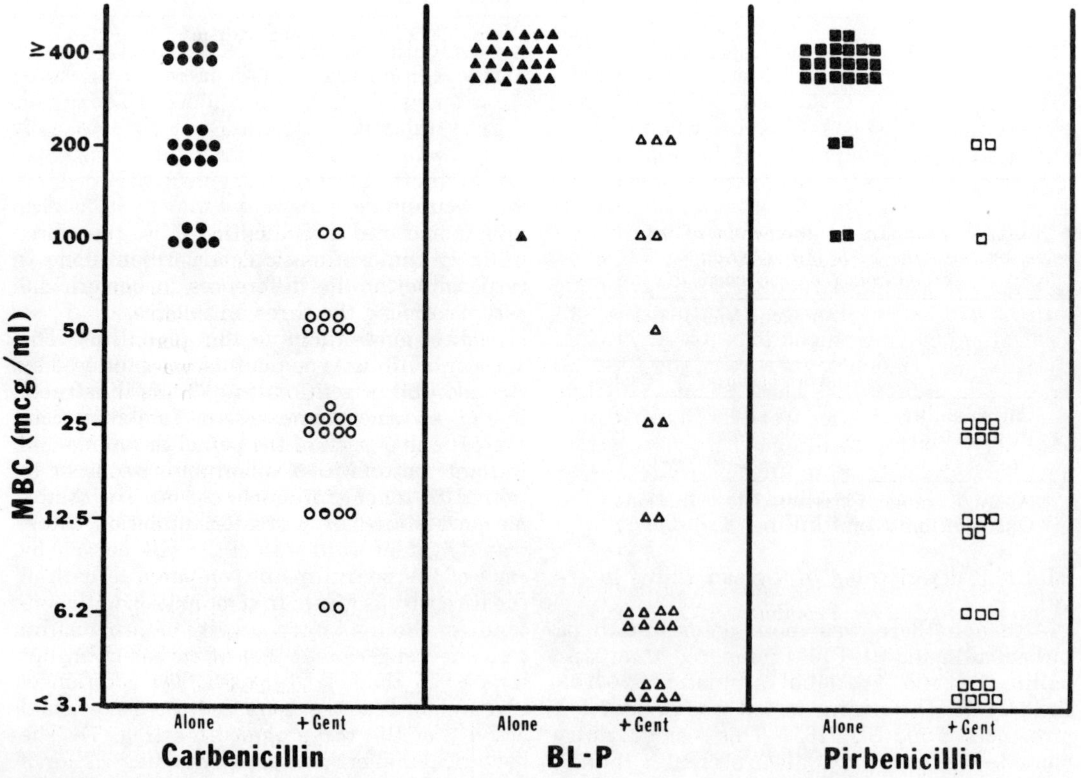

FIG. 7. *Comparison of the MBCs of the three penicillins alone and in combination with a subbactericidal concentration of 1.2 μg of gentamicin per ml against 24 isolates of P. aeruginosa.*

strains when used alone) to both pirbenicillin and BL-P1654 appeared somewhat superior to the effect of carbenicillin in combination with the aminoglycoside.

When concentrations likely to be achieved clinically were evaluated (up to 100 μg of each penicillin per ml and 5 μg of gentamicin per ml), the increased inhibitory effect of the penicillins resulting from adding gentamicin occurred for strains susceptible and/or moderately resistant to the aminoglycoside (Table 4). On the other hand, an increased inhibitory effect by the combination compared to the most effective antibiotic alone seldom occurred if the organism was highly resistant to the aminoglycoside antibiotic (MIC of gentamicin of ≥80 μg/ml) regardless of what penicillin was used in the combination. Only 12.5, 6.3, and 9.4% of these highly resistant strains showed an increased inhibitory effect when carbenicillin, pirbenicillin, and BL-P1654, respectively, were the semisynthetic penicillins in the combination.

DISCUSSION

Carbenicillin is highly effective against *P. aeruginosa* (2, 9, 16, 18, 25–27). Because of the great concentrations of carbenicillin required to inhibit these organisms, an undesirable sodium load with occasional circulatory congestion, frequent hypokalemia (11), occasional abnormalities of coagulation (4, 17), and, rarely, granulocytopenia (23) may be produced. Pirbenicillin, a monosodium salt, inhibits *P. aeruginosa* at concentrations that are generally one-fourth those of carbenicillin. Potentially, it may be clinically effective at lower doses and avoid some of these dose-related toxic effects.

With the standard tube dilution technique using 10^6 bacteria/ml as the inoculum, the concentrations of this compound required for cidal activity were much higher than those necessary for inhibition. The bactericidal end points for all three antibiotics were highly inoculum dependent, with the killing of *Pseudomonas* by pirbenicillin being more affected than that by carbenicillin but less than that by BL-P1654. Similarly, the rate of killing of *P. aeruginosa* by pirbenicillin was less than that by carbenicillin but greater than that by BL-P1654. The reasons for this are not readily apparent. Pirbenicillin is reported to be unstable in an alkaline pH (22). Since the metabolic products of *P. aeruginosa* create an alkaline environment in unbuffered amino acid-containing media, it has been suggested that this pH change causes deterioration of the antibiotic, therefore allowing the organisms to proliferate. Supporting this, Bodey has found marked antibiotic deterioration in unbuffered Mueller-Hinton broth. The regrowth of organisms resulting from this deterioration was prevented by replenishing the antibiotic in the media (3). Similarly, Retsema et al. (22) have found the differences between inhibitory and cidal concentrations to be minimal in buffered brain heart infusion broth. The present study, however, was performed in buffered Trypticase soy broth. Significant pH changes did not occur. Although deterioration of pirbenicillin was greater than the deterioration of carbenicillin, it was not sufficient by itself to explain the discrepancy between the inhibitory and cidal activity. Residual pirbenicillin at 24 h was always at least six times the inhibitory concentration of the organisms. For carbenicillin, the residual antibiotic-to-MIC ratio was less than 4, yet the cidal activity of carbenicillin was greater. Other factors, alone or in addition to antibiotic deterioration, must be responsible for these differences. Perhaps intracellular destruction of the antibiotics by *Pseudomonas* may be greater than that noted in the broth. Such destruction would certainly be inoculum dependent and may be influenced by pH and media differences.

P. aeruginosa are opportunistic invaders in patients with compromised host defenses (5–7, 15, 19, 25, 26). Bactericidal antibiotics appear desirable for the treatment of these infections. Carbenicillin is known to exhibit good in vitro bactericidal activity against *P. aeruginosa* (8, 24, 29) and is of proven efficacy alone and combined with gentamicin in the treatment of *P. aeruginosa* infections in compromised hosts (2, 9, 10, 25, 26). Whether or not pirbenicillin will be more or less bactericidal compared to carben-

TABLE 4. *Relationship of gentamicin susceptibility to the increased inhibitory effect produced by the three penicillin-gentamicin combinations in therapeutic concentrations against 135 strains of P. aeruginosa*

Gentamicin MIC (μg/ml)	No. of strains	No. (%) of strains showing increased inhibition		
		Carbenicillin	Pirbenicillin	BL-P1654
≤5, susceptible	89	89 (100)	89 (100)	89 (100)
10–40, moderately resistant	14	11 (76)	14 (100)	12 (86)
≥80, highly resistant	32	4 (12.5)	2 (6.3)	3 (9.4)

[a] Semisynthetic penicillin in the combination.

icillin in the clinical setting cannot be determined from these studies. However, careful observation is required to define this point if clinical trials are pursued.

Gentamicin clearly enhances the inhibitory and bactericidal ability of pirbenicillin, as it does for the other antipseudomonal penicillins. Theoretically, the aminoglycoside-penicillin combination may reduce the emergence of resistant *P. aeruginosa* during therapy. These features lend support to the use of combined penicillin-aminoglycoside therapy in serious systemic infections caused by *P. aeruginosa* unless the organisms are found to be highly resistant to the aminoglycoside component of the combination (13).

LITERATURE CITED

1. **Bennett, J. V., J. L. Brodie, E. J. Benner, and W. M. Kirby.** 1966. Simplified accurate method for antibiotic assay of clinical specimens. Appl. Microbiol. 14:170–177.
2. **Bodey, G. P., V. Rodriguez, and J. M. Luce.** 1969. Carbenicillin therapy of gram-negative bacilli infections. Am. J. Med. Sci. 257:408–414.
3. **Bodey, G. P., V. Rodriquez, and S. Weaver.** 1976. Pirbenicillin, a new semisynthetic penicillin with broad-spectrum activity. Antimicrob. Agents Chemother. 9:668–674.
4. **Brown, C. H., E. A. Natelson, W. Bradshaw, T. W. Williams, and C. P. Alfrey.** 1974. The hemostatic defect produced by carbenicillin. N. Engl. J. Med. 291:265–270.
5. **Curtin, J. A., R. G. Petersdorf, and I. L. Bennett, Jr.** 1961. Pseudomonas bacteremia: review of ninety-one cases. Ann. Intern. Med. 54:1077–1107.
6. **DuPont, H. L., and W. W. Spink.** 1969. Infections due to gram-negative organisms: an analysis of 860 patients with bacteremia at the University of Minnesota Medical Center 1958–1966. Medicine 48:307–332.
7. **Freid, M. A., and K. L. Vosti.** 1968. The importance of underlying disease in patients with gram-negative bacteremia. Arch. Intern. Med. 121:418–423.
8. **Holmes, K. K., H. Clark, F. Silverblatt, and M. Turck.** 1970. Emergence of resistant in *Pseudomonas* during carbenicillin therapy, p. 391–397. Antimicrob. Agents Chemother. 1969.
9. **Jordan, M. C., H. C. Standiford, and W. M. Kirby.** 1970. Carbenicillin in treatment of severe infections due to Pseudomonas. J. Infect. Dis. 122 (Suppl.):S96–103.
10. **Klastersky, J., R. Cappel, and D. Daneau.** 1973. Therapy with carbenicillin and gentamicin for patients with cancer and severe infections caused by gram-negative rods. Cancer 31:331–336.
11. **Klastersky, J., B. Vanderkelen, D. Daneau, and M. Mathieu.** 1973. Carbenicillin and hypokalemia (letter). Ann. Intern. Med. 78:774–775.
12. **Kluge, R. M., H. C. Standiford, B. Tatem, V. M. Young, W. H. Greene, S. C. Schimpff, F. M. Calia, and R. B. Hornick.** 1974. Comparative activity of tobramycin, amikacin, and gentamicin alone and with carbenicillin against *Pseudomonas aeruginosa*. Antimicrob. Agents Chemother. 6:442–446.
13. **Kluge, R. M., H. C. Standiford, B. Tatem, et al.** 1974. The carbenicillin-gentamicin combination against *Pseudomonas aeruginosa* – correlation of effect with gentamicin sensitivity. Ann. Intern. Med. 81:584–587.
14. **Kurtz, S., K. Holmes, and M. Turk.** 1975. Disparity between inhibitory and killing effects of BL-P1654. Antimicrob. Agents Chemother. 7:215–218.
15. **Levine, A. S., S. C. Schimpff, R. G. Graw, Jr., et al.** 1974. Hematologic malignancies and other marrow failure states: progress in the management of complicating infectious. Semin. Hematol. 11:141–202.
16. **Lyons, R. W., G. F. Thornton, and V. T. Andriole.** 1970. Carbenicillin: clinical and laboratory studies. J. Infect. Dis. 122(Suppl.):S104–113.
17. **McClure, P. D., et al.** 1970. Carbenicillin induced bleeding disorder (letter). Lancet ii:1307–1308.
18. **Marks, M., and T. Eickhoff.** 1970. Carbenicillin: a clinical and laboratory evaluation. Ann. Intern. Med. 73:179–187.
19. **Myerowitz, R. L., A. A. Medeiros, and T. F. O'Brien.** 1971. Recent experience with bacillemia due to gram negative organisms. J. Infect. Dis. 124:239–246.
20. **Overturf, G. D., R. Ressler, and J. Wilkins.** 1974. Comparative in vitro evaluation of BL-P1654 and carbenicillin against *Pseudomonas*. Antimicrob. Agents Chemother. 6:643–646.
21. **Price, K. E., F. Leitner, M. Misiek, R. Chisholm, and T. A. Pursiano.** 1971. BL-P1654, a new broad-spectrum penicillin with marked antipseudomonal activity, p. 17–29. Antimicrob. Agents Chemother. 1970.
22. **Retsema, J. A., A. R. English, and J. E. Lynch.** 1976. Laboratory studies with a new broad-spectrum penicillin, pirbenicillin. Antimicrob. Agents Chemother. 9:975–982.
23. **Reyes, M. P., M. Palutke, and A. M. Lerner.** 1973. Granulocytopenia associated with carbenicillin. Five episodes in two patients. Am. J. Med. 54:413–418.
24. **Sanders, C. C., and W. E. Sanders, Jr.** 1975. BL-P1654: a bacteriostatic penicillin? Antimicrob. Agents Chemother. 7:435–440.
25. **Schimpff, S., W. H. Greene, V. M. Young, and P. H. Wiernick.** 1974. Significance of *Pseudomonas aeruginosa* in the patient with leukemia or lymphoma. J. Infect. Dis. 130(Suppl):S24–31.
26. **Schimpff, S., W. Satterlee, V. M. Young, and A. Serpick.** 1971. Empiric therapy with carbenicillin and gentamicin for febrile patients with cancer and granulocytopenia. N. Engl. J. Med. 284:1061–1065.
27. **Smith, C. B., J. N. Wilfert, P. E. Dans, et al.** 1970. *In vitro* activity of carbenicillin and results of treatment of infections due to pseudomonas with carbenicillin singly and in combination with gentamicin. J. Infect. Dis. 122(Suppl):S14–25.
28. **Van Scoy, R. E., E. Warren, and J. A. Washington II.** 1971. In vitro antimicrobial activity of a new semisynthetic penicillin, BL-P1654 (6-[*R*-α-(guanylureido)phenylacetamido]-penicillanic acid), p. 12–16. Antimicrob. Agents Chemother. 1970.
29. **Wald, E. R., H. C. Standiford, B. A. Tatem, F. M. Calia, and R. B. Hornick.** 1975. BL-P1654, ticarcillin, and carbenicillin: in vitro comparison alone and in combination with gentamicin against *Pseudomonas aeruginosa*. Antimicrob. Agents Chemother. 7:336–340.

ANTIMICROBIAL AGENTS AND CHEMOTHERAPY, Mar. 1977, p. 449-450
Vol. 11, No. 3
Printed in U.S.A.

Resistance Plasmid Transfer by *Serratia marcescens* in Urine

DENNIS R. SCHABERG,* ANITA K. HIGHSMITH, AND INA K. WACHSMUTH

Bacterial Diseases Division, Bureau of Epidemiology, Center for Disease Control, Atlanta, Georgia 30333

Received for publication 8 November 1976

Resistance plasmids were transferred in urine from a multi-drug-resistant *Serratia marcescens* to *Escherichia coli*. Transfer of resistance to kanamycin, tetracycline, chloramphenicol, streptomycin, ampicillin, and carbenicillin occurred readily after 4 h of incubation at room temperature (25°C). The urinary catheter collection bag is postulated as a potential site for extraintestinal resistance plasmid transfer in the *Enterobacteriaceae*, especially for pathogens such as *Serratia*, which do not frequently colonize the intestinal tract.

Serratia marcescens is predominately a nosocomial pathogen and frequently has a high level of antimicrobial resistance (2). *Serratia* often derives resistance to antimicrobial agents from resistance (R) plasmids (5). An unusually resistant strain was the cause of a large outbreak of nosocomial infections in Nashville, Tenn., and most of the resistance of that strain was plasmid mediated (6). Although it could have been a naturally occurring strain that was subsequently introduced into the hospital, another explanation is that a partially resistant *Serratia* strain acquired one or more R-plasmids in the hospital, which then mediated the majority of the strain's drug resistance.

The postulated site for R-plasmid transfer between most gram-negative bacilli is the gastrointestinal tract. For *S. marcescens* this is less likely, since intestinal colonization with this organism is rarely demonstrated (4). In the Nashville investigation, we did not detect gastrointestinal colonization with *Serratia* in any instance despite the use of selective media (6).

The lack of intestinal colonization suggested the possibility that extraintestinal R-plasmid transfer might have been involved in contributing to the resistance of this strain. Numerous extraintestinal sites for transfer were possible, but because of the marked predilection of this strain for the urinary tract, we investigated the possibility that urine of catheterized patients might be a site for R-plasmid transfer among gram-negative bacteria.

MATERIALS AND METHODS

All *Serratia* isolates from patients with urinary tract infections in the Nashville outbreak were serotype O1:H7 and phage type 186 (6). The antibiotic resistance patterns of all isolates were determined by a standardized disk technique (1). Levels of resistance to antimicrobial agents were determined by a standard twofold dilution method using Mueller-Hinton broth (BBL).

R-plasmid transfer was determined by a modification of the method of Schroeder et al. (7), using ATCC 26772 *Escherichia coli* K-12, F^- (Lac^+ Nal) as the recipient strain. Donor strains were *S. marcescens* N35 and N61, which were multiply resistant but susceptible to nalidixic acid. A control strain, *S. marcescens* N10, which was multiply resistant including nalidixic acid, was plated simultaneously on all plates to insure that each plate would support growth of transconjugants.

A single colony each of R-donor *Serratia* and recipient *E. coli* were inoculated into 5 ml of sterile urine obtained from catheterized patients and incubated at room temperature (25°C) overnight. Mating cultures were prepared by adding 0.5 ml of the donor and 0.5 ml of the recipient overnight urine growth to 4 ml of sterile urine. After mixing, the cultures were incubated at room temperature. At 0, 4, 8, 12, and 24 h of incubation, 0.1 ml of the mixture and appropriate controls was spread on MacConkey agar containing nalidixic acid (25 μg/ml) and either tetracycline (8 μg/ml), streptomycin (25 μg/ml), gentamicin (15 μg/ml), or ampicillin (10 μg/ml), which was used for counterselection of transconjugants. After overnight incubation at 37°C, potential transconjugant colonies that grew on the selective plates were picked for biochemical identification and antimicrobial susceptibility testing.

RESULTS

R-plasmid transfer in urine was readily demonstrated between *S. marcescens* and *E. coli*. Transfer frequency was 2.6×10^{-6} per donor cell at 4 h of incubation and 1.6×10^{-5} per donor cell at 8 h. The pattern of resistance transferred was similar regardless of selecting drug (Table 1). Resistance to gentamicin, tobramycin, and colistin was not transferred to any of the transconjugants. A consistant observation in all experiments was a reduction in zone size around the 30-μg cephalothin disk from 22 to 24 mm in

TABLE 1. *Minimum inhibitory concentration of antibiotics for recipient, donor, and transconjugants mated in urine*

Antibiotic	Recipient, *E. coli* K-12 26772	R-donor		Transconjugant	
		S. marcescens N-35	*S. marcescens* N-61	26772/N-35	26772/N-61
Nalidixic acid	500.0	3.9	1.9	500.0	500.0
Kanamycin	3.9	500.0	250.0	500.0	500.0
Tetracycline	0.4	62.5	15.6	62.5	62.5
Gentamicin	0.4	250.0	1.9	3.9	0.9
Chloramphenicol	3.9	125.0	62.5	500.0	250.0
Streptomycin	3.9	250.0	250.0	250.0	125.0
Tobramycin	0.4	15.6	7.8	3.9	3.9
Ampicillin	3.9	>1,000.0	>1,000.0	>1,000.0	>1,000.0
Carbenicillin	3.9	>1,000.0	>1,000.0	>1,000.0	>1,000.0
Cephalothin	15.6	>1,000.0	>1,000.0	62.5	125.0

the recipient *E. coli* to 14 to 16 mm in the transconjugant. The donor *Serratia* gave no zone around cephalothin disks. The minimum inhibitory concentration of cephalothin for *E. coli* K-12 was 15.6 μg/ml. For the transconjugants, minimum inhibitory concentrations were 62.5 and 125 μg/ml, whereas that for the R-donor *Serratia* was >1,000 μg/ml.

DISCUSSION

The problem of drug-resistant nosocomial infections, especially those caused by gram-negative rods, is assuming increased importance. The contribution of plasmid-mediated resistance to the overall spectrum of drug resistance in these pathogens is well known. Extraintestinal R-plasmid transfer might account for a portion of this resistance.

Smith has shown that R-plasmid transfer in the intestinal tract can occur, but that unusual circumstances are necessary (8). Urine, on the other hand, is a good growth medium, and bag urine in catheterized patients is free of even the local antibacterial properties of the urinary bladder. Catheterized patients are frequently acutely ill and frequently receive antimicrobial therapy. This therapy would select for those strains that acquire resistance. In addition, bag urine is emptied at infrequent intervals, usually once at the end of an 8-h shift or "whenever full." We have shown R-plasmid transfer occurring within 4 h at room temperature. Multiple organisms are frequently cultured from urine of catheterized patients. This mixed-culture setting would provide an opportunity within the hospital for exchange of genetic information. Also, urine collection bags are usually not changed and complete emptying is difficult, so residual urine could provide an inoculum that would multiply rapidly to concentrations optimal for R-plasmid transfer.

R-plasmid transfer in urine among *Enterobacteriaceae* can occur. How frequently this occurs in the actual hospital setting requires further study. Like Gardner and Smith (3), we feel that, once established, multi-drug-resistant strains persist because of cross-infection, colonization, and selection by drug therapy and other factors. However, the control measures directed at preventing cross-infection may have an additional benefit. Proper insertion of catheters and care directed at minimizing the introduction of bacteria into the urinary drainage system may have as an added benefit the prevention of the opportunity for a drug-resistant strain to transfer its R-plasmids to other bacteria that might be present simultaneously in the urine.

LITERATURE CITED

1. **Bauer, A. W., W. M. M. Kirby, J. C. Sherris, and M. Turck.** 1966. Antibiotic susceptibility testing by a standardized single disc method. Am. J. Clin. Pathol. 45:493–496.
2. **Cooksey, R. C., E. R. Bannister, and W. E. Farrar.** 1975. Antibiotic resistance patterns of clinical isolates of *Serratia marcescens*. Antimicrob. Agents Chemother. 7:396–399.
3. **Gardner, P., and D. H. Smith.** 1969. Studies on the epidemiology of resistance (R) factors. Ann. Intern. Med. 71:1–9.
4. **Maki, D. G., C. G. Hennekens, C. W. Phillips, W. V. Shaw, and J. V. Bennett.** 1973. Nosocomial urinary tract infection with *Serratia marcescens:* an epidemiologic study. J. Infect. Dis. 128:579–587.
5. **Medeiros, A. A., and T. F. O'Brien.** 1969. Contribution of R factors to the antibiotic resistance of hospital isolates of *Serratia*, p. 30–35. Antimicrob. Agents Chemother. 1968.
6. **Schaberg, D. R., R. H. Alford, R. Anderson, J. J. Farmer, M. A. Melly, and W. Schaffner.** 1976. An outbreak of nosocomial multiply resistant *Serratia marcescens infections:* evidence of interhospital spread. J. Infect. Dis. 134:181–188.
7. **Schroeder, S. A., P. M. Terry, and J. V. Bennett.** 1968. Antibiotic resistance and transfer factor in *Salmonella*. United States, 1967. J. Am. Med. Assoc. 205:903–906.
8. **Smith, H. W.** 1969. Transfer of antibiotic resistance from animal and human strains of *Escherichia coli* to resident *E. coli* in the alimentary tract of man. Lancet i:1174–1176.

ANTIMICROBIAL AGENTS AND CHEMOTHERAPY, Mar. 1977, p. 451-454
Vol. 11, No. 3

Printed in U.S.A.

Comparison of the Actions of 5-Fluorouracil and Ftorafur in *Escherichia coli*

PRISCILLA P. SAUNDERS* AND LIAN-YU CHAO

Department of Developmental Therapeutics, The University of Texas System Cancer Center, M.D. Anderson Hospital and Tumor Institute, Houston, Texas 77030

Received for publication 21 September 1976

The actions of 5-fluorouracil (FU) and Ftorafur (NCS 148958) were compared in *Escherichia coli* B3 to determine if Ftorafur can act in ways other than through the production of FU. Very high concentrations of Ftorafur relative to FU were necessary to achieve a comparable inhibition of cell growth. Inhibition by both agents could be reversed by uracil. An FU-resistant strain and an Ftorafur-resistant strain were isolated and found to be cross-resistant to Ftorafur and FU, respectively.

A derivative of 5-fluorouracil (FU), 1-(2-tetrahydrofuranyl)5-fluorouracil (Ftorafur [NSC 148958]), has been synthesized in the Soviet Union and shown to be an effective antitumor agent. The spectrum of antineoplastic activity of Ftorafur is similar to FU, but it appears to be less myelosuppressive (2). It has been suggested that the cytotoxic activity of Ftorafur in murine L1210 leukemia cells may reflect cleavage of the drug with the subsequent release of FU (5). In this report we describe experiments that were designed to compare the mechanisms of action of FU and Ftorafur in *Escherichia coli* B3. Three types of comparative experiments were carried out: (i) growth inhibition; (ii) reversal of growth inhibition by uracil; and (iii) isolation of drug-resistant strains and determination of cross-resistance.

MATERIALS AND METHODS

Chemicals. Ftorafur was obtained through T. L. Loo from the Drug Research and Development Branch of the National Cancer Institute, Bethesda, Md. All other chemicals were purchased from appropriate commercial sources.

Growth of cells. *E. coli* B3, a thymidine-requiring strain, was grown in a previously described minimal medium (7) that was supplemented with 2 μg of thymidine per ml. Growth curves were routinely carried out in 250-ml nephelometer flasks (19 by 130 mm, with side arms) containing 10 ml of medium and additions as described. Incubation was at 37°C in a New Brunswick G-77 water bath shaker. The media were inoculated with an overnight culture such that the absorption at 420 nm was 0.07 to 0.15. An absorption reading of 0.1 was equal to 4.2×10^7 colony-forming units per ml. Thereafter, absorption readings were taken every 30 min at 420 nm with a Bausch and Lomb Spectronic 20 colorimeter.

Isolation of drug-resistant strains. Two sublines of *E. coli* B3, one capable of full growth in 10 μg of FU per ml of medium and a second exhibiting full growth in 200 μg of Ftorafur per ml, were obtained by serial cultivation of the parent strain in increasing concentrations of the respective drugs. Pure colonies were isolated by streaking onto nutrient agar. The stability of the phenotype was tested by carrying each strain for several transfers in the absence of drug. The susceptibility of each strain to varying concentrations of the agent was then tested as described above.

RESULTS AND DISCUSSION

For simplicity, *E. coli* B3 was chosen for these experiments to assure that thymidylate synthetase would not, in this case, be a primary target. (The organism requires thymidine.) Thus, any observed inhibition by FU would presumably reflect formation of FU ribonucleotides and incorporation into ribonucleic acid. In these forms, FU has been demonstrated to interfere with several cell functions in *E. coli*, including cell wall synthesis (8), ribosome maturation (1), and the fidelity of translation (6).

The growth curves of Fig. 1 and 2 show the comparative inhibitory activities of FU and Ftorafur toward *E. coli* B3. Very low concentrations of FU, 0.05 to 0.2 μg/ml, dramatically inhibited the cultures. Ftorafur, on the other hand, was active only at very high levels (25 to 200 μg/ml). It is possible that this inhibition arose from spontaneous cleavage of Ftorafur, resulting in the formation of FU, especially since very low levels of FU (0.05 μg/ml) can produce significant inhibition. The following experiments were performed to clarify this point.

Since the synthesis of deoxyribonucleic acid should not be affected by FU in this system, the inhibition produced should be reversible by uracil. When a culture of strain B3 was exposed

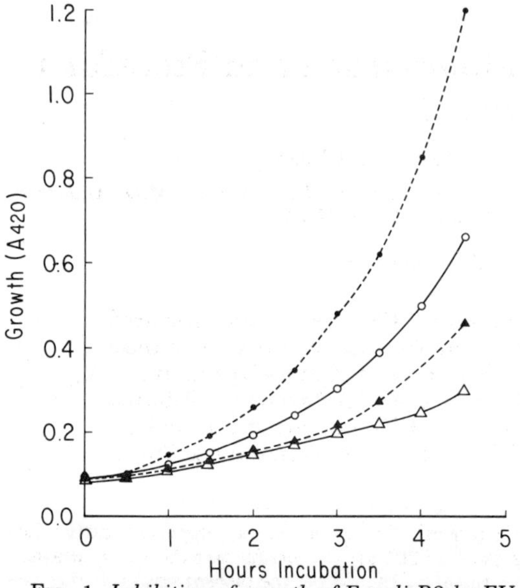

FIG. 1. *Inhibition of growth of E. coli B3 by FU. Cultures were grown as described in minimal medium supplemented with thymidine and varying concentrations of FU. Symbols: ●, control; ○, ▲, and △, 0.05, 0.08, and 0.20 μg of FU per ml in the culture medium, respectively.*

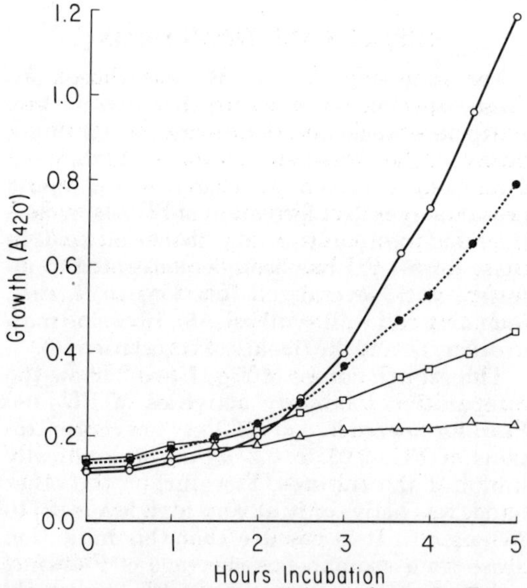

FIG. 2. *Inhibition of growth E. coli B3 by Ftorafur. The experiments were executed as described for Fig. 1. Symbols: ○, control; ●, □, and △, 25, 75, and 200 μg of Ftorafur per ml in the culture medium.*

to a highly inhibitory concentration of FU (10 μg/ml), the presence of 20 μg of uracil per ml almost entirely abolished the effect (Fig. 3A). The fact that a nearly complete reversal occurred suggests that uracil was preferentially used by the cell. In a comparable experiment with Ftorafur (Fig. 3B), uracil again effected a complete reversal of the inhibition, suggesting similarities in the action of the two agents.

If the action of Ftorafur arises from a spontaneous cleavage that produces FU, it should be possible to enhance the inhibitory activity of the compound by preincubation. Figure 4 shows

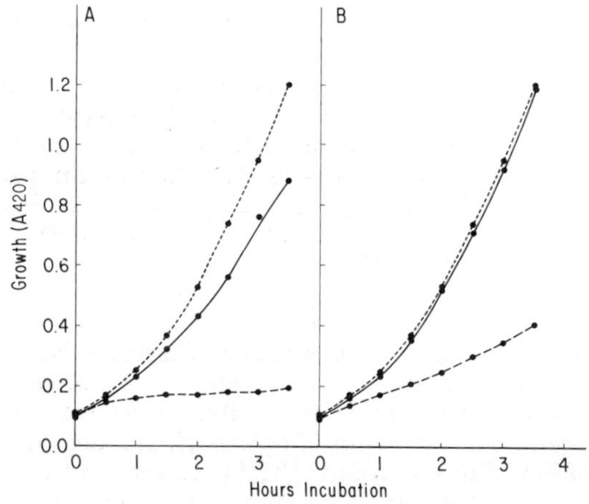

FIG. 3. *Reversal of FU (A) and Ftorafur (B) inhibition of growth by uracil. Cultures were grown as for Fig. 1 with the following additions: ●---●, control (no additions); ● – – ●, 10 μg of ml FU per ml (A) or 100 μg of Ftorafur per ml (B); ●——●, 10 μg of FU per ml plus 20 μg of uracil per ml (A) or 100 μg of Ftorafur per ml plus 20 μg of uracil per ml (B).*

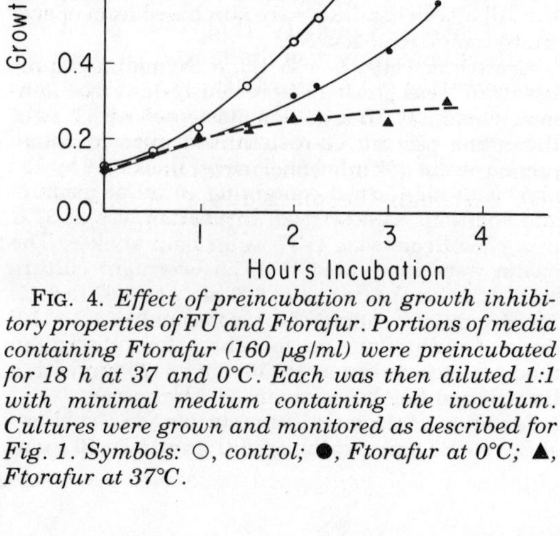

FIG. 4. *Effect of preincubation on growth inhibitory properties of FU and Ftorafur. Portions of media containing Ftorafur (160 μg/ml) were preincubated for 18 h at 37 and 0°C. Each was then diluted 1:1 with minimal medium containing the inoculum. Cultures were grown and monitored as described for Fig. 1. Symbols: ○, control; ●, Ftorafur at 0°C; ▲, Ftorafur at 37°C.*

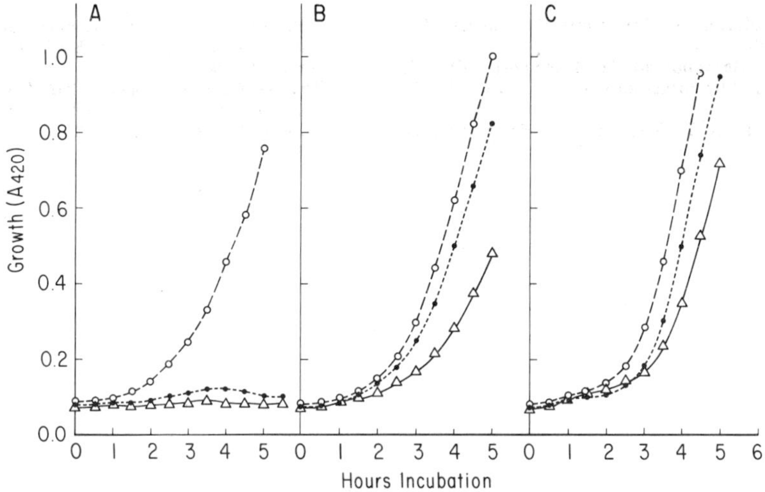

FIG. 5. *Resistance of E. coli B3 (A), an Ft-resistant strain (B), and an FU-resistant strain (C) to FU and Ftorafur. Cultures were grown as for Fig. 1. Symbols: Control cultures (○) contained no drug; FU concentration in each case was 10 μg/ml (△); Ftorafur concentration was 200 μg/ml (●).*

the results of preincubation of Ftorafur in medium without cells. After preincubation for 18 h and subsequent incubation with cells, the inhibitory activity of Ftorafur was greatly enhanced. When a similar experiment was carried out with FU (not shown), there was no change in drug activity. Although this observation has no bearing on other possible modes of action of Ftorafur, it does substantiate the spontaneous cleavage hypothesis.

Another means of detecting similarities or dissimilarities in the mode of action of drugs is to isolate drug-resistant strains and determine the degrees of cross-resistance to potentially related agents. An FU-resistant strain was isolated from *E. coli* B3 as described in Materials and Methods. This strain could grow normally in the presence of at least 10 μg of FU per ml (Fig. 5C), a level which is extremely toxic to the parent strain, *E. coli* B3 (Fig. 5A). When the FU-resistant strain was challenged with a toxic concentration of Ftorafur (200 μg/ml) the strain was found to be equally resistant (Fig. 5C). Likewise, a Ftorafur-resistant strain was cross-resistant to a high concentration of FU (Fig. 5B). Although the mechanisms of the resistance demonstrated by these strains are not known, the observation that they are indeed cross-resistant suggests again that FU and Ftorafur share similar mechanisms of action in *E. coli*.

The comparative experiments described here indicate that Ftorafur acts only as a release form of 5-fluorouracil in this system. All attempts to observe inhibitory activity unattributable to FU have been negative. Repeated attempts were made to detect enzymatic cleavage of Ftorafur, both with crude cell-free preparations of bacteria and purified pyrimidine nucleoside phosphorylase; all were unsuccessful. Since the spontaneous cleavage of Ftorafur to form FU can occur at a very slow rate in solution (unpublished observation), the inhibition observed toward *E. coli* probably reflects the formation of FU in this way.

The antitumor activity and toxicity of Ftorafur in man may be attributable, in part, to the spontaneous cleavage reaction. It is, however, probable that the agent is metabolized in the liver. Definition of the products of this metabolism, their rates of formation, and their cytotoxic activity, if any, will clarify this question.

ACKNOWLEDGMENTS

This work was supported by Public Health Service grants CA 12429 and CA 11520 from the National Cancer Institute.

LITERATURE CITED

1. **Andoh, T., and E. Chargaff.** 1965. Formation and fate of abnormal ribosomes *E. coli* cells treated with 5-fluorouracil. Proc. Natl. Acad. Sci. U.S.A. **58**:1181–1189.
2. **Carter, S. K., and M. Slavik.** 1976. Investigational drugs under study by the United States National Cancer Institute. Cancer Treatment Rev. **3**:43–60.
3. **Fujita, H., K. Ogawa, T. Sawabe, and K. Kimura.** 1972. Metabolism of N_1-(2′-tetrahydrofuryl)-5-fluorouracil (FT-207). Jpn. J. Cancer Clin. **18**:917–922.
4. **Heidelberger, C., N. K. Chaudhuri, P. Danneberg, D. Mooren, L. Griesbach, R. Duchinsky, R. J. Schnitzer, E. Pleven, and T. Scheiner.** 1957. Fluorinated pyrimidines, a new class of tumor-inhibitory compounds. Nature (London) **179**:663–666.
5. **Horwitz, J. P., J. J. McCormick, K. D. Philips, V. M. Maher, J. R. Otto, D. Kessel, and J. Zemlicka.** 1975. In vitro evaluation of the R and S isomers of 1-

(tetrahydrofuran-2-yl)-5-fluorouracil. Cancer Res. 35:1301–1304.
6. **Rosen, B., F. Rothman, and M. G. Weigert.** 1969. Miscoding caused by 5-fluorouracil. J. Mol. Biol. 44:363–375.
7. **Saunders, P. P., R. E. Bass, and G. F. Saunders.** 1968. Properties of 5-fluorouracil-containing ribonucleic acid and ribosomes from *Bacillus subtilis*. J. Bacteriol. 96:525–532.
8. **Tomasz, A., and E. Borek.** 1962. The mechanism of an osmotic instability induced in *E. coli* K-12 by 5-fluorouracil. Biochem. J. 1:543–552.

Antimicrobial Agents and Chemotherapy, Mar. 1977, p. 455–461
Vol. 11, No. 3

Terminal Stages in the Biosynthesis of Tylosin

E. T. SENO,* R. L. PIEPER, and F. M. HUBER

Biochemical Development Division, Eli Lilly and Company, Indianapolis, Indiana 46206

Received for publication 1 November 1976

Tylosin, a macrolide antibiotic, was co-produced with four structurally similar antibiotics in fermentation cultures of *Streptomyces fradiae*. Macrocin, desmycosin, lactenocin, and relomycin were found to be components of a common pathway that functions in tylosin biosynthesis. Data obtained by the addition of the purified ^{14}C-labeled antibiotics to cultures of *S. fradiae* revealed that macrocin and desmycosin were direct precursors of tylosin, whereas lactenocin was an immediate precursor of both macrocin and desmycosin. Incubation of these cultures with [^{14}C]tylosin resulted in an equivalent distribution of radioactive label between relomycin and an unidentified component. The kinetics of incorporation of label into the two species were similar, suggesting that both were derived directly from tylosin. A system that supported that methylation of macrocin to tylosin by cell-free extracts of *S. fradiae* was developed. A proposed scheme defining the terminal stages of tylosin biosynthesis is presented.

Tylosin, a macrolide antibiotic synthesized by *Streptomyces fradiae*, was first described by McGuire et al. in 1961 (10). Subsequently, macrocin, a related antibiotic, was detected in cultures of this organism (5). Relomycin, a similar compound, was reported as a fermentation product of *Streptomyces hygroscopicus* (14), and it has also been observed in cultures of *S. fradiae*. It was further demonstrated that relomycin could be obtained by either microbiological (2) or chemical (14) reduction of tylosin. Other investigations have revealed the occurrence of desmycosin and lactenocin in tylosin-producing fermentations (E. T. Seno, R. L. Pieper, and F. M. Huber, unpublished observations). These antibiotics were originally described by Hamill and co-workers (4, 5) as hydrolysis products of tylosin and macrocin, respectively. The structures of tylosin and these related compounds are presented in Fig. 1 (11). This report describes the terminal stages of tylosin biosynthesis with specific regard to the interactions occurring among tylosin-like compounds.

MATERIALS AND METHODS

Culture conditions. *S. fradiae* was propagated on agar slants containing: cerelose, 1%; phytone, 1%; Meer agar, 2.5%; biotin, 0.0001%; and sodium thiosulfate, 0.1%. Slant cultures were incubated at 28°C for 10 days and then stored at 4°C. Seed cultures were obtained by the addition of a *S. fradiae* spore suspension to 600 ml of liquid medium containing: cerelose, 1.5%; cornsteep liquor, 1.0%; yeast extract, 0.625%; and calcium carbonate, 0.38%. After incubation for 48 h, this culture was used to inoculate Erlenmeyer flasks containing a previously described medium (P. G. Caltrider and H. B. Hayes, U.S. Patent 3,433,711, 1969). A 10.0% (vol/vol) concentration of inoculum was used for this stage. Fermentations were carried out either in flasks (50 ml) with 10 or 15 ml of culture or in flasks (500 ml) with 90 ml of culture. All cultures were incubated at 28°C on a 2-in [ca. 5.08-cm] throw gyratory shaker at 250 rpm.

Quantitative methodology. The concentration of tylosin-like compounds in a filtered fermentation broth was determined as previously described (12). When these substances were present in nonaqueous solvents, their concentration was estimated spectrophotometrically by measuring their absorbance at 290 nm and comparing them to known concentrations of standard materials. The relative amount of each tylosin-like substance in filtered fermentation broth was estimated by quantitative thin-layer chromatography. Microliter samples of broth were spotted on silica gel plates (20 by 20 cm) and developed in a system containing ethyl acetate and diethylamine (95:5). When it was desirable to resolve components having no mobility in this system, a second developing solvent consisting of ethyl acetate, diethylamine, and methanol (79:5:20) was employed. The plates were then analyzed on a Schoeffel thin-layer plate scanner for material absorbing at 283 nm.

Radioactivity determinations. The radioactivity associated with individual tylosin components was estimated by scraping the appropriate zone from chromatography plates into vials. The macrolide compounds were then eluted with 1 ml of methanol, after which a 10-ml quantity of Toluscint was added to each vial. Counting was done in a Nuclear-Chicago liquid scintillation counter. The location of radioactive materials on thin-layer plates was determined by radioautography. All plates were exposed to Kodak BB-54 medical X-ray film for 2 to 4 weeks prior to film development.

Incorporation of radioactive substrates. A 25-μCi

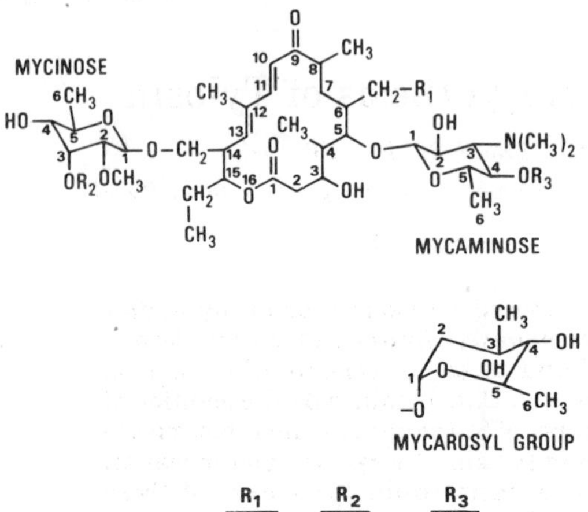

	R_1	R_2	R_3
TYLOSIN	$-CHO$	$-CH_3$	MYCAROSYL
DESMYCOSIN	$-CHO$	$-CH_3$	$-H$
MACROCIN	$-CHO$	$-H$	MYCAROSYL
RELOMYCIN	$-CH_2OH$	$-CH_3$	MYCAROSYL
LACTENOCIN	$-CHO$	$-H$	$-H$

FIG. 1. *Chemical structures of the tylosin fermentation components.*

portion of L-[*methyl*-^{14}C]methionine in sterile aqueous solution was added to 100 ml of culture at the indicated times after inoculation. Samples were mixed with acetone and filtered through Whatman no. 1 filter paper. The filtrates were evaporated to dryness, and the residues were dissolved in a minimal volume of methanol. The total concentration of tylosin and tylosin-like materials and the distribution of radioactive label among the tylosin components were determined as described in the preceding sections.

Preparation of radioactive antibiotics. Labeled tylosin-like antibiotics were prepared by the addition of 12.5 μCi each of D-[U-^{14}C]glucose, L-[*methyl*-^{14}C]methionine, and [2-^{14}C]sodium propionate to each of four 90-ml cultures at 90 h postinoculation. After incubation for 29 h at 25°C on a gyratory shaker, the broth was harvested by the addition of 3 volumes of acetone. The whole broth-acetone mixture was filtered through Whatman no. 42 paper. The filter cake was washed twice with 70% aqueous acetone, and the wash was combined with the filtrate. The acetone was removed in vacuo, the pH of the remaining solution was adjusted to 9.3, and the tylosin was extracted into 3 volumes of chloroform. The extract was evaporated to dryness, and the residue was dissolved in 100 ml of amyl acetate. The labeled macrolide antibiotics were extracted from the amyl acetate into 0.5 M phosphate buffer at pH 4.5. The pH was adjusted to 8.5, and the macrolide components were reextracted into chloroform. The chloroform solution was applied to a silica gel (Merck 7734) column prepared in chloroform and developed with a 1:1 mixture of ethyl acetate-acetone. Tylosin was eluted from the column in the early fractions and was followed by a partially resolved mixture of macrocin and relomycin. The fractions containing the [^{14}C]tylosin were pooled and evaporated to dryness, and the residue was dissolved in methanol.

Fractions containing [^{14}C]macrocin and [^{14}C]relomycin were pooled and dried in vacuo, and the residue was dissolved in a small volume of ethyl acetate. [^{14}C]macrocin was separated from [^{14}C]-relomycin and residual [^{14}C]tylosin by chromatography on a column of activated aluminum oxide (Woelm, activity grade I) prepared in ethyl acetate. The column was developed with an 80:20 mixture of ethyl acetate-ethanol. Fractions containing the [^{14}C]macrocin were pooled and evaporated to dryness, and the residue was dissolved in methanol.

[^{14}C]lactenocin was prepared by mild acid hydrolysis of [^{14}C]macrocin. The labeled macrocin was dissolved in 20 ml of distilled water, and the pH was adjusted to 2.0 with dilute sulfuric acid. Hydrolysis was complete in 19 h at 28°C, yielding a component with the chromatographic mobility of lactenocin. Treatment of the developed thin-layer plate with xanthydrol reagent indicated the presence of free mycarose, thus confirming the hydrolysis reaction. The pH of the hydrolysate was adjusted to 8.5, and the [^{14}C]lactenocin was extracted into chloroform. The chloroform was removed in vacuo, and the residue was dissolved in methanol.

[^{14}C]desmycosin was derived from [^{14}C]tylosin by the same method used in the preparation of [^{14}C]lactenocin from [^{14}C]macrocin.

Incorporation of [^{14}C]tylosin fermentation components. Biosynthetic studies employing labeled materials were carried out in shake flasks (50 ml) with culture volumes of 10 to 15 ml. [^{14}C]desmycosin was added to the cultures as an aqueous solution, whereas all other labeled substances employed in these studies were dissolved in methanol. The quantity of methanol introduced into the culture did not exceed 2.5% by volume. Sample collection and preparation were as described under "Incorporation of radioactive substrates."

Methylation of macrocin to tylosin by cell-free extracts of *S. fradiae*. Cells of *S. fradiae* were obtained from tylosin-producing cultures by centrifugation at 17,000 × *g* for 15 min in a Sorvall RC-2 centrifuge. The cells were washed twice in 0.02 M potassium phosphate buffer (pH 6.5) containing 0.85% NaCl and 0.02% Tween 80. The pellet derived from centrifugation was resuspended in an equal volume of the same buffer, and the cells were broken in a French pressure cell at 20,000 lb/in^2. The soluble fraction was obtained as the supernatant after centrifugation at 12,000 × *g* for 10 min. The cells were maintained at 4°C throughout the preparation of the extract.

The methylation reaction mixture contained in a volume of 200 μl: 100 μg of $MgCl_2 \cdot 6H_2O$; 50 μl of 3.3 mM tris(hydroxymethyl)aminomethane buffer (pH 7.0); 64 μg of macrocin in 20 μl of ethanol; 1.4 μg of *S*-[*methyl*-^{14}C]adenosylmethionine or 2.6 μg of L-[*methyl*-^{14}C]methionine and 17.8 μg of dipotassium adenosine 5′-triphosphate; 110 μl of cell extract. The mixture was incubated at 22°C, and the reaction was stopped by the addition of 1 ml of amyl acetate and 20 μl of 6 N NaOH. Solvent-extractable radioactivity and radioactivity associated with tylosin were determined as previously described. Protein was estimated by the method of Lowry et al. (7).

Radioactive isotopes. All radioactive chemicals employed in this study were purchased from the New England Nuclear Corp.

RESULTS

Course of antibiotic synthesis. The time course of antibiotic synthesis in a liquid culture at 28°C is illustrated in Fig. 2. Tylosin was detectable at approximately 30 h post-inoculation and its concentration increased linearly until 120 h. At this point, the synthetic rate significantly decreased. Macrocin and relomycin were first detected between 70 and 80 h. Relomycin continued to increase through the remainder of the fermentation, whereas macrocin attained peak concentration at 140 h.

Incorporation of L-[*methyl*-^{14}C]methionine into tylosin-related substances. Previous reports have indicated that the methyl groups on the sugar moieties of erythromycin were derived from methionine (1, 8, 13). These findings were later extended to include methylation of mycarose, a sugar present in the tylosin molecule (3). Therefore, it seemed likely that the methyl group of methionine could be incorporated into tylosin and its related factors.

Figure 3 illustrates the pattern of incorporation of radioactive label into tylosin, macrocin, and relomycin when L-[*methyl*-^{14}C]methionine was introduced into the fermentation at 68 h. Macrocin rapidly accumulated the label and was the most highly radioactive component at 15 min. Its activity peaked at 1 h and steadily declined thereafter. Tylosin also exhibited a high initial rate of incorporation, but it continued to accumulate radioactive label until 50 h after the addition of the isotope. The appearance of label in relomycin was initially slow, but its rate of incorporation was enhanced at about the time that tylosin attained its maximal activity.

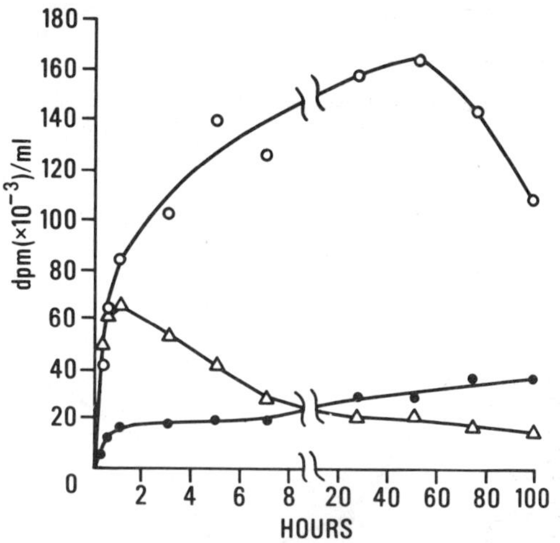

FIG. 3. *Incorporation of radioactive label into tylosin (○), macrocin (△), and relomycin (●) after addition of L-[methyl-^{14}C]methionine.*

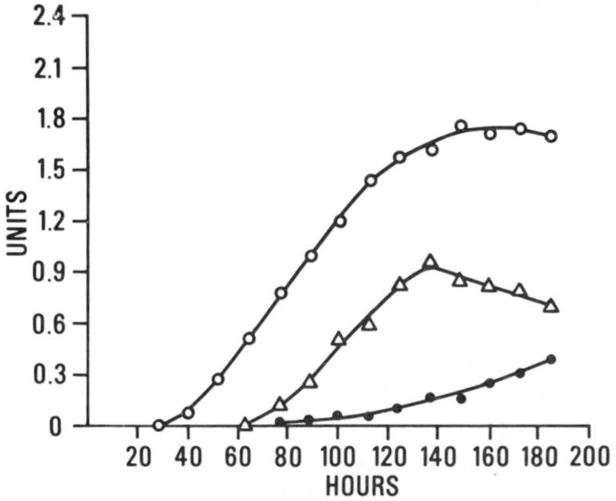

FIG. 2. *Time course of synthesis of tylosin (○), macrocin (△), and relomycin (●) in submerged cultures of S. fradiae.*

Incorporation of [^{14}C]tylosin fermentation components. Desmycosin has been infrequently observed in tylosin fermentation. In those instances where it did occur, it appeared very late in the cycle and in relatively small quantity. Table 1 illustrates the results obtained when [^{14}C]desmycosin was introduced into a tylosin fermentation at 116 h. After incubation at 30°C for 22 h, virtually all of the radioactivity originally present in the [^{14}C]desmycosin was associated with tylosin. The label present in tylosin components other than desmycosin and tylosin remained essentially unchanged over the period of incubation.

Macrocin differs from tylosin in the absence of a methyl group at the 3′-hydroxyl position of the mycinose residue. When [^{14}C]macrocin was introduced into fermentation cultures at 42 h, its radioactivity steadily decreased, with a concomitant increase in labeled tylosin (Fig. 4). After 95 h at 28°C, essentially all of the radioactivity was recovered in tylosin and relomycin, the latter having incorporated about one-fifth of the total label. The total radioactivity in tylosin, macrocin, and relomycin remained virtually constant throughout the period of incubation.

Relomycin is an inevitable component of tylosin fermentation. Early data obtained from the examination of antibiotic concentration changes during the fermentation suggested that relomycin was produced at the expense of

TABLE 1. *Distribution of radioactive label among tylosin fermentation components after addition of [14C]desmycosin*

Time after addition (h)	Radioactivity (dpm/ml)				
	Desmycosin	Tylosin	Macrocin	Relomycin	Total
0	13,721	2,016	2,334	1,292	19,363
22	2,275	14,286	2,687	1,305	20,553

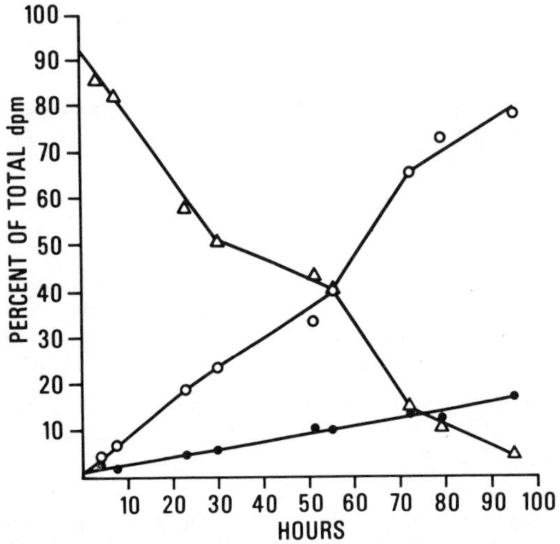

FIG. 4. *Incorporation of radioactive label into tylosin (○) and relomycin (●) after addition of [14C]macrocin (△).*

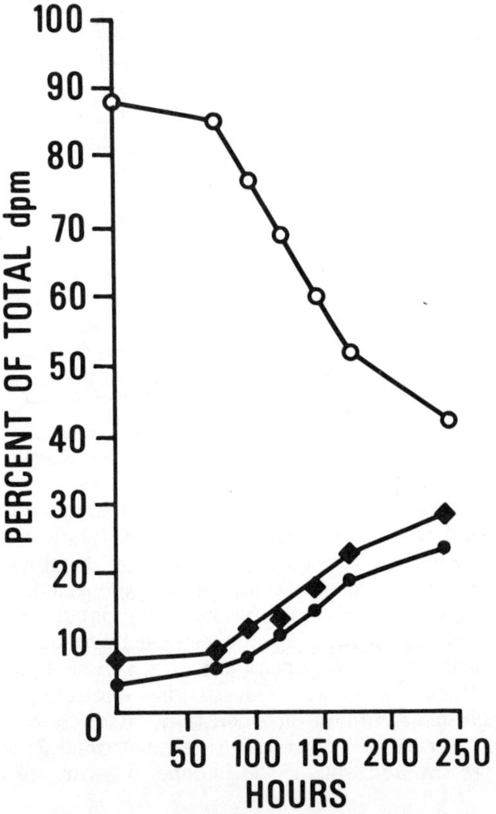

FIG. 5. *Incorporation of radioactive label into relomycin (●) and an unidentified component (◆) after addition of [14C]tylosin (○).*

tylosin. This hypothesis was confirmed by observing the fate of [14C]tylosin in liquid cultures of *S. fradiae*. Labeled tylosin, upon extended incubation at 32°C, lost about 46% of its radioactivity (Fig. 5). Approximately one-half of this label was recovered in relomycin; the other half was associated with material remaining at the origin after thin-layer chromatography. The rates of incorporation of radioactive label into both species were nearly equal.

The tylosin components reported thus far were those that occur with some measurable frequency in the tylosin fermentation. Lactenocin has been detectable only in broths of fermentations carried out at low temperature. When [14C]lactenocin was added at 63 h to a tylosin-producing culture, the initial response was a sharp increase in the concentrations of desmycosin and macrocin (Table 2). Within 24 h after the addition of the labeled lactenocin, the specific radioactivities of desmycosin and macrocin attained peak values, after which the activity in each component rapidly declined (Fig. 6). The label in tylosin continued to increase for an additional 24 h and thereafter remained relatively constant.

Methylation of macrocin in cell-free extracts of *S. fradiae*. To study the conversion of macrocin to tylosin in more detail, a cell-free system that was capable of supporting the methylation of macrocin by *S*-[*methyl*-14C]adenosylmethionine or by L-[*methyl*-14C]methionine and adenosine 5′-triphosphate (Table 3) was developed. The data reveal that the incorporation of the labeled methyl group into tylosin was totally dependent on the presence of macrocin. Similarly, adenosine 5′-triphosphate was required in the system employing L-methionine as the methyl donor.

TABLE 2. *Composition of tylosin fermentation broth after addition of [14C]lactenocin*

Time after addition (h)	% Total concn				
	Tylosin	Desmycosin	Relomycin	Macrocin	Lactenocin
0	36.5	0	0	0	63.5
23	55.6	20.8	0	3.8	19.9
47	53.4	12.1	0.9	12.9	20.7
72	64.1	5.0	1.4	11.9	17.6
96	65.7	6.3	2.4	12.0	13.5
169	62.6	11.0	12.2	10.1	4.2
188	64.5	9.8	18.9	4.3	2.5

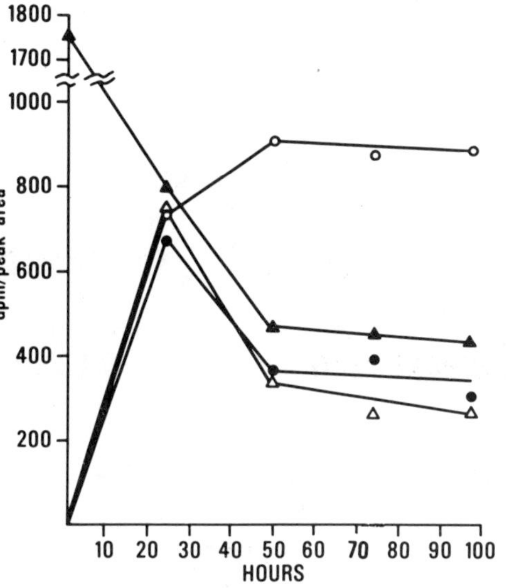

FIG. 6. *Distribution of radioactive label among tylosin fermentation components after addition of [14C]lactenocin. Values represent the ratio of disintegrations per minute to the peak area of each factor as determined from the thin-layer chromatography scan.*

DISCUSSION

This investigation was undertaken to determine whether tylosin and the tylosin-like compounds observed in fermentation cultures of *S. fradiae* were components of a common biosynthetic pathway. Early studies of the effect of temperature on tylosin synthesis had indicated that the concentrations of desmycosin, macrocin, and lactenocin in fermentation broths were enhanced at lower temperatures, whereas the accumulation of relomycin was favored at higher incubation temperatures. These observations suggested that if a common pathway were involved, the former three components were likely to be precursors of tylosin whereas the latter was likely to be an end product of the pathway. The data obtained from studies on the incorporation of label from L-[*methyl*-14C]methionine into several of these factors were consistent with this hypothesis (Fig. 3). The relatively rapid turnover of radioactive label in macrocin suggests that it is a transient intermediate in the pathway. The slower sustained accumulation of radioactivity in tylosin and relomycin indicates that they are more stable species with lower rates of turnover.

That macrocin is a direct precursor to tylosin was demonstrated by the nearly complete transfer of label from [14C]macrocin to tylosin after the introduction of this radioactive component into a fermentation culture of *S. fradiae* (Fig. 4). The relationship between macrocin and tylosin is analogous to that existing between erythromycin C and erythromycin A, the former being a demethyl form of the latter. Erythromycin C has been shown to be a precursor of erythromycin A in fermentation cultures of *Streptomyces erythreus* (9).

[14C]desmycosin was converted to tylosin upon introduction into the fermentation broth at 30°C (Table 1). This reaction, involving the addition of mycarose to the mycaminose residue of desmycosin, occurs readily under these conditions. The conservation of a label characterizing this conversion suggests that desmycosin is a direct precursor to tylosin.

The production of tylosin in cultures of *S. fradiae* is always associated with the later appearance of relomycin. The tendency of relomycin to accumulate upon extended incubation had suggested that this antibiotic was formed from tylosin, a reaction involving reduction of the tylosin aldehyde group to an alcohol function (14). Jensen et al. had reported that tylosin appeared before relomycin in cultures of *S. hygroscopicus* (6). The addition of tylosin to these cultures was observed to enhance production of relomycin. Feldman and his collaborators have demonstrated that several species of *Streptomyces* and one *Nocardia* species were capable of converting tylosin to relomycin (2). [14C]tylosin was converted to two components in fermentations of *S. fradiae*, one of which was clearly relomycin (Fig. 5). The identity of the other component is, as yet, unknown. This substance is considerably more polar than the known tylosin-like antibiotics, as judged by its lack of mobility in the thin-layer chromatography system. The kinetics of incorporation of label from [^{14}C]tylosin into relomycin and the unidentified factor were virtually identical throughout the incubation period (Fig. 5), suggesting a direct, equimolar conversion of tylosin to the two species. It is conceivable that the reduction of the tylosin aldehyde is coupled to a second reaction, perhaps one involving oxidation of the aldehyde to a carboxyl function. The test of this hypothesis awaits the identification of the unknown compound.

Lactenocin was originally described as the product of the hydrolytic cleavage of the mycarose residue of macrocin (5). Since methylation of lactenocin at the 3′-hydroxyl position of mycinose would form desmycosin and the addition of mycarose to the 4′-hydroxyl position of its mycaminose residue would yield macrocin, it was postulated that lactenocin could serve as a common precursor to both of these intermediates. These reactions have been demonstrated in the conversions of macrocin to tylosin and desmycosin to tylosin, respectively. The hypothesis was confirmed by examining the fate of [^{14}C]lactenocin in tylosin-producing cultures. The rapid accumulation of desmycosin after lactenocin addition was especially revealing, since this component is rarely detected in fermentation broths under these conditions (Table 2). The relatively high specific radioactivities of desmycosin and macrocin after addition of the labeled intermediate strongly suggests that they are formed from lactenocin (Fig. 6). Lactenocin, therefore, occupies a pivotal position in the tylosin biosynthetic pathway, since it is methylated to form desmycosin and glycosylated to produce macrocin. The rather large incorporation of label into tylosin reflects the precursor roles that were previously demonstrated for desmycosin and macrocin (Table 1; Fig. 4).

The evidence presented in this report is consistent with the scheme detailed in Fig. 7, which defines the terminal steps in tylosin biosynthesis. Two principal types of reactions occur just prior to tylosin formation: the addition of mycarose to the 4′-hydroxyl position of the mycaminoase residue and the methylation of the 3′-hydroxyl position of the mycinose residue. The sequence of the two reactions in the desmycosin branch of the pathway is the re-

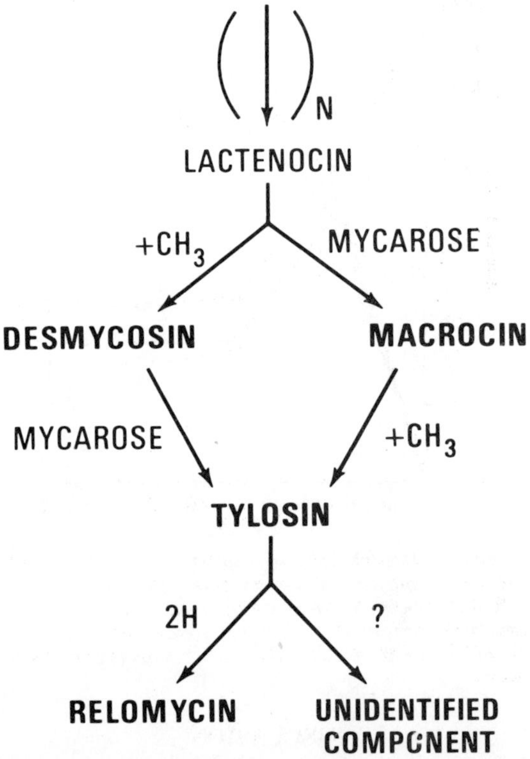

FIG. 7. *Proposed scheme for terminal steps in tylosin biosynthesis.*

TABLE 3. *Methylation of macrocin to tylosin in a cell extract of S. fradiae*[a]

System	Conditions	Dpm/ml in tylosin
S-[*methyl*-^{14}C]adenosylmethionine	Complete	49,960
S-[*methyl*-^{14}C]adenosylmethionine	Complete	50,090
S-[*methyl*-^{14}C]adenysylmethionine	Minus macrocin	350
S-[*methyl*-^{14}C]adenosylmethionine	Minus macrocin	260
L-[*methyl*-^{14}C]methionine-ATP[b]	Complete	5,430
L-[*methyl*-^{14}C]methionine-ATP[b]	Complete	6,850
L-[*methyl*-^{14}C]methionine-ATP[b]	Minus ATP	180
L-[*methyl*-^{14}C]methionine-ATP[b]	Minus ATP	110
L-[*methyl*-^{14}C]methionine-ATP[b]	Minus macrocin	240
L-[*methyl*-^{14}C]methionine-ATP[b]	Minus macrocin	220

[a] The reaction mixture was incubated at 22°C for 2.5 h.
[b] ATP, Adenosine 5′-triphosphate.

verse of that occurring via the macrocin route to tylosin.

The conversions of the radioactive tylosin pathway intermediates to their respective products were found to occur with varying rates and over extended periods of time. This was especially pronounced in the conversion of [^{14}C]tylosin to relomycin and the unidentified species. It is likely that the rate-determining step in these reactions is the uptake of the exogenous precursor. As such, the observed rates of conversion probably reflect the differential rates of uptake of the respective intermediates rather than the rates of the corresponding enzymatic reactions.

ACKNOWLEDGMENTS

We thank C. H. Nash III, G. M. Wild, and P. P. Gray for their helpful consultations.

LITERATURE CITED

1. **Corcoran, J. W.** 1961. Actinomycete antibiotics. II. Participation of the methionine methyl group in the biogenesis of L-cladinose, a branched chain monosaccharide. J. Biol. Chem. **236**:PC27–PC28.
3. **Feldman, L. I., I. K. Dill, C. E. Holmlund, H. A. Whaley, E. L. Patterson, and N. Bohonos.** 1964. Microbiological transformations of macrolide antibiotics, p. 54–57. Antimicrobial Agents Chemotherapy. 1963.
3. **Grisebach, H., H. Achenbach, and W. Hofheinz.** 1961. Biogenesis of macrolides. Origin of the branched methyl groups in cladinose and mycarose. Tetrahedron Lett. **7**:234–237.
4. **Hamill, R. L., M. E. Haney, M. Stamper, and P. F. Wiley.** 1961. Tylosin, a new antibiotic. II. Isolation, properties, and preparation of desmycosin, a microbiologically active degradation product. Antibiot. Chemother. **11**:328–334.
5. **Hamill, R. L., and W. M. Stark.** 1964. Macrocin, a new antibiotic, and lactenocin, an active degradation product. J. Antibiot. **17**:133–139.
6. **Jensen, A. L., M. A. Darken, J. S. Schultz, and A. J. Shay.** 1964. Relomycin: flask and tank fermentation studies, p. 49–53. Antimicrobial Agents Chemotherapy. 1963.
7. **Lowry, O. H., N. J. Rosebrough, A. L. Farr, and R. J. Randall.** 1951. Protein measurement with the Folin phenol reagent. J. Biol. Chem. **193**:265–275.
8. **Majer, J., M. Puža, L. Doležilovà, and Z. Vaněk.** 1961. Methylation stages in the biosynthesis of erythromycin sugars. Chem. Ind., p. 669–670.
9. **Martin, J. R., and A. W. Goldstein.** 1969. Final steps in erythromycin biosynthesis, p. 1112–1116. *In* Proceedings of the Sixth International Congress of Chemotherapy, Vol. 2. University of Tokyo Press, Tokyo.
10. **McGuire, J. M., W. S. Boniece, C. E. Higgens, M. M. Hoehn, W. M. Stark, J. Westhead, and R. N. Wolfe.** 1961. Tylosin, a new antibiotic. I. Microbiological studies. Antibiot. Chemother. **11**:320–327.
11. **Morin, R. B., M. Gorman, R. L. Hamill, and P. V. Demarco.** 1970. The structure of tylosin. Tetrahedron Lett. **54**:4737–4740.
12. **Roudebush, H.** 1965. An automatic extraction procedure for the quantitative determination of the antibiotic, tylosin. Ann. N.Y. Acad. Sci. **130**:582–588.
13. **Vaněk, Z., J. Majer, J. Liebster, K. Veres, and L. Doležilova.** 1959. Studies on the biosynthesis of erythromycin with the aid of ^{14}C labeled substrates, M. Herold and Z. Gabriel (ed.), p. 143–144. *In* Proceedings of the Symposium on Antibiotics (Prague) Státní Zdravotnické Nakladatelství, Prague.
14. **Whaley, H. A., E. L. Patterson, A. C. Dornbush, E. J. Backus, and N. Bohonos.** 1964. Isolation and characterization of relomycin, a new antibiotic, p. 45–48. Antimicrobial Agents Chemotherapy. 1963.

ANTIMICROBIAL AGENTS AND CHEMOTHERAPY, Mar. 1977, p. 462-469 Vol. 11, No. 3

Printed in U.S.A.

Bioavailability of Tetracycline and Doxycycline in Fasted and Nonfasted Subjects

PETER G. WELLING,* PATRICIA A. KOCH, CURTIS C. LAU, AND WILLIAM A. CRAIG

University of Wisconsin Center for Health Sciences, School of Pharmacy and Department of Medicine, and the Veterans Administration Hospital, Madison, Wisconsin 53706*

Received for publication 22 November 1976

The influence of various test meals and fluid volumes on the relative bioavailability of commercial formulations of doxycycline hyclate and tetracycline hydrochloride was studied in healthy human volunteers. Serum levels of tetracycline were uniformly reduced by approximately 50% by all test meals, whereas serum levels of doxycycline were reduced by 20%. The reduction of tetracycline serum levels will likely be of clinical significance. The bioavailability of each drug was almost identical from an oral solution and from capsules in fasted subjects. The rate of doxycycline absorption was reduced when capsules were administered with a small volume of water, but the overall efficiency of absorption of both drugs was essentially independent of co-administered fluid volume. The use of 8-h serum data provides a reliable estimate of drug bioavailability for tetracycline and, to a lesser extent, for doxycycline.

Although the tetracycline antibiotics may be bactericidal to some microorganisms at high concentrations, their activity is primarily bacteriostatic (14). It is therefore important that circulating levels of these compounds be maintained above the minimum inhibitory concentration (MIC) for pathogenic organisms during a course of treatment. In view of this, there has been considerable interest in factors influencing the absorption of tetracyclines after oral doses and the degree to which these factors affect circulating levels of antibiotic.

Inhibition of absorption of the tetracyclines due to chelation by heavy-metal ions is extensively documented (8, 12, 16, 20, 21). Inhibition by antacid preparations is also well established. The latter effect appears to be due to a combined influence of heavy-metal ion chelation and also a decreased dissolution rate of tetracycline (2) or the dosage form in which it is contained (9). Milk and other dairy products inhibit the absorption of tetracyclines to varying degrees. Rosenblatt and associates (22) reported that doxycycline absorption was reduced by about 20% in the presence of skimmed milk, whereas the absorption of demethylchlortetracycline was reduced by about 70%. Mattila and associates (18) reported 50 to 60% reduction in bioavailability of tetracycline, oxytetracycline, and methacycline in the presence of whole milk whereas the absorption of doxycycline was not significantly affected. Interactions influencing the absorption of tetracyclines have recently been reviewed (19).

In view of the above, and also the superior tissue distribution (5, 10) and apparently longer biological half-life of doxycycline (11, 22), this lipid-soluble compound appears to have several advantages over other tetracyclines. From the results obtained with dairy products and also specific heavy metals, it is generally considered that food has less influence on the absorption of doxycycline than that of other tetracyclines. In this study, the influence of solid test meals and fluid volumes on the bioavailability of doxycycline and tetracycline was examined in healthy human volunteers under controlled conditions.

MATERIALS AND METHODS

Subjects were four male and two female healthy volunteers. Male subjects were aged between 21 and 36 years (mean, 26) and weighed between 66 and 98 kg (mean, 77). The two female subjects were aged 19 and 22 years and weighed 55 and 70 kg. All subjects were shown by medical examination to be in good physical condition with normal blood and urine laboratory values. There were no histories of drug allergies.

Protocols. The protocols followed were similar to those described previously (26; P. G. Welling, H. Huang, P. A. Koch, W. A. Craig, and P. O. Madsen, J. Pharm. Sci., in press). Subjects were advised to take no drugs for 1 week preceding the study and no drugs other than the required doses of doxycycline and tetracycline during the study. Subjects were fasted overnight before each treatment and were permitted to eat no food, apart from test meals, until 4 h after dosing. On the morning of a treatment, subjects drank 250 ml of water on arising, at least 1 h before dosing. Drugs were administered at 8 a.m., and blood samples (~4 ml) were taken from a forearm vein into Vacutainers containing no anticoagulant immediately before and at 0.5, 1, 2, 3, 4, 6, 8, 24, and 32 (tetracycline) or 48 (doxycycline) h after dosing. Serum was separated and deep-frozen until assayed. Assays were done within 48 h of sampling.

Treatments. The tetracycline study immediately preceded the doxycycline study. All subjects received all treatments in both studies with one exception. One male subject vomited when taking doxycycline on an empty stomach. This subject was therefore replaced by another of similar age, weight, and height for the three doxycycline fasting treatments. Subjects received single 500-mg doses of tetracycline (hydrochloride) (Achromycin, lot 416-411, Lederle) as two 250-mg capsules or single 200-mg doses of doxycycline (hyclate) (Vibramycin, lot 51408, Pfizer) as two 100-mg capsules. Test meals were prepared and standardized as described previously (26). Each drug was administered as the following treatments: treatment 1, two capsules with 250 ml of water immediately after a standard high-carbohydrate meal; treatment 2, two capsules with 250 ml of water immediately after a standard high-fat meal; treatment 3, two capsules with 250 ml of water immediately after a standard high-protein meal; treatment 4, two capsules with 25 ml of water on an empty stomach; treatment 5, two capsules with 250 ml of water on an empty stomach; and treatment 6, the contents of two capsules dissolved in 250 ml of water taken on an empty stomach.

All subjects received the same treatment at the same time, and at least 2 weeks were allowed between each treatment. Capsules were swallowed whole.

Assay. Serum tetracycline and doxycycline concentrations were determined by the spectrofluorometric method of Kohn (17) as modified by Wilson and associates (27). Assays were carried out using 0.5 ml of serum, and volumes of all solutions and reagents used in the assay were suitably adjusted. Fluorescence was read on a Perkin-Elmer model MPF-4 instrument. The excitation wavelength was maintained at 395 nm, and emission was read at 525 nm. Both excitation and emission slits were set at 10 nm. Fluorescent response was linear over the concentration ranges of 0.1 to 5.0 μg/ml and 0.4 to 7.0 μg/ml for tetracycline and doxycycline, respectively. Standard solutions of both compounds were prepared and measured with each batch of unknowns to allow for slight instrument drift.

Interpretation of results. Individual serum antibiotic levels were fitted to equation 1, which is appropriate to the pharmacokinetic one-compartment open model, as described previously (25, 26; P. G. Welling et al., in press).

$$C = \frac{FD}{V}\left(\frac{k}{k-K}\right)\left(e^{-Kt} - e^{-kt}\right) \qquad (1)$$

In this equation, C is the concentration of drug in serum at any time t after dosing, F is the fraction of the dose D that is ultimately absorbed into the circulation, V is the apparent distribution volume of antibiotic in the body, and k and K are first-order rate constants for drug absorption and elimination, respectively. Fitting of individual data sets to the equation was improved in many cases by incorporating a lag time, t_0, to represent the time elapsed between dosing and appearance of antibiotic in serum. Statistical comparisons were carried out as described previously (25, 26; P. G. Welling et al., in press).

RESULTS

Serum levels. Mean serum concentrations of the two tetracyclines, together with statistical comparisons between treatments, are given in Tables 1 and 2, and the data are summarized in Fig. 1 and 2. Similar serum profiles were obtained from all fasting treatments with both agents. Absorption was delayed slightly when capsules were administered with a small volume of water. This delay, reflected in the absorption rate constant and time of peak height (Tables 3 and 4), was significant ($P < 0.05$) for doxycycline but not for tetracycline.

Serum levels of tetracycline after the high-carbohydrate and high-fat test meals were reduced to about one-half those in fasted subjects. Serum levels were reduced further after the high-protein meal, but differences in serum levels between nonfasting treatments were significant only at 3 and 6 h.

Serum levels of doxycycline were reduced by approximately 20% in nonfasted subjects. Differences between fasting and nonfasting levels were significant during the first 4 h after dosing, but not at later times. Doxycycline serum levels after the high-protein meal appeared to be somewhat lower than other nonfasting levels during the first 4 h after dosing, but the differences were not significant.

Results of the pharmacokinetic analysis are summarized in Tables 3 and 4. The adequacy of the simple one-compartment open model to describe the serum level profiles is indicated by the high coefficients of determination, r^2. Despite the large differences in tetracycline serum levels in fasted and nonfasted subjects, there were no significant differences between treatments in absorption rate constants or times of peak serum levels. With doxycycline, however, significant differences in these parameters were observed in some cases between fasting and nonfasting subjects.

The major differences in the effects of food on both drugs were those associated with overall absorption efficiency. For tetracycline, peak serum levels, areas under serum level curves from the time of dosing until 2, 8, and 32 h and to infinite time, and FD/V values (the fraction of dose absorbed expressed as a concentration in its overall distribution volume) were all significantly greater in fasted than in nonfasted subjects. With doxycycline, however, despite a

TABLE 1. *Tetracycline serum levels (±1 standard deviation)*

Treatment	Serum levels								
	0.5 h	1 h	2 h	3 h	4 h	6 h	8 h	24 h	32 h
1. Carbohydrate	0.1 ± 0.1	0.3 ± 0.1	0.7 ± 0.4	2.2 ± 0.5	2.6 ± 0.8	1.9 ± 0.9	1.2 ± 0.6	0.3 ± 0.2	0 ± 0
2. Fat	0.2 ± 0.2	0.4 ± 0.2	0.9 ± 0.4	2.0 ± 0.2	2.3 ± 0.7	2.5 ± 0.9	1.3 ± 0.5	0.4 ± 0.1	0 ± 0
3. Protein	0.1 ± 0.2	0.3 ± 0.1	0.5 ± 0.4	1.3 ± 0.4	1.8 ± 1.1	1.5 ± 0.7	1.1 ± 0.6	0.3 ± 0.2	0.1 ± 0.1
4. Fasting, low volume	0.7 ± 0.9	2.4 ± 0.6	3.4 ± 0.4	3.9 ± 0.2	4.1 ± 0.2	3.9 ± 0.4	3.4 ± 0.2	0.8 ± 0.3	0.2 ± 0.2
5. Fasting, high volume	0.4 ± 0.3	1.6 ± 0.6	3.4 ± 0.4	4.1 ± 0.5	4.4 ± 0.3	3.6 ± 0.6	2.7 ± 1.1	0.7 ± 0.5	0.3 ± 0.2
6. Fasting, solution	0.6 ± 0.2	2.3 ± 0.9	3.8 ± 0.7	4.3 ± 0.5	4.4 ± 0.6	3.6 ± 0.8	2.8 ± 1.0	0.4 ± 0.2	0.3 ± 0.1
Paired *t* test[a]	5 > 1 6 > 1–3	4–6 > 1–3	4–6 > 1–3	1, 2 > 3 4–6 > 1–3	4–6 > 1–3	2 > 1, 3 4–6 > 1–3	4–6 > 1–3	NSD[b]	NSD

[a] Significant at $P < 0.05$.
[b] NSD, no significant differences.

TABLE 2. *Doxycycline serum levels (±1 standard deviation)*

Treatment	Serum levels								
	0.5 h	1 h	2 h	3 h	4 h	6 h	8 h	24 h	48 h
1. Carbohydrate	0.2 ± 0.3	0.6 ± 0.4	1.2 ± 0.6	3.0 ± 1.3	4.0 ± 1.1	3.7 ± 2.3	3.6 ± 2.5	1.2 ± 0.4	0.7 ± 0.4
2. Fat	0.2 ± 0.2	0.3 ± 0.4	1.3 ± 0.7	2.5 ± 1.1	3.5 ± 1.1	3.6 ± 1.1	3.0 ± 0.9	1.2 ± 0.2	0.4 ± 0.2
3. Protein	0.1 ± 0.2	0.4 ± 0.5	1.0 ± 0.7	1.7 ± 1.2	2.6 ± 1.1	3.8 ± 1.2	3.5 ± 0.9	1.7 ± 0.5	0.6 ± 0.2
4. Fasting, low volume	0.6 ± 0.5	1.7 ± 1.5	3.5 ± 2.2	5.0 ± 1.9	5.4 ± 1.1	4.8 ± 0.9	4.0 ± 0.9	2.2 ± 0.8	0.5 ± 0.3
5. Fasting, high volume	0.8 ± 0.8	2.3 ± 1.6	4.4 ± 1.8	4.9 ± 1.9	4.8 ± 1.9	3.6 ± 1.4	3.0 ± 1.2	1.5 ± 0.5	0.3 ± 0.3
6. Fasting, solution	1.0 ± 0.5	2.5 ± 1.4	5.1 ± 1.5	5.0 ± 1.6	4.7 ± 1.6	3.6 ± 1.2	2.9 ± 1.2	1.3 ± 0.3	0.8 ± 0.2
Paired *t* test[a]	4, 5 > 3 6 > 1–3	4 > 3 5, 6 > 1–3	4–6 > 1–3	4–6 > 1–3	1, 2, > 3 4 > 1–3 5 > 2, 3	NSD[b]	4 > 2, 5, 6	NSD	6 > 2, 5

[a, b] See Table 1.

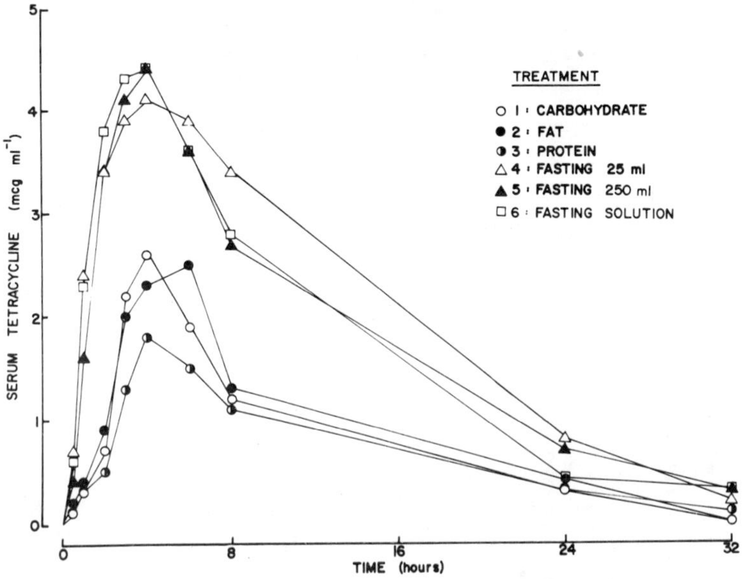

FIG. 1. *Average serum levels of tetracycline.*

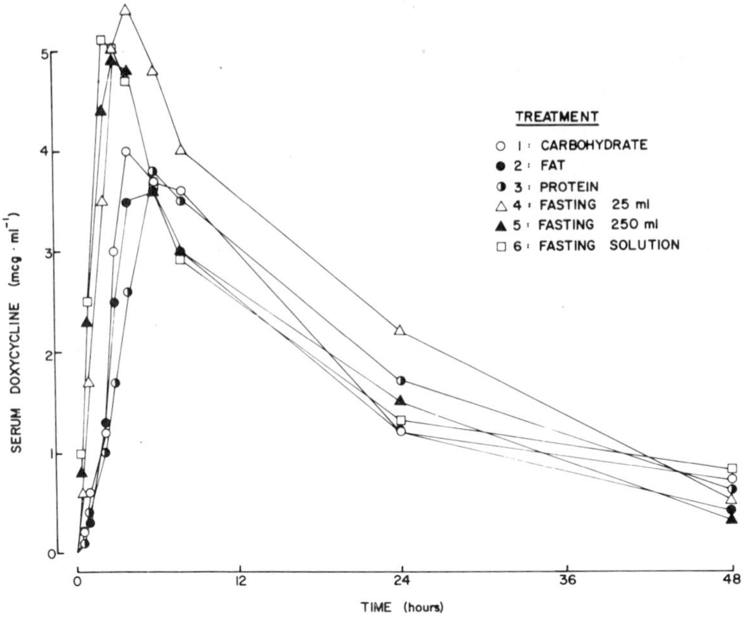

FIG. 2. *Average serum levels of doxycycline.*

tendency for these parameter values to be larger from the fasting treatments, differences in values between fasted and nonfasted treatments frequently failed to reach significant levels.

Serum levels, peak level values, times of peak levels, and serum half-lives in fasted subjects in this study were similar to previously reported values. Serum half-lives of doxycycline were somewhat shorter than those reported by some previous workers (11, 22), but were similar to those recently obtained by Ao and associates in normal individuals (1). The accuracy of some of the reported longer doxycycline half-lives has been questioned by Gibaldi (13).

TABLE 3. *Tetracycline pharmacokinetic parameters (±1 standard deviation)*

Treatment	Parameter												
	k (h^{-1})	$t_{1/2}$(abs) (h)	K (h^{-1})	$t_{1/2}$(elim) (h)	FD/V (μg/ml)	t_0 (h)	Areas (μg/ml × h)				r^{2c}	Peak ht (μg/ml)	Time of peak ht (h)
							0 → 2 h[a]	0 → 8 h[a]	0 → 32 h[a]	0 → ∞[b]			
1	0.47	1.6	0.13	5.6	3.4	0.5	0.7	11.9	24.4	27.0	0.90	2.6	3.8
	±0.16	±0.5	±0.03	±1.6	±1.2	±1.6	±0.2	±3.9	±9.8	±10.7	±0.04	±0.8	±0.4
2	0.49	1.9	0.11	6.2	3.6	0.45	0.9	12.8	28.3	31.7	0.94	2.7	4.7
	±0.33	±0.8	±0.01	±0.7	±1.1	±1.3	±0.3	±2.8	±6.2	±8.5	±0.04	±0.7	±1.5
3	0.50	1.8	0.10	7.2	2.5	0.5	0.5	9.0	23.5	25.5	0.92	2.0	4.5
	±0.76	±1.0	±0.02	±2.0	±1.2	±0.0	±0.4	±3.1	±10.0	±11.8	±0.05	±1.0	±1.2
4	0.52	1.6	0.11	8.1	6.4	0	3.2	27.0	66.5	74.7	0.99	4.1	4.2
	±0.33	±0.9	±0.02	±4.5	±1.3		±0.7	±1.0	±4.9	±18.9	±0.01	±0.2	±1.0
5	0.72	0.97	0.11	6.7	5.8	0.37	3.1	25.4	56.6	55.7	0.98	4.5	3.8
	±0.08	±0.12	±0.03	±1.5	±0.8	±0.7	±0.7	±3.3	±17.8	±12.5	±0.02	±0.3	±0.4
6	0.54	1.3	0.11	6.1	6.3	0	4.1	27.3	56.1	56.6	0.98	4.5	3.7
	±0.07	±0.2	±0.01	±0.6	±0.1		±1.0	±5.2	±14.7	±13.2	±0.01	±0.6	±0.5
Paired t test	NSD[d]	NSD	NSD	NSD	4–6	1–3, 5	4–6	4–6	4–6	4–6	NSD	4–6	NSD
					>1–3	>4, 6	>1–3	>1–3	>1–3	>1–3		>1–3	

[a] Calculated by trapezoidal rule.
[b] Calculated from FD/VK.
[c] $(\Sigma obs_2 - \Sigma dev_2)/\Sigma obs_2$.
NSD, No significant difference.

TABLE 4. *Doxycycline pharmacokinetic parameters (±1 standard deviation)*

Treatment	Parameter												
	k (h^{-1})	$t_{1/2}$ (abs) (h)	K (h^{-1})	$t_{1/2}$ (elim) (h)	FD/V (μg/ml)	t_0 (h)	Areas (μg/ml × h) 0 → 2 h[a]	0 → 8 h[a]	0 → 48[a]	0 → ∞[b]	r^{2c}	Peak ht (μg/ml)	Time of peak ht (h)
1	0.37	2.2	0.065	11.0	6.0	0.33	1.1	21.6	83.9	89.6	0.92	4.9	4.7
	±0.12	±1.0	±0.010	±2.2	±3.6	±0.26	±0.7	±8.9	±40.1	±48.8	±0.02	±2.1	±2.0
2	0.29	2.9	0.070	10.1	5.5	0.33	1.0	20.0	72.1	78.6	0.94	4.0	5.0
	±0.18	±1.2	±0.010	±1.8	±1.3	±0.41	±0.6	±7.0	±14.4	±17.2	±0.07	±1.1	±1.1
3	0.26	3.1	0.054	14.2	5.5	0.58	0.9	20.4	89.4	106.8	0.94	4.0	6.0
	±0.11	±1.3	±0.017	±5.3	±1.6	±0.49	±0.7	±8.7	±8.7	±37.6	±0.05	±0.9	±1.3
4	0.31	2.0	0.082	8.8	7.7	0	5.3	35.2	112.9	108.4	0.97	5.7	4.3
	±0.10	±0.9	±0.029	±2.9	±0.6		±1.3	±6.3	±26.9	±46.6	±0.01	±1.1	±1.4
5	0.78	1.0	0.067	11.0	5.8	0.08	4.4	28.9	87.4	85.3	0.96	5.1	3.2
	±0.35	±0.3	±0.020	±3.2	±2.3	±0.20	±2.1	±10.8	±30.2	±30.6	±0.02	±2.0	±1.0
6	1.03	0.85	0.062	12.6	5.7	0	5.2	31.1	90.3	90.4	0.95	5.2	2.7
	±0.48	±0.41	±0.024	±4.9	±2.5		±1.6	±8.8	±21.1	±16.5	±0.03	±1.5	±0.8
	5	1-3				1, 3							1-4
	>1-3	>5				>4, 6							>6
Paired t test	6	1-4	NSD[d]	NSD	4 >2,	3 > 5	4-6	4-6	4	NSD	NSD	4, 6	2-4
	>1-4	>6			3, 5, 6		>1-3	>1-3	>2, 6			>2, 3	>5
													3
													>4

[a-d] See Table 3.

DISCUSSION

The results obtained in this study show that, although the absorption of orally dosed doxycycline and tetracycline is impaired in the presence of food, the degree of impairment is far greater in the case of tetracycline. The small influence of food on doxycycline absorption is advantageous in view of the gastric irritation that may occur when this drug is taken on an empty stomach. Subjects in this study frequently reported transient nausea within 30 min of taking doxycycline in the fasting treatments, and one subject had to be withdrawn because of this. These symptoms did not occur when doxycycline was taken with food and were not observed at all with tetracycline.

The results also show that, for both drugs, inhibition of absorption is largely independent of the type of meal. It is interesting that the high-protein meal, which contained a higher proportion of heavy-metal ions, tended to produce somewhat lower serum levels of both tetracycline and doxycycline than did the other nonfasting treatments.

In other studies we demonstrated impaired absorption of amoxicillin trihydrate (P. G. Welling et al, in press) and, to a lesser extent, theophylline (25) when these drugs were administered in solid dosage forms with small accompanying water volumes. This may be attributed to their relatively low water solubility. Both doxycycline and tetracycline were administered as water-soluble salts in the present study, and changes in water volumes had only a small influence on their overall serum level profiles.

Several dosing and sampling methods have been used to measure the bioavailability of tetracycline drug products. Brice and Hammer (6) and Blair and associates (4) compared the bioavailability of various oxytetracycline products based on serum or blood level data collected through 6 h after single doses. Davis and associates (7) measured blood and urine tetracycline levels during a 96-h multiple-dosage regimen and concluded that single-dose studies using relatively short sampling periods may be inadequate for accurate bioavailability testing. Barr and associates (3), however, showed that results obtained from single-dose studies, using 10-h serum or 48-h urine sampling periods, accurately predicted tetracycline serum levels during multiple doses of various commercial products.

The present study utilized only single doses, but comparisons of data based on short and long postdosing intervals are instructive. Correlation coefficients between areas under serum level curves and also between 2-h, 8-h and peak serum levels and 0- to 32-h or 0- to 48-h areas are given in Table 5. With tetracycline, good correlations were obtained between all listed parameters, and it appears reasonable to suggest that the use of serum levels or areas under serum level curves measured at short postdosing time intervals provides a reliable estimate of tetracycline bioavailability characteristics. Agreement between the various parameters is not quite as good with doxycycline, but 8-h serum levels and 8-h areas correlate quite well with the 0- to 48-h areas.

Clinical significance. The in vitro MICs of most tetracyclines to susceptible bacteria range from 0.2 to 12.5 μg/ml (15, 23). Organisms with an MIC of 0.5 μg/ml or less are considered highly susceptible, those with an MIC of 0.5 to 2.5 μg/ml are considered moderately susceptible, and those with an MIC of 2.5 to 5 μg/ml are considered slightly susceptible. Doxycycline tends to be more active against many pathogens than tetracycline (22).

Based on our single-dose data, the mean tetracycline serum levels during a multiple-dosage regimen of 250 mg every 6 h would be approximately 4.5 μg/ml if the drug were dosed on an empty stomach (24). If the same regimen were followed but the doses were taken with meals, mean serum levels would drop to 2.4 μg/ml. The nonfasting regimen might thus result in insufficiently high circulating levels of antibiotic for activity against less susceptible organisms.

With doxycycline, the mean serum levels ob-

TABLE 5. *Correlations among areas under serum level curves and also between serum levels and areas from 0 to 48 h (doxycycline) and 32 h (tetracycline)*

Parameter	Correlation coefficient	
	Doxycycline	Tetracycline
Area 0 → 2 h vs. area 0 → 8 h	0.75	0.93
Area 0 → 2 h vs. area 0 → 48 (32) h	0.35	0.89
Area 0 → 8 h vs. area 0 → 48 (32) h	0.77	0.95
Peak serum level vs. area 0 → 48 (32) h	0.87	0.83
2-h serum level vs. area 0 → 48 (32) h	0.46	0.87
8-h serum level vs. area 0 → 48 (32) h	0.88	0.98

tained during a multiple-dosage regimen of 200 mg/day would be approximately 4.4 μg/ml if the drug were dosed on an empty stomach. If the doses were taken with meals this value would drop only slightly, to 4.0 μg/ml. This small reduction in serum levels is unlikely to cause therapeutic failures. Thus the reduction in serum levels due to food observed in this study is likely to be of clinical significance for tetracycline but not for doxycycline.

ACKNOWLEDGMENTS

This investigation was supported by Public Health Service Grant GM 20327 from the National Institute of General Medical Sciences and by a grant from Pfizer, Inc.

LITERATURE CITED

1. **Ao, N. K., O. P. Teneja, V. N. Bhatia, and D. S. Aggarwal.** 1974. Serum concentration and urinary excretion of doxycycline in normal subjects and patients with renal insufficiency. Chemotherapy **20**:129–140.
2. **Barr, W. H., J. Adir, and L. Garrettson.** 1971. Decrease of tetracycline absorption in man by sodium bicarbonate. Clin. Pharmacol. Ther. **12**:779–784.
3. **Barr, W. H., L. M. Gerbracht, K. Letcher, M. Plaut, and N. Strahl.** 1971. Assessment of the biologic availability of tetracycline products in man. Clin. Pharmacol. Ther. **13**:97–108.
4. **Blair, D. C., R. W. Barnes, E. L. Wildner, and W. J. Murray.** 1971. Biological availability of oxytetracycline capsules. J. Am. Med. Assoc. **215**:251–254.
5. **Blanchard, P., M. Rudhardt, and J. Fabre.** 1975. Behaviour of doxycycline in the tissues. Chemotherapy **21**(Suppl. 1):8–18.
6. **Brice, G. W., and H. T. Hammer.** 1969. Therapeutic nonequivalence of oxytetracycline capsules. J. Am. Med. Assoc. **208**:1189–1190.
7. **Davis, C. M., J. V. Vandersarl, and E. W. Kraus.** 1973. Tetracycline inequivalance: the importance of 96-hour testing. Am. J. Med. Sci. **265**:69–74.
8. **Dearborn, E. H., J. T. Litchfield, Jr., H. J. Eisner, J. J. Corbett, and C. W. Dunnett.** 1957. The effects of various substances on the absorption of tetracycline in rats. Antibiot. Med. Clin. Ther. **4**:627–641.
9. **Elliott, G. R., and M. F. Armstrong.** 1972. Sodium bicarbonate and oral tetracycline. Clin. Pharmacol. Ther. **13**:459.
10. **Eneroth, C. M., C. Lundberg, and B. Wretlind.** 1975. Antibiotic concentrations in maxillary sinus secretions and in the sinus mucosa. Chemotherapy **21**(Suppl. 1):1–7.
11. **Fabre, J., J. S. Pitton, J. P. Kunz, S. Rozbroj, and R. M. Hungerbühler.** 1966. Distribution and excretion of doxycycline in man. Chemotherapia **11**:73–85.
12. **Finland, M.** 1958. Antibiotic blood level enhancement. Antibiot. Med. Clin. Ther. **5**:359–363.
13. **Gibaldi, M.** 1967. Pharmacokinetics of absorption and elimination of doxycycline in man. Chemotherapia **12**:265–271.
14. **Goodman, L. S., and A. Gilman. (ed).** 1970. The pharmacological basis of therapeutics, p. 1253–1258. MacMillan Co., New York.
15. **Hirsch, H. A., and M. Finland.** 1960. Comparative activity of four tetracycline analogs against pathogenic bacteria *in vitro*. Am. J. Med. Sci. **239**:288–294.
16. **Kakemi, K., H. Sezaki, H. Ogata, and T. Nadai.** 1968. Absorption and excretion of drugs. XXXVI. Effect of Ca^{2+} on the absorption of tetracycline from the small intestine (1). Chem. Pharm. Bull. **16**:2200–2205.
17. **Kohn, K. W.** 1961. Determination of tetracyclines by extraction of fluorescent complexes. Application to biological materials. Anal. Chem. **33**:862–866.
18. **Mattila, M. J., P. J. Neuvonen, G. Gothoni, and C. R. Hackman.** 1972. Interference of iron preparations and milk with the absorption of tetracyclines, p. 128–133. *In* S. B. de C. Baker and G. A. Neuhaus (ed.), Exerpta Medica International Congress Series no. 254: Toxicological problems of drug combinations.
19. **Neuvonen, P. J.** 1976. Interactions with the absorption of tetracyclines. Drugs **11**:45–54.
20. **Neuvonen, P. J., G. Gothoni, R. Hackman, and K. af Björksten.** 1970. Interference of iron with the absorption of tetracyclines in man. Br. Med. J. **4**:532–534.
21. **Neuvonen, P. J., and H. Turakka.** 1974. Inhibitory effect of various iron salts on the absorption of tetracycline in man. Eur. J. Clin. Pharmacol. **7**:357–360.
22. **Rosenblatt, J. E., J. E. Barrett, J. L. Brodie, and W. M. M. Kirby.** 1967. Comparison of in vitro activity and clinical pharmacology of doxycycline with other tetracyclines, p. 134–141. Antimicrob. Agents Chemother. 1966.
23. **Steigbigel, N. H., C. W. Reed, and M. Finland.** 1968. Absorption and excretion of five tetracycline derivatives in normal young men. Am. J. Med. Sci. **255**:296–312.
24. **Wagner, J. G., J. I. Northam, C. D. Alway, and O. S. Carpenter.** 1965. Blood levels of drug at the equilibrium state after multiple dosing. Nature (London) **207**:1301–1302.
25. **Welling, P. G., L. L. Lyons, W. A. Craig, and G. A. Trochta.** 1975. Influence of diet and fluid on bioavailability of theophylline. Clin. Pharmacol. Ther. **17**:475–480.
26. **Welling, P. G., L. L. Lyons, F. L. S. Tse, and W. A. Craig.** 1976. Propoxyphene and norpropoxyphene: influence of diet and fluid on plasma levels. Clin. Pharmacol. Ther. **19**:559–565.
27. **Wilson, D. M., M. Lever, E. A. Brosnan, and A. Stillwell.** 1972. A simplified tetracycline assay. Clin. Chim. Acta **36**:260–261.

ANTIMICROBIAL AGENTS AND CHEMOTHERAPY, Mar. 1977, p. 470–474
Vol. 11, No. 3

Comparison of In Vitro Activity of Cephalexin, Cephradine, and Cefaclor

NANCY J. BILL AND JOHN A. WASHINGTON II*
Mayo Clinic and Mayo Foundation, Rochester, Minnesota 55901

Received for publication 27 October 1976

Inhibitory activity of cephalexin, cephradine, and cefaclor was compared by the WHO-ICS agar dilution technique. Cefaclor was substantially more active against staphylococci, streptococci, gonococci, meningococci, *Haemophilus*, *Escherichia coli*, *Klebsiella pneumoniae*, *Citrobacter diversus*, *Proteus mirabilis*, salmonellae, and shigellae than was cephalexin, which in turn was more active than cephradine. Cefaclor appeared to be less resistant to staphylococcal penicillinase than did the other two agents. None of these cephalosporins was active against *Enterobacter*, *Serratia*, indole-positive *Proteeae*, *Pseudomonas*, or *Bacteroides fragilis*.

Cefaclor, 3-chloro-7-D-(2-phenylglycinamido)-3-cephem-4-carboxylic acid, is a new orally effective cephalosporin. The purpose of this study was to compare its activity in vitro with that of cephalexin and cephradine.

MATERIALS AND METHODS

Organisms. Most of the organisms used in this study were recent isolates from the Clinical Microbiology Laboratory of the Mayo Clinic, Rochester, Minn. Stock cultures of clinical isolates of salmonellae, shigellae, and providenciae that had been stored on nutrient agar slants and overlayed with oil were used. Clinical isolates of anaerobic bacteria used for testing had been stored at −72°C in 10% skim milk (BBL). Ampicillin-resistant strains of *Haemophilus influenzae* were obtained from the Center for Disease Control, Atlanta, Ga.

Two reference strains of bacteria, *Staphylococcus aureus* (ATCC 25923) and *Escherichia coli* (ATCC 25922), and a strain of *Pseudomonas aeruginosa* were used in each trial as controls when determining minimum inhibitory concentrations (MICs).

All organisms were subcultured to solid media to check for purity before being inoculated into appropriate broth media for testing.

Antibiotics. Standard laboratory powders of cephalexin monohydrate and cefaclor (compound 99638) were kindly provided by Eli Lilly Laboratories for Clinical Research, Indianapolis, Ind. Cephradine was kindly provided by Smith, Kline, and French Co., Philadelphia, Pa.

Susceptibility studies. MICs were determined by the agar dilution method (13). Generally, Mueller-Hinton agar (MHA) containing each antibiotic diluted according to the WHO-ICS scheme (2) was inoculated with, unless indicated otherwise, a standardized inoculum of 10^4 colony-forming units (CFU) by using the replicator device of Steers et al. (9). For testing streptococci other than group D, 5% defibrinated sheep blood was added to the MHA. The plates were examined after 18 h of incubation at 35°C. The MIC was interpreted as the lowest concentration of antibiotic yielding no growth, a barely visible haze, or no more than one discrete colony.

MHA supplemented with 1% IsoVitaleX (BBL) and 2% hemoglobin solution (Difco) was used to test *Neisseria* and *Haemophilus* (14). The inocula were prepared by scraping growth from chocolate blood agar plates into Mueller-Hinton broth. The turbidity of each suspension was adjusted to match that of a one-half McFarland no. 1 standard. A 1:10 dilution of the adjusted suspension was then delivered onto the surfaces of the agar plates with an inocula replicator apparatus (9). To test the effect of increasing the inoculum size of *Haemophilus*, the turbidity of the suspension was adjusted to match a no. 4 McFarland standard, and the suspension was directly inoculated onto the agar plates with the replicator device. After inoculation, the plates were incubated at 35°C in 5% CO_2 for 18 h. The MICs were interpreted by the same criteria as above.

The MICs of anaerobic bacteria were determined according to the agar dilution procedure described in the *Wadsworth Anaerobic Bacteriology Manual* (10). In this method, three to four colonies of the anaerobe were inoculated into supplemented thioglycolate medium without indicator (BBL-135C) which was enriched with hemin (5 μg/ml) before sterilization, plus $NaHCO_3$ (1 mg/ml) and vitamin K_1 (0.1 μg/ml) added just before use. After anaerobic overnight incubation in a GasPak jar (BBL) at 35°C, the culture was diluted with brucella broth containing 5% Fildes enrichment (Difco) and vitamin K_1 (0.1 μg/ml) so that its turbidity matched that of one-half the turbidity of the no. 1 McFarland standard. Using the inocula replicator device, the adjusted broth culture was applied to plates of brucella agar base containing serial twofold dilutions of antibiotic at final concentrations ranging from 0.125 to 128 μg/ml and supplemented with vitamin K_1 (10 μg/ml) and 5% laked blood. The plates were incubated at 35°C in GasPak jars (BBL) for approximately 48 h. The

MICs of each strain were read as the lowest concentration of drug yielding no growth, a barely visible haze, or no more than one discrete colony.

Minimum bactericidal concentrations (MBCs) were performed according to the method described by Washington (12). Inoculum was prepared by subculturing portions of four or five isolated colonies of the organism into 5 ml of Mueller-Hinton broth and incubating the suspension for approximately 6 h. After the turbidity of the suspension was adjusted to match that of a no. 1 McFarland standard, it was diluted 1:10 to yield an inoculum of about 10^7 CFU/ml and 1:1,000 to yield an inoculum of about 10^5 CFU/ml. Each of the tubes was inoculated with 0.5 ml of the adjusted broth culture. MICs were read after 18 h of incubation at 35°C as the lowest concentration of antibiotic completely inhibiting visible growth. For the bactericidal phase, 0.5-ml aliquots from those tubes exhibiting no visible growth were used to prepare pour plates with brain heart infusion agar, which were read after 72 h of incubation at 35°C.

RESULTS

The susceptibilities of gram-positive cocci and gram-negative bacilli to the three cephalosporins are shown in Table 1. Cefaclor was generally more active than cephalexin or cephradine against both penicillin-susceptible and penicillin-resistant strains of *S. aureus* and *S. epidermidis*. At 2 μg/ml, cephalexin, cephradine, and cefaclor inhibited 17, 9, and 32%, respectively, of penicillin-resistant strains of *S. aureus* and 50, 25, and 80%, respectively, of penicillin-susceptible strains. At 4 μg/ml, 95% of penicillin-susceptible strains of *S. aureus* were inhibited by cefaclor, in contrast to 80% of strains inhibited by the other two antibiotics. At least 93% of penicillin-resistant strains of *S. aureus* were inhibited by cephalexin and cefaclor at 8 μg/ml, in contrast to 84% inhibited by cephradine at this level. The effects of inoculum size of *S. aureus* on the activities of the three cephalosporins are noted in Fig. 1. A factor for each antibiotic was calculated by dividing the MIC obtained with an inoculum of 10^7 CFU/ml by that obtained with an inoculum of 10^5 CFU/ml, as described elsewhere by Sabath et al. (7). The factors for cephalexin, cephradine, and cefaclor were ≤8, ≤16, and ≤64, respectively. Cefaclor was highly effective against group A and group B streptococci and inhibited all strains tested at 0.25 and 2.0 μg/ml, respectively. All strains of *Streptococcus pneumoniae* were inhibited by 1.0 μg/ml. All of the 21 strains of pathogenic *Neisseria* were inhibited by 0.25 μg of cefaclor per ml, whereas 4 μg of cephalexin and 4 to 8 μg of cephradine per ml were required to achieve the same results.

TABLE 1. *Susceptibility of gram-positive and gram-negative bacilli to cephalosporins*

Organism	No. of strains	MIC_{90} (μg/ml)[a]		
		Cephalexin	Cephradine	Cefaclor
Staphylococcus aureus (penicillin resistant)	82	8	16	8
S. aureus (penicillin susceptible)	20	8	8	4
S. epidermidis (penicillin resistant)	34	32	32	32
S. epidermidis (penicillin susceptible)	18	4	4	2
Streptococcus, group A	17	0.5	0.5	0.25
Streptococcus, group B	20	4	2	2
Streptococcus, group D	67	128	128	64
S. pneumoniae	15	4	2	0.5
Neisseria gonorrhoeae	16	2	2	0.25
N. meningitidis	7	4	8	0.25
Escherichia coli	195	16	16	8
Klebsiella pneumoniae	51	8	16	8
Enterobacter aerogenes	16	>128	>128	>128
E. cloacae	25	>128	>128	>128
Serratia marcescens	14	>128	>128	>128
Proteus mirabilis	32	>128	>128	>128
Proteus (indole positive)	32	>128	>128	>128
Salmonella	21	8	16	2
Shigella	20	8	16	8
Citrobacter diversus	6	64	64	8
C. freundii	6	>128	>128	>128
Providencia stuartii	18	>128	>128	>128
Pseudomonas aeruginosa	70	>128	>128	>128
P. maltophilia	6	>128	>128	>128

[a] Lowest concentration inhibiting at least 90% of strains tested.

The lowest concentrations of the three cephalosporins inhibiting at least 90% of facultatively anaerobic gram-negative bacilli are also shown in Table 1. At 4 μg/ml, cefaclor was more effective than cephalexin or cephradine against *E. coli,* with 83, 35, and 5%, respectively, of the 195 strains inhibited at this concentration. Cephalexin and cefaclor were more effective than cephradine against *E. coli* at 8 μg/ml, with 84, 93, and 55%, respectively, of the strains being inhibited. Similar results were obtained for *Klebsiella pneumoniae*. The three cephalosporins had little or no effect on *Enterobacter aerogenes, E. cloacae, Serratia marcescens,* indole-positive *Proteus, Citrobacter freundii, Providencia stuartii,* and *Pseudomonas. Citrobacter diversus, Salmonella,* and *Shigella* were highly susceptible to cefaclor, with 83, 95, and 75%, respectively, being inhibited with 2 μg/ml. To obtain similar results, a four- to eightfold increase in the concentrations of cephalexin and cephradine was required for this purpose. *Proteus mirabilis* was more susceptible to cefaclor than cephalexin and cephradine, although 32 μg of cefaclor per ml was required to inhibit 75% of the 32 strains tested.

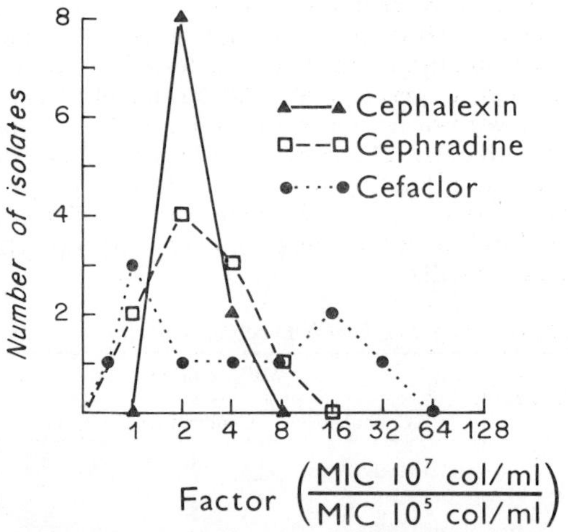

FIG. 1. *Effect of inoculum size on MIC of three cephalosporins for 10 strains of S. aureus.*

The effects of inoculum size and the effect of the presence of β-lactamase on the susceptibility of *H. influenzae* to cephalexin, cephradine, and cefaclor are shown in Table 2. A significant inoculum effect was demonstrated for all three antibiotics with both β-lactamase-positive and β-lactamase-negative *H. influenzae*. The presence of β-lactamase did not affect the activity of cefaclor but did affect the activity of cephalexin and cephradine. Inhibition of *H. influenzae* was achieved with only 2 μg of cefaclor per ml, in contrast to 8 μg of cephalexin and 16 μg of cephradine per ml needed for β-lactamase-negative organisms, and 32 μg of cephalexin and 64 μg of cephradine per ml needed for β-lactamase-positive organisms.

The activities of the three antibiotics against *Bacteroides fragilis, B. melaninogenicus,* and anaerobic gram-positive cocci are listed in Table 3. Cephalexin, cephradine, and especially cefaclor had little effect on *B. fragilis*. At 64 μg/ml, both cephalexin and cephradine inhibited 83% of the 18 strains of *B. fragilis,* whereas cefaclor inhibited only 11%. *B. melaninogenicus* was more susceptible to the cephalosporins than was *B. fragilis,* particularly if the strains of *B. melaninogenicus* were inhibited by penicillin at concentrations of ≤0.5 μg/ml. Cephalexin, cephradine, and cefaclor required 1, 2, and 0.5 μg/ml, respectively, for inhibition of *B.*

TABLE 2. *Susceptibility of Haemophilus influenzae to cephalosporins*

β-lactamase	Inoculum size (CFU/ml)	No. of strains	Antibiotic	Cumulative % inhibited at increasing concn (μg/ml)										
				0.12	0.25	0.5	1	2	4	8	16	32	64	128
+	10^4	15	Cephalexin						67	87	93	100		
			Cephradine							67	93	93	100	
			Cefaclor			7	73	100						
+	10^6	10	Cephalexin					10	10	10	20	50	60	60
			Cephradine								30	40	40	60
			Cefaclor						10	20	20	30	30	30
−	10^4	10	Cephalexin						50	100				
			Cephradine							50	100			
			Cefaclor			30	90	100						
−	10^6	10	Cephalexin						20	30	40	80	80	80
			Cephradine							10	40	40	70	80
			Cefaclor					10	40	40	40	50	50	50

TABLE 3. *Susceptibility of anaerobic bacteria to cephalosporins*

Organism	No. of strains	Antibiotic	Cumulative % inhibited at increasing concn (μg/ml)										
			≤0.12	0.25	0.5	1	2	4	8	16	32	64	128
Peptococcus	17	Cephalexin	12	18	29	29	53	76	82	82	82	94	100
		Cephradine	12	18	29	35	47	76	76	82	88	94	100
		Cefaclor	29	35	53	71	76	82	82	88	94	100	
Peptostreptococcus	10	Cephalexin	10	10	20	30	40	70	70	80	90	100	
		Cephradine	10	20	20	30	40	70	70	80	90	100	
		Cefaclor	10	20	30	40	60	70	80	80	80	80	100
Bacteroides fragilis	18	Cephalexin							6	11	44	83	94
		Cephradine							6	11	61	83	89
		Cefaclor										11	72
B. melaninogenicus (penicillin MIC, ≤0.5)	4	Cephalexin	25	25	25	100							
		Cephradine	25	25	25	75	100						
		Cefaclor	25	75	100								
B. melaninogenicus (penicillin MIC, >0.5)	5	Cephalexin					60	80	100				
		Cephradine					40	100					
		Cefaclor						40	40	80	100		

melaninogenicus with MIC values to penicillin of <0.5 μg/ml and 8, 4, and 32 μg/ml, respectively, for inhibition of *B. melaninogenicus* with MIC values to penicillin of >0.5 μg/ml. Of the three antibiotics, cefaclor appeared to be slightly more effective against the anaerobic gram-positive cocci that were tested. At 2 μg/ml, cephalexin, cephradine, and cefaclor inhibited 53, 47, and 76%, respectively, of the 17 strains of *Peptococcus* and 40, 40, and 60%, respectively, of the 10 strains of *Peptostreptococcus*.

Neither cefaclor nor cephradine produced 100% killing of 10^5 and 10^7 CFU of penicillin-susceptible and penicillin-resistant strains of *S. aureus* per ml at concentrations of ≤128 μg/ml. With one exception, neither cefaclor nor cephradine produced 99.9% killing of staphylococci in an inoculum of 10^7 CFU/ml. With one strain, cephradine produced 99.9% killing at 32 μg/ml. The MBC values of cefaclor against three strains of *E. coli* were the same as, two times (in the first two instances) and eight times the MIC values, respectively. With three strains of *K. pneumoniae,* the MBC values were four times the MIC values in two instances and twice the MIC value in one instance.

DISCUSSION

Against both penicillinase- and non-penicillinase-producing strains of *S. aureus,* cefaclor was at least three times as active as cephradine at 2 μg/ml and at least one and a half times as active as cephalexin at this concentration. The effects of inoculum size of *S. aureus* on the activities of the three cephalosporins varied substantially (Fig. 1), with cephalexin being the least affected by penicillinase-producing strains and cefaclor being the most affected by such strains; cephradine was intermediate between the two. Similar studies by Sabath et al. (7) have shown that cephalexin was only slightly less resistant to staphylococcal penicillinase than was cephalothin. These data disagree with those reported by Fong et al. (3), who assayed for residual cephalosporin activity in broth cultures of *S. aureus* and found that cephalexin was completely inactivated by staphylococcal penicillinase within 12 h, in contrast to cephalothin, which underwent little inactivation. They also found that cephradine, which was not tested by Sabath et al. (7), was degraded more slowly than cephalexin, with 18% of the original concentration being measurable at 12 h. Cephradine was found to be more resistant than cephalexin to crude β-lactamase derived from *S. aureus* by Hubsher et al. (4).

At 2 μg/ml, cefaclor inhibited all β-lactamase-positive and -negative strains of *H. influenzae* at the generally recommended inoculum of 10^4 CFU/ml (11), in contrast to cephalexin and cephradine, which required substantially greater concentrations to achieve the same order of activity and which were also considerably affected by *Haemophilus* β-lactamase. None of the cephalosporins inhibited a significant number of the strains of *H. influenzae* at the higher inoculum size. Our results with cephalexin and cephradine are similar to those reported by Emerson et al. (1). Whether or not cefaclor's greater activity against both β-lactamase-positive and -negative strains at the lower inoculum is clinically significant remains to be seen.

Cefaclor was also significantly more active against gonococci and meningococci than the other two agents and inhibited all strains at 0.25 μg/ml. The MIC values of cefaclor were at least 1/16 of those of the other two cephalosporins; however, no β-lactamase-positive strains of *Neisseria gonorrhoeae* were studied. In general, cephalosporins have demonstrated broad ranges of MIC values against these two species of *Neisseria*.

Cefaclor was substantially more active than cephalexin and cephradine against *E. coli, K. pneumoniae, P. mirabilis,* salmonellae, shigellae, and *C. diversus*. All three antibiotics were essentially inactive against *Enterobacter, Serratia,* indole-positive species of the *Proteeae, Citrobacter freundii,* and species of *Pseudomonas*.

Klastersky et al. (5) and Scholand et al. (8) have previously reported that the antibacterial activity of cephradine was nearly identical to that of cephalexin. McGowan et al. (6), however, reported that cephradine was less active than cephalexin against blood culture isolates of *E. coli, Klebsiella,* and *P. mirabilis*. The methodologies used in each of these studies differed considerably from one another and in varying degrees from the reference WHO-ICS method (2, 11). It was, therefore, of interest to us to try to resolve these different results by testing each of the cephalosporins with the reference method. In general, we agree with McGowan et al. (6) that cephradine is less active than cephalexin. Moreover, our results demonstrate that neither antibiotic is as active as cefaclor against gram-positive and gram-negative aerobic and facultatively anaerobic bacteria.

All three cephalosporins were active at clinically achievable serum levels (8 to 16 μg/ml) against most anaerobic cocci, but they were essentially inactive at these levels against *Bacteroides fragilis*. With *B. melaninogenicus* their activity correlated closely with the penicillin susceptibility of the strains tested. The four strains that were inhibited by $\leq$0.5 μg of penicillin per ml were also inhibited by 1, 2, and 0.5 μg of cephalexin, cephradine, and cefaclor per ml, respectively. The five strains requiring $>$0.5 μg of penicillin per ml for inhibition required 8, 4, and 32 μg of cephalexin, cephradine, and cefaclor per ml, respectively, for complete inhibition.

In conclusion, we have found cefaclor to be substantially more active than cephalexin, which in turn was more active than cephradine, against staphylococci, streptococci, gonococci, meningococci, and certain species of the *Enterobacteriaceae*. Cefaclor was also highly active against both β-lactamase-positive and -negative strains of *H. influenzae* at the recommended inoculum size. Clinical studies are required to substantiate cefaclor's value in the therapy of infections due to these susceptible species.

ACKNOWLEDGMENT

This work was supported by a grant from the Lilly Research Laboratories, Eli Lilly and Co., Indianapolis, Ind.

LITERATURE CITED

1. **Emerson, B. B., A. L. Smith, A. L. Harding, and D. H. Smith.** 1975. *Haemophilus influenzae* type B susceptibility to 17 antibiotics. J. Pediatr. **86**:617–620.
2. **Ericsson, H. M., and J. C. Sherris.** 1971. Antibiotic sensitivity testing: report of an international collaborative study. Acta Pathol. Microbiol. Scand. Sect. B Suppl. **217**:1.
3. **Fong, I. W., E. R. Engelking, and W. M. Kirby.** 1976. Relative inactivation by *Staphylococcus aureus* of eight cephalosporin antibiotics. Antimicrob. Ag. Chemother. **9**:939–944.
4. **Hubsher, J. A., H. H. Gadebusch, and A. G. Itkin.** 1976. Double-blind comparison of cephradine and cephalexin in the treatment of skin and soft-tissue infections due to *Staphylococcus aureus*. Curr. Ther. Res. Clin. Exp. **19**:579–588.
5. **Klastersky, J., D. Daneau, and D. Weerts.** 1973. Cephradine: antibacterial activity and clinical effectiveness. Chemotherapy **18**:191–204.
6. **McGowan, J. E., Jr., C. Garner, C. Wilcox, and M. Finland.** 1974. Antibiotic susceptibility of gram-negative bacilli isolated from blood cultures: results of tests with 35 agents and strains from 169 patients at Boston City Hospital during 1972. Am. J. Med. **57**:225–238.
7. **Sabath, L. D., C. Garner, C. Wilcox, and M. Finland.** 1975. Effect of inoculum and of beta-lactamase on the anti-staphylococcal activity of thirteen penicillins and cephalosporins. Antimicrob. Ag. Chemother. **8**:344–349.
8. **Scholand, J. F., G. R. Hodges, R. J. Fass, and S. Saslaw.** 1974. Clinical evaluation of cephradine, a new oral cephalosporin. Am. J. Med. Sci. **267**:111–116.
9. **Steers, E., E. L. Foltz, and B. S. Graves.** 1959. An inocula replicating apparatus for routine testing of bacterial susceptibility to antibiotics. Antibiot. Chemother. **9**:307–311.
10. **Sutter, V. L., V. L. Vargo, and S. M. Finegold.** 1975. Wadsworth anaerobic bacteriology manual, 2nd ed., p. 60–62. Wadsworth Hospital Center, Los Angeles.
11. **Thornsberry, C., and L. A. Kirven.** 1974. Antimicrobial susceptibility of *Haemophilus influenzae*. Antimicrob. Ag. Chemother. **6**:620–624.
12. **Washington, J. A., II.** 1974. Laboratory procedures in clinical microbiology. Little, Brown and Co., Boston.
13. **Washington, J. A., II, and A. L. Barry.** 1974. Dilution test procedures, p. 410–417. *In* E. H. Lennette, E. H. Spaulding, and J. P. Truant (ed.), Manual of clinical microbiology, 2nd ed. American Society for Microbiology, Washington, D.C.
14. **Washington, J. A., II, R. J. Snyder, and P. C. Kohner.** 1976. Spurious ampicillin resistance by testing *Haemophilus influenzae* with agar containing supplement C. Antimicrob. Ag. Chemother. **9**:199–200.

ANTIMICROBIAL AGENTS AND CHEMOTHERAPY, Mar. 1977, p. 475-481
Vol. 11, No. 3
Printed in U.S.A.

Effects of 2-Deoxy-D-Glucose and 3-Deazauridine Individually and in Combination on the Replication of Japanese B Encephalitis Virus

DANIEL R. WOODMAN* AND JIMMY C. WILLIAMS

Department of Microbiology, Naval Medical Research Institute, National Naval Medical Center, Bethesda, Maryland 20014

Received for publication 9 November 1976

We have tested the potencies of the competitors of glucose, 2-deoxy-D-glucose, and of uridine, 3-deazauridine, on the inhibition of Japanese B encephalitis virus multiplication in BHK-21 cell cultures. The relative effectiveness of the viral inhibitors were evaluated individually and in combination in relation to cytotoxicity as a measure of the selectivity of inhibition. When the drugs were administered individually, the antiviral activity was masked by the cytotoxic effect on the host. By combining the two drugs, it was possible to inhibit Japanese encephalitis virus production at noncytotoxic concentrations. The effects of 2-deoxy-D-glucose and 3-deazauridine on the growth inhibition of BHK-21 cells in cultures were only additive, while they were clearly synergistic on the inhibition of Japanese encephalitis virus production. Thus, it was possible to achieve an increased antiviral effect without a significant increase in cytotoxicity. Although the precise biochemical mechanism of the antiviral activity of these antimetabolites in combination is not known, our results indicate the potential value of this approach in viral chemotherapy.

A considerable amount of biochemical information has been gathered on the mode of action of antiviral drugs, but such information has not yet been reflected in improved chemotherapy of viral infections. In general, the conclusion has been drawn that viral infections do not respond well to chemotherapy, largely because viruses depend upon the synthetic mechanisms of the host cells. Therefore, any compound that effectively reduces the number of viral particles is likely to cause severe toxic side effects. Of the agents that have been tested on a variety of enveloped ribonucleic acid (RNA) viruses, the glucose competitor, 2-deoxy-D-glucose (2-DG), has probably been the most promising, largely because it interferes with the synthesis of viral glycoprotein (5, 7, 10). Another compound that possesses significant antiviral activity against RNA viruses is the antipyrimidine, 3-deazauridine (3-deazaUR). Although 3-deazaUR greatly restricts host as well as viral RNA synthesis at high concentration, this compound has antiviral activity at noncytotoxic levels (9, 11, 16).

Unfortunately, both 2-DG and 3-deazaUR exhibit severe cytotoxic side effects when administered in the high concentrations required for substantial antiviral activity. In this paper we describe preliminary studies in vitro in which we examined the feasibility of combining these two drugs to reduce the replication of Japanese B encephalitis virus (JEV) without greatly affecting the host cells. The relationship of the metabolic sites inhibited by the two agents under discussion are summarized in Fig. 1. Administration of 2-DG and its subsequent incorporation into host as well as viral glycoproteins causes toxic effects and a reduction in viral particles (for review, see reference 15). The antipyrimidine, 3-deazaUR, when phosphorylated to the triphosphate level, 3-deazauridine 5′-triphosphate (3-deazaUTP), exhibits strong competitive inhibition of the synthesis of cytidine 5′-triphosphate (CTP), thereby restricting host and viral RNA synthesis (11, 16). A consideration of the pathways suggested to us that 2-DG might potentiate the effect of 3-deazaUR and thus affect viral replication. This combination of drugs, at a low concentration, should be reasonably antiviral while not being cytotoxic. The effects of these combinations on antiviral activity and cytotoxicity were tested in the baby hamster kidney cell line (BHK-21) infected with JEV.

MATERIALS AND METHODS

Virus strain. The Nakayama strain of JEV (12) was used throughout this investigation. Virus seed was prepared from the harvest of a single passage in brains of suckling NIH-Nmri CV mice and stored at −70°C until used.

Cell cultures and media. BHK-21 clone 13 cell cultures from the American Type Culture Collection provided an in vitro assay system for both the titration of JEV (1, 8) and cytotoxicity evaluations. Stock cell cultures were grown in Eagle minimum essential medium (2) with Earle balanced salt solution (EMEM), supplemented with 10% tryptose phosphate broth and 10% heat-inactivated dialyzed fetal calf serum ($EMEM_{90}DFCS_{10}$). The cells were subcultured and passed in EMEM with the substitution of various metabolites for glucose as shown in Table 1. The cells were infected as nonconfluent monolayers (40,000 to 60,000 viable BHK-21 cells per 1 ml of maintenance medium) in each well of 24 well-dishes (Costar, Cambridge, Mass.). The maintenance medium contained the components of growth medium except that the level of fetal calf serum was reduced to 1% ($EMEM_{99}DFCS_{1}$).

Cytotoxicity tests. The cytotoxicities of 2-DG and 3-deazaUR were determined for each modification of growth ($DFCS_{10}$) and maintenance ($DFCS_{1}$) media used in this study by viability staining (eosin Y exclusion) and by microscopic examination. Growth medium was used to test inhibitor cytotoxicity (Table 2). Although maintenance medium was used for the cultures that served as controls for virus yield reduction tests with either 2-DG or 3-deazaUR, differences in cytotoxicity attributable to the concentration of serum were negligible. The cytotoxic dose

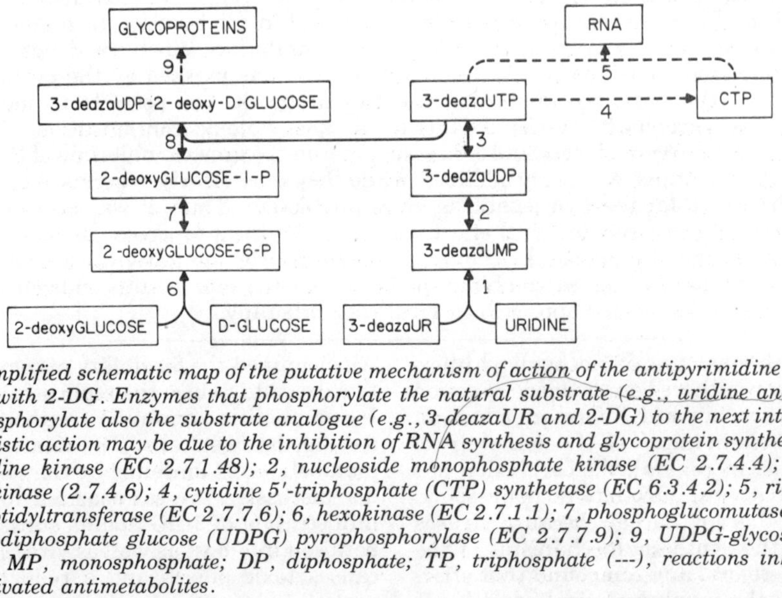

FIG. 1. *Simplified schematic map of the putative mechanism of action of the antipyrimidine 3-deazaUR in combination with 2-DG. Enzymes that phosphorylate the natural substrate (e.g., uridine and glucose) are known to phosphorylate also the substrate analogue (e.g., 3-deazaUR and 2-DG) to the next intermediate (15, 16). A synergistic action may be due to the inhibition of RNA synthesis and glycoprotein synthesis. Abbreviations: 1, uridine kinase (EC 2.7.1.48); 2, nucleoside monophosphate kinase (EC 2.7.4.4); 3, nucleoside diphosphate kinase (2.7.4.6); 4, cytidine 5'-triphosphate (CTP) synthetase (EC 6.3.4.2); 5, ribonucleic acid (RNA) nucleotidyltransferase (EC 2.7.7.6); 6, hexokinase (EC 2.7.1.1); 7, phosphoglucomutase (EC 2.7.5.1); 8, uridine 5'-diphosphate glucose (UDPG) pyrophosphorylase (EC 2.7.7.9); 9, UDPG-glycosyltransferase; UR, uridine; MP, monosphosphate; DP, diphosphate; TP, triphosphate (---), reactions inhibited by the respective activated antimetabolites.*

TABLE 1. *BHK-21 cell multiplication and JEV replication in modified EMEM containing increasing glucose levels*

Glucose (mg/liter)	Viable cell count[a] and JEV titer[b] in media: D-Galactose (900 mg/liter)[c]		D-Galactose (900 mg/liter), sodium pyruvate (550 mg/liter)[c]		Mannose (1,000 mg/liter)[c]		Mannose (1,000 mg/liter), sodium pyruvate (550 mg/liter)[c]	
	BHK-21[a]	JEV[b]	BHK-21[a]	JEV[b]	BHK-21[a]	JEV[b]	BHK-21[a]	JEV[b]
0	5.3	1.0	1.8	1.9	1.8	0.68	10.0	1.7
0.1	5.7	1.2	1.9	1.1	2.8	0.65	9.6	1.8
1	5.0	1.4	1.6	1.8	5.0	0.8	9.8	1.7
10	5.4	1.0	1.7	1.5	4.0	1.1	10.0	1.9
100	9.5	1.2	2.9	1.6	4.1	1.1	8.5	2.0
1000	10.7	1.1	6.8	1.7	4.5	1.0	10.0	2.0

[a] Viable cell count × 10^5 48 h after seeding 2 × 10^5 cells/ml of $EMEM_{90}DFCS_{10}$ in 1-ml wells.

[b] JEV titer × 10^6 PFU/ml 48 h after infection of BHK-21 cells at a multiplicity of infection of 10:1 in $EMEM_{99}DFCS_{1}$.

[c] Additional metabolites of EMEM.

TABLE 2. *Relative effectiveness of 2-DG and 3-deazaUR on the reduction of JEV titer and cytotoxic dose in EMEM and in modified EMEM without glucose*

Media	2-Deoxy-D-glucose			3-Deazauridine		
	MED_{50} (μM)[a]	Cytotoxic dose (μM)[b]	PER[c]	MED_{50}	Cytotoxic dose	PER
EMEM (glucose)	500	900	1.8	20	30	1.5
Modified EMEM (no glucose)						
D-(+)-Galactose (900 mg/liter)	500	800	1.6			
Sodium pyruvate (550 mg/liter)	500	1,500	3.0			
D-(+)-Galactose (900 mg/liter) and sodium pyruvate (550 mg/liter)	150	1,000	6.6			
Mannose (1,000 mg/liter)	300	2,400	8.0			
Mannose (1,000 mg/liter) and sodium pyruvate (550 mg/liter)	300	2,750	9.2	20	4	0.2

[a] Forty-eight-hour minimum effective dose (MED_{50}) based upon PFU reductions in maintenance medium.
[b] Forty-eight-hour cytotoxicity based upon viability determinations in growth medium.
[c] Physiologically effective range = cytotoxic dose/MED_{50}.

was considered to be that amount of compound, either alone or in combination, which reduced the viable cell count by 50% in growth media by 48 h.

Plaque assay. JEV plaque titrations were conducted in confluent monolayers of BHK-21 cell cultures. Serial 10-fold dilutions of JEV samples were prepared in pH 7.4 phosphate-buffered saline containing 0.75% bovine serum albumin fraction V (Calbiochem). Overlay medium contained a final concentration of 0.8% agarose (Seaken, Microbiological Associates, Inc.) in Gey's medium. Infected cultures were incubated at 37°C in a humidified 5% CO_2 atmosphere for 96 h before neutral red staining.

Virus yield reduction tests. Cultures were inoculated with 10 plaque-forming units (PFU) of JEV per viable cell, absorbed for 90 min at 37°C, and then rinsed twice with pH 7.4 phosphate-buffered saline. The appropriate maintenance medium containing increasing concentrations of either 2-DG (Aldrich Chemical Co.) or 3-deazaUR (ICN Corp., Irvine, Calif.) was then added to the cell cultures as well as to control uninfected cells. The cultures were incubated at 37°C in a humidified 5% CO_2 atmosphere for 48 h, and supernatant fluids were sampled at 12-h intervals. Viral titers expressed as PFU per cell were determined by plaque assays on BHK-21 cell cultures. The antiviral activity of a given concentration of either 2-DG or 3-deazaUR was determined as the percentage of control PFU obtained without either compound. The amount that reduced the number of PFU by 50% was defined as the minimal effective dose (MED_{50}) (3). Various combinations of 2-DG and 3-deazaUR were likewise evaluated for antiviral and cytotoxic effects.

RESULTS

Glucose requirement for cell multiplication and viral replication. When uninfected BHK-21 cells were subcultured with $EMEM_{90}DFCS_{10}$ either in the absence of glucose or in 0.1 to 1 mg of glucose/liter, the total number of cells doubled between 24 and 48 h. Significant growth after 48 h required at least 100 mg of glucose per liter. With a multiplicity of infection of 10 PFU, there was a definite requirement for glucose for optimal JEV replication. Viral assays for each glucose concentration at 24, 48, and 72 h indicated that JEV replication was always maximal at 48 h and the effect of the glucose level was also most evident at 48 h. Although there was some indication that JEV replicated in the absence of glucose or in the presence of small concentrations of glucose, maximum levels were reached only when the glucose concentration was either 100 or 1,000 mg/liter.

Effect of other carbon sources. Cell multiplication in $EMEM_{90}DFCS_{10}$ and JEV replication in $EMEM_{99}DFCS_1$ obtained with increasing glucose concentrations in the presence of various carbon sources are presented in Table 1. In the case of galactose, galactose plus sodium pyruvate, and mannose, the cell count approximately doubled as the concentration of glucose was increased. However, with a combination of mannose and sodium pyruvate the cell count was approximately the same at all concentrations of glucose. The titer of JEV, on the other hand, with the possible exception of the mannose medium, was not significantly stimulated by increasing the glucose concentration. Increasing serum levels from 1 to either 5 or 10% did not result in a significant change in JEV titers.

Antimetabolite effectiveness. The effects of 2-DG and 3-deazaUR on BHK-21 cells and JEV replication are summarized in Table 2. The data presented are the means of triplicate experiments. The cytotoxic dose was measured in $EMEM_{90}DFCS_{10}$ and the MED_{50} in $EMEM_{99}DFCS_1$. The potency of an inhibitor of viral replication can best be judged by the ratio of cytotoxic level to MED_{50}, expressing the physiologically effective range (PER), which is a measure of the selectivity of inhibition. A large PER reflects relatively high viral inhibition with respect to cytotoxicity. In complete EMEM and in modified EMEM containing galactose, the PER with 2-DG was small (<2) because of its cytotoxicity. When glucose was replaced by pyruvate, galactose plus pyruvate, mannose, or mannose plus pyruvate, the PER increased to 3.0, 6.6, 8.0, and 9.2, respectively.

The effect of increasing the concentration of 2-DG on cell viability and JEV production are presented in greater detail in Fig. 2. The results can be summarized as follows. (i) The cytotoxicity concentrations of 2-DG were markedly different in the four media. When mannose, galactose, and pyruvate-containing media were compared to glucose, the BHK-21 cells were protected from the effects of 2-DG most effectively by mannose. Toxicity levels were significantly lower ($P < 0.05$) at 0.6, 1.2, and 2.4 mM 2-DG. (ii) The reduction in yield of JEV was not greatly different in the four media. Hence, these results suggest that the reduction in yield of JEV by 2-DG in glucose-, pyruvate-, and galactose-containing media may have been due in part to the cytotoxic effects of 2-DG on the BHK-21 cells. Mannose, on the other hand, undoubtedly protected the host cell from the effects of 2-DG, whereas the reduction in yield of JEV was not altered.

The cytotoxic effect of 3-deazaUR was 30-fold greater than that of 2-DG in glucose medium. Surprisingly, its cytotoxicity, in contrast to 2-DG, was much greater in mannose-sodium pyruvate medium. Thus, there was an almost 700-fold ratio in the toxicity of the two compounds in the mannose-pyruvate medium. The MED_{50} was approximately the same in the two media. The PER was low in the glucose medium, approximately the same as for 2-DG, and very low (0.2) in the mannose-pyruvate medium.

Reversal of 2-DG inhibition by metabolite replacement. The effect of replacing 2-DG (0.5 mM) with various metabolites at 6, 12, 24, and

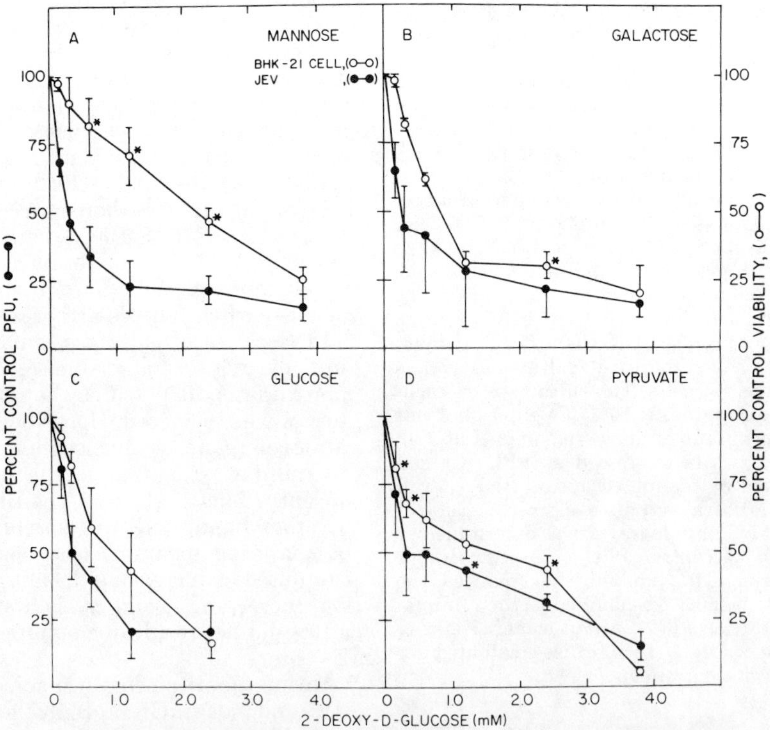

FIG. 2. *JEV yield reduction per infected BHK-21 cell at 48 h by 2-DG in 1 ml of modified maintenance EMEM. JEV titers in the presence of 2-DG were compared with PFU from controls consisting of infected cell cultures containing none of the antimetabolite. Total viable cell counts at 48 h from the uninfected wells containing increasing concentrations of 2-DG in modified maintenance media were compared to cell counts in control wells which contained no 2-DG. Metabolic concentrations were glucose (1 g/liter), galactose (900 mg/liter), pyruvate (550 mg/liter), or mannose (1 g/liter). Each point represents the mean ± standard error of the mean of four or more separate tests. Means that are significantly different from the glucose medium ($P < 0.05$) are indicated by an asterisk (*). (100% = 20 JEV/cell.)*

36 h after JEV infection of BHK-21 cells in $EMEM_{99}DFCS_1$ was most evident when metabolite replacement was accomplished at 24 h. Mannose most efficiently reversed viral inhibition by 2-DG, whereas differences in the effectiveness of galactose, pyruvate, and glucose were relatively small (Fig. 3). When replacement was made at 36 h (data not shown) comparable results were obtained, but the yield of JEV was reduced possibly because of the considerable amount of JEV removed with the medium change at 36 h. Results with infected control cultures containing no 2-DG indicated that any change of medium after 12 h reduced infectious virus production. In uninfected controls in which 2-DG medium was replaced with various carbon sources, glucose most effectively increased the number of viable BHK-21 cells at both 6-h (180%) and 24-h (100%) replacement. The 6-h mannose replacement was less effective (110%), whereas galactose was even poorer (85%).

Antiviral effect of 3-deazaUR and 2-DG in combination. To test the hypothesis that 3-deazaUR could potentiate the growth inhibitory effects of 2-DG on JEV, combination experiments were carried out. The effects of four different 3-deazaUR concentrations were tested alone and in the presence of three concentrations of 2-DG (Table 3). In every experiment the combination of the two drugs inhibited JEV replication to an extent greater than expected from purely additive effects while showing an inhibition of BHK-21 cell growth approximately the same or somewhat less than the additive effect. Hence, these two agents when used in combination display a considerable degree of synergism in JEV inhibition. Increasing concentrations of 3-deazaUR in the presence of a constant concentration of 2-DG brought about a significant decrease in the concentration of 3-deazaUR required to reduce the MED_{50} (Fig. 4).

The MED_{50} of the agents in combination in EMEM and in mannose-pyruvate medium indicates that 3-deazaUR was slightly more inhibitory of JEV replication in EMEM than in glu-

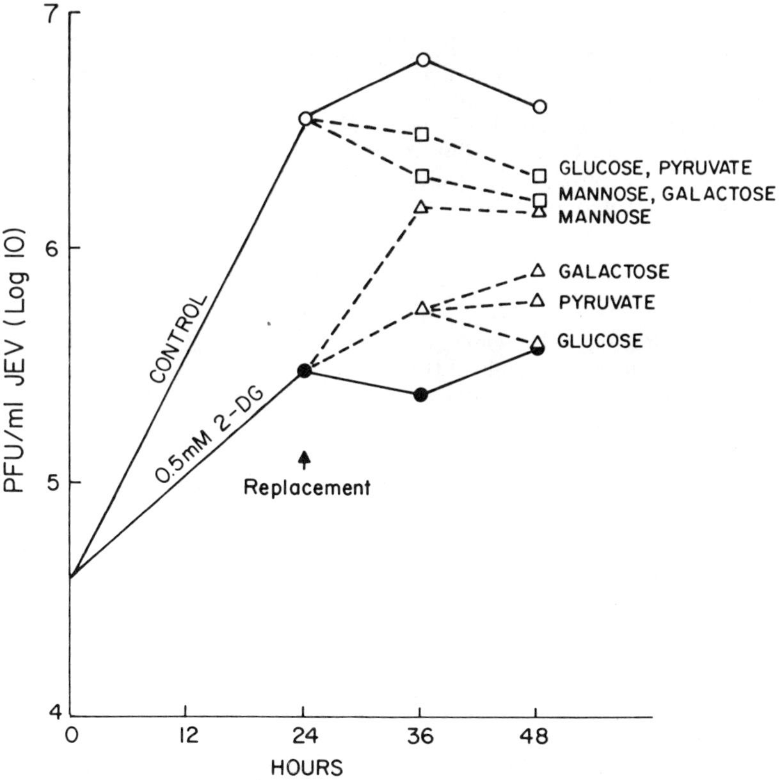

FIG. 3. *Effect of replacing 0.5 mM 2-DG with various metabolites 24 h after JEV infection of BHK-21 cell cultures maintained on EMEM. Metabolite concentrations in maintenance media were glucose (1 g/liter), sodium pyruvate (550 mg/liter), galactose (900 mg/liter), or mannose (1 g/liter). JEV titers in the presence of 0.5 mM 2-DG (●), with metabolite replacements containing no 2-DG (△), control without 2-DG (○), and control with metabolite replacement (□).*

TABLE 3. *Synergistic interaction of 2-DG and 3-deazaUR on JEV replication in glucose medium*

Agent	Concn (μM) of: 2-DG	Concn (μM) of: 3-deazaUR	Count as % of untreated controls in presence of: 2-DG (a)	3-deazaUR (b)	2-DG + 3-deazaUR: Predicted[a] (c)	2-DG + 3-deazaUR: Measured (d)
BHK-21	75	2.0	96	77	74	78
	150	2.0	85	77	65	68
	333	2.0	73	77	56	64
	75	4.0	96	73	70	74
	150	4.0	85	73	62	63
	75	20.0	96	55	53	55
	150	20.0	85	55	47	55
	150	40.0	85	40	34	46
JEV	75	2.0	78	62	48	31[b]
	150	2.0	54	62	33	20[b]
	333	2.0	43	62	27	18[b]
	75	4.0	78	58	45	20[b]
	150	4.0	54	58	31	11[b]
	75	20.0	78	54	42	20[b]
	150	20.0	54	54	29	11[b]
	150	40.0	54	34	18	5[b]

[a] Summation as defined by Webb (19), i.e., c = (a times b)/100. The letters refer to the numbers in the labeled columns.

[b] Significant potentiation, i.e., d < 0.7 times c.

cose-free medium (Fig. 4). Both lines in Fig. 4 indicate the enhanced antiviral activity demonstrated by the combination of noncytotoxic levels of 2-DG and 3-deazaUR in either EMEM or glucose-free medium. BHK-21 cell viability data computed for each compound, individually and in combination, indicated no significant cytotoxicity.

DISCUSSION

The production of viral glycoproteins and viral RNA via host-mediated mechanisms is a prerequisite for the subsequent assembly of the viral particle. The pivotal position of uridine 5′-triphosphate (UTP) and CTP as common precursors for RNA and the relative importance of UTP and glucose in glycosylation reactions was emphasized in Fig. 1. Multiple inhibition of sites immediately preceding RNA and glycoprotein synthesis would greatly facilitate the action of each competitive inhibitor. If the pool of competing natural substrate can be depleted via a judicious combination of antimetabolites, this should greatly enhance the effectiveness of the inhibitors. Clearly, the depletion of the CTP pool via the competitive action of 3-deazaUTP on CTP synthetase and the subsequent depletion of the UTP pools through the incorporation of 2-DG and 3-deazaUTP into the sugar nucleotides might potentiate the effect of 2-DG on JEV production. Our experiments were designed to test this prediction and our results have confirmed it for studies in vitro.

The uridine analogue 3-deazaUR and the antimetabolite 2-DG have both been shown to inhibit the production of infectious RNA viruses (5, 7, 9–11). The precise step of inhibition by 2-DG is not known; however, if the group B arboviruses are first assembled as immature forms containing two membrane glycoproteins, the incorporation of 2-DG might prevent assembly and/or subsequent maturation of JEV to the infectious form (6, 14, 17, 18). Recently, the nucleoside-diphosphate derivatives of 2-DG in BHK-21 cells have been identified as uridine

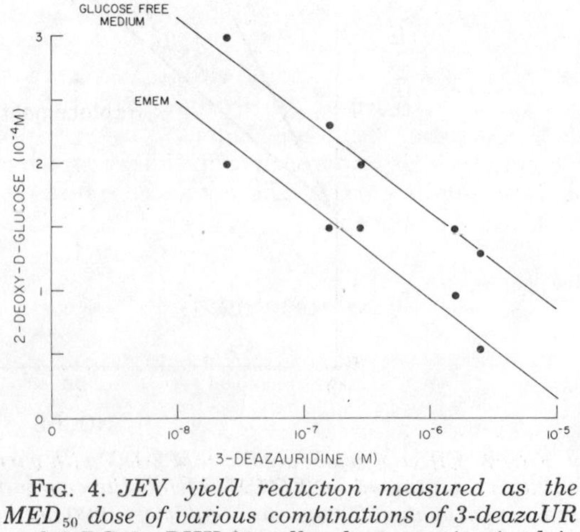

FIG. 4. *JEV yield reduction measured as the MED_{50} dose of various combinations of 3-deazaUR and 2-DG in BHK-21 cell cultures maintained in either EMEM or glucose-free medium.*

diphosphate-2-deoxy-D-glucose (UDP-2-DG) and guanidine diphosphate-2-deoxy-D-glucose (GDP-2-DG) (13). The discovery of the activated intermediates of ^{14}C-labeled 2-DG in BHK-21 cells indicates that the corresponding nucleoside diphosphate derivatives of UDP-2-DG and GDP-2-DG can be expected to contribute to the inhibition of the transglycosylation reactions during arboviral infections (4, 7). The viral inhibitory activity of 3-deazaUR, shown to occur during viral replication, was reversed by the naturally occurring pyrimidine nucleoside (9). Metabolic studies have shown that 3-deazaUR, phosphorylated by leukemia L-1210 cells, exerts its inhibitory activity by interfering with the activity of the CTP synthetase (11). Shannon et al. (16) showed that 3-deazaUR possessed a broad spectrum of antiviral activity against several important human RNA viruses. Although the precise biochemical mechanisms of these two drugs are not known, their combination could be expected to interfere with both glycoprotein and RNA synthesis in a synergistic manner.

Our studies of the inhibition of the production of JEV in BHK-21 cells by either 2-DG or 3-deazaUR alone or in combination were limited to determinations of infectivity. Although each of these compounds was shown to possess some antiviral activity against JEV at noncytotoxic concentrations, the levels of inhibition observed with combinations of 2-DG and 3-deazaUR were synergistic. Since it was possible to achieve this increased antiviral effect without any significant increase in cytotoxicity, our results demonstrate the potential feasibility of this approach to antiviral chemotherapy. Ours is the first attempt to study the combination of these two drugs against viral infections. Since JEV is an important human pathogen, and no effective treatment for the disease has been described, our studies should be extended to the animal model in order to evaluate the treatment potential for man. Indeed, our results indicate that this approach to antiviral chemotherapy might parallel the advances made in cancer chemotherapy.

ACKNOWLEDGMENTS

We wish to express our thanks to Robert Nye and Richard Grays for their excellent technical assistance. We also wish to thank Emilio Weiss for his constructive and helpful reviews of the manuscript.

This investigation was supported by the Navy Medical Research and Development Command, Research Task no. MPN03.12.5031.

LITERATURE CITED

1. **Diercks, F. H., and W. McD. Hammon.** 1958. Hamster kidney cell tissue cultures for propagation of Japanese B encephalitis virus. Proc. Soc. Exp. Biol. Med. **97**:627–632.
2. **Eagle, H.** 1959. Amino acid metabolism in mammalian cell cultures. Science **130**:432–437.
3. **Ehrlich, J., B. J. Sloan, F. A. Miller, and H. E. Machamer.** 1956. Searching for antiviral materials from microbial fermentations. Ann. N.Y. Acad. Sci. **130**:5–16.
4. **Froger, C., and P. Louisot.** 1972. Glycoprotein biosynthesis in arbovirus infected cells. II. Study of microsomic mannosyl transferase activity. Int. J. Biochem. **3**:613–622.
5. **Gandhi, S. S., P. Stanley, J. M. Taylor, and D. O. White.** 1972. Inhibition of influenza viral glycoprotein synthesis by sugars. Microbios **5**:41–50.
6. **Kaluza, G., M. F. G. Schmidt, and C. Scholtissek.** 1973. Effect of 2-deoxy-D-glucose on the multiplication of Semliki Forest virus and reversal of the block by mannose. Virology **54**:179–189.
7. **Kaluza, G., C. Scholtissek, and R. Rott.** 1972. inhibition of the multiplication of enveloped RNA viruses by glucosamine and 2-deoxy-D-glucose. J. Gen. Virol. **14**:251–259.
8. **Karabatsos, N., and S. M. Buckley.** 1967. Susceptibility of the baby hamster kidney cell line (BHK-21) to infection with arboviruses. Am. J. Trop. Med. Hyg. **16**:99–105.
9. **Khare, G. P., R. W. Sidwell, J. H. Huffman, R. L. Tolman, and R. K. Robins.** 1972. Inhibition of RNA virus replication *in vitro* by 3-deazacytidine and deazauridine. Proc. Soc. Exp. Biol. Med. **140**:880–884.
10. **Klenk, H. D., C. Scholtissek, and R. Rott.** 1972. Inhibition of glycoprotein biosynthesis of influenza virus by D-glucosamine and 2-deoxy-D-glucose. Virology **49**:723–734.
11. **McPartland, R. P., M. C. Wang, A. Bloch, and H. Weinfeld.** 1974. Cytidine 5′-triphosphate synthetase as a target for inhibition by the antitumor agent 3-deazauridine. Cancer Res. **34**:3107–3111.
12. **Mitamura, R.** 1936. Uber das Virus der epidemischen Enzephalitis (Sommerenzephalitis) mit besonderer Berucksichtigung seiner immunologischen Eigenschaften und seiner Beziehung zu einem Virus-Stamm der Winterenzephalitis. Trans. Soc. Pathol. Jpn. **26**:429–452.
13. **Schmidt, M. F. G., R. T. Schwarz, and C. Scholtissek.** 1974. Nucleoside-diphosphate derivatives of 2-deoxy-D-glucose in animal cells. Eur. J. Biochem. **49**:237–247.
14. **Scholtissek, C.** 1973. Glycoprotein synthesis of enveloped viruses. Adv. Biosci. **11**:193–204.
15. **Scholtissek, C.** 1975. Inhibition of the multiplication of enveloped viruses by glucose derivatives. Curr. Top. Microbiol. Immunol. **70**:101–119.
16. **Shannon, W. M., G. Arnett, and F. M. Schabel, Jr.** 1972. 3-Deazauridine: inhibition of ribonucleic acid virus-induced cytopathogenic effects in vitro. Antimicrob. Agents Chemother. **2**:159–163.
17. **Shapiro, O., W. E. Brandt, and P. K. Russell.** 1972. Change involving a viral membrane glycoprotein during morphogenesis of group B arboviruses. Virology **50**:906–911.
18. **Shapiro, D., K. A. Kos, and P. K. Russell.** 1973. Japanese encephalitis virus glycoproteins. Virology **56**:88–94.
19. **Webb, J. L.** 1963. Enzyme and metabolic inhibitors, vol. 1. Academic Press Inc., New York.

Antimicrobial Agents and Chemotherapy, Mar. 1977, p. 482-490
Vol. 11, No. 3

Comparative Growth Rates of Selected Anaerobic Species in Four Commonly Used Broth Media

WILLIAM SOTTILE II[1]* AND R. J. ZABRANSKY

Microbiology Research Laboratory, Department of Pathology, Mount Sinai Medical Center, Milwaukee, Wisconsin 53201

Received for publication 1 June 1976

Generations times (g_t) of selected anaerobic species were compared in four culture media commonly used for anaerobic bacteria to evaluate these media for growing inocula for anaerobic antibiotic susceptibility determinations. Twenty-two clinical isolates of *Bacteroides fragilis, Fusobacterium* spp., *Clostridium perfringens,* and *Clostridium* spp. were tested in Schaedler broth, supplemented Lombard-Dowell broth, supplemented thioglycolate broth, and supplemented peptone-yeast extract-glucose broth. Growth curves were performed in an anaerobic chamber; changes in cell density were followed by viable count procedures and, in some cases, turbidometric procedures. The clostridia did not appear to have significantly different g_t values in different media. The g_t values for the five clostridial species tested ranged from 18 to 45 min. The fusobacteria also showed no apparent differences in g_t values in the four media; values ranged from 51 to 60 min. The two subspecies of *B. fragilis* tested showed no significant differences in g_t values when compared with each other in the same media. The combined data, however, indicated that the growth rate in Schaedler broth was faster than in the other media (average g_t, 45.1 min), whereas the growth rate in peptone-yeast extract-glucose was slower (average g_t, 58.2 min). The growth rates in supplemented thioglycolate and supplemented Lombard-Dowell broth (average g_t, 53.6 min and average g_t, 51.0 min, respectively) were not significantly different.

Considerable advances have been made in routine isolation and identification of clinically significant anaerobic bacteria from clinical specimens. After isolation and identification, there are three primary techniques that may be used for antimicrobial susceptibility testing of anaerobic bacteria: (i) broth dilution, (ii) agar dilution, and (iii) agar diffusion. Each technique has numerous modifications and proponents (e.g., references 11, 16, 18, 19). Unfortunately, none of these techniques is nationally standardized as is the agar diffusion technique for aerobic susceptibility testing (National Committee for Clinical Laboratory Standards, Approved standard: ASM-2. Performance standards for antimicrobial disk susceptibility tests, Villanova, Pa. 1975). Regardless of the susceptibility testing technique used, it is important to standardize the initial inoculum because the in vitro antimicrobial susceptibility of an organism can be significantly affected by organism concentration (2, 7, 16). Currently used procedures for anaerobic susceptibility testing use a variety of growth media and inoculum standardization methods; some investigators (1, 8, 11, 15, 16) use the no. 1 MacFarland nephelometric standard or a 50% dilution of the same standard (10) as in the aerobic disk diffusion method, whereas other investigators (4, 5, 12, 13, 17, 18) use various dilutions for 18- to 24-h broth cultures. In using a nephelometric standard to standardize inocula, one must assume that different cultures with the same turbidity have approximately the same number of colony-forming units (CFU) per milliliter. Use of a diluted 18- to 24-h culture for an inoculum source presumes that all cultures will have approximately the same CFU-per-milliliter density at the time the sample is taken. Neither possibility has been adequately documented for anaerobic bacteria.

We thought, therefore, that it would be appropriate to investigate the effects of various broth culture media on the growth of anaerobic isolates routinely recovered in a clinical laboratory. It was the objective of this study to compare four commonly used broth media designed for anaerobes that could be used to grow the inoculum for subsequent antimicrobial suscep-

[1] Present address: Department of Pathology, Chicago Osteopathic Hosptial, Chicago, IL 60615.

tibility testing. The criteria for comparison of each medium to support rapid growth was the generation time (g_t) for selected anaerobes isolated from clinical specimens.

MATERIALS AND METHODS

Organisms. All bacterial cultures were obtained from the clinical microbiology laboratory at Mount Sinai Medical Center, Milwaukee, Wis., through routine isolation procedures for clinical specimens (3, 19) except one isolate, *Bacteroides fragilis* subsp. *fragilis* ATCC 25285, which was provided by T. Wilkins. Each isolate was identified by the procedures outlined by Dowell and Hawkins (6) and was assigned an accession number representing the clinical specimen from which the isolate was derived. The organisms used in the study were as follows: *Bacteroides fragilis* subsp. *fragilis*, 5 isolates; *Bacteroides fragilis* subsp. *thetaiotaomicron*, 4 isolates; *Fusobacterium* species, 4 isolates; *Clostridium perfringens*, 5 isolates; *C. bifermentans*, 1 isolate; *C. cadaveris*, 1 isolate; *C. ramosum*, 1 isolate; and *C. innoculum*, 1 isolate. These particular organisms were chosen because they represent the more frequently encountered, rapidly growing isolates seen in our laboratory.

Media. Four media were used for comparative growth curve studies. They were as follows: (i) Schaedler broth (BBL) without modification; (ii) thioglycolate broth without indicator (Difco) supplemented with 0.5% horse serum (GIBCO) and 1% vitamin K_1-hemin (VK-H) solution (9); (iii) Lombard-Dowell broth supplemented with 0.5% glucose (G. L. Lombard and J. C. McLaughlin, Abstr. Annu. Meet. Am. Soc. Microbiol. 1974, M334, p. 122); and (iv) peptone-yeast extract-glucose (PYG) broth supplemented with 1% VK-H solution (9). Ascites fluid (16) or horse serum (19) is frequently added to thioglycolate broth as a supplement to enhance the growth of fastidious organisms, and we believed it appropriate to include such a supplement in this study. VK-H solution was added to thioglycolate broth so that all media would contain comparable amounts of these growth supplements. Glucose was added to Lombard-Dowell broth so that all media would have comparable amounts of the same fermentable carbohydrate. Two-hundred milliliters of each broth medium was dispensed into 300-ml side arm flasks or, alternatively, 15 ml was dispensed into screw-cap tubes (16 by 150 mm). All media were autoclaved for 15 min at 121°C at 15 lb/in^2; after cooling to 40 to 50°C, all liquid media were promptly placed in an anaerobic chamber until used.

Viable counts were done on Columbia agar (BBL) plates supplemented with 0.5% yeast extract (Difco), 1% VK-H solution (9), and 5% defibrinated sheep blood (GIBCO). After hardening, plates were promptly placed in an anaerobic chamber until used. Both broth and plate media were allowed to become reduced for 24 h before use.

Anaerobic system and instrumentation. All procedures (inoculation, incubation, dilution, spread plating, and reincubation) were done in an anaerobic glove box (Coy Manufacturing, Ann Arbor, Mich.) with an atmosphere of 80% nitrogen, 10% hydrogen, and 10% carbon dioxide. Anaerobic conditions were maintained with a palladium-coated catalyst (Englehard Industries, East Newark, N.J.). All equipment was kept in the glove box for the duration of the study. Turbidity measurements were made within the anaerobic chamber with a Klett-Summerson colorimeter (Klett Manufacturing Co., New York) using a no. 66 red filter (Klett Manufacturing Co.). In the resultant turbidity measurement, 1 Klett unit equals 0.002 optical density units. Broth cultures and inoculated plates were incubated at 37°C in an incubator (Thelco model Z) within the anaerobic chamber.

Growth curve studies. The inoculum for each study was grown for 18 to 24 h in Schaedler broth within the glove box and then diluted in saline so that the inoculated test media would contain a 5×10^{-4} dilution of the inoculum broth. In practice, the inoculated test media contained about 5×10^3 CFU/ml in the late-log or early-stationary phase of growth.

Two kinds of growth curve studies were undertaken. For in-depth studies, representative isolates were selected for each group, and their growth cycles were followed by both turbidometric and viable count procedures in each of the four broth media, (these strains are indicated by an asterisk in Tables 1, 2, and 4). Turbidity measurements (Klett units) in side arm flasks and samples for viable count within the flasks were taken at 2-h intervals during the lag, logarithmic, and early-stationary phases of growth; longer sampling intervals were used thereafter. The in-depth growth studies were repeated within 1 week. The reproducibility of g_t values for a given strain in a given medium was within 10%.

Abbreviated studies were done in screw-cap tubes. Only viable count procedures were used and only during the logarithmic phase of growth. In these cases, samples were taken at the appropriate time intervals suggested by the preliminary and more detailed studies.

Samples for determinations of CFU per milliter were taken with a Selecta-pipette (Clay-Adams, New Jersey) and diluted in 0.85% saline. Blood agar plates were inoculated in duplicate with 0.1 ml of a given dilution and spread over the agar surface with a glass spreader. The time involved in sampling, diluting, and spreading was less than 7 min for each sample. Preliminary studies indicated that this procedure had no significant effect on the number of viable cells over a 7-min time period in an anaerobic atmosphere.

Calculation of g_t values. Linear regression of sampling time (t_x) on $\log_{10}$ CFU per mililliter observed for that sample was used to construct a regression line, from which the g_t could be calculated. This was done to minimize random error due to any given CFU-per-mililliter determination.

Data points for the early- and or late-logarithmic phases of growth were included in the analysis as long as the correlation coefficient for the regression remained above 0.950. The g_t, defined as minutes per generation, was calculated on the basis of the formula: $g_t = (t_f - t_i) \div [(\log_{10} CFU_f/ml - \log_{10}$

$CFU_i/ml) \div \log_{10}2]$, where CFU_f/ml and CFU_i/ml are the final and initial CFU per milliliter, respectively, and t_f and t_i are the times at which the final and initial samples were taken.

Statistical analysis. One-way analysis of variance or Student's t test was used, where appropriate, to determine whether observed differences in mean g_t values were statistically significant. The one-way analysis of variance was used to test the significance of differences between three or more sample means. Unless otherwise stated, the 95% confidence level ($\alpha = 0.05$) was chosen as the threshold for determination of significant differences between mean values. The reader is referred to standard texts on statistics for details concerning the performance of these tests.

RESULTS

The g_t values for five isolates of *C. perfringens* on each of the four media are shown in Table 1. Each isolate is denoted by its accession number in the left-hand column. Although it would appear that the average g_t was longest in supplemented thioglycolate broth, the analysis of variance indicates that there is no significant difference in growth rate of *C. perfringens* in any of the four media at the 95% confidence level. Values for g_t of four other clostridial species appear in Table 2. Except for *C. perfringens*, the other clostridia were tested only once in each medium, and it cannot be stated whether the observed differences in g_t values for a given organism are significantly different in different media. However, when the average g_t values observed for one organism are compared with those of another organism, some significant differences can be found. Specifically, the mean g_t values for *C. ramosum* and *C. cadaveris*, 32 and 33 min, respectively, are not significantly different, whereas the mean g_t value for *C. innoculum*, 46 min, is significantly different from those observed for *C. ramosum* or *C. cadaveris*. Furthermore, the mean g_t value for *C. perfringens*, 25 min, appears to be significantly less than that of *C. ramosum* and significantly more than that of *C. bifermentans*, 18 min.

In contrast to *C. perfringens*, the two subspecies of *B. fragilis* that were studied show statistically significant differences in g_t values in different media. Analysis of variance of the observed g_t values in different media. Analysis of variance of the observed g_t values for *B. fragilis* subsp. *fragilis*, listed in Table 3, indicated that one or more of the average g_t values were significantly different from the others.

TABLE 1. *g_t values of Clostridium perfringens*[a]

Isolate accession no.	g_t (min/doubling) in: Schaedler broth (avg = 23.9, SD = 4.2)	Thioglycolate[b] (avg = 26.6, SD = 7.1)	Lombard broth[b] (avg = 23.6, SD = 3.8)	PGY[b] (avg = 24.2, SD = 0.4)
1058-1*	23.6	31.0	19.0	24.2
3708-6	22.1	21.2	26.9	24.7
3544-6	31.2	36.9	20.6	23.6
4640-1	22.4	23.6	27.5	24.3
4839-1	20.4	20.5	24.1	24.1

[a] Asterisk indicates that generation times for this isolate were calculated from data taken during "in-depth" studies where all phases of growth were monitored. Generation times for isolates without asterisk were calculated from abbreviated studies in which only logarithmic growth was monitored.

[b] Plus appropriate supplements.

TABLE 2. *Comparison of g_t values for five Clostridium species*[a]

Medium	g_t (min/doubling) for: *C. innoccum* (avg = 45.8, SD = 1.8)	*C. rasmosum** (avg = 32.5, SD = 0.3)	*C. cadaveris* (avg = 32.7, SD = 1.9)	*C. perfringens*[b] (avg = 24.6, SD = 4.3)	*C. bifermentans** (avg = 18.4, SD = 2.7)
Schaedler broth	44.4	32.8	35.5	23.9	14.8
Thioglycolate broth[c]	44.1	32.2	32.2	26.6	20.9
Lombard broth[c]	46.7	32.4	31.3	23.6	17.9
PYG[c]	47.8	32.7	31.9	24.2	20.0

[a] Asterisk indicates that generation times for this isolate were calculated from data taken during "in-depth" studies where all phases of growth were monitored. Generation times for isolates without asterisk were calculated from abbreviated studies where only logarithmic growth was monitored.

[b] Average and standard deviation for *C. perfringens* were taken from the data in Table 1.

[c] Plus the appropriate supplements.

Similarly, an analysis of variance of the g_t values for *B. fragilis* subsp. *thetaiotaomicron*, listed in Table 4, indicated that there were statistically significant differences in the growth rates among the four different media.

A summary of the data used to compare the two *B. fragilis* subspecies on a medium-by-medium basis appears in Table 5. The results of testing indicated that there were no significant differences in the growth rates of the two subspecies in any given medium tested, even though the growth rates in different media are significantly different. Upon combining the g_t data for subspecies, also noted in Table 5, an analysis of variance indicated that one or more of the average g_t values in the four media were significantly different from the others at the 99.0% confidence level. The average g_t value for both subspecies is shortest in Schaedler broth and longest in supplemented PYG. By deleting the data for one of the media exhibiting either the longest or shortest average g_t value, the remaining media can be tested for significant differences. After deleting the data for Schaedler broth and performing an analysis of variance on the three remaining media, the results indicated that one or all of the average g_t values were still significantly different. Similarly,

TABLE 3. *g_t values of Bacteroides fragilis subsp. fragilis*

Isolate accession no.	g_t (min/doubling) in: Schaedler broth (avg = 46.6, SD = 4.4)	Thioglycolate[a] (avg = 55.0, SD = 6.7)	Lombard broth[a] (avg = 50.4, SD = 5.5)	PYG[a] (avg = 57.3, SD = 1.8)
3326-1	46.5	51.1	42.8	55.0
3468-4	46.5	45.3	49.7	58.3
3492-1	44.0	58.0	58.0	lost
3585-1	53.7	59.2	48.8	59.0
ATCC 25285	42.2	61.4	52.5	56.7

[a] Plus appropriate supplements.

TABLE 4. *g_t values of Bacteroides fragilis subsp. thetaiotaomicron*[a]

Isolate accession no.	g_t (min/doubling) in: Schaedler broth (avg = 43.4, SD = 3.7)	Thioglycolate[b] (avg = 51.9, SD = 4.6)	Lombard broth[b] (avg = 51.9, SD = 0.8)	PYG[b] (avg = 59.2, SD 9.2)
2957–9*	41.6	50.7	52.2	50.9
3139–1	43.1	50.2	51.8	51.7
3708–1	40.1	48.1	50.5	67.8
807–4	48.6	58.5	52.3	66.3

[a] Asterisk indicates that generation times for this isolate were calculated from data taken during "in-depth" studies where all phases of growth were monitored. Generation times for isolates without an asterisk were calculated from abbreviated studies where only logarithmic growth was monitored.
[b] Plus appropriate supplements.

TABLE 5. *Summary of comparative statistical data for Bacteroides fragilis subsp. fragilis and B. fragilis subsp. thetaiotaomicron*

Subspecies	Schaedler broth	Thioglycolate	Lombard broth	PYG
g_t				
Bacteroides fragilis subsp. *fragilis*	43.3	51.9	51.7	59.1
B. fragilis subsp. *thetaiotaomicron*	46.6	55.0	50.4	57.3
Significant differences between subspecies[a]	None	None	None	None
Average g_t[b] for both subspecies combined	45.1	53.6	51.0	58.2
SD	4.2	5.7	4.2	6.2

[a] Determined by Student's *t* test.
[b] Average g_t values were computed from all the entries for each medium listed in Tables 3 and 4.

after deleting the data for supplemented PYG and repeating the analysis in the first three media, the results indicated that one or all of the average g_t values were significantly different. This suggests that both the average g_t in Schaedler broth and average g_t in supplemented PYG were significantly different from the two intermediate values. Testing the difference between average g_t in supplemented thioglycolate broth and the average g_t of both subspecies in supplemented Lombard-Dowell broth combined indicated that there was no significant difference between these two.

Thus, it would appear from the data that the significant differences at the 95% confidence level between media for both subspecies of *B. fragilis* combined were as follows: (i) Schaedler broth, generation time = 45.1 min (standard deviation [SD] = 4.2 min); (ii) thioglycolate and Lombard-Dowell broth, generation time = 52.3 min (SD = 5.0 min); and (iii) PYG, generation time = 58.2 min (SD = 6.2 min).

An analysis of variance of the g_t data for the *Fusobacterium* species, listed in Table 6, indicated no significant differences in average g_t values among any of the four media. However, we believe that, because of the small sample size and wide apparent ranges in g_t values, our conclusions about this genus must remain tentative. Isolates 360-1, 3872-2, and F-2 were all *F. nucleatum*, whereas isolate F-1 was *F. necrophorum*. The standard inoculum in all of the growth studies was about 5 × 10^3 CFU/ml, which may have been too low for the fusobacteria to rapidly initiate growth. In three cases, the isolates simply did not grow in some of the test media during the time samples were being taken.

Examples of the turbidity and viable count data plotted against time for *C. perfringens* (1058-1), *C. ramosum*, and *B. fragilis* subsp. *thetaiotaomicron* (2957-9) appear in Fig. 1, 2, and 3, respectively. In Fig. 1, it is apparent that turbidity of *C. perfringens* does not appreciably increase until the number of cells reaches approximately 10^7 to 10^8 CFU/ml, which is about the end of logarithmic growth for this organism. Furthermore, the stationary-phase density is about 10^8 to 10^9 CFU/ml, and appears rather stable over a 10- to 12-h period. The turbidity and viable count curves behave differently for *C. ramosum* (Fig. 2). Again, turbidity does not increase appreciably until the number of cells is about 10^6 to 10^7 CFU/ml, which occurs toward the end of the logarithmic growth. However, in this case, the viable cell count appears to drop slightly within the range of 10^8 to 10^9 CFU/ml, whereas the turbidity tends to increase at a more gradual rate than is evident during logarithmic growth. In the third example, *B. fragilis* subsp. *thetaiotaomicron* (Fig. 3), the turbidity in three of the media does not appreciably increase until the cell population has reached a stationary phase of growth with approximately 10^9 CFU/ml. In contrast, the turbidity in Schaedler broth began to increase in the mid-logarithmic phase of growth and did not begin to taper off until the stationary phase of growth was established. In all three examples presented, the viable counts were more predictable in terms of growth in different media than the comparable turbidity measurements.

DISCUSSION

The standardization of an antimicrobial susceptibility testing procedure for anaerobic bacteria will depend ultimately upon an understanding of the physiological requirements and responses of these organisms. It is recognized that any given procedure will not be satisfactory for all anaerobic organisms, just as the aerobic disk diffusion technique is not suitable for all aerobic and facultative organisms. For this reason, we chose to study the least fastidious organisms with rapid rates of growth, which are also the organisms most commonly isolated from clinical specimens. Our objective has been to compare four commonly used anaerobic culture media in terms of their ability

TABLE 6. *g_t values of Fusobacterium spp.*

Isolate accession no.	g_t (min/doubling) in:			
	Schaedler broth (avg 51.7, SD = 3.1)	Thioglycolate[a] (avg = 54.9, SD = 5.4)	Lombard broth[a] (avg = 57.3, SD = 7.9)	PGY[a] (avg = 60.1, SD = 12.3)
360-1	53.9	57.2	62.5	67.0
3872-2	54.6	58.8	60.6	67.5
F-1	48.3	lost	48.0	45.9
F-2	49.8	48.7	lost	lost

[a] Plus appropriate supplements.

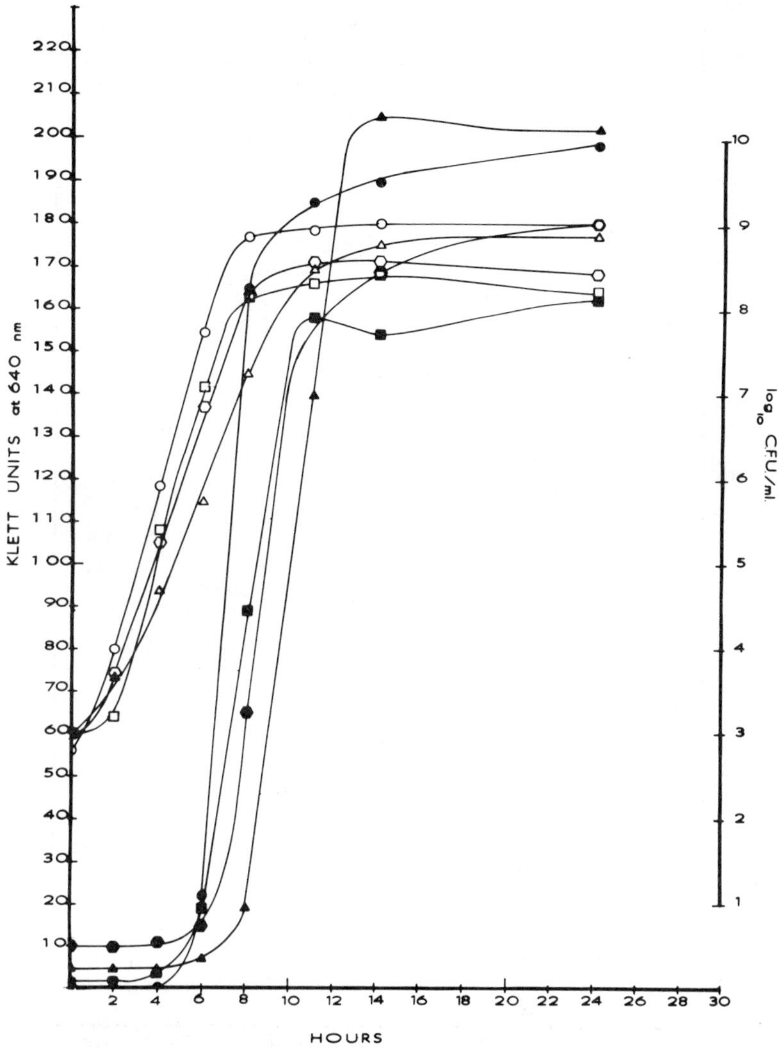

FIG. 1. *Growth curves of Clostridium perfringens in four culture media. Open symbols represent CFU/ml; closed symbols represent Klett turbidity values. Symbols: Schaedler broth (○, ●), supplemented thioglycolate broth (△, ▲), supplemented Lombard-Dowell broth (□, ■), supplemented PYG broth (⬡, ⬢).*

to support rapid growth, and to determine which single medium, if any, would support the most rapid growth.

The only species for which we could detect significant differences in g_t values in different media were the two subspecies of *B. fragilis*. All species tested grew in Schaedler broth as well, if not better than, in the other media tested.

Stalons et al. (14) have published a study similar to ours using a wider variety of media and organisms; however, their criterion for comparison was the "percent of change in turbidity calculated after a 24-h incubation period." From the three examples presented above (Fig. 1–3), it can be seen that an organism may grow at approximately the same rate and have the same number of organisms in different media, but produce strikingly different turbidometric responses. The examples above demonstrate that turbidity may or may not increase during logarithmic growth and, consequently, does not accurately reflect the number of organisms in the four different media. Although turbidity is a function of cell concentration, it can be influenced by size, shape, and presence or absence of cellular inclusions. Casual observation of some isolates

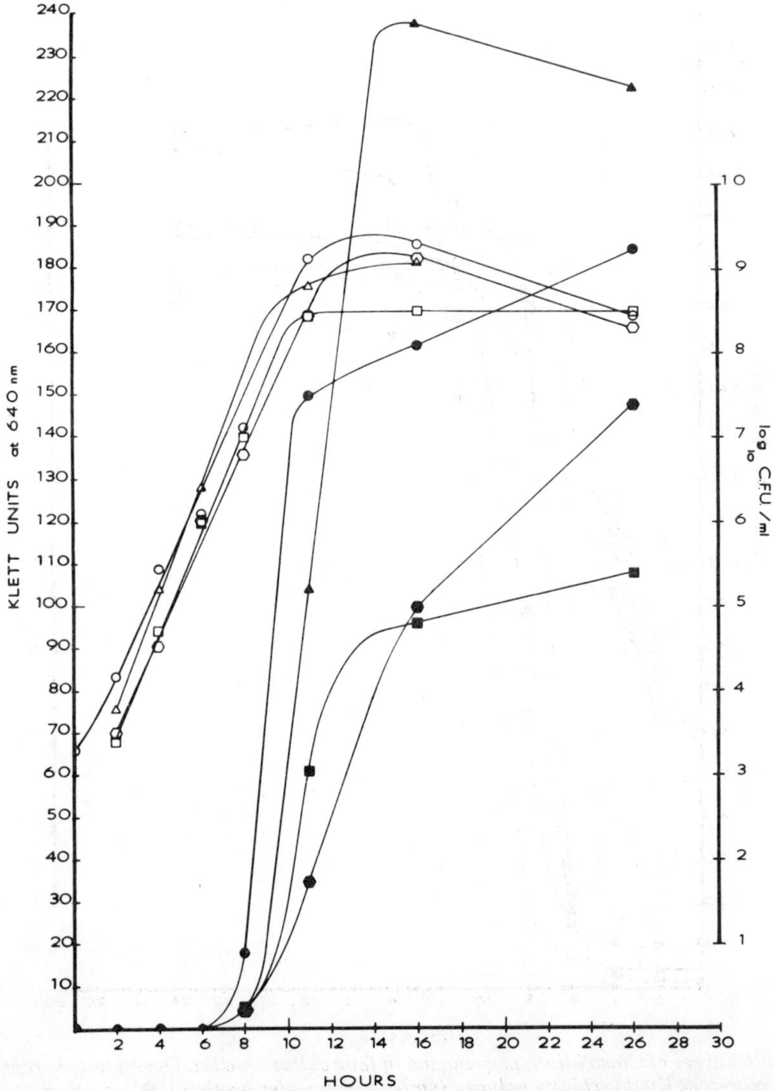

FIG. 2. *Growth curves of Clostridium ramosum in four culture media. Open symbols represent CFU/ml; closed symbols represent Klett turbidity values. Symbols: Schaedler broth (○, ●), supplemented thioglycolate broth (△, ▲), supplemented Lombard-Dowell broth (□, ■), supplemented PYG broth (⬡, ⬢).*

over the growth cycle disclosed some change in overall size and Gram-staining characteristics, but none of these effects appeared to be particularly characteristic of any given medium. We, therefore, do not think that turbidity is a satisfactory basis on which to compare bacterial growth, unless the relationship between turbidity and CFU per milliliter is actually known. Nevertheless, despite the differences in approach to the problem of comparative growth rates, our results are in general agreement with those of Stalons et al.

Ericsson and Sherris (7) cite results obtained with different aerobic cultures. Their data indicate the cultures in stationary-growth stages may show differences of up to 1,000-fold in viable counts within individual species. In contrast, we observed a rather narrow range for different species. Early-stationary-phase counts for most species tested routinely fell between 1×10^8 and 5×10^9 CFU/ml, regardless of the growth and medium used.

We propose that an appropriate dilution of an early-stationary-phase culture grown in Schae-

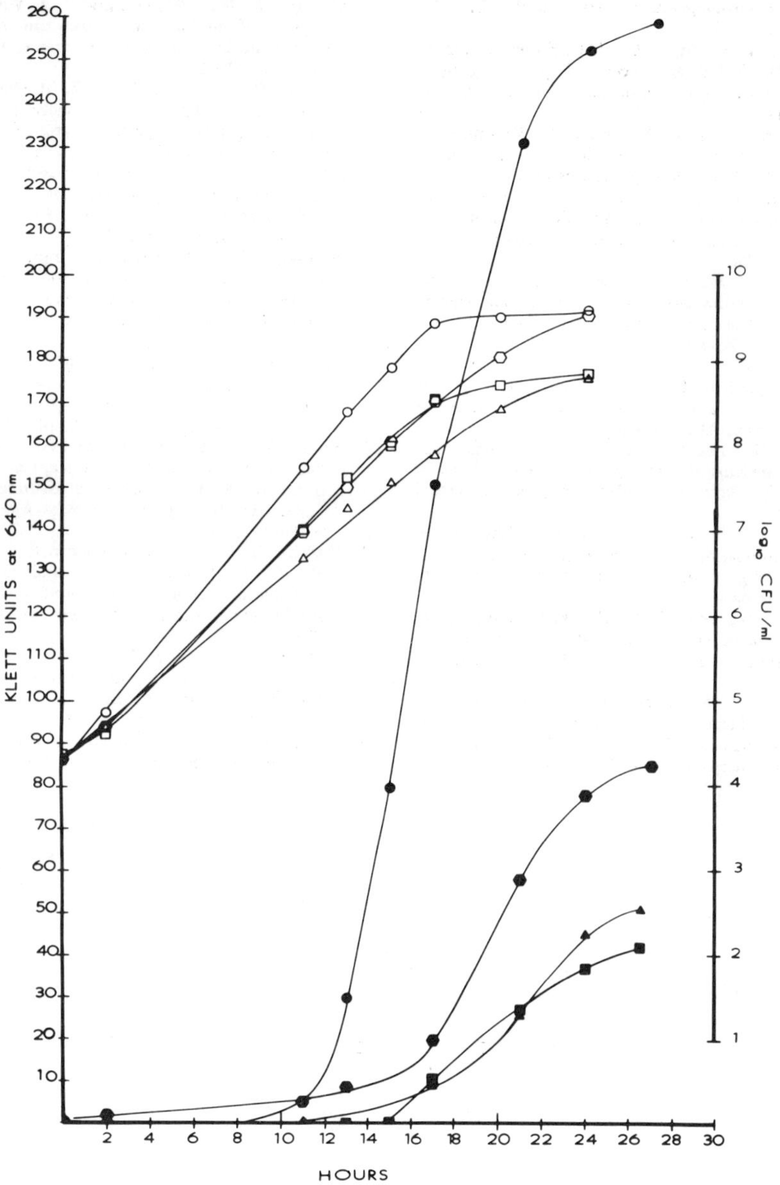

FIG. 3. *Growth curves of Bacteroides fragilis subsp. thetaiotaomicron in four culture media. Open symbols represent CFU/ml; closed symbols represent Klett turbidity values. Symbols: Schaedler broth (○, ●), supplemented thiogylcolate broth (△, ▲), supplemented Lombard-Dowell broth (□, ■), supplemented PYG broth (⬡, ⬢).*

dler broth would provide a more satisfactory inoculum for anaerobic susceptibility testing than would adjustment of turbidity to agree with a turbidity standard. The use of an "overnight" culture as an inoculum source has been used with acceptable results by other investigators (4, 5, 12, 14, 17, 18).

ACKNOWLEDGMENT

The technical assistance of Kenneth Hauser is greatly appreciated.

LITERATURE CITED

1. **Barry, A. L., and C. D. Fay.** 1974. Evaluation of four disc diffusion methods for antimicrobic susceptiblity

tests with anaerobic gram negative bacilli. Clin. Pathol 61:592–598.
2. **Bauer, A. W., W. M. M. Kirby, J. C. Sherris, and M. Turck.** 1966. Antibiotic susceptibility testing by a standardized single disk method. Am. J. Clin. Pathol. 45:493–496.
3. **Blair, J. E., E. H. Lennette, and J. P. Traunt (ed).** 1975. Manual of clinical microbiology, 2nd ed. American Society for Microbiology, Bethesda, Md.
4. **Blazevic, D. J.** 1975. Evaluation of the modified broth-disk method for determining antibiotic susceptibilities of anaerobic bacteria. Antimicrob. Agents Chemother. 7:721–723.
5. **Dornbusch, K., C. E. Nord, and B. Olsson.** 1975. Antibiotic susceptibility testing of anaerobic bacteria by standardized disc diffusion method with special reference to *Bacteroides fragilis*. Scand. J. Infect. Dis. 7:59–66.
6. **Dowell, V. R., and T. M. Hawkins (ed.).** 1968. Laboratory methods in anaerobic bacteriology. Center for Disease Control, Atlanta, Ga.
7. **Ericsson, H. M., and J. C. Sherris.** 1971. Antibiotic sensitivity testing. Report of an international collaborative study. Acta. Path. Microbiol. Scand. Sect. B 217(Suppl.).
8. **Hauser, K. J., J. A. Johnston, and R. J. Zabransky.** 1975. Economical agar dilution techniques for susceptibility testing of anaerobic bacteria. Antimicrob. Agents Chemother. 7:7–12.
9. **Holdeman, L. V., and W. E. C. Moore (ed.).** 1973. Anaerobe laboratory manual, 2nd ed. Virginia Polytechnic Institute Anaerobe Laboratory, Blacksburg, Va.
10. **Overman, S. V., D. W. Lambe, and J. V. Bennett.** 1974. Proposed standardized method for testing and interpreting susceptibility of *Bacteroides fragilis* to tetracycline. Antimicrob. Agents Chemother. 5:357–361.
11. **Rahimi, A., W. J. Martin, and J. A. Washington.** 1974. Effects of medium and inoculum on antimicrobial susceptibility of anaerobic bacteria. Am. J. Clin. Pathol. 62:425–427.
12. **Rotilie, C. A., R. J. Fass, R. B. Prior, and R. L. Perkins.** 1975. Microbilution technique for antimicrobial susceptibility testing of anaerobic bacteria. Antimicrob. Agents Chemother. 7:311–315.
13. **Schoutens, E., and E. Yourassowsky.** 1974. Speed of bactericidal action of penicillin G, ampicillin, and carbenicillin on *Bacteroides fragilis*. Antimicrob. Agents Chemother. 6:227–231.
14. **Stalons, D. R., C. Thornsberry, and V. R. Dowell.** 1974. The effect of culture medium and carbon dioxide concentration on the growth of anerobic bacteria commonly encountered in clinical specimens. Appl. Microbiol. 27:1098–1104.
15. **Sutter, V. L., Y-Y. Kwok, and S. M. Finegold.** 1972. Standardized antimicrobial disc susceptibility testing of anaerobic bacteria I. Susceptibility of *Bacteroides fragilis* to tetracycline. Appl. Microbiol. 23:268–275.
16. **Sutter, V. L., Y-Y. Kwok, and S. M. Finegold.** 1973. Susceptibility of *Bacteroides fragilis* to six antibiotics determined by standardized antimicrobial disc susceptibility testing. Antimicrob. Agents Chemother. 3:188–193.
17. **Wilkins, T. D., L. V. Holdemann, I. J. Abramson, and W. E. C. Moore.** 1972. Standardized single-disc method for antibiotic susceptibility testing of anaerobic bacteria. Antimicrob. Agents Chemother. 1:451–459.
18. **Wilkins, T. D., and T. Thiel.** 1973. Modified broth-disk method for testing the antibiotic susceptibility of anaerobic bacteria. Antimicrob. Agents Chemother. 3:350–356.
19. **Zabransky, R. J.** 1970. Isolation of anaerobic bacteria from clinical specimens. Mayo Clin. Proc. 45:256–264.

ANTIMICROBIAL AGENTS AND CHEMOTHERAPY, Mar. 1977, p. 491-499
Vol. 11, No. 3
Printed in U.S.A.

Inhibition of Initiation, Elongation, and Termination of Eukaryotic Protein Synthesis by Trichothecene Fungal Toxins

ERIC CUNDLIFFE[1] AND JULIAN E. DAVIES*

Department of Biochemistry, College of Agricultural and Life Sciences, University of Wisconsin-Madison, Madison, Wisconsin 53706

Received for publication 7 June 1976

The 12,13-epoxytrichothecenes, specific inhibitors of protein synthesis in eukaryotes, can be subdivided further in terms of their mode of action. In addition to the I-type (initiation inhibitors) and E-types (elongation inhibitors), we found that some E-types apparently exhibit inhibition of chain termination at low concentrations. The nature of substituents on C4 may determine the type of inhibitory activity observed.

The 12,13-epoxytrichothecenes (sesquiterpenoid fungal toxins) inhibit protein synthesis in eukaryotes but not in bacteria (for a comprehensive review, see reference 1). After the original demonstration that nivalenol inhibits protein synthesis in reticulocyte extracts (14), a number of these compounds have been shown to inhibit in vitro the "fragment reaction"—that is, an assay for ribosomal peptidyl transferase activity studied in isolation from other reactions normally involved in protein synthesis (3). However, when tested in systems synthesizing protein, either in vivo (7) or in vitro (10), it became clear that the trichothocenes fall into (at least) two functional groups. Thus (7), some trichothecenes inhibit the initiation of protein synthesis, whereas others inhibit either elongation or termination (or both). Other workers (12, 15) have concluded that trichodermin (a trichothecene) is a specific inhibitor of polypeptide chain termination, although it is clear that the drug can inhibit, under particular conditions in vitro, assays for both elongation and termination of polypeptides (13).

Here, we report that those trichothecenes which do not inhibit the initiation of protein synthesis can be divided into two further groups according to their actions in vivo. They include "E-types," which inhibit polypeptide chain elongation, and "T-types," which apparently inhibit chain termination preferentially at relatively low concentrations. Both E-types and T-types inhibit elongation of protein chains at higher concentrations. We also find differences between the actions of different "I-type" trichothecenes (inhibitors of polypeptide chain initiation) in intact H-HeLa cells.

[1] Present address: Department of Pharmacology, Cambridge University Medical School, Cambridge CB2 2QD, England.

MATERIALS AND METHODS

Growth of H-HeLa cells. All procedures were as described previously (7), including the change of growth medium (to remove amino acids and serum) prior to attempting to incorporate radioactive amino acids into proteins of intact cells. In all experiments, H-HeLa cells were growing exponentially at 37°C at densities of 3×10^5 to 4×10^5 cells per ml when used.

Sampling of H-HeLa cells and preparation of lysates. Ten milliliters of cells was pipetted into an equal volume of frozen, crushed, isotonic TMNa buffer [10 mM tris(hydroxymethyl)aminomethane, 15 mM $MgCl_2$ and 140 mM NaCl, adjusted with HCl to pH 7.6 at 20°C, and allowed to thaw at 0°C]. The cells were collected by centrifugation at $10,000 \times g$ for 5 min at 4°C in a Sorvall SS34 rotor. Pellets were then resuspended in 0.3 ml of TMNa buffer (containing 140 mM NaCl or 500 mM NaCl—see figure legends and text as appropriate), and lysis was facilitated by adding Nonidet P-40 (0.5%, vol/vol, final concentration). Lysis occurred rapidly at 0°C and, at this time, pancreatic ribonuclease (10 μg/ml, final concentration) was added to certain lysates (see legend to Fig. 3). Incubation with ribonuclease was continued at 0°C for 10 min before analysis of lysates on sucrose density gradients.

Sucrose density gradient analysis. Each lysate of H-HeLa cells (0.3 ml) in TMNa buffer (containing either 140 mM NaCl or 500 mM NaCl) was layered onto a sucrose density gradient (5-ml total volume, ranging from 10 to 30%, wt/vol, sucrose) made up in TMNa buffer of composition identical to that in which the lysate was prepared. Centrifugation was either for 40 min at 35,000 rpm or for 110 min at 40,000 rpm (see figure legends) at 3°C in the Spinco SW50.1 rotor. After centrifugation, the absorbance of components in the gradients was monitored continuously at 254 nm in a gradient analyzer (Isco model DUA-2) pumping at 1 ml/min and with a chart speed of 20 mm/min.

Toxins. These were used dissolved in dimethyl sulfoxide (Me_2SO) so that the final concentrations of Me_2SO in reaction mixtures never exceeded 1% (vol/vol). In controls, Me_2SO did not contribute to any of the effects reported here.

Incorporation of leucine into protein in vivo. Cultures of H-HeLa cells were transferred to a medium lacking amino acids and serum (see reference 7) and were incubated in that medium at 37°C for 15 min before use. Then, L-[^{14}C]leucine (342 mCi/mmol, 0.25 μCi/ml, final concentration) was added together with a particular trichothecene (see Fig. 1 and Table 1) and incubation was continued at 37°C. Samples of 1 ml each were taken at various times into 1 ml of 10% (wt/vol) trichloroacetic acid held at 90°C for 20 min and then cooled in ice. Precipitated material was collected on Whatman GF/C glass-fiber disks, which were washed three times with 5% (wt/vol) trichloroacetic acid, dried, and prepared for liquid scintillation counting according to standard procedures (7).

RESULTS

Effects of trichothecenes on protein synthesis in intact H-HeLa cells. Trichothecene toxins, particularly those previously classified by us as "I-types" (7) are potent inhibitors of protein synthesis in H-HeLa cells. As shown in Table 1, these toxins virtually halted protein synthesis within 2 to 3 min when employed at final concentrations of 1 μg/ml. The table also shows the effects of T-2 toxin upon protein synthesis when used at lower concentrations over a time course of 10 min.

Other trichothecenes, known to inhibit either elongation or termination of protein chains (7), are less potent inhibitors in intact H-HeLa cells (Fig. 1). Trichodermin inhibits protein synthesis by around 50% at 0.5 μg/ml (final concentration) and does so completely at around 20 μg/ml. In comparison with trichodermin, trichodermol is a less potent inhibitor, and other compounds such as 4-epitrichodermol are without inhibitory effect. The structures of various trichothecenes are given in Fig. 6.

Effects of trichothecenes on profiles of ribosomes and polyribosomes in intact H-HeLa cells. (i) We first examined a group of trichothecene toxins which were known to inhibit polypeptide chain elongation or termination or both (7). Their effects upon polyribosome profiles are given in Fig. 2—control profiles did not change significantly during the time courses employed (data not given). As seen in Fig. 2a, d, f, and h, trichodermin, trichodermol, and trichothecin all preserved polyribosomes at control sizes (although there was some buildup in amounts of smaller polyribosomes) when the toxins were used at high concentrations. Vomitoxin and trichodermone also gave similar effects when used at 20 to 50 μg/ml for up to 30 min (data not given). However, when used at concentrations not sufficient to stop protein synthesis, the trichothecenes were distinguishable according to whether they caused a buildup of large polyribosomes (vomitoxin and trichodermol—Fig. 2b and f) or a breakdown of polyribosomes (trichodermin and trichothecin—Fig. 2c and g). At drug concentrations around 10 μg/ml, trichodermone resembled trichodermol and caused a buildup of polyribosomes (data not given).

Profiles such as those shown in Fig. 2 (obtained by analysis in 140 mM NaCl) allow one to observe the size distributions of polyribosomes, but it is difficult to quantitate the data, since materials are distributed throughout the gradients, and variable amounts of polyribosomes are pelleted. Accordingly, we decided to

TABLE 1. *Effects of various trichothecenes on incorporation of [^{14}C]leucine into protein in intact H-HeLa cells*[a]

Incubation time (min)	[^{14}C]leucine incorporated (cpm) with: None	Verrucarin A 1 μg/ml	Verrucarin A 50 μg/ml	Roridin A (1 μg/ml)	T-2 toxin 1 μg/ml	T-2 toxin 0.5 μg/ml	T-2 toxin 0.1 μg/ml	HT-2 toxin (1 μg/ml)	DAS (1 μg/ml)
1	6,690	5,828	4,532						
1.5	11,460	7,571		8,689	6,989			7,576	8,120
3	16,018	8,354	5,426						
5	25,798	8,756	5,838						
7	41,899	12,426		12,473	12,538			20,932	14,700
10	58,834	12,977		12,388	12,741			21,870	14,911
	62,643				14,299	16,835	28,309		

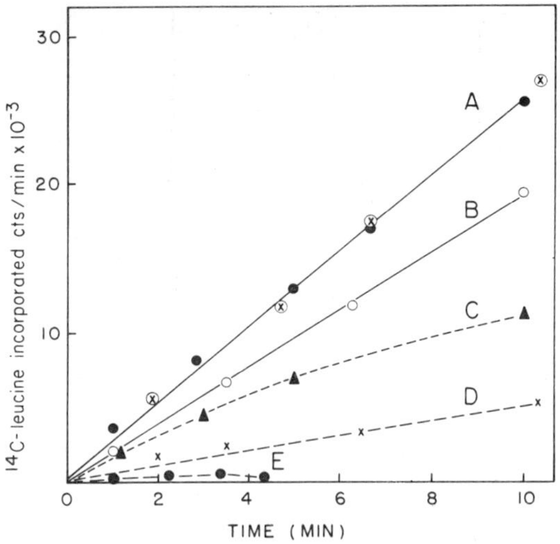

FIG. 1. *Effects of trichodermol and trichodermin on incorporation of [^{14}C]leucine into protein in intact H-HeLa cells. Drug added together with isotope at zero time. (A) Incorporation in control (●) or with 10 μg/ml of 4-epitrichodermol (○); (B) trichodermol (1 μg/ml added; (C) trichodermin (0.5 μg/ml) added; (D) trichodermol (10 μg/ml) added; (E) trichodermin (30 μg/ml) added. Final concentrations of drugs are given.*

analyze our lysates in 500 mM NaCl (see Materials and Methods) in which free 80*S* ribosomes are unstable and dissociate into 60*S* and 40*S* subunits. Also, we degraded polyribosomes to 80*S* monosomes, which are stable in 500 mM NaCl, by the action of pancreatic ribonuclease. Typical results are given in Fig. 3, in which ribosomal material possessing a sedimentation coefficient of 80*S* represents material present as polyribosomes before ribonuclease digestion. By comparing the areas under the various absorbance peaks recorded, we calculated that about 60% of the ribosomes present in control lysates were usually associated with messenger ribonucleic acid (mRNA) (63% in Fig. 3a). After incubation of H-HeLa cells with partially inhibitory concentrations of trichodermol (Fig. 3d) or trichodermone (Fig. 3e), 67 and 76%, respectively, of the ribosomes were estimated to have been present as polyribosomes. The corresponding values after incubation of H-HeLa cells with trichodermin were 51% when the drug was present at low concentrations (Fig. 3b) and 55% when high concentrations were employed (Fig. 3c). These results again indicate that low concentrations of trichodermol and trichodermone cause a buildup of polyribosomes, in agreement with the data presented in Fig. 2. Contrariwise, trichodermin usually causes a certain amount of polyribosome degradation.

(ii) In a second series of experiments, we examined a group of trichothecene toxins (I-types), which apparently inhibit polypeptide chain initiation in eukaryotes (7). Previously (7), we showed the effects upon polyribosome

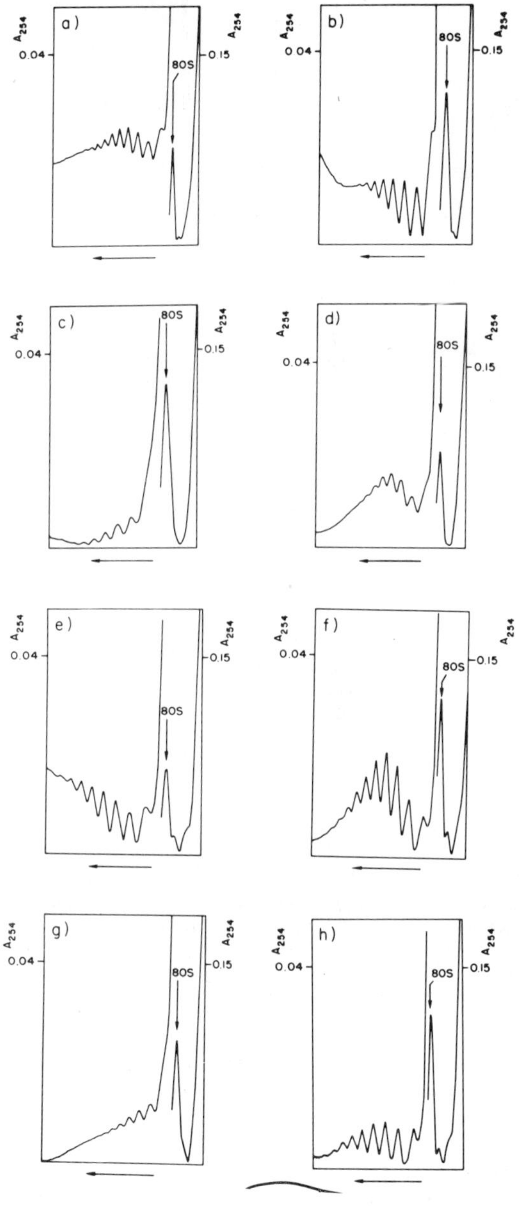

FIG. 2. *Effects of trichothecenes upon polyribosomes of H-HeLa cell. Cells were incubated with the following toxins for the times indicated. (a) None—control; (b) vomitoxin, 5 μg/ml, for 3 min; (c) trichodermin, 0.5 μg/ml, for 3 min; (d) trichodermin, 10 μg/ml, for 20 min; (e) trichodermol, 1 μg/ml, for 30 min; (f) trichodermol, 25 μg/ml, for 30 min; (g) trichothecin, 2 μg/ml, for 30 min; (h) trichothecin, 50 μg/ml for 30 min. Lysates and gradients contained 140 mM NaCl, and centrifugation was at 35,000 rpm for 40 min.*

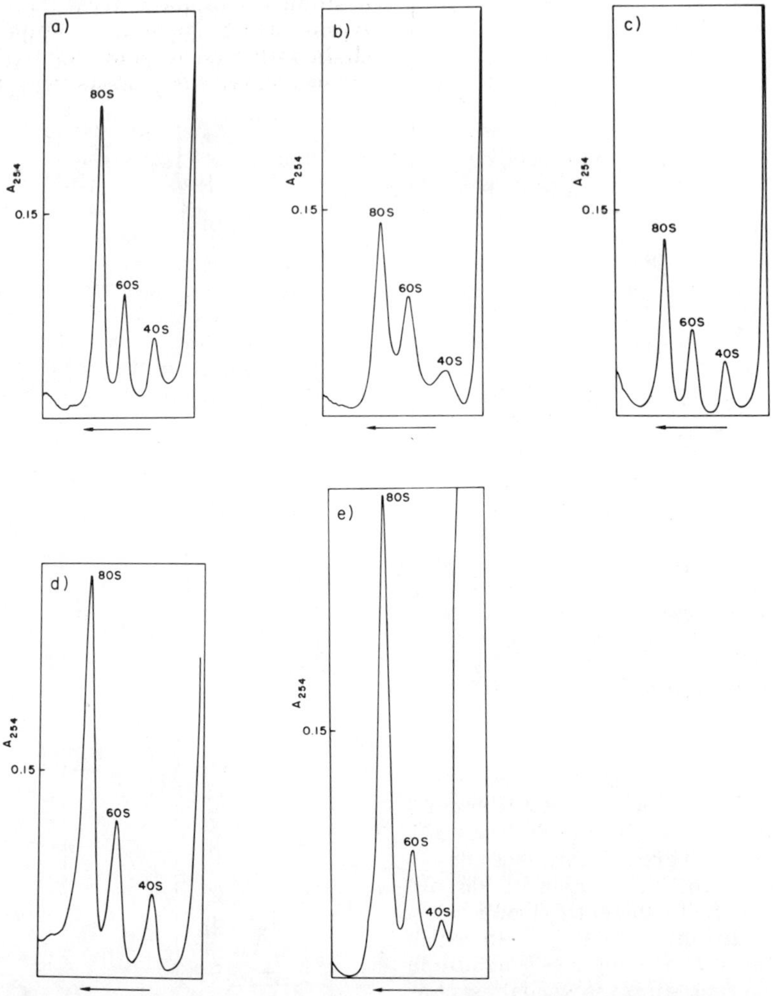

FIG. 3. *Effects of trichothecenes upon the polyribosome content of H-HeLa cells. Cells were incubated with toxins for the times indicated: (a) none—control; (b) trichodermin, 0.5 μg/ml, for 15 min; (c) trichodermin, 50 μg/ml, for 14 min; (d) trichodermol, 5 μg/ml, for 15 min; (e) trichodermone, 10 μg/ml, for 20 min. Lysates and gradients contained 500 mM NaCl, and centrifugation was at 40,000 rpm for 110 min after treatment of lysates with ribonuclease.*

profiles of incubating H-HeLa cells for 1 min with T-2 toxin, nivalenol, or verrucarin A at drug concentrations of 15 or 25 μg/ml. Here we reexamined the effects of these compounds, together with those of HT-2 toxin, roridin A, and diacetoxyscirpenol (DAS), over a wide range of drug concentrations and over longer periods of treatment. Except DAS, this group of compounds were inseparable in their effects and caused total degradation of the polyribosomes of H-HeLa cells within 2 to 3 min of drug addition, regardless of the amount of drug employed. Typical results obtained with verrucarin A are given in Fig. 4, together with the "aberrant" behavior of DAS. The latter toxin behaved like other I-types in the concentration range 1 to 5 μg/ml and caused complete and rapid breakdown of polyribosomes (Fig. 4c). However, when DAS was employed at 100 μg/ml (an exceedingly high concentration), polyribosomes were only partially degraded (Fig. 4d), in contrast to the effects observed with other I-types at similar concentrations.

Finally, we decided to examine more closely the character of any "initiation complexes" that might survive the treatment of H-HeLa cells with I-type trichothecenes. We prepared and analyzed lysates of such treated cells in 500 mM NaCl to dissociate free 80*S* ribosomes to subunits and to leave only mRNA-associated particles able to sediment faster than 60S. As shown in Fig. 5a, control lysates contain only a very few 80S monosomes, and there is no evidence of any other material sedimenting faster than 60S in such a gradient. (Under these conditions, "disomes" are pelleted in the sucrose gradients.) After exposure of HeLa cells to I-type trichothecenes, two different situations were encountered. With some I-types (e.g., nivalenol, T-2 toxin, and HT-2 toxin), ribosome profiles very similar to those observed in control lysates were observed (Fig. 5b). There was no obvious accumulation of any material sedimenting faster than 80S, and (data not given) there was no evidence for pelleted ribosomal materials. However, when H-HeLa cells were incubated with verrucarin A or roridin A (at whatever concentration), absorbance profiles with an extra peak (peak 2 in Fig. 5c), corresponding to material sedimenting faster than 80S monosomes (peak 1 in Fig. 5c), were obtained. This novel material was clearly sedimenting at a rate between those expected for monosomes or disomes. When samples were taken from gradients similar to that represented in Fig. 5c, digested mildly with ribonuclease, and reanalyzed on sucrose gradients, the results shown in Fig. 5d and e were obtained. As expected, the sedimentation properties of 80S monosomes (peak 1 in Fig. 5c) were

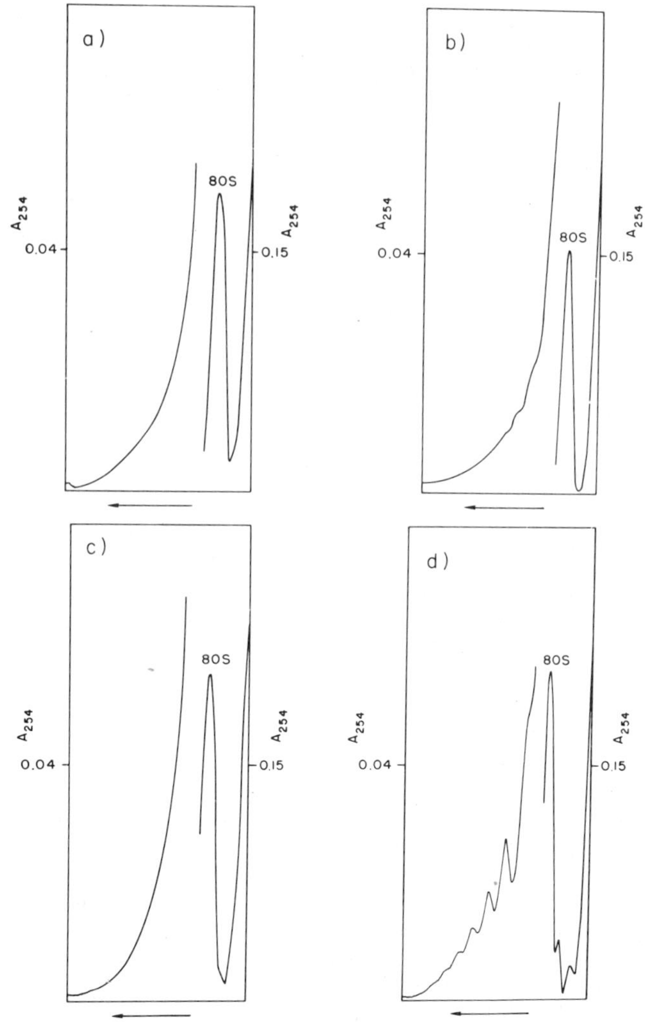

FIG. 4. *Effects of verrucarin A and DAS upon polyribosome profiles in intact H-HeLa cells. Cells were incubated with toxins as indicated: (a) verrucarin A, 5 µg/ml, for 2 min; (b) verrucarin A, 100 µg/ml, for 2 min; (c) DAS, 5 µg/ml, for 10 min; (d) DAS, 100 µg/ml, for 30 min. Lysates and gradients contained 140 mM NaCl. Centrifugation was at 35,000 rpm for 40 min.*

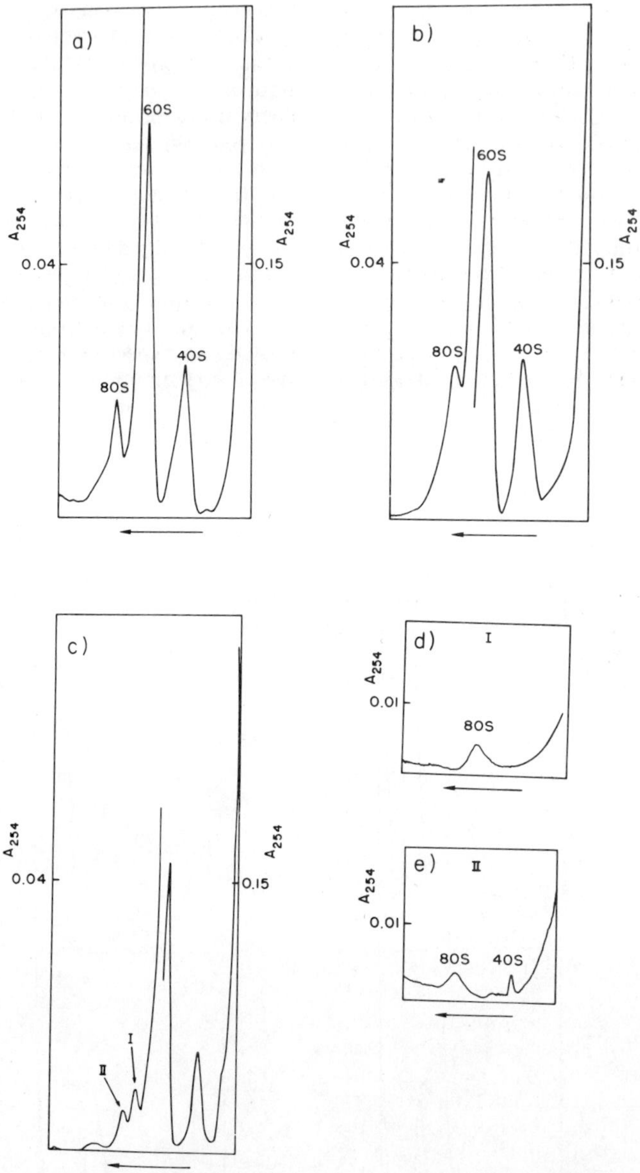

FIG. 5. *Nature of the ribosome-mRNA complexes surviving exposure of intact H-HeLa cells to nivalenol or roridin A. Cells were incubated with toxins as indicated: (a) none—control; (b) nivalenol, 1 µg/ml, 10 min; (c) roridin A, 5 µg/ml, 3 min. Lysates and gradients contained 500 mM NaCl and centrifugation was at 40,000 rpm for 110 min. Materials sedimenting in peaks 1 and 2 of Fig. 5c were collected, treated with ribonuclease, and reanalyzed: (d) and (e), respectively.*

not apparently affected by this treatment, whereas that material which previously sedimented faster than 80*S* (peak 2 in Fig. 5c) now gave rise to particles sedimenting at 80*S* and 40*S*. Peak 2 (Fig. 5c), therefore, apparently contained both 80*S* ribosomes and 40*S* ribosomal subunits attached to single strands of mRNA; structures of this type have previously been observed by others (8) and were referred to as "1.5 mers."

DISCUSSION

In intact cells and in many (but not all) cell-free systems, proteins are synthesized by polyribosomes, and not by individual ribosomes translating mRNA molecules. Therefore, much can be learned about the action of an inhibitor of protein synthesis by observing its effects upon the absorbance profiles of polyribosomes and, in particular, by comparing the effects of different concentrations of the inhibitor (for a review, see reference 6). Although it is not possible to make absolutely rigorous predictions in all cases, the following minimal statements appear, to us, to be valid.

(i) A drug that inhibits only the initiation of protein synthesis (i.e., an I-type) will, at all inhibitory concentrations, allow elongation and termination of polypeptide chains to proceed and will therefore cause breakdown of polyribosomes. Whether breakdown is complete or not will depend upon whether protein synthesis is totally inhibited, but breakdown should greatly exceed 50% at certain drug concentrations and should not be diminished by the addition of extra drug. The precise state of inhibited ribosomes is not predicted by this model: thus, an I-type drug may bind to free ribosomes or subunits thereof (the larger subunit in the case of trichothecenes) and may prevent their association with mRNA during initiation. Alternatively (or coincidentally), the drug may bind to mRNA-associated ribosomes to yield inhibited initiation complexes.

(ii) A drug that inhibits only the termination of polypeptide chains (i.e., a T-type) will not, at any concentration, cause breakdown of polyribosomes. Whether polyribosomes would be maintained at control sizes or increased in size in the presence of such an inhibitor would depend upon how fully the mRNA was laden with ribosomes, at the time of addition of the drug.

(iii) A drug that inhibits polypeptide chain elongation (an E-type) will, at minimal inhibitory concentrations, cause some degradation of polyribosomes but will preserve polyribosomes at levels nearer those in controls, when employed at higher concentrations. This category includes drugs that inhibit only elongation reactions and also those that affect mRNA-bound ribosomes at random. Thus, an E-type may also inhibit either initiation or termination (especially in cell-free assay systems) but will not do so specificaly. Polyribosome breakdown caused by E-types is readily distinguishable from that due to I-types, since the former cannot exceed 50% of the initial polyribosomes (see [6]) and is reduced when the drug concentration is increased.

Here, we have shown (Figs. 2b and e, 3d and e) that certain trichothecenes cause extensive buildup of large polyribosomes within H-HeLa cells when used at concentrations that inhibit protein synthesis incompletely. These drugs are trichodermol, trichodermone, and vomitoxin (4-deoxytrichodermol, see Fig. 6), and we suggest that, under these conditions, they are acting primarily as inhibitors of polypeptide chain termination (i.e., T-types). At totally inhibitory levels, however, these toxins tend to preserve polyribosomes at levels similar to those observed in controls, under which conditions they are acting (secondarily) as E-type inhibitors. However, in contrast to other workers (12, 15), we do not conclude that trichodermin is a T-type inhibitor under any conditions in vivo. Using trichodermin (Fig. 2c and 3b) it is easy to set up conditions under which polyribosomes are partially degraded in H-HeLa cells and also (Fig. 2d and 3c) to show that raising the drug concentration diminishes this effect. This type of behavior is very similar to that of

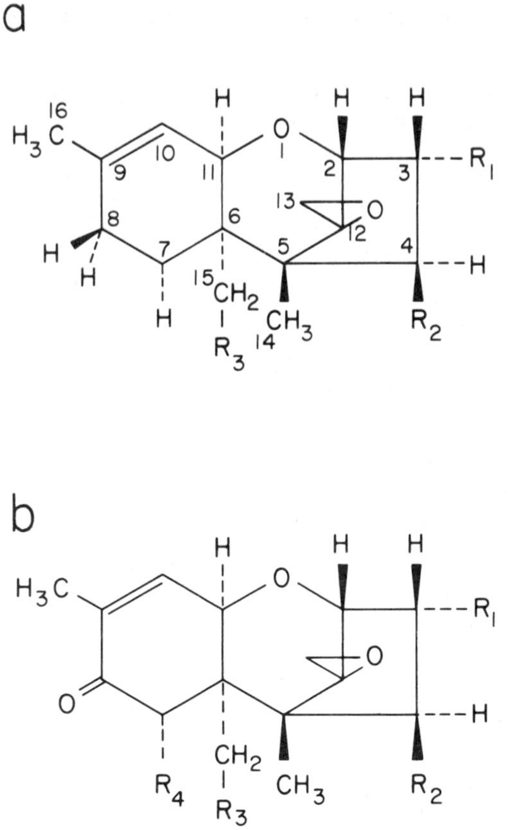

FIG. 6. *Structures of various 12,13-epoxytrichothecenes. (a) For trichodermin,* $R_1 = R_3 = H$*,* $R_2 = O.CO.CH_3$*; for trichodermol,* $R_1 = R_3 = H$*,* $R_2 = OH$*; for trichodermone,* $R_1 = R_2 = H$*,* $R_2 = O$*; for vomitoxin,* $R_1 = R_2 = R_3 = H$*; for diacetoxyscirpenol,* $R_1 = OH$*,* $R_2 = R_3 = O.CO.CH_3$*. (b) For trichothecin,* $R_1 = R_3 = R_4 = H$*,* $R_2 = O.CO.CH{:}\ CH.CH_3$*; for trichothecolone,* $R_1 = R_3 = R_4 = H$*,* $R_2 = OH$*; for fusarenone X,* $R_1 = R_3 = R_4 = OH$*,* $R_2 = O.CO.CH_3$*; for nivalenol,* $R_1 = R_2 = R_3 = R_4 = OH$*.*

chloramphenicol, chlortetracycline, and various other antibiotics in bacterial systems (E. Cundliffe, unpublished data; see also reference 6) and is that expected of an E-type inhibitor. As indicated in Fig. 2g and h, trichothecin resembles trichodermin in our assays, and we conclude that this toxin also is an E-type rather than a T-type.

As previously suggested by others (4), the E-type effects observed here with trichodermin or trichothecin or both, might also result from preferential inhibition of the initiation of protein synthesis at low drug concentrations, with a strong secondary effect upon elongation at slightly higher drug levels. It remains to be seen, therefore, whether all E-type trichothecenes are, in fact, semispecific inhibitors of initiation. However, recent evidence that the dissociation constant for the binding of trichodermin to free 80*S* ribosomes is one-third that for the binding of the drug to polyribosomes (M. Cannon, A. Jimenez, and D. Vazquez, manuscript in preparation) indicates that trichodermin, at least, probably behaves in this way.

We have also reexamined certain trichothecenes, previously classified by us as I-types (7), that caused rapid and extensive degradation of polyribosomes in vivo. Some of these compounds, T-2 toxin (11), fusarenone X, and diacetoxyscirpenol (9) did not inhibit any of the reactions peculiar to polypeptide chain initiation when added to reticulocyte extracts; rather, they inhibited formation of either the first peptide bond (T-2 toxin) or the second peptide bond (fusarenone X and diacetoxyscirpenol). Accordingly, we examined closely the nature of mRNA-associated ribosomal material present in H-HeLa cells after exposure to I-types, after first confirming that these compounds (diacetoxyscirpenol excepted) caused virtually complete degradation of polyribosomes over a wide range of drug concentrations (Fig. 4). Breakdown products were analyzed (Fig. 5) on sucrose gradients containing 500 mM NaCl, under which "high salt" conditions free 80*S* ribosomes are unstable and dissociate into 60*S* and 40*S* subunits. As shown in Fig. 5, some I-types (e.g., nivalenol—Fig. 5b; also, T-2 toxin and HT-2 toxin, data not given) degrade polyribosomes to leave only 80*S* monosomes associated with mRNA. We will refer to these inhibitors as I_2-types. Other trichothecenes, namely verrucarin A and roridin A, caused the accumulation of ribosomal structures not normally present in control lysates, in addition to 80*S* monosomes (Fig. 5c). These novel structures appeared to consist of 80*S* monosomes and 40*S* initiation complexes attached to the same mRNA strand (Fig. 5e). To distinguish verrucarin A and roridin A from I_2-type inhibitors, they will be referred to here as I_1-types.

These results suggest that I_1-type trichothecenes can, to some extent, prevent the formation of 80*S* initiation complexes, in addition to inhibiting the function of ribosomes already attached to mRNA. Clearly, however, any mRNA-bound ribosomes that are affected must be at or near the 5′ end of mRNA cistrons, since we have no evidence that disomes or larger structures survive under these conditions. Similarly, I_2-types must also be restricted in their action to ribosomes at or near the 5′ end of the mRNA, although there is no evidence that these compounds prevent the formation of 80*S* initiation complexes (10, 12; also, Fig. 5b). It remains to be seen to what extent the 80*S* monosomes, which persist in H-HeLa cells after treatment with either I_1- or I_2-type inhibitors, consist of inhibited initiation complexes, as opposed to ribosomes bearing short, nascent oligopeptides. This raises the possibility that some, or all, I-types might be better regarded as pseudospecific inhibitors whose ability to bind to active ribosomes might be determined by lengths of the nascent peptides being carried. A superficially similar situation is observed with lincomycin, the streptogramins, and certain macrolide antibiotics in bacterial systems and has been commented upon previously (5, 7, 10). It should also be noted that formation of "1.5 mers" has been observed in reticulocyte extracts treated with pactamycin (8) and is therefore not a consequence of the action of drugs that bind exclusively to the larger ribosomal subunit. Curiously, we have never observed these structures in control lysates (Fig. 5a).

One drug, DAS, previously classified as I-type, deserves separate mention. As shown in Fig. 4c and d, DAS caused complete breakdown of polyribosomes, even at 5 μg/ml, a concentration five times greater than that required to stop protein synthesis in vivo within 2 to 3 min (Table 1). In this respect, DAS behaved as an I-type. However, polyribosomes were extensively preserved when H-HeLa cells were exposed to higher levels of DAS. This indicates that DAS has a secondary effect upon polypeptide chain elongation at very high concentrations, a conclusion that is supported by other observations concerning the action of the compound (10; L. L. Liao, S. B. Horwitz, and A. P. Grollman, Fed. Proc. 5:1915, 1975).

It appears, therefore, that DAS is intermediate in its action between that of an I-type, such as T-2 toxin, and an E-type, such as trichodermin. A large group of trichothecene toxins (excluding the T-types) thus appear to comprise a functional series according to the relative potencies of their inhibitory effects on the initiation and the elongation steps in eukaryotic protein synthesis.

We have previously suggested (7) that the presence of oxygen-containing substituents on C15 of the trichothecene ring system may be crucial in specifying I-type as opposed to E- or T-type activity. We now suggest that the nature of substituents on C4 may determine E-type versus T-type activity (Fig. 6). Thus, T-types possess on C4 either a hydroxyl group (trichodermol), a keto group (trichodermone), or no substituent (vomitoxin); in contrast, trichodermin and trichothecin (both E-types) carry substituted hydroxyl groups on C4 (Fig. 6a and b). Another indication that this is a critical portion of the molecule comes from Fig. 1, in which 4-epitrichodermol (Fig. 6a) is shown to be inactive.

We also note that nivalenol and fusarenone X, both classified as I-types, carry C4 substituents which might be expected, according to our hypothesis, to specify T-type and E-type activities, respectively (Fig. 6). Evidently, their I-type activity, determined by substitution on C15, is dominant as it is in verrucarin A and roridin A, which possess macrocyclic rings linking C4 and C15 (1). DAS (Fig. 6) also affords an example of the dominance of I-type over E-type determinants, the latter only being expressed at very high drug concentrations.

After completion of this work, we learned that other workers share our view that trichodermin is not a termination inhibitor (4); they conclude that trichodermin may be a defective I-type which, at all inhibitory concentrations, partially inhibits elongation. Our data are entirely compatible with their conclusion and it remains to be seen whether any experimental situation can be devised to distinguish conclusively between their conclusion and ours regarding the action of trichodermin.

ACKNOWLEDGMENTS

This work was supported by grants or awards from the following bodies, to whom we are extremely grateful: Public Health Service, National Institute of Health Allergy and Infectious Diseases (AI1248) and Lilly Research Foundation (to J.E.D.); Medical Research Council of Great Britain and Wellcome Trust (to E.C.).

LITERATURE CITED

1. **Bamburg, J. R., and F. M. Strong.** 1971. 12,13-Epoxytrichothecenes, p. 207–292. *In* S. Kadis, A. Ciegler, and S. J. Ajl (ed.), Microbial toxins, vol. 7. Academic Press Inc., New York.
2. **Barbacid, M., and D. Vazquez.** 1974. Binding of [acetyl-^{14}C] trichodermin to the peptidyl transferase center of eukaryotic ribosomes. Eur. J. Biochem. **44:**437–444.
3. **Carrasco, L., M. Barbacid, and D. Vazquez.** 1973. The trichodermin group of antibiotics, inhibitors of peptide bond formation by eukaryotic ribosomes. Biochim. Biophys. Acta **312:**368–376.
4. **Carter, C. J., M. Cannon, and K. E. Smith.** 1976. Inhibition of protein synthesis in reticulocyte lysates by trichodermin. Biochem. J. **154:**171–178.
5. **Cundliffe, E.** 1969. Antibiotics and polyribosomes. II. Some effects of lincomycin, spiramycin and streptogramin A *in vivo*. Biochemistry **8:**2063–2066.
6. **Cundliffe, E.** 1972. Antibiotic inhibitors of ribosome function, p. 278–379. *In* Molecular basis of antibiotic action. John Wiley and Sons, Ltd., London.
7. **Cundliffe, E., M. Cannon, and J. Davies.** 1974. Mechanism of inhibition of eukaryotic protein synthesis by trichothecene fungal toxins. Proc. Natl. Acad. Sci. U.S.A. **71:**30–34.
8. **Kappen, L. S., H. Suzuki, and I. H. Goldberg.** 1973. Inhibition of reticulocyte peptide-chain initiation by pactamycin: accumulation of inactive ribosomal initiation complexes. Proc. Natl. Acad. Sci. U.S.A. **70:**22–26.
9. **Mizuno, S.** 1975. Mechanism of inhibition of protein synthesis initiation by diacetoxyscirpenol and fusarenone X in the reticulocyte lysate system. Biochim. Biophys. Acta **383:**207–214.
10. **Schindler, D.** 1974. Two classes of inhibitors of peptidyl transferase activity in eukaryotes. Nature (London) **249:**38–41.
11. **Smith, K. E., M. Cannon, and E. Cundliffe.** 1975. Inhibition at the initiation level of eukaryotic protein synthesis by T-2 toxin. FEBS Lett. **50:**8–12.
12. **Stafford, M. E., and C. S. McLaughlin.** 1973. Trichodermin, a possible inhibitor of the termination process of protein synthesis. J. Cell Physiol. **82:**121–128.
13. **Tate, W. P., and C. T. Caskey.** 1973. Peptidyl transferase inhibition by trichodermin. J. Biol. Chem. **248:**7970–7972.
14. **Ueno, Y., M. Hosoya, Y. Morita, I. Veno, and T. Tatsuno.** 1968. Inhibition of the protein synthesis in rabbit reticulocyte by nivalenol, a toxic principle isolated from *Fusarium nivale*–growing rice. J. Biochem. (Tokyo) **64:**479–485.
15. **Wei, C.-M., B. S. Hansen, M. H. Vaughan, and C. S. McLaughlin.** 1974. Mechanism of action of the mycotoxin trichodermin, a 12,13-epoxytrichothecene. Proc. Natl. Acad. Sci. U.S.A. **71:**713–717.

ANTIMICROBIAL AGENTS AND CHEMOTHERAPY, Mar. 1977, p. 500-513 Vol. 11, No. 3

Printed in U.S.A.

Cytochemical and Biochemical Studies of Yeasts After In Vitro Exposure to Miconazole

SONJA DE NOLLIN,* H. VAN BELLE, F. GOOSSENS, F. THONE, AND M. BORGERS
Laboratories of Cell Biology and Biochemistry, Janssen Pharmaceutica, Research Laboratories, 2340 Beerse, Belgium

Received for publication 7 July 1976

Yeast cells exposed to different doses of the antimycotic agent miconazole revealed important cytochemical changes in the topographic distribution of the phosphatases. A strong effect was observed on the behavior of oxidative and peroxidative enzymes. Decreased cytochrome *c* oxidase and peroxidase activity and increased catalase activity were seen after treatment with a fungistatic dose of miconazole, whereas a complete disappearance of these enzymes was observed after treatment with a minimal fungicidal dose of miconazole. This was in complete agreement with the quantitative biochemical data. A hypothesis is advanced concerning the possible involvement of peroxidase and catalase in the mechanism of action of this drug.

Miconazole, (1-{2-(2,4-dichlorophenyl)-2-[2,4-dichlorophenyl)methoxy]ethyl} - 1H - imidazole nitrate (Janssen Pharmaceutica), is an imidazole nitrate that has demonstrated broad-spectrum activity against most pathogenic fungi and gram-positive bacteria (7, 10, 18, 19, 36). The studies on the uptake and utilization of substances in *Candida albicans* by Van den Bossche (37) indicated that miconazole induced changes in the permeability of the plasmalemma and the cell wall. At the ultrastructural level, *C. albicans* cells show changes in a dose-dependent manner when grown in the presence of 10^{-8} to 10^{-4} M concentrations of miconazole. These changes range from slight alterations in the cell periphery and increase in the number of peroxisomes and lipid globules, to progressive cytoplasmic deterioration, prominent shape changes, and complete cellular necrosis (11, 12; S. De Nollin, Ph.D thesis, University of Brussels, Brussels, Belgium, 1976). Recent investigations with scanning and transmission electron microscopy (12) on *C. albicans* cultures treated with a fungicidal dose of miconazole (10^{-4} M) have shown that the sequence of alterations differs totally from that obtained with lower-dose treatments.

The cytochemistry of untreated yeast cells has already been described by several authors (2, 3, 13, 22, 40; S. De Nollin, Ph.D. thesis, 1976). In earlier experiments (16, 13), we tried to optimize the preparatory conditions for the cytochemical examination of yeasts cells by using a modification of the conventional procedure for preservation. This yields, besides a good micromorphology of the cells, sufficient enzyme activities and allows an adequate penetration of substrates and captation ions during the incubation. For the biochemical studies, Van Belle, Goossens, and Van Roy (in preparation) have recently developed a method for obtaining adequate homogenization of the very rigid cells of yeast, thereby yielding reliable enzyme activities that are directly proportional to the number of cells (more than 99.9% of the cells are thoroughly homogenized). Using these modifications of the cytochemical and biochemical preparative techniques, we have tried in this study to evaluate the effects of miconazole on the activities and the distribution pattern of phosphohydrolases and of oxidative and peroxidative enzymes in *C. albicans* and *Saccharomyces cerevisiae*. Our particular aim was to see whether there was any correlation between the observed morphological changes and the behavior of a number of enzymes (localized in different subcellular organelles) in order to get a better insight into the possible mode of action of this antifungal drug.

MATERIALS AND METHODS

Culture conditions. *C. albicans* RV 4688 and *S. cerevisiae* 17787 were maintained on Sabouraud glucose agar at 25°C. Casein hydrolysate (0.5%), yeast extract (0.5%), and glucose (0.5%) (CGY) medium was used in all experiments as a broth. For each experiment, a loopful of *C. albicans* or *S. cerevisiae* was transferred to 4.5 ml of Sabouraud glucose broth and incubated under stationary conditions for 24 h at 37°C. Cells were then inoculated in the CYG medium at a concentration of 2×10^5 cells/ml.

Treatment with miconazole. Immediately after inoculation, the cultures of *C. albicans* were exposed to fungistatic (10^{-6} M) or minimal fungicidal (10^{-5} M) doses of miconazole, whereas the cultures of *S.*

cerevisiae were exposed to the minimal fungicidal dose (2×10^{-8} M) of miconazole. *C. albicans* and *S. cerevisiae* were incubated as shake cultures in Erlenmeyer flasks at 37 and 30°C, respectively. Miconazole was dissolved in dimethyl sulfoxide. The final concentration of dimethyl sulfoxide in the cultures was 0.05%. Control cultures containing an equal amount of solvent were incubated at the same time. The cells were harvested at various points in time.

Biochemistry. (i) Homogenization of the cells. The cells were harvested, washed twice with saline, and finally taken up in the extraction buffer to a fixed absorbance (*A*) (0.250 ± 0.020 at 550 nm for a 1/50 dilution) before homogenization. The buffer was a 20 mM phosphate buffer, pH 7.0, containing 0.2% Brij-35; 4 ml of this suspension was then homogenized with 2 g of washed sand in a specially constructed device three times for 10 s each (*S. cerevisiae*) or nine times for 10 s each (*C. albicans*) with intervals of 1 min for cooling. The stroke distance was 83 mm, and the velocity was 40 strokes per s, with cooling performed with tap water (10°C). The enzymatic activities were determined on the supernatant fluid after centrifugation of the homogenate for 2.5 min (Eppendorf microcentrifuge).

In a series of preliminary homogenization tests, time, grain size of the sand, buffer, and cell concentration were found to be optimal (Van Belle, Goossens and Van Roy, in preparation). Only 0.01% of the cells remained viable as indicated from the colony-forming units determination.

(ii) Determination of enzymatic activities. Alkaline phosphatase (AlPase) activity was measured in 1 M *N*-ethylaminoethanol and 10 mM substrate as described recently for serum (35). Acid phosphatase (AcPase) was determined according to (4), but using an 0.1 M acetate buffer, pH 5.0, and a final volume of 2.1 ml.

Cytochrome *c* oxidase and peroxidase were determined by the method of Chantrenne (10), with slight modifications. The cytochrome *c*, reduced with dithionite, was desalted on a Sephadex G-25 column and kept at −20°C until used (the ratio, A_{550}/A_{565}, was >10). The oxidase activity was recorded for 1 min at 25°C and then inhibited by the addition of NaN_3 (5×10^{-3} M, final concentration). Subsequent addition of H_2O_2 (final concentration, 1.2×10^{-6} M) allowed the measurement of the peroxidase activity. A change in *A* of 0.021 corresponds to the oxidation of 1 μmol of cytochrome *c* in the reaction mixture.

Catalase was measured according to the ultraviolet method described by Bergmeyer (4). The decomposition of 1 μmol of H_2O_2 in the final reaction mixture results in a decrease in A_{240} of 0.0154.

Cytochemistry. (i) Preparation procedure. The detailed procedure has been described earlier (6, 13). Cells, harvested after 24 h of incubation, were pelleted by low-speed centrifugation and suspended in a few drops of rat serum. After centrifugation, the supernatant fluid was discarded, and 3% glutaraldehyde (buffered to pH 7.4 with 0.1 M sodium cacodylate) was gently added without disturbing the pellet. Solidification of the pellets proceeded at 4°C for 15 min. To obtain an instantaneous and adequate fixation, the pellets were frozen in a drop of fixative placed on the microtome table. Sections 7.5 μm thick were prepared and immersed in the same fixative solution at 4°C for 30 min. The sections were then washed for a minimum of 2 h in 0.1 M sodium cacodylate, supplemented with 0.22 M sucrose, and incubated in the appropriate medium listed below.

In addition, the following variation in the fixation procedure was used for the localization of catalase: the 7.5-μm sections were fixed for 24 h in a 4% formol solution containing 1% $CaCl_2$ (29). After a 1-min wash, the sections were incubated in the catalase medium as described below.

After incubation in the various media, the sections were postfixed in 2% O_sO_4, buffered in 0.05 M Veronal acetate buffer containing 0.12 M sucrose, quickly processed through a graded series of cold ethanol, and routinely embedded in Epon. Ultrathin sections were examined in an electron microscope (Philips EM 300), either unstained or stained with uranium acetate and lead citrate.

(ii) Incubation media for enzyme localization. The AlPase medium with β-glycerophosphate as substrate at pH 9.0, as described by Hugon and Borgers (23), was used. Mg^{2+} was added to a 5 mM concentration. The incubation time was 45 min at 37°C. Aminophylline, 10 mM, was used as AlPase inhibitor (13). For AcPase, β-glycerophosphate and nitrophenylphosphate (NOP) were used as substrates at pH 5.0 according to the Barka and Anderson technique (1). The incubation time was 30 min at 37°C. NaF (10 mM) was used as inhibitor. In the specific phosphatase assay, the activity against adenosine 5′-triphosphate (ATP) was tested at pH 7.2 and 8.5 using the medium of Wachstein and Meisel (42) modified as described by Borgers et al. (5). Incubation time was 30 min at 37°C. Cytochrome *c* oxidase was determined by the method of method of Seligman et al. (31). Incubation time was 1 h at 37°C. NaCN (10^{-3} M) was used as an inhibitor. Cytochrome *c* peroxidase activity at neutral pH was investigated using the diaminobenzidine (DAB) procedure of Graham and Karnovsky (20), without addition of exogenous cytochrome *c*. NaCN (10^{-2} M) was used as an inhibitor. Incubation time was 30 min at 37°C. Peroxidatic activity of catalase was investigated according to the methods of Fahimi (15) and Novikoff and Goldfischer (24) at pH 9.0 and 9.4, respectively. The latter medium contained 5.6 mM DAB and 17.4 mM H_2O_2. Aminotriazole (20 mM) was used as a catalase inhibitor. Incubation times were 1 and 2 h at 37°C.

RESULTS

Biochemical investigations were carried out to quantify the enzyme activities of control cells, as well as miconazole-treated cells, of *S. cerevisiae* and *C. albicans* at different stages of growth. There was no inhibitory effect on the activities of hydrolytic, oxidative, and peroxidative enzymes by miconazole, nor by the solvent, if either was added to the measuring medium.

AlPase. Yeast cells of both species studied show an exponential phase of growth beginning at 2 to 3 h after inoculation and lasting for 8 to 9

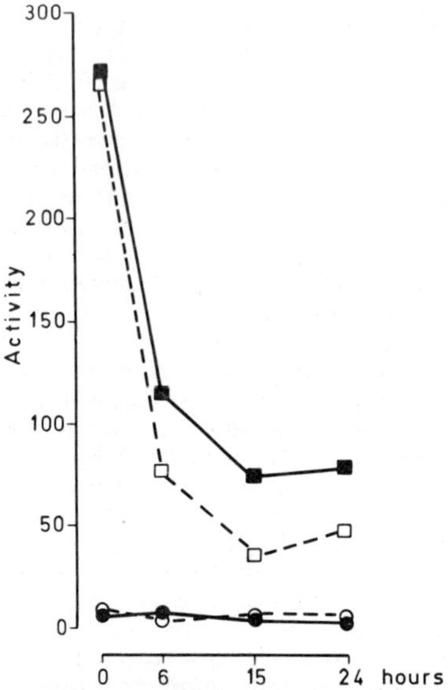

FIG. 1. *Nonspecific phosphatases (nanomoles of substrate hydrolyzed per minute per milligram of protein) of S. cerevisiae cells grown in CYG medium at 30°C. The values represent the mean of five determinations (the standard error is not plotted for the sake of clarity). Symbols: (●) AcPase activity of control cells; (○) AcPase activity of the cells exposed to a minimal fungicidal dose (2 × 10^{-8} M) of miconazole; (■) AlPase activity of control cells; (□) AlPase activity of cells exposed to a minimal fungicidal dose (2 × 10^{-8} M) of miconazole.*

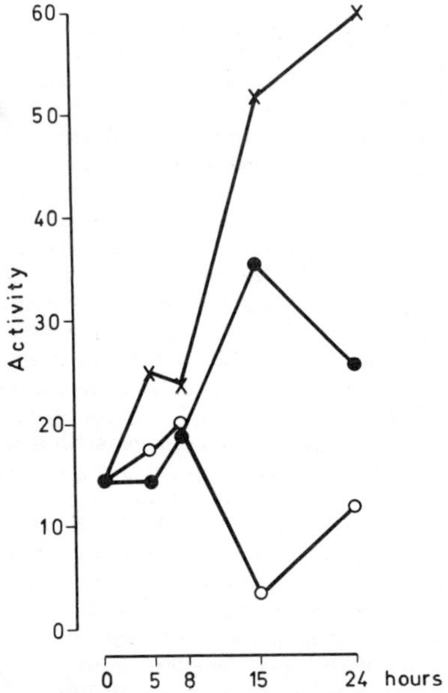

FIG. 2. *AlPase (nanomoles of substrate hydrolyzed per minute per milligram of protein) of C. albicans cells grown in CYG medium at 37°C (mean of seven determinations). Symbols: (●) AlPase activity of control cells; (×) AlPase activity of cells exposed to a fungistatic dose (10^{-6} M) of miconazole; (○) AlPase activity of cells exposed to a minimal fungicidal dose (10^{-5} M) of miconazole.*

h (38). As seen in Fig. 1, the AlPase of *S. cerevisiae* showed a decrease in activity during the growth of the control cells. After exposure to miconazole in a minimal fungicidal concentration (i.e., 2 × 10^{-8} M for *S. cerevisiae*), the activity of AlPase was diminished from the exponential phase of growth (6 h) onwards.

The AlPase of *C. albicans* showed an optimal activity after 15 h of growth (Fig. 2). After treatment with a fungistatic dose of miconazole (i.e., 10^{-6} M for *C. albicans*), a significant increase in activity was noted. The exposure of the minimal fungicidal dose (10^{-5} M) resulted in a marked decrease in AlPase activity.

Cytochemical experiments were carried out in parallel with the biochemical studies. As previously described (13), the AlPase activity in *C. albicans* control cells was confined to the limiting membrane of the central vacuole (Fig. 3). Cells of cultures exposed to 10^{-6} or 10^{-5} M miconazole for 24 h showed the enzymatic reaction product both on the vacuolar membrane and the vacuolar content, and the reaction was augmented strongly in proportion to the level of cellular damage (Fig. 4). Lomasomal structures were completely negative, even if they were localized in close proximity to the central vacuole. The activity displayed at neutral pH with ATP as substrate was always confined to the central vacuole, similar to AlPase activity.

FIG. 3. *AlPase. C. albicans control cell. Besides some small vacuoles (vac), most of the membranous structures (arrows) present in the cytoplasm show the reaction product. The plasmalemma (pl) and the other organelles such as mitochondria (m), cell wall (cw), and lomasomal structures (lo) are negative. (×22,600)*

FIG. 4. *AlPase. C. albicans cells exposed to 10^{-6} M miconazole. The limiting membrane and contents of the vacuole (vac) are covered with the precipitate. Abbreviations: Mitochondria (m), plasmalemma (pl), cell wall inclusions (i). (×20,000)*

FIG. 5. *AcPase. C. albicans control cell. With NOP as substrate, the reaction product (arrow) is localized exclusively inside the vacuole (vac). (×59,400)*

FIG. 6. *AcPase. C. albicans cells exposed to 10^{-6} M miconazole. With NOP as substrate, the precipitate is seen over the vacuolar content (vac), as well as on the plasmalemma (pl). (×30,000)*

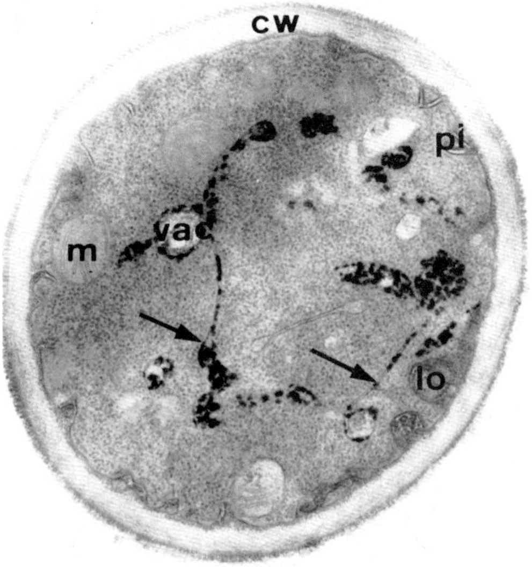

3

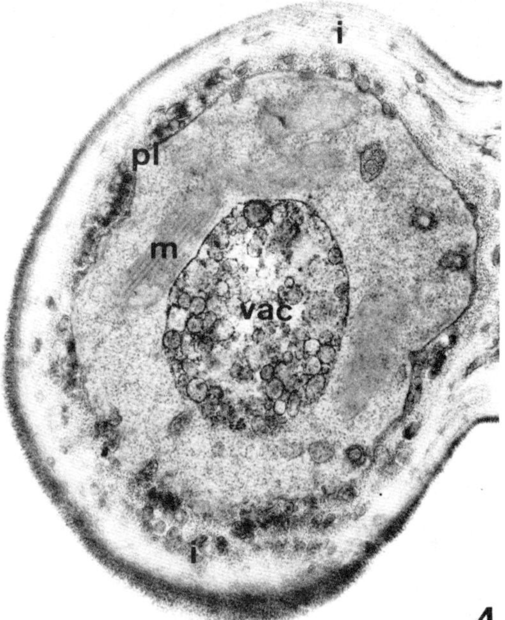

4

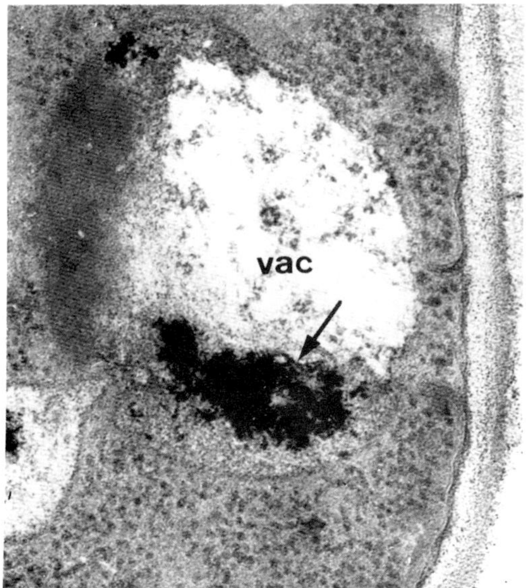

5

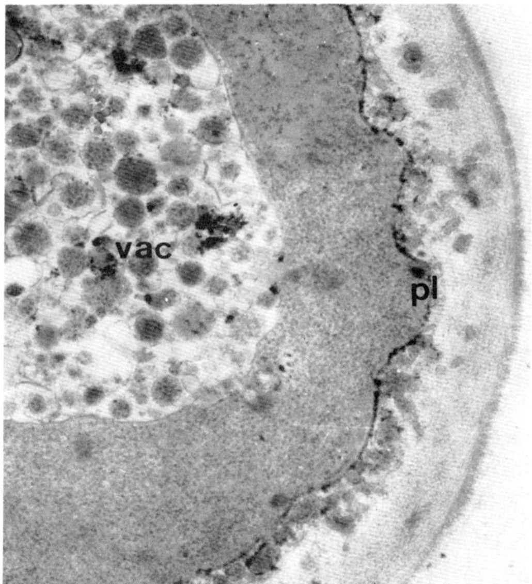

6

After exposure to miconazole, the precipitate was localized not only to the limiting membrane of the vacuole, but also to the vacuolar content. The activity at pH 8.5 with ATP was significantly lower than that at neutral pH.

AcPase. Quantitative determinations of AcPase in *S. cerevisiae* revealed a low and constant level of activity during growth of the control cultures. There seemed to be no effect of the drug on the activity of this enzyme, when added at a 2×10^{-8} M concentration (Fig. 1). As with *S. cerevisiae*, the low and rather constant rate of AcPase activity of *C. albicans* was not markedly influenced by drug interaction.

In the electron microscope, the reaction with β-glycerophosphate as substrate yielded only very few cells with a light deposition of reaction product (weak enzyme activity) in the vacuole, both in control and miconazole-treated cultures. On the other hand, with NOP as substrate, practically all cells of the control cultures demonstrated activity in the central vacuole (Fig. 5). After exposure to miconazole, the precipitate remained in the vacuole, but in addition, the plasmalemma was uniformly covered with the reaction product (Fig. 6). This latter localization was never seen in control cells. When the incubation was carried out at pH 6.0, the reaction was visibly lowered. The addition of 10 mM NaF to the incubation medium completely inhibited the precipitation of the reaction product.

Cytochrome *C* oxidase. The activity of the cytochrome *c* oxidase (Fig. 7), already present in *S. cerevisiae* cells in the lag phase, increased during growth. After exposure to 2×10^{-8} M miconazole for 6 h, cytochrome *c* oxidase activity was still present in amounts comparable to those of the control cells. The marked increase of this enzyme as seen in the control cells, however, was not present after treatment. After 24 h of growth, a marked decrease in the cytochrome *c* oxidase activity was observed. In *C. albicans* (Fig. 9), this enzyme presented an optimum in activity after 8 h. After exposure to miconazole, drastic dose-related changes were seen. At 10^{-6} M, the optimum in activity, as seen in the control cells after 8 h, was completely absent. The addition of 10^{-5} M miconazole to the culture resulted in a complete absence of this enzyme.

By cytochemistry, the activity of cytochrome *c* oxidase was localized on the mitochondrial cristae in the control cells (Fig. 10). In cells exposed to the fungistatic dose of miconazole (10^{-6} M), the distribution of the reaction product was rather similar, although present in lower amounts (Fig. 11). The reaction was completely absent when NaCN was added to the incubation medium. The exposure to the minimal fungicidal dose (10^{-5} M) resulted in a complete absence of activity on the mitochondrial cristae (Fig. 12).

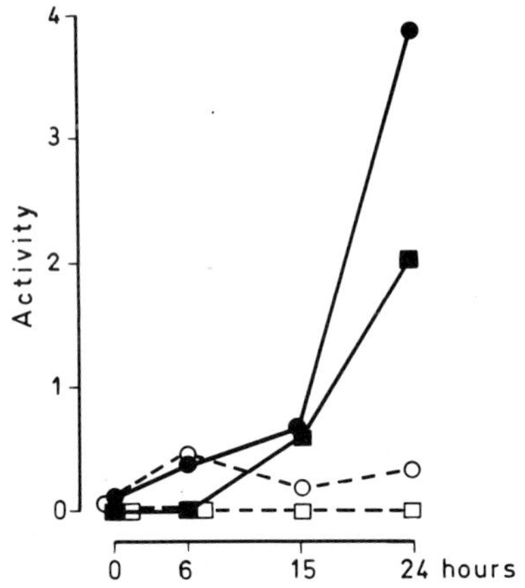

FIG. 7. *Oxidative and peroxidative enzymes (Δ per minute per milligram of protein) of S. cerevisiae cells grown in a CYG medium at 30°C (mean of five determinations). Symbols: (●) Cytochrome c peroxidase activity of control cells; (○) cytochrome c oxidase activity of cells exposed to a minimal fungicidal dose (2×10^{-8} M) of miconazole; (■) catalase activity of control cells; (□) catalase activity of cells exposed to a minimal fungicidal dose (2×10^{-8} M) of miconazole.*

Cytochrome *c* peroxidase. Under the culture condition used, cytochrome *c* peroxidase activity could not be quantitatively demonstrated in this strain of *S. cerevisiae*. In *C. albicans*, the optimum in activity appeared after 15 h (i.e., the early stationary phase) of growth. Strong inhibition of cytochrome *c* peroxidase activity was noted with the fungistatic dose, whereas after exposure to the minimal fungicidal dose, the enzyme activity was not detectable (Fig. 13).

Cytochemically, this enzyme was localized on the mitochondrial membranes (Fig. 14). After exposure to 10^{-6} M miconazole, the majority of the cells showed mitochondria in which the amount of reaction product was considerably decreased. Most of the cristae still showed the osmiophilic dye, whereas the outer membranes were devoid of reaction product (Fig. 15). Addition of 10 mM NaCN to the incubation medium resulted in complete inhibition. Aminotriazole (20 mM) had no influence on this mitochondrial cytochrome *c* peroxidase activity. In cells exposed to 10^{-5} M miconazole, no reaction product was demonstrated in the mitochondria (Fig. 16).

Catalase. In *S. cerevisiae*, paralleling the increase of cytochrome *c* oxidase, catalase activity also increased with time, although it was not present in the inoculum cells. After exposure to 2×10^{-8} M miconazole, no catalase activity was detectable (Fig. 7). This paralleled the strong inhibition of growth (Fig. 8). As for the control cells of *C. albicans*, the profile of the catalase activity was comparable to that of the cytochrome *c* peroxidase. A strong increase in catalase activity was evident after exposure to the fungistatic dose of miconazole (10^{-6} M), but no catalase activity was demonstrated after treatment with the minimal fungicidal dose (10^{-5} M) (Fig. 17). All the peroxisomes of the control cells showed a catalase-positive reaction (Fig. 18) when fixation and incubation were performed according to Roels et al. (29) and Novikoff and Goldfischer (24). This activity was completely inhibited after addition of 20 mM aminotriazole to the incubation medium, whereas the interfering cytochrome *c* peroxi-

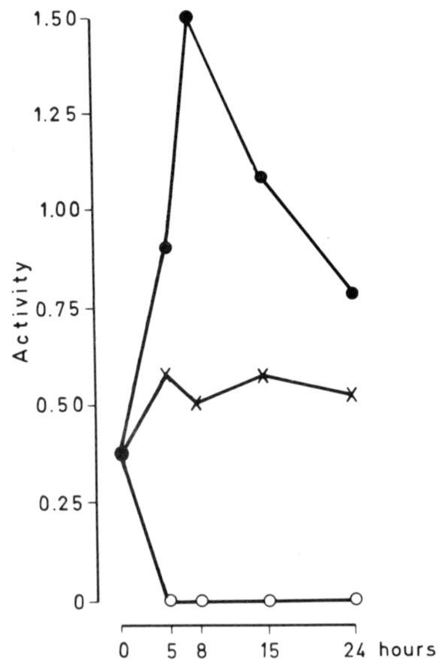

FIG. 9. *Cytochrome c oxidase (Δ per minute per milligram of protein) of C. albicans cells grown in CYG medium at 37°C (mean of seven determinations). Symbols: (●) Cytochrome c oxidase activity of control cells; (×) cytochrome c oxidase activity of cells exposed to a fungistatic dose (10^{-6} M) of miconazole; (○) cytochrome c oxidase activity of cells exposed to a minimal fungicidal dose (10^{-5} M) of miconazole.*

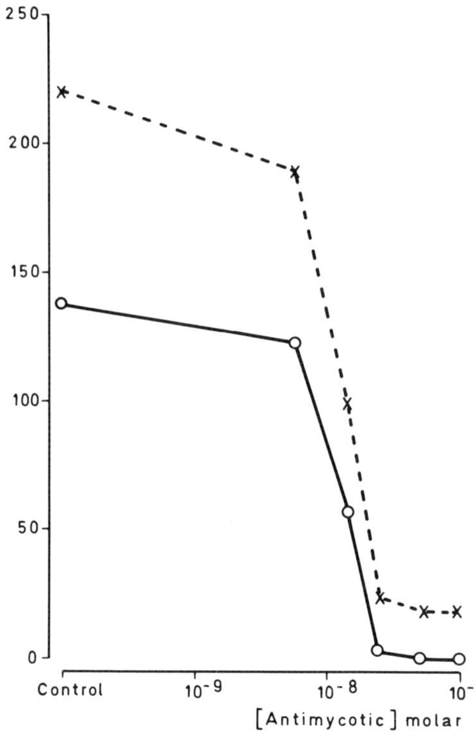

FIG. 8. *Correlation between inhibition of the growth (24 h) and disappearance of catalase activity in S. cerevisiae at different concentrations of miconazole. Symbols: (○) Catalase activity of S. cerevisiae grown for 24 h whether or not exposed to miconazole (Δ A × 1,000 per minute per 0.5 mg of acetone powder); (×) S. cerevisiae grown for 24 h in a CYG medium whether or not exposed to miconazole. Growth is expressed by milligrams of acetone powder per 50 ml of medium.*

dase activity on the mitochondria remained unchanged (Fig. 19). After exposure of cultures to the fungistatic dose (10^{-6} M), peroxisomes became very numerous and all showed a strong catalase activity (Fig. 20 and 21), and again aminotriazole (20 mM) completely inhibited the catalase activity in these peroxisomes. When the cells were exposed to 10^{-5} M miconazole, no positive peroxisomes could be found (Fig. 22).

DISCUSSION

Hydrolases. From the biochemical data obtained on *C. albicans*, it appears that the AlPase activity strongly increases after exposure to a fungistatic dose of miconazole. Our cytochemical experiments reveal that the AlPase is no longer confined to the limiting membrane of the vacuole, but is also present in the vacuolar content. The AlPase activity inside the vacuole may be derived from fragments of the vacuolar envelope, which progressively accumulate in the vacuole during the uptake of lytic cytoplasmic particles. The exposure to a minimal fungicidal dose results in a decrease in AlPase activity in *C. albicans* and *S. cerevisiae*. Although the exact role of the AlPase has not yet been elucidated, a transport function of nutritive substances and cell metabolites has been attrib-

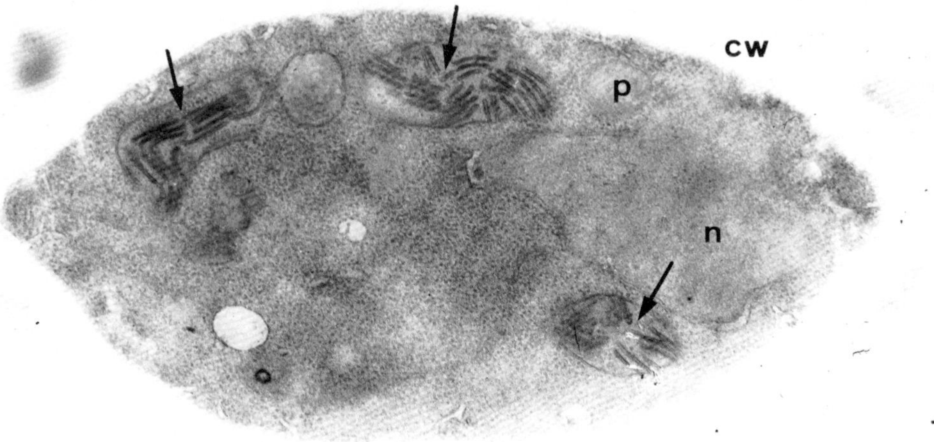

10

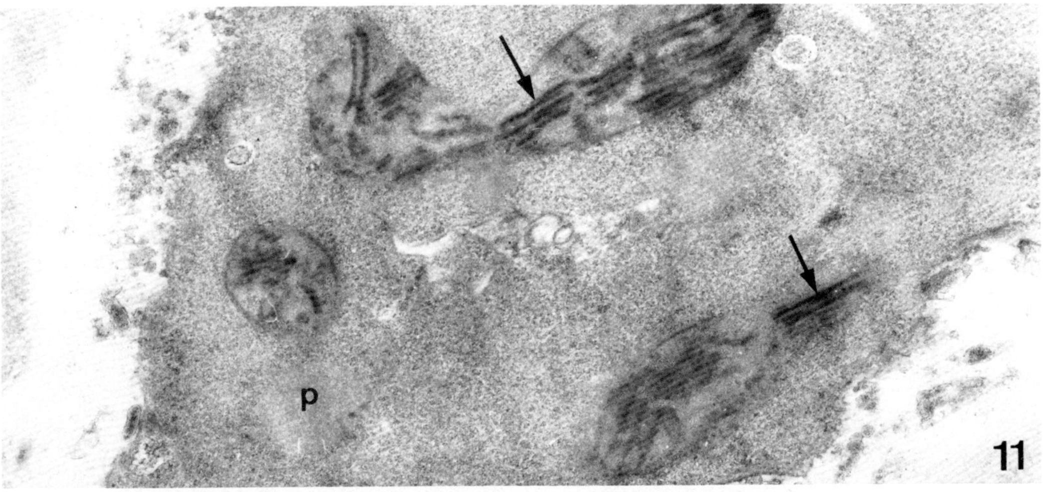

11

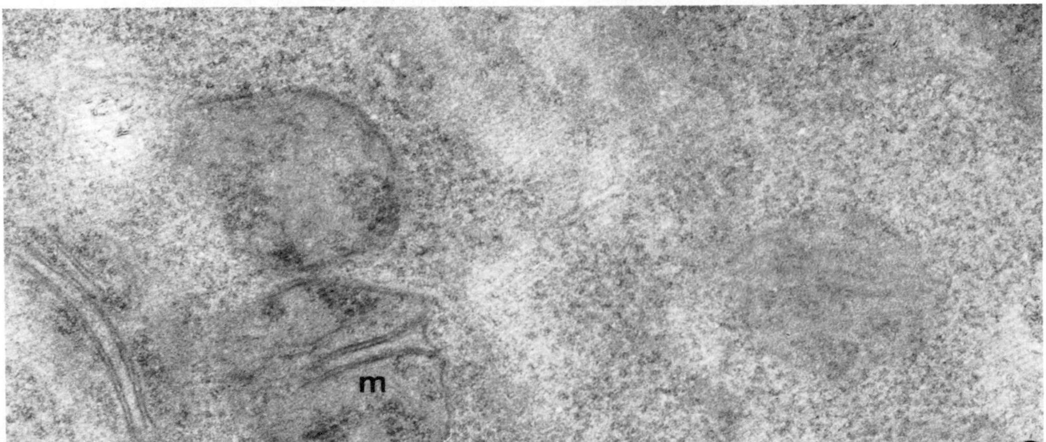

12

uted to this enzyme. The increase in AlPase, found after exposure to a fungistatic dose, may be due to increased catabolism as a consequence of a cellular defense mechanism and to a concomitant intracellular accumulation of organic phosphates. The rise in cell volume and the production of membranous structures and vesicles might be a morphological expression of an increased cell metabolism.

An increase in activity towards the specific substrate ATP is seen, which is analogous to the profile of the AlPase activity after treatment with a fungistatic dose. The fact that the activity towards ATP was visibly lowered at alkaline pH indicates that the activity found cannot be attributed exclusively to a nonspecific AlPase activity, but probably to an adenosine triphosphatase or a polyphosphatase activity that shows a pH optimum in the neutral range.

Marked alterations in the distribution of AcPase activity are observed after exposure of the cells to miconazole. Although the total amount of activity of this enzyme remains unchanged, drastic changes are seen in its topographical distribution. Using NOP as substrate, the AcPase activity is found not only in the vacuolar system but also on the plasmalemma. This localization is never found using β-glycerophosphate as substrate. These results can be seen in the light of the findings of Bowen and Ryder (8), who demonstrated AcPase on several extralysosomal sites with NOP and prefer this substrate for demonstrating cellular lysis. AcPase activity on the plasmalemma is also shown in another yeast species, cultured under different experimental circumstances by Van Rijn et al. (40). In view of our biochemical results, which demonstrate no increase in AcPase activity, the "unusual" localization seen after exposure to different doses of miconazole can only be explained by an unmasking or an activation of the fixed enzyme or by a dislocation of the enzyme from the vacuole to the plasmalemma. Because of the similar sensitivity to fluoride, the AcPase present on the plasmalemma seems to be of the same nature as the enzyme present in the vacuole.

Oxidative and peroxidative enzymes. Concerning cytochrome *c* oxidase, a quantitative

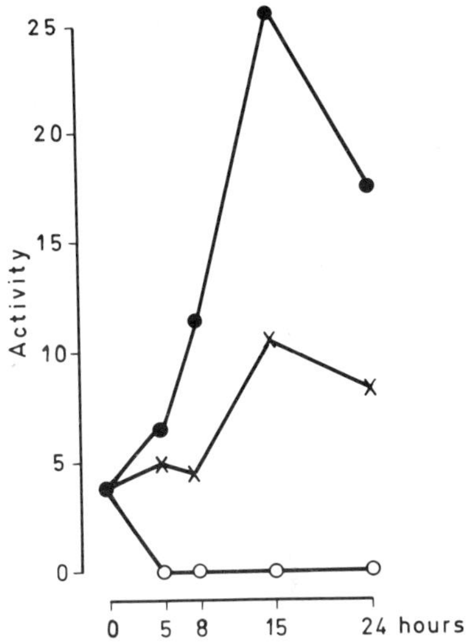

FIG. 13. *Cytochrome c peroxidase (Δ per minute per milligram of protein) of C. albicans cells grown in CYG medium at 37°C (mean of seven determinations). Symbols: (●) Cytochrome c peroxidase activity of control cells; (×) cytochrome c peroxidase activity of cells exposed to a fungistatic dose (10^{-6} M) of miconazole; (○) cytochrome c peroxidase activity of cells exposed to a minimal fungicidal dose (10^{-5} M) of miconazole.*

difference is found biochemically between *S. cerevisiae* and *C. albicans* under control conditions: the enzyme is already present in the inoculum cells of *C. albicans* and shows an optimum in activity in the exponential phase of growth. The inoculum cells of *S. cerevisiae* also show this enzyme activity, but the increase in activity takes place in the early stationary phase. This species difference is even more pronounced as regards cytochrome *c* peroxidase: under the culture conditions used, this strain of *S. cerevisiae* is apparently devoid of cytochrome *c* peroxidase activity at each phase of growth. Inoculum cells of *C. albicans*, on the other hand, already have cytochrome *c* peroxidase present, and cells in the early stationary phase demonstrate a strong increase. This difference in the time of appearance of maximal cytochrome *c* oxidase and peroxidase activities could be explained by the need for cytochrome *c* oxidase

FIG. 10. *Cytochrome c oxidase. C. albicans control cell. The mitochondrial cristae are the only reactive sites (arrows). Abbreviations: Nucleus (n); cell wall (cw); peroxisomes (p). (×25,600)*

FIG. 11. *Cytochrome c oxidase. C. albicans cell exposed to 10^{-6} M miconazole. The cristae (arrows) are reactive. Peroxisomes (p) and other organelles are unreactive. (×43,200)*

FIG. 12. *Cytochrome c oxidase. C. albicans cells exposed to 10^{-5} M miconazole. The mitochondria (m) are completely devoid of reaction product. (×68,800)*

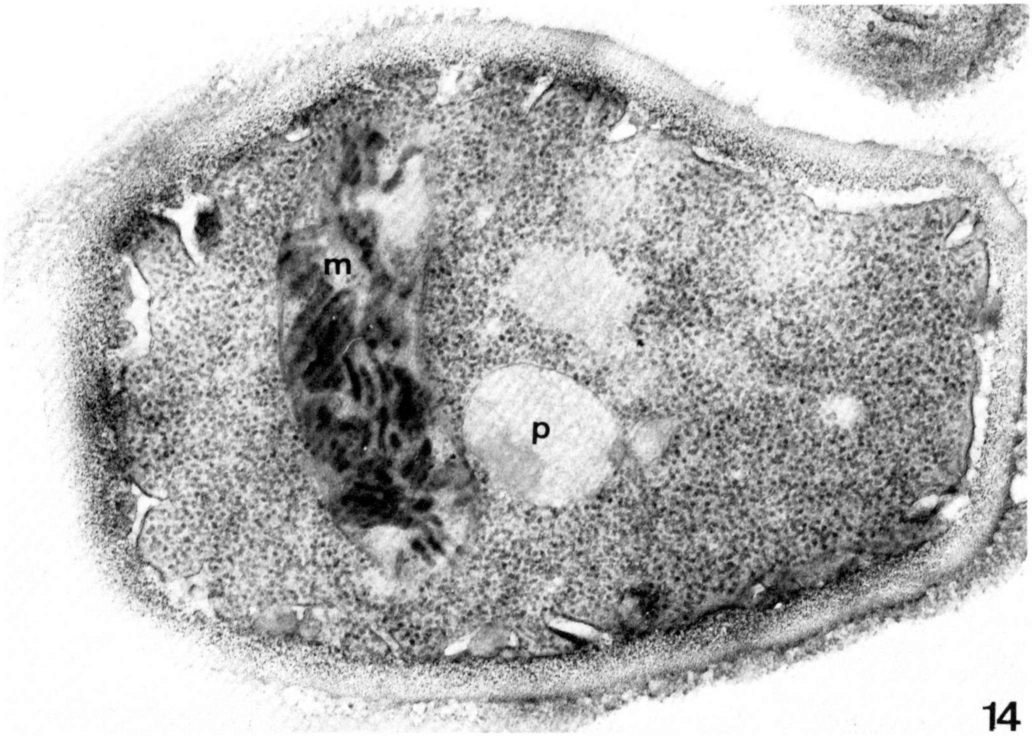

14

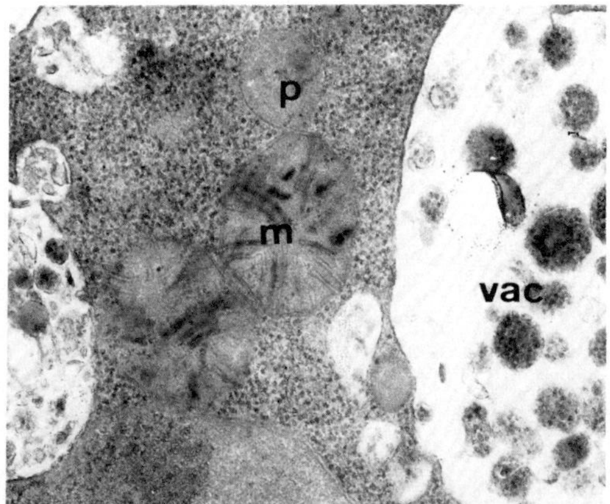

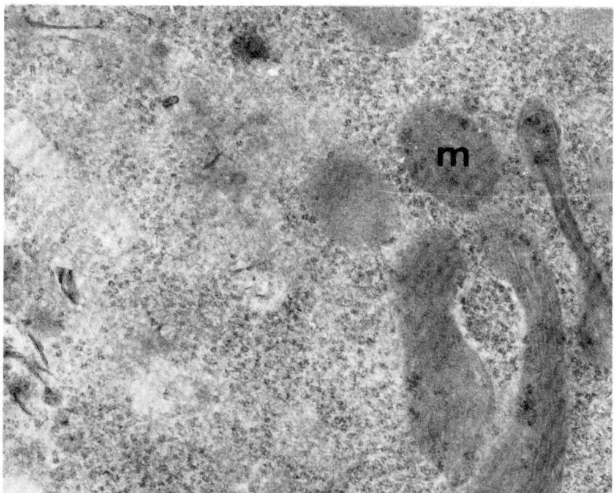

during this initial phase of growth, when the cells need large quantities of oxygen to provide the energy for growth and division. Between 8 and 15 h of growth, there is apparently a change in the cellular metabolism from anabolic processes (requiring high activity of cytochrome *c* oxidase) to catabolic processes. The latter appear to result in the production of hydrogen peroxide (through the action of oxidase or oxidases, since it is at that time that cytochrome *c* peroxidase and catalase activities begin to rise.

The different behavior of the oxidative and peroxidative enzymes of *S. cerevisiae* may be explained by the facultative aerobic condition of this species (27). In the present study, catalase activity is not found in the inoculum cells of both yeast species. The activity appears in an earlier stage of growth in *C. albicans* than in *S. cerevisiae,* but in *S. cerevisiae* the activity is doubled after 24 h of growth. The oval-round structures that resemble mammalian peroxisomes have been reported earlier to be catalase negative in *C. albicans* (13). However, this appears to be due to suboptimal preservation of this enzyme under the conditions used. With an adapted methodology (24, 29), these bodies become positive. Catalase-positive peroxisomes have already been described by several authors in other yeast species and under other growth conditions (16, 22, 25, 26, 28, 33, 34, 39). In our experiments, the peroxisomal activity is totally abolished in the presence of aminotriazole. Vorisek and Volfova (41) describe the relative insensitivity of the catalase of *C. biodinii* to aminotriazole if it is added to the measuring medium. These authors assume, therefore, that the DAB reaction in the mitochondria, which is also insensitive to aminotriazole, is caused by a catalase and a peroxidase. The experiments of Van Belle, Goossens, and Van Roy (in preparation) confirm this in vitro insensitivity of catalase. It is most likely that the difference between the biochemically "isolated" enzyme and the cytochemically "fixed" enzyme is due to the fact that aminotriazole exerts its inhibitory action on the peroxidase activity of catalase only (demonstrated by cytochemical means with a DAB reaction) and not on the catalytic activity

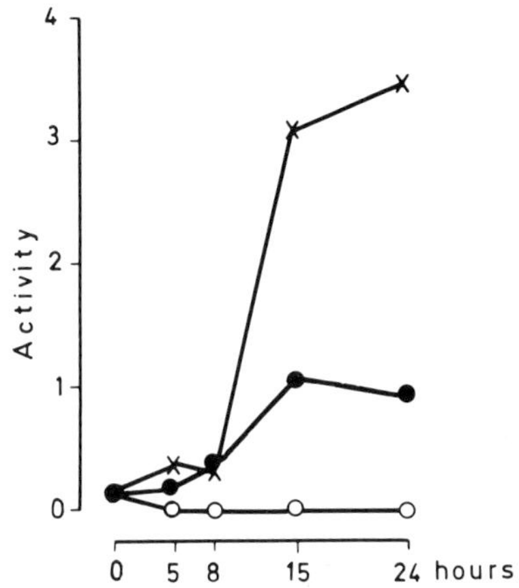

FIG. 17. *Catalase (Δ per minute per milligram of protein) of C. albicans cells grown in CYG medium at 37°C (mean of seven determinations). Symbols: (●) Catalase activity of control cells; (×) catalase activity of cells exposed to a fungistatic dose (10^{-6} M) of miconazole; (○) catalase activity of cells exposed to a minimal fungicidal dose (10^{-5} M) of miconazole.*

(demonstrated biochemically). This indicates that the reaction, after cytochemical incubation in a catalase medium, localized on the mitochondrial membranes, is caused by peroxidase activity, whereas catalase is localized in the peroxisomes of the cell.

After exposure to 10^{-6} and 10^{-5} M miconazole, the partial to complete inhibition of cytochrome *c* oxidase and peroxidase, as seen cytochemically, is in perfect correlation with our biochemical findings. From this, it appears that these enzymes are extremely sensitive to the drug. Since cytochrome *c* peroxidase is present in *C. albicans,* with high activity and with a specific localization in the mitochondria, one may assume that this enzyme plays a very important role in the oxidative metabolism of the cell.

As for catalase, Pritchard and Hudson (28) suggest that the massive cell death that is seen when oxygen under high pressure is put into the culture is due to an intracellular accumulation of peroxide. The loss in cell viability is preceded by a marked increase in catalase activity, followed by a steep decrease in activity.

FIG. 14. *Cytochrome c peroxidase. C. albicans control cell. The cristae, as well as the limiting membrane, of a mitochondrion (m) are strongly reactive. Note the absence of reaction product in a peroxisome (p). (×43,200)*

FIG. 15. *Cytochrome c peroxidase. C. albicans cell exposed to 10^{-6} M miconazole. In this cell, the mitochondrial activity (m) is rather weak. Abbreviations: Nucleus (n); peroxisomes (p); vacuole (vac). (×50,400)*

FIG. 16. *Cytochrome c peroxidase. C. albicans cell exposed to 10^{-5} M miconazole. The mitochondria (m) are totally devoid of reaction product. (×36,400)*

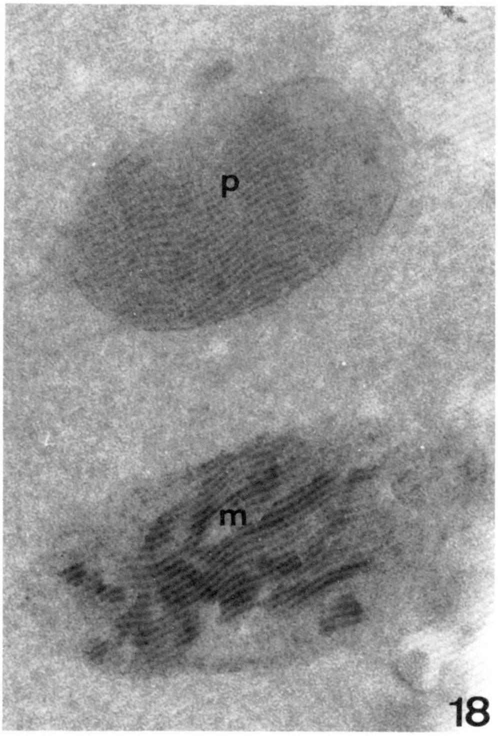
p
m
18

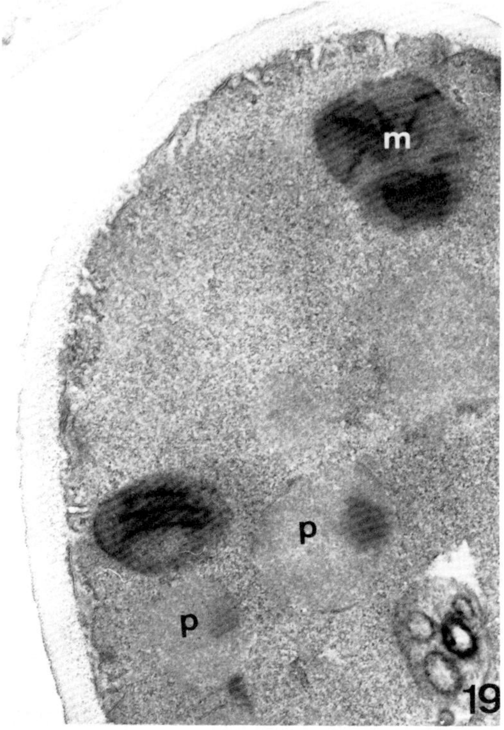
m
p
p
19

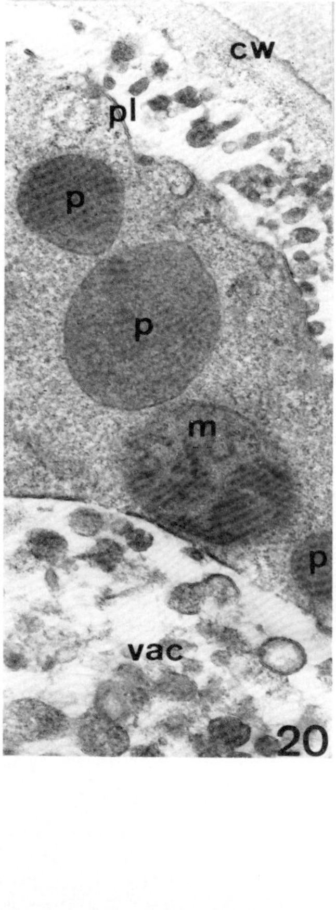
cw
pl
p
p
m
p
vac
20

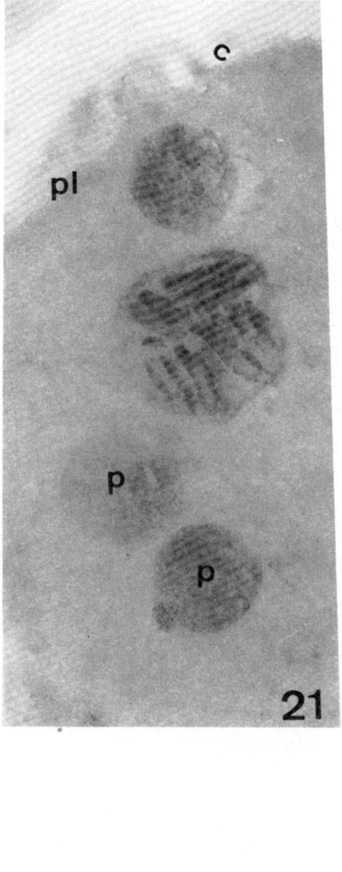
c
pl
p
p
21

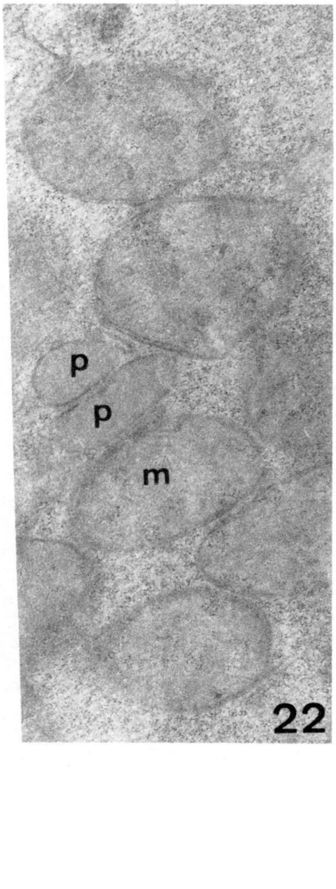
p
p
m
22

They believe that the increased catalase activity points to a possible protective mechanism that is related to the ability of the cells to survive long periods of treatment under oxygen at high pressure. Gifford and Pritchard (17) demonstrate further that when oxygen under high pressure is put into the culture in a "catalase-rich" phase of the cells, the cells are able to survive the exposure.

In view of the pronounced and specific effect of miconazole on the oxidative and peroxidative enzymes, as compared with the effect on hydrolases, we attach great importance to this observation, which might point to a possible mechanism of action of the drug. Since there is no direct effect of miconazole on the enzyme activities tested in the measuring medium, the early effects on the oxidative and peroxidative enzymes during growth suggest that miconazole interferes with the synthesis of these enzymes. The effects of benzimidazole on the synthesis of cytochrome oxidase have been studied by Schmitt-Verhulst et al. (30), who demonstrated that the presence of 9×10^{-3} M benzimidazole in aerobic cultures of *S. cerevisiae* partially blocks mitochondrial protein synthesis. When added to anaerobic cultures, the adaptation of these organisms to oxygen is blocked when oxygen is put into the culture. According to these authors, benzimidazole should have a direct effect on the synthesis of cytochrome oxidase by inhibiting the biosynthesis of cytochrome aa_3. Cytochrome oxidase appears to be very sensitive to the presence of oxygen in the medium (21, 28 30, 32).

On the other hand, it might be that, by activating the peroxide-generating system, the enzymes responsible for the breakdown of peroxide (peroxidase and catalase) are destroyed. The latter possibility is suggested by the work of Erman and Yonetani (14), who claim that cytochrome *c* peroxidase is very sensitive to the peroxide concentration, in the sense that peroxide does oxidize the heme group and various amino acid residues of cytochrome *c* peroxidase.

From the foregoing results, a hypothesis is formulated on the mechanism of action of miconazole (Fig. 23). The activities of cytochrome *c* peroxidase and catalase are indicative of the elimination and hence the production of peroxide in the normal yeast cell. The oxidative enzymes responsible for the production of peroxide in *C. albicans* are not well determined, although recently obtained data (M. Borgers, S. De Nollin, F. Thoné, and H. Van Belle, J. Histochem. Cytochem., in press) indicate that reduced nicotinamide adenine dinucleotide (NADH) might oxidase be involved. The treatment with a fungistatic dose of miconazole results in a strong inhibition of cytochrome *c* peroxidase. If one admits that the oxidative metabolic processes continue normally, or even at an increased level, as indicated by our preliminary experiments on NADH oxidase, the intracellular peroxide concentration may rise to levels that induce a strong catalase activity, thereby rescuing the cell from peroxide intoxication. After exposure to the minimal fungicidal dose of miconazole, the activities of cytochrome *c* peroxidase and catalase disappear completely, whereas NADH oxidase appears to be still very active. In this situation, the intracellular peroxide concentration may reach oxide concentration may reach levels that are incompatible with the viability of the cell.

Several additional observations (S. De Nollin, thesis, 1976) support this hypothesis. (i) The morphology of the mitochondria in *C. albicans* cells treated for a short time with a fungicidal dose of miconazole (10^{-4} M) reveals changes resembling the alterations of hypoxic mitochondria. (ii) The experiments on *S. cerevisiae* 17787, a strain very susceptible to miconazole and showing no cytochrome *c* peroxidase activity under our culture conditions, reveal an extremely sensitive catalase (complete inhibition with 2×10^{-8} M miconazole). There is a direct correlation between growth inhibition and the disappearance of catalase. (iii) *C. albicans* seems to be relatively nonsusceptible to

FIG. 18. *Catalase. C. albicans control cell. No counterstaining. A catalase-positive peroxisome (p) is situated near a mitochondrion (m) showing interfering cytochrome c peroxidase activity. (×86,400)*

FIG. 19. *Catalase. C. albicans control cell. The peroxisomes (p) are completely negative after incubation in the presence of 20 mM aminotriazole. The interfering activity of cytochrome c peroxidase on the mitochondria (m) remains unchanged. (×47,250)*

FIG. 20. *Catalase. C. albicans cell exposed to 10^{-6} M miconazole. The three peroxisomes (p) present on this section are strongly catalase reactive. Mitochondria (m) showing interfering cytochrome c peroxidase activity. Abbreviations: Vacuole (vac); cell wall (cw); plasmalemma (pl). (×41,500)*

FIG. 21. *Catalase. C. albicans cell exposed to 10^{-6} M miconazole. No counterstaining. Note the reactive peroxisomes (p). There is no activity on the cell wall (cw) and the plasmalemma (pl). (×58,300)*

FIG. 22. *Catalase. C. albicans cell exposed to 10^{-5} M miconazole. No activity remains on the peroxisomes (p). The cytochrome c peroxidase activity on the mitochondria (m) has also disappeared. (×58,300)*

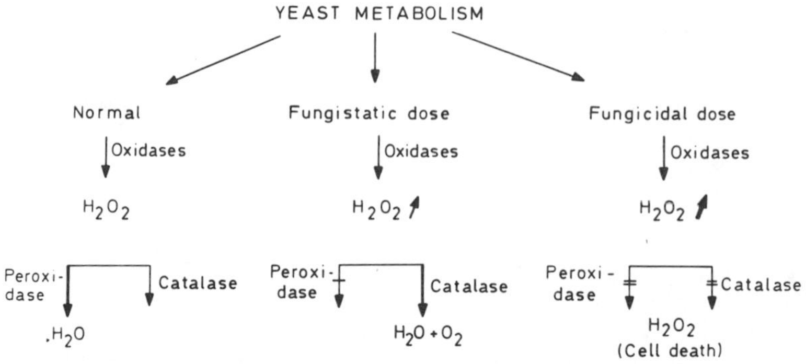

FIG. 23. *Schematic presentation of the hypothetical mechanism of action of the antimycotic miconazole.*

miconazole when the drug is added to nondiluted cells in stationary phase. Since miconazole has no direct effect on catalase or cytochrome *c* peroxidase activities, but only on their synthesis, it is likely that the cells that are already equipped with these enzymes are able to break down the produced hydrogen peroxide, even in the presence of the drug. (iv) The results of Van den Bossche (unpublished data) indicate that *S. cerevisiae* RV 11786, grown anaerobically and thus lacking oxidative and peroxidative enzymes, are relatively nonsusceptible to miconazole treatment.

ACKNOWLEDGMENTS

We wish to thank J. Van Cutsem for preparing the cultures. We are also grateful to P. Drochmans for his valuable criticism.

LITERATURE CITED

1. **Barka, T., and P. Anderson.** 1962. Histochemical methods for acid phosphatase using hexasonium pararosanilin as coupler. J. Histochem. Cytochem. **10:**741–753.
2. **Bauer, H., and E. Sigarlakie.** 1973. Cytochemistry on ultrathin frozen sections of yeast cells. J. Microsc. (Oxford) **99:**205–218.
3. **Bauer, H., and E. Sigarlakie.** 1975. Localization of alkaline phosphatase in *Saccharomyces cerevisiae* by means of ultrathin frozen sections. J. Ultrastruct. Res. **50:**208–215.
4. **Bergmeyer, H. U.** (ed.) 1974. Methods of enzymatic analysis. Academic Press, Inc., New York.
5. **Borgers, M., J. Schaper, and W. Schaper.** 1971. Localization of specific phosphatase activities in canine coronary blood vessels and heart muscle. J. Histochem. Cytochem. **19:**526–539.
6. **Borgers, M., and S. De Nollin.** 1974. The preservation of subcellular organelles of *C. albicans* using conventional fixatives. J. Cell Biol. **62:**574–581.
7. **Botter, A.** 1971. Topical treatment of nail and skin infections with miconazole, a broad-spectrum antimycoticum. Mykosen **14:**187–191.
8. **Bowen, I. D., and T. A. Ryder.** 1976. Use of the p-nitrophenyl phosphate method for the demonstration of acid phosphatase during starvation and cell autolyses in the planarian *Polycelis tenuis Iijina*. Histochemistry **8:**319–329.
9. **Brugmans, J. P., J. Van Cutsem, and D. Thienpont.** 1970. Treatment of long-term tinea pedis with miconazole. Arch. Dermatol **102:**428–432.
10. **Chantrenne, H.** 1955. Peroxydases induites par l'oxygène chez la levure. Biochim. Biophys. Acta **18:**58–62.
11. **De Nollin, S., and M. Borgers.** 1974. The ultrastructure of *Candida albicans* after *in vitro* treatment with miconazole. Sabouraudia **12:**341–351.
12. **De Nollin, S., and M. Borgers.** 1975. Scanning electron microscopy of *Candida albicans* after *in vitro* treatment with miconazole. Antimicrobiol. Agents Chemother. **7:**704–711.
13. **De Nollin, S., F. Thonè, and M. Borgers.** 1975. Enzyme cytochemistry of *Candida albicans*. J. Histochem. Cytochem. **23:**758–765.
14. **Erman, J. E., and R. Yonetani.** 1975. The oxidation of cytochrome c-peroxidase by hydrogen peroxide. Characterization of products. Biochim. Biophys. Acta **393:**343–349.
15. **Fahimi, H. D.** 1969. Cytochemical localization of peroxidatic activity of catalase in rat hypatic microbodies (peroxisomes). J. Cell Biol. **43:**275–288.
16. **Fukui, S., A. Tanaka, S. Kawamoto, S. Yasuhara, Y. Teranishi, and M. Osumi.** 1975. Ultrastructure of methanol-utilizing yeast cells: appearance of microbodies in relation to high catalase activity. J. Bacteriol. **123:**317–328.
17. **Gifford, G. D., and G. G. Pritchard.** 1969. Toxicity of hyperbaric oxygen to yeasts displaying periodic enzyme synthesis. J. Gen. Microbiol. **56:**143–149.
18. **Godefroi, E. F., J. Heeres, J. Van Cutsem, and P. A. J. Janssen.** 1969. The preparation and antimycotic properties of derivatives of l-phenetyl-imidazole. J. Med. Chem. **12:**784–791.
19. **Godts, P., P. Vermylen, and J. Van Cutsem.** 1971. Clinical evaluation of miconazole nitrate in the treatment of vaginal Candidiasis. Arzneim. Forsch. **21:**256–257.
20. **Graham, R. C., Jr., and M. J. Karnovsky.** 1966. The early stages of absorption of injected horseradish peroxidase in the proximal tubules of mouse kidney; ultrastructural cytochemistry by a new technique. J. Histochem. Cytochem. **14:**291–302.
21. **Groot, G. S. P., and R. O. Poyton.** 1975. Oxygen control of cytochrome c-oxidase synthesis in isolated mitochondria from *Saccharomycés cerevisiae*. Nature (London) **255:**238–240.
22. **Hoffmann, H. P., A. Szabo, and C. J. Avers.** 1970. Cytochemical localization of catalase activity in yeast peroxisomes. J. Bacteriol. **104:**581–584.
23. **Hugon, J., and M. Borgers.** 1966. Ultrastructural local-

ization of alkaline phosphatase activity in the absorbing cells of the duodenum of mouse. J. Histochem. Cytochem. 14:629-640.

24. **Novikoff, A. B., and S. Goldfischer.** 1969. Visualisation of peroxisomes and mitochondria with diaminobenzidine. J. Histochem. Cytochem. 17:675-680.
25. **Osumi, M., N. Miwa, Y. Teranishi, A. Tanaka, and S. Fukui.** 1974. Ultrastructure of *Candida* yeasts grown on n-alkanes. Appearance of microbodies and its relationship to high catalase activity. Arch. Microbiol. 99:181-201.
26. **Osumi, M., F. Fukuzumi, Y. Teranishi, A. Tanaka, and S. Fukui.** 1975. Development of microbodies *Candida tropicalis* during incubation in a n-alkane medium. Arch. Microbiol. 103:1-11.
27. **Polakis, E. S., W. Bartley, and G. Meck.** 1964. Changes in the structure and enzyme activity of *S. cerevisiae* in response to changes in the environment. Biochem. J. 90:369-374.
28. **Pritchard, G. G., and M. A. Hudson.** 1967. Changes in catalase activity in higher plants and fungi treated with oxygen at high pressure. Nature (London) 214:945-946.
29. **Roels, F., E. Wisse, B. De Prest, and J. van der Meulen.** 1975. Cytochemical discrimination between catalases and peroxidases using diaminobenzidine. Histochemistry 41:281-312.
30. **Schmitt-Verhulst, A.-M., F. Bex, and A. A. Sels.** 1973. Studies on the mechanism of the oxygen-induced synthesis of cytochrome oxidase in yeast. Specific effects of benzimidazole on cytochrome-oxidase anabolism. Eur. J. Biochem. 36:185-194.
31. **Seligman, A., M. Karnovsky, H. Wasserkrug, and J. Hanker.** 1968. Non-droplet ultrastructural demonstration of cytochrome oxidase activity with a polymerizing osmiophilic reagent, diaminobenzidine (DAB). J. Cell Biol. 38:1-14.
32. **Sels, A. A.** 1969. Origin of the increase in adaptability at oxygen of yeast pretreated with benzimidazole. Biochem. Biophys. Res. Commun. 34:740-747.
33. **Teranishi, Y., S. Kawamoto, A. Tanaka, M. Osumi, and S. Fukui.** 1974. Induction of catalase activity by hydrocarbons in *Candida tropicalis* pK 233. Agr. Biol. Chem. 38:1221-1225.
34. **Todd, M. M., and E. L. Vigil.** 1972. Cytochemical localization of peroxidase activity in *Saccharomyces cerevisiae*. J. Histochem. Cytochem. 20:344-349.
35. **Van Belle, H.** 1976. Alkaline phosphatase. II. Conditions affecting determination of total activity in serum. Clin. Chem. 22:977-981.
36. **Van Cutsem, J., and D. Thienpont.** 1972. Miconazole, a broad-spectrum antimycotic agent with antibacterial activity. Chemotherapy 17:392-404.
37. **Van den Bossche, H.** 1974. Biochemical effects of miconazole on fungi. I. Effects on the uptake and/or utilization of purines, pyrimidines, nucleosides, amino acids and glucose by *Candida albicans*. Biochem. Pharmacol. 23:887-899.
38. **Van den Bossche, H., G. Willemsens, and J. M. Van Cutsem.** 1975. The action of miconazole on the growth of *Candida albicans*. Sabouraudia 13:63-73.
39. **Van Dijken, J. P., M. Veenhuis, N. J. Kreger-Van Rij, and W. Harder.** 1975. Microbodies in methanol-assimilating yeasts. Arch. Microbiol. 102:41-44.
40. **Van Rijn, H. J., W. A. Linnemans, and P. Boer.** 1975. Localization of acid phosphotase in protoplasts from *Saccharomyces cerevisiae*. J. Bacteriol. 123:1144-1149.
41. **Vorisek, J., and O. Volfova.** 1975. Catalase activity in methanol-oxidizing *Candida biodinii* 11Bh and its cytochemical localization. FEBS Lett. 52:246-250.
42. **Wachstein, M., and E. Meisel.** 1957. Histochemistry of hepatic phosphatase at a physiologic pH with reference to the demonstration of bile canaliculi. Am. J. Clin. Pathol. 27:13-23.

ANTIMICROBIAL AGENTS AND CHEMOTHERAPY, Mar. 1977, p. 514-520
Vol. 11, No. 3

Printed in U.S.A.

Mobilization of Morganocin 174 Plasmid and Kinetics of Morganocin Production in *Proteus* and *Escherichia coli* Hosts

J. A. WILLIAMS

Microbial Genetics Unit, South African Medical Research Council, Department of Microbiology, University of Pretoria, Pretoria, South Africa

Received for publication 3 August 1976

Morganocin 174 is coded by a plasmid, Mor174. The plasmid is not self-transmissible but may be mobilized by resistance factor R772. Morganocin synthesis in all *Proteus* and *Providencia* strains carrying Mor174 was characterized by a longer lag period after induction and higher titers than in *Escherichia coli* B(Mor174). The low titers obtained in *E. coli* B(Mor174) are due to a heat-stable inhibitor produced by this strain. Synthesis of morganocin is not constitutive and may be induced by ultraviolet irradiation or mitomycin C. Morganocin production is not influenced by the growth medium of the organism.

Bacteriocins are antibiotic molecules produced by a wide range of organisms (see 23). Many are coded for by plasmids which have been identified by isolation (25), elimination (16, 27), or mobilization as a result of their sex factor activity (22) or that of a mobilizing plasmid (29). Several bacteriocins have been purified and characterized to varying degrees, and their mode of action has been established (see 9). Ease of purification depends on the concentration of bacteriocin synthesized, which, although measured in arbitrary units, varies considerably (see 11). The amount of bacteriocin produced may be influenced by the growth conditions of the organism. Staphylococcin 1580 and bacteriocins of *Streptococcus mutans* were synthesized more readily on semisolid media (17, 24), although a method has been described for production of *S. mutans* bacteriocins in liquid culture (6). Synthesis of colicin K (7) is influenced by the pH of the culture medium. Production of many bacteriocins is enhanced by treatment with inducing agents such as mitomycin C (MC) (13), ultraviolet irradiation (14), heat (8, 18), or transient inhibition of protein synthesis (2, 18). The rise in bacteriocin titer may be a result of a gene dosage effect due to amplification of the bacteriocinogenic plasmid in the cell (10, but see 9) or derepression of protein synthesis (19).

Proteus morganii 174 produces a bacteriocin (morganocin 174) in limited quantity and irregularly. The amount spontaneously present in the supernatant fluid of overnight cultures varied from 0 to 8 arbitrary units/ml. The host strain is lysogenic and occasionally lyses after induction, with resultant intracellular protein contamination of the bacteriocin (unpublished data). This investigation was done in an attempt to enhance the production of morganocin 174 to facilitate purification. A variety of media and inducing agents were investigated.

MATERIALS AND METHODS

Bacterial strains. Bacterial strains are listed in Table 1. A total of 973 locally isolated gram-negative strains was used to test the activity spectrum of the morganocin.

Media. *Proteus* and *Providencia* strains were grown in the nutrient broth of Coetzee and Sacks (4) or in defined medium (DM) made up as follows. A 375-ml aqueous solution, containing 10 g of NH_4SO_4, 10 mg of $MgSO_4$, 500 mg of sodium citrate, and 10 g of Casamino Acids, and 600 ml of 0.5 M potassium phosphate buffer, pH 7 (unless otherwise stated), were autoclaved separately and then combined and supplemented with 10 ml of 20% glucose and 5 ml each of 0.1% stock solutions of nicotinic acid, methionine, and calcium pantothenate to make 1 liter of medium. The effect of pH on morganocin production was investigated by using medium buffered with 0.3 M potassium phosphate at pH 6 and 7. The high ionic strength could be expected to decrease ionic interaction between morganocin and cell debris while maintaining the pH of the medium during the time of production. The pH measured after 96 h of growth had not changed by more than 0.2 pH unit. The high ionic strength had no effect on the growth of the bacteria (not shown). For *Escherichia coli* B, broth was antibiotic medium 3 (Difco), and DM was M-9 medium supplemented with 1.0% Casamino Acids. For morganocin production on semisolid media, defined media supplemented with 0.6% Difco agar (DM agar) and Hershey agar (30) containing 0.4% agar were used. For double-agar layer plates, Hershey agar containing 1.1% agar in the bottom layer and 0.4% agar in the top layer was used. Transconjugants were selected on McConkey agar (Difco) supplemented with the following antibiotics

TABLE 1. *Bacterial strains and plasmid*

Organism	Properties	Origin
P. morganii 174	Produces morganocin 174	Locally isolated
P. morganii 163	Indicator for morganocin 174	Locally isolated
P. morganii 163 *str*^{r}	Spontaneous mutant resistant to 1 mg of streptomycin per ml	Williams (unpublished data)
P. morganii 165	Indicator for morganocin 174	Locally isolated
P. morganii 165 *mor*^{r}	Spontaneous mutant selected for nonadsorption of morganocin 174	Williams (unpublished data)
P. morganii 165 *nal*^{r}	NG[a] mutant (1) resistant to 50 μg of nalidixic acid per ml All *P. morganii* strains resistant to 100 μg of ampicillin per ml	Williams (unpublished data)
P. mirabilis 5006 *nal*^{r}	Mutant of PM5006 resistant to 50 μg of nalidixic acid per ml	Coetzee (3)
P. mirabilis 5006 *str*^{r}(R772)	Derivative of PM5006 spontaneously resistant to 1 mg of streptomycin per ml and carrying the resistance plasmid R772	Coetzee (unpublished data)
Providencia P29	NCTC 9211	Coetzee et al. (5)
Providencia P29 *nal*^{r}	NG mutant (1) resistant to 50 μg of nalidixic acid per ml	Williams (unpublished data)
E. coli B		
E. coli B *str*^{r}	Spontaneous mutant resistant to 1 mg of streptomycin per ml	
Plasmid		
R772	Carries marker for kanamycin resistance (K)	Hedges (13)

[a] NG, Nitrosoguanidine.

as required: streptomycin, 1 mg/ml; kanamycin, nalidixic acid, and ampicillin, 50 μg/ml each.

Conjugation. Broth-grown cultures were mated according to Coetzee (3). For autonomous transfer of morganocinogeny, conjugation mixtures were treated after 2 h with 10^{10} killing units of morganocin for 1 h and then plated on media counterselective to the donor. When donors contained R772, transconjugants were initially selected for kanamycin resistance and then for simultaneous acquisition of morganocinogeny by replicating onto plates seeded with indicator organisms (2×10^7 colony-forming units) in a soft top layer. Before being replicated onto, these plates were chilled for 1 h at 4°C to reduce soft-agar tackiness. Morganocin-producing colonies show halos of inhibition of the indicator organism. This technique was also used to determine loss of the plasmid due to defective segregation.

Induction of morganocin. Cultures in the logarithmic phase of growth containing approximately 5×10^7 colony-forming units/ml in defined medium were induced. After 2 to 96 h, aliquots were centrifuged at $10{,}000 \times g$ for 10 min, and the supernatant liquid was tested for bacteriocin activity. The following induction procedures were used: with ultraviolet irradiation, washed bacteria resuspended in saline were irradiated to 99% mortality and diluted 1:100 in fresh DM; with MC 0.5 μg/ml was added to midlog cultures; cyclic adenosine 5′-monophosphate (cAMP) and dibutyryl cAMP, respectively, were added to a final concentration of 1 mM together with 0.5 μg of MC per ml. To test the effect of chloramphenicol, overnight cultures in DM were treated with 150 μg of chloramphenicol per ml for 2 h and then diluted 1:100 into warm DM. For morganocin synthesis in semisolid medium, midlog cells containing 0.5 μg of MC per ml were embedded in DM agar or Hershey agar at a concentration of 5×10^7 colony-forming units/ml, incubated at 37°C for 48 h, frozen at −20°C for 2 h, and thawed for 30 min at 37°C. After centrifugation at $10{,}000 \times g$ for 20 min, the supernatant was assayed for morganocin activity.

Bacteriocin assay. Double-agar layer plates seeded with 10^7 colony-forming units of indicator organism in the top layer were spotted with 0.02-ml aliquots of serially diluted morganocin. The titer in arbitrary units was expressed as the reciprocal of the highest dilution that gave a clear zone of inhibition. A more accurate measure of morganocin activity was made by addition of morganocin to indicator cells and titrating for surviving bacteria after 20 min. The number of killing units was determined from the Poisson distribution, $P/P_0 = e^{-n}$.

Lacunae. Morganocin-synthesizing bacteria were

identified by the lacunae method of Ozeki et al. (21) with *P. morganii* 163 *str*[r] as indicator. For improved visualization of lacunae, background growth was stained with 2,3,5-triphenyltetrazolium chloride (tetrazolium). Plates containing appropriate dilutions of producer organisms and 10^7 to 5×10^7 indicator cells were chilled for 4 h at 4°C, incubated for 12 h at 25°C, flooded with 5 to 10 ml of 0.1% aqueous solution of tetrazolium, and incubated for a further 1 h in a level position at 37°C. For optimal staining the seeded agar layer must be of even thickness and stained while the indicator organisms are still actively metabolizing.

Host range. Hershey agar lawns seeded with test organism in the top layer were spotted with crude morganocin and examined the following day for growth inhibition.

Column chromatography. A Pharmacia column (90 by 1.5 cm) was packed with Sephadex G200 in 0.01 M potassium phosphate buffer, pH 7, 0.1 M KCl, and the void volume was determined with blue dextran 2000. One milliliter of crude colicin was applied, and 2-ml fractions were collected and assayed for morganocin activity.

Chemicals. cAMP was obtained from Nutritional Biochemicals Corp. (Cleveland, Ohio); N^6, N^6, $O^{2'}$-dibutyryl cAMP from Calbiochem (San Diego, California); MC from Kyowa Hakko Kogyo (Tokyo); 2,3,5-triphenyltetrazolium chloride and trypsin from Merck (Darmstadt); Pronase from Miles-Seravac (Cape Town); and lysozyme from British Drug Houses (London).

RESULTS

Properties of morganocin 174. The inhibition spectrum of morganocin 174 on a variety of independently isolated gram-negative bacterial strains was investigated (Table 2). Apart from two *Proteus mirabilis* strains, activity was limited to *P. morganii* strains, 74% of which were susceptible. Molecular exclusion chromatography of crude morganocin on Sephadex G200 revealed an activity peak which eluted after the void volume, indicating a molecular weight of less than 800,000. The stability of morganocin to various inactivating agents is shown in Table 3. It was concluded that morganocin 174 is a proteinaceous bacteriocin rather than a defective phage.

TABLE 2. *Spectrum of morganocin 174 activity on gram-negative organisms*

Organism	No. of strains	
	Tested	Susceptible
P. morganii	97	72
P. rettgeri	127	0
P. mirabilis	309	2
P. vulgaris	296	0
Providencia	35	0
E. coli	69	0
Klebsiella	40	0

TABLE 3. *Susceptibility of morganocin 174 to inactivating agents*

Treatment	Morganocin titer after treatment (killing units/ml)	Inactivation (%)
Control	1.08×10^9	
Trypsin[a]	3.03×10^8	72
Pronase[b]	0.00	100
Lysozyme[c]	1.25×10^9	0
Chloroform[d]	5.40×10^8	50
50°C, 30 min	1.05×10^9	0
60°C, 5 min	3.00×10^8	72

[a] 100 μg/ml in 0.02 M potassium phosphate buffer (pH 8.0) at 25°C for 15 min.

[b] 100 μg/ml in 0.07 M phosphate buffer (pH 7.4) at 37°C for 15 min.

[c] 100 μg/ml in 0.07 M phosphate buffer (pH 7.0) (0.017 M NaCl) at 25°C for 15 min.

[d] 25% (vol/vol) $CHCl_3$ shaken for 1 min, centrifuged to facilitate phase separation and the aqueous phase titrated. Medium similarly treated had no effect on indicator organism.

Conjugal transfer of morganocinogeny. An attempt was made to transfer morganocin activity by conjugation. *P. morganii* 165, which is susceptible to morganocin 174, was chosen as recipient, since, after allowing for expression of immunity, crude morganocin could be used to counterselect morganocin-negative organisms. No morganocinogenic 165 clones were found in four experiments. However, when the kanamycin resistance plasmid R772 was introduced into *P. morganii* 174 and this strain was used as donor, morganocinogenic clones were regularly found among transconjugants selected for antibiotic resistance (Table 4). The similar transfer frequencies to *P. morganii* 165 *nal*[r] and *P. morganii* 165 *nal*[r] *mor*[r] suggest that it is unlikely that the absence of transconjugants in the cross *P. morganii* 174 × *P. morganii* 165 *nal*[r] might be due to the lethal effect of morganocin spontaneously produced by the donor. Morganocinogeny and kanamycin resistance segregated independently in the transconjugants (Table 5). The high frequency of defective segregation of morganocinogeny in *E. coli* B(Mor174) (Fig. 1) contrasted with its apparent absence in the original host, *P. morganii* 174, where no morganocin-negative clones were found among 10,000 investigated. The latter results may, however, be misleading due to the possibility that spontaneously produced morganocin 174 would have been lethal to any segregant. It was concluded that morganocin 174 is coded for by non-self-transmissible plasmid (Mor174), which could be mobilized by R772.

TABLE 4. *Conjugal transfer of morganocinogeny*

Donor	Recipient	Frequency of R772 transfer[a]	Cotransfer of morganocinogeny (%)
P. morganii 174	*P. morganii* 165 *nal*^{r}	$<1 \times 10^{-9}$	
P. mirabilis 5006 *str*^{r}(R772)	*P. morganii* 174	2.3×10^{-6}	
P. morganii 174(R772)	*P. morganii* 165 *nal*^{r}	1.1×10^{-5}	32
P. morganii 174(R772)	*P. morganii* 165 *nal*^{r}, *mor*^{r}	1.3×10^{-5}	35
P. morganii 174(R772)	*P. mirabilis* 5006 *nal*^{r}	5.7×10^{-7}	30
P. morganii 174(R772)	*Providencia* P29 *nal*^{r}	5.2×10^{-3}	15
P. morganii 174(R772)	*E. coli* B *str*^{r}	1.1×10^{-5}	28

[a] Frequency/donor cell.

TABLE 5. *Defective segregation of R722 and morganocinogeny*

Organism	Defective segregants (%)[a]		
	R772^{-} Mor174^{+}	R772^{+} Mor174^{-}	R772^{-} Mor174^{-}
P. morganii 174(R772)	0.89	0.00	0.00
P. morganii 165 *nal*^{r} *mor*^{r} (R772 Mor174)	0.06	0.10	0.00
P. mirabilis 5006 *nal*^{r}(R772 Mor174)	0.15	0.10	0.00
Providencia P29 *nal*^{r}(R772 Mor174)	0.16	0.36	0.04
E. coli B *str*^{r}(R772 Mor174)	0.00	43.90	0.00

[a] Percentage of defective segregants after overnight growth in broth.

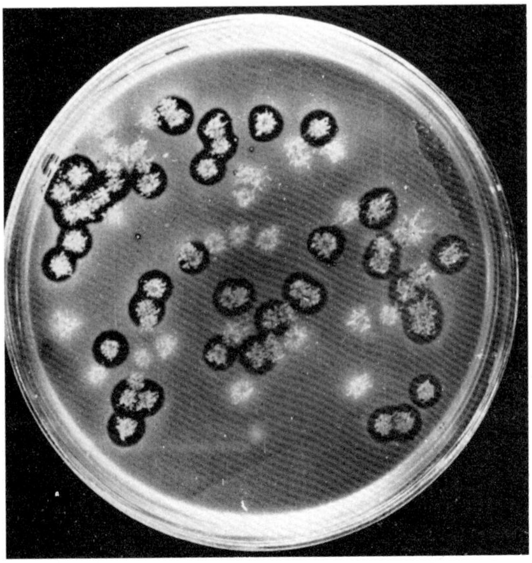

FIG. 1. *Replica plate showing E. coli B (Mor174) colonies with halos of inhibition and defective segregants.*

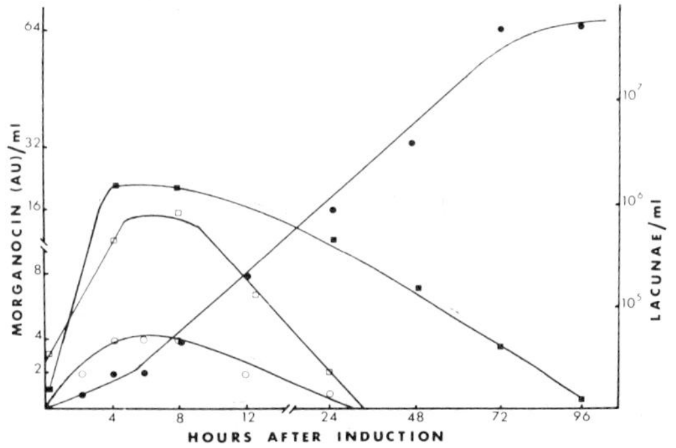

FIG. 2. *Kinetics of morganocin synthesis and appearance of lacunae after induction with 0.5 μg of MC per ml. Symbols: (●) P. morganii 165 mor*^{r} *(Mor174) morganocin; (■) P. morganii 165 mor*^{r} *(Mor174) lacunae; (○) E. coli B (Mor174) morganocin; (□) E. coli B (Mor174) lacunae.*

Kinetics of morganocin synthesis. Figure 2 shows the morganocin titer and number of *P. morganii* 165 mor^{r}(Mor174)- and *E coli* B(Mor174)-producing cells monitored for 96 h after induction with MC. In *P. morganii* 165 *mor*^{r} (Mor174), although the maximum number of lacunae appeared after 6 to 8 h, the morganocin titer increased to a plateau 72 to 96 h after induction. Other *Proteus* and *Providencia* hosts (not shown) showed the same behavior. In *E. coli* B(Mor174) the appearance of a maximal number of lacunae was synchronal with the highest morganocin titer.

Effect of growth media on morganocin synthesis. Synthesis of morganocin 174 in defined medium consisting of dialyzable components was compared to that in broth (Table 6). Both pH 6 and pH 7 based media yielded titers of morganocin 174 comparable to those obtained in broth. To investigate the possibility of in-

TABLE 6. *Effect of host and medium on morganocin 174 production*

Organism	Time (h)	Morganocin titer (arbitrary units/ml)				
		Broth	DM (pH 6)	DM (pH 7)	DM agar	Hershey agar
P. morganii 174	72[a]	32	32	32	32	64
P. morganii 165 *mor*^{r}(Mor174)	72	64	64	64	64	32
P. mirabilis 5006(Mor174)	72	32	32	32	32	32
Providencia P29(Mor174)	72	32	64	64	32	64
E. coli B(Mor174)	4	4	ND[b]	8	8	4

[a] Hours after induction with 0.5 μg of MC per ml.
[b] ND, Not determined.

TABLE 7. *Effect of inducing agents on production of morganocin 174*

Organism	Maximum morganocin titer (arbitrary units/ml[a])					
	UV[b]	MC	cAMP	Dibutyryl cAMP	CM	None
P. morganii 174	8	32	32	32	16	4
P. morganii 165 *mor*^{r}(Mor174)	8	64	32	32	16	4
P. mirabilis 5006(Mor174)	8	32	32	64	32	2
Providencia P29(Mor174)	4	64	32	32	32	2
E. coli B(Mor174)	2	8	4	8	4	1

[a] Organisms were grown in DM.
[b] Inducing agent. UV, ultraviolet; CM, chloramphenicol.

creased yields in semisolid agar, organisms were grown in DM supplemented with 0.4% agar and in Hershey agar. Log-phase cultures were induced and incorporated into the agar. No significant increase in titer over that found in liquid culture was found. The morganocin titer yielded by *E. coli* B(Mor174) was consistently lower than that produced by *Proteus* and *Providencia* strains containing the plasmid.

Morganocin induction. Organisms in the logarithmic phase of growth were subjected to a variety of inducing agents (Table 7). Although the treatments caused some increase in morganocin titer, best results were obtained with MC. Neither cAMP nor dibutyryl cAMP enhanced the effect of MC.

Inhibition of morganocin 174 activity by *E. coli* B(Mor174). The similarity in the number of lacunae in MC-induced *Proteus* strains and *E. coli* B(Mor174) was not reflected by morganocin titers in the supernatant fluid. To investigate the possibility that morganocin produced by *E. coli* B(Mor174) may be inactivated by the production of an inhibitory substance, the supernatant fluid of a culture of *E. coli* B(Mor174), 48 h after induction, was mixed with a known titer of morganocin 174. The inactivation of morganocin 174, shown in Table 8, indicated that *E. coli* B(Mor174) produced a heat-stable inhibitory factor. The greater inhibition of morganocin activity by the *E. coli* B(Mor174) culture indicated that some of the inhibiting factor was cell bound.

TABLE 8. *Inactivation of morganocin 174 activity by E. coli B(Mor174)*

Treatment of morganocin[a]	Morganocin titer (arbitrary units/ml) remaining
Saline	64
E. coli B(Mor174) supernatant fluid	16
E. coli B(Mor174) supernatant fluid, 100°C, 10 min	16
E. coli B(Mor174) culture[b]	8

[a] Morganocin was diluted 1:1 as indicated and titrated after 12 h at 37°C.
[b] Supernatant fluid was titrated after treatment.

Localization of morganocin 174. Table 9 shows the localization of morganocin 6 and 96 h after induction by MC. At 6 h the original host, *P. morganii* 174, showed an even distribution of intracellular, cell wall-bound, and extracellular morganocin, whereas the other strains, being receptorless, had increased titers in the extracellular fluid at the expense of the cell-bound fraction. At 96 h all *Proteus* strains show very little morganocin intracellularly, with an accumulation of the bacteriocin in the medium. The relatively high percentage of intracellular morganocin in *E. coli* B(Mor174) is misleading

TABLE 9. *Location of morganocin 174 after MC induction*

Organism[a]	Time after induction (h)	Morganocin (%)		
		Extracellular[b]	Cell wall bound[c]	Intracellular[d]
P. morganii 174	6	45	35	20
	96	56	41	3
P. morganii 165 *mor*^{r}(Mor174)	6	52	19	29
	96	79	18	3
P. mirabilis 5006(Mor174)	6	54	19	27
	96	90	3	7
E. coli B(Mor174)	6	61	13	26
	96	51	29	20

[a] Organisms were grown in DM.
[b] Morganocin in supernatant fluid after centrifugation.
[c] Morganocin in 1 M NaCl wash of pelleted cells.
[d] Morganocin was released after sonic disruption of NaCl-washed cells.

due to the low morganocin titer of this strain at 96 h. It is notable that even in morganocin-resistant, and presumably receptorless, strains, a significant amount of morganocin was bound to the cell wall.

DISCUSSION

Mobilization of morganocinogeny by the R factor R772 and subsequent independent segregation of kanamycin resistance and morganocinogeny in transconjugants indicate that the morganocin is plasmid coded. In accordance with the nomenclature for bacteriocinogenic plasmids, this plasmid has been called Mor174. Hardy et al. (11), on the basis of criteria such as molecular weight, copy number per chromosome, mode of replication, and amount of cell-bound colicin, distinguished two groups of colicinogenic plasmids. From these preliminary observations Mor174 appears to resemble the EK-like plasmids rather than the BIV group in that approximately half the morganocin was free in the culture medium. A further similarity with this group is the non-self-transmissible nature of Mor174.

Colicin K synthesized in *P. mirabilis* had an activity 50 times that synthesized in *E. coli* (15). Transfer of Mor174 to different hosts made it possible to investigate the effect of the intracellular environment on morganocin synthesis. Apart from a slight increase in the amount of free morganocin produced by *Proteus* and *Providencia* strains lacking a receptor, no difference in morganocin production was observed. In contrast, the amount of morganocin synthesized in *E. coli* B(Mor174) was consistently lower. Although the intracellular environment may be significant, the low titer of morganocin 174 produced by *E. coli* B(Mor174) is due to the synthesis of a heat-stable inhibitor. The high rate of segregation of Mor174 in *E. coli* B(Mor174) may indicate a difference in the mode of replication of the plasmid in this host.

In contrast to some other bacteriocins (7, 17, 24), synthesis of morganocin was not influenced by the growth media investigated. The protracted accumulation of morganocin in *Proteus* cultures reflected its stability in the media, in contrast to the bacteriocin produced by *P. morganii* MR336, which had to be stabilized by addition of sodium sulfite (27). A long lag period after induction (maximum production 36 to 48 h after induction) has also been described for streptococcin A (28).

Synthesis of morganocin by Mor174 is not constitutive since morganocin titers could be increased by induction. Although cAMP has been found to enhance colicin El production (20), no effect on morganocin synthesis was observed. To circumvent the possibility that this resulted from a lack of uptake of cAMP, the more readily absorbed dibutyryl cAMP (26) was investigated. Since similar results were obtained, it appears that these agents do not influence morganocin production.

Transfer of Mor174 has enabled the formation of a morganocinogenic strain, *P. morganii* 165 *mor*^{r} (Mor174), which produces higher extracellular titers than the original host, *P. morganii* 174, and does not lyse on induction with MC (not shown). Growth of this organism in DM will facilitate isolation and characterization of the morganocin.

ACKNOWLEDGMENTS

I wish to thank K. Krizsanovich-Williams for critical discussion and help in preparation of the manuscript.

LITERATURE CITED

1. **Adelberg, E. A., M. Mandel, and G. C. C. Chen.** 1965. Optimal conditions for mutagenesis by N-methyl-N'-

nitro-N-nitrosoguanidine in *Escherichia coli* K12. Biochem. Biophys. Res. Commun. **18**:788–795.
2. **Ben-Gurion, R.** 1970. Chloramphenicol and puromycin as inducers of colicinogenic bacteria. Biochem. Biophys. Res. Commun. **40**:1281–1288.
3. **Coetzee, J. N.** 1975. Chromosome transfer in *Proteus mirabilis* mediated by a hybrid plasmid. J. Gen. Microbiol. **86**:133–146.
4. **Coetzee, J. N., and T. G. Sacks.** 1960. Transduction of streptomycin resistance in *Proteus mirabilis*. J. Gen. Microbiol. **23**:445–455.
5. **Coetzee, J. N., J. A. Smit, and O. W. Prozesky.** 1966. Properties of Providence and *Proteus morganii* transducing phages. J. Gen. Microbiol. **44**:167–176.
6. **Delisle, A. L.** 1975. Production of bacteriocins in a liquid medium by *Streptococcus mutans*. Antimicrob. Agents Chemother. **8**:707–712.
7. **Goebel, W. F., G. T. Barry, and T. Shedlovsky.** 1956. Colicine K. I. The production of colicine K in media maintained at constant pH. J. Exp. Med. **103**:577–580.
8. **Gromkova, R. H.** 1971. Induction of colicin Ia at high temperature. J. Bacteriol. **106**:720–723.
9. **Hardy, K. G.** 1975. Colicinogeny and related phenomena. Bacteriol. Rev. **39**:464–515.
10. **Hardy, K. G., and G. G. Meynell.** 1972. A model relating the replication and expression of colicin factor E2-P9. Genet. Res. **20**:331–334.
11. **Hardy, K. G., G. G. Meynell, J. E. Dowman, and B. G. Spratt.** 1973. Two major groups of colicin factors: their evolutionary significance. Mol. Gen. Genet. **125**:217–230.
12. **Hedges, A. J.** 1974. R factors from *Proteus mirabilis* and *P. vulgaris*. J. Gen. Microbiol. **87**:301–311.
13. **Iijima, T.** 1962. Studies on the colicinogenic factor in *Escherichia coli* K12. Induction of colicin production by mitomycin C. Biken J. **5**:1–8.
14. **Jacob, F., L. Siminovitch, and E. Wollman.** 1952. Sur la biosynthèse d'une colicine et sur son mode d'action. Ann. Inst. Pasteur (Paris) **83**:295–315.
15. **Jesaitis, M. A.** 1970. The nature of colicin K from *Proteus mirabilis*. J. Exp. Med. **131**:1016–1038.
16. **Jetten, A. M., and G. D. Vogels.** 1973. Characterization and extrachromosomal control of bacteriocin production in *Staphylococcus aureus*. Antimicrob. Agents Chemother. **4**:49–57.
17. **Jetten, A. M., G. D. Vogels, and F. de Windt.** 1972. Production and purification of a *Staphylococcus epidermidis* bacteriocin. J. Bacteriol. **112**:235–242.
18. **Kennedy, C. K.** 1971. Induction of colicin production by high temperature inhibition of protein synthesis. J. Bacteriol. **108**:10–19.
19. **Monk, M., and R. C. Clowes.** 1965. The regulation of colicin synthesis and colicin transfer in *Escherichia coli* K12. J. Gen. Microbiol. **36**:385–392.
20. **Nakazawa, A., and T. Tamada.** 1972. Stimulation of colicin El synthesis by cyclic 3′,5′-adenosine monophosphate in mitomycin C-induced *Escherichia coli*. Biochem. Biophys. Res. Commun. **46**:1004–1010.
21. **Ozeki, H., B. A. D. Stocker, and H. de Miargerie.** 1959. Production of colicine by single bacteria. Nature (London) **184**:337–339.
22. **Ozeki, H., B. A. D. Stocker, and S. M. Smith.** 1962. Transmission of colicinogeny between strains of *Salmonella typhimurium* grown together. J. Gen. Microbiol. **28**:671–687.
23. **Reeves, P.** 1972. The bacteriocins. Springer-Verlag, Berlin.
24. **Rogers, A. H.** 1972. Effect of the medium on bacteriocin production among strains of *Streptococcus mutans*. Appl. Microbiol. **24**:294–295.
25. **Roth, T. F., and D. Helinski.** 1967. Evidence for circular DNA forms of a bacterial plasmid. Proc. Natl. Acad. Sci. U.S.A. **58**:650–657.
26. **Shapiro, L., N. Agabian-Keshishian, A. Hirsch, and O. M. Rosen.** 1972. Effect of dibutyryladenosine 3′,5′-cyclic monophosphate on growth and differentiation in *Caulobacter crescentus*. Proc. Natl. Acad. Sci. U.S.A. **69**:1225–1229.
27. **Smit, J. A., H. C. de Klerk, and J. N. Coetzee.** 1968. Properties of a *Proteus morganii* bacteriocin. J. Gen. Microbiol. **54**:67–75.
28. **Tagg, J. R., A. S. Dajani, L. W. Wannamaker, and E. D. Gray.** 1973. Group A streptococcal bacteriocin. Production, purification, and mode of action. J. Exp. Med. **138**:1168–1183.
29. **Timmis, K.** 1972. Purification and characterization of colicin D. J. Bacteriol. **109**:12–20.
30. **Winkler, U., W. Rüger, and W. Wackernagel.** 1972. Bakterien- Phagen-und Molekulargenetik. Springer-Verlag, Berlin.

ANTIMICROBIAL AGENTS AND CHEMOTHERAPY, Mar. 1977, p. 521-527 Vol. 11, No. 3

Inhibition of Cellular and Viral Protein Synthesis by 3-Methyleneoxindole

SERGIO L. ABREU[1] AND JEAN LUCAS-LENARD*

Biochemistry and Biophysics Section, University of Connecticut, Storrs, Connecticut 06268

Received for publication 12 October 1976

The effect of 3-methyleneoxindole (MO) on mengovirus and L-cell protein synthesis was investigated. MO was found to inhibit mengovirus multiplication and the incorporation of radioactive amino acids into both viral and cellular proteins. These results suggest that the antiviral effect of this compound is not specific but rather stems from its inhibition of the cellular translational machinery upon which mengovirus depends. We have also found that MO inhibits natural messenger ribonucleic acid (mengovirus and globin messenger ribonucleic acid) translation in cell-free extracts from Ehrlich ascites tumor cells but has no significant effect on polyuridylic acid translation. Additional data which suggest that MO inhibits protein synthesis at the level of initiation are shown.

It has been reported (21) that 3-methyleneoxindole (MO) can selectively inhibit the replication of herpesvirus, mengovirus, poliovirus, and Sindbis virus. MO has been shown to be an oxidation product of the plant hormone indole-3-acetic acid (20), and it has been claimed that it is an obligatory intermediate in the indole-3-acetic acid-induced elongation of wheat coleoptiles (4).

Our interest in MO stems solely from its reported selectivity in interfering with viral, but not cellular, protein synthesis (19, 21). A compound with such properties could be advantageous in the study of the mechanism by which certain viruses shut off host protein synthesis while their own protein-synthetic processes remain active. Our efforts in this latter area have centered on the molecular interactions of mengovirus with permissive host cells (1, 6, 13).

The experimental approaches taken here were shaped by the reported results of Tuli and co-workers (19, 21). In a series of experiments using whole cells, they reported that: (i) the antiviral action of MO is not mediated by interferon; (ii) MO is not virucidal; (iii) viral ribonucleic acid (RNA) synthesis is not affected by antiviral concentrations of MO; and (iv) the ability of poliovirus messenger RNA (mRNA) to attach to ribosomes is decreased, but the same concentration of MO does not prevent HeLa cell polysome formation.

In an attempt to specifically determine the value of this compound as a tool in studies of cell-virus protein synthesis interactions and, in general, as a useful agent in studies on cellular protein synthesis regulation, we studied its effects on cellular and viral protein synthesis in whole cells and cell extracts.

MATERIALS AND METHODS

Synthesis of MO. 3-Bromooxindole-3-acetic acid was prepared by the reaction of *N*-bromosuccinimide (Aldrich Chemical Co.) and indole-3-acetic acid (Aldrich Chemical Co.) as detailed by Hinman and Bauman (9). This compound is rapidly debrominated and decarboxylated to yield MO (9) upon dissolving in aqueous solutions. The spectral characteristics of our MO are seen in Fig. 1. They conform to those previously reported for this compound (10), exhibiting maxima at 247 and 253 nm.

Cells. L cells of strain 929 were grown as monolayer cultures in Eagle minimum essential medium (MEM) (Earle salts) containing 9% fetal bovine serum. The cells were grown in either 100-mm plastic petri dishes for studies of amino acid incorporation or in 60-mm petri dishes for virus titer assays. Ehrlich ascites tumor cells were propagated as previously described (1).

Virus growth, purification, and plaque assays. Mengovirus (S variant) was grown in Ehrlich ascites tumor cells, harvested, and purified for mRNA extraction as described earlier (1). To plaque assay the virus, monolayer cultures in 60-mm plastic petri dishes were washed with phosphate-buffered saline at 37°C. Then, 0.3 ml of each viral dilution was applied, and the virus was allowed to adsorb for 45 min at room temperature. At this time, the unadsorbed virus was removed by aspiration from the cultures, and 5 ml of MEM containing 0.8% agarose and 3% fetal bovine serum was added. After 48 h at 37°C, the plaques were quantitated.

Incorporation of radioactive amino acids into uninfected and mengovirus-infected cells in the pres-

[1] Laboratory of Reproductive Physiology, University of Pennsylvania, Philadelphia, PA 19174.

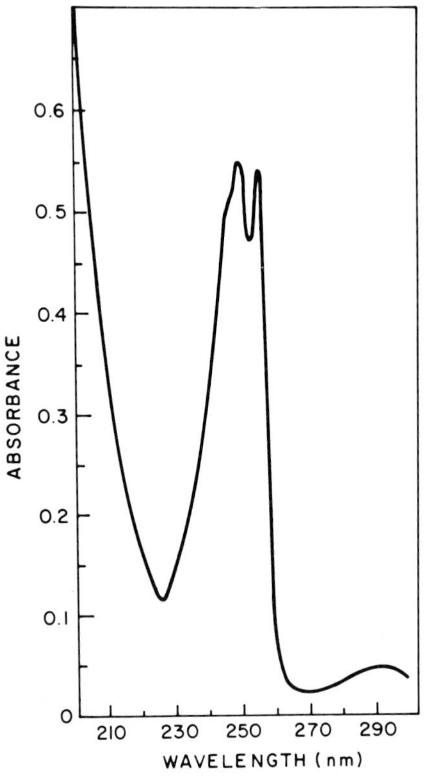

FIG. 1. *Spectral characteristics of MO. Ultraviolet spectrum of a 20 μM solution (in distilled H_2O) of MO measured with a Cary recording spectrophotometer.*

ence or absence of MO. Monolayer cultures of L cells in 100-mm petri dishes were infected with mengovirus at a multiplicity of infection of 20 plaque-forming units per cell, and the uninfected controls were mock infected with phosphate-buffered saline. After the adsorption period, 10 ml of MEM-9% fetal bovine serum (10 μM in MO) was added. At 3 h after adsorption, the medium was aspirated, and 10 ml of the same medium containing 10 μM MO was added.

At 6 h after adsorption, the medium was removed once more, and the monolayer cultures were washed with 10 ml of prewarmed (37°C) MEM without amino acids and containing 10 μM MO. After removal of this medium, 3 ml of MEM without amino acids (10 μM in MO) and 50 μCi of a ^{3}H-labeled amino acid mixture per ml (New England Nuclear, NET-250) supplemented with six non-radioactive amino acids (asparagine, cysteine, glutamine, histidine, methionine, and tryptophan) at a concentration of 100 μM were added. The cells were labeled for 0.5 h and then chased for 1 h with MEM containing amino acids, 5% fetal bovine serum, and 10 μM MO.

Another experimental group consisted of mengovirus-infected cells and mock-infected cells, neither of which received MO but were otherwise treated using the same protocol. All experiments were carried out in duplicate. A second set of experiments utilizing 40 μM MO was performed similarly.

Analyses of the incorporation of ^{3}H-labeled amino acids into whole cells. At the end of the chase period, the media were aspirated, and 1 ml of a buffer containing 10 mM HEPES (*N*-2-hydroxyethylpiperazine-*N'*-2-ethanesulfonic acid, pH 7.6), 2 mM dithiothreitol (DTT), 1 mM magnesium acetate, 10 mM KCl, and 0.5% Nonidet P-40 was added to each plate. After exposure to this hypotonic medium for 10 min at 4°C, the cells were scraped off the plates. Duplicate experiments were pooled and centrifuged at 15,000 × *g* for 10 min. At this point, the samples were treated in either of two ways, depending on the aim of the experiment. In one case, 20 μl from the pooled supernatants was placed in test tubes and 200 μg of bovine serum albumin was added to each as carrier. A 2-ml portion of a 10% trichloroacetic acid solution was then added to each sample, the suspension was heated at 95°C for 15 min and cooled in ice, and the precipitate was collected on 0.45-μm membrane filters (Millipore). The dried filters were placed in a Triton-based scintillation mixture and counted in a liquid scintillation counter.

If the proteins were to be subjected to polyacrylamide gel electrophoresis, 10 volumes of cold acetone was added to the supernatant fluids to precipitate the protein and the suspension was stored at −20° overnight. After low-speed centrifugation, the pellets were washed twice with acetone, thoroughly dried, and dissolved in 500 μl of a gel electrophoresis sample buffer (see below). The samples were heated at 95°C for 5 min, and a 5-μl portion was placed on slab gels as described below.

Sodium dodecyl sulfate-polyacrylamide slab gel electrophoresis. Five microliters of the sample in 2.3% sodium dodecyl sulfate, 10% glycerol, 5% 2-mercaptoethanol, and 62.5 mM tris(hydroxymethyl)-aminomethane (pH 6.8) were analyzed electrophoretically by the methods of Laemmli (11) and Studier (18). A slab gel consisting of a 4.5% acrylamide stacking gel and a discontinuous gradient (7.5, 10, and 12.5% polyacrylamide) separating gel was used. Electrophoresis was carried out at 80 V for 5 h. The slabs containing ^{3}H-labeled protein were processed for fluorography as described by Bonner and Laskey (5). Autoradiography was performed with Kodak Royal X-OMAT X-ray film, and the film was exposed for 2 days at −70°C.

Cell-free translation. Preincubated cell-free systems derived from uninfected Ehrlich ascites tumor cells were prepared as previously described (1), except that the final Mg^{2+} concentration in the reaction mixture was 2.0 mM and spermidine was added to 0.4 mM. The reaction volume was 50 μl except as noted. Also, a 0.25-μCi portion of [^{14}C]leucine (280 mCi/mmol) supplemented with the other 19 amino acids at a concentration of 10^{-6} M each was present. When "DTT-minus" cell-free systems were used, the cell extract was prepared in the presence of 2 mM DTT (1) but was dialyzed against 100 volumes of HKMT buffer (1) without DTT and two changes of buffer. The reaction mixtures were incubated for 1 h at 37°C, terminated by the addition of 10% trichloroacetic acid, and processed as described above. When polyuridylic acid [poly(U)] was the messagenger,

150,000 cpm of precharged [^{3}H]phenylalanyl-transfer RNA per reaction mixture was added.

Preparation of mRNA's. Preparation of mengo mRNA was performed as described (1). Globin mRNA was extracted from a frozen rabbit reticulocyte lysate, the kind gift of W. C. Merrick, as follows. The thawed lysate was centrifuged at 30,000 × *g* for 10 min. The supernatant fluid was adjusted to 0.1 M in NaCl, 20 mM in ethylenediaminetetraacetic acid, and 0.5% in sodium dodecyl sulfate and then extracted three times with an equal volume of hot (45°C) phenol-chloroform (1:1) saturated with 0.1 M NaCl and 1 mM ethylenediaminetetraacetic acid. The RNA was precipitated from the final aqueous layer by the addition of 0.2 volume of 1.0 M NaCl and 2 volumes of 95% ethanol and stored overnight at −20°C. The polyadenylic acid-containing globin mRNA was purified by oligothymidylic acid-cellulose (Collaborative Research, Inc.) chromatography as described by Aviv and Leder (2).

RESULTS

Antiviral activity of MO. The addition of MO to the growth medium right after virus adsorption (time zero) resulted in the inhibition of viral growth (Fig. 2). More than 1 log inhibition was seen at 6 h after adsorption, as revealed by plaque assay. The inhibition was maintained for an additional 2 h, but by 10 h there was less than a log difference between the MO-treated and untreated cells. By 24 h, no significant difference in virus yield was observed. When MO was added at zero time and then again at 6 h after infection, the virus yield was depressed nearly 2 logs compared to the control samples. This difference was maintained up to 10 h after infection, and at 24 h postinfection, the virus yield was still significantly lower.

This transient inhibition of virus production elicited by MO was also reported by Tuli et al. (21), who considered the transitory nature of the inhibition to be a consequence of the reduction of MO to 3-methyloxindole by either reduced nicotinamide adenine dinucleotide- or reduced nicotinamide adenine dinucleotide phosphate-linked enzyme systems. They have shown that the enzyme-mediated reduction of MO to 3-methyloxindole takes place in plant cells (20), bacteria (8), and animal cells (21). The results summarized in Fig. 2 are in general agreement with their findings (21).

Effect of MO on cellular and viral protein synthesis. We wished to determine if the inhibition of growth of mengovirus results directly from the inhibition of viral functions or indirectly from the inhibition of cellular functions necessary for viral growth. Because Tuli et al. (19,21) found that MO does not inhibit either viral or cellular RNA synthesis, we focused our attention on its effects on protein synthesis. Tuli and co-workers (21) reported that the in-

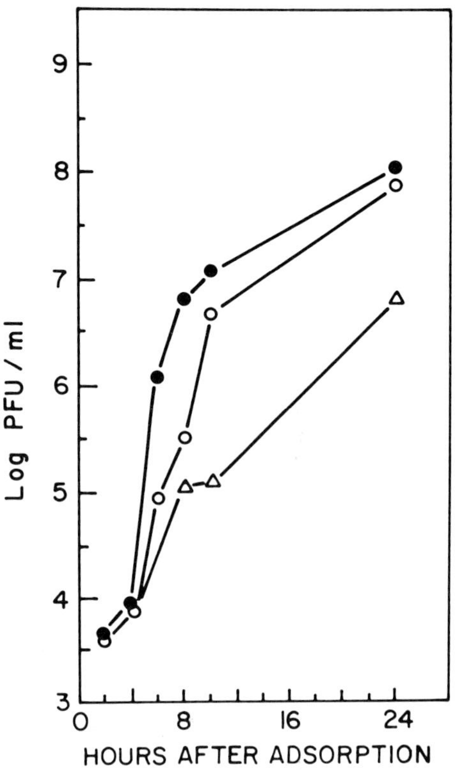

FIG. 2. *Inhibition of mengovirus growth by MO. Monolayers of L cells were infected with mengovirus at a multiplicity of infection of 20 and treated with MO as shown. At the indicated time points, the infected cells and medium were frozen. The cells were frozen and thawed three times prior to determining infectivity. Symbols: ●, no MO added; ○, MO (10 μM final concentration) added immediately after adsorption (zero time); △, MO (10 μM final concentration) added at zero time and 6 h after adsorption.*

corporation of L-[^{14}C]glucose into trichloroacetic acid-insoluble products (which would presumably include protein) was similar in MO-treated and untreated cells. From this result, they concluded that antiviral concentrations of MO do not inhibit major host-specified functions. In our experiments, the incorporation of radioactive amino acids into protein was examined as a more specific assay of protein synthesis.

Uninfected or virus-infected cells were exposed to MO at the beginning of the experimental period and at 3 and 6 h after infection or mock infection. The growth medium was replenished with MO because of the lability of MO, as demonstrated in Fig. 2 and by Tuli et al. (21). It was thought that an analysis of the effect of MO on viral and cellular protein synthesis ought to be carried out under conditions in which its activity would still be present.

At 6 h after infection or mock infection, the

cells were labeled with a ^{3}H-labeled amino acid mixture for 30 min and then chased for 1 h with an unlabeled amino acid mixture. The reactions were stopped and analyzed as described in Materials and Methods. Table 1 shows that MO at a concentration of 10 μM inhibited the incorporation of amino acids into protein in both mengovirus-infected and uninfected L cells. Virtually all protein synthesis with 40 μM MO was stopped in both uninfected and infected cells.

The inhibition of both viral and cellular protein synthesis with 10 μM MO was further analyzed by sodium dodecyl sulfate-polyacrylamide gel electrophoresis. Figure 3b demonstrates the protein pattern obtained on gels from cells that

TABLE 1. *Effect of MO on cellular and viral protein synthesis*

Expt	MO (μM)	^{3}H-labeled amino acid incorporation (cpm/μl of sample taken)	% Inhibition
1. Mengovirus-infected cells	0	34,572	
Mengovirus-infected cells	10	14,034	60
Uninfected cells	0	69,791	
1A. Uninfected cells	10	38,340	45
2. Mengovirus-infected cells	0	32,811	
Mengovirus-infected cells	40	914	97
2A. Uninfected cells	0	39,000	
Uninfected cells	40	2,450	94

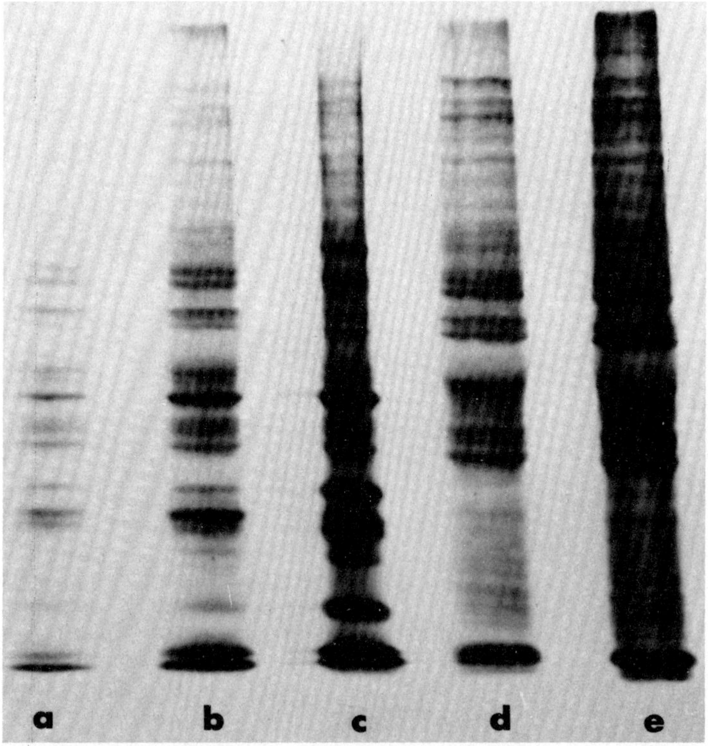

FIG. 3. *Polyacrylamide gel electrophoretic analysis of the effect of MO on cellular and viral protein synthesis in L cells. L-cell monolayers were incubated with or without 10 μM MO as indicated. At 6 h postinfection, the cells were pulsed and chased with a mixture of ^{3}H-labeled amino acids and analyzed as described under Materials and Methods. (a) Amino acid incorporation into protein in mengovirus-infected cells treated with 10 μM MO; (b) same as in (a) but with no MO added; (c) 20 μl of a [^{14}C]mengovirus polypeptide marker prepared as described previously (15); (d) amino acid incorporation into protein in uninfected L cells treated with 10 μM MO; (e) same as in (d) but not treated with MO.*

were infected with mengovirus and labeled as described above. This pattern was similar to that shown in Fig. 3c, which represents a ^{14}C-labeled viral protein marker. Comparison of Fig. 3a (with MO) and Fig. 3b (without MO) shows that the synthesis of all the viral proteins was inhibited by MO. The labeling pattern of cellular proteins from uninfected cells is depicted in Fig. 3e, and the effect of MO on this pattern is shown in Fig 3d. In this case, a decreased labeling was also observed, confirming that MO inhibits both cellular and viral protein synthesis (Table 1).

If the growth medium was not replenished with MO at the indicated time periods, there was no effect of 10 μM MO on either host or viral protein synthesis, except at early times after infection or mock infection (data not shown). This corroborates the data in Fig. 2.

Effect of MO on protein synthesis in a cell-free system. The inhibition of protein synthesis by MO was further explored by studying its effect on translation using extracts from Ehrlich ascites tumor cells to supply the necessary components for protein synthesis. The translation of both globin and mengovirus mRNA was reduced by approximately 50% in the extract containing 100 μM MO (Table 2). Poly(U) translation, on the other hand, was decreased by only 12%.

The effect of different amounts of MO on globin mRNA, mengovirus RNA, and poly(U) translation was also examined. Figure 4 illustrates that the inhibition of incorporation of amino acids into globin and mengovirus proteins was similar for all of the concentrations of MO tested. Approximately 50% inhibition was obtained with 100 μM MO. With 500 μM MO, the translation of both globin and mengovirus mRNA's was drastically reduced. A residual activity, amounting to about 15% of the total activity, remained even after the addition of 1 mM MO. In contrast to these results, the trans-

TABLE 2. *Effect of MO on mRNA translation by Ehrlich ascites tumor cell extracts*

Additions	MO (μM)	[^{14}C]leucine or [^{14}C]phenylalanine incorporated (cpm/50-μl reaction mixture
No mRNA	0	6,443
1.2 μg of mengo mRNA	0	61,284
1.0 μg of globin mRNA	0	41,774
No poly(U)	0	1,044
10 μg of poly(U)	0	88,317
No mRNA	100	5,018
1.2 μg of mengo mRNA	100	29,730
1.0 μg of globin mRNA	100	20,004
No poly(U)	100	995
10 μg of poly(U)	100	77,660

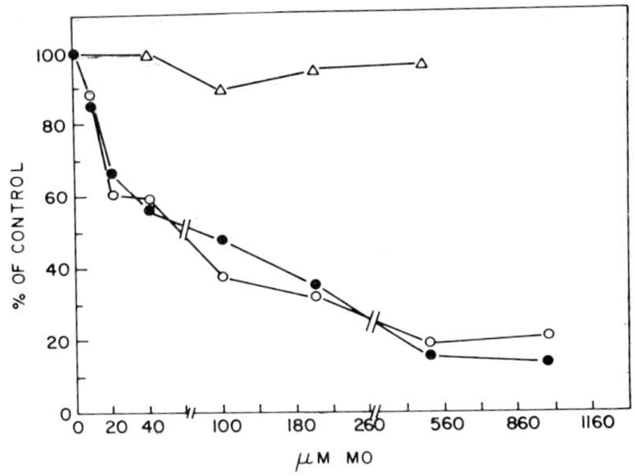

FIG. 4. *Cell-free translation inhibition by various MO concentrations. The indicated concentrations of MO were added to the reaction mixtures at the onset of incubation. The conditions were the same as described in Materials and Methods. Symbols:* ●, *Mengovirus mRNA (1.0 μg) translation;* ○, *globin mRNA (1.0 μg) translation;* △, *poly(U) translation.*

lation of poly(U) was never reduced more than 10% of the control sample (Fig. 4 and Table 2) throughout the concentration range of MO inhibitory for natural RNA translation.

Whole cells exhibited a much greater sensitivity to this compound, with 10 μM MO reducing both cellular and viral protein synthesis about 50% (Table 1 and Fig. 3). The apparent lesser sensitivity of the cell-free extract to MO might possibly be explained by the presence of 2 mM DTT in the extract or because the MO reductase system in Ehrlich ascites tumor cell extracts is particularly active. MO has been reported to form adducts with compounds that contain free SH groups, thereby losing its biological activities (17). An attempt to remove the DTT from the extract by dialysis of the extract against DTT-free buffer, however, did not increase the sensitivity of the incorporation reaction to MO (data not shown). This could result from the presence of residual amounts of DTT in the extract, which would decrease the activity of the MO. Extracts prepared in the absence of a reducing agent were only weakly active in protein synthesis, and so a cell-free system without DTT could not be tested. In view of the similarity of the MO effect in cell-free extracts with and without DTT, all subsequent experiments were carried out in cell-free systems with DTT.

Effect of MO on the kinetics of amino acid incorporation. MO was added to the cell-free system at different times during incubation to determine which step in protein synthesis it affects. Figure 5 shows that the addition of MO at zero time resulted in a 54% reduction in the

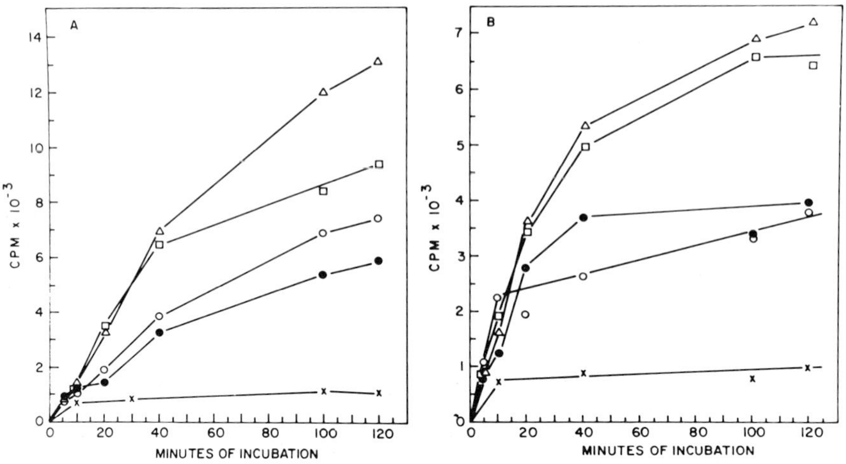

FIG. 5. *Effect of MO on the kinetics of amino acid incorporation in cell-free extracts. A 100-μl reaction mixture was made 500 μM in MO at 0, 10, or 50 min after the start of the incubation period at 37°C. At the indicated times, 15 μl of each reaction mixture was withdrawn, precipitated with 10% trichloroacetic acid, and analyzed as described in Materials and Methods. (A) Mengovirus mRNA (2.0 μg) translation; (B) globin mRNA (2.0 μg) translation. Symbols: x, background incorporation, no mRNA added;* ○, *MO added at zero time;* ●, *MO added at 10 min of incubation;* □, *MO added after 50 min of incubation;* △, *no MO added.*

incorporation of [^{14}C]leucine programed by mengovirus RNA and a 50% reduction in the incorporation of this amino acid directed by globin mRNA. When MO was added after 10 min of incubation, globin and mengovirus mRNA translations were reduced by 45 and 47%, respectively. The addition of MO after 50 min of incubation resulted in a 22% inhibition of mengovirus mRNA-directed amino acid incorporation and a 10% reduction of globin RNA translation. The fact that there was very little inhibition if MO was added late in the incubation period suggested that MO was affecting an early event in translation, possibly polypeptide chain initiation. This possibility was further studied by comparing these results to those of a similar experiment utilizing a known inhibitor of initiation, aurintricarboxylic acid (ATA) (12, 16, 22). Figure 6 shows that ATA significantly decreased the incorporation of [^{14}C]leucine into protein only if added up to 20 min of incubation. Beyond that time, the addition of ATA had little effect. Therefore, initiation is likely to be taking place only during the first 20 min, a time consistent with that previously reported for similar cell-free systems (7, 14). A comparison of Fig. 5 and 6 shows that the effects on amino acid incorporation of MO and ATA are somewhat similar, suggesting that MO may act at the level of initiation.

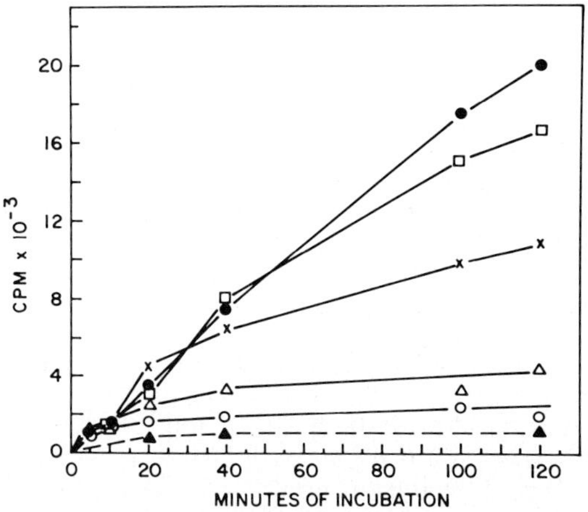

FIG. 6. *Effect of ATA on the kinetics of [^{14}C]leucine incorporation in cell-free extracts. A 100-μl reaction mixture was made 100 μM in ATA at 0, 10, 20, or 50 min after the start of the incubation period at 37°C. Where indicated, 2 μg of mengovirus mRNA was present in each reaction. All analyses proceeded as in Materials and Methods. Symbols:* ▲, *background incorporation;* ○, *ATA added at zero time;* △, *ATA added at 10 min of incubation; x, ATA added at 20 min;* □, *ATA added at 50 min;* ●, *no ATA added.*

DISCUSSION

Tuli and co-workers (19, 21) have reported that MO has a differential effect on viral and cellular protein synthesis. Furthermore, evidence which indicated that the differential inhibition was effected by the binding of MO to ribosomes, specifically to ribosomal RNA, was presented (19). This binding supposedly rendered the ribosomes unable to associate with viral mRNA's. Our interest in the mechanism(s) involved in the differential shut-off of host protein synthesis by picornavirus infection (3) led us to the present investigation. We thought that an understanding of the mechanism of action of MO might give us a clue as to how viruses shut off host protein synthesis.

We have found, as reported by Tuli et al. (21), that MO inhibits viral growth and that this effect is transient (Fig. 2). However, we have no evidence that this inhibition is taking place by a mechanism that acts selectively on viral mRNA translation. On the contrary, our evidence clearly shows that MO inhibits both cellular and viral protein synthesis equally. This was demonstrated both in whole cells (Fig. 3 and Table 1) and in extracts of Ehrlich ascites tumor cells (Fig. 4 and Table 2). Thus, the effect of MO on viral growth can be explained by its action on the cell's translational machinery on which the virus depends.

The lack of a significant inhibitory effect of MO on poly(U) translation (Fig. 4 and Table 2) suggests that MO acts at an early stage of translation, possibly at initiation. The similarity of the results of the experiments in Fig. 5 and 6, in which MO and the initiation inhibitor ATA were added at different times after the start of the incorporation reaction, further suggests an effect at the level of initiation.

The reported binding of MO to ribosomal RNA (19) could be the mechanism by which MO inhibits protein synthesis. It is possible that neither cellular nor viral messages interact with ribosomes if MO is already bound to them. A lack of mRNA binding would result in an inhibition at the site of initiation.

In summary, we have not found this compound to be an effective tool for the study of the mechanism by which viruses shut off host cell protein synthesis. However, because of its selective inhibition of natural mRNA translation and its possible specificity for the initiation step, it merits further investigation.

ACKNOWLEDGMENTS

We would like to gratefully acknowledge Ron Pape for his essential advice in the synthesis of MO and thank Michael Jaye for preparing the [^{14}C]mengovirus protein marker.

This work was supported by Public Health Service grant RO1 CA 12144 from the National Cancer Institute. This work has benefited from the use of the Cell Culture Facility, which was supported by Public Health Service grant CA-14733 from the National Cancer Institute.

LITERATURE CITED

1. **Abreu, S. L., and J. Lucas-Lenard.** 1976. Cellular protein synthesis shut off by mengovirus: translation of nonviral and viral mRNA's in extracts from uninfected and infected Ehrlich ascites tumor cells. J. Virol. **18**:182–194.
2. **Aviv, H., and P. Leder.** 1972. Purification of biologically active globin messenger RNA by chromatography on oligothymidylic acid-cellulose. Proc. Natl. Acad. Sci. U.S.A. **69**:1408–1412.
3. **Baltimore, D.** 1969. The replication of picornaviruses, p. 101–176. *In* H. B. Levy (ed.), The biochemistry of viruses. Marcel Dekker, Inc., New York.
4. **Basu, P. S., and V. Tuli.** 1972. The binding of indole-3-acetic acid and 3-methyleneoxindole to plant macromolecules. Plant Physiol. **50**:507–509.
5. **Bonner, W. M., and R. A. Laskey.** 1974. A film detection for tritium-labelled proteins and nucleic acids in polyacrylamide gels. Eur. J. Biochem. **46**:83–88.
6. **Colby, D. S., V. Finnerty, and J. Lucas-Lenard.** 1974. Fate of mRNA of L cells infected with mengovirus. J. Virol. **13**:858–869.
7. **Eggen, K. L., and A. J. Shatkin.** 1972. In vitro translation of cardiovirus ribonucleic acid by mammalian cell-free extracts. J. Virol. **9**:636–645.
8. **Fukuyama, T. T., and H. S. Moyed.** 1964. Inhibition of cell growth by photooxidation products of indole-3-acetic acid. J. Biol. Chem. **239**:2392–2397.
9. **Hinman, R. L., and C. P. Bauman.** 1964. Reactions of N-bromosuccinimide and indoles. A simple synthesis of 3-bromooxindoles. J. Org. Chem. **29**:1206–1215.
10. **Hinman, R. L., C. P. Bauman, and J. Lang.** 1961. The conversion of indole-3–acetic acid to 3-methyleneoxindole in the presence of peroxidase. Biochem. Biophys. Res. Commun. **5**:250–254.
11. **Laemmli, U. K.** 1970. Cleavage of structural proteins during the assembly of the head of bacteriophage T4. Nature (London) **227**:680–685.
12. **Lebleu, B., G. Marbaix, J. Werenne, A. Burny, and G. Huez.** 1970. Effect of aurintricarboxylic acid and NaF on the binding of globin messenger RNA to reticulocyte 40S ribosomal subunits. Biochem. Biophys. Res. Commun. **40**:731–739.
13. **Manak, M., S. L. Abreu, and J. Lucas-Lenard.** 1975. Association of mengovirus proteins with host cell native 40S ribosomal subunits. In *In vitro* transcription and translation of viral genomes. INSERM **47**:387–396.
14. **Mathews, M. B., and A. Korner.** 1970. Mammalian cell-free protein synthesis directed by viral ribonucleic acid. Eur. J. Biochem. **17**:328–338.
15. **Nakai, K., and J. Lucas-Lenard.** 1976. Processing of mengovirus precursor polypeptides in the presence of zinc ions and sulfhydryl compounds. J. Virol. **18**:918–925.
16. **Stewart, M. L., A. P. Grollman, and M. T. Huang.** 1971. Aurintricarboxylic acid: inhibitor of initiation of protein synthesis. Proc. Natl. Acad. Sci. U.S.A. **68**:97–101.
17. **Still, C. C., T. T. Fukuyama, and H. S. Moyed.** 1965. Inhibitory oxidation products of indole-3-acetic acid: mechanism of action and route of detoxification. J. Biol. Chem. **240**:2612–2618.
18. **Studier, F. W.** 1973. Analysis of bacteriophage T7 early RNAs and proteins on slab gels. J. Mol. Biol. **79**:237–248.
19. **Tuli, V.** 1974. Mechanism of the antiviral action of 3-methyleneoxindole. Antimicrob. Agents Chemother. **5**:485–491.
20. **Tuli, V., and H. S. Moyed.** 1967. Inhibitory oxidation products of indole–3-acetic acid: 3-hydroxymethyl-onindole and 3-methyleneoxindole as plant metabolites. Plant Physiol. **42**:425–430.
21. **Tuli, V., H. S. Moyed, D. Stevenson, and I. Gordon.** 1974. Antiviral activity of 3-methyleneoxindole. Antimicrob. Agents Chemother. **5**:479–484.
22. **Whitelam, J. M., and H. Naora.** 1974. Interaction of informational macromolecules with ribosomes. VIII. Restoration of RNA-binding ability of 40S ribosome subunit and effect of aurintricarboxylic acid. Biochim. Biophys. Acta **349**:178–188.

ANTIMICROBIAL AGENTS AND CHEMOTHERAPY, Mar. 1977, p. 528-533 Vol. 11, No. 3

Plasmid-Mediated Beta-Lactamase Production in *Neisseria gonorrhoeae*

LYNN P. ELWELL,* MARILYN ROBERTS, LEONARD W. MAYER, AND STANLEY FALKOW

Department of Microbiology and Immunology, University of Washington School of Medicine, Seattle, Washington 98195

Received for publication 6 December 1976

Several β-lactamase-producing, penicillin-resistant strains of *Neisseria gonorrhoeae* were examined for R plasmids. Penicillin-resistant strains isolated from men returning from the Far East and their contacts contained a 4.4×10^6-dalton plasmid in common. Transformation studies and the isolation of a spontaneous penicillin-susceptible segregant showed that the structural gene for β-lactamase was part of the 4.4×10^6-dalton plasmid. An additional penicillin-resistant gonococcal strain isolated in London was found to harbor a 3.2×10^6-dalton R plasmid. Deoxyribonucleic acid (DNA)-DNA duplex studies revealed that the penicillin-resistant gonococcal isolates contained a significant portion (about 40%) of the transposable DNA sequence, TnA, which includes the β-lactamase gene commonly found on R plasmids of the *Enterobacteriaceae* and *Haemophilus influenzae*.

It has been known for some time that the R plasmids of enteric species enjoy a very broad host range (1, 14). The recent finding (reviewed in 4, 6, 28) that certain plasmid-mediated antibiotic resistance genes reside upon discrete sequences of deoxyribonucleic acid (DNA) that have the capacity to transpose from plasmid to plasmid has further demonstrated that the range of plasmid-mediated antibiotic resistance genes might be even broader than that of the whole plasmid genome. Therefore, plausible mechanisms exist by which pathogenic microorganisms, previously antibiotic susceptible, may be converted to stable antibiotic resistance by the direct extension of an entire R plasmid or by the simple addition of only a segment of DNA to a preexisting indigenous plasmid gene pool (6, 15, 19).

Previous studies from this laboratory (21) and others (3, 24, 30) have established that most strains of *Neisseria gonorrhoeae* contain plasmid species that are cryptic in the phenotypic sense. For example, our examination of 30 antibiotic-susceptible gonococcal isolates showed that 28 strains harbored a multicopy $(2.6 \pm 0.2) \times 10^6$-dalton (2.6 MDal) plasmid, and 1 strain contained a 24.5-MDal plasmid species, whereas 1 strain was plasmid free (13; L. P. Elwell and S. Falkow, *in* R. Roberts, ed., *The Gonococcus*, in press). The demonstration of a widespread plasmid gene pool in gonococci together with the emergence, epidemiology, and molecular nature of R plasmids mediating ampicillin resistance in *Haemophilus influenzae* (11, 12) led us to speculate (15) that gonococci were likely candidates to acquire plasmid-mediated penicillin resistance specified by a β-lactamase. Consequently, the recent isolation of β-lactamase-producing strains of *N. gonorrhoeae* (2, 25, 26) prompted us to examine them for the presence of a novel DNA species that might represent an R plasmid.

In this study we report the detection of plasmid species from three penicillin-resistant clinical isolates of *N. gonorrhoeae*. We further demonstrate that these plasmids probably represent a direct or indirect extension of the plasmid gene pool of enteric species to gonococci.

MATERIALS AND METHODS

Bacterial strains. Penicillin-resistant strains of *N. gonorrhoeae* were kindly supplied by Clyde Thornsberry, Center for Disease Control, Atlanta, Ga. The strains, CDCO1, CDC66, CDC67, and CDC36N, were recent representative isolates from United States military personnel recently returned from the Far East as well as a sexual contact (3, 25). The IPL strain was originally isolated in London from the vagina of a woman with a pelvic inflammatory disease (26). The gonococcal strains F62 and KH45 were antibiotic-susceptible laboratory strains whose plasmid complement have been previously characterized (21; Elwell and Falkow, in press). Penicillinase production of the parental strains as well as selected transformants was detected by using the chromogenic cephalosporin method (23). Resistant strains were maintained on modified Kellogg agar (21) supplemented with 1 μg of penicillin G per ml.

Agarose gel electrophoresis of DNA. Plasmid

DNA was initially detected and characterized by the agarose gel electrophoretic method (22). The strains of *N. gonorrhoeae* were grown overnight in 30 ml of modified GC medium (Difco) supplemented as described by Mayer et al. (21). Cleared lysates were prepared (16, 22) and, after ribonuclease digestion and phenol extraction, the clear aqueous phase was adjusted to 0.2 M sodium acetate (final concentration) and precipitated with ethanol. The precipitate was dissolved in 0.2 ml of TES buffer [50 mM NaCl-5mM ethylenediaminetetraacetic acid (EDTA)-30 mM tris(hydroxymethyl)aminomethane (Tris) (pH 8)] and electrophoresed in a 0.7% agarose gel dissolved in Tris-borate buffer (pH 8.2) (89 mM Tris base-2.5 mM sodium EDTA-89 mM boric acid). DNA was visualized by staining with ethidium bromide and viewing the gel under long-wave ultraviolet light. Plasmid DNA of known molecular weight was included in each gel as a standard (22).

Preparation of plasmid DNA. Unlabeled covalently closed circular (CCC) plasmid DNA was prepared as previously described (19). [^{3}H]thymine-labeled RSF1050 plasmid DNA was prepared from *Escherichia coli* 1485 as described by Heffron et al. (18, 19).

DNA contour length. Plasmid DNA was spread onto parlodion-coated electron microscope grids by the Kleinschmidt technique (10). Molecular weights of the plasmids were calculated as previously described (18, 19).

DNA-DNA hybridization studies. Unlabeled whole-cell DNA from penicillin-resistant and -susceptible strains of *N. gonorrhoeae* was prepared by the method of So et al. (29). For DNA-DNA duplex studies, approximately 0.01 μg of ^{3}H-labeled, sheared, denatured RSF1050 plasmid DNA was incubated with 150 μg of unlabeled, sheared, denatured DNA from each of the indicated organisms. DNA reassociation was performed in 0.21 M NaCl at 68°C for 240 min. At the end of the incubation period, samples were assayed by the S_1 endonuclease technique (7).

RESULTS

Detection of R plasmid in *N. gonorrhoeae*. Figure 1 shows the agarose gel electrophoresis of ethanol-precipitated plasmid DNA from cleared lysates of selected *N. gonorrhoeae* strains. The prominent band of linear chromosomal DNA migrates to a characteristic position in such gels and may obscure CCC plasmid species of about 10×10^6 to 15×10^6 daltons, depending upon its width (22). Figures 1A and B contain lysates extracted from the antibiotic-susceptible laboratory strains KH45 and F62 and show the presence of previously characterized CCC plasmids of 24.5 and 2.6 MDal, respectively. The faint DNA band in Fig. 1B, appearing between the 2.6-MDal CCC plasmid species and the chromosomal band, represents the open circular (OC) form of the 2.6-MDal plasmid. The identification of this intermediate band as the OC form of the 2.6-MDal plasmid species was deducted from the direct electron microscopic examination of molecules extracted from this band as well as the direct observation of the banding patterns of known 2.6-MDal CCC and OC species (see also 22). Figures 1C and D contain lysates extracted from independently isolated penicillin-resistant strains CDC66 and CDC67 contracted by military personnel in the Far East. The lysate of strain CDC66 (Fig. 1C) shows the CCC and OC forms of the 2.6-MDal indigenous plasmid and an additional plasmid species that migrates in the agarose gel at a position (relative to the molecular weight standard [Fig. 1H]) characteristic of a CCC molecule with a molecular mass of 4.4 MDal. The lysate of strain CDC67 (Fig. 1D) contains both the 2.6- and 24.5-MDal plasmids typical of gonococci, but also contains a 4.4-MDal plasmid species. The association of the 4.4-MDal molecular species with the penicillin-resistant phenotype was materially strengthened by examining the lysate extracted from a penicillin-resistant strain, CDC01 (Fig. 1F), isolated from a case contact and a spontaneous pencillin-susceptible derivative of CDC01 (Fig. 1E). It may be seen that the lysates from these two strains differ in only one aspect, namely, the 4.4-MDal plasmid species.

The lysate extracted from the penicillin-resistant IPL strain isolated in London from a patient with pelvic inflammatory disease is shown in Fig. 1G. The IPL strain was found to contain the 2.6-MDal plasmid and a unique plasmid species that, migrated at a position, relative to the molecular weight standards (Fig. 1H), for a CCC molecule with a molecular mass of 3.2 MDal.

The number and molecular mass of the plasmid species in the gonococcal isolates were verified by isolating purified CCC DNA from each strain and measuring the contour lengths of OC species seen in the electron microscope. The results were in excellent agreement with the agarose gel data. Relative to the indigenous gonococcal plasmid, which was taken as a molecular mass of 2.6 MDal (21, 24, 30), the molecular masses of the unique plasmid species present in the Far East and London strains were calculated to be 4.3 ± 0.15 and 3.2 ± 0.2 MDal, respectively, based on measurements of at least 10 molecules. In subsequent studies we have been able to transform, by using the method of Cohen et al. (5), a suitable *E. coli* recipient to ampicillin resistance (Ap^r) with purified plasmid DNA from the penicillin-resistant strains CDC36N and IPL. The resulting *E. coli* Ap^r transformants derived from CDC36N DNA contained a single plasmid species corresponding

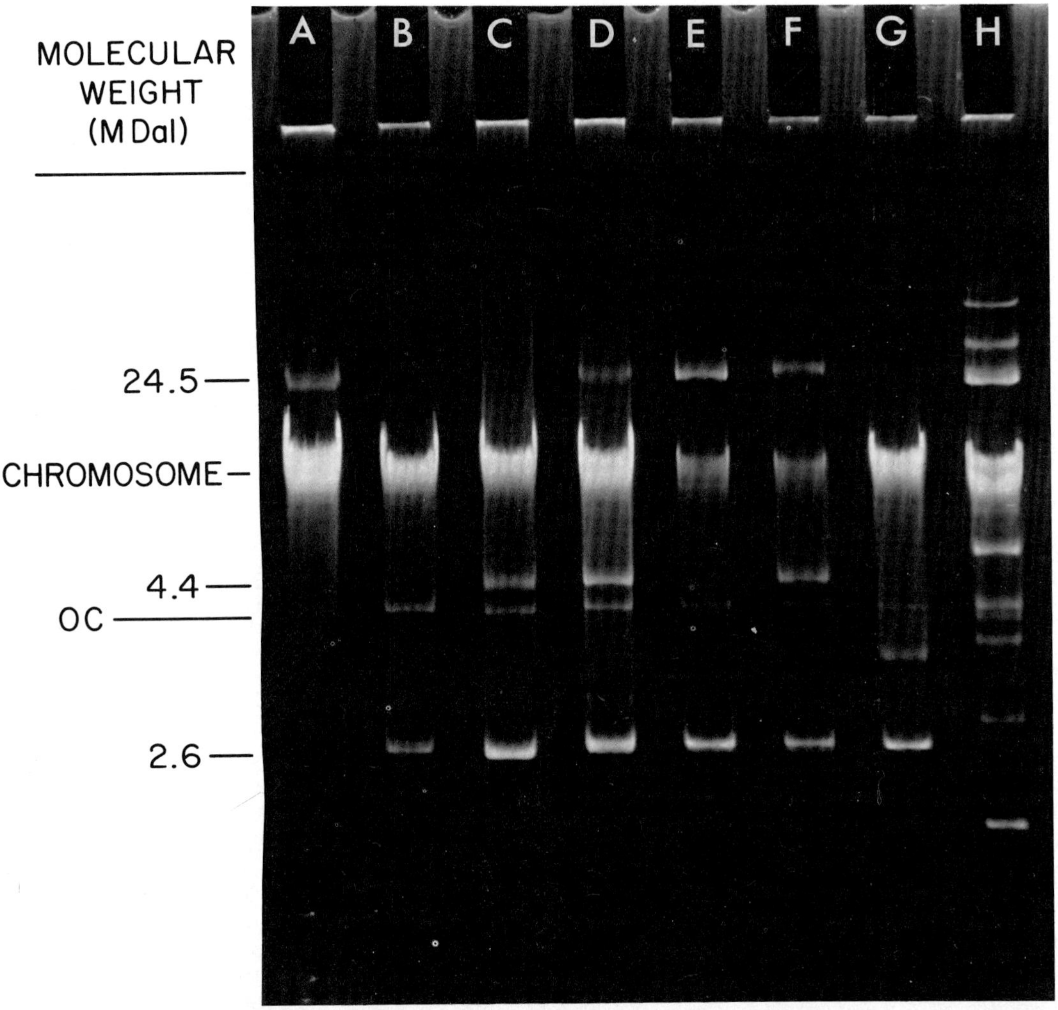

FIG. 1. *Agarose gel electrophoresis of ethanol-precipitated DNA from cleared lysates of penicillin-susceptible (Pen^s) and penicillin-resistant (Pen^r) N. gonorrhoeae strains. (A) Strain KH45 (Pen^s) containing the 24.5 × 10^6-dalton cryptic plasmid; (B) strain F62 (pen^s) containing the 2.6 × 10^6-dalton cryptic plasmid; (C) strain CDC66 (Pen^r), Far East isolate; (D) strain CDC67 (Pen^r), Far East isolate; (E) spontaneous Pen^s derivative of strain CDC01; (F) strain CDC01 (Pen^r), from case contact of patient infected in the Far East; (G) strain IPL (Pen^r), London, England, isolate; (H) standard plasmid DNAs, ranging in size from 62 × 10^6 (uppermost band) to 1.9 × 10^6 daltons (lowest band). OC refers to the open circular form of the 2.6 × 10^6-dalton cryptic plasmid.*

to 4.3 MDal, whereas the *E. coli* Ap^r transformants obtained with IPL DNA contained a single plasmid species of 3.2 MDal. The complete molecular characterization of these plasmids is currently in progress (M. Roberts, L. P. Elwell, and S. Falkow, manuscript in preparation). Nevertheless, the preliminary data presented here provide sufficient evidence to conclude that the penicillin resistance of the Far East and London gonococcal isolates is plasmid mediated.

Origin of β-lactamase genes residing on gonococcal plasmids. Although gonococci relatively resistant to penicillin have been known for a number of years (reviewed in 15), the penicillin-resistant gonococci isolated from the Far East and London were unlike any previously described strains in that they elaborated a β-lactamase that conferred resistance to penicillin, ampicillin, and cephaloridine, similar to the TEM β-lactamase of enteric species (2, 26, C. Thornsberry, personal communication; unpublished data from this laboratory). It is well established that among R plasmids within species of the family *Enterobacteriaceae*, the gene specifying the TEM β-lactamase resides upon a common transposable 3.2×10^6-dalton sequence of DNA (3, 4, 6, 17-19). The ability of this DNA sequence, TnA, to be excised from one plasmid and become inserted into a recipient plasmid has been suggested as an explanation for the ubiquity of the TEM β-lactamase gene among R plasmids of the *Enterobacteriaceae* and other bacterial species (15, 17-19). It seemed of considerable interest, therefore, to determine whether any, or all, of the TnA DNA sequence was present in the penicillin-resistant strains of *N. gonorrhoeae*. To study this possibility, DNA-DNA duplex studies were performed.

Whole-cell DNA was prepared from the *N. gonorrhoeae* Far East isolates CDC66 and CDC67, the London isolate IPL, as well as the laboratory strains F62 and KH45. [^{3}H]thymine-labeled RSF1050, a 4.9-MDal ColE1 plasmid derivative containing the entire TnA sequence (29), was hybridized against the unlabeled gonococcal whole-cell DNA. RSF1050 served as a particularly convenient probe for TnA since this sequence comprised about 50% of the entire plasmid genome (F. Heffron, P. Bedinger, J. Champoux, and S. Falkow, submitted for publication). Table 1 shows the results of the hybridization experiments. Labeled RSF1050 plasmid DNA shared no DNA sequences in common with the drug-susceptible strains of *N. gonorrhoeae* harboring either the 24.5- or 2.6-MDal indigenous plasmids. In contrast, all of the penicillin-resistant strains tested contained DNA that bound 20 to 22% of the RSF1050 nucleotide sequence. As indicated in Table 1, ^{3}H-labeled RSF1050 was hybridized against whole-cell DNA extracted from *H. influenzae* (RSF007). The plasmid RSF007 has previously been shown to contain the entire TnA sequence by heteroduplex analysis (11); therefore, the reaction between RSF1050 and *H. influenzae* (RSF007) was assumed to reflect only TnA-TnA interaction. On the basis of a relative DNA sequence homology of 51% in the case of an R plasmid containing the entire TnA segment, it can be estimated that both the 4.4- and 3.2-MDal gonococcal R plasmids contain 39 to 43% of the TnA sequence. To determine whether the homology shared by RSF1050 and the gonococcal R plasmids was specifically in the TnA segment and not another portion of RSF1050, hybridization experiments were carried out with ^{3}H-labeled PMB8 plasmid DNA. PMB8, which is RSF1050 minus TnA, showed no significant nucleotide base sequence homology with unlabeled DNA derived from the penicillin-resistant *N. gonorrhoeae* isolates. Heteroduplex studies are in progress to substantiate these hybridization data.

TABLE 1. *Hybridization between ^{3}H-labeled RSF1050 plasmid DNA and whole-cell DNA*

Source of unlabeled DNA	Relative DNA sequence homology with ^{3}H-labeled RSF1050 plasmid DNA (%)[a]
E. coli W1485 (RSF1050)	100
H. influenzae (RSF007)	51
N. gonorrhoeae F62 (Pen^s)[b]	1
N. gonorrhoeae 45 (Pen^s)	1
N. gonorrhoeae 67 (Pen^r)	22
N. gonorrhoeae 66 (Pen^r)	20
N. gonorrhoeae IPL (Pen^r)	20

[a] The degree of DNA-DNA duplex formation was assayed by the S1 endonuclease method (7). In every case, the degree of duplex formation was calculated relative to the homologous reaction. The actual extent of binding in the homologous reaction was 75 to 78%. All other reactions were normalized to this value set at 100%. Each value shown is an average of three separate determinations. The RSF007 plasmid resident in *H. influenzae* has been previously shown to contain the entire TnA DNA sequence (11). The reaction between RSF1050 and *H. influenzae* (RSF007) was assumed to reflect only TnA-TnA interaction. The reaction between RSF1050 and the gonococcal isolates was also assumed to reflect only TnA-TnA reaction.

[b] Pen^s, Penicillin susceptible; Pen^r, penicillin resistant.

DISCUSSION

The sudden appearance of plasmid-mediated penicillin resistance among strains of *N. gonorrhoeae* in both the Far East and London bears a striking similarity to the earlier emergence of ampicillin-resistant strains of *H. influenzae* (20). Antibiotic resistance in *Haemophilus* strains has occurred by virtue of several independent events, as evidenced by the characterization of two genetically distinct R plasmids from ampicillin-resistant isolates (11, 12, 15). Similarly, antibiotic resistance in *N. gonorrhoeae* appears to be more complex than merely the dissemination of a single R plasmid-containing strain. This conclusion is suggested by the plasmid pattern observed in the lysates of the Far East strains CDC66 and CDC67 since one harbors the 24.5-MDal indigenous plasmid and the other does not (Fig. 1C and D). Both of these isolates carry the 4.4-MDal R plasmid as well as the 2.6-MDal indigenous plasmid. Furthermore, the IPL strain isolated in London presumably represents a third independent resistant strain. Preliminary auxotyping of selected penicillin-resistant isolates (D. Rose, and M. Roberts, unpublished data) supports the conclusion that many of the strains are unrelated and that resistance has occurred by independent genetic events.

A number of investigators (reviewed in 1, 14, 31) have noted that the R plasmid pool of enteric bacteria has been increasing sharply, particularly over the past decade. As the pool of R plasmid-containing enteric bacteria has increased, so has the possibility that R plasmids might emerge that could better cross biological barriers and so, perhaps, enter bacterial species and genera apparently widely different from their original enterobacterial hosts (1, 31). We believe the emergence of penicillin resistance in gonococci provides yet another example of the direct or indirect extension of the enteric R plasmid pool. The R plasmids specifying β-lactamase characterized in *H. influenzae* were shown to contain, in one case, the entire TnA segment and, in another case, at least one-third of the transposable TnA sequence that is found on a wide variety of enteric R plasmids (11, 12, 15). Similarly, in this study we have shown that R plasmids of gonococci likewise contain a significant portion (about 40%) of the TnA sequence. The possibility that a relationship exists between the emergence of plasmid-mediated resistance in *N. gonorrhoeae* and *H. influenzae* is currently under study. Whatever the relationship, the evidence that both of these formerly antibiotic-susceptible pathogens have been recently penetrated by R plasmids, perhaps of enteric origin, has profound implications. For example, a survey of selected strains of *N. meningitidis* for the presence of extrachromosomal DNA has shown that this bacterial species does not ordinarily contain plasmid DNA (Elwell and Falkow, in press). Since *N. gonorrhoeae* and *N. meningitidis* are known to be closely related, we believe that there is cause for concern that meningococci may soon acquire plasmid-mediated drug resistance.

Whether the plasmids carrying a portion of TnA now residing in *N. gonorrhoeae* were directly acquired from some unknown enteric species by conjugation or whether the R plasmids were, in effect, generated by the translocation of the ubiquitous TnA sequence into resident neisserial plasmid species is not clear from currently available data. The relationship between indigenous gonococcal plasmids and gonococcal R plasmids is currently being investigated. A 4.4-MDal plasmid is probably not self-transmissible (14); however, it may be more than fortuitous that the 24.5-MDal cryptic plasmid co-resides with the R plasmid in three of the seven ampicillin-resistant strains we have examined thus far. This large indigenous plasmid was found in only 1 of over 30 antibiotic-susceptible gonococcal isolates that we had previously examined (Elwell and Falkow, in press), and it is tempting to speculate that this large plasmid is mobilizing the smaller R plasmid during conjugation. This possibility is currently being investigated.

Continued surveillance of resistance in *H. influenzae* has provided suggestive evidence that, after the initial breach of some sort of genetic barrier leading to the emergence of R plasmids bearing ampicillin resistance, there have followed in rapid succession R plasmids specifying resistance to tetracycline (8), kanamycin (9), and linked tetracycline and chloramphenicol resistance (B. Van Klingeren, J. Van Embden, and M. Dessens-Kroon, in press). If we look to the future of antimicrobial therapy of gonococcal infections, the experience with *H. influenzae* provides a disquieting precedent.

ACKNOWLEDGMENTS

We are grateful to C. Thornsberry, Center for Disease Control, Atlanta, Ga., for calling our attention to and providing us with the penicillin-resistant strains of *N. gonorrhoeae*.

This work was supported by Public Health Service grant AI00191-03 from the National Institute of Allergy and Infectious Diseases. L. P. Elwell was supported by Public Health Service grant AI05328-01 from the National Institute of Allergy and Infectious Diseases.

LITERATURE CITED

1. **Anderson, E. S.** 1968. The ecology of transferable drug resistance in the *Enterobacteriaceae*. Annu. Rev. Microbiol. 22:132–180.
2. **Ashford, W. A., R. G. Golash, and V. G. Hemming.** 1976. Penicillinase-producing *Neisseria gonorrhoeae*. Lancet 22:657–658.
3. **Bennett, P. M., and M. H. Richmond.** 1976. The transposition of a discrete piece of deoxyribonucleic acid carrying an *amp* gene between replicons in *Escherichia coli*. J. Bacteriol. **126**:1–6.
4. **Cohen, S. N.** 1976. Transposable genetic elements and plasmid evolution. Nature (London) **263**:731–738.
5. **Cohen, S. N., A. C. Y. Chang, and L. Hsu.** 1972. Nonchromosomal antibiotic resistance in bacteria: genetic transformation of *Escherichia coli* by R-factor DNA. Proc. Natl. Acad. Sci. U.S.A. **69**:2110–2114.
6. **Cohen, S. N., and D. J. Kopecko.** 1976. Structural evolution of bacterial plasmids: role of translocating genetic elements and DNA sequence insertions. Fed. Proc. 35:2031–2036.
7. **Crosa, J. H., D. J. Brenner, and S. Falkow.** Use of a single-strand specific nuclease for analysis of bacterial and plasmid deoxyribonucleic acid homo- and heteroduplexes. J. Bacteriol. **115**:904–911.
8. **Dang Van, A., G. Beith, and D. H. Bouanchaud.** 1975. Resistance plasmidique à la tetracycline chez *H. influenzae*. C.R. Acad. Sci **280**:1321–1323.
9. **Dang Van, A., F. Goldstein, J. F. Acar, and D. H. Bouanchaud.** 1975. A transferable kanamycin resistance plasmid isolated from *Haemophilus influenzae*. Ann. Microbiol. (Paris) **126**:397–399.

10. **Davis, R. W., M. Simon, and N. Davidson.** 1971. Electron microscope heteroduplex methods for mapping region of base sequence homology in nucleic acids, p. 413-427. *In* L. Grossman and K. Moldave (ed.), Methods in enzymology, vol. 21. Academic Press Inc., New York.
11. **de Graaff, J., L. P. Elwell, and S. Falkow.** 1976. Molecular nature of two beta-lactamase-specifying plasmids isolated from *Haemophilus influenzae* type b. J. Bacteriol. **126**:439-446.
12. **Elwell, L. P., J. de Graaff, D. Seibert, and S. Falkow.** 1975. Plasmid-linked ampicillin resistance in *Haemophilus influenzae* type b. Infect. Immun. **12**:404-410.
13. **Engelkirk, P. G., and D. E. Schoenhard.** 1972. Physical evidence of a plasmid in *Neisseria gonorrhoeae*. J. Infect. Dis. **127**:197-200.
14. **Falkow, S.** 1975. Infectious multiple drug resistance. Pion Ltd., London.
15. **Falkow, S., L. P. Elwell, J. de Graaff, F. Heffron, and L. Mayer.** 1976. A possible model for the development of plasmid-mediated penicillin resistance in the gonococcus, p. 120-133. *In* R. D. Catterall and C. S. Nicol (ed.), Sexually transmitted diseases. Academic Press Inc., London.
16. **Guerry, P., D. J. LeBlanc, and S. Falkow.** 1973. General method for the isolation of plasmid deoxyribonucleic acid. J. Bacteriol **116**:1064-1066.
17. **Hedges, R. W., and A. Jacob.** 1974. Transposition of ampicillin resistance from RP4 to other replicons. Mol. Gen. Genet. **132**:31-40.
18. **Heffron, F. C., C. Rubens, and S. Falkow.** 1975. Translocation of a plasmid DNA sequence which mediates ampicillin resistance: molecular nature and specificity of insertion. Proc. Natl. Acad. Sci. U.S.A. **72**:3623-3627.
19. **Heffron, R., R. Sublett, R. W. Hedges, A. Jacob, and S. Falkow.** 1975. Origin of the TEM beta-lactamase gene found on plasmids. J. Bacteriol. **122**:250-256.
20. **Khan, W., S. Ross, W. Rodriguez, G. Controri, and A. K. Saz.** 1974. *Haemophilus influenzae* type b resistant to ampicillin. A report of two cases. J. Am. Med. Assoc. **229**:298-301.
21. **Mayer, L. W., K. K. Holmes, and S. Falkow.** 1974. Characterization of plasmid deoxyribonucleic acid from *Neisseria gonorrhoeae*. Infect. Immun. **10**:712-717.
22. **Meyers, J., D. Sanchez, L. P. Elwell, and S. Falkow.** 1976. A simple agarose gel electrophoretic method for the identification and characterization of plasmid deoxyribonucleic acid. J. Bacteriol. **127**:1529-1537.
23. **O'Callaghan, C. H., A. Morris, S. M. Kirby, and A. H. Shindler.** 1972. Novel method for detection of β-lactamase by using a chromogenic cephalosporin substrate. Antimicrob. Agents Chemother. **1**:283-288.
24. **Palchaudhuri, S., E. Bell, and M. R. J. Salton.** 1975. Electron microscopy of plasmid deoxyribonucleic acid from *Neisseria gonorrhoeae*. Infect. Immun. **11**:1141-1146.
25. Penicillinase-producing *Neisseria gonorrhoeae*. 1976. Morbid. Mortal. Week. Rep. 25:261.
26. **Phillips, I.** 1976. Beta-lactamase-producing penicillin-resistant gonococcus. Lancet **2**:656-657.
27. **Rubens, C., F. Heffron, and S. Falkow.** 1976. Transposition of a plasmid dexoyribonucleic acid sequence that mediates ampicillin resistance: independence from host *rec* functions and orientation of insertion. J. Bacteriol. **128**:425-434.
28. **Saunders, J.** 1975. Transposable resistance genes. Nature (London)**258**:384.
29. **So, M., J. H. Crosa, and S. Falkow.** 1974. Polynucleotide sequence relationships among Ent plasmids and the relationship between Ent and other plasmids. J. Bacteriol. **121**:234-238.
30. **Stiffler, P. W., S. A. Lerner, M. Bohnhoff, and J. A. Morello.** 1975. Plasmid deoxyribonucleic acid in clinical isolates of *Neisseria gonorrhoeae*. J. Bacteriol. **122**:1293-1300.
31. **World Health Organization.** 1976. Public health aspect of antibiotic-resistant bacteria in the environment. World Health Organization Regional Office for Europe, Copenhagen.

ANTIMICROBIAL AGENTS AND CHEMOTHERAPY, Mar. 1977, p. 534-540 Vol. 11, No. 3

Printed in U.S.A.

Effect of Ethambutol on the Viable Cell Count in *Mycobacterium smegmatis*

JAMES O. KILBURN* AND JOSEPH GREENBERG

Center for Disease Control, Atlanta, Georgia 30333

Received for publication 8 September 1976

Soon after a strain of *Mycobacterium smegmatis* was exposed to ethambutol (EMB), the number of viable cells increased dramatically above the number in a drug-free control. This rapid rise did not occur when the culture was maintained at 4°C instead of 37°C, when an EMB-resistant mutant was used, when auxotrophs were exposed in medium lacking nutrients essential for growth, nor when the levo form of EMB was used. EMB caused no increase in deoxyribonucleic acid synthesis, nor in septum formation of dividing cells. Treated cells changed morphologically, resulting in a lower surface area-to-volume ratio. Whereas EMB did not eliminate cell clusters, the cluster size decreased markedly as detected by filtration and Coulter counter measurements. We concluded that EMB causes a reduced surface-to-volume ratio, leading to reduced cell cohesion and a consequent reduction in cluster size, reflected in an increase in colony-forming units.

Ethambutol (EMB) is an effective antituberculosis drug and, in combination with isoniazid, is commonly used in many chemotherapeutic regimens. EMB is effective only against mycobacteria (3). Only the D isomer shows activity (5). Forbes et al. (1) noted an increase in viable cell counts, above those in drug-free control, in a culture of *Mycobacterium smegmatis* exposed to EMB. This unexplained rapid rise and its relationship to cell viability were examined.

MATERIALS AND METHODS

Bacteria and growth conditions. Both EMB-susceptible and the EMB-resistant mutants (resistant to 3 μg of EMB/ml) were grown in liquid 7H-9 medium (Difco). The albumin-dextrose enrichment was omitted, and 0.05% Tween 80 (Atlas Powder Co., Wilmington, Del.) and 0.2% glycerol were substituted. Cultures were grown at 37°C in a shaking water bath to an optical density (OD) of 0.5. Before use, they were diluted with fresh 7H-9 medium to an OD = 0.1 or 0.025, corresponding to 1.5×10^7 and 2.5×10^6 colony-forming units (CFU) per ml, respectively. The numbers of CFU were determined by serial dilution plate counts on Dubos- Middlebrook agar (Difco). The plates were incubated at 37°C for 2 days before the colonies were counted. In filtration experiments, 5-ml culture samples were aseptically filtered through 5.0-μm Metricel membrane filters (Gelman Instrument Co., Ann Arbor, Mich.).

Electronic cell counting. Cell size distribution in EMB-treated and control cultures was determined in a Coulter counter, model TAII, equipped with an X-Y recorder (Coulter Electronics, Inc., Hialeah, Fla.). The aperture setting was 30 μm, and Isoton was used as the diluent.

Electron microscopy. Samples of control and EMB-treated *M. smegmatis* were centrifuged at 9,000 × g for 30 min, and the pellets were resuspended in 2 ml of distilled water. A drop of each suspension was added to Formvar-coated copper grids and negatively stained with 2% aqueous uranyl acetate (pH 4.0) for 15 s. The grids were blotted dry, examined, and photographed with a Philips model 200 transmission electron microscope operating at an accelerating voltage of 60 kV.

Measurement of DNA synthesis. A modified membrane-filter technique of Roodyn and Mandel (4) was used. A 60-ml culture (OD = 0.1) was exposed for 60 min to 0.6 m Ci of [*methyl*-^{3}H]thymidine (2.0 Ci/mmol, New England Nuclear, Boston, Mass.). The cells were washed two times by centrifuging in the cold at 18,000 × *g* for 15 min and resuspending the cells in equal volumes of cold medium. After the final wash, the culture was divided into two equal parts, and 0.25 μg of EMB/ml was added to half. Both were incubated at 37°C. Incorporation of label into deoxyribonucleic acid (DNA) was determined by pipetting 1.0-ml samples into an equal volume of 10% trichloroacetic acid and maintaining the mixture for 15 min in an ice bath. The samples were then collected on membrane filters (0.45-μm, Millipore Corp., Bedford, Mass.) and washed with 15 ml of cold 1.0% trichloroacetic acid. Total cell counts were determined by collecting 1.0-ml samples on membrane filters and washing the samples with 15 ml of cold 1.0% trichloroacetic acid. After air-drying, the filters were added to vials containing 10 ml of toluene-based Spectrofluor (Amersham/Searle, Des Plaines, Ill.), and the radioactivity was determined in an Isocap/300 liquid scintillation counter (Searle Analytic, Des Plaines, Ill.). Nonincorporated counts were determined by subtracting incorporated counts (trichloroacetic acid-insoluble) from the total counts.

RESULTS

Effect of EMB on cell viability. *M. smegmatis* at a concentration of approximately 2×10^6 organisms/ml was treated in growth medium with EMB concentrations from 0.1 to 3.0 μg/ml (Fig. 1). There was no discernible difference between cultures treated with 0.1 μg/ml and the untreated controls. At concentrations of 0.25 μg/ml, there was a rapid rise in CFU discernible in 2 h and reaching a peak at about 4 h. Thereafter, there was a decline in CFU until after 24 h, at which time cultures treated with 0.25 and 0.5 μg of EMB/ml increased in CFU. Treatment with 1.5 μg and 3.0 μg of EMB/ml resulted in death; there were fewer CFU after 48 h than there were at 0 h. The following should also be noted in Fig. 1: (i) from 0 to 12 h the kinetics of CFU was identical for concentrations of EMB from 0.25 to 3.0 μg/ml; (ii) the untreated culture did not reach the same density of CFU as cultures treated with $\geq$ 0.25 μg of EMB/ml until after 12 h, whereas it took untreated cells 8 h longer to reach the CFU density achieved by the treated cultures in 4 h.

Figure 2 shows CFU when the original cell density was about 2×10^7/ml, which is 10 times that used in the experiments shown in Fig. 1; the EMB concentration was 3 μg/ml. Though the early kinetics—the rapid, almost 10-fold rise in CFU, followed by a slight decline between 2 and 4 h—was the same as with less-dense cell populations, there was recovery, and CFU increased in numbers after 6 h at the higher cell density. At lower cell densities, the CFU declined progressively after 4 h with no evidence of recovery (Fig. 1). The data in Fig. 1 and 2 clearly show that although the rapid rise always preceeded cell death in populations treated with EMB, some recovery was possible after the rapid rise. The amount of recovery was a function of both the concentration of EMB and of the density of the cell population.

Conditions affecting the rapid rise. The rapid rise was not detected when cells were treated with 3 μg of the levo form of EMB/ml, which is not effective in killing mycobacteria (data not shown).

A mutant of *M. smegmatis,* selected for re-

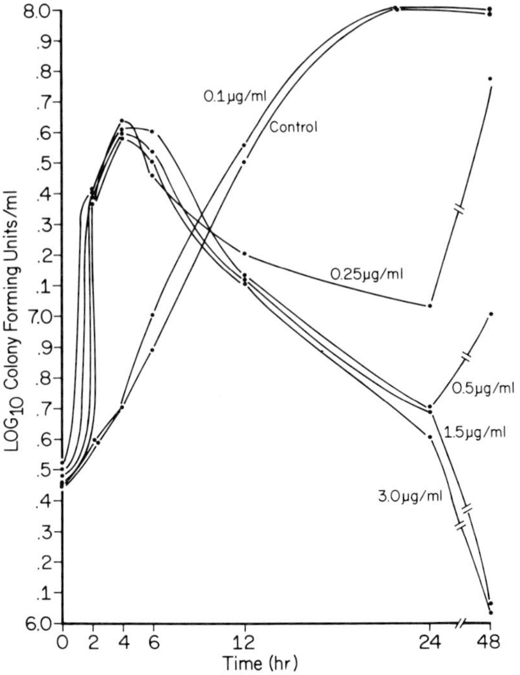

FIG. 1. *Dose response of a low-density cell population. An initial cell density of 2.5×10^6 CFU/ml was exposed to concentrations of EMB ranging from 0.1 to 3.0 μg/ml; samples were removed, diluted, and plated at the indicated times.*

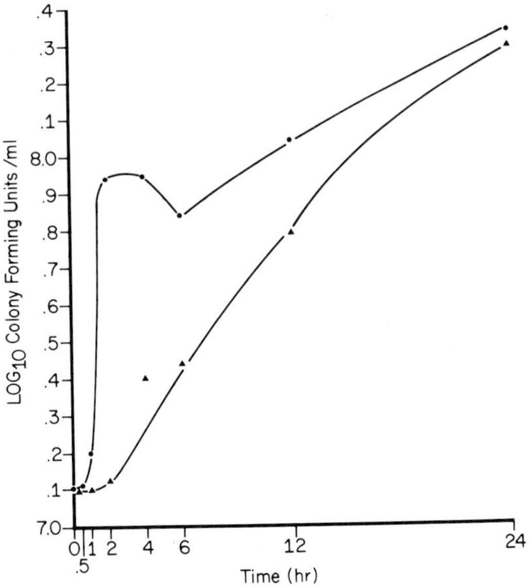

FIG. 2. *Effect of 3.0 μg of EMB/ml on a high-density cell population. An initial cell density of 1.5×10^7 CFU/ml was exposed to 3.0 μg of EMB/ml (closed circles) and treated as in Fig. 1. Samplings at 0.5 and 1.0 h are included. The control is represented by closed triangles.*

sistance to 3 μg of EMB/ml, exhibited no rapid rise until exposed to 12 and 24 μg of EMB/ml (Fig. 3).

The rapid rise requires metabolizing cells, as is evidenced by its absence in cultures treated with 3 μg of EMB/ml and maintained at 4°C (data not shown). Furthermore, an auxotrophic mutant, P22, treated with 3 μg of EMB/ml of medium lacking the essential amino acids, leucine, arginine, and histidine, did not exhibit the rapid rise (Fig. 4).

Static cultures exhibited the same rapid rise as shaken cultures, indicating that the physical effects of shaking did not cause the rapid rise (data not shown).

From these data, it may be concluded that the rapid rise observed to begin between 30 to 60 min after exposure of cells to EMB is not a physical effect and depends on a stereospecific form of the drug reacting with actively metabolizing cells.

Effect of EMB on DNA synthesis. Since the rapid rise is elicited only in metabolizing cells, it is possible that EMB initiates rapid cell division. The data for untreated controls in Fig. 1 indicate that, under the conditions of the exper-

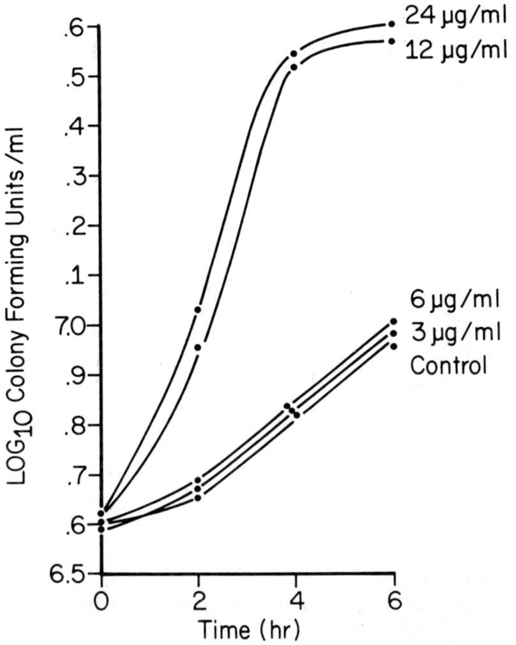

FIG. 3. *Effect of EMB concentration on the rapid rise in EMB-resistant mutant cells. The EMB-resistant mutant was selected by plating a susceptible population on Dubos-Middlebrook agar containing 3 μg of EMB/ml. Liquid cultures of the EMB-resistant mutant were exposed to the indicated EMB concentrations, and platings were made at the indicated times.*

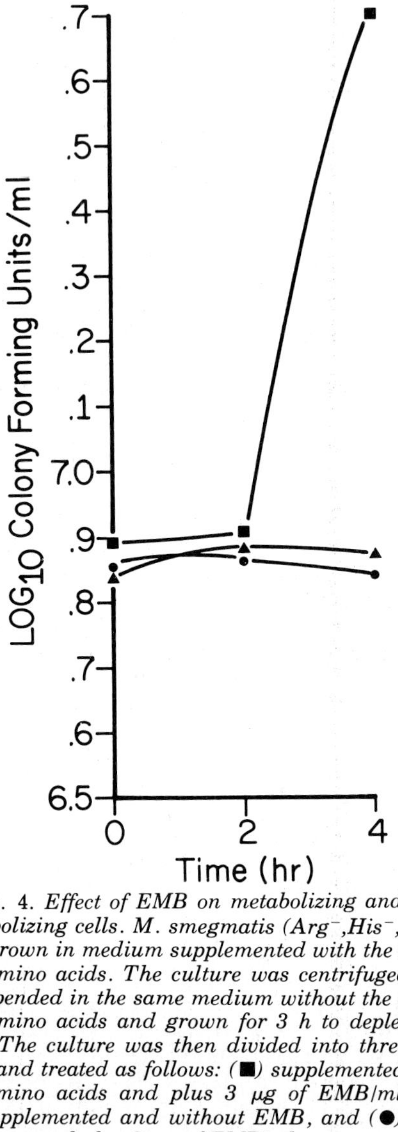

FIG. 4. *Effect of EMB on metabolizing and nonmetabolizing cells. M. smegmatis (Arg^-,His^-,Leu^-) was grown in medium supplemented with the essential amino acids. The culture was centrifuged and resuspended in the same medium without the essential amino acids and grown for 3 h to deplete the pool. The culture was then divided into three portions and treated as follows: (■) supplemented with the amino acids and plus 3 μg of EMB/ml, (▲) nonsupplemented and without EMB, and (●) nonsupplemented plus 3 μg of EMB/ml.*

iment, the generation time for *M. smegmatis* is about 4 h. To accomodate the hypothesis that EMB increases the rapidity of cell division, the generation time would have to be 2 h and would be reflected in an increased rate of DNA synthesis. Therefore, cells preloaded with [^{3}H]thymidine and exposed to EMB should incorporate this precursor from the pool to the acid-insoluble fraction more rapidly than the untreated cells. As seen in Fig. 5, this did not occur. Therefore, the rapid rise is not attributible to an increased rate of cell division.

Effect of EMB on cell morphology. Another possibility explaining the rapid rise is that indi-

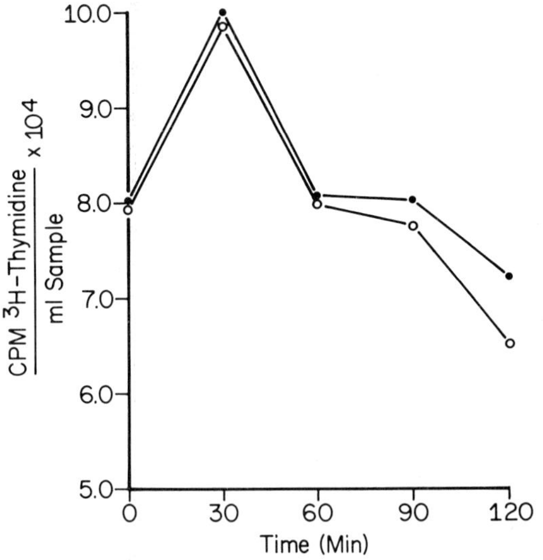

FIG. 5. *Effect of EMB on [³H]thymidine incorporation. An initial cell concentration of 1.5 × 10⁷ CFU/ml was preloaded with [³H]thymidine as described in Materials and Methods. Half was exposed to 0.25 μg of EMB/ml (open circles); the other half served as control (closed circles). One-milliliter samples were removed at the indicated times and assayed for label incorporation. The "pool" content at time 0 was 5.0 × 10⁴ CPM/ml.*

vidual cells of *M. smegmatis* are actually multinucleate filaments, requiring only the formation of septa to mature and to separate as individual CFU. EMB could accelerate the process of septation and dechaining. This hypothesis would require that each cell "unit" is potentially ≥10 CFU. To examine this possibility, cells treated with 3 μg of EMB/ml for 4 h were compared with untreated cells in an electron microscope. A sufficient number of cells could be examined at a magnification of ×9,000 to detect septation or a large number of small cells. Representive fields of treated and untreated cells are shown in Fig. 6. Cell clusters occurred in both preparations. No evidence of very small cells could be found in either the treated or untreated preparation, and no convincing evidence of incipient septation was observed in the control preparation. What was observed was that the treated cells were shorter and wider than the control. The average dimension of 10 untreated cells was 3.5 × 0.48 μm, of the treated cells, 2.2 × 0.65 μm. Treating both as ideal cylinders, the volumes of the treated and control cells are almost identical. However, the surface area of the treated cells is ≤80% that of the controls.

Effect of EMB on cluster size. The possibility that the rapid rise associated with EMB was attributible to the breaking up of clusters of cells was examined. Despite the fact that the variant of *M. smegmatis* used in these experiments was "smooth" and that Tween 80 was used in the liquid culture medium, the cells, treated with EMB or not, tended to cluster. This can be seen in the electron microscope pictures (Fig. 6) and could be seen through a light microscope in liquid drops of culture in which there was no distortion from drying. Nevertheless, that EMB treatment does reduce the size of clusters can be seen from the next two experiments.

In the first experiment, a culture treated with 3 μg of EMB/ml was compared with an untreated culture by passing a sample, at times given in Table 1, through a 5-μm membrane filter. The filtrates were appropriately diluted and plated for viable cell counts. About 10% of the cells in the untreated culture could pass through the filter, and this percentage remained the same through 6 h of growth and a tripling of the viable unit count. In the treated culture, the proportion of filterable cells doubled (22%) relative to the control within 2 h, increased slightly more (25%) at 4 h, but dropped to less than the control at 6 h (5%). These results are like the kinetics of the whole population shown in Fig. 1 and Table 1, in which there was a rapid rise of viable cells up to 4 h followed by a drop. Clearly, the increase in cells filterable through a 5-μm filter does not account for the 12- to 15-fold increase in total viable cells in the treated population. This leads to the conclusion that the increase in viable units in the treated culture is not attributable to an increase in single cells, all of which would have passed through the filter. It suggests rather that larger units are being deaggregated to smaller units, but still only a small portion of these are small enough to pass through the filter.

When units were selected by filtration through a 5-μm filter before their treatment with 0.25 μg of EMB/ml, it was observed (Fig. 7) that no significant rapid rise occurred and, unlike the situation with the general population, no recovery occurred after 24 h. This suggests that there is little deaggregation of small units and that some protection from the lethal effects of EMB is afforded cells in larger clusters.

The idea that EMB reduces the size of clusters of cells is confirmed by examining size distributions in a Coulter counter in cultures treated with 3 μg of EMB/ml for 4 h as compared with the untreated culture. As the data in Table 2 show, the volume sizes of units in the untreated culture varied over a 256-fold range;

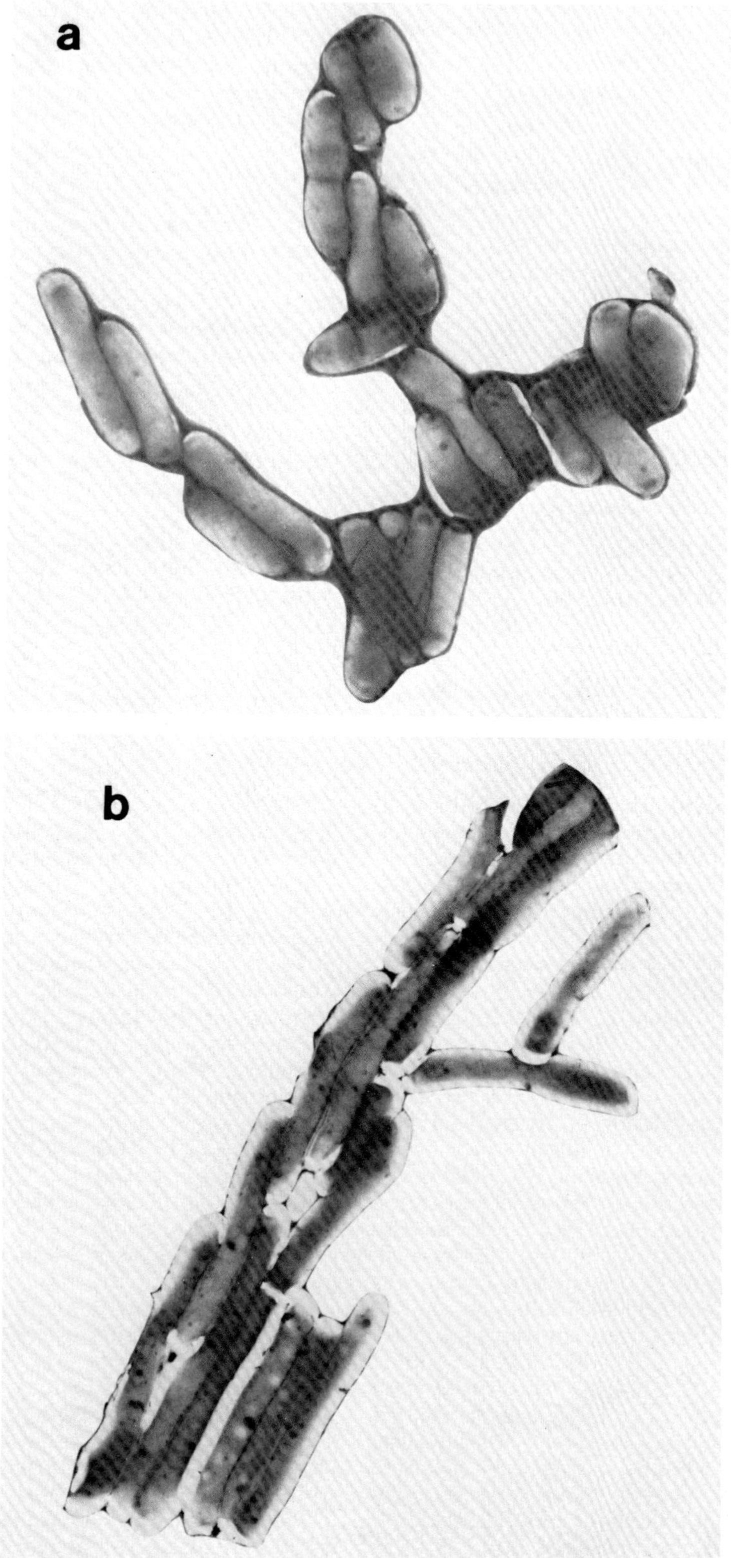
a
b

TABLE 1. *Comparison of untreated total and untreated filterable populations to EMB-treated total and filterable populations*

Time (h)	Populations			
	Untreated total	Untreated filterable	Treated total	Treated filterable
0	5.7×10^{6} [a]	6.1×10^{5}	5.7×10^{6}	6.1×10^{5}
2	5.4×10^{6}	5.0×10^{5}	6.7×10^{7}	1.5×10^{7}
4	9.5×10^{6}	9.2×10^{5}	6.8×10^{7}	1.7×10^{7}
6	1.6×10^{7}	1.6×10^{6}	4.8×10^{7}	2.3×10^{6}

[a] Expressed as CFU/ml of culture. The treated culture was exposed to 3 μg of EMB/ml. Five-milliliter samples were filtered through 5-μm Gelman membrane filters at the given times. The filtrates, along with total population samples, were diluted and plated as previously described.

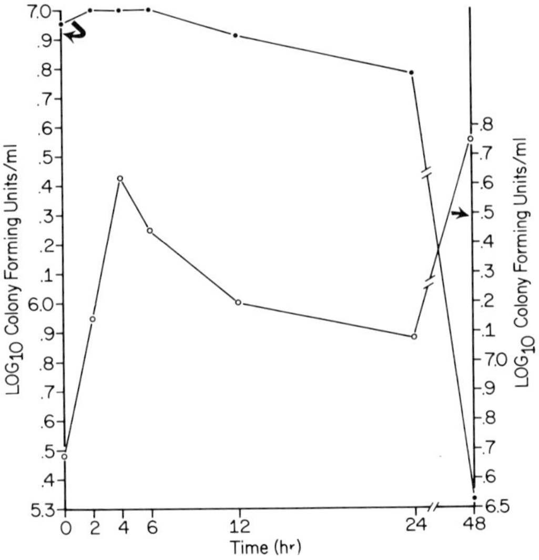

FIG. 7. *Comparison of preselected cells to a nonselected population after exposure to EMB. Cells were selected for size by passing 100 ml of an overnight culture through a 5-μm membrane filter. The filtrate was concentrated by centrifuging and resuspending in 20 ml of fresh medium. The nonselected population (open circle) was an overnight culture diluted with fresh medium to a cell density of approximately 1.5×10^7 CFU/ml. Both cultures were exposed to 0.25 μg of EMB/ml, sampled, and plated at the indicated times. The arrows indicate the correct axis.*

more than half the population was in cluster units larger than 16 times the smallest measurable units. In the treated culture, the largest clusters were only 32 times the smallest units,

TABLE 2. *Comparison of particle-volume distribution (expressed as percent) in EMB-treated and untreated populations*

Volume (μm^3)	Cultures[a]	
	Untreated (%)	Treated (3 μg of EMB/ml) (%)
0.52	7.0	13.0
1.047	10.0	33.0
2.094	16.0	30.0
4.189	20.0	17.0
8.378	17.0	5.0
16.760	12.0	2.0
33.510	10.0	0
67.020	4.0	0
134.00	4.0	0

[a] Both treated and untreated cultures were diluted to an initial cell density of 1.5×10^7 CFU/ml. A 0.5-ml sample was removed from each culture after 4 h of incubation, diluted with 20 ml of Isoton, and run through a Coulter counter with an aperture setting of 30 μm.

and almost half the population (46%) was in units smaller than twice the minimum. Assuming that each cluster produces a colony and assuming no difference in the total number of viable cells in the two populations, it is clear that the reduction in cluster size can account for the rapid rise in viable colonies in the treated population. The fact that even the treated cells tend to cluster obscures the kinetics of killing by EMB, since even one viable cell in a cluster will probably yield a viable colony.

DISCUSSION

The picture that emerged from these experiments is the following: within 2 h after exposure to EMB the shape of the treated cells changed; they became shorter and wider. Although their volume did not change, their surface area lessened. It is reasonable to consider clumping a function of adhesion which depends on surface area. A reduction of surface area would contribute to the breaking up of clumps of cells to smaller units. This was reflected in a rapid rise in the number of units which, when plated, form a colony.

The change in shape of EMB-treated cells was so readily apparent even in the light microscope, that no experimental attempt was made to explain the failure of Gale and McLain (2) to observe this in their electron microscope preparations. It is noted, however, that these investigators used a much higher concentration of EMB (1,000 μg/ml) for a much longer time (10 h) than we did. Furthermore, their electron

FIG. 6. *Comparison of EMB-treated (a) and untreated (b) M. smegmatis. Culture was exposed to 3 μg of EMB/ml for 4 h. Note the change in the EMB treated to a more spherical shape. The magnification is ×9,000.*

microscope preparations were fixed and sectioned as opposed to negative staining used in the present study.

Alternative explanations that have been considered for the rapid rise in CFU are not supported by the data. There is no evidence of a rapid increase in DNA synthesis, which might indicate that EMB stimulates cell division. Nor was any evidence found that EMB causes the fragmentation into single CFU of multinucleated cells. In fact, no evidence was found for the extremely large or extremely small cells in an untreated population that would be necessary to support the fragmentation hypothesis. The idea that EMB causes a reduction in the size of clumps is suggested by the data from the Coulter counter, demonstrating that large, multicell clumps in untreated cultures are dispersed into smaller clusters. The large clusters become sufficiently dispersed to account for the increase in numbers of colonies formed during EMB treatment.

No explanation is yet offered for the change in shape of treated cells. This is being further investigated, particularly the possibility that EMB causes some change in a structural component of the cell wall which results in a relaxation of its rigidity. The results reported in this paper offer some guidelines to further studies. Clearly, the effects of EMB are not simply physical and dispersal of clumps is not the result of shaking. The L-form of EMB does not cause dispersal or cell death, so the effect is sterospecific. Dispersal was not observed at 4°C, nor in an auxotrophic mutant deprived of its essential amino acids, nor in a mutant resistant to EMB. With regard to the last observation, when the concentration of EMB was increased sufficiently to approach that needed to kill cells, dispersal occurred. Cell death occurs in susceptible and resistant cells only at doses slightly larger than the dose required to cause dispersal of clumps. Much of the kinetics of the survival of mycobacteria treated with EMB is obscured by complications arising from the fact that the cells are clumped and, even when dispersed, do not present a uniform population of single cells. The picture is further obscured by the yet unexplained observation that survival is a function of the density of the population.

ACKNOWLEDGMENTS

We thank Janice C. Bullard, Gonococcal Research Section, Venereal Disease Branch, Bacteriology Division, for performing the electron microscope examinations and the Viral Pathology Branch, Virology Division, Center for Disease Control, for use of the Philips electron microscope. We also thank Martin Forbes, Lederle Laboratories, Pearl River, New York, for providing the ethambutol and K. Suga, National Institutes of Health, Tokyo, Japan, for the *M. smegmatis* auxotroph, and Gary Johnson of Coulter Electronics, Inc., Hialeah, Fla., for the electronic cell counting.

LITERATURE CITED

1. **Forbes, M., N. Kuck, and E. Peets.** 1962. Mode of action of ethambutol. J. Bacteriol. 84:1099–1103.
2. **Gale, G. R., and H. H. McLain.** 1963. Effect of ethambutol on cytology of *Mycobacterium smegmatis*. J. Bacteriol. 86:749–756.
3. **Karlson, A. G.** 1961. The *in vitro* activity of ethambutol (dextro-2,2[1]-(ethylene-diimino) di-1-butanol) against tubercle bacilli and other microorganisms. Am. Rev. Respir. Dis. 84:905–906.
4. **Roodyn, D. B., and H. G. Mandel.** 1960. A simple membrane fractionation method for determining the distribution of radioactivity in chemical fractions of *Bacillus cereus*. Biochem. Biophys. Acta 41:80–88.
5. **Wilkinson, R. G., R. Shepherd, J. Thomas, and C. Baughn.** 1961. Stereospecificity in a new type of synthetic antituberculous agent. J. Am. Chem. Soc. 83:2212–2213.

ANTIMICROBIAL AGENTS AND CHEMOTHERAPY, Mar. 1977, p. 541-552 Vol. 11, No. 3

Printed in U.S.A.

Comparison of the Effects of Mecillinam and 6-Aminopenicillanic Acid on *Proteus mirabilis*, *Escherichia coli*, and *Staphylococcus aureus*

VICTOR LORIAN* AND BARBARA ATKINSON

Division of Microbiology and Epidemiology, Department of Pathology, The Bronx-Lebanon Hospital Center, Bronx, New York 10456, and The Albert Einstein College of Medicine, Bronx, New York 10461

Received for publication 20 July 1976

Single strains of *Proteus mirabilis, Escherichia coli,* and *Staphylococcus aureus* were grown on filter membranes placed on agar containing concentration series of mecillinam (FL 1060), 6-aminopenicillanic acid (6-APA), or ampicillin. *P. mirabilis* and *E. coli* were also exposed to combinations of mecillinam or 6-APA with ampicillin. Colony-forming units were counted, and cells were examined by interference phase-contrast and transmission electron microscopy. Mecillinam and 6-APA were very effective in reducing the viability of the two gram-negative species, but they were less effective against *S. aureus*. Combinations of mecillinam and 6-APA with ampicillin acted synergistically against the gram-negative bacilli. When the antibiotics were presented consecutively, their effects on viability were usually no greater than the effects of the individual antibiotics acting alone. When *P. mirabilis* and *E. coli* were exposed to mecillinam alone or in combination with ampicillin, the cells became rounded. 6-APA alone or in combination with ampicillin produced elongated polymorphic cells in these species. The most unusual morphological effects were ultrastructural. Mecillinam and, to a lesser extent, 6-APA produced inward growth of numerous pairs of trilamellar membranous structures within the cells. It is possible that these membranes represent the growth initiation of aberrant cross walls. Both mecillinam and 6-APA produced multiple, thick cross walls in *S. aureus*.

Mecillinam (FL 1060), a β-amidinopenicillanic acid derivative, differs from the other known penicillanic acid derivatives in its antibacterial spectrum (1, 7, 19, 23) and in its mode of action (16). Mecillinam is very active against *Escherichia coli* and other gram-negative rods, and it acts synergistically with ampicillin (1, 7, 23). Whereas subinhibitory concentrations of most penicillins turn *E. coli* and other gram-negative bacilli into filaments (2–4, 14), mecillinam produces ovoidal forms and no filaments (6, 17, 21). Subinhibitory concentrations of 6-aminopenicillanic acid (6-APA) also produce ovoidal forms in *E. coli* and *Proteus mirabilis* (14, 21), and 6-APA acts synergistically with ampicillin (L.D. Sabath, personal communication).

The present paper reports the effects of mecillinam and 6-APA on the morphology and viability of *E. coli, P. mirabilis,* and *Staphylococcus aureus*. Combinations of mecillinam or 6-APA with ampicillin were also tested on *P. mirabilis* and *E. coli*.

MATERIALS AND METHODS

Strain 209P (FDA) of *S. aureus,* strain K-12 of *E. coli,* and a strain of *P. mirabilis* isolated from urine (9) were grown for 24 h in Trypticase soy broth (BBL) at 37°C. The minimum inhibitory concentrations (MIC) of 6-APA, mecillinam, and ampicillin were determined for each strain by using a twofold agar dilution method (22).

Trypticase soy agar plates (BBL) containing concentration series of single drugs were prepared. For each organism, the drug concentration ranged, in a series of twofold dilutions, from 4× the MIC to 1/128 of the MIC. Mecillinam and 6-APA were also tested in combination with ampicillin for their effects on *P. mirabilis* and *E. coli*. Filter membranes (no. PHWP047SO, Millipore Corp., Bedford, Mass.) were placed on Trypticase soy agar, prewarmed for 1 h at 37°C, and inoculated with 0.1 ml of a 1:10 Trypticase soy broth dilution of a 24-h broth culture of one of the organisms. The inoculated membranes were incubated on drug-free agar at 37°C for 90 min. They were then transferred to agar containing the antibiotics and incubated at 37°C for another 6 h. Some membranes, after exposure to mecillinam, were transferred back onto drug-free agar and incubated at 37°C for an additional 4 h. Inoculated control membranes were transferred from drug-free agar to drug-free agar at the same time that the test membranes were transferred from drug-free agar to agar containing antibiotic.

In an effort to examine the nature of the synergistic effect, each component of the combination treatment was presented consecutively. *P. mirabilis* and

E. coli were exposed to ampicillin for 1 h and then to 6-APA or mecillinam for 5 h. The reverse sequences were also carried out; that is, both species were exposed to 6-APA or mecillinam for 1 h and then to ampicillin for 5 h.

To select the samples appropriate for ultrastructural examination, the organisms on each membrane were inspected by interference phase-contrast microscopy, and the number of colony-forming units (CFU) per membrane was counted. One concentration of mecillinam and one concentration of 6-APA that produced representative morphological changes in *P. mirabilis* were selected and one concentration of mecillinam that produced morphological changes in *S. aureus* was selected; the organisms grown on these membranes were examined by electron microscopy. The bacterial cells were fixed for 1 h in 5% glutaraldehyde in 0.067 M phosphate buffer, pH 7.4. They were centrifuged, rinsed in buffer, and fixed for 30 min in 1% osmic acid in chromate buffer, pH 7.4. The bacteria were then treated with 0.5% uranyl and lead salts. Details of the CFU counting and the electron microscopy fixation procedures were described previously (11).

RESULTS

The viability curves for *P. mirabilis* and *E. coli* treated with decreasing concentrations of mecillinam, 6-APA, ampicillin, and combinations of mecillinam and 6-APA with ampicillin are shown in Fig. 1. *S. aureus* viability in the presence of mecillinam and 6-APA is shown in Fig. 2. There were large quantitative differences between the drug concentrations and the magnitude of the viability responses of *E. coli* and *P. mirabilis*.

When *P. mirabilis* was grown on Trypticase

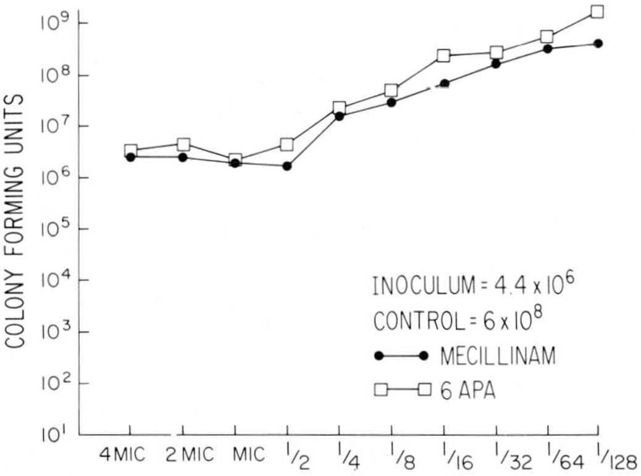

FIG. 2. *Effect of mecillinam and 6-APA on the viability of S. aureus. The MICs were: mecillinam, 100 μg/ml; 6-APA, 25 μg/ml.*

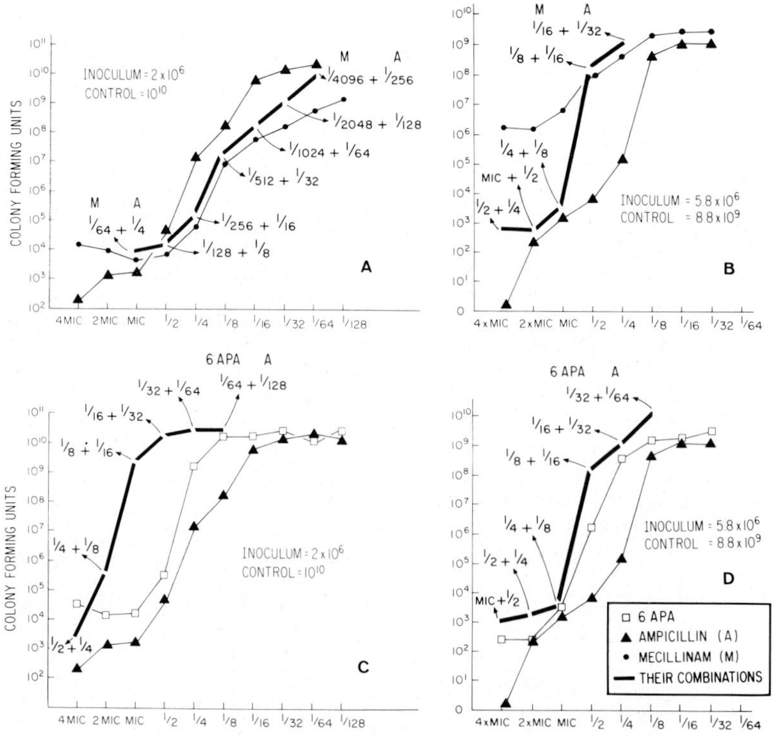

FIG. 1. *Effect of mecillinam, 6-APA, and their combinations with ampicillin on the viability of P. mirabilis (A and D) and E. coli (B and C). The MICs were: P. mirabilis to ampicillin, 3 μg/ml; 6-APA, 100 μg/ml; mecillinam, 800 μg/ml; E. coli to ampicillin, 12 μg/ml; 6-APA, 100 μg/ml; mecillinam, 0.5 μg/ml.*

soy agar containing 1/8 of the MIC of mecillinam, the CFU per membrane were 1.7×10^7; CFU per membrane for the control were 10^{10}. Interference phase-contrast microscopy showed that this treatment turned *P. mirabilis* into round cells 7 to 12 μm in diameter (Fig. 3). The reversibility of this response was indicated when *P. mirabilis* exposed to 1/8 of the MIC of mecillinam for 6 h was transferred to drug-free agar, incubated for 4 h at 37°C. The number of CFU increased to 10^8, and the organisms returned to rodlike forms.

P. mirabilis grown on Trypticase soy agar containing 1/4 of the MIC of 6-APA for 6 h had a CFU count of 1.6×10^9; the control had a CFU count of 10^{10}. Although some organisms resem-

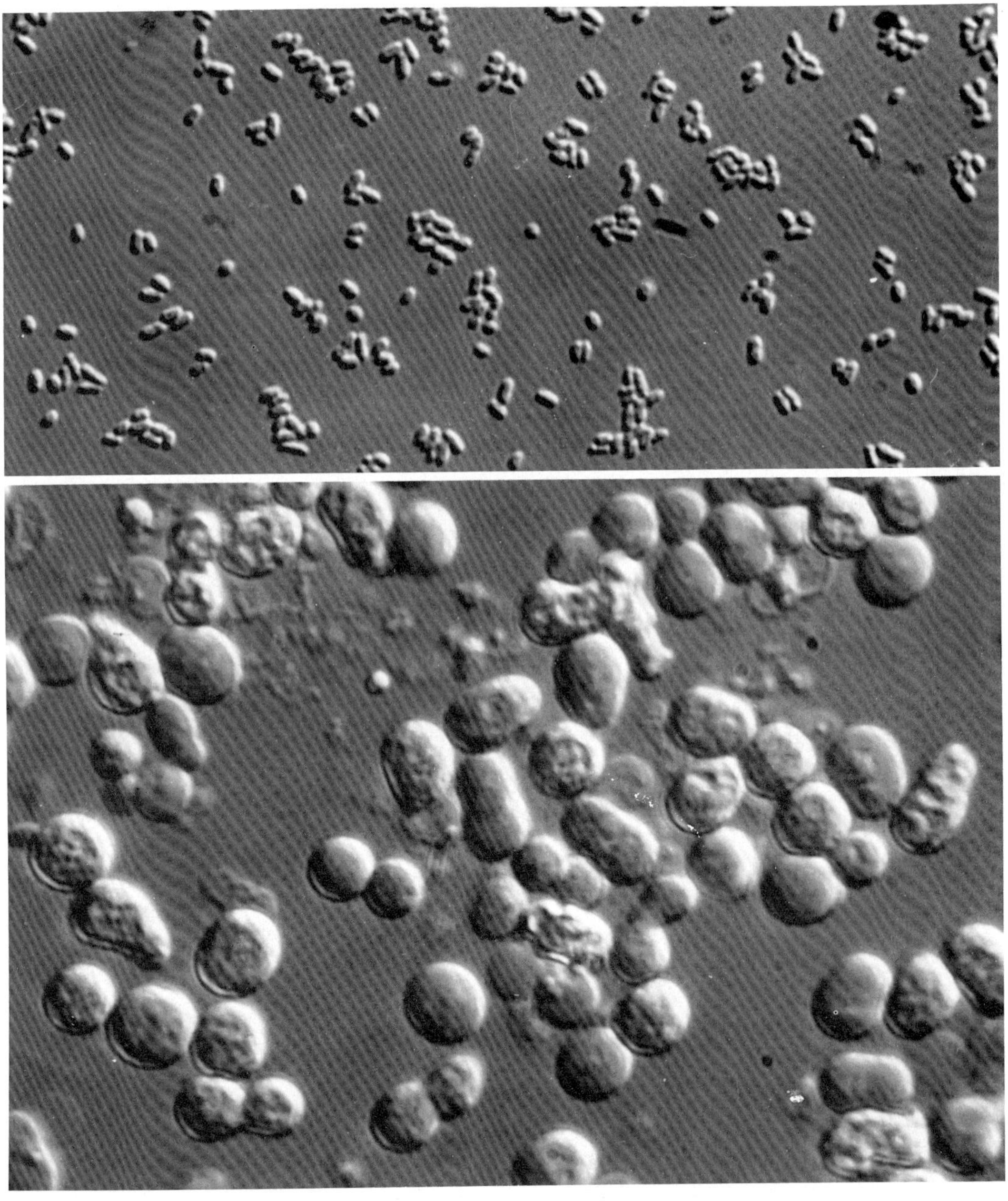

FIG. 3. *(Top) P. mirabilis grown on drug-free agar. (Bottom) Agar containing 1/8 of the MIC (100 µg/ml) of mecillinam produced round and ovoid cells. Interference phase contrast (×1,200).*

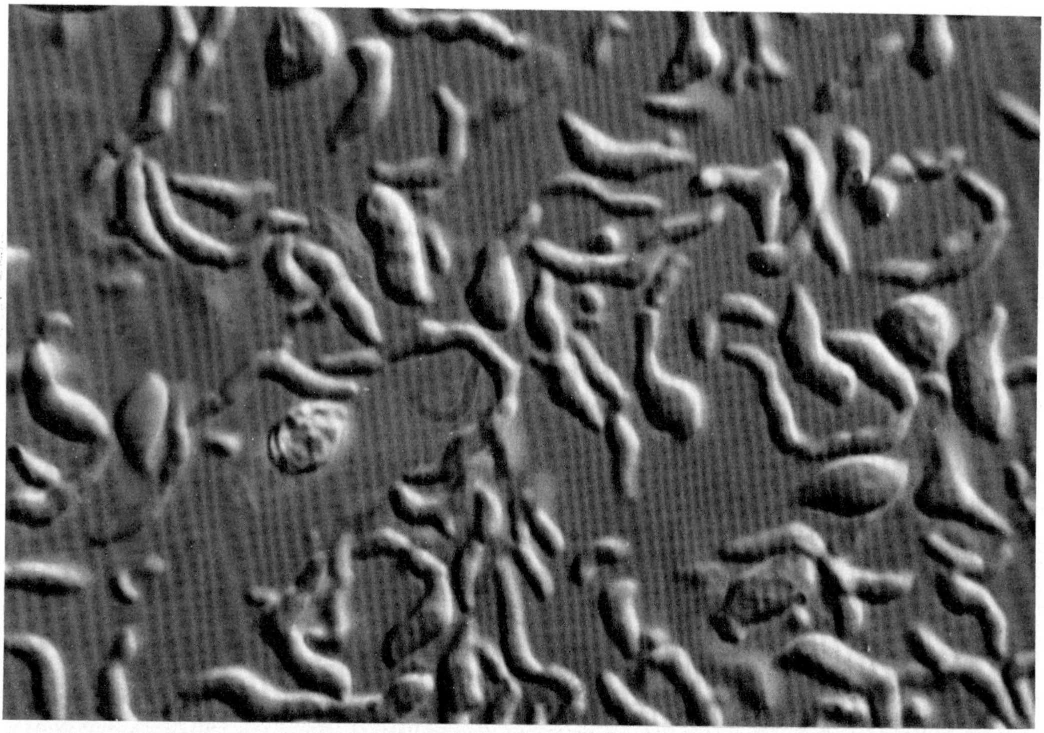

FIG. 4. *P. mirabilis grown on agar containing 1/4 of the MIC of 6-APA (25 μg/ml) produced elongated polymorphic cells and some round cells. Interference phase contrast (×1,162).*

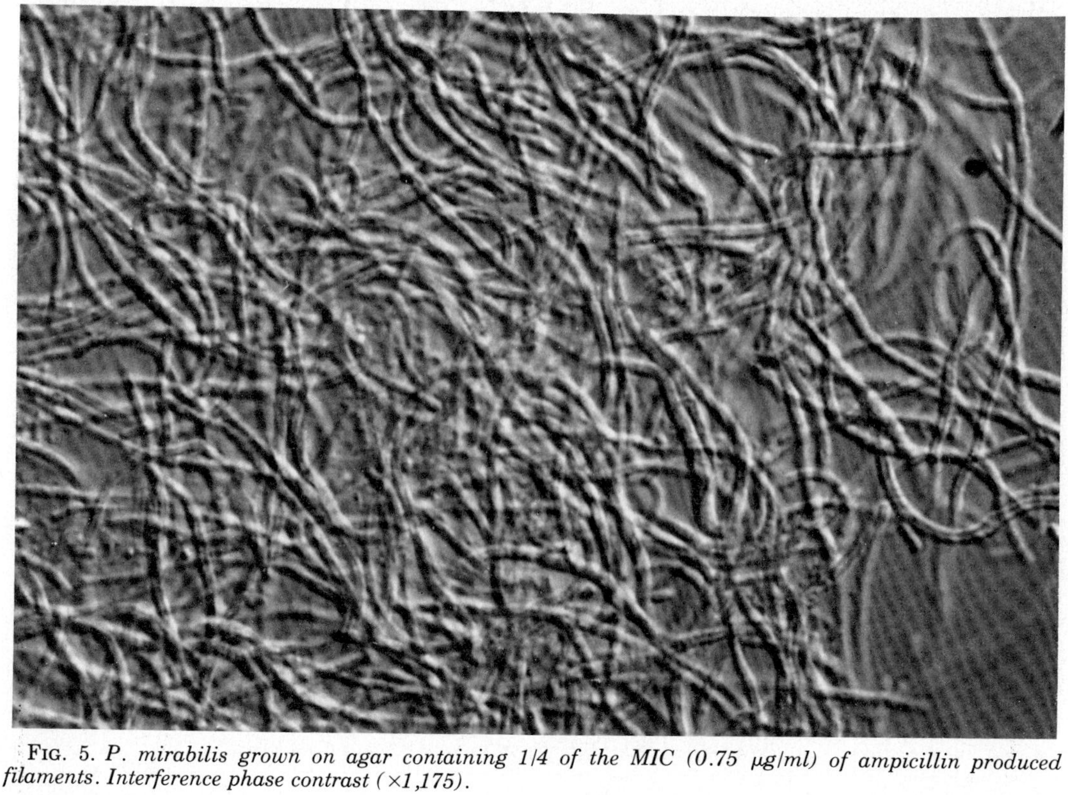

FIG. 5. *P. mirabilis grown on agar containing 1/4 of the MIC (0.75 μg/ml) of ampicillin produced filaments. Interference phase contrast (×1,175).*

bled the round cells produced by mecillinam, most 6-APA-treated bacilli became elongated polymorphic cells 8 to 15 μm long and 2 to 5 μm wide (Fig. 4).

Ampicillin treatment (1/4 of the MIC) of *P. mirabilis* reduced CFU per membrane to 1.5 × 10^7. Figure 5 shows the filaments produced by this treatment. The morphology of *P. mirabilis* exposed to ampicillin in combination with mecillinam or 6-APA resembled round cells or elongated polymorphic cells, respectively.

The morphological responses of *E. coli* to all three antibiotics and to the ampicillin combinations with mecillinam and 6-APA were very similar to the responses of *P. mirabilis* discussed above.

The *S. aureus* grown on Trypticase soy agar containing 1/4 of the MIC of mecillinam or 6-APA produced 2 × 10^7 or 1.4 × 10^7 CFU/membrane, respectively. Compared with a CFU count of 6 × 10^8 for the control, this indicated a weak antibacterial effect. Both drugs produced cells with irregular forms (Fig. 6).

The synergistic effect of combining mecillinam with ampicillin was striking for *P. mirabilis*. Viability was reduced to 1 log below control levels when 1/2,048 of the mecillinam MIC was combined with 1/128 of the ampicillin MIC. These concentrations were also the lowest that produced morphological changes (Table 1). The synergistic effect was also seen with *E. coli* (Table 1, Fig. 1).

Consecutive exposure of *P. mirabilis* or *E. coli* to ampicillin/6-APA or ampicillin/mecilli-

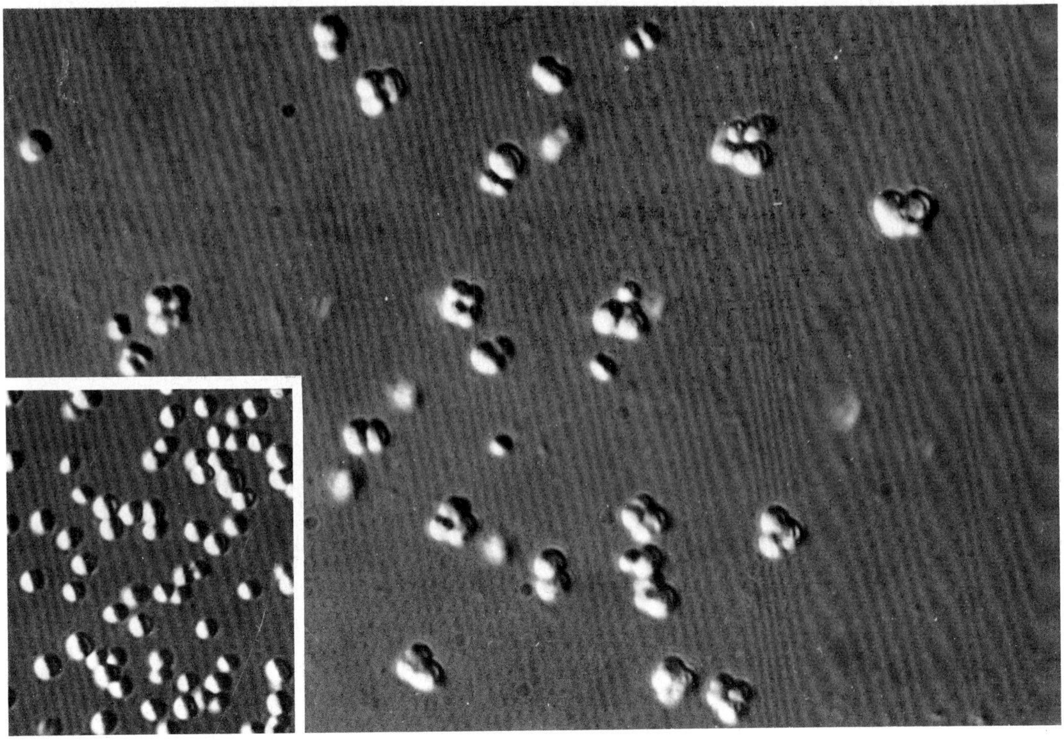

FIG. 6. *S. aureus grown on agar containing 1/4 of the MIC (25 μg/ml) of mecillinam produces cells with irregular forms. Inset is control grown on drug-free agar. Interference phase contrast (×1,200).*

TABLE 1. *Lowest concentration of drug to produce a change in morphology*

Species	Mecillinam μg/ml	Mecillinam Fraction of MIC	6-APA μg/ml	6-APA Fraction of MIC	Ampicillin μg/ml	Ampicillin Fraction of MIC	Ampicillin (am) plus mecillinam (mec) μg/ml	Ampicillin (am) plus mecillinam (mec) Fraction of MIC	Ampicillin (am) plus 6-APA (ap) μg/ml	Ampicillin (am) plus 6-APA (ap) Fraction of MIC
P. mirabilis	0.80	1/1,024	6.2	1/16	0.38	1/8	0.022 am 0.400 mec	1/128 1/2,048	0.38 am 25.00 ap	1/8 1/4
E. coli	0.05	1/8	12.5	1/8	1.50	1/8	0.75 am 0.05 mec	1/16 1/8	0.75 am 12.50 ap	1/16 1/8
S. aureus	6.20	1/16	0.75	1/16						

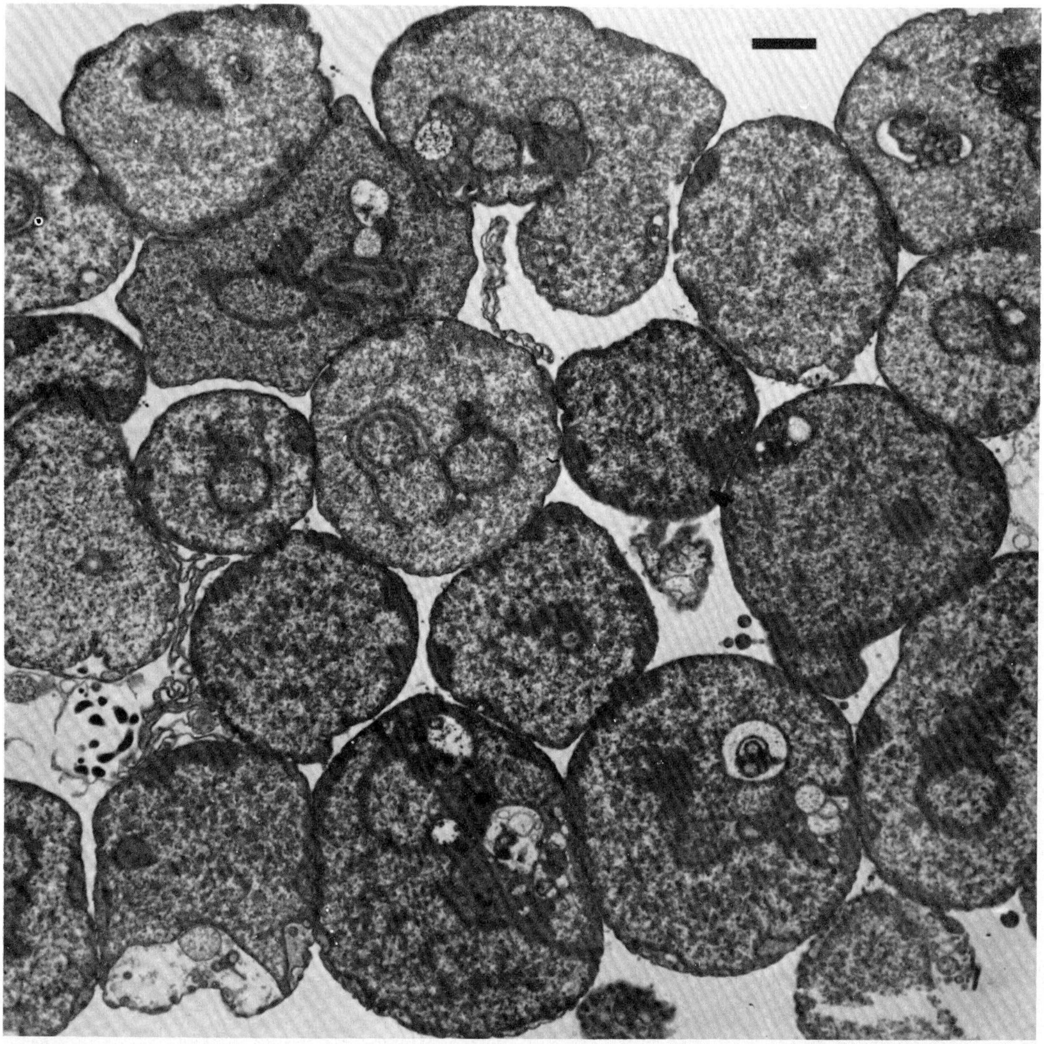

FIG. 7. *P. mirabilis grown on agar containing 1/8 of the MIC (100 μg/ml) of mecillinam. Most cells contain some membranous structures (×8,100). Bar, 1 μm.*

nam did not produce a synergistic decrease in viability. Table 2 shows that the viability effects were, in every case except one, equal to or less than the viability reductions produced by the drugs separately. The one exception, 1-h exposure to mecillinam and 5-h exposure to ampicillin, produced the same response as the response seen after exposure to the mecillinam/ampicillin combination, that is, a 5-log reduction compared to the control.

Electron microscopy of *P. mirabilis* exposed to mecillinam at a concentration of 1/8 of the MIC showed round cells with cell walls that appeared as a dense layer of 10 to 15 nm. Most of the cells contained paired trilamellar membranes, some of which appeared to be membranous intrusions of the peripheral cytoplasmic membrane (Fig. 7 and 8). Many of the membranes were surrounded by clusters of ribosomes in greater density than in the rest of the cell (Fig. 9). Electron microscopy of *P. mirabilis* exposed to 6-APA showed elongated cells of various irregular shapes. The cell wall was of normal appearance; some cells contained membranous structures (Fig. 10 and 11).

Electron microscopy of the filaments induced in *P. mirabilis* by ampicillin showed a normal cell wall and some decrease in density of the ribosomes compared with the control. The effect has been described previously (15).

TABLE 2. *Effect of consecutive exposure of P. mirabilis and E. coli to mecillinam or 6-APA and ampicillin*

Species	Exposure				CFU/membrane
	1 h		5 h		
	Antibiotic	μg/ml	Antibiotic	μg/ml	
P. mirabilis					
Inoculum, 1.7 × 10^7 per membrane	Mecillinam	6.2	Ampicillin	0.38	2.8 × 10^5[a]
Control at 1.5 h, 3.2 × 10^7 per membrane	6-APA	25	Ampicillin	0.38	3.9 × 10^9
Control at 7.5 h (1.5 + 6), 1.6 × 10^{10} per membrane	Ampicillin	0.38	Mecillinam	6.2	5.5 × 10^8[b]
	Ampicillin	0.38	6-APA	25	6 × 10^9
E. coli					
Inoculum, 7.0 × 10^6 per membrane	Mecillinam	0.1	Ampicillin	1.5	2.7 × 10^8
Control at 1.5 h, 2.5 × 10^7 per membrane	6-APA	25	Ampicillin	1.5	1.8 × 10^9
Control at 7.5 h (1.5 + 6), 4.5 × 10^{10} per membrane	Ampicillin	1.5	Mecillinam	0.1	7.5 × 10^8
	Ampicillin	1.5	6-APA	25	4.2 × 10^9

[a] Round cells with irregular surfaces.
[b] Round cells with smooth surfaces.

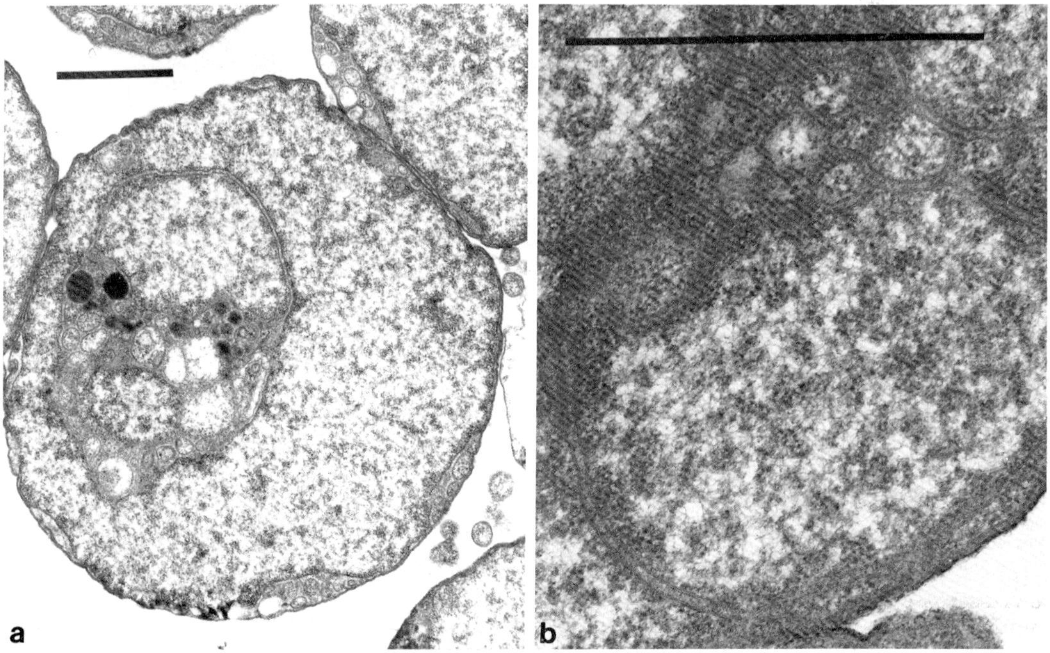

FIG. 8. *P. mirabilis grown on agar containing 1/8 of the MIC (100 μg/ml) of mecillinam. (a) Membranes are surrounded by a dense zone of ribosomes. Some opaque material as well as some vacuoles are present (×14,880). (b) A pair of intruding membranes, which appear to be a continuation of the peripheral cytoplasmic membrane, are surrounded by a dense zone of ribosomes (×55,800). Bar, 1 μm.*

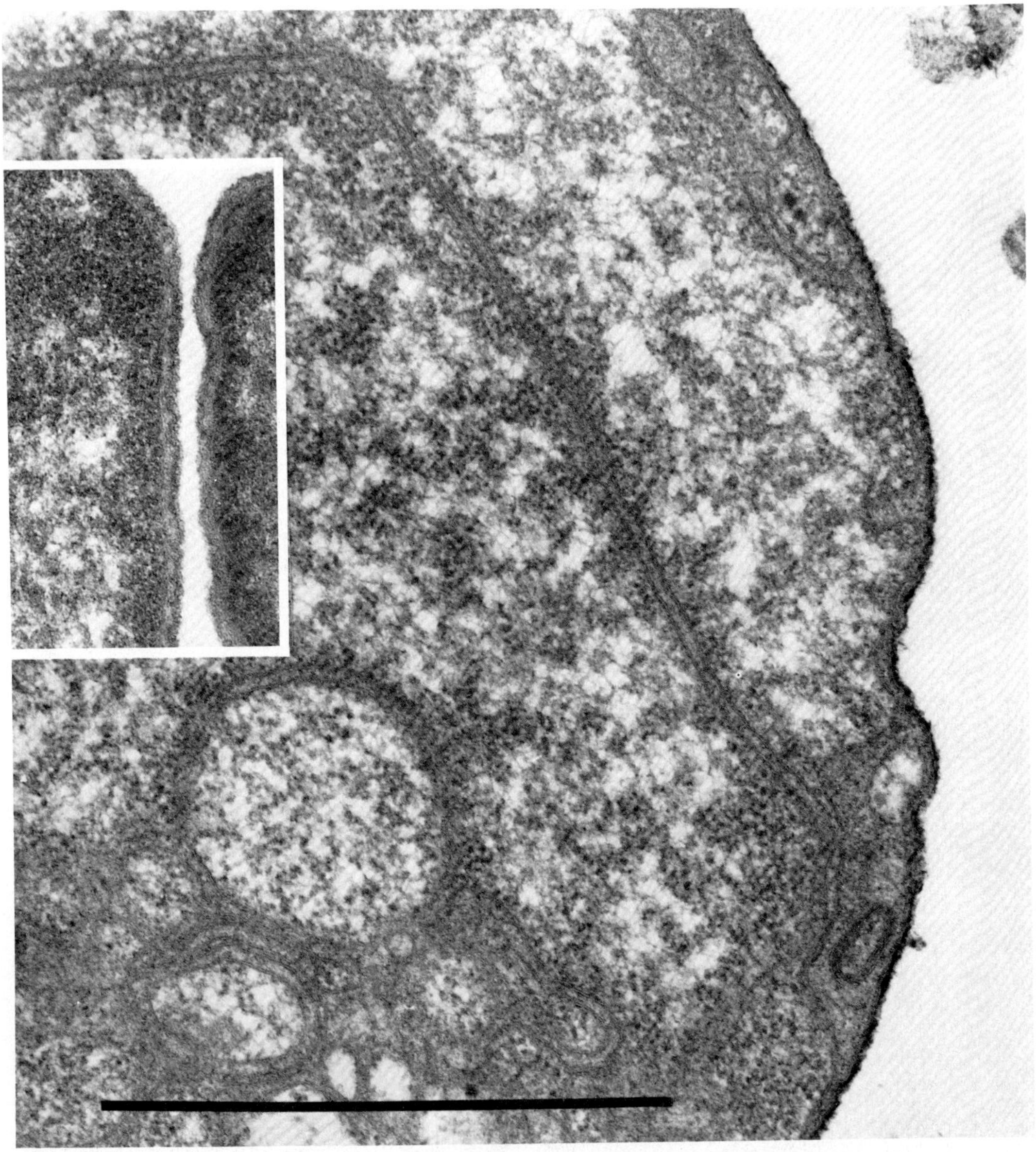

FIG. 9. *P. mirabilis grown on agar containing 1/8 of the MIC (100 μg/ml) of mecillinam. A pair of membranes surrounded by ribosomes traverses the cell in a septum-like manner (×77,400). Inset is control grown on drug-free agar. Bar, 1 μm.*

On electron microscopy, *S. aureus* exposed to mecillinam or 6-APA had changed into large cells of 1.5 to 3.5 μm in diameter. These cells were crisscrossed by thick cross walls 0.1 to 0.4 μm wide (Fig. 12).

DISCUSSION

The synergism of mecillinam with β-lactam antibiotics against *Enterobacteriaceae* has been well documented (1, 7, 23). The results of the present study show that for the strain of *P. mirabilis* investigated, the lowest active synergistic combination of mecillinam and ampicillin (as a fraction of the MIC) involves lower concentrations of mecillinam than have been reported previously. In fact, the lowest mecillinam concentration that, in combination with ampicillin, produced an effect on the structure

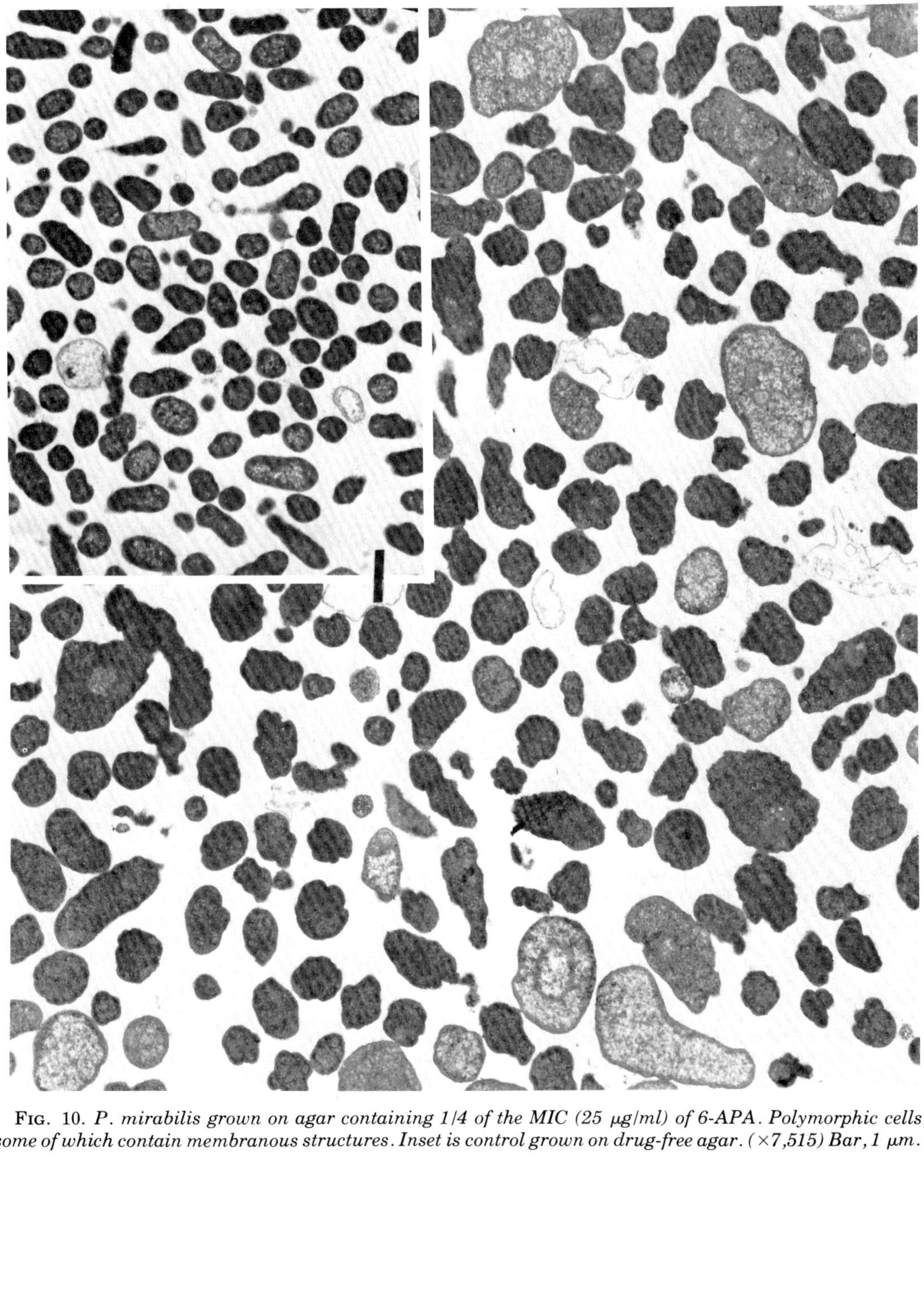

FIG. 10. *P. mirabilis grown on agar containing 1/4 of the MIC (25 μg/ml) of 6-APA. Polymorphic cells, some of which contain membranous structures. Inset is control grown on drug-free agar. (×7,515) Bar, 1 μm.*

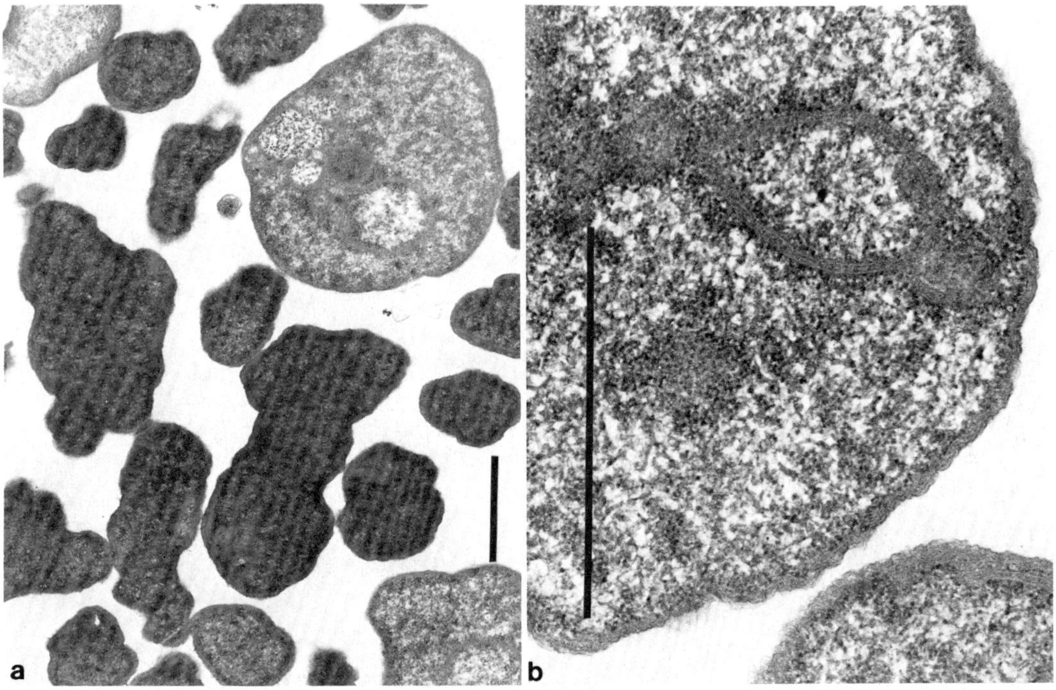

FIG. 11. *P. mirabilis grown on agar containing 1/8 of the MIC (12.5 μg/ml) of 6-APA. (a) One oval cell and other polymorphic cells. Two cells contain some membranous structure (×13,920). (b) A normal cell wall and a membranous structure (×52,200). Bar, 1 μm.*

and growth rate of *P. mirabilis* was the smallest fraction of the MIC of any drug ever investigated in this laboratory (10, 11, 13, 14).

The consecutive exposure of *P. mirabilis* and *E. coli* to the synergistically effective drugs had, with one exception, the same or less effect on viability that each drug acting separately had. This indicates that the simultaneous action of both drugs is necessary to produce the synergistic effect.

The effects of β-lactam antibiotics on the morphology of *E. coli* appear to be related to the affinity of these drugs for three different proteins (20). The morphological changes induced by mecillinam, 6-APA, and ampicillin in the *P. mirabilis* strain used in the present study suggest that a similar mechanism may also be present in this species.

It has been shown that the exposure of *S. aureus* to subinhibitory concentrations of penicillin or oxacillin leads to the formation of large cells containing many thick cross walls (11, 12). In this study, subinhibitory concentrations of mecillinam and 6-APA had the same effect. Because the structural effects of mecillinam and 6-APA are the same as those of penicillin, the mode of action on *S. aureus* may also be similar to that of penicillin.

Polymyxin is known to produce alterations of the cytoplasmic membrane in gram-negative bacteria (5). In this study, the most unusual structural alterations produced by mecillinam and, to some extent, by 6-APA were the pairs of trilamellar membranes inside the cells. Many of these membranes appeared to grow inward as an intrusion from the periphery of the cytoplasmic membrane. One might suggest that these membranes are deteriorating structures inside a dying organism. However, the quantity of membrane in some cells was greater than can be accounted for by the sloughing off of cytoplasmic membrane alone. Furthermore, the regional clustering of ribosomes in the vicinity of the membranes suggested a recent or ongoing transfer of proteins into functional membranes (8, 18). Finally, the 1-log increase in CFU after 4 h of growth on drug-free agar showed that these organisms are not dying cells. It is possible that these paired membranes represent the growth initiation of aberrant cross walls. No other β-lactam antibiotic has shown this effect.

ACKNOWLEDGMENTS

We wish to thank Herbert Dembitzer for the electron microscopy and for his help in interpreting the micrographs

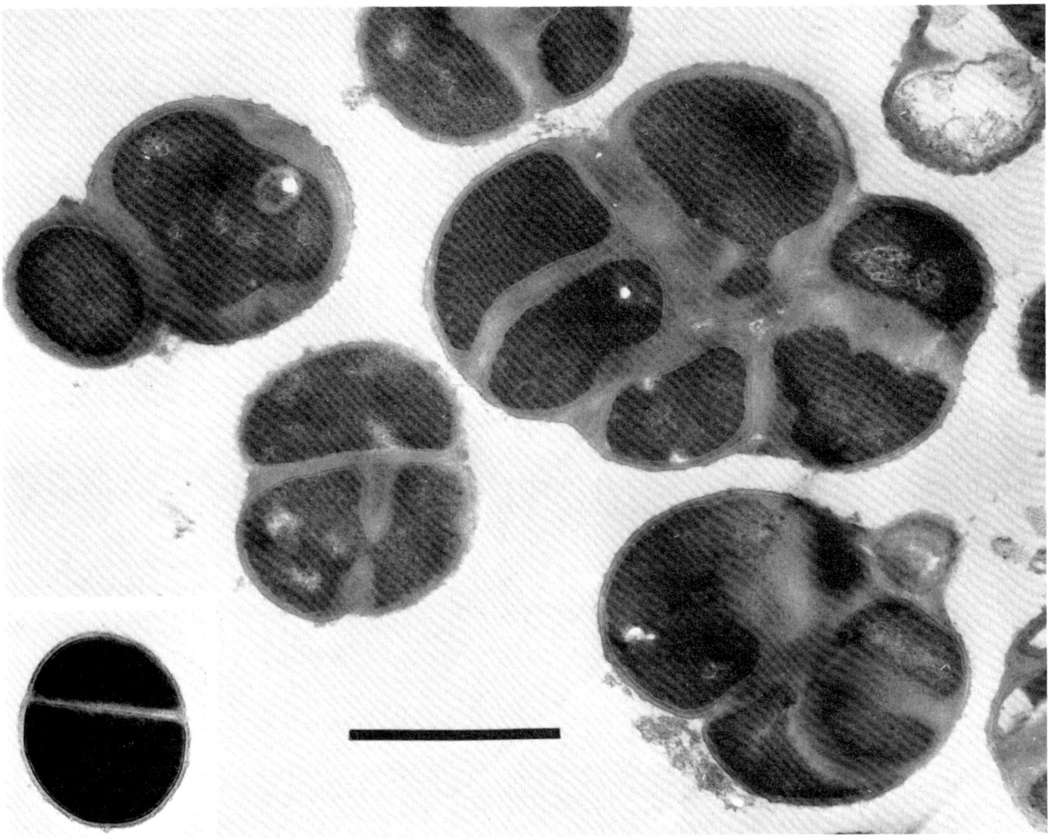

FIG. 12. *S. aureus grown on agar containing 1/4 of the MIC (200 μg/ml) of mecillinam produced large cells containing multiple, wide cross walls (×21,160). Inset is control grown on drug-free agar. Bar, 1 μm.*

and R. G. E. Murray and Milton Salton for their suggestions regarding the membranous structures seen in the electron micrographs.

LITERATURE CITED

1. **Baltimore, R. S., J. O. Klein, C. Wilcox, and M. Finland.** 1976. Synergy of mecillinam (FL 1060) with penicillins and cephalosporins against *Proteus* and *Klebsiella*, with observations on combinations with other antibiotics and against other bacterial species. Antimicrob. Agents Chemother. **9**:701–705.
2. **Duguid, J. P.** 1946. The sensitivity of bacteria to the action of penicillin. Edinburgh Med. J. **53**:401–412.
3. **Fleming, A., A. Voureka, I. R. H. Kramer, and W. H. Hughes.** 1950. The morphology and motility of *Proteus vulgaris* and other organisms cultured in the presence of penicillin. J. Gen. Microbiol. **4**:257–269.
4. **Gardner, A. D.** 1940. Morphological effects of penicillin on bacteria. Nature (London) **146**:837–838.
5. **Gilleland, H. E., Jr., and R. G. E. Murray.** 1976. Ultrastructural study of polymyxin-resistant isolates of *Pseudomonas aeruginosa*. J. Bacteriol. **125**:267–281.
6. **Greenwood, D., and F. O'Grady.** 1973. FL1060: a new beta-lactam antibiotic with novel properties. J. Clin. Pathol. **26**:1–6.
7. **Gruneberg, E., R. Cleeland, G. Beskid, and W. F. DeLorenzo.** 1976. In vivo synergy between 6β-amidinopenicillanic acid derivatives and other antibiotics. Antimicrob. Agents Chemother. **9**:589–594.
8. **Leive, L. (ed.).** 1973. Bacterial membranes and walls. M. Dekker, Inc., New York.
9. **Lennette, E. H., E. H. Spaulding, and J. P. Truant (ed.).** 1974. Manual of clinical microbiology, 2nd ed. American Society for Microbiology, Washington, D.C.
10. **Lorian, V.** 1975. Some effects of subinhibitory concentrations of antibiotics on bacteria. Bull. N.Y. Acad. Med. **51**:1046–1055.
11. **Lorian, V.** 1975. Some effects of subinhibitory concentrations of penicillin on the structure and division of staphylococci. Antimicrob. Agents Chemother. **7**:864–870.
12. **Lorian, V., and B. Atkinson.** 1976. Effects of subinhibitory concentrations of antibiotics on cross walls of cocci. Antimicrob. Agents Chemother. **9**:1043–1055.
13. **Lorian, V., and B. Poppola.** 1972. The effect of nitrofurantoin on the morphology of gram negative bacilli. J. Infect. Dis. **125**:187–189.
14. **Lorian, V., and L. D. Sabath.** 1972. Penicillins and cephalosporins: differences in morphologic effects. J. Infect. Dis. **125**:560–564.
15. **Lorian, V., L. D. Sabath, and M. Simonescu.** 1975. Decrease in ribosomal density of *Proteus mirabilis* exposed to subinhibitory concentrations of ampicillin or cephalothin (38888). Soc. Exp. Biol. Med. **149**:731–735.

16. **Matsuhashi, S., K. Tatsuyuki, P. M. Blumberg, P. Linnett, E. Willoughby, and J. L. Strominger.** 1974. Mechanism of action and development of resistance to a new amidino penicillin. J. Bacteriol. **117**:578–587.
17. **Melchior, N. H., J. Blom, L. Tybring, and A. Birth-Andersen.** 1973. Light and electron microscopy of the early response of *Escherichia coli* to a 6 beta-amidinopenicillanic acid (FL 1060). Acta Pathol. Microbiol. Scand. **81**:393–407.
18. **Mindich, L.** 1973. *In* L. Leive (ed.), Bacterial membranes and walls, p. 1–27. Marcel Dekker, Inc., New York.
19. **Neu, H.** 1976. Mecillinam, a novel penicillanic acid derivative with unusual activity against gram-negative bacteria. Antimicrob. Agents Chemother. **9**:793–799.
20. **Spratt, B. G.** 1975. Distinct penicillin binding proteins involved in the division, elongation, and shape of *Escherichia coli* K 12. Proc. Natl. Acad. Sci. U.S.A. **72**:2999–3003.
21. **Spratt, B. G., and A. B. Pardee.** 1975. Penicillin binding proteins and cell shape in *E. coli*. Nature (London) **254**:516–517.
22. **Steers, E., E. L. Folz, and B. S. Graves.** 1959. Inocula replicating apparatus for routine testing of bacterial susceptibility to antibiotics. Antibiot. Chemother. **9**:307–311.
23. **Tybring, L., and N. H. Melchior.** 1975. Mecillinam (FL 1060), a 6β-amidinopenicillanic acid derivative: bacterial action and synergy in vitro. Antimicrob. Agents Chemother. **8**:271–276.

ANTIMICROBIAL AGENTS AND CHEMOTHERAPY, Mar. 1977, p. 553-558
Vol. 11, No. 3

Printed in U.S.A.

Characterization of an R-Plasmid Associated with Ampicillin Resistance in *Shigella dysenteriae* Type 1 Isolated from Epidemics

JORGE H. CROSA,* JORGE OLARTE, LEONARDO J. MATA, LINDA K. LUTTROPP, AND MARIA E. PEÑARANDA

Department of Microbiology, School of Medicine, University of Washington, Seattle, Washington 98195; Laboratorio de Bacteriologia Intestinal, Hospital Infantil de México, Mexico City, Mexico; and Instituto de Investigaciones en Salud, University of Costa Rica, San Jose, Costa Rica*

Received for publication 4 December 1976

Ampicillin-resistant strains of *Shigella dysenteriae* type 1 isolated in epidemics in Mexico, Central America, and Bangla Desh were examined for the presence of plasmid deoxyribonucleic acid (DNA) by gel electrophoresis. All strains contained a heterogeneous population of plasmids. Transfer experiments to *Escherichia coli* K-12 indicated that the ampicillin resistance determinant (Ap^r) was located on a 5.5-megadalton (Mdal) plasmid identical in all Shiga strains examined, as judged by DNA hybridization and by its molecular properties. This 5.5-Mdal plasmid contained the ampicillin transposon (TnA) sequences. There was not a high degree of homology between the Shiga Ap^r plasmid DNA and DNA obtained from Ap^r *Salmonella typhi* strains isolated from typhoid epidemics in Mexico, previous to the dysentery outbreaks. Although low, the degree of reassociation observed indicated that probably part of the TnA sequence was present in *S. typhi* DNA. The DNA hybridization experiments showed, in addition, that there was a high degree of homology among Ap^r plasmids isolated from different enterobacteria, and this identity was confirmed by restriction endonuclease activity. These results together with their similarities in molecular and replicative properties indicate that the Ap^r plasmids, as was suggested for the Sm^r Su^r plasmids, possibly evolved once and then epidemiologically spread in the *Enterobacteriaceae*.

Shigella dysenteriae type 1 was the causative organism in the 1970 epidemics of dysentery in Central America (12) and Mexico (16). The isolated Shiga bacillus strains were resistant to chloramphenicol, tetracycline, streptomycin, and sulfonamides, but uniformly susceptible to ampicillin. Subsequently, an outbreak of dysentery occurred in Mexico in a hospital ward lodging children under treatment for tuberculosis. This time the causative organism was Shiga bacillus, which was resistant to ampicillin in addition to the other drugs (14). In the period between 1972 and 1974 several ampicillin-resistant strains of *S. dysenteriae* type 1 were also isolated in outbreaks that occurred in Central America (17) and Bangla Desh (18). In at least two cases (14, 17) the ampicillin resistance could be transferred independently from the other drug resistances from *S. dysenteriae* to *Escherichia coli* K-12, suggesting that an independent R-plasmid might be involved. Our present communication is to report the isolation, molecular characterization, and epidemiological implications of the R-plasmid associated with ampicillin resistance in *S. dysenteriae* type 1.

MATERIALS AND METHODS

Bacterial strains. The ampicillin-resistant strains of *S. dysenteriae* type 1 were: strain 51B isolated in a Mexican epidemic, strain 762 isolated in a Costa Rican outbreak, and strain CDC 6986 (obtained from the Center for Disease Control, Atlanta, Ga.) isolated in a Bangla Desh epidemic. *Salmonella typhi* strains JM and P12 and *E. coli* K-12 W 1485-1 thy^- Nx^r (SF 148) were described previously (6, 14).

Bacterial conjugation. Crosses between multiply resistant *S. dysenteriae* type 1 and *E. coli* K-12 Nx^r were carried out by mixing 5 ml of log-phase cultures of both donor and recipient into 25 ml of Pennassay broth and incubating at 37°C without shaking for 10 h. Samples were plated on MacConkey agar containing the appropriate antibiotics at a concentration of 20 μg/ml. Colonies were restreaked several times on antibiotic plates before further processing. When needed, the antibiotic minimal inhibitory concentration was determined by the method of Bauer et al. (3).

Determination of plasmid DNA content. The

presence of plasmid deoxyribonucleic acid (DNA) was determined by an agarose electrophoretic method (13). Strains were grown overnight in 30 ml of brain heart infusion broth. Lysates were prepared (13) and after digestion with ribonuclease and extraction with phenol (once) and chloroform (twice), the clear aqueous phase was adjusted to 0.3 M sodium acetate and precipitated with twice the volume of precooled ethanol (−20°C) overnight at −20°C. After centrifugation at −10°C at 10,000 rpm for 20 min, the precipitate was resuspended in 0.2 ml of TES buffer [50 mM tris(hydroxymethyl)aminomethane (Tris)-hydrochloride-5 mM ethylenediaminetetraacetate (EDTA)-50 mM NaCl (pH 8)]. A sample was electrophoresed in a 0.7% agarose gel in Tris-borate buffer (89 mM Tris base–2.5 mM disodium EDTA–89 mM boric acid). DNA was visualized by staining with ethidium bromide and viewing the fluorescence produced by the intercalated dye when illuminated with an ultraviolet light source. The preparation of ^{3}H-labeled plasmid DNA and unlabeled whole-cell DNA as well as the analysis of plasmid DNA in cesium chloride-ethidium bromide and sucrose density gradients was described previously (7, 8).

DNA hybridization. DNA-DNA hybridizations were carried out essentially as described previously (6). Approximately 0.01 μg of ^{3}H-labeled, sheared, denatured plasmid DNA was incubated with 150 μg of unlabeled, sheared, denatured whole-cell DNA from each of the indicated organisms. DNA reassociation was performed in 0.42 M NaCl at 70°C for 22 min.

The degree of homology was assessed by the S1 nuclease method of Crosa et al. (6).

RESULTS

Molecular characterization of plasmids in *S. dysenteriae* type 1. Resistance to ampicillin (Ap^r) was reported to be independently transferred from resistance to chloramphenicol (Cm^r), tetracycline (Tc^r), streptomycin (Sm^r), and sulfonamides (Su^r) from *S. dysenteriae* type 1 to *E. coli* K-12 (14, 17). These results suggested that the Ap^r determinant was carried on an independent plasmid from the one carrying the Cm Tc Sm Su determinants. When both plasmids in *E. coli* K-12 were tested for their transfer properties to other *E. coli* K-12 strains, it was found that the plasmid carrying the Cm Tc Sm Su determinants was conjugative, whereas the Ap^r plasmid was not conjugative but mobilizable by the conjugative R plasmid (unpublished data).

To analyze the molecular nature of the *Shigella* plasmids, we began by examining agarose gel electrophoresis patterns of DNA isolated from the Shiga and exconjugant *E. coli* strains isolated from the conjugal crosses with *Shigella*. The rationale for this method is that covalently closed circular (CCC) plasmid DNA molecules band in agarose gels according to their size, whereas the chromosome DNA (which is sheared due to manipulations during its preparation) forms a broader band at a specific region (13).

All three multiple resistant *Shigella* strains show quite a number of bands in addition to that of the chromosome (Fig. 1), which indicates the presence of several different plasmids in each strain. By comparison with a molecular weight standard, it is possible to calculate the molecular weight of the Shiga plasmids that are listed in the legend to Fig. 1. Although there are several different plasmid sizes in each Shiga strain, there is only one plasmid band that all three Shiga strains have in common, that corresponding to a molecular species of 5.5 megadaltons (Mdal). When the DNA obtained from the *E. coli* exconjugants is analyzed, it becomes easier to assign drug resistance determinants to plasmids. The 80-Mdal band is identified as the multiple drug resistance conjugative plasmid, and the 5.5-Mdal band is the nonconjugative Ap^r plasmid. The Bangla Desh strain does not show the 80-Mdal band, but it has two bands of 62 and 52 Mdal instead. The rest of the *Shigella* plasmids remain cryptic in the phenotypic sense.

To further characterize the Shiga Ap^r plasmid, ^{3}H-labeled plasmid DNA obtained from exconjugants 1 and 2 was purified on a CsCl-ethidium bromide density gradient and fractions from the CCC peak were pooled and rerun in a second CsCl-ethidium bromide gradient. This time the fractions corresponding to the CCC peak were pooled, isopropanol treated to remove the ethidium bromide and then dialyzed against 6 mM Tris-0.1 mM EDTA (pH 7.5). The purified plasmid DNA was then analyzed on 5 to 20% sucrose density gradients and by electron microscopy to determine the molecular weight. The results are in close agreement with those obtained by gel electrophoresis of partially purified plasmid DNA (Table 2), indicating that the Ap^r plasmid is 5.5 Mdal in size in all of these strains.

Polynucleotide sequence relationships among Ap^r plasmids. We used the S1 nuclease method (6) to assess the DNA homology among the Ap^r plasmid isolated from different sources.

We hybridized ^{3}H-labeled Ap^r plasmid DNA with unlabeled DNA extracted from the *Shigella* strains and from the *E. coli* exconjugants containing either the Ap^r plasmid, the conjugative R plasmid, or both together. DNA extracted from the *Shigella* strains, independent of the geographical source of the epidemic, shared a high level of homology with the Ap^r plasmid isolated from the Mexican strain. This is also true when DNAs from *E. coli* exconju-

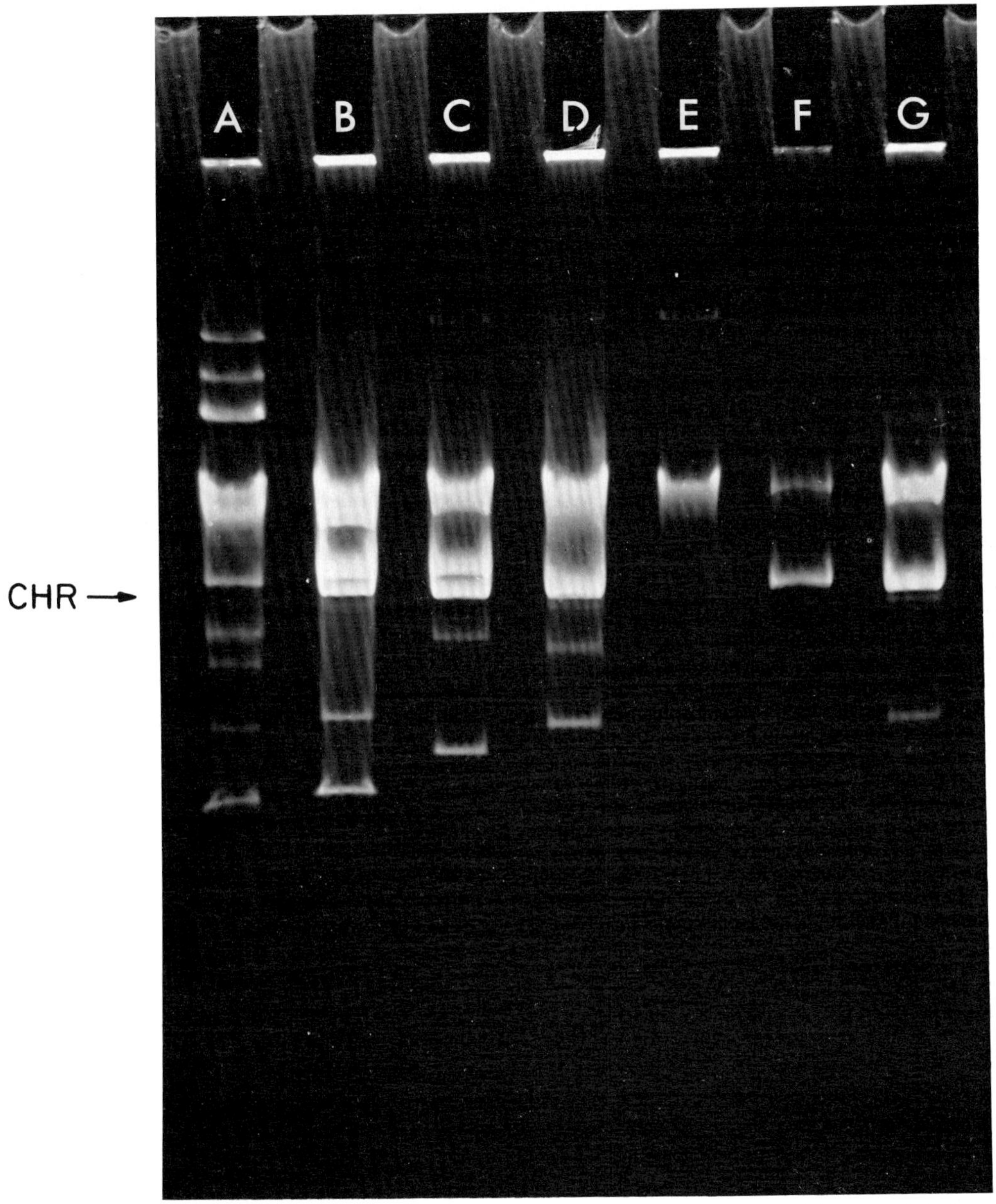

FIG. 1. *Agarose gel electrophoresis of ethanol-precipitated DNA from bacterial lysates. (A) Standard plasmid DNAs ranging in molecular weights from 62 Mdal (uppermost band) to 1.8 Mdal (lowest band). CHR, Band position of the chromosomal DNA. (B) Lysate from S. dysenteriae type 1 strain M6982 Cm^r Tet^r Sm^r Su^r Ap^r isolated in the Bangla Desh epidemics. Molecular weights of plasmids present (in Mdal): 62, 52, 6.1, 5.5, 4.85, 2.65, and 1.85. (The 62-, 52- and 4.85-Mdal bands are barely visible.) (C) Lysate from S. dysenteriae type 1 strain 762 Cm^r Tet^r Sm^r Su^r Ap^r isolated in Costa Rica. Molecular weights of plasmids present (in Mdal): 80, 6.1, 5.5, 4.4, 4.1, and 2.2. (D) Lysate from S. dysenteriae type 1 strain 51B Cm^r Tc^r Sm^r Su^r Ap^r isolated in Mexican epidemic. Molecular weights of plasmids present (in Mdal): 80, 5.5, 4.6, 3.7, and 2.5. (E) Lysate from an E. coli K-12 (exconjugant no. 1; obtained from cross between S. dysenteriae type 1 (Mexico) and E. coli K-12 W1485-1 Nx^r) Cm^r Tet^r Sm^r Su^r and Ap^s. Molecular weights of plasmids present (in Mdal): 80. (F) Lysate from an E. coli K-12 (exconjugant no. 5; obtained from cross between S. dysenteriae type 1 (Mexico) and E. coli K-12 W1485-1 Nx^r) Ap^r (Cm^s Tc^s Sm^s Su^s). (G) Lysate from an E. coli K-12 (exconjugant no. 25; obtained from cross between S. dysenteriae type 1 (Mexico) and E. coli K-12 W1485-1 Nx^r) Cm^r Tet^r Sm^r Su^r Ap^r. Molecular weights of plasmids present (in Mdal): 80, 5.5, and 4.6. The band present at the position of 20 Mdal corresponds to form II (open circular) DNA of the 5.5-Mdal plasmid.*

TABLE 1. *Hybridization between ^{3}H-labeled RJHC5 Ap^r plasmid DNA and whole-cell DNA*

Source of unlabeled DNA	Relative DNA sequence homology with ^{3}H-labeled RJHC5 Ap^r DNA[a] (%)
E. coli K-12 exconjugant 1 (Ap^r Mexico)	100
E. coli K-12 exconjugant 2	0
E. coli K-12 exconjugant 3	89
E. coli K-12 exconjugant 4 (Ap^r Costa Rica)	98
E. coli K-12 exconjugant 5 (Ap^r Bangla Desh)	94
S. dysenteriae type 1 (Mexico)	91
S. dysenteriae type 1 (Costa Rica)	87
S. dysenteriae type 1 (Bangla Desh)	91
E. coli K-12 (RSF1030) (originally from *S. panama*)	98
E. coli K-12 (RJHC2) (originally from *C. freundii* Ind 6A)	93
E. coli K-12 (Sa-1)	51
E. coli K-12 (Sa)	0
S. typhi JM	23
S. typhi P12	30
E. coli K-12 W1485-1	0

[a] The degree of DNA-DNA duplex formation was assayed by the S1 endonuclease method (6). The actual extent of reassociation for the homologous reaction was in average 87%. All other reactions were normalized to this value set at 100%. Each value shown is an average of three separate determinations.

gants containing only the Ap^r plasmid from either the Mexican, Costa Rican, or Bangla Desh epidemics are analyzed. DNA extracted from *E. coli* exconjugants containing the *Shigella* conjugative R-plasmid shared only 1.5% of its sequences with the Ap^r plasmid, whereas exconjugants containing both conjugative and nonconjugative Ap^r R-plasmids were as expected, highly related to the Ap^r plasmid.

The DNA-DNA hybridization experiments show not only the identity among the different *Shigella* Ap^r plasmids but also their high relation to RSF1030 and RJHC2, two Ap^r nonconjugative, 5.5-Mdal plasmids carrying determinants for Ap^r and isolated, respectively, from *Salmonella panama* (4) and *Citrobacter freundii* (unpublished data). It is now well established that, among R-plasmids present in the *Enterobacteriaceae*, the gene specifying TEM β-lactamase resides upon a 3×10^6-dalton sequence of DNA that is capable of excising itself from one plasmid and inserting itself into another (5, 10, 11). To determine whether any or all of the TnA segment was present in the ampicillin-resistant strains of *S. dysenteriae*, DNA-DNA hybridization experiments with Sa-1, a W plasmid containing the TnA sequences, and its counterpart, Sa, which does not carry the TnA sequences (10, 11), were carried out. Results indicate that about 50% of the Ap^r plasmid sequences are shared in common with Sa-1, but no homology was detected with Sa; i.e., about 3 Mdal of the 5.5-Mdal Shiga Ap^r plasmid

TABLE 2. *Comparison of replication properties of the Ap^r plasmids*

Origin of Ap^r plasmid	Designation	Mol wt (Mdal)[a]	No. of copies in *E. coli* K-12[b]	Replication in chloramphenicol[c]	Polymerase I requirement[d]
S. dysenteriae type 1 (Mexico)	RJHC5	5.5	39	90	+
S. dysenteriae type 1 (Costa Rica)	RJHC8	5.5	31	101	+
S. dysenteriae type 1 (Bangla Desh)	RJHC7	5.5	30	97	+
S. panama	RSF1030	5.5	35	100	+
C. freundii	RJHC2	5.5	35	110	+

[a] Molecular weights were determined by centrifugation on 5 to 20% neutral sucrose gradients as described previously (7).

[b] Number of copies per chromosome equivalent was determined as described previously (8).

[c] *E. coli* K-12 W1485-1 containing an Ap^r plasmid was prelabeled with [^{14}C]thymine (0.6 μCi/ml; 3.6 μg/ml) in minimal medium (7) until a concentration of 5×10^8 cells/ml was achieved. At this time cells were centrifuged at 25°C and resuspended in minimal medium without any label and containing 170 μg of chloramphenicol per ml. After 2.5 h in the presence of chloramphenicol, [^{3}H]thymine (55 μCi/ml; 2 μg/ml) was added and incubation was continued for 10 h. Cleared lysates were prepared and spun in a CsCl-ethidium bromide gradient (8). The ratio of ^{3}H to ^{14}C in the plasmid peak for RSF1030 was taken arbitrarily as 100%, and the rest of the values were normalized to this figure.

[d] The requirement of polymerase I for replication was determined by transformation of plasmid DNA into *E. coli* K-12 MM383, a thermosensitive *polA*$^-$ mutant, and by determining the amount of plasmid replicated at the nonpermissive temperature.

DNA must be the TnA sequences. There is not a high degree of homology between the Shiga Ap^r plasmid and DNA obtained from Ap^r *S. typhi* strains isolated from typhoid epidemics previous to the dysentery outbreaks in Mexico. Although low, the degree of reassociation observed would indicate that probably part of the TnA sequences are present in ampicillin-resistant *S. typhi*. Figure 2 shows the identical *Hin*cII restriction endonuclease banding pattern for the 5.5-Mdal Ap^r plasmids from *S. panama, C. freundii,* and *S. dysenteriae,* confirming the homology of all three plasmids.

Replication properties of the Ap^r plasmids. Table 2 shows a comparision of the replication properties of the *Shigella* Ap^r plasmid with those of RSF1030 and RJHC2. All Ap^r plasmids replicate as a multicopy pool in *E. coli* cells. They also replicate in the absence of protein synthesis, accumulating RNA-containing CCC DNA. All of them require for their replication a functional chromosomal *polA* product.

DISCUSSION

Ampicillin has been considered the drug of choice for treatment of patients seriously ill with dysentery. The finding of high-level ampicillin-resistant *S. dysenteriae* type 1 strains in geographically widespread dysentery epidemics is of great concern when one considers the serious nature of this disease.

Genetic evidence for the presence of two plasmids, one carrying determinants for resistance to chloramphenicol, tetracycline, sulfonamides, and streptomycin and transfer properties and a separate one with determinants for ampicillin resistance, was presented recently (14, 17). We have now shown that all *S. dysenteriae* type 1 strains have a different and heterogeneous plasmid population, although a unique nonconjugative 5.5-Mdal plasmid has been associated with the ampicillin-resistant strains, irrespective of the geographical source of the epidemics. The rest of the drug resistance determinants are carried (at least in the Costa Rican and Mexican strains) on an 80-Mdal conjugative R-plasmid. Thus, the ampicillin resistance in *S. dysenteriae* type 1 is part of a class 2 transfer system (1).

Interestingly, our DNA-DNA hybridization studies show not only the identity among the different *Shigella* Ap^r plasmids but also their high relation to RSF1030 and RJHC2, two nonconjugative 5.5-Mdal plasmids isolated, respectively, from *S. panama* and *C. freundii* (unpublished data). This identity is confirmed by the restriction endonuclease analysis and by the similarities of the replicative properties of all Ap^r plasmids.

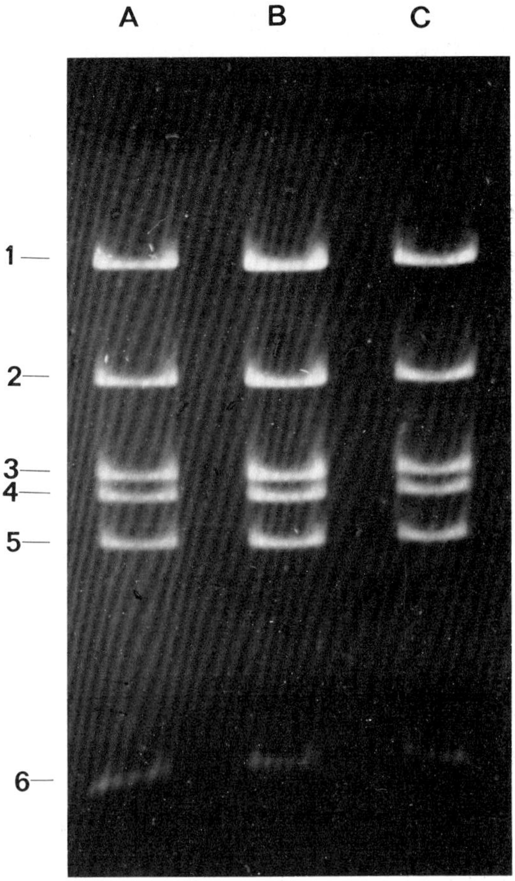

FIG. 2. *HincII restriction endonuclease patterns obtained with* Ap^r *plasmids from different enterobacteria. Reactions were carried out in 10 mM Tris-hydrochloride pH 7.9, 7 mM* $MgCl_2$*, 6 mM 2-mercaptoethanol, 60 mM NaCl and purified plasmid DNA in a final volume of 30 μl. Reactions were initiated by the addition of 1 μl of HincII restriction endonuclease (New England Biolab, 2,000 U/ml), incubated at 37°C for 90 min, and halted by adding 5 μl of a mixture containing 7% sodium dodecyl sulfate and 33% glycerol plus 0.04% bromophenol blue. The gel system consisted of 1.5% agarose in a Tris-borate buffer, pH 8.3 (see Materials and Methods). The gels were run at 100 V, 50 mA, at room temperature until the bromophenol blue reached the bottom of the gel. The gel was removed, stained, and photographed as described in Materials and Methods. HincII restrictions patterns for: (A) Citrobacter freundii* Ap^r *plasmid (RJHC 2); (B) Shigella dysenteriae* Ap^r *plasmid (RJHC 5); and (C) Salmonella panama* Ap^r *plasmid (RSF 1030).*

Our results with the Ap^r plasmids are similar to those obtained with the Sm^r Su^r plasmids, which were interrelated (2) but not phylogenetically related to the Ap^r plasmids (Crosa, unpublished data). It is highly likely, then, that the Ap^r plasmids, as it was suggested for the

Sm^r Su^r plasmids (2), have also evolved once and then epidemiologically spread.

It has been established that certain drug resistance genes reside upon sequences of DNA that have the capacity of translocating themselves from one plasmid to another (5, 10, 11). The ability of drug resistance genes to migrate between DNA molecules helps explain the rapid evolution of R-plasmids that possess a varied antibiotic resistance phenotype. Among the enterics, the structural gene for TEM-type β-lactamase is situated on a 3 $\times$ 10^6-dalton translocatable segment of DNA, so-called TnA (5, 10, 11). Our DNA-DNA hybridization experiments show that the TnA segment is present in the Ap^r plasmid. The translocation of Ap^r to an ancestor cryptic plasmid and then mobilization due to their coexistence with drug resistance transfer factors would furnish an additional explanation for the ubiquity of the Ap^r plasmid. There is not a high degree of homology between the Shiga Ap^r plasmid and DNA obtained from the Ap^r *S. typhi* strains isolated from typhoid epidemics previous to the dysentery outbreaks in Mexico. Although low, the degree of reassociation observed indicates that some sequences are held in common between the Shiga Ap^r plasmid and the *Salmonella* DNA (probably part of the TnA sequence).

It is noteworthy that plasmids carrying part of the enteric TnA translocon were also found to be responsible for the ampicillin resistance of recently isolated strains of nonenteric bacteria, such as *Haemophilus influenzae* (9) and *Neisseria gonorrhoeae* (L. Elwell, M. Roberts, L. Mayer, and S. Falkow, manuscript submitted for publication). We are presently investigating whether the same segment of TnA is present in all three bacteria.

ACKNOWLEDGMENTS

We are indebted to S. Falkow for helpful discussions, criticisms and careful reading of this manuscript.

This investigation was supported by grants from the National Science Foundation (PMC 75-14174), Food and Drug Administration (contract 223-73-7210), U.S. Agency for International Development, and the Consejo Nacional de Investigaciones Cientificas y Tecnologicas of Costa Rica.

LITERATURE CITED

1. **Anderson, E. S., and E. Natkin.** 1972. Transduction of resistance determinants and R factors of the Δ transfer system by phage P1kc. Mol. Gen. Genet. **114**:261–265.
2. **Barth, P. T., and N. J. Grinter.** 1974. Comparison of the deoxyribonucleic acid molecular weights and homologies of plasmids conferring linked resistance to streptomycin and sulfonamides. J. Bacteriol. **120**:618–630.
3. **Bauer, A. W., W. M. M. Kirby, J. C. Sherris, and M. Turk.** 1966. Antibiotic susceptibility testing by a standard single disk method. Ann. J. Clin. Pathol. **45**:493–496.
4. **Bouanchard, D. H., and Y. A. Chabbert.** 1969. Stable coexistence of three resistance factors (fi) in *Salmonella panama* and *Escherichia coli* K12. J. Gen. Microbiol. **58**:107–113.
5. **Cohen, S. N., and D. J. Kopecko.** 1976. Structural evolution of bacterial plasmids. Role of translocating genetic elements and DNA sequence insertions. Fed. Proc. **35**:2031–2036.
6. **Crosa, J. H., D. J. Brenner, and S. Falkow.** 1973. Use of a single-strand specific nuclease for analysis of bacterial and plasmid deoxyribonucleic acid homo- and heteroduplexes. J. Bacteriol. **115**:904–911.
7. **Crosa, J. H., L. K. Luttropp, and S. Falkow.** 1975. Nature of R factor replication in the presence of chloramphenicol. Proc. Natl. Acad. Sci. U.S.A. **73**:654–658.
8. **Crosa, J. H., L. K. Luttropp, F. Heffron, and S. Falkow.** 1975. Two replication initiation sites on R plasmid DNA. Mol. Gen. Genet. **140**:39–50.
9. **de Graaff, J., L. P. Elwell, and S. Falkow.** 1976. Molecular nature of two beta-lactamase-specifying plasmids isolated from *Haemophilus influenzae* type b. J. Bacteriol. **126**:439–446.
10. **Hedges, R. W., and A. Jacob.** 1974. Transposition of ampicillin resistance from RP4 to other replicons. Mol. Gen. Genet. **132**:31–40.
11. **Heffron, F., R. Sublett, R. W. Hedges, A. Jacob, and S. Falkow.** 1975. Origin of the TEM beta-lactamase gene found on plasmids. J. Bacteriol. **122**:250–256.
12. **Mata, L. J., E. J. Gangarosa, A. Caceres, D. R. Perera, and M. L. Mejicanos.** 1970. Epidemic Shiga bacillus dysentery in Central America. I. Etiologic investigation in Guatemala in 1969. J. Infect. Dis. **122**:170–180.
13. **Meyers, J., D. Sanchez, L. P. Elwell, and S. Falkow.** 1976. Simple agarose electrophoretic method for the identification and characterization of plasmid deoxyribonucleic acid. J. Bacteriol. **127**:1529–1537.
14. **Olarte, J.**, L. Filloy, and E. Galindo. 1976. Resistance of *Shigella dysenteriae* type 1 to ampicillin and other antimicrobial agents: strains isolated during a dysentery outbreak in a hospital in Mexico City. J. Infect. Dis. **133**:572–575.
15. **Olarte, J., and E. Galindo.** 1973. *Salmonella typhi* resistant to chloramphenicol, ampicillin, and other antimicrobial agents: strains isolated during an extensive typhoid fever epidemic in Mexico. Antimicrob. Agents Chemother. **4**:597–601.
16. **Olarte, J., G. Varela, and E. Galindo.** 1971. Infeccion por *Shigella dysenteriae* 1 (Bacilo de Shiga) en Mexico. Bol. Med. Hosp. Infant. Mex. (Span. Ed.) **28**:605–612.
17. **Peñaranda,** M. E., and L. J. Mata. 1976. Transfer of ampicillin resistance from *Shigella dysenteriae* type 1 to *Escherichia coli*. Lancet **ii**:1295–1296.
18. **Rahaman, M. M., I. Hug, C. R. Dey, A. K. G. M. Kibriya, and G. Curlin.** 1974. Ampicillin-resistant Shiga bacillus in Bangla Desh. Lancet **i**:406–407.

ANTIMICROBIAL AGENTS AND CHEMOTHERAPY, Mar. 1977, p. 559-562 Vol. 11, No. 3

Printed in U.S.A.

NOTES

Ampicillin-Induced Morphological Alterations of *Haemophilus influenzae* Type b

RICHARD D. KLEIN AND G. H. LUGINBUHL*

Department of Microbiology, North Carolina State University, Raleigh, North Carolina 27607

Received for publication 29 October 1976

Inhibitory levels of ampicillin induced filamentation of growing *Haemophilus influenzae* ATCC 19418 within 30 min. Filaments became swollen and interrupted by regular periodic saccular outpouchings along the major axis. The degree of filamentation was dependent upon ampicillin concentration and time.

The beta-lactam antibiotics, which inhibit peptidoglycan biosynthesis, have been demonstrated to induce a variety of morphological changes in gram-positive and gram-negative bacteria (3, 4, 7). These changes include spheroplasting, filament formation, and lysis. *Haemophilus influenzae* has been reported to form spheroplasts in the presence of bacteriostatic concentrations of ampicillin (1).

In the present study the morphological effects of ampicillin on *H. influenzae* type b were examined by light and scanning electron microscopy. *H. influenzae* type b (ATCC 19418), an ampicillin-susceptible, beta-lactamase-negative strain (minimum inhibitory concentration [MIC], 0.1 μg/ml), was grown overnight at 37°C in brain heart infusion broth (Difco) with 1% Difco supplement C (BHIC) on a rotary shaker. The culture was diluted 1:10 in BHIC, and 0.45 ml of this dilution was added to 8.55 ml of fresh BHIC and incubated for 2 h at 37°C on a rotary shaker. One milliliter of appropriate concentrations of ampicillin (Parke Davis oral suspension) was added to give final ampicillin concentrations of 0.1, 1, and 10 times the MIC. No ampicillin was added to one tube as a control. At 30 min and 4 h, samples were removed and processed for light and scanning electron microscopy. Bacterial suspensions on glass slides were air dried, heat fixed, and stained with crystal violet. Samples for scanning electron microscopy were filtered through 0.45-μm Nucleopore filters, dehydrated through 100% ethanol, critical point dried, and observed in an ETEC scanning electron microscope.

Light microscopy of the untreated control culture revealed a uniform population of coccobacilli. When incubated for 30 min with ampicillin at a concentration 10 times the MIC, bacillary cells two to three times larger than the control were observed. After 4 h at this concentration, large, swollen, elongated cells were prevalent. These cells were irregular and displayed circular distortions or saccular outpouchings of apparent cellular material along the major axis of the cell.

As examined by scanning electron microscopy (Fig. 1), the untreated control cells were coccobacillary in nature and smooth surfaced and ranged from 0.7 to 1 μm in length. After 30 min of incubation with 10 times the MIC of ampicillin (Fig. 2), the cells displayed a rough surface and were elongated, ranging from 1 to 3 μm in length. Obvious septum formation had taken place between some cells (Fig. 3). After 4 h of incubation with 10 times the MIC of ampicillin (Fig. 4), elongated filaments were present. These filaments were smooth surfaced and frequently intertwined. No evidence of septum formation was observed. Periodic saccular outpouchings were present along the filaments (Fig. 5). The diameter of these spherical saccular outpouchings was not consistent. At concentrations of 0.1 and 1 times the MIC of ampicillin the morphological changes were less evident. At both concentrations, after 30 min, 4 h, and 24 h of exposure, the cells were not appreciably elongated, ranging from 1 to 3 μm in length. The only dramatic change noted was an increased roughness of the cell surface. At 24 h, ampicillin at 10 times the MIC is bactericidal, killing greater than 99.9% of the cells, whereas the lower concentrations of ampicillin, 0.1 and 1 times the MIC, are not bactericidal.

A variety of gram-negative organisms have been demonstrated to form filaments in the presence of beta-lactam antibiotics. *Proteus mirabilis* (6) and *Proteus vulgaris* (3) produce filaments in response to carbenicillin and penicillin, respectively. The same phenomenon has

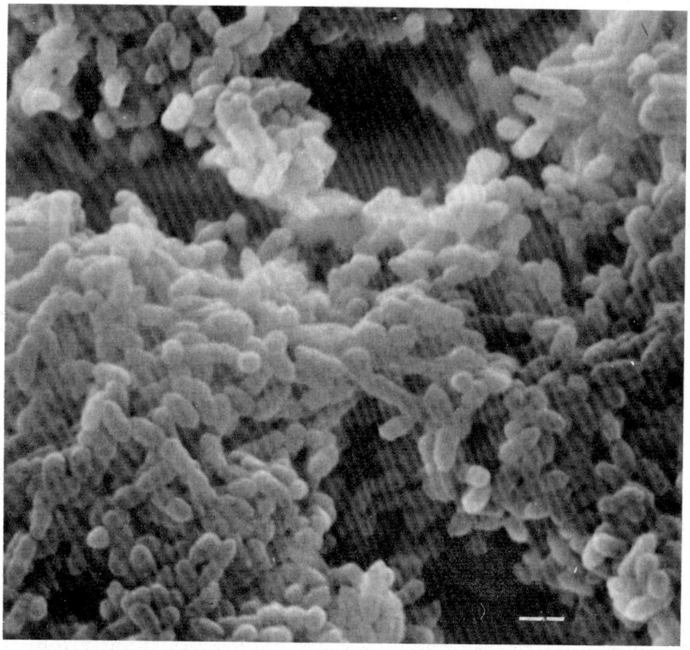

FIG. 1. *Scanning electron micrograph of untreated control cells. Bar, 1 μm.*

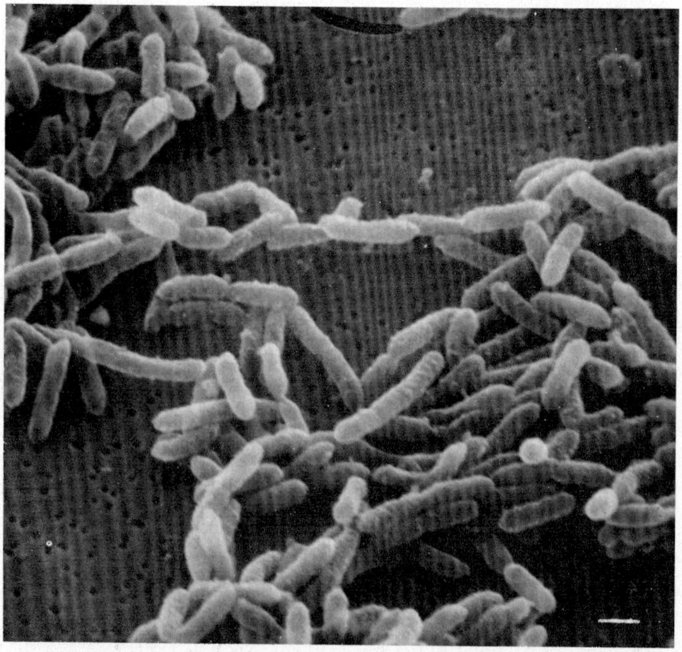

FIG. 2. *H. influenzae after 30 min of incubation with 10 times the MIC of ampicillin. Cells are elongated. Bar, 1 μm.*

been reported for *Enterobacter cloacae* (7) and *Escherichia coli* (5) with cefoxitin and cephalexin, respectively. In addition, filaments of *H. influenzae* have been reported by light microscopy after exposure to bacteriostatic concentrations of ampicillin (1).

In each of these studies the presence of saccular outpouchings of the filament was noted.

Saccular outpouching of *H. influenzae* filaments may result from the inhibition of septum formation at ampicillin concentrations greater than the MIC. This is suggested by the presence of obvious septation between cells after a 30-min exposure to 10 times the MIC (Fig. 3) in contrast to the absence of septation after a 4-h exposure to this concentration (Fig. 4, 5). In

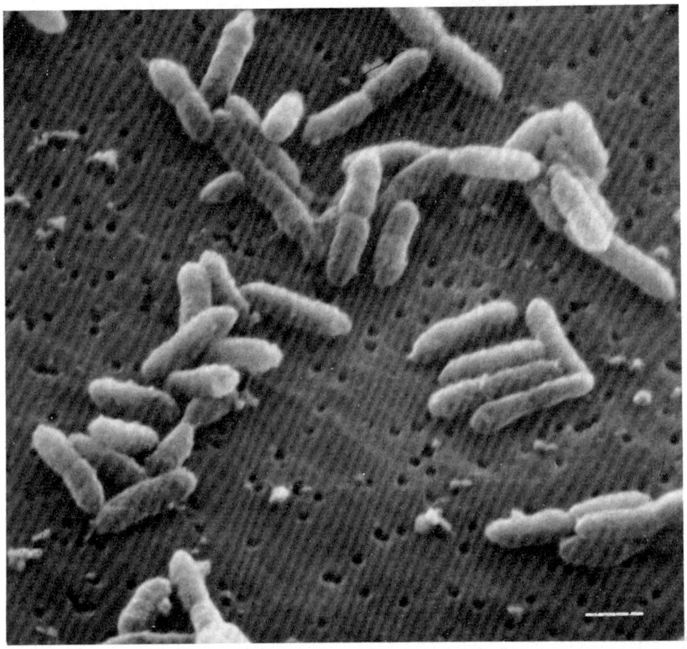

FIG. 3. *H. influenzae after 30 min of incubation with 10 times the MIC of ampicillin. Septum formation has been completed between some cells. Bar, 1 μm.*

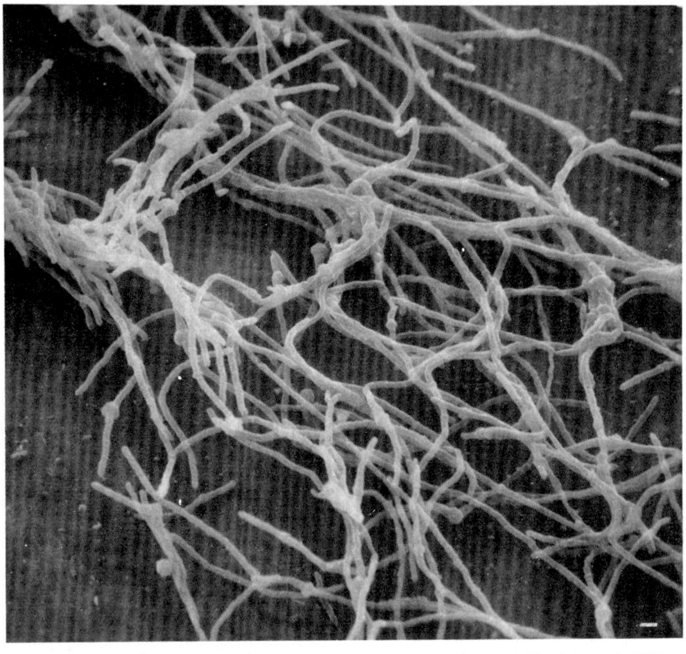

FIG. 4. *H. influenzae after 4 h of incubation with 10 times the MIC of ampicillin. Filamentous forms predominate. Bar, 1 μm.*

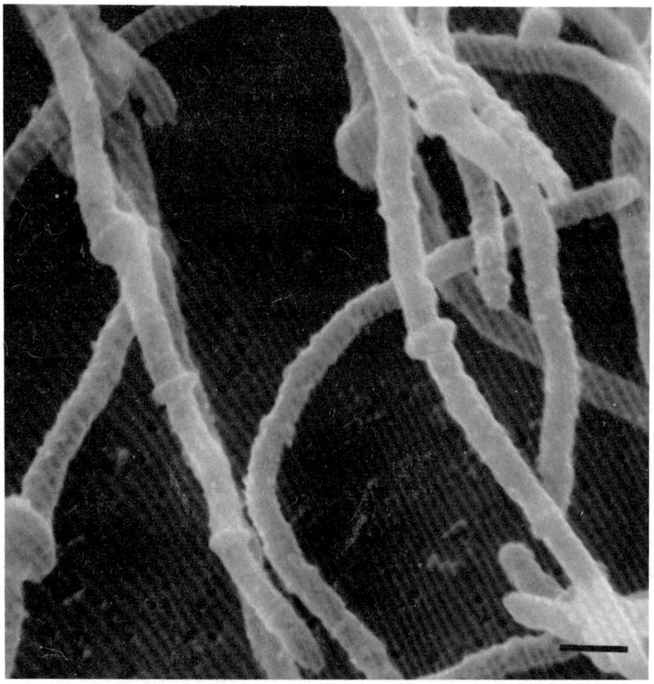

FIG. 5. *H. influenzae after 4 h of incubation with 10 times the MIC of ampicillin. Periodic saccular outpouchings along the filaments. Bar, 1 μm.*

addition, transmission electron microscopy of *E. cloacae* treated with cefoxitin revealed that the resulting filaments and saccular outpouchings were multinucleate and nonseptate (7). Similar results were noted when *E. cloacae* was treated with benzylpenicillin or cephalothin. In a report on the effects of carbenicillin on *Pseudomonas pseudomallei*, Dilworth et al. (2) observed by transmission electron microscopy the presence of saccular outpouchings on the resulting filaments at sites where transverse septa would occur. A similar situation is reported here in *H. influenzae* with ampicillin. Dilworth et al. (2) further suggest that the presence of beta-lactam antibiotics preferentially inhibits the formation of transverse septa, as opposed to cell wall peptidoglycan in general. Although conclusive evidence has not been obtained, this process could readily result in the formation of multinucleate, nonseptate filaments.

This investigation was supported in part by the Faculty Research and Professional Development Fund of North Carolina State University and by the North Carolina Agriculture Experiment Station.

LITERATURE CITED

1. **Bottone, E. J., Z. Brandman, and S. S. Schneierson.** 1976. Spheroplasts of *Haemophilus influenzae* induced by cell wall-active antibiotics and their effect upon the interpretation of susceptibility tests. Antimicrob. Agents Chemother. **9**:327–333.
2. **Dilworth, C. R., M. Franklin, and G. N. Bance.** 1974. Morphological and cytological effects of carbenicillin on *Pseudomonas pseudomallei*. Can. J. Microbiol. **20**:1229–1233.
3. **Fleming, A., A. Voureka, I. R. H. Kramer, and W. H. Huges.** 1950. The morphology and motility of *Proteus vulgaris* and other organisms cultured in the presence of penicillin. J. Gen. Microbiol. **4**:257–269.
4. **Lorian, V., and B. Atkinson.** 1976. Effects of subinhibitory concentrations of antibiotics on cross walls of cocci. Antimicrob. Agents Chemother. **9**:1043–1055.
5. **Nishino, T., and S. Nakazawa.** 1973. Cephalexin-induced morphological alterations in the surface structures of *Staphylococcus aureus* and *Escherichia coli* demonstrated by scanning electron microscopy. Jpn. J. Microbiol. **17**:383–392.
6. **Prior, R. B., and R. L. Perkins.** 1974. Artifacts induced by preparation for scanning electron microscopy in *Proteus mirabilis* exposed to carbenicillin. Can. J. Microbiol. **20**:794–795.
7. **Zimmerman, S. B., and E. O. Stapley.** 1976. Relative morphological effects induced by cefoxitin and other beta-lactam antibiotics in vitro. Antimicrob. Agents Chemother. **9**:318–326.

ANTIMICROBIAL AGENTS AND CHEMOTHERAPY, Mar. 1977, p. 563-565
Vol. 11, No. 3

Action of the *N*-Trifluoroacetyl Analogue of D-Chloramphenicol

K. B. FREEMAN
Department of Biochemistry, McMaster University, Hamilton, Ontario

Received for publication 29 November 1976

The *N*-trifluoroacetyl analogue of chloramphenicol was found to inhibit the growth of *Escherichia coli* less than chloramphenicol, rather than more as previously reported by others. It also inhibits protein synthesis by *E. coli* and rat liver mitochondria less.

Chloramphenicol is a potent inhibitor of protein synthesis in whole-cell and cell-free systems of bacteria (1, 16) and in mitochondria (8, 11). It also inhibits deoxyribonucleic acid synthesis (23) and mitochondrial reduced nicotinamide adenine dinucleotide (NADH) oxidation (6) of mammalian cells and causes two types of bone marrow depression (18, 22). The reversible bone marrow depression has been ascribed to an inhibition of mitochondrial protein synthesis (8, 22). As it would be desirable to have an analogue of chloramphenicol that inhibits bacterial but not mitochondrial protein synthesis and that does not cause the hematological side effects, the action of many analogues on whole-cell and cell-free systems has been examined (3, 8, 10, 13, 17, 19). Generally, the inhibition of bacterial cell-free and mitochondrial protein-synthesizing systems are similar but cell permeability affects the action of some analogues against intact bacteria. Recently, it has been reported that the *N*-trifluoroacetyl analogue of chloramphenicol inhibited the growth of *Escherichia coli* more than chloramphenicol (10). We have, therefore, examined the effect of this analogue in *E. coli*, mammalian cells, and cell-free systems derived from them.

E. coli B/r was grown on Pennassay broth (Difco) and growth was followed by measuring light transmitted at 600 nm. Mouse L cells were grown as described previously (5).

Bacterial protein synthesis was measured by determining the incorporation of [^{3}H]leucine into hot acid-insoluble material using both *E. coli* and *E. coli* cell-free systems as described previously (8) with midlog phase cells. Protein synthesis was determined in whole cells by a 10-min incubation at 30°C in 50 μl of minimal growth medium containing 8×10^7 cells/ml, 0.2% glucose, and 0.85 mM L-[4,5-^{3}H]leucine (32 mCi/mmol). Protein synthesis by an S30 extract of *E. coli* was determined in incubations of 110 μl containing 8 μCi of L-[^{3}H]leucine (38 Ci/mmol)/ml and 0.3 mg of protein at 37°C for 20 min (8). Mitochondrial protein synthesis was measured by a modification (20) of earlier procedures (9). Incubations were at 30°C for 30 min with 17 μCi of L-[^{3}H]leucine (38 Ci/mmol) per ml. Mitochondria were also incubated with 0.1% digitonin (1.1 mg of digitonin/mg of mitochondrial protein) in a medium in which the adenosine 5'-diphosphate and succinate usually present were replaced by 2.3 mM adenosine 5'-triphosphate, 10 mM creatine phosphate, and approximately 50 μg of creatine kinase/ml.

NADH oxidase of four-times-washed rat liver mitochondria which had been frozen and thawed three times (7), the solubility of the trifluoroacetyl analogue in water and ethanol (7), radioactive counting (8), and protein determination (13) were performed as have been described previously. The source of materials has been described previously (5, 7, 8) except for the *N*-trifluoroacetyl analogue of chloramphenicol which was a gift of C. Hansch, Pomona College, Claremont, Calif.

The effect of chloramphenicol and its trifluoroacetyl analogue on the growth of *E. coli* and protein synthesis by whole bacteria, *E. coli* extracts, and rat liver mitochondria are shown in Fig. 1A–D, along with the level of antibiotic required for 50% inhibition. In all cases the trifluoroacetyl analogue was less inhibitory than chloramphenicol. The lesser inhibition in the *E. coli* cell-free system indicates that the results with whole cells cannot be explained by a lack of permeability to the analogue. Similarly, with mitochondria incubated in 0.1% digitonin (1.1 mg of digitonin/mg of mitochondrial protein), conditions in which the mitochondria should be disrupted (14), the trifluoroacetyl analogue was less inhibitory to protein synthesis as shown in Fig 1D. In contrast to the *N*-trifluoroacetyl analogue, the *p*-

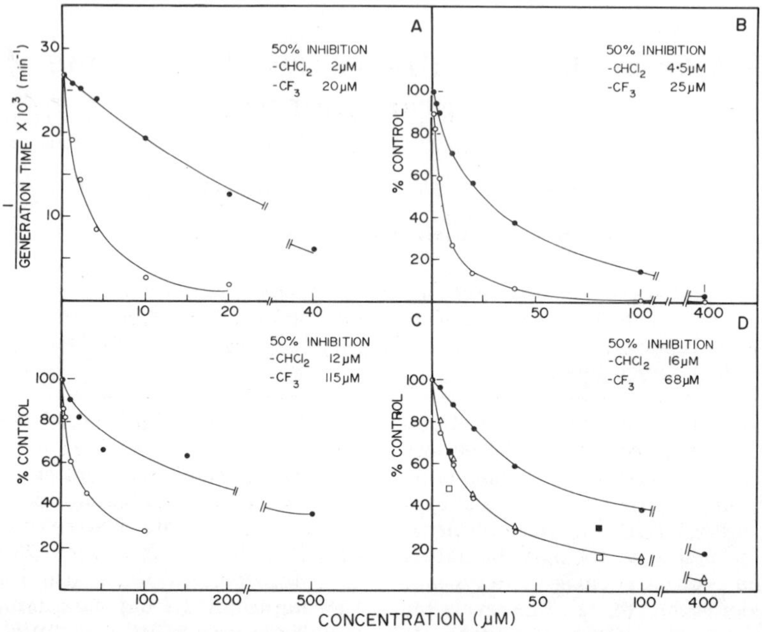

FIG. 1. *Effect of chloramphenicol and its trifluoroacetyl analogue on the growth of E. coli (A), protein synthesis by E. coli (B), E. coli extracts (C), and mitochondria (D). The controls were (A) a generation time of 37.2 min, (B) an incorporation of 1.8 $\times 10^4$ cpm/10^8 cells per 10 min, (C) an incorporation of 1.8 $\times 10^4$ cpm per mg of protein per 20 min, and (D) an incorporation of 6.0 $\times 10^4$ cpm per mg of protein per 30 min. The values for 50% inhibition are given in each case. For E. coli cell-free protein synthesis the value given is for 60% inhibition, which is halfway between 100% and 20%, the approximate level of maximum inhibition. Symbols: ○, □, Chloramphenicol; ●, ■, trifluoroacetyl analogue; △, p-sulfamoyl analogue. The square symbols represent mitochondrial protein synthesis in the presence of 0.1% digitonin. The control value was 7.6 $\times 10^3$ cpm per mg of mitochondrial protein which was 55% of the amount in the absence of digitonin.*

sulfamoyl analogue inhibited mitochondrial protein synthesis as much as chloramphenicol (Fig. 1D).

The trifluoroacetyl analogue inhibited NADH oxidation of frozen-thawed rat liver mitochondria 50% at 1.9 mM compared with 1 mM with chloramphenicol. The lesser inhibition by the trifluoroacetyl is a reflection of its lower relative solubility in ethanol (1.68 $\times 10^3$ mmol/liter) compared with water (90 mmol/liter) than chloramphenicol (7) as would be expected from previous results (7). The effect of the trifluoroacetyl analogue and the sulfamoyl analogue of chloramphenicol on the growth of mouse L cells is shown in Fig. 2. The sulfamoyl analogue has the same effect on mitochondrial protein synthesis as chloramphenicol (8; Fig.1D), but inhibits NADH oxidation less (7). Although the trifluoroacetyl analogue inhibited growth more at first than the sulfamoyl analogue, the cells grew about the same number of generations before growth ceased.

This study was initiated because of a report that the trifluoroacetyl analogue of chloramphenicol was a stronger inhibitor of the growth of *E. coli* than chloramphenicol (10). This has not been confirmed. Garrett (personal communication) has rechecked his results and found that the earlier results arose from a misreading of the notation of the concentration of the analogue resulting in an apparent 10-fold greater inhibition. From the results of the present study and those of others (3, 4, 13, 17), it is suggested that any change in the dichloroacetyl side chain of chloramphenicol will decrease its inhibitory activity in both mitochondrial and bacterial cell-free protein-synthesizing systems. It has been suggested that chloramphenicol inhibits the peptidyl transferase reaction on bacterial ribosomes by inhibiting the binding of the aminoacyladenylyl terminus of charged transfer ribonucleic acid to ribosomes (3, 15). If this is correct, the stereochemical requirement for a dichloroacetyl side chain or its charge distribution may be critically important. In contrast, the *p*-nitro group can be replaced in some cases with no change in inhibitory strength (2, 8). The lesser inhibition of protein synthesis by mitochondria and *E. coli* extracts by the trifluoroacetyl analogue supports earlier

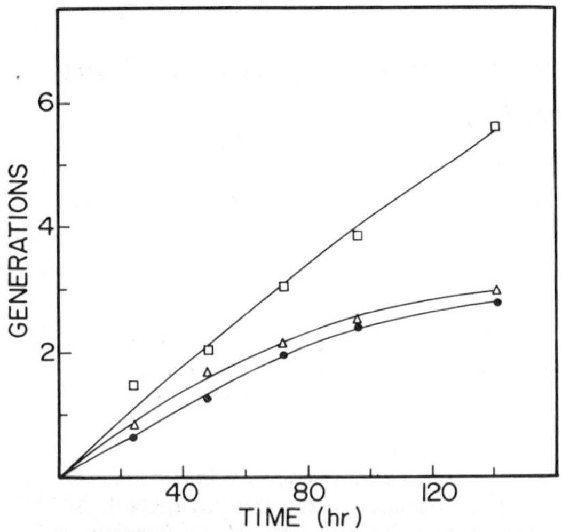

FIG. 2. *Effect of the sulfamoyl and the trifluoroacetyl analogue of chloramphenicol on the growth of L cells. The antibiotics were present at 0.28 mM. Symbols: □, Control; △, sulfamoyl analogue; ●, trifluoroacetyl analogue.*

studies with analogues that suggested a similar binding site for chloramphenicol on bacterial and mitochondrial ribosomes (8, 17).

We had previously found that the inhibition of growth of mammalian cells by chloramphenicol was due to the inhibition of mitochondrial protein synthesis and of NADH oxidation (5). The trifluoroacetyl analogue also inhibited the growth of mouse L cells as would be expected from its inhibition of mitochondrial protein synthesis. It is likely, then, that only an analogue that entered bacteria but not mammalian cells or mitochondria would have no hematological side effects.

This work was supported by grant MT-1940 from the Medical Research Council of Canada. I wish to thank T. M. Williams, D. Rupka, and H. Patel for excellent technical assistance.

LITERATURE CITED

1. **Brock, T. D.** 1961. Chloramphenicol. Bacteriol. Rev. **25**:32–48.
2. **Contreras, A., M. Barbacid, and D. Vazquez.** 1974. Binding to ribosomes and mode of action of chloramphenicol analogs. Biochim. Biophys. Acta **349**:376–388.
3. **Coutsogeorgopoulos, C.** 1966. On the mechanism of action of chloramphenicol in protein synthesis. Biochim. Biophys. Acta **129**:217–220.
4. **Coutsogeorgopoulos, C.** 1967. Inhibitors of the reaction between puromycin and polylysyl-RNA in the presence of ribosomes. Biochem. Biophys. Res. Commun. **27**:46–52.
5. **Fettes, I. M., D. Haldar, and K. B. Freeman.** 1972. Effect of chloramphenicol on enzyme syntheses and growth of mammalian cells. Can. J. Biochem. **50**:200–209.
6. **Freeman, K. B., and D. Haldar.** 1968. The inhibition of mammalian mitochondrial NADH oxidation by chloramphenicol and its isomers and analogs. Can. J. Biochem. **46**:1003–1008.
7. **Freeman, K. B.** 1970. Effects of chloramphenicol and its isomers and analogs on the mitochondrial respiratory chain. Can. J. Biochem. **48**:469–478.
8. **Freeman, K. B.** 1970. Inhibition of mitochondrial and bacterial protein synthesis by chloramphenicol. Can. J. Biochem. **48**:479–485.
9. **Haldar, D., and K. B. Freeman.** 1969. Importance of the osmolarity of the incubation medium on amino acid incorporation into protein by isolated rat liver mitochondria. Biochem. J. **111**:653–663.
10. **Hansch, C., K. Nakamoto, M. Gorin, P. Denisevich, E. R. Garrett, S. M. Hemanachak, and C. H. Won.** 1973. Structure activity relationship of chloramphenicols. J. Med. Chem. **16**:917–922.
11. **Kroon, A. M.** 1965. Protein synthesis in mitochondria. III. On the effects of inhibitors on the incorporation of amino acids into protein by intact mitochondria and digitonin fractions. Biochim. Biophys. Acta **108**:275–284.
12. **Lowry, O. H., N. J. Rosebrough, A. L. Farr, and R. J. Randall.** 1951. Protein measurement with the Folin phenol reagent. J. Biol. Chem. **193**:265–275.
13. **Manyan, D. R., G. K. Arimura, and A. A. Yunis.** 1975. Comparative metabolic effects of chloramphenicol analogues. Mol. Pharmacol. **11**:520–527.
14. **Matlib, M. A., and P. J. O'Brien.** 1975. Compartmentation of enzymes in the rat liver mitochondrial matrix. Arch. Biochem. Biophys. **167**:193–202.
15. **Pestka, S.** 1970. Studies on the formation of transfer ribonucleic acid-ribosome complexes. VIII. Survey of the effects of antibiotics on N-acetyl-phenylalanyl-puromycin formation: possible mechanism of chloramphenicol action. Arch. Biochem. Biophys. **136**:80–88.
16. **Rendi, R., and S. Ochoa.** 1962. Effect of chloramphenicol on protein synthesis in cell-free preparations of *Escherichia coli*. J. Biol. Chem. **237**:3711–3713.
17. **Ringrose, P. S., and R. W. Lambert.** 1973. The action of novel chloramphenicol analogs on prokaryotic and eukaryotic systems. Biochim. Biophys. Acta **299**:374–384.
18. **Snyder, M. J., and T. E. Woodward.** 1970. Chloramphenicol. Med. Clin. North Am. **54**:1187–1198.
19. **Vazquez, D.** 1966. Binding of chloramphenicol to ribosomes: the effect of a number of antibiotics. Biochim. Biophys. Acta **114**:277–288.
20. **Wallace, R. B., T. M. Williams, and K. B. Freeman.** 1975. Mitochondrial protein synthesis in a mammalian cell-line with a temperature-sensitive leucyl-tRNA synthetase. Eur. J. Biochem. **59**:167–173.
21. **Yunis, A. A., U. S. Smith, and A. Restrepo.** 1970. Reversible bone marrow suppression from chloramphenicol: a consequence of mitochondrial injury. Arch. Intern. Med. **126**:272–275.
22. **Yunis, A. A.** 1973. Chloramphenicol-induced bone marrow suppression. Semin. Hematol. **10**:225–234.
23. **Yunis, A. A., D. R. Manyan, and G. K. Arimura.** 1973. Comparative effect of chloramphenicol and thiamphenicol on DNA and mitochondrial protein synthesis in mammalian cells. J. Lab. Clin. Med. **81**:713–718.

ANTIMICROBIAL AGENTS AND CHEMOTHERAPY, Mar. 1977, p. 566-568
Vol. 11, No. 3

Antimicrobial Susceptibilities of *Yersinia enterocolitica* Biotype 4, Serotype O:3

S. HAMMERBERG, S. SORGER, AND M. I. MARKS[1] *

McGill University-Montreal Children's Hospital Research Institute and Departments of Pediatrics (Infectious Disease) and Microbiology, Montreal, Quebec H3H 1P3 Canada

Received for publication 29 October 1976

Agar dilution antimicrobial susceptibility tests were carried out against recent clinical isolates of *Yersinia enterocolitica* biotype 4, serotype O:3. Aminoglycosides and co-trimoxazole were the most active drugs. All isolates were resistant to ampicillin, carbenicillin, cloxacillin, and erythromycin.

Yersinia enterocolitica is being isolated with increasing frequency from children with gastroenteritis. At the present time there are few data pertaining to antimicrobial chemotherapy and the quantitative in vitro susceptibilities of this organism to antimicrobial agents (2, 3, 5). The present study was undertaken to expand upon the few existing reports of other groups (2, 3, 5). The comparative in vitro activity of 16 single antimicrobials and 1 drug combination of these were studied against recent clinical isolates from ill children; the effects of different media and inocula on the agar dilution minimum inhibitory concentrations (MIC) for this organism were also examined briefly.

Twenty-three isolates of *Y. enterocolitica* were obtained from 22 ill children at the Montreal Children's Hospital from 1974 to 1976. These strains were all cultured from stool specimens with the exception of a swab from an appendix. Identification was carried out using the differential characteristics defined by Sonnenwirth (6). Biological and serological typing were performed by S. Toma (Public Health Laboratories, Toronto). All isolates were biotype 4, serotype O:3, the predominant serotype associated with clinical infection in humans in Canada (8).

The agar dilution replicator technique of Steers et al. (7) was used for MIC determinations. Mueller-Hinton agar (MH; Difco) adjusted to pH 7.4 was used for all drugs, and additional sets of sulfamethoxazole (SMZ)-trimethoprim (TMP) (alone and in combination) plates were prepared with Diagnostic Sensitivity Test (DST) agar (Oxoid DST broth with 12 g of agar [Difco] per liter) for comparative purposes (4). A stock solution of each drug was prepared and serial twofold dilutions in distilled water (0.5 ml) were added to 9.5 ml of agar for each dilution plate. The effects of two inocula, an undiluted overnight growth in MH broth (approximately 10^8 colony-forming units [CFU]/ml by colony count) and a 10^{-3} dilution of this suspension, were compared. After inoculation, plates were incubated for 16 to 18 h at 37°C and the results were recorded. The MIC of all drugs except SMZ alone was defined as the lowest drug concentration at which no growth was visible on the surface of the agar. The MIC of SMZ was defined as the lowest concentration at which there was an 80% or sudden reduction in growth.

Disk diffusion susceptibility tests (1) were carried out with the following antibiotics (antibiotic concentration of disk in parentheses): ampicillin (10 μg), kanamycin (30 μg), gentamicin (10 μg), cephalothin (30 μg), SMZ/TMP (23.75/1.25 μg), sisomicin (10 μg), amikacin (10 μg), and netilmicin (10 μg).

The agar dilution test results are illustrated in Table 1 and Fig. 1. When one considers the higher achievable serum concentrations of kanamycin and amikacin, all strains had similar susceptibilities to the six aminoglycosides tested: gentamicin, kanamycin, netilmicin, sisomicin, amikacin, and tobramycin. Chloramphenicol was less active than the aminoglycosides and similar to tetracycline and rifampin.

All isolates were resistant to ampicillin, carbenicillin, cloxacillin, and erythromycin. Susceptibility to cephalothin ranged from moderate resistance (MIC, 25 μg/ml) to complete resistance (MIC >100 μg/ml).

The above results were similar with both inocula tested (10^8 and 10^5 CFU/ml); however, the lighter inoculum produced more clear-cut end points than the undiluted, overnight growth.

TMP and SMZ were examined alone and in combination on both MH and DST agar with undiluted and diluted inocula. The clearest re-

[1] Address reprint requests to: Montreal Children's Hospital, Montreal, Quebec, H3H 1P3, Canada.

sults were obtained with the 10^5-CFU/ml inoculum and are illustrated in Fig. 1. The inoculum effect for SMZ MICs performed on both DST and MH agar was extreme. All isolates had an MIC of >400 μg of SMZ per ml when the inoculum was from an undiluted overnight growth but 3.12 to 6.25 μg/ml with the 10^5 inoculum. MH agar proved to be superior to DST agar for TMP susceptibilities as clearly defined end points were obtained only on this medium and only with the 10^5-CFU/ml inoculum. The inoculum effect was sufficient to alter the susceptibility pattern from susceptible to resistant as in the case of SMZ. When SMZ and TMP were combined in a 20:1 ratio, marked synergism resulted, reducing the MIC of the former at least fourfold and the latter at least eightfold. All isolates were susceptible to a ratio of 1.56 μg of SMZ per ml and 0.078 μg of TMP per ml.

Disk susceptibility tests carried out on 8 of 17 drugs gave results corresponding to those agar dilution MICs where an inoculum of 10^5 CFU/ml was used.

The results of this study demonstrate that aminoglycosides and co-trimoxazole are the most active antimicrobials in vitro against. *Y. enterocolitica*. Although the isolates tested in this study were slightly more resistant to TMP alone and more susceptible to SMZ than reported by Gutman et al., the SMZ-TMP combination results were similar (2). Our results with cloxacillin, tetracycline, kanamycin, gentamicin and ampicillin correlated well with those reported by Hausnerová et al. (3) who also studied *Y. enterocolitica* biotype 4 strains. In contrast to their report where 12% were susceptible to cephalothin (MIC, <10 μg/ml), none of our strains were susceptible to this drug; our strains were also more resistant to carbenicillin. This inconsistency could be attributed to the fact that their strains were isolated from 1967 to 1972 when these two β-lactam drugs were relatively new. The isolates from our hospital appear to be extremely homogeneous in their antibiotic susceptibility pattern as well as biotype and serotype. No other biotype or serotype has been isolated in this hospital up to the present time.

TABLE 1. *Susceptibilities of 23 isolates of Y. enterocolitica to 14 antibiotics (agar dilution, inoculum-replicating method, 10^5-CFU/ml inoculum)*

Antimicrobial	Range of MIC (μg/ml)
Gentamicin	0.78–1.56
Netilmicin	0.78–1.56
Sisomicin	0.78–1.56
Tobramycin	0.78–3.12
Amikacin	1.56–6.25
Kanamycin	3.12–6.25
Tetracycline	6.25
Chloramphenicol	6.25
Rifampin	6.25
Erythromycin	25
Cloxacillin	50–100
Ampicillin	25–100
Cephalothin	25–>100
Carbenicillin	200

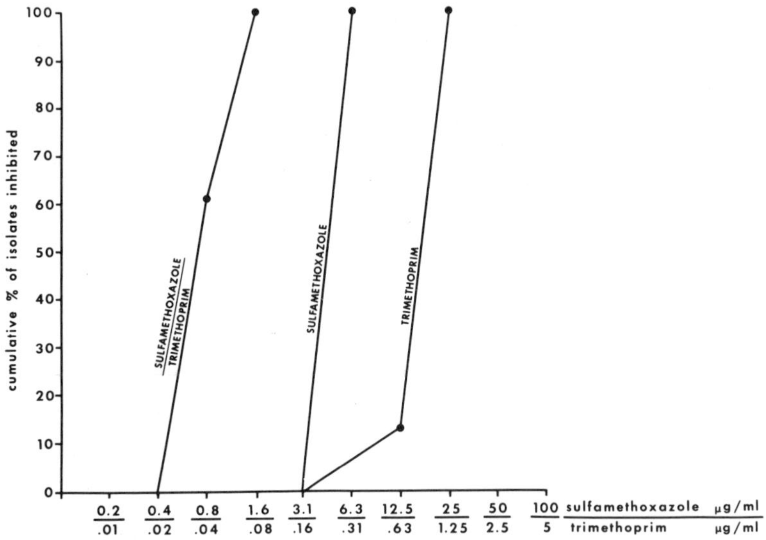

FIG. 1. *Susceptibilities of 23 clinical isolates of Y. enterocolitica to SMZ and TMP, alone and in combination. (Method as in Table 1).*

We recommend the use of MH agar and a 10^5-CFU/ml inoculum (a 10^{-3} dilution of an overnight growth in MH broth) for agar dilution MICs with the drugs tested; a Steers replicator delivers approximately 0.002 ml, thus the inoculum deposited on the agar surface is 2×10^2 CFU. A standardized disk diffusion test correlates well with the quantitative test. These in vitro results suggest co-trimoxazole or aminoglycoside antibiotics may have clinical usefulness in the therapy of *Y. enterocolitica* infections.

LITERATURE CITED

1. **Barry, A. L., F. Garcia, and L. D. Thrupp.** 1970. An improved single-disk method for testing the antibiotic susceptibility of rapidly-growing pathogens. Am. J. Clin. Pathol. 53:149–158.
2. **Gutman, L. T., C. M. Wilfert, and T. Quan.** 1973. Susceptibility of *Yersinia* enterocolitica to trimethoprim-sulfamethoxazole. J. Infect. Dis. 128(Suppl): 538.
3. **Hausnerová, S., O. Hausner, and V. Paučkova.** 1973. Antibiotic sensitivity of *Yersinia enterocolitica* strains isolated in two regions of Czechoslovakia, p. 76–80. *In* Contributions to microbiology and immunology, vol. 2. Yersinia, Pasteurella and Francisella. Karger, Basel.
4. **Marks, M. I., and G. Weinmaster.** 1975. Influence of media and inocula on the in vitro susceptibility of *Hemophilus influenzae* to co-trimoxazole, ampicillin, penicillin and chloramphenicol. Antimicrob. Agents Chemother. 8:657–663.
5. **Nilehn, B.** 1967. Studies on *Yersinia enterocolitica*. Acta Pathol. Microbiol. Scand. 69:83–91.
6. **Sonnenwirth, A. C.** 1974. *Yersinia*, p. 222–229. *In* E. H. Lennette, E. H. Spaulding, and J. P. Truant (ed.), Manual of clinical microbiology, 2nd ed. American Society for Microbiology, Washington, D.C.
7. **Steers, E., E. L. Foltz, and B. S. Graves.** 1959. An inocula replicating apparatus for routine testing of bacterial susceptibility to antibiotics. Antibiot. Chemother. 9:307–311.
8. **Toma, S., and L. Lafleur.** 1974. Survey on the incidence of *Yersinia enterocolitica* infection in Canada. Appl. Microbiol. 28:469–473.

ANTIMICROBIAL AGENTS AND CHEMOTHERAPY, Mar. 1977, p. 569–570
Vol. 11, No. 3

Microbial Formation of 4-Thiouracil

L. DOLAK,* W. T. SOKOLSKI, S. MIZSAK, D. W. STROMAN, AND O. K. SEBEK
The Upjohn Research Laboratories, Kalamazoo, Michigan 49001

Received for publication 28 October 1976

A soil organism identified as *Streptomyces libani* var. *soldani* was found to produce 4-thiouracil. The product was isolated in a yield of 150 μg/ml of filtered beer and characterized by C-13 magnetic resonance and high-resolution mass spectroscopy. The product has a broad antibacterial spectrum but low specific activity.

4-Thiouracil inhibits the growth of *Lactobacillus casei* (1), causes an almost complete regression of mammary carcinoma 755 in mice (1), and is weakly active against the leukemia SR-61 system (3). Chemical synthesis of 4-thiouracil was reported in 1908 (5) and that of its nucleoside in 1958 (2). The nucleoside is present as a minor component of transfer ribonucleic acid in *Escherichia coli* (4).

We are reporting here an efficient method of microbial formation of 4-thiouracil as an alternative to the chemical synthesis.

Inoculum of *Streptomyces libani* subsp. *soldani*, NRRL 8174, was prepared by inoculating the organism into a medium containing 2.5% glucose and 2.5% Pharmamedia (Traders Oil Mill Co., Fort Worth, Tex.), adjusted to pH 7.2. The taxonomic identification of the organism was carried out by Alma Dietz (manuscript in preparation). After a 3-day incubation on a rotary shaker (250 rpm, 28°C), 5 ml of the heavily grown mycelium was inoculated into 100 ml of the fermentation medium consisting of 0.5 g of tryptone, 1 g of Brer Rabbit molasses, 1 g of glycerol, and 0.25 g of yeast extract (pH 6.4) per 500-ml Erlenmeyer flask and incubated as above.

The formation of the 4-thiouracil was determined by assaying filtered fermentation beer daily for its activity against *Bacillus subtilis*. In Table 1 we define one biounit as the amount of the antibiotic in 80 μl of filtered beer that gives a 20-mm-diameter zone of inhibition when applied on a filter paper disk (12.7 mm in diameter), placed on a layer of nutrient agar (thickness, 3 mm), inoculated with *B. subtilis* UC 564, and incubated overnight at 37°C.

A medium of the following composition was used in isolating the antibiotic: 1% glucose (technical grade), 2% dextrin, 0.1% yeast extract, and 1% tryptone adjusted to pH 7.0. One liter of this medium was dispensed in 100-ml portions in 500-ml wide-mouth Erlenmeyer flasks, inoculated with 5% inoculum volume, and incubated on a shaker at 28°C for six days. At the end of this period, the contents of the flasks were pooled (pH 7.8) and filtered. The clear filtrate (750 ml) was adjusted to pH 7.0 with hydrochloric acid and extracted twice with equal volumes of ethyl acetate. The organic phase was washed with brine and dried with magnesium sulfate; the solvent was removed on a rotary evaporator. The residue (166.0 mg) was dissolved in 5 ml of a mixture of ethyl acetate and methanol (10:1, vol/vol), injected into a size C Merck prepacked silica gel column, and eluted isocratically with ethyl acetate at a rate of 5 ml/min, collecting 25-ml fractions.

The antibiotic-containing fractions (fractions 23–28) were pooled and concentrated to give 112.2 mg of a yellow solid for a yield of 150 μg/ml of filtered beer.

The product gave a high-resolution mass spectrum, which showed a parent ion at *m/e* 128.0055 (calculated for $C_4H_4N_2OS$ = 128.0044). The carbon magnetic resonance spectrum (d_6-dimethyl sulfoxide, internal tetramethylsilane) was obtained on a Varian CFT-20 spectrometer.

TABLE 1. *Formation of 4-thiouracil*

Day	Broth pH	Biounits/ml
1	5.4	5
2	5.7	9
3	6.6	22
4	6.8	26
5	6.5	21

TABLE 2. *The ^{13}C chemical shifts of 4-thiouracil*

Shift (ppm)	Multiplicity	Assignment
111.7	D	C-5
138.1	D	C-6
148.7	S	C-2
191.3	S	C-4

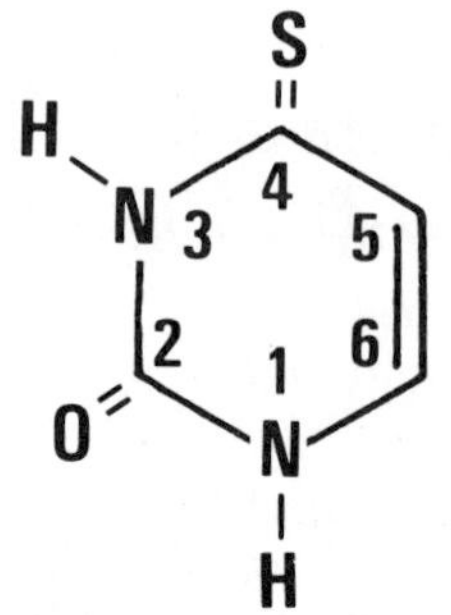

FIG. 1. *Structure of 4-thiouracil.*

TABLE 3. *Antibacterial spectrum of 4-thiouracil*

Organism	Inhibition zone[a] (diam in mm)
Proteus vulgaris UC 93	41
Salmonella schottmuelleri UC 126	41
Salmonella gallinarum UC 265	37
Pseudomonas fluorescens UC 2049	36
Escherichia coli UC 51	35
Bacillus subtilis UC 564	30
Sarcina lutea UC 130	26
Staphylococcus aureus UC 80	23
Bacillus cereus UC 3145	22

[a] Zone of inhibition produced by the application of 100 μg of 4-thiouracil on a paper disk (12.7 mm in diameter), which has been placed on a layer of nutrient agar (thickness, 3 mm) inoculated with the test organism.

Noise decoupled and off-resonance data are given in Table 2.

The isolated product was not separable from synthetic 4-thiouracil (Fig. 1) on Analtech silica gel plates with ethyl acetate-methanol (10:1, vol/vol) or with pure ethyl acetate. The ultraviolet, infrared, and proton magnetic resonance spectra and elemental analysis were consistent with those expected for 4-thiouracil.

Antibiotic activity was evaluated by using agar diffusion tests and by determination of minimum inhibitory concentrations in brain heart infusion.

4-Thiouracil was found to have broad-spectrum activity in agar diffusion tests. Zones of inhibition were larger with gram-negative than with gram-positive bacteria (Table 3), but its minimum inhibitory concentrations as determined by dilution in brain heart infusion broth were 250 to 1,000 μg/ml.

We thank P. G. Lemaux for initial fermentation experiments, L. Baczynskyj for the mass spectral data, and G. E. Zurenko for the minimum inhibitory concentration determinations of the product.

LITERATURE CITED

1. **Elion, G. B., S. Bieber, H. Nathan, and G. H. Hitchings.** 1958. Uracil antagonism and inhibition of mammary adenocarcinoma 755. Cancer Res. 18:802–817.
2. **Fox, J. J., D. van Praag, I. Wempsen, I. L. Doerr, L. Cheong, J. E. Knoll, M. L. Eidinoff, A. Bendich, and G. B. Brown.** 1958. Thiation of nucleosides. II. Synthesis of 5-methyl-2′-deoxycytidine and related pyrimidine nucleosides. J. Am. Chem. Soc. 81:178–187.
3. **Hoshi, A., M. Saneyoshi, and K. Kuretani.** 1971. Antitumor activity of 2- and 4-substituted derivatives of pyrimidine and their ribonucleosides. Pharmacometrics 5:441–443.
4. **Lipsett, M. N.** 1965. The isolation of 4-thiouridylic acid from the soluble ribonucleic acid of *Escherichia coli*. J. Biol. Chem. 240:3975–3978.
5. **Wheeler, H. L., and L. M. Liddle.** 1908. Researches on pyrimidines. XL. The thio derivatives of uracil and the preparation of uracil in quantity. Am. Chem. J. 40:547–558.

ANTIMICROBIAL AGENTS AND CHEMOTHERAPY, Mar. 1977, p. 571-573
Vol. 11, No. 3

Stimulation of Interferon Production in Mice and in Mouse Spleen Leukocytes by Analogues of BL-20803

PAUL SIMINOFF* AND R. R. CRENSHAW

Departments of Microbiology Research and Medicinal Chemistry, Bristol Laboratories, Division of Bristol-Myers Company, Syracuse, New York 13201

Received for publication 4 October 1976

Various structural analogues of the interferon inducer BL-20803 exhibited close agreement between ability to stimulate interferon production in the intact mouse and in cultures of spleen adherent leukocytes.

In several reports we have suggested that the interferon-eliciting activity of the low-molecular-weight compound BL-20803 is directed at certain leukocytes, of which the adherent (A) spleen cell is the paradigm (2, 3). Among the lines of evidence offered, we have shown that spleen A cells, when recovered from mice treated with the compound and then cultured in vitro, actively produced interferon. Furthermore, direct exposure of spleen A cells to BL-20803 elicted about 2.5 to 8 times as much interferon as did treatment of spleen nonadherent cells. Finally, pretreatment of mice with rabbit antiserum to mouse spleen A cells inhibited their subsequent interferon response to BL-20803 by at least 65%.

The synthesis in our laboratories of a large number of analogues of BL-20803 (compound 5 in Table 1), which have varying abilities to elicit interferon in mice (1), has provided us an additional opportunity to test the involvement of the spleen A cell in the animals' interferon responses by comparing interferon production in the whole animal and in spleen A cell cultures stimulated by the various analogues. In an exact correlation, there would be the same rank order of activity between in vivo and in vitro treatment. The data in Table 1 compare the ability of compounds to stimulate interferon in the mouse in terms of minimal effective dose (MED) with interferon stimulation of isolated A cells at two concentrations of compounds, 3.1 and 0.78 μg/mg. In general, those compounds most active in vivo were the most potent interferon inducers in vitro. None of the compounds that failed to stimulate A cells were active in the intact animal. On the other hand, a few of the analogues, e.g., compounds 15, 16, 17, 19, and 24, appeared to elicit at least a small amount of interferon from A cells but had no discernible stimulating effect in intact mice. In the particular case of compound 17, the in vitro activity was as pronounced as the activities of those analogues that were unequivocally stimulatory in the intact mouse. It seemed likely that these results reflected interference by somatic processes with the compound's interaction with the target cells in adequate concentration or in an active form. As mouse blood is known to be rich in esterases, it seemed possible that in the body the methyl ester at the 7 position of compound 17 was converted to the corresponding carboxylic acid, thus forming the known inactive compound 18 (see Table 1). We tested this possibility in the following way.

A stock solution of compound 17 was prepared in phosphate-buffered saline at pH 7.2 containing 1.8 mg of compound per ml. A 0.5-ml portion of the solution was distributed to separate tubes, each containing an equal volume of (i) unheated mouse serum, (ii) mouse serum that had been heated to 56°C for 30 min, or (iii) phosphate-buffered saline. All samples were incubated at 36°C for 30 min. Portions of 0.1 or 0.2 ml were diluted in RPMI medium containing 10% fetal bovine serum, and various dilutions were added to A cell cultures to test their ability to stimulate interferon. These dilutions were selected such that at least one dilution would contain a concentration of compound 17 within its nontoxic, active range of approximately 0.4 to 6 μg/ml, as has already been reported for BL-20803 (2). At equal dilutions of 1/270, there appeared to be more active compound in the heated mouse serum than in the unheated serum, as indicated in Table 2 by the threefold greater amount of interferon stimulated by the heated serum sample. More precise quantitation was not possible because this biological test has two limitations: (i) at high or borderline toxic levels, the compound either abolished or depressed interferon yields; and (ii) only that amount of compound in excess of the binding capacity of the serum contributed to biological activity (0.5 ml of serum could bind at least 100 μg of compound 17).

TABLE 1. *Interferon-stimulating ability of BL-20803 (compound 5) and its analogues*

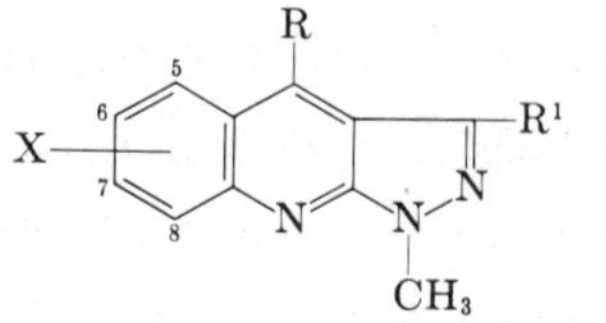

Compound no.	R	R^1	X	Interferon stimulation: Mouse MED (mg/kg)	A cells ($U/10^6$ cells): 3.1 μg/mg	A cells ($U/10^6$ cells): 0.78 μg/mg
1	$HN(CH_2)_3N(CH_3)_2$	CH_3	5,7-di-CH_3O	25 to 50	20	67
2	$HN(CH_2)_3N(CH_3)_2$	CH_3	6,7-di-CH_3	50	28	14
3	$HN(CH_2)_3N(CH_3)_2$	CH_3	6,7-di-CH_3O	50	27	10
4	$HN(CH_2)_3N(CH_3)_2$	CH_3	7-CH_3O	50	>95	57
5	$HN(CH_2)_3N(CH_3)_2$	CH_3	H	200	42	5
6	$HN(CH_2)_5N(CH_3)_2$	CH_3	H	200	41	10
7	$HN(CH_2)_6N(CH_3)_2$	CH_3	H	200	20	10
8	$HN(CH_2)_3N(CH_3)_2$	CH_3	7-CH_2OH	200	7	3.4
9	$HN(CH_2)_3N(CH_3)_2$	CH_3	6-C_2H_5	200	7	<1.5
10	$HN(CH_2)_3N(CH_3)_2$	CH_3	6-F	400	10	2
11	$HNCH_2CHOHCH_2N(C_2H_5)_2$	CH_3	7-Cl	400	16	7
12	S-$(CH_2)_3N(CH_3)_2$	CH_3	H	>50[a]	<1	<1
13	$HNCH_2$-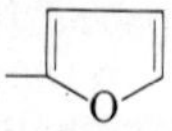	CH_3	H	>100[b]	<2	<2
14	$HN(CH_2)_3N(CH_3)_2$	CH_3	5-Cl,8-CH_3O	>100[c]	1.8	<1
15	$HN(CH_2)_3N(CH_3)_2$	CH_3	7-CF_3	>100[b]	3	2.7
16	$HN(CH_2)_3N(CH_3)_2$	CH_3	7-OH	>300	7	3.6
17	$HN(CH_2)_3N(CH_3)_2$	CH_3	7-CO_2CH_3	>300	40	14
18	$HN(CH_2)_3N(CH_3)_2$	CH_3	7-COOH	>300	<3	<3
19	$HN(CH_2)_3N(CH_3)_2$	Cl	H	>400	15	<3
20	NH_2	CH_3	H	>400	<3	<3
21	$HN(CH_2)_3N(CH_3)_2$	CH_3	6-$CH_3\overset{O}{\overset{\|}{C}}$-NH	>400	<3	<3
22	$HN(CH_2)_3N(CH_3)_2$	CH_3	5-NO_2	>400	<3	<3
23	H	CH_3	7-CH_3CH_2NH	>400	2	2
24	$HN(CH_2)_3N(CH_3)_2$	CH_3	5-NH_2	>400	3.4	2
25	H	CH_3	5-$NH(CH_2)_3N(CH_3)_2$	>400	1.6	1

[a] Toxic at 100 mg/kg.
[b] Toxic at 300 mg/kg.
[c] Toxic at 200 mg/kg.

The remaining 0.8 to 0.9 ml of unheated and heated mouse serum samples of compound 17 were lyophilized, and the residues were each extracted with chloroform containing 10% (vol/vol) triethylamine. As shown by vapor-phase chromatographic analysis, the unheated and heated serum samples contained 68 and 273 μg of unaltered ester, respectively. The residue from the unheated serum sample remaining after extraction was suspended in chloroform containing *N,N*-dimethylformamide, and this supernatant was shown to contain less than 1 μg of compound 17. The suspension was then acidified with 1 N hydrochloric acid and treated with diazomethane to convert any carboxylic acid present to the corresponding methyl ester. The mixture was evaporated, and the residue was extracted as above with chloroform-triethylamine. By vapor-phase chromatographic analysis, this residue now contained 215 μg of compound 17. Thus, active esterases in the unheated serum converted a significant proportion of the available compound 17 to the inactive 7-carboxyl derivative, compound 18. The 68 μg of unaltered ester detected in the unheated serum sample probably represented the

TABLE 2. *Effect of mouse serum on the ability of compound 17 to stimulate interferon production by mouse spleen A cells*

Sample	Dilution	Interferon production (U/10^6 cells)
Unheated mouse serum	1/30	Toxic
	1/90	Toxic
	1/270	20.8
Heated mouse serum	1/90	Toxic
	1/270	61.9
	1/810	10.7
Phosphate-buffered saline	1/270	12.3[a]
	1/810	12.3
	1/2,430	2.9

[a] This sample was partially toxic to the spleen A cells.

amount by which the hydrolytic capacity of the esterases was exceeded. In another study, we found that 300 μg of compound 17 was completely inactivated by the enzymatic activity contained in 0.5 ml of unheated mouse serum.

The results support our general conclusion from prior studies that the spleen A cell, possibly representative of a certain class of fixed macrophages, is readily stimulated by BL-20803 to produce interferon. This observation is now extended to other active, structurally related compounds. The A cell response appears to be a more sensitive indication of a compound's interferon-inducing potential than the intact mouse, obviously due to the optimum conditions in the in vitro culture system for unimpeded contact between compound and target cell. The structural specificity of the BL-20803 series of compounds is also emphasized by the loss of activity resulting from the relatively small change in the substituent grouping when the 7-methyl ester is converted to the 7-carboxyl derivative.

LITERATURE CITED

1. **Crenshaw, R. R., G. M. Luke, and P. Siminoff.** 1976. Interferon inducing activities of derivatives of 1,3-dimethyl-4-(3-dimethylaminopropylamino)-1H-pyrazolo [3,4-b] quinoline and related compounds. J. Med. Chem. **19**:262–275.
2. **Siminoff, P.** 1975. In vivo and in vitro stimulation of mouse spleen leukocytes by BL-20803, a low-molecular-weight interferon inducer. Infect. Immun. **12**:1051–1057.
3. **Siminoff, P.** 1976. Target cells for interferon induction by BL-20803. J. Infect. Dis. **133**(Suppl.):A37–A42.

ANTIMICROBIAL AGENTS AND CHEMOTHERAPY, Mar. 1977, p. 574-576 Vol. 11, No. 13

Printed in U.S.A.

Cerulenin-Inhibited Cells of *Staphylococcus aureus* Resume Growth When Supplemented with Either a Saturated or an Unsaturated Fatty Acid

ROBERT A. ALTENBERN

Pathology Division, United States Army Medical Research Infectious Diseases, Fort Detrick, Frederick, Maryland 21701

Received for publication 5 October 1976

In the presence of an inhibitory concentration of cerulenin, cells of *Staphylococcus aureus* can resume growth when supplemented with either a saturated or an unsaturated fatty acid. A requirement for both types of acids for growth could not be demonstrated.

The antibiotic cerulenin has been shown to inhibit, reversibly, fatty acid biosynthesis by interfering with the action of β-ketoacyl-acyl carrier protein synthetase (4). Several studies (5, 8) have demonstrated that both a saturated fatty acid (SFA) and an unsaturated fatty acid (UFA) or branched-chain saturated acid are required to reverse the inhibition by cerulenin of either *Escherichia coli* or *Bacillus subtilis*. Although the minimal inhibitory concentration of cerulenin for *Staphylococcus aureus* (6) and the failure of cerulenin to block induction of tetracycline resistance in *S. aureus* (2) have been reported, no data on restoration of growth of *S. aureus* cells inhibited by cerulenin have appeared. In this article, it is shown that although an SFA and a UFA together do promote growth of cerulenin-inhibited cells of *S. aureus*, single supplementation with certain SFAs or UFAs permits resumption of growth in the presence of cerulenin.

S. aureus ATCC 14458 was grown in NAK medium (1) at 37°C on a shaker for 24 h. Tubes (18 by 150 mm) containing 5 ml of NAK medium plus graded amounts of cerulenin (Makor Chemicals, Ltd., Jerusalem, Israel) and supplemented with various concentrations of SFAs and/or UFAs were inoculated with 0.05 ml of the 24-h culture. The tubes were then incubated at an angle on a shaker at 37°C. At 30-min intervals, the absorbance at 600 nm was measured on a Coleman Jr. spectrophotometer to determine mass doubling time(s). Subsequently, the absorbance of a 1:5 dilution in water of 21-h cultures measured the final growth density. There was no attempt made to determine colony-forming units per milliliter during exponential growth or at the final density attained. It is possible that under the varied fatty acid supplementation reported in this note, cell size and cell viability may affect the number of colony-forming units per unit of optical density. Cerulenin and fatty acids were added as ethanolic solutions. All fatty acids were purchased from Sigma Chemical Co., St. Louis, Mo.

Preliminary experiments (Fig. 1) showed that the minimal inhibitory concentration of cerulenin for this strain of *S. aureus* was about 100 μg/ml, in good agreement with 100 μg/ml reported by Omura et al. (6) for another strain and 125 μg/ml used by Chopra (2).

The effect of graded amounts of oleic acid in the presence of several constant levels of pal-

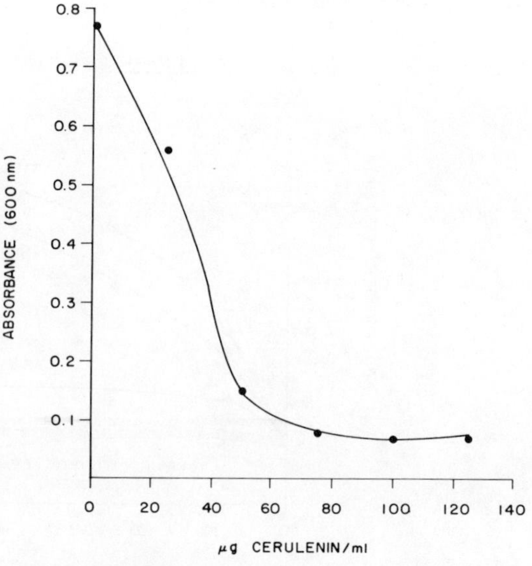

FIG. 1. *Final growth density of a 1:5 dilution of S. aureus in the presence of various concentrations of cerulenin.*

mitic acid on final growth density of *S. aureus* strain 14458, in NAK medium containing 100 μg of cerulenin per ml, is presented in Fig. 2. The concentration levels of palmitic acid were 8, 24, and 40 μg/ml. Oleic acid was added so that the ratios of SFAs to UFAs (micrograms per milliliter) were 25, 8, 2, and 1 at each level of the palmitic. There was no evidence in this and other experiments that there was an optimal ratio for growth. It is clear that with a constant level of palmitate, oleic acid in increasing amounts promoted greater growth. Similar experiments with palmitic plus elaidic acids or stearic plus oleic acids yielded nearly identical results. Of interest was the observation that palmitic acid alone supported considerable growth, and that the final growth density was a function of palmitic acid concentration.

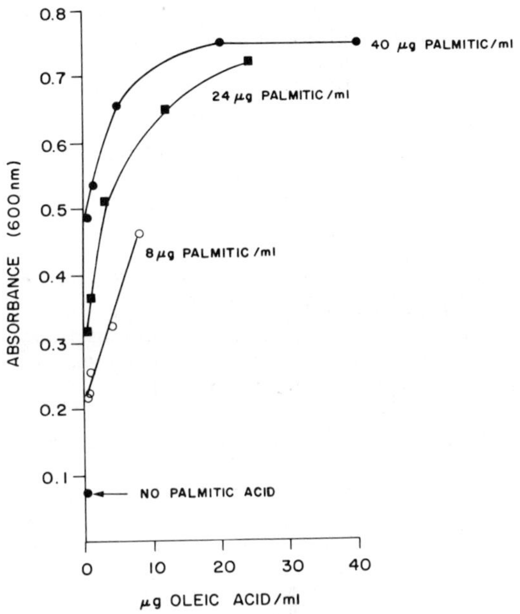

FIG. 2. *Growth of S. aureus in cerulenin medium containing 8, 24, or 40 μg of palmitic acid per ml and graded concentrations of oleic acid.*

Consequently, the ability of various SFAs or UFAs to support growth of *S. aureus* in NAK medium containing 100 μg of cerulenin per ml was determined (Fig. 3). Only palmitic and stearic acids of the SFAs, with the possible exception of arachidic acid, allowed appreciable growth in the presence of cerulenin. Petroselinic, elaidic, and oleic acids were the only UFAs stimulating growth. Such UFAs as arachidonic, palmitoleic, and docosahexaenoic acid were growth inhibitory in the lowest concentration tested (1.6 μg/ml).

Determination of mass doubling times from regular measurements of absorbance during exponential growth showed that most rapid growth was supported by palmitic acid, followed by stearic, arachidic, and the UFAs (Table 1). It appears that only those acids with a 16-, 18-, or 20-carbon chain were effective.

In almost all respects, the response of *S. aureus* to cerulenin inhibition closely matched results obtained with *E. coli* (5) and *B. subtilis* (8). For *S. aureus*, inoculation of media containing 100 μg of cerulenin per ml resulted in a

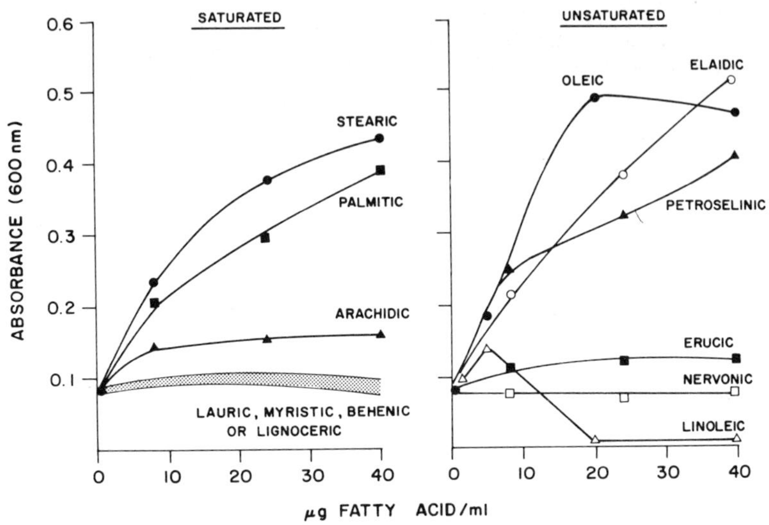

FIG. 3. *Support of growth of S. aureus in cerulenin medium by single supplementation with SFAs or UFAs.*

TABLE 1. *Mass doubling time for S. aureus growing in medium containing cerulenin and certain fatty acids*[a]

Fatty acid	Mass doubling time (min) in fatty acid (μg/ml):					
	1.6	5.0	8.0	20	24	40
Palmitic			82		70	76
Stearic			128		103	85
Arachidic			115		115	115
Elaidic			133		135	128
Petroselinic			133		154	154
Oleic	153	155		130		150

[a] Mass doubling time in unsupplemented medium was 42 min.

slow increase in absorbance up to about 3 h of incubation, at which time all growth ceased. The presence of effective fatty acids allowed growth at a maximum rate of 50 to 60% of the rate in cerulenin- and fatty acid-free medium.

It is concluded that *S. aureus* can grow in the minimal inhibitory concentration of cerulenin when supplemented with either palmitic or stearic acid and can dispense with the expected requirement for a UFA. The C_{15}, C_{17}, and C_{19} iso or ante-iso fatty acids comprise at least 85% of the total fatty acids of the membrane phospholipids of *S. aureus* grown under commonly used conditions (7) and seem to confer the desired degree of fluidity to the membrane lipids, since the amount of straight-chain SFAs or UFAs is minimal. It is estimated that *E. coli* requires for growth a minimum of 10% of the total fatty acid supplement as a SFA or UFA (3). Such a requirement cannot be demonstrated for *S. aureus* with the spectrum of acids used in this study. It is possible that *S. aureus* can carry out oxidative desaturation of palmitic or stearic acids to satisfy a hidden requirement for UFA or, conversely, that UFAs can be reduced to furnish a saturated acid. However, identical results were obtained when incubation was carried out statically and without aeration, although final growth densities were considerably lower than those for aerated (shaken) cultures. In any event, *S. aureus* does not display a stringent requirement for an exogenous supply of both an SFA and a UFA for growth in the presence of cerulenin.

LITERATURE CITED

1. **Altenbern, R. A.** 1976. Enterotoxin B formation by fermentation mutants of *Staphylococcus aureus*. Can. J. Microbiol. 22:182–188.
2. **Chopra, I.** 1975. Induction of tetracycline resistance in *Staphylococcus aureus* in the absence of lipid synthesis. J. Gen. Microbiol. **91:**433–436.
3. **Cronan, J. E., Jr., and E. P. Gelmann.** 1975. Physical properties of membrane lipids: biological relevance and regulation. Bacteriol. Rev. **39:**232–256.
4. **D'Agnolo, G., I. S. Rosenfeld, J. Amaya, S. Omura, and P. R. Vagelos.** 1973. Inhibition of fatty acid synthesis by the antibiotic cerulenin. Specific inactivation of β-ketoacyl-acyl carrier protein synthetase. Biochim. Biophys. Acta **326:**155–166.
5. **Goldberg, I., J. R. Walker, and K. Bloch.** 1973. Inhibition of lipid synthesis in *Escherichia coli* cells by the antibiotic cerulenin. Antimicrob. Agents Chemother. **3:**549–554.
6. **Omura, S., M. Katagiri, J. Awaya, T. Furukawa, I. Umezawa, N. Oi, M. Mizoguchi, B. Aoki, and M. Shindo.** 1974. Relationship between the structures of fatty acid amide derivatives and their antimicrobial activities. Antimicrob. Agents Chemother. **6:**207–215.
7. **Theodore, T. S., and C. Panos.** 1973. Protein and fatty acid composition of mesosomal vesicles and plasma membranes of *Staphylococcus aureus*. J. Bacteriol. **116:**571–576.
8. **Wille, W., E. Eisenstadt, and K. Willecke.** 1975. Inhibition of de novo fatty acid synthesis by the antibiotic cerulenin in *Bacillus subtilis*: effects on citrate-Mg^{2+} transport and synthesis of macromolecules. Antimicrob. Agents Chemother. **8:**231–237.

ANTIMICROBIAL AGENTS AND CHEMOTHERAPY, Apr. 1977, p. 577-579 Vol. 11, No. 4

In Vitro Activity of Cinoxacin, Ampicillin, and Chloramphenicol Against *Shigella* and Nontyphoid *Salmonella*

ETHAN RUBINSTEIN* AND BRACHA SHAINBERG

Sheba Medical Center, Tel-Aviv University, Sackler School of Medicine, Tel-Hashomer, Israel

Received for publication 1 November 1976

The in vitro antibacterial activity of cinoxacin was compared with that of ampicillin and chloramphenicol against 26 strains of nontyphoid *Salmonella* and 44 strains of *Shigella*. Cinoxacin was found to have a lower minimal inhibitory concentration than ampicillin and chloramphenicol against all *Salmonella* and *Shigella sonnei* strains. Cinoxacin had minimal inhibitory concentrations similar to those of chloramphenicol but lower than those of ampicillin against *Shigella flexneri* and *S. boydii* strains.

Cinoxacin, 1-ethyl-4(1H)-oxo-(1,3)diaxdo(4,5-g)cinnoline-3-carboxylic acid, is a new antibacterial agent (6) with activity similar to that of nalidixic acid and oxolonic acid, which are effective in vitro against *Salmonella* and *Shigella* strains (1, 4).

Because of the emergence of chloramphenicol- and ampicillin-resistant *Shigella* and *Salmonella* strains, we tested cinoxacin against recent isolates of nontyphoid *Salmonella* and *Shigella* strains and compared its activity with that of ampicillin and chloramphenicol.

MATERIALS AND METHODS

Twenty-six strains of nontyphoid *Salmonella* and 44 strains of *Shigella* isolated recently in Israel were tested. The strains were typed by the *Shigella* and *Salmonella* reference laboratories of the Ministry of Health. Included were nine strains of *Salmonella typhimurium*, five strains of *S. heidelberg*, four strains of *S. anatum*, two strains of *S. dublin*, and one strain each of *S. carmel*, *S. sofia*, *S. muenchen*, *S. newport*, *S. blackley*, and *S. lille*. The *Shigella* strains included: 12 *S. sonnei*, 14 *S. flexneri*, 18 *S. boydii*. All strains were kept in lyophilized form. Organisms were incubated overnight at 37°C in Mueller-Hinton broth before testing.

Antibacterial activity was determined by antibiotic dilution methods performed in Mueller-Hinton agar by use of a Steers replicator device (5). The inoculum used was a 10^{-2} dilution of an overnight broth culture of each strain tested. The minimal inhibitory concentration (MIC) was defined as the lowest concentration of the drug that inhibited macroscopic colonial growth.

Stock solutions containing 1,000 μg of cinoxacin or 1,000 μg of ampicillin per ml were prepared in phosphate buffer (pH 7). Chloramphenicol was dissolved in dimethyl sulfoxide and water to a concentration of 500 μg/ml. All stock solutions were stored at −20°C and used within 2 weeks.

RESULTS

The mean MIC of cinoxacin for inhibition of *Salmonella typhimurium* was 2.8 μg/ml (range, 1.5 to 4.5 μg/ml). The mean MIC of ampicillin was 51.2 μg/ml (range, 2.5 to >100 μg/ml). Four of the nine strains tested were resistant to 100 μg of ampicillin per ml. The mean MIC of chloramphenicol was 14.8 μg/ml (range, 3.1 to 50 μg/ml). The mean MIC for *S. heidelberg* was 2 μg/ml (range, 1 to 3.5 μg/ml). The mean MIC of ampicillin was 22 μg/ml (range, 2.5 to >100 μg/ml). One strain was resistant to 100 μg of ampicillin per ml. The mean MIC of chloramphenicol was 28.5 μg/ml (range, 0.35 to >100 μg/ml). One strain was resistant to 100 μg of chloramphenicol per ml. The mean MIC of cinoxacin against *S. anatum* was 2.5 μg/ml; that of ampicillin was 38.12 μg/ml, and that of chloramphenicol was 33.5 μg/ml. In this group there was one isolate resistant to ampicillin and one resistant to chloramphenicol.

Of the group including *S. dublin*, *S. carmel*, *S. sofia*, *S. muenchen*, *S. newport*, *S. blackley*, and *S. lille*, the mean MIC of cinoxacin was 3 μg/ml. The mean MIC of ampicillin was 28.75 μg/ml, and that of chloramphenicol was 11.87 μg/ml. The cumulative percentage of all *Salmonella* isolates inhibited by cinoxacin, ampicillin, and chloramphenicol is shown in Fig. 1.

Whereas nine of our *Salmonella* strains were resistant to 100 μg of ampicillin or chloramphenicol per ml, all strains were susceptible to 4.5 μg or less of cinoxacin per ml. Except for one strain each of *S. heidelberg* and *S. sofia*, against which the MIC of chloramphenicol was lower than that of cinoxacin, for all strains tested, the MIC of cinoxacin was lower than that of either ampicillin or chloramphenicol. The mean MIC of cinoxacin against all *Salmonella* strains was 2.8 μg/ml, whereas that of ampicillin was 36.5 μg/ml and that of chloramphenicol was 19.5 μg/ml.

***Shigella* strains.** The mean MIC of cinoxacin against *Shigella sonnei* was 1.31 μg/ml (range, 0.7 to 3.1 μg/ml). The mean MIC of ampicillin was 14.7 μg/ml (range, 4.5 to 25 μg/ml). The mean MIC of chloramphenicol was 19 μg/ml (range, 0.7 to >100 μg/ml). Two strains were resistant to at least 100 μg of chloramphenicol per ml.

The mean MIC of cinoxacin against *S. flexneri* was 1.34 (range, 0.7 to 1.5 μg/ml). The mean MIC of ampicillin was 10.7 μg/ml (range, 1.5 to 25 μg/ml). The mean MIC of chloramphenicol was 2.24 μg/ml (range, 0.5 to 4.5 μg/ml). The mean MIC of cinoxacin against *S. boydii* was 2.27 μg/ml (range, 1 to 2.5 μg/ml). The mean MIC of ampicillin was 29.3 μg/ml (range, 7.5 to >100 μg/ml). Three strains were resistant to 100 μg of ampicillin per ml. The mean MIC of chloramphenicol was 2.62 μg/ml (range, 0.7 to 3.1 μg/ml).

The cumulative percentage of all *Shigella* strains inhibited by cinoxacin, ampicillin, and chloramphenicol is shown in Fig. 2. The mean MIC of cinoxacin against all 44 strains of *Shigella* was 1.71 μg/ml, that of ampicillin was

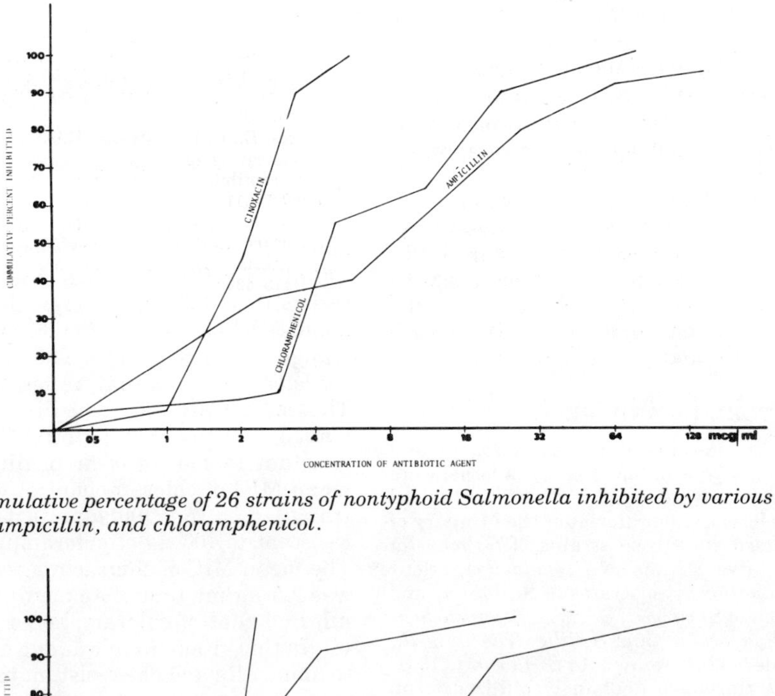

FIG. 1. *Cumulative percentage of 26 strains of nontyphoid Salmonella inhibited by various concentrations of cinoxacin, ampicillin, and chloramphenicol.*

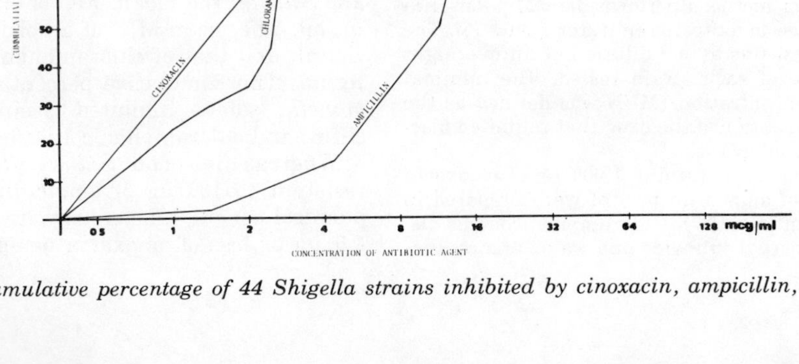

FIG. 2. *Cumulative percentage of 44 Shigella strains inhibited by cinoxacin, ampicillin, and chloramphenicol.*

12.4 μg/ml, and that of chloramphenicol was 6.9 μg/ml. None of the strains was resistant to cinoxacin, whereas five strains were resistant to 100 μg of either ampicillin or chloramphenicol per ml. For nine strains of *Shigella*, the MIC of cinoxacin was equal to or higher than that of either chloramphenicol or ampicillin.

DISCUSSION

Our results demonstrate that cinoxacin is significantly more active in vitro than ampicillin and chloramphenicol against *Salmonella typhimurium*, *S. heidelberg,* and *S. anatum* and against a variety of other *Salmonella* species. Cinoxacin is significantly more active in vitro than either ampicillin or chloramphenicol against *Shigella sonnei*, but cinoxacin and chloramphenicol are equally active against strains of *S. flexneri* and *S. boydii*. Ampicillin was less active than chloramphenicol and cinoxacin against *S. flexneri* and *S. boydii*.

The recent increase in *Shigella* and *Salmonella* strains resistant to chloramphenicol and ampicillin requires new agents active against these pathogens.

Moorhead and Parry found an 88.5% cure rate among patients with *S. sonnei* dysentery treated with nalidixic acid (2). Haltalin et al. (1) found nalidixic acid to be inferior to ampicillin in the treatment of severe shigellosis susceptible to ampicillin, but recommended nalidixic acid for treatment of ampicillin-resistant shigella dysentery. We believe that because of the favorable in vitro activity of cinoxacin against *Shigella* and *Salmonella* strains and because of the paucity of its side effects (3), clinical trials with cinoxacin are warranted in cases of shigella gastroenteritis.

LITERATURE CITED

1. **Haltalin, K. C., J. D. Nelson, and H. T. Kusmiesz.** 1973. Comparative efficacy of nalidix acid and ampicillin for severe shigellosis. Arch. Dis. Child. 48:305–312.
2. **Moorhead, P. J., and A. E. Parry.** 1965. Treatment of sonne dysentery. Br. Med. J. 2:913–916.
3. **Panwalka, A. P., H. Giamarellou, and G. J. Jackson.** 1976. Efficacy of cinoxacin in urinary tract infections. Antimicrob. Agents Chemother. 9:502–505.
4. **Sanford, J. P., N. N. Linh, E. Kutscher, K. Arnold, and K. Gould.** 1976. Oxolonic acid in the treatment of typhoid fever due to chloramphenicol-resistant *Salmonella typhi*. Antimicrob. Agents Chemother. 9:387–392.
5. **Steers, E., E. L. Plotz, and B. S. Groves.** 1959. Inocula replicating apparatus for routine testing of bacterial susceptibility to antibiotics. Antibiot. Chemother. 9:307–311.
6. **Wick, W. F., D. A. Preston, W. A. White, and R. S. Gordee.** 1973. Compound 64716, a new synthetic antibacterial agent. Antimicrob. Agents Chemother. 4:415–420.

ANTIMICROBIAL AGENTS AND CHEMOTHERAPY, Apr. 1977, p. 580-584 Vol. 11, No. 4
 Printed in U.S.A.

Effect of Antibiotics on Chemotaxis of Human Leukocytes

ARNE FORSGREN* and DAVID SCHMELING[1]

Department of Clinical Bacteriology, University of Lund, General Hospital, S-214 01 Malmö, Sweden

Received for publication 27 September 1976

The effect of 20 different antibiotics on chemotaxis by human neutrophils was studied. Human leukocytes incubated with chloramphenicol, rifampin, sodium fusidate, and tetracyclines in vitro showed markedly depressed migration. The mechanisms by which these antibiotics affect leukotaxis are discussed.

Leukotaxis may be defined as the directional migration of leukocytes toward a chemotactic stimulus and is believed to represent the means by which a massive influx of polymorphonuclear leukocytes occurs in an area of inflammation (30). The attraction of polymorphonuclear leukocytes is brought about by a series of effector substances involving complement components (27), bacterial culture filtrates (14, 28), extracts from the leukocytes themselves (6), and tissues infected with virus (25, 31).

The possible role of drugs on the inflammatory system has received increasing attention. Martin et al. (18, 19) recently reported an inhibitory effect of tetracycline on leukocyte migration, which was discovered during a serial study of leukotaxis using human leukocytes and sera. The purpose of the present study was to extend earlier studies on the effects of antibiotics other than tetracyclines on the chemotaxis of human neutrophils.

MATERIALS AND METHODS

Antibiotics. A wide range of antibiotics was tested: sulfametoxazol (Kabi AB, Sweden, batch 10708-52), trimethoprim (Syraprim, Burroughs Wellcome Co., batch 55034), nalidixic acid (Winthrop Laboratories, batch K1 1770), nitrofurantoin (Pharmacia Fine Chemicals, Sweden, batch T 8533), ampicillin (aminobenzylpenicillin, Astra AB, Sweden, batch 175), benzylpenicillin (Astra AB, Sweden, batch 61062-01), carboxybenzylpenicillin sodium (Fugacillin, Astra AB, Sweden, batch 50428-02), cefazolin sodium (Lilly Research Centre Ltd., batch 7 KK43), cephalothin sodium (Lilly Research Centre Ltd., batch 215-DJ2-1), doxycycline hyclate (Pfizer, batch 312-58709), lymecycline (Carlo Erba, Italy, batch 6 D 5154 9764), tetracycline chloride (Dumex, batch 308296), gentamicin sulfate (San Bolagen AB, Sweden, batch 6694), kanamycin (Ferrosan, Sweden, batch 03205 Z9), chloramphenicol succinate (Carlo Erba, Italy, batch 730767), erythromycin (Upjohn, batch 2324 W), clindamycin hyclate (Cleocin, Upjohn, batch U-21251 FIEK 55), rifampin (Ferrosan, Sweden, batch 4422:T) and sodium fusidate (Leo Pharmaceutical Products, Denmark, batch 22194). Fresh stock solutions were prepared for all experiments, both in water, for use in the agarose medium, and in tissue culture medium 199, for preincubation with leukocytes.

Leukocytes. Heparinized venous blood was drawn from healthy volunteers. Erythrocytes were allowed to sediment by gravity at room temperature for a period of about 1 h. The leukocyte-rich plasma was then removed, and the concentration of polymorphonuclear leukocytes was adjusted to 10^7/ml of plasma.

Chemotaxis studies. Leukocyte chemotaxis was studied by a modification of the method described by Nelson et al. (21). Briefly, agarose plates were prepared containing 0.5 ml of 10× tissue culture medium 199 (Flow Laboratories), 0.15 mmol of HEPES (*N*-2-hydroxyethyl piperazine-*N'*-2-ethanesulfonic acid buffer (Schwarz/Mann, Div. of Becton Dickinson & Co., Orangeburg, N. Y.), 0.5 ml of 5% agarose (Litex, Glostrup, Denmark), and the desired concentration of the antibiotics to be tested. The pH of the medium was adjusted to 7.4 before addition of the agarose. Five milliliters of the agarose solution was then transferred to a tissue culture dish (60 by 15 mm; 3002, Falcon, Oxnard, Calif.) and allowed to harden. Wells with a diameter of 3 mm and spaced 3 mm apart were cut. Each plate contained five series of three wells.

In most experiments, 0.5 ml of a plasma suspension containing 10^7 polymorphonuclear leukocytes per ml was preincubated with 0.5 ml of the various antibiotic solutions in 1× tissue culture medium 199 (National Bacteriological Laboratory, Stockholm, Sweden) for 30 min in a shaking water bath at 37°C. After centrifugation for 10 min at 200 × *g*, the cell pellet was resuspended in a small portion of the supernatant to give a final concentration of 10^8 polymorphonuclear leukocytes per ml.

Cell suspensions preincubated with antibiotics were added to the middle wells in three of the five well sets in the agarose plates with the corresponding concentration of antibiotics. The remaining two middle wells were filled with 10 μl of plasma, containing 10^8 polymorphonuclear leukocytes per ml, which had been kept free of any antibiotic contact. The five inner wells were all filled with 10 μl of a chemotactically active *Escherichia coli* culture filtrate (28), and the outer wells were filled with 10 μl

[1] Present address: Department of Pediatrics, University of Minnesota Medical School, Minneapolis, MN 55455.

of 1× tissue culture medium. Incubation was carried out for a period of 3 h at 37°C in a humidified atmosphere containing 5% CO_2 in air. The plates were then fixed and stained, and the chemotaxis was quantitated by measurement of a greatly enlarged projection of the migration patterns; i.e., the number of millimeters from the wells was measured.

Results were calculated as percentages of control values that were obtained using cells preincubated with tissue culture medium without antibiotics and tested for chemotactic capacity in plates lacking antibiotic content but otherwise identical to the test plates. Plate variation was checked by comparing migration zones for the cells that had not been preincubated with an antibiotic. The reproducibility of the method was determined: 100 ± 7.78 (standard deviation); 0.9431 (standard error).

RESULTS

Rifampin. Figure 1 shows the result of one typical experiment out of five. When normal human polymorphonuclear leukocytes were incubated with rifampin for 30 min and then placed in an agarose gel not containing rifampin, the directional migration (leukotaxis) toward an *E. coli* filtrate was significantly inhibited and, at a rifampin concentration of 25 μg per ml, the chemotactic movement after 3 h of incubation was only 50% of that obtained with cells that had been preincubated with tissue culture medium without antibiotics. When rifampin was included in the agarose gel used for the chemotaxis experiment in the same concentration as in the medium used for preincubation, an even more pronounced effect was seen and, at a rifampin concentration of 2.5 μg per ml, the chemotaxis movement was 50% of the control value obtained with cells that had been preincubated in tissue culture medium and tested in a gel without antibiotics.

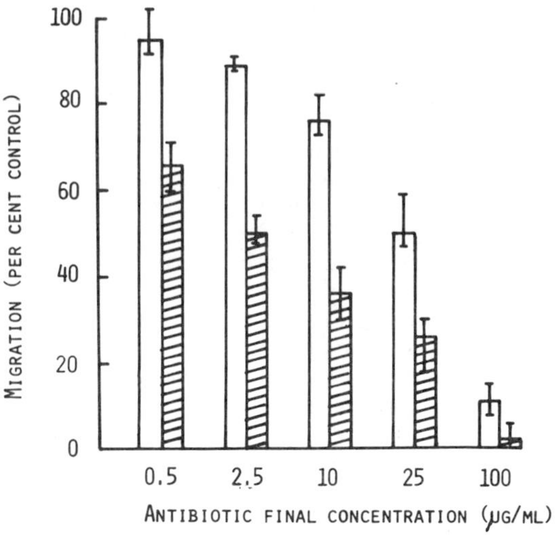

FIG. 1. *Chemotaxis of normal human polymorphonuclear leukocytes preincubated with rifampin and then concentrated and placed in agarose gel (mean and range of three determinations). Open bars indicate the chemotaxis in gels that were free of antibiotics, and the shaded bars represent the chemotaxis of neutrophils in antibiotic-containing gels. Symbols: (□) cells preincubated with rifampin, (▨) cells preincubated with and placed in gels containing rifampin.*

Tetracyclines. Figure 2 demonstrates the effect of three different tetracyclines on chemotaxis. The results signify a series of experiments using polymorphonuclear leukocytes from different healthy volunteers. The neutrophils were preincubated with the drugs and then added to chemotaxis plates containing the corresponding antibiotic concentration. At therapeutically attainable concentrations, the effect of tetracyclines was slight. However, at higher concentrations (25 to 100 μg/ml), the effect was striking, especially with doxycycline, for which (at a concentration of 100 μg per ml) the neutrophils did not move on the chemotaxis plate. Control cells not preincubated with antibiotics but placed in agarose plates containing antibiotics showed the same degree of migration as those incubated in antibiotic-free plates. This shows that the preincubation with tetracyclines was necessary for an effect on chemotaxis and also that the effect detected was an effect on the cells and not merely an effect of tetracyclines on the agarose plate.

Chloramphenicol and fusidic acid. Figure 3 shows a representative experiment with chlor-

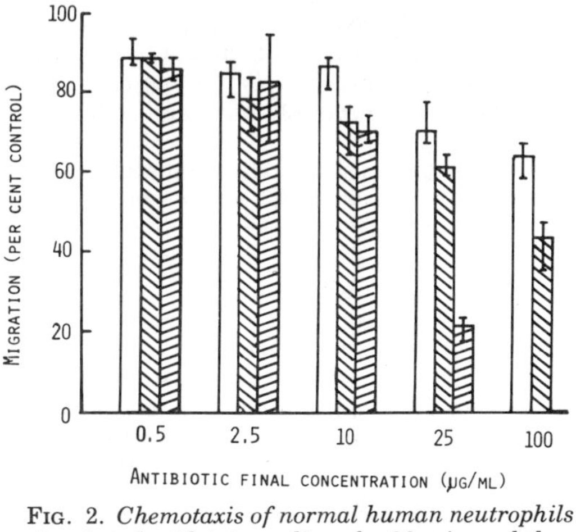

FIG. 2. *Chemotaxis of normal human neutrophils preincubated with tetracyclines for 30 min and then concentrated and tested in agarose gels containing the same concentration of the corresponding antibiotic (mean and range of three determinations). Symbols: (□) tetracycline chloride, (▧) lymecycline, (▨) doxycycline.*

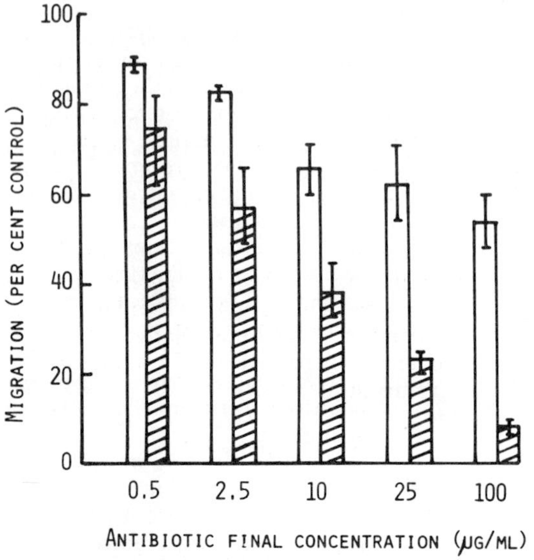

FIG. 3. *Effects of chloramphenicol and fusidic acid on chemotaxis of normal human neutrophils that were preincubated with different concentrations of the drugs and then tested in plates containing the corresponding antibiotic concentrations (mean and range of three determinations). Symbols: (□) chloramphenicol, (▨) fusidic acid.*

amphenicol and sodium fusidate similar to that described above for tetracyclines. The figure reflects a very strong depressive effect of sodium fusidate on neutrophil chemotaxis and, at a level of 10 μg per ml, the chemotactic migration was only 38% of control values. The corresponding figure for chloramphenicol was 66%. At higher concentrations, a more marked effect was shown with both drugs and, at 25 and 100 μg per ml, the observed chemotaxis values were 62 and 54, respectively, 23 and 8% of control values for chloramphenicol and sodium fusidate.

Other antibiotics. For the remaining antibiotics tested, chemotaxis values were generally within 15% of the control values, a range that we considered nonindicative of any significant depressive effect upon chemotactic migration. Exceptions included a slightly depressive effect by clindamycin, erythromycin, and nitrofurantoin in the highest concentration (100 μg/ml) tested. For penicillins and cephalosporins, no appreciable effect on chemotaxis could be detected. Nor was there any effect of sulfa, Syraprim, gentamicin, kanamycin, colistin, or nalidixic acid.

DISCUSSION

Chemotaxis and phagocytosis are both important steps in the major defence mechanism against pyogenic infections. Very few studies on the effect of antibiotics on chemotaxis of polymorphonuclear leukocytes have been reported (18, 19).

Rifampin is of special interest, due to its capacity to penetrate leukocytes and destroy intracellular microorganisms in vitro and probably in vivo (17). Hoeprich et al. (13) previously demonstrated that rifampin did not interfere with phagocytosis and intracellular killing. However, Urbanitz et al. (26), when comparing the function of monocytes from 15 patients with tuberculosis under treatment with rifampin, detected a significantly impaired phagocytosis of immunoglobulin G-coated erythrocytes. Several authors have reported on the influence of rifampin upon immunological reactions (11, 23, 24).

In the present study, a significant effect of rifampin on the chemotaxis of human polymorphonuclear leukocytes was obtained. The effect was most pronounced when human cells, which had been preincubated with rifampin for 30 min, were applied in a gel plate containing the same concentration of the drug, but cells that were preincubated with rifampin and then applied to a gel without antibiotics were also significantly inhibited. Rifampin has been shown to inhibit deoxyribonucleic acid-dependent ribonucleic acid (RNA) polymerase activity (12) in susceptible bacterial cells. However, the basis for the effect of rifampin on chemotaxis, as reported in this paper, is unknown.

Many reports are available concerning the effects of tetracycline on the phagocytic system (1, 13, 20). Most recently, in a study by Forsgren et al. (8), it was demonstrated that polymorphonuclear leukocytes incubated in vitro with tetracycline hydrochloride or doxycycline showed a decreased capacity to phagocytize yeast and bacteria. Furthermore, leukocytes harvested from healthy volunteers after ingestion of tetracycline also demonstrated decreased phagocytic capacity. By scanning electron microscopy, Gnarpe and Leslie (10) could detect distinct surface alterations in human leukocytes; they noted that bacteria adhered to, but were not ingested by, the leukocytes when doxycycline was present. Gnarpe and Leslie (10) attributed the inhibitory effect of tetracycline to antibiotic complex binding of membrane-bound divalent cations. Those ions are necessary for both the phagocytic and chemotactic function of polymorphonuclear leukocytes (3, 9, 32).

Martin et al. (18, 19) reported on inhibiting effect of tetracyclines on leukotaxis. The present study confirms their findings. The incubation of human blood cells with tetracyclines results in considerably higher concentrations intracellularly than in the surrounding medium (22). The differences in ability to impair chemotaxis between doxycycline in high concentrations and other tetracyclines might be due to the fact that doxycycline is more lipid soluble (5) than the other tetracyclines.

Earlier studies on the effect of chloramphenicol on phagocytic cells have failed to show any effect at therapeutic concentrations of the drug. Lehrer (16), Downey and Pisana (7), and Odegaard and Lamvik (33) could only detect an effect on phagocytosis by chloramphenicol at very high concentrations of the drug. Kernbaum (15), however, reports no depression of phagocytosis by human neutrophils with high concentrations (1 mg/ml) of chloramphenicol. However, it has been suggested that chloramphenicol inhibits antibody production by interfering with some early phase of the response, and it was hypothesized that the interference involves messenger RNA (2). The basis for the effect of chloramphenicol on human neutrophil leukocytes, as described in this paper, has not been further studied, but it seems to be most pronounced for concentrations of the drug that are above therapeutic levels.

Fusidic acid is, like chloramphenicol, an inhibitor of protein synthesis. Fusidic acid inhibits the transfer of transfer-RNA-bound amino acids to ribosomes. In the chemotaxis system, used by us, sodium fusidate had a pronounced effect on chemotaxis, even in therapeutic levels. The basis for this effect warrants further studies.

Carruthers (4) reported that drugs which inhibit RNA and protein synthesis, such as puromycin at 10^3 M and actinomycin D at 10 μg per ml, had a slight inhibitory effect on random migration of neutrophils but a complete inhibitory effect on directional migration. It is of great interest that all antibiotics tested in this investigation with a strong inhibitory effect on human leukotaxis have an inhibitory effect on either transcription or protein synthesis. Thus, it is possible that a protein(s) necessary for the chemotactic response is synthesized on contact of the cell with chemotactic factors and that this synthesis can be blocked at the level of transcription or later, thus blocking the response of the cell.

Clindamycin and erythromycin, which also inhibit protein synthesis, seemingly had no effect on the chemotaxis of polymorphonuclear leukocytes, except at higher concentrations, where a decreasing effect was seen. As might be expected, no effect was found when the beta-lactam antibiotics benzylpenicillin, ampicillin, Fugacillin, cefazolin, and cephalothin were tested. Penicillin G was tested in phagocytosis systems by Downey and Pisana (7) and Kernbaum (15) without any detectable effect. Gentamycin and trimethoprim have been reported by Kernbaum (15) to have no detectable effect on phagocytosis. Nor could we detect any effect on chemotaxis. Sulfonamides have been reported to inhibit myeloperoxidase-mediated bactericidal reactions of polymorphonuclear leukocytes. However, there have been no reports on the effect of sulfonamides on phagocytic uptake and chemotaxis. This study reveals no effect of sulfonamides on chemotaxis. Nor could any effect on chemotaxis be detected for nalidixic acid and nitrofurantoin.

ACKNOWLEDGMENTS

This work was supported by grants from the Swedish Medical Research Council.

LITERATURE CITED

1. **Altura, B. M., S. G. Hershey, M. Ali, and C. Thaw.** 1966. Influence of tetracycline on phagocytosis, infection and resistance to experimental shock: relationship to microcirculation. J. Reticuloendothel. Soc. **3**:447–457.
2. **Ambrose, C. T., and A. H. Coons.** 1963. Studies on antibody production. VII. Inhibitory effect of chloramphenicol on synthesis of antibody in tissue culture. J. Exp. Med. **117**:1075–1088.
3. **Bryant, R. E.** 1969. The effect of divalent cation depletion on phagocytosis of staphylococci. Yale J. Biol. Med. **41**:303–310.
4. **Carruthers, B. M.** 1967. Leukocyte mobility. II. Effect of absence of glucose in the medium: effect of presence of deoxyglucose, dinitrophenyl, puromycin, actinomycin D and trypsin on the response to chemotactic substance: effect of segregation of cells from chemotactic substance. Can. J. Physiol. Pharmacol. **45**:269–280.
5. **Colazzi, J. L., and P. R. Klink.** 1969. pH-partition behavior of tetracyclines. J. Pharm. Sci. **58**:1184–1189.
6. **Cornely, H. P.** 1966. Reversal of chemotaxis in vitro and chemotactic activity of leukocyte fractions. Proc. Soc. Exp. Biol. Med. **122**:831–835.
7. **Downey, R. J., and J. C. Pisana.** 1965. Some effects of antimicrobial compounds on phagocytosis in vitro. J. Reticuloendothel. Soc. **2**:75–88.
8. **Forsgren, A., D. Schmeling, and P. G. Quie.** 1974. Effect of tetracycline on the phagocytic function of human leukocytes. J. Infect. Dis. **130**:412–415.
9. **Gimber, P. E., and G. W. Rafter.** 1969. The effect of Escherichia coli endotoxin with leukocytes. Arch. Biochem. **135**:14–20.
10. **Gnarpe, H., and D. Leslie.** 1974. Tetracycline and host defense mechanisms. Doxycycline interference with phagocytosis of Escherichia coli. Microbios 10A:127–138.
11. **Grassi, G. G., and E. Pozzi.** 1972. Effect of rifampicin on delayed-hypersensitivity reactions. J. Infect. Dis. **126**:542–544.
12. **Hartmann, G., K. O. Honikel, F. Knüsel, and J. Nüesch.** 1967. The specific inhibition of the DNA-directed RNA-synthesis by rifamycin. Biochim. Biophys. Acta **145**:843–844.
13. **Hoeprich, P. D., and C. H. Martin.** 1970. Effect of tetracycline, Polymyxin B, and rifampin on phagocy-

tosis. Clin. Pharmacol. Ther. 11:418-422.
14. **Keller, H. U., and E. Sorkin.** 1967. Studies on chemotaxis. V. On the chemotactic effect of bacteria. Int. Arch. Allergy Appl. Immunol. 31:505-517.
15. **Kernbaum, S.** 1974. Pouvoir candidacide des polynucleaires et chemotherapieppe antibacterienne. Pathol. Biol. 22:789-794.
16. **Lehrer, R. I.** 1973. Effects of colchicine and chloramphenicol on the oxidative metabolism and phagocytic activity on human neutrophils. J. Infect. Dis. 127:40-48.
17. **Mandell, G. L., and T. K. Vest.** 1972. Killing of intraleukocytic Staphylococcus aureus by Rifampin: In-vitro and in-vivo studies. J. Infect. Dis. 125:486-490.
18. **Martin, R. R., W. Glenn, R. Couch, and V. Knight.** 1973. Chemotaxis of human leukocytes: Responsiveness of Mycoplasma pneumoniae. J. Lab. Clin. Med. 81:520-529.
19. **Martin, R. R., G. Warr, H. Yeager, R. Couch, and V. Knight.** 1974. Effect of tetracycline on chemotaxis. J. Infect. Dis. 129:110-116.
20. **Munoz, J., and R. Geister.** 1950. Inhibition of phagocytosis by aureomycin. Proc. Soc. Exp. Biol. Med. 75:367-370.
21. **Nelson, R. D., P. G. Quie, and R. L. Simmons.** 1975. Chemotaxis under agarose: a new and simple method for measuring chemotaxis and spontaneous migration of human polymorphonuclear leukocytes and monocytes. J. Immunol. 115:1650-1656.
22. **Park, J. K., and R. C. Dow.** 1970. The uptake and localization of tetracycline in human blood cells. Br. J. Exp. Pathol. 51:179-182.
23. **Paunesco, E., M. Stoinescu, A. Serbescu, R. Musateanu, C. Zaharescu, A. Indriesm, and V. Patru.** 1971. Recherches biochemiques et immunologiques, concernant les effect secondaires de la rifampicine. Fitzologia 20(Suppl.): 33.
24. **Serrou, B., C. Solassal, H. Joyeux, H. Pujol, and C. Romieu.** 1972. Immunosuppressive effect of rifampicin. Transplantation 14:654-655.
25. **Snyderman, R., C. Wohlenberg, and A. L. Notkins.** 1972. Inflammation and viral infection: chemotactic activity resulting from the interaction of antiviral antibody and complement with cells infected with herpes simplex virus. J. Infect. Dis. 126:207-209.
26. **Urbanitz, D., E. Gregoritz, I. Fechner, and R. Gross.** 1974. Reduced phagocytosis of monocytes from patients with tuberculosis under treatment. Klin. Wschr. 52;544-548.
27. **Ward, P. A., C. G. Cochrane, and H. J. Müller-Eberhard.** 1965. The role of serum complement in chemotaxis of leukocytes in vitro. J. Exp. Med. 122:327-346.
28. **Ward, P. A., I. H. Lepow, and L. S. Newman.** 1968. Bacteriol factors chemotactic for polymorphonuclear leucocytes. Am. J. Pathol. 52:725-736.
29. **Ward, P. A.** 1968. Chemotaxis of polymorphonuclear leukocytes. Biochem. Pharmacol. (Suppl.) 99.
30. **Ward, P. A.** 1972. Insubstantial leucotaxis. J. Lab. Clin. Med. 6:873-877.
31. **Ward, P. A., S. Cohen, and T. D. Flanagan.** 1972. Leucotactic factors elaborated by virus-infected tissues. J. Exp. Med. 135:1095-1103.
32. **Wilkinson, P. C.** 1975. Leukocyte locomotion and chemotaxis. The influence of divalent cations and cation ionophoresis. Exp. Cell. Res. 93:420-426.
33. **Ødegaard, A., and J. Lamvik.** 1976. The effect of phenylbutazone and chloramphenicol on phagocytosis of radiolabelled Candida albicans by human monocytes cultured in vitro. Acta Pathol. Microbiol. Scand. Sect. C 84:37-44.

ANTIMICROBIAL AGENTS AND CHEMOTHERAPY, Apr. 1977, p. 585-588
Vol. 11, No. 4

R Plasmids from Asian Strains of *Vibrio cholerae*

R. W. HEDGES,* J. L. VIALARD, N. J. PEARSON, AND F. O'GRADY

Bacteriology Department, Royal Postgraduate Medical School, London, W12 OHS England; Bacteriology Department, Pasteur Institute, Paris 75015 France; and Microbiology Department, University of Nottingham, Nottingham, NG5 1PH England*

Received for publication 20 October 1976

Five R plasmids transferred from Asian strains of *Vibrio cholerae* all proved to be members of compatibility group C. A non-self-transmissible plasmid, stable in *V. cholerae*, was mobilized for transfer to *Escherichia coli* K-12 and found to be unstably inherited in that host. Plasmids of group C and P transferred to a wild *V. cholerae* strain were stably inherited.

The seventh cholera pandemic has been the result of the westward spread of the E1 Tor biotype of *Vibrio cholerae* from Indonesia (3). Initially these bacteria were apparently uniformly susceptible to antibiotics but, once the pandemic spread was accomplished, antibiotic-resistant strains were reported from several different parts of the world. In several cases, this resistance was apparently due to the presence of antibiotic resistance plasmids (R plasmids).

The occurrence of these plasmid-carrying (R+) strains was sporadic and the antibiotics to which they conferred resistance differed from case to case, suggesting that the acquisition of an R factor by *V. cholerae* cells has occurred on different occasions and in different parts of the world.

Kuwahara et al. (12) in the Philippines and Rizzo et al. (17) in Apulia seem to have observed the transfer of R plasmids from unknown donor strains into pathogenic strains of *V. cholerae* in infected humans.

Despite this diversity of origins, Hedges and Jacob (11) noted that all the plasmids reported from *V. cholerae* isolates were either known to belong to compatibility group C or determined resistance phenotypes, which suggested that they might belong to this group. This generalization was based on the properties of a very small number of plasmids, so we have sought further antibiotic-resistant cultures of *V. cholerae* to test the conclusion.

MATERIALS AND METHODS

Bacteria. The *V. cholerae* strains are listed in Table 1, and additionally, strain V63P$^-$ was used which requires adenine, leucine, and arginine for growth (6). Also *rif*^{r} and *nal*^{r} derivatives of the above strains resistant to 50 μg of rifampin per ml or 15 μg of nalidixic acid per ml were employed.

The *Escherichia coli* K-12 strains used were: J53, F$^-$ *pro met*; J53-1, F$^-$ *pro met nal*^{r}; J53-2, F$^-$ *pro met rif*^{r}; J62, F$^-$ *pro his trp lac*; C600-2, F$^-$ *thr leu thi lac rif*^{r}.

Plasmids. R40a, R55, and R57b, plasmids of compatibility group C (4), the equivalent of *com6* (1), were used. R40a confers resistance to ampicillin, kanamycin, and sulfonamides and the latter two confer resistance to ampicillin, chloramphenicol, gentamicin, kanamycin, and sulfonamides. RP4, a plasmid of compatibility group P conferring resistance to ampicillin, tetracycline, and kanamycin was used (5).

Techniques for plasmid transfer to *E. coli* and determination of compatibility were described in references 1, 2, 6, and 7. Transfer between strains of *V. cholerae* was attempted using a *rif*^{r} mutant of the donor and a *nal*^{r} mutant of the recipient strain, usually V63P$^-$. Apparent transcipients were tested for susceptibility to rifampin and amino acid requirement.

RESULTS

Resistant strains of *V. cholerae*. Strains of *V. cholerae* resistant to therapeutically used drugs were found during a survey of 1,156 strains from worldwide sources. The origins of the strains are described elsewhere (15). Several of the isolates that were initially found to be resistant to one or more drugs were, upon subsequent testing, found to be fully susceptible. That several R factors are unstable in *V. cholerae* has been reported by Yokota et al. (21). Those strains which retained antibiotic resistance are listed in Table 1.

All these strains were tested for ability to transfer resistances to *E. coli* K-12 strains J53-2 and C600-2. Five cultures, E14, F1, P78, L171, and L172 were effective donors (Table 1). All other strains failed to transfer their resistances.

Transmissible R factors. The antibiotic resistance properties determined by the five plasmids in *E. coli* K-12 are shown in Table 2. As

TABLE 1. *Antibiotic-resistant strains for Vibrio cholerae*

Original strain no.	Nottingham no.	Origin	Minimal inhibitory concn[a]						Resistance pattern[a]	Resistances transferred to *E. coli*
			Am	Cm	Su	Tc	St[b]	Ka[b]		
A27	JA27	Philippines (J)	1	32	>256	0.5	R	S	St Cm Su	
C24	JC24	Philippines (J)	2	32	>256	32	R	S	St Tc Cm Su	St Tc Cm (Su?)[c] R1146
C28	JC28	Philippines (J)	2	32	>256	1	R	S	St Cm Su	
H1	JH1	Philippines (J)	1	32	>256	4	R	S	St Cm Su	
6397	28	Philippines (G)	256	0.25	4	0.5	S	S	Am	
C21	C21	Philippines (G)	2	32	>256	128	R	S	St Tc Cm Su	
C24	C24	Philippines (G)	2	32	>256	128	R	S	St Tc Cm Su	
552	P64	Philippines (S)	2	32	4	2	R	S	St Cm	
3505	P78	Philippines (S)	2	4	>256	64	R	S	St Tc Cm Su	St Tc Cm Su R1144
5506	A80	Calcutta	2	32	>256	2	R	S	St Cm Su	
5482	A148	Calcutta	256	0.5	8	2	S	S	Am	
13/69	BA39	W. Bengal	1	0.5	64	0.5	R	S	St Su	
8/75	F1	Thailand	>256	16	4	64	R	R	Am St Tc Cm Ka	Am St Tc Cm Ka[d] R1143
1249	E14	Indonesia	2	16	>256	32	R	S	St Tc Cm Su	St Tc Cm Su R1145
	L171	Indonesia	2	0.5	>256	32–64	R	S	St Tc Su	St Tc Su Lac R1166
	L172	Indonesia	2	0.5	>256	32–64	R	S	St Tc Su	St Tc Su Lac R1167

[a] Abbreviations: Am, Ampicillin; Cm, chloramphenicol; Su, sulfafurazole; Tc, tetracycline; St, streptomycin; Ka, kanamycin.
[b] Resistances tested by multodisk.
[c] Mobilized by R40a.
[d] Ampicillin resistance is due to production of a TEM-1β-lactamace (13; M. Mathew, personal communication).

TABLE 2. *Minimal inhibitory concentrations (MIC) of antibacterial agents for V. cholerae and E. coli strains*

Strain	MIC (μg/ml)[a] of antibiotics				
	Sp[b]	St	Tc	Cm	Ka
J53-2	10	2.5	<1.25	<1.25	<1.25
J53-2 (R1143)	>100	>100	25	>100	>100
J53-2 (R1144)	>100	25	50	50	<1.25
J53-2 (R1145)	10[c]	25	50	100	<1.25
J53-1 (R40a) (R1146)	100	25	100	100	>100
J53-2 (R1166)	25	10	25	<1.25	<1.25
J53-2 (R1167)	50	10	25	<1.25	<1.25
P78[d]	>100	50	25	10	<1.25
P78 (R40a)[d]	10	5	<1.25	1.25	>100

[a] In Direct Sensitivity Testing agar (Oxoid, CM261).
[b] Abbreviations: Sp, Spectinomycin; St, streptomycin; Tc, tetracycline; Cm, chloramphenicol; Ka, kanamycin.
[c] Since R1145 determines resistance to streptomycin but not to spectinomycin, we presume that it determines synthesis of streptomycin phosphotransferase, whereas the R factors that confer resistance to both antibiotics probably carry genes for streptomycin, spectinomycin adenyltransferase (8).
[d] A spontaneous rifampin-resistant mutant of P78.

may be seen, the level of chloramphenicol resistance determined by these R factors in *E. coli* is very markedly greater than that shown by the original host strains (Table 1).

The compatibility properties of the plasmids were determined by testing their ability to coexist with representatives of the known plasmid compatibility groups. R1143 was shown to be incompatible with R57b, and R1144, R1145, R1166, and R1167 were incompatible with R40a. All five were capable of excluding, and subject to exclusion by, R factors of group C. Thus, all are members of group C (4).

Both R1166 and R1167 confer lactose fermentation ability upon *E. coli* J62. Plasmids of this group which determine this metabolic ability have been described (9).

When J53(R40a) was mated with a rifampin-resistant mutant of P78 the rate of transfer was very low, less than one transcipient per 10^{10} donors, indicating that, as in *E. coli*, R1144 determined powerful surface exclusion. A single R40a$^+$ colony was obtained; this clone had lost tetracycline and chloramphenicol resistances. Thus, we conclude that in *V. cholerae* (as in *E. coli*) R1144 is incompatible with R40a and that the low level of chloramphenicol resistance of P78 is due to the presence of the resident plasmid.

Nontransmissible resistances of strain JC24. *V. cholerae* strain JC24 was resistant to streptomycin, tetracycline, chloramphenicol, and sulfonamides, and these resistances are stably inherited. JC24 was, however, unable to transfer this resistance either to *E. coli* or to other *V. cholerae* strains.

R40a was transferred to a rifampin-resistant mutant of JC24 with an efficiency (10^{-5} to 10^{-6} per donor) sufficiently high to suggest that JC24 has no surface exclusion ability. After entry of R40a into the strain, there was no elimination of the resistance.

When JC24 Rif^r(R40a) was incubated with *E. coli* J53-1 there was efficient transfer of R40a but very little mobilization of the resistances to JC24. However, a single clone of J53-1 was obtained which had acquired tetracycline resistance. The efficiency of transfer of tetracycline resistance was less than one per 10^{10} donors.

This clone was resistant to streptomycin, tetracycline, and chloramphenicol (as well as possessing the ampicillin, kanamycin, and sulfonamide resistances attributable to R40a). It was designated J53-1(R40a)(R1146).

The R40a-determined resistances were stable, but those of R1146 were highly unstable. Cultures grown overnight in drug-free broth at 37°C contained one-quarter to one-third of the cells that lacked the R1146-determined resistances. We therefore conclude that the R1146 replication mechanism functions efficiently in *V. cholerae* but only very inefficiently in *E. coli* K-12.

When J53-1(R40a)(R1146) was allowed to conjugate with J62, the R40a markers were transferred with a frequency approaching 10^{-4} per donor and usually without R1146. Of 24 kanamycin-resistant transcipients, all lacked the R1146 markers. When the mating was performed and selection was made for tetracycline-resistant transcipients, the transfer rate was less than 10^{-6} per donor. All carried R40a as well as R1146.

Stability of plasmids in *V. cholerae*. Yokota et al. (21) introduced *fi*$^+$ and *fi*$^-$ plasmids into a strain of *V. cholerae* and found that most of these were very unstably inherited. We therefore examined the stability of JC24rif^r(R40a) and a strain of JC24rif^r into which RP4 had been transferred. Both plasmids were stably inherited and overnight cultures grown in drug-free broth regularly contained more than 99% R$^+$ cells.

Stability in *V. cholerae* of several plasmids belonging to group C has also been described by Rahal et al. (K. Rahal, G. R. Gerbaud, and D. H. Bouanchaud, Abstr. Annu. Meet. Am. Soc. Microbiol. 1974, G149, p. 44). Conversely, they observed that plasmids belonging to a large number of different groups were lost at high frequency in *V. cholerae* "El Tor."

DISCUSSION

Our results confirm the impression that the R plasmid set of *V. cholerae* is dominated by plasmids of compatibility group C. The five self-transmissible R plasmids from our collection of strains all exhibit this compatibility.

Plasmids of group C have been found in a wide range of genera including *Pseudomonas, Proteus, Providencia,* and *Klebsiella* (20). In *Providencia* they are by far the most abundant type of R factor (9). Thus, it is not surprising that they are to be found in *Vibrio*. More surprising is the failure to find R plasmids of compatibility group P in this genus. RP4 is readily transmissible to, stably inherited in, and able to express resistance in *V. cholerae*. So, there seems no reason to doubt that such plasmids will sooner or later be found in *Vibrio*.

It is hard to avoid the conclusion that certain bacterial groups, notably the coliform bacteria with deoxyribonucleic acid of ~50% guanine + cytosine, were easily able to produce a large range of R plasmid groups. Perhaps, they were preadapted by virtue of carrying a variety of plasmids determining colicinogenicity, fermentation genes, etc., onto which resistance genes could be transposed. Other groups of bacteria, e.g., the *Proteus*-Providence (40% guanine + cytosine deoxyribonucleic acid) group seem to have had greater difficulty in generating a set of R factors. Thus the R factor set of *Proteus rettgeri* (2), *Proteus mirabilis*, and *Proteus vulgaris* (10) contain plasmids of groups imperfectly adapted to these bacteria, e.g., F_{II} plasmids that dissociate.

However, R factors specific for these genera

are evolving. Some are capable of functioning efficiently in other genera, but are, in nature, found only in particular genera. Thus, plasmids of compatibility group T have been found in *P. vulgaris* in Japan (19), *Providencia* in the United Kingdom (10), and *P. rettgeri* in South Africa (2), but never in any strain outside this group.

A more highly adapted class is represented by plasmids of compatibility group V. These have only been detected in strains of *P. mirabilis* in Asia. (They are transmissible to *E. coli* but are unstably inherited; apparently their replication mechanism is not coordinated with that of the alien host [10].)

Finally, a few R factors have been described that are transmissible between strains of *P. mirabilis* but not to *E. coli* (14, 18).

V. cholerae may, in this respect, resemble the *Proteus* group in that its plasmid set contains R factors of a group well known for its wide host range and also plasmids whose replication cycle is so specifically adapted to these bacteria that inheritance is unstable in *E. coli*.

It may not be a coincidence that most of the plasmids of group C have been observed in *V. cholerae* strains at the fringe of the spread of the current pandemic, e.g., Algeria (16) and European U.S.S.R. (11), whereas the strain shown to carry the plasmid more highly adapted to *V. cholerae* was isolated in the Philippines, near the center of distribution of the pandemic.

LITERATURE CITED

1. **Chabbert, Y. A., M. R. Scavizzi, J. L. Witchitz, G. R. Gerbaud, and D. H. Bouanchaud.** 1972. Incompatibility groups and the classification of *fi*⁻ resistance factors. J. Bacteriol. 112:666–675.
2. **Coetzee, J. N., N. Datta, and R. W. Hedges.** 1972. R factors from *Proteus rettgeri*. J. Gen. Microbiol. 72:543–552.
3. **Cvjetanovic, B., and D. Barua.** 1972. The seventh pandemic of cholera. Nature (London) 239:137–138.
4. **Datta, N., and R. W. Hedges.** 1972. R factors identified in Paris, some conferring gentamicin resistance, constitute a new compatibility group. Ann. Inst. Pasteur Paris 123:879–883.
5. **Datta, N., R. W. Hedges, E. J. Shaw, R. B. Sykes, and M. H. Richmond.** 1971. Properties of an R factor from *Pseudomonas aeruginosa*. J. Bacteriol. 108:1244–1249.
6. **Datta, A., C. D. Parker, J. A. Wolheiter, and L. S. Baron.** 1973. Isolation and characterization of the fertility factor P of *Vibrio cholerae*. J. Bacteriol. 113:763–771.
7. **Dennison, S.** 1972. Naturally occurring R factor, derepressed for pilus synthesis, belonging to the same compatibility group as the sex factor F of *Escherichia coli* K-12. J. Bacteriol. 109:416–422.
8. **Hedges, R. W.** 1972. Resistance to spectinomycin determined by R factors of various compatibility groups. J. Gen. Microbiol. 72:407–409.
9. **Hedges, R. W.** 1974. R factors from Providence. J. Gen. Microbiol. 81:171–181.
10. **Hedges, R. W.** 1975. R factors from *Proteus mirabilis* and *P. vulgaris*. J. Gen. Microbiol. 87:301–311.
11. **Hedges, R. W., and A. E. Jacob.** 1975. A 98 megadalton R factor of compatibility group C in a *Vibrio cholerae* El Tor isolate from Southern U.S.S.R. J. Gen. Microbiol. 89:383–386.
12. **Kuwahara, S., S. Goto, M. Kimura, and H. Abe.** 1967. Drug sensitivity of El Tor *Vibrio* strains isolated in the Philippines in 1964 and 1965. Bull. W.H.O. 37:763–771.
13. **Matthew, M., and R. W. Hedges.** 1976. Analytical isoelectric focusing of R factor-determined β-lactomases: correlation with plasmid compatibility. J. Bacteriol. 125:713–718.
14. **Naide, Y., T. Kawamura, K. Makino, H. Tamura, and T. Watanabe.** 1967. Prevalence of transferable drug resistance in drug-resistant bacteria isolated from urinary tract infections in Japan. Jpn. J. Microbiol. 11:87–94.
15. **O'Grady, F., M. J. Lewis, and N. J. Pearson.** 1976. Global surveillance of antibiotic sensitivity of *Vibrio cholerae*. Bull. W.H.O. 54:181–185.
16. **Rahal, K., G. R. Gerbaud, and Y. A. Chabbert.** 1973. Caracterization d'un facteur de resistance transferable de *Vibrio cholerae* biotype El Tor. Ann. Microbiol. 124B:283–294.
17. **Rizzo, G., G. Leogrande, S. Barbuti, and E. Jatta.** 1975. Comportamento di stipiti di "*Vibrio cholerae*" del biotypo El Tor isolati in Puglia nel 1973, nei confronti di alcuni antibiotici e chemioterapici, from the symposium 'Il cholera in Puglia.' Annati Sclavo 17:473–479.
18. **Shafi, M. S., and N. Datta.** 1975. Infection caused by *Proteus mirabilis* strains with transferable gentamicin-resistance factors. Lancet i:1355–1357.
19. **Terawaki, Y., H. Takayasu, and T. Akiba.** 1967. Thermosensitive replication of a kanamycin resistance factor. J. Bacteriol. 94:687–690.
20. **Witchitz, J. L., and G. R. Gerbaud.** 1972. Classification de plasmids conferant la resistance a la gentamicine. Ann. Inst. Pasteur Paris 123:333–339.
21. **Yokota, T., T. Kasuga, M. Kaneko, and S. Kuwahara.** 1972. Genetic behavior of R factors in *Vibrio cholerae*. J. Bacteriol. 109:440–442.

Antimicrobial Agents and Chemotherapy, Apr. 1977, p. 589–593 Vol. 11, No. 4

Pseudomonas aeruginosa Strain Isolated in France That Carries a Plasmid Determining Carbenicillin Resistance

Y. MICHEL-BRIAND,* VILMA A. STANISICH,[1] AND M. JOUVENOT

Laboratoire de Bactériologie-Virologie, Faculté de Medecine et de Pharmacie, Place Saint-Jacques, 25030 Besancon, France, and Department of Bacteriology, Bristol University Medical School, Bristol BS8 1 TD, England*

Received for publication 8 October 1976

A plasmid, R56Be, derived from a clinical strain of *Pseudomonas aeruginosa* isolated in France in 1973 has been studied. This plasmid confers resistance only to carbenicillin, and although freely transferable between unrelated strains of *P. aeruginosa*, its transfer from *P. aeruginosa* to *Escherichia coli* K-12 was undetectable. R56Be could not be isolated as covalently closed circular deoxyribonucleic acid, but the plasmid could be transduced intact by phage F116L. This suggests that its molecular weight does not exceed that of the phage genome (ca. 40×10^6). In terms of its interaction with male and female sex-specific phages, its exclusion characteristics, and the main properties of β-lactamase determined by them, R56Be is similar to the previously characterized plasmid RP1-1.

Pseudomonas aeruginosa is an important opportunistic pathogen that has a marked resistance to many antibiotics, but it is usually sensitive to carbenicillin. However, in 1969, carbenicillin-resistant strains of *P. aeruginosa* were isolated from patients in a Burns Unit in Birmingham, England, and the resistance was shown to be plasmid mediated (6, 16). Similarly resistant strains have subsequently been isolated in different parts of the world, and the plasmids carried by them have been shown to comprise at least five incompatibility groups (2, 12–14, 26, 29). However, with the exception of RP1-1 (9) and R91 (27), both of which were derived from the Birmingham strains and confer resistance only to carbenicillin, these various plasmids confer a multiple resistance phenotype.

This study examines the nature of carbenicillin resistance in a strain of *P. aeruginosa* isolated from a patient in France. We show that resistance is determined by a conjugative plasmid whose transfer is confined to strains of *P. aeruginosa*. Moreover, a comparison of the properties of this new plasmid with those conferred by other carbenicillin resistance plasmids suggests that it is similar to the previously described plasmid RP1-1.

MATERIALS AND METHODS

Media. Oxoid Muller-Hinton medium was used as the nutrient agar and Oxoid heart brain infusion as the nutrient broth. The composition of the minimal medium was that described by Stanisich and Holloway (28). Antibiotic supplements to nutrient agar and minimal medium were as follows: carbenicillin, 500 μg/ml; streptomycin sulfate, 250 μg/ml; rifampin, 100 μg/ml.

Bacterial strains and plasmids. The properties and origin of the bacterial strains and plasmids used are shown in Table 1. Ps19 is a clinical isolate of *P. aeruginosa* that is prototrophic and does not carry resistance plasmids (N. A. C. Curtis, personal communication). Plasmid-carrying derivatives of various PAO strains were also used. R91-21 is a transfer-derepressed (*drd*) mutant of R91 (27). Such mutants also express an Spp_I phenotype. R18-1-1 and R91-16, respectively, are carbenicillin-susceptible mutants of R18-1 and a *drd* mutant (R91-5) of R91. RP1-2 is a Cb^s mutant of RP1 (4).

General methods. All bacterial strains were used in exponential growth phase. In mating experiments in nutrient broth, donor and recipient bacteria were mixed in a ratio of 5:1 and maintained at 37°C for the mating period, and samples of the mixture were plated onto the appropriate selective medium. Spot plate matings, spot assays for the determination of efficiency of phage plating, and the method for F116L-mediated transduction have been described previously (29).

Phages. The origins and properties of the phages used have been described previously (29). They were the RP1 donor-specific phages PRR1, PR4, PRD1, and Pf3, the temperate phages B3, B33, B39, and F116L, and the virulent phage E79. The clear plaque mutant G101c was also used.

Determination of substrate profile of β-lactamase and the isolation of plasmid DNA. The procedures for the growth of bacteria, induction of the β-lactamase, and the determination of its substrate profile were those previously described (17, 18). The isolation of plasmid deoxyribonucleic acid (DNA) as

[1] Present address: Department of Microbiology, La Trobe University, Bundoora 3083, Victoria, Australia.

TABLE 1. *Bacterial strains and plasmids*

Strain or plasmid	Genotype or phenotype[a]	Reference or source[b]
P. aeruginosa		
Ps19	Prototroph	N. A. C. Curtis
PAT900	*his-404 str-1100*	28
PAO8	*met-28 ilv-202 str-1*	10
PAO303	*argB18 chl-2*	11
PAO307	*argC54 chl-2*	11
PAO315	*argG9 chl-2*	11
PAO366	*argA36 chl-2*	11
PAO381	*leu-38 str-13* FP2$^+$	28
PAO1670	*ade-136 leu-8 chl-3 rif-1*	15
PAO2001	*argH32 str-39 chl-2*	15
PAO2003	*argH32 str-39 chl-2 rec-2*	15
PAO2637	Prototroph, *chl-2 fon-100*	29
E. coli		
W3110	Prototroph, *rif*	M. H. Richmond
Plasmids		
RP1	Cb^r Nm^r/Km^r Tc^r Spp$_I^+$ Tra$^+$ Inc P	6, 24
RP1-2	Cb^s Nm^r/Km^r Tc^r Spp$_I^+$ Tra$^+$ Inc P	4
RP1-1	Cb^r Spp$_{III}^+$ Tra$^+$	9, 24
R18-1-1	Cb^s Spp$_{III}^+$ Tra$^+$	P. M. Chandler
R91	Cb^r Tra$^+$	27
R91-16	Cb^s Spp$_I^+$ Tra$_{drd}^+$	P. M. Chandler
R91-21	Cb^r Spp$_I^+$ Tra$_{drd}^+$	27

[a] Genotypic symbols follow those proposed by Demerec et al. (5). *fon,* Resistance to phage F116L. Plasmid phenotypic designations follow those proposed by Novick et al. (20). Spp$_I^+$, Reduced plating of phage G101 (29); Spp$_{III}^+$, reduced plating of phages B33 and B39 (19).

[b] N. A. C. Curtis and M. H. Richmond are from the Department of Microbiology, Bristol University, Bristol U.K.; P. M. Chandler is from the Department of Genetics, Monash University, Monash, Australia.

the closed covalent circular form was carried out using the procedures of Grinsted et al. (6). [^{3}H]adenine was used to label the DNA of R$^+$ derivatives of PAO1670. The subline carrying RP1 was used as a control.

RESULTS

Derivation of R56Be. *P. aeruginosa* strain 56Be was isolated in 1973 from a patient in the hospital in Besançon, France. The strain was highly resistant to carbenicillin (>8 mg/ml), and also to terramycin (100 μg/ml), kanamycin (500 μg/ml), streptomycin (100 μg/ml), and mercuric chloride (25 μg/ml), but was susceptible to rifampin.

To determine whether the carbenicillin resistance (Cb^r) phenotype of this strain was transferable, matings were carried out with the recipient PAO1670 (Rif^r). Cb^r transconjugants were selected on nutrient agar containing carbenicillin and rifampin and occurred at a frequency of about 10^{-4}/donor per 3-h mating. The transconjugants displayed only the Cb^r phenotype of the donor parent (20 colonies tested), and one derivative from each mating was chosen for further study after ensuring that it had not been lysogenized by phages carried by the donor strain.

The possession by this PAO1670 derivative of a conjugative plasmid was confirmed in subsequent matings with PAO2001 (*arg-32 str-39*) and its recombination-deficient subline PAO2003 (*arg-32 str-39 rec-2*). Cb^r transconjugants were recovered from all matings at frequencies of between 1.2×10^{-2} and 3.8×10^{-4}/donor per 30-min mating, but transfer of the chromosomal allele *arg-32*$^+$ was not observed ($<10^{-8}$/donor). The latter result contrasted with the behavior of an FP2$^+$ donor (PAO381) that gave prototrophic progeny with the Rec$^+$ strain (1.3×10^{-3}/donor) but not with the Rec$^-$ strain ($<10^{-8}$/donor). It was concluded, therefore, that the Cb^r determinant was plasmid borne and that the inheritance of this plasmid did not depend on the host recombination system. Similar mating experiments were carried out between the PAO1670 derivative and recipients that carried arginine mutations at either the 8-, 18-, 32-, or 54-min location on the PAO chromosome (B. W. Holloway, personal communication), but none yielded prototrophic progeny at frequencies greater than 10^{-8}/donor. This confirmed the finding with the *arg-32* recipient that the plasmid was poor in initiating transfer of the PAO chromosome.

The Cb^r determinant of the PAO1670 derivative was readily transferable to *P. aeruginosa* strains PAT and Ps19 (frequency, 4×10^{-1} to 4×10^{-3}/donor per 3-h mating) and was stable in these strains. In contrast, no transfer could be detected to *Escherichia coli* K-12 ($<10^{-8}$/donor). It appears, therefore, that *P. aeruginosa* 56Be carries a plasmid designated R56Be that confers resistance to carbenicillin. The formal demonstration that this determinant is on a conjugative plasmid is given below.

Characterization of R56Be. The properties of R56Be and the phenotype it confers in *P. aeruginosa* PAO were studied in a variety of tests.

(i) Curing. The stability of R56Be was determined by growing the PAO1670 derivative, and the clinical isolate, in the presence of various "curing" agents. These included sodium dodecyl sulfate (2%) and subinhibitory concentrations of acriflavine, mitomycin C, and ethidium bromide. The bacteria were grown for 20 to 25 generations and, when necessary, diluted so that the cell density did not exceed about 5×10^7 bacteria/ml. Of 500 to 2,000 colonies tested from each treatment, Cb^s derivatives were isolated in only one instance, from the mitomycin C treatment of strain 56Be (3/1,800). These had the serological and pyocin types of the parent strain and could possibly have represented plasmidless derivatives. Clearly, however, R56Be is generally resistant to curing whether carried by the wild-type strain or by strain PAO.

(ii) Transduction. The $R56Be^+$ subline of *P. aeruginosa* PAO8 was used as donor in phage F116L-mediated transduction to PAO1670 (*ade-136 leu-8*). Cb^r and *ade-136*$^+$ transductants were obtained at a frequency of 5×10^{-7}/plaque-forming unit. All the Cb^r transductants were found to be resistant to lysis by phage B33 (50 tested), and these phenotypes could be transferred in subsequent matings to PAO2637 (*fon-100*). Since this strain is resistant to phage F116L, we can be sure that transfer occurs by conjugation. This suggests that the Cb^r and Spp_{III}^+ determinants (see Table 1 and below) occur on a conjugative plasmid, R56Be, that can be transduced intact by phage F116L. It is likely, therefore, that the size of this plasmid does not exceed 40×10^6 daltons, the size of the phage genome (23).

(iii) Molecular properties. Repeated attempts to isolate closed covalent circular DNA from whole-cell lysates of PAO1670 sublines carrying R56Be were not successful. The same experimental procedures could, however, be used to isolate plasmid DNA from an analogous subline carrying RP1 (6). Since the transduction experiments suggested that R56Be were not exceptionally large plasmids, we conclude that its inability to be isolated as closed covalent circular DNA probably reflects some difference in its mode of replication or maintenance in the cell. In this respect, R56Be is similar to the *Pseudomonas* plasmid RP1-1 (9) and the J-group plasmids of *E. coli* K-12 (8), none of which have yet been isolated as closed covalent circular DNA.

(iv) Interaction with bacteriophages. Krishnapillai (15) has shown that R plasmids can interfere with the plating of certain phages. We therefore compared the responses of PAO8 and its $R56Be^+$ subline to a variety of temperate and virulent phages. Included for comparison were analogous strains carrying the resistance plasmids RP1-1 and R91 (Table 1). Bacteria carrying R56Be and RP1-1 were similar in their reduced plating of the serologically related phages B33 and B39 (19; Table 2). This contrasted with the behavior of $R91^+$ and $RP1^+$ bacteria; the former plated all the phages, whereas the latter showed a reduced plating of phage G101c.

Strains carrying R56Be or RP1-1 were also similar in their responses to donor-specific phages. Phages Pf3 and PRR1 only infect bacteria carrying P-group plasmids such as RP1, whereas phages PR4 and PRD1 have a broader host range that includes bacteria carrying RP1-1 and R91 (21, 22, 27, 29). Preliminary experiments showed that none of these phages could produce plaques on bacteria carrying R56Be or RP1-1 (Table 2). However, an increase in the Titer of phages PR4 and PRD1, but not of Pf3 or PRR1, could be detected if these phages were cultured with the R^+ host in liquid medium (Table 2). This suggests that R56Be, RP1-1, and R91 (from previous studies [27]) all carry the

TABLE 2. *Propagation of male and female sex-specific phages on R^+ lines of P. aeruginosa PAO*

Plasmid in host	Efficiency of plating[a]			Increase in phage titer in liquid culture[b]	
	G101c	B33, B39	Pf3, PRR1 PRD1, PR4	Pf3, PRR1	PR4, PRD1
None	1	1	$<10^{-8}$	0	0
R56Be	1	10^{-6}	$<10^{-8}$	0	10^4
RP1-1	1	10^{-6}	$<10^{-8}$	0	10^4
RP1	10^{-4}	1	1	10^3	10^4
R91	1	1	$<10^{-8}$	ND	ND

[a] Determined by spot phage assays.

[b] R^+ bacteria (10^7 to 10^8 cells/ml) in nutrient broth were infected with phage (final titer, 10^4 to 10^5 plaque-forming units), and the mixture was incubated for approximately 6 h at 37°C with shaking. After centrifugation, the phage titer of the supernatant was determined. ND, Not done.

gene(s) necessary for the propagation of phages PR4 and PRD1, but that these are normally repressed.

(v) Exclusion phenotype. RP1-1, R91, and R56Be confer resistance only to carbenicillin, so that their mutual incompatibility properties cannot easily be determined. Their exclusion phenotypes could, however, be studied by using Cb^s derivatives of RP1, R91, and R18-1 (a plasmid that is probably identical to RP1-1 [24]). In matings between these various strains, exclusion was evident in the homologous combinations involving $RP1^+$ or $R91^+$ bacteria and also in that between $RP1\text{-}1^+$ and $R18\text{-}1\text{-}1^+$ strains (Table 3). R18-1-1 also excluded R56Be, but in all other combinations the plasmid transfer frequencies were similar to those obtained in matings with the R^- strain. Although not conclusive, the exclusion exhibited between $R56Be^+$ and $R18\text{-}1\text{-}1^+$ bacteria suggests that this plasmid probably belongs to the same incompatibility group. R56Be is found to be compatible with RP1-2(Inc P1) on the basis of the Cb, Km, and Tc resistance phenotypes of the transcipients.

(vi) Carbenicillin resistance. The carbenicillin resistance of *P. aeruginosa* strain 56Be is due to a β-lactamase (18). PAO8 sublines carrying R56Be or RP1-1 were each found to constitutively produce a β-lactamase that had a similar substrate profile against various penicillins (Table 4). It must be noted that the recipient strain PAO8, deprived of plasmid, does not produce any constitutive enzyme detectable by our titration method. The plasmid-mediated enzymes were also similar in isoelectric point (5.6) and could not be distinguished by isoelectric focusing (M. Matthew, personal communication). The K_m value of the R56Be and RP1-1 enzymes against carbenicillin was 38.1 and 33.3 μM, respectively. Thus, the two plasmids determine a β-lactamase with similar properties and thus would belong to type IIIa.

DISCUSSION

In this study, we have examined the nature of carbenicillin resistance in a multiresistant clinical isolate of *P. aeruginosa*. Strain 56Be was isolated in 1973, and only carbenicillin resistance occurs on a conjugative plasmid (56Be). This plasmid is readily transferable between unrelated strains of *P. aeruginosa* and is stable in these hosts.

The resistance of 56Be depends on the synthesis of a β-lactamase of type IIIa. M. Matthew (personal communication) has shown that the β-lactamases determined by RP1-1, R56Be, R91, and RP1, which represent three different incompatibility types, are all indistinguishable by isoelectric focusing, suggesting their overall similarity. Other studies have shown that the *bla* gene of RP1 and RP1-1 occurs on a translocatable element (TnA) (1, 7), and although this aspect has not yet specifically been investigated, it is likely that this same unit occurs on R56Be and R91.

The stable transfer of R56Be is apparently confined to strains of *P. aeruginosa,* and no transfer was detected in our experiments using

TABLE 3. *Surface exclusion in matings between R^+ lines of P. aeruginosa PAO*

Plasmid in donor	Cb^r transconjugants/donor[a]			
	None[b]	RP1-2	R91-16	R18-1-1
R56Be	3×10^{-1}	2.1×10^{-1}	8×10^{-2}	4×10^{-3}
RP1-1	7×10^{-3}	5×10^{-3}	6×10^{-3}	1.4×10^{-4}
R91-21	9×10^{-1}	1.7×10^{-1}	1.7×10^{-5}	6×10^{-1}
RP1	8×10^{-2}	1.7×10^{-4}	3×10^{-1}	1.4×10^{-2}

[a] Determined by spot plate matings; the selective medium was nutrient agar supplemented with streptomycin and carbenicillin. Donors were R^+ derivatives of PAO1670 and recipients were derivatives of PAO8.
[b] Plasmid in recipient.

TABLE 4. *Substrate profiles of the β-lactamase produced by R^+ lines of P. aeruginosa PAO8*

Strain with or without plasmid	Substrate profile[a] against:					
	Benzylpenicillin	Ampicillin	Carbenicillin	Cloxacillin	Cefaloridin	Cefalexin
PAO8	0	0	0	0	0	0
PAO8 (56Be)	100	84	12	3	240	0
PAO8 (RP1-1)	100	88	12	2	196	0

[a] Enzyme activity was measured by the microacidimetric method (18). The substrate concentration of β-lactamase saturation was 0.24 mM; it was 6.58 mM for cefaloridin. All figures are relative to the V_{max} for benzylpencillin (arbitrarily = 100).

an *E. coli* K-12 recipient. However, M. Moillo-Batt (personal communication) has found that this plasmid can be transferred to certain *E. coli* K-12 derivatives, but that the subsequent replication in this host is poor. Such a response has previously been reported for plasmid RP1-1 (25). In all the comparisons carried out, R56Be and RP1-1 behaved similarly, and the two plasmids were distinguishable in several respects from both R91 and RP1.

As far as we are aware, this is the first report of the isolation of plasmids similar to RP1-1 outside the United Kingdom. It may be that plasmids of this type occur commonly in populations of *Pseudomonas* but remain undetected in the clinical environment unless they acquire resistance determinants by either translocation or recombination events with other genetic elements. The frequency of such plasmids can be underestimated due to the relative stability in the wild host: the curing problems and the difficulty in mobilizing the plasmid.

ACKNOWLEDGMENTS

We thank M. Matthew for isoelectric point determinations and examination of the β-lactamases by isoelectric focusing. One of us (Y.M.B.) thanks M. H. Richmond for the hospitality of his laboratory. The gift of carbenicillin and rifampin from Beecham Sevigné and Lepetit Labs is gratefully acknowledged.

Financial support for this work was from the Institut National de la Santé et de la Recherche Médicale and the Medical Research Council (U.K.).

LITERATURE CITED

1. **Bennett, P. M., and M. H. Richmond.** 1976. Translocation of a discrete piece of DNA carrying an *amp* gene between replicons in *Escherichia coli*. J. Bacteriol. 126:1-6.
2. **Chabbert, Y. A., M. P. Scavizzi, J. L. Witchitz, G. R. Gerbaud, and D. H. Bouanchaud.** 1972. Incompatibility groups and the classification of *fi*⁻ resistance factors. J. Bacteriol. 112:666-675.
3. **Chandler, P. M., and V. Krishnapillai.** 1974. Isolation and properties of recombination deficient mutants of *Pseudomonas aeruginosa*. Mutat. Res. 23:15-23.
4. **Curtis, N. A. C., M. H. Richmond, and V. A. Stanisich.** 1973. R factor mediated resistance to penicillins which does not involve a β-lactamase. J. Gen. Microbiol. 79:163-165.
5. **Demerec, M., E. A. Adelberg, A. J. Clark, and P. E. Hartman.** 1966. A proposal for a uniform nomenclature in bacterial genetics. Genetics 54:61-76.
6. **Grinsted, J., J. R. Saunders. L. C. Ingram, R. B. Sykes, and M. H. Richmond.** 1972. Properties of an R factor which originated in *Pseudomonas aeruginosa* 1822. J. Bacteriol. 110:529-537.
7. **Hedges, R. W., and A. E. Jacob.** 1974. Transposition of ampicillin resistance from RP4 to other replicons. Mol. Gen. Genet. 132:31-40.
8. **Hedges, R. W., A. E. Jacob, N. Datta, and J. N. Coetzee.** 1975. Properties of plasmids produced by recombination between R factors of groups J and F_{II}. Mol. Gen. Genet. 140:289-302.
9. **Ingram, L. C., R. B. Sykes, J. Grinsted. J. R. Saunders, and M. H. Richmond.** 1972. A transmissible resistance element from a strain of *Pseudomonas aeruginosa* containing no detectable extrachromosomal DNA. J. Gen. Microbiol. 72:269-279.
10. **Isaac, J. H., and B. W. Holloway.** 1968. Control of pyrimidine biosynthesis in *Pseudomonas aeruginosa*. J. Bacteriol. 96:1732-1741.
11. **Isaac, J. H. and B. W. Holloway.** 1972. Control of arginine biosynthesis in *Pseudomonas aeruginosa*. J. Gen. Microbiol. 73:427-438.
12. **Kawakami, Y., F. Mikoshiba, S. Nagasaki, H. Matsumoto, and T. Tasaki.** 1972. Prevalence of *Pseudomonas aeruginosa* strains possessing R factors in a hospital. J. Antibiot. 25:607-609.
13. **Kontomichalou, P., and E. Papachristou.** 1974. Multiresistance plasmids in *Pseudomonas aeruginosa* highly resistant to gentamicins. *In* International symposium on multiple drug resistance, Tokyo.
14. **Korfhagen, T. R., and J. C. Loper.** 1975. RPL11, an R factor of *Pseudomonas aeruginosa* determining carbenicillin and gentamicin resistance. Antimicrob. Agents Chemother 7:69-73.
15. **Krishnapillai, V.** 1974. The use of bacteriophages for differentiating plasmids of *Pseudomonas aeruginosa*. Genet. Res. 23:327-334.
16. **Lowbury, E. J. L., A. Kidson, H. A. Lilly, G. A. Ayliffe, and R. J. Jones.** 1969. Sensitivity of *Pseudomonas aeruginosa* to antibiotics: emergence of strains highly resistant to carbenicillin. Lancet ii:448-452.
17. **Michel-Briand, Y., and L. Bruand.** 1972. Etude de la production de β-lactamase pour la carbénicilline chez trente souches de *Pseudomonas aeruginosa*. C. R. Acad. Sci. 275:503-506.
18. **Michel-Briand, Y., and M. Jouvenot.** 1975. Mise en évidence d'un facteur de résistance à la carbéncilline chez *Pseudomonas aeruginosa*. C. R. Acad. Sci. 280:2397-2400.
19. **Morgan, T. M., and V. A. Stanisich.** 1975. Properties of phage B33: a female-specific bacteriophage of *Pseudomonas aeruginosa*. J. Gen. Virol. 30:73-79.
20. **Novick, R. P., R. C. Clowes, S. N. Cohen, R. Curtiss III, N. Datta, and S. Falkow.** 1976. Uniform nomenclature for bacterial plasmids: a proposal. Bacteriol. Rev. 40:168-189.
21. **Olsen, R. H., J. S. Siak, and R. H. Gray.** 1974. Characterization of PRD1, a plasmid-dependent broad host range DNA bacteriophage. J. Virol. 14:689-699.
22. **Olsen, R. H., and D. A. Thomas.** 1973. Characterization and purification of PRR1, and RNA phage specific for the broad host range *Pseudomonas* R1822 drug resistance plasmid. J. Virol. 12:1560-1567.
23. **Pemberton, J. M.** 1973. F116L: a DNA bacteriophage specific for the pili of *Pseudomonas aeruginosa* strain PAO. Virology 55:558-560.
24. **Richmond, M. H., and B. W. Holloway.** 1973. R factors used for genetic studies in strains of *Pseudomonas aeruginosa* and their origin. Genet. Res. 21:103-105.
25. **Richmond, M. H., and A. Moillo-Batt.** 1975. Alternative methods for survival of R plasmids in a "new" bacterial host. Proc. Soc. Gen. Microbiol. 3:26.
26. **Smith, D. I., R. Gomez Lus, M. C. Rubio Calvo, N. Datta, A. E. Jacob, and R. W. Hedges.** 1975. Third type of plasmid conferring gentamicin resistance in *Pseudomonas aeruginosa*. Antimicrob. Agents Chemo. 8:227-230.
27. **Stanisich, V. A.** 1974. Properties and host range of male-specific bacteriophages of *Pseudomonas aeruginosa*. J. Gen. Microbiol. 84:332-342.
28. **Stanisich, V. A., and B. W. Holloway.** 1972. A mutant sex factor of *Pseudomonas aeruginosa*. Genet. Res. 19:91-108.
29. **Stanisich, V. A., and J. M. Ortiz.** 1976. Similarities between plasmids of the P-incompatibility group derived from different bacterial genera. J. Gen. Microbiol. 94:281-289.

ANTIMICROBIAL AGENTS AND CHEMOTHERAPY, Apr. 1977, p. 594-598 Vol. 11, No. 4

Penetration of Cefazolin, Cephaloridine, and Cefamandole into Interstitial Fluid in Rabbits

CLAUDE CARBON, ALAIN CONTREPOIS, NILS BRION, AND SUZANNE LAMOTTE-BARRILLON*

Service de Médecine Interne, Hôpital Louis Mourier, F 92701 Colombes Cédex, Université Paris VII, France

Received for publication 27 October 1976

We compared the penetration of three cephalosporins into interstitial fluid. Interstitial fluid was obtained in rabbits from Silastic tissue cages. Cefazolin, cephaloridine, and cefamandole were administered by the intramuscular route (30 mg/kg per injection). Peak blood levels and interstitial concentrations were studied after a single injection. Interstitial levels were also compared in a three-injection study (one injection every 12 h) and in a cumulative effect study (six injections), in which the interval between injections was established for each drug on the basis of its common therapeutic use. After a single injection, cephaloridine activity was detected more rapidly and attained higher levels than the other two drugs within the first 4 h. However, 2 h after the third injection, cefazolin levels in tissue fluid were higher than with cephaloridine. Cefamandole consistently gave the lowest interstitial levels. With all three drugs, detectable concentrations were present in interstitial fluid at a time when no detectable antibiotic was found in serum. In the six-injection study, the interstitial levels obtained with cefazolin were significantly higher than those observed with the other drugs. Our data suggest that cefazolin is a drug of choice due to its high extravascular levels.

Cephalosporins appear to have comparable in vitro antibacterial activity, although susceptibility to inactivation by bacterial penicillinase may vary from drug to drug. In some instances, however, the antibacterial activity of one cephalosporin derivative has been shown to be superior to another against a few susceptible bacterial species. To our knowledge, it is difficult to demonstrate through clinical studies—on the sole record of survival of patients after an infectious process—that one cephalosporin derivative is therapeutically more effective than the others. The preferred agent should combine the best pharmacokinetic and antibacterial features, i. e., high blood concentrations, long serum half-life, large apparent volume of distribution, low rate of side effects, possible administration through the intramuscular (i.m.) route, and the lowest minimal inhibiting concentrations.

The purpose of our study was to provide new pharmacokinetic data for clinical choice. After i.m. injections, the concentrations of three cephalosporins were compared in an extravascular space. An animal model was used to obtain interstitial tissue fluid. Cefazolin, cephaloridine, and cefamandole were selected for study on the following grounds: (i) Cefazolin has been described as the preferred agent for both therapeutic and economic reasons (10, 12; W. M. M. Kirby, J. B. DeMaine, and W. S. Serill, Postgrad. Med. J. 47:41, 1971), but some authors have questioned its diffusibility because of its high level of serum protein binding (15). (ii) Cefamandole pharmacology is similar to that of cephalothin (8), but this drug has been shown to be active in vitro against some *Enterobacter* and indole-positive *Proteus* strains that are not usually susceptible to other cephalosporins and to be more effective against *Haemophilus* species (11). (iii) Cephaloridine has been reported to be less than 30% bound in human serum (14) and is frequently used in prophylaxis.

MATERIALS AND METHODS

Animal model and interstitial tissue fluid. The investigations were carried out in female rabbits (Fauve de Bourgogne; weight range, 3.8 to 4.2 kg). Interstitial fluid was obtained as described by Chisholm et al. in dogs (7). "Tissue cages" were made from Silastic tubing (Silastic drains, Scurasil 72035, Rhône Poulenc Medical, Paris). Each tissue cage, provided with four holes (5-mm diameter), was 40 mm long and 13 mm in diameter and was closed at each end by vulcanization with self-vulcanizing silicone elastomer (Scurasil 20-350, Rhône Poulenc Medical, Paris). The abdominal skin of each rabbit was shaved, swabbed with merthiolate and then with absolute alcohol, and draped. After infiltration with 2% lidocaine, an incision (40 to 50 mm long) was made in the skin. A subcutaneous space was made by dissection, and the tissue cage was inserted beneath the skin. The incision was closed with surgical silk and protected with dressing. After 4 weeks, the animals were used for the experiment.

Exchanges between plasma and tissue cage fluid were studied after injection of ^{82}Br (20 μCi), either intravenously or into tissue cage fluid. Normal renal function was assessed by determination of serum creatinine in all rabbits.

Antibiotics. Cefamandole nafate, sodium cefazolin, and cephaloridine in 1-g ampoules for injection and standard laboratory powders for assay were supplied by Eli Lilly and Co.

Single i.m. injection. A 30-mg/kg dose of cefamandole, cefazolin, or cephaloridine was injected into the thigh of five rabbits for each drug. Interstitial fluid was withdrawn from the tissue cage by needle aspiration at 30 min and at 1, 2, 4, 8, and 12 h. Blood samples were collected from a femoral catheter at 0.5, 1, 2, 4, 6, and 8 h.

Cumulative effect study. Three 30-mg/kg doses of cefamandole, cefazolin, or cephaloridine were injected i.m. every 12 h (respectively, at 0 h, 12 h, and 24 h) in rabbits for each drug. Blood samples were collected just before injection. Interstitial fluid samples were taken at 1, 2, 12, and 26 h.

Cumulative saturation effect study in simulated therapeutic conditions. A 30-mg/kg dose of cefamandole, cephaloridine, or cefazolin was injected i.m. every 6, 8, and 12 h, respectively, in five rabbits for each drug. Six injections of each antibiotic were made to each rabbit. Interstitial fluid samples were collected just before the next injection.

Assay procedure. Blood samples were first allowed to clot and then centrifuged at 3,500 rpm for 15 min; the serum was stored like the interstitial fluid, at −30°C. Standards for the assay of serum samples were prepared in normal rabbit serum. Standards for the assay of interstitial fluid samples were prepared with rabbit serum diluted threefold in 0.15 M phosphate buffer (pH 7.4). Concentrations of antibiotics were determined by diffusion in nutrient agar according to the method of Bennett et al. (4) with *Bacillus subtilis* ATCC 6633 as the test organism.

Protein binding. Protein binding was determined by an ultrafiltration method using 100% pooled rabbit serum adjusted to physiological temperature and pH, with an antibiotic concentration of 20 μg/ml (3).

Serum half-life. For the pharmacokinetic analysis, the serum half-life of each antibiotic was calculated from the serum concentrations obtained after intravenous injection at the time when blood levels declined exponentially during the late elimination phase. The formula used was $T^{1}/_{2} = \ln 2/Ke$, where ln2 is the natural logarithm of 2 and Ke is the slope of the regression line determined by the method of least squares (9).

Statistical analysis. Statistical studies were carried out by analysis of variance using time as the block factor (16). A significant interaction appeared between time and antibiotics. The Student *t*-test was used to compare, two by two, the interstitial antibiotics levels at 1, 2, 12, and 26 h. For that test, the residual variance and its degree of freedom were used. The Student's *t*-test was also used to compare, two by two, the interstitial concentrations obtained at 2 and 26 h with each drug in the cumulative effect study.

RESULTS

Interstitial fluid. Mean values of main biological components of the fluid were similar to those obtained by Calnan et al. (6). Initial concentrations of total protein in the cage fluid, which were similar to those in serum, declined (after approximately 3 weeks) to a steady level of 30% of serum protein concentrations (Table 1).

Studies with ^{82}Br. Rapid diffusion of ^{82}Br from plasma to tissue fluid and vice versa was demonstrated: when injected intravenously, ^{82}Br appeared in tissue fluid within 5 min. Equilibrium was obtained at approximately 60 min. After injection into the Silastic cage, ^{82}Br was detected within 3 min in plasma.

Single i.m. injection. After a 30-mg/kg i.m. dose, peak blood levels occurred at 0.5 h for cefazolin, cephaloridine, and cefamandole. Peak levels in serum (± standard deviation) were significantly higher for cefazolin (35.10 ± 1.27 μg/ml) than for cephaloridine (25.83 ± 1.04 μg/ml) and cefamandole (18.77 ± 6.44 μg/ml). Average concentrations of the three drugs in serum are shown in Fig. 1. No drug activity was detectable in serum 12 h after i.m. injection with all three antibiotics.

Interstitial fluid concentrations achieved after a single i.m. injection of each drug are shown in Fig. 2. Cephaloridine appeared more rapidly in interstitial fluid and gave significantly higher levels than the other two drugs within the first 4 h. Twelve hours after i.m. injection, all three antibiotics were still detectable in interstitial fluid; interstitial fluid levels at that time were significantly higher for cefazolin than for the other two derivatives ($P <$ 0.01).

TABLE 1. *Comparison of physicochemical properties of arterial blood and interstitial tissue fluid in rabbits*

Determination	Arterial blood[a]	Interstitial tissue fluid[a]
Protein (g/100 ml)	5.7 ± 0.5	1.9 ± 0.5
Albumin/globulins	0.92	2.23
Na (meq/liter)	138 ± 3	138 ± 4
K (meq/liter)	4.4 ± 0.3	3.9 ± 0.3
Cl (meq/liter)	100 ± 2	105 ± 3
pH	7.43 ± 0.04	7.31 ± 0.03
Urea (g/100 ml)	0.038 ± 0.005	0.035 ± 0.006
Cells		100/ml

[a] Mean values ± standard deviation.

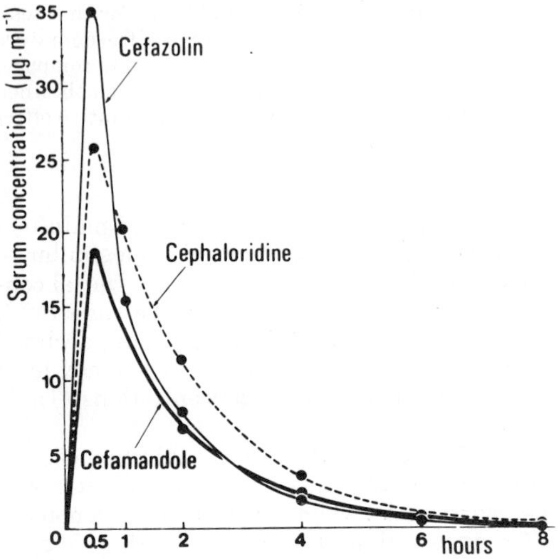

FIG. 1. *Average (± standard error) serum concentrations of cefazolin, cephaloridine, and cefamandole after a single i.m. injection (30 mg/kg) in rabbits.*

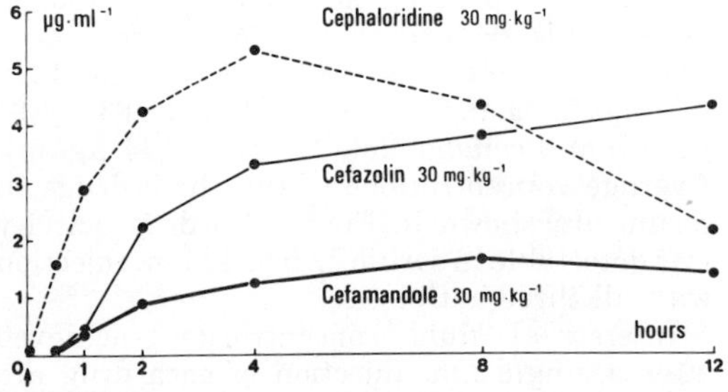

FIG. 2. *Interstitial fluid concentrations of cefazolin, cephaloridine, and cefamandole after a single i.m. injection (30 mg/kg) in rabbits.*

Cumulative effect study. For all three compounds, interstitial concentrations measured 2 h after the third injection (26 h) were significantly higher than those obtained 2 h after the first injection (2 h) (Fig. 3).

The concentrations achieved in interstitial fluid at 1, 2, 12, and 26 h after the administration of three injections given, respectively, every 12 h were compared. The results of these comparisons are shown in Table 2.

Cefamandole always gave the lowest concentrations. As indicated above, cephaloridine produced higher levels at 1 and 2 h. Cefazolin, however, induced significantly higher concentrations 2 h after the third injection (26 h).

Cumulative and saturation effect in simulated therapeutic conditions. The effect on interstitial concentrations of six i.m. injections

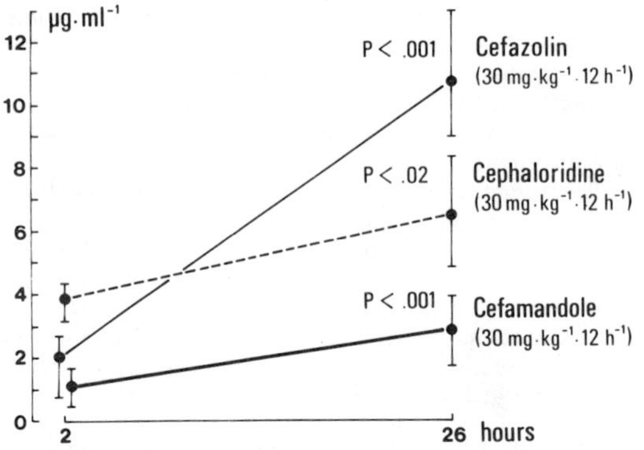

FIG. 3. *Cumulative effect of three i.m. injections (30 mg/kg every 12 h). Comparison of the interstitial concentrations (± standard error) obtained 2 h after the first injection (2 h) and 2 h after the third injection (26 h) of cefazolin, cephaloridine, and cefamandole in rabbits.*

administered at various intervals for each antibiotic is reported in Fig. 4. A saturation effect seemed to occur with all three antibiotics: rapidly (two injections) with cephaloridine, at a level of approximatively 5 μg/ml, and after the fifth injection for cefamandole and cefazolin, at levels of approximatively 4 and 9.5 μg/ml, respectively.

Serum half-life. The half-life of the three drugs after intravenous injection in rabbits was 32 min for cefazolin, 24 min for cephaloridine, and 23 min for cefamandole. The correlation coefficients of the regression lines plotted on a semilogarithmic scale with a straight line were $\geq$ 0.99.

Protein binding. The protein binding of the three antibiotics measured in 100% rabbit serum under simulated physiological conditions was 92.5% for cefazolin, 39.5% for cephaloridine, and 88% for cefamandole.

DISCUSSION

The same dose, 30 mg/kg, was used for all three cephalosporins. In the first part of this experiment, the animals received the drug at identical time intervals in order to study the diffusion into interstitial fluid under the same conditions. In the second part, an attempt was made to reproduce human therapeutic conditions as closely as possible.

In the single injection study, the rapid penetration of cephaloridine (0.5 h) and the higher levels obtained at 1, 2, and 4 h can be explained by the low degree of protein binding of this agent. Many authors have emphasized the importance of protein binding in determining the distribution of antibiotics in vivo (2, 15). Our

TABLE 2. *Cumulative effect study*[a]

Drug pair	Concn (μg/ml) at:			
	1 h	2 h	12 h	26 h
Cefazolin Cephaloridine	0.47 ± 0.27[b] 2.83 ± 0.50	2.26 ± 0.80 4.25 ± 0.77	4.30 ± 0.75 2.71 ± 0.59	10.76 ± 3.4 6.52 ± 1.7
Degree of significance	$P < 0.001$	$P < 0.01$	$P < 0.01$	$P < 0.05$
Cefazolin Cefamandole	0.47 ± 0.27 0.32 ± 0.27	2.26 ± 0.80 0.85 ± 0.44	4.30 ± 0.75 1.39 ± 0.71	10.76 ± 3.4 2.92 ± 0.98
Degree of significance	NS[c]	$P < 0.01$	$P < 0.01$	$P < 0.01$
Cephaloridine Cefamandole	2.83 ± 0.50 0.32 ± 0.27	4.25 ± 0.77 0.85 ± 0.44	2.17 ± 0.59 1.39 ± 0.71	6.52 ± 1.7 2.92 ± 0.98
Degree of significance	$P < 0.001$	$P < 0.001$	NS	$P < 0.02$

[a] Injections, 30 mg/kg i.m., were given at 0, 12, and 24 h. Comparison, two by two, of the concentrations of cefazolin, cephaloridine, and cefamandole in interstitial fluid in rabbits. Each drug was administered to five rabbits.
[b] ± Standard deviation.
[c] NS, Not significant, $P < 0.05$.

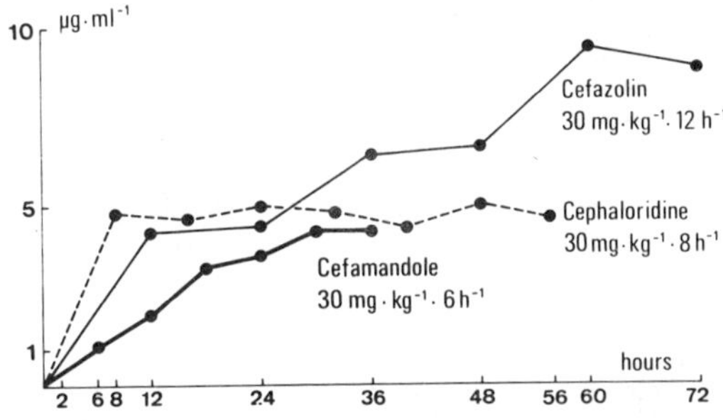

FIG. 4. *Cumulative effect of six i.m. injections of cefazolin (30 mg/kg every 12 h), cephaloridine (30 mg/kg every 8 h), and cefamandole (30 mg/kg every 6 h) on interstitial fluid concentrations measured just before the next injection in rabbits.*

determinations of the extent of protein binding in rabbits for cefazolin and cephaloridine are in the same range as those obtained by Nishida et al. (13). They are somewhat higher than in man. Barza and Weinstein (1) have shown an inverse correlation between the percentage of penetration into fibrin clots and the extent of binding of our penicillins. It appeared from their study that the degree of penetration is closely related to the relative levels of free drug in the blood. It is not well defined whether the peak level or the area under the curve of free drug is the most important determinant of penetration. In this part of our study, the very high concentrations observed with cefazolin in tissue fluid at 12 h after a single i.m. injection are somewhat at variance with what is generally accepted regarding the influence of protein binding on the diffusion of the drug. Cefazolin is highly bound, and Regamey et al. (14) have postulated a potential limitation of this drug related to its high level of serum protein binding. In our study, we have shown that cefazolin is likely to give high interstitial concentrations. Waterman et al. have demonstrated that binding of antibiotics by serum proteins does not restrict such agents to the intravascular space (19). The late high levels of cefazolin can be accounted for by its blood peak and half-life, which are, respectively, higher and longer than for cephaloridine. Cefamandole is relatively highly bound and gives the lowest blood levels. Consequently, this drug produces the lowest interstitial fluid concentration.

With all three drugs, late sustained interstitial levels were measured at a time (12 h) when no concentration of the drug was detectable in the blood. This finding has been described by many authors on similar animal models (1, 5, 7, 17, 18). Calnan et al. claimed that the fluid obtained under these conditions is indeed representative of body interstitial fluid (6). The presence of protein in the tissue fluid raises many questions. The extent to which cephalosporins bind to protein within the interstitial fluid has been demonstrated to be weak (19). It does not seem to affect the antibiotic behavior outside the vascular compartment (19). Our findings—and those of the aforementioned authors—

parallel the results reported by Barza et al. for fibrin clots rather than for their "interstitial fluid." We do not claim that this animal model closely approximates the physiological situation, but the tissue cage model provides some basis for comparison between different drugs in the same pharmacological group.

In the three-injection study (every 12 h), the cumulative effect of each drug in the interstitial fluid seems to be related to the late sustained levels. The higher interstitial levels of cefazolin over cephaloridine obtained 2 h after the third injection are probably due to a greater cumulative effect of cefazolin. It should be pointed out that this comparison was not carried out under strictly comparable conditions: the intervals between injections were identical, whereas the half-life of cephaloridine is shorter than that of cefazolin. In the six-injection study, cefazolin, administered in the same total dose, produced the highest interstitial concentrations over a much longer period of time. Therefore, within the limits of this animal study, it appeared that cefazolin might be the preferred agent in prophylactic treatment and probably in long-term therapeutic use.

ACKNOWLEDGMENTS

We are indebted to C. Mariel and D. Barral for discussion and criticisms and to D. Lanchon for a review of the English text.

LITERATURE CITED

1. **Barza, M., and L. Weinstein.** 1974. Penetration of antibiotics into fibrin loci in vivo. I. Comparison of penetration of Ampicillin into fibrin clots, abscesses, and "interstitial fluid." J. Infect. Dis. 129:59–65.
2. **Barza, M., T. Samuelson, and L. Weinstein.** 1974. Penetration of antibiotics into fibrin loci. II. Comparison of nine antibiotics: effect of dose and degree of protein binding. J. Infect. Dis. 129:66–72.
3. **Bennett, J. V., and W. M. M. Kirby.** 1965. A rapid, modified ultrafiltration method for determining serum protein binding and its application to new penicillin. J. Lab. Clin. Med. 66:721–732.
4. **Bennett, J. V., E. J. Benner, and W. M. M. Kirby.** 1966. Simplified, accurate method for antibiotic assay of clinical specimens. Appl. Microbiol. 14:170–177.
5. **Bodin, N. O., B. Ekström, U. Forsgren, L. P. Jalar, L. Magni, C. H. Ramsay, and B. Sjöberg.** 1975. Bacampicillin, a new orally well-absorbed derivative of ampicillin. Antimicrob. Agents Chemother. 8:518–525.
6. **Calnan, J. S., J. J. Pflug, G. D. Chisholm, and L. M. Taylor.** 1972. Pathophysiology of tissue fluid. Proc. R. Soc. Med. 65:715–719.
7. **Chisholm, G. D., P. M. Waterworth, J. S. Calnan, and L. P. Garrod.** 1973. Concentration of antibacterial agents in interstitial tissue fluid. Br. Med. J. 1:569–573.
8. **Fong, W. I., E. D. Ralph, E. R. Engelking, and W. M. M. Kirby.** 1976. Clinical pharmacology of cefamandole as compared with cephalothin. Antimicrob. Agents Chemother. 9:65–69.
9. **Goldstein, A., L. Aranov, and S. Kilman.** 1968. Principles of drug action, the basis of pharmacology, p. 142–196. Harper & Row, Publishers, New York.
10. **Moellering, R. C., and M. N. Swartz.** 1976. The newer cephalosporins. N. Engl. J. Med. 294:24–28.
11. **Neu, H. C.** 1974. Cefamandole, a cephalosporin antibiotic with an unusually wide spectrum of activity. Antimicrob. Agents Chemother. 6:177–182.
12. **Nightingale, C. H., S. Douglas, X. Greene, and R. Quintiliani.** 1975. Pharmacokinetics and clinical use of cephalosporin antibiotics. J. Pharm. Sci. 64:1889–1927.
13. **Nishida, M., T. Matsubara, T. Murakawa, Y. Mine, and Y. Yokota.** 1970. Cefazolin, a new semisynthetic cephalosporin antibiotic. II. In vitro and in vivo antimicrobial activity. J. Antibiot. 23:137–148.
14. **Regamey, C., R. C. Gordon, and W. M. M. Kirby.** 1974. Cefazolin VS cephalothin and cephaloridine. A comparison of their clinical pharmacology. Arch. Intern. Med. 133:407–410.
15. **Rolinson, C. S.** 1967. The significance of protein binding of antibiotics in vitro and in vivo, p. 254–283. *In* A. P. Waterson (ed.), Recent advances in medical microbiology. Churchill, London.
16. **Snedecor, G. W., and W. G. Cochran.** 1972. Statistical methods, 6th ed. The Iowa State University press, Ames.
17. **Tight, R., R. Prior, R. Perkins, and C. Rotilie.** 1975. Fluid and penicillin G dynamics in polyethylene chambers implanted subcutaneously in rabbits. Antimicrob. Agents Chemother. 8:495–497.
18. **Waterman, N. G., and L. G. Kastan.** 1972. Interstitial fluid and serum antibiotic concentrations. Arch. Surg. 105:192–196.
19. **Waterman, N. G., M. J. Raff, L. Scharfenberger, and P. A. Barnwell.** 1976. Protein binding and concentrations of cephaloridine and cefazolin in serum and interstitial fluid of dogs. J. Infect. Dis. 133:642–647.

ANTIMICROBIAL AGENTS AND CHEMOTHERAPY, Apr. 1977, p. 599-604 Vol. 11, No. 4

Comparative Activity of Ampicillin and Cefuroxime Against Three Types of *Haemophilus influenzae*

R. B. SYKES,* A. GRIFFITHS, AND D. M. RYAN

Glaxo Research Ltd., Greenford, Middlesex, UB6 OHE, England

Received for publication 23 November 1976

On the basis of their susceptibility to ampicillin, strains of *Haemophilus influenzae* can be divided into three types: type 1 are normally susceptible strains, type 2 produce stable spheroplasts from low inocula, and type 3 are β-lactamase producers. Because of the production of spheroplasts, standard broth and agar dilution techniques have failed to differentiate between the responses of type 2 and 3 strains to ampicillin, or to identify the superiority of cefuroxime over ampicillin against the β-lactamase-producing strains. Disk susceptibility tests with heavily seeded plates were also difficult to interpret. To overcome these problems, we developed a medium that supports the growth of *H. influenzae,* but not survival of spheroplasts, thereby reducing the complicating influence of spheroplast formation. Utilization of the medium made it possible to identify β-lactamase-producing strains via both minimal inhibitory concentration and disk susceptibility techniques, as well as the superiority of cefuroxime over ampicillin against such strains. In vivo experiments showed that cefuroxime and ampicillin are equally active against infections with type 1 and 2 strains, but that cefuroxime is superior to ampicillin against infections with type 3 β-lactamase-producing strains.

Until relatively recently, *H. influenzae* has remained remarkably stable in regard to its susceptibility to antibiotics (22). Ampicillin, chloramphenicol, and the tetracyclines have proved generally effective against the organism. However, over the last few years, an increasing number of reports have described the appearance of antibiotic-resistant strains (3, 5, 6, 8–10, 16, 19).

Infection due to ampicillin-resistant strains of *H. influenzae* has become an increasingly serious and widespread problem (1, 4, 18). The primary cause of ampicillin resistance appears to be the production of a β-lactamase that is capable of hyrolyzing a number of penicillin and cephalosporin substrates (7, 13, 17).

We have also found strains of *H. influenzae* which, tested by the conventional minimal inhibitory concentration (MIC) technique, show increased resistance to ampicillin but do not produce a β-lactamase. The apparent resistance of these strains resides in their ability to form osmotically stable spheroplasts at low inoculum concentrations. Thus, on the basis of their susceptibility to ampicillin, strains of *H. influenzae* are of three types. Type 1 includes normally susceptible strains, type 2 strains produce stable spheroplasts at low inocula, and type 3 strains are β-lactamase producers.

By using representative strains of the three types of *H. influenzae*, we compared the activities of ampicillin and cefuroxime, a β-lactamase-stable cephalosporin (14). Tests have been carried out using a commercially available nutrient medium and a contrived medium of low osmolality in which the spheroplasts of *H. influenzae* fail to survive.

MATERIALS AND METHODS

Organisms. All studies were carried out using six strains of each type of *H. influenzae*. Isolates were all derived from clinical material and given to us by P. Cavanagh, Public Health Laboratory, Stafford, England.

Media. The nutrient broth was Oxoid no. 2 (osmolality, 260 mOsmol/kg). The nutrient agar was Oxoid blood agar base. Dextrose phosphate broth contained bacteriological peptone (Difco), 4 g, dipotassium hydrogen phosphate, 5 g, and 4 g of glucose per liter (osmolality, 115 mOsmol/kg). To prepare the agar, agar (Difco) was added at a concentration of 1.5%. All media were supplemented with 5% Fildes and yeast extract (osmolality, 30 mOsmol/kg), prepared by adding equal volumes of Fildes extract (Oxoid) and 20% yeast extract (Difco). Cultures on solid media were incubated at 37°C in a CO_2 incubator (CO_2 concentration, 5 to 8%). Cultures in broth were grown in an air incubator at 37°C.

Susceptibility tests. Dilutions of antibiotics were prepared in the appropriate medium. Organisms grown for 6 h in liquid culture in a rotary shaking incubator at 37°C were diluted to give the required inoculum levels. Results were determined by both macroscopic and microscopic examination after 18 h of incubation at 37°C.

Osmolality. Osmolality was determined using a digimatic osmometer (Advanced Instruments Inc., Needham Heights, Mass.).

Protection tests. The animals used were albino Charles River female mice, weighing 18 to 20 g. Mice were challenged by the intraperitoneal route with the test organisms suspended in 0.2 ml of 2% dried bakers' yeast. The challenge dose was approximately 10 to 100 times the mean lethal dose, and the majority of untreated animals died within 24 h of challenge. Five animals were used at each of the serial threefold dose concentrations of antibiotic tested, which were given subcutaneously (0.2 ml per animal) at 1 and 5 h after challenge. The number of animals surviving on day 5 was used to calculate the median effective dose by logit transformation of the dose-response curve.

RESULTS

(i) MIC determinations. The activity of ampicillin and cefuroxime against the three types of *H. influenzae* is shown in Table 1. Both antibiotics were highly active against the type 1 strains but, above inocula of 10^5 colony-forming units (CFU), spheroplast formation was observed. With the type 2 strains, spheroplast formation was observed at low inoculum levels, leading to an apparent increase in the MIC.

Cefuroxime was highly active against the type 3 strains, but spheroplasts were present at the high inoculum levels. Ampicillin, however, showed a response similar to that seen against the type 2 strains, with increased resistance at the low inoculum levels but, in the case of the type 3 strains, no spheroplast formation was observed.

(ii) Disk susceptibility tests. Two sets of nutrient agar plates were inoculated by flooding with 6-h broth cultures of *H. influenzae*, undiluted and diluted 1:100, respectively, and antibiotic disks (30 μg) of ampicillin and cefuroxime were applied to each. Type 1 strains gave large, clear zones with ampicillin and cefuroxime on the lightly seeded plates but hazy zones on the heavily seeded plates. With the type 2 strains, zones were difficult to read at both inoculum levels (Fig. 1a and b), spheroplasts being responsible for the hazy zones. Against the β-lactamase-producing strain (Fig. 2a and b), a reduced zone was seen for ampicillin on the lightly seeded plate, compared with a large, clear cefuroxime zone. No zones were visible on the heavily seeded plates.

The spheroplasts of *H. influenzae* induced by β-lactam antibiotics are almost unique in their remarkable osmotic stability. Roberts and colleagues (16) reported that *H. influenzae* spheroplasts were highly resistant to osmotic lysis. They suggested that to overcome the "spheroplast problem," a light inoculum should be used in testing *H. influenzae* for susceptibility to β-lactam antibiotics. With the emergence of resistant strains, such a method may have many pitfalls.

With these points in mind, we set out to find a medium that could support the growth of *H. influenzae* but in which spheroplasts could not survive. Dextrose phosphate medium fulfilled these requirements. With this medium, we repeated the comparison between ampicillin and cefuroxime against the three types of *H. influenzae*.

(i) MIC determinations. Ampicillin and cefuroxime showed high antibacterial activity against *H. influenzae* type 1 and 2 strains even at the high inoculum levels (Table 2). Against the type 3 strains, cefuroxime was highly active, whereas ampicillin resistance was still apparent (Table 2).

(ii) Disk susceptibility tests. Ampicillin and cefuroxime disks produced clear zones against *H. influenzae* type 1 and 2 strains at both inoculum concentrations (Fig. 3a and b). Against the β-lactamase-producing strain (Fig. 4a and b), ampicillin showed reduced activity on the lightly seeded plate and no activity at the

TABLE 1. *Activity of ampicillin and cefuroxime against H. influenzae—nutrient broth and nutrient agar*

H. influenzae	MIC ampicillin/MIC cefuroxime (μg/ml) with CFU in inoculum:				
	10	10^3	10^5	10^6	10^7
Nutrient broth					
Type 1	0.25/0.25	0.25/0.5	0.5/0.5	16[a]/2[a]	>250[a]/>250[a]
Type 2	0.5/0.5	4[a]/8[a]	8[a]/16[a]	31[a]/31[a]	>250[a]/>250[a]
Type 3	0.5/0.25	2/0.5	31/0.5	>250/2[a]	>250/>250[a]
Nutrient agar					
Type 1	0.25/0.5	0.5/0.5	31[a]/31[a]	>250[a]/>250[a]	>250[a]/>250[a]
Type 2	0.5/0.5	2[a]/2[a]	31[a]/31[a]	>250[a]/>250[a]	>250[a]/>250[a]
Type 3	4/0.5	4/0.5	250/62[a]	>250/>250[a]	>250/>250[a]

[a] Spheroplasts predominant cell type.

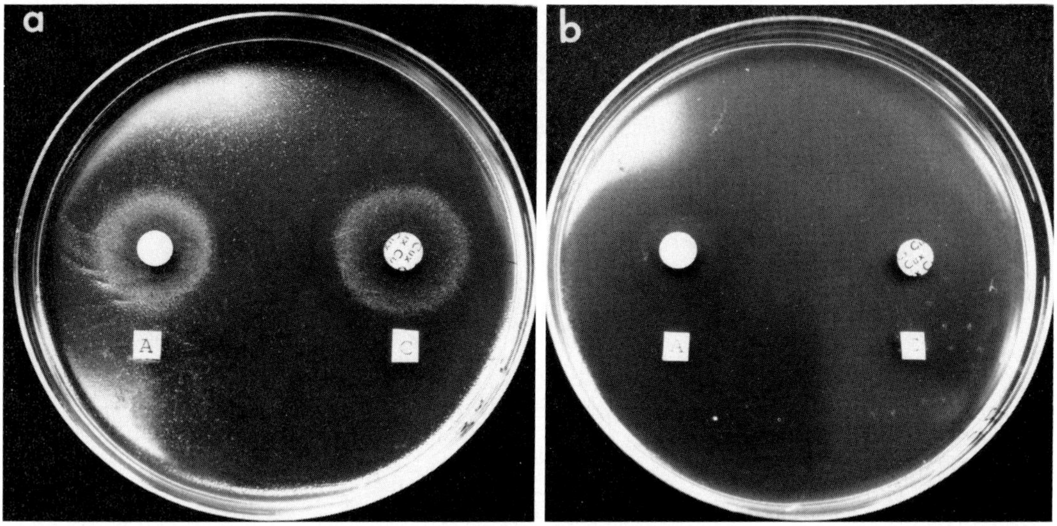

FIG. 1. *Disk susceptibility of H. influenzae type 2 to ampicillin (A) and cefuroxime (C) on enriched nutrient agar. (a) Light inoculum; (b) heavy inoculum.*

TABLE 2. *Activity of ampicillin and cefuroxime against H. influenzae—dextrose phosphate medium*

H. influenzae	MIC ampicillin/MIC cefuroxime (μg/ml) with CFU in inoculum:				
	10	10^3	10^5	10^6	10^7
Dextrose phosphate broth					
Type 1		0.5/0.25	0.5/0.5	1/0.5	1/1
Type 2		0.25/0.25	1/0.25	1/0.25	2/1
Type 3		4/0.25	16/0.5	125/0.5	>250/1
Dextrose phosphate agar					
Type 1	0.1/0.25	0.1/0.25	0.25/0.5	0.25/1	0.25/1
Type 2	0.25/0.25	0.25/0.5	0.5/1	1/1	2/1
Type 3	2/0.5	4/0.5	16/0.5	125/0.5	>250/0.5

heavy inoculum. Cefuroxime, on the other hand, showed clear zones at both inoculum levels.

In vivo studies. Protection tests in mice infected with each of the *H. influenzae* types showed ampicillin and cefuroxime to be equally effective against type 1 and 2 strains and cefuroxime to be 20 times more effective than ampicillin against the β-lactamase producer (Table 3).

DISCUSSION

Susceptibility testing of *H. influenzae* to β-lactam antibiotics with the conventional macroscopic determination of end point can lead to highly misleading results. Technical difficulties result from the ability of *H. influenzae* to form osmotically stable spheroplasts (2, 11, 12, 15).

The isolation of β-lactamase-producing strains of *H. influenzae* and the necessity of detecting these strains at an early stage of investigation has put greater emphasis on susceptibility testing procedures. With conventional techniques, we have encountered difficulties in differentiating between β-lactamase-producing strains and those strains of *H. influenzae* that form stable spheroplasts at low inoculum concentrations. Also, the superior activity of cefuroxime over ampicillin against β-lactamase-producing strains is not obvious by such techniques.

These difficulties have been overcome by the use of a medium in which the normal bacillary form of the organism can grow, but in which the spheroplasts do not survive. With this medium, either in a liquid or solid form, the importance of the inoculum size is greatly reduced, since spheroplasts no longer interfere with the interpretation of results. In the presence of am-

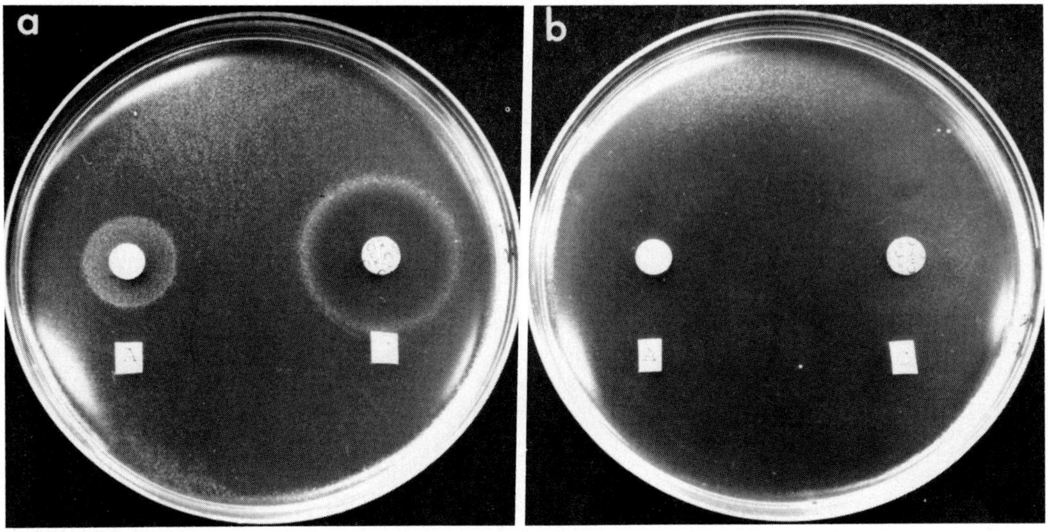

FIG. 2. *Disk susceptibility of H. influenzae type 3 to ampicillin (A) and cefuroxime (C) on enriched nutrient agar. (a) Light inoculum; (b) heavy inoculum.*

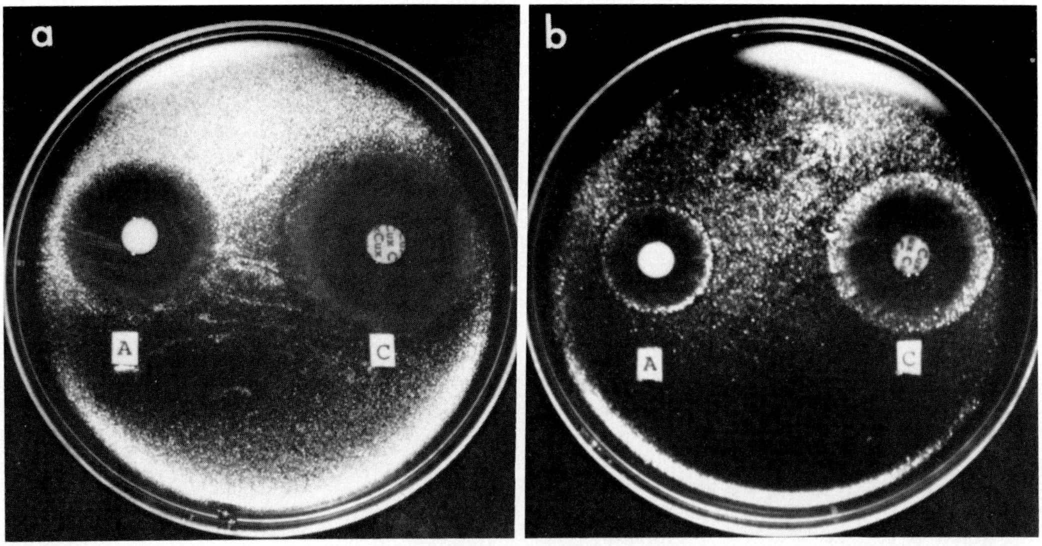

FIG. 3. *Disk susceptibility of H. influenzae type 2 to ampicillin (A) and cefuroxime (C) on dextrose phosphate medium. (a) Light inoculum; (b) heavy inoculum.*

picillin, β-lactamase-producing strains of *H. influenzae* are easily recognized on this medium, both by MIC and disk susceptibility tests. The superior activity of cefuroxime over ampicillin against such strains is also readily evident.

The in vitro results correlate well with the in vivo findings, in which cefuroxime, equally active as ampicillin against the type 1 and 2 strains of *H. influenzae,* is superior in activity to ampicillin against the β-lactamase-producing strain.

Cefuroxime should be an extremely useful β-lactam antibiotic for treating infections caused by *H. influenzae,* irrespective of their susceptibility to ampicillin.

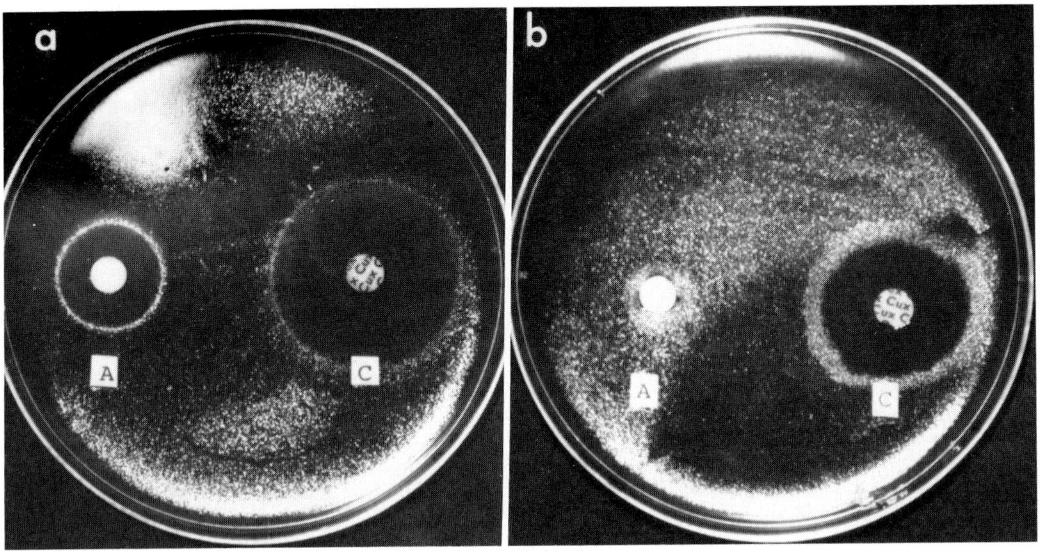

FIG. 4. *Disk susceptibility of H. infuenzae type 3 to ampicillin (A) and cefuroxime (C) on dextrose phosphate medium. (a) Light inoculum; (b) heavy inoculum.*

TABLE 3. *Protection tests on experimentally infected mice*

Haemophilus type	Median effective dose in mg/kg dose of:	
	Ampicillin	Cefuroxime
1	3	5
2	3	3
3	30	1.5

ACKNOWLEDGMENTS

We would like to thank D. Kedgley for kindly taking the photographs and W. Penn for making the osmolality determinations.

LITERATURE CITED

1. **Anonymous.** Ampicillin-resistant *Haemophilus influenzae* meningitis. 1974. Morbidity Mortality Week. Rep. 23:202–207.
2. **Bottone, E. J., Z. Brandman, and S. S. Schneirson.** 1976. Spheroplasts of *Haemophilus influenzae* induced by cell wall active antibiotics and their effect upon the interpretation of susceptibility tests. Antimicrob. Agents Chemother. 9:327–333.
3. **Cavanagh, P., C. A. Morris, and N. J. Mitchell.** 1975. Chloramphenicol resistance in Haemophilus species. Lancet 1:696.
4. **Clymo, A. B., and L. A. Harper.** 1974. Ampicillin-resistant *Haemophilus influenzae* meningitis. Lancet 1:453–454.
5. **Dang Van, A., G. Bieth, and D. H. Bouanchaud.** 1975. Tetracycline resistance plasmids from *Haemophilus influenzae*. C.R. Acad. Seances. Paris t. 280, Ser. D, p. 1321–1323.
6. **Emerson, B. B., A. L. Smith, A. L. Harding, and D. H. Smith.** 1975. *Haemophilus influenzae* Type B susceptibility to 17 antibiotics. Paediatrics 86:617–620.
7. **Farrar, E. W., and N. M. O'Dell.** 1974. β-lactamase activity in ampicillin-resistant *Haemophilus influenzae*. Antimicrob. Agents Chemother. 6:625–629.
8. **Gunn, B. A., J. B. Woodall, and J. F. Jones.** 1974. Ampicillin-resistant *Haemophilus influenzae*. Lancet 2:845.
9. **Kammer, R. B., D. A. Preston, J. R. Turner, and L. C. Hawley.** 1975. Rapid detection of ampicillin-resistant *Haemophilus influenzae* and their susceptibility to sixteen antibiotics. Antimicrob. Agents Chemother. 8:91–94.
10. **Manten, A., B. Van Klingeren, and M. Dessons-Kroon.** 1976. Chloramphenicol resistance in *Haemophilus influenzae*. Lancet 1:702.
11. **Marks, M., and G. Weinmaster.** 1975. Influence of media and inocula on the *in vitro* susceptibility of *Haemophilus influenzae* to co-trimoxazole, ampicillin, penicillin and chloramphenicol. Antimicrob. Agents Chemother. 8:657–663.
12. **McLinn, E. S., J. D. Nelson, and K. C. Haltalin.** 1970. Antimicrobial susceptibility of *Haemophilus influenzae*. Paediatrics 45:827–838.
13. **Medeiros, A. A., and T. F. O'Brien.** 1975. Ampicillin-resistant *Haemophilus influenzae* Type B possessing a TEM-type β-lactamase, but little permeability barrier to ampicillin. Lancet 1:716–718.
14. **O'Callaghan, C. H., R. B. Sykes, D. M. Ryan R. D. Foord, and P. W. Muggleton.** 1976. Cefuroxime – a new cephalosporin antibiotic. J. Antibiot. 29:29–37.
15. **Roberts, D. E., A. Ingold, S. V. Want, and R. J. May.** 1974. Osmotically stable L forms of *Haemophilus influenzae* and their significance in testing sensitivity to penicillins. J. Clin. Pathol. 27:560–564.
16. **Schiffer, M. S., J. MacLowry, R. Schneerson, and J. B. Robbins.** 1974. Clinical, bacteriological and immunological characterisation of ampicillin-resistant *Haemophilus influenzae* Type B. Lancet 2:257–259.
17. **Sykes, R. B., M. Matthew, and C. H. O'Callaghan.**

1975. R-factor mediated β-lactamase production by *Haemophilus influenzae*. J. Med. Microbiol. 8:437–441.

18. **Tomeh, M. O., S. E. Starr, J. E. McGowan, P. M. Terry, and A. J. Nahmias.** 1974. Ampicillin-resistant *Haemophilus influenzae* type B infection. J. Am. Med. Assoc. **229:**295–297.

19. **Williams, J. D., and J. Andrews.** 1974. Sensitivity of *Haemophilus influenzae* to antibiotics. Br. Med. J. **1:**134–137.

20. **Yourassowsky, E., E. Schoutens, M. P. Vanderlinden, and M. R. Prudhomme.** 1975. Susceptibility of Haemophilus to antibiotics: present status. Infection **3:**15–18.

ANTIMICROBIAL AGENTS AND CHEMOTHERAPY, Apr. 1977, p. 605-608 Vol. 11, No. 4

Penicillin Resistance and Penicillinase Production in Clinical Isolates of *Bacteroides melaninogenicus*

PATRICK R. MURRAY[1]* AND JON E. ROSENBLATT

Mayo Clinic and Mayo Foundation, Rochester, Minnesota 55901

Received for publication 4 December 1976

The minimum inhibitory concentrations (MIC) of penicillin and six other antimicrobials were determined for 50 clinical isolates of *Bacteroides melaninogenicus*. Agar dilution susceptibilities were performed using supplemented brucella blood agar and the proposed National Committee for Clinical Laboratory Standards standard method for anaerobes; results with the two methods were comparable. A penicillin concentration ≥0.8 μg/ml was needed to inhibit 56% of the isolates, whereas 100% were susceptible to 0.1 μg of clindamycin per ml. All isolates with penicillin MIC values ≥0.8 μg/ml produced β-lactamase using a slide method. A micro-iodometric assay was used to quantitate β-lactamase production in six isolates. The β-lactamase activity of *B. melaninogenicus* was comparable to that of a *Staphylococcus aureus* isolate but was not inducible, and the specific amount produced correlated only partially with penicillin MIC values. A clinical review of patients from whom the β-lactamase-producing strains of *B. melaninogenicus* were isolated did not suggest any increased virulence in these strains or an unexpectedly poor clinical response to appropriate therapy.

The susceptibility of anaerobes to antimicrobial agents is, in most instances, predictable. Generally, penicillin G is effective against anaerobes, with the exception of *Bacteroides fragilis* and some strains of *Fusobacterium varium* and *Clostridium* species (2, 3). The mechanism of *B. fragilis* resistance to penicillin is unknown, although it may be related to the production of β-lactamase. This enzyme is more active against cephalosporins than penicillins, is present in very low concentrations, and is associated with the bacterial cell membranes and released only with the disruption of the cell (1, 6, 7). β-Lactamase production by other anaerobes had not been detected until A. S. Hackman and J. Wong (Abstr. Annu. Meet. Am. Soc. Microbiol. 1976, A9, p. 2) recently reported the isolation of β-lactamase-producing strains of *Bacteroides melaninogenicus*. Although *B. melaninogenicus* is commonly considered to be susceptible to penicillin, previous studies from our laboratory demonstrated that a concentration of penicillin of 12.5 μg/ml or greater was required for the inhibition of 17% of the clinical isolates of *B. melaninogenicus* (5, 8). These data and the report of Hackman and Wong (above) prompted us to investigate further the antimicrobial susceptibilities of *B. melaninogenicus* and to determine the frequency and significance of β-lactamase production in our isolates.

[1] Present address: Microbiology Laboratory, Division of Laboratory Medicine, Barnes Hospital, St. Louis, MO 63110.

MATERIALS AND METHODS

B. melaninogenicus isolates were recovered from clinical specimens submitted to our clinical microbiology laboratory between October 1975 and May 1976. Isolation and identification of the isolates were performed according to the methods detailed in the Virginia Polytechnic Institute (4) and the Wadsworth (9) anaerobe laboratory manuals. Subcultures of the isolates were made at the time of identification, and equal volumes of skim milk (Baltimore Biological Laboratory, Cockeysville, Md.) and the culture in thioglycolate broth (enriched with hemin, 5 μg/ml, and vitamin K, 0.1 μ/ml) were mixed and stored at −60°C.

Antimicrobial susceptibility testing was performed in an anaerobic chamber by the agar dilution method as described by Sutter et al. (9). The antimicrobial agents in appropriate dilutions in sterile distilled water were incorporated into a brucella agar base enriched with 5% whole defibrinated sheep blood and vitamin K, 0.1 μg/ml. The concentration of metronidazole was calculated on a dry-weight basis; the remaining antimicrobials were diluted on the basis of the specific activity. Susceptibility tests were also performed using the proposed National Committee for Clinical Laboratory Standards standard method for anaerobes. The results were comparable for the two methods.

β-Lactamase production by isolates of *B. melaninogenicus* was determined by two methods, the slide modification of the iodometric method (J. E. Rosenblatt and A. M. Neumann, Prog. Abstr. Intersci. Conf. Antimicrob. Agents Chemother., 15th, Washington, D.C., Abstr. 388, 1975) and the quantitative micro-iodometric assay described by Sykes and Nordström (10). For the slide iodometric assay, a heavy loopful of colonies was removed from a blood agar plate and emulsified on a slide in a drop of phosphate-buffered saline (pH 6.4) containing iodine (3 mg/ml), potassium iodide (15 mg/ml), and aqueous pencillin G (50 mg/ml). One drop of 0.4% starch in water was then added, and the mixture was observed for 5 min. Although the mixture may initially be purple-colored, a positive reaction will be white or colorless within 5 min. The inoculum for the micro-iodometric assay of β-lactamase was prepared with isolates of *B. melaninogenicus* that were grown for 48 h in brucella broth supplemented with hemin and vitamin K. Each broth was then divided into two aliquots; penicillin G (100 μg/ml) was added to one aliquot in an attempt to induce β-lactamase production and the broths were reincubated for 4 h. The broths were then centrifuged, and the bacterial pellets were washed twice in phosphate-buffered saline at pH 5.9 and frozen at −60°C. Before the determination of enzyme activity, the bacteria were frozen and thawed three times and adjusted to an absorbance of 0.25 at 620 nm. The quantitative assay of β-lactamase activity was expressed in units defined as the amount of enzyme that hydrolyzed benzylpenicillin at the rate of 1 μmol/min at 30°C and pH 5.9.

RESULTS

Fifty isolates representing all three subspecies of *B. melaninogenicus* were recovered from various clincal sources. The minimum inhibitory concentrations (MICs) of seven antibiotics against 46 or 50 of these isolates are presented in Table 1. A penicillin concentration of 0.8 μg/ml was needed to inhibit 48% of the isolates. Fifty micrograms of carbenicillin per milliliter inhibited 100% of the isolates. At 3.1 μg/ml, cephalothin inhibited 46% of the isolates, and all isolates tested were susceptible to 0.1 μg of clindamycin per ml. Only 43% of the isolates were inhibited by 3.1 μg of tetracycline per ml, whereas 6.2 μg of chloramphenicol per ml inhibited all the isolates. All but 1 of the 46 isolates were inhibited by 3.1 μg of metronidazole per ml. In the isolates reported herein, resistance to β-lactam antibiotics was not associated with resistance to other antibiotics.

All isolates with penicillin MIC values ≥0.8 μg/ml and cephalothin MIC values ≥1.6 μg/ml produced detectable β-lactamase using the slide method (Table 2). Twenty-seven of the 28 isolates with carbenicillin MIC values ≥0.8 μg/ml produced β-lactamase. There was no difference in the qualitative production of β-lactamase among the three *B. melaninogenicus* subspecies.

β-Lactamase production was quantitated by the micro-iodometric assay for six isolates of *B. melaninogenicus* that had penicillin MIC values ranging from 0.1 to 50 μg/ml (Table 3). The β-lactamase activity of *B. melaninogenicus* was equal to or greater than that of the *Staphylococcus aureus* isolate not induced by pre-exposure to penicillin. In addition, β-lactamase production by isolates of *B. melaninogenicus* was not inducible with penicillin, whereas β-lactamase production by *S. aureus* was inducible. The specific amount of β-lactamase produced correlated only partially with the MIC values of penicillin.

TABLE 1. *Inhibitory activity of antibiotics against isolates of B. melaninogenicus*

Antibiotic	No. of isolates tested	Cumulative % inhibited at concn (μg/ml) of: 0.8	3.1	6.2	50
Penicillin	50	48	62	74	98
Carbenicillin	46	43	72	85	100
Cephalothin	46	41	46	46	93
Clindamycin	50	100			
Tetracycline	46	28	43	54	93
Chloramphenicol	46	26	85	100	
Metronidazole	46	67	98	98	100

DISCUSSION

Previous studies from our laboratory (5, 8) have characterized the in vitro antimicrobial susceptibilities of anaerobes isolated from clinical material and have provided data with which to compare the results reported in the present study. The isolates of *B. melaninogenicus* examined in the present study and in the earlier

TABLE 2. *Correlation of penicillin and cephalothin MICs and β-lactamase activity (slide test) in isolates of B. melaninogenicus*

MIC (μg/ml)	Penicillin[a] No. tested	Penicillin[a] No. with β-lactamase activity	Cephalothin[b] No. tested	Cephalothin[b] No. with β-lactamase activity
0.1	21	0	9	0
0.2	1	0	5	0
0.4			4	0
0.8	2	2	1	0
1.6	1	1	1	1
3.1	6	6	1	1
6.2	6	6		
12.5	7	7	7	7
25	3	3	8	8
50	2	2	7	7
100	1	1	2	2
>100			1	1

[a] Fifty-six percent with β-lactamase activity.
[b] Fifty-nine percent with β-lactamase activity.

TABLE 3. *Quantitation of β-lactamase activity (micro-iodometric assay) in isolates of B. melaninogenicus*

Isolate	Penicillin MIC (μg/ml)	β-Lactamase activity (IU × 10^{-3})	
		Without penicillin pre-exposure	With penicillin pre-exposure
S. aureus	1.0	0.59	1.72
B. melaninogenicus subsp.			
intermedius	0.1	ND[a]	ND
melaninogenicus	1.6	0.78	0.81
asaccharolyticus	6.2	1.19	1.16
asaccharolyticus	25	0.95	0.99
intermedius	50	1.43	1.40
melaninogenicus	50	0.61	0.59

[a] ND, Not detectable.

studies were highly susceptible to clindamycin, chloramphenicol, and, with one exception reported herein, metronidazole. An increase in resistance to tetracycline was found. Only 43% of the isolates in this study were inhibited at 3.1 μg/ml or less, compared with 79% of the isolates of *B. melaninogenicus* reported in 1972. The β-lactam antibiotics were not as effective in the current study, compared with the earlier results. Although the production of β-lactamase was not examined in previous studies, 38 and 50% of the isolates of *B. melaninogenicus* reported in 1972 and 1974, respectively, had penicillin MIC values ≥0.8 μg/ml, the concentration at which β-lactamase production was detected in the present study. In contrast, 28 of 50 (56%) of the current isolates had penicillin MIC values ≥0.8 μg/ml. Less than 0.8 μg of carbenicillin per ml inhibited 50 and 39% of the isolates reported in 1974 and herein, respectively. Less than 1.6 μg of cephalothin per ml was effective against 69% of the isolates reported in 1972 and 41% of those studied herein. Although the decreased effectiveness of the β-lactam antibiotics could be the result of technical differences in antimicrobial susceptibility testing, it is significant that more than half of the isolates of *B. melaninogenicus* examined in this study produced β-lactamase with activity against both penicillins and cephalosporins.

β-Lactamase production was initially detected with the slide modification of the starch agar iodometric method and was observed in all three subspecies of *B. melaninogenicus*. In contrast to the report of Hackman and Wong (Abstr. Annu. Meet. Am. Soc. Microbiol. 1976, A9, p. 2), the amount of enzyme produced was similar for the three subspecies and was substantially greater than we have detected in isolates of *B. fragilis*, although similar to that detected in *S. aureus*. As has been noted with *B. fragilis*, the enzyme activity was not inducible with penicillin and was only roughly correlated with the MIC values.

To determine the effect of β-lactamase production by *B. melaninogenicus* on the management of anaerobic infections, the clinical histories of 28 patients from whom β-lactamase-producing isolates had been recovered were reviewed. In 14 of the 28 patients, we were unable to determine the clinical significance of the isolate; and in the other 14 patients, the isolate was from a source where infection was either obvious or likely. Of the latter 14 patients, 12 were appropriately treated with an effective antimicrobial agent or surgical drainage and debridement (or both) when indicated. Of these 12 patients, 6 received clindamycin and 4 received therapeutic doses of a penicillin plus surgery. Two other patients were surgically treated but did not receive adequate antibiotic therapy. One patient with an isolate from two separate blood cultures had a self-limiting bacteremia, and another with endometritis was treated only with cephalothin (MIC = 50 μg/ml). Thus, this brief clinical review did not suggest any increased virulence for β-lactamase-producing isolates of *B. melaninogenicus* nor any evidence of poor clinical response to appropriate treatment, including penicillin therapy.

This study shows that most (56%) of the clinical isolates of *B. melaninogenicus* produce β-lactamase. The clinical significance of this finding is in doubt because the enzyme does not appear to be inducible, and our brief clinical review did not suggest a poor clinical outcome in patients yielding these isolates. However, because approximately 25 and 40% of our isolates had penicillin MIC values ≥12.5 and 6.2 μg/ml, respectively, knowledge of specific susceptibility results seems to be important. When these data are not routinely available, the simple slide iodometric test can detect β-lactamase-producing isolates of *B. melaninogenicus*.

LITERATURE CITED

1. **Anderson, J. D., and R. B. Sykes.** 1973. Characterization of a β-lactamase obtained from a strain of *Bacteroides fragilis* resistant to β-lactam antibiotics. J. Med. Microbiol. 6:201–206.
2. **Finegold, S. M., J. G. Barlett, A. W. Chow, D. J. Flora, S. L. Gorbach, E. J. Harder, and F. P. Tally.** 1975. Management of anaerobic infections. Ann. Intern. Med. 83:375–389.

3. **Finegold, S. M., V. L. Sutter, H. R. Attebery, and J. E. Rosenblatt.** 1974. Isolation of anaerobic bacteria, p. 365–375. *In* E. H. Lennette, E. H. Spaulding, and J. P. Truant (ed.), Manual of Clinical Microbiology, 2nd ed. American Society for Microbiology, Washington, D.C.
4. **Holdeman, L. V., and W. E. C. Moore.** 1972. Anaerobe laboratory manual. Virginia Polytechnic Institute and State University, Blacksburg, Va.
5. **Martin, W. J., M. Gardner, and J. A. Washington II.** 1972. In vitro antimicrobial susceptibility of anaerobic bacteria isolated from clinical specimens. Antimicrob. Agents Chemother. **1**:148–158.
6. **Olsson, B., C.-E. Nord, and T. Wadström.** 1976. Formation of beta-lactamase in *Bacteroides fragilis:* cell-bound and extracellular activity. Antimicrob. Agents Chemother. **9**:727–735.
7. **Pinkus, G., G. Veto, and A. I. Braude.** 1968. *Bacteroides* penicillinase. J. Bacteriol. **96**:1437–1438.
8. **Staneck, J. L., and J. A. Washington II.** 1974. Antimicrobial susceptibilities of anaerobic bacteria: recent clinical isolates. Antimicrob. Agents Chemother. **6**:311–315.
9. **Sutter, V. L., V. L. Vargo, and S. M. Finegold.** 1975. Wadsworth anaerobic bacteriology manual, 2nd ed. Regents of the University of California, Los Angeles.
10. **Sykes, R. B., and K. Nordström.** 1972. Microiodometric determination of β-lactamase activity. Antimicrob. Agents Chemother. **1**:94–99.

ANTIMICROBIAL AGENTS AND CHEMOTHERAPY, Apr. 1977, p. 609-614 Vol. 11, No. 4

Printed in U.S.A.

Netilmicin and Gentamicin: Comparative Pharmacology in Humans

LOUISE J. RIFF* AND GAIL MORESCHI

*Department of Medicine, University of Illinois at the Medical Center, Chicago, Illinois 60680, and Research and Education Division, West Side Veterans Administration Hospital, Chicago, Illinois 60612**

Received for publication 19 October 1976

Thirteen male subjects received 1 mg of either gentamicin or netilmicin per kg, first intramuscularly and then intravenously. After the intramuscular dose, concentrations of gentamicin in the serum were more variable than those of netilmicin. After the intravenous dose, the distribution phase of netilmicin was twice as rapid as gentamicin. The average half-times of the elimination phase were similar, but there was marked variability among the subjects receiving gentamicin. Serum clearance of netilmicin was more rapid than that of gentamicin and could not be attributed to renal elimination. The data indicate that, after intramuscular administration, netilmicin may produce more predictable blood levels than gentamicin and suggest that the body distribution of netilmicin may differ from that of gentamicin.

Netilmicin is a new semisynthetic aminoglycoside (32). Netilmicin is *N*-ethyl sisomicin, with the substituent attached to 2-deoxystreptamine. Another aminoglycoside in clinical use with a substitution on 2-deoxystreptamine is amikacin, a hydroxyaminobutyric acid derivative of kanamycin A. In vitro testing in our laboratory and others (8-10, 20, 23, 27, 31) indicates that the activity of netilmicin against *Enterobacteriaceae*, *Pseudomonas*, and *Staphylococcus*, in general, approximates that of gentamicin. Serum concentrations in animals and humans are comparable to those of gentamicin (27).

Netilmicin appears to have two advantages. First, like amikacin, it is effective against some organisms resistant to gentamicin, including indole-negative proteus and strains that produce aminoglycoside-adenylating enzymes (16, 23). Second, animal studies indicate that netilmicin has significantly less oto- and nephrotoxicity than does gentamicin (19, 27; R. E. Brummett and K. E. Fox, Fed. Proc. 35:621, 1976). If reduced toxicity is also found in humans, it will strongly influence the relative usefulness of this agent.

Netilmicin is now in the early stages of therapeutic evaluation, and expanded information concerning its pharmacology will be of benefit to physician investigators and their patients. For this reason, we have investigated the disposition of netilmicin in humans.

MATERIALS AND METHODS

Thirteen adult male graduate students were used in our study. The subjects underwent a complete medical history and psychological evaluation; physical examination; determination of base line blood chemistries (chloride, carbon dioxide, potassium, sodium, blood urea nitrogen and glucose, total protein, serum albumin, calcium, inorganic phosphorus, cholesterol, uric acid, creatinine, total bilirubin, alkaline phosphatase, creatine phosphokinase, lactic dehydrogenase, serum glutamic oxaloacetic transferase); complete blood count; urinalysis, including microscopic urinalysis and determination of creatinine clearance. All subjects were judged free from any recognizable illness by the above parameters. The experimental design of the project and the drugs used were explained, and informed consent was obtained from each individual. The study was approved by the Human Investigation Committee of the University.

With a preselected division of two groups, six gentamicin and seven netilmicin, the men were randomly assigned, single blind, to either group. The men receiving gentamicin had an average weight of 69.4 kg (range, 56 to 90 kg), and those receiving netilmicin had an average weight of 77.5 kg (range, 70 to 90 kg). None of the individuals was obviously under- or overweight. For the subjects receiving gentamicin the mean body surface area was 1.84 m^2, and for those receiving netilmicin it was 1.94 m^2. The mean age for both groups was 24 years (range, 22 to 27 years). Two of the men withdrew from the project after the intramuscular (i.m.) dose because of time pressures related to final examinations. Parenteral gentamicin, 40 mg/ml, and parental netilmicin, 100 mg/ml, were supplied specifically for this study by Schering Corp., Bloomfield, N.J. Each drug was given in a dose of 1 mg/kg of subject weight, first by i.m. injection into the deltoid and then by intravenous (i.v.) administration into a forearm vein, with a minimum of 1 week between doses (range, 7 to 41 days). The i.v. dose was given over 3 to 5 min in a side arm rider of 50 ml of normal saline. Before and after each dose, a general symptom review, blood pressure, oral temperature, and complete urinalysis were obtained. The morning after a dose, the subject returned for urinalysis, evaluation of auditory and labyrinthine function, blood chemistries, and complete blood count. A 16-h overnight urine collection was used to determine creatinine clearance.

For the i.m. injection, blood samples for serum drug concentration were obtained predose and at 10, 20, 30, 40, 60, and 90 min and 2, 3, 4, 5 or 6, and 7.5 h after drug administration. For the i.v. dose, blood samples were obtained predose, at 10-min intervals for h 1, 20-min intervals for h 2, at hourly intervals until 6 h, and at 7.5 h. Blood samples were collected in red-top Vacutainer-brand tubes, which are silicon coated, but do not contain anticoagulant. Urine was collected immediately prior to the dose, and the total urinary output from each subject was collected in timed portions; urinary concentrations of drug were measured at 1, 2, 4, 6, 8, 16, and 24 h after each dose.

Laboratory. Serum samples were separated, frozen at −20°C, and assayed within 1 to 6 days. Portions of urine collections were treated similarly. Assays were performed by the agar well diffusion technique (18, 26), using Mueller-Hinton agar (Difco) seeded with *Bacillus subtilis* spores. Standards for either gentamicin or netilmicin were used on each assay plate in concentrations of 1.2, 2.5, 5, 10, and 20 μg/ml. Portions of a stock solution of laboratory standard assay powder (gentamicin and netilmicin, supplied by Schering Corp., Bloomfield, N.J.) at 2,000 μg/ml of water were stored at −20°C. The standard solutions were freshly diluted in 100% human serum (Grand Island Biological Co., Grand Island, N.Y.) immediately prior to assay. Each urine assay plate contained standards of 3.1, 6.2, 12.5, 25, and 50 μg of the appropriate drug per ml, prepared by diluting stock solution in phosphate buffer, pH 8.0, that had previously been determined to give the same diffusion characteristics as human urine. Each serum and urine sample was determined in triplicate.

Analysis. The formulas and methods of Wagner (30) and Greenblatt and Koch-Weser (14) were used for the pharmacokinetic analyses. The "stripping" technique was used to determine the rate constants for the serum concentration curves after i.v. administration. The statistical analyses used are those of Batson (3).

RESULTS

i.m. administration. Figure 1 shows the average and range of observed serum concentrations for 8 h after i.m. administration of a 1-mg/kg dose. For most of the time points, the subjects given gentamicin exhibited a broader range of serum concentrations than did those receiving netilmicin.

The average peak serum concentration was identical for both drugs, 3.76 μg/ml. However, the time to achieve peak serum concentration was different for the two drugs. For four of the six subjects receiving gentamicin, the peak serum concentration occurred at 20 min, one occurred at 10 min, and one occurred at 40 min. Of the seven subjects who received netilmicin, one occurred at 30 min, and six had peak serum concentrations at 40 min.

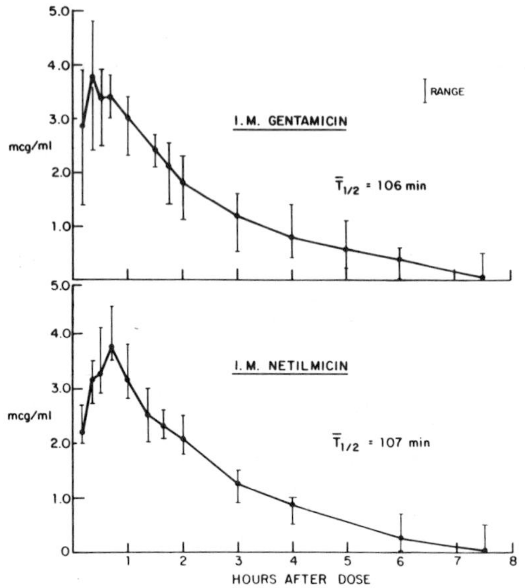

FIG. 1. *Average and range of serum concentrations after i.m. administration of netilmicin (seven subjects) and gentamicin (six subjects). The dose for each drug was 1 mg/kg of body weight.*

After the peak concentration was achieved, the elimination half-life ($T_{1/2}$) was the same for both drugs. The individual $T_{1/2}$ values, based on $n = 7$ to 11 points for each subject, demonstrated more variability for gentamicin than for netilmicin. For gentamicin, the $T_{1/2}$ ranged from 64 to 131 min; for netilmicin, the $T_{1/2}$ ranged from 79 to 117 min. The average time from the injection of dose to 50% of the peak level was approximately 2 h (126 min) for gentamicin and 2.5 h (147 min) for netilmicin.

i.v. administration. Figure 2 shows representative subjects who received gentamicin and netilmicin by i.v. "slow bolus" over 3 to 5 min, with actual (not "stripped") values plotted on semilog graph paper. Although not shown in the figure, serum concentrations were sampled until 450 min (7.5 h). The individual serum concentration curves were based on 14 to 17 determination points for each subject. Table 1 shows the mean values and range of serum concentrations at representative time points for the subjects in each group.

When the serum concentration plots were

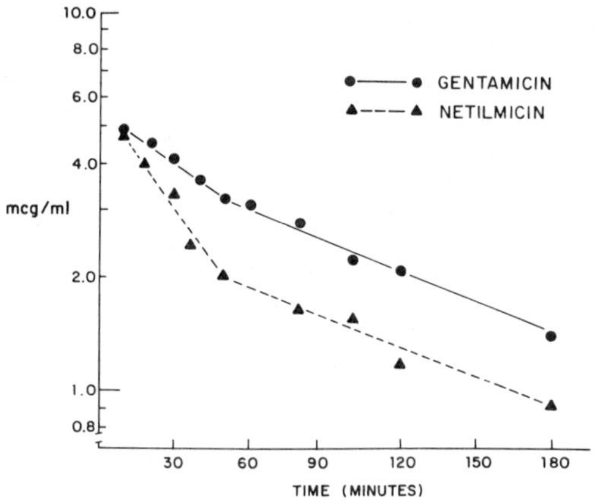

FIG. 2. *Serum concentrations after i.v. slow bolus in a subject receiving gentamicin as compared with one receiving netilmicin. The dose for each drug was 1 mg/kg.*

TABLE 1. *Average (and range) serum concentrations after i.v. slow-bolus administration of gentamicin and netilmicin (1 mg/kg)*

Time (min.)	Serum concn (μg/ml)	
	Gentamicin	Netilmicin
10	5.0 (4.2–6.0)[a]	4.8 (4.1–6.3)
20	4.5 (3.8–5.8)	3.9 (2.8–5.0)
30	4.0 (3.4–5.3)	3.4 (2.6–4.2)
40	3.6 (2.9–4.5)	2.9 (2.3–3.5)
60	3.0 (2.2–4.1)	2.3 (1.7–2.9)
80	2.5 (1.9–3.3)	1.9 (1.6–2.2)
100	2.2 (1.7–3.2)	1.7 (1.3–1.9)
120	1.9 (1.1–2.5)	1.5 (1.1–1.7)
180	1.2 (0.6–1.9)	0.9 (0–1.1)
240	0.8 (0.5–1.1)	0.4 (0–0.8)
360	0.3 (0–0.8)	0

[a] Numbers in parentheses indicate ranges.

examined individually, all subjects evidenced a biphasic curve, as illustrated by the subjects shown in Fig. 2. The initial portion of the curve, the α segment, or distribution phase, was markedly and consistently distinctive for the individuals receiving netilmicin as compared with those receiving gentamicin. For the group receiving gentamicin, the $T_{1/2\alpha}$ averaged 23.8 min (range, 20.6 to 27.4 min). The $T_{1/2\alpha}$ for the netilmicin group averaged 9.2 min (range, 6.4 to 10.4 min). The differences in $T_{1/2}$ values for the α phase are significant ($P = <0.01$).

For the second portion of the curve, the β segment or elimination phase, the average half-times were not different for gentamicin and netilmicin. The subjects receiving gentamicin displayed more variability in the half-time of the β phase than did those receiving netilmicin. The $T_{1/2\beta}$ for the subjects receiving gentamicin averaged 119.5 min (range, 94 to 160 min), and the $T_{1/2\beta}$ for the netilmicin group averaged 103.4 min (range, 91 to 119 min).

Urine recovery of drug. Figure 3 shows the average and range of urine recovery of both drugs after i.m. and i.v. administration at three representative time points, 2, 8, and 24 h. When the two routes of administration were compared for each drug individually, the i.v. dose resulted in greater urine recovery of both drugs at all time periods.

At 2 h after the administration of gentamicin, an average of 51% of the dose appeared in the urine when the drug was given i.v., as compared with 24% when the same dose was given to the same subject by the i.m. route. This difference is statistically significant ($P = <0.05$). The urine recovery of drug progressively increased after both i.m. and i.v. doses, and a differential of approximately 30% greater recovery after i.v. administration of gentamicin persisted for all time points. The urine recoveries after i.m. versus i.v. administration of gentamicin were significantly different at 8 and 24 h (for both time periods, $P = <0.05$). As shown in Fig. 3, the ranges of urine recovery for gentamicin were mutually exclusive for each method of administration.

When the two routes of administration for netilmicin were examined, the urine recovery at 2 h after an i.v. dose was approximately 13% greater than after an i.m. dose. This difference progressively diminished until, at 24 h after a dose, there was very little difference in urine recovery of netilmicin, regardless of the route of administration.

At 2 h after an i.m. dose, slightly more netilmicin was recovered than gentamicin (29 versus 24%). The average urinary netilmicin re-

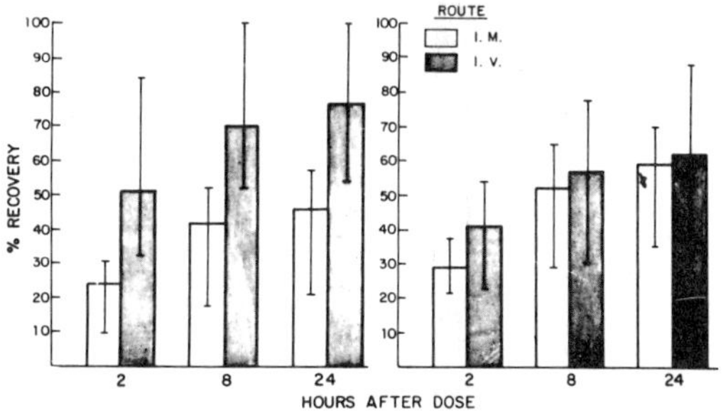

FIG. 3. *Cumulative urine recovery of aminoglycosides expressed as a percentage of the administered dose. (Left) Average of five subjects given 1 mg of gentamicin per kg by the i.m. and i.v. routes; (Right) six subjects given 1 mg of netilmicin per kg. I, Range of subjects.*

covery after i.m. administration showed a progressively greater increase as compared with gentamicin at 8 h (52 versus 42%) and 24 h (59 versus 46%). None of these values was significantly different. After i.v. administration, the average gentamicin recovery was greater than netilmicin recovery at all time periods. At 2 h after the i.v. dose, the average recovery of gentamicin was 51% of the administered dose; at 8 and 12 h, gentamicin recovery averaged 70 and 76% of the dose given. After i.v. administration of netilmicin, urine recovery at 2, 8, and 12 h averaged 41, 57, and 62% of the administered dose.

During the first 2 h after the i.m. dose of both drugs, urinary concentrations of the antibiotic ranged from approximately 15 to 60 μg/ml. During the first 2 h after the i.v. dose, urine concentrations of both drugs ranged from approximately 20 to 150 μg/ml. For both drugs, the urinary concentrations varied inversely with urinary output.

Distribution and clearance. The total volume of distribution (V_d) of drug for each individual was calculated by the formula: V_d = [Dose(mg)]/[β (area under serum concentration curve from T = 0 to T = ∞ = [Dose (mg)]/[$\beta(A/\alpha + B/\beta)$]. The total V_d was divided by the weight of the subject to convert the value to V_d per kilogram of body weight. The average V_d per kilogram of body weight for gentamicin was 222 ml, and for netilmicin it was 267 ml. These values are significantly different (P = <0.05).

A creatinine clearance was obtained for each subject on the day the i.v. dose was given. The serum clearance of administered drug was calculated by using the formula: Cl = $\beta \times V_d$ (14, 30).

The relationship of creatinine clearance and drug clearance for the two groups is shown in Table 2. There was no difference in creatinine clearance for the group receiving gentamicin as compared with netilmicin, nor was there any difference between creatinine clearance and the clearance of gentamicin. However, netilmicin was cleared from serum at a substantially higher rate than creatinine (P = <0.01). This was observed for each subject who received netilmicin. When the range of clearance of netilmicin was compared with the range of clearance of gentamicin, there was no overlap. For the subjects who received gentamicin, the range of drug clearance was 60 to 127 ml/min, and for netilmicin it was 122 to 162 ml/min. When the t test for unequal sample sizes is used, the differences between the clearance of netilmicin and gentamicin are significant (P = <0.01).

TABLE 2. *Relationships of creatinine clearance and drug clearance for the groups receiving either gentamicin or netilmicin*

Subjects receiving:	Mean creatinine clearance (ml/min)	Mean drug clearance (ml/min)
Gentamicin	108.2	98.6 (±12.4)[a]
Netilmicin	95.8	140.0 (±6.4)

[a] Numbers in parentheses indicate mean standard deviations.

Tolerance and toxicity. Both drugs were tolerated very well. None of the subjects experienced pain or discomfort from the i.m. or the i.v. administration of either drug. None of the physical parameters or symptoms that were checked before and after drug administration showed a meaningful change. Fluctuations in creatinine clearance, blood counts, and chemistries were all within normal limits and showed no consistent upward or downward trends.

During the second portion of the study (i.v. administration), it was noted that the 4- to 6-h postdose blood samples from three subjects appeared to have abnormal clotting (clotting did not appear to proceed as usual and did not have the customary morphology when complete). One of the subjects received gentamicin, and the other two received netilmicin. Evaluation of clotting parameters was performed by our special coagulation laboratory. One of these subjects, who received netilmicin, was discovered to have a mild deficiency of factor VIII (36 to 40% of normal). On repeated evaluations over the next 3 months, his partial thromboplastin time varied between normal and slightly prolonged. An explanation was not found for the other two subjects. It was the opinion of the coagulation specialist that we were viewing excessive erythrocyte "fallout," and not incomplete clotting. No other individuals in the study had an unusual appearance of blood clots or showed evidence of any coagulation abnormality.

DISCUSSION

The behavior of netilmicin in humans appears to differ from gentamicin in several respects. After i.m. administration, the average peak concentrations of netilmicin and gentamicin in the serum were the same, but the times from injection to peak serum concentration were notably different. The rapidity of peak levels of gentamicin in the serum differs from earlier observations (6, 12, 25). The rapidity may be due to the evaluation of lean, healthy, young subjects, who have neither diminished blood supply to muscles concurrent with aging nor other factors (intercurrent disease, prolonged bed rest, etc.) that may decrease muscle perfusion.

The time difference between peak levels may be either the effect of differences in the concentration of injected material, a characteristic of the compounds themselves, or a distortion due to small sample size. The latter seems unlikely because of the consistency of the differences between the drugs. Although medications given by i.m. injection generally follow a concentration gradient in diffusion from the i.m. site, at least one drug in clinical use does not: atropine has been reported to be more rapidly absorbed when given in a dilute solution and a larger volume (29).

In the comparison of amikacin and kanamycin (formulated as 260 and 250 mg/ml, respectively), Clarke et al. (7) found that, after i.m. injection, antibiotic concentration reached peak levels between 45 min and 2 h (J. T. Clarke, personal communication). Categorization of peak times according to drug was not given; however, from the data presented, it appears that kanamycin levels peaked approximately 30 min earlier than did amikacin levels and then sustained a plateau. If netilmicin and amikacin, both of which possess side chains on 2-deoxystreptamine, are absorbed from an i.m. site at a different rate (i.e., slower) than the analogous compounds gentamicin and kanamycin, then the alteration in the 2-deoxystreptamine moiety may confer pharmacological differences as well as microbiological ones. Whether apparent differences in absorption of gentamicin and netilmicin are due to structural differences in the two compounds or whether aminoglycosides as a class behave differently from other i.m. medications and mimic the behavior of atropine is unknown. If the differences are related to concentration of injected material, then the phenomenon may well be observed in patients: for clinical use, gentamicin is formulated as 40 mg/ml, and netilmicin is formulated as 100 mg/ml. The observation may be worthy of further investigation.

Even in a young, healthy population, gentamicin continues to display marked variability in peak serum concentration after i.m. injection (2, 11, 13, 15, 17, 24, 28). The variability in the peak level of gentamicin was almost twice that of netilmicin. In addition, there was a twofold range of variability in the $T_{1/2}$ among subjects who received gentamicin. These observations emphasize the need for monitoring the blood levels of gentamicin, even in patients with normal renal function (2, 22, 24, 25).

The i.v. dose of both drugs, given over 3 to 5 min, resulted in serum concentrations that were in an acceptable range and not excessively high. This is consistent with the observations of Mendelson et al. (21), who used higher doses of gentamicin in patients than our subjects received. Although the i.v. slow bolus appears to be relatively safe, it may have a major disadvantage as a routine method of administration to patients. An average of half the administered dose of gentamicin appeared in the urine within 2 h after the rapid i.v. dose. Obviously, a drug that is rapidly excreted is not available for tissue distribution.

The serial blood levels after the i.v. slow-bolus dose demonstrated a biphasic curve for both drugs. Although the average β phase was similar for both drugs, the α phase of netilmicin was considerably more rapid than gentamicin. The rapid plasma disappearance of netilmicin could be due to several causes, such as: metabolism of the drug, very rapid urinary excretion, or movement out of the vascular compartment to elsewhere in the body. Although metabolism is possible, it is unlikely in view of the knowledge of other aminoglycosides. The urinary recovery of netilmicin after the i.v. dose was less than the urinary recovery of gentamicin administered i.v., and the urine recovery of netilmicin was almost the same regardless of the route of administration. These observations, combined with the fact that the α phase of netilmicin exceeds that of gentamicin, suggest that the extravascular distribution of netilmicin appears independent of the route of administration. The converse appears true for gentamicin. That is, a large urinary output and a slow α phase after an i.v. dose suggest less extravascular distribution than with netilmicin.

There were no adverse reactions directly attributable to either of the drugs; however, an unusual observation regarding the blood clots in the samples from three subjects was noted. One subject was discovered to have a factor VIII deficiency, a congenital defect that was previously unsuspected (1; F. Rodriguez-Erdmann, submitted for publication). Other than for this individual, we have no explanation for the abnormal appearance of the clots in some samples after the i.v. doses. The phenomenon was observed with gentamicin as well as with netilmicin. Although it is entirely possible that some extraneous factor (such as excess silicon coating of the sample tubes) caused the phenomenon, unusual effects have been observed with drugs that have been in use for long periods of time (4, 5). The occurrence is reported here to inform other investigators of the possibility.

In summary, a comparison of gentamicin with netilmicin showed that netilmicin had a slower onset to peak concentration in serum and less variance in peak level after i.m. administration, a faster disappearance from serum after i.v. administration, a greater V_d, less variability in the $T_{1/2}$ phase, and a lesser recovery in urine than gentamicin. Our observations suggest that therapeutic levels of netilmicin may be more easily predicted in patients than levels of gentamicin. The rate differences and the urinary recovery data suggest that netilmicin may have a greater extravascular distribution than gentamicin. Future studies should also be directed toward determining the tissue distribution of netilmicin.

ACKNOWLEDGMENTS

We are grateful to Lawrence Isaac, Department of Pharmacology, for encouragement and guidance during the study and for critical review of the data and the manuscript, Doug Lewis for technical help, and Thomas Mizen for his invaluable assistance. We appreciate the support of Franz Rodriguez-Erdmann in the definitive coagulation analyses and evaluation and thank George Jackson for review of the manuscript. We acknowledge the excellent technical assistance of Al Simonaitis.

G. M. was a Public Health Service trainee under grant AI-00208-115 from the National Institute of Allergy and Infectious Diseases. Support was also provided by the Schering Corp., Bloomfield, N.J.

LITERATURE CITED

1. **Aggeler, P. M., H. S. Hoag, R. O. Wallterstein, and D. Whissell.** 1961. The mild hemophilias. Am. J. Med. 30:84–94.
2. **Barza, M., R. B. Brown, and D. Shen.** 1975. Predictability of blood levels of gentamicin in man. J. Infect. Dis. 132:165–174.
3. **Batson, H. C.** 1966. Statistics in the medical sciences. Chicago Medical Book Co., Chicago.
4. **Bell, W. R.** 1976. Editorial: thrombocytopenia occurring during heparin therapy. New Engl. J. Med. 295:276–277.
5. **Bell, W. R., P. A. Tomasula, B. M. Alving, and T. P. Duffy.** 1976. Thrombocytopenia occurring during the administration of heparin. A prospective study in 52 patients. Ann. Intern. Med. 85:155–160.
6. **Black, J., B. Calesnick, D. Williams, and M. J. Weinstein.** 1964. Pharmacology of gentamicin, a new board-spectrum antibiotic, p. 138–147. Antimicrob. Agents Chemother. 1963.
7. **Clarke, J. T., W. M. M. Kirby, R. D. Libke, and C. Regamey.** 1974. Comparative pharmacokinetics of amikacin and kanamycin. Clin. Pharmacol. Ther. 15:610–616.
8. **Flournoy, D. J.** 1976. Sisomicin versus netilmicin: in vitro susceptibility testing. Antimicrob. Agents Chemother. 10:864–865.
9. **Fu, K. P., and H. C. Neu.** 1976. In vitro synergistic effect of netilmicin, a new aminoglycoside antibiotic. Antimicrob. Agents Chemother. 10:511–518.
10. **Fu, K. P., and H. C. Neu.** 1976. In vitro study of netilmicin compared with other aminoglycosides. Antimicrob. Agents Chemother. 10:526–534.
11. **Galioto, G., C. Grassi, G. Manara, and P. Santarelli.** 1974. Studies on tolerance and blood levels of gentamicin in old subjects. Int. J. Clin. Pharmacol. 10:95–100.
12. **Goldstein, A., L. Aronow, and S. M. Kalman.** 1974. principles of drug action: the basis of pharmacology, 2nd ed. John Wiley and Sons, New York.
13. **Goodman, E., J. Gelder, R. Holmes, A. Hull, and J. Sanford.** 1975. Prospective comparative study of variable dosage and variable frequency regimens for administration of gentamicin. Antimicrob. Agents Chemother. 8:434–438.
14. **Greenblatt, D. J., and J. Koch-Weser.** 1975. Clinical pharmacokinetics. New Engl. J. Med. 293:702–705, 964–970.
15. **Hull, H., and F. Sarubbi.** 1976. Gentamicin serum concentrations: pharmacokinetic predictions. Ann. Intern. Med. 85:183–189.
16. **Kabins, S., C. Nathan, and S. Cohen.** 1976. In vitro comparison of netilmicin, a semisynthetic derivative of sisomicin, and four other aminoglycoside antibiotics. Antimicrob. Agents Chemother. 10:139–145.
17. **Kaye, D., M. E. Levison, and E. D. Labovitz.** 1974. The unpredictability of serum concentrations of gentamicin: pharmacokinetics of gentamicin in patients with normal and abnormal renal function. J. Infect. Dis. 130:150–154.
18. **Litwack, K.** 1969. Discussion on chemistry and microbiology of gentamicin. J. Infect. Dis. 119:381–382.
19. **Luft, F. C., M. H. Yum, and S. A. Kleit.** 1976. Comparative nephrotoxicities of netilmicin and gentamicin in rats. Antimicrob. Agents Chemother. 10:845–849.
20. **Marks, M. I., S. Hammerberg, G. Greenstone, and B. Silver.** 1976. Activity of newer aminoglycosides and carbenicillin, alone and in combination, against gentamicin-resistant *Pseudomonas aeruginosa*. Antimicrob. Agents Chemother. 10:399–410.
21. **Mendelson, J. J. Portnoy, V. Dick, and M. Black.** 1976. Safety of the bolus administration of gentamicin. Antimicrob. Agents Chemother. 9:633–638.
22. **Noone, P., T. M. C. Parsons, J. R. Pattison, R. C. B. Slack, D. Garfield-Davies, and K. Hughes.** 1974. Experience in monitoring gentamicin therapy during treatment of serious gram-negative sepsis. Br. Med. J. 1:477–481.
23. **Rahal, J., M. Simberkoff, K. Kagan, and N. Moldover.** 1976. Bactericidal efficacy of Sch 20569 and amikacin against gentamicin-sensitive and -resistant organisms. Antimicrob. Agents Chemother. 9:595–599.
24. **Riff, L.** 1973. Pseudomonas bacteremia: evaluation of factors influencing response to therapy. Acta. Pathol. Microbiol. Scand. 81:79–88.
25. **Riff, L. J., and G. G. Jackson.** 1971. Pharmacology of gentamicin in man. J. Infect. Dis. 124:(Suppl.):98–105.
26. **Sabath, L. D., J. I. Casey, P. A. Ruch, L. L. Stumpf, and M. Finland.** 1971. Rapid microassay for circulating nephrotoxic antibiotics, p. 83–90. Antimicrob. Agents Chemother. 1970.
27. **Schering Corporation.** 1975. Investigator's brochure for Sch 20569. Schering Corp., Bloomfield, N.J.
28. **Schimpff, S., W. Saterlee, V. M. Young, and A. Serpick.** 1971. Empiric therapy with carbenicillin and gentamicin for febrile patients with cancer and granulocytopenia. New Engl. J. Med. 284:1061–1065.
29. **Schriftman, H., and A. Kondritzer.** 1957. Absorption of atropine from muscle. Am. J. Physiol. 191:591–594.
30. **Wagner, J. G.** 1975. Fundamentals of clinical pharmacokinetics. Drug Intelligence Publications, Hamilton, Ill.
31. **Watanakunakorn, C.** 1976. Comparative in vitro activity of Sch 20656, netilmicin, gentamicin, and tobramycin. Antimicrob. Agents Chemother. 10:382–383.
32. **Weinstein, M. J., J. A. Marquez, R. T. Testa, G. H. Wagman, E. M. Oden, and J. A. Waitz.** 1970. Antibiotic 6640, a new micromonospora produced aminoglycoside antibiotic. J. Antibiot. 23:551–554.

ANTIMICROBIAL AGENTS AND CHEMOTHERAPY, Apr. 1977, p. 615-618 Vol. 11, No. 4

Printed in U.S.A.

Influence of Antioxidants on the Bioactivity of Amphotericin B

FRED A. ANDREWS,* WILLIAM H. BEGGS, AND GEORGE A. SAROSI

General Medical Research Service, Veterans Administration Hospital, Minneapolis, Minnesota 55417

Received for publication 3 December 1976

Four antioxidants, propyl gallate, butylated hydroxyanisole, butylated hydroxytoluene, and D-α-tocopherol acid succinate were found to stabilize amphotericin B and to prolong its antifungal activity against *Candida albicans*. Although each of the antioxidants was effective in this respect, propyl gallate and butylated hydroxyanisole were better than butylated hydroxytoluene and D-α-tocopherol acid succinate. None of the antioxidants alone adversely affected normal cell growth. It is suggested that amphotericin B instability is due, at least in part, to lability of the carbon-carbon double bonds of the polyene moiety toward autoxidation. By protecting the drug molecule with an antioxidant, it is possible to significantly lower the quantity of AB necessary to obtain particular antifungal effects.

Amphotericin B (AB), in spite of its instability (6, 10, 11, 16, 21) and high toxicity (11, 13, 14, 20), is the most important single antibiotic for treatment of the systemic mycoses (1). Since AB is a polyunsaturated molecule containing seven conjugated carbon-carbon double bonds (11), it is not surprising that the drug is unstable. One would expect the molecule to autoxidize in the presence of air (either under anhydrous or solvated conditions) with the formation of free radicals, hydroperoxides, peroxides, oxiranes, and carbonyl compounds, as is typical of unsaturated lipids (19). Formation of these highly reactive intermediates would not only reduce the effective drug concentration in solution but would also quite likely contribute to its toxicity, as has been shown for a number of unsaturated lipids (2, 8, 9, 12, 15, 18).

If instability of AB involves autoxidation of the conjugated double bonds, the addition of an antioxidant to a yeast culture treated with AB should improve stability and therefore biological activity of the antibiotic. There are isolated reports in which it has been observed that antioxidants can retard decomposition of polyenes (3, 4, 16). However, we are not aware of any published work in which the possibility that antioxidants can improve the biological activity of AB (or other polyenes) has been systematically investigated. In the present study, we have tested the effect of four well-known primary antioxidants – butylated hydroxyanisole (BHA), *n*-propyl gallate (PG), butylated hydroxytoluene (BHT) and D-α-tocopherol acid succinate (VE) – in a *Candida albicans*-AB system.

MATERIALS AND METHODS

Test organism. *C. albicans* ATCC 11651 was purchased from the American Type Culture Collection, Rockville, Md. Stock cultures were maintained on Sabouraud dextrose agar (Difco) and passed at weekly intervals.

Antibiotic. AB in the form of Fungizone was purchased from E. R. Squibb & Sons, Princeton, N.J. This product was supplied as a sterile lyophilized powder containing 50 mg of AB, 41 mg of sodium desoxycholate, and 25.2 mg of sodium phosphates as buffer. Stock solutions of the drug were prepared in sterile deionized water. In each experiment, freshly prepared solutions, protected from light, were used.

Antioxidants. The four primary antioxidants, PG, BHA, BHT, and VE, were purchased from Sigma Chemical Co., St. Louis, Mo. Each compound was dissolved and diluted in dimethyl sulfoxide (Me_2SO). Concentrations of antioxidant stock solutions were such that the volumes of Me_2SO added to cell suspensions were $\leq 1\%$ of the total volume. At a concentration of 1%, Me_2SO alone or in combination with 0.1 μg of sodium desoxycholate per ml had no observable effect on either the growth of *C. albicans* or on the bioactivity of AB.

Culture medium. The synthetic liquid medium used in these studies had the same composition as that described by Shadomy (17) and contained 6.7 g of yeast nitrogen base (Difco), 1.5 g of L-asparagine, and 10.0 g of dextrose in 1 liter of distilled water. For our purposes, however, the medium was adjusted to pH 7 before filter sterilization.

Experimental. *C. albicans* was grown in synthetic liquid medium at 37°C with rotary shaking (150 rpm). Cultures grown for 12 to 16 h were diluted in fresh medium to a calculated optical density (OD) at 420 nm of 0.008, which represents 3×10^5 to 5×10^5 colony-forming units/ml, as determined by standard dilution and plate count techniques.

In the initial screening experiments designed to compare the four antioxidants, 20-ml portions of cell suspension containing either no drug or 0.10 μg of AB per ml were added to 50-ml Erlenmeyer flasks containing various amounts of the specific antioxidants such that the final concentrations ranged from 0 to 8.0 μg/ml. The mixtures of cells, antibiotic, and antioxidant were then incubated for 24 to 29 h at 37°C with shaking in the dark, and OD values were read on a spectrophotometer (Coleman model 6C) at 420 nm. Three control flasks were included in each experiment: flask 1 contained cells only, flask 2 contained cells plus 8.0 μg of antioxidant per ml, and flask 3 contained cells plus 0.10 μg of AB per ml.

In growth experiments designed to show the enhanced effects of antioxidants on the antifungal activity of AB in more detail, three concentrations of AB were used, with the incorporation of a constant ratio of drug to antioxidant. *C. albicans* cultures were diluted as described above, and 75-ml volumes of cell suspension were placed in 500-ml Nephelo-Culture flasks (Bellco) containing sufficient antioxidant to give the desired final concentrations. Drug was then added at 0.025, 0.05, or 0.10 μg of AB per ml. Controls included 75-ml volumes of cell suspension with either no additions, AB alone at the three different concentrations, or antioxidants alone at 0.60 μg/ml. A drug/antioxidant ratio of 1:6 was

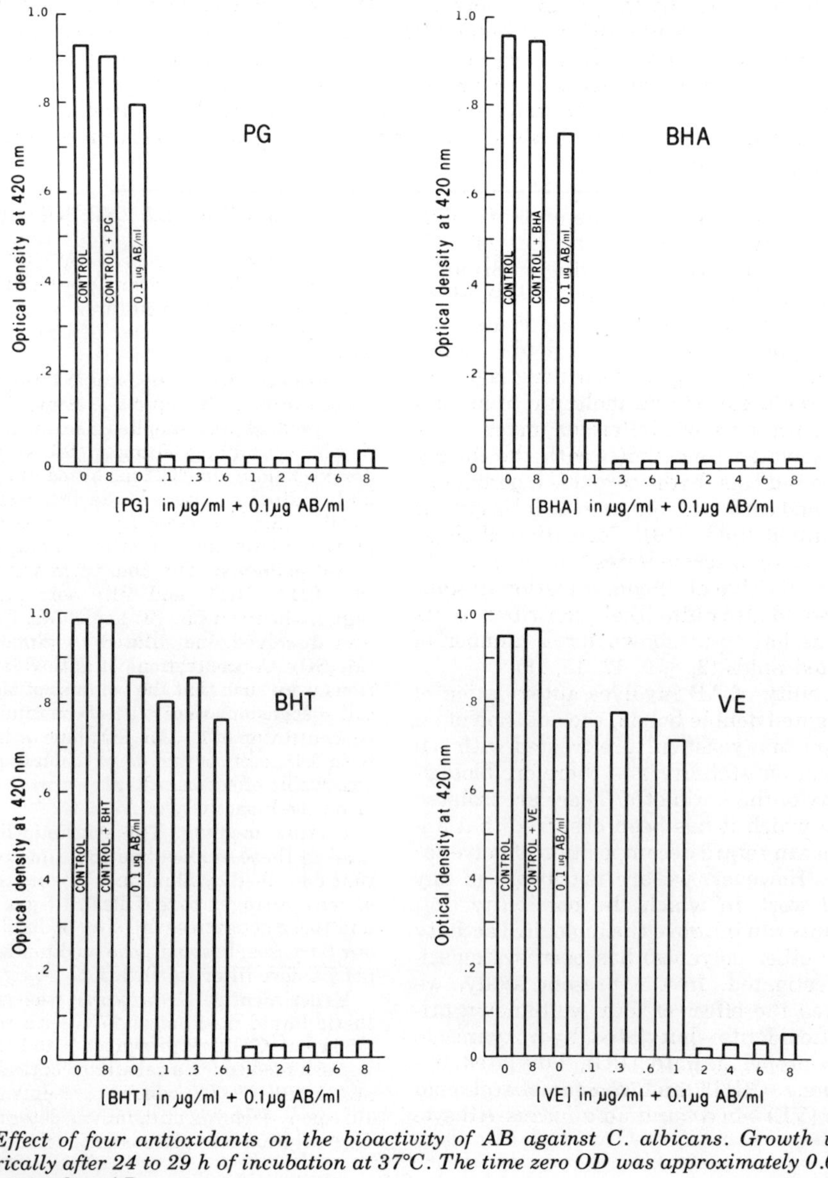

FIG. 1. *Effect of four antioxidants on the bioactivity of AB against C. albicans. Growth was assayed turbidimetrically after 24 to 29 h of incubation at 37°C. The time zero OD was approximately 0.008. Control cultures contained no AB.*

maintained (e.g., 0.10 μg of AB plus 0.60 μg of BHA per ml). The flasks were incubated with shaking at 37°C in the dark and OD values were read at time intervals over a 72-h incubation period.

RESULTS

Growth data shown in Fig. 1 support the contention that primary antioxidants preserve the structural integrity of AB and prolong its biological activity. PG and BHA were highly effective over the entire range of concentrations tested. Growth in cultures treated with 0.10 μg of AB per ml alone approached that of the controls in 24 to 29 h, but when PG or BHA was also present at 0.10 to 8.0 μg/ml, growth remained completely inhibited. BHT did not protect AB from loss of activity below 1.0 μg/ml, and the lowest effective concentration for vitamin E was approximately 2.0 μg/ml. Since each compound has a different oxidation-reduction potential, variations in effectiveness would be expected. None of the antioxidants alone, at a level of 8.0 μg/ml, adversely affected cell growth.

To further demonstrate the improved antifungal effect of AB on *C. albicans* in the presence of an antioxidant, detailed growth experiments were conducted with three different concentrations of AB and a constant ratio of drug to antioxidant (1:6). In these studies, the effects of the two agents alone and in combination were measured turbidimetrically over prolonged incubation periods. Data for the antioxidant BHA are shown in Fig. 2. It can be noted that AB at 0.025, 0.05, and 0.10 μg/ml inhibited growth for varying periods of time that were directly proportional to the initial drug concentrations used. On a microgram basis, AB to BHA ratios of 1:6 approximately doubled the time period that each level of drug completely prevented growth. It should also be noted that growth in the presence of BHA alone at a level of 0.60 μg/ml was the same as in the control culture containing no drug or antioxidant. In identical experiments using PG instead of BHA, the results were even more dramatic as shown in Fig. 3. The combination of 0.05 μg of AB and 0.30 μg of PG per ml of cell suspension appeared to be as effective as 0.10 μg of AB plus 0.60 μg of BHA per ml (Fig. 2), thus indicating the superiority of PG as an antioxidant under the test conditions used. Although it is not shown in Fig. 2 and 3, 0.10 μg of AB plus 0.60 μg of BHA per ml and 0.05 μg of AB plus 0.30 μg of PG per ml inhibited cell growth as well as did 0.20 μg of AB per ml alone.

DISCUSSION

The data presented above and the observations of Rickards et al. (16) leave little doubt that the instability of AB is due, at least in part, to lability of its polyene structure to autoxidation. The drug appears to behave much like an unsaturated lipid in the presence of molecular oxygen in that the molecule is stabilized and its bioactivity is preserved by primary antioxidants.

It is reasonable to assume that peroxidation of AB occurs in a relatively short time in the presence of air, and our data suggest that the intermediates resulting from this process are not biologically active. Since neither the lactone ring nor the other functional groups are

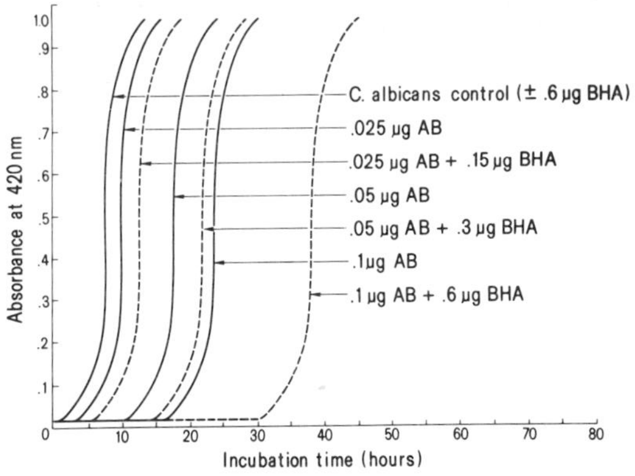

FIG. 2. *Growth inhibition of C. albicans by three different concentrations of AB and the effects of BHA on the duration of inhibition. The time zero absorbance (OD) was approximately 0.008. Growth was measured turbidimetrically and plotted as a function of time. Numbers represent micrograms of AB or BHA per milliliter of cell suspension.*

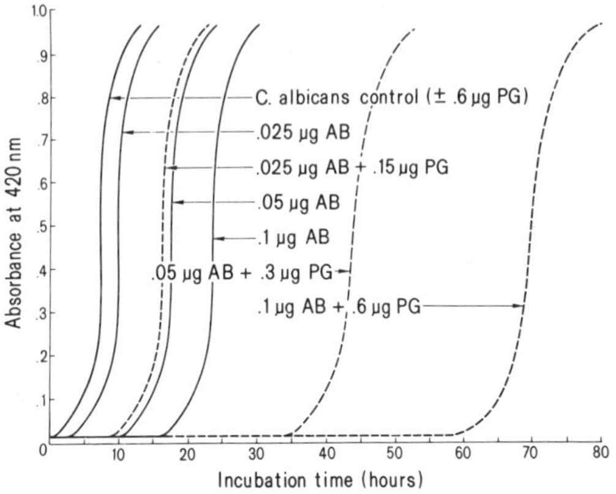

FIG. 3. *Growth inhibition of C. albicans by three different concentrations of AB and the effects of PG on the duration of inhibition. The time zero absorbance (OD) was approximately 0.008. Growth was measured turbidimetrically and plotted as a function of time. Numbers represent micrograms of AB or PG per milliliter of cell suspension.*

affected by small amounts of added antioxidants, it is reasonable to assume that the polyene region of the AB molecule is primarily responsible for instability under rather mild conditions.

PG, BHA, and BHT are widely used as antioxidants in the food and pharmaceutical industries and are generally regarded as safe for human consumption (5, 7). Similarly, VE is nontoxic, but is a less effective antioxidant than the other three considered here. Since these compounds are well tolerated by animals and humans and since they can stabilize and prolong the biological activity of AB, antioxidants may find practical application in AB chemotherapy. It might be possible to design effective treatment regimens on the basis of low-dose AB in combination with an antioxidant, thereby reducing AB toxicity. Although the possibility is purely speculative at this point, an antioxidant might also reduce toxicity by preventing the formation and interaction of highly reactive peroxides with tissue proteins, as is the case with other peroxidized lipids in vivo (8, 18).

LITERATURE CITED

1. **Abernathy, R. S.** 1973. Treatment of systemic mycoses. Medicine 52:385–394.
2. **Andrews, F. A., J. Bjorksten, F. B. Trenk, A. S. Henick, and R. B. Koch.** 1965. The reaction of an autoxidized lipid with proteins. J. Am. Oil Chem. Soc. 42:779–781.
3. **Belenkii, B. C., S. N. Solovev, A. I. Filippova, A. A. Nevinskii, A. M. Mamtsis, and S. B. Kogan.** 1966. Photo- and thermoinactivation of sodium nystatin. Antibiotikii 11:112–117.
4. **Bonner, D. P., W. Mechlinski, and C. P. Schaffner.** 1975. Stability studies with amphotericin B and amphotericin B methyl ester. J. Antibiotics 28:132–135.
5. **Branen, A. L.** 1975. Toxicology and biochemistry of butylated hydroxyanisole and butylated hydroxytoluene. J. Am. Oil Chem. Soc. 52:59–63.
6. **Cheung, S. C., G. Medoff, D. Schlessinger, and G. S. Kobayashi.** 1975. Stability of amphotericin B in fungal culture media. Antimicrob. Agents Chemother. 8:426–428.
7. **Chipault, J. P.** 1961. Antioxidants for use in foods, p. 477–542. *In* W. O. Lundberg (ed.), Autoxidation and antioxidants, vol. 2. Interscience Publishers, New York.
8. **DiLuzio, N. R.** 1973. Antioxidants, lipid peroxidation and chemical-induced liver injury. Fed. Proc. 32:1875–1881.
9. **Fitch, C. D.** 1968. The red blood cell in the vitamin E-deficient monkey. Am. J. Clin. Nutr. 21:51–56.
10. **Hamilton-Miller, J. M. T.** 1973. The effect of pH and of temperature on the stability and bioactivity of nystatin and amphotericin B. J. Pharm. Pharmacol. 25:401–407.
11. **Hamilton-Miller, J. M. T.** 1973. Chemistry and biology of polyene macrolide antibiotics. Bacteriol. Rev. 37:166–196.
12. **Holman, R. T., and S. I. Greenberg.** 1958. A note on the toxicities of methyl oleate peroxide and ethyl linoleate peroxide. J. Am. Oil Chem. Soc. 35:707.
13. **Lampen, J. O.** 1969. Amphotericin B and other polyene antifungal antibiotics. Am. J. Clin. Pathol. 52:138–146.
14. **Miller, R. P., and J. H. Bates.** 1969. Amphotericin B toxicity. Ann. Intern. Med. 71:1089–1095.
15. **Oski, F. A., and L. A. Barness.** 1968. Hemolytic anemia in vitamin E deficiency. Am. J. Clin. Nutr. 21:45–50.
16. **Rickards, R. W., R. M. Smith, and B. T. Golding.** 1970. Macrolide antibiotic studies. XV. The autoxidation of the polyenes of the filipin complex and lagosin. J. Antibiot. 23:603–612.
17. **Shadomy, S.** 1969. In vitro studies with 5-fluorocytosine. Appl. Microbiol. 17:871–877.
18. **Tappel, A. L.** 1973. Lipid peroxidation damage to cell components. Fed. Proc. 32:1870–1874.
19. **Uri, N.** 1961. Physico-chemical aspects of autoxidation, p. 55–77. *In* W. O. Lundberg (ed.), Autoxidation and antioxidants, vol. 1. Interscience Publishers, New York.
20. **Utz, J. P.** 1968. Clinical applications and side effects of antifungal drugs, p. 242–250. *In* G. E. W. Wolstenholme and R. Portec (ed.), CIBA Foundation Symposium on Systemic Mycoses. Churchill, London.
21. **Zhdanovich, Y. V., G. B. Lokshin, and A. D. Kusovkov.** 1967. Mechanism for inactivation of polyene antibiotics. IV. Isolation and identification of low molecular weight products of nystatin inactivation. Khim. Farm. Zh. 1:42–47.

ANTIMICROBIAL AGENTS AND CHEMOTHERAPY, Apr. 1977, p. 619-624 Vol. 11, No. 4
 Printed in U.S.A.

Plasmid-Mediated Aminoglycoside Phosphotransferase of Broad Substrate Range That Phosphorylates Amikacin

PATRICE COURVALIN AND JULIAN DAVIES*

Department of Biochemistry, College of Agricultural and Life Sciences, University of Wisconsin-Madison, Madison, Wisconsin 53706

Received for publication 29 December 1976

A plasmid-mediated aminoglycoside phosphotransferase that phosphorylates amikacin has been detected in clinical isolates of *Staphylococcus aureus*. This enzyme does not confer detectable amikacin resistance to the strains.

The discovery of aminoglycoside-modifying enzymes in antibiotic-resistant bacteria has prompted considerable research on these enzymes, their role in resistance, and their origins and on the evolution of the plasmids that code for them. Although only a small number of amino or hydroxyl groups (four to six) on aminoglycoside molecules are modified, a large number of enzymes catalyze these modifications. Thus, at least three different enzymes have been reported to acetylate the 3-amino group of deoxystreptamine (3), and three phosphotransferases have been described that modify the 3′-hydroxyl group of neomycin, kanamycin, and related antibiotics (J. Dowding and J. Davies, *Microbiology—1974,* p. 179-186, 1975). The enzymes differ in substrate range and physical properties.

We wish to describe a new 3′-phosphotransferase that differs from the aminoglycoside phosphotransferases described thus far. This 3′-phosphotransferase activity has been detected in antibiotic-resistant clinical isolates of *Staphylococcus aureus* and, in addition to neomycin and kanamycin, phosphorylates amikacin; amikacin is a derivative of kanamycin A that has been chemically altered to block modification at several sites, including phosphorylation at the 3′ position. Surprisingly, although these strains possess an amikacin-modifying enzyme, they remain susceptible to the antibiotic.

MATERIALS AND METHODS

Bacterial strains and plasmids. The sources and properties of the staphylococci and their plasmids are listed in Table 1. Plasmid-free *S. aureus* strains RN450(9) and 209P were obtained from R. P. Novick and Y. A. Chabbert, respectively. Plasmid RN1956 was introduced into *S. aureus* RN450 by transduction.

Enzymatic assays. The extracts for assay were prepared as follows. A 100-ml amount of an exponential culture in broth was harvested and washed once in 10 mM tris(hydroxymethyl)aminomethane (Tris)-hydrochloride (pH 7.2)-1 mM ethylenediaminetetraacetate and resuspended in 2 ml of 10 mM Tris-hydrochloride (pH 7.8)-10 mM $MgCl_2$-25 mM NH_4Cl-0.6 mM β-mercaptoethanol. The cells were treated for 30 min at 37°C with 100 μg of lysostaphin per ml (Sigma) and then subjected to two 30-s bursts from a sonicator at 60-W output. The resulting suspension was centrifuged at 105,000 × *g* for 45 min, and the supernatant was removed and used in enzyme assays as described previously (5). The time course of phosphorylation of antibiotics was determined by increasing the volume of the reaction mixture and removing samples for counting at the indicated times.

Minimal inhibitory concentrations. The method of Steers et al. (9) was used for the determination of minimal inhibitory concentrations.

Antibiotics. The antibiotics were provided by the following laboratories: kanamycins A, B, and C and amikacin, Bristol; neomycin B and spectinomycin, Upjohn; paromomycin and butirosin, Parke-Davis; lividomycin A, Kowa; ribostamycin, Meiji; tobramycin, Lilly; streptomycin, Pfizer.

RESULTS

During the course of our studies on enzyme-mediated resistance to aminoglycoside antibiotics, we have examined a large number of clinical isolates of both gram-negative and gram-positive bacteria. To our surprise, many *S. aureus* strains were found to contain an activity that catalyzed the phosphorylation of amikacin in addition to the usual substrates for aminoglycoside phosphotransferases (Fig. 1). The strains and their resistance phenotypes are shown in Table 1.

Amikacin is a derivative of kanamycin A that has a hydroxyaminobutyric acid substituent (HABA) at position 1 of the deoxystreptamine ring (Fig. 2). The presence of this substituent normally blocks modification of kanamycin at the 3′-hydroxyl, 2″-hydroxyl and 3-amino groups, thus providing an antimicrobial agent that is effective against strains containing en-

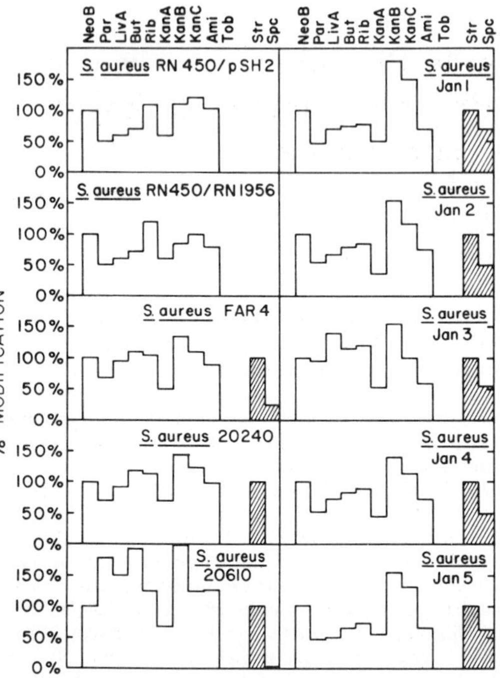

FIG. 1. *Substrate profiles of enzymes extracted from S. aureus strains. Phosphorylation (plain area) or adenylylation (hatched area) are expressed relative to neomycin B or streptomycin as 100%, respectively. Same abbreviations as in Table 2.*

zymes that modify these sites. Aminoglycoside phosphotransferases of gram-negative strains do not phosphorylate amikacin.

We assume that amikacin is modified at the 3′-hydroxyl group; none of the 3′-deoxyaminoglycosides (e.g. tobramycin, Fig. 1) is a substrate for phosphorylation by the *S. aureus* extracts. The fact that both butirosin and lividomycin A are phosphorylated (Fig. 1) indicates that the enzymes are type III aminoglycoside phosphotransferases.

In view of the fact that the *S. aureus* strains are resistant to kanamycin A and susceptible to amikacin, although the phosphotransferase modifies both antibiotics (Fig. 1), we have examined these molecules as substrates for the enzyme. Figure 3 shows kinetics of phosphorylation at different concentrations of the two drugs.

There is one other unusual property of the strains that we have examined. *S. aureus* FAR 4 and JAN 3 are highly resistant to spectinomycin and weakly resistant to streptomycin; strain FAR 4-Neo^s is highly resistant to spectinomycin and fully susceptible to streptomycin. *S. aureus* 20240 is highly resistant to streptomycin but susceptible to spectinomycin, whereas all the other strains were resistant to both drugs (Table 2). When crude extracts of these strains were examined for streptomycin and spectinomycin-modifying enzymes, with the exception of strain FAR 4-Neo^s, they were found to contain a streptomycin-adenylylating activity that was less effective against spectinomycin as substrate (Fig. 1). No phosphorylation of streptomycin has been detected in these strains.

In gram-positive bacteria such as *S. aureus*, plasmid-coded resistance to β-lactam antibiotics and chloramphenicol results from the inducible expression of modifying enzymes that detoxify all of the drug in the culture medium (2). By contrast, in gram-negative bacteria (4) and in streptococci (P. Courvalin et al., manuscript in preparation), plasmid-mediated aminoglycoside–aminocyclitol-modifying enzymes do not express resistance by gross inactivation of the antibiotic; modification of a small amount of the drug prevents further uptake of the antibiotic by the cell, by an unknown mechanism (4). When *S. aureus* strains FAR 4 and RN450/RN1956 were grown in the presence of streptomycin or neomycin B, respectively, no detectable change in the antibiotic concentration was found by microbiological methods; the antibiotic remained unchanged. Measurements of aminoglycoside–aminocyclitol-adenylylating or aminoglycoside-phosphorylating enzyme activities in strains grown with or without antibiotic revealed the presence of substantial modifying activities in all cases. Thus, the aminoglycoside–aminocyclitol-modifying enzymes in *S. aureus* (as well as in streptococci; P. Courvalin et al., manuscript in preparation), like their counterparts in gram-negative bacteria, are synthesized constitutively; however, we cannot eliminate the possibility that superinduction of the constitutive level occurs in the presence of the drug.

In *S. aureus* strains RN450/pSH2 (10), RN450/RN1956, and FAR 4 the amikacin-phosphorylating activity is plasmid mediated; the streptomycin-adenylylating enzyme in strain FAR 4 is also plasmid linked (Table 1) (P. Courvalin and M. Fiandt, manuscript in preparation). Strains 20240 and 20610 each contain at least two different plasmids and were not studied further (Table 1); it is not known if one or both of the plasmids code for the phosphotransferase and the adenylyltransferase.

DISCUSSION

A new plasmid-determined 3′-phosphotransferase has been detected in a number of inde-

TABLE 1. *Properties of the staphylococcal strains and plasmids*

S. aureus strain/plasmid	Phenotype[a]	Genotype[b]	Plasmid content		
			No.	Mol wt (Mdal)[c]	Source
RN450/pSH2	Neo	APH	1	10.1	S. Cohen (10)
RN450/RN1956	Neo	APH	1	10.6	R. P. Novick
FAR 4-Neo^s/pWA2	Em$_c$ Su		1	1.9	R. W. Lacey (6)
FAR 4/pWA1, pWA2	Neo Str Em$_i$ Su Fa	APH SAdT	2	11.7 1.9	R. W. Lacey (6)
20240	Neo Str Pc Tc Su	APH SAdT	≥2[c]	ND[d]	J. W. Griffith
20610	Neo Str Pc Tc Em$_c$ Cm Su	APH SAdT	≥2[c]	ND	K. Casson
JAN 1	Neo Str Pc Mc Tc Em$_c$ Su	APH SAdT	ND		J. Witchitz
JAN 2	Neo Str Pc Mc Tc Em$_c$	APH SAdT	ND		J. Witchitz
JAN 3	Neo Str Pc Em$_i$	APH SAdT	ND		J. Witchitz
JAN 4	Neo Str Pc Mc Tc Em$_c$ Su	APH SAdT	ND		J. Witchitz
JAN 5	Neo Str Pc Mc Tc Em$_c$ Cm Su Rif	APH SAdT	ND		J. Witchitz

[a] Neo, Neomycin; Str, streptomycin; Pc, penicillin; Mc, methicillin; Tc, tetracycline; Em$_i$, erythromycin inducible; Em$_c$, erythromycin constitutive; Cm, chloramphenicol; Su, sulfonamide; Rif, rifampin; Fa, fusidic acid. Susceptibility tests were performed by a standard agar diffusion method (1).

[b] APH, Aminoglycoside phosphotransferase; SAdT, streptomycin adenylyltransferase.

[c] P. Courvalin and M. Fiandt, manuscript in preparation.

[d] ND, Not done.

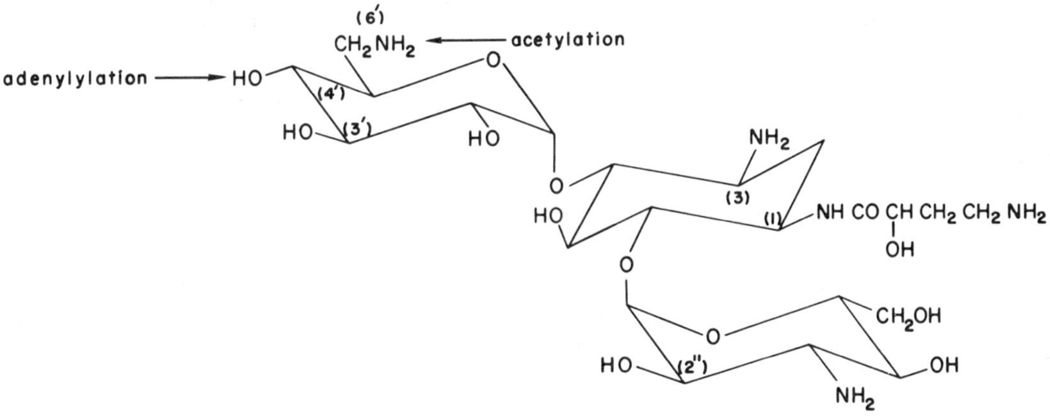

FIG. 2. *Structure of amikacin. The arrows indicate the previously known sites of modification.*

pendent clinical isolates of *S. aureus* obtained from a variety of different sources. This phosphotransferase is distinct from those previously described since it catalyzes the modification of the 3′-hydroxyl group of amikacin. Amikacin (1-*N*-HABA kanamycin A) is an important semisynthetic aminoglycoside that has a broad spectrum of activity; it is effective against most kanamycin-resistant strains of *Escherichia coli*, *Klebsiella pneumoniae*, *Pseudomonas aeruginosa*, and *S. aureus*. The modification at the 1-amino group normally blocks phosphorylation of the 3′-hydroxyl group. The reason for the "blocking" capacity of the hydroxyaminobutyric acid side chain is not known; it presumably alters the conformation of the molecule so that it is no longer a substrate for the modifying enzymes. Until recently, no enzyme of the aminoglycoside phosphotransferase class had been found to modify amikacin. A gentamicin-phosphorylating enzyme (2″-phosphotransferase) that modifies amikacin weakly has been detected in gentamicin-resistant *S. aureus* strains (F. H. Kayser, Prog. Abstr. Intersci. Conf. Antimicrob. Agents Chemother., 16th, Chicago, Ill., abstr. 204, 1976; Davies et al., unpublished observation). A 3′-phosphotransferase from *S. aureus* and *S. epidermidis*, which appears to be similar to the enzyme described in this study, has been described recently (Kayser, Progr. Abstr. Intersci. Conf. Antimicrob. Agents Chemother, 16th, Chicago, Ill., abstr. 204, 1976).

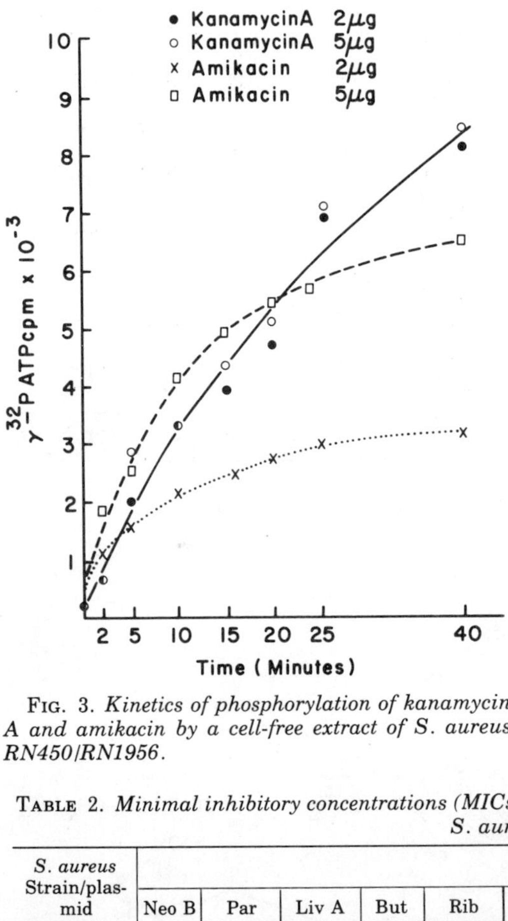

FIG. 3. *Kinetics of phosphorylation of kanamycin A and amikacin by a cell-free extract of S. aureus RN450/RN1956.*

It should be noted that the 1-*N*-HABA substitution does not block all 3′-phosphorylating enzymes, since aminoglycoside phosphotransferase II is capable of phosphorylating butirosin (which can be considered a 1-*N*-HABA ribostamycin).

The new phosphotransferase we have described has the widest substrate range of any 3′-phosphotransferase and is different from other phosphotransferases. It does not cross-react with antisera prepared against aminoglycoside phosphotransferase II (D. Smith, unpublished observation), nor is there any detectable homology at the deoxyribonucleic acid level with the aminoglycoside phosphotransferase gene(s) from the butirosin-producing *Bacillus circulans*, as studied by electron microscopy heteroduplex analysis (P. Courvalin et al., unpublished observation). It has a substrate range quite different from aminoglycoside phosphotransferases isolated from the neomycin-producing *Streptomyces fradiae* and the butirosin-producing *B. circulans* (5); the latter do not phosphorylate amikacin but can modify the HABA-substituted antibiotic butirosin. From the number of different 3′-phosphotransferase enzymes, it would appear that extensive divergent evolution has occurred.

There is one interesting and paradoxical

TABLE 2. *Minimal inhibitory concentrations (MICs) of various aminoglycoside-aminocyclitol antibiotics for S. aureus strains*

S. aureus Strain/plasmid	MIC (μg/ml)[a]											
	Neo B	Par	Liv A	But	Rib	Kan A	Kan B	Kan C	Ami[b]	Tob	Str	Spc
RN450	1	1	2	2	4	2	0.5	8	1 (1–1)	0.5	4	32
RN450/pSH2	256	512	2,048	128	4,096	2,048	512	>1,024	4 (4–4)	0.5	4	32
RN450/RN1956	512	512	2,048	512	4,096	4,096	512	>1,024	8 (8–8)	2	8	32
FAR 4-Neo[s]/pWA2	≤0.5	1	2	2	2	2	0.5	8	1 (1–1)	≤0.25	1	2,048
FAR 4/pWA1, pWA2	16	512	>4,096	16	2,048	256	64	>1,024	1 (1–1)	≤0.25	128	>4,096
209P	≤0.5	≤0.5	2	1	2	2	0.5	8	2	≤0.25	1	32
20240	256	4,096	>4,096	128	4,096	1,024	512	>1,024	8	≤0.25	>4,096	32
20610	32	1,024	>4,096	32	2,048	512	128	>1,024	4	≤0.25	>4,096	2,048
JAN 1	128	4,096	>4,096	64	>4,096	1,024	512	>1,024	8	≤0.25	>4,096	>4,096
JAN 2	256	2,048	>4,096	64	>4,096	1,024	512	>1,024	8	≤0.25	>4,096	2,048
JAN 3	16	512	2,048	32	2,048	256	256	>1,024	2	≤0.25	64	>4,096
JAN 4	256	2,048	>4,096	64	>4,096	1,024	256	>1,024	8	≤0.25	>4,096	>4,096
JAN 5	256	4,096	>4,096	128	>4,096	2,048	256	>1,024	8	0.5	>4,096	2,048

[a] Neo B, Neomycin B; Par, paromomycin; Liv A, lividomycin A; But, butirosin; Rib, ribostamycin; Kan A, kanamycin A; Kan B, kanamycin B; Kan C, Kanamycin C; Ami, amikacin; Tob, tobramycin; Str, streptomycin; Spc, spectinomycin.

[b] Average of two independent determinations.

property of the new 3′-phosphotransferase of *S. aureus*. Amikacin is an excellent substrate for the enzyme (Fig. 1), but all the strains are susceptible (Table 2)! Does this mean that enzymatic modification (inactivation) of aminoglycoside antibiotics is an artifact not related to the determination of resistance? This is unlikely since the same enzyme modifies and determines resistance to high levels of neomycin B and kanamycins A, B, and C (Fig. 1, Table 2).

Enzymatic modification of aminoglycoside antibiotics determines resistance, not by inactivation of the drug but (presumably) by establishing a block to transport or entry of the aminoglycoside into the cell (4). We can, perhaps, explain the amikacin susceptibility of these *S. aureus* strains, in spite of the presence of an amikacin-modifying enzyme, in either of the following ways. (i) Amikacin, although structurally related to kanamycin, is transported into the cell by a separate transport mechanism that is not affected by the phosphorylation of amikacin that takes place inside the cell. (ii) Amikacin and kanamycin are transported by the same transport system, but 3′-phosphorylation of amikacin occurs at a slow rate that is not sufficient to affect the transport of the antibiotic; the drug still enters the cell, binds to ribosomes, and inhibits protein synthesis and growth. Modification of kanamycin and neomycin leads to the establishment of a block in the transport of these antibiotics, with concomitant resistance.

Other explanations may be possible, but we favor the latter. Consistent with this model is the fact that modification of amikacin is concentration dependent and occurs at a slower rate than that of kanamycin A (Fig. 3); these experiments, with a crude enzyme preparation, indicate that the K_m for amikacin phosphorylation is substantially higher than that for kanamycin A. This phenomenon has also been observed with several *E. coli* strains, carrying aminoglycoside phosphotransferase I, that are resistant to neomycin and kanamycin but susceptible to the related aminoglycoside seldomycin; the enzyme extracted from these strains is capable of phosphorylating seldomycin but at a slower rate than neomycin and kanamycin (D. Smith, unpublished observation). In *P. aeruginosa* gentamicin acetyltransferase I determines resistance to gentamicin and not tobramycin but is capable of modifying both drugs in extracts; kinetic studies with the pure enzyme have shown that there is a fivefold difference in K_m for gentamicin C_{1a} and tobramycin (J. W. Williams and D. B. Northrop, Fed. Proc. 35:1705, 1976). The enzymatic modification of an aminoglycoside antibiotic is not sufficient alone to establish resistance; the rate of modification, coupled with an effect on transport of the antibiotic into the cell, must determine the expression of this resistance. Another possibility is that amikacin 3′-phosphate is an inhibitor of the enzyme.

There is another unusual characteristic of the *S. aureus* strains that we have examined. They contain a streptomycin adenylyltransferase that modifies streptomycin and spectinomycin in extracts and determines various phenotypic responses to streptomycin and spectinomycin; susceptibility to streptomycin may also be due to a rate phenomenon, as described above. The mechanism of resistance to spectinomycin in these strains remains to be explained, it may be associated with *O*-adenylylation, but strain 20240, although it possesses such activity, is susceptible to this drug. Strain FAR 4-Neo^s does not possess streptomycin-adenylylating or -phosphorylating activity and is highly resistant to spectinomycin.

The discovery of this new plasmid-mediated 3′-phosphorylating enzyme shows that potential resistance mechanisms to antibiotics such as amikacin already exist in the bacterial population. A 4′-adenylylating enzyme that determines resistance to amikacin, tobramycin, and kanamycin has also been detected in *S. aureus* (7). Since it is obvious that extensive genetic interchange occurs between resistance plasmids, we must anticipate the possibility that amikacin-modifying and resistance-determining enzymes, such as the aminoglycoside phosphotransferase described here, may, in due course, appear in gram-negative bacteria and restrict the useful life of antibiotics such as amikacin.

ACKNOWLEDGMENTS

We are extremely grateful to Cecile Carlier and Dagmar Hochkeppel for expert assistance in certain experiments.

This work was supported by grants from the National Institutes of Health (AI 10076, National Institute of Allergy and Infectious Diseases), National Science Foundation (BMS7202264), and Merck Sharp and Dohme.

LITERATURE CITED

1. **Bauer, A. W., W. M. M. Kirby, J. C. Sherris, and M. Turck.** 1966. Antibiotic susceptibility testing by a standardized single disc method. Am. J. Clin. Pathol. 45:493–496.
2. **Benveniste, R., and J. Davies.** 1973. Mechanisms of antibiotic resistance in bacteria. Annu. Rev. Biochem. 42:471–506.
3. **Biddlecombe, S., M. Haas, J. Davies, G. H. Miller, D. F. Rane, and P. J. L. Daniels.** 1976. Enzymatic modification of aminoglycoside antibiotics: a new 3-*N*-acetylating enzyme from a *Pseudomonas aeruginosa* isolate. Antimicrob. Agents Chemother. 9:951–955.
4. **Davies, J. E., and R. E. Benveniste.** 1974. Enzymes that inactivate antibiotics in transit to their targets. Ann. N.Y. Acad. Sci. 235:130–136.
5. **Haas, M., and J. E. Dowding.** 1975. Aminoglycoside-modifying enzymes, p. 611–628. *In* J. H. Hash (ed.),

Methods in enzymology, vol. 43. Academic Press Inc., New York.

6. **Lacey, R. W., E. Lewis, and V. T. Rosdahl.** 1974. Evolution of plasmids *in vivo* in a strain of *Staphylococcus aureus*. J. Med. Microbiol. 7:117–125.
7. **Le Goffic, F., A. Martel, M. L. Capman, B. Baca, P. Goebel, H. Chardon, C. J. Soussy, J. Duval, and D. H. Bouanchaud.** 1976. New plasmid-mediated nucleotidylation of aminoglycoside antibiotics in *Staphylococcus aureus*. Antimicrob. Agents Chemother. 10:258–264.
8. **Novick, R. P.** 1967. Properties of a cryptic high-frequency transducing phage in *Staphylococcus aureus*. Virology 33:155–166.
9. **Steers, E., E. L. Foltz, B. S. Graves, and J. Riden.** 1959. An inocula replicating apparatus for routine testing of bacterial susceptibility to antibiotics. Antibiot. Chemother. 9:307–311.
10. **Stiffler, P. M., H. M. Sweeney, M. Schneider, and S. Cohen.** 1974. Isolation and characterization of a kanamycin resistance plasmid from *Staphylococcus aureus*. Antimicrob. Agents Chemother. 6:516–520.

Antimicrobial Agents and Chemotherapy, Apr. 1977, p. 625-630 Vol. 11, No. 4

Printed in U.S.A.

Therapeutic Evaluation of Minocycline and Tetracycline for Mixed Anaerobic Infection in Mice

GALE B. HILL

Departments of Obstetrics and Gynecology, and Microbiology and Immunology, Duke University Medical Center, Durham, North Carolina 27710

Received for publication 12 November 1976

Minocycline has demonstrated greater in vitro activity against anaerobic bacteria than its parent compound, tetracycline. In vivo therapeutic efficacy of the two drugs was tested against a mixed anaerobic infection in a mouse model. *Fusobacterium necrophorum* plus *F. nucleatum* injected intraperitoneally produced progressive intrahepatic and occasional extrahepatic abscesses, which were measured at autopsy. Three treatment regimens were tested, single daily doses of antibiotic being administered by oral gavage: four doses begun at 2 or 24 h after challenge and 14 doses begun 3 weeks after challenge when abscesses were well developed. Autopsy was not performed until several weeks after completion of treatment to assess long-term effects. Based on the number of mice without lesions, the median effective dose (ED_{50}) in milligrams per kilogram per dose for minocycline was significantly lower than that for tetracycline with each regimen tested. With the 2-h (immediate therapy) regimen and the 24-h-delayed therapy regimen, minocycline was 30 and 6 times, respectively, more effective against hepatic abscesses than tetracycline on a weight basis. With each antibiotic, abscesses outside the liver were more resistant to therapy, although again minocycline was more effective. In the treatment of developed abscesses (3-week-delayed regimen), minocycline was effective (ED_{50} <16 mg/kg), whereas tetracycline was ineffective (ED_{50} >256 mg/kg). Minocycline has demonstrated greater therapeutic efficacy in vivo than tetracycline in this experimental infection, which is similar, in certain aspects, to human anaerobic infection. These data support further evaluation of the clinical usefulness of minocycline.

Increased recognition of the importance of anaerobic bacteria in human infection has intensified the search for antibiotics active against these organisms (2-5). In the past, tetracycline has been effective in treatment of anaerobic infection, but a variety of medically significant anaerobic bacteria have become increasingly resistant to the drug. Presently, approximately two-thirds of clinical isolates of *Bacteroides fragilis* are resistant (1, 13). In vitro data indicate that minocycline, a tetracycline derivative, has significantly greater activity against anaerobic and aerobic bacteria than the parent compound or other analogues (1, 12). The drug also has improved pharmacokinetic characteristics. Since it is more lipophilic than other tetracyclines, it is readily absorbed by tissues and gives rise to higher tissue levels of antibiotic (7, 9). Improved efficacy of minocycline versus tetracycline has been demonstrated in vivo in treatment of experimental infections with tetracycline-resistant staphylococci and other aerobic pathogens in mice (10).

Since a broader choice of antibiotics active against anaerobic bacterial infection is desirable, in this study the therapeutic efficacy in vivo of minocycline was compared with that of tetracycline in a standardized anaerobic infection, consisting primarily of liver abscesses, in mice. The model infection, which has been described previously (6), mimics common characteristics of human anaerobic infection. This mixed infection with two anaerobic species produces deep-seated abscesses that are chronic and progressive within the viscera. The present evaluation of minocycline and tetracycline was directed towards determining therapeutic, in addition to prophylactic, efficacy.

MATERIALS AND METHODS

Bacterial culture. Human clinical isolates of *Fusobacterium necrophorum* NCDC 9432 and *Fusobacterium nucleatum* NCDC 10206 were maintained as frozen samples prepared from cultures of lyophilized stocks. For each experiment, a frozen sample was inoculated into fluid thioglycolate medium (no.

135C, Baltimore Biological Laboratories, Cockeysville, Md.) supplemented with 0.2% yeast extract, menadione (0.5 μg/ml), hemin (5 μg/ml), and 10% rabbit serum. After one further transfer, growth was harvested at 20 h. The concentration of viable bacteria used for injection was determined by spreading duplicate 0.1-ml samples of 10-fold dilutions of broth cultures on the surface of blood agar plates. These were incubated, and plates containing 30 to 300 colonies were counted. Plates were prepared with brucella agar (Baltimore Biological Laboratories) supplemented with menadione (0.5 μg/ml), hemin (5 μg/ml), and 5% defibrinated sheep blood. All media were immediately placed under anaerobic conditions for storage after preparation. Inoculation, incubation (37°C), and harvesting of cultures were performed within an anaerobic glove chamber (Coy Manufacturing Co., Ann Arbor, Mich.) containing 85% nitrogen, 10% hydrogen, and 5% carbon dioxide.

Antibiotics. Minocycline-hydrochloride and tetracycline-hydrochloride (Lederle Laboratories Division, American Cyanamid Co.) solutions were prepared fresh daily in sterile distilled water. Doubling dilutions of each antibiotic were administered to mice by oral gavage. The correct dose (range, 4 to 256 mg/kg) was determined by weighing each mouse before treatment and by administering 0.1 ml of antibiotic dilution per 10 g of body weight.

In vitro susceptibility tests. The minimum inhibitory concentration (MIC) of tetracycline and minocycline for *F. necrophorum* and *F. nucleatum* was determined by a broth dilution test (14). Each MIC test was performed in duplicate on two occasions.

Experimental animals. Male, inbred, A/J mice (The Jackson Laboratory, Bar Harbor, Me.) were used at 10 to 12 weeks of age. Animals were given laboratory chow and water ad libitum. They were held 2 weeks after shipment to stabilize their health before use in experiments.

Infection model. The infection model (6) is briefly outlined here as it pertains to this study. Broth cultures of *F. necrophorum* and *F. nucleatum* were mixed in a 1:1 ratio, and 0.5 ml was injected intraperitoneally into mice. Mucin was not utilized for these inocula. The number of organisms injected ranged from 1×10^8 to 5×10^8 throughout these experiments.

On the day after challenge, untreated control mice appeared ill, with a ruffled coat, eyes partially or totally closed, and an increased respiratory rate. At autopsy, mice revealed a heavy growth of both anaerobic species around the liver and particularly below the diaphragm. Many control animals had positive blood cultures with the injected anaerobic species. Depending on the challenge dose, some mice (infrequently to a maximum of approximately one-third in these experiments) died of septicemia and peritonitis within several days. Fewer deaths occurred after 2 to 3 weeks. If animals were sacrificed and autopsied at 1 week, intrahepatic and perihepatic lesions were primarily visible, but abscesses were also located in the abdomen, mesentery, or scrotum and occasionally in the thoracic cavity. Although some of the lesions outside the liver spontaneously resolved during the first 1 to 2 weeks after challenge, after approximately 3 weeks, the number of abscesses remained quite constant, and these exhibited progressive enlargement. After several weeks, the majority of lesions were intrahepatic, with fewer abscesses in other sites. At approximately 5 weeks, one to three intrahepatic abscesses, which measured between 4 and 8 mm in diameter, were usually present. These increased to approximately 1 cm in diameter by 8 to 10 weeks. The liver and particularly the spleen were enlarged. The injected anaerobic species were present within these abscesses in high concentration and were verified by Gram stain smears and aerobic and anerobic culture. Sparse growth of other organisms was detected only rarely.

Experimental design and analysis. The therapeutic effectiveness of minocycline and tetracycline were evaluated as follows. Mice were challenged with the mixed *Fusobacterium* inoculum and were randomized into the following groups: antibiotic test groups consisting of 10 to 15 animals per antibiotic dilution and an untreated infection control group consisting of two to three times the number of animals in each antibiotic test group. Two groups of drug control mice (5 to 10 per group) were injected with sterile broth and were administered the highest concentration of each of the antibiotics, 256 mg/kg, on the same schedule as the drug-treated infected mice. The infected control animals were given water (oral gavage) on the same dosage schedule.

Three different antibiotic regimens were tested, each in duplicate on separate occasions. After completion of a drug regimen, animals were held an additional 2.5 to 4 weeks before the results of therapy were evaluated at autopsy. This delay permitted observation of more long-term effects of treatment versus nontreatment. The test and control animals were autopsied at the same time, and the number and size of abscesses present in each animal were recorded (pathology score). A score of 0 was assigned when no lesions were found. Although assignment of pathology scores, which consider both the number and size of abscesses present in each mouse rather than simply a positive or negative score for any lesions, is probably a more sensitive measurement, analysis of these data is more complicated. Since differences could be discerned by comparing the number of mice negative for lesions among the matched antibiotic groups, this information was used for probit analysis to obtain the median effective dose (ED_{50}) in milligrams per kilogram per injection for each antibiotic.

RESULTS

In vitro susceptibility. MICs expressed as micrograms of minocycline and of tetracycline per milliliter were: 0.0188 and 0.075, respectively, against *F. necrophorum* and 0.0375 and 0.15, respectively, against *F. nucleatum*.

Treatment immediately after challenge. The effect of administering antibiotic shortly after infection of mice with *F. necrophorum* and *F. nucleatum* was tested. The initial dose was administered 2 h after challenge, and three additional doses were given at 24-h intervals on consecutive days. Mice were autopsied 4.5 weeks after challenge. Animals were evaluated on the basis of: (i) liver abscesses and (ii) abscesses at any site (i.e., intra-abdominal, scrotal, thoracic, with or without concurrent liver abscess), since tetracycline is known to reach high concentrations in the liver. With 256 mg/kg, minocycline completely protected mice, and with 4 mg/kg, protection was 62% (Table 1). Corresponding doses of tetracycline protected 67 and 20%, respectively. At each dose, the antibiotics, in general, protected fewer mice when extrahepatic lesions were considered in addition to hepatic ones than when hepatic lesions alone were graded. The ED_{50} (Table 2) for minocycline was significantly less than that for tetracycline for liver abscesses alone or for abscesses at all sites.

Treatment delayed for 1 day after challenge. On the second antibiotic regimen, the effect of delaying initiation of therapy for 24 h after infection was tested. Again, four doses at 24-h intervals were administered. Mice were autopsied at 3.5 weeks after challenge. With this 24-h-delayed regimen, higher doses of each drug were required to treat liver abscesses and, in particular, abscesses at all sites, but minocycline was significantly more effective by weight than tetracycline (Table 2). Minocycline was as effective for lesions at any site as was tetracycline for liver abscesses alone. Tetracycline was ineffective in preventing extrahepatic abscesses.

Treatment delayed for 3 weeks after challenge. The effect of allowing abscesses to develop for 3 weeks before initiating antibiotic therapy was tested. Animals were administered single daily doses for a 2-week period (14 treatments). Mice were autopsied 7.5 weeks after challenge. On this schedule, minocycline was effective (Table 2), whereas tetracycline was ineffective at the highest dose tested (256 mg/kg). This degree of effectiveness (minocycline) was not anticipated against well-established abscesses so that the lowest concentrations tested were 16 and 8 mg/kg in the two experiments. The ED_{50} of minocycline, therefore, is indicated in Table 2 as being less than 16 mg/kg, but the extrapolated ED_{50} for minocycline on this regimen was 1 mg/kg for treating liver abscesses and abscesses at all sites.

Splenic enlargement. Infected mice, in general, had enlarged spleens. The splenic weights

TABLE 1. *Effect of minocycline and tetracycline on mixed F. necrophorum and F. nucleatum infection in mice*

Antibiotic[a]	Abscess site	% Mice negative for lesions[b] at dose (mg/kg per injection) of:						
		256	128	64	32	16	8	4
Minocycline	Liver only	100	94	84	85	89	74	62
	All lesions	100	88	84	85	89	53	52
Tetracycline	Liver only	67	53	47	67	40	33	20
	All lesions	61	47	37	67	20	29	13

[a] Antibiotics administered by oral gavage at 2, 24, 48, and 72 h after challenge.
[b] Combined data from two tests, 10 to 15 mice per group in each test. Infected nontreated control mice: 29/33 (88%) positive for liver abscesses, 30/33 (91%) positive for abscesses at any site.

TABLE 2. *Activities of minocycline and tetracycline on three different treatment schedules against mixed F. necrophorum and F. nucleatum infection in mice*

Antibiotic[a]	Abscess site	Median effective dose[b] (mg/kg per injection) on schedule of:		
		4 Treatments (from 2 to 72 h)	4 Treatments (from 24 to 96 h)	14 Treatments (from 3 to 5 weeks)
Minocycline	Liver only	1.4 (0.03–4.4)	11.2 (5.6–18.2)	<16
	All lesions	3.6 (0.6–7.4)	66.1 (36.3–169)	<16
Tetracycline	Liver only	42.7 (15.5–186)	67.6	>256
	All lesions	89.1 (38.9–646)	>256	>256

[a] Antibiotics administered by oral gavage.
[b] Median effective doses were determined from combined data from two separate tests on each schedule. Numbers in parentheses are 95% confidence limits. A total of 20 to 25 mice were committed to each dilution of antibiotic tested.

of minocycline- and tetracycline-treated mice at autopsy were compared to test whether these data would serve as a further index of infection and of response to each antibiotic. To obtain the most critical analysis of any differences, the splenic weights compared were from mice administered concentrations of antibiotic that were in between the ED_{50} values (for liver lesions) derived for minocycline and tetracycline with each treatment regimen (Tables 2 and 3). The splenic weights (Table 3) generally reflected the greater therapeutic activity of minocycline, as indicated by its lower ED_{50} for each regimen. Minocycline-treated mice, in general, had significantly smaller spleens than those of tetracycline-treated mice administered equivalent doses. Although the combined data (two experiments) from mice administered 8 mg/kg on the immediate regimen (Table 3) were not significant, one of these duplicate experiments, when analyzed individually, demonstrated significantly smaller ($P = 0.05$, rank sum test) splenic weights for minocycline-treated mice compared with those given tetracycline.

DISCUSSION

The therapeutic regimens tested in the present studies were designed to simulate clinical usage of antibiotics, whereas drug efficacy studies are often performed with single doses of antibiotics being administered immediately after bacterial challenge. The immediate treatment regimen can be considered analogous to the rapid initiation of antibiotic therapy incident to sudden contamination of the peritoneal cavity after trauma or bowel surgery. The 24-h-delayed regimen was initiated at a time when mice had bacteremia and appeared quite ill. This regimen might represent the treatment of symptoms in postoperative infectious complications or the early stages of a ruptured viscus. The third therapy regimen (3-week delay) simulated the more extensive medical treatment required for a well-established disease process as, for example, a patient presenting with an intrahepatic or intra-abdominal abscess. Autopsies were delayed for several weeks after termination of therapy to allow for resolution of treated abscesses and redevelopment or an increase in size of inadequately treated lesions. The absence of lesions would, therefore, be related more to a permanent effect than to continued inhibitory activity.

On each of the three regimens, minocycline was demonstrated to be significantly more effective by weight than tetracycline. Although positive/negative data for lesions were used for analysis, it was apparent that the pathology scores closely paralleled these values. Minocycline-treated mice generally had fewer and smaller lesions than mice given the same dose of tetracycline. The lower ED_{50} values of each antibiotic in treating only hepatic abscesses in contrast to abscesses at any site probably relate to the affinity of tetracyclines for the liver, resulting in higher antibiotic concentrations.

Wilkins and Smith (15) tested four antibiotics useful against anaerobic infections in a lethal subcutaneous infection model initiated in mice with a sheep foot rot strain of *F. necrophorum*. Different combinations of the route of

TABLE 3. *Effect of minocycline and tetracycline on spleen size of mice infected with F. necrophorum and F. nucleatum*

Antibiotic regimen	Drug dose per injection (mg/kg)	Mean spleen wt at autopsy (g ± standard deviation)		P^a value
		Minocycline	Tetracycline	
Immediate therapy	16	0.09 ± 0.05[b]	0.22 ± 0.07	$P < 0.001$
		0.13 ± 0.03	0.16 ± 0.05	
	8	0.08 ± 0.05	0.13 ± 0.05	$0.1 < P < 0.2$
		0.16 ± 0.03	0.15 ± 0.10	
24-h-delayed therapy	64	0.13 ± 0.02	0.22 ± 0.07	$P < 0.001$
		0.16 ± 0.03	0.19 ± 0.04	
	32	0.18 ± 0.04	0.24 ± 0.06	$P < 0.05$
		0.08 ± 0.04	0.15 ± 0.11	
3-week-delayed therapy	64	0.12 ± 0.05	0.19 ± 0.03	$P < 0.01$
		0.13 ± 0.04	0.13 ± 0.02	
	16	0.11 ± 0.04	0.18 ± 0.09	$P < 0.005$
		0.13 ± 0.05	0.16 ± 0.06	

[a] *P* values by Wilcoxon and Mann-Whitney rank sum test on combined data from duplicate experiments.

[b] Mean splenic weights from mice, corresponding to each of the two (duplicate) experiments, are presented separately.

infection, antibiotics, and dosing schedules were tested. On the most effective regimen, tetracycline was more active (ED_{50} of 5 mg/kg) compared with clindamycin (11.1 mg/kg), penicillin G (11.8 mg/kg), and lincomycin (52.9 mg/kg). Minocycline was not tested. Kuck (8) compared minocycline with other antibiotics in infections initiated with human clinical isolates of *F. necrophorum* alone. A subcutaneous model similar to that of Wilkins and Smith (15) and an intraperitoneal model similar to that of Hill et al. (6) were employed. Drug efficacy was based on the number of animals without macroscopic lesions 10 to 14 days after challenge. These lesions generally healed spontaneously, but occasionally, they were progressive. With the antibiotic regimens tested, minocycline was the most active drug on a weight basis, whereas clindamycin was more active on the basis of serum concentration. Doxycycline and ampicillin were much less active, and tetracycline, penicillin G, and cephalexin were ineffective at the doses tested. Comparison of serum concentrations and the ED_{50} values of minocycline and clindamycin in mice indicated that antibiotic levels readily achievable in humans would be effective against the organism. Although less effective than minocycline, tetracycline was found in the present studies and in tests by Wilkins and Smith (15) to be considerably more active than in Kuck's studies, in which the ED_{50} was never less than 256 mg/kg, even with tetracycline administered twice daily. The basis for this difference is not clear, since the two strains of *F. necrophorum* tested by Kuck (8) were susceptible in vitro to tetracycline (0.25 and 0.06 μg/ml).

In the present studies, the greater activity of minocycline over that of tetracycline might be predicted on the basis of in vitro susceptibility data, which showed that, against both organisms, minocycline was approximately four times more active than tetracycline. The in vivo activity of an antibiotic, however, is often not predictable by in vitro susceptibility data, a point demonstrated by the present data and other studies (8, 15). In addition, Redin (10) has demonstrated that, with an equivalent oral dose, minocycline achieves approximately four times higher plasma concentrations than tetracycline. The activity of minocycline in the present study, however, was even greater with the immediate regimen and the 3-week-delayed regimen than would have been predicted on the basis of in vitro susceptibility and plasma level data.

The in vivo model utilized in this evaluation of drug efficacy was similar in certain aspects to infections in humans with anaerobic bacteria. Approximately one-half or more of liver abscesses involve anaerobes, and fusobacteria, particularly *F. necrophorum* (formerly designated as *Sphaerophorus necrophorus*), are common isolates (11). Extrahepatic abscesses within the abdomen have an even higher incidence, over 90%, of anaerobic bacteria (3). Although in vitro susceptibility tests have demonstrated less inhibition of anaerobic bacteria with minocycline compared with that observed with clindamycin or chloramphenicol, alternate drugs are often desirable. Minocycline may be clinically useful, therefore, in a variety of settings, but in vitro susceptibility should be ascertained before its use in serious disease. The present data further encourage the potential clinical usefulness of minocycline for anaerobic infections.

ACKNOWLEDGMENTS

The valuable technical assistance of Ouida Ayers and Clinton Moorman is gratefully acknowledged.

I thank Dennis Tolley and Lawrence Myers of the Department of Community Health Sciences (Biostatistics) for their help in the statistical analysis.

This investigation was supported by a grant from Lederle Laboratories, Pearl River, N.Y.

LITERATURE CITED

1. **Chow, A. W., V. Patten, and L. B. Guze.** 1975. Comparative susceptibility of anaerobic bacteria to minocycline, doxycycline, and tetracycline. Antimicrob. Agents Chemother. 7:46–49.
2. **Finegold, S. M., J. G. Bartlett, A. W. Chow, D. J. Flora, S. L. Gorbach, E. J. Harder, and F. P. Tally.** 1975. Management of anaerobic infections. Ann. Intern. Med. 83:375–389.
3. **Gorbach, S. L., and J. G. Bartlett.** 1974. Anaerobic infections. N. Engl. J. Med. 290:1177–1184.
4. **Gorbach, S. L., and J. G. Bartlett.** 1974. Anaerobic infections. N. Engl. J. Med. 290:1237–1245.
5. **Gorbach, S. L., and J. G. Bartlett.** 1974. Anaerobic infections. N. Engl. J. Med. 290:1289–1294.
6. **Hill, G. B., S. Osterhout, and P. C. Pratt.** 1974. Liver abscess production by non-spore-forming anaerobic bacteria in a mouse model. Infect. Immun. 9:599–603.
7. **Kelly, R. G., and L. A. Kanegis.** 1967. Metabolism and tissue distribution of radioisotopically labeled minocycline. Toxicol. Appl. Pharmacol. 11:171–183.
8. **Kuck, N. A.** 1975. Effect of minocycline and other antibiotics on *Fusobacterium necrophorum* infections in mice. Antimicrob. Agents Chemother. 7:421–425.
9. **Macdonald, H., R. G. Kelly, E. S. Allen, J. F. Noble, and L. A. Kanegis.** 1973. Pharmacokinetic studies on minocycline in man. Clin. Pharmacol. Ther. 14:852–861.
10. **Redin, G. S.** 1967. Antibacterial activity in mice of minocycline, a new tetracycline, p. 371–376. Antimicrob. Agents Chemother. 1966.
11. **Sabbaj, J., V. L. Sutter, and S. M. Finegold.** 1972. Anaerobic pyogenic liver abscess. Ann. Intern. Med. 77:629–638.
12. **Steigbigel, N. H., C. W. Reed, and M. Finland.** 1968. Susceptibility of common pathogenic bacteria to seven tetracycline antibiotics in vitro. Am. J. Med.

Sci. 255:179–195.
13. **Sutter, V. L., Y. Y. Kwok, and S. M. Finegold.** 1972. Standardized antimicrobial disc susceptibility testing of anaerobic bacteria. I. Susceptibility of *Bacteroides fragilis* to tetracycline. Appl. Microbiol. 23:268–275.
14. **Sutter, V. L., and J. A. Washington, Jr.** 1974. Susceptibility testing of anaerobes, p. 436–438. *In* E. H. Lennette, E. H. Spaulding, and J. P. Truant (ed.), Manual of clinical microbiology. American Society for Microbiology, Washington, D.C.
15. **Wilkins, T. D., and L. DS. Smith.** 1974. Chemotherapy of an experimental *Fusobacterium* (*Sphaerophorus*) *necrophorum* infection in mice. Antimicrob. Agents Chemother. 5:658–662.

ANTIMICROBIAL AGENTS AND CHEMOTHERAPY, Apr. 1977, p. 631-637
Vol. 11, No. 4

Susceptibility of Anaerobic Bacteria to Metronidazole, Ornidazole, and Tinidazole and Routine Susceptibility Testing by Standardized Methods

JÜRG WÜST
Institute for Medical Microbiology, University of Zurich, CH-8028 Zurich, Switzerland

Received for publication 1 December 1976

A total of 114 strains of anaerobic bacteria were examined for their susceptibility to metronidazole, ornidazole, and tinidazole by measuring the minimum inhibitory concentration (MIC) and minimum bactericidal concentration in different media. All strains, with the exception of the isolates of *Propionibacterium acnes*, were inhibited by 3.1 μg each and killed by 6.3 μg each of all three nitroimidazole compounds per ml. No significant differences in MIC values were found among metronidazole, ornidazole, and tinidazole. Only minor differences were detected by comparing MIC values obtained in brain heart infusion agar with and without sheep blood, brucella agar, and Mueller-Hinton agar (both containing blood). When the strains were tested by the modified broth-disk method proposed by the Anaerobe Laboratory of the Virginia Polytechnic Institute (VPI), there was good correlation with the MIC values (97.4% agreement for metronidazole and 94.7% for ornidazole and tinidazole). For routine testing, use of a 30-μg-class disk of either nitroimidazole derivative is proposed for the broth-disk method, resulting in a final concentration of 6 μg/ml in the test tubes, a concentration easily attainable in body fluids. In contrast to the broth-disk method, there was very poor correlation between inhibition zone diameters by the standardized VPI agar diffusion test and MIC values.

Metronidazole and related nitroimidazole derivatives, including ornidazole and tinidazole, are receiving increasing attention in the treatment of anaerobic infections. This interest rests on the results of intensive in vitro susceptibility evaluations (2–4, 9, 10, 20, 24, 26, 28, 32) and limited but promising trials of these agents in patients infected with various anaerobic bacteria (14, 19, 31, 39).

All in vitro data have been obtained by determination of minimal inhibitory concentrations (MIC), a procedure that is not suitable for routine testing in the clinical laboratory, unless a sufficient number of strains have to be tested every day.

Currently, there are several methods proposed for routine susceptibility testing of anaerobic bacteria (5, 8, 21, 25, 29, 36, 37). The purpose of this study was to investigate the reliability of susceptibility testing of anaerobes against metronidazole, ornidazole, and tinidazole by two routine procedures proposed by the Anaerobe Laboratory of the Virginia Polytechnic Institute (VPI), Blacksburg, Va., namely, the modified broth-disk method proposed by Wilkins and Thiel (37) and the agar diffusion method of Wilkins et al. (36). In addition, the influence of media most used in anaerobic bacteriological work on the results of MIC determinations was evaluated, since Chow et al. (3) have found higher MIC values on Mueller-Hinton agar than authors using other media (2, 4, 9, 24, 26, 28, 32).

MATERIALS AND METHODS

Bacterial strains. Of the 114 strains examined in this study, 9 were provided from VPI and 105 were isolated from clinical specimens at the Institute for Medical Microbiology of the University of Zurich. They were identified according to the criteria outlined by Holdeman and Moore (13). Identification of subspecies of *Bacteroides fragilis* was performed by considering acid production from mannitol, rhamnose, and trehalose and indole production; carbohydrate fermentation was considered positive only if a pH of less than 5.75 was achieved (L. V. Holdeman, personal communication).

The isolated strains comprised the following species: 39 *B. fragilis* (2 *B. fragilis* subsp. *distasonis*, 28 *B. fragilis* subsp. *fragilis*, 6 *B. fragilis* subsp. *thetaiotaomicron*, 1 *B. fragilis* subsp. *vulgatus*, and 2 *B. fragilis* strains that could not be subspecified), 2 *Bacteroides melaninogenicus* subsp. *asaccharolyticus*, 2 *Fusobacterium mortiferum*, 3 *Fusobacterium necrophorum*, 7 *Fusobacterium nucleatum*, 1 *Fuso-*

bacterium varium, 7 *Peptococcus asaccharolyticus*, 8 *Peptococcus magnus*, 2 *Peptococcus prevotii*, 7 *Peptostreptococcus anaerobius*, 4 *Veillonella* sp., 1 *Eubacterium cylindroides*, 1 *Eubacterium lentum*, 7 *Propionibacterium acnes*, 1 *Clostridium butyricum*, 1 *Clostridium chauvoei*, 1 *Clostridium novyi* A, 9 *Clostridium perfringens*, 3 *Clostridium ramosum*, 6 *Clostridium sporogenes*, 1 *Clostridium tertium*, 1 *Clostridium* sp. The strains were maintained at room temperature in chopped-meat broth (13).

Media. Throughout the experiments, prereduced, anaerobically sterilized media were used. These were prepared according to methods described by Holdeman and Moore (13). The basic media were supplemented brain heart infusion (BHI) broth and chopped-meat carbohydrate (CMC) broth. The basal peptone-yeast extract medium used for testing biochemical reactions contained 0.5% peptone (Difco) and 0.5% Trypticase (BBL) instead of 1% peptone (W. E. C. Moore, personal communication).

The media used for MIC determinations were: BHI agar (Difco), supplemented with 0.5% yeast extract (Difco), with and without 5% citrated sheep blood (BHIA); brucella agar (kindly supplied by Pfizer Overseas, Inc., New York) with 5% sheep blood; Mueller-Hinton agar (BBL), supplemented with 0.5% yeast extract (Difco) and 5% sheep blood. All media for MIC determinations were supplemented with menadione (0.5 μg/ml) and hemin (5 μg/ml).

Antimicrobial agents. Metronidazole and ornidazole were kindly supplied by P. Angehrn, Hoffmann-La Roche & Co. AG, Basel, Switzerland, and tinidazole was supplied by E. Milek, Pfizer AG, Zurich, Switzerland.

Stock solutions containing 1,000 μg of each antimicrobial agent per ml were prepared in distilled water, filter-sterilized (Millipore, 0.22 μm), and kept frozen at -20°C.

MIC determinations. MIC determinations were performed according to Blazevic (1). For the agar dilution technique, plates were prepared containing serial twofold dilutions of each antimicrobial agent from 100 to 0.1 μg/ml. The plates were held overnight at room temperature in GasPak jars (BBL) or prepared on the day of the experiment. Prior to use, they were dried with the lids slightly opened, at 37°C.

All strains were checked for purity by subculturing to an anaerobic blood agar plate. One colony was inoculated into CMC broth. After overnight incubation at 37°C, a 1:100 dilution was made in BHI broth. The agar plates were inoculated with a device similar to the Steers replicator (27), resulting in an inoculum of approximately 2×10^3 to 2×10^4 bacteria per spot. Only 19 organisms were replicated at a time to avoid prolonged exposure to air. Anaerobic control plates without antimicrobial agents were inoculated last to ensure that viable organisms were present throughout the experiment and that the strains were able to grow on the media (35). The plates were incubated in GasPak jars at 37°C for 48 h. Plates incubated aerobically and in an atmosphere with 10% CO_2 were included as additional controls. After incubation, the MIC was determined as the lowest concentration of the antimicrobial agent showing no growth, a barely visible haze, or one discrete colony (7). One strain of *B. fragilis* subsp. *fragilis* was included in each experiment to determine the reproducibility of the method.

MIC determinations of nine swarming clostridia were performed separately for each strain and each concentration of metronidazole, ornidazole, and tinidazole, using the cups of disposable plastic trays as miniaturized petri dishes. These experiments were performed only with BHIA, and therefore these strains were excluded from the comparative evaluation of the different media.

Determination of the MBC. The minimal bactericidal concentration (MBC) in BHIA without blood was determined by replica plating (6). The velvet surface of a sterilized pad was pressed against the primary BHI master plate and then to a BHIA plate without antimicrobial agent. The MBC was defined as the lowest concentration showing no growth or only one single colony in the subculture after 48 h of incubation at 37°C in GasPak jars.

Disks for susceptibility testing. Disks containing 10 and 30 μg of antimicrobial agent were prepared by adding 10 μl of a 1,000-μl/ml solution and 20 μl of a 1,500-μl/ml solution, respectively, to 6-mm filter paper disks. The disks were dried for about 16 h at 37°C and stored at 4°C together with a desiccant.

Broth-disk method. The broth-disk method described by Wilkins and Thiel (37) was strictly followed. One drop of an overnight culture in CMC broth was added to 5 ml of BHI broth. A disk containing 30 μg of metronidazole, ornidazole, or tinidazole was added, resulting in a final concentration of 6 μg/ml of the respective antimicrobial agent. A control culture without antimicrobial agent was included for each strain. Incubation was at 37°C for 18 to 24 h. Susceptibility was defined as either absence of growth or less than 50% of the turbidity of the control culture. When there was growth in the tubes, indicating resistance, the strain was subcultured anaerobically and aerobically to exclude the possibility of contamination.

Agar diffusion test. The method for the agar diffusion test described by Wilkins et al. (36) was used. A 1.5-ml portion of an 18- to 24-h culture at maximal turbidity in CMC broth was added to 10 ml of melted and cooled (50°C) supplemented BHIA (13). The contents were mixed by inversion and poured into standard 90-mm petri dishes. After the agar had solidified, filter-paper disks containing 10 and 30 μg of metronidazole, ornidazole, and tinidazole were applied. After incubation at 37°C in GasPak jars for 18 to 24 h, the zone diameters were measured with a ruler. Some strains of *B. fragilis* exhibited an inner area of light growth around the disk, with a clear area of inhibition outside this hazy growth. In these instances, the outer zone of inhibition was measured.

RESULTS

The cumulative percentages of anaerobic bacterial strains inhibited and killed at various concentrations of metronidazole, ornidazole, and tinidazole are summarized in Table 1. All strains except the isolates of *P. acnes* were inhibited by 3.1 μg each and killed by 6.3 μg each of all three nitroimidazoles per ml. For most strains the MBC was equal to the MIC; in some instances the MBC was one or two twofold dilutions higher than the MIC. In a few rare cases the MBC was one dilution step lower than the MIC, indicating that the antimicrobial agent became effective only after several generations (22) or that the microorganisms were killed by exposure to oxygen during the transfer.

Table 2 contains the geometric means of the MICs of metronidazole, ornidazole, and tinidazole in the different media tested. A two-way analysis of variance showed no significant difference betwen the three antimicrobial agents in all four media ($P > 5\%$). Whereas no difference was detected between BHIA with and without blood ($P > 5\%$), the geometric means of the MICs in brucella agar with 5% sheep blood and Mueller-Hinton agar with 5% sheep blood were slightly higher ($P < 1\%$) than in BHIA.

Table 3 compares the results obtained by the broth-disk test and the agar dilution method. Three organisms considered as susceptible to metronidazole according to the MICs were classified as resistant by the broth-disk method. For ornidazole and tinidazole there were six strains each showing similar behavior. These false resistance results in the broth-disk test were primarily found in testing clostridia; in addition, there was one strain of *F. necrophorum* resistant to all three nitroimidazoles in the broth-disk test. Upon repetition, part of the strains again showed false growth in the broth disk test tubes. When the tests were repeated with a 1:100 dilution of the CMC broth culture as inoculum, no false resistant classifications were encountered any more.

In general, the results of the broth-disk method were easy to read. The tubes showed either heavy growth or were clear. With some *B. fragilis* strains there was a slight turbidity in the drug-containing tubes, but it was easy to ascertain a marked difference from the heavily grown control tube without drug. Difficulties

TABLE 1. *Inhibitory and bactericidal effect of metronidazole, ornidazole, and tinidazole on anaerobic bacteria*

Organisms	No. of strains tested	Antimicrobial agent	Cumulative percent of isolates inhibited/killed at various concn (μg/ml)[a]							
			≤0.1	0.2	0.4	0.8	1.6	3.1	6.3	>100
Bacteroides fragilis	39	Metronidazole		15/15	38/31	62/67	97/90	100/100		
		Ornidazole	3/5	18/15	44/44	72/79	97/95	100/97	100/100	
		Tinidazole	3/3	28/23	56/56	74/82	92/95	100/97	100/100	
Bacteroides melaninogenicus	2	Metronidazole	100/100							
		Ornidazole	100/100							
		Tinidazole	100/100							
Fusobacterium sp.	13	Metronidazole	62/62	85/85	92/100		100/100			
		Ornidazole	62/54	85/85	92/92	100/100				
		Trinidazole	62/54	85/77	92/92		100/100			
Clostridium perfringens	9	Metronidazole		33/33	44/44	89/89	100/100			
		Ornidazole		11/22	56/44	100/89	100/100			
		Tinidazole		11/11	56/33	89/78	100/100			
Clostridium sp. (other)	14/5[b]	Metronidazole	14/0	64/0		86/60	100/80	100/100		
		Ornidazole	14/0	57/0	71/0	93/80	100/100			
		Tinidazole	14/0	57/0	64/0		93/80	100/100		
Peptococcus sp. and *Peptostreptococcus* sp.	24	Metronidazole	4/8	58/50	71/67	92/88	100/96	100/100		
		Ornidazole	4/4	50/46	92/79	100/96	100/100			
		Tinidazole	4/8	42/25	75/58	96/92	100/100			
Veillonella sp.	4	Metronidazole				100/100				
		Ornidazole			50/50	100/100				
		Tinidazole			50/50	50/100	100/100			
Eubacterium sp.	2	Metronidazole			50/50	100/50	100/100			
		Ornidazole			50/50	100/100				
		Tinidazole			50/50		100/100			
Propionibacterium acnes	7	Metronidazole								100/100
		Ornidazole								100/100
		Tinidazole								100/100
Total	114/105[b]	Metronidazole	11/11	39/32	53/46	75/74	93/88	94/93		100/100
		Ornidazole	12/11	36/30	62/54	83/83	93/91	94/92	94/93	100/100
		Tinidazole	12/11	38/27	62/53	75/74	90/90	94/92	94/93	100/100

[a] In BHIA without blood.

[b] MIC determinations of nine swarming clostridia were performed separately in small petri dishes. Therefore, the MBC assay could not be performed by the method used.

were encountered with five *Peptococcus* and *Peptostreptococcus* species (i.e., 4.3% of the strains tested), which showed only very fair growth in the control tube. Prolonged incubation for another 24 h produced growth sufficient to read, although this procedure does not conform to the test described originally and has to be interpreted with caution, because of possible inactivation of the antimicrobial agent.

Figure 1 shows the relationship of zone diameters around a 10-μg metronidazole disk and MIC values in BHIA without blood. Twenty-six organisms (22.8%) that grew slowly in CMC broth and did not produce confluent growth in the pour plates, or produced indistinct zones, were excluded as proposed by Wilkins et al. (36). These strains comprised mainly *Peptococcus* sp. and some clostridia other than *C. perfringens*. Due to the extensive spread of diameters at the various MIC values and the relative narrow range of MICs, no regression line was calculated and drawn (7, 16, 18). The problems met in reading the diffusion tests were mainly cloudy zones due to the dense inoculum or organisms that grew well close to the disk but were inhibited further away from the disk (33). The complications of spreading were also encountered when 30-μg disks were used and with ornidazole and tinidazole as well as with metronidazole.

The reproducibility of the agar diffusion and the agar dilution method (see Table 4) was tested by performing the assays on different days with the same strain of *B. fragilis* subsp. *fragilis*. Direct numerical comparisons of the extent of variability of the two test procedures cannot be made, because the results were obtained in two systems not directly transferable (7).

TABLE 2. *Comparison of MIC values of metronidazole, ornidazole, and tinidazole against anaerobic bacteria in different media*[a]

Antimicrobial agent	MIC (μg/ml) in:[b] BHIA Without blood	BHIA With blood	BA	MHA
Metronidazole	0.56	0.55	0.87	0.72
Ornidazole	0.50	0.49	0.84	0.59
Tinidazole	0.54	0.53	0.79	0.60

[a] Geometric means of the MIC values of 105 strains.

[b] BA, Brucella agar with 5% sheep blood; MHA, Mueller-Hinton agar with 5% sheep blood.

DISCUSSION

There is controversy over the questions of whether the susceptibility testing of anaerobic bacteria should be performed routinely or whether the management of anaerobic infections should rely upon published susceptibility patterns for the different bacterial species (11, 16, 26, 34). I believe that routine testing should be done for clinically significant anaerobes from sources not contaminated with normal flora, since the susceptibility pattern of various anaerobes against several antimicrobial agents is known to change (12, 15–17, 21, 28, 30). For

TABLE 3. *Comparison of results with the broth-disk and the agar dilution methods*

Antimicrobial agent	Resistant strains[a]: No. of strains	Resistant strains[a]: No. of false susceptible readings[b]	Susceptible strains[a]: No. of strains	Susceptible strains[a]: No. of false resistant readings[b]	Overall agreement (%) between the two methods	Strains with false reaction in broth-disk test: Species	MIC (μg/ml)[c]
Metronidazole	7	0	107	3	97.4	*Clostridium perfringens*	0.8
						Clostridium sp.	0.8
						Fusobacterium mortiferum	0.4
Ornidazole	7	0	107	6	94.7	*Clostridium perfringens*	0.4 (2 strains)
						Clostridium perfringens	0.8 (2 strains)
						Clostridium sp.	0.8
						Fusobacterium mortiferum	0.8
Tinidazole	7	0	107	6	94.7	*Bacteroides fragilis*	0.4
						Clostridium perfringens	0.4
						Clostridium perfringens	0.8
						Clostridium perfringens	1.6
						Clostridium sp.	1.6
						Fusobacterium mortiferum	1.6

[a] According to MIC in BHIA without blood.

[b] In broth-disk test.

[c] In BHIA without blood.

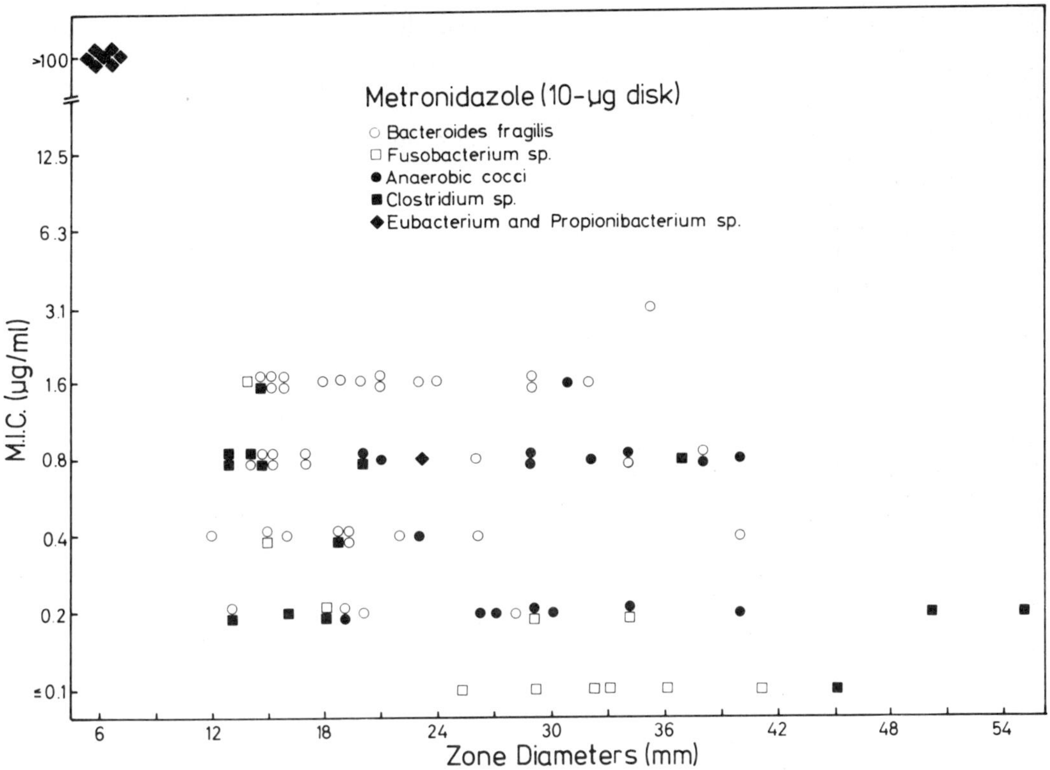

FIG. 1. *Lack of correlation of MIC values in BHIA without blood and inhibition zone diameters of anaerobic bacteria around 10-μg metronidazole disks. Similar patterns were found when ornidazole and tinidazole were tested and when 30-μg disks were used instead of 10-μg disks for all three nitroimidazoles.*

TABLE 4. *Reproducibility of antimicrobial susceptibility tests*[a]

Antimicrobial agent	Agar diffusion test (zone diam, mm)			Agar dilution test (MIC, μg/ml)		
	Mean	Standard deviation	Range	Mean	Standard deviation	Range
Metronidazole	22.2	2.8	17–25	0.73	0.47	0.4–1.6
Ornidazole	19.3	2.7	15–22	0.53	0.21	0.4–0.8
Tinidazole	18.7	2.5	15–22	0.80	0.44	0.4–1.6

[a] A strain of *B. fragilis* subsp. *fragilis* was tested seven times on different days.

instance, several strains with an unusual susceptibility pattern have been isolated in our laboratory over a period of only a few months, e.g., *C. perfringens* resistant to penicillin (MIC, 25 μg/ml in BHI broth, determined with an inoculum of approximately 10^5 bacteria/ml) or chloramphenicol (MIC, 50 μg/ml) and *B. fragilis* resistant to chloramphenicol (MIC, 100 μg/ml).

The broth-disk method of Wilkins and Thiel (37) is easy to perform and has been found to give reliable results (1, 37). When this method was used for testing susceptibility to metronidazole, ornidazole, and tinidazole and the results were compared with MIC values, growth in the tubes gave contradictory results in 2.6% of the tests with metronidazole and in 5.3% of the tests with the latter two drugs. This problem was encountered mainly with a few clostridial strains and could be overcome by using a 1:100 dilution of the original inoculum in CMC broth. A possible explanation of this phenomenon may be found in the observation by Plant and Edwards (22), who have shown that growth of *Clostridium bifermentans* was inhibited by metronidazole and tinidazole only after 3 to 4 h of incubation, a period long enough to result in dense growth when 1 drop of an overnight CMC broth culture is added to 5 ml of BHI broth.

This initial growth phase in the presence of the nitroimidazole drug has, however, not been uniformly observed by other workers using *C. perfringens* and *B. fragilis* (23; R. Lüthy, F. Weber, and W. Siegenthaler, Prog. Abstr. Intersci. Conf. Antimicrob. Agents Chemother., 16th, Chicago, Ill., Abstr. 454, 1976). For clostridia, therefore, a 1:100 dilution of a CMC broth culture is recommended as the inoculum for the broth-disk test.

A level of 6 μg/ml was chosen to differentiate between susceptible and resistant organisms, because such a concentration and a higher level of all three nitroimidazoles in serum are easily obtained (4, 23, 24, 28, 31, 32; additional data were provided by Hoffmann-La Roche and Co. AG and Pfizer AG). The level of 6 μg/ml also takes into account the deviation in disk content allowed by the Food and Drug Administration, i.e., 67 to 150% of the labeled value (37).

Because no significant differences in MIC values of metronidazole, ornidazole, and tinidazole could be detected, use of only one representative disk in the modified broth-disk test is recommended (class disk).

In contrast to the modified broth-disk test, very poor correlation was found betwen zone size in the agar diffusion test (36) and MIC values. For a given MIC value, the range of zone diameters obtained was very large. A similar observation has been made by Reynolds et al. (24) using a different diffusion test procedure. Due to the lack of strains with an intermediate susceptibility, no standard zone diameters representing susceptibility or resistance can be given at present. The reproducibility of the agar diffusion test was low, and when the same strain of *B. fragilis* was tested several times, the standard deviation was about double the standard deviation allowed by Sutter et al. (29) with their method. Therefore, the agar diffusion test cannot be recommended, at least for the time being, for detection of strains resistant to the nitroimidazole compounds, with the exception of extremely resistant bacteria such as *P. acnes* which show no inhibition zone at all.

The results of MIC determinations were essentially identical in the various test media, BHI agar with and without blood, brucella agar, and Mueller-Hinton agar (both with blood).

The current study has shown that the modified broth-disk test provides a reliable and comparatively uncomplicated approach to measuring drug susceptibilities of various anaerobic bacteria. Clinical laboratories should be encouraged to apply this method to isolates of medically important anaerobic organisms. Metronidazole, or another nitroimidazole, should be included among the agents evaluated in these tests. The results of such determinations could play an important role in the treatment of infections with a group of organisms that is exhibiting changing patterns of drug susceptibility.

ACKNOWLEDGMENTS

I thank F. H. Kayser and P. Santanam for critically reviewing the manuscript, J. Iten for skillful technical assistance, P. Landis for preparing the prereduced media, and L. Ruegg for help in preparing the manuscript.

LITERATURE CITED

1. **Blazevic, D. J.** 1975. Evaluation of the modified broth-disk method for determining antibiotic susceptibilities of anaerobic bacteria. Antimicrob. Agents Chemother. 7:721–723.
2. **Busch, D. F., V. L. Sutter, and S. M. Finegold.** 1976. Activity of combinations of antimicrobial agents against *Bacteroides fragilis*. J. Infect. Dis. 133:321–328.
3. **Chow, A. W., V. Patten, and L. B. Guze.** 1975. Susceptibility of anaerobic bacteria to metronidazole: relative resistance of non-spore-forming gram-positive bacilli. J. Infect. Dis. 131:182–185.
4. **Dornbusch, K., and C.-E. Nord.** 1974. In vitro effect of metronidazole and tinidazole on anaerobic bacteria. Med. Microbiol. Immunol. 160:265–267.
5. **Dornbusch, K., C.-E. Nord, and T. Wadström.** 1974. Biochemical characterization and in vitro determination of antibiotic susceptibility of clinical isolates of *Bacteroides fragilis*. Scand. J. Infect. Dis. 6:253–258.
6. **Elek, S. D., and G. R. F. Hilson.** 1954. Combined agar diffusion and replica plating techniques in the study of antibacterial substances. J. Clin. Pathol. 7:37–44.
7. **Ericsson, H. M., and J. C. Sherris.** 1971. Antibiotic sensitivity testing. Report of an international collaborative study. Acta Pathol. Microbiol. Scand. Suppl. 217:1–90.
8. **Fass, R. J., R. B. Prior, and C. A. Rotilie.** 1975. Simplified method for antimicrobial susceptibility testing of anaerobic bacteria. Antimicrob. Agents Chemother. 8:444–452.
9. **Ferguson, I. R., and L. L. Smith.** 1976. *Bacteroides fragilis* and nitroimidazoles. J. Antimicrob. Chemother. 2:220–221.
10. **Finegold, S. M., J. G. Bartlett, A. W. Chow, D. J. Flora, S. L. Gorbach, E. J. Harder, and F. P. Tally.** 1975. Management of anaerobic infections. Ann. Intern. Med. 83:375–389.
11. **Gorbach, S. L., and J. G. Bartlett.** 1974. Anaerobic infections. N. Engl. J. Med. 290:1177–1184, 1237–1245, 1289–1294.
12. **Hamilton-Miller, J. M. T.** 1975. Antimicrobial agents acting against anaerobes. J. Antimicrob. Chemother. 1:273–289.
13. **Holdeman, L. V., and W. E. C. Moore (ed.).** 1975. Anaerobe laboratory manual, 3rd ed. Virginia Polytechnic Institute and State University, Blacksburg.
14. **Ingham, H. R., G. E. Rich, J. B. Selkon, J. H. Hale, C. M. Roxby, M. J. Betty, R. W. G. Johnson, and P. R. Uldall.** 1975. Treatment with metronidazole of three patients with serious infections due to *Bacteroides fragilis*. J. Antimicrob. Chemother. 1:235–242.
15. **Kislak, J. W.** 1972. The susceptibility of *Bacteroides fragilis* to 24 antibiotics. J. Infect. Dis. 125:295–299.

16. **Laslie, W. W., and D. W. Lambe, Jr.** 1976. Susceptibility testing of anaerobic bacteria with 100-μg carbenicillin disks. Antimicrob. Agents Chemother. 10:112-118.
17. **Martin, J. W., M. Gardner, and J. A. Washington II.** 1972. In vitro antimicrobial susceptibility of anaerobic bacteria isolated from clinical specimens. Antimicrob. Agents Chemother. 1:148-158.
18. **Metzler, C. M., and R. M. DeHaan.** 1974. Susceptibility tests of anaerobic bacteria: statistical and clinical considerations. J. Infect. Dis. 130:588-594.
19. **Mitre, R. J., and E. B. Rotheram, Jr.** 1974. Anaerobic septicemia from thrombophlebitis of the internal jugular vein. J. Am. Med. Assoc. 230:1168-1169.
20. **Nastro, J. L., and S. M. Finegold.** 1972. Bactericidal activity of five antimicrobial agents against *Bacteroides fragilis*. J. Infect. Dis. 126:104-107.
21. **Overman, S. B., D. W. Lambe, and J. V. Bennett.** 1974. Proposed standardized method for testing and interpreting susceptibility of *Bacteroides fragilis* to tetracycline. Antimicrob. Agents Chemother. 5:357-361.
22. **Plant, C. W., and D. I. Edwards.** 1976. The effect of tinidazole, metronidazole and nitrofurazone on nucleic acid synthesis in *Clostridium bifermentans*. J. Antimicrob. Chemother. 2:203-209.
23. **Ralph, E. D., and W. M. M. Kirby.** 1975. Unique bactericidal action of metronidazole against *Bacteroides fragilis* and *Clostridium perfringens*. Antimicrob. Agents Chemother. 8:409-414.
24. **Reynolds, A. V., J. M. T. Hamilton-Miller, and W. Brumfitt.** 1975. A comparison of the in vitro activity of metronidazole, tinidazole and nimorazole against gramnegative anaerobic bacilli. J. Clin. Pathol. 28:775-778.
25. **Stalons, D. R., and C. Thornsberry.** 1975. Broth-dilution method for determining the antibiotic susceptibility of anaerobic bacteria. Antimicrob. Agents Chemother. 7:15-21.
26. **Staneck, J. L., and J. A. Washington II.** 1974. Antimicrobial susceptibilities of anaerobic bacteria: recent clinical isolates. Antimicrob. Agents Chemother. 6:311-315.
27. **Steers, E., E. L. Foltz, B. S. Graves, and J. Riders.** 1959. An inocula replicating apparatus for routine testing of bacterial susceptibility to antibiotics. Antibiot. Chemother. 9:307-311.
28. **Sutter, V. L., and S. M. Finegold.** 1975. Susceptibility of anaerobic bacteria to carbenicillin, cefoxitin, and related drugs. J. Infect. Dis. 131:417-422.
29. **Sutter, V. L., V. L. Vargo, and S. M. Finegold.** 1975. Wadsworth anaerobic bacteriology manual, 2nd ed. Anaerobic Bacteriology Laboratory, Wadsworth Hospital Center and the Department of Medicine, Los Angeles.
30. **Tally, F. P., A. Y. Armfield, V. R. Dowell, Jr., Y. Y. Kwok, V. L. Sutter, and S. M. Finegold.** 1974. Susceptibility of *Clostridium ramosum* to antimicrobial agents. Antimicrob. Agents. Chemother. 5:589-593.
31. **Tally, F. P., V. L. Sutter, and S. M. Finegold.** 1975. Treatment of anaerobic infections with metronidazole. Antimicrob. Agents Chemother. 7:672-675.
32. **Whelan, J. P. F., and J. H. Hale.** 1973. Bactericidal activity of metronidazole against *Bacteroides fragilis*. J. Clin. Pathol. 26:393-395.
33. **Wilkins, T. D.** 1974. Antibiotic susceptibility testing of anaerobic bacteria, p. 451-455. *In* A. Balows, R. M. DeHaan, V. R. Dowell, Jr., and L. B. Guze (ed.), Anaerobic bacteria: role in disease. Charles C Thomas, Springfield, Ill.
34. **Wilkins, T. D., and M. D. Appleman.** 1976. Review of methods for antibiotic susceptibility testing of anaerobic bacteria. Lab. Med. 7:12-15.
35. **Wilkins, T. D., S. L. Chalgren, F. Jimenez-Ulate, C. R. Drake, Jr., and J. L. Johnson.** 1976. Inhibition of *Bacteroides fragilis* on blood agar plates and reversal of inhibition by added hemin. J. Clin. Microbiol. 3:359-363.
36. **Wilkins, T. D., L. V. Holdeman, I. J. Abramson, and W. E. C. Moore.** 1972. Standardized single-disc method for antibiotic susceptibility testing of anaerobic bacteria. Antimicrob. Agents Chemother. 1:451-459.
37. **Wilkins, T. D., and T. Thiel.** 1973. Modified broth-disk method for testing the antibiotic susceptibility of anaerobic bacteria. Antimicrob. Agents Chemother. 3:350-356.
38. **Willis, A. T., C. L. Bullen, I. R. Ferguson, et al.** 1974. Metronidazole in the prevention and treatment of bacteriodes infections in gynaecological patients. Lancet ii:1540-1543.
39. **Willis, A. T., I. R. Ferguson, P. M. Jones, et al.** 1976. Metronidazole in the prevention and treatment of bacteroides infections following appendicectomy. Br. Med. J. 1:318-321.

ANTIMICROBIAL AGENTS AND CHEMOTHERAPY, Apr. 1977, p. 638-644
Vol. 11, No. 4
Printed in U.S.A.

Growth Inhibition of *Escherichia coli* W by D-Norvalyl-D-Alanine: an Analogue of D-Alanine in Position 4 of the Peptide Subunit of Peptidoglycan

F. C. NEUHAUS,* S. GOYER, AND D. W. NEUHAUS

Department of Biochemistry and Molecular Biology, Northwestern University, Evanston, Illinois 60201

Received for publication 30 November 1976

Position 4 analogues of D-alanine in the peptide subunit of uridine 5'-diphosphate-*N*-acetylmuramyl-Ala[1]-DGlu[2]-Lys[3]-DAla[4]-DAla[5] have a significant inhibitory effect on penicillin-sensitive peptidoglycan synthesis in *Gaffkya homari* (C. V. Carpenter, S. Goyer, and F. C. Neuhaus, 1976). The specificity profile of this in vitro system has been used as a basis for designing analogues with potential antibacterial activity. To circumvent the specificity determinants exerted by D-alanine:D-alanine ligase (adenosine 5'-diphosphate), attention was directed to DD-dipeptides of the type D-alanyl-analogue-D-alanine as a method for incorporating analogues into position 4 of the peptide subunit in vivo. Of the three dipeptides, DAbu-DAla, DNva-DAla, and DVal-DAla, only DNva-DAla (5×10^{-4} M) inhibited the growth of *Escherichia coli* W in the presence of 5×10^{-6} M D-cycloserine. This concentration of D-cycloserine did not inhibit growth, but it potentiated the bactericidal activity of the dipeptide. The lack of antibacterial activity observed with DAbu-DAla and DVal-DAla was correlated with the poor ability of these dipeptides to be taken up via the dipeptide transport system of this organism. Prevention of lysis induced by DNva-DAla plus D-cycloserine by certain dipeptides and not by others supported this correlation. It is proposed that the D-norvalyl residue of the dipeptide is incorporated in vivo into position 4 of the peptide subunit of peptidoglycan, and that this subunit is not an effective substrate in the reaction(s) catalyzed by the penicillin-susceptible enzyme(s) of cross-linked peptidoglycan synthesis.

The design of potential analogues of D-alanine that inhibit the assembly of cross-linked, functional peptidoglycan requires that they be incorporated into a precursor where they can exert their effect. Inhibition of the cross-linking reaction by such analogues would lead to the synthesis of a polymer that is unable to function in normal wall formation. Amino acid residues 4 and 5 of the peptide moiety of peptidoglycan play an important role in cross-linking. Analogues of D-alanine in position 4 have a significant in vitro inhibitory effect on penicillin-sensitive peptidoglycan synthesis in *Gaffkya homari* (1). For example, if D-alanine in this position is replaced by D-norvaline, less than 2% of the in vitro synthetic activity is observed. Thus, incorporation of analogues of D-alanine into position 4 of the peptide moiety may provide a useful tool for controlling bacterial growth.

Because of the specificity determinants of D-alanine:D-alanine ligase, it is not possible for the cell to utilize D-norvaline for the synthesis of D-norvalyl-D-alanine (DNva-DAla) (8, 9). However, since uridine 5'-diphosphate-*N*-acetylmuramyl (UDP-MurNAc)-Ala-DGlu-Lys: DAla-DAla ligase will utilize DNva-DAla, it is possible to incorporate the analogue into position 4 via the dipeptide (11). The potential antibacterial action of this analogue in this position will require that the dipeptide, DNva-DAla, be transported by the cell.

The transport of dipeptides by *Escherichia coli* is catalyzed by a dipeptide system that has a high specificity for amino acid residues of the L configuration (2, 5, 6, 13, 14). However, prevention of lysis by D-cycloserine with DAla-DAla implies that this dipeptide is also taken up from the medium (P. Chambers, J. Bing, J. Lynch, F. C. Neuhaus, and R. W. Brockman, Bacteriol. Proc., p. 119, 1963). Kessel and Lubin (5) observed that DAla-DAla is an inhibitor of Gly-Gly transport. These results suggest that DAla-DAla is transported via the dipeptide system that accumulates Gly-Gly, and that this system may play a role in the uptake of the dipeptide analogues of DAla-DAla.

The purpose of these experiments is to examine the effect of analogues of DAla-DAla, with emphasis on DNva-DAla, on the growth of *E. coli* W. The inhibition of growth by this analogue can be related to the proposal that the D-norvalyl and D-alanyl residues of the dipeptide are incorporated into positions 4 and 5, respectively, of the peptide subunit of peptidoglycan, and that this subunit is not an effective donor substrate in the reaction catalyzed by the penicillin-sensitive transpeptidase. The uptake of DNva-DAla appears to be catalyzed by the dipeptide transport system; thus, this system plays a significant role in the antibacterial action of this dipeptide.

(A preliminary report of this work has been presented [F. C. Neuhaus, C. V. Carpenter, and S. Goyer, Prog. Abstr. Intersci. Conf. Antimicrob. Agents Chemother., 16th, Abstr. 118, 1976).

MATERIALS AND METHODS

Materials. We are indebted to Roger Harned of the IMC Chemical Group for generous samples of D-cycloserine. The DD-dipeptides were synthesized by Herman Plaut and are available from Vega-Fox. In addition, Leon Barstow of Vega-Fox has synthesized a sample of DNva-DAla used in this project. D-[^{14}C]alanine and [^{14}C]Gly-[^{14}C]Gly were purchased from Amersham/Searle. Chloramphenicol was obtained from Sigma Chemical Co. Membrane filters (0.45 μm pore size) were the product of Gelman Corp. All other materials were reagent grade. D[^{14}C]Ala-D[^{14}C]Ala was prepared according to the method described by Neuhaus and Struve (11).

Strains and medium. *E. coli* W ATCC 9637 was maintained in vacuo at -20°C. The minimal medium for growing these strains was: 0.1% NH_4Cl, 0.3% $NaH_2PO_4 \cdot H_2O$, 0.6% K_2HPO_4, 0.02% $MgSO_4$, 0.05% NaCl, and 0.4% glucose. Minimal medium minus glucose will be designated buffer A. The cultures for the growth experiments (10 ml) were grown at 37°C on a New Brunswick Gyrotory shaker (setting, 80). Bacterial growth was monitored turbidimetrically by measuring the absorbance of the culture at 650 nm in a spectrophotometer (Bausch and Lomb Spectronic 20) against medium.

Measurement of dipeptide uptake. For transport experiments, the bacteria were grown in 500-ml cultures to a turbidity of 0.4 in minimal medium containing 0.4% glucose. Chloramphenicol was then added to the culture to make a concentration of 200 μg/ml; the culture was maintained for an additional 30 min at 37°C. The cells were harvested, washed, and resuspended in buffer A (4°C) containing 200 μg of chloramphenicol per ml to give 200 mg (wet weight) per ml. The cell suspension was maintained at 4°C until used (<4 h).

The procedure for measuring the uptake of labeled dipeptides by nongrowing cells was similar to the method described by Wargel et al. (16). A portion (6×10^9 cells in 150 μl) of the cell suspension was added to 750 μl of minimal growth medium (glucose) that contained chloramphenicol (200 μg/ml), and the suspension was maintained at the accumulation temperature for 5 min. From this suspension, 600 μl was added to 400 μl of medium (chloramphenicol) containing the labeled dipeptide (5×10^{-5} M). Samples (200 μl) were removed at the desired time, and the cells were collected on a damp 0.45-μm-pore-size membrane filter. The cells were washed with buffer A (10 ml) at 25°C, and the damp membrane filter and cells were dissolved in 1 ml of ethyl acetate. The amount of radioactivity was determined according to the procedure described by Patterson and Greene (12).

RESULTS

Effect of DNva-DAla on growth. The effect of increasing concentrations of DNva-DAla in the presence of 5×10^{-6} M D-cycloserine is illustrated in Fig. 1A. Under these conditions, this concentration of D-cycloserine does not inhibit bacterial growth, but it is required for potentiating the inhibition by this dipeptide at the concentration used. D-Cycloserine is used to limit the activity catalyzed by alanine racemase and D-alanine:D-alanine ligase (adenosine 5′-diphosphate [ADP]) (10). The minimal inhibitory concentration of DNva-DAla is 2×10^{-4} M. For comparison, in the absence of D-cycloserine, 2×10^{-3} M D-Nva-DAla is required to effect the same degree of inhibition (Fig. 1B). The addition of 1×10^{-3} M DNva-DAla at different times to the bacterial culture in the presence of 5×10^{-6} M D-cycloserine results in the cessation of growth, followed by lysis of the culture (Fig. 2).

The specificity of growth inhibition is summarized in Table 1. Of the dipeptides tested, only DNva-DAla inhibits bacterial growth at 5×10^{-4} M in the presence of 5×10^{-6} M D-cycloserine. When equimolar concentrations of D-norvaline and D-alanine (5×10^{-4} M) replace DNva-DAla, growth inhibition was not observed. Thus, DNva-DAla would appear to exert a specific inhibition that results in lysis of the culture.

Prevention of D-cycloserine-induced lysis. Growth of *E. coli* W in concentrations of D-cycloserine higher than 7.5×10^{-6} M results in lysis of the bacterial culture. Chambers et al. (1963) observed that this inhibition is prevented by DAla-DAla. These results suggested that *E. coli* could utilize this dipeptide for the synthesis of UDP-MurNAc-pentapeptide. Prevention of lysis by a dipeptide would appear to be a good indication of those dipeptides that are transported and utilized for the synthesis of functional peptidoglycan. Of the dipeptides tested, D-alanyl-D-α-amino-n-butyric acid (DAla-DAbu) and DAla-DNva are as effective as DAla-DAla in preventing the inhibitory effect resulting from

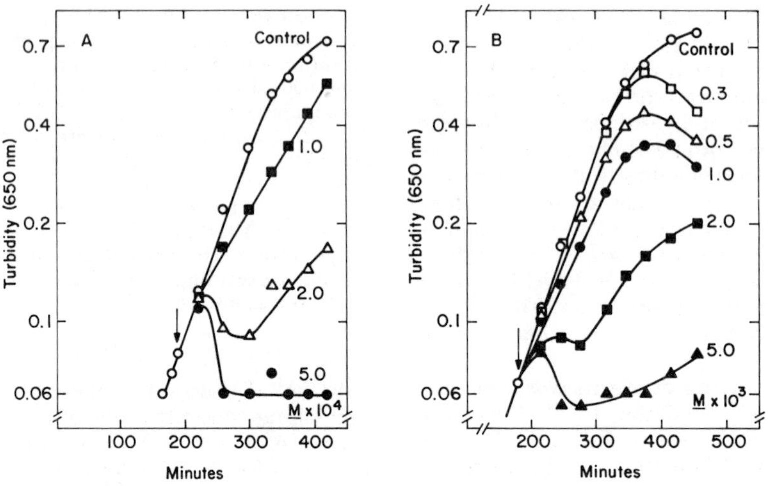

FIG. 1. *Growth studies with E. coli W. Effect of increasing concentrations of* DNva-DAla *in the presence of 5* $\times 10^{-6}$ *M* D-*cycloserine (A) and in the absence of* D-*cycloserine (B). (A) Concentrations of* DNva-DAla *were:* 1×10^{-4} *M (■),* 2×10^{-4} *M (△), and* 5×10^{-4} *M (●); (B) concentrations were:* 3×10^{-4} *M (□),* 5×10^{-4} *M (△),* 1×10^{-3} *M (●),* 2×10^{-3} *M (■) and* 5×10^{-3} *M (▲).*

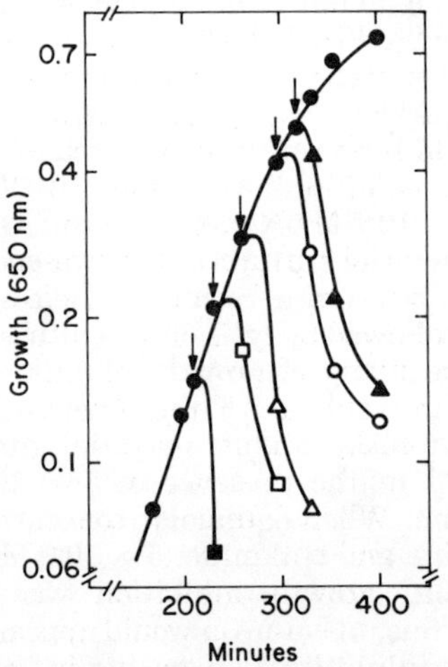

FIG. 2. *Growth inhibition and lysis of E. coli W.* DNva-DAla *(1 mM) was added at the indicated time to samples of E. coli W growing in the presence of 5* $\times 10^{-6}$ *M* D-*cycloserine.*

TABLE 1. *Specificity of growth inhibition by* DD-*dipeptides*

Dipeptide addition	Growth response (turbidity)[a]
None	0.72
DNva-DAla	0.07
DAla-DNva	0.68
DAla-DVal	0.73
DVal-DAla	0.70
DAla-DAbu	0.70
DAbu-DAla	0.68
DAla-DAla	0.70

[a] Turbidity represents the growth response 200 min after the addition of 5×10^{-4} M dipeptide in the presence of 5×10^{-6} M D-cycloserine.

D-cycloserine action (Table 2) (the prevention of D-cycloserine-induced lysis with DAla-DAbu and not DAbu-DAla confirms observations made by R. W. Brockman [personal communication]). DAbu-DAla has a limited ability to antagonize the action of D-cycloserine. In contrast, DAla-DVal, DVal-DAla, and DNva-DAla have no effect in preventing the bactericidal activity. Three interpretations of these results may be considered. Peptides that show no activity are either not transported, or are ineffective in replacing the DAla-DAla requirement for UDP-MurNAc-pentapeptide synthesis, or are utilized for the synthesis of nonfunctional peptidoglycan.

Prevention of DNva-DAla-induced lysis. The addition of either DAla-DAla (Fig. 3A) or D-alanine (Fig. 3B) antagonizes the effect exerted by DNva-DAla. Prevention of lysis with DD-dipeptides that are analogues of DAla-DAla is summarized in Table 3. Except for DVal-DAla and DAla-DVal, each of the peptides has some ability to prevent DNva-DAla-induced lysis when tested at equimolar concentrations. An interesting feature of this experiment is that DAla-DNva prevents the lytic action induced by DNva-DAla. In Table 3 (experiment 2), additional specificity studies reveal that the prevention is not restricted to dipeptides of the DD-configuration. Gly-Gly, LAla-LAla, and LNva-

LAla have some ability to prevent the inhibitory activity exerted by DNva-DAla. Two interpretations of these data may be considered. The antagonizing dipeptide either inhibits the uptake of DNva-DAla or it effectively competes with DNva-DAla for addition to UDP-MurNAc-tripeptide in the reaction catalyzed by UDP-MurNAc-tripeptide:DAla-DAla ligase, resulting in a functional subunit. However, since specificity studies with this enzyme eliminate LL-dipeptides as substrates for this enzyme (4, 11), it would appear that these dipeptides inhibit the uptake of DNva-DAla.

TABLE 2. *Prevention of D-cycloserine-induced lysis*

Dipeptide addition	Growth response (turbidity)[a]
None	0.02
DAla-DAla	0.64
DAla-DAbu	0.62
DAla-DNva	0.68
DAla-DVal	0.02
DNva-DAla	0.02
DAbu-DAla	0.32
DVal-DAla	0.03
Gly-Gly	0.58

[a] Dipeptide (5×10^{-4} M) was added to *E. coli* W in minimal medium containing 5×10^{-5} M D-cycloserine. This concentration of D-cycloserine gave complete lysis. The turbidity represents the growth response 220 min after the addition of the dipeptide.

Transport of DNva-DAla. An analysis of the transport system that is responsible for the accumulation of DAla-DAla may provide a basis for interpreting the specificity studies described above. *E. coli* has a specific transport system for dipeptides (2, 6, 13, 14). Payne (13) concludes that dipeptide transport "appears to have a stereospecific requirement for L-residues." However, Kessel and Lubin (5) observed that DAla-DAla is an inhibitor of Gly-Gly uptake. These results suggest that DAla-DAla may be accumulated via the dipeptide transport system. The uptake of DAla-DAla by *E. coli* KMBL-146 has been briefly described (7). To establish the role of the dipeptide transport system for the accumulation of these DD-dipeptides, a series of experiments was initiated with two labeled dipeptides, D[^{14}C]Ala-D[^{14}C]Ala and [^{14}C]Gly-[^{14}C]Gly.

In Fig. 4A, the uptake of D[^{14}C]Ala-D[^{14}C]Ala is illustrated. The addition of azide (0.01 M) reduces the uptake of this dipeptide. The addition of either LAla-LAla or Gly-Gly markedly inhibits the uptake of D[^{14}C]Ala-D[^{14}C]Ala. The DD-dipeptide, DNva-DAla (10 mM), inhibits the transport of this labeled dipeptide by 80%. In a similar experiment, the time course of [^{14}C]Gly-[^{14}C]Gly uptake was examined (Fig. 4B). DAla-DAla (10 mM) and DNva-DAla (10 mM) significantly reduce the accumulation of this dipeptide. LAla-LAla is a very effective inhibitor of

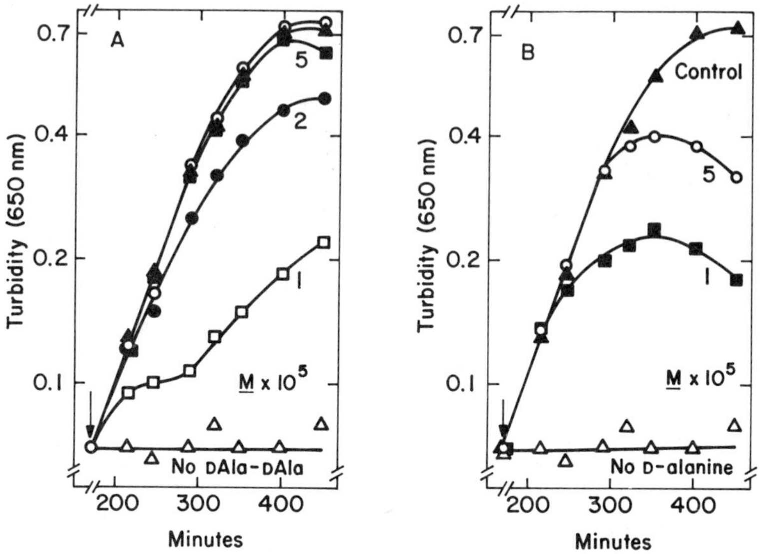

FIG. 3. *Prevention of DNva-DAla-induced lysis with DAla-DAla (A) and D-alanine (B). (A) Concentrations of DAla-DAla were: 1×10^{-5} M (□), 2×10^{-5} M (●), 5×10^{-5} M (■), and 1×10^{-4} M (▲); (B) concentrations of D-alanine were 1×10^{-5} M (■) and 5×10^{-5} M (○). These growth studies were performed in the presence of 5×10^{-6} M D-cycloserine, and the concentration of DNva-DAla in each sample except the control (A, ○; B, ▲) was 5×10^{-4} M.*

both DAla-DAla uptake and Gly-Gly uptake. On the basis of these results, it would appear that Gly-Gly and DAla-DAla are transported by a common system, a result that is implied from the inhibition data presented by Kessel and Lubin (5).

Each of the analogue dipeptides has been tested as an inhibitor of either D[^{14}C]Ala-D[^{14}C]Ala or [^{14}C]Gly-[^{14}C]Gly uptake (Table 4). It will be assumed that dipeptides which inhibit the uptake of either labeled dipeptide are also substrates for the dipeptide transport system. This assumption is necessary since labeled analogues of DAla-DAla are not readily available. As summarized in Table 4, DNva-DAla, DAla-DAbu, and DAla-DNva are relatively better inhibitors of D[^{14}C]Ala-D[^{14}C]Ala uptake than are DAla-DVal, DVal-DAla, and DAbu-DAla. With [^{14}C]Gly-[^{14}C]Gly as the labeled dipeptide, DAla-DAla, DNva-DAla, DAla-DNva, and DAla-DAbu are better inhibitors of dipeptide uptake than are DVal-DAla, DAla-DVal, and DAbu-DAla. The similarity in inhibition profiles indicates that DAla-DAla, DNva-DAla, DAla-DNva, and DAla-DAbu are transported via the dipeptide transport system described by Kessel and Lubin (5).

TABLE 3. *Prevention of DNva-DAla-induced lysis*

Dipeptide addition	Growth response (turbidity)[a]
Expt 1	
Control	0.64
DNva-DAla	0.05
DNva-DAla + DAbu-DAla	0.38
DNva-DAla + DAla-DAbu	0.53
DNva-DAla + DAla-DNva	0.48
DNva-DAla + DAla-DVal	0.10
DNva-DAla + DVal-DAla	0.08
DNva-DAla + DAla-DAla	0.64
Expt 2	
Control	0.69
DNva-DAla	0.08
DNva-DAla + Gly-Gly	0.66
DNva-DAla + LAla-LAla	0.31
DNva-DAla + LNva-LAla	0.48

[a] Turbidity represents the growth response in the presence of 5×10^{-6} M D-cycloserine 210 min after the addition of 5×10^{-4} M DNva-DAla and 5×10^{-4} M dipeptide.

DISCUSSION

The successful incorporation of a D-alanine analogue into position 4 of the peptide subunit of peptidoglycan is dependent on the specificity determinants of a variety of enzyme and transport systems. Each of these exerts its discrimination against the potential analogue. In our studies of D-alanine:D-alanine ligase, it was evident that this enzyme has a high degree of

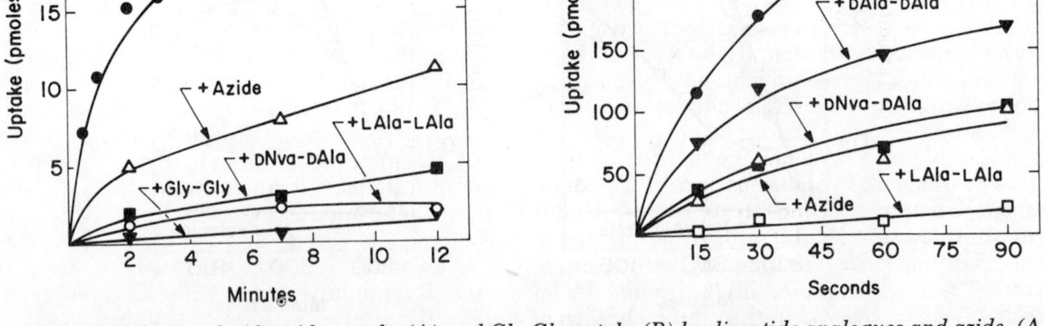

FIG. 4. *Inhibition of DAla-DAla uptake (A) and Gly-Gly uptake (B) by dipeptide analogues and azide. (A) Concentration of D[^{14}C]Ala-D[^{14}C]Ala was 50 μM; (B) concentration of [^{14}C]Gly-[^{14}C]Gly was 50 μM. The concentration of sodium azide was 10 mM. In (A), either 10 mM DNva-DAla (■), 10 mM LAla-LAla (○), or 10 mM Gly-Gly (▼) was added; in (B), either 10 mM DAla-DAla (▼), 10 mM DNva-DAla (■), or 10 mM LAla-LAla (□) was added. The accumulation temperature for the experiments in (A) was 25°C and in (B) it was 15°C. The procedure is described in Materials and Methods.*

TABLE 4. *Inhibition of uptake of DAla-DAla and Gly-Gly*

Dipeptide addition	Inhibition (%)	
	D[^{14}C]Ala-D[^{14}C]Ala	[^{14}C]Gly-[^{14}C]Gly
DVal-DAla	5	12
DAla-DVal	9	2
DAbu-DAla	28	10
DAla-DAla		27
DNva-DAla	70	41
DAla-DNva	65	40
DAla-DAbu	70	38
LAla-LAla	98	96
Gly-Gly	96	

[a] Uptake was measured with either 50 μM D[^{14}C]Ala-D[^{14}C]Ala or 50 μM [^{14}C]Gly-[^{14}C]Gly in the presence of 5 mM dipeptide. In the case of D[^{14}C]Ala-D[^{14}C]Ala, uptake was measured for 1 min at 25°C. In the case of [^{14}C]Gly-[^{14}C]Gly, uptake was measured for 15 s at 15°C.

specificity for the *N*-terminal residue, the precursor of the D-alanine residue in position 4 of the peptide subunit (8, 9). To circumvent these specificity determinants, attention was directed to DD-dipeptides that have the *N*-terminal D-alanine analogue. Specificity studies with UDP-MurNAc-Ala-DGlu-Lys:DAla-DAla ligase indicated that changes in the *N*-terminal residue of the dipeptide, e.g., D-α-amino-*n*-butyric acid and D-norvaline, would not affect the activity catalyzed by this enzyme (11). Thus, the use of DD-dipeptides of the type D-alanyl-analogue-DAla was considered as a potential method for incorporating an analogue into position 4 of the peptide subunit in vivo.

Incorporation of either D-α-amino-*n*-butyric acid, D-norvaline, or D-valine into residue 4 of the peptide subunit relative to incorporation into residue 5 significantly inhibits the in vitro synthesis of penicillin-sensitive peptidoglycan in membrane wall preparations from *G. homari* (1). Thus, three dipeptides, DAbu-DAla, DNva-DAla, and DVal-DAla have been considered for potential antibacterial activity. Of the three, only DNva-DAla has the ability to inhibit growth under the conditions tested. To potentiate the activity, a concentration of D-cycloserine that does not inhibit growth was added to the medium. It was assumed that this concentration was sufficient to limit the amount of DAla-DAla synthesized in the alanine branch of peptidoglycan synthesis but would allow the same rate of growth as in the control. The lack of antibacterial activity observed with DAbu-DAla and DVal-DAla can be correlated with the relatively poorer ability of these dipeptides to inhibit the uptake of DAla-DAla and Gly-Gly. Thus, it is presumed that these analogues are not transported via the dipeptide system to a significant extent under the conditions tested. On the other hand, DNva-DAla, which inhibits the uptake of DAla-DAla and Gly-Gly, does have significant antibacterial activity. Our data suggest that this dipeptide is transported as effectively as DAla-DAla, DAla-DAbu, and DAla-DNva.

Prevention of D-cycloserine-induced lysis by DD-dipeptides provides an independent method of testing for those dipeptides that are transported and utilized for the synthesis of functional peptidoglycan. In addition to DAla-DAla, DAla-DAbu and DAla-DNva prevent the lysis induced by D-cycloserine. These results imply that the three dipeptides satisfy the dipeptide requirement for UDP-MurNAc-pentapeptide synthesis. Since DAla-DVal lacks the ability to prevent lysis induced by D-cycloserine, it is presumed that DAla-DVal is not taken up. Although DNva-DAla appears to be transported, no prevention of D-cycloserine-induced lysis is observed. It is presumed that the defective peptidoglycan with residue 4 replaced by D-norvaline is synthesized and that this glycan does not participate in cross-linked peptidoglycan synthesis (1).

Prevention of DNva-DAla-induced lysis by DD-dipeptides provides an indication of those dipeptides that effectively compete with DAla-DAla for transport into the bacterium. In addition, Gly-Gly, LAla-LAla, and LNva-LAla were effective in preventing the action of DNva-DAla. The specificity of the dipeptide transport system suggests that LL-dipeptides and Gly-Gly will compete effectively with DNva-DAla and thus prevent the uptake of this DD-dipeptide. DAla-DNva prevents the inhibitory action of DNva-DAla. On the other hand, DAla-DVal cannot prevent the action of DNva-DAla because it does not compete for the transport system. Thus, the interpretation of the growth experiments relies on the definition of the specificity profile of the transport system. The antibacterial activity of the DD-dipeptide not only reflects the specificity determinants of the relevant enzyme systems, but it also must reflect the specificity determinants exerted by the transport system.

Analogues of DAla-DAla with *C*-terminal substituents have been synthesized and tested for antibacterial activity (3, 15). None of these compounds showed significant antibacterial activity. On the basis of our specificity studies, it is doubtful that analogues with changes in the *C*-terminal residue would have been ligated to UDP-MurNAc-tripeptide. Alternatively, if they had been added to the -tripeptide, the analogue would have been incorporated into position 5 rather than into position 4. Incorporation of an analogue into position 5 does not have a major effect on the cross-linked peptidoglycan synthesis relative to incorporation of an analogue into position 4 in *G. homari* (1).

ACKNOWLEDGMENTS

We are indebted to Carolyn V. Carpenter for discussions of the ideas that led to these experiments and to William A. Weppner for discussions of the data.

The investigation was supported by Public Health Service grant AI-04615 from the National Institute of Allergy and Infectious Diseases.

LITERATURE CITED

1. **Carpenter, C. V., S. Goyer, and F. C. Neuhaus.** 1976. Steric effects on penicillin-sensitive peptidoglycan synthesis in a membrane-wall system from *Gaffkya homari*. Biochemistry 15:3146–3152.
2. **De Felice, M., J. Guardiola, A. Lamberti, and M. Iaccarino.** 1973. *Escherichia coli* K-12 mutants altered in the transport systems for oligo- and dipeptides. J. Bacteriol. 116:751–756.
3. **Gale, G. R., and A. B. Smith.** 1973. Insensitivity of bacteria to proposed antimetabolites of D-alanyl-D-alanine. J. Bacteriol. 114:460–461.
4. **Ito, E., and J. L. Strominger.** 1962. Enzymatic synthesis of the peptide in bacterial uridine nucleotides. II. Enzymatic synthesis and addition of D-alanyl-D-alanine. J. Biol. Chem. 237:2696–2703.
5. **Kessel, D., and M. Lubin.** 1963. On the distinction between peptidase activity and peptide transport. Biochim. Biophys. Acta 71:656–663.
6. **Levine, E. M., and S. Simmonds.** 1962. Further studies on metabolic uptake by serine-glycine auxotrophs of *Escherichia coli*. J. Biol. Chem. 237:3718–3724.
7. **Lugtenberg, E. J. J., and A. van Schijndel-van Dam.** 1973. Temperature-sensitive mutant of *Escherichia coli* K-12 with an impaired D-alanine:D-alanine ligase. J. Bacteriol. 113:96–104.
8. **Neuhaus, F. C.** 1962. The enzymatic synthesis of D-alanyl-D-alanine. I. Purification and properties of D-alanyl-D-alanine synthetase. J. Biol. Chem. 237:778–786.
9. **Neuhaus, F. C.** 1962. The enzymatic synthesis of D-alanyl-D-alanine. II. Kinetic studies on D-alanyl-D-alanine synthetase. J. Biol. Chem. 237:3128–3135.
10. **Neuhaus, F. C.** 1967. The antibiotics D-cycloserine and *O*-carbamyl-D-serine, p. 40–83. *In* D. Gottlieb and P. D. Shaw (ed.), Antibiotics: mechanism of action, vol. 1. Springer-Verlag, Heidelberg.
11. **Neuhaus, F. C., and W. G. Struve.** 1965. Enzymatic synthesis of analogs of the cell-wall precursor. I. Kinetics and specificity of uridine diphospho-*N*-acetylmuramyl-L-alanyl-D-glutamyl-L-lysine: D-alanyl-D-alanine ligase (ADP) from *Streptococcus faecalis* R. Biochemistry 4:120–131.
12. **Patterson, M. S., and R. C. Greene.** 1965. Measurement of low energy beta-emitters in aqueous solution by liquid scintillation counting of emulsions. Anal. Chem. 37:854–857.
13. **Payne, J. W.** 1976. Peptides and micro-organisms. Adv. Microb. Physiol. 13:55–113.
14. **Payne, J. W., and C. Gilvarg.** 1971. Peptide transport. Adv. Enzymol. 35:187–244.
15. **Smissman, E. E., A. Terada, and S. El-Antably.** 1976. Synthesis of inhibitors of bacterial cell wall biogenesis. Analogs of D-alanyl-D-alanine. J. Med. Chem. 19:165–167.
16. **Wargel, R. J., C. A. Shadur, and F. C. Neuhaus.** 1970. Mechanism of D-cycloserine action: transport systems for D-alanine, D-cycloserine, D-alanine and glycine. J. Bacteriol. 103:778–788.

ANTIMICROBIAL AGENTS AND CHEMOTHERAPY, Apr. 1977, p. 645-650 Vol. 11, No. 4

Therapy of Antimicrobial-Resistant Typhoid Fever

THOMAS BUTLER,* NGUYEN NGOC LINH,[1] KEITH ARNOLD, MICHAEL D. ADICKMAN, DUONG MINH CHAU, AND MACH MUOI MUOI

Division of Geographic Medicine, Department of Medicine, Case Western Reserve University and University Hospitals, Cleveland, Ohio 44106; the Division of Infectious Diseases, Department of Medicine, Johns Hopkins University School of Medicine and Hospital, Baltimore, Maryland 21205; the Cho-Quan Hospital, Saigon, South Vietnam; and the Department of Medicine, University of Oklahoma Health Sciences Center, Oklahoma City, Oklahoma, 73190*

Received for publication 11 November 1976

Antimicrobial-resistant typhoid fever in Saigon was studied by examining in vitro antimicrobial susceptibilities of *Salmonella typhi* strains and conducting a randomized clinical trial of ampicillin and trimethoprim-sulfamethoxazole (TMP-SMZ). Isolates of *S. typhi* were obtained from blood or stool cultures of 90 patients. Of 87 isolates tested for antimicrobial susceptibility, 65 (75%) were resistant (R) to chloramphenicol, streptomycin, sulfonamide, and tetracycline, and 22 (25%) were susceptible (S). The drug resistance was transferable to *Escherichia coli* and was found in 11 different Vi-phage types. All isolates were susceptible to ampicillin and to TMP-SMZ. Agar dilution studies of TMP and SMZ showed synergistic inhibition of growth in all 18 S isolates and in 12 of 48 R isolates tested. The clinical trial of ampicillin and TMP-SMZ showed that both drugs were equally effective. Treatment failure with both drugs was more frequent in patients with S isolates than in patients with R isolates. Therefore, in an area where antimicrobial-resistant typhoid fever exists, patients with R isolates should receive either ampicillin or TMP-SMZ, but patients with S isolates should be treated with chloramphenicol.

Between 1971 and 1974 antimicrobial-resistant (R) typhoid fever emerged in Vietnam and became the predominant form of the disease (11, 14, 27). The causative strains of *Salmonella typhi* belonged to multiple Vi-phage types and were highly resistant to chloramphenicol, streptomycin, sulfonamides, and tetracycline. This multiple antimicrobial resistance was mediated by an R-factor (infectious antibiotic resistance factor), identical to the R-factor associated with the concomitant epidemic of typhoid fever in Mexico (6, 8, 25, 29, 41).

The treatment of antimicrobial-resistant typhoid fever has posed a dilemma. Alternatives to chloramphenicol, which have been shown to be clinically effective, include ampicillin and trimethoprim-sulfamethoxazole (TMP-SMZ) (1, 4, 16, 21, 22, 23, 31, 33, 35, 36, 39). TMP-SMZ offered promise because of favorable results in the treatment of antimicrobial-susceptible typhoid fever (4, 16, 21, 22, 33, 39). Other reports, however, contained reservations concerning treatment failures and toxicity (18, 34, 35). Furthermore, the objection was raised that use of a drug containing a sulfonamide to treat disease caused by a sulfonamide-resistant organism is not rational (5). The following studies were designed to evaluate therapy by performing in vitro antimicrobial studies and by conducting a randomized clinical trial of ampicillin and TMP-SMZ.

[1] Deceased April 1975. We dedicate this work to his bereaved family and his exemplary devotion to the treatment and prevention of infectious diseases in Vietnam.

MATERIALS AND METHODS

Microbiological. Two milliliters of blood obtained at the time of admission was placed into Vacutainers containing supplemented peptone broth and penicillinase. Stool swabs were streaked onto blood agar and salmonella-shigella agar. *S. typhi* was identified by standard methods, including agglutination by antisera to group D (26). All isolates of *S. typhi* were sent to the Enteric Reference Laboratory, London, for Vi-phage typing and antibiotic resistance transfer studies.

Antimicrobial susceptibilities were determined by the Kirby-Bauer method (10). Additional agar dilution studies for susceptibility to TMP, SMZ, and a combination (1 part TMP to 20 parts SMZ) were done with Mueller-Hinton agar containing 7.5% lysed horse blood and drugs (13). Overnight broth cultures were diluted to 10^{-3} and placed onto the agar in streaks measuring 1 mm by 10 mm. The lowest concentrations of drugs in which less than 10 colonies appeared in a streak was defined as the minimum inhibitory concentration (MIC). Synergism of the combination of TMP and SMZ (in a ratio of 1 part TMP to 20 parts SMZ by weight) was defined as a threefold or greater reduction in the MIC of TMP by the addition of SMZ. All antimicrobial studies were performed on isolates transported to Baltimore on Cary-Blair medium; the results were, therefore, not available for application to patient care.

Acute and convalescent sera from patients with suspected typhoid fever, whose cultures were negative for *S. typhi*, were tested by a standard serological test for agglutination of *Salmonella* O antigen (17). Criteria used for a positive diagnosis were either a fourfold increase between acute and convalescent phases or a titer ≥160 at any time during the illness.

Clinical. Patients who were suspected of having typhoid fever were admitted to the study. The initial diagnosis was based on two or more of the following: a history of fever for more than 1 week, a rectal temperature ≥38.5°C, abdominal tenderness, splenomegaly, and rose spots. Rectal temperatures were recorded twice daily and changes in clinical status noted.

Therapeutic studies. During 1973 and 1974 therapy was not controlled but was chosen by individual physicians. In 1975 the final 20 patients were randomly assigned to receive either ampicillin or TMP-SMZ (Septrin was a gift of The Wellcome Foundation Limited). Both drugs were given intravenously during the first 3 to 5 days and then, after improvement had been noted, oral therapy was started. Ampicillin was administered in a dosage of approximately 100 mg/kg per day (4 g for most patients) in four equally divided doses. Injectable TMP-SMZ containing 320 mg of TMP and 1,600 mg of SMZ was given intravenously daily to adults in two evenly divided doses. Half of this dose was given to children under 12 years old. The oral dosage was the same. A patient was considered afebrile when the rectal temperature reached ≤38°C and remained at this level for at least 48 h.

RESULTS

Diagnostic studies. A diagnosis of typhoid fever was confirmed in 101 patients. Blood cultures were positive for *S. typhi* in 89 patients. Stool cultures were positive in only 7 patients and 6 of these had concomitantly positive blood cultures. Diagnoses were made serologically in 11 patients with negative cultures.

Antimicrobial susceptibilities. All 87 strains tested by the Kirby-Bauer method were susceptible to ampicillin, cephalothin, and colistin. By agar dilution testing all strains were inhibited by 0.1 to 1.0 μg of TMP per ml. Twenty-two were also susceptible (S) to chloramphenicol, streptomycin, sulfonamides, and tetracycline. The remaining 65, or 75% of all tested strains, were resistant (R) to these four drugs. These multiple-resistant strains transferred their resistance to recipient *Escherichia coli* and, thus, possessed R-factors. The MICs of SMZ for the R strains were ≥100 μg/ml in all instances. Thus, the concentrations of SMZ (0.2 to 20 μg/ml) used in combination with TMP were not inhibitory for the R strains and a combination resulting in a threefold or greater susceptibility to TMP clearly constituted synergistic inhibition. The S strains displayed greater degrees of inhibition. Table 1 shows that 30 of 66 strains tested were synergistically inhibited by TMP and SMZ. Six of the 18 S strains showed a 10-fold decrease in the MIC of TMP with the addition of SMZ. Although 12 of the 48 R strains were synergistically inhibited, they never showed more than a threefold decrease.

Phage types. Of the 17 different Vi-phage types detected in 82 tested strains of *S. typhi*, antimicrobial resistance was present in 11 different phage types (Table 2). Six phage types were present in only S strains, and five phage types were included in both R and S strains.

Antimicrobial treatment. Chloramphenicol

TABLE 1. *Amount of synergism[a] with trimethoprim (TMP) and sulfamethoxazole (SMZ) in antimicrobial-resistant (R) and antimicrobial-susceptible (S) strains of S. typhi*

Anitmicrobial susceptibility	No. of strains		
	No synergism	3-fold synergism	10-fold synergism
R	36	12	0
S	0	12	6

[a] Amount of synergism is the decrease in the MIC of TMP for an organism caused by the addition of SMZ to TMP in a ratio of 20 parts SMZ to 1 part TMP by weight.

TABLE 2. *Distribution of Vi-phage types in 82 strains of S. typhi.*

Vi-phage type	Antimicrobial susceptibility	
	Resistant	Susceptible
56	27	2
UVS	0	1
UVS (1)	4	7
UVS (2)	12	0
UVS (3)	3	0
UVS (4)	1	0
DVS	1	0
DVS9	0	4
A	1	1
B2	0	2
D6	3	1
E1	0	1
E7	2	0
E10	0	2
M1	1	1
37	0	3
Vi-negative variant	2	0

was frequently used to treat patients in 1973 before the prevalence of antimicrobial resistance was recognized. In 1974 ampicillin and TMP-SMZ were used, and the choice was based on staff physicians' preferences. Table 3 shows the numbers of patients treated with each drug. A patient was included when the drug was the initial treatment or was later added and used for at least 5 days. Nine patients, including one fatal case, received two drugs and are counted twice in Table 3. Eight patients died. Chloramphenicol was used to treat 16 patients, of whom 3 died. *S. typhi* was recovered from 2 of these cases and both had R isolates. Although ampicillin and TMP-SMZ were effective in vitro against all isolated strains of *S. typhi*, the overall mortality rate in these two treatment groups combined was 6 of 71 or 8.5%. Furthermore, the patients treated with ampicillin or TMP-SMZ who were infected with S strains of *S. typhi* had a higher mortality rate (2 out of 14 or 14%) than the patients infected with R strains (3 out of 46 or 6.5%). This difference, however, was not statistically significant ($P >$ 0.05 by an exact test [9]).

The results of the randomized treatment of 20 patients are shown in Table 4. Excluding the deaths, the median number of days until defervescence in the group treated with ampicillin was 5.5 and with TMP-SMZ 5.0 days. One death occurred in each treatment group. Therefore, no clear differences in the responses to the two drugs were observed. When the patients in both treatment groups are combined, it is apparent that six of seven patients with R isolates were afebrile within 7 days of treatment, whereas four of six patients with S isolates had unsatisfactory responses, including two deaths and two with fever persisting longer than 7 days. Although these differences were not statistically significant, these poor responses of patients infected with S isolates may suggest that S isolates are less susceptible in vivo to these drugs than are R isolates.

DISCUSSION

The almost simultaneous appearance of widespread typhoid fever caused by antimicrobial-resistant *S. typhi* in 1972 in both Vietnam and Mexico has forced physicians to reevaluate therapy and has caused concern for travelers going to these countries (42). In both countries the afflicted patients were reported to respond poorly to chloramphenicol (11, 14, 27, 41). All strains of antimicrobial-resistant *S. typhi* iso-

TABLE 3. *Relationship of therapy to antimicrobial resistance and mortality in 78 patients with typhoid fever*

Antibiotic	No. of patients[a]			No. of deaths[a]		
	Total	With R strains	With S strains	Total	With R strains	With S strains
Chloramphenicol	16	9	6	3	2	0
Ampicillin	27	17	4	3	1	1
TMP-SMZ[b]	44	29	10	3	2	1

[a] R, Resistant; S, susceptible.
[b] TMP-SMZ, Trimethoprim-sulfamethoxazole.

TABLE 4. *Randomized treatment of 20 confirmed cases of typhoid fever with ampicillin or trimethoprim-sulfamethoxazole (TMP-SMZ)*

Patient no.	Ampicillin		Patient no.	TMP-SMZ	
	Diagnosis[a]	Days febrile[b]		Diagnosis[a]	Days febrile[b]
103	1,280 → 2,560	5.5	102	*S. typhi* S	4.0
104	80 → 160	5.5	106	*S. typhi* S	11.0
105	*S. typhi* R	3.5	113	*S. typhi* S	Died day 8
107	*S. typhi* R	3.5	116	640 → 2,560	2.0
111	20,480 → 10,240	5.5	117	*S. typhi* R	9.5
114	320 → 320	4.5	118	*S. typhi* R	5.5
115	*S. typhi* R	5.5	122	640 → 1,280	4.5
119	640 → 1,280	4.5	124	*S. typhi* R	3.5
120	*S. typhi* S	10.5	125	*S. typhi* R	6.0
121	*S. typhi* S	Died day 8			
123	*S. typhi* S	5.5			

[a] Diagnosis established either by positive blood culture for *S. typhi* (S, susceptible; R, resistant) or a titer of *Salmonella* O agglutinins ≥160. Titers are designated as acute → convalescent.
[b] Days after initiation of treatment until rectal temperatures ≤38°C were recorded for 48 h or longer.

lated from these patients were shown to possess an R-factor carrying information for resistance to chloramphenicol, streptomycin, sulfonamide, and tetracycline. This R-factor has been assigned to group H_1 and has also been found in resistant strains of *S. typhi* from Mexico, India, and Thailand (6, 20, 24, 38). Besides these similarities, there were important differences between disease patterns in Vietnam and Mexico. In Mexico there was an epidemic of typhoid fever which originated in the State of Hidalgo, and all Vi-phage types of *S. typhi* were the same degraded Vi (A) phage type, indicating a point source outbreak (33). A year later the epidemic was waning and now seems to be over. In Saigon, on the other hand, typhoid fever was hyperendemic, and the antibiotic resistance emerged in several different Vi-phage types (14), which have been expanded to 11 different types in the present study. After the appearance of the R-factor in 1971, there were remarkably similar proportions of resistant cases to total cases throughout Saigon, where three major hospitals reported resistance in 59 to 71% of cases in 1972 to 1973 (1). In the present study, spanning the years 1973 to 1975, there was a 75% frequency of antimicrobial resistance, and there were no indications of a diminishing frequency of resistance at the conclusion of our work in Saigon.

The acquisition of R-factors by *S. typhi* has been related to indiscriminant antibiotic usage in the environment (8). Nonpathogenic bacteria such as *E. coli* harbor the R-factors because of selective antibiotic pressure (2). *S. typhi* come into contact with R-factor-bearing bacteria and, during mitosis, conjugation of two bacteria occurs and the R-factor is transferred. In Mexico the R-factor transfer needed to have occurred only once because all R-factor-bearing isolates belonged to the same Vi-phage type, a stable genetic property of *S. typhi*. In Vietnam this presumed transfer of the R-factor must have occurred at least 11 times from other bacteria into the recipient strains of *S. typhi*. It follows from the multiple Vi-phage types in Saigon that the antimicrobial-resistant form of typhoid fever will persist longer than in Mexico and perhaps as long as antibiotics continue to be used indiscriminantly there.

The R strains of *S. typhi* isolated from these patients appeared fully virulent and produced the classical spectrum of illness associated with typhoid fever (28, 37). The mortality rate of 9% in this study is comparable to the preantibiotic era in the United States, when the mortality was reported to be 9 to 13% (37, 43). It is also significantly higher than an average mortality of 4.5% reported after the introduction of chloramphenicol (43). However, in developing countries where nutrition and medical facilities are substandard, the mortality rate of typhoid fever treated with chloramphenicol in unselected hospitalized patients may be as high as 15%, despite the absence of chloramphenicol resistance (7).

All strains of *S. typhi* tested for susceptibility to TMP by an agar dilution method had MICs of TMP from 0.1 to 1.0 μg/ml. Addition of SMZ resulted in synergistic inhibition of the combination for all of the tested strains without the R-factor. With the agar dilution technique used in this study, 12 of 48 R strains also were synergistically inhibited. Another study of TMP-SMZ, performed with isolates of antimicrobial-resistant *S. typhi* in Mexico, showed no synergism against the R strains studied (19). This disparity in results may have been caused by biological differences in the R-factors or by differences in techniques and definitions of synergism. Our results indicate that, despite the presence of sulfonamide resistance, synergistic inhibition by TMP and SMZ occurred. This agrees with in vitro studies of other bacteria resistant to sulfonamides. Thus, SMZ may reduce the synthesis of dihydrofolate in sulfonamide-resistant organisms to a level that allows TMP to reduce its conversion to tetrahydrofolate to a critically low level (12).

The results of treatment of typhoid fever with ampicillin and TMP-SMZ in this study revealed that both drugs were effective, especially in treating patients with R organisms. On the other hand, six patients with S isolates in the randomized trial included two deaths and two with fever persisting beyond 7 days. Although the number of patients is small, these findings suggest that S strains of *S. typhi* may respond less well in vivo to ampicillin and TMP-SMZ than the R strains. In contrast to our study, Gilman et al. found that patients in Mexico with S isolates of *S. typhi* had more rapid clinical responses to TMP-SMZ than did patients with R isolates (19). When comparing the results of these studies, important differences must be noted. Our study included toxic patients with complications who would have been excluded from their study, and our patients received intravenous drugs initially, whereas Gilman et al. used only oral drugs.

Newer antibiotics have been used to treat typhoid fever. Amoxicillin and cefazolin have been used successfully in patients with R strains (15, 19, 32) and S strains [30, 34a, 40]. Nevertheless, chloramphenicol was shown to be superior to ampicillin and TMP-SMZ for typhoid fever caused by S strains (36). Our results suggesting unsatisfactory responses in patients with S strains both to ampicillin and to TMP-SMZ make it imperative that susceptibility testing be done in areas where antimicrobial resistance has been reported in order that chloramphenicol can be given to patients with S strains.

ACKNOWLEDGMENTS

These studies were supported in part by grant no. RDRF S92-544-75-G233 from the Department of the Army and grants from The Rockefeller Foundation, The Wellcome Foundation Limited, and the Andrew W. Mellon Foundation for support of postdoctoral scholars.

We are grateful for the assistance of E. S. Anderson, Nguyen Dinh Tiep, Tran van Bang, Nguyen Huu Tu, Vu thi Dan, Do thi Minh Tam, and L. S. Bernstein, and for the technical assistance of Amalia Franco and Tran Kim Anh.

LITERATURE CITED

1. **Anonymous.** 1974. Chloramphenicol-resistant strains of *Salmonella typhi*. Week Epidemiol. Rec. 9:75.
2. **Anonymous.** 1974. Plasmids. Lancet 1:249.
3. **Anonymous.** 1975. Typhoid fever in Mexico. Lancet 1:1230.
4. **Akinkugbe, O. O., E. A. Lewis, D. Montefiore, and O. A. Okubadejo.** 1968. Trimethoprim and sulfamethoxazole in typhoid. Br. Med. J. 3:721–722.
5. **Anderson, E. S.** 1973. Chloramphenicol-resistant *Salmonella typhi*. Lancet ii:1494–1495.
6. **Anderson, E. S.** 1975. The problem and implications of chloramphenicol resistance in the typhoid bacillus. J. Hyg. 74:289–299.
7. **Anderson, K. E., S. W. Joseph, R. Nasution, Sunoto, T. Butler, P. F. D. Van Peenan, G. S. Irving, J. S. Sarosa, and R. H. Watten.** 1976. Febrile illnesses resulting in hospital admission: a bacteriological and serological study in Jakarta, Indonesia. Am. J. Trop. Med. Hyg. 25:116–121.
8. **Anderson, E. S., and H. R. Smith.** 1972. Chloramphenicol resistance in the typhoid bacillus. Br. Med. J. 3:329–331.
9. **Bailey, N. T. J.** 1969. Statistical methods in biology, p. 56–66. English University Press Ltd., London.
10. **Bauer, A. W., W. M. M. Kirby, J. C. Sherris, and M. Turk.** 1966. Antibiotic susceptibility testing by a standardized single disc method. Am. J. Clin. Pathol. 45:493–496.
11. **Brown, J. D., D. H. Mo, and E. R. Rhoades.** 1975. Chloramphenicol-resistant *Salmonella typhi* in Saigon. J. Am. Med. Assoc. 231:162–166.
12. **Bushby, S. R. M.** 1973. Trimethoprim-sulfamethoxazole: *in vitro* microbiological aspects. J. Infect. Dis. 128:S442–S462.
13. **Bushby, S. R. M.** 1975. Sensitivity testing with trimethoprim-sulfamethoxazole. Med. J. Aust. 1(Suppl.):10–18.
14. **Butler, T., N. N. Linh, K. Arnold, and M. Pollack.** 1973. Chloramphenicol-resistant typhoid fever in Vietnam associated with R factor. Lancet ii:983–985.
15. **Calderon, E.** 1974. Amoxicillin in the treatment of typhoid fever due to chloramphenicol-resistant *Salmonella typhi*. J. Infect. Dis. 129:S219–S221.
16. **Cardoso, N.** 1972. Double-blind trial with chloramphenicol and the combination trimethoprim-sulfamethoxazole in typhoid. S. Afr. Med. J. 46:1286–1287.
17. **Edwards, P. R., and W. H. Ewing.** 1962. Identification of *Enterobacteriaceae*, 2nd ed. Burgess Publishing Co., Minneapolis.
18. **Geddes, A. M., R. Fothergill, J. A. D. Goodall, and P. R. Dorken.** 1971. Evaluation of trimethoprim-sulfamethoxazole compound in treatment of Salmonella infections. Br. Med. J. 3:451–454.
19. **Gilman, R. H., M. Terminel, M. M. Levine, P. Hernandez-Mendosa, E. Calderone, V. Vasquez, E. Martinez, M. J. Snyder, and R. B. Hornick.** 1975. Comparison of trimethoprim-sulfamethoxazole and amoxicillin in therapy of chloramphenicol-resistant and chloramphenicol-sensitive typhoid fever. J. Infect. Dis 132:630–636.
20. **Grindley, N. D. F., G. O. Humphreys, and E. S. Anderson.** 1973. Molecular studies of R factor compatibility groups. J. Bacteriol. 115:387–398.
21. **Hassan, A., S. Hathout, Y. Safwat, M. Erian, M. F. A. Wahab, K. Sorensen, J. Sippel, and Z. Farid.** 1975. A comparative evaluation of the treatment of typhoid fevers with co-trimoxazole and chloramphenicol in Egypt. J. Trop. Med. Hyg. 78:50–53.
22. **Kamat, S. A.** 1970. Evaluation of therapeutic efficacy of trimethoprim-sulfamethoxazole and chloramphenicol in enteric fevers. Br. Med. J. 3:320–322.
23. **Kaye, D., H. Rocha, L. Eyckmous, A. Prata, and E. W. Hook.** 1967. Comparison of parenteral ampicillin and parenteral chloramphenicol in the treatment of typhoid fever. Ann. N. Y. Acad. Sci. 145:423–428.
24. **Lampe, R. M., P. Mansuwan, and C. Duangmani.** 1974. Chloramphenicol-resistant typhoid. Lancet i:623–624.
25. **Lawrence, R. M., E. Goldstein, and P. D. Hoeprich.** 1973. Typhoid fever caused by chloramphenicol-resistant organisms. J. Am. Med. Assoc. 224:861–863.
26. **Lennette, E. H., E. H. Spaulding, and J. P. Truant (ed.).** 1974. Manual of clinical microbiology, 2nd ed. American Society for Microbiology, Washington, D.C.
27. **Linh, N. N.** 1974. Typhoid fever treated with chloramphenicol and co-trimoxazole. Lancet i:1222.
28. **Osler, W.** 1967. Typhoid fever, p. 17–105. *In*. A. M. Harvey and V. A. McKusick (ed.), Osler's textbook revisited. Appleton-Century-Crofts, New York.
29. **Overturf, G., K. I. Marton, and A. W. Mathies.** 1973. Antibiotic resistance in typhoid fever. N. Engl. J. Med. 289:463–465.
30. **Pillay, N., E. B. Adams, and D. North-Coombes.** 1975. Comparative trial of amoxycillin and chloramphenicol in treatment of typhoid fever in adults. Lancet ii:333–334.
31. **Robertson, R. P., M. F. A. Wahab, and F. O. Raasch.** 1968. Evaluation of chloramphenicol and ampicillin in Salmonella enteric fever. N. Engl. J. Med. 278:171–176.
32. **Sanford, J. P., N. N. Linh, E. Kutscher, K. Arnold, and K. Gould.** 1976. Oxolinic acid in the treatment of typhoid fever due to chloramphenicol-resistant strains of *Salmonella typhi*. Antimicrob. Agents Chemother. 9:387–392.
33. **Sardesai, H. V., R. S. Karandikar, and R. G. Harshe.** 1973. Comparative trial of co-trimoxazole and chloramphenicol in typhoid fever. Br. Med. J. 1:82–83.
34. **Scragg, J. N., and C. J. Rubidge.** 1971. Trimethoprim and sulfamethoxazole in typhoid fever in children. Br. Med. J. 3:738–741.

34a. **Scragg, J. N., and C. J. Rubidge.** 1975. Amoxyallin in the treatment of typhoid fever in children. Am. J. Trop. Med. Hyg. 24:860–865.

35. **Snyder, M. J., J. Perroni, O. Gonzalez, C. Palomino, C. Gonzalez, S. Music, H. L. DuPont, R. B. Hornick, and T. E. Woodward.** 1973. Trimethoprim-sulfamethoxazole in the treatment of typhoid and paratyphoid fevers. J. Infect. Dis. 128:S734–S737.
36. **Snyder, M. J., O. Gonzalez, C. Palomino, S. J. Music, R. B. Hornick, J. Perroni, W. E. Woodward, C. Gonzalez, H. L. DuPont, and T. E. Woodward.** 1976.

Comparative efficacy of chloramphenicol, ampicillin, and co-trimoxazole in the treatment of typhoid fever. Lancet ii:1155–1157.

37. **Stuart, B. M., and R. L. Pullen.** 1946. Typhoid. Clinical analysis of three hundred and sixty cases. Arch. Intern. Med. 78:629–661.
38. **Thorne, G. M., and W. E. Farrar.** 1974. Superinfection compatibility of R factors in *Shigella dysenteriae* type 1 from Central America and *Salmonella typhi* from Mexico. J. Infect. Dis. 130:284–287.
39. **Uwaydah, M., R. Matossian, and M. Balabanian.** 1975. Co-trimoxazole compared to chloramphenicol in the treatment of enteric fever. Scand. J. Infect. Dis. 7:123–126.
40. **Uwaydah, M.** 1976. Cefazolin in the treatment of acute enteric fever. Antimicrob. Agents Chemother. 10:52–56.
41. **Vazquez, V., E. Calderon, and R. Rodriquez.** 1972. Chloramphenicol-resistant strains of *Salmonella typhi*. N. Engl. J. Med. 286:1220.
42. **Weissman, J. B., P. A. Rice, D. J. Krogstad, W. B. Baine, and E. J. Gangarosa.** 1973. Risk of severe intestinal infections to the traveler in Mexico. J. Infect. Dis. 128:574–578.
43. **Woodward, T. E., and J. E. Smadel.** 1964. Management of typhoid fever and its complications. Ann. Intern. Med. 60:144–157.

ANTIMICROBIAL AGENTS AND CHEMOTHERAPY, Apr. 1977, p. 651-655 Vol. 11, No. 4
 Printed in U.S.A.

Assay of Gentamicin in Serum by High-Pressure Liquid Chromatography

JOHN P. ANHALT

Department of Laboratory Medicine, Mayo Clinic and Mayo Foundation, Rochester, Minnesota 55901

Received for publication 26 November 1976

A procedure is described that uses high-pressure liquid chromatography for assay of gentamicin in serum. The technique involves extraction of gentamicin from serum by using a CM-Sephadex column and analysis by reverse-phase, ion-pair chromatography. Continuous-flow, post-column derivatization with *o*-phthaladehyde is used to form fluorescent products for detection. The possible scope of this method for analysis of other aminoglycoside antibiotics is illustrated by application to sisomicin and netilmicin.

High-pressure liquid chromatography is well suited for the analysis of polar, water-soluble compounds. These characteristics are common to many antibiotics, and procedures for analysis of some of these in serum have been developed (2, 3, 6). To attain the necessary sensitivity, detection was based upon ultraviolet absorption in each of these procedures. Aminoglycoside antibiotics, however, present a special problem in that they are not easily detected by this method. One approach to this problem would be to derivatize the antibiotic to give a more easily detectable compound. Under alkaline conditions, *o*-phthalaldehyde reacts rapidly with primary amines to give fluorescent products (1, 7). Chromatographic analysis of kanamycin using continuous-flow, post-column derivatization with this reagent has been reported (5). This procedure, however, was not applied to determinations in serum.

I wish to report the application of high-pressure liquid chromatography to analysis of gentamicin in serum.

MATERIALS AND METHODS

The purified gentamicin components C_1, C_{1a}, and C_2 were kindly provided by J. Allan Waitz (Schering Corp., Bloomfield, N.J.). Gentamicin sulfate (USP reference standard), sisomicin sulfate, and netilmicin (Sch 20569) were also obtained from Schering Corp. *o*-Phthalaldehyde (Fluoropa, Durrum) was obtained from Pierce Chemical Co., Rockford, Il. The 2-mercaptoethanol was from Sigma Chemical Co., St. Louis, Mo. Methanol was obtained from Burdick and Jackson Laboratories, Muskegon, Mich. Sodium pentanesulfonate was obtained from Eastman Kodak Co., Rochester, N.Y. CM-Sephadex (C-25) was from Pharmacia Fine Chemicals, Inc., Piscataway, N.J. Human serum was obtained from a healthy volunteer. Water was deionized and glass distilled. All other chemicals were of reagent grade.

***o*-Phthalaldehyde reagent (OPA).** Potassium borate buffer was prepared by the titration of boric acid (24.7 g, 0.4 mol) dissolved in 900 ml of water with concentrated potassium hydroxide solution to pH 10.40, followed by dilution to 1.0 liter. OPA was prepared by dissolving *o*-phthalaldehyde (60 mg) in 1 ml of methanol, followed by addition of 2-mercaptoethanol (0.2 ml). The solution was gently mixed until complete decolorization occurred. Potassium borate buffer (100 ml) was then added with vigorous stirring. The solution was placed in the supply vessel for OPA, flushed several times with nitrogen, and used within 2 days.

Antibiotic solutions. All antibiotic concentrations were calculated on the basis of activity. Stock solutions containing 1,000 μg of antibiotic per ml were prepared in 0.1 M phosphate buffer, pH 8.0, and stored at −20°C. Appropriate dilutions of the stock solutions were made with water. A serum solution containing 10 μg of gentamicin per ml was prepared by addition of an appropriate amount of aqueous standard containing 100 μg/ml of serum. Additional dilutions of this solution in serum were made to obtain other concentrations.

Apparatus. The chromatographic equipment was constructed from commercially available components. A Tracor model 990 pump (Tracor Instruments, Austin, Tex.) was used to deliver mobile phase. A Schoeffel model 970 fluorometer (Schoeffel Instrument Corp., Westwood, N.J.) was used to detect fluorescent products formed by continuous-flow, post-column derivatization with OPA. Fluorescence excitation was at 340 nm, and a KV418 filter was used for emission. Photomultiplier voltage was varied between 1,000 and 1,100 V, depending on the sensitivity required. OPA was supplied to a mixing tee from a pressurized glass vessel. A Cheminert fitting (CJ3031, Laboratory Data Control, Riviera Beach, Fla.) was used for the mixing tee, and a delay coil consisting of a Teflon tube (2.0 m by 0.6 mm ID) was used between the mixing tee and detector. Analysis was performed by using a μ-Bondapak C_{18} column (30 cm by 3.9 mm ID) (Water Associates, Milford, Mass.) with a precolumn (4.3 cm by 4.2 mm ID) packed with Micropart C_{18} phase-bonded silica gel (5 μm; Applied Science Laboratories, State College, Pa.). Detector signal was processed and recorded by using a CDS 101 computing integrator (Varian, Palo Alto, Calif.) and a model 7123A recorder (Hewlett-Packard Co., Avondale, Pa.). Samples were injected by using a Valco CV-6-VHPa-C20 injection valve with a 15-μl injection loop modified for variable volume injection (Glenco Scientific, Houston, Tex).

Chromatographic conditions. Mobile-phase compositions are expressed as the ratio of components, by volume, added to give the final solution. No correction was made for volume changes as a result of mixing. Predominantly aqueous mobile phases were degassed before use by vacuum filtration through a Millipore type HA (0.45 μm) membrane filter (Millipore Corp., Bedford, Mass); solutions that were predominantly methanol were filtered through a solvent-resistant type FH (0.5 μm) filter. The mobile phase used for analyses contained 0.2 M Na_2SO_4, 0.02 M sodium pentanesulfonate, and 0.1% (vol/vol) acetic acid in a water-methanol (97:3) mixture. Column flow rate was 2 ml/min at 184 atm. OPA flow rate was about 0.5 ml/min.

Serum preparation. Gentamicin was separated from interfering compounds in serum by ion-exchange gel chromatography. A short (1.5-cm) column with a bed volume of 1 ml was prepared from CM-Sephadex (C-25), using 0.2 M Na_2SO_4 as the initial buffer. Serum (400 μl) was applied to this column and then eluted in succession with 1 ml and 4 ml of initial buffer. The eluting buffer was changed to 0.01 M NaOH in 0.2 M Na_2SO_4, and 600 μl of this buffer was added. After the column had drained completely, a second volume of alkaline buffer (400 μl) was added and the eluate was collected. This fraction was used for chromatographic analysis. Volume injected was 15 μl.

RESULTS

Analysis of aqueous standards. The chromatogram of an aqueous sample containing 2.5 μg of each of the purified gentamicin components per ml is shown in Fig. 1. Individual components were used to determine the order and position of elution. The small peaks occurring before and after gentamicin C_{1a} presumably represent minor components of the gentamicin complex (Fred Sancilio, Schering Corp., personal communication). Three injections of this mixture were made to demonstrate reproducibility (Table 1). Figures 2 and 3 show chromatograms of sisomicin (10 μg/ml) and netilmicin (10 μg/ml), respectively. The apparent impurities evident in the chromatogram of netilmicin were present in repeat analyses of this material and are as yet unidentified.

Analysis of gentamicin in serum. A chromatogram of the gentamicin-containing fraction from a serum sample containing 1.0 μg of gentamicin per ml is shown in Fig. 4. For comparison, the chromatogram obtained from gentamicin-free serum at the same sensitivity is shown in Fig. 5. There are no peaks in this chromatogram that would interfere with the gentamicin components, sisomicin, or netilmicin. The detector sensitivity used for these determinations was approximately four times that used to obtain the chromatogram in Fig. 1, and long-term fluctuations in base line were probably due to variations in the OPA flow rate.

The recovery of gentamicin added to serum was determined by comparing the component

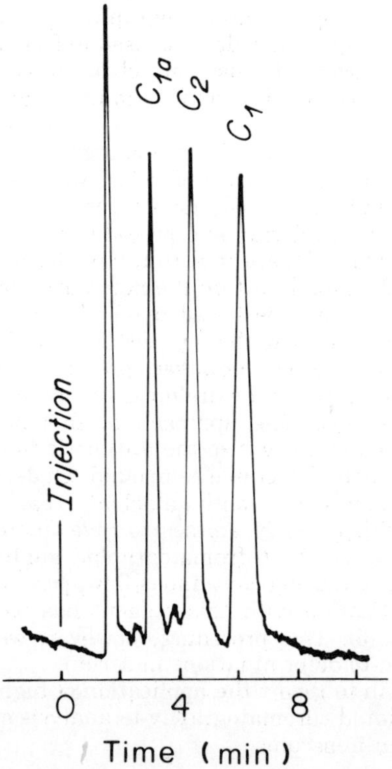

FIG. 1. *Chromatogram of a mixture of gentamicin components C_{1a}, C_2, and C_1 (2.5 μg/ml in each component). Volume injected: 15 μl. Chart speed: 0.25 inch/min.*

TABLE 1. *Comparison of peak heights for three analyses of a standard mixture of gentamicin components*

Injection	Peak height[a]		
	C_{1a}	C_2	C_1
1	1.00	1.00	1.00
2	0.95	0.96	0.95
3	0.94	0.97	0.93

[a] The peak height for each component is given relative to the first injection.

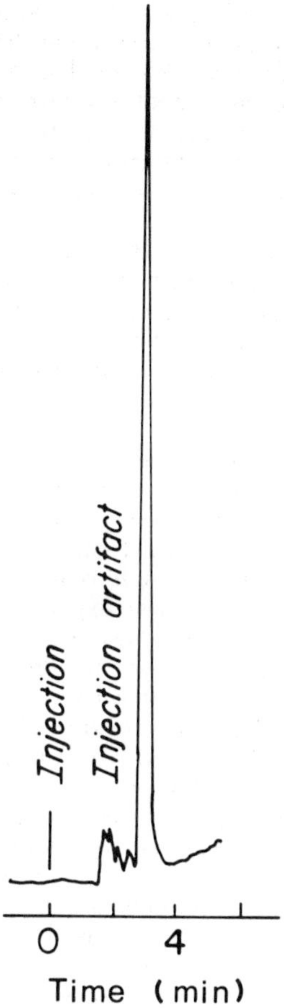

FIG. 2. *Chromatogram of sisomicin (10 μg/ml). Volume injected: 10 μl. Chart speed: 0.25 inch/min.*

peak heights from a serum sample containing 10 μg of gentamicin per ml with the results obtained from an aqueous standard of the same concentration. These results (Table 2) indicate that recovery is greater than 95% and that no significant change in relative peak height occurs as a result of the extraction procedure.

Serum samples containing 1.0, 2.0, 3.0, 5.0, and 10.0 μg of gentamicin per ml were prepared and analyzed in order to determine the standard curve shown in Fig. 6. For each concentration, duplicate injections were made, and the sums of the component peak heights were averaged. A linear least-squares regression analysis gave a coefficient of correlation (r) of 0.997.

DISCUSSION

Thin-layer chromatography (10) and ion-exchange chromatography (8) have been used to separate the gentamicin components; however, reverse-phase chromatography using a C_{18}

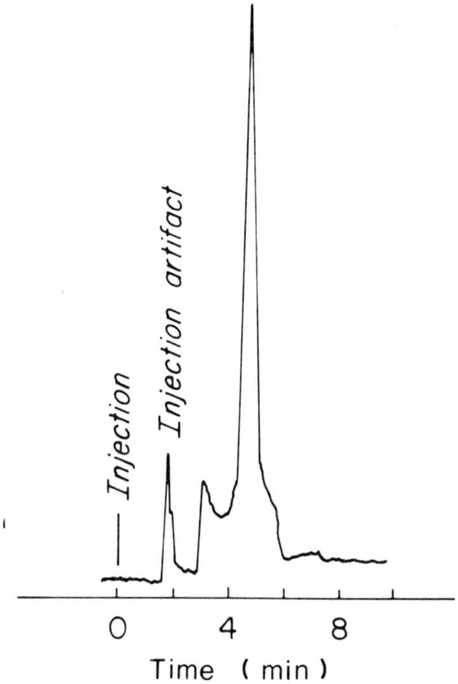

FIG. 3. *Chromatogram of netilmicin (10 μg/ml). Volume injected: 10 μl. Chart speed: 0.25 inch/min.*

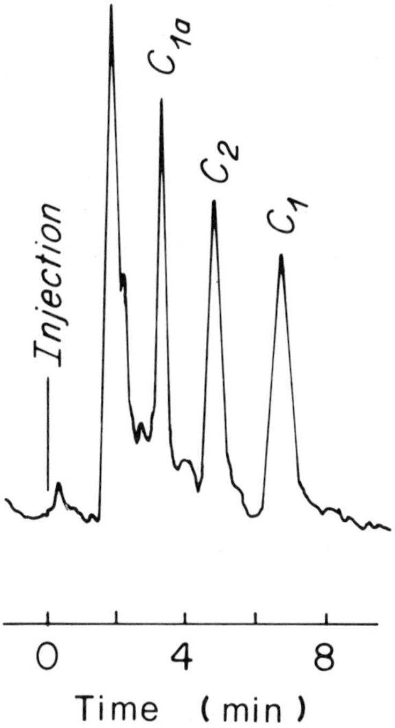

FIG. 4. *Chromatogram obtained from serum containing 1.0 μg of gentamicin per ml. Volume injected: 15 μl. Chart speed: 0.25 inch/min.*

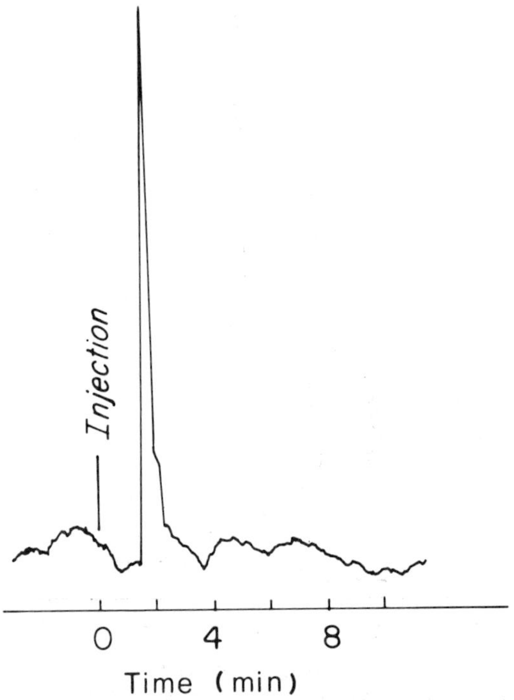

FIG. 5. *Chromatogram obtained from gentamicin-free serum. Volume injected: 15 μl. Chart speed: 0.25 inch/min.*

TABLE 2. *Recovery of gentamicin from serum*

Component	Peak height ratio (serum/water)[a]
C_{1a}	1.04
C_2	0.96
C_1	0.95
Sum	0.99

[a] Average of two determinations.

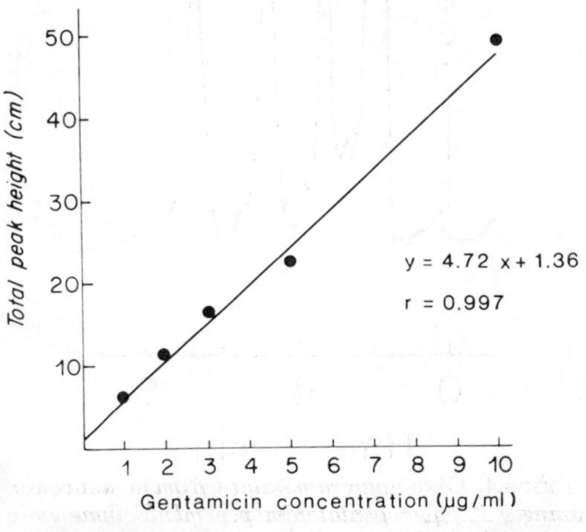

FIG. 6. *Standard curve for gentamicin in serum. Each point represents the average of two determinations.*

phase-bonded microparticulate silica gel column was chosen for this study. This type of column usually provides rapid separations that are related to the nonpolar differences between similar polar molecules. In addition, retention of charged compounds can be affected by ion-pair formation with a suitable reagent in the mobile phase (9). The separations demonstrated in this study, therefore, are probably due to ion-pair formation between protonated aminoglycoside molecules and pentanesulfonate anions, with differences in the interaction of nonpolar groups with the reverse-phase column accounting for the observed order of elution.

The mobile-phase composition, particularly with regard to incorporation of 0.2 M Na_2SO_4, was critical. In the early phases of this study, chromatography was attempted with various sodium sulfonate ion-pair reagents, but without Na_2SO_4 added. These experiments resulted in skewed peaks, poor resolution of the gentamicin components, and mobile phases with high methanol concentrations. Increased concentration of ion-pair reagent in reverse-phase chromatography should result in increased retention time (9); however, a paradoxical decrease in retention time occurred. Since a polyvalent cation, such as gentamicin, would exist largely as undissociated ion pairs in a low-ionic-strength mobile phase (4), this effect was probably related to increased dissociation of gentamicin ion pairs as a result of increased ionic strength. With 0.2 M Na_2SO_4 in the mobile phase, the expected increase in retention time with increased ion-pair reagent concentration was observed.

The extraction experiments with serum (Table 2) indicate that almost quantitative recovery of gentamicin is possible by using a CM-Sephadex column. Since no dilution of specimen occurs in this procedure, a 2.5-fold concentration can be accomplished if 1.0 ml, instead of 400 μl, of serum is extracted (unpublished data).

A standard curve (Fig. 6) shows linear response over at least a 10-fold range in concentration. The procedure used for this study, however, did not incorporate an internal standard. Therefore, results might have been affected by such variables as evaporation, nonspecific adsorption of drug to glass surfaces, and variation in the volume of eluate collected.

LITERATURE CITED

1. **Benson, J. R., and P. E. Hare.** 1975. *o*-Phthalaldehyde: fluorogenic detection of primary amines in the picomole range. Comparison with fluorescamine and ninhydrin. Proc. Natl. Acad. Sci. U.S.A. 72:619–622.
2. **Blair, A. D., A. W. Forrey, B. T. Meijsen, and R. E. Cutler.** 1975. Assay of flucytosine and furosemide by

high-pressure liquid chromatography. J. Pharm. Sci. 64:1334–1339.
3. **Cooper, M. J., M. W. Anders, and B. L. Mirkin.** 1973. Ion-pair extraction and high-speed liquid chromatography of cephalothin and deacetylcephalothin in human serum and urine. Drug Metab. Dispos. 1:659–662.
4. **Hine, J.** 1962. Physical organic chemistry, p. 73–75. McGraw-Hill, New York.
5. **Mays, D. L., R. J. Van Apeldoorn, and R. G. Lauback.** 1976. High-performance liquid chromatographic determination of kanamycin. J. Chromatogr. 120:93–102.
6. **Nilsson-Ehle, I., T. T. Yoshikawa, M. C. Schotz, and L. B. Guze.** 1976. Quantitation of antibiotics using high-pressure liquid chromatography: tetracyline. Antimicrob. Agents Chemother. 9:754–760.
7. **Roth, M.** 1971. Fluorescence reaction for amino acids. Anal. Chem. 43:880–882.
8. **Thomas, A. H., and S. D. Tappin.** 1974. Separation of gentamicin complex by ion-exchange chromatography. J. Chromatogr. 97:280–283.
9. **Wahlund, K.-G.** 1975. Reversed-phase ion-pair partition chromatography of carboxylates and sulfonates. J. Chromatogr. 115:411–422.
10. **Wilson, W. L., G. Richard, and D. W. Hughes.** 1973. Chemical determination of component ratio and potency of gentamicin complex. J. Pharm. Sci. 62:282–284.

ANTIMICROBIAL AGENTS AND CHEMOTHERAPY, Apr. 1977, p. 656-660
Vol. 11, No. 4

Susceptibility of Clinical Isolates of Cytomegalovirus to Human Interferon

BOSKO POSTIC* AND JOHN N. DOWLING

Department of Medicine, University of Pittsburgh School of Medicine, and the Medical Service, the Oakland Division of the Veterans Administration Hospital, Pittsburgh, Pennsylvania 15240*

Received for publication 22 November 1976

Human cell culture-derived interferon was shown to inhibit human cytomegalovirus in vitro. A prototype strain, Davis, and six clinical isolates of cytomegalovirus were tested. All six isolates showed uniform susceptibility to interferon, exceeding that of the Davis strain by two- to fourfold. The latter virus was found to be 32 to 4 times less susceptible than the sensitive indicator, vesicular stomatitis virus. However, the laboratory finding of susceptibility to an antiviral material may not relate to its clinical effectiveness.

Human cytomegalovirus (CMV) causes a broad spectrum of clinical illness (21). The devastating effects of congenital disease have long been recognized. More recently, subtle sequelae, including decreased mentation and auditory impairment, have been described, even among children with subclinical presentation at birth (18). Although acquired CMV infection is generally benign, significant morbidity and mortality occurs, especially in organ transplant recipients and immunosuppressed patients (16, 20; S. Suwansirikul, N. Rao, J. N. Dowling, and M. Ho, Arch. Intern. Med., in press).

Therapeutic trials have been attempted with a number of agents. CMV is inhibited in cell culture by the nucleoside analogues, 5-iodo-2'-deoxyuridine, adenine arabinoside, and cytosine arabinoside (7). In practice, these compounds may transiently suppress urinary excretion of CMV, but generally fail to eradicate the virus or alter the natural course of the disease (4, 5, 13, 15, 19). Administration of massive interferon doses may also affect CMV excretion in the urine. Viruria was completely inhibited in three of nine patients with congenital or acquired infection treated by Emodi et al. (6), and in five patients, viruria was transiently suppressed. Viremia was not affected. Arvin et al. (3) obtained transient suppression of viruria in only one of six courses of therapy, but the doses of interferon employed were lower. No clinical response was appreciated in these trials, but this was difficult to evaluate.

These results are not surprising in view of the relative nonsusceptibility of CMV to interferon in cell culture. Early work by Glasgow et al. (8) demonstrated that CMV is more resistant to the antiviral action of interferon than other viruses, including Sindbis, vaccinia, and vesicular stomatitis virus (VSV), to which it was compared. However, the amount of interferon employed was relatively small. The antiviral effect of interferon against CMV needs to be reassessed in view of the massive doses now available for human administration. In this study, the in vitro inhibition of CMV by human interferon was characterized quantitatively. The antiviral effect on the Davis strain of CMV was compared with that observed with VSV. In addition, the susceptibility of six clinical isolates of CMV was determined.

MATERIALS AND METHODS

Viruses. The Indiana strain of VSV was used as indicator for the assay of interferon (1). CMV of the Davis strain was originally obtained from Thomas H. Weller (Harvard School of Public Health, Boston, Mass.) and had undergone numerous passages in human embryo fibroblast cells in this laboratory. Clinical isolates of CMV were obtained from the buffy coat or urine of patients, as described in preceding studies (2, 10).

Cell culture. MA-184 (Microbiological Associates, Bethesda, Md.) human foreskin cell monolayers were produced in tissue culture tubes. For the growth and maintenance of cultures, as well as viruses and interferon dilutions, medium 199 was supplemented with 2% newborn calf serum, 0.2% $NaHCO_3$, penicillin, streptomycin, and nystatin at 100 U, 100 μg, and 50 U per ml, respectively.

Human interferon. Human interferon was prepared by the hyperinduction procedure (9) in FS-4 cells kindly supplied by Jan Vilcek. Two batches of interferon were prepared. Their titers were 40,000 and 25,000 IU, respectively, in MA-184 cell cultures by the microassay of Armstrong (1), adapted for human interferon (11). The interferon units determined by this assay are contained in 0.1 ml. The microwells were each seeded with 20,000 MA-184 cells and used in assays 48 to 72 h later. The standard human interferon, G-023-901-527, distributed by the Research Resources Branch, National Institutes of Health, had a titer of 23,000 U in the microassay. A local standard human leukocytic interferon, with a geometric mean titer of 2,560 reference units, was used in each experiment to standardize the test titers obtained by the microassay (1, 11, 12, 17).

Inhibition of cytopathic effect (CPE). Human interferon was applied to MA-184 cultures in appropriate dilutions by adding 1 ml to each tube, which had been seeded with 200,000 cells 48 to 72 h previously. After the time intervals designated in Results, the medium with interferon was drained, and the cultures were infected with either VSV or CMV. The infectivity of the inoculum, contained in 0.1 ml, was determined by parallel titration in the same cell culture system and expressed as the mean tissue culture infective dose ($TCID_{50}$). The virus was absorbed for 15 h in cultures on a stationary rack at 37°C, and the tubes were fed with medium alone or medium containing interferon. During incubation at 37°C, medium was changed weekly. Tubes infected with CMV were examined for the characteristic CPE at least three times weekly for 6 weeks. Infection with VSV resulted in total destruction of control monolayers by 72 h; these cultures were examined daily. Monolayers were scored for CPE on a scale of 0 to 4+. Protection in interferon-treated cultures was judged as less than 1+ (25%) CPE in the cell sheet at the time when untreated controls first showed 3+ to 4+ (75 to 100%) CPE. Interferon titers in this system refer to 1 ml and represent reciprocals of highest dilutions that protected the cells. Cultures receiving the high interferon dose required for protection from CMV showed no cytotoxicity when examined in the microassay by the quantitative elution of the methylrosaniline dye (1).

CMV yield reduction. MA-184 cultures were inoculated with 0.1 ml, containing 100 $TCID_{50}$ of the Davis strain. After adsorption, the inoculum was aspirated, and each tube was washed with 10 ml of medium and fed either with medium alone (controls) or medium containing interferon. At intervals, four controls and four test tubes were removed from the incubator, frozen, and thawed, and their contents were pooled, as "controls" or "treated," and clarified by low-speed centrifugation. The infectivity of the supernatants was determined by titration in sets of four MA-184 culture tubes per 10-fold dilution and expressed as $TCID_{50}$ per 0.1 ml.

RESULTS

The effect of human interferon was examined first by inhibition of the CPE produced by the Davis strain in MA-184 cultures. The batch of interferon used in this experiment had a titer of 40,000 U by the microassay (1, 11). Since this method could not be applied to CMV, inhibition of CPE was attempted in duplicate sets of interferon-treated tubes. These were infected with VSV and CMV (Davis) for the purpose of comparison. To examine the relationship of timing of interferon treatment to infection, cultures were treated prior to, after, and before and after inoculation of virus, as detailed under Table 1. The infection due to VSV was completed (i.e., complete CPE was evident in untreated cultures) by 48 h, whereas the comparable CMV effect was evident by 28 days. The interferon titers determined in this experiment are shown in Table 1. As expected, VSV was more susceptible to the antiviral action of interferon than CMV. The relative potency of interferon in favor of VSV was greatest when treatment preceded infection. By comparison of groups 1 and 2, inhibition of VSV and CMV was 32 and 4 times greater, respectively, when interferon treatment preceded, rather than followed, infection. Since the interferon was removed from group 1 cultures at the time of challenge with CMV, it is clear that the antiviral effect persisted for several weeks. The combined treatment (group 3) was the most effective in protecting the cells from either virus. However, application of interferon after infection, which was the least sensitive method of treatment, was used in further experiments with CMV. This timing was considered to be more applicable to therapeutic attempts in established and chronic human infections.

The effect of the challenge dose of CMV on the antiviral effect of interferon was examined in two experiments. Cell cultures were inoculated with infectious virus in a volume of 0.1 ml. The inocula were determined by parallel titration. Infected cultures were incubated with twofold dilutions of interferon which, undiluted, contained 25,000 reference units per 0.1 ml. The protective dilutions are shown in Table 2. It is evident from the more complete experiment 2 that the increase in the challenge dose

TABLE 1. *Results of concurrent titrations of human interferon with VSV or CMV (Davis)*

Treatment[a]		Titer[b] measured with:		Relative[c] potency
Group	Interferon versus infection	VSV	CMV	
1	Before	4,096	128	32
2	After	128	32	4
3	Before and after	8,192	512	16

[a] Groups of human foreskin cell cultures (MA-184) were treated with interferon: 1, 18 h prior to; 2, continuously after; and 3, prior and after infection with 100 $TCID_{50}$ of VSV or CMV.

[b] Reciprocal of highest dilution of interferon inhibiting the viral CPE.

[c] Titer to VSV/CMV.

TABLE 2. *Effect of the CMV (Davis) challenge dose on the titer of human interferon*[a]

Log_{10} $TCID_{50}$	Interferon titer[b]	
	Expt 1	Expt 2
1.0	ND	256
2.0	128	128
3.0	128	64
4.0	<128	16
5.0	ND	8

[a] MA-184 cell cultures were infected with graded doses of virus. One hour later, interferon treatment was begun.

[b] Reciprocal of highest dilution protecting the cells from the viral cytopathic effect; ND, not done.

required a lower dilution (i.e., higher dose) of interferon to produce the antiviral effect. Also, the 100-$TCID_{50}$ inoculum yielded the same interferon titer of 1:128 in experiments 1 and 2, and 1:100 in a trial with a 2 log_{10} inoculum only, indicating fair reproducibility. This challenge was selected for subsequent experiments.

To confirm the antiviral effect of interferon by another method, the yields of CMV were measured in interferon-treated and untreated cultures. MA-184 cultures were infected with 100 $TCID_{50}$ of the Davis strain. Subsequently one set was fed with medium (control) and another was given 2,500 reference units of human interferon, as determined by the microassay (1, 11). This exogenous interferon had a titer of 1:16 by the CPE inhibition method with the Davis strain. Samples, consisting of four tubes from each set, were frozen, thawed, and pooled at various times during incubation. Infectious CMV content was determined by titration in MA-184 cell cultures. The results of this experiment are shown in Table 3. It is evident that the treated cultures had a reduced yield of infectious CMV, amounting to 2 log_{10} observed after 24 and 28 days of incubation. The observed antiviral effect was not due to the transfer of exogenous interferon into assay cultures, since its activity would have been effectively diluted with inocula beyond the dilution of 10^{-1}.

To examine the susceptibility of six clinical isolates of CMV to human interferon, stock virus suspensions were made by passing the original suspension of each isolate once in MA-184 cell cultures. When the cultures showed evidence of CPE, the cells were disrupted by a freeze-thaw cycle, and the supernatants were collected after low-speed centrifugation. The inoculum of each isolate was adjusted so that it contained 100 $TCID_{50}$. After infection of MA-184 monolayers, twofold dilutions of interferon were added to the culture tubes. The undiluted preparation contained 25,000 U/0.1 ml. The cultures were observed for 6 weeks for CPE. The results are shown in Table 4. It is evident that all CMV isolates were inhibited in a comparable way. The interferon susceptibility of these clinical isolates appears to exceed by two- to fourfold that of the Davis strain, since the latter yielded a titer of 128 in a parallel titration (experiment 1 in Table 2). Thus, CMV isolates originating from two different hospitals and six individual patients showed little variation in their susceptibility to the antiviral effect of interferon.

DISCUSSION

Human CMV enjoyed, until recently, the reputation of nonsusceptibility to the antiviral action of interferon. Glasgow and co-workers found that CPE due to CMV in human foreskin tissue was somewhat retarded by 120 U of interferon, in contrast to the complete protection achieved against VSV and Sindbis virus (8). In the same study, viruria in a chronic human carrier of CMV was not altered by the low circulating levels of interferon induced by live measles vaccine. Lang et al. demonstrated an interferon-mediated protection of human em-

TABLE 3. *Reduction of the yield of CMV (Davis) in interferon-treated human cell culture*

Interferon	Log_{10} $TCID_{50}$ of CMV on day[a]				
	4	16	20	24	28
0 (Control)	0[b]	0	1.0	3.0	2.0
2,500 U	0	0	0	1.0	0

[a] Yield per 0.1 ml of fluid from MA-184 cultures infected with 100 $TCID_{50}$ of virus on day 1. The inoculum was washed off before treatment with interferon.

[b] 0 relates to <1 $TCID_{50}$ per 0.1 ml.

TABLE 4. *Susceptibility of human CMV isolates to interferon*

Isolate		Patient		Interferon[b]
No.	Site	Group	Condition[a]	
1	Buffy coat	Adult	RT	512
2	Urine	Adult	RT	256
3	Urine	Adult	RT	512
4	Urine	Adult	RT	512
5	Urine	Child	OH	256
6	Urine	Child	OH	512

[a] RT, After renal transplant; OH, after open heart surgery.

[b] MA-184 cell cultures were incubated with interferon 1 h postinfection with 100 times the $TCID_{50}$ of the listed CMV suspensions. The reciprocal of the highest inhibitory dilution is shown.

bryonic fibroblasts against challenge with extracellular, but not intracellularly contained, CMV (14). These observations were extended by A. R. Holmes, L. Rasmussen, and T. C. Merigan (Fed. Proc., p. 624, 1976) who used potent human leukocytic interferon. An inoculum of CMV-infected cells required up to 300-fold increment in the interferon dose required for protection, compared with extracellular virus. With either inoculum, the increase in the infectious dose was associated with decreases in susceptibility to interferon. The most sensitive measurements of the antiviral action of interferon were decreases in the yield of infectious CMV and the intracellular inclusion formation. The production of CPE was somewhat less sensitive.

More recently, human leukocytic interferon was administered in massive and repeated doses of $\geq 10^5$ U daily to several patients with congenital or acquired CMV infections (3, 6). The responses varied. In some patients, viruria was completely inhibited, and in others, the effect was transient or not evident. The interferon susceptibilities of the particular clinical CMV isolates were not determined.

The present study addressed the relative susceptibility of clinical CMV isolates to interferon. The susceptibility of the Davis strain was first demonstrated by the inhibition of CPE in human foreskin cells and in the same assay system, to that observed with VSV, a sensitive indicator. Depending on the timings of the interferon treatment of cells and virus challenge, VSV was 4 to 32 times more susceptible (Table 1).

Data contained in Table 1 indicate also that the titration of interferon by CPE inhibition is less sensitive than the microassay. This comparison could be made with the (prophylactic) treatment group 1, challenged with VSV, which is also used in the microassay. The relationship between the microassay titer of 40,000 and that of 4,096 by the CPE assay in tubes suggests a tenfold lower sensitivity for the latter, assuming that the different volumes, 0.1 and 1.0 ml, as well as the obvious difference in the number of cells in the respective assays, allow a direct comparison. The CPE inhibition method for estimating interferon effect could be applied to both CMV and VSV, and it was therefore useful, despite the loss in sensitivity.

The method of CPE inhibition was found to depend on the dose of extracellular virus, which was the only type of challenge used in the current study. This finding is in keeping with those by Holmes and co-workers (above). Likewise, the inhibitory effect of interferon on the yield of infectious CMV was confirmed.

For the testing of clinical isolates, the interferon-mediated inhibition of CPE was selected because of relative ease and shorter time required for performance. Based on three separate experiments, in which the same interferon was titrated with 100 $TCID_{50}$ of CMV, the method was judged to be reproducible. Clinical CMV isolates were propagated only once after original isolation, so as to obviate the possibility of a change in interferon susceptibility. In parallel assays, all were found to be at least twice as susceptible to interferon as the Davis strain. By extrapolation from findings in Table 1, the clinical isolates were only 2 to 16 times less susceptible than VSV. It is far more difficult to predict whether these findings correlate with effectiveness in vivo. Arvin and associates found that doses producing a serum interferon level of 400 did not decrease the amount of CMV in the urine of a patient, whereas in others, lower levels did (3). In interpreting the finding relative to serum levels of interferon, one should bear in mind that the units refer to a sensitive assay with VSV. A decrease in interferon effectiveness can be expected when one considers CMV instead of the sensitive indicator (Table 1). Also, due to the intracellular character of virus infection, the serum level of a drug may not appropriately monitor its therapeutic efficacy.

In conclusion, six clinical isolates of human CMV were found to be susceptible to interferon when tested in the laboratory. This encourages further trials with interferon in patients with CMV infections, since the efficacy of treatment cannot be assured by laboratory results alone.

ACKNOWLEDGMENTS

This study was supported by the Monsour Medical Foundation, Jeannette, Pa., and the Medical Research Service of the Veterans Administration.

We thank Monto Ho for his advice and review of the manuscript, Lucille Ople Guevarra for excellent technical assistance, and Debbie Zozom and Susan Vozel for devoted secretarial support.

LITERATURE CITED

1. **Armstrong, J. A.** 1971. Semi-micro, dye-binding assay for rabbit interferon. Appl. Microbiol. 21:723–725.
2. **Armstrong, J. A., G. C. Tarr, L. A. Youngblood, J. N. Dowling, A. R. Saslow, J. P. Lucas, and M. Ho.** 1976. Cytomegalovirus infection in children undergoing open-heart surgery. Yale J. Biol. Med. 49:83–91.
3. **Arvin, A. M., A. S. Yeager, and T. C. Merigan.** 1976. Effect of leukocyte interferon on urinary excretion of cytomegalovirus by infants. J. Infect. Dis. 133 (Suppl.):A205–A210.
4. **Barton, B. E., and J. O'H. Tobin.** 1970. The effect of iodoxuridine on the excretion of cytomegalovirus in congenital infection. Ann. N.Y. Acad. Sci. 172:90–95.
5. **Ch'ien, L. T., N. J. Cannon, R. J. Whitley, A. G.**

Diethelm, W. E. Dismukes, C. W. Scott, R. A. Buchanan, and C. A. Alford, Jr. 1974. Effect of adenine arabinoside on cytomegalovirus infections. J. Infect. Dis. 130:32-39.

6. **Emodi, G., R. O'Reilly, A. Muller, L. K. Everson, U. Binswanger, and M. Just.** 1976. Effect of human exogenous leukocyte interferon in cytomegalovirus infections. J. Infect. Dis. 133(Suppl.):A199-A204.
7. **Fiala, M., A. W. Chow, K. Miyasaki, and L. B. Guze.** 1974. Susceptibility of herpesviruses to three nucleoside analogues and their combinations and enhancement of the antiviral effect at acid pH. J. Infect. Dis. 129:82-85.
8. **Glasgow, L. A., J. B. Hanshaw, T. C. Merigan, and J. K. Petralli.** 1967. Interferon and cytomegalovirus *in vivo* and *in vitro*. Proc. Exp. Soc. Biol. Med. 125:843-849.
9. **Havel, E. A., and J. Vilcek.** 1972. Production of high-titered interferon in cultures of human diploid cells. Antimicrob. Agents Chemother. 2:476-484.
10. **Ho, M., S. Suwansirikul, J. N. Dowling, L. A. Youngblood, and J. A. Armstrong.** 1975. The transplanted kidney as a source of cytomegalovirus infection. N. Engl. J. Med. 293:1109-1112.
11. **Ho, M., Y. H. Tan, and J. A. Armstrong.** 1972. Accentuation of production of human interferon by metabolic inhibitors. Proc. Soc. Exp. Biol. Med. 139:259-262.
12. **Ke, Y. H., J. A. Armstrong, M. K. Breinig, L. Ople, B. Postic, and M. Ho.** 1970. The assay and standardization of rabbit interferons. Symp. Ser. Immunobiol. Stand. 14:131-144.
13. **Kraybill, E. N., J. L. Sever, G. B. Avery, and N. Movassaghi.** 1972. Experimental use of cytosine arabinoside in congenital cytomegalovirus infection. J. Pediatr. 80:485-487.
14. **Lang, D. J., M. T. Thomas, and I. Gresser.** 1969. Protection par l'interferon de cellules embryonnaires humaines contre l'infection par le virus cytomegaligue. C. R. Acad. Sci. Paris 268:D3137-D3139.
15. **McCracken, G. H., and J. P. Luby.** 1972. Cytosine arabinoside in the treatment of congenital cytomegalic inclusion disease. J. Pediatr. 80:488-495.
16. **Myers, J. D., H. C. Spencer, J. C. Watts, M. B. Gregg, J. A. Stewart, R. H. Troupin, and E. D. Thomas.** 1975. Cytomegalovirus pneumonia after human marrow transplantation. Ann. Intern. Med. 82:181-188.
17. **Postic, B., C. J. Schleupner, J. A. Armstrong, and M. Ho.** 1969. Two variants of sindbis virus which differ in interferon induction and serum clearance. I. The phenomenon. J. Infect. Dis. 120:339-347.
18. **Reynolds, D. W., S. Stagno, K. G. Stubbs, A. D. Dahle, M. M. Livingston, S. S. Saxon, and C. A. Alford.** 1974. Inapparent congenital cytomegalovirus infection with elevated cord IgM levels. N. Engl. J. Med. 290:291-196.
19. **Rytel, M. W., and H. M. Kauffman.** 1976. Clinical efficacy of adenine arabinoside in therapy of cytomegalovirus infections in renal allograft recipients. J. Infect. Dis. 133:202-205.
20. **Spencer, E. S.** 1974. Clinical aspects of cytomegalovirus infection in kidney-graft recipients. Scand. J. Inect. Dis. 6:315-323.
21. **Weller, T. H.** 1971. The cytomegaloviruses: ubiquitous agents with protean clinical manifestations. N. Engl. J. Med. 285:203-214, 267-274.

ANTIMICROBIAL AGENTS AND CHEMOTHERAPY, Apr. 1977, p. 661-668 Vol. 11, No. 4

Printed in U.S.A.

Macrolide Resistance in *Staphylococcus aureus*: Induction of Macrolide-Resistant Protein Synthesis

NORRIS E. ALLEN

The Lilly Research Laboratories, Eli Lilly and Company, Indianapolis, Indiana 46206

Received for publication 12 October 1976

Induction of resistance to macrolide-, lincosamide-, and streptogramin B-type antibiotics in *Staphylococcus aureus* was studied by monitoring the appearance of erythromycin A (EM)-resistant [^{14}C]leucine incorporation. Examination of the induction process revealed saturation kinetics and a time course much like that reported for penicillinase in gram-positive bacteria. Induction kinetics in exponentially growing cells were sigmoidal and appeared to reach a maximum and constant rate when growth reached stationary phase. Since the induction of EM-resistant colony-forming ability was complete within 60 min, ribosome modification cannot be limited to a fraction of the population and must occur in essentially every cell. However, EM-resistant growth was expressed in cells where less than half the [^{14}C]leucine-incorporating activity was resistant to EM. This suggests that resistance requires that only a threshold level of ribosome modification be exceeded and that, once exceeded, resistance is dominant to sensitivity.

Inducible resistance to erythromycin A (EM) has been described for certain clinically isolated strains of *Staphylococcus aureus* (2,3; B. Weisblum, *in Microbiology–1974*, p. 199-206, American Society for Microbiology, Washington, D.C.). Exposure to subinhibitory concentrations of EM induces resistance to high concentrations of EM plus other macrolide-, lincosamide-, and streptogramin B-type (MLS) antibiotics (2, 3, 21), all of which bind specifically to the 50*S* ribosomal subunit and inhibit ribosome function (14, 20). EM does not induce resistance to nonmacrolide 50*S* ribosome inhibitors other than those cited or to 30*S* inhibitors (21). Inducible resistance to macrolides and lincosamides also has been reported in clinically isolated strains of *Streptococcus pyogenes* (4, 24).

Macrolide resistance (i.e., resistance to MLS antibiotics) in *S. aureus* is due to an alteration of the 50*S* ribosomal subunit (20). Specifically, N^6,N^6-dimethyl adenine has been detected in 23*S* ribosomal ribonucleic acid (RNA) of inducible strains grown under inducing conditions and in constitutively resistant mutants grown in the absence of any inducer (6, 7). Ribosomes from resistant cells show a decreased binding affinity for EM (7, 22), and ribosome reconstitution experiments have established that methylation of ribosomal RNA is a cause rather than a result of resistance (8).

Although methylation of ribosomal RNA provides an attractive explanation for the mode of macrolide resistance, little information is available to explain the specific mechanism of the induction process. Protein and RNA synthesis are required for induction, but synthesis of deoxyribonucleic acid is not (19, 22). Moreover, induced resistance is reversible and is lost when resistant cells are transferred and grown in an inducer-free medium (19, 22). These findings suggest classical induction, but the possibility that macrolide resistance is induced via a direct interaction between EM and the ribosome cannot be ruled out.

In this paper, the measurement of induced EM-resistant protein synthesis is described. The method requires measuring rates of EM-resistant [^{14}C]leucine incorporation after exposure to subinhibitory concentrations of EM. Unlike measuring EM-resistant growth, this technique reflects directly the functional change due to the induced ribosomal alteration. In an accompanying paper (1), this method is used to survey MLS antibiotics, including EM derivatives, for inducer activity.

MATERIALS AND METHODS

Strains. *S. aureus* 1206, kindly supplied by B. Weisblum, has been described previously (Weisblum, *Microbiology–1974*, p. 199-206). This strain demonstrates a partial requirement for leucine (unpublished findings, this laboratory).

S. aureus 1206-C4 is a generalized constitutively macrolide-resistant mutant according to the nomenclature of Weisblum and Demohn (21). The mutant was isolated in this laboratory from *S. aureus* 1206 as a resistant clone growing on agar supplemented with 10 μg of niddamycin per ml. Constitutive methylating activity was not tested.

Media. Synthetic growth medium contained (in grams per liter): K_2HPO_4, 7; KH_2PO_4, 2; $MgSO_4 \cdot 7H_2O$, 0.1; $(NH_4)_2SO_4$, 1; and sodium citrate, 0.5. It was supplemented after autoclaving with appropriate stock solutions to give (final concentration): glucose, 2 g/liter; calcium pantothenate, (0.2 mg/liter; pyrodoxine-hydrochloride, 0.2 mg/liter; niacinamide, 0.2 mg/liter; inositol, 0.2 mg/liter; thiamine-hydrochloride, 0.2 mg/liter; *para*-aminobenzoic acid, 0.2 mg/liter; riboflavin, 0.05 mg/liter; biotin, 0.002 mg/liter; folic acid, 0.02 mg/liter; adenine, 1.5 mg/liter; guanine, 1.5 mg/liter; xanthine, 1.5 mg/liter; hypoxanthine, 1.5 mg/liter; thymine 1.5 mg/liter; uracil, 1.5 mg/liter; cytosine, 1.5 mg/liter; and each of 20 amino acids (50 mg/liter).

Antibiotic medium no. 1 (Difco) or Trypticase agar (BBL) was used for antibiotic disk diffusion assays.

Antibacterial activity. Antibiotic sensitivity was indicated by a zone of inhibition around antibiotic-containing disks (20 μg/disk) placed on seeded agar and incubated for 18 h at 37°C. Inducible resistance to an antibiotic was indicated by a distorted zone of inhibition when placed adjacent to EM (21). Constitutive resistance was indicated by the absence of a zone of inhibition.

Induction of resistance. Both log-phase and stationary-phase cells were used to measure induction of EM resistance. The methods used in each experiment are given in the appropriate figure legends.

Incorporation of [^{14}C]leucine. The relative capacity of cells to synthesize protein in the presence or absence of EM was determined by measuring the incorporation of [^{14}C]leucine, using cells washed once and resuspended in phosphate-buffered saline (0.05 M potassium phosphate in 0.15 M sodium chloride, pH 6.9) to a density of 0.06 to 0.12 mg of whole-cell protein per ml.

Reactions contained, in a total volume of 1.0 ml: 0.05 M potassium phosphate (pH 6.9); 0.15 M sodium chloride; 0.001 M glucose; 0.05 μg of 19 amino acids not including leucine; 0.05 μCi of [^{14}C]leucine (280 mCi/mmol); and 0.06 to 0.12 mg of cell protein. After a preincubation period of 5 min at 37°C, reactions were initiated with the addition of [^{14}C]leucine. Unless otherwise indicated, reactions were run in duplicate and incubated for 1 min in a 37°C water bath. EM-resistant [^{14}C]leucine incorporation was measured by adding EM to the reaction mixture at a final concentration of 140 μM (100 μg/ml). These conditions provide a rapid assay of EM-resistant incorporation unaffected by changes due to cell growth.

Reactions were stopped by adding ice-cold 10% trichloroacetic acid supplemented with 10 mM (cold) leucine. Tubes were heated at 90°C for 15 min, and the precipitates were collected by filtration on Whatman GF/C glass-fiber filters. The filters were washed three times with 5% trichloroacetic acid containing (cold) leucine, dried, and counted by liquid scintillation spectrometry.

EM and other antibiotics were prepared as 1- to 5-mg/ml methanol-water stock solutions. The maximum level of 0.2% methanol in the reaction mixture had no measurable effect on rates of [^{14}C]leucine incorporation.

Uptake of [^{14}C]leucine. Cells and reaction mixtures were exactly as described for measuring acid-insoluble incorporation of [^{14}C]leucine except that each reaction contained 200 μg of chloramphenicol per ml to stop protein synthesis. After 1 min of incubation at 37°C, cells were rapidly collected on membrane filters (0.45 nm, type HA; Millipore Corp.) at room temperature, immediately washed three times with 5-ml portions of phosphate-buffered saline, dried, and counted.

Protein determination. Whole-cell protein was determined on cells grown in synthetic broth, washed, and resuspended in phosphate-buffered saline. Protein was extracted with trichloroacetic acid and solubilized according to the procedures of Winshell and Shaw (23). Solubilized protein was measured by the method of Lowry et al. (10).

Antibiotics. Antibiotics used in this study and their sources were: methymycin, vernamycin Bα (Squibb); oleandomycin, triacetyloleandomycin, carbomycin (Pfizer); narbomycin (Ciba-Geigy); lankamycin, desacetyllankamycin (Taisho); pikromycin (Farbenfabriken-Bayer); megalomycin, rosamycin (Schering); niddamycin (Farbwerke Hoechst AG); spiramycin (Rhone-Poulenc); chalcomycin, viridogrisein (Parke-Davis); shincomycin A (Tohoku); cirramycin A and B (Bristol); josamycin (Yamanouchi); propionylmaridomycin (Takeda); relomycin (Lederle); mydecamycin (Meiji Sheika Kaisha); leucomycin (Toyo Jozo); lincomycin, clindamycin, celesticetin (Upjohn); griseomycin (University of Louvain, Louvain, Belgium); chloramphenicol (Calbiochem); erythromycin, tylosin, desmycosin, benzylpenicillin G (Eli Lilly).

RESULTS

Antibiotic sensitivity. When the 30 MLS antibiotics listed in Table 1 were tested against *S.*

TABLE 1. *MLS antibiotics*

12-membered-ring macrolides	16-membered-ring macrolides
Methymycin	Carbomycin
	Niddamycin
14-membered-ring macrolides	Spiramycin
	Tylosin
Erythromycin A	Desmycosin
Oleandomycin	Chalcomycin
Triacetyloleandomycin	Shincomycin A
Narbomycin	Cirramycin A
Lankamycin	Cirramycin B
Desacetyllankamycin	Josamycin
Pikromycin	Propionylmaridomycin
Griseomycin	Relomycin
Megalomycin	Mydecamycin
	Rosamycin
Lincosamides	Leucomycin
Lincomycin	
Clindamycin	Streptogramin-B types
Celesticetin	Vernamycin Bα
	Viridogrisein

aureus 1206, a zone of inhibition was observed around each antibiotic disk except those containing EM, desacetyllankamycin, megalomycin, and celesticetin. With the exception of the latter four antibiotics, placing drug-containing disks adjacent to a disk containing EM (21) resulted in distorted zones of inhibition. Desacetyllankamycin, megalomycin, and celesticetin behaved like EM and caused distorted zones of inhibition when disks containing these drugs were placed adjacent to lincomycin.

These results suggest that at least three antibiotics in addition to EM are capable of inducing resistance and that induced *S. aureus* 1206 is cross-resistant to a variety of MLS antibiotics (Table 1). This pattern of resistance supports and extends a previous report (21) showing that *S. aureus* 1206 is inducibly resistant to at least 10 MLS antibiotics. *S. aureus* 1206-C4 was isolated as a niddamycin-resistant mutant and demonstrated constitutive resistance to the 30 antibiotics in Table 1, but remained sensitive to nonmacrolide antibiotics.

Inhibition of protein synthesis. Incorporation of [^{14}C]leucine by *S. aureus* 1206 grown without prior exposure to inducing levels of EM is illustrated in Fig. 1. Incorporation was sensitive to the same minimal levels of EM (0.14 to 1.4 μM) required to inhibit growth of this strain (22). Maximum but incomplete inhibition was obtained with 140 μM EM. EM may be unable to completely inhibit incorporation because it has little effect on ribosomes actively synthesizing peptides (18). Since the time course of incorporation in the presence or absence of EM was linear during the first 2 min of the reaction (Fig. 1), initial rates of incorporation in the presence of EM were used to estimate EM resistance in subsequent experiments.

[^{14}C]leucine incorporation by *S. aureus* 1206 was sensitive to other MLS antibiotics providing that cells were grown in the absence of EM (Table 2). In contrast, incorporation by the constitutively resistant mutant was essentially insensitive to these drugs.

Induction of EM resistance in dividing cells. Although *S. aureus* 1206 was sensitive to EM and other MLS antibiotics when grown under noninducing conditions, rates of [^{14}C]leucine incorporation in the presence of 140 μM EM (EM-resistant incorporation) increased after exposing mid-log-phase cells to 0.014 μM EM. A differential plot where rates of EM-resistant incorporation are expressed relative to the increase in cell mass is illustrated in Fig. 2. The maximum differential rate occurred as the culture approached higher turbidities. At a turbidity of 1.4 the cells were entering stationary phase, so that maximum induction appeared to coincide with a diminution in growth rate. Without added inducer, the rate of EM-resistant incorporation remained unchanged. Identical kinetics were observed in a separate

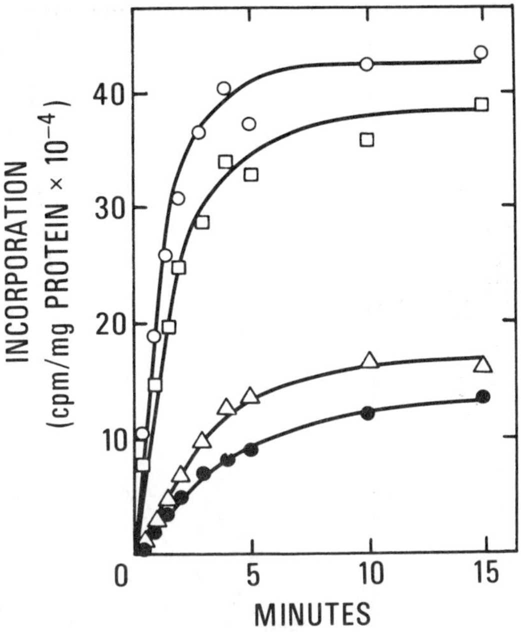

FIG. 1. *Sensitivity of protein synthesis in uninduced S. aureus 1206 to EM. Cells were grown to early stationary phase in synthetic broth (approximately 0.15 mg of protein per ml), harvested, washed once, and resuspended in phosphate-buffered saline. [^{14}C]leucine incorporation (see Materials and Methods) was measured in reactions containing: 0 (○), 0.14 (□), 1.4 (△), and 140 or 700 (●) μM EM.*

TABLE 2. *Antibiotic sensitivity of protein synthesis in inducible and constitutive S. aureus*[a]

Antibiotic[b]	Inducible strain[c]		Constitutive strain[d]	
	[^{14}C]leucine incorporation	% of control	[^{14}C]leucine incorporation	% of control
None	251	100	261	100
Erythromycin	58	23	258	99
Megalomycin	21	8	235	90
Tylosin	33	13	245	94
Carbomycin	22	9	188	72
Lincomycin	32	13	250	96

[a] Cells were grown under noninducing conditions, and [^{14}C]leucine incorporation was measured as described in the legend to Fig. 1.

[b] Each antibiotic was tested at 100 μg/ml.

[c] *S. aureus* 1206. Incorporation is expressed as counts/minute per milligram of protein × 10^{-3}.

[d] *S. aureus* 1206 C4. Incorporation is expressed as in footnote *c*.

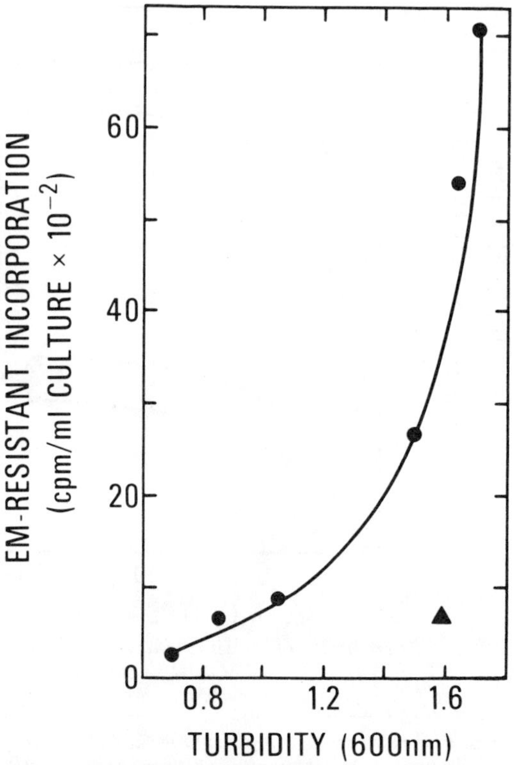

FIG. 2. *Differential plot of induction of EM-resistant incorporation. Synthetic broth was inoculated with an overnight culture of S. aureus 1206 and grown at 37°C to mid-exponential phase. EM was added to the growing culture to give a final concentration of 0.014 μM, and incubation was continued. A companion culture received no EM. Samples were taken periodically over a 2-h period for measuring turbidity and macrolide-resistant protein synthesis. [^{14}C]leucine incorporation was measured on washed cells as described in Materials and Methods, except that glucose was omitted from the mixture and reactions were incubated for 2 min. Symbols: (●) Rates of EM-resistant [^{14}C]leucine incorporation after addition of inducer; (▲) rate of EM-resistant [^{14}C]leucine incorporation after 2 h of incubation without inducer.*

experiment where inducer was added to early-log-phase cells (data not shown).

The effect of inducer concentration on EM-resistant incorporation is shown in Fig. 3. The concentration of EM required for maximum induction was between 0.03 and 0.06 μM, with higher concentrations being less effective due to inhibition of protein synthesis and induction (see Fig. 1 and references 19 and 22). Weisblum et al. (22) reported similar concentration optima for induction of colony-forming ability on EM-supplemented agar.

Induction of EM resistance in slowly growing or resting cells. Figure 4 illustrates the induction of EM resistance using stationary-phase cells. Both the rate and maximum level of EM-resistant incorporation increased relative to the uninhibited rates during the 2-h induction period.

Initial rates of incorporation (Table 3) indicated that EM-resistant incorporation increased more than eightfold, whereas control (uninhibited) incorporation increased only twofold. (EM resistance is expressed as a percentage of the uninhibited rate in order to adjust for changes in rates of protein synthesis occurring during induction.) In repeated experiments (data not shown), the level of EM-resistant incorporation by cell suspensions incubated for 120 min without inducer remained between 10 and 20% of the uninhibited rate.

In Fig. 5, rates of EM-resistant incorporation are plotted against time of induction. The data for this figure were taken from two separate experiments and include the data in Table 3. Induction kinetics under these conditions appeared linear.

Changes in amino acid transport. Induction of EM-resistant [^{14}C]leucine incorporation is assumed to reflect a ribosomal alteration. Similar changes in rates of incorporation might occur if induced resistance led to an alteration that resulted in increased transport of the radioactive amino acid. The experiment summarized in Table 4 indicated that the uptake of [^{14}C]leucine was slightly reduced in the presence of EM. However, the extent of this reduction as well as the level of leucine uptake remained essentially unchanged during the 120-min induction period and cannot account for the increases in EM-resistant [^{14}C]leucine incorporation.

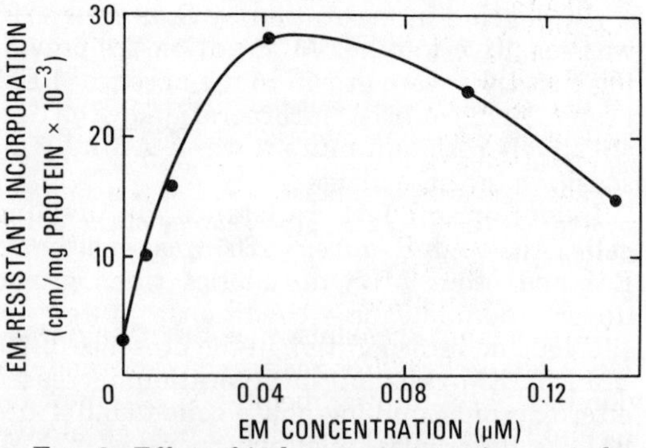

FIG. 3. *Effect of inducer concentration on induction of EM-resistant incorporation. EM was added at the concentrations shown to exponentially growing S. aureus 1206 as described in Fig. 2, and incubation was continued for 2 h. EM-resistant [^{14}C]leucine incorporation was measured on washed cells as described in Materials and Methods.*

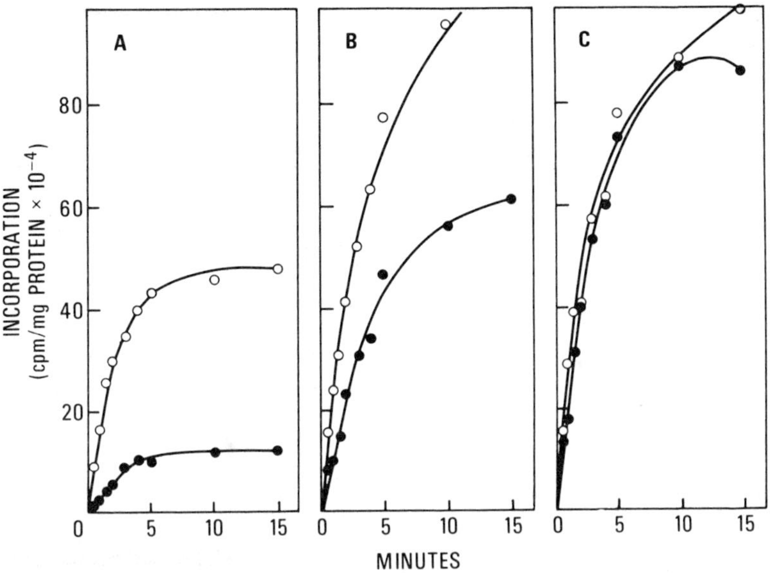

FIG. 4. *Induction of EM-resistant incorporation in slowly growing or resting cells. S. aureus 1206 was grown to early stationary phase in synthetic broth, at which time cells were washed once and resuspended in fresh broth to a cell density of 0.24 mg of protein per ml. The cell suspension was preincubated for 30 min, EM (0.04 μM) was added as inducer, and incubation was continued. Samples were taken before, 60 min after, and 120 min after adding EM. There was less than a 35% increase in cell mass during the 2-h incubation. Measurement of [¹⁴C]leucine incorporation was as described in Materials and Methods. (A) Incorporation by uninduced cells; (B) incorporation after 60 min of induction; (C) incorporation after 120 min of induction. Symbols: (○) Uninhibited [¹⁴C]leucine incorporation; (●) [¹⁴C]leucine incorporation in the presence of 140 μM EM.*

TABLE 3. *Effects of induction on rates of uninhibited and EM-resistant incorporation*[a]

Induction time (min)	[^{14}C]leucine incorporation[b]		% EM-resistant incorporation[c]
	−EM	+EM	
0	162	23.3	14.4
60	207	100	48.3
120	275	198	72.0

[a] Data were taken from the experiment illustrated in Fig. 4.

[b] Initial rates were calculated from the linear portions of the curves in Fig. 4. Incorporation is expressed as in Table 2.

[c] EM resistance is expressed as EM-resistant incorporation calculated as a percentage of the uninhibited rate.

EM-resistant translation of functional protein. Cells induced for resistance grow and divide in EM-containing media (19, 22), indicating indirectly that the induced change allows synthesis of functional protein in the presence of antibiotic. The experiment illustrated in Fig. 6 further rules out the possibility that EM-resistant incorporation of [^{14}C]leucine might represent synthesis of nonfunctional protein. It is readily apparent that penicillinase was synthesized in the presence of 140 μM EM by cells preinduced for EM resistance but not by uninduced cells. In the absence of EM, induced and uninduced cells synthesized equal amounts of enzyme.

EM-resistant colony formation. Induction of EM-resistant colony-forming ability was compared with the induction of EM-resistant [^{14}C]leucine incorporation. Induction of resistant colony-forming ability was complete within 60 min, yet resistant incorporation was less than 40% of the uninhibited rate in these cells (Table 5). Although these findings imply that ribosome modification must occur in all cells, the actual rate of modification may not be reflected by the apparent rate of induced EM-resistant colony formation.

DISCUSSION

Our current understanding of the induction of macrolide resistance in *S. aureus* has come from studies that, for the most part, were based on the ability of induced cells to grow in media containing high concentrations of EM (20). This methodology, especially the disk method (21), has been effectively used to establish that EM induces resistance to all MLS antibiotics. How-

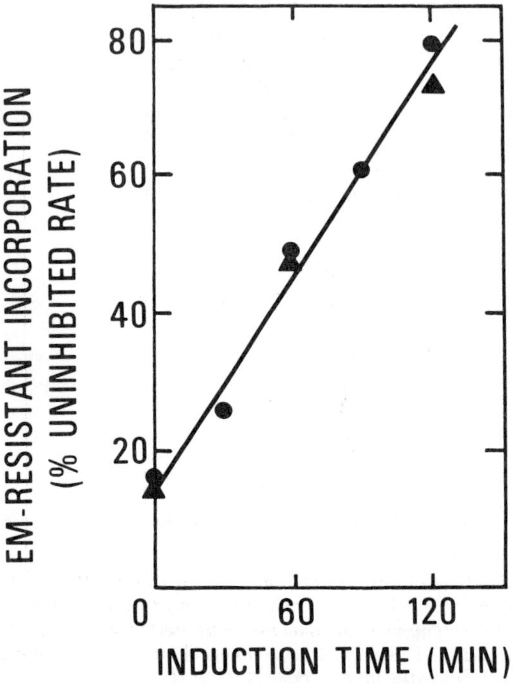

FIG. 5. *Time course of induction. Rates of EM-resistant [^{14}C]leucine incorporation calculated as percentage of the uninhibited rates are plotted against time of exposure to inducer. Results from two separate experiments are presented: (▲) data taken from Table 3; (●) data from a separate experiment conducted as described in the legend to Fig. 4.*

TABLE 4. *Effect of induction on transport of [^{14}C]leucine*[a]

Induction time (min)	[^{14}C]leucine uptake[b]		Uptake ratio[c]
	−EM	+EM	
0	692	552	0.80
30	754	578	0.77
60	605	530	0.88
90	607	506	0.83
120	710	641	0.90

[a] Induction conditions as described in Fig. 4.
[b] Uptake is expressed as counts/minute per milligram of protein × 10^{-2}.
[c] Ratio of uptake in presence of EM to uptake in the absence of EM.

ever, a close examination of the induction kinetics has been difficult since assay of resistance has depended on growth measurements.

In contrast to measuring the induction of an enzyme such as β-galactosidase, where a gene product can be followed directly, antibiotic-resistant growth is at least several steps removed from the induced change. Furthermore, since the resistant phenotype is lost during growth in the absence of inducer (19, 22), the assays for

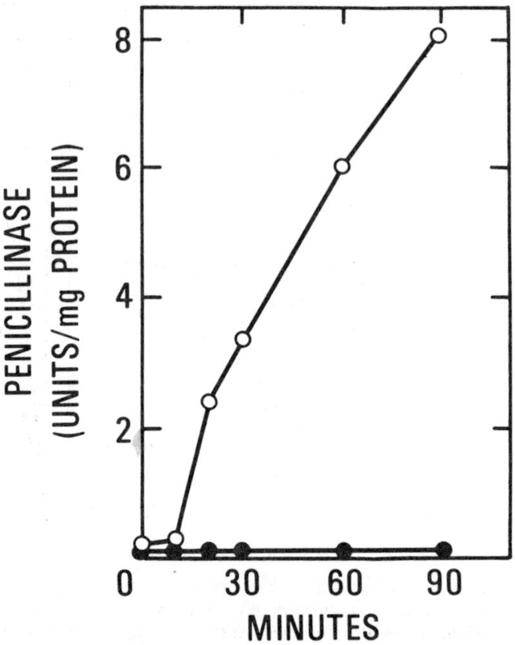

FIG. 6. *EM sensitivity of induced penicillinase synthesis in cells induced and uninduced for EM resistance. S. aureus 1206 was induced for 2 h as described in Fig. 4. A parallel culture was handled identically but received no inducer. After a 2-h incubation, induced and uninduced cells were harvested and resuspended to a cell density of 0.06 mg of protein per ml in fresh synthetic broth supplemented with 0.1% yeast extract plus 140 μM EM. Benzylpenicillin G was added to each flask at 1 μg/ml to induce penicillinase, and the cultures were incubated for another 90 min. Three-milliliter samples were removed as indicated, chloramphenicol (200 μg/ml) was added, and penicillinase activity was measured iodometrically according to Perret (11). One unit of enzyme activity is defined as that amount of enzyme needed to hydrolyze 1.0 μmol of benzylpenicillin G in 1 h at 30°C. Values were corrected for background constitutive enzyme levels. Symbols: (○) Penicillinase produced in the presence of 140 μM EM by cells induced for EM resistance or (●) by cells uninduced for EM resistance.*

TABLE 5. *Induction of EM-resistant incorporation and EM-resistant colony-forming units (CFU)*

Induction time (min)[a]	% EM-resistant incorporation[b]	% EM-resistant CFU/ml[c]
0	18	1.1
30	25	91
60	38	109

[a] EM resistance was induced in *S. aureus* 1206 as described in Fig. 4.
[b] Calculated as described in Table 3.
[c] Determined on the same cells by diluting and plating onto tryptone-glucose agar (22) with and without 140 μM EM and expressed as a percentage of the total population.

resistance have required the continued presence of inducer. The reduced ability of ribosomes from resistant cells to bind EM and other macrolide antibiotics has been used to demonstrate induced resistance (13, 16, 22), as has the increased resistance of these ribosomes to inhibition by macrolide antibiotics in cell-free protein synthesis (15). Nevertheless, these methods do not easily allow for monitoring induction kinetics. In the present communication, rates of [^{14}C]leucine incorporation by whole cells in the presence of 140 μM EM have been used to measure induction. Since this technique will reflect changes at the ribosome level, it should be a closer approximation of the induced event than is a measure of EM-resistant growth.

The studies of Weisblum and co-workers (6–8) indicate that both induced and constitutive resistance is due to the presence of N^6,N^6-dimethyl adenine in 23*S* ribosomal RNA. Although alternative models are possible, inducible resistance is most simply explained as induced synthesis of an enzyme capable of N^6,N^6-dimethylation of adenine (Weisblum, *Microbiology–1974*, p. 199–206). Rates of EM-resistant [^{14}C]leucine incorporation are assumed to reflect the functional change due to induced methylation of RNA, and the extent of this ribosomal modification may or may not be directly proportional to the amount of methylating enzyme produced.

Experiments reported here tend to rule out alternative explanations for the observed increases in EM-resistant [^{14}C]leucine incorporation. For example, induction of EM-resistant incorporation was accompanied by EM-resistant synthesis of penicillinase, indicating that incorporation measured in the presence of EM represents synthesis of functional rather than nonsense protein. Further, changes in amino acid transport cannot readily account for the observed changes in incorporation. Nor is it likely that resistance is due to a decreased uptake of EM, since although uptake of EM by resistant cells is reduced (22), this reduction could be explained as a decreased affinity of the ribosome for the drug, resulting in reduced accumulation (13, 25). There is no evidence to support the induction of an altered transport system to exclude macrolide antibiotics, nor has an EM-inactivating enzyme been detected in *S. aureus* (25).

Several aspects of EM resistance induction, including concentration of inducer required, the inhibitory effects of high concentrations of inducer, and the time course of induction, bear a resemblance to the induction of penicillinase in gram-positive bacteria (5, 9, 12, 17). The induction of EM resistance follows saturation kinetics, and the time course is similar to that reported by Leggate and Holms (9) for penicillinase induction in *S. aureus*. Both systems are characterized by an increasing differential rate of induction during logarithmic growth that appears to be maximum and constant when cells enter stationary growth. The kinetic similarities are consistent with the proposal that EM induces synthesis of an N^6,N^6-adenyl dimethylase.

The induction kinetics are subject to numerous interpretations, all of which are speculative at this point. The low differential rate at the start of induction in exponentially growing cells could be due to a rate-limiting step or steps in the ribosome modification process. A rate-limiting step could occur in the synthesis of a methylase-specific messenger RNA, or the methylation reaction itself could be limited by some step in ribosome formation. In fact, Lai and Weisblum (Fed. Proc. 31:455, 1972) showed that a precursor of the 50*S* subunit rather than the mature ribosome served as the substrate for methylation. Thus, a rate-limiting step in the maturation of 50*S* subunits could be rate limiting for induced methylation. It is unlikely that the initial low differential rate is due to induction of a system required for inducer transport since no such lag was observed when stationary-phase cells were induced. In the latter case, induction was linear.

The simultaneous measurement of EM-resistant colony formation and EM-resistant [^{14}C]leucine incorporation (Table 5) during induction revealed several interesting properties of the induction process. Although less than 40% of the [^{14}C[leucine-incorporating activity was resistant to EM after induction for 60 min, the entire culture had acquired EM-resistant colony-forming ability. Weisblum et al. (22) likewise demonstrated complete induction of EM-resistant growth in 60 min with this strain, which indicates that ribosome modification is not limited to a fraction of the cell population and occurs in essentially every cell. Furthermore, since EM-resistant colony-forming ability is observed when ribosome modification is less than complete, the expression of resistant growth must be dominant over sensitivity. If sensitivity were dominant, growth of cells where less than 40% of protein synthesis is resistant to EM should be inhibited by this drug.

Since cells showing low levels of EM-resistant incorporation are nevertheless able to grow in the presence of EM, the expression of EM-resistant colony-forming ability may require that only a threshold level of ribosome modification be exceeded. For example, methylation of only one of the two or more proposed methylatable sequences in 23S ribosomal RNA (6) could be sufficient to allow expression of EM-resistant colony-forming ability. Alternatively, if the number of methylated ribosomes rather than the extent of methylation is critical, methylation of only a few ribosomes might be enough, especially since in situ induction can continue during outgrowth on EM-containing agar (22). Since induction occurs in stationary-phase cells, the earlier prediction (22) that resistant growth requires methylation of 50 to 75% of the ribosomes may be overestimated. Regardless of what the threshold level is, differences in methylation have been suggested previously (22) to explain differences in macrolide binding to ribosomes. Ribosomal 50S subunits from a constitutively resistant mutant were almost completely resistant to EM or lincomycin binding, whereas subunits isolated from induced cells were able to bind at least half as much EM or lincomycin as did uninduced sensitive cells. The extent of EM-resistant incorporation reported here for the induced strains and for the constitutive mutant are consistent with these binding studies. Incomplete methylation could help explain why ribosomes from the induced cells were not totally insensitive to EM binding (22) or to EM inhibition of [^{14}C]leucine incorporation (Table 5). Thus, although EM-resistant colony-forming ability seems to be maximally induced within 60 min, the true rate of ribosome modification may be different and may be more accurately reflected by rates of induction of EM-resistant [^{14}C]leucine incorporation.

ACKNOWLEDGMENTS

I thank Ken Christy and Janet Epp for their assistance in portions of this work.

LITERATURE CITED

1. **Allen, N. E.** 1977. Macrolide resistance in *Staphylococcus aureus*: inducers of macrolide resistance. Antimicrob. Agents Chemother. 11:669–674.
2. **Chabbert, Y.** 1956. Antagonisme in vitro entre l'erythromycine et la spiramycine. Ann. Inst. Pasteur Paris 90:787–790.
3. **Hashimoto, H., H. Oshima, and S. Mitsuhashi.** 1968. Drug resistance of staphylococci. IX. Inducible resistance to macrolide antibiotics in *Staphylococcus aureus*. Jpn. J. Microbiol. 12:321–327.
4. **Hyder, S. L., and M. M. Streitfeld.** 1973. Inducible and constitutive resistance to macrolide antibiotics and lincomycin in clinically isolated strains of *Streptococcus pyogenes*. Antimicrob. Agents Chemother. 4:327–331.
5. **Imsande, J.** 1970. Regulation of penicillinase synthesis: evidence for a unified model. J. Bacteriol. 101:173–180.
6. **Lai, C. J., J. E. Dahlberg, and B. Weisblum.** 1973. Structure of an inducibly methylatable mucleolide sequence in 23S ribosomal ribonucleic acid from erythromycin-resistant *Staphylococcus aureus*. Biochemistry 12:457–460.
7. **Lai, C. J., and B. Weisblum.** 1971. Altered methylation of ribosomal RNA in an erythromycin-resistant strain of *Staphylococcus aureus*. Proc. Natl. Acad. Sci. U.S.A. 68:856–860.
8. **Lai, C. J., B. Weisblum, S. R. Fahnestock, and M. Nomura.** 1972. Alteration of 23S ribosomal RNA and erythromycin-induced resistance to lincomycin and spiramycin in *Staphylococcus aureus*. J. Mol. Biol. 74:67–72.
9. **Leggate, J., and W. H. Holms.** 1968. Gratuitous synthesis of β-lactamase in *Staphylococcus aureus*. J. Bacteriol. 96:2110–2117.
10. **Lowry, O. H., N. J. Rosebrough, A. L. Farr, and R. J. Randall.** 1951. Protein measurement with the Folin phenol reagent. J. Biol. Chem. 193:265–275.
11. **Perret, C. J.** 1954. Iodometric assay of penicillinase. Nature (London) 174:1012–1013.
12. **Richmond, M. H.** 1969. Enzymic adaptation in bacteria: its biochemical and genetic basis, p. 105–154. *In* P. N. Campbell and G. D. Greville (ed.), Essays in biochemistry, vol. 4. Academic Press Inc., New York.
13. **Saito, T., H. Hashimoto, and S. Mitsuhasi.** 1969. Drug resistance of staphylococci. Formation of erythromycin-ribosome complex. Decrease in the formation of erythromycin-ribosome complex in erythromycin-resistant strains of *Staphylococcus aureus*. Jpn. J. Microbiol. 13:119–121.
14. **Saito, T., M. Shimizu, and S. Mitsuhashi.** 1971. Macrolide resistance in staphylococci. Ann. N.Y. Acad. Sci. 182:267–278.
15. **Shimizu, M., T. Saito, and S. Mitsuhashi.** 1970. Macrolide resistance in *Staphylococcus aureus*. Correlation between spiramycin binding to ribosomes and inhibition of polypeptide synthesis in a cell-free system. Jpn. J. Microbiol. 14:215–219.
16. **Shimizu, M., T. Saito, and S. Mitsuhashi.** 1970. Macrolide resistance in *Staphylococcus aureus*. Decrease of spiramycin binding to 50S ribosomal subunit in macrolide-resistant strains of staphylococci. J. Antibiot. 23:467–468.
17. **Swallo, D. L., and P. H. A. Sneath.** 1962. Studies on staphylococcal penicillinase. J. Gen. Microbiol. 28:461–469.
18. **Tai, P. C., B. J. Wallace, and B. D. Davis.** 1974. Selective action of erythromycin on initiating ribosomes. Biochemistry 13:4653–4659.
19. **Weaver, J. R., and P. A. Pattee.** 1964. Inducible resistance to erythromycin in *Staphylococcus aureus*. J. Bacteriol. 88:574–580.
20. **Weisblum, B.** 1971. Macrolide resistance in *Staphylococcus aureus*, p. 217–238. *In* S. Mitsuhashi (ed.), Drug action and drug resistance in bacteria, vol. I: Macrolide antibiotics and lincomycin. University Park Press, Baltimore.
21. **Weisblum, B., and V. Demohn.** 1969. Erythromycin-inducible resistance in *Staphylococcus aureus*: survey of antibiotic classes involved. J. Bacteriol. 98:447–452.
22. **Weisblum, B., C. Siddhikol, C. J. Lai, and V. Demohn.** 1971. Erythromycin-inducible resistance in *Staphylococcus aureus*: requirements for induction. J. Bacteriol. 106:835–847.
23. **Winshell, E., and W. V. Shaw.** 1969. Kinetics of induction and purification of chloramphenicol acetyltransferase from chloramphenicol-resistant *Staphylococcus aureus*. J. Bacteriol. 98:1248–1257.
24. **Yagi, Y., A. E. Franke, and D. B. Clewell.** 1975. Plasmid-determined resistance to erythromycin: comparison of strains of *Streptococcus faecalis* and *Streptococcus pyogenes* with plasmid homology and resistance inducibility. Antimicrob. Agents Chemother. 7:871–873.
25. **Yamagishi, S., Y. Nakajima, M. Inoue, and Y. Oka.** 1971. Decrease in accumulation of macrolide antibiotics as a mechanism of resistance in *Staphylococcus aureus*. Jpn. J. Microbiol. 15:39–52.

Antimicrobial Agents and Chemotherapy, Apr. 1977, p. 669-674 Vol. 11, No. 4

Macrolide Resistance in *Staphylococcus aureus*: Inducers of Macrolide Resistance

NORRIS E. ALLEN

The Lilly Research Laboratories, Eli Lilly and Company, Indianapolis, Indiana 46206

Received for publication 12 October 1976

Several macrolide-, lincosamide-, and streptogramin B-type (MLS) antibiotics were tested as inducers of erythromycin A (EM)-resistant [^{14}C]leucine incorporation. Only 14-membered-ring macrolides having a glycosidically linked 6-deoxy sugar at the C-3 position of the lactone ring and the structurally dissimilar lincosamide, celesticetin, showed inducer activity. Modifications of EM at the C-4'' position of cladinose can apparently destroy the inducer property but do not affect the inhibitory properties of the antibiotic. The findings clearly show that inducer and inhibitor activities can be dissociated and are consistent with the concept that distinct binding/receptor sites are utilized for inhibition of ribosome function and induction of resistance.

Macrolide resistance in certain strains of *Staphylococcus aureus* can be induced by exposure to subinhibitory concentrations of erythromycin A (EM) (1, 19). Several antibiotics besides EM reportedly induce macrolide resistance in *S. aureus*. For example, oleandomycin (7, 8), lankamycin (7), desacetyllankamycin (7), leucomycin (11), carbomycin (14), and lincomycin (14) have been reported to induce resistance in strains isolated from diverse sources. Among clinical isolates, published descriptions of inducibly resistant *S. aureus* indicate only EM, oleandomycin, the lankamycins, and megalomycin as inducers of macrolide resistance (5, 7-9, 18). These compounds are all 14-membered-ring macrolide antibiotics. In contrast, mutants of clinical strains that can be induced by diverse MLS antibiotics, including 14- and 16-membered-ring macrolides (11) and lincomycin (14), have been isolated in the laboratory. One mutant is described as inducible by high temperature (13). Apparently, both strain and drug specificities are determining factors in the induction of macrolide resistance.

EM and its derivatives are the only reported inducers of macrolide resistance in *S. aureus* 1206 (16, 19). It was recently reported (14) that a mutant of this strain had lost EM inducibility but could be induced by either lincomycin or carbomycin. This report, coupled with the observation that celesticetin and several macrolides other than EM induced zone distortion when placed adjacent to lincomycin (1), suggested that several antibiotics might induce macrolide resistance in *S. aureus* 1206.

MLS antibiotics and EM derivatives were surveyed for ability to induce EM-resistant [^{14}C]leucine incorporation. The results indicate that several 14-membered-ring macrolides and celesticetin induce resistance in *S. aureus* 1206. Furthermore, a single modification of the EM molecule appears to eliminate inducer capability without affecting the inhibitory properties of the antibiotic.

MATERIALS AND METHODS

The inductive capacity of MLS antibiotics was measured by growing *S. aureus* 1206 to early stationary phase in synthetic broth as described (1). Cells were washed once and resuspended in fresh broth to a cell density of approximately 0.24 mg of protein per ml. After preincubation at 37°C for 30 min, inducers were added at the desired concentration. Incubation of the cell suspension was continued for 2 h, and [^{14}C]leucine incorporation in the presence and absence of 140 μM EM was measured on duplicate aliquots exactly as described before (1). Each of the antibiotics tested for inducer activity was also assayed for inhibition of [^{14}C]leucine incorporation as described (1), using cells incubated for 2 h without added antibiotics.

Sources of the antibiotics used have been cited previously (1), and EM derivatives were kindly furnished by E. Massey of the Lilly Research Laboratories. Antibiotic stock solutions were routinely prepared in methanol-water at 1 to 5 mg/ml. The maximum level of methanol present during induction was 0.1%, and there was no inhibition of [^{14}C]leucine incorporation or induction by methanol at this concentration. The EM derivatives were generally less soluble than the other antibiotics and were dissolved in undiluted methanol. Equivalent amounts of methanol were added to the untreated controls.

RESULTS

MLS antibiotics. MLS antibiotics were tested at 0.14, 1.4, and 14 μM for their ability to induce EM-resistant [^{14}C]leucine incorporation

(Table 1). The inhibitory activity of each compound was simultaneously determined at 1.4, 14, and 140 μM. Induced EM-resistant incorporation is expressed as a percentage of the uninhibited rate since exposure to many compounds for 120 min resulted in lowered rates of [^{14}C]leucine incorporation. The inhibitory effects of 16-membered-ring macrolides at 14 μM precluded any estimate of induction.

The data in Table 1 were accumulated from five separate experiments. In each experiment, EM was tested as an inducer along with an uninduced control, and standard errors are included with these data. In the absence of exogenous inducer, EM-resistant incorporation was approximately 16% of the uninhibited rate. An increase in resistant incorporation above this level indicates induction by the given antibiotic.

Among the 14-membered-ring macrolides,

TABLE 1. *Inducer activity of MLS antibiotics*

Antibiotic	Concn (μM)	Inducer activity[a]	Inhibitor activity[b]	Antibiotic	Concn (μM)	Inducer activity[a]	Inhibitor activity[b]
None	0	16 ± 1.2[c]		12-membered-ring macrolides			
14-membered-ring macrolides				Methymycin	0.14	20	
Erythromycin A	0.14	76 ± 1.5			1.4	16	7
	1.4	52 ± 3.6	64 ± 2.5		14	18	1
	14	23 ± 1.8	76 ± 1.3		140		2
	140		78 ± 1.3	16-membered-ring macrolides			
Oleandomycin	0.14	26		Carbomycin	0.14	18	
	1.4	45	31		1.4	INH[d]	23
	14	20	59		14	INH	84
	140		55		140		89
Triacetyloleandomycin	0.14	19		Spiramycin	0.14	19	
	1.4	44	19		1.4	13	18
	14	38	48		14	INH	82
	140		60		140		83
Megalomycin	0.14	21		Tylosin	0.14	17	
	1.4	66	17		1.4	INH	27
	14	58	76		14	INH	84
	140		90		140	INH	84
Lankamycin	0.14	13		Niddamycin	0.14	17	
	1.4	17	4		1.4	INH	80
	14	40	22		14	INH	84
	140		30		140		85
Desacetyllankamycin	0.14	20		Streptogramin B types			
	1.4	66	4				
	14	66	11	Vernamycin Bα	0.14	18	
	140		34		1.4	18	8
					14	18	27
Narbomycin	0.14	13			140		38
	1.4	15	<1				
	14	12	<1	Lincosamides			
	140		<1				
				Lincomycin	0.14	18	
Pikromycin	0.14	18			1.4	14	44
	1.4	21	3		14	14	80
	14	9	5		140		85
	140		9				
				Celesticetin	0.14	34	
					1.4	51	<1
					14	71	10
					140		61

[a] Inducer activity is the rate of EM-resistant [^{14}C]leucine incorporation expressed as a percentage of the uninhibited rate. Each antibiotic listed was tested for inducer activity at three concentrations as described in Materials and Methods. After the 120-min induction, cells were washed free of inducer and incorporation of [^{14}C]leucine was measured in the presence and absence of 140 μM EM as described (1). The rate of [^{14}C]leucine incorporation in the presence of 140 μM EM, expressed as a percentage of the rate of incorporation in the absence of EM, reflects the extent of induction by each antibiotic. Uninduced, control cells were incubated 120 min without added antibiotics. [^{14}C]leucine incorporation by these cells in the presence of 140 μM EM was 16 ± 1.2% of the uninhibited rate; i.e., incorporation was inhibited by 84%.

[b] Inhibitor activity is the percentage of inhibition of [^{14}C]leucine incorporation. Each antibiotic listed was tested for inhibition of protein synthesis at three concentrations as described (1), using cells incubated for 120 min without added inducer.

[c] Standard errors from five determinations.

[d] INH, No measurement of EM-resistant [^{14}C]leucine incorporation due to inhibitory effects of inducer.

EM, oleandomycin, triacetyloleandomycin, megalomycin, lankamycin, and desacetyllankamycin showed inducer activity. Griseomycin was not tested. EM was clearly the most potent inducer and was also the most active inhibitor of [^{14}C]leucine incorporation. The decreased levels of induced resistance at EM concentrations exceeding 0.14 μM resulted from inhibition of the induction process (17).

Narbomycin and pikromycin both failed to induce resistance, but they also failed to inhibit [^{14}C]leucine incorporation. Induced resistance to both compounds was readily demonstrated by the disk test (1), implying that they inhibit ribosome function as do other MLS antibiotics (17). Additional experiments with narbomycin (data not presented) showed no inductive capacity even at 700 μM. Methymycin, a 12-membered-ring macrolide, also failed to induce resistance or inhibit [^{14}C]leucine incorporation, but higher concentrations were not evaluated.

No 16-membered-ring macrolide induced macrolide resistance. At 1.4 μM, most of these compounds destroyed greater than 80% of the [^{14}C]leucine-incorporating activity. Because these antibiotics were such potent inhibitors of protein synthesis, it was possible that even at the lowest concentration tested their capacity to inhibit exceeded their capacity to induce. In further testing, lower noninhibitory concentrations (0.0014 and 0.014 μM) of carbomycin and tylosin were nevertheless unable to induce resistance (data not shown).

Neither vernamycin Bα nor lincomycin induced resistance, but celesticetin, a derivative of lincomycin (6), showed good inducer activity. Although not as active as an inducer as EM at 0.14 μM, celesticetin appeared to be a more effective inducer at higher concentrations since its ability to inhibit protein synthesis and thus induction was less than that of EM.

EM derivatives. Eighteen derivatives of EM were compared for inducer activity using the disk method (18). The derivatives are listed in Table 2 and the structure of EM is given in Fig. 1. Each of the derivatives demonstrated antibacterial activity when tested against *Sarcina lutea* by the disk diffusion test (data not shown). All but two compounds induced macrolide resistance in *S. aureus* 1206; the 4''-tosyl and 4''-mesyl derivatives of the cyclic carbonate were the only compounds unable to induce noticeable zone distortion.

Several derivatives, including the 4''-tosyl cyclic carbonate, were compared as inducers of EM-resistant [^{14}C]leucine incorporation (Table 3). The unmodified cyclic carbonate was a strong inhibitor of protein synthesis and was also a potent inducer. Further modification yielding the 4''-tosyl derivative preserved the inhibitory properties of this molecule but resulted in a derivative unable to induce resistance at the concentrations tested. The comparable mesyl derivative was not tested further, but all other derivatives tested showed inducer activity.

DISCUSSION

MLS antibiotics constitute a diverse and structurally dissimilar group of compounds. The macrolides contain a characteristic 12-, 14-, or 16-membered-ring lactone with one, two, or three 6-deoxy sugar substitutions. The size of the lactone ring and the number and position of the attached deoxy sugars are used to classify these antibiotics. With the exception of possible similarities between EM and lincomycin based on a comparison of molecular models (16), the macrolides are structurally distinct from the lincosamides and the streptogramin B-type antibiotics.

Although structurally diverse, the MLS antibiotics demonstrate functional relatedness. Competition between lincomycin and EM for binding to the same, overlapping, or related sites on the ribosome is well established (2, 6). In *S. aureus*, induced EM resistance is accompanied by resistance to all MLS antibiotics (1, 16), and a constitutive mutation confers resistance to the same drugs (1). The present study reveals that several macrolide antibiotics plus celesticetin can induce EM resistance in *S. aureus* 1206. Thus, the functional relatedness of these antibiotics is extended to include inducer as well as inhibitor function.

Work from other laboratories (8, 10, 12) has indirectly suggested that the inductive capacity of macrolide antibiotics may be due, in part, to the structure and position of the 6-deoxy sugars. The results from the present study support this idea and further suggest a critical role for the sugar attached at the C-3 position of the lactone ring, e.g., cladinose in EM (Fig. 1). The evidence for the importance of this sugar and the size of the lactone ring in induction of resistance in *S. aureus* by macrolide antibiotics is considerable.

First, only 14-membered-ring macrolides containing a C-3-linked 6-deoxy sugar were active as inducers. No 12- or 16-membered-ring macrolide tested induced zone distortion (1) or EM-resistant [^{14}C]leucine incorporation (Table 1). The 12- and 16-membered-ring macrolides have different sugar arrangements and no C-3-linked deoxy sugar. Second, the two 14-membered-ring macrolides that did not induce, narbomycin and pikromycin, are unique in not containing an attached 6-deoxy sugar at the C-3

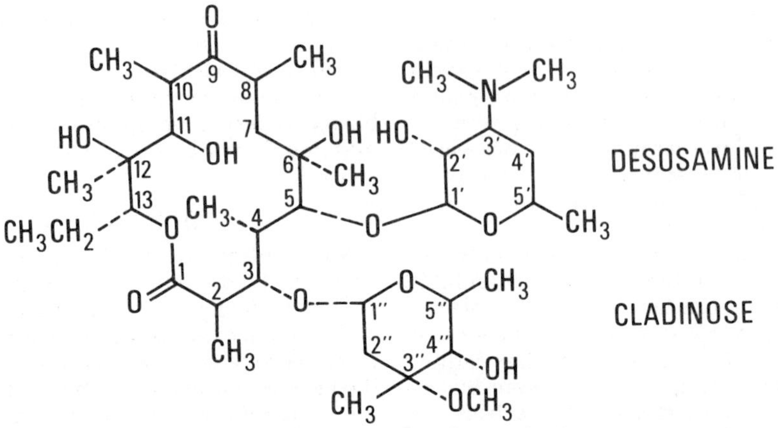

FIG. 1. *Structure of erythromycin A.*

TABLE 2. *Erythromycin derivatives*

Erythromycin A	6,9-Hemiketal
Erythromycin B	6,9,12-Spiroketal
Erythromycin C	11,12-Cyclic carbonate
N-oxide	11,12-Cyclic carbonate-8-hydroxy
Des-*N*-methyl	2′-Benzoyl
8-Hydroxy	3′-De(dimethylamino)
9-Hydrazone	4″-Tosyl-11,12-cyclic carbonate
9-Ketoxime	4″-Mesyl-11,12-cyclic carbonate
9(s)-Dihydro	
9(s)-Erythromycylamine	
9(r)-Erythromycylamine	

position. These two antibiotics differ only by a single hydroxyl on the lactone ring. It should be pointed out that interpretation of the negative inducer response is complicated by the inability of both antibiotics to inhibit [^{14}C]leucine incorporation, although neither compound behaved as an inducer in the disk test.

Third, both lankamycin and desacetyllankamycin showed inducer activity, but the desacetyl form was a more active inducer than the acetylated antibiotic. Lankamycin is acetylated at the C-4″ position of arcanose, which is the 6-deoxy sugar attached to the lactone ring at the C-3 position. Omura et al. (7) reported identical findings for these two antibiotics using another method to measure induction.

Fourth, using the disk method to detect inducer activity among EM derivatives, all but two compounds were strong inducers. The 4″-tosyl and 4″-mesyl derivatives of EM cyclic carbonate were unable to induce zone distortion. The tosylated derivative failed to induce EM-resistant [^{14}C]leucine incorporation, whereas the unmodified cyclic carbonate was as active an inducer as EM (Table 2; 8). Furthermore, inhibition of protein synthesis by the cyclic carbonate was equal to or greater than that shown by EM. Since the 4″-tosyl cyclic carbonate retains inhibitory activity, it is clear that reduced transport cannot account for the reduction in inducer activity. Thus, the loss of inductive capacity can be attributed to the modification at the C-4″ position of cladinose (see Fig. 1).

Other workers have shown that the monoglycosides of EM (minus cladinose or desosamine)

TABLE 3. *Inducer activity of EM derivatives*

Derivative	Concn (μM)	Inducer activity[a]	Inhibitor activity[b]
None	0	14	
Erythromycin A	0.14	77	
	1.4	45	64
	14	28	64
	140		66
2′-Benzoyl	0.14	35	
	1.4	72	37
	14	76	54
	140		71
3′-De(dimethylamino)	0.14	23	
	1.4	19	23
	14	33	13
	140		27
11,12-Cyclic carbonate	0.14	82	
	1.4	49	68
	14	38	69
	140		72
4″-Tosyl-11,12-cyclic carbonate	0.14	14	
	1.4	10	75
	14	14	86
	140		98

[a, b] See Table 1.

and the aglycone (minus both sugars) were either inactive or had severely diminished inducer activity (8, 10, 12). Moreover, Ono et al. (8) reported that introduction of an acetyl group in the C-4″ position of EM resulted in decreased inducer activity but had a negligible effect on antibacterial activity. Taken together, the data clearly indicate that inducer and inhibitor activities of EM can be dissociated.

Fifth, induction by leucomycin using the mutant described by Saito et al. (11) was affected by modification of mycarose at the C-4″ position. Although leucomycin is a 16-membered-ring macrolide and the sugar arrangement is not the same as in EM, removal of mycarose or deacetylation at the C-4″ appeared to eliminate inducer activity.

Celesticetin's ability to induce macrolide resistance was unexpected since this antibiotic is structurally dissimilar to EM and other 14-membered-ring macrolides. Whether a structural similarity exists between celesticetin and EM analogous to the similarity between lincomycin and EM proposed to explain identical or related ribosome binding sites (16) remains to be determined. At any rate, induction by celesticetin means that inducibility in *S. aureus* is not limited to a narrow spectrum of closely related structural types and proves that induction of resistance in natural isolates of *S. aureus* is not strictly a property of macrolides. A closer similarity with inducibly macrolide-resistant streptococci, some of which can be induced by numerous MLS antibiotics (3, 4, 20), is suggested. The fact that only MLS antibiotics will induce raises the interesting possibility that the binding or receptor site(s) on the hypothetical regulatory protein may recognize the same molecular structures as does the ribosomal binding site(s).

Tanaka and Weisblum (14) described a mutant of *S. aureus* that had lost EM inducibility but that could be induced by either lincomycin or carbomycin. They theorized that this phenotype may have resulted from a reversal of the relative potency these antibiotics had for inhibition and induction. In other words, other MLS antibiotics may be potential inducers, but fail because their capacity to inhibit is so much greater. The finding that celesticetin can induce resistance in *S. aureus* is consistent with this proposal, since although higher concentrations of this antibiotic are required for induction, celesticetin's capacity to inhibit ribosome function appears to be much less than that of EM. The inability of the 4″-tosyl cyclic carbonate of EM to induce resistance is further evidence that modification can alter the relative potency an antibiotic has for induction and inhibition.

Finally, clinically isolated inducibly macrolide-resistant staphylococci have been classified on the basis of whether they could be induced by EM only or by EM and oleandomycin (5, 8). EM was previously reported as the only inducer in *S. aureus* 1206 (16). It can be concluded from the studies reported here that numerous MLS antibiotics can potentially induce resistance but go undetected because they have a much stronger affinity for ribosome inhibition or because detection may require a sensitive measure of induction. The possibility that mutations can lead to a changed inducer spectrum coupled with the disclosure of inducible macrolide resistance in streptococci (3, 4, 20) warns that any classification of strains based solely on response to inducers would be an oversimplification at this time.

ACKNOWLEDGMENTS

I thank Ken Christy and Janet Epp for their assistance in portions of this work.

LITERATURE CITED

1. **Allen, N. E.** 1976. Macrolide resistance in *Staphylococcus aureus*: induction of macrolide-resistant protein synthesis. Antimicrob. Agents Chemother. **11**:661–668.
2. **Chang, F. N., and B. Weisblum.** 1967. The specificity of lincomycin binding to ribosomes. Biochemistry **6**:836–843.
3. **Hyder, S. L., and M. M. Streitfeld.** 1973. Inducible and constitutive resistance to macrolide antibiotics and lincomycin in clinically isolated strains of *Streptococcus pyogenes*. Antimicrob. Agents Chemother. **4**:327–331.
4. **Malke, H.** 1974. Genetics of resistance to macrolide antibiotics and lincomycin in natural isolates of *Streptococcus pyogenes*. Mol. Gen. Genet. **135**:349–367.
5. **Mitsuhashi, S., H. Oshima, M. Inoue, and Y. Yamaguchi.** 1971. Resistance to macrolide antibiotics and lincomycin in *Staphylococcus aureus*, p. 23–40. *In* S. Mitsuhashi (ed.), Drug action and drug resistance, vol. I: Macrolide antibiotics and lincomycin. University Park Press, Baltimore.
6. **Monro, R. E., R. Fernandez-Munoz, M. L. Celma, and D. Vazquez.** 1971. Mode of action of lincomycin and related antibiotics, p. 305–336. *In* S. Mitsuhashi (ed.), Drug action and drug resistance in bacteria, vol. I: Macrolide antibiotics and lincomycin, University Park Press, Baltimore.
7. **Omura, S., S. Namiki, M. Shibata, T. Muro, and J. Sawada.** 1970. Studies on the antibiotics from *Streptomyces spinochromogenes* var. *kujimyceticus*. V. Some antimicrobial characteristics of kujimycin A and kujimycin B against macrolide resistant staphylococci. J. Antibiot. **23**:448–460.
8. **Ono, H., M. Inoue, J. C. H. Mao, and S. Mitsuhashi.** 1975. Drug resistance in *Staphylococcus aureus*. Induction of macrolide resistance by erythromycin, oleandomycin and their derivatives. Jpn. J. Microbiol. **19**:343–347.
9. **Osono, T., and H. Umezawa.** 1971. Josamycin, a new

macrolide antibiotic of resistance non-inducing type, p. 41-120. *In* S. Mitsuhashi (ed.), Drug action and drug resistance in bacteria, vol. I: Macrolide antibiotics and lincomycin. University Park Press, Baltimore.
10. **Pestka, S., R. Vince, R. LeMahieu, F. Weiss, L. Fern, and J. Unowsky.** 1976. Induction of erythromycin resistance in *Staphylococcus aureus* by erythromycin derivatives. Antimicrob. Agents Chemother. 9:128-130.
11. **Saito, T., H. Hashimoto, and S. Mitsuhashi.** 1970. Macrolide resistance in *Staphylococcus aureus*. Isolation of a mutant in which leucomycin is an active inducer. Jpn. J. Microbiol. 14:473-478.
12. **Saito, T., M. Shimizu, and S. Mitsuhashi.** 1971. Macrolide resistance in staphylococci, p. 239-266. *In* S. Mitsuhashi (ed.), Drug action and drug resistance in bacteria, vol. I: Macrolide antibiotics and lincomycin. University Park Press, Baltimore.
13. **Shimizu, M., T. Saito, and S. Mitsuhashi.** 1970. Macrolide resistance in *Staphylococcus aureus*. Relation between spiramycin-binding to ribosome and inhibition of polypeptide synthesis in a heat inducible-resistant mutant. Jpn. J. Microbiol. 14:155-162.
14. **Tanaka, T., and B. Weisblum.** 1974. Mutant of *Staphylococcus aureus* with lincomycin- and carbomycin-inducible resistance to erythromycin. Antimicrob. Agents Chemother. 5:538-540.
15. **Weaver, J. R., and P. A. Pattee.** 1964. Inducible resistance to erythromycin in *Staphylococcus aureus*. J. Bacteriol. 88:574-580.
16. **Weisblum, B.** 1971. Macrolide resistance in *Staphylococcus aureus*, p. 217-238. *In* S. Mitsuhashi (ed.), Drug action and drug resistance in bacteria, vol. I: Macrolide antibiotics and lincomycin. University Park Press, Baltimore.
17. **Weisblum, B., and J. Davies.** 1968. Antibiotic inhibitors of the bacterial ribosome. Bacteriol. Rev. 32:493-528.
18. **Weisblum, B., and V. Demohn.** 1969. Erythromycin-inducible resistance in *Staphylococcus aureus*: survey of antibiotic classes involved. J. Bacteriol. 98:447-452.
19. **Weisblum, B., C. Siddhikol, C. J. Lai, and V. Demohn.** 1971. Erythromycin-inducible resistance in *Staphylococcus aureus*. Requirements for induction. J. Bacteriol. 106:835-847.
20. **Yagi, Y., A. E. Franke, and D. B. Clewell.** 1975. Plasmid-determined resistance to erythromycin: comparison of strains of *Streptococcus faecalis* and *Streptococcus pyogenes* with regard to plasmid homology and resistance inducibility. Antimicrob. Agents Chemother. 7:871-873.

ANTIMICROBIAL AGENTS AND CHEMOTHERAPY, Apr. 1977, p. 675-678 Vol. 11, No. 4

Printed in U.S.A.

Measurement of Polyene Antibiotic-Mediated Erythrocyte Damage by Release of Hemoglobin and Radioactive Chromium

E. B. SIEGEL[1]

Waksman Institute of Microbiology, Rutgers University, New Brunswick, New Jersey 08903

Received for publication 7 October 1976

Polyene antifungal antibiotics produce various degrees of membrane damage in sheep erythrocytes in vitro. Mediocidin, filipin, amphotericin B, and candicidin were found to result in greater damage than nystatin, pimaricin, and amphotericin B methyl ester. The degree of sensitivity of the cells varied by 100-fold for mediocidin verus amphotericin B methyl ester as measured by curves of hemoglobin release versus drug concentration. In erythrocytes prelabeled with radioactive chromium, release of the isotope through polyene-damaged cell membranes was found to occur at lower drug concentrations than measurable hemoglobin release, and the percentage of isotope released at the highest drug dose was consistently greater than the percentage of hemoglobin released. Thus, the isotope assay is a more sensitive indicator of polyene-induced membrane damage in the test system. These significant differences in release of molecules through polyene-induced membrane lesions indicate the complex nature of the binding and further interactions of this class of drugs with the plasma membrane.

Polyene antifungal antibiotics have been shown to induce the rapid lysis of rat and human erythrocytes in the presence of isotonic saline (6). The extent of hemolysis was dependent on the antibiotic/cell concentration ratio. Further, a critical threshold ratio of antibiotic molecules to cell surface area was established (7). It has been shown that the mode of action of the polyene antifungals involves the binding of drug molecules to cell membrane sterols, with the attendant distortion of the membrane and leakage of essential metabolites (9). Eventually, loss of protein occurs through the altered cell membrane. It has also been observed that heptaenes containing an aromatic moiety, such as candicidin (CAND), are generally more active than those without such a moiety, such as amphotericin B (AB) (11).

Minor changes in structure can radically affect the biological activity of a polyene. Amphotericin B methyl ester (AME) is a recently synthesized compound (1), possessing equal antifungal activity to the parent compound, AB, but with a greatly increased solubility in aqueous media and decreased in vivo toxicity (5).

In homeothermic animals, the selectivity of membrane transport of K^+ over Na^+ ions into the cell is on the order of 25:1 (2). This figure cannot be taken as the real rest-state selectivity since the absolute membrane selectivity for K^+ over Na^+ is much higher. This ratio refers to the presence of the ions in the cell cytoplasm and the suspending medium outside the plasma membrane. Chromium-51 (^{51}Cr) is a 0.33-MeV gamma radiation-emitting isotope with a half-life of 28.7 days. It is taken up, in the form of sodium chromate ($Na_2{}^{51}CrO_4$), by animal cells and erythrocytes in much the same way as potassium and is selectively concentrated, by active transport, against the normal-concentration gradient in aqueous solutions. Since the cell's sodium-potassium pump is involved in this process, any damage to the cell membrane will result in release of the isotope, thus rendering it available to scintillation counting in the supernatant of a pelleted cell suspension. ^{51}Cr isotope assays for cell toxicity have been used in recent years in tumor cell-antibody systems (10, 13), virus-cell antigen-antibody systems (3, 8), and lymphocyte-cell systems (4, 12, 14). In the studies described below, sheep erythrocytes were labeled with the gamma-emitting isotope ^{51}Cr in the form of radioactive sodium chromate, and the release of the isotope and/or hemoglobin was studied after damage to the cell membrane with filipin (FIL), mediocidin

[1] Present address: Biological Sciences Research Center of the Child Development Institute, Division of Health Affairs, University of North Carolina, Chapel Hill, NC 27514.

(MED), AB, AME, CAND, PIM, and NYS. I hoped to further illuminate the mechanism of membrane damage by polyenes by comparing the release of ^{51}Cr and hemoglobin in drug-treated erthrocytes.

MATERIALS AND METHODS

Erythrocytes. Fresh sheep erythrocytes were obtained as a 20% suspension in Alsever solution from Microbiological Associates, Inc., 100 ml at a time. They were washed in Dulbecco phosphate-buffered saline by centrifugation at 1,000 × *g* and 4°C, followed by resuspension. This procedure was repeated three times. Cell density was adjusted so that 0.2 ml of suspension, lysed with 2.2 ml of distilled water, gave an optical density of 0.700 at 541 nm. The pH of all suspensions was kept rigidly at pH 6.8.

Polyene antifungal antibiotics. Polyenes were obtained in crystalline form, purified by liquid chromatography, from Daniel P. Bonner and Wietold Mechlinski of Carl Schaffner's laboratory, Waksman Institute of Microbiology, Rutgers University. The drugs were stored at −20°C until use. After use they were stored as frozen solutions at −20°C for up to 7 days; after this time they were not reused. AME, AB, FIL, MED, NYS, and CAND were dissolved in highly purified dimethyl sulfoxide. PIM was dissolved in dimethyl fluoride.

Treatment of erythrocytes. Aliquots of a freshly prepared erythrocyte suspension were treated with polyene drugs in the following manner: 0.2 ml of the cell suspension was added to each of a number of glass disposable culture tubes (12 by 75 mm) and allowed to equilibrate at 24°C. Freshly prepared solutions of polyene antibiotic diluted in dimethyl sulfoxide or dimethyl fluoride were added by Hamilton microsyringe in 2-μl volumes. The drugs were diluted in such a manner that a 2-μl volume would contain a quantity of drug equivalent to the final concentration (in micrograms per milliliter) desired. (Thus, if the drug dose required was 10 μl, 2 μg of drug would be added in 2 μl of solution to the 0.2 ml of erythrocyte suspension.) The tubes were agitated and allowed to incubate at 24°C for 30 min.

Hemoglobin release assay. Tubes of treated erythrocytes were filled with 2.2 ml of Dulbecco phosphate-buffered saline except the distilled-water blanks, which received 2.2 ml of deionized, distilled water. All tubes were centrifuged at 1,000 × *g* and 4°C for 10 min, and the supernatant was analyzed for optical density at 541 nm. The distilled-water blank was considered to represent 100% hemoglobin release; a no-drug blank, treated only with dimethyl sulfoxide or dimethyl fluoride, represented 0% hemoglobin release. The following formula was utilized to calculate percentage of hemoglobin release:

$$\%\ \text{hemoglobin release} = \frac{OD_2\ (\text{drug sample}) - OD_1\ (\text{blank})}{OD_3\ (\text{distilled-}H_2O\ \text{blank})}$$

where OD is optical density. Results for each experiment were then graphed linearly. The concentration of a drug resulting in release of 50% of the value obtained after treatment of the cell suspension in distilled water was defined as the 50% release value of the drug.

Combined ^{51}Cr and hemoglobin release assay for erythrocytes. An assay, utilizing prelabeled erythrocytes, was developed in order to examine the comparative sensitivities of ^{51}Cr and hemoglobin release as a measure of erythrocyte membrane damage by the polyene drugs. A washed suspension of 10^8 to 2×10^9 cells/ml was incubated with an equal volume of balanced salt solution containing 100 to 300 μCi of ^{51}Cr per ml at 37°C, with gentle agitation every 5 min for the first 30 min. The cells were then washed five times by centrifugation and resuspension and used immediately. Ten million (4×10^8) erythrocytes/0.2 ml were dispensed into glass culture tubes.

After dispensing, the erythrocytes were treated, as described above, with various doses of polyenes. After resuspension and centrifugation, 0.4 ml out of the total 2.2 ml of each sample was assayed in a Packard Tri-Carb liquid scintillation counter, and the rest was assayed for optical density at 541 nm. The results were graphed as percentage of hemoglobin release and percentage of ^{51}Cr release versus drug concentration.

RESULTS

The standard time of incubation was 30 min from the moment of addition of drug to the erythrocyte suspension. This period of time was found to be sufficient for virtually 100% of the maximum damage to be imposed on the cell membrane by any of the polyenes utilized in these experiments. This experimental finding did not vary from drug to drug or from concentration to concentration for any particular drug, regardless of the specific hemolytic capability of a particular polyene. In other words, any drug dose of any polyene was found to exert its maximum degree of damage within 30 min of the time of application, whatever the final percent release value attained.

The drug concentrations resulting in 50% total hemoglobin release for sheep erythrocytes treated with seven polyene antifungal antibiotics under controlled conditions are given in Table 1. It is evident that MED, FIL, AB, and CAND were the most damaging agents to the cell membrane, followed by NYS, PIM, and AME. These 50% values were taken from the curves of percent release versus drug concentration made after each experiment (Fig. 1, lower curve). They represent the means of five separate determinations each; it was found that, under the same conditions of temperature, pH, buffer, and time of incubation, response to drug treatment agreed within a few percentage points. Since the drugs were obtained from the same source each time, batch variation was eliminated (although with AB, NYS, AME, and FIL it was found that different batches of drug from the same sources differed only slightly in their hemolytic ability). Different erythrocyte batches were found to be quite similar in membrane fragility and sensitivity to a particular series of polyenes; in any case, all erythrocytes were obtained from the same source.

Comparative release of ^{51}Cr and hemoglobin from erythrocytes. The comparative release of isotope from prelabeled erythrocytes and that of hemoglobin from the same cells was examined after treatment with AME, AB, CAND, and PIM. Drug concentrations producing 50% release are shown in Table 2. An approximately twofold-lower concentration of drug was required for 50% release of the isotope in the cases of AME, AB, and PIM than for 50% release of hemoglobin. For CAND the ^{51}Cr release technique was found to be approximately threefold more sensitive than that of hemoglobin release. Figure 1 represents the curves of the release of the two indicators in sheep erythrocytes treated with CAND: at 2.5 μg/ml the difference between the two curves was significant at the 0.001 level. For PIM (Fig. 2) the significance was at the 0.001 level at drug concentrations of 75 μg/ml.

DISCUSSION

The twofold difference in drug concentration needed to give a 50% release of isotope versus

TABLE 1. *Release of hemoglobin from sheep erythrocytes damaged by seven polyene antifungal antibiotics*

Drug	Drug concn (μg/ml) leading to 50% hemoglobin release
AME	200
FIL	2.3
AB	3.2
MED	2.0
PIM	100
NYS	50
CAND	4.0

TABLE 2. *Release of chromium-51 and hemoglobin from sheep erythrocytes damaged by four polyene antifungal antibiotics*

Drug	Drug concn (μg/ml) leading to:	
	50% ^{51}Cr release	50% hemoglobin release
AME	95	200
AB	1.8	3.2
CAND	1.25	4.0
PIM	50	100

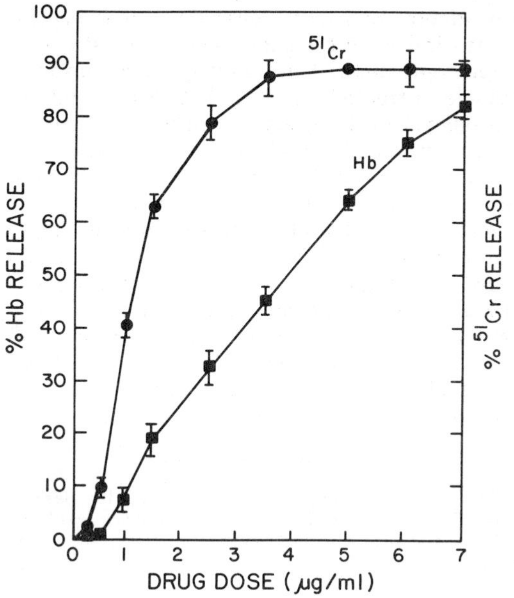

FIG. 1. *Graph of percentage of hemoglobin and ^{51}Cr release versus drug concentration for sheep erythrocytes treated with candicidin. Results are for sheep erythrocytes after treatment with graduated doses of the polyene. Symbols: (●) ^{51}Cr release; (■) hemoglobin release.*

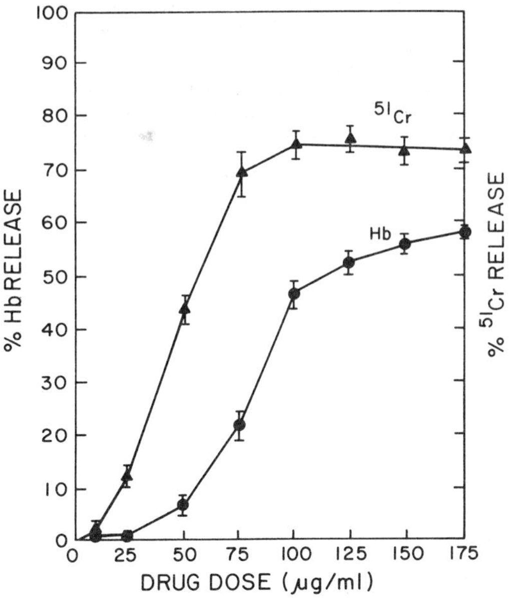

FIG. 2. *Graph of percentage of hemoglobin and ^{51}Cr release versus drug concentration for sheep erythrocytes treated with pimaricin. Results are for the sheep erythrocytes after treatment with graduated doses of the polyene. Symbols: (▲) ^{51}Cr release; (●) hemoglobin release.*

hemoglobin from polyene-treated sheep erythrocytes indicates the more sensitive nature of the isotopic method in quantifying membrane damage in treated cells (Table 2, Fig. 1 and 2). The significantly greater release of labeled chromium (and, by implication, that of K^+ ions) as compared with the much larger hemoglobin molecule indicates the complex nature of the lesions produced and the membrane damage and disruption incurred by the binding of polyene antifungal antibiotics to erythrocytes. The use of labeled compounds in this manner, combined with assays of endogenous release of such molecules as hemoglobin, could be a powerful tool for the study of membrane dynamics and mechanisms of cytotoxicity in animal cells.

ACKNOWLEDGMENTS

This work was supported by Public Health Service grants GM507 (from the National Institute of General Medical Sciences) and CA05234 (from the National Cancer Institute).

LITERATURE CITED

1. **Bonner, D. P., W. Mechlinski, and C. P. Schaffner.** 1972. Polyene macrolide derivatives. III. Biological properties of polyene macrolide ester salts. J. Antibiot. 25:261-262.
2. **Brewer, A. K., and R. A. Passwater.** 1972. Physics of the cell membrane. Part 1. The role of double-bond energy states. Am. Lab., April 1974, p. 59-74.
3. **Bries, A. M., C. Wahlenberg, J. Rosenthal, N. Mage, and A. L. Natkins.** 1971. Inhibition or enhancement of immunological injury of virus-infected cells. Proc. Natl. Acad. Sci. U.S.A. 68:3073-3077.
4. **Harada, M., G. Pearson, H. Pettigrew, L. Redmon, and T. Orr.** 1973. Enhancement of normal lymphocyte cytotoxicity by sera with high antibody titers against H-2 or virus-associated antigens. Cancer Res. 33:2886-2893.
5. **Keim, G. R., J. W. Pautsiaka, J. Kupan, and C. N. Keysser.** 1973. Amphotericin B methyl ester hydrochloride and amphotericin B: comparative acute toxicity. Science 179:584-585.
6. **Kinsky, S. C.** 1963. Comparative responses of mammalian erythrocytes and microbial protoplasts to polyene antibiotics and vitamin A. Arch. Biochem. Biophys. 102:180-188.
7. **Kinsky, S. C., J. Auruch, M. Permutt, H. B. Rogers, and H. H. Schander,** 1962. The lytic effect of polyene antifungal antibiotics on mammalian erythrocytes. Biochem. Biophys. Res. Commun. 9:503-507.
8. **Kjellen, L., and J. Anherst,** 1973. Cytotoxicity of adenovirus-antibody aggregates: sensitivity to different cell strains, and inhibition by hexon antiserum and by complement. J. Virol. 12:25-32.
9. **Lampen, J. O.** 1966. Interference by polyene antifungal antibiotics (especially Nystatin and Filipin) with specific membrane functions. Symp. Soc. Gen. Microbiol. 16:111-130.
10. **Pancake, S. J., and A. T. Mara.** 1974. Comparison of SV40 induced antigens on the surface of cultivated cells by a cytolytic microassay. Virology 59:323-327.
11. **Pansy, F. E.** 1972. Comparative chemotherapeutic activity of heptaene macrolide antifungal antibiotics in experimental candidases. J. Antibiot. 25:405-408.
12. **Rosenberg, E. B., J. L. McCoy, S. S. Green, F. C. Donnelly, D. F. Siwanski, P. H. Levine, and R. B. Herberman.** 1974. Destruction of human lymphoid tissue–culture cell lines by human peripheral lymphocytes in ^{51}Cr-release cellular cytotoxicity assays. J. Natl. Cancer Inst. 52:345-352.
13. **Rubens, R. D., and R. Dulbecco.** 1974. Augmentation of cytotoxic drug action by antibodies directed at cell surface. Nature (London) 248:81-82.
14. **Sharma, B., and P. I. Terasaki.** 1974. *In vitro* immunization to cultured human tumor cells. Cancer Res. 34:115-118.
15. **Utahara, R.** 1954. On a new antifungal substance, mediocidin, and three other antifungal substances of *Streptomyces* with characteristic absorption maxima. J. Antibiot. 74:120-124.

ANTIMICROBIAL AGENTS AND CHEMOTHERAPY, Apr. 1977, p. 679-682
Vol. 11, No. 4

Comparative Susceptibility of Anaerobic Bacteria to Ticarcillin, Cefoxitin, Metronidazole, and Related Antimicrobial Agents

DAVID K. HENDERSON, ANTHONY W. CHOW,* AND LUCIEN B. GUZE

Department of Medicine, Harbor General Hospital, Torrance, California 90509; Research and Medical Services, Veterans Administration Hospital (Wadsworth), Los Angeles, California 90073; and University of California School of Medicine, Los Angeles, California 90024*

Received for publication 7 October 1976

The in vitro antimicrobial activity of two newer agents, ticarcillin and cefoxitin, against 204 recent clinical isolates of anaerobic bacteria was determined by an agar dilution technique, and compared to their related compounds carbenicillin, cephalothin, and penicillin, as well as metronidazole, clindamycin, and chloramphenicol. Ticarcillin was similar to carbenicillin, and cefoxitin was more active than cephalothin. At readily achievable blood concentrations of each antimicrobial agent, ticarcillin was slightly less active than clindamycin against *Bacteroides fragilis*. Cefoxitin was superior to cephalothin and penicillin against *B. fragilis*. Penicillin remained highly active against all obligate anaerobes other than *B. fragilis*. Metronidazole, while highly effective against *B. fragilis* and *Clostridium perfringens*, was only intermediately effective against anaerobic gram-positive cocci and relatively inactive against nonsporulating anaerobic gram-positive bacilli. Further evaluation of the clinical efficacy of ticarcillin, carbenicillin, and cefoxitin against anaerobic infections is indicated.

With the increasing awareness of potential serious side effects of clindamycin (3, 15, 18) and chloramphenicol (16), effective and nontoxic alternative agents are clearly needed for the therapy of severe anaerobic infections.

We evaluated the in vitro activity of two newer antimicrobial agents, ticarcillin and cefoxitin, against 204 recent clinical isolates of obligate anaerobes and compared these results to their related compounds, carbenicillin, cephalothin, and penicillin, as well as to clindamycin, chloramphenicol, and metronidazole. Both of these newer agents have been reported to have broad spectrum activity against obligate anaerobes (5, 10, 14); however, only a limited number of strains has been studied previously.

MATERIALS AND METHODS

The isolates examined in this study, obtained from inpatients of Harbor General Hospital 1971 through 1975, are listed according to genus, species, and subspecies in Table 1. Identification and speciation were determined in prereduced anaerobically sterilized (PRAS) differential media, according to the method of Holdeman and Moore (6). A pH meter was used for recording carbohydrate fermentation reactions, and fatty acid analysis of fermentation products was performed with the AnaBac gas-liquid chromatograph. Clinical isolates were stored in 20% skim milk and frozen at −75°C until ready for susceptibility testing.

Susceptibility testing for all antimicrobial agents was determined on Mueller-Hinton agar (Difco), which had been adjusted to pH 7.2, and enriched with 10% defibrinated sheep blood and 0.01% (vol/vol) vitamin K-hemin. Twofold serial dilutions of ticarcillin (Beecham-Massengil), carbenicillin (Roerig), cefoxitin (Merck, Sharp & Dohme), cephalothin (Lilly), penicillin (USP), clindamycin (Upjohn), chloramphenicol (USP), and metronidazole (Searle) sensitivity powders were added. Test organisms in skim milk were inoculated into PRAS chopped-meat glucose, streaked for purity and growth characteristics, and subcultured in PRAS thioglycolate glucose broth. This subculture was incubated for 48 h and adjusted to a MacFarland no. 1 nephelometer standard (1), previously determined to approximate 10^6 to 10^7 organisms per ml by colony counting in roll tubes with PRAS media. Inocula (0.0025 ml) were delivered with a Steers replicating apparatus (13). Plates were then incubated at 37°C in anaerobic jars after air had been evacuated and replaced with a gas mixture containing 80% nitrogen, 10% hydrogen, and 10% carbon dioxide. Anaerobic, microaerophilic (incubated in a candle jar), and aerobic plates without antibiotics were used for controls, and a reference strain with known minimum inhibitory concentrations (MIC) was included in each test to demonstrate reproducibility. All results were read at 48 h, and the MIC recorded was the least antimicrobial concentration that yielded no visible growth.

RESULTS

The median and range of MIC of all eight antimicrobial agents against various obligate anaerobes tested are summarized in Table 2. Due to paucity of strains representing certain species or subspecies of isolates, data have been grouped and analyzed according to genus designation for most isolates. Relative activities of various antimicrobial agents (expressed as ra-

TABLE 1. *Genera and species of 204 obligate anaerobes tested*

Organism	No. tested	Organism	No. tested
Bacteroides fragilis	85	*Peptococcus*	37
subsp. fragilis	29	*P. asaccharolyticus*	13
subsp. vulgatus	17	*P. prevotii*	12
subsp. thetaiotaomicron	16	*P. magnus*	12
subsp. distasonis	13	*Peptostreptococcus*	29
subsp. ovatus	5	*P. anaerobius*	14
"Other"	5	*P. micros*	13
Bacteroides (not *fragilis*)	15	*P. intermedius*	2
B. melaninogenicus	8	*Clostridium perfringens*	9
B. capillosus	3	*Actinomyces naeslundii*	4
B. oralis	1	*Propionibacterium acnes*	8
B. corrodens	1	*Eubacterium*	11
B. amylophilus	1	*E. lentum*	10
B. pneumosintes	1	*E. aerofaciens*	1
Fusobacterium	3	*Veillonella parvula*	3
F. nucleatum	2		
F. naviforme	1		

TABLE 2. *Ranges of susceptibility of anaerobic bacteria to selected antimicrobial agents*

Genus/species (no. of isolates tested)		Median minimum inhibitory concn and range (μg/ml)			
		Ticarcillin	Carbenicillin	Cefoxitin	Cephalothin
Bacteroides fragilis	(85)	34.9 (≤3.1–800)	31.6 (6.2–800)	7.7 (2–≥128)	81.3 (8–≥128)
Bacteroides (miscellaneous)	(15)	≤1.8 (≤3.1–6.2)	≤1.8 (≤3.1–6.2)	0.5 (≤0.25–16)	3.0 (0.5–≥128)
Fusobacterium	(3)	≤3.1 (≤3.1–6.2)	≤3.1 (≤3.1–6.2)	≤0.25 (≤0.25–2)	0.75 (0.5–1)
Peptococcus	(37)	≤1.6 (≤3.1)	≤1.7 (≤3.1–12.5)	0.31 (≤0.25–64)	0.56 (≤0.25–≥128)
Peptostreptococcus	(29)	≤1.9 (≤3.1–50)	≤1.9 (≤3.1–50)	0.67 (≤0.25–32)	≤0.25 (≤0.25–16)
Clostridium	(9)	≤1.9 (≤3.1–12.5)	≤1.9 (≤3.1–12.5)	0.42 (≤0.25–2)	0.75 (≤0.25–2)
Actinomyces	(4)	≤1.5 (≤3.1)	≤1.5 (≤3.1)	2.0 (0.5–32)	4.0 (2–≥128)
Eubacterium	(11)	≤2.7 (≤3.1–25)	≤3.1 (≤3.1–25)	2.0 (≤0.25–8)	1.0 (≤0.25–≥128)
Propionibacterium	(8)	≤1.5 (≤3.1)	≤1.5 (≤3.1)	1.3 (0.5–4)	0.30 (≤0.25–0.5)
Veillonella	(3)	9.3 (6.2–12.5)	12.5 (6.2–25)	0.5 (≤0.25–4)	0.5 (≤0.25–16)
		Penicillin	Clindamycin	Chloramphenicol	Metronidazole
Bacteroides fragilis	(85)	14.4 (≤0.16–>80)	0.69 (≤0.02–≥10)	8.6 (≤0.1–25)	0.88 (≤0.2–≥100)
Bacteroides (miscellaneous)	(15)	≤0.13 (≤0.16–>80)	≤0.02 (≤0.02–5.0)	4.3 (≤0.1–50)	0.64 (≤0.2–≥100)
Fusobacterium	(3)	≤0.10 (≤0.16)	0.06 (≤0.02–0.08)	1.2(≤0.1–1.6)	≤0.13 (≤0.20)
Peptococcus	(37)	≤0.12 (≤0.16–20)	0.38 (≤0.02–>10)	3.1(≤0.1–25)	0.71 (≤0.2–≥100)
Peptostreptococcus	(29)	≤0.10 (≤0.16–10)	0.05 (≤0.02–0.62)	1.3(≤0.1–12.5)	2.3 (≤0.2–≥100)
Clostridium	(9)	≤0.10 (≤0.16–0.31)	1.25 (≤0.02–5.0)	4.0(1.6–12.5)	0.67 (≤0.2–1.6)
Actinomyces	(4)	≤0.16 (≤0.16–0.62)	0.31 (≤0.02–1.25)	2.4(0.8–6.25)	25.0 (0.8–≥100)
Eubacterium	(11)	≤0.21 (≤0.16–1.25)	0.08 (≤0.02–1.25)	4.0(≤0.1–12.5)	1.2 (≤0.2–≥100)
Propionibacterium	(8)	≤0.08 (≤0.16)	0.08 (≤0.02–1.25)	2.7(0.8–6.25)	>100 (>100)
Veillonella	(3)	≤0.08 (≤0.16)	0.12 (≤0.02–0.16)	9.4(0.8–6.25)	9.4 (≤0.2–12.5)

tios of antimicrobial concentrations readily achievable in plasma to concentrations required to inhibit growth of 90% of isolates) are also summarized in Table 3.

Against *B. fragilis*, ticarcillin was equally active as carbenicillin, with a similar median MIC and comparable relative activity. Cefoxitin was far superior to cephalothin. At readily achieved blood concentrations, the relative activity of ticarcillin against *B. fragilis* was slightly less active than clindamycin and metronidazole, but higher than the remaining agents.

With the exception of cephalothin and metronidazole, relative activities of all antimicrobial agents tested were more than adequate against obligate anaerobes other than *Bacteroides*.

Metronidazole demonstrated variable activity against obligate anaerobes other than *B. fragilis*, and was least active against *Propionibacterium*, *Actinomyces*, *Peptostreptococcus*, and *Peptococcus*.

DISCUSSION

Recent awareness of the potential serious complications of clindamycin (3, 8, 15) as well as chloramphenicol (16) has prompted an intensive search for alternative antimicrobial agents with excellent activity against obligate anaerobes, especially *B. fragilis*. Additionally, an increasing number of obligate anaerobes has been noted to be resistant to chloramphenicol (7) as well as clindamycin (12). For these reasons, the in vitro activity of several potentially useful, newer antimicrobial agents was tested and compared.

Carbenicillin has been reported as an effective and relatively safe agent in the therapy of certain anerobic infections (4). In the present study, however, it was slightly less active than clindamycin and metronidazole against *B. fragilis* at readily achievable blood concentrations.

Ticarcillin, a newer semisynthetic penicillin, which has been demonstrated to be more active in vitro against certain aerobic gram-negative bacilli than carbenicillin (2, 9), also appears to be comparable to carbenicillin for all species of obligate anaerobes tested. With respect to *B. fragilis*, ticarcillin was slightly less active than clindamycin and metronidazole, but was more active than chloramphenicol, cefoxitin, cephalothin, and penicillin.

Cefoxitin, while inferior to ticarcillin against *B. fragilis* in vitro, was comparable to ticarcillin, carbenicillin, clindamycin and chloramphenicol against the remaining obligate anaer-

TABLE 3. *Relative activities of various antimicrobial agents against diverse genera and species of anaerobic bacteria*[a]

Genus/species (No. of isolates tested)		RACP/MIC$_{90}$ (μg/ml)[b]			
		Ticarcillin	Carbenicillin	Cefoxitin	Cephalothin
Bacteroides fragilis	(85)	100/97.7 (1.0)	100/95.8 (1.0)	16/25.8 (0.6)	16/>128 (<0.1)
Bacteroides (misc.)	(15)	100/≤3.0 (≥33.3)	100/≤3.0 (≥33.3)	16/10.0 (1.6)	16/>128 (<0.1)
Fusobacterium	(3)	100/5.7 (17.5)	100/5.7 (17.5)	16/1.7 (9.4)	16/0.92 (17.3)
Peptococcus	(37)	100/≤2.8 (≥35.7)	100/≤3.0 (≤33.3)	16/3.3 (4.8)	16/10.4 (1.5)
Peptostreptococcus	(29)	100/6.2 (16.1)	100/9.6 (10.4)	16/6.7 (2.3)	16/2.1 (7.6)
Clostridium	(9)	100/4.04 (24.8)	100/4.04 (24.8)	16/1.1 (14.5)	16/1.7 (9.4)
Actinomyces	(4)	100/≤2.8 (≥35.7)	100/≤2.8 (≥35.7)	16/25.6 (0.6)	16/>128 (<0.1)
Eubacterium	(11)	100/9.0 (11.1)	100/12.1 (8.2)	16/5.8 (2.7)	16/30.4 (0.5)
Propionibacterium	(8)	100/≤2.8 (≥35.7)	100/≤2.8 (≥35.7)	16/3.2 (5.0)	16/0.46 (34.7)
Veillonella	(3)	100/11.5 (8.7)	100/21.2 (4.7)	16/3.4 (4.7)	16/13.6 (1.1)

Genus/species (No. of isolates tested)		Penicillin	Clindamycin	Chloramphenicol	Metronidazole
Bacteroides fragilis	(85)	16/55 (0.3)	5/2.2 (2.3)	12.5/16.8 (0.7)	12.5/3.6 (3.5)
Bacteroides (misc.)	(15)	16/30 (0.5)	5/0.47 (10.6)	12.5/10.9 (1.1)	12.5/>100 (<0.1)
Fusobacterium	(3)	16/≤0.14 (≥114.3)	5/0.07 (71.4)	12.5/1.48 (8.4)	12.5/≤0.18 (≥69.4)
Peptococcus	(37)	16/0.57 (28.0)	5/3.3 (1.5)	12.5/9.7 (1.3)	12.5/>100 (<0.1)
Peptostreptococcus	(29)	16/≤0.14 (≥114.3)	5/0.24 (20.8)	12.5/4.4 (2.8)	12.5/>100 (<0.1)
Clostridium	(9)	16/0.24 (66.6)	5/2.8 (1.8)	12.5/6.9 (1.8)	12.5/1.36 (9.2)
Actinomyces	(4)	16/0.50 (32.0)	5/1.1 (4.5)	12.5/5.1 (2.4)	12.5/>100 (<0.1)
Eubacterium	(11)	16/0.60 (26.6)	5/0.91 (5.5)	12.5/9.1 (1.4)	12.5/95 (0.1)
Propionibacterium	(8)	16/≤0.15 (≥106.6)	5/0.75 (6.6)	12.5/5.5 (2.3)	12.5/>100 (<0.1)
Veillonella	(3)	16/≤0.14 (≥114.3)	5/0.15 (33.3)	12.5/11.6 (1.1)	12.5/11.6 (1.1)

[a] Expressed as ratios of concentrations readily obtained in plasma (RACP) to concentrations required to inhibit growth of 90% of isolates (MIC$_{90}$).

[b] Figure in parenthesis, calculated index.

obes tested. Its strikingly improved activity compared with cephalothin and penicillin is undoubtedly related to its resistance against beta-lactamase of *B. fragilis* (10, 11).

These in vitro data indicate that ticarcillin, carbenicillin, and cefoxitin may be useful alternative agents for clindamycin and chloramphenicol in the treatment of serious anaerobic infections, and further clinical studies with these agents are clearly warranted.

LITERATURE CITED

1. **Bailey, W. R., and E. G. Scott (ed.).** 1970. Diagnostic Microbiology. C. V. Mosby, St. Louis.
2. **Bodey, G. P., and B. Deerhake.** 1971. In vitro studies of α-carboxyl-3-thienylmethyl penicillin, a new semisynthetic penicillin. Antimicrob. Agents Chemother. 21:61–65.
3. **Cohen, L. E., C. J. McNeill, and R. F. Wells.** 1973. Clindamycin-associated colitis. J. Am. Med. Assoc. 223:1379–1380.
4. **Fiedelman, W., and C. C. Webb.** 1975. Clinical evaluation of carbenicillin in the treatment of infection due to anaerobic bacteria. Curr. Ther. Res. 18:441–451.
5. **Finegold, S. M., J. G. Bartlett, A. W. Chow, D. J. Flora, S. L. Gorbach, E. J. Harder, and F. P. Tally.** 1975. Management of anaerobic infections. Ann. Intern. Med. 83:375–389.
6. **Holdeman, L. V., and W. E. C. Moore (ed.)** 1972. Anaerobe laboratory manual. Virginia Polytechnic Institute Anaerobe Laboratory, Blacksburg.
7. **Kagnoff, M. F., and D. Armstrong.** 1971. Antibiotics for Bacteroides sepsis (letter to the editor). Ann. Intern. Med. 75:316–317.
8. **Keusch, G. T., and D. H. Present.** 1976. Summary of a workshop of clindamycin colitis. J. Infect. Dis. 133:578–588.
9. **Neu, H. C., and E. B. Winshell.** 1971. In vitro studies of a semisynthetic penicillin 6-[D(-)-α-carboxy-3-thienylacetamido] penicillin acid (BRL 2288), active against *Pseudomonas,* p. 385–389. Antimicrob. Agents Chemother. 1970.
10. **Norrby, R., J. E. Brorsson, and S. Seeberg.** 1976. Comparative study of the in vitro antibacterial activity of cefoxitin, cefuroxime, and cephaloridine. Antimicrobe. Agents Chemother. 9:506–510.
11. **Onishi, H. R., D. R. Daoust, S. B. Zimmerman, D. Henoun, and E. O. Staphley.** 1974. Cefoxitin, a semisynthetic antibiotic resistant to beta-lactamase inactivation. Antimicrob. Agents Chemother. 5:38–48.
12. **Salaki, J. S., R. Black, F. P. Tally, and J. W. Kislak.** 1976. *Bacteroides fragilis* resistant to the administration of clindamycin. Am. J. Med. 60:426–428.
13. **Steers, E., E. L. Foltz, B. S. Graves, and J. Riden.** 1959. Inocula-replicating apparatus for routine testing of bacterial susceptibility to antibiotics. Antibiot. Chemother. 9:307–311.
14. **Tally, F. P., N. V. Jacobus, J. G. Bartlett, and S. L. Gorbach.** 1975. Susceptibility of anaerobes to cefoxitin and other cephalosporins. Antimicrob. Agents Chemother. 7:128–132.
15. **Tedesco, F. J., R. W. Barton, and D. H. Alders.** 1974. Clindamycin-associated colitis, a prospective study. Ann. Intern. Med. 81:429–433.
16. **Wallerstein, R. O., P. K. Conoit, and C. K. Kasper.** 1969. Statewide study of chloramphenicol therapy and fatal aplastic anemia. J. Am. Med. Assoc. 208:2045–2050.

ANTIMICROBIAL AGENTS AND CHEMOTHERAPY, Apr. 1977, p. 683-687 Vol. 11, No. 4

Printed in U.S.A.

Indirect Mouse Model for the Evaluation of Potential Antiviral Compounds: Results with Venezuelan Equine Encephalomyelitis Virus

RALPH W. KUEHNE,* WALLACE L. PANNIER, AND EDWARD L. STEPHEN

United States Army Medical Research Institute of Infectious Diseases, Fort Detrick, Frederick, Maryland 21701

Received for publication 15 November 1976

An indirect mouse model was utilized to evaluate the antiviral activity of several compounds against Venezuelan equine encephalomyelitis (VEE) virus infection in mice. Mice were given various dosages of lysine-stabilized polyriboinosinic acid-polyribocytidylic acid, a tilorone analogue, kethoxal, or mepacrine before and/or shortly after receiving one of several dose levels of attenuated strain TC-83 VEE virus. Twenty-one days later, the same mice were rechallenged intracranially with virulent Trinidad donkey strain VEE virus. Susceptibility to rechallenge was interpreted as evidence of drug effectiveness in completely preventing the initial immunizing virus infection. In contrast, if a drug lacked antiviral effectiveness, the initial attenuated infection stimulated sufficient immunity to protect mice against the virulent rechallenge. Both of the interferon inducers, lysine-stabilized polyriboinosinic acid-polyribocytidylic acid and tilorone analogue 11,567, possessed significant ($P < 0.01$) antiviral activity based upon this indirect model, whereas mepacrine and kethoxal were inactive. Results using the indirect method were confirmed by using the conventional direct method for evaluating the effectiveness of potentially useful antiviral compounds. The indirect mouse model described should prove useful for studying drug efficacy against certain viruses that are lethal only by intracranial inoculation.

Antiviral chemotherapy has become potentially feasible in recent years as a result of extensive empirical screening programs (1, 2, 6). However, only a few selected compounds have been successful in clinical trials (9, 17, 24). The lack of satisfactory in vivo experimental models has in some cases hindered progress in proceeding to clinical trials in man (22, 24). Because chemotherapy has great potential to control certain viral diseases (2, 10, 17), we have undertaken studies to evaluate the in vivo antiviral activity of a number of selected compounds in the laboratory mouse. The compounds were selected especially for their previously described biological activity in both in vitro and in vivo test systems (11, 16, 31; G. D. Mayer, A. C. Hagan, and F. Bray, Fed. Proc. 32:704, 1973). This report describes (i) a new, indirect method for the evaluation of potential and antiviral compounds against viruses that are lethal only by intracranial inoculation, and (ii) results of investigations to assess the effectiveness of several antiviral compounds against Venezuelan equine encephalomyelitis (VEE) virus infection in the laboratory mouse.

MATERIALS AND METHODS

Animals. Weanling (18 to 25 days old) outbred albino Swiss male mice (ICR) were obtained from Flow Laboratories, Dublin, Va. The mice were housed four to six per cage, fed, and given water ad libitum.

Viruses. Live, attenuated VEE vaccine virus (TC-83) was used to immunize mice in these studies and has been described previously (27). TC-83 vaccine, lot 3, run 9, supplied by Merrill-National Laboratories, Swiftwater, Pa., was reconstituted with modified Hanks balanced salt solution containing 0.5% human serum albumin. When administered subcutaneously (s.c.), this attenuated virus is not lethal and can immunize mice against subsequent intracranial (i.c.) challenge with virulent virus (26). The Trinidad donkey strain of virulent VEE virus was used as a rechallenge virus for mice used in indirect tests and as a primary challenge for mice used in the direct test (20). The virus was originally isolated in guinea pigs and has been maintained by 13 serial passages in embryonated chicken eggs and 2 passages in primary chicken fibroblast cells. This strain of VEE virus produces fatal paralytic disease in mice when inoculated by s.c., intraperitoneal (i.p.), or i.c. routes. Inocula were diluted in modified Hanks balanced salt solution containing 2% fetal calf serum.

Animal techniques. (i) Indirect method: the theory of the indirect VEE model is based on the assumption that mice will not be immunized by a live, attenuated virus (TC-83) if an antiviral compound prevents replication of the attenuated virus to the extent that it cannot produce protective immunity; thus, successfully treated mice are susceptible to rechallenge using the virulent strain of VEE virus. In this model, death of the mouse indicates a successful earlier treatment. Mice were initially given either 500 or 5,000 guinea pig i.p. median immunizing doses ($GPIPID_{50}$) of attenuated TC-83 VEE virus administered s.c. Evaluation of antiviral activity was based on decreased percentage of survivors in drug-treated groups of mice after i.c. rechallenge with 1,000 plaque-forming units (PFU) of Trinidad VEE virus 21 days after the inoculation of TC-83 VEE virus. (ii) Direct method: in the direct VEE mouse model, the antiviral compound acts directly on an otherwise lethal virus, limits its replication, and prevents death of the host. Subcutaneous virus inoculations with 0, 10, 100, and 1,000 PFU of the virulent Trinidad donkey strain of VEE virus were used to establish infections in the direct method studies. Successful antiviral activity by this method was assessed by increased percentage of survivors in drug-treated mice at 14 days. All survivors were rechallenged at 21 days with 1,000 PFU of Trinidad VEE virus by the s.c. route to determine whether drug treatment prevented an immunizing infection in surviving animals.

Compounds. (i) Kethoxal: β-ethoxy-α-ketobutyraldehyde monohydrate, supplied as 54% aqueous concentrate from G. E. Underwood, The Upjohn Co., Kalamazoo, Mich.; (ii) lysine-stabilized polyriboinosinic-polyribocytidylic acid [poly (ICLC)]: a complex of poly(I)·poly(C) with poly-1-lysine and carboxymethylcellulose (16), received from H. B. Levy, National Institute of Health, Bethesda, Md.; (iii) mepacrine: 3-chlor-7-methoxy-9-(1-methyl-4-diethylaminobutylamino)acridine dihydrochloride, received from M. H. Heiffer, Walter Reed Army Institute of Research, Washington, D.C.; and (iv) tilorone analogue RMI 11,567DA: 2,8-bis[2-(dimethylamino)acetyl]-dibenzofuran dihydrochloride, received from G. D. Mayer, Merrill-National Laboratories, Cincinnati, Ohio. All compounds were dissolved in pyrogen-free 0.85% NaCl solution prior to use. Dosages ranged from 1 to 250 mg/kg. Compounds were administered on a milligrams-per-kilogram basis. In both the direct and indirect studies, tilorone analogue 11,567 was given 24 h before the time of virus inoculation, and poly(ICLC) was given 24 h before and again at the time of virus inoculation. Kethoxal was administered 2 h before and 24 h after virus inoculation in the direct method studies, and at 8 and 24 h after virus inoculation in the indirect method studies. Mepacrine was given 8 h before virus in the direct method studies, and 2 h before and 24 h after virus in the indirect method studies. All compounds were administered i.p. with the exception of poly(ICLC), which was given s.c. Each study included appropriate control groups of infected, untreated mice and uninfected, treated mice.

Statistical analysis of data. Independent comparisons were made for each virus dose by partitioning the overall chi-square for the given virus dose into independent chi-squares with single degrees of freedom (29). For a given comparison among dose levels, the ratio of dead to total animals in the untreated group was compared with the ratio of dead to total animals in the lowest-drug-dosage group. If no significance ($P < 0.01$) was found, the two ratios were averaged and compared with the response to the next higher dose (29). This averaging of responses for comparison with the next higher dose of drug was continued until a significant ($P < 0.01$) difference was found between the response of mice at a higher dosage level and that of previous groups in which no significant difference was noted. Data from two replicate experiments were not significantly different and were combined.

RESULTS

Results using the indirect method, by which the antiviral effects of poly(ICLC), analogue 11,567, kethoxal, or mepacrine on attenuated VEE virus infection of mice are manifested by susceptibility to lethal rechallenge, are presented in Table 1. Preliminary trials indicated that dosages equal to or greater than 500 mg of 11,567 per kg, 120 mg of kethoxal per kg or 250 mg of mepacrine per kg were significantly ($P < 0.01$) toxic to mice, and that an immunizing dose of 50 $GPIPID_{50}$ of TC-83 was not adequate for sufficient immunization of untreated control mice to demonstrate significant effects of treatment. Prophylactic treatment with 1 or 3 mg of poly(ICLC) per kg was effective against 500 or 5,000 $GPIPID_{50}$ of TC-83 virus, resulting in significantly reduced survival in each treatment group following virulent challenge 21 days after immunization with TC-83 virus. All concentrations (31.3 to 250 mg/kg) of analogue 11,567 were also significantly effective against 500 or 5,000 $GPIPID_{50}$ of TC-83 virus. Kethoxal or mepacrine was ineffective.

Table 2 shows results of studies to assess the effects of prophylactic administration of potential compounds on Trinidad VEE virus infection in mice as determined by survival (direct method). Significant antiviral activity was detected with both 1 and 3 mg of poly(ICLC) per kg against 10, 100, and 1,000 PFU of Trinidad VEE virus. None of the dose levels of either kethoxal or mepacrine showed significant antiviral activity against any of the challenge levels of virus. Survivors of all studies were uniformly susceptible to rechallenge with 1,000 PFU of Trinidad VEE virus.

DISCUSSION

The concept of an indirect model for use in chemotherapy studies appears to be valid, since similar conclusions regarding the antiviral activity of several compounds are obtained using both the direct and indirect VEE mouse models. In previous studies with the direct method, tilorone analogue 11,567 exhibited effective antiviral activity against virulent VEE virus infection in mice when given prophylactically: 125 mg/kg showed significant activity against 100 PFU of virus, and 250 mg/kg was significantly active against 100 and 1,000 PFU of Trinidad VEE virus (15). Significant in vivo activity of poly(ICLC) against VEE virus infection in mice confirms previous findings by others using the direct model with nonstabilized poly(I)·poly(C) (30). In addition, we have shown that prophylactic treatment of mice with analogue 11,567 or poly(ICLC) successfully controlled a TC-83 VEE virus infection that normally stimulates development of immunity.

The protective action of both 11,567 and poly(ICLC) is presumed to be due to the induction of endogenous interferon (4, 18, 19, 23). Both virulent Trinidad and attenuated TC-83 strains of VEE virus are susceptible to the antiviral activity of interferon (13). Although tilorone and structurally related compounds increase concentrations of interferon in serum in rodents, but not in monkeys or man (14; H. E. Kaufman and Y. Centifanto, J. Clin. Invest. 50:53a, 1971), some antiviral activity of analogue 11,567 has been observed against TC-83 in monkeys (G. D. Mayer, A. C. Hagan, and F. Bray, Fed. Proc. 32:704, 1973). Although it has been reported that interferon cannot be induced in Vero cells (5), recent in vitro studies (W. L. Pannier, unpublished data) have shown that (per ml) 50 μg of either tilorone or its analogues or poly(ICLC) results an 80% reduction in Trinidad VEE virus plaques in Vero cell cultures,

TABLE 1. *Effect of prophylactic administration of poly(ICLC), tilorone analogue 11,567, kethoxal, or mepacrine on immunization of mice with TC-83 VEE virus as determined by susceptibility to lethal challenge (indirect method)*

Drug (mg/kg)	% Deaths (dead/total) after challenge with virulent virus with $GPIPID_{50}$ of TC-83 virus: 500	5,000
No drug	22 (8/37)	3 (1/30)
Poly(ICLC)		
1	95[a] (56/59)	89[a] (24/27)
3	100[a] (58/58)	61[a] (17/28)
11,567		
31.3	58[a] (35/60)	41[a] (11/27)
62.5	76[a] (45/58)	27[a] (8/30)
125	91[a] (49/54)	69[a] (20/29)
250	96[a] (48/50)	71[a] (17/24)
Kethoxal		
60	34 (20/58)	4 (1/27)
Mepacrine		
31.3	43 (25/58)	14 (4/28)
62.5	42 (25/59)	17 (5/29)
125	47 (24/51)	7 (2/27)

[a] $P < 0.01$ compared with untreated infected mice.

TABLE 2. *Effect of prophylactic administration of poly(ICLC), kethoxal, or mepacrine on virulent VEE virus infection of mice as determined by survival (direct method)*

Drug (mg/kg)	% Survival (survivors/total) 14 days postchallenge with PFU of virus: 0	10	100	1,000
Poly(ICLC)				
0	100 (30/30)	50 (15/30)	20 (6/30)	0 (0/30)
1	97 (29/30)	93[a] (28/30)	90[a] (27/30)	83[a] (25/30)
3	100 (30/30)	100[a] (30/30)	100[a] (30/30)	[a] (26/30-
Kethoxal				
0	100 (10/10)	80 (8/10)	50 (5/10)	0 (0/10)
40	100 (10/10)	80 (8/10)	20 (2/10)	0 (0/10)
60	100 (10/10)	50 (5/10)	50 (5/10)	0 (0/10)
Mepacrine				
0	100 (10/10)	40 (4/10)	0 (0/10)	0 (0/10)
62.5	100 (10/10)	50 (5/10)	0 (0/10)	0 (0/10)
125	90 (9/10)	60 (6/10)	0 (0/10)	0 (0/10)

[a] $P < 0.01$ compared with untreated infected mice.

with no evidence of cytopathic effects. Protection in the absence of detectable interferon may be due to some other unknown mechanisms, such as cellular immunity, production of lymphokines, or insensitivity of the interferon assay methodology.

Although no detectable activity can be seen with kethoxal against VEE infection in mice in the present studies, in vitro virucidal activity has been reported by others against numerous viruses including Sindbis, influenza A and B, and Western equine encephalomyelitis (WEE) (21, 31). Mepacrine has been reported to exert antiviral activity against the causative viruses of Rift Valley fever, herpes febrilis, lymphocytic choriomeningitis, St. Louis encephalomyelitis, louping ill, WEE, and Eastern equine encephalomyelitis in mice when treatment was initiated before, or soon after, infection (11), but no significant activity was found against VEE virus infection in mice in our studies by either the direct or indirect method of evaluation.

In the development of usable experimental animal model systems with a human disease-producing virus, investigators have tended to limit the therapeutic potential of some compounds by selecting virus strains with a short incubation period and high mortality and administering high dosages by an unnatural route of infection into a host selected for maximum susceptibility (22). Such fulminating diseases produced in response to massive doses of host-adapted virus progress rapidly, often with extensive and irreversible damage to the host. Potential antiviral activity of a given drug tested against such overwhelming infections might conceivably be partially or totally obscured (7). The use of such unrealistically demanding models to screen candidate antiviral compounds might yield essentially negative results (22). Subclinical infections, on the other hand, may provide a more sensitive and conceivably more realistic approach to drug evaluation (7).

We have described a novel and effective model for in vivo evaluation of potential antiviral compounds based on the prophylaxis of asymptomatic infection detectable directly by immunological response. VEE virus was selected for initial studies to assess the validity of this indirect method because this infection enables a comparison to be made with the more conventional direct method of measuring antiviral activity. The indirect model more closely resembles conditions of natural infections and may be applied to yellow fever, Tacaribe, certain strains of WEE, and any other viruses, inoculated peripherally, which are only lethal for the laboratory mouse when inoculated by the i.c. or other unnatural route.

The utilization of the serological response as a measure of prevention of subclinical infection in absence of overt disease is not in itself a new approach (8). Others have successfully employed the measurement of antibody in clinical trial evaluations of antiviral compounds in volunteers challenged with live, attenuated viruses (12, 28). An enlarged application of this basic principle to the study of experimental animal infections with potential utility in the search for antiviral agents was proposed by Engle et al. (7) and by Davies et al. (3).

A compound with potentially useful antiviral activity may well be overlooked by overwhelming the animal with virus or by testing a single dose of the compound. The importance of varying dose levels of both virus and potential antiviral compounds is borne out in these and previous studies (15), since it is possible to make the virus dose sufficiently high so that drug effectiveness is reduced and, conversely, drug dose can be increased so that toxic manifestations reduce beneficial effects of therapy. We concur with the suggestion of Sidwell et al. (25) that additional criteria besides in vitro or in vivo activity or both be used in the evaluation of potential antiviral compounds, including antiviral activity in a reasonable and orderly dose response, and decreasing activity when an effective dose regimen of compound is used against progressively increasing concentrations of the infectious agent.

ACKNOWLEDGMENTS

We gratefully acknowledge Glen A. Higbee for the statistical analysis of our data, Duane E. Hilmas, Peter B. Jahrling, and Harry Rozmiarek for their critical review, and Debra A. Stevens for typing the manuscript.

LITERATURE CITED

1. **Bucknall, R. A.** 1973. The continuing search for antiviral drugs. Adv. Pharmacol. Chemother. 11:295–319.
2. **Buthala, D. A.** 1965. Experience gained in screening synthetic antiviral compounds. Ann. N. Y. Acad. Sci. 130:17–23.
3. **Davies, W. L., R. R. Grunert, and C. E. Hoffmann.** 1966. Influenza virus growth and antibody response in amantadine-treated mice. J. Immunol. 95:1090–1094.
4. **De Clercq, E., and T. C. Merigan.** 1971. Bis-DEAE-fluorenone: mechanism of antiviral protection and stimulation of interferon production in the mouse. J. Infect. Dis. 123:190–199.
5. **Desmyter, J., J. L. Melnick, and W. E. Rawls.** 1968. Defectiveness of interferon production and of rubella virus interference in a line of African green monkey kidney cells (Vero). J. Virol. 2:955–961.
6. **Dice, J. R., W. A. Rightsel, F. M. Schabel, Jr., and I. W. McLean, Jr.** 1965. Experiences in developing po-

tential antiviral compounds. Ann. N. Y. Acad. Sci. 130:24–30.
7. **Engle, C. G., J. W. Frankel, and J. Gelzer,** 1970. Quantitative assessment of virus inhibition by indirect techniques *in vivo*. Ann. N. Y. Acad. Sci. 173:139–150.
8. **Goulet, N. R., K. W. Cochran, and G. C. Brown.** 1960. Differential and specific inhibition of ECHO viruses by plant extracts. Proc. Soc. Exp. Biol. Med. 103:96–100.
9. **Haff, R. F.** 1970. The future: antiviral drugs or vaccines. Ann. N. Y. Acad. Sci. 173:210–214.
10. **Herrmann, E. C., Jr.** 1970. Introductory remarks. Ann. N. Y. Acad. Sci. 173:9.
11. **Hurst, W. E., J. M. Peters, and P. Melvin.** 1952. The action of mepacrine and trypan red in a number of virus diseases. Br. J. Pharmacol. 7:473–481.
12. **Jackson, G. G., R. L. Muldoon, and L. W. Akers.** 1964. Serological evidence for prevention of influenzal infection in volunteers by an anti-influenzal drug adamantanamine hydrochloride, p. 703–707. Antimicrob. Agents Chemother. 1963.
13. **Jordan, G. W.** 1973. Interferon sensitivity of Venezuelan equine encephalomyelitis virus. Infect. Immun. 7:911–917.
14. **Kaufman, H. E., Y. M. Centifanto, E. D. Ellison, and D. C. Brown.** 1971. Tilorone hydrochloride: human toxicity and interferon stimulation. Proc. Soc. Exp. Biol. Med. 137:357–360.
15. **Kuehne, R. W., W. L. Pannier, and E. L. Stephen.** 1977. Evaluation of various analogues of tilorone hydrochloride against Venezuelan equine encephalomyelitis virus in mice. Antimicrob. Agents Chemother. 11:92–97.
16. **Levy, H. B., G. Baer, S. Baron, C. E. Buckler, C. J. Gibbs, M. J. Iadarola, W. T. London, and J. Rice.** 1975. A modified polyriboinosinic-polyribocytidylic acid complex that induces interferon in primates. J. Infect. Dis. 132:434–439.
17. **Maugh, T. H., II.** 1976. Chemotherapy: antiviral agents come of age. Science 92:128–132.
18. **Mayer, G. D., and R. F. Krueger.** 1970. Tilorone hydrochloride: mode of action. Science 169:1214–1215.
19. **Merigan, T. C., E. De Clercq, M. S. Finkelstein, L. Clever, S. Walker, and D. J. Waddell.** 1970. Clinical studies employing interferon inducers in man and animals. Ann. N. Y. Acad. Sci. 173:746–759.
20. **Randall, R., and J. W. Mills.** 1944. Fatal encephalitis in man due to the Venezuelan virus of equine encephalomyelitis in Trinidad. Science 99:225–226.
21. **Renis, H. E.** 1970. Antiviral studies with kethoxal. Ann. N. Y. Acad. Sci. 173:527–535.
22. **Schabel, F. M.** 1965. Virus chemotherapy—why and how. Ala. J. Med. Sci. 2:149–154.
23. **Schafer, T. W., and R. Z. Lockart, Jr.** 1970. Interferon required for viral resistance induced by poly I·poly C. Nature (London) 226:449–450.
24. **Sidwell, R. W.** 1976. Viral diseases: a review of chemotherapy systems, p. 31–53. *In* H. H. Gadebusch (ed.), Chemotherapy of infectious diseases. CRC Press, Cleveland, Ohio.
25. **Sidwell, R. W., G. J. Dixon, S. M. Sellers, and F. M. Schabel, Jr.** 1968. In vivo antiviral properties of biologically active compounds. II. Studies with influenza and vaccinia viruses. Appl. Microbiol. 16:370–392.
26. **Spertzel, R. O., D. E. Hilmas, J. R. Brown, and D. W. Mason.** 1975. Response of irradiated mice to live-virus (TC-83) immunization. Infect. Immun. 11:481–487.
27. **Spertzel, R. O., and D. E. Kahn.** 1971. Safety and efficacy of an attenuated Venezuelan equine encephalomyelitis vaccine for use in *Equidae*. J. Am. Vet. Med. Assoc. 159:731–738.
28. **Stanley, E. D., R. E. Muldoon, L. W. Akers, and G. G. Jackson.** 1965. Evaluation of antiviral drugs: the effect of amantadine on influenza in volunteers. Ann. N. Y. Acad. Sci. 130:44–51.
29. **Steel, R. G. D., and J. H. Torrie.** 1960. Principles and procedures of statistics. McGraw-Hill Book Co., New York.
30. **Tazulakhova, E. B., A. S. Novokhatsky, and F. I. Yershov.** 1973. Interferon induction by, and antiviral effect of poly (rI)-poly (rC) in experimental viral infection. Acta Virol. 17:487–492.
31. **Underwood, G. E., and S. D. Weed.** 1961. The effect of carbonyl compounds on poliovirus. Virology 13:138–139.

ANTIMICROBIAL AGENTS AND CHEMOTHERAPY, Apr. 1977, p. 688-694 Vol. 11, No. 4

Printed in U.S.A.

Tobramycin: Maternal-Fetal Pharmacology

BETTY BERNARD,* SALVADOR J. GARCIA-CÁZARES,[1] CHARLES A. BALLARD, LAURI D. THRUPP, ALLEN W. MATHIES, AND PAUL F. WEHRLE

*Departments of Pediatrics and Obstetrics and Gynecology, and the Hastings Infectious Disease Laboratory, University of Southern California School of Medicine, and the Los Angeles County/University of Southern California Medical Center, Los Angeles, California 90033**

Received for publication 5 October 1976

To investigate the maternal-fetal transfer of tobramycin (TBM) and its distribution in the fetus, a single dose of 2 mg/kg was administered intramuscularly to 35 pregnant patients (13 first trimester, 22 second trimester) 0.5 to 34 h before hysterectomy. TBM concentration was assayed microbiologically in maternal serum, fetal tissues (placenta, brain, lung, liver, and kidney), and fluids (amniotic, cerebrospinal fluid [CSF], urine, and serum). Mean maternal serum half-life (1.54 h) and mean peak serum concentration of TBM were within ranges reported for nonpregnant adults. In fetal serum, half-life was 5.2 h, and TBM levels did not exceed 0.58 μg/ml. For intervals up to 34 h, the mean TBM concentration in placental tissues was 1.4 μg/g. Concentration differences related to fetal maturation were found for fetal CSF, amniotic fluid, and fetal kidney. No antimicrobial activity was found in the fetal CSF of >16 weeks' gestation. TBM was present predominantly in the second trimester amniotic fluid specimens. Fetal kidney concentrations reached 7.2 μg/g at 34 h after maternal drug administration. Higher TBM concentrations were related to advanced maturation of the fetal kidney. Second trimester fetal urine concentrations for TBM ranged from 0.1 to 3.4 μg/ml, and the fetal urinary half-life was 3.7 h. Knowledge of fetal pharmacology is essential for weighing the fetal benefits or risks of antimicrobial therapy for the infected gravid patient.

Tobramycin (tobramycin sulfate [Nebcin]; TBM) is one of the more recently identified components of the nebramycin complex introduced by Stark et al. (12) in 1967. Nebramycin is known to have eight factors, of which TBM is factor 6. These are water-soluble, basic compounds that fall into the general class of aminoglycosidic antibiotics produced by fermentation biosynthesis with *Streptomyces tenebrarius*.

TBM sulfate was released for clinical use in the United States in 1975. Its particular effectiveness is in the inhibition of *Pseudomonas* species, including those resistant to other aminoglycosides. The clinical benefits and risks of maternal therapy for the conceptus are often overlooked because of a paucity of human data. This study was undertaken to investigate the maternal-fetal transfer of TBM and its distribution in the human fetus of 9 to 20 weeks' gestation.

(Presented in part at the American Pediatric Society-Society for Pediatric Research, San Francisco, Calif., May 1973.)

[1] Present address: Instituto Nacional de Perinatologia, Vosgos y Montes Urales, Lomas de Chapultepec, Mexico 10, D.F.

MATERIALS AND METHODS

Thirty-five healthy gravid patients were admitted from July 1972 to June 1973 for elective therapeutic abortion and sterilization by hysterectomy. After informed consent was obtained, a single 2-mg/kg intramuscular dose of TBM was administered to the patients before surgery. Thirteen patients were in the first (I) trimester, and 22 were in the second (II) trimester. The time interval between administration of TBM to the patient and the clamping of the uterine arteries at delivery will be referred to as an "interval" in this report. This interval varied from 2 to 20.5 h for the trimester I patients and from 40 min to 34 h for trimester II patients. Thirty-four fetuses, from 9 to 20 weeks' gestation, were available for sampling.

Gestational age was calculated from day 1 of the last normal menstrual period. When the date of the last menstrual period was uncertain, fetal weight and foot length were used to estimate gestational age (13).

Maternal serum samples were taken before the intramuscular administration and at 1, 2, 4 and 8 h after the injection of TBM. A delivery time sample was obtained at the time of uterine artery clamping.

After surgical removal of the uterus, its contents were dissected under sterile conditions. Total amniotic fluid volume was measured, and an aliquot was taken for sampling. The placenta was separated, weighed, and sampled. The fetus was weighed and then measured for crown-heel, crown-rump, and foot length. Fetal blood, urine, and cerebrospinal fluid (CSF) samples were obtained by needle aspiration. Fetal brain, lung, liver, and kidney tissue samples were acquired by dissection. Complete sampling of all fetal tissues and fluids was not technically possible in fetuses of less than 12 weeks' gestation. All specimens were frozen at −20°C until time of TBM assay.

TBM concentrations in maternal and fetal tissues and fluids were determined in duplicate by microbiological assay (1) with a modified standard cylinder plate method and *Bacillus subtilis* (ATCC 6633) on AM11 agar (Difco, 0593-01, Detroit, Mich.). The lowest detectable TBM concentrations were the following: 0.06 μg/ml for fetal urine and in maternal and fetal serum; 0.1 μg/ml for fetal CSF and amniotic fluid; 0.4 μg/g for placenta; and 0.08 μg/g for fetal brain, kidney, lung, and liver. Control curves of fetal tissues and fluids were made from a pool of six antibiotic-free fetuses.

STATISTICS

The two-sample rank test (the Mann-Whitney *U* test) was used to measure the significance of differences between any two groups of data, and significance levels were judged at $P < 0.01$. A regression line, determined by the method of least squares, was obtained from individual TBM concentrations in tissues and fluids and extrapolated to theoretical time zero. The time at which the sample concentration was one-half the concentration at theoretical time zero was defined as the half-life ($t_{1/2}$) with the following equation: $t_{1/2} = (-\log_e 2)/\beta$, where β is the rate constant for decrease in concentration in tissues or fluids with time.

RESULTS

Maternal serum. Maternal serum concentrations of TBM at 1, 2, 4, and 8 h, plus those at delivery time only up to an 11-h interval, are shown in Fig. 1. TBM was not detected in the delivery time maternal serum samples of the 15 gravid patients who delivered after the 11-h interval (Table 1). A mean maternal peak serum concentration of 4.0 μg/ml occurred at 1 h and $t_{1/2}$ was 1.54 h. Since no significant difference by trimester was found for $t_{1/2}$ or peak serum concentrations, the 35 patients could be considered as one group and are represented by the regression line in Fig. 2a ($r = 0.93$).

Placenta. TBM appeared in the first placental sample at 40 min and remained detectable until the last sample, taken at 34 h (Table 1). In all but 2 of the 29 samples, concentrations were above 1 μg/g, with an overall mean concentration of 1.4 μg/g. Although not significant, a definite trend toward increasing TBM concen-

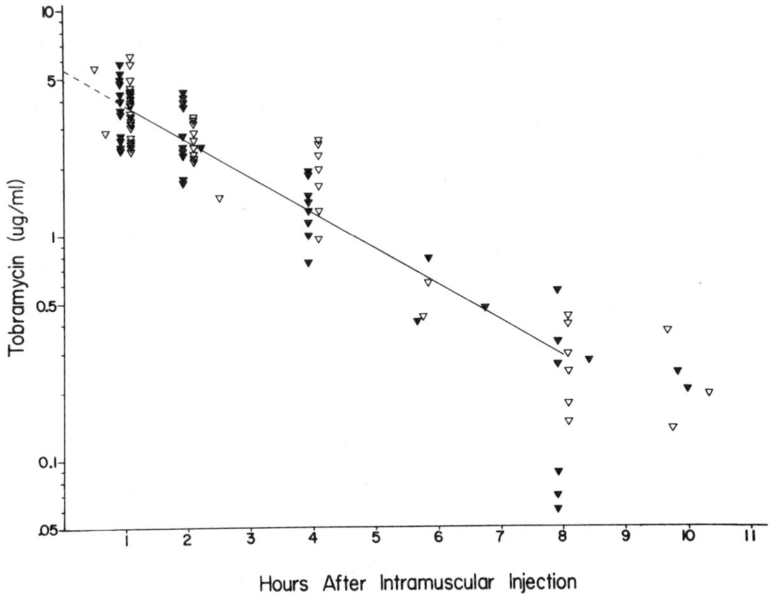

Fig. 1. *Maternal serum concentrations after a single 2-mg/kg injection of tobramycin to 35 healthy gravid patients who were 9 to 20 weeks' gestation. The symbols represent individual TBM concentrations of individual maternal serum samples at 1, 2, 4, and 8 h, plus the scattered samples taken at the time of clamping the uterine artery. The solid line represents a linear regression of the mean maternal serum concentration, and the dotted line represents the extension of this line to a theoretical time zero ($r = 0.93$). Symbols: (▼) Trimester I patients, (▽) trimester II patients.*

TABLE 1. *TBM concentrations after a single intramuscular dose of 2 mg/kg administered to 35 healthy gravidas 9 to 20 weeks' gestation*

Gestational age (weeks)	Interval[a] (h)	TBM concn in: Maternal serum at delivery (μg/ml)	Fetal tissues and body fluids: Placenta (μg/g)	Fetal serum (μg/ml)	Kidney (μg/g)	Urine (μg/ml)	Amniotic fluid (μg/ml)	CSF (μg/ml)
Trimester I patients								
12	2:00	2.8	1.04		1.2		0	0
11	2:13	2.05					0	0.2
11	4:00	1.0					0	0.3
12	4:00	1.45	1.92	0.56	2.4		0	0.2
12	5:40	0.42	1.6	0.28			0	0.2
9	5:50	0.8						
9	6:45	0.48					0.2	
11	8:25	0.28	1.6	0.25			0	0.7
11	9:50	0.25	1.5	2.56	0		0	
11	10:00	0.21	1.2	0	0.8			0.5
13	16:35	0	1.6	0	1.2	0	0.2	0
13	19:35	0	1.0	0	0	0.1	0.1	0.1
9	20:35	0		0				
Trimester II patients								
20	0:40	2.9	1.16	0	0	0.27	0	0
15	2:30	1.5		0.58	1.0	3.4	0	0
20	4:00	1.3	1.52	0.28	1.9		0.3	0
17	5:45	0.44	1.6	0.14	2.4	2.3	0.3	0
17	5:50	0.62	1.2	0.34	2.2		0.1	0
14	8:05	0.15	2.0	0.17	0.8		0.2	0
17	9:05	0	0.9	0.32	1.8		0.1	0
20	9:40	0.38	1.3	0.2		2.2	0.2	0
19	9:45	0.14	1.0	0.1	3.0	1.8	0.3	0
20	10:20	0.2	1.2	0.1	4.6	1.0	0.5	0
15	11:45	0	1.3	0	1.7	1.0	0.2	0
16	12:00	0	1.8	0.08	2.6	0.7	0.5	0.2
20	12:00	0	0.5	0.07	4.8	1.3	0.5	0
20	16:00	0	1.1	0.06	2.0	0.3	0.3	0
17	16:22	0	1.7		3.3	0.6	0.3	0
20	17:00	0	1.5	0.1	6.6	0.6	0.6	0
20	18:30	0	1.1		3.7	0.4	0.4	0
15	19:25	0	1.6	0	1.5	0.2	0.2	0.1
14	20:00	0	1.1	0	2.2	0.1	0.2	0
20	20:00	0	1.0	0	4.0		0.2	0
19	21:35	0	1.6	0	3.2	0.2	0.4	0
20	34:00	0	2.8		7.2	0	0.13	0

[a] Interval = hours between maternal TBM administration and clamping of uterine arteries.

trations with an increasing interval can be seen in Fig. 2b. There was no correlation of placental TBM concentration with duration of gestation, maternal serum concentration, or fetal tissue or fluid levels.

Fetal serum. TBM was detected in 19 fetal serum samples at delivery time. These concentrations are represented in Fig. 2c. The time when TBM first appeared in fetal serum, 2.5 h after maternal injection, was also the time when the highest TBM concentrations were observed. All fetal serum concentrations were less than 0.6 μg/ml and undetectable by a 17-h interval. The $t_{1/2}$ determined from these individual samples is 5.25 h ($r = 0.69$). No difference in TBM concentrations in fetal serum could be related to gestational age.

Fetal kidney. The highest and most persistent TBM concentration was demonstrated in the fetal kidney (Fig. 2d). TBM was present as early as 2 h and as late as 34 h in 24 of 27 samples analyzed. At more than 9 h after maternal antibiotic injection, 53% of the trimester II fetal kidney samples had TBM concentrations of 3 μg/g or more, a clinically therapeutic concentration. Two 20-week fetal kidney samples had 6.6 and 7.2 μg of TBM per g at 17 and 34 h, respectively. A significant correlation be-

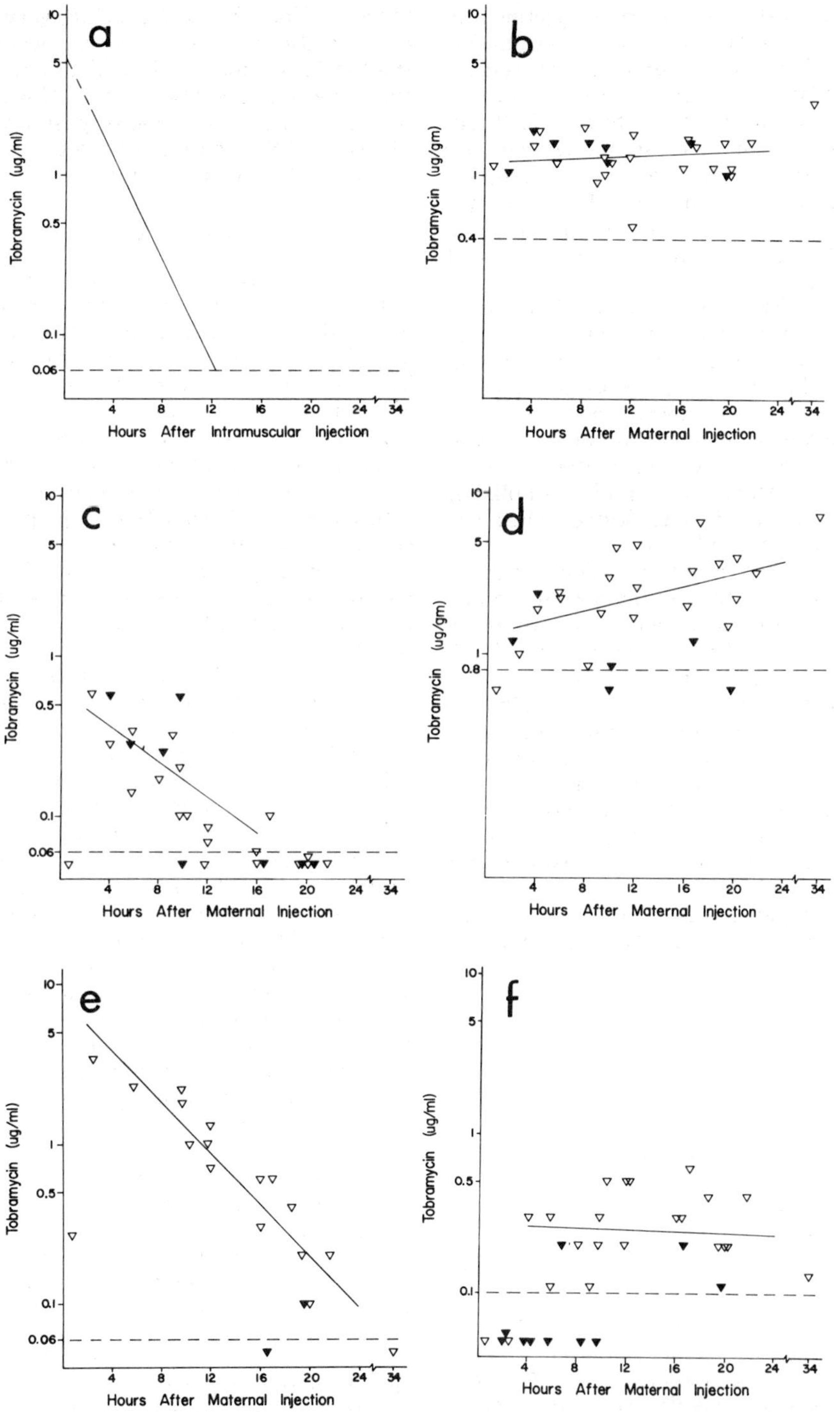

FIG. 2. *Tobramycin concentrations in: (a) maternal serum ($r = 0.93$; $t_{1/2} = 1.54$ h); (b) placenta (mean, 1.4 μg/g); (c) fetal serum ($r = 0.69$; $t_{1/2} = 5.25$ h); (d) fetal kidney ($r = 0.54$); (e) fetal urine ($r = 0.92$; $t_{1/2} = 3.7$ h); (f) amniotic fluid (mean, 0.25 μg/ml), after a single intramuscular dose administered to 35 gravid patients 9 to 20 weeks' gestation. The solid lines represent the regression line or mean concentration as determined from the individual values represented by the triangular symbols in figures (b) through (f). The interrupted horizontal lines indicate the lowest detectable concentrations of tobramycin for that tissue or fluid. Symbols: (▼) Samples from trimester I of pregnancy, (▽) samples from trimester II of pregnancy.*

tween the interval from maternal injection and fetal kidney concentration can be seen in Fig. 2d ($r = 0.54$). When gestational age was related to the fetal kidney TBM concentration, the correlation coefficient improved to $r = 0.79$. An even more significant correlation coefficient of $r = 0.82$ was found when multiple regression analysis was used to relate (i) TBM concentration in fetal kidney, (ii) the interval after maternal TBM injection, and (iii) the weeks of gestation (Fig. 3).

Fetal urine. Fetal urine was available from 19 fetuses of more than 12 weeks' gestation. TBM appeared promptly in the first sample taken at 40 min. The highest concentration, 3.4 μg/ml, occurred at an interval of 2.5 h. After this peak, a steady decline in concentration was observed. A $t_{1/2}$ of 3.7 h was calculated ($r = 0.92$; Fig. 2e). No relationships could be established between fetal urine and fetal kidney TBM concentrations or gestational age.

Amniotic fluid. In fetuses older than 13 weeks' gestation, antimicrobial activity in amniotic fluid was first detected at a 4-h interval. An overall mean TBM concentration of 0.25 μg/ml was sustained until the 21.6-h interval. In trimester II samples, TBM was found in fetal urine before it appeared in amniotic fluid samples (Fig. 2f). At or beyond a 4-h interval, only three of eight trimester I amniotic fluid samples revealed TBM activity, whereas all of 20 trimester II samples had aminoglycoside present, indicating a significant relationship to gestational age (Table 1).

CSF and other tissues. Of 27 fetal brain samples, none contained TBM in detectable

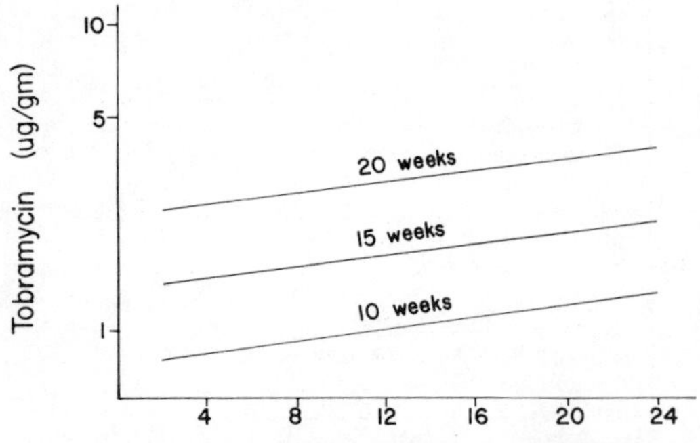

FIG. 3. *Predicted regression curves for tobramycin concentrations in fetal kidneys of 10, 15, and 20 weeks' gestation after a single 2-mg/kg intramuscular injection to 35 gravid patients, 9 to 20 weeks' gestation.* ($Log_n Y' = -1.3525 + 0.024X + 0.11037$, *where* X = *time in hours after TBM administration to the gravid patient and* Y = *gestational age in weeks,* $Rx \cdot Yz = 0.82$.)

concentrations. In the fetal CSF, very low TBM concentrations (0.1 to 0.7 μg/ml) were found at the 2- to 20-h interval in 9 of 15 fetuses of less than 17 weeks' gestation. No TBM was detected in the 16 fetuses of 17 weeks' gestation or more (Table 1). TBM could not be detected in any of the 32 fetal lung or 33 fetal liver specimens.

DISCUSSION

Our data, from the single sampling of 34 different fetuses in the early weeks of pregnancy, demonstrated enough consistency to establish biological curves and provide a meaningful indicator of the kinetics and distribution of TBM in the conceptus.

During the first 20 weeks of pregnancy, the maternal plasma volume increases 30% (2), and renal plasma flow and glomerular filtration rate increase 30% to 50% (6). In spite of these changes, the mean maternal peak serum concentration and serum $t_{1/2}$ were found to be within the ranges reported for healthy, nonpregnant adults when similar doses were used (3, 11).

In the placental tissue samples from fetuses in the first half of pregnancy, a mean tissue TBM concentration of 1.4 μg/g was maintained for at least 24 h; this concentration bore no relationship to presence of TBM in maternal serum. If we can assume that micrograms per grams of tissue are equivalent to micrograms per milliliter of body fluids for bacteriological inhibition, then TBM may prove useful in the treatment of placental infections, since in vitro bacterial inhibitory concentrations of TBM range from 0.4 to 0.8 μg/ml for *Staphylococcus aureus* and 0.8 to 3.1 μg/ml for *Pseudomonas* species, *Escherichia coli,* and *Klebsiella pneumoniae* (9, 10). Investigations addressing the question of whether higher placental concentrations can be produced by larger or repetitive doses may define a limited or linear capacity to handle TBM.

After it had crossed the placenta to the fetus, TBM was cleared from the fetal serum within 17 h, with a $t_{1/2}$ of 5.25 h. Kaplan and co-workers (5) reported that the TBM serum $t_{1/2}$ for small premature infants is 8.7 h. If the longer fetal serum $t_{1/2}$ of the premature infant is attributable to immature renal function, then the shortened fetal serum $t_{1/2}$ may reflect the role of the placenta in the fetal clearance of TBM.

TBM was not found in the CSF of the fetuses older than 16 weeks' gestation. A mechanism limiting the entry of this aminoglycoside into the CSF seems to be established at this stage of maturation (4).

Fetal renal tissue concentrations of TBM were high and were found to increase significantly for as long as 34 h, whereas both fetal serum and urine concentrations steadily declined to nondetectable levels by 17 and 21.6 h, respectively. Luft and Kleit (7) reported prolonged renal parenchymal accumulation in adult rats after a single dose of several aminoglycosidic antibiotics. Dissection of the adult rat kidneys revealed 85% of the TBM to be in the cortex, which consists mostly of proximal tubules and where histological evidence of gentamicin toxicity has been described. With advancing gestational age, the human fetal kidney has a more defined cortical structure (14). This may explain the significant differences in TBM concentration in the fetal kidneys of 10 weeks' gestation as compared with those 20 weeks of age. The absolute or relative tissue concentration of TBM that would cause fetal renal toxicity is not known for any stage of fetal maturation. One wonders whether TBM, a potentially nephrotoxic aminoglycoside, could be used more safely in trimester I because of the lower concentrations found in the younger fetal kidney or whether it could be equally or more toxic because of the greater degree of renal immaturity. If, in our studies, the fetal kidney could attain such high and sustained levels after administration of a single therapeutic dose to the gravid patient, then might higher renal tissue concentrations be reached when multiple doses of TBM are administered? This has been shown to occur with other antibiotics by Philipson and co-workers (8). They reported a considerably higher increase in fetal kidney concentration of both erythromycin (500 mg) and clindamycin (450 mg) after multiple doses compared with single doses of the same agents administered to pregnant patients.

Thirty percent of the human fetal glomeruli appear to be relatively mature histologically by 16 weeks' gestation (14). Fetal urine concentrations of TBM were 5 to 10 times greater than those found in simultaneous fetal serum samples. If TBM is primarily excreted by glomerular filtration, our results are consistent with active renal glomerular TBM excretion in the fetus of 13 or more weeks' gestation.

TBM did not appear in the amniotic fluid until it was present in the urine; this is consistent with the premise that the presence of the antibiotic in amniotic fluid is primarily related to renal excretion. One might expect TBM to accumulate in amniotic fluid; however, rather inexplicable static levels were found in amniotic fluid, which is known to undergo a dynamic turnover.

Although it has been traditional to sample body fluids for evidence of drug concentrations in a toxic range, our findings in the fetal kidney give rise to a serious skepticism about the equatability of such an approach since, with the longer intervals, the fetal kidney had increasing mean concentrations of TBM, whereas fetal serum and urine levels were decreasing to undetectable amounts. Tissue sampling for drug levels may be a more appropriate, although usually inaccessible, approach to extending the understanding of the pharmacology of certain therapeutic agents. Further investigation of the perinatal pharmacology of this and other drugs is imperative to obtain the data necessary for treating the infected gravid patient and her fetus with the increasing number of available antimicrobials.

ACKNOWLEDGMENTS

We wish to express our sincere appreciation and gratitude to Lorraine Wittman and Paul F. Thielen for technical assistance, and to Michaeline Abate for statistical analysis.

This study was supported by a grant from Eli Lilly & Co., Indianapolis, Ind.

LITERATURE CITED

1. **Bennett, J. V., J. L. Brodie, E. J. Benner, and W. M. M. Kirby.** 1966. Simplified, accurate method for antibiotic assay of clinical specimens. Appl. Microbiol. 14:170–177.
2. **Berlin, N. I., C. Goetsch, G. M. Hyde, and R. J. Parsons.** 1953. The blood volume in pregnancy as determined by p^{32} labeled red blood cells. Surg. Gynecol. Obstet. 97:173–176.
3. **Black, H. R., and R. S. Griffith.** 1974. Comparative pharmacology of tobramycin and gentamicin in adult volunteers, p. 24–30. *In* Tobramycin: selected proceedings from the Eighth International Congress of Chemotherapy, Athens, September 8–15, 1973. Excerpta Medica, New York.
4. **Evans, C. A. N., J. M. Reynolds, M. L. Reynolds, N. R. Saunders, and M. B. Segal.** 1974. The development of a blood-brain barrier mechanism in foetal sheep. J. Physiol. 238:371–386.
5. **Kaplan, J. M., G. H. McCracken Jr., M. L. Thomas, L. J. Horton, and N. Davis.** 1973. Clinical pharmacology of tobramycin in newborns. Am. J. Dis. Child. 125:656–660.
6. **Lindheimer, M. D., and A. I. Katz.** 1973. Pregnancy and the kidney. J. Reprod. Med. 11:14–18.
7. **Luft, F. C., and S. A. Kleit.** 1974. Renal parenchymal accumulation of aminoglycoside antibiotic in rats. J. Infect. Dis. 130:656–659.
8. **Philipson, A., L. D. Sabath, and D. Charles.** 1973. Transplacental passage of erythromycin and clindamycin. N. Engl. J. Med. 288:1219–1221.
9. **Ries, K., M. E. Levison, and D. Kaye.** 1973. In vitro evaluation of a new aminoglycoside derivative of kanamycin, a comparison with tobramycin and gentamicin. Antimicrob. Agents Chemother. 3:532–533.
10. **Schoutens, E., and E. Yourassowsky.** 1974. Tobramycin: clinical and microbiological evaluation, p. 94–101. *In* Tobramycin: selected proceedings from the Eighth International Congress of Chemotherapy, Athens, September 8–15, 1973. Excerpta Medica, New York.

11. **Simon, V. K., E. U. Mösinger, and V. Malerczy.** 1973. Pharmacokinetic studies of tobramycin and gentamicin. Antimicrob. Agents Chemother. 3:445–450.

12. **Stark, W. M., M. M. Hoehn, and N. G. Knox.** 1968. Nebramycin, a new broad spectrum antibiotic complex. I. Detection and biosynthesis, p. 314–323. Antimicrob. Agents Chemother. 1967.

13. **Trolle, D.** 1947. Age of the foetus determined from its measures. Acta Obstet. Gynecol. Scand. 27:327–332.

14. **Vernier, R. L., and F. G. Smith, Jr.** 1968. Fetal and neonatal kidney, p. 225–260. *In* N. S. Assali (ed.), Biology of gestation, vol. 2. Academic Press Inc., New York.

ANTIMICROBIAL AGENTS AND CHEMOTHERAPY, Apr. 1977, p. 695-697
Vol. 11, No. 4

Printed in U.S.A.

Susceptibility of *Clostridium perfringens* Isolated from Human Infections to Twenty Antibiotics

JOSEPH D. SCHWARTZMAN, L. BARTH RELLER,* AND WEN-LAN L. WANG

Departments of Pathology and Medicine, University of Colorado Medical Center, Denver, Colorado 80262, and Veterans Administration Hospital, Denver, Colorado 80220*

Received for publication 19 November 1976

The proper choice of antibiotic for *Clostridium perfringens* infections in patients allergic to penicillin is not clear; the usual recommendations and recent in vitro studies disagree. We tested the susceptibility of 57 strains of *C. perfringens* to eight penicillins, seven cephalosporins, two tetracyclines, clindamycin, chloramphenicol, and rifampin by the agar dilution method. All strains were inhibited by (per milliliter) 4 μg or less of any of the penicillins, chloramphenicol, or clindamycin and 8 μg or less of any of the cephalosporins tested. Penicillin G and amoxicillin inhibited all strains at 0.12 μg or less per ml. Only 54% of the strains were inhibited by 1 μg of tetracycline per ml. Penicillin G remains the drug of first choice for infections with *C. perfringens*; it need not be added to a regimen containing a penicillinase-resistant penicillin given parenterally in high doses. The cephalosporins should be considered as alternative drugs for penicillin-allergic patients. Clindamycin and chloramphenicol are also effective. Tetracyclines cannot be depended upon in clostridial infections without in vitro testing, which is impracticable for initial empirical therapy.

Penicillin G is the antibiotic of first choice for treating cellulitis, sepsis, and myonecrosis caused by *Clostridium perfringens* (1, 2, 8, 11, 18). Although erythromycin and tetracycline are the alternative drugs usually recommended (1, 2, 8, 11, 18), 10 to 30% of *C. perfringens* are resistant to tetracycline, and a few strains are also resistant to erythromycin (6, 8, 9, 13). Cephalosporins and penicillinase-resistant and other semisynthetic penicillins are used for contaminated wounds after severe trauma and for suspected sepsis in patients with cancer, who are also at a higher risk for clostridial infections (3, 4, 14). Because of both scanty information about many of these agents and the need for a safe antibiotic for penicillin-allergic patients, we studied the activity of 20 antibiotics against strains of *C. perfringens* isolated from human infections or feces.

MATERIALS AND METHODS

Strains of bacteria. Fifty-seven isolates of *C. perfringens* type A were collected from the following institutions: University of Colorado Medical Center, 18 strains; Center for Disease Control (CDC), 12 strains; University of Minnesota Hospital, 10 strains; University of Utah Medical Center, 7 strains; University of California-Los Angeles Health Sciences Center, 6 strains; and University of Oregon Health Sciences Center, 4 strains. All strains of *C. perfringens* produced a double zone of hemolysis on sheep-blood agar, were nonmotile, grew at 46°C, fermented lactose, had no visible spores, produced lecithinase that was inhibited by type A antiserum (Burroughs Wellcome Co., Research Triangle Park, N.C.), and liquefied gelatin. Fifty-five of the strains were isolated from clinical specimens; two were recovered from normal feces.

Antibiotics. Antibiotic solutions were prepared in distilled water with standard powders of known potency provided by the following firms: amoxicillin (Hoffmann-LaRoche, Inc., Nutley, N.J.); cloxacillin and dicloxacillin (Bristol Laboratories, Syracuse, N.Y.); methicillin, oxacillin, and ticarcillin (Beecham-Massengill, Inc., Bristol, Tenn.); nafcillin (Wyeth Laboratories, Philadelphia, Pa.); penicillin G, doxycycline, and tetracycline (Pfizer Laboratories, New York, N.Y.); cefamandole, cephalexin, cephaloridine, and cephalothin (Eli Lilly & Co., Indianapolis, Ind.); cefazolin and cephradine (Smith Kline & French Laboratories, Philadelphia, Pa.); cefoxitin (Merck, Sharp & Dohme, West Point, Pa.); chloramphenicol (Parke, Davis & Co., Detroit, Mich.); clindamycin (The Upjohn Co., Kalamazoo, Mich.); and rifampin (CIBA-Geigy and Co., Summit, N.J.). Stock solutions of antibiotics were prepared fresh or stored at −70°C for a maximum of 4 weeks before use.

Susceptibility testing. Agar dilution tests were done by the method of Sutter and Washington (15). Antibiotics were diluted in twofold steps above and below 1 μg/ml in Brucella agar (Pfizer) supplemented with 5% laked sheep blood and vitamin K_1 (10 μg/ml). The inoculum was adjusted to a no. 1 MacFarland turbidity standard (3×10^8 colony-forming units) and then diluted with prereduced Carey-Blair buffer, so that each spot delivered by the multipoint inoculator contained between 10^4 and 10^5 organisms. The viable counts were confirmed by the method of Miles and Misra (10). Tests were done in triplicate, and a control strain of *C. perfringens* (CDC no. 15443) was included with each experiment. Growth was defined as more than one discrete colony on at least two out of three spots after incubation at 35°C in an anaerobic glove box in an atmosphere of 85% N_2, 5% CO_2, and 10% H_2 for 24 and 48 h.

RESULTS

End points at 24 and 48 h were similar, except that 12% of the minimal inhibitory concentrations (MIC) at 48 h were one dilution step higher. The MIC of the control strain of *C. perfringens* was always within one twofold-dilution step of the MIC reported by the CDC or our earlier results for antibiotics not tested by the CDC. The results shown in Table 1 are those obtained at 24 h.

Penicillin G and amoxicillin had the lowest MIC. One hundred percent of the strains were inhibited by 0.12 μg of either antibiotic per ml. All the semisynthetic penicillins and cephalosporins tested were active against *C. perfringens* at concentrations readily achieved in human serum with usual doses. Chloramphenicol and clindamycin were also active over a narrow range against all strains. In contrast, 19% of strains were resistant to 4 μg of tetracycline per ml. Rifampin inhibited all but one strain at 0.015 μg/ml; the remaining strain was 500-fold more resistant.

TABLE 1. *Antibiotic susceptibility of C. perfringens (57 strains)*

Class and antibiotic	Cumulative % susceptible to indicated concn (μg/ml)				
	0.5	1	2	4	8
Penicillins					
Amoxicillin	100				
Penicillin G	100				
Ticarcillin	91	100			
Methicillin	61	100			
Nafcillin	95	98	100		
Oxacillin	98		100		
Cloxacillin	86	96	98	100	
Dicloxacillin	81	95	96	100	
Cephalosporins					
Cefamandole	100				
Cephaloridine	98	100			
Cefoxitin	39	91	100		
Cephalothin	14	67	98	100	
Cefazolin	74	84	89	96	100
Cephalexin	32	70	82	93	100
Cephradine	42	67	82	93	100
Miscellaneous					
Chloramphenicol	0	11	100		
Clindamycin	75	85	98	100	
Doxycycline	82	89	96	98	100
Rifampin	98				100
Tetracycline	46	56	74	81	91

DISCUSSION

Our results for penicillin G agree with those of others who used similar methods (6, 8, 9, 13). The semisynthetic penicillins tested were also active against *C. perfringens*. Any of the penicillins we tested should constitute effective therapy against *C. perfringens*. Our findings with cephalosporins agree with published results for cefamandole, cephalexin, cephaloridine, and cephalothin (16, 17). Cefazolin, cefoxitin, and cephradine showed activity comparable to the other cephalosporins. Our results with chloramphenicol and clindamycin were similar to those of others (6, 8, 9, 13). We also found resistance to tetracyclines among strains of *C. perfringens* (6, 8, 9, 13). About half of our strains were inhibited by 1 μg of tetracycline per ml, but 64 μg/ml was required to inhibit 100% of strains; 21% of strains required more than 1 μg of doxycycline per ml.

Tetracyclines may be chemically inactivated in environments having low oxidation-reduction potentials (7). Erythromycin is much less active, if at all, at a low redox potential and an acid pH (12). The acidosis and anaerobic environment in myonecrosis caused by *C. perfringens* (19) would contraindicate the use of these drugs on theoretical grounds. Penicillin, ampicillin, and cephalothin are not appreciably affected by different pH conditions in media (13).

In conclusion, our data support the efficacy of all the penicillins tested against *C. perfringens*. Neither tetracycline nor erythromycin should be considered as an alternative drug for infection with *C. perfringens*, unless susceptibility can be demonstrated by appropriate testing. In most penicillin-allergic patients, a cephalosporin would be both safe and effective treatment for *C. perfringens* (5, 18); clindamycin and chloramphenicol would be alternative drugs.

ACKNOWLEDGMENTS

We thank David B. Weeks for technical help.

This work was supported by grant CA-15823 from the National Cancer Institute and by a grant-in-aid from Lilly Research Laboratories, Eli Lilly & Co.

LITERATURE CITED

1. **Altemeier, W. A., and W. D. Fullen.** 1971. Prevention and treatment of gas gangrene. J. Am. Med. Assoc. 217:806–813.
2. **Anonymous.** 1976. Antimicrobial drugs of choice, p. 14–20. *In* M. Abramowicz (ed.), Handbook of antimicrobial therapy. The Medical Letter on Drugs and Therapeutics, New Rochelle, N.Y.

3. **Anonymous.** 1972. Antimicrobial prophylaxis in surgery. Med. Lett. Drugs Ther. 14:25–27.
4. **Boggs, D. R., E. Frei III, and L. B. Thomas.** 1958. Clostridial gas gangrene and septicemia in four patients with leukemia. N. Engl. J. Med. 259:1255–1258.
5. **Dash, C. H.** 1975. Penicillin allergy and the cephalosporins. J. Antimicrob. Chemother. 1(Suppl.):S107–S118.
6. **Dornbusch, K., C.-E. Nord, and A. Dählback.** 1975. Antibiotic susceptibility of *Clostridium* species isolated from human infections. Scand. J. Infect. Dis. 7:127–134.
7. **Ingham, H. R., J. B. Selkon, A. A. Codd, and J. H. Hale.** 1970. The effect of carbon dioxide on the sensitivity of *Bacteroides fragilis* to certain antibiotics *in vitro*. J. Clin. Pathol. 23:254–258.
8. **Johnstone, F. R. C., and W. H. Cockcroft.** 1968. *Clostridium welchii* resistance to tetracycline. Lancet i:660–661.
9. **Martin, W. J., M. Gardner, and J. A. Washington II.** 1972. In vitro antimicrobial susceptibility of anaerobic bacteria isolated from clinical specimens. Antimicrob. Agents Chemother. 1:148–158.
10. **Miles, A. S., and S. S. Misra.** 1938. The estimation of the bactericidal power of the blood. J. Hyg. 38:732–749.
11. **Parker, M. T.** 1969. Postoperative clostridial infections in Britain. Br. Med. J. 3:671–676.
12. **Rosenblatt, J. E., and F. Schoenknecht.** 1972. Effect of several components of anaerobic incubation on antibiotic susceptibility test results. Antimicrob. Agents Chemother. 1:433–440.
13. **Sapico, F. L., Y.-Y. Kwok, V. L. Sutter, and S. M. Finegold.** 1972. Standardized antimicrobial disc susceptibility testing of anaerobic bacteria: in vitro susceptibility of *Clostridium perfringens* to nine antibiotics. Antimicrob. Agents Chemother. 2:320–325.
14. **Schimpff, S. C., S. Landesman, D. M. Hahn, H. C. Standiford, C. L. Fortner, V. M. Young, and P. H. Wiernik.** 1976. Ticarcillin in combination with cephalothin or gentamicin as empiric antibiotic therapy in granulocytopenic cancer patients. Antimicrob. Agents. Chemother. 10:837–844.
15. **Sutter, V. L., and J. A. Washington II.** 1975. Susceptibility testing of anaerobes, p. 436–438. *In* E. H. Lennette, E. H. Spaulding, and J. P. Truant (ed.), Manual of clinical microbiology. American Society for Microbiology, Washington, D.C.
16. **Traub, W. H.** 1971. The susceptibility of *Clostridium perfringens* type A to cephalosporin C antibiotics *in vitro*. Chemotherapy 16:11–17.
17. **Washington, J. A., II.** 1976. The *in vitro* spectrum of the cephalosporins. Mayo Clin. Proc. 51:237–250.
18. **Weinstein, L., and M. A. Barza.** 1973. Gas gangrene. N. Engl. J. Med. 289:1129–1131.
19. **Willis, A. T.** 1969. Clostridia of wound infection, p. 41–156. Butterworths, London.

Antimicrobial Agents and Chemotherapy, Apr. 1977, p. 698–700
Copyright © 1977 American Society for Microbiology

Vol. 11, No. 4
Printed in U.S.A.

Levels of Carbenicillin, Ticarcillin, Cephalothin, Cefazolin, Cefamandole, Gentamicin, Tobramycin, and Amikacin in Human Serum and Interstitial Fluid

JAMES S. TAN* and SARA JANE SALSTROM

Infectious Disease Service, Department of Medicine, Akron City Hospital, Akron, Ohio 44309

Received for publication 20 October 1976

The ability of eight antibiotics (carbenicillin, ticarcillin, cefamandole, cephalothin, cefazolin, gentamicin, tobramycin, and amikacin) to enter human interstitial fluid was evaluated by the skin window technique. All of the antibiotics tested, except cefazolin, which has the highest percentage of protein binding, diffused into the interstitial fluid quite well. This study confirms our previous observation on the effect of high-percentage protein binding on diffusion of a drug into the minimally inflamed extravascular space.

A method of measuring antibiotic levels in human interstitial fluid (ITF), using a skin window technique, has been described previously (9). Using this technique, we have determined the diffusibility of eight other antibiotics into human ITF.

MATERIALS AND METHODS

Volunteers. Written informed consent was obtained from male adult volunteers.

Antibiotics. (i) Carbenicillin and ticarcillin. A double-crossover study was performed using these two drugs. Twelve volunteers were included in the study. Six volunteers were given 3 g of one drug over 30 min by intravenous infusion, and the remaining six were given 3 g of the other drug. The study was repeated after 1 week, and the volunteers received the drug that they had not received previously.

(ii) Cephalothin, cefazolin, and cefamandole. Twelve volunteers participated in this study. Twelve received cefamandole, 10 received cephalothin, and 12 received cefazolin. Each volunteer was given a 1-g intravenous dose over a 30-min period.

(iii) Amikacin, gentamicin, and tobramycin. A triple-crossover study was performed. Four volunteers were given 1.7 mg of gentamicin per kg, 1.7 mg of tobramycin per kg, or 7.5 mg of amikacin per kg. Each of the drugs was given intramuscularly. In parts 2 and 3 of the study, each volunteer was given whichever drug he had not previously received. Each part of the study was carried out at a 1-week interval.

Serum samples. Venous blood was obtained before and at 1, 2, 3, and 4 h after antibiotic administration. The sera were separated after 45 min at 24°C and immediately frozen.

ITF samples. The technique of obtaining ITF by using a skin window chamber has been described (9). These skin window fluid samples were removed completely, and the chambers were refilled with sterile isotonic saline at pH 6.0 within 5 min after the hourly venous blood samples were obtained.

Assay of antibiotics. All of the antibiotics were assayed by using the agar well method of Bennett et al. (1). The test organism for ticarcillin and carbenicillin was *Pseudomonas aeruginosa*. *Bacillus subtilis* spore suspension (Difco Laboratories, Detroit, Mich.) was used as the test organism for the other antibiotics in the study.

RESULTS

Carbenicillin and ticarcillin. The mean peak serum and skin window fluid levels of carbenicillin and ticarcillin were observed at 1 h after intravenous administration (Table 1). The serum and skin window fluid as well as the skin window fluid-to-serum ratios (W/S ratios) were almost identical throughout the 4-h study. The percentage of protein binding of both drugs was approximately 50% (5), which may be considered as intermediate. The W/S ratios of carbenicillin and ticarcillin fall between those of nafcillin (9) and flucloxacillin (9), which have high percentages of protein binding, and those of amoxicillin (7) and ampicillin (7), which have low percentages of protein binding.

Cefamandole, cephalothin, and cefazolin. All of these cephalosporin antibiotics showed peak concentrations in serum at 1 h. Unlike the other two agents, peak cefazolin skin window fluid levels were noted 2 h after intravenous administration. Cefazolin, which has the highest percentage of protein binding (6) among the cephalosporin drugs studied (3), showed the lowest W/S ratio.

Gentamicin, tobramycin, and amikacin. Each of the drugs achieved peak skin window fluid levels 2 h after intramuscular administration. The mean peak levels of gentamicin and tobramycin in serum were found at 1 h, and that of amikacin was found at 2 h. The W/S

TABLE 1. *Mean drug concentrations in skin window fluids and sera for the eight antibiotics tested*

Drug administered	Mean drug concn (μg/ml) ± SE[a] at h after drug administration:				Ratio of mean concn (W/S ratio) at h after drug administration:			
	1	2	3	4	1	2	3	4
Carbenicillin	13.67 ± 6.60[b]	10.80 ± 5.90	5.27 ± 3.09	2.60 ± 1.84	0.1382	0.2213	0.2373	0.2394
	98.90 ± 17.20	48.80 ± 15.37	22.20 ± 9.89	10.86 ± 5.27				
Ticarcillin	11.71 ± 5.90	10.92 ± 4.64	5.16 ± 2.51	2.10 ± 0.71	0.1283	0.2318	0.2163	0.1842
	91.20 ± 13.75	47.10 ± 6.40	23.80 ± 7.91	11.40 ± 5.67				
Cefamandole	2.45 ± 0.94	1.38 ± 0.40	0.55 ± 0.18	0.10 ± 0.07	0.1306	0.2782	0.3197	0.2083
	19.44 ± 5.64	4.96 ± 1.77	1.72 ± 0.87	0.48 ± 0.30				
Cephalothin	2.00 ± 1.06	0.83 ± 0.37	*[c]	*[c]	0.2797	1.000		
	7.15 ± 2.20	0.83 ± 0.27	0.19 ± 0.07					
Cefazolin	2.61 ± 2.80	4.27 ± 1.30	1.87 ± 0.24	1.23 ± 0.86	0.0420	0.1054	0.0869	0.0884
	62.00 ± 2.82	40.50 ± 0.70	21.50 ± 1.41	13.90 ± 1.55				
Gentamicin	1.36 ± 1.03	1.81 ± 0.77	1.07 ± 0.48	0.62 ± 0.33	0.1689	0.3088	0.2955	0.2384
	8.05 ± 1.93	5.86 ± 2.65	3.62 ± 1.19	2.60 ± 0.94				
Tobramycin	0.84 ± 0.61	1.44 ± 0.53	0.91 ± 0.49	0.53 ± 0.38	0.1078	0.2239	0.2116	0.2208
	7.79 ± 2.02	6.43 ± 3.46	4.30 ± 1.31	2.40 ± 1.02				
Amikacin	2.16 ± 1.53	4.22 ± 2.11	3.36 ± 1.70	2.11 ± 1.23	0.0892	0.1714	0.1741	0.1825
	24.21 ± 9.30	24.62 ± 4.72	19.29 ± 5.90	11.56 ± 4.03				

[a] SE, Standard error.
[b] Numerator = skin window fluid; denominator = serum.
[c] *, Most specimens had undetectable antibiotic activity.

ratios of gentamicin and tobramycin were comparable, and those of amikacin were slightly lower. All three drugs are poorly bound to serum proteins, but their W/S ratios were not higher than carbenicillin and ticarcillin.

DISCUSSION

Although the absolute antibiotic concentration in the ITF is more important clinically than is the W/S ratio, the diffusibility as measured by the W/S ratio provides a better means of comparison among different groups of antibiotics.

The diffusibility of the penicillins into ITF, using the skin window technique, appears to be related to the percentage of protein binding, as noted (7, 9). Significantly poor diffusibility was noted only with nafcillin and flucloxacillin, both of which have approximately 10% or less of the free form in human serum (9).

The proportions of ticarcillin and carbenicillin bound to serum proteins are quite comparable. Our present study showed that their W/S ratios are almost identical.

Like that of the penicillins, the diffusibility of the cephalosporins into skin window fluid in our study is related to the percentage of protein binding. Cefazolin, which is bound to the serum proteins more than the others, had a lower W/S ratio. Cephalothin apparently did not follow the general rule since it has the highest W/S ratio. This apparent discrepancy is due to the relatively rapid fall of serum cephalothin activity within an hour. This finding is probably a result of rapid renal clearance of serum cephalothin and a slower clearance of extravascular cephalothin.

The percentages of gentamicin, tobramycin, and amikacin bound to serum protein are low, i.e., 0 (4), 0 (4), and 3.6% (2), respectively. These three antibiotics, which have low percentages of protein binding, did not enter the ITF any better than did the penicillins or cephalosporins, with protein binding of less than 90%. Other factors not included in the present investigation may contribute to this discrepancy.

Our earlier report showed that the amount of protein in the fluid during the 5-h study was low and, hence, did not represent true inflammatory exudate (9). In this type of ITF, the percentage of protein binding did not appear to hinder diffusibility, except for those antibiotics that were highly protein bound, i.e., nafcillin, flucloxacillin, and cefazolin. In another study in which *Staphylococcus aureus* was instilled into the canine pericardium to induce inflammatory exudate, the ability of the antibiotics to enter this fluid was not related to protein binding (8).

The skin window model showed that antibiotics that have a higher percentage of protein binding did not diffuse well into noninflamed ITF. This observation raises doubts about using a highly protein-bound antibiotic as a prophylactic agent against extravascular infections, especially if the ITF levels have not been shown to be adequate.

ACKNOWLEDGMENT

This research was supported by Eli Lilly & Co., Bristol Laboratories, and Beecham Massengill Laboratories.

LITERATURE CITED

1. **Bennett, J. V., J. L. Brodie, E. J. Benner, and W. M. M. Kirby.** 1966. Simplified, accurate method for antibiotic assay of clinical specimens. Appl. Microbiol. 14:170–177.
2. **Clarke, J. R., R. D. Libke, C. Regamey, and W. M. M. Kirby.** 1974. Comparative pharmacokinetics of amikacin and kanamycin. Clin. Pharmacol. Ther. 15:610–616.
3. **Fong, I. W., E. D. Ralph, E. R. Engelking, and W. M. M. Kirby.** 1976. Clinical pharmacology of cefamandole as compared with cephalothin. Antimicrob. Agents Chemother. 9:65–69.
4. **Gordon, R. C., C. Regamey, and W. M. M. Kirby.** 1973. Serum protein binding of aminoglycoside antibiotics. Antimicrob. Agents Chemother. 2:214–216.
5. **Libke, R. D., J. T. Clarke, E. D. Ralph, R. P. Luthy, and W. M. M. Kirby.** 1975. Ticarcillin vs carbenicillin: clinical pharmacokinetics. Clin. Pharmacol. Ther. 17:441–446.
6. **Moellering, R. C., Jr., and M. N. Swartz.** 1976. The newer cephalosporins. N. Engl. J. Med. 294:24–28.
7. **Tan, J. S., T. Bannister, and J. P. Phair.** 1974. Levels of amoxicillin and ampicillin in human serum and interstitial fluid. J. Infect. Dis. 129(Suppl.):S146–148.
8. **Tan, J. S., J. C. Holmes, N. O. Fowler, G. T. Manitsas, and J. P. Phair.** 1974. Antibiotic levels in pericardial fluid. J. Clin. Invest. 53:7–12.
9. **Tan, J. S., A. Trott, J. P. Phair, and C. Watanakunakorn.** 1972. A method for measurement of antibiotics in human interstitial fluid. J. Infect. Dis. 126:492–497.

ANTIMICROBIAL AGENTS AND CHEMOTHERAPY, Apr. 1977, p. 701-707 Vol. 11, No. 4

Chemotherapy of Genital Herpes Simplex Virus Type 2 Infections of Female Hamsters

HAROLD E. RENIS

Department of Experimental Biology, The Upjohn Company, Kalamazoo, Michigan 49001

Received for publication 22 November 1976

The antiviral activity of 1-β-D-arabinofuranosylcytosine (ara-C, cytarabine, Cytosar), 5-iodo-2'-deoxyuridine (IdUrd), 9-β-D-arabinofuranosyladenine (ara-A), and disodium phosphonoacetate (PAA) have been compared in herpes simplex virus type 2 (HSV-2)-infected primary rabbit kidney cells and in female hamsters with genital HSV-2 infection. In vitro, ara-C and IdUrd were more active than ara-A, and PAA was least active. In female hamsters with genital HSV-2 infection, intravaginal treatment with PAA or ara-A was more effective than either ara-C or IdUrd. PAA was more active than ara-A when treatment was initiated early (1 h) after infection. The activity of PAA was greatly reduced if initiation of treatment was delayed for 24 h. Both PAA and ara-A reduced the virus titers of the vagina and protected hamsters from death when the drugs were given by either the intravaginal or subcutaneous route, with intravaginal treatment being more effective.

Genital herpesvirus infections, primarily caused by herpes simplex virus type 2 (HSV-2), are transmitted by venereal contact (9, 26). The infection can be painful and recurrent. If lesions are present late during the gestation period, the neonate is at high risk, resulting in disease with high morbidity and mortality (25). Furthermore, HSV-2 has been implicated in the etiology of cervical carcinoma (2, 4, 23).

At the present time, there is no effective treatment for genital HSV infections. However, several agents with antiherpes activity in other systems have been studied in herpes genitalis. Topical application of certain heterocyclic dyes, followed by exposure to light, has been proposed as a method for treating this disease (5). However, in subsequent studies with proflavine (34), or in a double-blind study with neutral red (24), it was not possible to demonstrate efficacy.

We have recently described the experimental genital infection of female hamsters with HSV-2 (30). In the studies described herein, several drugs with reported antiherpes activity have been compared in vitro and in female hamsters with genital HSV-2 infection.

MATERIALS AND METHODS

Virus. Stocks of HSV-2 (strain 35D) were supplied by L. T. Chien, University of Tennessee. The virus had a titer of 7.5×10^5 to 1.0×10^6 plaque-forming units per 0.5 ml on primary rabbit kidney monolayers.

In vitro antiviral activity. Contiguous monolayers of primary rabbit kidney cells were infected by incubating 0.5 ml of stock virus with drained monolayers (60-mm plastic petri dishes, Falcon) for 60 min at 37°C. The monolayers were washed and refed with 4.5 ml of Eagle medium containing 3% fetal bovine serum. The drugs were prepared in Hanks solution, and 0.5 ml of the appropriate dilution was added to each plate, resulting in the concentrations indicated. The cultures were harvested to −70°C when approximately 50 to 75% of the cells in the control cultures showed evidence of cytopathology. The virus titers of the frozen-thawed cultures were determined by the plaque method on rabbit kidney monolayers.

Genital infection of female hamsters. The method of infecting hamsters with HSV-2 has been described (30). Briefly, female hamsters obtained from Charles River Lakeview (Newfield, N.J.) were housed in stainless-steel cages in a room containing male hamsters. The hamsters were infected within 1 week of arrival and at that time weighed 45 to 50 g. The vaginas were washed with 2 ml of saline about 1 h before inoculation of 0.1 ml of HSV-2 intravaginally.

Drug treatment. The drugs were obtained from commercial sources, except for disodium phosphonoacetate (PAA), which was generously provided by H. I. Skulnick of these laboratories. For the in vivo studies, the drugs were prepared in saline (0.9% NaCl) solution. For vaginal therapy, 0.1 ml of drug was delivered intravaginally using a tuberculin syringe fitted with a Temflex no. 24 vinyl-covered 22-gauge needle. Drugs were given three times each day at 8 a.m., noon, and 4 p.m. The drug concentration was 20 mg/ml.

For systemic treatment, the drugs were prepared at the appropriate concentration in saline solution and given by subcutaneous injection. Drug treatments were given twice each day (8 a.m. and 4 p.m.).

Fifteen hamsters comprised each group.

Vaginal swabs. Cotton-tipped swabs on 1/8-inch (ca. 0.3 cm) wooden dowels, wetted with Hanks solution, were used to swab the vaginas. The swabs were placed in tubes containing 2 ml of Eagle medium-3% fetal bovine serum. The samples were stored at −40°C until the time of virus assay by the plaque method on primary rabbit kidney cells.

RESULTS

Figure 1 compares the HSV-2 yields from primary rabbit kidney monolayers treated with different concentrations of 1-β-D-arabinofuranosylcytosine (ara-C), 5-iodo-2′-deoxyuridine (IdUrd), 9-β-D-arabinofuranosyladenine (ara-A), and PAA. These data show that ara-C was more active than the other compounds included in this study, and that PAA was the least inhibitory. None of the compounds was cytotoxic under these conditions. The effect of treating hamsters infected vaginally with HSV-2 by the topical application of drug is shown in Fig. 2. In this study, 13 of 15 hamsters treated with saline died (mean survival time [MST], 9.6 days). ara-C and IdUrd had little effect on the disease process. In both cases, 80% of the animals died and the MST was 10.9 and 11.5 days, respectively. ara-A treatment extended the MST to 15.6 days, but only 4 of the 15 hamsters survived the infection. PAA was most effective of the agents tested, in that 80% of the hamsters were protected with this drug. When the drug solutions were adjusted to pH 7, the resulting antiviral activity was nearly the same.

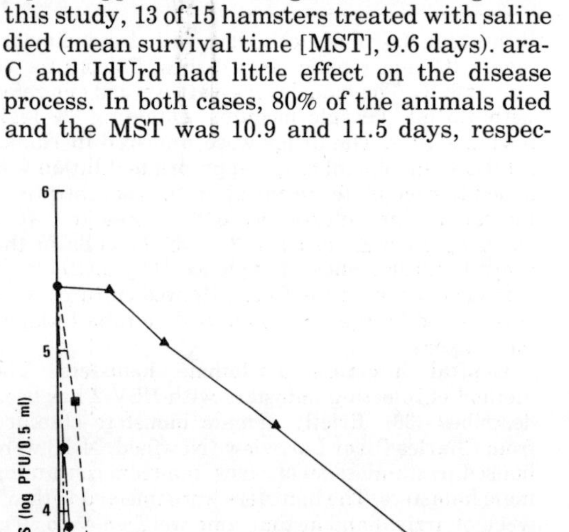

FIG. 1. *Virus (HSV-2) yields from infected primary rabbit kidney monolayers treated with different concentrations of ara-C (●), IdUrd (○), ara-A (■), and PAA (▲).*

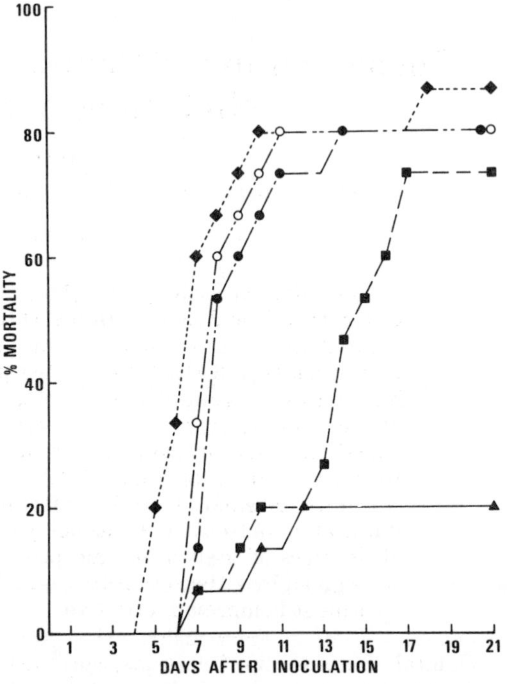

FIG. 2. *Effect of intravaginal treatment with saline (◆), ara-C (○), IdUrd (●), ara-A (■), and PAA (▲) on genital HSV-2 infection of female hamters. Each hamster received 15 treatments beginning on day 0.*

Vaginal swabs were taken from those animals depicted in Fig. 2 at 120 h after virus inoculation, i.e., 16 h after the final drug treatment. Titration of these samples (Table 1) showed that both ara-C and ara-A treatment reduced the virus titers, compared with the saline-treated animals, by nearly 1 log. IdUrd was less effective. PAA was the most effective drug in this series in that virus could not be recovered from any of the vaginal swabs taken at this time. Even though the virus titers of the ara-A-treated hamsters were similar to those of the ara-C-treated group, ara-A treatment was considerably more beneficial in delaying death than was either ara-C or IdUrd (Fig. 2).

Figure 3 compares the activity of PAA and ara-A when therapy was initiated at different times after virus inoculation. In this study, drug was administered for 4 days, rather than the 5 days described in Fig. 2. When treatment

TABLE 1. *Effect of intravaginal drug treatment on vaginal HSV-2 virus titers at 120 h after virus inoculation*

Treatment	Nv/Nt[a]	Mean[b]	S.D.[c]	ΔMean
Saline	9/12[d]	2.37	1.56	
Drug (20 mg/ml)				
ara-C	8/15	1.39	1.58	−0.98*[e]
ara-A	8/15	1.41	1.52	−0.95*
IdUrd	10/15	1.83	1.55	−0.54 (NS)
PAA	0/15	0		−2.37**

[a] Nv refers to the number of hamsters shedding virus, and Nt is the total number of hamsters in the group.
[b] Mean indicates the log of the mean of the virus titers.
[c] S.D., Standard deviation.
[d] Three hamsters were dead.
[e] * indicates $P < 0.05$, ** indicates $P < 0.01$, and NS is nonsignificant.

was initiated on day 0 (1 h after virus inoculation), ara-A treatment resulted in 33% survivors with an MST of 16 days, whereas PAA treatment resulted in 60% survivors with an MST of 17.3 days (Fig. 3A). This should be compared with saline treatment after which none of the hamsters survived and the MST was 7.9 days. If treatment was delayed for 24 h after inoculation (Fig. 3B), ara-A increased the percentage of hamsters surviving from 13.3% for the saline-treated controls to 40%, and the MST was increased from 9.3 days for the saline-treated controls to 18.3 days. PAA was less active when treatment was delayed; only 13% of the hamsters survived and the MST was 11 days, or about 2 days longer than that for saline-treated groups.

The virus titers of the vaginal swabs from 10 hamsters in each group taken 16 h after the final drug treatment (Table 2) showed that ara-A reduced the virus titers but not the number of animals shedding virus, compared with the saline-treated group, whether the therapy was initiated 1 or 24 h after virus inoculation. The difference in the titers between the ara-A- and saline-treated groups were 1.4 and 1.25 logs when therapy was initiated 1 or 24 h after virus inoculation, respectively. When PAA treatment was initiated at 1 h, virus was recovered from only one of 10 hamsters. Delaying PAA treatment until 24 h after virus inoculation greatly reduced the antiviral activity; seven of nine hamsters shed virus, and the mean virus titer was about 1 log less than that for the saline-treated group: this difference was not significant.

Figure 4 compares the effect of treating hamsters with ara-A or PAA by the intravaginal route (part A) versus the subcutaneous (part B) route. At the doses used, both ara-A and PAA appeared to be more effective when given intravaginally than when given subcutaneously. For example, vaginal treatment with ara-A increased the number of survivors from 6.7% for the saline-treated group to 53.3%. The MSTs were 9.8 and 18.1 days, respectively, for saline and ara-A. Vaginal treatment with PAA was most effective in that 93% of the hamsters survived.

When the drugs were given subcutaneously, 33% of the hamsters survived with ara-A (250 mg/kg) treatment, and the MST was 16.8 days. Treatment with PAA (400 mg/kg) by the same route resulted in 46.7% survivors, with an MST of about 16 days, whereas 13.3% of the saline-treated animals survived, and the MST was 10.5 days. The ara-A and PAA concentrations used for subcutaneous treatment were previously shown to be effective in HSV-infected hamsters (32) and mice (18, 31), respectively.

The course of the vaginal infection in hamsters treated vaginally or subcutaneously with ara-A or PAA (Fig. 4) was followed by daily virus titrations of vaginal swabs from 10 ham-

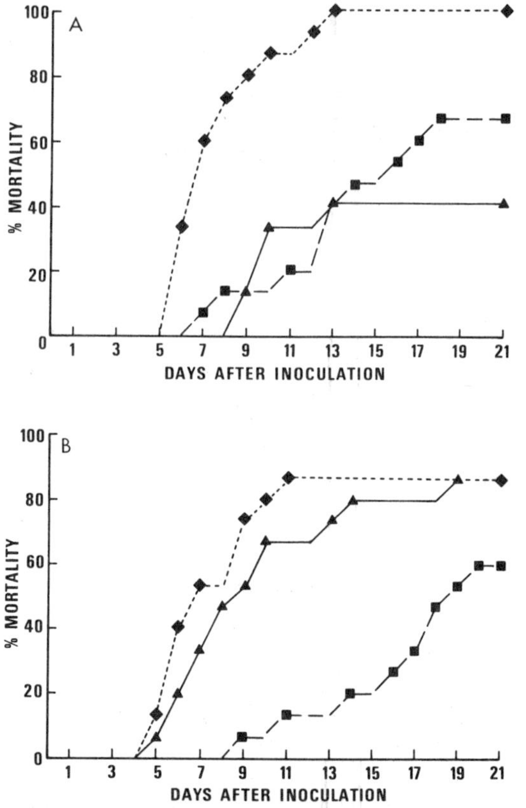

FIG. 3. *Effect of initiating drug therapy 1 h (A) or 24 h (B) after virus inoculation on genital HSV-2 infection of female hamsters. Each hamster received 12 treatments with saline (◆), ara-A (■), or PAA (▲).*

TABLE 2. *Vaginal HSV-2 virus titers from hamsters treated with saline, ara-A, or PAA according to the schedule in Fig. 3* [a]

Determination	Treatment (day 0)			Treatment (day 1)		
	Saline	ara-A	PAA	Saline	ara-A	PAA
Nv/Nt	9/10	8/10	1/10	8/9 [b]	7/10	7/9
Mean	2.45	1.07	0.05	2.98	1.73	2.03
S.D.	1.45	0.89	0.15	1.20	1.39	1.26
ΔMean		−1.39**	−2.40**		−1.25*	−0.95 (NS)
Survivors	0/15	5/15 (33%)	9/15 (60%)	2/15 (13%)	6/15 (40%)	2/15 (13%)
MST	7.9	16	17.3	9.3	18.3	11.1

[a] Vaginal swabs were taken 16 h after the final drug treatment. See Table 1 for definitions of symbols.
[b] Nine of ten hamsters survived at this time.

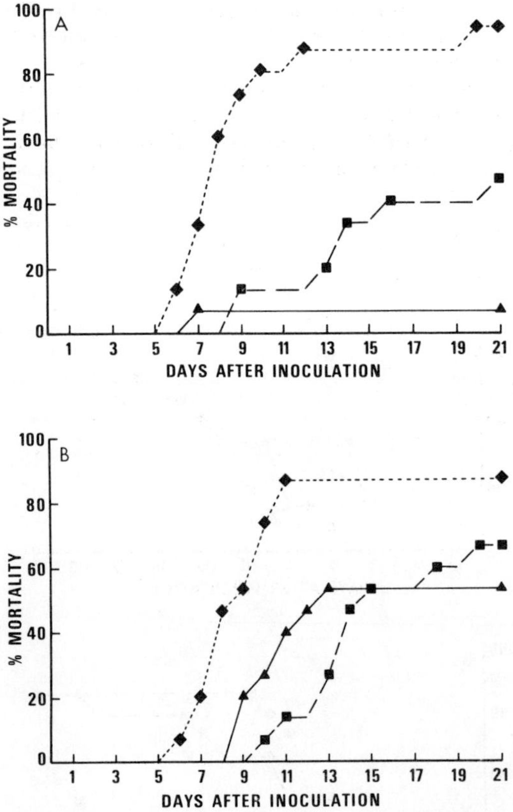

FIG. 4. *Effect of treating hamsters with saline (◆), ara-A (■), or PAA (▲) on genital HSV-2 infection. (A) Intravaginal treatment was given three times a day on days 0 through 4. (B) Subcutaneous treatment (PAA at 400 mg/kg, ara-A at 250 mg/kg) was given twice a day on days 0 through 4.*

sters in each group. Vaginal treatment with ara-A reduced the number of hamsters shedding virus from 10 for the saline-treated group to 5 to 6 (Table 3). Except for the swabs taken 72 h after inoculation, the means of the logs of the virus titers were significantly less than saline with the ara-A treatment. Vaginal treatment with PAA resulted in nearly complete protection from HSV infection, as determined by the vaginal swab virus titers.

When ara-A was administered subcutaneously, the vaginal virus titers were significantly less than the control, except for the 96-h samples (Table 3). The number of hamsters shedding virus at 120 and 144 h was decreased. Subcutaneous treatment with PAA decreased the number of hamsters shedding virus from 6 of 10 at 24 h to 1 of 10 at 72 h. At all times studied, the virus titers were significantly less than in the saline-treated group. In spite of the reduction in the number of hamsters shedding virus during this period of observation, nearly half of the animals died during the following 2 weeks.

DISCUSSION

The compounds included in the present study were selected because of demonstrated antiviral activity for HSV in vitro and in animals by the topical application directly to the site of the herpesvirus infection.

The relative in vitro antiviral activity for HSV-1 and HSV-2 for some of the compounds studied herein has been somewhat controversial. For example, ara-A was found to be more inhibitory than IdUrd for HSV-2 in chicken embryo cells and, further, it was observed that HSV-1 was more susceptible to either drug than HSV-2 (20). Person et al. (29) showed that the antiviral activity of ara-A and IdUrd for HSV-2 was dependent upon the host cell; e.g., HSV-2 was considerably less susceptible to IdUrd in chicken embryo cells than in HeLa cells. Fiala et al. (6) showed that ara-C was more active than ara-A, and IdUrd was less active for several strains of HSV-2 in WI-38 cells. These studies were extended by Marks (22), who showed that IdUrd was somewhat less active than ara-C, but both compounds were more active than ara-A in primary cultures from rabbit kidney or rat brain infected with several isolates of HSV-1 and HSV-2. The results presented herein agree with the latter studies, indicating that ara-C is the most active compound, followed by IdUrd and ara-A. PAA was the least active compound in the in vitro studies.

When these same drugs were applied topically to female hamsters with genital HSV-2 infection, PAA was the most active compound; ara-A was less active than PAA but more active than either ara-C or IdUrd. Treatment with ara-C and IdUrd did not increase the number of survivors and only slightly extended the MST. Hamsters treated with ara-C yielded less virus from vaginal swabs than did those treated with IdUrd, but neither drug significantly reduced the number of hamsters yielding virus. ara-A treatment extended the MST and increased the number of hamsters that survived infection. Approximately 50 to 80% of the hamsters treated with ara-A yielded virus, and the virus titers were reduced. PAA treatment, when drug therapy was initiated 1 h after virus inoculation, resulted in 80 to 93% survivors. Treatment with PAA under these conditions was highly effective in reducing the number of hamsters from which virus could be recovered in the vaginal swabs. In the above studies, the drugs were prepared in saline, and other vehicles were not used.

A topical antiherpes activity of IdUrd was first described by Kaufman, who used rabbits with herpes keratitis (12), and later in clinical keratitis (15). In addition, it has been shown that IdUrd in dimethyl sulfoxide is effective when applied topically to HSV infections of guinea pig skin (35) and in man (21). ara-C is topically active against experimental herpes keratitis in rabbits (36) and in man (14); however, ara-C is not used in clinical keratitis because of its corneal toxicity (13).

Sloan (32) has reviewed the antiviral activity of ara-A in animals with experimental herpesvirus infections, and Hyndiuk and Kaufman (10) have shown that ara-A is effective against ocular herpes simplex infections. It has recently been shown that topical application of ara-A was effective in treating herpetic eye disease in patients intolerant of or resistant to IdUrd (28). Systemic administration of ara-A to patients with cutaneous HSV-1 infections resulted in dramatic improvement, whereas the effect on HSV-2 lesions was less dramatic (3). ara-A has also been shown to be effective in immunosuppressed patients with varicella zoster (1, 11, 37). However, in a double-blind study comprised of 32 men with virologically proven herpes progenitalis, topical ara-A (3% in petrolatum vehicle) was not effective in altering the quantitative virology or the clinical course of the disease (8). ara-A, given intraperitoneally at 500 mg/kg to newborn mice inoculated intranasally with HSV-2, suppressed virus replication for 2 days and increased the MST by 2 days but did not increase the number of mice surviving the infection (16). Subcutaneous treatment with ara-A protected mice with

TABLE 3. *Vaginal HSV-2 titers from hamsters treated intravaginally or subcutaneously with saline, ara-A, or PAA*[a]

h postinfection	Saline			ara-A				PAA			
	Nv/Nt	Mean	S.D.	Nv/Nt	Mean	S.D.	ΔMean	Nv/Nt	Mean	S.D.	ΔMean
Intravaginal treatment											
24	10/10	2.66	0.92	6/10	1.08	1.03	−1.58**	0/10	0.0		−2.66**
48	10/10	3.46	0.80	5/10	1.39	1.52	−2.07**	0/10	0.0		−3.46**
72	10/10	2.56	1.04	6/10	1.88	1.61	0.69 (NS)	1/10	0.03	0.07	−2.53**
96	10/10	3.36	0.78	6/10	1.87	1.59	−1.48**	0.10	0.0		−3.36**
120	9/10	2.64	1.12	6/10	1.19	1.03	−1.45**	0.10	0.0		−2.64**
144	7/8[b]	2.08	1.15	6/10	1.00	1.02	−1.09**	0.10	0.0		−2.08**
Subcutaneous treatment											
24	10/10	3.07	0.95	7/10	1.52	1.24	−1.55**	6/10	1.26	1.14	−1.81**
48	10/10	3.68	0.57	8/10	1.71	1.16	−1.98**	4/10	0.63	0.89	−3.05**
72	10/10	2.54	0.81	7/10	1.68	1.38	−0.86*	1/10	0.33	0.93	−2.22**
96	9/10	2.44	1.51	7/10	1.69	1.40	−0.76 (NS)	1/10	0.36	1.14	−2.08**
120	10/10	2.91	0.93	4/10	0.69	0.97	−2.22**	1/10	0.27	0.87	−2.64**
144	9/9[c]	2.33	0.94	1/10	0.05	0.15	−2.28**	2/10	0.64	1.28	−1.69**

[a] Ten hamsters comprised each group. See Table 1 for definitions of symbols.
[b] Two dead.
[c] One dead.

HSV-1 or HSV-2 encephalitis (33). ara-A has been found to protect mice from cutaneous HSV infection if the drug is given intradermally at the site of infection (19) or intraperitoneally (17). ara-A treatment intraperitoneally of adult female mice with genital HSV-2 infection resulted in an extension of the MST without affecting the vaginal virus titers or the final mortality (27). Subsequently, it was observed that intravaginal ara-A treatment of mice with vaginal HSV-2 infection did not alter the virus replication in the vagina, nor did ara-A decrease the final mortality, whereas PAA was highly effective if given early after infection (E. R. Kern, J. C. Overall, and L. A. Glasgow, Prog. Abstr. Intersci. Conf. Antimicrob. Agents Chemother., 15th, Washington, D.C., Abstr. 239, 1975). The conflict concerning the reported efficacy of ara-A in mice with vaginal HSV-2 infections and the present studies with vaginally infected hamsters may be due to differences in the susceptibility of HSV-2 used for inoculation or the disposition of ara-A in the two animal species.

PAA was originally shown by Shipkowitz et al. (31) to be active when applied topically or given orally to mice with cutaneous HSV-2 infection. Subsequently, it was shown that intraperitoneal treatment was effective in mice with cutaneous HSV-1 infections (18). PAA was also effective when administered as drops to the eyes of rabbits with experimental keratitis (7) and when applied topically to the skin of mice with cutaneous HSV-1 lesions (38). Of interest is the observation that PAA, in the latter study, was effective only if treatment was initiated before 24 h after virus inoculation (38). PAA was similarly effective in mice inoculated intraperitoneally or vaginally, but only when drug treatment, given by the systemic or topical route, was initiated within 24 h after inoculation (E. R. Kern, J. C. Overall, and L. A. Glasgow, Prog. Abstr. Intersci. Conf. Antimicrob. Agents Chemother., 15th, Washington, D.C., Abstr. 239, 1975). In the studies reported herein, it was also observed that PAA was highly effective (using vaginal virus titers or mortality as criteria for antiviral activity) if topical drug treatments were initiated on the day of infection, but not if therapy was delayed for 1 day. ara-A was nearly as effective whether treatment was initiated on the day of infection or 24 h later.

In the present studies, no correlation existed between the in vitro antiviral activity and the activity resulting from the intravaginal treatment of female hamsters with genital HSV-2 infection. In fact, an inverse relationship existed: ara-C and IdUrd, the most inhibitory compounds in vitro, were the least active in hamsters, and ara-A and PAA, the least active in vitro, were the most active in hamsters. Both ara-A and PAA were effective in reducing vaginal virus titers and protecting hamsters from death when given parenterally (subcutaneously), as well as intravaginally, in this model. PAA appeared to be more active when given intravaginally. However, as in the other model infections (38; E. R. Kern, J. C. Overall, and L. A. Glasgow, Prog. Abstr. Intersci. Conf. Antimicrob. Agents Chemother., 15th, Washington, D.C., Abstr. 239, 1975) PAA was maximally active when drug treatment was initiated early after infection. ara-A retained activity even when therapy was initiated 24 h after virus inoculation.

ACKNOWLEDGMENTS

I wish to acknowledge the technical assistance of Barbara A. Court, E. B. Swynenberg, and F. T. Maida, as well as P. Good for the statistical analysis of the data.

LITERATURE CITED

1. **Aronson, M. D., C. F. Phillips, D. W. Gump, R. J. Albertini, and C. A. Phillips.** 1976. Vidarabine therapy for severe herpesvirus infections. J. Am. Med. Assoc. 235:1339–1342.
2. **Aurelian, L.** 1973. Virions and antigens of herpesvirus type 2 in cervical carcinoma. Cancer Res. 33:1539–1547.
3. **Chien, L. T., R. J. Whitley, L. J. Charamella, R. A. Buchanan, N. J. Cannon, W. E. Dismukes, and C. A. Alford.** 1975. Clinical and virologic studies with systemic administration of adenine arabinoside in severe, progressive, mucocutaneous herpes simplex virus infections, p. 205–224. *In* D. Pavan-Langston, R. A. Buchanan and C. A. Alford (ed.), Adenine arabinoside: an antiviral agent. Raven Press, New York.
4. **Duff, R., and F. Rapp.** 1971. Properties of hamster embryo fibroblasts transformed *in vitro* after exposure to ultraviolet-irradiated herpes simplex virus type 2. J. Virol. 8:469–477.
5. **Felber, T. D., E. B. Smith, J. N. Knox, C. Wallis, and J. L. Melnick.** 1973. Photodynamic inactivation of herpes simplex. Report of a clinical trial. J. Am. Med. Assoc. 223:289–292.
6. **Fiala, M., A. W. Chow, K. Miyasaki, and L. B. Guze.** 1974. Susceptibility of herpesviruses to three nucleoside analogues and their combinations and enhancement of the antiviral effect of acid pH. J. Infect. Dis. 129:82–85.
7. **Gerstein, D. D., C. R. Dawson, and J. O. Oh.** 1975. Phosphonoacetic acid in the treatment of experimental herpes simplex keratitis. Antimicrob. Agents Chemother. 7:285–288.
8. **Goodman, E. L., J. P. Luby, and M. T. Johnson.** 1975. Prospective double-blind evaluation of topical adenine arabinoside in male herpes progenitalis. Antimicrob. Agents Chemother. 8:693–697.
9. **Hutfield, D.** 1968. Herpes genitalis. Br. J. Vener. Dis. 44:241–250.
10. **Hyndiuk, R. A., and H. E. Kaufman.** 1967. Newer compounds in therapy of herpes simplex keratitis. Arch. Ophthalmol. 78:600–605.

11. **Johnson, M. T., J. P. Luby, R. A. Buchanan, and D. Mikulec.** 1975. Treatment of varicella-zoster virus infections with adenine arabinoside. J. Infect. Dis. **131**:225–229.
12. **Kaufman, H. E.** 1962. Clinical cure of herpes simplex keratitis by 5-iodo-2′-deoxyuridine. Proc. Soc. Exp. Biol. Med. **109**:251–252.
13. **Kaufman, H. E., J. A. Capella, E. D. Maloney, J. E. Robbins, G. M. Cooper, and M. H. Uotila.** 1964. Corneal toxicity of cytosine arabinoside. Arch. Ophthalmol. **72**:535–540.
14. **Kaufman, H. E., and E. D. Maloney.** 1963. IDU and cytosine arabinoside in experimental herpetic keratitis. Arch. Ophthalmol. **69**:626–629.
15. **Kaufman, H. E., E. Martola, and C. Dohlman.** 1962. Use of 5-iodo-2′-deoxyuridine (IDU) in treatment of herpes simplex. Arch. Ophthalmol. **68**:235–239.
16. **Kern, E. R., J. C. Overall, Jr., and L. A. Glasgow.** 1975. Herpesvirus hominis infection in newborn mice. Comparison of the therapeutic efficacy of 1-β-D-arabinofuranosylcytosine with 9-β-D-arabinofuranosyladenine. Antimicrob. Agents Chemother. **7**:587–595.
17. **Klein, R. J., A. E. Friedman-Kien, and E. Brady.** 1974. Herpes simplex virus skin infection in hairless mice: treatment with antiviral compounds. Antimicrob. Agents Chemother. **5**:318–322.
18. **Klein, R. J., and A. E. Friedman-Kien.** 1975. Phosphonoacetic acid-resistant herpes simplex virus infection in hairless mice. Antimicrob. Agents Chemother. **7**:289–293.
19. **Lieberman, M., T. W. Schafer, and P. E. Came.** 1973. Chemotherapy of cutaneous herpesvirus infections of hairless mice. J. Invest. Dermatol. **60**:203–206.
20. **Lowry, S. P., J. L. Melnick, and W. E. Rawls.** 1971. Investigation of plaque formation in chick embryo cells as a biological marker for distinguishing herpes virus type 2 from type 1. J. Gen. Virol. **10**:1–9.
21. **MacCallum, F. O., and B. E. Juel-Jensen.** 1966. Herpes simplex virus skin infection in man treated with iodoxuridine in dimethyl sulfoxide. Results of a double-blind controlled trial. Br. Med. J. **2**:805–807.
22. **Marks, M. I.** 1974. Variables influencing the *in vitro* susceptibilities of herpes simplex viruses to antiviral drugs. Antimicrob. Agents Chemother. **6**:34–38.
23. **Melnick, J. L., and W. E. Rawls.** 1970. Herpesvirus type 2 and cervical carcinoma. Ann. N. Y. Acad. Sci. **174**:993–998.
24. **Myers, M. G., M. N. Oxman, J. E. Clark, and K. A. Arndt.** 1975. Failure of neutral red photodynamic inactivation in recurrent herpes simplex virus infection. N. Engl. J. Med. **293**:945–949.
25. **Nahmias, A. J., C. A. Alford, and S. B. Korones.** 1970. Infection of the newborn with herpesvirus hominis. Adv. Pediatr. **17**:185–226.
26. **Nahmias, A. J., W. R. Dowdle, Z. M. Naib, W. E. Josey, D. McLone, and G. Domescik.** 1969. Genital infection with type 2 herpesvirus hominis. A commonly occurring veneral disease. Br. J. Vener. Dis. **45**:294–298.
27. **Overall, J. C., E. R. Kern, and L. A. Glasgow.** 1975. Treatment of herpesvirus hominis type 2 infections in mice with adenine arabinoside, p. 95–110. *In* D. Pavan-Langston, R. A. Buchanan, and C. A. Alford (ed.), Adenine arabinoside: an antiviral agent. Raven Press, New York.
28. **Pavan-Langston, D.** 1975. Clinical evaluation of adenine arabinoside and iodoxuridine in the treatment of ocular herpes simplex. Am. J. Ophthalmol. **80**:495–502.
29. **Person, D. A., P. J. Sheridan, and E. C. Herrmann, Jr.** 1970. Sensitivity of types 1 and 2 herpes simplex virus to 5-iodo-2′-deoxyuridine and 9-β-D-arabinofuranosyladenine. Infect. Immun. **2**:815–820.
30. **Renis, H. E.** 1975. Genital infection of female hamsters with herpesvirus hominis type 2 (HVH-2). Proc. Soc. Exp. Biol. Med. **150**:723–727.
31. **Shipkowitz, N. L., R. R. Bower, R. N. Appell, C. W. Nordeen, L. R. Overby, W. R. Roderick, J. B. Schleicher, and A. M. VonEsch.** 1973. Suppression of herpes simplex virus infection by phosphonoacetic acid. Appl. Microbiol. **26**:264–267.
32. **Sloan, B. J.** 1975. Adenine arabinoside: chemotherapy studies in animals, p. 45–94. *In* D. Pavan-Langston, R. A. Buchanan, and C. A. Alford (ed.), Adenine arabinoside; an antiviral agent. Raven Press, New York.
33. **Sloan, B. J., F. A. Miller, and I. W. McLean.** 1973. Treatment of herpes simplex virus types 1 and 2 encephalitis in mice with 9-β-D-arabinofuranosyladenine. Antimicrob. Agents Chemother. **3**:74–80.
34. **Taylor, P. K., and N. R. Doherty.** 1975. Comparison of the treatment of herpes genitalis in men with proflavine photoinactivation, iodoxuridine ointment, and normal saline. Br. J. Vener. Dis. **51**:125–129.
35. **Tomlinson, A. H., and F. O. Maccallum.** 1968. The effect of 5-iodo-2′-deoxyuridine on herpes simplex virus infections in guinea pig skin. Br. J. Exp. Pathol. **49**:277–282.
36. **Underwood, G. E.** 1962. Activity of 1-β-D-arabinofuranosylcytosine hydrochloride against herpes simplex keratitis. Proc. Soc. Exp. Biol. Med. **111**:660–664.
37. **Whitley, R. J., L. T. Chien, R. Dolin, G. J. Galasso, and C. A. Alford, Jr.** 1976. Adenine arabinoside therapy of herpes zoster in the immunosuppressed. N. Engl. J. Med. **294**:1193–1199.
38. **Wohlenberg, C. R., M. A. Walz, and A. L. Notkins.** 1976. Efficacy of phosphonoacetic acid on herpes simplex virus infection of sensory ganglia. Infect. Immun. **13**:1519–1521.

ANTIMICROBIAL AGENTS AND CHEMOTHERAPY, Apr. 1977, p. 708-711 Vol. 11, No. 4

Printed in U.S.A.

Cefazaflur, a New Parenteral Cephalosporin: In Vitro Studies

GEORGE W. COUNTS,* DAVID GREGORY, DOLORES ZELEZNIK, AND MARVIN TURCK

Department of Medicine, University of Washington and Harborview Medical Center, Seattle, Washington 98104

Received for publication 10 December 1976

Cefazaflur was tested in vitro against 262 strains of bacteria. Inhibitory and bactericidal concentrations were determined with two inoculum sizes of bacterial cells in Mueller-Hinton broth and nutrient broth. Agar dilution studies also were performed. When tested in agar, 5.0 μg or less of cefazaflur per ml inhibited almost all strains of *Staphylococcus aureus*, *Escherichia coli*, *Klebsiella*, and *Proteus mirabilis*. The drug was less active against *Enterobacter* and indole-positive *Proteus*, and 7.5 μg of antibiotic per ml inhibited approximately two-thirds to one-fourth of the strains. A concentration of 50 μg of cefazaflur per ml was required for inhibition of the enterococci. There was negligible activity against *Pseudomonas*. The drug demonstrated less activity in broth than in agar, and a major inoculum effect was seen with some strains. For example, with a lower inoculum, 2.5 μg of cefazaflur per ml killed all strains of *E. coli*, whereas with the higher inoculum, 7.5 μg of cefazaflur per ml, inhibited 64% and killed only 8% of strains. The activity of the drug for some strains was greater in Mueller-Hinton broth; for others, it was greater in nutrient broth. There were considerable differences in the results of the broth and agar studies for some species when the same medium was employed. Because of differences in activity found with different media, inocula, and method of testing, an evaluation of the eventual usefulness of cefazaflur must await the results of in vivo studies.

Cefazaflur, SKF 59962, is a new parenteral cephalosporin containing a 7-trifluoromethylthioacetyl group at the 7-acyl position (3). Drug concentrations in the serum of experimental animals were found to be similar to those obtained with comparable doses of cephalothin, although cefazaflur demonstrated greater in vitro activity than cephalothin against some genera of organisms, including isolates of *Enterobacter* (1).

The purpose of this study was to evaluate the antibacterial activity of cefazaflur in in vitro studies utilizing several different test conditions.

MATERIALS AND METHODS

Minimum inhibitory concentrations (MICs) and minimum bactericidal concentrations (MBCs) were determined using Mueller-Hinton (MH) broth (MHB; Difco) and nutrient broth (NB; Difco) according to previously described methods (4, 6). In broth dilution studies, the MBC was defined as the lowest concentration of drug yielding 10 colony-forming units or less when about 0.005 ml of broth from each clear tube was subcultured onto agar without antibiotic. Two different inocula containing 10^6 and 10^8 viable organisms per ml were used. Agar dilution MICs were determined with Mueller-Hinton agar (MHA) and nutrient agar (NA). The MIC in agar, obtained using a Steers replicator (5), was defined as the lowest concentration of drug that produced 3 or fewer colony-forming units on an agar plate after an 18-h incubation at 37°C. A total of 262 isolates were studied, including 53 strains of *Enterobacter* species, which represented 27 *Enterobacter cloacae*, 13 *Enterobacter aerogenes*, 4 *Enterobacter hafnia*, 4 *Enterobacter agglomerans*, and 5 *Enterobacter liquefaciens*. Thirty indole-positive *Proteus* isolates, which included 13 *Proteus morganii*, 11 *Proteus vulgaris*, and 6 *Proteus rettgeri*, were used. A laboratory reference strain of *Escherichia coli* inhibited by 1.0 μg of cefazaflur per ml was used as a control organism in all experiments.

RESULTS

Agar dilution. The results of studies determined in agar are presented in Table 1. There were no consistent differences among results obtained with various species of *Enterobacter* and indole-positive *Proteus* isolates, and the results are composited for each genus. The drug had negligible activity against *Pseudomonas aeruginosa*, and at least 50 μg of cefazaflur per ml was required to inhibit more than half of enterococcal isolates in agar. The drug was very active against strains of *E. coli*, *Proteus mirabilis*, *Klebsiella pneumoniae*, and *Staphylococcus aureus*, and 2.5 μg of cefazaflur per ml inhibited nearly all strains that had been tested with both inoculum sizes of bacterial cells. Ta-

TABLE 1. *Agar dilution MICs using inocula of 10^6 and 10^8 organisms/ml in MHA and NA*

Organism	Medium	Inoculum (organisms/ml)	Cumulative % of strains inhibited by an MIC (μg/ml) of: ≤0.5	1.0	2.5	5	7.5	10	15	20	25	50	100	250
Enterobacter	MHA	10^6	2	28	57	68	73	73	75	79	81	85	87	94
		10^8	2	9	36	53	57	60	66	66	73	75	77	85
	NA	10^6	2	2	15	24	32	36	40	45	49	55	77	79
		10^8	0	0	4	15	19	26	32	32	38	47	55	79
Proteus, indole positive	MHA	10^6	7	10	13	13	57	67	80	83	90	100	100	100
		10^8	3	3	10	10	27	27	50	53	60	90	90	10
	NA	10^6	10	27	37	50	73	83	93	93	93	100	100	100
		10^8	0	13	17	30	30	40	73	77	77	83	100	100
P. mirabilis	MHA	10^6	3	40	90	100	100	100	100	100	100	100	100	100
		10^8	3	27	83	100	100	100	100	100	100	100	100	100
	NA	10^6	97	97	100	100	100	100	100	100	100	100	100	100
		10^8	73	83	100	100	100	100	100	100	100	100	100	100
E. coli	MHA	10^6	87	100	100	100	100	100	100	100	100	100	100	100
		10^8	57	100	100	100	100	100	100	100	100	100	100	100
	NA	10^6	77	100	100	100	100	100	100	100	100	100	100	100
		10^8	63	97	100	100	100	100	100	100	100	100	100	100
Klebsiella	MHA	10^6	80	90	100	100	100	100	100	100	100	100	100	100
		10^8	73	87	97	100	100	100	100	100	100	100	100	100
	NA	10^6	63	93	97	100	100	100	100	100	100	100	100	100
		10^8	47	77	97	97	100	100	100	100	100	100	100	100
S. aureus	MHA	10^6	97	100	100	100	100	100	100	100	100	100	100	100
		10^8	97	97	100	100	100	100	100	100	100	100	100	100
	NA	10^6	97	97	100	100	100	100	100	100	100	100	100	100
		10^8	97	97	100	100	100	100	100	100	100	100	100	100

ble 1 also shows the results obtained when cefazaflur was tested in the two media. With *Enterobacter* strains, there was considerably more activity in MHS than in NA. For example, 15 μg of cefazaflur per ml inhibited approximately 70% of strains in MHA, whereas only 35% were similarly inhibited in NA. With indole-positive *Proteus* isolates, the drug was slightly more active in NA than in MHA, especially when tested at lower concentrations of antibiotic.

Broth dilution. Figures 1 and 2 show the results of studies that were determined in MHB and NB tested against 10^6 and 10^8 organisms/ml. In both broth media, cefazaflur demonstrated only modest activity against *Enterobacter* isolates. With the lower inoculum, 250 μg of antibiotic per ml inhibited about half of the strains and killed only 15 to 40%. There was insignificant activity with the higher inoculum when drug concentrations of up to 250 μg of cefazaflur per ml were used. Results with indole-positive strains of *Proteus* were essentially comparable in the two media. For example, 50 μg of cefazaflur per ml was required to inhibit approximately half of the strains when tested against the lower inoculum. For strains of *E. coli* and *Klebsiella*; MBCs that had been determined with 10^8 inoculum were considerably higher than MICs and MBCs that had been obtained with the lower inoculum of bacterial cells. In NB, a marked disparity between inhibition and killing was observed with strains of *P. mirabilis* and *Klebsiella* when tested with the higher inoculum. This difference in killing was less apparent in MHB.

Examples of representative observations obtained when comparing cefazaflur in agar and broth media are depicted in Fig. 3. Although 50 μg of cefazaflur per ml inhibited approximately 80% of *Enterobacter* strains when tested in agar, this concentration of antibiotic when studied in broth inhibited 25% at the lower inoculum, and none of the isolates was susceptible at the higher inoculum. Similarly, with isolates of indole-positive *Proteus*, 50 μg of cefazaflur per ml inhibited nearly all strains which had been tested in agar at both inoculum sizes of bacterial cells. However, 50 μg of cefazaflur per ml in a broth medium inhibited only 40% with the lower inoculum and none with the higher inoculum of bacterial cells. A difference was also observed with *E. coli* where MBCs were appreciably higher when the higher inoculum had been used in broth.

DISCUSSION

These in vitro studies with cefazaflur reveal that results were considerably influenced by several variables in methodology. First, the drug was very active against *S. aureus* and most isolates of *Enterobacteriaceae* when tested in agar. Second, a significant difference was demonstrated with *Enterobacter* when results

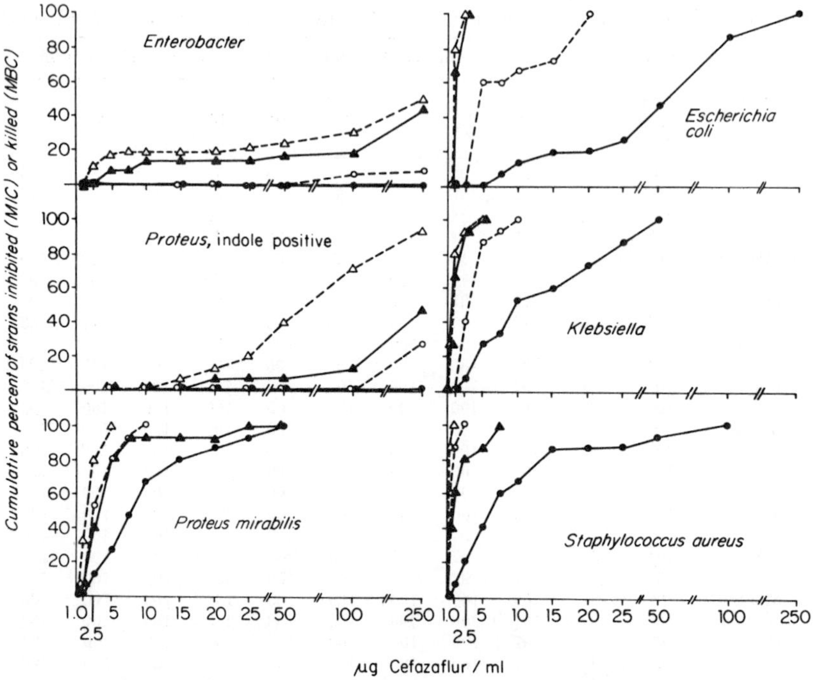

FIG. 1. *Cumulative percentage of isolates inhibited (MIC) or killed (MBC) by cefazaflur tested in MHB with an inocula of 10^6 and 10^8 organisms/ml. Symbols:* △, *MIC of 10^6 organisms/ml;* ▲, *MBC of 10^6 organisms/ml;* ○, *MIC of 10^8 organisms/ml;* ●, *MBC of 10^8 organisms/ml.*

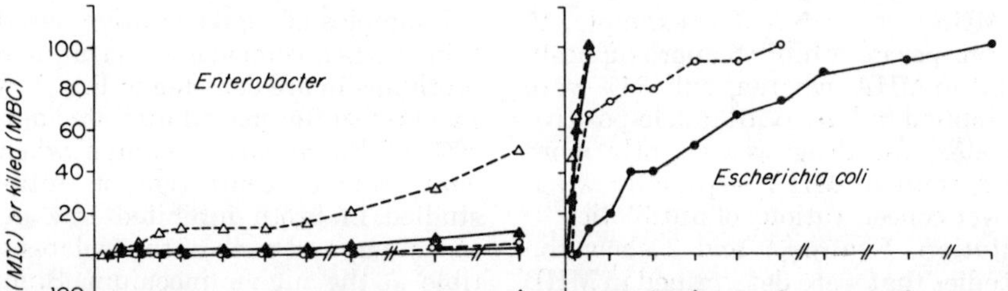

FIG. 2. *Cumulative percentage of isolates inhibited (MIC) or killed (MBC) by cefazaflur tested in NB with inocula of 10^6 and 10^8 organisms/ml. Symbols:* △, *MIC of 10^6 organisms/ml;* ▲, *MBC of 10^6 organisms/ml;* ○, *MIC of 10^8 organisms/ml;* ●, *MBC of 10^8 organisms/ml.*

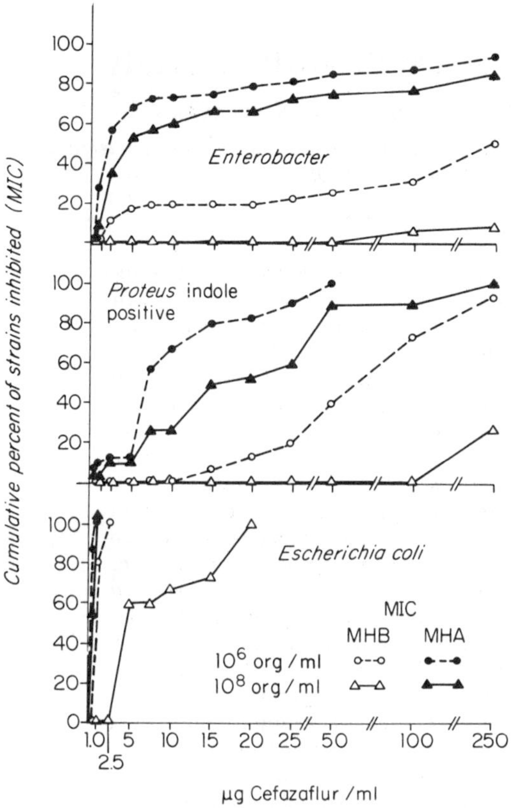

FIG. 3. *Cumulative percentage of isolates of Enterobacter, indole-positive Proteus, and E. coli inhibited (MIC) by cefazaflur in MHA compared to MHB with a bacterial inocula of two different sizes.*

that had been obtained with one medium were compared to those which had been obtained with another. Moreover, in MH medium, the results were quite different when the same strains of *Enterobacter* were tested by agar dilution and not by a broth dilution technique. Third, a significant inoculum effect was demonstrated when most isolates were tested in broth. For example, with an inoculum of 10^6 organisms/ml the drug exerted impressive activity, both inhibitory and killing, for some organisms, but it failed to inhibit or kill a significant percentage of organisms when a higher inoculum was employed.

Of the several variables that may influence the results of in vitro studies with antibiotics, it is by no means certain which test conditions most accurately predict potential clinical efficacy. Among these variables are inoculum size, pH, concentration of various ions, the presence or absence of serum in broth testing, and testing in solid versus liquid media. A marked effect of pH on in vitro activity of 16 of 17 cephalosporins was recently reported (M. Laverdiere and L. D. Sabath, Prog. Abstr. Intersci. Conf. Antimicrob. Agents Chemother., 16th, Chicago, Ill., Abstr. 319, 1976). It was noted that those antibiotics increased their activity 1- to 32-fold when the pH of the medium was decreased from 7.4 to 5.5. The initial pH of the MH medium used in our studies was 7.4 and that of nutrient was 6.8. Cefazaflur was not consistently more active in nutrient than in MH medium. There was no difference in calcium or magnesium concentrations, and we did not include serum in our studies or measure residual drug activity after incubation with organisms.

The activity of cefazaflur against *Enterobacter* strains tested in agar was similar to results reported from our laboratory with cefamandole (2). When tested in broth, cefamandole was somewhat more active than cefazaflur or cefoxitin against these same *Enterobacter* isolates (2). The higher MBCs for cefazaflur found with *P. mirabilis* and *Klebsiella* strains when tested with the higher inoculum of bacterial cells in NB also were observed to some extent with both cefamandole and cefoxitin.

In conclusion, cefazaflur demonstrated good antibacterial activity against many isolates of *Enterobacteriaceae* and *S. aureus*. However, because of the differences in activity found with different media, inocula, and method of testing, an evaluation of the eventual usefulness of cefazaflur must await the results of in vivo studies.

LITERATURE CITED

1. **Actor, P., J. V. Uri, J. R. Guarini, I. Zajac, L. Phillips, C. S. Sachs, R. M. DeMarinis, J. R. E. Hoover, and J. A. Weisbach.** 1975. A new parenteral cephalosporin. SK&F 59962: *In vitro* and *in vivo* antibacterial activity and serum levels in experimental animals. J. Antibiot. (Tokyo) 28:471–476.
2. **Adams, H. G., G. A. Stilwell, and M. Turck.** 1976. In vitro evaluation of cefoxitin and cefamandole. Antimicrob. Agents Chemother. 9:1019–1024.
3. **DeMarinis, R. M., J. R. E. Hoover, G. L. Dunn, P. Actor, J. V. Uri, and J. A. Weisbach.** 1975. A new parenteral cephalosporin. SK&F 59962: 7-trifluoromethylthioacetamido-3-(1-methyl-1H-tetrazol-5-ylthiomethyl)-3-cephem-4-carboxylic acid. Chemistry and structure activity relationships. J. Antibiot. (Tokyo) 28:463–470.
4. **Reller, L. B., W. W. Karney, H. N. Beaty, K. K. Holmes, and M. Turck.** 1973. Evaluation of cefazolin, a new cephalosporin antibiotic. Antimicrob. Agents Chemother. 3:488–497.
5. **Steers, E., E. L. Foltz, and B. S. Graves.** 1959. An inocula replicating apparatus for routine testing of bacterial susceptibility to antibiotics. Antibiot. Chemother. 9:307–311.
6. **Turck, M., K. N. Anderson, R. H. Smith, J. F. Wallace, and R. G. Petersdorf.** 1965. Laboratory and clinical evaluation of a new antibiotic–cephalothin. Ann. Intern. Med. 63:199–211.

ANTIMICROBIAL AGENTS AND CHEMOTHERAPY, Apr. 1977, p. 712-717 Vol. 11, No. 4

Side Effects of Minocycline: A Double-Blind Study

W. LEE FANNING,[1] DIETER W. GUMP,* AND ROBERT A. SOFFERMAN

Department of Medicine, Division of Infectious Diseases, and the Department of Surgery, Division of Otolaryngology, University of Vermont College of Medicine, Burlington, Vermont 05401*

Received for publication 19 October 1976

We studied the incidence and type of side effects of minocycline in a double-blind study. A total of 45 volunteers (18 men and 27 women) were given minocycline, and 44 volunteers (23 men and 21 women) were given placebo. The men in both the minocycline and placebo groups were significantly ($P < 0.0001$) larger than the women in the comparable groups. Minocycline dosage was 100 mg every 12 h for 5 days, and placebo was administered in an identical manner. Minocycline serum concentrations were determined in 12 volunteers at 1, 2, 4, and 6 h after the morning doses on days 1, 3, and 5 of the study. Side effects were recorded by volunteers in diaries and also through daily interviews and were evaluated by examination and electronystagmography. Peak minocycline serum concentrations were seen by day 3 and correlated with the peak onset of side effects. These concentrations were significantly higher in women than in men. Vestibular side effects occurred in 70.4% of the women on minocycline and significantly ($P < 0.0001$) exceeded the rate of the women on placebo (9.5%). Only loss of balance was significantly ($P < 0.05$) increased in the men taking minocycline as contrasted with men on placebo. Electronystagmography generally revealed no abnormalities. Side effects were usually not severe: four volunteers in the minocycline group and two in the placebo group discontinued their capsules because of side effects. It is concluded that women experience an unacceptably high incidence of side effects from minocycline, and this may be related to their higher serum concentrations, which in turn may relate to their smaller size.

Minocycline has been shown to be an effective drug for meningococcal prophylaxis (8). Many recent reports, however, have indicated a high incidence of side effects from minocycline (3, 6, 10, 15), and the Center for Disease Control now recommends rifampin for meningococcal prophylaxis (4). Recent studies showing a high incidence of side effects were, however, retrospective and not double blind. Therefore, this double-blind study was undertaken to document the frequency and character of side effects associated with minocycline.

MATERIALS AND METHODS

Volunteers. A total of 89 healthy volunteers were selected after history, physical examination, white blood count, differential, hematocrit, urinalysis, and a negative pregnancy test. The volunteers consisted of students and university and hospital employees. Hematological tests and urinalyses were repeated at the conclusion of the study. Persons allergic to tetracycline, those taking antacids, or those who had a past history of vertigo or light-headedness were excluded from the study. A full disclosure consent form outlining all the possible side effects of the drug was signed by each volunteer. The study protocol and consent forms were reviewed and approved by the University of Vermont Human Experimentation Committee.

Volunteers were randomly assigned into the placebo or the minocycline group in a double-blind fashion. The study utilized the out-patient facilities of the Clinical Research Center at the University of Vermont. The medications were supplied in identical packets for each volunteer indicating the order in which each capsule would be taken over the course of 5 days. The 45 volunteers in the minocycline group received 100-mg capsules at 8:00 a.m. and 8:00 p.m. for 5 consecutive days, and the 44 volunteers in the placebo group received placebo capsules in a similar manner.

Volunteers were seen once a day to evaluate side effects, but it was up to the volunteer to mention any problems, and only then were further questions asked concerning the complaint and related side effects. Used medication packets were turned in each day from the previous day. Volunteers were given recording sheets that divided the day into six hourly intervals to record the onset of side effects while at home. Side effects were scored for both duration and severity each day as follows. Duration: (i) symptoms lasting less than 2 min; (ii) symptoms lasting from 2 min to 1 h; (iii) symptoms lasting from 1 to 6 h; (iv) symptoms lasting for more than 6 h; and

[1] Present address: 100 Wendell Ave., Pittsfield, MA 01201.

severity: (i) minimal, noticeable symptom, but no limitation of daily activity; (ii) mild, slight limitation of daily activity; (iii) moderate, definite limitation of daily activity, but still active; (iv) severe, limitation of activity to bed or chair.

The mean age of both the minocycline and placebo groups was 27 years, and ages ranged from 19 to 52 years in the minocycline group and from 18 to 52 years in the placebo group. There were 48 women and 41 men overall with 27 women and 18 men in the minocycline group and 21 women and 23 men in the placebo group. The mean surface area in the placebo group was 1.97 m^2 for the men and 1.63 m^2 for the women and, in the minocycline group, 1.89 m^2 for the men and 1.61 m^2 for the women. The difference in surface area between men and women in both groups was significant ($P < 0.0001$, Student's t test).

Bioassay. Twenty volunteers (twelve minocycline and eight placebo) had blood drawn at 1, 2, 4, and 6 h after the 8:00 a.m. capsule on days 1, 3, and 5 to determine concentrations of minocycline in their serum. Urine assays were done on the morning of day 5 at 7:30 a.m. for the presence or absence of antibacterial activity as a measure of volunteer compliance. The bioassay for serum and urine minocycline concentrations were done using a standard agar diffusion assay employing *Bacillus subtilis* spores, American Type Culture Collection 6633 (14).

ENG testing. Prior to the study, 40 of the 89 volunteers had screening electronystagmograms (ENGs) consisting of spontaneous direct current recording from the horizontal leads with eyes closed and bithermal water calorics. Testing was done with a dual channel Instrumentation and Control Systems Incorporated ENG recorder. All sedative medications and alcoholic beverages were discontinued 24 h prior to testing. During the study week, symptomatic volunteers with dizziness, light-headedness, or tinnitus were given complete ENGs, and the tests were repeated on subsequent days if symptoms persisted. We also examined symptomatic volunteers for neurological abnormalities.

The complete ENG examination included spontaneous recordings for horizontal and vertical nystagmus, visually induced eye movements (pendular tracking, optokinetic nystagmus and gaze testing), positional tests, and bithermal water calorics. Except for the visual tests, all recordings were performed with eyes closed. The slow phase velocity for each caloric test was averaged for that ENG, and comparisons were then made between premedication, medication, and postmedication readings. All volunteers with significant abnormalities on ENG during the study period had repeat ENGs performed a minimum of 3 days after the last dose of medication. All ENGs were read before the drug code was broken.

RESULTS

Table 1 presents the incidence of side effects for men and women volunteers in the minocycline and placebo groups. With the exception of loss of balance ($P < 0.05$), the male subjects did not experience any significant increase in side effects. However, women subjects noted a significant increase in many different symptoms including light-headedness ($P < 0.0001$), lack of ability to concentrate ($P < 0.0001$), loss of balance ($P < 0.01$), nausea ($P < 0.002$), and dizziness ($P < 0.01$). Vestibular symptoms (light-headedness, loss of balance, dizziness, and tinnitus combined) occurred in 70.4% of the women taking minocycline as contrasted with only 9.5% on placebo, a markedly significant ($P < 0.0001$) increase. It was also evident that women taking minocycline had significantly

TABLE 1. *Side effects in placebo and minocycline groups divided according to sex*

Side effect	No. experiencing side effects with:				P values[a]			
	Placebo		Minocycline					
	Men (n = 23)	Women (n = 21)	Men (n = 18)	Women (n = 27)	M vs. M	W vs. W	M vs. W	M vs. W
Light-headed	3 (13.0)[b]	1 (4.8)	3 (16.7)	18 (66.7)	NS	<0.0001	NS	<0.002
Lack of concentration	1 (4.3)	0 (0)	2 (11.1)	9 (33.3)	NS	<0.0001	NS	NS
Loss of balance	0 (0)	1 (4.8)	2 (11.1)	9 (33.3)	<0.05	<0.01	NS	NS
Nausea	3 (13.0)	1 (4.8)	3 (16.7)	12 (44.4)	NS	<0.002	NS	<0.05
Dizzy (vertigo)	2 (8.7)	1 (4.8)	1 (5.6)	9 (33.3)	NS	<0.01	NS	<0.01
Euphoria	0 (0)	0 (0)	1 (5.6)	2 (7.4)	NS	NS	NS	NS
Vomiting	1 (4.3)	0 (0)	0 (0)	2 (7.4)	NS	NS	NS	NS
Weakness	1 (4.3)	1 (4.8)	2 (11.1)	1 (3.7)	NS	NS	NS	NS
Headache	4 (17.4)	3 (14.3)	5 (27.8)	7 (25.9)	NS	NS	NS	NS
Skin rash	2 (8.7)	1 (4.8)	1 (5.6)	2 (7.4)	NS	NS	NS	NS
Visual problems	1 (4.3)	0 (0)	0 (0)	2 (7.4)	NS	NS	NS	NS
Tinnitus	0 (0)	1 (4.8)	0 (0)	2 (7.4)	NS	NS	NS	NS
Vestibular symptoms[c]	4 (17.4)	2 (9.5)	5 (27.8)	19 (70.4)	NS	<0.0001	NS	<0.005
All side effects	11 (47.8)	3 (14.3)	11 (61.1)	22 (81.5)	NS	<0.0001	<0.005	NS

[a] Four comparisons are presented: men in the placebo group versus men in the minocycline group (M vs. M), women in the placebo group versus women in the minocycline group (W vs. W), men versus women in the placebo (M vs. W), and men versus women in the minocycline group (M vs. W). NS, not significant. P values were computed by a test of proportions using the arc sine transformation.

[b] Numbers in parentheses signify percentages.

[c] Combination of light-headedness, loss of balance, dizziness, and tinnitus.

higher rates of light-headedness, nausea, dizziness, and vestibular symptoms than did men in the minocycline group. Finally, men in the placebo group had a higher rate (47.8%) of all side effects than did women (14.3%) in the same group.

Seventy percent (23/33) of side effects began between the second and third day with 6% (2/33) of side effects occurring in the first 24 h and 24% (8/33) beginning after the third day. Seventy-five percent (18/24) of side effects that continued after stopping the minocycline were gone by 48 h, but 25% (6/24) continued for 3 days or more. None of the volunteers had symptoms disappear before actually stopping the drug.

The symptomatic volunteers in the minocycline group had a significantly longer duration of side effects for all symptoms ($P < 0.01$) and vestibular symptoms ($P < 0.05$) than did the symptomatic volunteers in the placebo group (Table 2). However, the severity of side effects between these two groups did not differ. Four volunteers in the minocycline group and two in the placebo group discontinued their capsules because of severe side effects. Those in the minocycline group discontinued the capsules on day 4 or 5, and all had moderate or severe vestibular symptoms. The two who stopped taking the capsules in the placebo group had an influenza-like illness and, in one volunteer, this was serologically confirmed as influenza A.

There were five volunteers in the minocycline group with positive physical findings while they were symptomatic, and there were none in the placebo group. They included a positive Romberg, slight tremor, slight nystagmus, minimal postural hypotension, and a maculo-papular skin rash. Three volunteers in the minocycline group developed a vaginal yeast infection after the study week with none occurring in the placebo group.

Table 3 demonstrates that there was a significant ($P < 0.02$) fall in the white blood counts of the male volunteers taking minocycline compared with those of the men in the placebo group. The women taking minocycline also showed a decrease in white blood counts, but this change was not significant when compared with those of the women in the placebo group.

TABLE 2. *Analysis of duration and severity code of symptomatic volunteers*[a]

Determination	All side effects[b]		Vestibular side effects[b]	
	Duration (days)	Severity (days)	Duration (days)	Severity (days)
Placebo	2.21 ± 0.33[c]	1.43 ± 0.29	1.67 ± 0.49	1.50 ± 0.50
Minocycline	3.33 ± 0.17	2.00 ± 0.20	3.13 ± 0.24	1.88 ± 0.23
P value[d]	<0.01	NS[e]	<0.05	NS

[a] See text for the duration and severity codes.
[b] Number of volunteers with all side effects: 14 placebo and 33 minocycline. Number of volunteers with vestibular side effects: 6 placebo and 24 minocycline.
[c] Standard error of the mean.
[d] Student's *t* test.
[e] Not significant at the 0.05 level.

TABLE 3. *Minocycline and white blood count (WBC) before and after study period*

	Pre-WBC/mm³	Post-WBC/mm³	Mean Δ	*P*[a]
Men				
Minocycline (18)[b]	7,330 ± 2,680[c] (4,300–15,100)[d]	6,020 ± 1,420 (3,400–9,600)	−1,310 ± 2,766	0.02
Placebo (23)	5,670 ± 990 (4,300–8,300)	5,780 ± 1,480 (3,100–8,800)	+110 ± 1,119	
Women				
Minocycline (27)	5,640 ± 1,210 (3,600–9,300)	5,190 ± 1,150 (3,100–7,400)	−450 ± 1,171	NS
Placebo (21)	6,010 ± 1,430 (4,000–8,700)	6,050 ± 1,560 (3,700–9,600)	+40 ± 1,426	

[a] Two sample *t* tests.
[b] Numbers in parentheses signify number of volunteers in group.
[c] Plus or minus 1 standard deviation.
[d] Range.

Minocycline serum concentrations 1, 2, 4, and 6 h after the ingestion of 100 mg of drug revealed a peak at 2 h (Fig. 1). Serum concentrations demonstrated a progressive increase from day 1 to day 5, and the difference between day 1 and 5 was significant ($P < 0.001$). The mean peak concentration (2 h) for all 3 days in women versus men was significantly different with a higher mean for the women of 3.40 ± 0.33 standard error of the mean μg/ml and a mean for the men of 2.45 ± 0.25 standard error of the mean μg/ml ($P < 0.05$). Correlation of body surface area versus serum concentrations of minocycline revealed an inverse correlation of surface area to serum concentration ($P = 0.01$, Pearson correlation coefficient of −0.6334).

All volunteers in the minocycline group had evidence of minocycline in their urine on a first morning specimen of day 5. Three volunteers in the placebo group also had evidence of antibiotic activity in their urine, but in only one of the volunteers was this activity marked. This volunteer was discovered to have taken rifampin on day 4 of the study after exposure to a patient with meningococcal meningitis. She had no symptoms. The two other placebo urines with minimal antibiotic activity could not be explained.

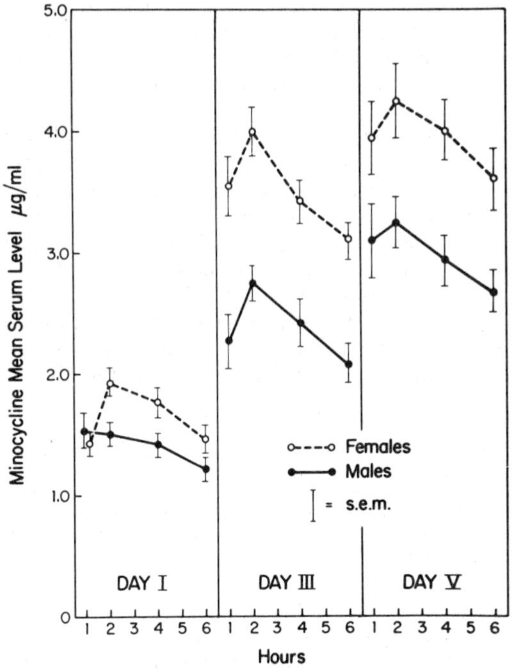

FIG. 1. *Mean serum concentrations of minocycline in 12 volunteers on days 1, 3, and 5. These volunteers received 100 mg of minocycline twice daily for the 5-day period, and the blood samples were obtained at 1, 2, 4, and 6 h after the ingestion of 100 mg of minocycline. The marked increase in serum levels between day 1 and 3 is evident and is a reflection of the 13.5-h half-life of the drug.*

Forty volunteers had screening ENGs prior to the study. All forty had normal bithermal water caloric tests. Twenty symptomatic volunteers had ENGs completed during the study period. Sixteen of the twenty volunteers had only one ENG during the 5-day study period, and four had multiple ENGs during that time. Four volunteers taking minocycline had abnormal ENGs, and all four demonstrated disorganized optikokinetic nystagmus, and three of the four improved in the posttreatment test. One volunteer demonstrated a hyperactive caloric response averaging 29° per s during the treatment phase returning to a normal average response of 18.9° per s after minocycline was stopped. Five volunteers taking minocycline had equivocal ENGs, three demonstrating slightly increased caloric responses and two manifesting equivocal slow spontaneous horizontal nystagmus. The remaining 11 volunteers had normal ENGs including the only individual on placebo. Abnormal ENG readings did not correlate well with neurological findings or severity of side effects, and several volunteers with the most severe vestibular symptoms had normal ENGs. There were too few volunteers who underwent both ENG and serum antibiotic concentration tests to correlate these two measurements.

DISCUSSION

Previous data on side effects produced by minocycline are confusing. Studies published in 1974 or before showed a low incidence of side effects with minocycline using a short prophylactic regimen (5, 7, 9, 12). The incidence of side effects varied from 0% to 36% with very few vestibular symptoms (dizziness or light-headedness) reported. Reports from 1974 and later showed an incidence of side effects of 73% to 90%, and the majority were vestibular (3, 4, 6, 10, 15). It is difficult to explain the change in the incidence, but differences between the earlier and later studies are apparent.

Most of the earlier studies were done in male, military personnel and were designed mainly to look at eradication of the meningococcal carrier state (5, 9, 15). It is interesting that the study of Devine (5) showed an increase in the frequency of side effects in males when the dosage was increased from 200 mg per 24 h to 400 mg per 24 h, but the frequency did not approach recent figures. A British report stated that side effects in women were 7 to 13 times higher than those in men using 300 mg of minocycline in one dose for gonococcal cervicitis or urethritis (11). In the U.S., using minocycline for meningococcal chemoprophylaxis, one group of observers also noted a higher reaction rate among women than among men, but the difference was not significant (11).

Our data definitely establish that vestibular and other side effects are significantly increased in women taking minocycline. In men, only loss of balance was increased, and this was at a borderline level of significance ($P < 0.05$). It may be that a major explanation for the increase in side effects observed with minocycline is due to the more extensive use in women and also to the greater attention now being paid to side effects.

We observed significantly higher serum concentrations of minocycline in women and feel this may be the explanation for their higher incidence of side effects. The women's higher serum levels are probably related to their smaller size. An analysis of the inverse correlation of body surface area with serum concentrations in the present study confirmed an earlier report of significant differences between peak serum concentrations in men and women when related to body surface area (2). Unfortunately, we determined antimicrobial serum concentrations in too few volunteers to permit an analysis of body surface and sex as independent factors affecting serum minocycline concentrations.

In the present study the men received a mean of 106 mg/m^2 per day of minocycline, and the women received 124 mg/m^2 per day. Recalculation of a female dosage regimen using the male dose of 106 mg/m^2 per day would yield a mean daily dose in women of 170 mg/day. It is not presently known whether reducing the dose in women would decrease the vestibular side effects.

The degree of leukopenia observed in the men in this study was slight but significant. Leukopenia has been associated with tetracycline administration but is rare (13).

The onset of symptoms in the symptomatic volunteers differs from other studies, which reported a high frequency of symptoms within the first 24 h (3, 10). Only 6% of our volunteers had the onset of their symptoms in the first 24 h with the onset occurring most often (70%) between the second and third day. The time of onset may be related to the fact that minocycline serum concentrations increased markedly from day 1 to day 3 (Fig. 1) as would be expected with a drug with a half-life of 13.5 h (2). Most symptoms appear to wane by 48 h (75%) after stopping minocycline, which is in agreement with other studies (10, 15). However, six volunteers had persistence of symptoms for 3 days or more after stopping the medication, and these were the volunteers with the most severe side effects. In two recent studies, a majority of those with symptoms could not complete the course of minocycline because of side effects (10, 15). In our study, only four volunteers in the minocycline group and two volunteers in the placebo group could not complete their medication because of vestibular side effects.

Minocycline has been shown to give levels in canine brains that are higher than doxycycline, tetracycline, or oxytetracycline, and this is probably due to its higher lipid solubility (1). This finding is of interest in view of the vestibular side effects. We used the ENG in hopes of objectively evaluating the vestibular symptoms, but ENG abnormalities were subtle and inconsistent. Forty-seven percent of symptomatic volunteers on minocycline demonstrated normal ENGs. Unfortunately, the ENG did not correlate well with severity of vestibular symptoms; several volunteers with severe symptoms had normal ENGs. The side effects may still be related to the brain levels of minocycline, but minocycline may affect cerebral areas to which the ENG is insensitive. The value of the ENG in predicting ENG abnormalities and the rapid return to normal suggests that the insult to the vestibular system is transient and not particularly severe.

The high frequency of vestibular side effects which we observed in women would argue against the use of minocycline for meningococcal prophylaxis (9). These symptoms might easily confuse the physician looking for the subtle early changes of meningococcal meningitis in the exposed patient. We would agree with the U.S. Public Health Service that rifampin should be used presently until another alternative prophylactic antibiotic is available (10).

ACKNOWLEDGMENTS

We are indebted to Susan Sykas for technical assistance and to Taka Ashikaga for biostatistical assistance.

This study was supported by a grant from the Parke, Davis & Co., the General Research Support Grant 05429-14 and Public Health Service grant M01 00109-13 from the Clinical Research Center.

LITERATURE CITED

1. **Barza, M., R. B. Brown, C. Shanks, C. Gamble, and L. Weinstein.** 1975. Relation between lipophilicity and pharmacological behavior of minocycline, doxycycline, tetracycline, and oxytetracycline in dogs. Antimicrob. Agents Chemother. 8:713–720.
2. **Bernard, B., E. J. Yin, and H. J. Simon.** 1971. Clinical pharmacologic studies with minocycline. J. Clin. Pathol. 11:332–348.
3. **Center for Disease Control.** 1975. Vestibular reactions to minocycline after meningococcal prophylaxis. Morbid. Mortal. Weekly Rep. 24:9–11.

4. **Center for Disease Control.** 1975. Vestibular reactions to minocycline – follow-up. Morbid. Mortal. Weekly Rep. 24:55-56.
5. **Devine, L. F., D. P. Johnson, C. R. Hagerman, W. E. Pierce, S. L. Rhode, and R. O. Peckinpough.** 1971. The effect of minocycline on meningococcal nasopharyngeal carrier state in naval personnel. Am. J. Epidemiol. 93:337-345.
6. **Fanning, W. L., and D. W. Gump.** 1976. Minocycline: distressing side effects. Arch. Intern. Med. 136:761-762.
7. **Frisk, A. R., and G. Tunevall.** 1969. Clinical evaluation of minocycline, p. 335-339. Antimicrob. Agents Chemother., 1968.
8. **Guttler, R. B., G. W. Counts, C. K. Avent, and H. N. Beaty.** 1971. Effect of rifampin and minocycline on meningococcal carrier rates. J. Infect. Dis. 124:199-205.
9. **Guttler, R. B., and H. Beaty.** 1972. Minocycline in the chemoprophylaxis of meningococcal disease. Antimicrob. Agents Chemother. 1:397-402.
10. **Jacobson, J. A., and B. Daniel.** 1975. Vestibular reactions associated with minocycline. Antimicrob. Agents Chemother. 8:453-455.
11. **Masterton, G., and C. B. Schofield.** 1976. Vestibular reactions to minocycline – Scotland. Morbid. Mortal. Weekly Rep. 25:31.
12. **Munford, R. S., A. J. Sussuarana de Vasconcelos, C. J. Phillips, D. S. Gelli, G. W. Gorman, J. B. Risi, and R. A. Feldman.** 1974. Eradication of carriage of *Neisseria meningitidis* in families: a study in Brazil. J. Infect. Dis. 129:644-649.
13. **Ory, E. M.** 1974. The tetracyclines, p. 102. *In* B. M. Kagan (ed.), Antimicrobial therapy. W. B. Saunders Co., Philadelphia.
14. **Sabath, L. D., and J. M. Matsen.** 1974. Assay of antimicrobial agents, p. 428-430. *In* E. H. Lennette, E. H. Spaulding, and J. P. Truant (ed.), Manual of clinical microbiology, 2nd ed. American Society for Microbiology, Washington, D.C.
15. **Williams, D. N., L. W. Laughlin, and Y. Lee.** 1974. Minocycline: possible vestibular side effects. Lancet ii:744-746.

ANTIMICROBIAL AGENTS AND CHEMOTHERAPY, Apr. 1977, p. 718-724 Vol. 11, No. 4

Printed in U.S.A.

Bacteriocin Production by Strains of *Bacteroides* Isolated from Human Feces and the Role of These Strains in the Bacterial Ecology of the Colon

S. J. BOOTH,* J. L. JOHNSON, AND T. D. WILKINS

Anaerobe Laboratory, Virginia Polytechnic Institute and State University, Blacksburg, Virginia 24061

Received for publication 16 November 1976

Several human fecal isolates of *Bacteroides* have been found to produce bacteriocins. The bacteriocin-producing strain T1-1 was studied in the most detail. Strain T1-1 belongs to the 0061-1 deoxyribonucleic acid (DNA) homology group of *Bacteroides*. This homology group phenotypically resembles *Bacteroides thetaiotaomicron* but has little DNA homology with it. The bacteriocin-producing strains T1-12 and T1-48 belong to the 3452-A DNA homology group. This group has DNA homology with *B. thetaiotaomicron* and *Bacteroides ovatus*. The bacteriocin-producing strain T1-42 remains unidentified in that it does not belong to any recognized DNA homology group of the saccharolytic intestinal bacteroides. The extracellular bacteriocin produced by strain T1-1 was specifically bactericidal for other bacteria within the genus *Bacteroides*. The highest bacteriocin titers (32 to 64) were produced in complex media, with only trace amounts being produced in a defined medium. The bacteriocin appeared to have a high molecular weight ($\geq$300,000) and was unusual because it was stable from pH 1 to 12 and only a 50% reduction in activity resulted after 15 min at 121°C in an autoclave. It was inactivated by trypsin and Pronase. Strain T1-1 was isolated from all three fecal samples obtained over a 25-week period from an individual who was part of a National Aeronautics and Space Administration mock Skylab flight. Strains T1-12, T1-48, and T1-42 were isolated only from the first fecal sample. Each of these strains was immune to the bacteriocins produced by the others. These strains were found to coexist in the colon with a larger population of non-bacteriocin-producing, bacteriocin-susceptible strains of *Bacteroides*.

Bacteriocins are produced by representatives of many groups of bacteria, including those found in the colon of man. It is of interest to know what influence the production of bacteriocins by one group of bacteria would have on other bacteria in the colon. The bacteriocins of *Escherichia coli* (colicins) have been investigated with respect to their possible influence on the normal human fecal flora (5, 7, 8, 16–19). However, *E. coli* represents less than 0.5% of the bacterial population of the colon, whereas the four major *Bacteroides* species found in the colon comprise about 25% of the bacterial flora (10, 14). There have been only a few reports on the production of bacteriocins by *Bacteroides* species (3, 4, 15) and none on the possible role of these bacteriocins on the bacterial ecology of the human colon.

In this investigation we have determined some biological and physical-chemical properties of a bacteriocin produced by a member of the 0061-1 deoxyribonucleic acid (DNA) homology group of *Bacteroides*. We have also found that bacteriocin-susceptible bacteroides coexist in the human colon in larger numbers than bacteriocin-producing strains.

MATERIALS AND METHODS

Bacterial strains and media. Fecal isolates of bacteroides were obtained by W. E. C. Moore and L. V. Holdeman from an astronaut during a mock Skylab flight (10). Although nine fecal samples were obtained between 10 May and 1 November, only the bacteroides isolated on 10 May, 19 September, and 1 November (samples designated as T1, T7, and T9 respectively) were used in this study. The present investigation was possible only because of the availability of the cultures from the study of Holdeman et al. (10). We would have like to study bacteriocin production by *Bacteroides* from subjects not under test conditions such as the mock Skylab flight, but have been unable to do this because of the tremendous expense of identifying organisms in several replicate samples from individuals. The conditions of the mock flight and factors affecting the fecal flora, including the Skylab diet, have been previously discussed (10). The food was quite varied and similar to a normal diet except it was frozen, canned, irradiated, or dehydrated. In general, changes in diet had little effect on the composition of the fecal flora. Stool samples were normal in character and frequency. Fecal sample T1 was obtained 43 days before beginning the Skylab diet while living at home, sample T7 was obtained after 56 days of Skylab confinement (but 78 days after beginning the Skylab diet), and sample T9 was obtained 24 days after returning to a normal diet at home. The fecal flora of the astronaut was judged normal since it was within the large person-to-person variations noted in previous studies (10, 14). All other anaerobic bacteria were obtained from the culture collection of the Virginia Polytechnic Institute and State University (VPI) Anaerobe Laboratory. Phenotypic characteristics were determined by methods described in the VPI *Anaerobe Laboratory Manual* (12). Identifications of strains used were based on characteristics of strains described previously (10–12, 14). Stock cultures were grown overnight at 37°C in chopped-meat broth and stored at room temperature. Inocula for all experiments were from 18- to 24-h cultures grown in supplemented brain heart infusion (BHI-S) broth. Facultative bacterial strains were obtained from the culture collection of the VPI Biology Department and were grown anaerobically in peptone yeast extract-glucose broth. The preparation of all media has been previously described (12).

The interrelationships of strains isolated from the astronauts were measured by DNA homology (J. L. Johnson, unpublished data). The bacteriocin-producing strain T1-1 belongs to the 0061-1 DNA homology group of *Bacteroides* (J. L. Johnson, submitted for publication). Organisms belonging to this group are phenotypically very similar to those in the *B. thetaiotaomicron* group. However, the 006-1 group has only a low level of DNA homology to *B. thetaiotaomicron*.

Screening for bacteriocin production and sensitivity. In the work by Holdeman et al. (10), 55 colonies were picked at random from dilutions of the fecal samples. We tested all the isolates identified as *Bacteroides* from samples T1, T7, and T9 for bacteriocin production and sensitivity by a modification of the method described by Brock et al. (6). Eighteen- to twenty-four-hour BHI-S cultures of bacteria were spotted onto the surface of BHI-S agar (1.5%) plates with a Steers replicator (21) and allowed to dry. After incubation at 37°C for 48 h in an anaerobic glove box (2) with an atmosphere of 85% N_2, 5% CO_2, and 10% H_2, the cells were killed by exposure to chloroform for 30 min. Residual chloroform was allowed to evaporate, and the plates were overlayed with 3.5 ml of BHI-S soft agar (0.7%) which had been inoculated with 0.2 ml of an 18- to 24-h BHI-S culture of the test organism. Zones of inhibition were usually visible after overnight incubation in an anaerobic glove box. Possible bacteriophage activity was determined by picking areas of inhibition and testing for the presence of bacteriophage by standard plaque assays (1).

Determination of optimal conditions for bacteriocin production in liquid media. *Bacteroides* VPI strain T1-1 was grown under oxygen-free N_2 or CO_2 in the following media to determine optimal conditions for bacteriocin production: BHI-S, peptone yeast extract, peptone yeast extract-glucose, chopped meat (12), and minimal medium (22). Mitomycin C (Sigma Chemical Co., St. Louis, Mo.) was added to BHI-S cultures at concentrations of 0.5, 1.0, and 2.0 μg/ml after 5 and 9 h of incubation to determine the inducibility of the bacteriocin. Comparative growth rates of the bacteriocin-producing and -susceptible strains were determined by growing cells at 37°C in BHI-S broth under O_2-free N_2. Growth was followed by determining the optical density at 650 nm (Spectronic 20, Bausch and Lomb, Rochester, N.Y.).

Bacteriocin production, concentration, and partial purification. For routine bacteriocin production, strain T1-1 was grown in 2.5-liter quantities of BHI-S at 37°C under oxygen-free nitrogen for 72 to 96 h. After centrifugation at 7,500 × *g* for 45 min, the supernatant was concentrated to approximately 25 ml by filtration through an Amicon XM300 filter utilizing a thin-channel cell (Amicon Corp., Lexington, Mass.). Low-molecular-weight medium components and metabolites were removed from the retained material by repeatedly adding an equal volume of either 0.01 M HEPES (*N*-2-hydroxyethyl piperazine-*N*'-2-ethanesulfonic acid) (Sigma Chemical Co.) containing 0.01 M $MgCl_2$, pH 7 (HEPES-$MgCl_2$ buffer) or 0.01 M sodium phosphate buffer and reconcentrating to 25 ml. When the retained material became clear (after seven to ten additions of buffer), the concentrated liquid was centrifuged at 16,000 × *g* for 30 min, and the supernatant was sterilized by membrane filtration (0.45-μm pore size; Millipore Corp., Bedford, Mass.) and stored at 4°C. To determine whether the bacteriocin dissociated into active subunits, the partially purified bacteriocin was concentrated an additional ninefold with a Minicon S125 concentrator (Amicon Corp.) and applied to a column (1.5 by 90 cm) of Sepharose 6B (Pharmacia, Uppsala, Sweden) equilibrated with one of the following buffers: 0.01 M HEPES, pH 7; 0.01 M HEPES-$MgCl_2$, pH 7; 0.01 M sodium phosphate, pH 7; or 0.1 M sodium phosphate, pH 5.5. Bacteriocin activity was assayed in each 2-ml fraction and the elution profiles were compared.

Bacteriocin assay. Bacteriocin titers were determined by spotting 0.05 ml of dilutions in HEPES-$MgCl_2$ buffer on the surface of BHI-S agar plates. The spots were allowed to dry before being overlayed with 3.5 ml of BHI-S soft agar inoculated with 0.2 ml of an overnight culture of indicator cells (*B. fragilis*, VPI 2393). The plates were incubated overnight at 37°C in an anaerobic glove box. The titer was considered to be the reciprocal of the highest dilution which gave a clear zone of inhibition. These ranged from 16 to 64. The number of bacteriocin arbitrary units (a.u.) per milliliter was defined as 20 times the numerical value of the titer.

Temperature and pH stability. The temperature stability of the T1-1 bacteriocin was determined by incubating 0.5-ml samples at pH 7 for 1 h at various temperatures. Samples were also autoclaved for 15 min at 15 lb/in^2 and 121°C. To test the pH stability of the bacteriocin, samples were adjusted to different pH values with either HCl or NaOH and incubated for 1 h at 37°C.

Enzyme susceptibility. Unless otherwise indicated, the inactivation by various enzymes was determined by incubation of the enzyme and partially purified bacteriocin for 2.5 h at 37°C at pH 7.5 in the presence of 0.01 M $MgCl_2$ and 0.01 M $CaCl_2$. The following enzymes were tested at the concentrations indicated: trypsin, 200 μg/ml; Pronase, 300 μg/ml; proteinase K, 100 μg/ml; pepsin, 300 μg/ml, pH 5.5; deoxyribonuclease, 10 μg/ml; ribonuclease, 5 μg/ml; phospholipase A, 100 μg/ml. Control experiments demonstrated that the enzymes were active. Pronase and deoxyribonuclease were purchased from Calbiochem, San Diego, Calif., and proteinase K was from EM Laboratories, Elmsford, N.Y. All other enzymes were purchased from Sigma Chemical Co.

Bactericidal effect of bacteriocin. *B. fragilis* VPI 2393 was grown in BHI-S for 3.5 h until it reached early log phase, at which time bacteriocin was added. Viability was determined by standard plate count procedures on BHIA plates incubated in an anaerobic chamber.

RESULTS

In a preliminary experiment 57 clinical and fecal isolates of *Bacteroides* were tested for both bacteriocin production and susceptibility. Twenty-two of these strains produced bacteriocins. These included 14 of 23 *B. fragilis* DNA homology group I, seven of eleven *B. fragilis* group II (J. L. Johnson, submitted for publication) and one of three which belonged to the 0061-1 homology group. None of the other seven homology groups tested produced bacteriocins, although a maximum of only four strains from each group was included. The susceptibility patterns of the strains varied widely. Except for three strains (two *B. fragilis* group I and one 0061-1) which were not susceptible to any of the bacteriocins, no two strains had identical patterns of susceptibility. We chose bacteriocin-producing strain VPI T1-1 for further study because it was one of approximately 450 fecal isolates obtained from one person over a 25-week period.

Bacteriocin production. Strain T1-1 was grown in several media (see Materials and Methods) to determine optimal conditions for bacteriocin production. The highest titers (32 to 64) were obtained when the cultures were incubated under N_2 in BHI-S or in chopped-meat broth. The BHI-S medium was selected for further work.

The bacteriocin was released from the cells during the logarithmic phase of growth (Fig. 1). Eight times as much activity was found in the culture supernatant as in sonicated cells. Also, bacteriocin production stopped when the cells entered the stationary phase of growth. No increase in bacteriocin titer was observed with the addition of mitomycin C under the conditions tested.

Partial characterization of T1-1 bacteriocin. Approximately 80% of the bacteriocin activity was retained after filtration of cell-free growth medium through an Amicon XM300 filter (nominal retention of 300,000 daltons). Adsorption of the bacteriocin to the filter was not detected. The specific activity of the bacteriocin preparation was about 960 a.u./mg of protein after concentration and removal of medium components by ultrafiltration. When this active fraction was applied to a column of Sepharose 6B, the activity eluted immediately after the void volume. The molecular weight therefore appeared to be very large (≥300,000). No bacteriophage-like particles or subunits were visible when negatively stained preparations were examined with the electron microscope.

Several other properties of the partially purified T1-1 bacteriocin were determined and are presented in Table 1. An unusual property for a substance with such a large molecular weight was its extreme heat resistance. There was no detectable loss in activity after heating at 100°C for 1 h and only a 50% reduction resulted after 15 min at 121°C in an autoclave. The bacteriocin was not dissociated by varying the pH or ionic strength as evidenced by its identical elution profiles from a Sepharose 6B column which had been equilibrated with various buffer solu-

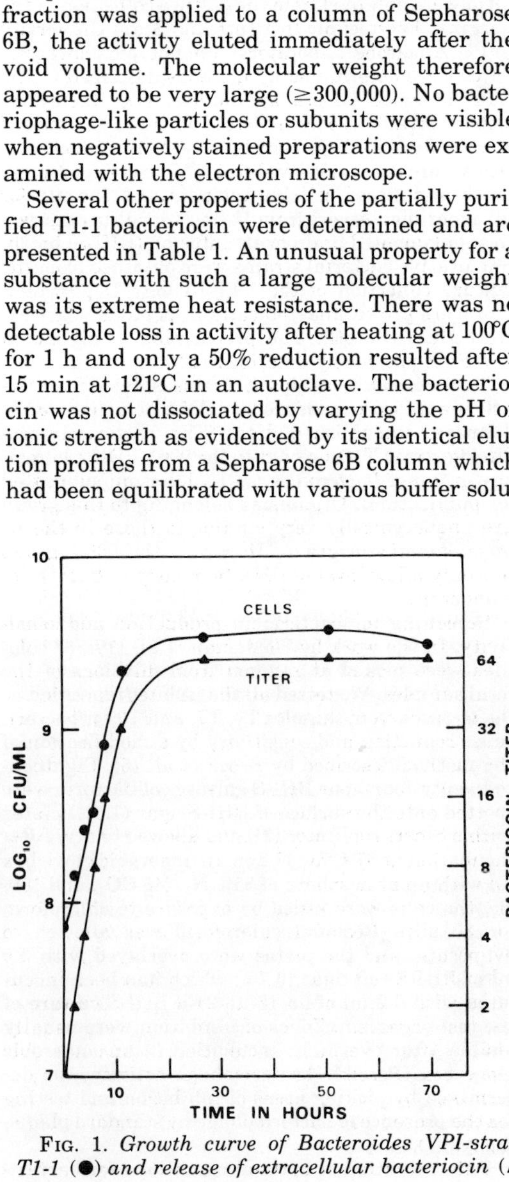

FIG. 1. *Growth curve of Bacteroides VPI-strain T1-1* (●) *and release of extracellular bacteriocin* (▲) *from cells.*

tions (Materials and Methods). The bacteriocin also was stable over a pH range from 1 to 12 (Table 1).

The bacteriocin appeared to be at least partially protein in nature. It was inactivated by trypsin and Pronase, although proteinase K and pepsin did not appear to affect the bacteriocin (Table 1). Incubation of the bacteriocin preparation with ribonuclease, deoxyribonuclease, and phospholipase A resulted in no change in activity.

Bactericidal effect of bacteriocin. Within 1 to 2 h after addition of the bacteriocin to a susceptible culture (VPI 2393) in the logarithmic phase of growth, the viability of the culture decreased (Fig. 2). At a cell concentration of 2×10^8 colony-forming units/ml, a bacteriocin concentration of 2.0 a.u./ml or higher was bactericidal. A concentration of 1.0 a.u./ml or lower did not kill the cells. The mechanism of killing has not been determined.

Host range of T1-1 bacteriocin. The bacteriocin from T1-1 was tested against 70 strains of bacteria representing 39 bacterial species and 17 genera other than *Bacteroides* (Table 2). None of these organisms was inhibited. However, most strains in each of the DNA homology groups of *B. fragilis* and related organisms were inhibited (Table 3). Most strains of *B. melaninogenicus* and *B. oralis* were also inhibited.

Ecological role of T1-1 bacteriocin in the colon. Because the bacteriocin of strain T1-1 was active only against other *Bacteroides* strains, it was of interest to determine what effect a bacteriocin-producing strain might have on other bacteroides in the colon. Eighteen strains of *Bacteroides* had been isolated from the first fecal sample (T1) from astronaut T (10; Table 4). Four of these, including T1-1, produced bacteriocins. From the T7 sample, obtained 19 weeks after T1, eight of the 23 *Bacteroides* isolated were bacteriocin-producers, and from the T9 sample (25 weeks after T1), 2 of the 22 *Bacteroides* isolated were bacteriocin-producers. The interrelationships of all of these *Bacteroides* were determined by DNA homology. When T1-1 was used as a DNA reference organism, all of the bacteriocin-producing organisms isolated from samples T7 and T9 were essentially identical to it. Two of the other three

TABLE 1. *Physical-chemical properties of T1-1 bacteriocin*

Treatment	Titer
None (control)	64
100°C (1 h)	64
Autoclave (15 min, 15 lb/in)	32
pH 1.0 (1 h)	32
pH 12.0 (1 h)	16
Trypsin	0
Pronase	0
Proteinase K	64
Pepsin	64
Ribonuclease	64
Deoxyribonuclease	64
Phospholipase A	64

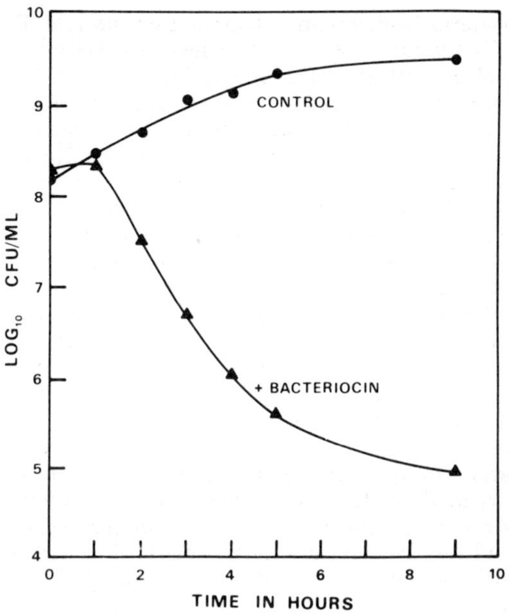

FIG. 2. *Bactericidal effect of T1-1 bacteriocin on log growing cells of VPI 2393: (●) control (no bacteriocin), (▲) 2 a.u. bacteriocin/ml. Bacteriocin was added at zero time.*

TABLE 2. *Bacteriocin-resistant bacteria*

Genus	No. of species tested	No. of strains tested
Propionibacterium	4	6
Clostridium	3	6
Fusobacterium	6	10
Bifidobacterium	4	6
Peptostreptococcus	2	3
Eubacterium	4	11
Streptococcus	1	2
Coprococcus	1	2
Lactobacillus	1	2
Escherichia	1	3
Shigella	2	3
Proteus	3	9
Klebsiella	1	1
Salmonella	3	3
Serratia	1	1
Enterobacter	1	1
Providencia	1	1

bacteriocin-producing strains from sample T1 (T1-12 and T1-48) had high levels of DNA homology with the 3452-A homology group (J. L. Johnson, submitted for publication). This is another unnamed group whose DNA preparations have about 35% homology with the reference DNAs of *B. thetaiotaomicron* and *B. ovatus*. The last bacteriocin-producing strain from sample T1 (T1-42) did not have homology to any of the DNA homology groups that have been delineated.

Each of the producing strains from the three fecal samples was tested for inhibitory activity against each of the other 62 fecal isolates of *Bacteroides* from these fecal samples. All 49 of the nonproducing strains were susceptible to all 14 of the bacteriocin-producing strains. However, the producing strains were not inhibited by any of the other bacteriocin-producing strains. Furthermore, the producing strains had nearly identical host ranges when tested against 140 other strains of *Bacteroides* (Table 3).

B. vulgatus was the most numerous of the bacteroides fecal isolates, representing 11, 3, and 10 of the isolates from fecal samples T1, T7, and T9, respectively. Using one of these as a reference, DNA homology experiments demonstrated that 17 of the other 23 were completely homologous to it. If one accepts this as evidence that these isolates are representative of a single strain, then the experiments demonstrate that this bacteriocin-susceptible strain was present throughout the 25-week survey period. The other six strains had about 70% homology to the reference strain and probably represent a second strain, which was also present throughout the test period.

TABLE 3. *Bacteriocin sensitivity among species and strains of Bacteroides*

Name or DNA homology group	No. tested	No. susceptible to:		
		T1-1	T1-12	T1-42
B. fragilis	42	39	39	41
B. vulgatus	9	8	8	8
B. thetaiotaomicron	7	7	7	7
B. ovatus	9	9	9	9
B. distasonis	11	11	11	11
0061-1	10	10	10	10
3452A	8	8	8	8
B. melaninogenicus	22	20	15	20
B. oralis	11	9	11	11
B. eggerthii	2	2	2	2
Subspecies a	9	8	8	8

TABLE 4. *Strains of Bacteroides isolated from an astronaut*

Fecal sample	Time (weeks)	Total no. of *Bacteroides* isolated	Total no. of bacteriocin producers	DNA homology group of producing strains
T1	0	18	4	0061-1 (1)[a] 3452A (2) Unidentified (1)
T7	19	23	8	0061-1
T9	25	22	2	0061-1

[a] Number in parenthesis refers to the number of bacteriocin-producing strains that belong to that DNA homology group. From sample T1; the bacteriocin producing strain belonging to the 0061-1 homology group was T1-1, the producing strains belonging to the 3452A homology group were T1-12 and T1-48. The unidentified producing strain was T1-42.

Growth rate experiments demonstrated that two of the three bacteriocin-producing strains had longer generation times than the susceptible strains. The generation times of five bacteriocin-susceptible strains of *Bacteroides* (each representing a different DNA homology group) from astronaut T ranged from 0.9 to 1.0 h when grown on BHI-S. The generation time of the bacteriocin-producing strain T1-42 was similar and had a value of 1.0 h. However, the bacteriocin-producing strains T1-1 and T1-12 had longer generation times of 2.6 and 5.7 h, respectively.

DISCUSSION

Bacteroides bacteriocins which were studied by Beerens et al. (4) specifically inhibited only species belonging to *Bacteroides* and the bacteriocins were susceptible to proteolysis (4, 15). This was also found to be the case with the bacteriocin of strain T1-1. Although the bacteriocins from several other bacteroides appear to be heat labile (3, 4), the T1-1 bacteriocin was able to withstand a temperature of 100°C for 1 h. The heat stability was unusual since the bacteriocin appeared to have a molecular weight above 300,000. We were not able to demonstrate lower molecular-weight subunits which might help explain its heat stability. Although we have not tested sufficient numbers of strains to develop a typing system based upon bacteriocin susceptibility, the wide variation in susceptibility patterns which was observed in the preliminary experiment suggests that bacteriocin typing of isolates should be possible for use in epidemiology and ecology studies.

Of the three fecal samples that were studied, the bacteriocin-producing strains of bacteroides were always a minority (9 to 35%) of the total bacteroides isolated. The non-bacteriocin-producing strains of bacteroides in these fecal samples were all susceptible to the bacteriocins of the producing strains. Furthermore, DNA homology experiments on those susceptible strains which were phenotypically identified as

B. vulgatus indicated that most were isolates of a single strain and that this strain persisted in the colon throughout the 25-week period. It might be expected that bacteriocin production would give an organism an advantage over bacteriocin-susceptible organisms to grow and persist in an ecological niche. If this is the case, then one would expect that the introduction of producing strains would result in their becoming the predominant organisms and that the susceptible organisms would find it very difficult to persist. Our results show that bacteriocin-susceptible strains of *Bacteroides* not only persist, but outnumber the bacteriocin-producing strains. The simultaneous presence of bacteriocin-producing and -susceptible strains of *E. coli* in the human colon has previously been demonstrated (7, 23). Others have found it difficult to demonstrate that colicins give *E. coli* a growth advantage in the normal human colon (5, 7, 16, 18, 23). However, it has recently been shown that the possession of the ColV plasmid, but not of ColE, confers increased ability of *E. coli* to survive in the alimentary tract (20). It appears that in the system studied by us, bacteriocin production by strains of *Bacteroides* does not give the producing strains a growth advantage over the susceptible strains. The bacteriocins from the three producing strains of *Bacteroides* in the first fecal sample inhibited all the other non-bacteriocin-producing *Bacteroides* strains from the three fecal samples in vitro. Yet, of the three bacteriocin-producing strains, only T1-1 remained at detectable levels throughout the 25-week experimental period. We cannot adequately explain why this strain remained at such low levels compared to the susceptible strains or why the other two bacteriocin-producing strains (T1-12 and T1-42) could not be detected in subsequent fecal samples. Although strains T1-1 and T1-12 had significantly longer generation times than did the bacteriocin-susceptible strains in BHI-S, this does not fully explain their low numbers in the feces since strain T1-42 had a generation time similar to the susceptible strains, yet it was detected only in the first fecal sample and at a low level. It is probable that both the bacteriocin-producing and -susceptible strains have different generation times in the colon than the ones determined experimentally in BHI-S. However, it would be difficult to duplicate the colonic environment for growth rate determination. Host factors, as suggested by Cooke et al. (7) and Holdeman et al. (10), may play a role in determining the composition of the fecal flora. The potential role of bacteriocins may be limited by their lability to proteases, their limited diffusability, the presence of inactivators, the limited or nonproduction in their environment, or other, as yet unknown, factors (7, 13). We found that the T1-1 bacteriocin was susceptive to proteases in vitro and that bacteriocin production was influenced by the growth medium. Although bacteriocin production by *Bacteroides* does not appear to give them a growth advantage over susceptible strains, we cannot rule out that bacteriocin production has no influence. It is conceivable that bacteriocin production allows the producing strains to persist, even at their low levels.

It is interesting to us that the bacteriocins of the three producing strains from the first fecal sample, each of which represents a distinct DNA homology group, not only have nearly identical host ranges, but are immune to the bacteriocins produced by the others. This suggests that the three strains produce the same or a very similar bacteriocin (6), which raises the question of the possible genetic transfer of bacteriocinogenic factors between strains of *Bacteroides*. Although plasmids have been detected in *Bacteroides*, their functions have not been determined (9). Experiments are currently underway in our laboratory to demonstrate genetic transfer between *Bacteroides*.

ACKNOWLEDGMENTS

We would like to acknowledge the excellent technical assistance of Roger Van Tassell. We also thank L. V. Holdeman and W. E. C. Moore for characterizing many of the bacteria used in this study.

This research was supported by Public Health Service grant AI-12137-02 from the National Institute of Allergy and Infectious Diseases.

LITERATURE CITED

1. **Adams, M. H.** 1959. Bacteriophages, p. 450–451. Interscience Publishers, New York.
2. **Aranki, A., and R. Freter.** 1972. Use of anaerobic glove box for the cultivation of strictly anaerobic bacteria. Am. J. Clin. Nutr. **25:**1329–1334.
3. **Beerens, H., and G. Baron.** 1965. Mise en évidence de bactériocines élaborées par les bactéries anaérobies a gram négatif appartenant au genre *Eggerthella*. Ann. Inst. Pasteur Paris **108:**255–256.
4. **Beerens, H., G. Baron, and M. M. Tahon.** 1966. Mise en évidence de substrances inhibitrices élaborées por les bactéries anaérobies non sporulees. Ann. Inst. Pasteur Lille **17:**1–20.
5. **Branche, W. C., Jr., V. M. Young, H. G. Robinet, and E. M. Massey.** 1964. Effect of colicine production of *Escherichia coli* in the normal human intestine. Soc. Exp. Biol. Med. **114:**148–201.
6. **Brock, T. D., B. Peacher, and D. Pierson.** 1963. Survey of the bacteriocines of enterococci. J. Bacteriol. **86:**702–707.
7. **Cooke, E. M., I. G. T. Hettiaratchy, and A. C. Buck.** 1972. Fate of ingested *Escherichia coli* in normal persons. J. Med. Microbiol. **5:**361–369.
8. **Emslie-Smith, A. H.** 1965. Observations on strains of *Escherichia coli* exhibiting ecological dynasticism in

the faecal flora of man. Ernaehrungforshung **10**:302–307.

9. **Guinez, D. G., and C. E. Davis.** 1975. Isolation of plasmid deoxyribonucleic acid from two strains of *Bacteroides*. J. Bacteriol. **124**:503–510.
10. **Holdeman, L. V., I. J. Good, and W. E. C. Moore.** 1976. Human fecal flora: variation in bacterial composition within individuals and a possible effect of emotional stress. Appl. Environ. Microbiol. **31**:359–375.
11. **Holdeman, L. V., and W. E. C. Moore.** 1974. New genus, *Coprococcus,* twelve new species, and emended descriptions of bacteria from human feces. Int. J. Syst. Bacteriol. **24**:260–277.
12. **Holdeman, L. V., and W. E. C. Moore. (ed.).** 1975. Anaerobe laboratory manual, 3rd ed., p. 27–36, 101–128, Virginia Polytechnic Institute and State University, Blacksburg.
13. **Kelstrup, J., and R. J.Gibbons.** 1969. Inactivation of bacteriocins in the intestinal canal and oral cavity. J. Bacteriol. **99**:888–890.
14. **Moore, W. E. C., and L. V. Holdeman.** 1974. Human fecal flora: the normal flora of 20 Japanese-Hawaiians. Appl. Microbiol. **27**:961–979.
15. **Podhaisky, C., and L. Reinhold.** 1970. Bacteriocinbildung und Bacteriocin sensibilitat bei *Bacteroides fragilis* und *Bacteroides thetaiotaomicron* aus Klinischem Material. Zentralbl. Bakteriol. Parasltenkd., Infektionskr. Hyg. Abt. 1 Orig. **215**:475–482.
16. **Robbins, M. L., A. M. Somer, and L. W. Parr.** 1957. Variation in the antibiotic producing bacterial flora of the human intestinal tract. J. Bacteriol. **74**:377–380.
17. **Sears, H. J., and I. Brownlee.** 1952. Further observations on the persistence of individual strains of *Escherichia coli* in the intestinal tract of man. J. Bacteriol. **63**:47–57.
18. **Sears, H. J., I. Brownlee, and J. K. Uchiyama.** 1950. Persistence of individual strains of *Escherichia coli* in the intestinal tract of man. J. Bacteriol. **59**:293–301.
19. **Sears, H. J., H. Jones, R. Saloum, I. Brownlee, and L. F. Lamoreaux.** 1956. Persistence of individual strains of *Escherichia coli* in man and dog under varying conditions. J. Bacteriol. **71**:370–372.
20. **Smith, H. W. and M. B. Huggins.** 1976. Further observations on the association of the colicine V plasmid of *Escherichia coli* with pathogenicity and with survival in the alimentary tract. J. Gen. Microbiol. **92**:335–350.
21. **Steers, E., E. L. Foltz, and B. S. Graves.** 1959. An inocula replicating apparatus for routine testing of bacterial susceptibility to antibiotics. Antibiot. Chemother. **9**:307–311.
22. **Varel, V. H., and M. P. Bryant.** 1974. Nutritional features of *Bacteriodes fragilis* subsp. *fragilis*. Appl. Microbiol. **18**:251–257.
23. **Vieu, J. F.** 1964. Applications de la bacteriocinogenie et des bacteriocines. Ann. Inst. Pasteur Paris **197** (Suppl. to no. 5):93–114.

Antimicrobial Agents and Chemotherapy, Apr. 1977, p. 725-734
Vol. 11, No. 1

Cefoxitin Resistance to Beta-Lactamase: a Major Factor for Susceptibility of *Bacteroides fragilis* to the Antibiotic

GARY DARLAND* AND JEROME BIRNBAUM
Merck Institute for Therapeutic Research, Rahway, New Jersey 07065

Received for publication 18 October 1976

Toluene-treated cell suspensions of *Bacteroides fragilis* were used to screen clinical isolates for the production of β-lactamase. Approximately one-third of the isolates possessed considerable cephalosporinase activity. A significant correlation was found between β-lactamase production and resistance to cephalosporin antibiotics. Several isolates were resistant to cefuroxime and cefamandole and produced enzymes capable of hydrolyzing these antibiotics. However, none of the 79 strains tested could hydrolyze the cephamycin derivative, cefoxitin. A large percentage (>90%) of the strains were susceptible to cefoxitin. Therefore, resistance to lactamase hydrolysis is a major factor for the effectiveness of cefoxitin against *B. fragilis*. Detailed studies of four isolates suggest that two different enzymes may be produced. Both are cephalosporinases but differ with regard to cellular distribution and substrate specificity. Cefoxitin is not a substrate for either enzyme, but it is an excellent competitive inhibitor ($K_i \approx 0.1$ μM).

Cephalosporins are broad-spectrum antibiotics with activity against most gram-positive and gram-negative bacteria. Among the exceptions to this general rule are members of the gram-negative species *Bacteroides fragilis*. Martin et al. (11) in a study of 195 clinical isolates, found that only 9% were susceptible to 25 μg or less of cephalothin per ml. Although cephaloridine has generally proven to be more effective, Kislak (9) found only 50% of 40 isolates to be sensitive to 25 μg or less per ml. These observations have since been confirmed by others (21, 22).

Recently, cefoxitin (a semisynthetic cephamycin analogue) was demonstrated to be considerably more effective against *B. fragilis* than the cephalosporins now in use (21, 22). Over 95% of the strains tested by the two groups were susceptible to 32 μg or less of cefoxitin per ml. Of the several hypotheses available to explain the effectiveness of cefoxitin against this group of bacteria, perhaps the most attractive is related to its stability to hydrolysis by β-lactamase.

The cephamycins in general and cefoxitin in particular have been demonstrated to be resistant to β-lactamases from a variety of gram-negative bacteria (5, 17). Onishi and co-workers (17) tested 91 isolates, mainly members of the family *Enterobacteriaceae,* and were able to demonstrate β-lactamase activity against cefoxitin by only seven cultures: three of *Enterobacter* sp., three of *Escherichia coli,* and one of *Klebsiella* sp. Cefoxitin has also been demonstrated to be resistant to the β-lactamases of *Yersinia enterocolitica* (4).

In 1973, two groups reported the presence of β-lactamase activity in *B. fragilis* (1, 6). Recently, Olsson et al. (16) confirmed the existence of lactamase in several isolates of *B. fragilis*, including four of the five subspecies. These workers provided evidence that the enzyme is synthesized during exponential growth and declines during the stationary phase. The substrate profile of the *B. fragilis* enzyme is typical for a cephalosporinase with a minimal amount of activity against penicillin (6, 16).

Weinrich and Del Bene (23) presented some data that suggest that cefoxitin is comparatively resistant to the action of the *B. fragilis* enzyme. The data in the present report provide stronger evidence for the resistance of cefoxitin to this cephalosporinase and establish that the antibiotic is an excellent competitive inhibitor of the enzyme. Furthermore, a survey of a large number of isolates revealed a highly significant correlation between the presence of β-lactamase in *B. fragilis* and resistance to cephalosporin antibiotics.

MATERIALS AND METHODS

Cultures. The strains used in this study were clinical isolates obtained from several laboratories, including Center for Disease Control, Atlanta, Ga.; University of California, Los Angeles, School of Medicine, Los Angeles, Calif.; University of Miami

Medical School, Miami, Fla.; University of Cincinnati Medical Center, Cincinnati, Ohio; Department of Clinical Microbiology, National Institutes of Health, Bethesda, Md.; and the Anaerobe Laboratory, Virginia Polytechnic Institute, Blacksburg, Va.

Upon receipt, the cultures were grown overnight and streaked on two plates of brucella agar (Baltimore Biological Laboratory [BBL], Cockeysville, Md.) supplemented with 5% sheep blood. One plate was incubated aerobically, and the other was incubated anaerobically in a GasPak jar (BBL). After the purity of the cultures was confirmed, they were grown for 48 h on slants of the same medium. The growth was washed from the surface with sterile skim milk and lyophilized. The culture numbers used in this paper refer to the culture collection of the Merck Sharp & Dohme Research Laboratories.

Media and maintenance of the cultures. The growth medium was Schaedler broth (SB) purchased from BBL. Except in the preliminary screening of culture, the medium was always prereduced anaerobically and sterilized under an atmosphere of 10% CO_2 and 90% N_2; traces of O_2 were removed by passing the gas over a heated copper column. In the preliminary experiments, the cultures were grown overnight (16 to 18 h) in SB in GasPak jars. While cultures were under active study, they were maintained by weekly transfers in SB.

Antibiotic susceptibility testing. The procedure used for antibiotic susceptibility testing was a modification of the agar dilution method recommended by Sutter (20). Serial twofold dilutions of the antibiotic were prepared in distilled water and added to freshly prepared agar-containing medium. The agar medium consisted of brucella agar (BBL) supplemented with 5% (vol/vol) sheep blood. The plates were prepared on the day they were to be used. Prior to incubation, the plates were dried for about 3 h in an anaerobe chamber under 10% CO_2 and 90% N_2. The inoculum was prepared by adjusting the optical density at 620 nm of an overnight culture in SB to approximately 0.1 by dilution with reduced SB. The inoculum was applied to the agar surface by using a Steers replicator. The minimum inhibitory concentration (MIC) was defined as the lowest concentration of antibiotic showing no distinct growth.

Assay for β-lactamase. The method used routinely for β-lactamase assay was a modification of the microiodometric assay of Novick (13) and Goldner et al. (8). Unless otherwise stated, the reaction was started by adding 0.1 ml of an enzyme preparation in 0.1 M sodium phosphate buffer (pH 7.0) to 0.1 ml of the twofold-concentrated substrate in the same buffer. Both reagents were equilibrated at 37°C for 5 to 10 min before mixing. The reaction was stopped, usually after 5 min, by addition of 5.0 ml of the starch-iodine indicator. The indicator was prepared by adding 0.8 ml of an iodine reagent (0.08 M iodine in 3.2 M potassium iodide) to 1 liter of a 0.1% (wt/vol) solution of soluble starch in 0.5 M sodium acetate buffer (pH 4.0). The amount of hydrolysis was determined by measuring absorbance at 620 nm in a Bausch & Lomb Spectronic 20 (Bausch & Lomb, Inc., Rochester, N. Y.) exactly 10 min after addition of the starch-iodine indicator. The decrease in absorbance relative to a substrate blank was compared with standard curves derived by using alkali-hydrolyzed antibiotics. Since the hydrolysis products of cephalosporins are not well characterized with regard to their ability to react with iodine, standard curves were prepared for each substrate. The amount of enzyme added to each reaction was adjusted so that less than 25% of the antibiotic was hydrolyzed during incubation. Under these conditions, hydrolysis was linear with regard to time. One enzyme unit is defined as the amount of enzyme hydrolyzing 1 μmol of substrate per min at 37°C and pH 7.0, with a substrate concentration of 1,000 μM.

Occasionally, the rates of hydrolysis obtained with the microiodometric assay were confirmed by direct spectrophotometric measurements in the ultraviolet region (14, 18). No significant discrepancies were noted.

Screening of isolates for β-lactamase activity. Overnight cultures of *B. fragilis* in SB were washed once with deionized water and resuspended in water to an optical density at 620 nm of 10 (approximately 5 mg [dry weight] per ml). The cell suspension was then treated with 0.2 volume of toluene for 30 min in an ice bath. The aqueous phase was removed and used as a source of enzyme. Later experiments showed that toluene treatment had no effect on enzyme activity, but the treatment was continued to facilitate comparison between experiments. The reaction was started by adding 0.10 ml of the toluene-treated cells to 0.10 ml of substrate in phosphate buffer. The final reaction mixture contained 50 μg of substrate per ml and 0.1 M sodium phosphate buffer (pH 6.7) in a final volume of 0.2 ml. The reaction was terminated with the starch-iodine indicator after 1 h at 37°C. Strains were considered positive for β-lactamase activity if more than 20% of the added substrate was hydrolyzed during incubation.

Preparation of cell extracts. Except in the experiments where the culture age was a variable, all cells were harvested in mid-log phase from prereduced, anaerobically sterilized SB. The cells were washed once in 0.1 M sodium phosphate buffer (pH 7.0) and suspended in 1/10 to 1/20 culture volumes of the same buffer. The cell suspensions were sonically oscillated for three 20-s intervals with a Branson sonifier set at 6 A. Where appropriate, the crude sonically treated materials were centrifuged at 30,000 × *g* for 30 min. The supernatant (S30) and pellet (P30) were both saved for enzyme assay. Protein was determined by the method of Lowry et al. (10).

Estimation of kinetic parameters. The S30 and P30 fractions were both used to estimate the K_m and V_{max} for several substrates. The K_m and V_{max}, expressed in micromolarity and in micromoles of substrate hydrolyzed per minute per milligram of protein, respectively, were estimated from a least-squares fit to Lineweaver-Burk plots with substrate concentrations in the range of 150 to 600 μM. The physiological efficiency, V_{max}/K_m, was obtained by taking the reciprocal of the slope obtained in Lineweaver-Burk plots.

Cefoxitin inhibition of β-lactamase. The substrate for studies of β-lactamase inhibition by cefoxitin was cephaloridine. Cephaloridine and cefoxitin at appropriate concentrations were mixed together in 0.1 ml of buffer and equilibrated at 37°C. The reaction was started as described above by adding 0.1 ml of enzyme.

RESULTS

Cephalosporin resistances and β-lactamase. The results of testing *B. fragilis* susceptibility to a variety of cephalosporin antibiotics are summarized in Table 1. It is clear that cefoxitin was the most active of the antibiotics tested, with 85 of 90 strains (94%) having MIC values of <32 μg/ml. The percentages of susceptible strains for the cephalosporin antibiotics were: cephaloridine, 51; cephalothin, 44; cefamandole, 43; cefuroxime, 45; and cefazolin, 50.

The results of preliminary screening for β-lactamase activity in strains of *B. fragilis* obtained from a number of clinical laboratories are summarized in Table 2. When the substrate was one of the cephalosporins (cefazolin, cefamandole, or cephaloridine) approximately one-half of the isolates tested hydrolyzed at least 5% of the added antibiotic under our standard assay conditions, and one-third of the strains degraded >20% of the cephalosporin. A somewhat lower percentage of strains hydrolyzed penicillin G. Only 2 of 79 isolates showed any activity against cefoxitin. The activity against cefoxitin was low and not reproducible in cell-free extracts.

If β-lactamase plays a role in the resistance of *B. fragilis* to cephalosporins, it would be expected that the strains possessing the enzyme would be more resistant than the isolates that did not. One way of testing this hypothesis is to perform a chi-square test for association between resistance and the presence or absence of the enzyme. The null hypothesis is that no differences exist. For the purposes of this analysis, the isolates were divided into three resistance categories for each antibiotic and were considered to have lactamase activity if >20% of any one cephalosporin was hydrolyzed in 1 h.

The data in Table 3 are strongly suggestive of a role for β-lactamase in resistance to cephalosporins. In the cases of cephaloridine, cefazolin, and cefamandole, a significant association between susceptibility to the antibiotic and possession of a β-lactamase was found. In the case

TABLE 2. *β-Lactamase activity in B. fragilis*

Substrate	No. of positive strains[a]/total tested
Cefoxitin	2/79
Cefamandole	27/79
Cefazolin	27/79
Cephaloridine	27/57
Penicillin G	12/58

[a] A 0.1-ml amount of a toluene-treated cell suspension obtained from an overnight culture was incubated with 0.1 ml of substrate (100 μg/ml) for 1 h at 37°C. Isolates were scored as positive if at least 20% of the added antibiotic was hydrolyzed. Cefuroxime was not included in the survey, due to a shortage of material.

TABLE 3. *Association of β-lactamase with susceptibility to β-lactam antibiotics*

Substrate	β-Lactamase activity[a]	No. of strains with MICs (μg/ml) of: >64	16 to 64	≤16	Statistical analysis[b]
Cefoxitin	+	1	10	19	χ^2 = 3.3;
	–	0	11	38	$P > 0.05$
Cefamandole	+	21	7	2	χ^2 = 14.9;
	–	13	25	11	$P < 0.001$
Cefazolin	+	22	0	8	χ^2 = 29.4;
	–	11	18	20	$P < 0.001$
Cephaloridine	+	25	5	0	χ^2 = 20.4;
	–	18	18	11	$P < 0.001$

[a] Strains were assumed to have β-lactamase if greater than 20% of any one of the substrates was hydrolyzed in 1 h at 37°C.

[b] Chi-square analysis with two degrees of freedom. $\alpha_{0.005,2}$ = 10.60.

TABLE 1. *Susceptibility of B. fragilis to cephalosporin antibiotics*[a]

Antibiotic	No. tested	Cumulative % susceptible to (μg/ml): ≤1	≤2	≤4	≤8	≤16	≤32	≤64
Cefoxitin	90	1	3	13	59	74	94	99
Cefazolin	90			9	14	33	50	69
Cefamandole	90				4	19	43	61
Cephaloridine	87	2		5	7	14	29	51
Cephalothin	55		2	5	7	13	25	44
Cefuroxime	31			13	29	39	45	48

[a] MICs were determined by agar dilution. Drops containing approximately 10^5 bacteria were spotted on antibiotic-containing media.

of cefoxitin, no statistical association could be demonstrated, due to the almost total resistance of the antibiotic to hydrolysis.

Intracellular distribution of β-lactamase. To determine whether or not *B. fragilis* has a permeability barrier that restricts assessibility of cephalosporins to the β-lactamase, enzyme activity in whole cells was compared to that of sonically treated cell suspensions (Table 4). As can be seen, the effect of sonic treatment was minimal. Enzyme activity increased by no more than a factor of 2 in any case. This indicates that crypticity is not a major factor and that the antibiotics are freely accessible to the enzyme in whole cells.

In one strain (MB3389), the β-lactamase was found associated with the particulate fraction obtained after centrifugation at 30,000 × *g* for 30 min. This led to attempts to demonstrate this phenomenon in other strains. Twenty isolates were selected to represent the various susceptibility patterns to β-lactam antibiotics. Nine of these isolates showed significant β-lactamase activity (Table 5). In six of nine strains, a large percentage (≥97%) of the enzyme activity resided in the soluble (S30) fraction, whereas in the three remaining isolates (MB3445, MB3388 and MB3389) a considerable amount of enzyme activity (33 to 51%) was found in the particulate fraction. Since the distribution of total protein between S30 and P30 fractions was similar to that of the other 17

TABLE 4. *Crypticity of β-lactamase activity*[a]

Strain	Treatment	Antibiotic hydrolyzed μmol/min per mg of protein[b]						
		CEX	CEM	CEZ	CEF	CET	CXM	PG
B3214	Cells	0	1.4	3.5	5.1	4.7	3.0	0.2
	Sonic extract	0	3.0	7.5	10.1	9.1	6.0	0.3
B3248	Cells	0	0.01	0.04	0.04	0.05	0.01	<0.001
	Sonic extract	<0.001	0.01	0.05	0.07	0.06	0.01	0
B3272	Cells	0	0.6	1.4	2.1	2.2	1.0	0
	Sonic extract	0	0.9	2.3	3.3	3.3	2.0	0.03
B3389	Cells	<0.001	0.4	1.6	1.1	0.5	1.3	0.15
	Sonic extract	<0.001	0.5	2.4	1.0	0.6	1.7	0.15

[a] Cultures were harvested in mid-log phase, washed once with buffer, and divided into two aliquots, one of which was sonically treated. Reaction mixtures were adjusted to contain equal amounts of protein.

[b] CEX, Cefoxitin; CEM, cefamandole; CEZ, cefazolin; CEF, cephaloridine; CET, cephalothin; CXM, cefuroxime; PG, penicillin G.

TABLE 5. *Intracellular distribution of β-lactamase*

Isolate	Strain	Fraction	Cephaloridine		Cefazolin		Cefoxitin
			Total activity (%)	U/mg of protein	Total activity (%)	U/mg of protein	U/mg of protein
MB3214	*B. fragilis* subsp. *fragilis*	S30	97	2.73	97	1.65	0
		P30	3	0.28	3	0.14	0
MB3272	*B. fragilis* subsp. *fragilis*	S30	98	1.05	98	0.84	0
		P30	2	0.09	2	0.08	0
MB3403	*B. fragilis* subsp. *fragilis*	S30	99	1.16	100	0.78	ND[a]
		P30	1	0.09	0	0	ND
MB3389	*B. fragilis* subsp. *distasonis*	S30	60	0.29	59	0.74	<0.01
		P30	40	0.75	41	1.97	<0.01
MB3445	*B. fragilis* subsp. *distasonis*	S30	49	0.22	61	0.34	0
		P30	51	0.78	39	0.76	0
MB3248	*B. fragilis* subsp. *ovatus*	S30	~100	0.10	100	0.10	0
		P30	0	<0.01	0	0	0
MB3426	*B. fragilis* subsp. *ovatus*	S30	~100	0.08	100	0.08	ND
		P30	0	<0.01	0	0	ND
MB3388	*B. fragilis*	S30	67	0.28	72	0.89	0
		P30	33	0.53	28	1.27	0
MB3402	*B. fragilis*	S30	98	1.72	98	1.18	<0.01
		P30	2	0.12	2	0.08	0

[a] ND, Not determined.

strains, it seems unlikely that the distribution of enzymes is an artifact of sonic treatment. Enzyme activity against cephaloridine and cefazolin was distributed similarly. Little or no reproducible activity was found in either fraction when cefoxitin was used as a substrate. It is worthy of note, however, that the three strains that had significant activity associated with the particulate fraction were the only strains tested that were resistant (MIC $\geq$ 32 μg/ml) to cefoxitin.

Synthesis of β-lactamase during growth. Olsson and co-workers (16) indicated that the β-lactamase content of *B. fragilis* is highly dependent on culture age. Our results with strain MB3272 (Fig. 1) confirm their observation. Enzyme activity increased rapidly during the early exponential phase, reached a plateau during late log to early stationary phase, and then decreased rapidly. The loss of cell-bound enzyme from stationary-phase cells may represent an actual destruction of enzyme. No enzyme activity could be demonstrated in the culture medium. Furthermore, experiments in which the crude S30 from stationary-phase cells was mixed with S30 from log-phase cells showed no evidence of an inhibitor.

The same basic data were obtained with three additional strains of *B. fragilis* (Fig. 2). The results were similar regardless of the substrate used to assay the enzyme. This suggests that the demonstration of β-lactamase in *B. fragilis* is highly dependent on culture age and that maximal specific activity can be obtained only during the mid-log phase.

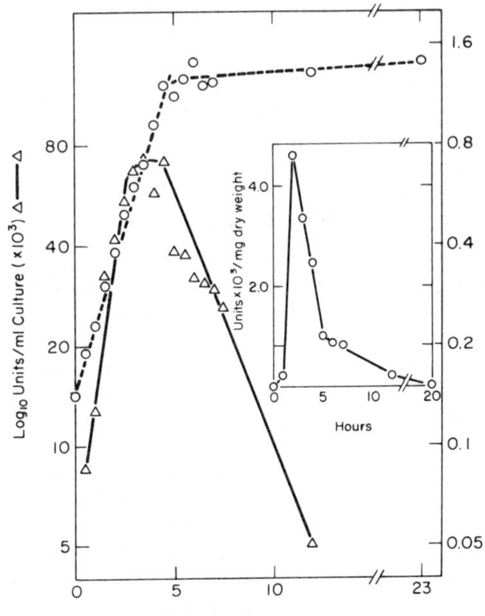

FIG. 1. *Production of β-lactamase during the growth of B. fragilis MB3272. Enzyme activity was determined in toluene-treated cell suspensions with cephaloridine as substrate. Insert: Plot of specific activity (units per milligram dry weight).*

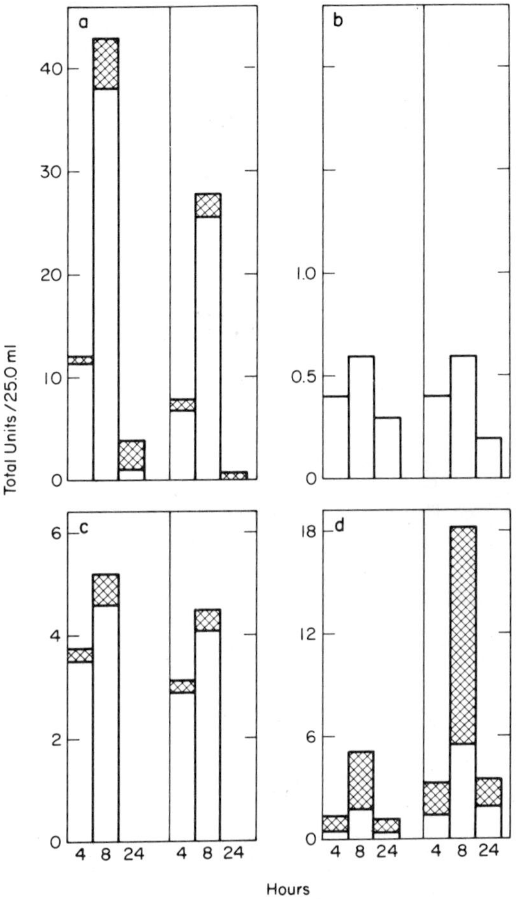

FIG. 2. *β-Lactamase activity in cell-free extracts at various times during growth. Cells were harvested from 25.0-ml cultures at the indicated times. Washed cells were sonically treated, and the soluble and particulate fractions were assayed for enzyme, using both cephaloridine (left) and cefazolin (right) as substrates. Both S30 (clear bars) and P30 (hatched bars) fractions were assayed. (a) MB3214; (b) MB3248; (c) MB3272; (d) MB3389.*

Substrate specificity of β-lactamase. The substrate specificities of the enzymes from five *B. fragilis* strains were determined in crude extracts. Assays with these extracts showed that the enzymes gave typical Michaelis-Menten kinetics. In the cases where substantial enzyme activity was demonstrable in the soluble and particulate fraction, both fractions were examined (Table 6).

Three of the strains examined (MB3214, MB3272, and MB3402) were remarkably simi-

TABLE 6. *Substrate specificity of B. fragilis β-lactamase in crude extracts*

Substrate	MB3214, S30			MB3272, S30			MB3402, S30		
	Relative V_{max} [a]	K_m [b]	V_{max}/K_m [c] ($\times 10^{-3}$)	Relative V_{max}	K_m	V_{max}/K_m ($\times 10^{-3}$)	Relative V_{max}	K_m	V_{max}/K_m ($\times 10^{-3}$)
Cephaloridine	100	700	8.8	100	700	3.3	100	600	5.4
Cefazolin	53	400	6.2	75	600	2.7	67	450	5.0
Cefuroxime	33	200	6.0	28	300	2.9	35	200	4.6
Cefamandole	16	70	9.3	24	60	5.2	22	80	9.2
Cephalothin	54	350	7.3	66	200	4.9	62	350	7.6
Penicillin G	3 [d]	ND [e]	– [f]	1	ND	–	1	ND	–
Cefoxitin [g]									

Substrate	MB3389, S30			MB3389, P30			MB3445, S30			NB3445, P30		
	Relative V_{max}	K_m	V_{max}/K_m ($\times 10^{-3}$)	Relative V_{max}	K_m	V_{max}/K_m ($\times 10^{-3}$)	Relative V_{max}	K_m	V_{max}/K_m ($\times 10^{-3}$)	Relative V_{max}	K_m	V_{max}/K_m ($\times 10^{-3}$)
Cephaloridine	100	60	8.0	100	60	16.0	100	100	3.9	100	250	5.0
Cefazolin	279	150	9.0	238	80	13.2	149	200	3.3	135	350	4.6
Cefuroxime	182	100	7.9	176	90	9.3	88	200	2.3	75	350	2.7
Cefamandole	32	50	4.1	46	60	7.5	35	150	1.3	25	200	1.7
Cephalothin	43	30	6.5	35	50	7.1	48	50	4.3	34	100	4.6
Penicillin G	7	ND	–	ND	ND	–	9	ND	–	15	ND	–
Cefoxitin [g]												

Strain, fraction (column groups above).

[a] V_{max} relative to cephaloridine = 100.
[b] K_m in micromolarity.
[c] Determined by calculating the reciprocal of the slope in a Lineweaver-Burk plot.
[d] V_{max} estimated at a 2,000 μM substrate concentration.
[e] ND, Not determined.
[f] No reaction after 1 h at 37°C and a 2,000 μM substrate concentration.
[g] No reaction with any strain.

lar in substrate specificity, with essentially identical K_m and relative V_{max} values for all substrates. The remaining two strains (MB3389 and MB3445) showed a different substrate profile, with cefazolin being more rapidly hydrolyzed than cephaloridine at saturation. Furthermore, in strain MB3389, cefuroxime was hydrolyzed more readily than cephaloridine. The relative activity of cefamandole and cephalothin was the same in all strains. The soluble and particulate fractions from the respective strains did not differ appreciably. In all cases, penicillin G was hydrolyzed very poorly, with an estimated V_{max} approximately 5% that of cephaloridine. No measurable activity could be demonstrated against cefoxitin with any of the preparations. In all cases the ratio of V_{max}/K_m, which was defined by Citri and Pollock (2) as the physiological efficiency, was relatively constant for all cephalosporins. This suggests that at low substrate concentrations the enzyme may be equally effective against all cephalosporins.

Inhibition of β-lactamase. The results in Fig. 3 demonstrate the ability of cefoxitin to inhibit β-lactamase in three strains of *B. fragilis*. In all three cases, cefoxitin proved to be an effective inhibitor of enzyme activity. Furthermore, there was no difference in the inhibition by cefoxitin in sonically treated cells versus whole cells. This suggests that not only is cefoxitin an effective inhibitor of *B. fragilis* β-lactamase, but also that it diffuses freely to the enzyme in intact cells.

The data suggest that cefoxitin is a competitive inhibitor of the β-lactamase. The V_{max} for cephaloridine was affected little, if at all, by varying the cefoxitin concentration (Fig. 4).

DISCUSSION

Based on screening of 79 clinical isolates, it is concluded that a β-lactamase(s) is produced by a significant proportion of *B. fragilis* strains. This is in basic agreement with Del Bene and Farrar (6), who found cephalosporinase activity in the 10 clinical isolates they examined. The activity in cell-free extracts (S30) was quite low, generally less than 0.2 U/mg of protein, with cephaloridine at 1,000 μM as substrate. Several strains, however, had 10 to 20 times this specific activity. It is reasonable to assume that the estimate of the percentage of strains that produce a lactamase is conservative. The screening of *B. fragilis* isolates for enzyme production was performed on overnight cultures. Due to the dependence of lactamase activity on culture age, it is likely that the estimate of β-lactamase production by strains of *B. fragilis* is

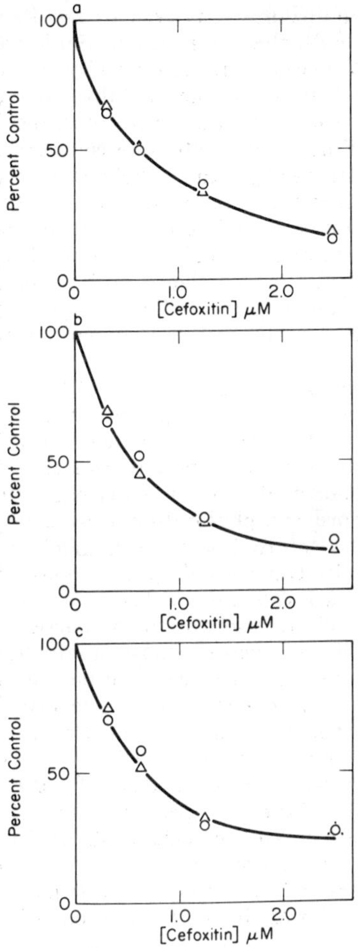

FIG. 3. *Inhibition of β-lactamase by cefoxitin. Cells were harvested, washed once with buffer in mid-log phase, and divided into two aliquots, one of which was sonically treated. A 0.1-ml amount of either whole cells or sonic extract was added to 0.1 ml of a mixture containing 2 mM cephaloridine and a variable amount of cefoxitin. The rate of cephaloridine hydrolysis was determined. Symbols: △, whole cells; ○, sonic extract (a) MB3214; (b) MB3272; (c) MB3389.*

minimal. Erroneous negative or low results are obtained when one waits to harvest the cells for enzyme assay at maximum cell density, i.e., stationary phase. An example of this may be found in the recent report of Weinrich and Del Bene (23), who used 18-h cultures for their study of β-lactamase. In general, their specific activities are much lower (sometimes 1/60) than those reported here for exponential-phase cells.

In addition to the strains represented in Fig. 1 and 2, 16 other isolates were examined, and in only three instances was the level of β-lactamase in late stationary-phase cells greater than 10% of the activity in log-phase cells. Olsson et al. (16) observed the same phenomenon and, in addition, stated that they were able to obtain maximum enzyme yields by maintaining exponential growth in a chemostat (C. E. Nord et

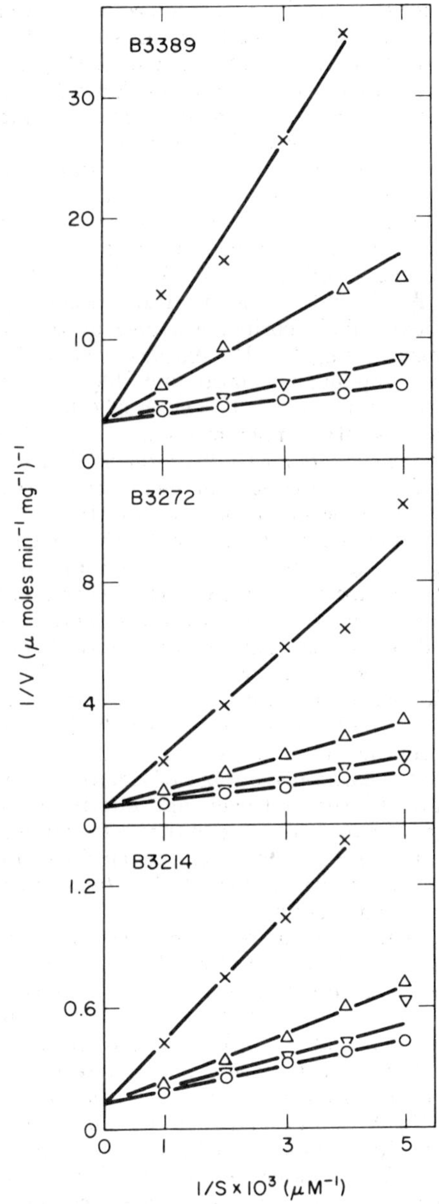

FIG. 4. *Competitive inhibition of β-lactamase by cefoxitin. Enzyme from the S30 fraction was added to a mixture containing varying amounts of cefoxitin and cephaloridine. Symbols: ×, 1 μM cefoxitin; △, 0.25 μM cefoxitin; ▽, 0.063 μM cefoxitin; ○, control (no cefoxitin).*

al., Prog. Abstr. Intersci. Conf. Antimicrob. Ag. Chemother. 15th, Washington, D.C., Abstr. 282, 1975).

The role of β-lactamase in resistance to an antibiotic is often difficult to assess. For example, Neu reported (12) that gram-negative aerobic organisms may often possess a β-lactamase that is very effective in the hydrolysis of cephalosporins, but they still remain susceptible to the antibiotics. The situation with *B. fragilis* seems more clear. The data in Table 3 demonstrate that there is a highly significant positive correlation between the presence of β-lactamase activity and the relative resistance of *B. fragilis* to cephalosporins. Cefoxitin, which is extremely resistant to the action of the enzyme, is the most active β-lactam antibiotic among the drugs tested against *B. fragilis*. Cephamycins A, B, and C, the naturally occurring 7-methoxycephalosporins, are also quite active against *B. fragilis* (H. Wallick and J. Birnbaum, unpublished data) and, like cefoxitin, are very resistant to the action of β-lactamase from a variety of microorganisms (5, 17). This provides support for the hypothesis that for *B. fragilis* the antibiotic must be extremely resistant or indifferent to the action of the β-lactamase to be active. For example, the enzyme(s) from *B. fragilis* had poor, but measurable, activity against penicillin G, yet the organism is known to be resistant to the antibiotic. Cefamandole and cefuroxime, which have been reported to be relatively resistant to attack by β-lactamase from gram-negative aerobic bacteria, were both quite susceptible to hydrolysis by the enzyme from *B. fragilis* (15), and, as expected, a large percentage of isolates were resistant to the antibacterial effects of both drugs. It may be concluded that cefoxitin resistance to the β-lactamase is a major factor in its superior activity against *B. fragilis*, compared to the cephalosporins.

Although the association between β-lactamase susceptibility and antibacterial action is very significant statistically, the relationship is not absolute. Several of our *B. fragilis* isolates were resistant to the cephalosporins even though no β-lactamase could be detected. This has been observed with the *Enterobacteriaceae* (12, 17, 18) as well and should not detract from the positive association between enzyme and susceptibility described above. The absolute role of β-lactamase in resistance to cephalosporins by *B. fragilis* will only be known when single-gene mutants deficient in this enzyme become available.

Del Bene and Farrar (6) found that breaking cells by freezing and thawing had a negligible effect on enzyme activity. Our results are consistent with this observation. Sonic treatment did not increase enzyme activity, as would be expected if some permeability barrier prevented the substrate from reaching the enzyme. Since no hydrolysis of cefoxitin could be demonstrated by either whole cells or sonic extracts no direct estimation of crypticity for this antibiotic is available. However, the inhibition of β-lactamase by cefoxitin showed a similar concentration dependence both in intact cells and in sonically treated cell suspensions, suggesting the absence of a major permeability barrier.

On the basis of substrate profile, the strains examined fell into two groups. In the first, consisting of the strains in which essentially all the enzyme was in the supernatant, the V_{max} for the substrates could be arranged in the following order: cephaloridine > cefazolin > cephalothin ≃ cefuroxime > cefamandole > penicillin G. In the second group, represented by strains MB3389 and MB3445, a considerable amount of enzyme was in the particulate fraction. Cefazolin was the most rapidly hydrolyzed cephalosporin in this case. In both groups, the enzyme was clearly a cephalosporinase, confirming earlier studies (1, 6). Other strains in which a single estimation of V_{max} was obtained at a substrate concentration of 1,000 μM fell into one of the two groups (data not shown). Although possibly coincidental, it is interesting that both members of the second group were members of *B. fragilis* subsp. *distasonis*.

From the Michaelis-Menten equation

$$-\frac{dS}{dt} = \frac{V_{max} S}{K_m + S}$$

it is easy to see that the physiological efficiency (V_{max}/K_m) as defined by Citri and Pollock (2) is a pseudo first-order rate constant when $S \ll K_m$. It seems reasonable to assume that in the natural state *B. fragilis* encounters only very low levels of cephalosporins. Under these circumstances, the physiological efficiency is a reasonable approximation to the stability of the antibiotics in the presence of lactamase. In this regard, it is of considerable interest that V_{max}/K_m was virtually identical for all cephalosporins, even though individual K_m and V_{max} values showed considerable variability. The exception to this generalization is cefoxitin, which was not hydrolyzed even at high substrate concentrations.

The kinetic data presented above were determined with a modified starch-iodine assay. Due to the diverse nature of the reaction products that result from the hydrolysis of the β-lactam ring of cephalosporins (18), standard curves had to be derived for each individual substrate. In all cases, a linear relationship was observed between the concentration of alkali-hydrolyzed cephalosporin and decrease in absorbance at 620 nm. The slopes for the various cephalosporins, however, varied dramatically. It should also be pointed out that in spite of the inherent limitations of the starch-iodine assay when applied to cephalosporins, the method remains one of the standard assays for β-lactamase activity against this class of β-lactams (8, 17, 19, 24).

In marked contrast to the cephalosporins tested, cefoxitin was not hydrolyzed by the β-lactamase from *B. fragilis*. In two cases, incubation was continued overnight, and still we were unable to demonstrate hydrolysis of cefoxitin relative to a substrate blank. Even in the six isolates with MICs greater than 32 μg of cefoxitin per ml, no enzymatic activity could be demonstrated with cefoxitin as a substrate. This result is in direct contrast to the finding of Weinrich and Del Bene (23). These workers have claimed that they can measure rates of hydrolysis of cefoxitin by *B. fragilis* β-lactamase that in some cases exceed those of cephamandole and even cephaloridine. This is indeed puzzling, since cephaloridine is recognized by most workers as being very susceptible to the action of most cephalosporinases. Furthermore, Weinrich and Del Bene used 18-h cultures for their source of enzyme, which gave very low specific activities. It seems surprising, therefore, that they could observe activity against cefoxitin with low-potency enzyme, whereas we could not observe any activity at all with a high-potency enzyme preparation. In this regard, our work is in agreement with that of Olsson et al. (16), who obtained similar specific activities with the cephalosporin substrates and no measurable hydrolysis of cefoxitin.

Not only is cefoxitin stable in solutions containing β-lactamase from *B. fragilis*, it has been shown to be an inhibitor of the enzyme (16). We have demonstrated here that the antibiotic is a competitive inhibitor of the enzyme (16). We show double reciprocal plots (7) where the K_i was estimated and found to be very low, i.e., about 0.3 μM for strains MB3272 and MB3214 and about 0.1 μM for strain MB3389. The fact that cefoxitin inhibits β-lactamase suggests that, in addition to its own antibacterial activity, it might be a useful synergen when used in conjunction with other β-lactam antibiotics. Similar suggestions have been made for certain synthetic penicillins (3, 14, 25).

Some of our observations do not agree with those reported by Olsson et al. (16). One major difference was our inability to demonstrate enzyme activity in the culture supernatant. Our culture medium interfered with our standard iodometric assay, and it was necessary to dialyze the medium overnight to eliminate this interference. It is conceivable that during dialysis the extracellular enzyme was inactivated. In spite of this difference, the main points of our data support, confirm, and extend those of Olsson et al. (16).

LITERATURE CITED

1. **Anderson, J. D., and R. B. Sykes.** 1973. Characterization of a β-lactamase obtained from a strain of *Bacteroides fragilis* resistant to β-lactam antibiotics. J. Med. Microbiol. 6:201–206.
2. **Citri, N., and M. R. Pollock.** 1966. The biochemistry and function of β-lactamase (penicillinase). Adv. Enzymol. Relat. Subj. Biochem. 28:237–323.
3. **Cole, M., S. Elson, and P. D. Fullbrook.** 1972. Inhibition of *Escherichia coli* and *Klebsiella aerogenes* by semisynthetic penicillins. Biochem. J. 127:295–308.
4. **Cornelis, G., and E. P. Abraham.** 1975. β-Lactamases from *Yersinia enterocolitica*. J. Gen. Microbiol. 87:273–284.
5. **Daoust, D. R., H. R. Onishi, H. Wallick, D. Hendlin, and E. O. Stapley.** 1973. Cephamycins, a new family of β-lactam antibiotics: antibacterial activity and resistance to β-lactamase degradation. Antimicrob. Agents Chemother. 3:254–261.
6. **Del Bene, V. E., and W. E. Farrar, Jr.** 1973. Cephalosporinase activity in *Bacteroides fragilis*. Antimicrob. Agents Chemother. 3:369–372.
7. **Dixon, M., and E. C. Webb.** 1964. Enzymes, 2nd ed. Academic Press Inc., New York.
8. **Goldner, M., D. G. Glass, and P. C. Fleming.** 1968. Characteristics of *Aerobacter* beta-lactamase. Can. J. Microbiol. 14:139–145.
9. **Kislak, J. W.** 1972. The susceptibility of *Bacteroides fragilis* to 24 antibiotics. J. Infect. Dis. 125:295–299.
10. **Lowry, O. H., N. J. Rosebrough, A. L. Farr, and R. J. Randall.** 1951. Protein measurement with the Folin phenol reagent. J. Biol. Chem. 193:265–275.
11. **Martin, W. J., M. Gardner, and J. A. Washington II.** 1972. In vitro antimicrobial susceptibility of anaerobic bacteria isolated from clinical specimens. Antimicrob. Agents Chemother. 1:148–158.
12. **Neu, H. C.** 1975. The role of β-lactamase in the resistance of gram-negative bacteria to penicillin and cephalosporin derivatives. Infect. Dis. Rev. 3:130–149.
13. **Novick, R. P.** 1962. Microiodimetric assay of penicillinase. Biochem. J. 83:236–240.
14. **O'Callaghan, C. H., and A. Morris.** 1972. Inhibition of β-lactamases by β-lactam antibiotics. Antimicrob. Agents Chemother. 2:442–448.
15. **O'Callaghan, C. H., R. B. Sykes, A. Griffiths, and J. E. Thornton.** 1976. Cefuroxime, a new cephalosporin antibiotic: activity in vitro. Antimicrob. Agents Chemother. 9:511–519.
16. **Olsson, B., C.-E. Nord, and T. Wadström.** 1976. Formation of beta-lactamase in *Bacteroides fragilis:* cell-bound and extracellular activity. Antimicrob. Agents Chemother. 9:727–735.
17. **Onishi, H. R., D. R. Daoust, S. B. Zimmerman, D. Hendlin, and E. O. Stapley.** 1974. Cefoxitin, a semisynthetic cephamycin antibiotic: resistance to beta-

lactamase inactivation. Antimicrob. Agents Chemother. 5:38–48.

18. **Ross, G. W., and C. O'Callaghan.** 1975. β-Lactamase assays, p. 69–85. *In* J. H. Hash (ed.), Methods in enzymology, vol. 43. Academic Press Inc., New York.
19. **Sawada, Y., S. Yaginuma, M. Tai, S. Iyobe, and S. Mitsuhashi.** 1976. Plasmid-mediated penicillin beta-lactamases in *Pseudomonas aeruginosa*. Antimicrob. Agents Chemother. **9**:55–60.
20. **Sutter, V. L.** 1974. Antibiotic susceptibility testing of anaerobes, p. 109–118. *In* A. Balows (ed.), Current techniques for antibiotic susceptibility testing. Charles C Thomas, Publisher, Springfield, Ill.
21. **Sutter, V. L., and S. M. Finegold.** 1975. Susceptibility of anaerobic bacteria to carbenicillin, cefoxitin and related drugs. J. Infect. Dis. **131**:417–422.
22. **Tally, F. P., N. V. Jacobus, J. G. Bartlett, and S. L. Gorbach.** 1975. Susceptibility of anaerobes to cefoxitin and other cephalosporins. Antimicrob. Agents Chemother. **7**:128–132.
23. **Weinrich, A. E., and V. E. Del Bene.** 1976. Beta-lactamase activity in anaerobic bacteria. Antimicrob. Agents Chemother. **10**:106–111.
24. **Yaginuma, S., N. Terakado, and S. Mitsuhashi.** 1975. Biochemical properties of a penicillin beta-lactamase mediated by R factor from *Bordetella bronchiseptica*. Antimicrob. Agents Chemother. 8:238–242.
25. **Zemelman, R., and E. Olivari.** 1972. Carbenicillin as inhibitor of β-lactamase from *Pseudomonas aeruginosa*. Nature (London) **235**:121–122.

ANTIMICROBIAL AGENTS AND CHEMOTHERAPY, Apr. 1977, p. 735-742 Vol. 11, No. 4

Bactericidal Factor Produced by *Haemophilus influenzae* b: Partial Purification of the Factor and Transfer of Its Genetic Determinant

R. A. VENEZIA,* P. M. MATUSIAK, AND R. G. ROBERTSON

Department of Microbiology, University of Rochester, School of Medicine and Dentistry, Rochester, New York 14642

Received for publication 7 October 1976

When aerobically grown on complex media, *Haemophilus influenzae* b and unencapsulated variants, Rb strains, produced a bactericidal factor that was active against other *Haemophilus* species and certain genera of the *Enterobacteriaceae*. A total of 341 clinical isolates of *Haemophilus* were tested for susceptibility to the factor. Ninety-three percent of *H. influenzae* (nontypable), 75% of *H. haemolyticus*, 71% of *H. parainfluenzae*, and 22% of *H. parahaemolyticus* were susceptible. *H. influenaze* b strains were resistant producers of the bactericidal factor and *H. influenzae* f strains were susceptible nonproducers. Only one strain each of *H. aegyptius* and *H. aphrophilus* was isolated and each was susceptible and resistant, respectively. 143 clinical isolates of the *Enterobacteriaceae* were tested and of those 82% of *Escherichia coli*, 85% of *Salmonella* sp., and all *Citrobacter* sp., *Shigella* sp., and *Yersinia* sp. were sensitive to the bactericidal factor produced by *H. influenzae* b. Attempts to isolate the bactericidal activity from mechanically disrupted, solubilized, or osmotically shocked cells failed to release active bactericidal factor. However, we partially purified the bactericidal factor from the spent culture medium of aerobically grown *H. influenzae* b by a series of extractions. The ability to produce the bactericidal factor was transferable to nonproducer strains without also genetically transforming for type b encapsulation. The converse was also true in that type b capsules were produced by transformed *H. influenzae* Rd strains but no bactericidal factor was detected from these strains. Additionally, nitrosoguanidine-induced mutants of *H. influenzae* b lost the ability to produce bactericidal factor without loss of their type-specific capsule, demonstrating that production of the bactericidal factor was genetically separable from production of the type capsule of *H. influenzae* b.

We have reported that *Haemophilus influenzae* b produces a bactericidal factor that is active against *Haemophilus* species and certain members of the *Enterobacteriaceae* but not against gram-positive bacteria (13). Preliminary characterization of the bactericidal factor showed that it was a heat-stable protein of between 50,000 and 100,000 daltons in size, as determined by membrane filter retention. It was produced throughout the growth cycle of *H. influenzae* when cultured aerobically. The bactericidal factor appeared to be different from "colicin-like" bacteriocins in that its production was not inducible by mitomycin C, it did not kill by "single-hit" kinetics and, as opposed to the strain specificity of bacteriocin production, we have observed that all *H. influenzae* b strains produced the factor. None of the clinical nontypable *H. influenzae* strains tested produced the bactericidal factor. It is interesting that *H. influenzae* Rb, i.e., type b strains that have lost the ability to produce a capsule, retained the capacity to produce the bactericidal factor. We have hypothesized that capsule production occurs independently of bactericidal factor production. In this report, we present data to support that hypothesis and look more extensively into the spectrum of activity among the *Haemophilus* species and the *Enterobacteriaceae*. Additionally, our attempts at the isolation of the bactericidal factor from bacterial cells and the spent culture medium suggest that it may be produced as an extracellular protein.

MATERIALS AND METHODS

Bacterial strains. The clinical isolates of the *Haemophilus* species and the *Enterobacteriaceae* were obtained from the Bacteriology Laboratory, Strong Memorial Hospital, Rochester, N.Y. *H. influenzae* b (105) and *H. influenzae* Rd (C25) were studied as the bactericidal factor producer and susceptible strains, respectively.

Media. Brain heart infusion (BHI) agar and 3.7% BHI broth (Difco) were prepared and supplemented with hemin (Kodak) and nicotinamide adenine dinucleotide (NAD; Sigma) as previously described (sBHI) (13).

Other media tested for supporting the production of the bactericidal factor included chocolate agar (Baktron), Trypticase soy broth (Difco), and 1.5% proteose peptone no. 3 (Difco), supplemented with 1.2% agar (Difco), 2 μg of NAD per ml, and 10 μg of hemin per ml. Additionally, IsoVitaleX (BBL) or GC supplement without antibiotics (Oxoid) was added as indicated according to the manufacturer's instructions.

The defined medium, utilizing the base medium described by Michalka and Goodgal (9), was modified by the addition of 0.2% milk casein hydrolysate (Difco), 0.01% glutamine (Sigma), 0.005% tryptophan (Sigma), 0.02% cystine (Sigma), 0.002% Tween 80 (Sigma), and 0.5% soluble starch (Difco) (final concentrations). In all cases, percent compositions were by weight/volume. We increased the glucose concentration to 0.5% and decreased the supplement of hemin to 10 μg/ml and that of NAD to 2 μg/ml (final concentrations). Strains of 105 and C25 were selected for growth on this medium.

Preparation of the bactericidal factor. Isolation of the partially purified bactericidal factor was accomplished by extraction of the spent culture of strain 105 grown in sBHI. The crude extract was obtained by the addition of $(NH_4)_2SO_4$, to 55% saturation, to the cell-free, spent culture medium at 0°C. After the mixture was stirred for 2 h, the precipitate was collected by centrifugation at 12,000 × *g* for 30 min at 4°C, and the supernatant fluid was dialyzed extensively against 50 mM tris(hydroxymethyl)aminomethane (Tris)-hydrochloride buffer, pH 7, until no free sulfate ion was detected by addition of 2% BaCl, pH 6. The retained fraction was extracted with an equal volume of chloroform-methanol (2:1, vol/vol). The interface that formed between the aqueous methanol and chloroform phases was collected by centrifugation at 3,000 × *g* for 5 min and washed twice with an upper phase (chloroform-methanol-Tris-hydrochloride buffer, 3:48:47) (11). The interface was resuspended in Tris-hydrochloride buffer to the original volume and dissolved by heating in a 100°C water bath for 15 min. The solution was centrifuged, and then the supernatant fluid was titrated with concentrated HCl until a precipitate formed at pH 3.2. It was left overnight at 4°C, and the precipitate was removed by centrifugation at 5,000 × *g* for 15 min at 4°C. The activity remained in the supernatant fluid and was stable at 4°C after filter sterilization. For long-term storage the bactericidal factor was maintained at −70°C. Protein estimates were performed according to Lowry (7). In some preparations the chloroform-methanol extraction was repeated. The assays for bactericidal activity have been previously described (13).

Gel electrophoresis. Polyacrylamide gel electrophoresis was performed using either of two sodium dodecyl sulfate (SDS) systems: Biophore precast gels and SDS buffer (Bio-Rad) or SDS-polyacrylamide gels according to Laemmli (8). All samples were concentrated by precipitation with nine parts of cold acetone, redissolved with an SDS-denaturing buffer (Bio-Rad), and heated for 4 min in a 100°C water bath. The gels were fixed and stained with Coomassie blue (3).

To isolate the bactericidal factor from unfixed gels, gel slices were homogenized in 2 ml of water and refrigerated overnight, and the acrylamide was pelleted by centrifugation at 1,500 × *g* for 10 min. The supernatant fluid was lyophilized and redissolved with water to 50% of the sample volume. The factor was precipitated with nine parts of cold acetone (14), and the precipitate, after pelleting at 1,500 × *g* for 10 min, was dissolved in Tris-hydrochloride buffer for assaying its activity.

Disruption of washed cells. *H. influenzae* b was grown in 1 liter of sBHI at 37°C with shaking at 200 rpm until early stationary phase (260 to 280 Klett units, filter 54). The cells were pelleted by centrifugation at 17,000 × *g* for 10 min, washed once in deionized water, and resuspended to give a heavy slurry with 0.01 M Tris-hydrochloride buffer, pH 8. All resuspensions were with that buffer unless otherwise indicated. The cell suspension was divided into four equal parts and kept at 0°C or frozen at −20°C until treatment. The spent culture from those cells was used for extraction of the bactericidal factor. Four types of cellular disruption were used on the cell suspension.

(i) Sonication. An aliquot of the cell suspension was sonically treated with a Bronwill Biosonic III (Bronwill Scientific, Rochester, N.Y.) in an ice bath until approximately greater than 80% cellular breakage was estimated by observation with a light microscope (3 min). The cellular debris was pelleted at 17,000 × *g* for 10 min at 4°C. Both the supernatant fluid and the resuspended debris were assayed for activity. One milliliter of a crude extract of the bactericidal factor was exposed to sonication for 1 min at 0°C to determine if activity was lost by this treatment.

(ii) Na_2CO_3 solubilization. The cells of a second aliquot were pelleted and resuspended in 25 ml of 1% Na_2CO_3, pH 11, according to Tunevall (12). The resulting highly viscous solution was dialyzed overnight at 4°C against Tris-hydrochloride buffer and treated with deoxyribonuclease I (Sigma) until viscosity decreased. The treated solution was heated to 80°C for 10 min and clarified by centrifugation at 9,000 × *g* for 30 min. Both the resuspended cellular debris and the deoxyribonuclease-treated supernatant fluid were tested for activity.

(iii) Heat disruption of cells. The cells from a third aliquot were resuspended in 5 ml of Tris-hydrochloride buffer and heated in a water bath at 65°C for 15 min. The lysed cellular suspension was assayed for activity.

(iv) Cell homogenization. Cells of the fourth aliquot were resuspended in 0.01 M Tris-hydrochloride buffer, pH 7.5 with 1 mM ethylenediaminetetraacetate, and disrupted by homogenization with acid-cleaned glass beads (0.10 to 0.11 mM) in a liquid CO_2-cooled Bronwill homogenizer. The resulting liquid was decanted and centrifuged at 5,000 × *g* for 10 min at 4°C. The supernatant fluid was heated to 65°C for 15 min. A precipitate was formed by addition of $(NH_4)_2SO_4$ to 55% saturation at 4°C, pelleted by centrifugation at 12,000 × *g* for 30 min at 4°C, dissolved to 10% of the original volume in Tris-hydrochloride buffer, and assayed for activity.

(v) Osmotic shock. Freshly grown cells from both midexponential and early stationary phases of growth were osmotically shocked according to Heppel (5). The released cellular fluid was concentrated by lyophilization and tested for activity.

Transformation of C25. A streptomycin-resistant mutant of strain 105 was selected as previously described (13). Transforming deoxyribonucleic acid (DNA) from 105 was isolated by the phenol extraction technique of Yasbin et al. (15). C25 cells were made competent, and the transformation reaction was according to the methods of Barnhart and Herriott (2). Competent cells and transformed cells were stored at −70°C in sBHI with 15% glycerol.

The streptomycin resistance marker was selected by plating transformants on sBHI agar containing 200 μg of streptomycin sulfate, grade B (Calbiochem), per ml.

Controls of transformation experiments either involved the use of deoxyribonuclease-treated DNA from strain 105 or no DNA was added to the transformation reaction.

NTG treatment of strain 105. Nitrosoguanidine (NTG; Aldrich) treatment of strain 105 was accomplished according to Adelberg et al. (1). Briefly, 0.33 mg of NTG per ml (final concentration), pH 6, was added to one part of 0.1 M sodium acetate, pH 5, and five parts of saline containing approximately 10^{10} cells/ml. The mixture was incubated for 10 min at 37°C, and the reaction was terminated with an equal volume of ice-cold BHI, resuspended in 100 ml of sBHI, and incubated at 31°C for 2.5 h (four to five generations). The cells were stored at −70°C in 15% glycerol. This gave a final cell concentration of 2×10^6 cells/ml.

The NTG-treated 105 cells were diluted to give 200 colonies per sBHI agar plate after 18 h of incubation at 37°C in a 10% CO_2 atmosphere. Single colonies were streaked onto an indicator lawn (C25). All colonies that failed to give zones of inhibition for three transfers were scored as *H. influenzae* b nonproducers of the bacteridical factor. Crude extracts from broth cultures of these mutants were assayed for bactericidal activity. Control cells were not treated with NTG.

RESULTS

H. influenzae grew on each of the media tested; however, bactericidal activity by strain 105 was observed only when grown on the complex media. Although all media allowed good to excellent growth of *H. influenzae* with capsule formation by type b strains, the defined medium would not support the production of bactericidal activity by strain 105 unless Oxoid GC supplement was added. In a similar experiment, GC supplement or IsoVitaleX had to be added to GC base medium, Trypticase soy medium, or the proteose peptone no. 3 medium. Only highly complex and enriched media supported the release or production of the bactericidal activity by strain 105. The crude extract of the bactericidal factor inhibited the indicator lawn grown on each of the media, indicating that no substances inhibitory to the bactericidal activity were present in those media tested.

The bactericidal activity produced by strain 105 was typical of that produced by other *H. influenzae* b strains. The bactericidal factor killed strains of *H. influenzae* (nontypable), *H. parainfluenzae*, and *H. haemolyticus* (Table 1). The least susceptible strains were *H. parahaemolyticus*; only one *H. aegyptius* and one *H. aphrophilus* was isolated and they were susceptible and resistant, respectively.

The members of the *Enterobacteriaceae*, which were susceptible to the bactericidal factor, were strains of *Escherichia coli* and closely related genera (Table 2). Lawns of 50 of 61 *E. coli* strains were susceptible to streaked overlays of strain 105 and crude extracts of the bactericidal factor. However, *Proteus* sp., *Enterobacter* sp., *Klebsiella* sp., and the other *Enterobacteriaceae* tested were uniformly resistant to the bactericidal activity.

The bactericidal factor was isolated from the spent culture of strain 105 grown in sBHI (Fig. 1). The extraction procedures resulted in a preparation containing active bactericidal factor that resolved as a single diffuse band on 12% polyacrylamide SDS gels (Fig. 2). When the band was cut from unstained gels and extraneous SDS was removed by precipitation in

TABLE 1. *Strains of Haemophilus species susceptible to the bactericidal factor*

Haemophilus sp.	No. of strains	No. susceptible	% Susceptible[a]
H. aegyptius	1	1	
H. aphrophilus	1	0	
H. haemolyticus	12	9	75
H. influenzae (nontypable)	121	113	93
H. influenzae type b	11	0	0
H. influenzae type f	3	3	100
H. parahaemolyticus	68	15	22
H. parainfluenzae	124	88	71

[a] An insignificant number of strains was isolated to give a meaningful calculation for percent susceptible.

TABLE 2. *Strains of Enterobacteriaceae susceptible to the H. influenzae b bactericidal factor*

Enterobacteriaceae	No. of strains	No. susceptible	% Susceptible[a]
Citrobacter sp.	5	5	100
E. coli	61	50	82
Salmonella sp.	13	11	85
Shigella sp.	7	7	100
Yersinia sp.	1	1	
Enterobacter sp.	29	0	0
Klebsiella sp.	33	0	0
Pectobacterium sp.	1	0	
Proteus sp.	33	0	0
Providencia sp.	5	0	0
Serratia sp.	7	0	0

[a] An insignificant number of strains was isolated to give a meaningful calculation for percent susceptible.

acetone, no activity was lost as compared with control samples treated in a similar manner with SDS and acetone. Although further determinations are in progress, we feel that we have obtained the bactericidal factor in a partially purified form after the three-step extraction procedure. The specific activity has increased approximately 16 times that of the crude extract (Table 3).

All four means of disruption and osmotic shock of the washed cells of strain 105 failed to release active bactericidal factor. None of the methods inactivated bactericidal activity when crude extracts were tested under similar conditions. The disruption of washed cells by use of a liquid CO_2-cooled Bronwill homogenizer resulted in the release of material that inhibited lawns of both strains C25 and 105. The activity of the inhibitory material was destroyed upon heating to 65°C for 15 min in a water bath. Both the lack of specificity of the bactericidal effect and its heat lability were inconsistent with those properties of the bactericidal factor. The technique of disruption was applied to midlog-phase cells and the results were the same. The washes from the cells did not contain any bactericidal activity.

The competent cells of strain C25 were transformed with DNA from a streptomycin-resistant 105 strain. The transformants were selected for streptomycin resistance and then tested for ability to produce bactericidal activity. Of 200 streptomycin-resistant transformants screened, none was as able to produce the bactericidal activity. However, when competent cells were treated with DNA isolated from strain 105 and subsequently grown in the presence of the bactericidal factor, transformants were obtained that could produce the bactericidal factor. All transformants were both producers of the bactericidal factor and resistant to it, but none was also transformed for a type b capsule. By use of anti-*H. influenzae* Rd rabbit serum, we were able to select for C25 strains transformed to type b capsule production, because anti-Rd rabbit serum would agglutinate Rd type strains and leave type b transformants in the supernatant fluid. These encapsulated transformants were not producers of the bactericidal factor and were sensitive to its activity. Control cells treated with deoxyribonuclease-degraded DNA, or no DNA, did not show transformation to streptomycin resistance, to production of the bactericidal factor, or to encapsulation. In addition, strains resistant to the bactericidal factor, but not producers of it, arose among both the transformed cells and control cells grown in the presence of the bactericidal factor.

When strain 105 was treated with NTG under the conditions described, 2 of 200 colonies resulted in mutants that were encapsulated but had lost the ability to produce the bactericidal factor both on sBHI agar and in broth. They remained resistant to the bactericidal activity. Control cells failed to produce spontaneous mutants.

DISCUSSION

The range of activity of the bactericidal factor produced by *H. influenzae* b varied among the *Haemophilus* species isolated. Certain species were observed to be very susceptible and these included *H. influenzae* (nontypable), *H. haemolyticus*, and *H. parainfluenzae*. *H. parahaemolyticus* was least susceptible, and an insufficient number of *H. aegyptius* and *H. aphrophilus* were isolated to made a determination. The number of encapsulated strains of *H. influenzae* was also low. However, all the type b strains were producers of the bactericidal factor and maintained the same spectrum of activity as test strain 105. In a previous study in which all six serotypes were tested, none other than type b produced or was resistant to the bactericidal factor (13). It was interesting to find that a large percentage of *E. coli* and related genera were susceptible to this bactericidal factor. The less closely related genera, i.e. *Klebsiella*, *Proteus*, and *Enterobacter*, were uniformly resistant. According to a recent report by Johnson (6), the *Enterobacteriaceae* can be divided into three groups or classifications based on biochemical, physiological, and morphological characters. From the results of their taxonomical study, *Escherichia, Shigella, Salmonella,* and *Yersinia* fell into one closely related group

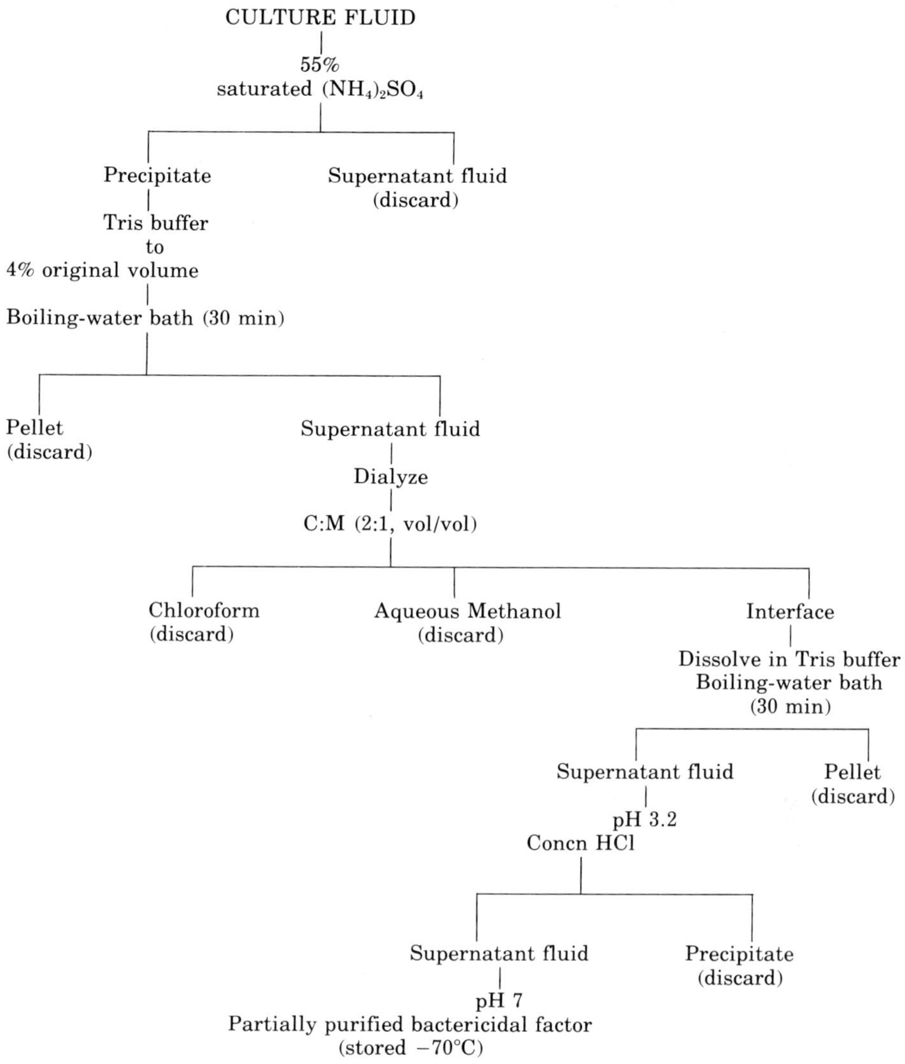

Fig. 1 Venezia et al.

FIG. 1. *Summary scheme of the purification of the bactericidal factor from culture fluid of H. influenzae b. C:M, Chloroform-methanol.*

differing from both the *Proteus-Providencia* group and a *Klebsiella*, *Serratia*, *Enterobacter* group. It is not surprising that genera of the group closely related to *E. coli* would all be susceptible to the same bactericidal factor. The exact reason for the spectrum of activity of the factor extending from the genus *Haemophilus* to those particular members of the *Enterobacteriaceae* is not readily apparent. However, we can suggest that similar receptor sites for the factor may exist on both the *Haemophilus* species and the *E. coli* group and quite possibly the metabolic response to the effect of the bactericidal factor may be similar. This is currently being investigated.

The bactericidal factor is readily extracted from the spent culture medium of aerobically grown *H. influenzae* b. However, we have observed that only when complex media were used for growth did production of the bactericidal factor occur. The *H. influenzae* strains grew on simple media when supplied with hemin and NAD. We observed good growth on both supplemented Trypticase soy broth and the defined medium, but *H. influenzae* b did not exhibit bactericidal activity unless each

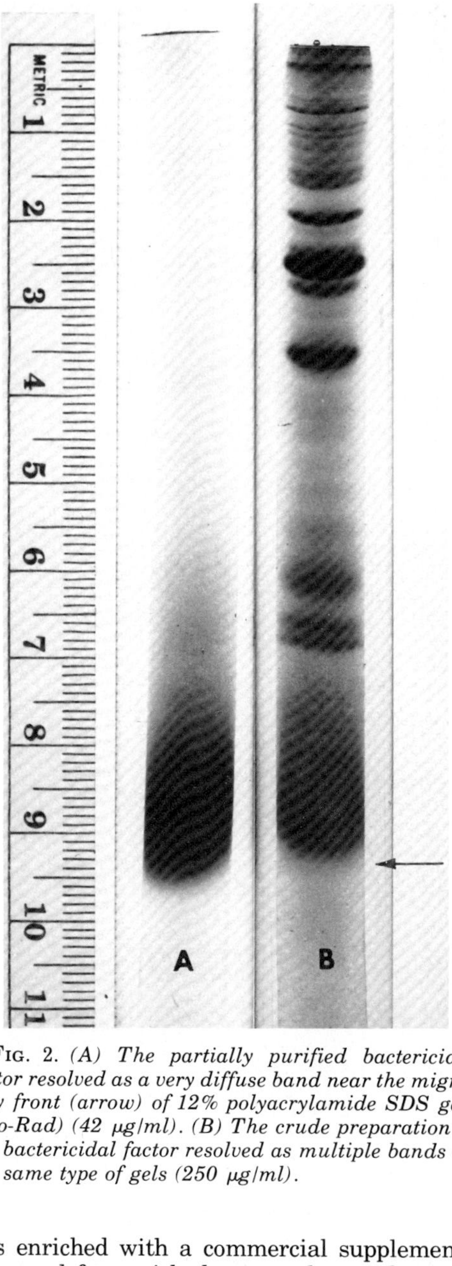

FIG. 2. *(A) The partially purified bactericidal factor resolved as a very diffuse band near the migratory front (arrow) of 12% polyacrylamide SDS gels (Bio-Rad) (42 μg/ml). (B) The crude preparation of the bactericidal factor resolved as multiple bands on the same type of gels (250 μg/ml).*

was enriched with a commercial supplement. The need for enriched or complex media suggests to us that the bactericidal factor may be a metabolic product requiring "luxuriant" growth conditions for either its production by the cell or its release into the culture medium.

We have attempted several methods for the isolation of the bactericidal factor from washed cells. The bactericidal factor in its extracellular form is resistant to heat or alkali conditions for short periods of time. When either the released cellular fluid or the cellular debris was concentrated and tested for bactericidal activity, none was observed. The failure to isolate active bactericidal factor from disrupted, solubilized, or osmotically shocked bacterial cells can be interpreted either as a lack of significant intracellular pools of the factor or as evidence that it exists in an inactive or characteristically different form within the cell. It seems unlikely that inactivation of the bactericidal factor occurred by the action of bacterial proteases. Enzymatic activity was kept to a minimum by maintaining the cells at less than 0°C prior to treatment and heat treating the lysates after treatment. In any case, solubilization of the cellular envelope by heat or alkali treatment would argue against enzymatic inactivation of the bactericidal factor. In addition, the bactericidal factor was not inactivated by any of the means of cell fractionation and remained active in control preparations when treated under similar conditions. Previously, we showed that the bactericidal factor is released into the growth medium throughout the growth cycle of *H. influenzae* b (13). No net increase in bactericidal activity was noted during the stationary phases of growth when autolysis was increased. The presence of the bactericidal factor in the medium throughout the entire growth curve, the requirement for complex growth medium, the sensitivity to proteolytic activity, and the inability to isolate active factor from washed cells suggest that the bactericidal factor may be an "exoprotein." Final determination as to the bactericidal factor's exoprotein nature will rest in demonstrating that during growth each cell is capable of producing and releasing it without damage to the cellular integrity.

We were unable to use either molecular-sieve or ion-exchange column chromatography for the purification of the bactericidal factor from crude extracts. This was attributed to inactiva-

TABLE 3. *Partial purification of the bactericidal factor from the culture supernatant fluid of H. influenzae b*

Fraction	Vol (ml)	Bactericidal activity[a] (%)	Protein (mg/ml)	Sp act[b]
Crude extract, $(NH_4)_2SO_4$	38.5	47	14.1	3.26
100°C, 30 min	33	50	14.8	3.39
Dialysis	34.5	54	8.0	6.75
Chloroform-methanol interface	19	47	0.96	48.96
pH 3.2	18.5	43	0.84	51.19

[a] Percentage of C25 killed after 10 min of incubation at room temperature with 100 μl of each fraction when added to 5 × 10^4 colony-forming units of C25 per ml.

[b] Bactericidal activity per milligram of total protein per milliliter.

tion of the factor or adsorption to the column supports. The bactericidal factor also displayed the unusual property of nonspecific binding to cellulose or cellulose-like derivatives. However, we have developed a series of extractions that lead to a partial purification of the factor.

The partially purified factor forms a single diffuse band on SDS-polyacrylamide gels after electrophoresis. The band migrates near the front on 12% gels and maintains all the bactericidal activity. This suggests that the molecular size of the factor is smaller than 14,000 daltons. However, we previously stated the factor was larger than 50,000 daltons based on retention by membrane filters. When the electrophoresis is performed without SDS, the bactericidal factor remains near the top of the 12% gels, and this indicates that aggregates of the molecule form in the absence of SDS. This also could explain the larger size estimated by the membrane filters. What clouds the issue is that the factor appears as a diffuse band atypical of SDS-denatured proteins on electrophoresis with SDS buffers. We suspect that the bactericidal factor may represent a class of molecules of approximately the same size. This heterogeneity would account for the diffuseness of the factor on SDS-containing gels. However, we cannot rule out the presence of acyl groups or other molecules bound to the protein of the bactericidal factor that contribute to this heterogeneity. For these reasons we prefer to state that the bactericidal factor is partially purified.

It is interesting that the bactericidal factor remains active after partitioning between organic and aqueous phases. This condition suggests that the bactericidal factor is an amphipathic molecule. This configuration would allow the molecule to accommodate its interface location without undergoing an irreversible unfolding of its molecular structure. In addition, Reynolds (10) has observed that SDS interacts with some proteins in a way suggestive of the hydrophobic interactions of proteins within a biological membrane. This may explain why the active site of the bactericidal factor remains intact after denaturation in the presence of SDS. In any case, these characteristics indicate that the bactericidal factor is an interesting molecule that warrants further investigation to test this hypothesis.

Since we have found that in addition to *H. influenzae* b strains *H. influenzae* Rb strains produce this bactericidal activity, it seemed unlikely that the activity was a consequence of encapsulation. We tested this by genetic transformation and mutagenesis. The selection for the streptomycin resistance marker was our monitor as to whether genetic transformation was occurring. This marker appeared to transform with the same frequency as reported by others (4). We were able to transfer by genetic transformation the ability to produce the bactericidal factor to a nonproducing strain without also transferring the capacity to produce a capsule. The converse was also true. In addition, *H. influenzae* b, when exposed to a mutagen, lost the bactericidal activity but maintained its characteristic capsule. This confirms the hypothesis, suggested by the observation that *H. influenzae* Rb strains produce the bactericidal activity, that production of the bactericidal factor is independent of encapsulation. Whether this proves to be useful as an epidemological marker for *H. influenzae* Rb strains will be determined by clinical laboratories that screen for bactericidal factor production in association with disease-causing *H. influenzae* strains.

ACKNOWLEDGMENTS

We thank the Diagnostic Laboratory, Strong Memorial Hospital, Rochester, N.Y., and in particular Barbara Doerflein, for their cooperation in obtaining strains used in this study.

This investigation was supported by U.S. Public Health Service training grant no. GM 00592 from the National Institute of General Medical Sciences.

LITERATURE CITED

1. **Adelberg, E. A., M. Mandel, and G. C. C. Cheir.** 1965. Optimal conditions for mutagenesis by N-methyl-N-nitro-N-Nitroso-Guanidine in *Escherichia coli* K-12. Biochem. Biophys. Res. Commun. 18:788–795.
2. **Barnhart, B. J., and R. M. Herriott.** 1963. Penetration of deoxyribonucleic acid into *Haemophilus influenzae*. Biochim. Biophys. Acta 76:25–39.
3. **Fairbanks, G., T. L. Steck, and D. F. H. Wallach.** 1971. Electrophoretic analysis of the major polypeptides of the human erthrocyte membrane. Biochemistry 10:2606–2617.
4. **Goodgal, S. H., and R. W. Herriott.** 1961. Studies on transformation of *Haemophilus influenzae*. I. Competence. J. Gen. Physiol. 44:1201–1227.
5. **Heppel, A.** 1971. The concept of periplasmic enzymes, p. 223-247. *In* L. I. Rothfield (ed.), Structure and function of biological membranes. Academic Press Inc., New York.
6. **Johnson, R., R. R. Colwell, R. Sakazaki, and K. Tamura.** 1975. Numerical taxonomy study of the *Enterobacteriaceae*. Int. J. Syst. Bacteriol. 25:12–37.
7. **Kabat, E. A., and M. M. Mayes.** 1961. Experimental immunochemistry, p. 556–558. Charles C Thomas Publishers, Springfield, Ill.
8. **Laemmli, U. K.** 1970. Cleavage of structural progeins during the assembly of the head of bacteriophage T4. Nature (London) 227:680–685.
9. **Michalka, J., and S. H. Goodgal.** 1969. Genetic and physical maps of the chromosome of *Haemophilus influenzae*. J. Mol. Biol. 45:407–421.
10. **Reynolds, J. A., and C. Tanford.** 1970. The gross conformation of protein-sodium dodecyl sulfate complexes. J. Biol. Chem. 245:5161–5165.
11. **Soto, E. F., J. M. Pasquini, R. Placido, and J. L. Latorre.** 1969. Fractionation of lipids and proteolipids from cat grey and white matter by chromatography

on an organaphilic dextran gel. J. Chromatogr. 41:400–409.

12. **Tunevall, G.** 1953. Studies on *Haemophilus influenzae. Haemophilus influenzae* antigens studied by the gel precipitation method. Acta. Pathol. Microbiol. Scand. 32:193–197.
13. **Venezia, R. A., and R. G. Robertson.** 1975. Bactericidal substance produced by *Haemophilus influenzae* b. Can. J. Microbiol. 21:1587–1594.
14. **Weber, K., and M. Osborne.** 1969. The reliability of molecular weight determinations by dodecyl sulfate-polyacrylamide gel electrophoresis. J. Biol. Chem. 211:4406–4412.
15. **Yasbin, R. E., G. A. Wilson, and F. E. Young.** 1975. Transformation and transfection in lysogenic strains of *Bacillus subtilis:* evidence for selective induction of prophage in competent cells. J. Bacteriol. 121:269–304.

ANTIMICROBIAL AGENTS AND CHEMOTHERAPY, Apr. 1977, p. 743-749
Vol. 11, No. 4

Printed in U.S.A.

Evaluation of the In Vitro Antifungal Activity of Allicin

YASUO YAMADA* AND KEIZŌ AZUMA

Department of Microbiology, Fujita-Gakuen University School of Medical Technology, Toyoake, Aichi 470-11, Japan

Received for publication 4 December 1976

Allicin was effective in vitro against *Candida, Cryptococcus, Trichophyton, Epidermophyton,* and *Microsporum*. The minimal inhibitory concentrations (MICs) of allicin against these organisms were 3.13 to 6.25 μg/ml by the agar dilution method and 1.57 to 6.25 μg/ml by the broth dilution method, using Sabouraud glucose (SG) medium. However decreased activity was demonstrated against *Aspergillus*. The MIC of allicin against various pathogenic fungi was affected considerably by differences in the experimental conditions, e.g., incubation time, inoculum size, type of medium, and medium pH. The MIC of allicin against *Candida, Cryptococcus,* and *Aspergillus* remained constant after more than 3 days of incubation, and that against *Dermatophytes* remained constant after more than 10 days of incubation. Decreasing the inoculum size increased the susceptibility to allicin. The antifungal activity of allicin was stronger on SG agar medium with a pH of 5.6 than on the same medium with a pH of 6.0 or higher. By microscopical observation, allicin induced morphological abnormalities in hyphae of *Trichophyton mentagrophytes* Morita. Percent germination of spores of the Morita strain at 24 h in SG agar medium was greatly decreased with an allicin concentration of 3.13 μg/ml, and the lethal dose for the spores was about four times higher than the fungistatic concentration. These results suggest that allicin inhibits both germination of spores and growth of hyphae.

An investigation of the literature showed that *Allium sativum,* the common garlic, has been endowed with therapeutic virtues both in legend and in scientific publications. Several investigators have observed the antibacterial activity of garlic extracts. In 1944, an extract of oil from garlic was obtained by steam distillation and by fractional distillation of the crushed cloves and named allicin; this substance possessed potent antibacterial activity against both gram-positive and gram-negative bacteria (1). It is a colorless oil that is approximately 2.5% soluble in water and relatively unstable; it has been assigned the structure: allyl-S-S-allyl (2).

$$\text{allyl-S-}\underset{\substack{\| \\ \text{O}}}{\text{S}}\text{-allyl}$$

In this report, the in vitro antifungal activity of allicin will be described.

MATERIALS AND METHODS

Organisms. *Candida albicans* 381 and Nakamura, *Cryptococcus neoformans* Duke, M-1, and 1814, *Aspergillus fumigatus* Kuboyama, N-2, and IFO 5840, *Trichophyton mentagrophytes* Morita, T-N-2, and T-N-4, *Trichophyton ferrugineum* T-N-1, *Trichophyton rubrum* Ishida and Suzuki, *Microsporum gypseum* Suzuki, and *Epidermophyton floccosum* Suzuki were used.

Stock cultures of *Candida, Cryptococcus,* and *Aspergillus* were grown at 37°C for 3 days on Sabouraud glucose (SG) agar medium, and those of *Trichophyton, Microsporum,* and *Epidermophyton* were grown at 25°C for 15 days on SG agar medium. They were maintained at room temperature.

Viable-cell suspensions of *Candida* or *Cryptococcus* were prepared by suspending viable cells harvested from 3-day-old SG agar slants in sterile saline.

Spore suspensions of *Aspergillus* or *Dermatophytes* were prepared by rubbing on the surface of 3- or 15-day-old SG agar slants with a loop after the addition of a solution of 0.5% (wt/vol) carboxymethylcellulose in sterile saline and filtered through two layers of gauze.

Cell or spore counts were made in a hemocytometer, and the suspension was adjusted to the desired strength by adding more sterile saline or 0.5% carboxymethylcellulose saline. A viable-cell suspension with 10^7 *Candida* or *Cryptococcus* cells per ml and spore suspensions with 10^7 *Aspergillus* or *Trichophyton* spores per ml, 10^6 *Microsporum* spores per ml, and 10^5 *Epidermophyton* spores per ml were used as standard suspensions in all experiments, unless stated otherwise.

Allicin. Allicin was extracted from the crushed cloves of *A. sativum* (4). The preparation used here was pure and had a d^{20} of 1.112, and n_D^{20} 1.561.

By calculation, analysis of allicin showed (for $C_6H_{10}OS_2$): molecular weight, 162; C, 44,44; H, 6.17; S, 39.51. Composition as found was: C, 44.35; H,

6.25; S, 39.70%. Before use, allian was diluted with water to the desired concentration and sterilized by filtering through a 0.22-μm-pore size membrane filter (Millipore Corp.).

Medium. SG agar medium and SG broth medium were used. The pH was 5.6.

Recording of radial growth of colonies. A 0.002-ml standard spore suspension of *T. mentagrophytes* Morita was inoculated by stabbing with a wire needle into the center of an SG agar plate containing the different concentrations of allicin, and the resultant colonies were measured along two diameters, crossing at right angles, marked on the back of the plates, and the average diameters of colonies were calculated. To determine the growth rate, this measurement was repeated at various intervals of time.

Germination test and morphological observation. A twofold-dilution series of allicin in molten SG agar medium at 45°C was prepared in 20-ml volumes in petri dishes, immediately added to a 0.1-ml standard spore suspension of *T. mentagrophytes* Morita, mixed well, and solidified in plates. The final concentration of allicin ranged from 0 to 12.5 μg/ml. After 24 h of incubation, square samples (10 by 10 mm) cut off from the plates were mounted in lactophenol cotton blue and examined microscopically. The number of germination of spores in a total of 500 was counted, and the percentage of germination was determined. A spore was considered to be germinated when the germ tube was as long as it was wide.

Morphological changes were observed at various intervals of time for 15 days of incubation.

Minimal inhibitory concentration (MIC). The agar dilution method used was as follows: a 0.01-ml viable-cell suspension of *Candida* or *Cryptococcus* was inoculated by making a 2-cm-long streak with a loop on an SG agar plate containing the different concentrations of allicin, and the plate was incubated at 37°C for 5 days. A 0.002-ml spore suspension of *Aspergillus* or *Dermatophytes* was inoculated by stabbing with a wire needle in the center of an SG agar plate containing the different concentrations of allicin, and the plate was incubated at 37 or 25°C for 5 or 15 days, respectively. The minimal concentration at which a colony did not grow after incubation at a suitable temperature for a set time was taken as the MIC. The broth dilution method was as follows: a twofold-dilution series of allicin in SG broth medium was prepared in 10-ml volumes in test tubes, inoculated with 0.05 ml of viable-cell or spore suspension, and incubated at a suitable temperature. The minimal concentration which caused complete inhibition of growth after a set time was taken as the MIC. The concentrations of allicin used were as follows: 0, 0.05, 0.1, 0.2, 0.39, 0.78, 1.56, 3.13, 6.25, 12.5, and 25.0 μg/ml.

Effect of pH on activity. The MIC of allicin against fungi on medium with different pH values was determined by the agar dilution method on SG agar medium adjusted to a final pH value of 5.6, 6.0, 6.5, and 7.5 with inoculum sizes of 0.01 or 0.002 ml of a standard viable-cell or spore suspension.

Effect of inoculum size on activity. The MIC of allicin against fungi with different inoculum sizes was determined by agar dilution method on SG agar medium (pH 5.6) with an inoculum size of 0.01 or 0.002 ml of 10^4, 10^5, 10^6, and 10^7 viable cells or spores per ml.

Fungicidal activity test. A series of test tubes containing 10 ml of SG broth medium incorporating from 0 to 25 μg of allicin per ml was prepared, inoculated with 0.1 ml of a standard spore suspension of *T. mentagrophytes* Morita, and incubated at 25°C for 10 days. Samples (10 ml) were taken after 10 days of exposure to the drug, washed twice with large volumes of sterile saline to remove unabsorbed allicin, and resuspended in 0.5 ml of sterile saline; 0.2-ml samples of this suspension were spread over each of the SG agar slants, and the survival or death of the spores was determined by the presence or absence of colonies that developed within 15 days of incubation.

RESULTS

Antimicrobial spectrum. The MIC of allicin against *Candida, Cryptococcus, Aspergillus, Trichophyton, Epidermophyton,* and *Microsporum* was measured by the broth and agar dilution methods with an inoculum of a standard viable-cell or spore suspension incubated for 5 or 15 days. The results are given in Table 1. The MIC value against *Candida, Cryptococcus, Trichophyton, Epidermophyton,* and *Microsporum* was as low as 3.13 to 6.25 μg/ml on SG agar medium, and as low as 1.57 to 6.25 μg/ml in SG broth medium, even after either 5 to 15 days of incubation. The MIC value against *Aspergillus* was 12.5 to 25 μg/ml by both broth and agar dilution methods after 5 days of incubation. The antimicrobial activity of allicin against *A. fumigatus* Koboyama and *Dermatophytes* was stronger on agar medium than in broth medium. The MIC value of allicin against fungi changed significantly between 1 and 15 days of incubation. However, the MIC against *Candida* and *Cryptococcus* (except *C. neoformans* Duke) by the broth dilution method and the MIC against *Aspergillus* by both broth and agar dilution methods remained constant after 3 days of incubation. The MIC value against dermatophytes by both broth and agar dilution methods remained constant after 10 days of incubation.

Effect of inoculum size on activity. The MIC of allicin against *Candida, Cryptococcus, Aspergillus, Trichophyton, Microsporum,* and *Epidermophyton* on SG agar medium (pH 5.6) with different inoculum sizes was determined by the agar dilution method (Tables 1 and 2). The activity of allicin against these fungi, except *C. albicans* 381, *T. mentagrophytes* Morita, T-N-2, and T-N-4, and *T. ferrugineum* T-N-1 increased as inoculum size decreased from 10^7

TABLE 1. *MICs of allicin against various pathogenic fungi*

Organism[a]	Medium[b]	MIC (μg/ml)				
		1 day	3 days	5 days	10 days	15 days
Candida albicans 381	A	3.13	6.25	6.25		
	B	3.13	6.25	6.25		
C. albicans Nakamura	A	1.57	1.57	3.13		
	B	0.20	3.13	3.13		
Cryptococcus neoformans Duke	A	–[c]	1.57	3.13		
	B	–	1.57	3.13		
C. neoformans 1814	A	–	1.57	3.13		
	B	–	3.13	3.13		
C. neoformans M-1	A	–	0.79	3.13		
	B	–	1.57	1.57		
Aspergillus fumigatus Kuboyama	A	6.25	12.5	12.5		
	B	12.5	25.0	25.0		
A. fumigatus N-2	A	3.13	25.0	25.0		
	B	3.13	25.0	25.0		
A. fumigatus IFO 5840	A	25.0	25.0	25.0		
	B	12.5	25.0	25.0		
Trichophyton mentagrophytes Morita	A	–	1.57	3.13	3.13	3.13
	B	–	3.13	6.25	6.25	6.25
T. mentagrophytes T-N-2	A	–	1.57	3.13	3.13	3.13
	B	–	1.57	3.13	3.13	3.13
T. mentagrophytes T-N-4	A	–	1.57	3.13	3.13	3.13
	B	–	0.79	3.13	6.25	6.25
T. ferrugineum T-N-1	A	–	0.79	3.13	3.13	3.13
	B	–	3.13	6.25	6.25	6.25
T. rubrum Suzuki	A	–	0.79	1.57	3.13	3.13
	B	–	3.13	6.25	6.25	6.25
T. rubrum Ishida	A	–	–	0.78	1.57	3.13
	B	–	1.57	1.57	3.13	3.13
Microsporum gypseum Suzuki	A	–	1.57	1.57	3.13	3.13
	B	–	3.13	6.25	6.25	6.25
Epidermophyton floccosum Suzuki	A	–	–	0.78	3.13	3.13
	B	–	1.57	3.13	6.25	6.25

[a] Inoculum size was 0.01 or 0.002 ml of a suspension of 10^7 viable cells or spores per ml, except for *Microsporum* and *Epidermophyton*: inoculum size was 0.002 ml of suspensions containing 10^6 and 10^5 spores per ml, respectively.

[b] A, SG agar medium, pH 5.6; B, SG broth medium, pH 5.6.

[c] –, No growth.

to 10^4 viable cells or spores per ml.

Effect of medium pH on activity. The MIC of allicin against *Candida, Cryptococcus, Aspergillus, Trichophyton, Epidermophyton,* and *Microsporum* on SG agar medium with a pH of 5.6 to 7.5 was determined by the agar dilution method with an inoculum consisting of a standard viable-cell or spore suspension (Tables 1 and 2). The MIC of allicin against these fungi, except *C. albicans* Nakamura, *A. fumigatus* N-2 and IFO 5840, and *T. rubrum* Suzuki, was higher on the medium with a pH of 6.0 or above than on that with a pH of 5.6.

Radial growth of colony. The effects of various additions of allicin on radial growth of colonies of *T. mentagrophytes* Morita on SG agar medium are shown in Fig. 1. From the growth curve drawn for each concentration of allicin, the length of the lag phase was determined: at 0.78 or 1.57 μg/ml, the lag phase increased by 1 or 2 days over that of the controls, and the radial growth of colonies at subinhibitory concentrations was considerably restricted in comparison with the controls.

Effect of inoculum size on radial growth of colony. The effect of inoculum size on radial growth of colonies of *T. mentagrophytes* Morita after 15 days of incubation on SG agar medium containing 0 to 3.13 μg of allicin per ml is shown in Fig. 2. The size of the colonies decreased both when inoculum size was decreased from 10^7 to 10^5 spores per ml and when allicin concentration was increased from 0 to 3.13 μg/ml.

Effect of allicin on germination. The percent germination of spores of *T. mentagrophytes* Morita after 24 h in the presence of allicin (incorporated into SG agar medium) was

TABLE 2. *Effect of inoculum size and medium pH on the MIC of allicin against various pathogenic fungi*

Organism	MIC (μg/ml)[a]						
	Inoculum size[b] (viable cells or spores/ml)			pH of SG agar medium[c]			
	10^4	10^5	10^6	6.0	6.5	7.0	7.5
Candida albicans 381	6.25	—[d]	6.25	6.25	—	6.25	12.5
C. albicans Nakamura	1.57	—	3.13	3.13	—	3.13	3.13
Cryptococcus neoformans Duke	1.57	—	3.13	3.13	—	3.13	6.25
C. neoformans 1814	1.57	—	3.13	3.13	—	6.25	12.5
C. neoformans M-1	0.78	—	3.13	3.13	—	6.25	12.5
Aspergillus fumigatus Kuboyama	1.57	—	3.13	12.5	—	12.5	25.0
A. fumigatus N-2	3.13	—	12.5	25.0	—	25.0	25.0
A. fumigatus IFO 5840	1.57	—	25.0	25.0	—	25.0	25.0
Trichophyton mentagrophytes Morita	—	3.13	3.13	6.25	6.25	12.5	—
T. mentagrophytes T-N-2	—	3.13	3.13	3.13	3.13	6.25	—
T. mentagrophytes T-N-4	—	3.13	3.13	6.25	6.25	12.5	—
T. ferrugineum T-N-1	—	3.13	3.13	6.25	6.25	12.5	—
T. rubrum Suzuki	—	1.57	3.13	3.13	3.13	3.13	—
T. rubrum Ishida	—	1.57	3.57	3.13	3.13	6.25	—
Microsporum gypseum Suzuki	1.57	3.13	1.13	3.13	3.13	6.25	—
Epidermophyton floccosum Suzuki	1.57	3.13	—	3.13	3.13	6.25	—

[a] Expressed as a value determined after 5 days of incubation against *Candida, Cryptococcus,* and *Aspergillus*, and as that after 15 days of incubation against *Dermatophytes*.
[b] Inoculum size was 0.01 or 0.002 ml of suspensions containing 10^4, 10^5, and 10^6 viable cells or spores per ml on SG agar medium (pH 5.6).
[c] Inoculum size was 0.01 or 0.002 ml of a suspension containing 10^7 viable cells or spores per ml, except for *Microsporum* and *Epidermophyton*: inoculum size was 0.002 ml of suspensions containing 10^6 and 10^5 spores per ml, respectively.
[d] —, Not tested.

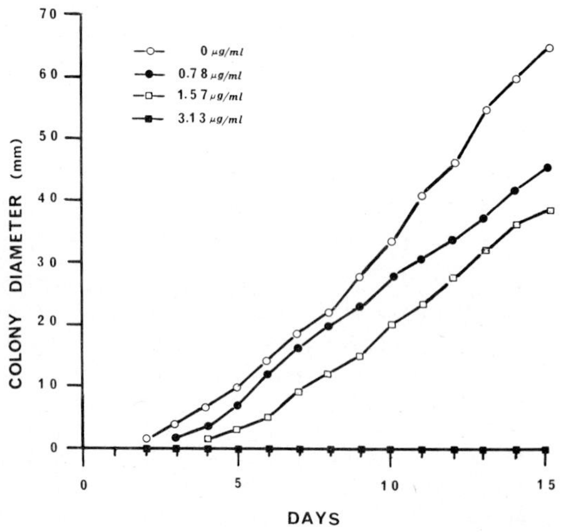

FIG. 1. *Effect of allicin on radial growth of colonies of Trichophyton mentagrophytes Morita on SG agar medium.*

determined by counting the number of germinating spores microscopically. The results are plotted in Fig. 3. Allicin markedly inhibited swelling and germination of spores at concentrations of 3.13 μg or more per ml. The numbers that were germinated decreased with increasing allicin concentration, until a concentration was reached at which no swelling of the spores occurred (12.5 μg/ml). After 24 h of incubation, the numbers of spores that germinated at subinhibitory concentrations of allicin increased, and a few germinated at a concentration that had been inhibitory for 24 h. This was probably due to the normal decomposition of allicin, but the small numbers of spores that germinated at high concentrations could not continue to develop into normal hyphae.

Effect of allicin on hyphae. Morphological effect of allicin on hyphae of *T. mentagrophytes* Morita was observed as follows: on normal SG agar medium, the germ tubes grew rapidly; they were long and regularly branched, and their tips appeared normal. But on SG agar medium containing 3.13 μg of allicin per ml, spherical hyphae or bamboo-joint-like hyphae occurred after 8 or 15 days of incubation, respectively (Fig. 4). These abnormal hyphae were shorter and thicker than those in the controls. They resulted from the noticeable inhibition of longitudinal extension of hyphae by allicin.

Fungicidal activity of allicin. At low concentrations, nystatin is fungistatic to *Aspergillus*

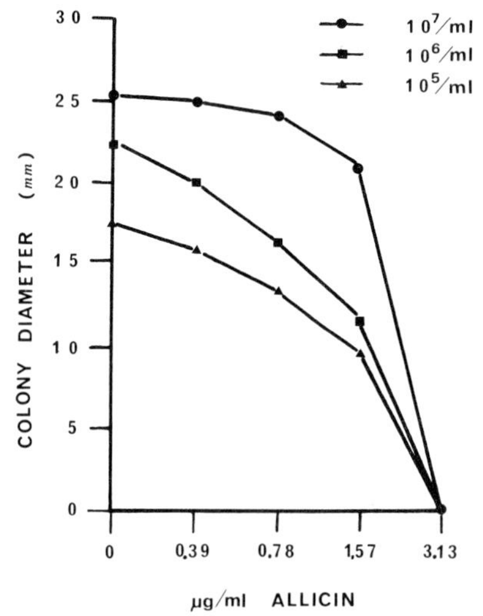

FIG. 2. *Effect of inoculum size on radial growth of colonies of Trichophyton mentagrophytes Morita at 15 days on SG agar medium containing various amounts of allicin. The inoculum size was 0.002 ml of a suspension containing 10^7 to 10^5 spores per ml.*

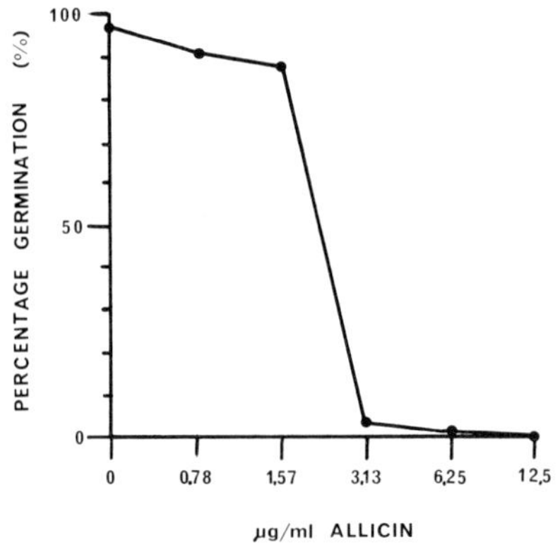

FIG. 3. *Percentage of germination of spores of Trichophyton mentagrophytes Morita after 24 h in SG agar medium containing various amounts of allicin.*

species, but at high concentrations it becomes fungicidal (5). Therefore, the following experiment was performed to determine the concentration of allicin at which this occurred with *T. mentagrophytes* Morita. After exposure to allicin concentrations ranging from 0 to 25 μg/ml in SG broth medium at 25°C for 10 days, the spores were removed from unabsorbed allicin by washing with sterile saline, inoculated onto each of SG agar slants, and incubated. The survival or death of the spores was determined by the presence or absence of colonies that developed on each of the slants within 15 days of incubation. The results are given in Table 3. No significant fungicidal action was noted at allicin concentrations ranging from 1.56 to 12.5 μg/ml, although growth on the slants was delayed from 1 to 4 days in comparison with the controls, but at concentration of 25 μg/ml no spores survived. Since the MIC of allicin against the Morita strain was 6.25 μg/ml in SG broth medium, we conclude that the fungicidal effect occurred at a concentration of allicin about four times higher than the fungistatic concentration.

DISCUSSION

Allicin was found to be highly effective in vitro against *Candida, Cryptococcus, Trichophyton, Epidermophyton,* and *Microsporum.* However, less activity was demonstrated against *Aspergillus*. The MIC value of allicin against these organisms was considerably affected by inoculum size, medium pH, type of medium, and incubation time; also, there were some differences in the MIC according to whether solid or liquid medium was used; i.e., more allicin was required to inhibit growth in liquid than in solid medium. This may have happened because allicin deteriorated more rapidly in liquid than in solid medium. Heavy inocula are known to be far less susceptible to fungicides than light inocula (3). The decreased susceptibility to allicin in medium with a pH of more than 5.6 may be partly a consequence of the further degradation of allicin at a pH value higher than 5.6 and partly a consequence of the decrease of acidity of medium. It is desirable to express the MIC of fungicides as a value determined after 5 days of incubation against *Candida, Cryptococcus,* and *Aspergillus* and as determined after 15 days of incubation against *Dermatophytes*.

Allicin affected germination of spores of *T. mentagrophytes* Morita and the morphology of the hyphae. The lengthening in the lag phase at concentrations approaching the inhibitory level resulted from the delay in swelling and germination of spores, and the restriction of the radial growth of fungal colony on SG agar medium containing allicin resulted from the noticeable inhibition of longitudinal extension of hyphae. The level of allicin necessary to inhibit spore germination was the same as that needed to inhibit hyphal growth. The small numbers of spores that germinated at the inhibitory concentration after 24 h developed into the hyphae with abnormal morphology and could not grow any longer during 15 days of incubation. This suggests a possible fungicidal effect.

In the fungicidal test, it was found that the

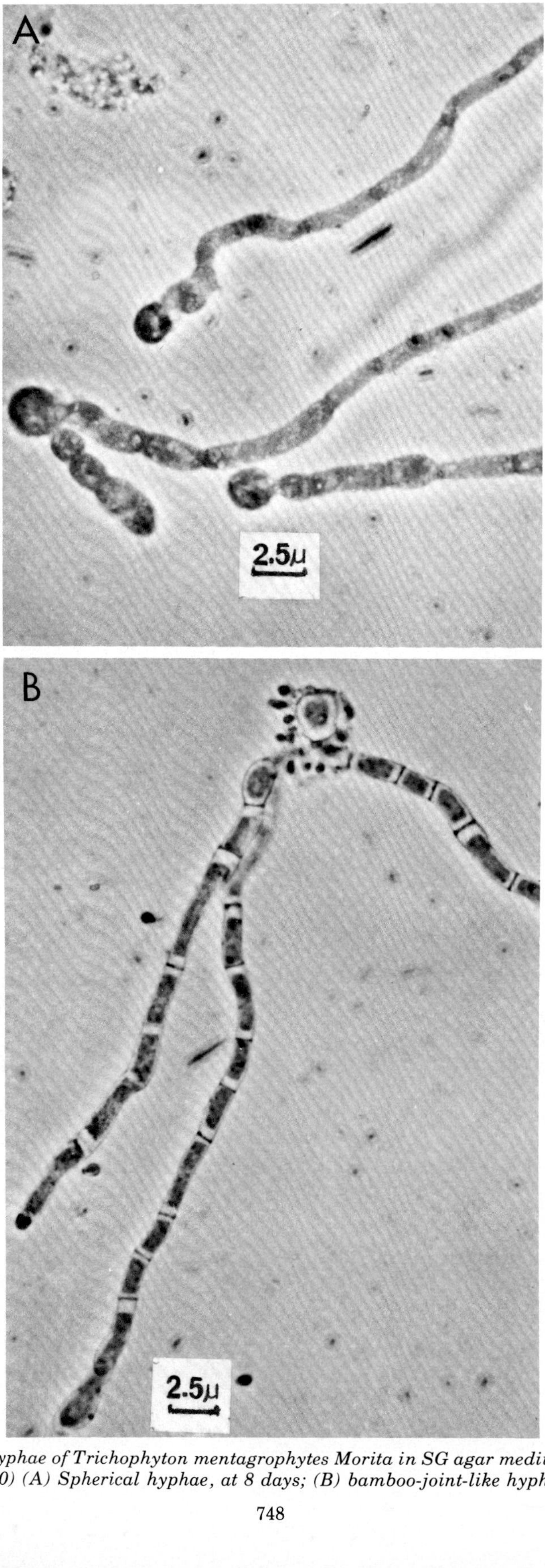

FIG. 4. *Abnormal hyphae of Trichophyton mentagrophytes Morita in SG agar medium containing 3.13 μg of allicin per ml. (×350) (A) Spherical hyphae, at 8 days; (B) bamboo-joint-like hyphae, at 15 days.*

TABLE 3. *Death of spores of Trichophyton mentagrophytes Morita caused by exposure to allicin in SG broth medium*[a]

Concn of allicin in SG broth medium (μg/ml)	Growth of colonies on SG agar slant[b] after days of incubation:														
	1	2	3	4	5	6	7	8	9	10	11	12	13	14	15
25.0	−	−	−	−	−	−	−	−	−	−	−	−	−	−	−
12.5	−	−	−	−	+[c]	+	+	+	+	+	+	+	+	+	+
6.25	−	−	+	+	+	+	+	+	+	+	+	+	+	+	+
3.13	−	−	+	+	+	+	+	+	+	+	+	+	+	+	+
1.56	−	−	+	+	+	+	+	+	+	+	+	+	+	+	+
0	−	+	+	+	+	+	+	+	+	+	+	+	+	+	+

[a] Exposure was for 10 days at 25°C.

[b] Survival or death of the spores after exposure to allicin was determined by the presence or absence of colonies that developed on SG agar slant within 15 days.

[c] +, Colonies present; −, no colonies.

spores were killed by allicin at a concentration only four times greater than that which caused fungistasis.

Cavallito et al. (1, 2) reported that an allicin solution has a pH of approximately 6.5 and shows immediate inactivation upon addition of an excess of any of the standard alkalis, although dilute acids have no effect, and that nonalkaline, aqueous, or nonaqueous solutions or dry preparations undergo a chemical change after standing at room temperature, resulting in an inactive liquid usually within 2 days. Yet, the data obtained with the fungicidal test suggest that the allicin added to the SG broth medium retained its activity for at least 10 days. At present, it is difficult to explain this discrepancy concerning the stability of allicin, but it may have occurred because allicin is comparatively stable in the presence of SG medium as well as in the presence of blood and artificial gastric juice (4) or because the adsorbed allicin on the spore or cell is more stable than free allicin in the medium.

Studies on the mechanism of action of allicin are now in progress. The details of these investigations will be published elsewhere.

ACKNOWLEDGMENTS

We are grateful to K. Fujita for his encouragement throughout this work, and to S. Kuroki, Y. Hoshino, K. Yonemitsu, and K. Kinukawa for their technical assistance.

LITERATURE CITED

1. **Cavallito, C. J., and J. H. Brailey.** 1944. Allicin, the antibacterial principle of *Allium sativum*. I. Isolation, physical properties and antibacterial action. J. Am. Chem. Soc. **66**:1950–1951.
2. **Cavallito, C. J., J. S. Buck, and C. M. Suter.** 1944. Allicin, the antibacterial principle of *Allium sativum*. II. Determination of the chemical structure. J. Am. Chem. Soc. **66**:1952–1954.
3. **Horesfall, J. G.** 1945. Fungicides and their action. *In* F. Verdoon (ed.), Annales cryptogamici et photopathologici, vol. 2. Chronica Bontanica Co., Waltham, Mass.
4. **Raghunandana, R. R., R. S. Srinivasa, and P. R. Venkatarman.** 1946. Investigations on plant antibiotics. I. Studies on allicin, the antibacterial principle of *Allium sativum* (garlic). J. Sci. Ind. Res. **1B**:31–35.
5. **Stanley, V. C., and M. P. English.** 1965. Some effects of nystatin on the growth of four *Aspergillus* species. J. Gen. Microbiol. **40**:107–118.

ANTIMICROBIAL AGENTS AND CHEMOTHERAPY, Apr. 1977, p. 750-752 Vol. 11, No. 4

NOTES

Evaluation of the Autobac 1 Susceptibility Testing System in a Clinical Diagnostic Laboratory

MIGUEL MOGYOROS, JOHN R. MORGAN, AND JOHN A. SMITH*

Divisions of Medical Microbiology and Medicine, and Department of Laboratories, University of Toronto, Mount Sinai Hospital, Toronto, Ontario, Canada M5G 1X5

Received for publication 31 August 1976

The Autobac 1 system was compared to the disk diffusion and agar dilution methods. Overall, there was good correlation; however, certain antibiotic/bacterial combinations gave unreliable results. In particular, unreliable results were obtained against staphylococci with penicillins, aerobic gram-negative rods with cephalothin, and enterococci with cephalothin and clindamycin.

The performance of Autobac 1 (Pfizer) was compared with the disk diffusion and agar dilution methods in a routine hospital microbiology laboratory.

Four hundred gram-negative and 300 gram-positive organisms were isolated from clinical specimens submitted to our laboratory. These were *Escherichia coli* (181), *Klebsiella* species (74), *Proteus* species (56), *Pseudomonas aeruginosa* (51), *Enterobacter* species (22), *Citrobacter* species (7), *Acinetobacter calcoaceticus* (3), *Salmonella* species (3), *Alcaligenes faecalis* (2), *Serratia marcescens* (1), *Staphylococcus aureus* (156), *Staphylococcus epidermidis* (53), *Enterococcus* (44), and beta-hemolytic streptococcus (37).

The materials and the methods used in this study were essentially those of a previously published collaborative study (4) with one important modification; i.e., in addition to the agar dilution breakpoints selected by Thornsberry et al. (4), we introduced alternative breakpoints for ampicillin, cephalothin, and kanamycin (see Table 2) based on data concerning obtainable drug concentrations in blood (1, 2, 3).

Autobac 1 and agar dilution–gram-negative bacteria. Agreement (Table 1) ranged between 57 and 98% with nine antibiotics tested against gram-negative organisms; there was over 90% agreement with five antibiotics. With each antibiotic, major and very major discrepancies were less than 5%. When the breakpoints of Thornsberry et al. (4) were applied to the agar dilution test, the agreement was only 57% with cephalothin, 74.75% with ampicillin, and 87.5% with kanamycin. However, when our breakpoints (Table 2) were applied, the agreements between results obtained with Autobac 1 and agar dilution technique changed to the following: cephalothin 79%, ampicillin 91.2%, and kanamycin 95.1% (Table 3). Thus, applying our breakpoints reduced the number of minor discrepancies without increasing the discrepancies in major and very major categories.

Autobac 1 and agar dilution–gram-positive bacteria. When the breakpoints of Thornsberry et al. (4) were used, many major discrepancies were seen (Table 3). This was particularly true of tests with penicillin G (16.66%) and ampicillin (11.66%). Thus, with respect to penicillin, 26 of 156 strains (16.6%) of *S. aureus* and 23 of 53 strains (43%) of *S. epidermidis* tested showed major discrepancies. Similarly, major discrepancies were seen with 17 of 156 (11%) strains of *S. aureus* and 15 of 53 (28%) strains of *S. epidermidis* tested with ampicillin. Minor discrepancies were common (14.66%) in the tests of cephalothin against the gram-positive group of

TABLE 1. *Comparison of agar dilution and Autobac 1 methods with 400 gram-negative bacteria*

Antibiotics	Discrepancies (%) Minor	Major	Very major	Agreement (%)
Ampicillin	21	4	0.25	74.75
Cephalothin	42.5	0	0.5	57
Kanamycin	10.75	0.25	1.5	87.5
Chloramphenicol	2.5	3.5	0.5	93.5
Tetracycline	0.75	0.25	4.25	92.75
Gentamicin	0.75	0.25	1	98
Nalidixic acid[a]	1.3	0	2.6	96.1
Colistin	3.75	0.25	4	92
Carbenicillin	7	1	3.5	88.5

[a] One-hundred and fifty strains tested.

TABLE 2. *Comparison of agar dilution and Autobac 1 against 400 gram-negative bacteria with ampicillin, cephalothin, and kanamycin and 300 gram-positive bacteria with cephalothin*

Bacterial group	Antibiotics	Discrepancies (%)[a]						Agreement (%)[a]	
		Minor		Major		Very major			
		(A)	(B)	(A)	(B)	(A)	(B)	(A)	(B)
Gram-negative group	Ampicillin	21	3	4	4.7	0.2	2	74.75	91.2
	Cephalothin	42.5	20	0	0.5	0.5	0.5	57	79
	Kanamycin	10.7	1.5	0.2	2.2	1.5	1.2	87.5	95.1
Gram-positive group	Cephalothin								
	All gram-positive organisms	14.6	1	0.3	0.3	0.3	6	85	93
	All gram-positive organisms except enterococci	3.1	0.4	0.4	0.4	0.4	3.1	96.1	96.1

[a] (A), Breakpoints of Thornsberry et al: ampicillin-susceptible ≤8, intermediate 16 and 32, resistant ≥64; cephalothin-susceptible ≤8, intermediate 16 and 32, resistant ≥64; kanamycin-susceptible ≤8, intermediate 16, resistant ≥32. (B), Our own breakpoints: ampicillin-susceptible ≤8 μg/ml, resistant ≥16 μg/ml; cephalothin-susceptible ≤16 μg/ml, resistant ≥32 μg/ml; kanamycin-susceptible ≤16 μg/ml, resistant ≥32 μg/ml.

TABLE 3. *Comparison of the agar dilution and Autobac 1 methods with 300 gram-positive bacteria*

Antibiotic	Discrepancies (%)			Agreement (%)
	Minor	Major	Very major	
Penicillin	0	16.66	0.66	82.68
Cephalothin				
All organisms	14.66	0.33	0.33	84.68
All organisms except enterococci	3.1	0.4	0.4	96.1
Ampicillin	2.33	11.66	0.66	85.35
Erythromycin	0	0.33	1.33	98.34
Tetracycline	1	0.33	2.33	96.34
Clindamycin				
All organisms	1.6	1	8	89.4
All organisms except enterococci	0.4	1.1	0.4	98.1
Methicillin	0.66	1	1.33	97.0
Chloramphenicol	0.66	0.66	0	98.68

bacteria. However, the use of our breakpoints (Table 2) dropped minor discrepancies to 1%, but very major discrepancies rose from 0.3 to 6%. Discrepancies were also reduced when the results of enterococci with cephalothin and clindamycin were excluded (Tables 2 and 3).

Autobac 1 and disk diffusion–gram-negative bacteria. There was an overall correlation that ranged from 86.25 to 99.34% (Table 4). Discrepancies were most commonly associated with cephalothin and ampicillin.

Autobac 1 and disk diffusion–gram-positive bacteria. Agreement among gram-positive organisms (Table 5) ranged from 83.1 to 97.67%. Correlations improved when tests of enterococci with penicillin G, cephalothin, and clindamycin were excluded. Five percent very major discrepancies were associated with ampicillin.

TABLE 4. *Comparison of the disk diffusion and Autobac 1 methods with 400 gram-negative bacteria*

Antibiotic	Discrepancies (%)			Agreement (%)
	Minor	Major	Very major	
Ampicillin	5.75	7.75	0.25	86.25
Cephalothin	8	1.5	1.25	89.75
Kanamycin	2.75	0.25	2.25	95
Chloramphenicol	5.5	1.5	0.25	92.75
Tetracycline	4	0	0.25	95.75
Gentamicin	0.25	1.25	1	97.5
Nalidixic acid[a]	0	0	0.66	99.34
Carbenicillin	3.25	1.25	0.75	94.75
Colistin	1.75	0	0.5	97.75

[a] One-hundred and fifty strains tested.

TABLE 5. *Comparison of disk diffusion and Autobac 1 methods with 300 gram-positive bacteria*

Antibiotics	Discrepancies (%)			Agreement (%)
	Minor	Major	Very major	
Penicillin				
All organisms	14.3	1	1.6	83.1
All organisms excluding enterococci	0.1	0.03	0.03	99.84
Cephalothin				
All organisms	4.3	0.66	2.6	92.44
All organisms excluding enterococci	0.8	0.8	0.8	97.6
Ampicillin	1.6	1.6	5	91.8
Erythromycin	2	0.66	3	94.34
Tetracycline	0.66	2.6	1.6	95.14
Clindamycin				
All organisms	1	0.66	10	88.34
All organisms excluding enterococci	0.4	0.8	1.5	97.3
Chloramphenicol	1	0.33	1	97.67

There was broad general agreement between our results and those of Thornsberry et al. (4). Our correlations between Autobac 1 and agar dilution were similar to theirs in tests with ampicillin and kanamycin against gram-negative bacteria, but the correlations were improved by applying our breakpoints, which further obviated the need to exclude pseudomonas/kanamycin results. We could not confirm the finding of Thornsberry et al. (4) with respect to cephalothin, which in our hands correlated poorly regardless of the breakpoint values used.

We experienced problems with enterococci, as did Thornsberry et al. (4), not only in tests with cephalothin but also with penicillin and clindamycin. We confirmed Thornsberry's observations on tests with penicillin against *S. epidermidis*, but we found a similar problem with penicillin against *S. aureus* and also with ampicillin against both species.

Our assessment indicated that Autobac 1 was reliable for tests of most gram-negative bacteria. We found it technically less exacting than other methods, but the need to retain an alternative system for testing strains of *Haemophilus, Neisseria,* and *Staphylococcus* was inconvenient.

ACKNOWLEDGMENTS

We would like to acknowledge the technical staff whose contribution made this study possible and also Pfizer Diagnostics, Canada.

LITERATURE CITED

1. **Dolvisio, J. T., J. C. LaPiana, and L. W. Dittert.** 1971. Pharmacokinetics of ampicillin trihydrate, sodium ampicillin and sodium dicloxacillin following intramuscular injection. J. Pharm. Sci. 60:715–719.
2. **Kunin, C. M.** 1966. Absorption, distribution, excretion and fate of kanamycin. Ann. N.Y. Acad. Sci. 132:811–818.
3. **Nightingale, C. H., D. S. Green, and R. Quintiliani.** 1975. Pharmacokinetics and clinical use of cephalosporin antibiotics. J. Pharm. Sci. 64:1899–1927.
4. **Thornsberry, C., T. L. Gavan, J. C. Sherris, A. Ballows, J. M. Matsen, L. D. Sabath, F. Schoenknecht, L. D. Thrupp, and J. A. Washington II.** 1975. Laboratory evaluation of a rapid, automated susceptibility testing system: report of a collaborative study. Antimicrob. Agents Chemother. 7:466–480.

ANTIMICROBIAL AGENTS AND CHEMOTHERAPY, Apr. 1977, p. 753-755 Vol. 11, No. 4

Mutagenicity and Antibacterial Activity of Hydroxamic Acids

CHING YUNG WANG* AND LANFONG H. LEE

Division of Clinical Oncology, Department of Human Oncology, University of Wisconsin Center for Health Sciences, Madison, Wisconsin 53706

Received for publication 16 November 1976

Hydroxamic acids demonstrated mutagenic and antibacterial activities. These activities appear to be dependent on the hydroxamic acid function and are probably due to the interaction with deoxyribonucleic acid.

Hydroxamic acids have been shown to be effective antifungal and antibacterial agents. Sorbic hydroxamic acid (2) and decanoylhydroxamic acid (3) demonstrated antifungal activities. Salicylhydroxamic acid had in vitro and in vivo antitubercular activity (8). Hase et al. (5) synthesized a series of alkyloxybenzoylhydroxamic acids and fatty acyl hydroxamic acids and found that some of these chemicals possessed antifungal activity. However, none of them was effective against enteric bacteria. Acetohydroxamic acid was an inhibitor of bacterial urease. It also inhibited ammonia and stone formation in the urinary tract during infections (4). The present study investigated the mutagenic and antibacterial activity of several hydroxamic acids with differing acyl groups.

The Ames spot test for chemical mutagenicity (1) was used for the present study. Fifty microliters of sterile dimethyl sulfoxide containing 1 mg of the tested chemical was spotted on the center surface of an agar plate containing *Salmonella typhimurium* strains TA100 or TA98 (7). The control plates were treated with the solvent only. After incubation at 37°C for 2 days, the revertant colonies that appeared were counted, and the clear inhibition zone produced by antibacterial activity was measured. Chemicals inducing more than twice the number of revertants found in the control plate were considered as mutagenic.

In the antibacterial tests, various strains of bacteria (Table 1) were grown in Difco nutrient broth for 6 h at 37°C. The culture was then diluted 100 times with fresh nutrient broth. One-half milliliter of dimethyl sulfoxide containing various amounts of test compounds was added to 4.5 ml of the diluted culture. After incubation at 37°C for 24 h, the minimal concentration for complete growth inhibition was recorded. The concentrations of hydroxamic acids in the medium were 1000, 500, 100, 50, 10, and 1 μg/ml. Minimal inhibitory concentrations of 10 μg/ml or less were considered as "effective," 50 to 100 μg/ml as "slightly effective," and 100 μg/ml or greater as "ineffective."

The results of mutation and antibacterial tests were presented in Table 1. All the hydroxamic acids tested except *p*-butoxyphenylacetohydroxamic acid produced clear antibacterial zones and mutations in both *S. typhimurium* strains TA100 and TA98. It appears that these mutagenic hydroxamic acids may interact with bacterial deoxyribonucleic acid. 2-Naphthoylhydroxamic acid was "effective" against *Streptococcus faecalis* and *Escherichia coli* and was "slightly effective" against *Bacillus cereus* and *Proteus morganii*. Benzoylhydroxamic acid, salicylhydroxamic acid, and indole-2-carbohydroxamic acid were "slightly effective" against some bacterial strains. *p*-Butoxyphenylacetohydroxamic acid lacked mutagenicity for *S. typhimurium* and was virtually ineffective against the tested bacteria.

Thus, hydroxamic acid function appears to be essential for the mutagenic and antibacterial activities of hydroxamic acids, whereas the acyl moiety appears to determine their potency. Although hydroxamic acids have been shown to be effective inhibitors of bacterial and plant urease (6), their antibacterial activity probably is not due to urease inhibition (5). It seems likely that the antibacterial activity is due to their interaction with bacterial deoxyribonucleic acid since hydroxamic acids were shown to have mutagenic and antibacterial effects in this study.

TABLE 1. *Antibacterial and mutagenic activity of hydroxamic acids*

Hydroxamic acid	Structure	Mutagenicity[a]	Minimal inhibitory concentration (μg/ml)							
			I[b]	II	III	IV	V	VI	VII	VIII
Benzoylhydroxamic acid	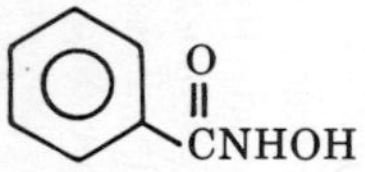	+	1,000	1,000	NA[c]	500	NA	1,000	100	100
Salicylhydroxamic acid	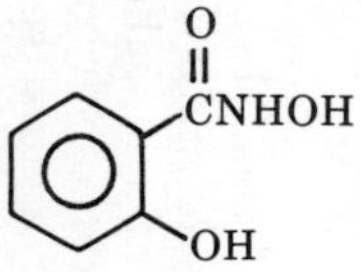	+	500	1,000	1,000	500	NA	NA	500	50
Benzoylaminoacetohydroxamic acid	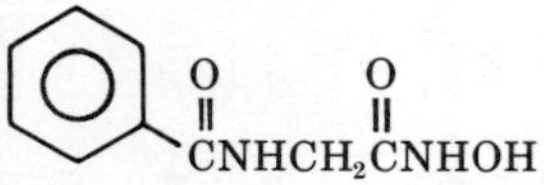	+	NA	NA	NA	NA	NA	NA	1,000	10
p-Butoxyphenylacetohydroxamic acid	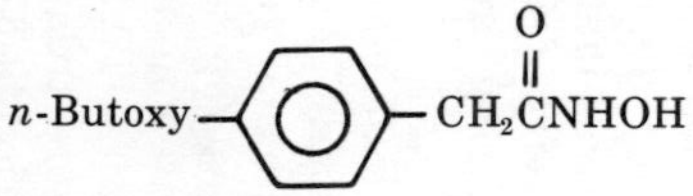	−	NA	NA	NA	NA	NA	NA	NA	500
Indole-2-carbohydroxamic acid	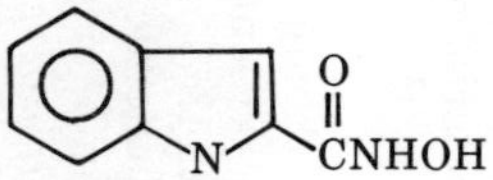	+	50	500	500	500	1,000	500	500	50
2-Naphthoylhydroxamic acid	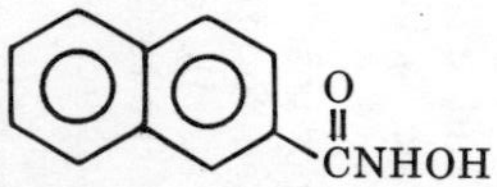	+	100	500	500	100	NA	500	10	10

[a] +, Mutagenic for *S. typhimurium* TA98 and TA100; −, not mutagenic.
[b] I, *Bacillus cereus*; II, *Corynebacterium xerosis*; III, *Klebsiella pneumoniae*; IV, *Proteus morganii*; V, *Pseudomonas aeruginosa*; VI, *Staphylococcus aureus*; VII, *Streptococcus faecalis*; VIII, *Escherichia coli*.
[c] NA, Not active at a dose of 500 μg/ml for *p*-butoxyphenylacetohydroxamic acid or 1,000 μg/ml for the other compounds. *p*-Butoxyphenylacetohydroxamic acid was not soluble at 1 mg/ml in the medium.

This investigation was supported by Public Health Service research grant CA 17449 from the National Cancer Institute.

We thank F. Baier for the assistance in the preparation of this manuscript.

LITERATURE CITED

1. **Ames, B. N.** 1971. The detection of chemical mutagens with enteric bacteria, p. 267–282. *In* A. Hollaender (ed.), Chemical mutagens: principles and methods for their detection, vol. 1. Plenum Press, New York.
2. **Dudman, W. F.** 1963. Sorbic hydroxamic acid, an antifungal agent effective over a wide pH range. Appl. Microbiol. **11**:362–364.
3. **Gale, G. R., F. Bernheim, and A. M. Welch.** 1962. Antifungal activity of decanoic hydroxamic acid. Proc. Soc. Exp. Biol. Med. **109**:188–192.
4. **Griffith, D. P., and D. M. Musher.** 1973. Prevention of infected urinary stones by urease inhibition. Invest. Urol. **11**:228–233.
5. **Hase, J., K. Kobashi, N. Kawaguchi, and K. Sakamoto.** 1971. Antimicrobial activity of hydroxamic acids. Chem. Pharm. Bull. **19**:363–368.
6. **Kobashi, K., K. Kumaki, and J. Hase.** 1971. Effect of acyl residues of hydroxamic acids on urease inhibition. Biochim. Biophys. Acta **227**:429–441.
7. **McCann, J., N. E. Singarn, J. Kobori, and B. N. Ames.** 1975. Detection of carcinogens as mutagens: bacterial tester strains with R factor plasmids. Proc. Natl. Acad. Sci. U.S.A. **72**:979–983.
8. **Urbanski, T.** 1950. Salicylhydroxamic acid as an antitubercular agent. Nature (London) **166**:267–268.

ANTIMICROBIAL AGENTS AND CHEMOTHERAPY, Apr. 1977, p. 756-759
Vol. 11, No. 4

Effects of Ionenes on Interferon Induction by Poly(Inosinic Acid)·Poly(Cytidylic Acid)

ERIK DE CLERCQ, BOREK JANIK,* AND RONALD G. SOMMER

*Rega Institute for Medical Research, University of Leuven, B-3000 Leuven, Belgium; and Miles Laboratories, Inc., Elkart, Indiana 46514**

Received for publication 26 November 1976

Depending on the spacing of their positive charges, ionenes, a class of quaternary ammonium polymers, increased the interferon-inducing activity of poly(inosinic acid)·poly(cytidylic acid) in mouse L-929 cells, whereas they did not enhance poly(inosinic acid)·poly(cytidylic acid) induced interferon production in primary rabbit kidney and human skin fibrolast cells.

Many polyamines have been shown to enhance the formation of interferon and resistance to viral infections induced by poly(inosinic acid)·poly(cytidylic acid) [$(I)_n \cdot (C)_n$] in a variety of cell systems (4, 9, 27). Diethylaminoethyl (DEAE)-dextran, the most widely studied polyamine, was found effective in a variety of cells such as chicken embryo (3, 13, 15), mouse L-(1, 5-7, 17), primary rabbit kidney (PRK) (29), human leukocytes (8), and human skin fibroblasts (HSF) (22, 26). However, attempts to potentiate the $(I)_n \cdot (C)_n$-induced interferon response by DEAE-dextran and other polyamines did not prove successful in all cell systems (9, 16).

Ionenes, quaternary polyamines of the general formula $[N(CH_3)_2\text{-}(CH_2)_x\text{-}N(CH_3)_2\text{-}(CH_2)_y]_z^{2+}\ Br^-_{2z}$ (2), were found to exert biological activity in a number of systems (23). Polyamines structurally similar to ionenes can enhance antitumor activity of (11) and interferon induction by double-stranded mycophage ribonucleic acid (RNA). (The numbers in ionene names refer to the x and y multiples of the methylene group repeating unit. The values of intrinsic viscosity, $[\eta]$, in 0.4 M KBr for 3,3-, 6,6-, and 6,10-ionene were 0.115, 0.298, and 0.335, respectively. The correlation of $[\eta]$ with molecular weight (M) (2) gives a molecular weight $M = 4.2 \times 10^4$ for 6,6-ionene. Values of molecular weight for 3,3- and 6,10-ionene can only be estimated due to unavailability of correlation parameters (2) as being of the same order but lower than that for 6,6-ionene.) We now report enhancement of the $(I)_n \cdot (C)_n$-induced interferon response in L-cells treated with ionenes.

The ionenes tested for their effects on interferon induction included 3,3-ionene, 6,6-ionene, and 6,10-ionene (M. R. Harnden, A. G. Brown, T. J. Sharpe, and R. A. Vere-Hodge, Am. Chem. Soc., 166th Meet., Chicago, Ill., Abstr. no. MEDI 48, 1973).

Treatment of L-929 cells (Table 1) with 10 μg of 6,10-ionene per ml for 1 h before their exposure to $(I)_n \cdot (C)_n$ markedly increased ($P < 0.01$) the production of interferon. At the same concentration, neither 3,3-ionene, 6,6-ionene, nor DEAE-dextran showed any significance ($P <$ 0.05) stimulatory effect. At 100 μg/ml, however, DEAE-dextran showed any significant ($P <$ tion ($P < 0.01$) while 6,10-ionene was cytotoxic. None of the compounds tested were stimulatory at 1 μg/ml.

When a treatment regimen similar to that used in L-929 cells (Table 1) was applied to primary rabbit kidney (PRK) or human skin fibroblast (HSF) cells, neither ionenes nor DEAE-dextran caused an increased interferon response. In fact, such treatment with ionenes or DEAE-dextran for 1 h before the addition of $(I)_n \cdot (C)_n$ tended to decrease the subsequent production of interferon at both 10-μg/ml and 100-μg/ml concentrations of the individual components (data not shown).

Other treatment regimens were then installed in attempts to increase the interferon production in PRK and HSF cells. The ionenes or DEAE-dextran were directly mixed with $(I)_n \cdot (C)_n$ at a 1:1 (wt/wt) ratio, and after the cells had been incubated with these mixtures, cycloheximide and actinomycin D were added (10, 28) to further stimulate interferon production ("superinduction") (Table 2). In PRK cells, the only significant difference observed ($0.01 < P < 0.05$) was between the treatments with 6,6-ionene and 6,10-ionene, whereby the former slightly decreased and the latter slightly increased interferon production. In HSF cells, the 3,3- and 6,6-ionenes depressed ($0.01 < P < 0.05$) interferon production, whereas neither 6,10-io-

TABLE 1. *Effect of ionenes on interferon-inducing capacity of $(I)_n \cdot (C)_n$ in mouse L-929 cells*

Polycation	Interferon yield (U/ml)[a, b]						
	1[c]	10				100	
3,3-Ionene	6	3	3	3	9	19	20
6,6-Ionene	10	10	10	3	4	10	6
6,10-Ionene	16	150		186	1,700	T[d]	T[d]
DEAE-dextran	20	45	16	10	6	2,500	500
Control[e]	20	20	20	3	3	20	20

[a] Confluent L-929 cell monolayers were treated with the ionenes or DEAE-dextran (Pharmacia), diluted in serum-free minimal essential medium (MEM) to the indicated concentrations, for 1 h at 37°C, then washed (3×) with MEM and exposed to $(I)_n \cdot (C)_n$ (P-L Biochemicals) at 10 μg/ml in MEM for 1 h at 37°C. The cells were washed again (3×) with MEM and further incubated with MEM containing 3% calf serum for 24 h at 37°C. The supernatant fluids were then collected and titrated for interferon by a vesicular stomatitis virus plaque inhibition assay in L-929 cells. The data represent individual interferon titer readings from different replicate experiments.

[b] The $\log_{10}$ values of interferon yields were subjected to studentized range statistics to determine whether or not the individual treatments with polycations differ significantly from each other or from the control with respect to interferon yields. The statistical significance is noted in the text.

[c] Polycation concentration (micrograms per milliliter).

[d] T, At 100 μg/ml, 6,10-ionene was toxic for the cells.

[e] The control experiments were carried out as shown in *a* except in the absence of polycation.

TABLE 2. *Effect of ionenes on interferon-inducing capacity of $(I)_n \cdot (C)_n$ in primary rabbit kidney (PRK) and human skin fibroblast cells (HSF)*

Polycation	Interferon yield (U/ml)[a, b]								
	PRK						HSF		
3,3-Ionene	3,000	1,500	3,000	6,000	6,000	1,000	20	50	100
6,6-Ionene	1,000	1,000	1,000	2,000	1,000	2,000	20	60	200
6,10-Ionene	3,000	1,500	15,000	10,000	6,000	10,000	100	150	500
DEAE-dextran		1,000	6,000	3,000	1,000	10,000	200	600	4,000
Control[c]	3,000	1,500	3,000	1,000	1,000	10,000	300	600	5,000

[a] Ionenes or DEAE-dextran and $(I)_n \cdot (C)_n$ were mixed in serum-free minimal essential medium (MEM) to yield a final concentration of 10 μg/ml for each component. The mixtures were first incubated for 1 h at 37°C and then applied onto the cells for another 1 h at 37°C. The cells were washed (3×) with MEM and further processed according to a "superinduction" schedule, i.e., PRK cells were treated consecutively with cycloheximide (2 μg/ml) for 3 h and actinomycin D (3 μg/ml) for 0.5 h; HSF cells were treated with cycloheximide (10 μg/ml) for 6 h, and actinomycin D (1 μg/ml) was added for the last 2 h of this 6-h incubation period. After removal of the metabolic inhibitors, PRK and HSF cells were washed (3×) with MEM and further incubated with MEM containing 3% calf serum for 24 h at 37°C. The supernatant fluids were then collected and titrated for interferon by a vesicular stomatitis virus cytopathogenicity inhibition assay in PRK cells (rabbit interferon) or HSF cells (human interferon). The data represent individual interferon titer readings from replicate experiments.

[b] See footnote *b* in Table 1.

[c] See footnote *e* in Table 1.

nene nor DEAE-dextran affected it. Interferon induction was also monitored in HSF cells which had been "primed" with interferon (10) or exposed to ultraviolet irradiation (19) and in HSF cells which had been primed and "superinduced." In none of these systems, however, did mixtures of ionenes (or DEAE-dextran) with $(I)_n \cdot (C)_n$ (each component at 10 μg/ml) prove more efficacious in eliciting interferon production than $(I)_n \cdot (C)_n$ alone (data not shown).

The results presented herein establish that polycations such as 6,10-ionene and DEAE-dextran, while potentiating the induction of interferon by $(I)_n \cdot (C)_n$ in some cell cultures, fail to do so in others. They further indicate that the spacing or density of the positive charges in the ionene is of critical importance, since only 6,10-ionene and not 3,3- and 6,6-ionenes proved effective in enhancing the interferon induction by $(I)_n \cdot (C)_n$ in L-cells. Quarternary polyamines readily complex with double-stranded RNA (11). The efficacy of ionenes to enhance interferon induction seems to be related to their avidity to complex. We observed (data not shown) that 6,10-ionene precipitates various polynucleotides at concentrations severalfold lower than do 3,3- or 6,6-ionene.

Although the exact mechanism by which DEAE-dextran or other polyamines potentiate interferon production has not been elucidated, DEAE-dextran is assumed to act by promoting the interaction of $(I)_n \cdot (C)_n$ with its putative receptor site (13, 22). DEAE-dextran greatly enhances the rate of uptake of $(I)_n \cdot (C)_n$ by the cells (1, 3). Ionenes, too, exhibit uptake-stimulating properties, whereby 6,10-ionene is by far more effective than 6,6- and 3,3-ionenes (12). In neither case, however, has it been determined with certainty whether this uptake represents penetration of the polynucleotide across the cell membrane or only a cell surface adsorption. DEAE-dextran and quarternary polyamines also protect various polynucleotides against hydrolysis by endonucleases (7, 11, 12, 22), which can be present in the serum (14, 20, 25) and/or associated with the cells (24). In general, the stimulatory effects of polycations seem to be exerted through neutralization of the negative cell surface charges and consequent destabilization of the cell membrane (18, 21) and through interaction with polynucleotides which may result in reduction of their repulsion from the cell surface (17), stabilization of their conformation, and protection against enzymatic degradation (11, 17, 21). Why a polycation cannot enhance $(I)_n \cdot (C)_n$ induced interferon production in every cell line and why the induction can be enhanced by one polycation and not by its homologue remains to be answered. It appears that more delicate complementarity requirements have to be met than simply the presence of negative charges on the cell surface or polynucleotide inducer and positive charges on the polycation. Our findings warn against generalizations based on the results obtained in one particular cell system regarding the effects of polycations on the interferon-inducing activity of double-stranded RNAs and the mechanism(s) involved.

ACKNOWLEDGMENTS

This work was supported by grants from the Belgian Fonds voor Geneeskundig Wetenschappelijk Onderzoek and the Katholieke Universiteit te Leuven (Fonds Derde Cyclus). The skilled technical assistance of Anita Van Lierde is gratefully acknowledged. We wish to thank A. Rembaum for a generous gift of ionenes.

LITERATURE CITED

1. **Bausek, G. H., and T. C. Merigan.** 1969. Cell interaction with a synthetic polynucleotide and interferon production *in vitro*. Virology 39:491–498.
2. **Casson, D., and A. Rembaum.** 1972. Solution properties of novel polyelectrolytes. Macromolecules 5:75–81.
3. **Colby, C., and M. J. Chamberlin.** 1969. The specificity of interferon induction in chick embryo cells by helical RNA. Proc. Natl. Acad. Sci. U.S.A. **63:**160–167.
4. **De Clercq, E.** 1974. Synthetic interferon inducers. Top. Curr. Chem. **52:**173–208.
5. **De Clercq, E., and P. De Somer.** 1975. Are cytotoxicity and interferon inducing activity of poly(I)·poly(C) invariably linked in interferon-treated L cells? J. Gen. Virol. **27:**35–44.
6. **Dianzani, F., P. Cantagalli, S. Gagnoni, and G. Rita.** 1968. Effect of DEAE-dextran on production of interferon induced by synthetic double-stranded RNA in L cell cultures. Proc. Soc. Exp. Biol. Med. **128:**708–710.
7. **Dianzani, F., S. Baron, C. E. Buckler, and H. B. Levy.** 1971. Mechanisms of DEAE-dextran enhancement of polynucleotide induction of interferon. Proc. Soc. Exp. Biol. Med. **136:**1111–1114.
8. **Falcoff, E., and R. Perez-Bercoff.** 1969. Intérferons humains induits *in vitro* par des polynucléotides synthétiques. Biochim. Biophys. Acta **174:**108–116.
9. **Field, K. A.** 1973. Interferon induction by polynucleotides, p. 149–176. *In* W. A. Carter (ed.), Selective inhibitors of viral functions. CRC Press, Cleveland, Ohio.
10. **Havell, E. A., and J. Vilcek.** 1972. Production of high-titered interferon in cultures of human diploid cells. Antimicrob. Agents Chemother. 2:476–484.
11. **Heyes, J., E. J. Catherall, and M. R. Harnden.** 1974. Antitumor evaluation of a ribonuclease resistant double-stranded RNA-polyquaternary ammonium complex (BRL 10739). Eur. J. Cancer **10:**431–435.
12. **Janik, B., and R. G. Sommer** 1976. Effect of polyamines on the uptake of poly(2′-fluoro-2′-deoxyuridylic acid) by a mammalian cell line. J. Supramol. Struct. 4:475–480.
13. **Kalmakoff, J. and F. J. Austin.** 1973. Induction of viral interference: effects of poly rl·rC and diethylaminoethyl-dextran on the activity of the antiviral protein. Infect. Immun. 8:63–67.
14. **Kao, P. C., J. D. Regan, and E. Volkin.** 1973. Fate of homologous and heterologous DNAs after incorporation into human skin fibroblasts. Biochim. Biophys. Acta 324:1–13.
15. **Long, W. F., and D. C. Burke.** 1971. Interferon production by double-stranded RNA: a comparison of induction by reovirus to that by a synthetic double-stranded polynucleotide. J. Gen. Virol. 12:1–11.
16. **Machida, H., A. Kuninaka, and H. Yoshino.** 1975. Interferon production and resistance to viral infection induced by poly I·poly C in chick embryo cells. II. Lack of enhancement by DEAE-dextran. Jpn. J. Microbiol. 19:65–68.
17. **Maes, R., W. Sedwick, and A. Vaheri.** 1967. Interaction between DEAE-dextran and nucleic acid. Biochim. Biophys. Acta 134:269–276.
18. **Mayhew, E., J. P. Harlos, and R. L. Juliano.** 1973. The effect of polycations on cell membrane stability and transport processes. J. Membr. Biol. 14:213–228.
19. **Mozes, L. W., E. A. Havell, M. L. Gradoville, and J. Vilcek.** 1974. Increased interferon production in human cells irradiated with ultraviolet light. Infect. Immun. 10:1189–1191.
20. **Nordlund, J. J., S. M. Wolff, and H. B. Levy.** 1970. Inhibition of biologic activity of poly I:poly C by human plasma. Proc. Soc. Exp. Biol. Med. 133:439–444.
21. **Pagano, J. S.** 1970. Biological activity of isolated viral nucleic acids. Prog. Med. Virol. 12:1–48.
22. **Pitha, P. M., and W. A. Carter.** 1971. The DEAE dextran:polyriboinosinate-polyribocytidylate complex: physical properties and interferon induction. Virology 45:777–781.
23. **Rembaum, A.** 1973. Biological activity of ionene polymers. Appl. Polym. Symp. 22:299–317.

24. **Shugar, D., and H. Sierakowska.** 1967. Mammalian nucleolytic enzymes and their localization. Progr. Nucleic Acid Res. Mol. Biol. 7:369–429.
25. **Stern, R.** 1970. A nuclease from animal serum which hydrolyzes double-stranded RNA. Biochem. Biophys. Res. Commun. 41:608–614.
26. **Tilles, J. G.** 1970. Diethylaminoethyl-dextran enhancement of interferon induction by a complexed polyribonucleotide. Proc. Soc. Exp. Biol. Med. 133:1334–1341.
27. **Tytell, A. A., and A. K. Field.** 1972. Interferons and host resistance with particular emphasis on induction by complexed polynucleotides. CRC Crit. Rev. Biochem. 1:1–32.
28. **Vilcek, J., and M. H. Ng.** 1971. Post-transcriptional control of interferon synthesis. J. Virol. 7:588–594.
29. **Vilcek, J., S. L. Barmak, and E. A. Havell.** 1972. Control of interferon synthesis: effect of diethylaminoethyl-dextran on induction by polyinosinic-polycytidylic acid. J. Virol. 10:614–621.

Antimicrobial Agents and Chemotherapy, Apr. 1977, p. 760–762 Vol. 11, No. 4

Printed in U.S.A.

Distribution of Sodium Cefazolin in Serum, Muscle, Bone Marrow, and Bone of Normal Rabbits

D. H. PITKIN, C. SACHS, I. ZAJAC, and P. ACTOR*

Research and Development Division, Smith Kline & French Laboratories, Philadelphia, Pennsylvania 19101

Received for publication 28 October 1976

Cefazolin levels were detected in bone and bone marrow of normal rabbits dosed intramuscularly, even in the absence of detectable levels in serum.

Sodium cefazolin, chemically 3-{[(5-methyl-1,3,4-thiadiazol-2-yl)thio]methyl}-8-oxo-7-[2-(1H-tetrazol-1-yl)acetamido]-5-thio-1-azabicyclo[4.2.0]oct-2-ene-2-carboxylic acid sodium hydrate, has been shown to be effective in vitro and in vivo in both animal and human infections (1–3). Although cefazolin has been reported to be of use in patients with bone and joint infections (1), only limited information is available as to the ability of this antibiotic to penetrate into bone and bone marrow. Consequently, this study was undertaken to determine the cefazolin content of selected tissues, including bone and bone marrow.

Twelve healthy, male New Zealand white rabbits were dosed intramuscularly with 50 mg of sodium cefazolin, dissolved in parenteral water for injection, per kg of body weight. Three rabbits were used in each of four treatment groups. Groups 1 and 2 each received a single dose of cefazolin, whereas groups 3 and 4 each received six loading doses at 9 a.m. and 3 p.m. on days 1, 2, and 3 plus a final dose on day 4. Tissue samples were obtained 1 h after dosing groups 1 and 3 and 3 h after dosing groups 2 and 4. Blood samples were obtained from the central artery of the ear; subsequently, all rabbits were sacrificed with sodium pentobarbital given intracardially. After sacrifice, the fore- and hindlimbs, from the side opposite that used for dosing, were removed surgically, and the muscle tissue was completely removed from each limb. After defleshing, the long bones were cracked and all of the marrow was removed. All tissues were rinsed with water to minimize contamination with blood. Muscle (1.0 g) and marrow (0.1 g) samples were weighed, ground in a Ten-Broeck homogenizer containing about 10 mg of glass beads (100 μm), and extracted for 1 h with pH 6 buffer at 4°C. Bone (1.0 g) samples were weighed, equilibrated to −70°C, pulverized in a mortar and pestle at −20°C, and extracted overnight with pH 6 buffer at 4°C. All samples were stored at −20°C until assayed. The procedure used to prepare bone samples for assay is a modification of the procedure reported by Norden for cephalothin (4).

All samples were assayed by using a disk agar diffusion assay employing *Bacillus subtilis* ATCC 6633 as an internal indicator. Six adsorbent paper disks (Schleicher and Schuell No. 740E; 6.35 mm), containing either a test or reference solution, were alternately placed on each assay plate. Assays were incubated overnight (serum assays at 30°C and other tissues at 23°C) before determining the diameter of the inhibition zone. After correcting for reference variation, a dose-response line was constructed, using data from the four assay plates at each of the five sodium cefazolin concentrations. The resulting regression line was computed by using the method of least squares.

Separate experiments were carried out with cefazolin-spiked tissue extracts to determine the percent recovery of cefazolin as well as the background activity of the tissue extracts (Table 1). The average recovery of cefazolin from these tissue extracts ranged from 73 to 84%. Bone samples were found to be free from nonspecific background activity, whereas muscle and bone marrow showed activities of 0.14 and 0.35 μg/sample, respectively. All final tissue determinations were adjusted to account for average recovery and background activity.

The data obtained in dosed rabbits is presented in Table 2. All samples obtained 1 h after dosing contained higher concentrations of sodium cefazolin as compared with those obtained at 3 h. Tissue loading was not observed; i.e., groups 1 and 3 or 2 and 4 gave equivalent results. Significant concentrations of antibiotic were found in the bone marrow, even in the absence of detectable levels in serum. Sodium cefazolin was detected in all bone samples obtained 1 h after the last dosing and in half of those obtained 3 h after the last dose. On the average, the tibias contained 1% of the serum content of sodium cefazolin observed at 1 h after dosing normal rabbits.

There appears to be a trend toward higher levels of cefazolin in samples obtained from rabbit forelimb as compared with hindlimb samples. This could reflect a difference in blood supply. Specific tests were not carried out to determine the possible contamination of tissue samples with blood. However, cefazolin tissue levels were obtained in the absence of serum levels, and extreme care was taken in the collection and handling of the samples.

Two additional rabbits were dosed with 50 mg of cephalothin per kg of body weight, using the regimen previously described for group 3. The antibiotic content of the defleshed tibias devoid of marrow was 0.6 μg/g at 1 h after dosing in each rabbit. This concentration is comparable to that reported by Norden (4).

The results obtained show that sodium cefazolin penetrates into rabbit bone and can be readily detected in marrow, even in the absence of detectable levels in serum. This finding is in agreement with that presented by Kopta and Lesken (J. A. Kopta and P. Lesken, Abstr. Assoc. Bone Joint Surgeons, 1975), who showed that antibiotic levels in bone remain high in rabbits with experimental osteomyelitis, even after serum levels have decreased. Since osteomyetilis may involve both marrow cavity and cortical bone, these results support the use of cefazolin in the treatment of bone infections. Limited data in humans obtained in eight patients with osteomyelitis show significant cancellus bone concentrations over an 8-h period after a 1-g dose of cefazolin (2). The levels obtained in our study with normal rabbit bone were lower and may not reflect the possible enhanced ability of cefazolin to penetrate into infected tissues.

Parsons, who recently reviewed the subject of antibiotics in bone, concludes that cefazolin seems to be the antibiotic of choice for prophylactic use in subjects undergoing total hip replacement (5). He has obtained cefazolin bone concentrations well above the minimal bactericidal concentration for *Staphylococcus aureus* and those gram-negative organisms causing postoperative prosthetic infections.

TABLE 1. *Recovery of cefazolin from tissue extracts to which known amounts of cefazolin were added*

Tissue	Sample wt (g)	No. of samples	Avg recovery (%)	Background activity (μg)[a]
Bone	1.0	4	84 (74–95)[b]	0
Bone marrow	0.1	4	73 (58–79)	0.35
Muscle	1.0	4	79 (57–100)	0.14

[a] Average of four bone samples, six marrow samples, and seven muscle samples.

[b] Numbers in parentheses indicate ranges.

TABLE 2. *Concentration of sodium cefazolin in selected rabbit tissues after single or multiple intramuscular dosing with 50 mg/kg*

Group	Rabbit	No. of doses	Time (h) of sacrifice after last dose	Serum (μg/ml)	Tissue concn (μg/ml): Muscle		Marrow		Bone	
					Fore	Hind	Fore	Hind	Fore	Hind
1	1	1	1	64.2	1.6	0.3	12.9	4.2	0.8	0.5
	2	1	1	82.6	6.8	0.7	33.2	13.4	1.1	0.5
	3	1	1	58.8	1.1	0.8	6.0	4.5	0.8	0.6
Avg				68.5	3.2	0.6	17.4	7.4	0.9	0.5
2	4	1	3	0	0	0	0.8	3.4	0	0.4
	5	1	3	0	0	0	1.2	2.7	0	0.2
	6	1	3	2.3	0	0	0.8	1.6	0	0.5
Avg				0.7	0	0	0.9	2.6	0	0.4
3	7	7	1	74.4	2.0	4.4	17.6	7.6	0.8	0.4
	8	7	1	65.4	0.6	0.5	17.0	8.6	0.6	0.4
	9	7	1	24.6	Trace	Trace	2.8	1.6	0.4	0.6
Avg				54.8	0.9	1.6	12.5	5.9	0.6	0.5
4	10	7	3	Trace	0	0	2.7	0.8	0	0
	11	7	3	Trace	0	0	4.0	1.6	0	0
	12	7	3	1.7	0	0	2.0	1.7	0	0
Avg				0.6	0	0	2.9	1.3	0	0

ACKNOWLEDGMENTS

We thank Joan David for her excellent technical assistance.

LITERATURE CITED

1. **Gold, J. A., J. J. McKee, and D. S. Ziv.** 1973. Experience with cefazolin: an overall summary of pharmacologic and clinical trials in man. J. Infect. Dis. 128-(Suppl.):S415–S421.
2. **Gould, S., P. Actor, J. J. McKee, and D. S. Ziv.** 1975. Cefazolin sodium: developmental review and update. Clin. Med. 82:23–28.
3. **Nishida, M., T. Matsubara, T. Murakawa, Y. Mine, Y. Yokota, S. Kuwahara, and S. Goto.** 1970. In vitro and in vivo evaluation of cefazolin, a new cephalosporin C derivative, p. 236–243. Antimicrob. Agents Chemother. 1969.
4. **Norden, C. W.** 1971. Experimental osteomyelitis. II. Therapeutic trials and measurement of antibiotic levels in bone. J. Infect. Dis. 124:565–571.
5. **Parsons, R. L.** 1976. Antibiotics in bone. Br. J. Antimicrob. Chemother. 2:228–231.

ANTIMICROBIAL AGENTS AND CHEMOTHERAPY, Apr. 1977, p. 763-764 Vol. 11, No. 4

Printed in U.S.A.

Mycobacterium chelonei Infection: Successful Treatment Based on a Radiometric Susceptibility Test

JULIO ARROYO AND GERALD MEDOFF*

Division of Infectious Diseases, Department of Medicine, Washington University School of Medicine, St. Louis, Missouri 63110

Received for publication 28 October 1976

A patient with *Mycobacterium chelonei* infection was treated with erythromycin stearate and streptomycin. The choice of antibiotics was based on a rapid radiometric susceptibility test developed in our laboratory.

The methods employed by most laboratories for antibiotic susceptibility testing of mycobacteria require 3 to 6 weeks for completion (2).

We described previously a method for measuring mycobacterial drug susceptibility that requires only 8 to 48 h for completion (1). The purpose of this communication is to describe a patient with *Mycobacterium chelonei* infection whose successful therapy was based on susceptibility tests done with this radiometric method.

Case report. Five months prior to admission to Barnes Hospital a 43-year-old woman with severe rheumatoid arthritis developed subcutaneous nodules on her left leg that were pruritic, erythematous, and slightly tender. Griseofulvin was given but had no effect on the lesions, which became more numerous and spread to the right leg. A biopsy of the affected skin showed caseating granulomas with acid-fast bacilli. Cultures grew mycobacteria after 1 week of incubation, which were identified as *M. chelonei* by the Barnes Hospital Bacteriology Laboratory and confirmed by the Center for Disease Control, Atlanta, Ga. The patient had no history of exposure to tuberculosis and denied receiving any trauma or parenteral injections in the involved areas. She was receiving 40 mg of triamcinolone diacetate per day for her rheumatoid arthritis and 300 mg of phentoin sodium per day for a seizure disorder, and this medication was continued.

Physical examination at the time of her admission to Barnes Hospital showed cushingoid features and musculoskeletal abnormalities consistent with the diagnosis of rheumatoid arthritis. She had several erythematous, slightly tender nodules, 1 to 1.5 cm in diameter, on both legs.

After a 1-week course of isoniazid, rifampin, and ethambutol, the patient was switched to streptomycin (1 g intramuscularly three times per week) and erythromycin stearate (3 g orally per day) on the basis of our susceptibility tests. Rifampin could not be used because of drug intolerance. Gradual improvement and eventual healing of the patient's lesions occurred over the subsequent 3 months. Streptomycin was discontinued after 3 months of therapy, and the patient remains on oral erythromycin. She has had no recurrence of her disease 6 months after discharge from the hospital.

Antibiotic susceptibility testing. The organism was maintained on Lowenstein-Jensen medium at 37°C in 5% CO_2 and subcultured every 7 days. Antibiotic susceptibility studies were performed using the radiometric method we have described (1) and the traditional indirect agar dilution method described by Canetti et al. (2) and modified by the National Center for Disease Control.

Figure 1 shows the effects of several antibiotics on the incorporation of [^{3}H]uracil into mycobacterial ribonucleic acid (RNA). Up to 20 μg of isoniazid and ethambutol per ml had little effect on RNA synthesis, whereas streptomycin, erythromycin, and rifampin effectively inhibited RNA synthesis. Amikacin, gentamicin, and kanamycin susceptibility curves were similar to streptomycin, and these data are not shown. In addition, Trimethoprim-Sulfa, penicillin, methicillin, and cephalothin were completely ineffective against this strain.

If we accept our previous criterion for antibiotic susceptibility of greater than a 50% inhibition of RNA synthesis, then the minimum inhibitory concentrations of these antibiotics are: 6 μg/ml for streptomycin, 2 μg/ml for erythromycin, and 1 μg/ml for rifampin. We also tested several drug combinations by our radiometric method, and the combination of erythromycin and streptomycin appeared to be the most active and better than either drug alone (Table 1). At 1 μg of erythromycin or

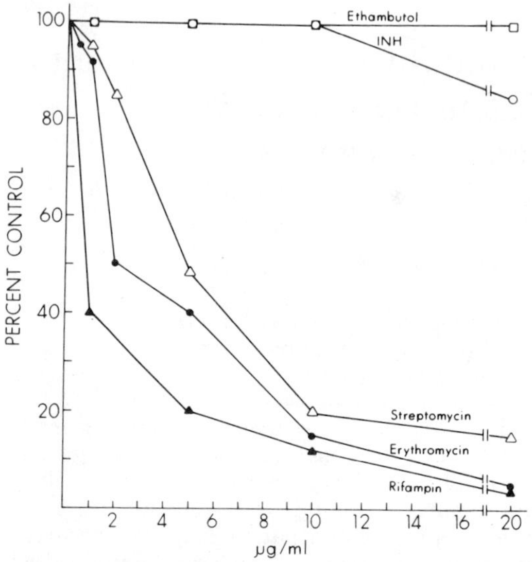

FIG. 1. *Percentage of control [^{3}H]uracil incorporation into RNA with increasing concentrations of drugs. Control was 52,784 cpm/ml.*

TABLE 1. *Effects of erythromycin and streptomycin combinations in [^{3}H]uracil incorporation into RNA of M. chelonei*[a]

Erythromycin (µg/ml)	[^{3}H]uracil incorporation (%) with streptomycin (µg/ml)		
	0	0.1	1.0
0	100	97	92
0.1	100	90	41
1.0	90	50	18

[a] Expressed as percentage of control cultures.

streptomycin per ml, the incorporation of ^{3}H was 90 and 92% for each drug, respectively. However, when 1 µg of each drug was combined, the uptake decreased to 18%.

The results obtained with the agar dilution method after 5 days of incubation showed that the organism was completely resistant to all of the antibiotics tested except streptomycin. Dosages of 2 and 10 µg of streptomycin per ml completely inhibited colony formation at 5 days, but, after 10 days of incubation, the plates had 5 to 10% of control colony counts.

Our patinet fulfilled all the clinical, pathological, and microbiological characteristics of *M. chelonei* soft tissue infection. Since we could find no previous experience with the natural course of this infection in compromised hosts, and since our patient had alarming spread of her lesions on both legs, we decided to treat her.

We chose to treat her with erythromycin and streptomycin on the basis of the radiometric susceptibility tests despite the disagreement with the traditional method of susceptibility testing. Rifampin could not be used because of drug intolerance. Although we cannot prove it, the rapidity of reversal of the progression of her abscess and the complete resolution of her skin lesions within 3 months strongly suggest to us that she responded to these antiobiotics; this is an encouraging indication of the potential value of the radiometric susceptibility test.

This work was supported by Public Health Service fellowship AI-00199 to Julio Arroyo, Training Grant AI-00459, and Grant AI-10622, from the National Institute of Allergy and Infectious Diseases, and by a grant from the John A. Hartford Foundation, Inc.

LITERATURE CITED

1. **Benitez, P., G. Medoff, and G. S. Kobayashi.** 1974. Rapid radiometric method of testing susceptibility of mycobacteria and slow-growing fungi to antimicrobial agents. Antimicrob. Agents Chemother. 6:29–33.
2. **Canetti, G., S. Froman, J. Grosset, P. Hauduroy, N. Langerova, H. T. Mahler, G. Meissner, D. A. Mitchison, and L. Sula.** 1963. Mycobacteria: laboratory methods for testing drug sensitivity and resistance. Bull. W.H.O. 29:565–578.

Antimicrobial Agents and Chemotherapy, Apr. 1977, p. 765-767 Vol. 11, No. 4

Efficacy of 5,6-Dihydro-5-Azathymidine Against Cutaneous Herpes Simplex Virus in Hairless Mice

GERALD E. UNDERWOOD and SHELDON D. WEED*

Experimental Biology, The Upjohn Company, Kalamazoo, Michigan 49001

Received for publication 9 November 1976

5,6-Dihydro-5-azathymidine, administered subcutaneously, was active both prophylactically and therapeutically against cutaneous herpesvirus infection of hairless mice. Activity was comparable to that obtained with adenine arabinoside.

A new nucleoside antibiotic, 5,6-dihydro-5-azathymidine (DHAdT), inhibited the replication of herpes simplex virus (HSV) in cell cultures and protected mice from lethal intravenous or intracerebral HSV challenge (H. E. Renis, B. A. Court, and E. E. Eidson, Abstr. Annu. Meet. Am. Soc. Microbiol. 1976, A22, p. 4). We had previously developed a model cutaneous HSV infection of hairless mice (7), which we (7, 8) and others (4–6) have used for the evaluation of antiviral agents. Studies with DHAdT, therefore, were extended to this cutaneous model.

The HWC strain of HSV (type 1) was isolated from a herpetic lip lesion and passed three times in rabbit kidney cell cultures. The virus had a titer of 10^7 plaque-forming units per ml when assayed on primary rabbit kidney cells. Hairless mice of the HRS/J strain were obtained from Jackson Laboratories, Bar Harbor, Me. To infect the mice, the lumbar area was lightly scratched with a hypodermic needle, and the undiluted virus suspension (about 10^6 plaque-forming units) was gently applied to the scratched area with a cotton swab (7). Development of cutaneous HSV lesions in hairless mice has been described (1, 7). Deaths, as well as lesion scores on surviving mice, were recorded daily. Lesions were scored on a 0 to 4 scale: 0, no lesion; 0.5, <2-mm length lesion; 1, 2- to 4-mm length lesion; 2, 5- to 8-mm length lesion; 3, 9- to 15-mm length lesion; and 4, >15-mm length lesion.

Lesion scores were significantly lower in all drug-treated groups than in the control group from days 4 through 6 (Table 1). A statistical comparison of mean lesion scores among the various treated groups was made on day 6, the

Table 1. *Average skin lesion scores and mortality of hairless mice infected with herpes simplex virus and treated with DHAdT in experiment 1* [a]

Group no.	Treatment			Average lesion score on day:							No. of survivors/total no. of mice (day 28)	Extended life-span (days)[c]
	Drug	mg/kg per dose	Started at:	3	4	5	6[b]	7	8	9		
1	DHAdT	400	−2 h	0.50	0.62|	0.82	1.88	2.90	3.20	4.00	1/20	2
2	DHAdT	200	−2 h	0.50	0.72|	1.08	2.60	3.75	4.00	4.00	0/20	2
3	Saline		−2 h	0.50	1.68|	2.18	3.63	4.00			0/20	
4	DHAdT	400	+21 h	0.50	0.75	1.05|	2.22	3.50	3.95	4.00	0/20	3
5	DHAdT	400	+45 h	0.50	0.78	1.12	2.70|	3.90	4.00	4.00	6/20	8

[a] Twenty 18 to 22-g male mice were used per group. Herpesvirus was inoculated cutaneously at 0 h on day 0. DHAdT in 0.1 ml of saline was administered subcutaneously daily at 8 a.m., 1 p.m., and 4 p.m. for 5 consecutive days. Only survivors were included in the calculation of lesion scores. Vertical bar indicates last day of treatment.

[b] Statistical comparisons among groups were made using rank sums (see reference 3). Significant differences ($P < 0.05$) in lesion severity on day 6 were as follows. (i) All drug-treated groups were less severely infected than the control group. (ii) Group 1 was less severely infected than groups 2 and 5. (iii) Group 4 was less severely infected than group 5.

[c] All drug-treated groups showed a significantly ($P < 0.05$) extended life-span compared to the control group, based on the Kolmogorov-Smirnov two-sample test (see reference 2).

final day on which any group received a drug (footnote *b*, Table 1). It should be noted that among the infected mice, the 2-day "therapeutic" group, group 5, had the best recorded prolonged life-span. This increased survival, obtained when the initiation of DHAdT treatment was delayed until 2 days after virus inoculation, is consistent with results reported for two other antiviral nucleosides, 5-iododeoxyuridine and adenine arabinoside (ara-A) (5). Mice cutaneously infected with lethal strains of HSV die of a generalized infection (1). A delay in starting treatment may allow skin lesions to progress more rapidly, but continuing treatment longer into the infection, as in group 5, may slow the spread of the virus to other tissues and, thereby, extend the survival time of these therapeutically treated mice. Viral pathogenesis studies will be required to determine whether this explanation is correct.

In a second experiment, the efficacy of DHAdT was compared to that obtained with equimolar amounts of ara-A, which had been previously reported to be highly effective in the cutaneous herpes mouse model (5, 6). As ara-A (Pfanstiehl Labs., Inc., Waukegan, Ill.), in con-

TABLE 2. *Average skin lesion scores on hairless mice treated with DHAdT or ara-A in experiment 2*[a]

Group no.	Treatment		Average lesion score on day:										
	Drug	mg/kg per dose	3	4	5	6	7	8	9	10	11	14	18
1	DHAdT	400	0.10	0.63	1.25	2.05	2.73	3.27	3.18	3.00	2.70	2.13	1.29
2	DHAdT	200	0.16	0.74	1.66	2.58	3.63	4.00	4.00	4.00	4.00		
3	DHAdT	100	0.15	0.63	1.25	2.68	3.65	4.00	4.00	4.00	4.00		
4	DHAdT	50	0.18	1.47	1.80	3.29	4.00	4.00					
5	DHAdT	25	0.36	1.16	2.06	3.27	3.83	4.00	4.00				
6	DHAdT	12	0.32	1.59	2.11	3.36	4.00	4.00					
7	Saline		0.29	1.74	2.53	3.67	4.00						
8	Ara-A	436	0.05	0.28	0.33	1.23	2.10	2.80	2.77	3.25	3.00		
9	Ara-A	218	0.03	0.47	0.66	1.95	2.89	3.64	3.78	3.33	3.33		
10	Ara-A	109	0.45	0.75	1.28	2.75	3.74	3.88	4.00	3.33	3.50	3.00	3.00
11	Ara-A	54	0.33	1.14	1.88	3.35	3.94	4.00	4.00	3.00	3.00	3.00	3.00
12	Ara-A	27	0.38	1.70	2.55	3.58	4.00						
13	Ara-A	14	0.52	1.78	2.70	3.61	4.00						
14	Saline		0.58	1.85	2.60	3.69	4.00						

[a] Twenty 16- to 18-g female mice were used per group. Herpesvirus was inoculated cutaneously on day 0. Treatment was started 7 h later. Drugs in 0.2 ml of saline were administered subcutaneously daily at 8 a.m. and 4 p.m. through day 11. Equimolar amounts of DHAdT and ara-A were used for each dosage level. Only survivors were included in calculation of lesion scores. Vertical bar indicates the last day of treatment.

TABLE 3. *Mortality of herpes-infected hairless mice treated with DHAdT or ara-A*[a]

Group no.	Treatment		Total no. of mice dead by day:															Surviving mice on day 28	Extended life-span (days)[b]
	Drug	mg/kg per dose	3	4	5	6	7	8	9	10	11	12	13	14	15	21	25		
1	DHAdT	400					2	5	9	10		12			13	15		5	13
2	DHAdT	200	1				4	11	14	18		19		20				0	2
3	DHAdT	100				1	3	14	18	19		20						0	1
4	DHAdT	50				3	8	14	20									0	1
5	DHAdT	25	2			9	14	19		20								0	NS
6	DHAdT	12	1			6	14	18	20									0	NS
7	Saline		1			5	18	20										0	
8	Ara-A	436						3	7	16	19	20						0	3
9	Ara-A	218		1				6	11	17		20						0	3
10	Ara-A	109					1	4	8	17	18						20	0	3
11	Ara-A	54					3	13	15	19								1	1
12	Ara-A	27				1	18	20										0	NS
13	Ara-A	14				2	17	20										0	NS
14	Saline					7	18	20										0	
15[c]	Saline		1			12	36	40										0	

[a] Determined with the same mice used in experiment 2 (Table 2).

[b] Each number in this column indicates a significantly ($P < 0.05$) extended life-span compared to control group, based on Kolmogorov-Smirnov two-sample test. NS, Not significantly different from control.

[c] Combination of groups 7 and 14. Group 15 was used for statistical calculations.

trast to the highly water-soluble DHAdT, is only sparingly soluble, it was finely ground and suspended in saline.

Both DHAdT and ara-A were active, gave consistent dose responses with respect to lesion development (Table 2) and mortality (Table 3), and showed a minimal effective level of approximately 50 mg/kg per dose when administered twice daily. Others (4-6) have reported higher survival rates in herpes-infected hairless mice that had been treated with ara-A. This may be due to the different strain of virus used or to a lower virus challenge; in our studies, all control mice died. Valid comparisons with the cutaneous herpes mouse model can be made only within a given experiment, in which conditions of infection and treatment are held constant. We conclude that ara-A and DHAdT showed about equal activity in our model under the specified experimental conditions.

Continuing treatment with DHAdT for 11.5 days in experiment 2, rather than stopping after 5 days as in the first experiment, showed no dramatic improvement in activity, based either on lesion score or mortality. It should be noted, however, that mice were treated twice daily in the second experiment as compared to three times per day in experiment 1. Optimal treatment schedule for DHAdT remains to be established.

We wish to thank P. I. Good for performing the statistical analyses.

LITERATURE CITED

1. **Constantine, V. S., R. D. Francis, and B. H. Mason.** 1971. Experimental zoster-like herpes simplex in hairless mice. J. Invest. Dermatol. 56:193-199.
2. **Conover, W. J.** 1971. Practical nonparametric statistics. John Willey & Sons, Inc., New York.
3. **Dunn, O. J.** 1964. Multiple comparisons using rank sums. Technometrics 6:241-252.
4. **Klein, R. J., and A. E. Friedman-Kien.** 1975. Phosphonoacetic acid-resistant herpes simplex virus infection in hairless mice. Antimicrob. Agents Chemother. 7:289-293.
5. **Klein, R. J., A. E. Friedman-Kien, and E. Brady.** 1974. Herpes simplex virus skin infection in hairless mice: treatment with antiviral compounds. Antimicrob. Agents Chemother. 5:318-322.
6. **Lieberman, M., T. W. Schafer, and P. E. Came.** 1973. Chemotherapy of cutaneous herpesvirus infection of hairless mice. J. Invest. Dermatol. 60:203-206.
7. **Underwood, G. E.** 1968. Kethoxal for treatment of cutaneous herpes simplex. Proc. Soc. Exp. Biol. Med. 129:235-239.
8. **Underwood, G. E., and F. R. Nichol.** 1971. Clinical evaluation of kethoxal against cutaneous herpes simplex. Appl. Microbiol. 22:588-592.

ANTIMICROBIAL AGENTS AND CHEMOTHERAPY, Apr. 1977, p. 768-770 Vol. 11, No. 4

^{125}I Radioimmunoassay of Netilmicin

PAUL STEVENS,* LOWELL S. YOUNG, AND WILLIAM L. HEWITT

Department of Medicine, Division of Infectious Diseases, University of California School of Medicine, Los Angeles, California 90024

Received for publication 26 November 1976

We report a radioimmunoassay for the new semisynthetic aminoglycoside netilmicin with a sensitivity of 480 pg per tube and a correlation coefficient of 0.94 between this radioimmunoassay and a microbioassay for measurement of netilmicin in serum.

Netilmicin is a new semisynthetic aminoglycoside produced by ethylation of the one amino group of the deoxystreptamine moiety of sisomicin. Like gentamicin, netilmicin is active against most clinically significant gram-negative bacilli (5). Although preliminary data suggest that netilmicin is less nephrotoxic in rats (7) than is gentamicin, it has the potential for oto- and nephrotoxicity. Methods to determine serum or body fluid levels of netilmicin could aid in management of human therapy by helping to avert untoward reactions, select adequate dosage regimens, and provide useful pharmacokinetic data.

Netilmicin (provided by Schering Corporation) was conjugated to porcine thyroglobulin by the carbodiimide reaction (4, 6), and New Zealand white rabbits were immunized with this conjugate as described previously (9, 10). Netilmicin antiserum was obtained 7 to 10 days after the booster injections and stored at −20°C.

Netilmicin was commercially iodinated by Diagnostic Products Corp., Los Angeles, Calif., using a modified Bolton and Hunter method. This procedure is similar to that recently described for the iodination of gentamicin (2). The netilmicin had an initial approximate specific activity of 200 to 250 Ci/mmol.

The radioimmunoassay (RIA) procedure used was similar to the RIA of amikacin (10) using ^{125}I-labeled antigen. For the assay, the reaction mixture consisted of the following: 200 μl of the diluted standard or samples, 100 μl of ^{125}I-labeled netilmicin, which contained anywhere from 30,000 to 60,000 cpm, and 100 μl of appropriately diluted rabbit antisera that would bind approximately 40 to 50% of ^{125}I-labeled netilmicin in the absence of unlabeled netilmicin. The tubes were incubated at 22°C for 30 min. To separate bound from free netilmicin, dextran-charcoal was used as described previously (10). The standard curve was constructed using logit-log graph paper (10). Values for unknown serum samples were interpolated from the standard curve. The RIA for netilmicin was compared with an agar diffusion microbioassay using *Klebsiella pneumoniae* as the seed organism (11). Twenty-five patient sera that covered a range from 1 to 10 μg of netilmicin per ml were selected. The sera were assayed simultaneously by both methods in duplicate on two different days, and the correlation coefficient (*r* value) was determined between the methods by least squares linear regression.

A typical standard curve of the RIA of netilmicin in which the logit of B/B_0 in percentage of relative bound ^{125}I-labeled netilmicin was plotted versus the logarithmic amount of netilmicin in nanograms per assay tube as shown in Fig. 1. The sensitivity of the assay was determined to be 480 pg per tube. This was based on a theoretical mean value which was two standard deviations (SD) below the mean of the maximum binding tube (B_0).

To assess precision, five replicate determinations were run on three samples that represented the low, middle, and high concentrations of clinically expected serum netilmicin levels. The samples with mean concentrations in micrograms per milliliters ± the SD with the coefficient of variation (CV) were as follows: low, 1.02 ± 0.04, CV 3.9%; middle, 4.42 ± 0.18, CV 4.1%; and high, 7.78 ± 0.25, CV 3.2%. Reproducibility of the assay was determined by assaying the same three representative samples in duplicate on five different assay days. The mean concentration in micrograms per milliliter ± SD with the CV was as follows: low, 1.2 ± 0.13, CV 13.3%; middle, 4.66 ± 0.42, CV 9.1%; and high, 8.48 ± 0.86, CV 10.2%.

There was no cross-reaction of the netilmicin antisera with the following antimicrobial agents at serum levels at least 20 times greater than would be expected therapeutically: tobramycin, amikacin, cephalothin, chloramphenicol, cefazolin, carbenicillin, or oxacillin. There was, however, a 3% cross-reaction with gentamicin and sisomicin.

The comparison of the RIA with the microbioassay, as determined by linear regression analysis, is depicted in Fig. 2. The correlation coefficient was 0.94 and was significant at $P < 0.00005$. The line of regression had the equation of $y = 0.94x + 0.96$. Statistically, therefore, there was no significant difference in the measurement of netilmicin between these two methods.

RIA is a rapid, sensitive and, more importantly, the most specific method for the determination of aminoglycosides in serum. The desirability of having more rapid and specific assay methods for aminoglycosides is obvious and has been discussed in previous investigations (8, 9). Clinically, the major advantage to this assay other than rapidity is its specificity which obviates the need for laboratory personnel to obtain information regarding other antimicrobial agents that the patient may be receiving.

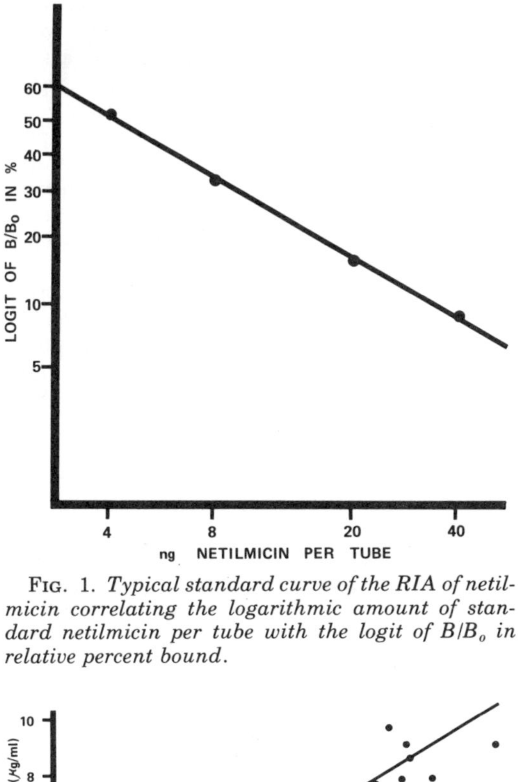

FIG. 1. *Typical standard curve of the RIA of netilmicin correlating the logarithmic amount of standard netilmicin per tube with the logit of B/B_0 in relative percent bound.*

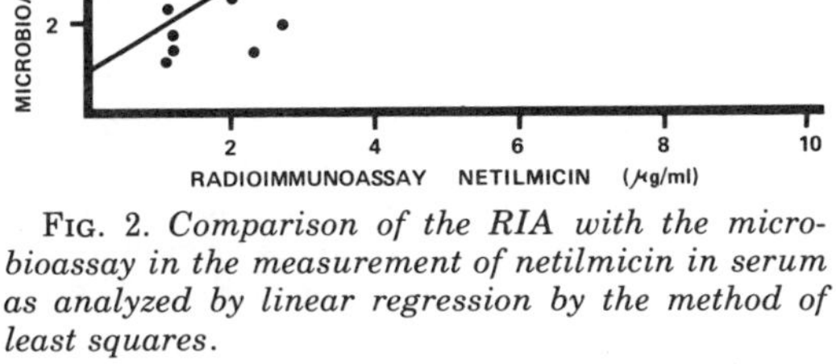

FIG. 2. *Comparison of the RIA with the microbioassay in the measurement of netilmicin in serum as analyzed by linear regression by the method of least squares.*

Unlike the extensive cross-reaction (70%) between kanamycin and antisera produced to the semisynthetic derivative of kanamycin, amikacin (10), we find little cross-reactivity (3%) between netilmicin antisera and its parent compound sisomicin. The possible reasons for this are numerous but most likely relate to the groups or portions of the aminoglycoside molecule that are immunodeterminant after the aminoglycoside molecule has been conjugated to porcine thyroglobulin.

Recent work has shown the usefulness of cross-reacting gentamicin antisera for dual use in an RIA for sisomicin (3). This novel use of cross-reacting antisera was primarily due to the reported 65% cross-reaction of gentamicin antisera with sisomicin. Analogous multiple use of netilmicin antisera for RIA of other aminoglycosides, while theoretically possible, is neither practical nor economical since the cross-reactivity of netilmicin antisera with gentamicin and sisomicin is only 3% and would require large amounts of antisera to obtain any type of useful standard curve.

The RIA reported here is precise and reproducible and well within limits of acceptable coefficients of variation for clinical laboratories. It correlates well with the microbiological assay, and the high degree of sensitivity of this method will permit quantification of concentrations not possible with microbiological and radioenzymatic techniques.

We acknowledge the expert technical assistance of Sandra Smaller. This study was supported by a grant from the Schering Corporation.

LITERATURE CITED

1. **Bolton, A. E., and W. M. Hunter.** 1973. The labelling of proteins to high specific activity by conjugation to a ^{125}I-containing acylating agent. Biochem. J. **133**:529–539.
2. **Broughton, A., and J. E. Strong.** 1976. Radioimmunoassay of iodinated gentamicin. Clin. Chim. Acta **66**:125–129.
3. **Broughton, A., J. E. Strong, and G. P. Bodey.** 1976. Radioimmunoassay of sisomicin. Antimicrob. Agents Chemother. **9**:247–250.
4. **Doleschall, G., and K. Lempert.** 1963. On the mechanism of carboxyl condensations of carbodiimides. Tetrahedron Lett. **18**:1195–1199.
5. **Fu, K. P., and H. C. Neu.** 1976. In vitro study of netilmicin compared with other aminoglycosides. Antimicrob. Agents Chemother. **10**:526–534.
6. **Goodfriend, T. L., L. Levine, and G. D. Fasman.** 1964.

Antibodies to bradykinin and angiotensin: a use of carbodiimides in immunology. Science 144:1344–1346.

7. **Luft, F. C., M. N. Yum, and S. A. Kleit.** 1976. Comparative nephrotoxicities of netilmicin and gentamicin. Antimicrob. Agents Chemother. **10**:845–849.
8. **Stevens, P., and L. S. Young.** 1976. Rapid assay of aminoglycosides by radioenzymatic techniques, pp. 64–72. *In* D. Schlessinger (ed.), Microbiology—1975, American Society for Microbiology, Washington, D. C.
9. **Stevens, P., L. S. Young, and W. L. Hewitt.** 1975. Radioimmunoassay, acetylating radioenzymatic assay and microbioassay of gentamicin: a comparative study. J. Lab. Clin. Med. **86**:349–359.
10. **Stevens, P., L. S. Young, and W. L. Hewitt.** 1976. ^{125}I-radioimmunoassay of amikacin and comparison with a microbioassay. J. Antibiot. **29**:829–832.
11. **Winters, R. E., K. D. Litwack, and W. L. Hewitt.** 1971. Relation between dose and levels of gentamicin in blood. J. Infect. Dis. **124** (Suppl.):S90–S95.

ERRATUM

Preparation of Isolated Intestinal Villi Useful for Studying Hydrolysis Rates of Penicillin and Cephalosporin Esters

WALTER E. WRIGHT* AND VERLE D. LINE

The Lilly Research Laboratories, Indianapolis, Indiana 46206

Volume 10, no. 5, p. 862, column 2, line 25: "about 0.5 mm" should read "about 0.5 cm."

Antimicrobial Agents and Chemotherapy, May 1977, p. 773-779
Vol. 11, No. 5

Permeability Barrier to Rifampin in Mycobacteria

J. HUI, N. GORDON, and R. KAJIOKA*

Laboratory Services Branch, Ministry of Health, Toronto, Ontario, Canada

Received for publication 11 January 1977

A strain of *Mycobacterium intracellulare* that exhibited natural resistance to rifampin was isolated. The ribonucleic acid polymerase was found to be susceptible to rifampin. Studies with Tween 80 suggested that a permeability barrier against rifampin was present in the intact organism. A type strain of *Mycobacterium smegmatis*, ATCC 607, considered resistant to rifampin also demonstrated a permeability barrier. The possibility that rifampin resistance in naturally occurring strains of mycobacteria and variable levels of resistance in strains of certain species of this organism are due to permeability barriers is discussed.

Rifampin is a highly potent inhibitor of the deoxyribonucleic acid (DNA)-dependent ribonucleic acid (RNA) polymerase of many procaryotic cells. Complex formation between rifampin and the β-subunit of the enzyme (11) results in blockage of initiation of transcription (9, 15). Resistant mutants fail to form complexes between the enzyme and rifampin (18). To date, mutations to rifampin resistance have been identified in the β-subunit gene locus (2, 6, 10).

The susceptibility of mycobacteria to rifampin has been well documented (7, 12, 21). Resistant mutants derived from these strains appear to be affected in the RNA polymerase. A number of species of mycobacteria are inherently resistant to rifampin. This resistance has also been attributed to a resistant polymerase (8, 21). Tsukamura (17) has presented evidence for an "obligatory" single-step event in the development of resistant mutants, clinically and experimentally, for *Mycobacterium tuberculosis* var. *hominis*, based on the failure to obtain mutants of intermediate resistance. Taken together, the evidence leads to the view that the action of rifampin on mycobacteria is directed specifically against the RNA polymerase, and those naturally resistant species originated from a single-step mutation leading to a change in the polymerase. However, somewhat at variance with this view is the observation that the naturally occurring populations of certain species of mycobacteria can be differentiated into a number of strains according to their degrees of resistance to rifampin. The minimum inhibitory concentrations of the strains of each species are distributed over a wide range (12). This gradation of resistance, such as in group III mycobacteria, suggests that the resistance of each population did not result from a mutation affecting the RNA polymerase, as this should have led to a uniformly maximal resistance according to the obligatory single-step concept.

We have investigated rifampin resistance in a group III organism, and our results are consistent with the view that the natural resistance of this species can be attributed to a permeability barrier. Moreover, the greater part of the natural resistance of all species of mycobacteria may possibly be attributed to permeability factors.

MATERIALS AND METHODS

Mycobacteria strains. The strains used in this study were *Mycobacterium intracellulare* strain AT 13786 and *M. tuberculosis* var. *hominis* strain 55429, both isolated from cases of human infection, and were propagated on Lowenstein-Jensen medium and clonally purified by repeated single-colony isolations on Middlebrook 7H10 medium containing glycerol and supplemented with albumin and dextrose. For each experiment a single colony was selected from stock culture plates of 50 to 100 colonies each and grown to the required density in suspension.

Culture methods. The medium for colony counts was essentially Middlebrook 7H10 supplemented with albumin (0.5%) and dextrose (0.2%) and including either glycerol or Tween 80 as explained in the text. Rifampin, whenever included, was added at the appropriate concentration to the sterile, liquified medium at 43°C immediately before the plates were poured. Stock cultures were grown on Middlebrook 7H10 medium containing glycerol, albumin, and dextrose.

Cultures were grown in suspension in Middlebrook 7H9 medium supplemented with albumin (0.5%) and dextrose (0.2%) and including glycerol and/or Tween 80 as explained in the text. Rifampin, when included, was added immediately before use.

Incubation for growth was at 37°C in all cases, liquid cultures were not agitated during incubation, and growth was monitored at 450 nm with the Spectronic 20 (Bausch & Lomb) colorimeter, after vortexing.

Reagents. Rifampin (Rimactan) was a gift from Ciba Pharmaceuticals. Tween 80 (polyoxyethylene [19] sorbitan monooleate) was a product of the Atlas Chemical Co. [^{14}C]adenosine 5′-triphosphate was obtained from New England Nuclear Corp.

Preparation and assay of RNA polymerase. To obtain cell-free DNA-dependent RNA polymerase, cultures of strain AT 13786 were grown in suspension, and the cells were collected by centrifugation at 5,000 rpm for 15 min in a GSA (Sorvall) rotor. The mucid pellet (0.45 g/500 ml of culture) was suspended in ice-cold buffer G (3) to 250 mg (wet weight)/ml. Cells were disrupted by passage through a Ribicell fractionater (Ivan Sorvall Inc.) at 4°C. Subsequent steps were done according to White et al. (20), and the fraction insoluble in 30 to 42% saturated ammonium sulfate was kept at −20°C in storage buffer (3). The activity of this fraction was 97.5% dependent on added DNA and incorporated 9 μmol of adenosine monophosphate per mg of protein at 37°C in 10 min into the trichloroacetic acid (5%)-insoluble fraction.

Polymerase assay. The incorporation mixture contained, in 0.25 ml: 0.5 mg of bovine serum albumin per ml (fraction V, Sigma); 0.15 M KCl; 40 mM tris(hydroxymethyl)aminomethane (pH 7.9 at 4°C); 10 mm $MgCl_2$; 8 mM spermidine HCl; 0.1 mM ethylenediaminetetraacetate; 0.1 mM dithiothreitol; 1 mM triphosphates (cytidine triphosphate, uridine triphosphate, and guanosine triphosphate); 200 μg of calf thymus DNA per ml (highly polymerized); and 0.1 μCi of [^{14}C]adenosine 5′-triphosphate (specific activity, 0.8 μCi/μmol). The reaction mixture was incubated at 37°C. The reaction was stopped by chilling and by the addition of 2 ml of cold 5% trichloroacetic acid. The trichloroacetic acid-insoluble fraction was collected on Whatman GF/C filters, washed with 3% trichloroacetic acid, dried, placed in Liquifluor scintillation fluid (New England Nuclear Corp.), and counted in the Packard Tri-Carb scintillation counter. When rifampin was included in the assay, DNA and the unlabeled nucleoside triphosphates were added after 3 min of preincubation of the reaction mixture with the drug.

RESULTS

Effects of rifampin on strain AT 13786. The survival of *M. intracellulare* AT 13786 against different concentrations of rifampin was measured by colony number. The results are given in Table 1. The surviving fraction, compared with the rifampin concentration, was almost 50% at 20 μg of rifampin per ml.

Although a cloned population was used, the culture appeared to respond heterogeneously to the drug.

A strain of *M. tuberculosis* tested simultaneously showed a high degree of susceptibility to rifampin, comparable to other results (7). This confirmed that conditions for the test were favorable for the action of the drug and served to standardize the effective biological dose level of the rifampin preparation used in these studies.

That strain AT 13786 possessed a substantial degree of natural resistance to rifampin was clearly evident.

Effect of rifampin on strain AT 13786 in the presence of Tween 80. Tween 80 is capable of reducing permeability barriers (1). Since strain AT 13786 did not use dextrose for growth unless Tween 80 was present (15), it was also rendered more permeable by this surfactant.

The susceptibility of strain AT 13786 to rifampin was measured with Tween in the medium. Under these conditions AT 13786 was over 50-fold more susceptible to rifampin than in the absence of Tween (Table 2). In fact, the minimum inhibitory concentration was below the standard of 1 μg/ml for 1% survivors generally accepted for therapeutic purposes.

These results suggested that the natural resistance exhibited by strain AT 13786 was due to a permeability barrier to rifampin.

Effect of rifampin on suspended cultures of strain AT 13786 in the presence of Tween. Strain AT 13786 grew well in suspension with Tween but poorly when glycerol was substituted for Tween. In the absence of Tween and glycerol, growth was either absent (Fig. 1) or limited to a very slight initial increase in opti-

TABLE 1. *Effect of rifampin on the survival of M. intracellulare strain AT 13786*[a]

Concn of rifampin (μg/ml)	Relative colony no.	
	AT 13786	*M. tuberculosis* 55429
0	100	100
0.1	100	0.8
0.5	100	0.034
1.0	100	0.00002
2.0	77	0.00002
4.0	69	0.00002
10	54	0.00002
20	48	0.00002

[a] Colonies were counted at 2 weeks for AT 13786 and 3 weeks for *M. tuberculosis*. Medium contained 0.5% glycerol.

TABLE 2. *Effect of rifampin on the survival of M. intracellulare strain AT 13786 exposed to Tween 80*[a]

Concn of rifampin (μg/ml)	Relative colony no.
0	100
0.01	100
0.05	74
0.1	87
0.5	36 (minute)
1	0.0000072
5	0.0000072
10	0.0000072

[a] Medium contained Tween 80 at 0.05%.

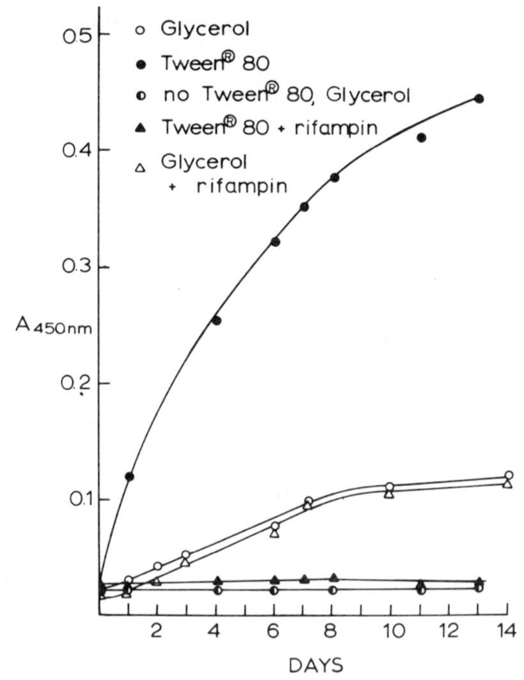

FIG. 1. *Inhibitory action of rifampin on AT 13786 in the presence of Tween 80. Cultures were grown in liquid media as described in the text. The Tween 80 concentration was 0.05%. The glycerol concentration was 0.2%. Rifampin was used at a final concentration of 1.0 μg/ml.*

cal density, as recorded for the studies illustrated in Fig. 2.

Cultures of AT 13786 were exposed to 1 μg of rifampin per ml in 7H9 liquid medium containing Tween (0.05%). Albumin and dextrose were included, but glycerol was absent. The susceptibility to low levels of rifampin could be engendered by Tween in liquid cultures of AT 13786 (Fig. 1). No growth was observed in the presence of rifampin and Tween. The absence of colony formers with 1 μg of rifampin per ml (Table 1) was due to a complete cessation of growth and not to a delayed appearance resulting from a reduced growth rate (i.e., total bacteriostasis).

Although growth was not prolific when glycerol was substituted for Tween, there was sufficient growth to reveal a lack of inhibition by 1 μg of rifampin per ml in glycerol in the absence of Tween. The cultures in glycerol appeared to grow equally well with or without rifampin (Fig. 1).

Nature of Tween effect on rifampin susceptibility of strain AT 13786. Because Tween 80 can be metabolized by mycobacteria (4, 5, 16, 22) and was found to stimulate the growth of strain AT 13786 suboptimally without any added carbon source (R. Kajioka, J. Hui, and N. Gordon, manuscript in preparation), it was of some interest to investigate whether other factors involving Tween besides permeability could account for its effect on rifampin susceptibility. A study was carried out to determine the effective medium concentration of Tween 80 and the role, if any, of Tween metabolism and growth. Suspended cultures were grown in liquid medium with different concentrations of Tween and with or without rifampin (1 μg/ml) and glycerol (0.2%). Because the rate of growth in glycerol without Tween is greatly reduced, and because growth under limiting, suboptimal conditions is not exponential, for purposes of comparison the index of growth was arbitrarily measured as the increase in optical density in 8 days and plotted against the concentration of Tween (Fig. 2). Tween up to 0.01% produced little enhancement of growth regardless of whether glycerol was included, although growth was faster with glycerol than without it. Rifampin had no effect at lower Tween levels, but inhibition rose rapidly from nil to maximum between 0.005 and 0.01% Tween. Although the effectiveness of rifampin was wholly dependent upon Tween concentration, there was no apparent proportionality between the degree of inhibition and concentration of Tween. Instead, a narrow range of Tween level existed, which determined the degree of rifampin action. In the same context, the maximum inhibition by rifampin occurred well before growth was significantly enhanced, and there

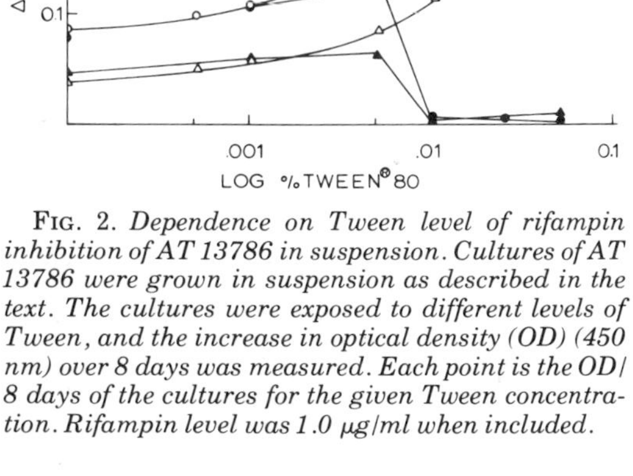

FIG. 2. *Dependence on Tween level of rifampin inhibition of AT 13786 in suspension. Cultures of AT 13786 were grown in suspension as described in the text. The cultures were exposed to different levels of Tween, and the increase in optical density (OD) (450 nm) over 8 days was measured. Each point is the OD/8 days of the cultures for the given Tween concentration. Rifampin level was 1.0 μg/ml when included.*

was no relationship apparent between the extent of inhibition and the degree of enhancement of growth of Tween. This was further substantiated by the observation that the Tween threshold for rifampin action was not different when a higher basal growth rate was maintained with glycerol.

These experiments suggested that a natural inaccessibility of the rifampin target site in the cell was overcome by Tween and that this barrier was sufficiently eliminated to allow rifampin action over a narrow range of Tween concentrations between 0.005 and 0.01%. They also indicated that neither the action of rifampin nor the barrier to its target (RNA polymerase) resulted from the metabolism of Tween by strain AT 13786 or the enhancement of growth by Tween.

The effect produced by Tween was neither permanent nor long lasting. When cultures grown in Tween 80 were exposed with minimum delay to rifampin (1 μg/ml) in the absence of Tween, they were again resistant.

Susceptibility of cell-free DNA-dependent RNA polymerase of strain AT 13786 to rifampin. The results of the preceding studies suggested that the resistance of strain AT 13786 to rifampin might be due to the RNA polymerase being inaccessible and that accessibility was developed as a result of the Tween action on the cell envelope.

This view was supported by the results of studies on cell-free extracts of DNA-dependent RNA polymerase. The activity of this enzyme from strain AT 13786 was highly sensitive to rifampin (Table 3, Fig. 3). Complete inhibition of [^{14}C]adenosine monophosphate incorporation was achieved with between 0.25 and 0.50 μg of rifampin per ml. The enzyme activity was virtually eliminated at a rifampin concentration some 40-fold lower than that required to inhibit the intact Tween-free organism to a 1% level of survival.

These experiments further confirmed that Tween was not enhancing the susceptibility of strain AT 13786 to rifampin by priming complex formation between the drug and polymerase (Table 4). The addition of Tween did not alter the degree of inhibition of [^{14}C]adenosine monophosphate incorporation by rifampin in the cell-free system.

Effect of Tween on the rifampin resistance of ATCC strain 607B (*Mycobacterium smegmatis*). ATCC strain 607B (*M. smegmatis*) exhibits substantial resistance to rifampin and has been placed in the category of resistant strains of mycobacteria (8, 21). However, resistance could be attributed to a rifampin barrier rather than to a naturally resistant polymerase, since resistance was substantially low-

TABLE 3. *RNA polymerase activity of cell-free extracts of AT 13786*[a]

Reaction mixture	[^{14}C]AMP incorporated (cpm)
Complete	702
− DNA	21
− Protein	7
+ Rifampin (1 μg/ml)	0

[a] Complete mixture included 200 μg of DNA per ml and 25 μg of protein per 0.25 ml. The equivalent cell number per reaction mixture was 9 × 10^{10} cells. AMP, Adenosine monophosphate.

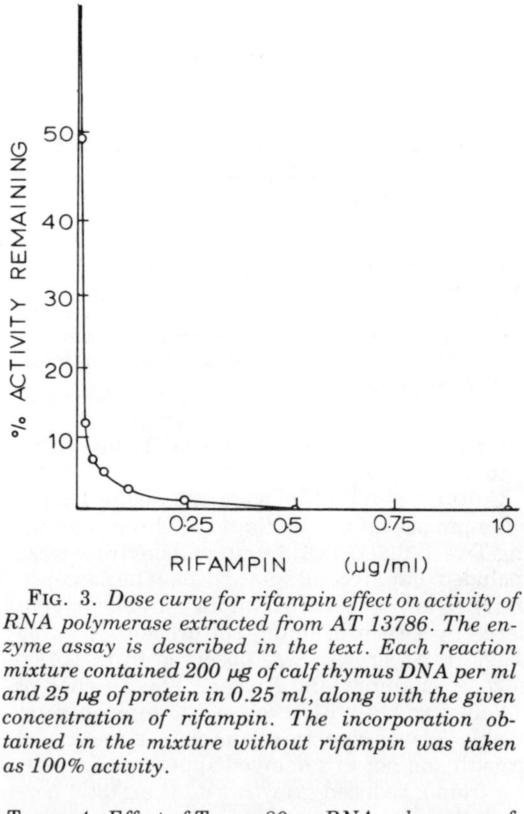

FIG. 3. *Dose curve for rifampin effect on activity of RNA polymerase extracted from AT 13786. The enzyme assay is described in the text. Each reaction mixture contained 200 μg of calf thymus DNA per ml and 25 μg of protein in 0.25 ml, along with the given concentration of rifampin. The incorporation obtained in the mixture without rifampin was taken as 100% activity.*

TABLE 4. *Effect of Tween 80 on RNA polymerase of AT 13786*[a]

Rifampin (μg/ml)	cpm incorporated	
	Tween[b]	No Tween
0	644	613
0.005	116	128
1.0	0	0

[a] Reaction mixture contained 200 μg of DNA per ml and 25 μg of protein in 0.25 ml.

[b] Tween 80 was included at 0.05%.

ered in the presence of Tween as a permeability agent (Fig. 4).

DISCUSSION

Our results demonstrated that strain AT 13786 possessed a rifampin-susceptible DNA-dependent RNA polymerase even though the cultures of this strain were relatively resistant to the inhibitory action of rifampin. In the intact cell, therefore, the enzyme was apparently inaccessible to rifampin. The presence of Tween allowed interaction between polymerase and rifampin to take place, as evidenced by the marked increase in susceptibility of the cultures to rifampin when Tween 80 was included in the medium. This effect was not dependent on a Tween-enhanced metabolic activity, or on the metabolism specifically of Tween 80. This suggested that the action of Tween might be attributed to a direct effect on the cell envelope.

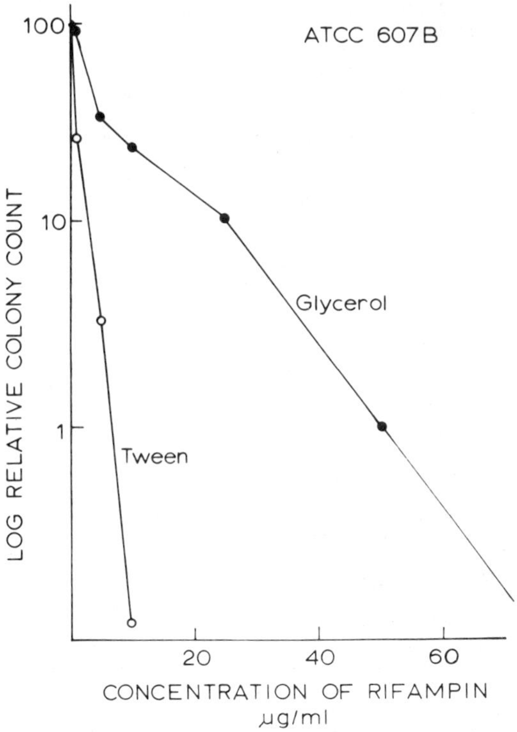

FIG. 4. *Enhancement of rifampin inhibition of strain ATCC 607B by Tween. The dose curve of rifampin was carried out on 7H10 medium as described in the text. The strain tested was M. smegmatis strain ATCC 607B, propagated in Lowenstein-Jensen medium and clonally purified on Middlebrook medium. Colonies were selected and dispersed into suspension, and dilutions were plated at different concentrations of rifampin. Symbols;* ●, *0.2% glycerol, no Tween;* ○, *0.05% Tween 80, no glycerol. Colonies were counted after 14 days of incubation at 37°C. The growth rate of ATCC 607B was similar on both glycerol and Tween media in the absence of rifampin.*

Tween enhances the permeability of mycobacteria (1) and, as a result of its action on the mycobacterial surface, reduces phage adsorption (13) and prevents the formation of cell aggregates. These properties are compatible with the interpretation of our results that strain AT 13786 was resistant to rifampin by virtue of a permeability barrier, and that Tween action on the cell envelope rendered it permeable to rifampin. Although the nature of the Tween-cell interaction altering permeability has not been established, Shands (14) observed the long ribbons of trilaminar lipopolysaccharide extracts of cell wall to become short segments with the leaflets pushed apart in the presence of Tween. The possible importance of hydrophobic bonds cannot be overlooked.

We cannot entirely discount at present an alternative hypothesis that disorganization of the membranes of strain AT 13786 led to, for all practical purposes, an inhibition of a hypothetical rifampin-modifying enzyme. Antibiotic-modifying enzymes are generally found in the cell envelope of drug-resistant organisms and are episome directed. To the best of our knowledge, rifampin-modifying enzymes have not been demonstrated in rifampin-resistant bacteria, and direct evidence for the existence of episomes in mycobacteria has not been presented.

In view of our results, the classification of strains of mycobacteria with respect to rifampin action into three groups (10), susceptible, resistant, and variable, was considered in light of permeability barriers. ATCC strain 607B (*M. smegmatis*) exhibits substantial resistance to rifampin and has been placed in the category of resistant strains (12, 21). However, the resistance could be attributed to a permeability barrier rather than to a naturally resistant polymerase, since, like strain AT 13786, resistance of ATCC strain 607B was substantially lowered in the presence of Tween as a permeability agent (Fig. 4). Although Jones and David (8) noted an inhibition of phage D29 replication by 1 µg of rifampin per ml which was resisted by the host, ATCC strain 607, suggesting that host resistance to rifampin lay in the polymerase and not in a permeability barrier, our results conform to these observations in that this level of rifampin allowed approximately 93% survivors of this mycobacteria in the absence of Tween. This would imply that a low level of permeability was present, sufficient to inhibit some growth. The transcription of the phage genome was apparently sensitive to low levels of rifampin.

These observations invite the speculation that the natural resistance of strains of mycobacteria, generally, might be attributed to a permeability barrier rather than to a rifampin-resistant polymerase. In those species exhibiting a wide variation of resistant strains, the variability might be due to different degrees of permeability to rifampin, which in turn might result from a multistep event in mutation. This is in contrast to the experimentally derived mutants whose resistance to rifampin has been mapped in the β-gene locus of RNA polymerase (2, 6, 10) and to resistant mutants appearing after rifampin therapy that develop by a single-step event (17).

A comparison of the minimum inhibitory concentration of strain ATCC 607 to that of strain AT 13786 (Table 2, Fig. 4) revealed that strain ATCC 607 was somewhat more resistant to rifampin. Since both populations are homogeneous, this may suggest that the polymerase of strain ATCC 607 is somewhat more resistant to rifampin or that the permeability barrier was not entirely overcome. Even in susceptible strains a residual barrier may exist. Hobby and Lenert found a twofold increase in susceptibility of rifampin-susceptible, clinically isolated strains of *M. tuberculosis* var. *hominis* when tested in Tween (7). A comparison of the susceptibility of the polymerases of different groups of organisms is of some interest. Ninety-nine percent inhibition of the activity of *Escherichia coli* RNA polymerase was achieved at approximately 0.6 μg of rifampin per ml by Wehrli et al. (19). The polymerase of strain AT 13786 was inhibited similarly at 0.25 μg of rifampin per ml. *Staphylococcus aureus* (19) and strain AT 13786 required the same level of rifampin (0.02 μg/ml) to achieve 90% inhibition of their polymerases. These comparisons suggest that the polymerases of different susceptible bacteria do not differ greatly in their susceptibility to rifampin.

The manner in which species such as the group III organisms evolved populations with different and widely varying susceptibilities to rifampin poses an interesting problem. Possibly a mutant with altered surface properties, either structural or enzymatic, possessed selective growth advantages over the rest of the population, as well as altered permeability. If the change occurred as a series of events, different mutant populations would emerge with different degrees of permeability and, therefore, a different degree of rifampin resistance in each population. In support of this view, we have noted changes in surface properties and permeability accompanied by selective growth advantages in high-frequency mutants of strain AT 13786 and in lysogenic strain ATCC 607 (Kajioka et al., in preparation). The consistent demonstration of rifampin susceptibility in some species may be due to genetic incompetence involving a deletion preventing mutations to impermeability.

ACKNOWLEDGMENT

We thank H. B. Smith for his continued support and encouragement.

LITERATURE CITED

1. **Aubert, E.** 1950. "Cold" stain for acid-fast bacteria. Can. J. Public Health 41:31–32.
2. **Babinet, C., and H. Condamine.** 1968. Mutants resistants a la Rifampicine modifies dans leur DNA-RNA polymerase. C. R. Acad. Sci. 267:231–232.
3. **Burgess, R. R.** 1969. A new method for the large scale purification of Escherichia coli deoxyribonucleic acid dependent ribonucleic acid polymerase. J. Biol. Chem. 244:6160–6167.
4. **Dubos, R. J.** 1947. The effect of lipids and serum albumin on bacterial growth. J. Exp. Med. 85:9–22.
5. **Dubos, R. J.** 1950. The effect of organic acids on mammalian tubercle bacilli. J. Exp. Med. 92:319–332.
6. **Ghysen, A., and M. Pironio.** 1972. Relationship between N function of bacteriophage λ and host RNA polymerase. J. Mol. Biol. 65:259–272.
7. **Hobby, G. L., and T. F. Lenert.** 1968. The antimicrobial activity of rifampin. Am. Rev. Respir. Dis. 97:713–714.
8. **Jones, W. D., and H. L. David.** 1971. Inhibition by rifampin of mycobacteriophage D29 replication in its drug-resistant host, *Mycobacterium smegmatis* ATCC 607. Am. Rev. Respir. Dis. 103:618–624.
9. **Lill, V., R. Santo, A. Sippel, and G. Hartmann.** 1970. Inhibitors of the RNA polymerase reaction. Colloq. Ges. Biol. Chem. 20:48–59.
10. **Mindlin, S. Z., T. S. Ilyina, T. A. Vocykova, and V. V. Velkov.** 1972. Genetic analysis of rifampin resistant mutants of Escherichia coli K12. Mol. Gen. Genet. 115:115–121.
11. **Rabussay, D., and W. Zillig.** 1969. A rifampicin resistant RNA polymerase from E. coli altered in the B-subunit. FEBS Lett. 5:104–106.
12. **Rynearson, T. K., J. S. Shrontis, and E. Wolinsky.** 1971. Rifampin: in vitro effect on atypical mycobacteria. Am. Rev. Respir. Dis. 104:272–274.
13. **Sellers, M. I., W. L. Baxter, and H. R. Runnels.** 1962. Growth characteristics of Mycobacteriophages D28 and D29. Can. J. Microbiol. 8:389–399.
14. **Shands, J. W., Jr.** 1971. The physical structure of bacterial lipopolysaccharides, p. 127–144. *In* S. J. Ajl et al. (ed.), Microbial toxins: a comprehensive treatise, vol. 4. Academic Press Inc., New York.
15. **Sippel, A., and G. Hartmann.** 1968. Mode of action of rifampicins on the RNA polymerase reaction. Biochim. Biophys. Acta 157:218–219.
16. **Stinson, M. W., and M. Solotorovsky.** 1971. Interaction of Tween 80 detergent with mycobacteria in synthetic medium. Am. Rev. Respir. Dis. 104:717–727.
17. **Tsukamura, M.** 1972. The pattern of resistance development to rifampin in *Mycobacterium tuberculosis*. Tubercle 53:111–117.
18. **Wehrli, W., F. Knusel, K. Schmid, and M. Staehelin.** 1968. Interaction of rifamycin with bacterial RNA polymerase. Proc. Natl. Acad. Sci. U.S.A. 61:667–673.

19. **Wehrli, W., F. Knusel, and M. Staehelin.** 1968. Action of rifamycin on RNA polymerase from sensitive and resistant bacteria. Biochem. Biophys. Res. Commun. 32:284–288.

20. **White, R. J., G. C. Lancini, and L. G. Silvestri.** 1971. Mechanism of action of rifampin on *Mycobacterium smegmatis*. J. Bacteriol. 108:737–741.

21. **Woodley, C. L., J. O. Kilburn, H. L. David, and V. A. Silcox.** 1972. Susceptibility of mycobacteria to rifampin. Antimicrob. Agents Chemother. 2:245–249.

22. **Youmans, A. D., and G. P. Youmans.** 1954. Studies on the metabolism of Mycobacterium tuberculosis. IV. The effect of fatty acids on the growth of M. tuberculosis var. hominis. J. Bacteriol. 67:731–737.

ANTIMICROBIAL AGENTS AND CHEMOTHERAPY, May 1977, p. 780–784
Copyright © 1977 American Society for Microbiology

Vol. 11, No. 5
Printed in U.S.A.

Amoxicillin Therapy of Acute Urinary Infections in Adults

A. R. RONALD,* F. A. JAGDIS, G. K. M. HARDING, S. A. HOBAN, P. L. MUIR, AND M. J. GURWITH

Departments of Medicine and Medical Microbiology, University of Manitoba, and the Health Sciences Centre, Winnipeg, Manitoba R3E OZ3, Canada*

Received for publication 22 November 1976

Fifty-two patients, 48 females and 4 males, with suspected urinary infection were treated with amoxicillin. Twenty-two females with presumed bladder infection were treated with amoxicillin, 250 mg three times a day for 7 days; 26 females and 4 males with presumed renal infection were treated with amoxicillin, 500 mg three times a day for 14 days. Five patients were immediate treatment failures, with positive urine cultures during therapy. All five patients had been infected with amoxicillin-resistant urinary pathogens. Three patients, treated as for bladder infections, reinfected during 6 weeks of follow-up, and only one relapsed. Two patients, treated as for renal infections, reinfected, whereas four relapsed. During therapy, amoxicillin-susceptible gram-negative rods were eradicated from the periurethral area in all but one patient. Of 28 patients studied, 19 acquired a predominant growth of either resistant aerobic gram-negative rods or *Candida albicans* from periurethral cultures. Our findings suggest that these two regimens of amoxicillin achieve satisfactory cure rates in urinary infection, but both regimens significantly alter the normal periurethral flora.

The hydroxylation of the phenyl side chain of ampicillin has resulted in amoxicillin, a penicillin with an antibacterial spectrum similar to ampicillin but more completely absorbed after oral administration (11). Several studies have reported the use of this agent in the treatment of urinary infection (3, 5, 6, 10). However, the optimal duration and dose of therapy to eradicate infection is undetermined. This report concerns itself with an evaluation of two different regimens in patients with acute urinary infection: (i) a "low-dose" regimen of 250 mg three times a day for 1 week in women with probable bladder infection, and (ii) a "high-dose" regimen of 500 mg three times a day for 2 weeks in patients with probable renal infection.

MATERIALS AND METHODS

Patient selection. Fifty-two adults, 48 females and 4 males, were studied. All patients gave verbal informed consent to be included in the study. Most patients were first seen with acute urinary symptoms at the Emergency Room or Primary Health Care Unit of the Health Sciences Centre, and amoxicillin treatment was begun immediately after urine cultures and periurethral swabs were obtained. No patient was known to have renal calculi or urological disease that would compromise successful therapy with an antimicrobial agent. All the patients had normal renal function, with a serum creatinine of less than 1.5 mg/100 ml. Patients with a previous history of untoward reaction to any of the penicillins were excluded from participation in the study. Pregnant patients were also excluded. Twenty-six females with a history of fever, chills, and flank pain, with costovertebral angle tenderness, symptoms and signs indicative of upper urinary tract infection were given amoxicillin 500 mg three times a day for 14 days; patients without these findings but with frequency, dysuria, and suprapubic pain were given amoxicillin 250 mg three times a day for 7 days. All four male patients had upper urinary tract symptoms and were treated with the high-dose 2-week course. Six women had less acute bladder symptoms and, after two positive urine cultures, their infections were treated as bladder infections with the low-dose one-week regimen.

To assess the immediate response to therapy, patients were requested to return at the end of 1 week of therapy and at 2 and 6 weeks after therapy to determine drug efficacy in the cure of infection. At each visit, the patient was specifically questioned about side effects and symptoms of infection, and a urine culture was obtained.

A modified Fairley bladder wash-out procedure was performed in nine women to localize the site of infection with greater accuracy (2). Unfortunately, most patients had to be treated at the time when they were first seen with acute symptoms, and no localization procedures were carried out.

Collection of specimens. Periurethral specimens were collected at each visit from female patients, with the patient on the examining table in the lithotomy position. A research nurse wearing sterile gloves spread the labia apart exposing the urethral meatus. With a cotton-tipped applicator, a specimen was collected by a circular motion around the entire urethra. The swab was inserted into a screw-capped glass tube containing 5 ml of physiological saline. Finally, a clean, voided midstream urine specimen was collected.

Bacteriological techniques. The tube containing the periurethral swab was blended in a Vortex mixer at high speed for 1 min, and portions of 0.001 and 0.01 ml of the suspension and the urine were inoculated onto sheep blood agar, MacConkey agar, and chocolate agar. After 24 h of incubation at 37°C, colony counts were determined on all organisms isolated from the swab and urine. Susceptibility tests were performed on all urinary pathogens with a single disk diffusion method with an inoculum of 5×10^7 organisms per ml on Mueller-Hinton agar (1). Minimum inhibitory concentrations (MICs) of amoxicillin were determined on Mueller-Hinton agar with the Steers replicator device and an inoculum of 10^6 organisms per ml (8). Susceptible organisms had an MIC of ≤ 50 μg of amoxicillin per ml. Actually, all but one were susceptible to 6.25 μg or less per ml. Resistant organisms were not inhibited by 100 μg of amoxicillin per ml. All *Escherichia coli* isolates from periurethral and urine specimens were serotyped with antisera to the O somatic antigens (4).

Bacteriuria was defined as the presence of more than 100,000 organisms per ml of urine in a single clean, voided midstream urine in 30 patients who developed acute urinary symptoms and by two cultures positive for over 100,000 organisms of the same species in 12 patients with less severe symptoms.

RESULTS

The results of therapy are summarized in Table 1. Nineteen of the 22 females entered in the "low-dose bladder study" had bacterial urinary infection. In retrospect, three patients with symptoms considered to be due to bacterial cystitis had a negative urine culture, and *Trichomonas vaginalis* infection was subsequently found in one and moniliasis was observed in the other two. These patients were then treated appropriately and were not included further in the study. Four of the 19 patients were infected with organisms resistant to amoxicillin. Three of these patients were immediate treatment failures, since the organisms persisted during therapy, and two patients had continuing symptoms. Infection recurred in four patients either during or within 6 weeks of completing amoxicillin therapy. One patient with a *Streptococcus faecalis* urinary infection had a relapse with the same organism within 1 week after therapy. Three patients reinfected, each with an organism resistant to amoxicillin. Six weeks after completion of low-dose amoxicillin therapy, 11 of the 19 patients were free of bacteriuria without additional therapy. Of the 15 patients infected with susceptible organisms, 11 (73%) were cured at 6 weeks.

Six patients in the low-dose study group had untoward effects. Two patients developed symptomatic moniliasis, and four had mild gastrointestinal symptoms. However, none of these patients discontinued therapy.

After initial evaluation, 26 female patients were entered into the study under the upper tract infection category and were treated with 2 weeks of amoxicillin, 500 mg three times a day. Unfortunately, seven of these patients had negative cultures. This included two patients who, in retrospect, were seen to be ill with acute pelvic inflammatory disease. In one, *Neisseria*

TABLE 1. *Summary of amoxicillin therapy in urinary infection in females*

Determination	Lower tract infection: amoxicillin, 250 mg three times a day for 7 days	Upper tract infection: amoxicillin, 500 mg three times a day for 14 days
No. of symptomatic patients entering the study	22	26
No. with bacteriuria	19	19
Infecting organism		
E. coli	15	11
Klebsiella sp.	0	1
Enterobacter sp.	0	1
Proteus mirabilis	0	2
Group D streptococci	2	1
Group B streptococci	1	1
Staphlyococcus epidermidis	1	2
Results of therapy		
Immediate failures[a]	3	2
Reinfections[b]		
During therapy	1	0
Within 6 weeks	2	2
Relapses[c]	1	4
Cures at 6 weeks	11	6
Inadequate follow-up	1	5
Untoward effects		
Rash	0	1
Moniliasis	2	3
Gastrointestinal intolerance	4	1

[a] Failure is defined as a positive culture during therapy for the same pretherapy infecting pathogen. All failures were due to organisms which had an amoxicillin MIC of ≥ 100 μg/ml prior to therapy.

[b] Reinfection is defined as the appearance of a new species or a different serotype of *E. coli*.

[c] Relapse is defined as the recurrence of the same species or serotype of *E. coli* within 2 weeks of completing therapy.

gonorrhoeae was isolated from a cervical culture. Both patients improved on amoxicillin but are not included in the evaluation of therapeutic efficacy. No specific diagnoses were made in the other five patients to account for their symptoms. Five of these 19 patients had upper tract infection by the bladder wash-out technique. Two of the 19 were infected with amoxicillin-resistant organisms, and in both instances the organism persisted during therapy. Five patients who initially responded to therapy, with negative urine cultures during therapy, failed to return for follow-up. Of the 12 patients with susceptible organisms who did return, four relapsed within 2 weeks of completing therapy with the initial infecting organism. In three of these patients, *E. coli*, and, in one, *Proteus mirabilis*, was the infecting pathogen. After relapse, two of these four patients were given a 6-week course of amoxicillin, 1.5 g/day. One was cured with this course of therapy and one again had a relapse with the same serotype of *E. coli*. Two patients reinfected with an amoxicillin-resistant *Klebsiella* sp. during the 6 weeks of follow-up. Of the 14 females with adequate follow-up, initially treated with 2 weeks of amoxicillin, 500 mg three times a day, six were free of bacteriuria without additional therapy at 6 weeks after completion of therapy.

All patients with amoxicillin-susceptible organisms responded satisfactorily to therapy, with rapid improvement in upper tract symptoms. Five patients with an elevated temperature at the onset of therapy became afebrile within 48 h.

Five patients had side effects on the high-dose regimen. One patient had urticaria, one had severe nausea and vomiting with epigastric distress, two had vulvar pruritis, and one noted soft stools. The patient with urticaria and the patient with epigastric distress both discontinued taking amoxicillin before completion of therapy.

Four male patients with amoxicillin-susceptible *E. coli* urinary infection were treated for 14 days with 500 mg three times a day. All four tolerated the medication well and had negative urine cultures during therapy. After discontinuation of therapy, two patients relapsed with their initial infecting strain, and two remained free of infection during 6 weeks of follow-up.

Organisms resistant to ampicillin, as determined by the Bauer-Kirby (1) high-content single disk diffusion technique, had an amoxicillin MIC of 50 μg or more per ml. Five of the six patients with amoxicillin-resistant organisms in this study had persistent positive cultures during therapy and were immediate therapeutic failures.

Paired periurethral swabs were obtained before treatment and at the completion of therapy from 28 patients. Eight of 15 treated with the low-dose regimen and 5 of 13 treated with the high-dose regimen had positive periurethral cultures before therapy, with the same gram-negative rod present in the voided urine culture.

Table 2 summarizes the results of the periurethral swabs at the completion of therapy. In every instance, susceptible *Enterobacteriaceae* disappeared from the perineum during high-dose therapy and persisted in only one patient during low-dose therapy. Eight of the 15 patients on the low-dose regimen acquired amoxicillin-resistant enteric pathogens or *C. albicans*. Two patients acquired resistant *E. coli*, and four acquired resistant *Klebsiella* sp. Eleven of the 13 patients on the high-dose regimen were colonized during therapy with resistant gram-negative organisms. The amoxicillin-resistant organisms appearing during therapy always differed in either species or serotype from the pretherapy susceptible periurethral organisms. All five patients who reinfected during or within 6 weeks of completion of therapy became reinfected with amoxicillin-resistant organisms present on periurethral cultures at the time of or before their recurrence.

DISCUSSION

This study confirms the efficacy of amoxicillin in the treatment of urinary infection in females infected with susceptible organisms. The patient population in this study consisted, for the most part, of acutely symptomatic, healthy females with normal renal function and no underlying urological disease. Although localization of infection on clinical criteria is fraught with error, we have found that 78% of women with upper tract symptoms have organisms emanating from their upper tracts (2). Localization by the bladder wash-out technique cannot be carried out routinely in acutely ill patients, and the test for the detection of antibody-coated bacteria (9) only became available in our hospital after this study was completed. Most acutely ill patients are treated for renal or bladder infection solely on the basis of clinical parameters.

Earlier studies from this center have shown that a short therapeutic regimen is adequate to cure proven bladder infections in the majority of females (7). In this study, a 1-week low-dose oral amoxicillin regimen eradicated the infection in 13 of 14 patients with susceptible patho-

TABLE 2. *Enterobacterial and candidal periurethral colonization during amoxicillin therapy*

Determination	Amoxicillin dose (three times a day)	
	250 mg for 7 days	500 mg for 14 days
No enterobacterial or candidal colonization prior to or during therapy	3	1
Periurethral culture negative pretherapy but positive during therapy with resistant *Enterobacteriaceae* or *Candida*	4	7
Resistant *E. coli*	1	2
Resistant *Klebsiella* sp.	1	3
Resistant *Klebsiella* sp. and *C. albicans*	1	1
C. albicans	1	1
Periurethral culture positive for susceptible *Enterobacteriaceae* pretherapy which were eliminated and replaced with resistant organisms	4	4
Resistant *E. coli*	1	1
Resistant *E. coli* and *Klebsiella* sp.	0	2
Resistant *Klebsiella* sp.	2	1
C. albicans	1	0
Periurethral culture positive for *Enterobacteriaceae* pretherapy which were eliminated and not replaced	2	0
Susceptible *Enterobacteriaceae* present before therapy persisted throughout therapy	1	0
Resistant *Enterobacteriaceae* present before therapy persisted throughout therapy	1	1

gens and presumed bladder infections. A longer duration or a higher dose of amoxicillin would not have provided any additional benefit to these 13 patients.

A two-week course of 1.5 g of amoxicillin per day eradicated infection in 8 of 12 adequately followed patients who were infected with susceptible strains that were presumed to originate in the upper urinary tract. It is our impression from ongoing studies that about 75% of patients with acute uncomplicated upper tract infection are cured by a 2-week course of an oral antimicrobial agent if the infecting organism is susceptible and cultures during therapy are negative. The numbers are too small in the present group to conclude that amoxicillin differs from other oral agents.

Four of the 48 women treated with amoxicillin complained of vulvar pruritis, and in every instance. *C. albicans* was present on culture. One patient developed an urticarial rash, one had severe epigastric distress, and five noted soft, frequent stools. Without careful double-blind prospective studies, this level of drug intolerance cannot be said to be different from that associated with ampicillin.

Although superinfection with resistant organisms is a recognized complication of antimicrobial chemotherapy, only recently has their role in predisposing the urinary tract to resistant reinfections received serious study. Alteration of the colonic and periurethral flora precedes recurrence with resistant organisms (12). An optimal therapeutic regimen should cure the target infection with little disruption of bacterial ecology. We hypothesized that low-dose therapy for 1 week with a well-absorbed oral antimicrobial agent excreted unchanged in the urine would cure bladder infections without altering periurethral flora. Although amoxicillin eradicated the infection in 13 of 14 women with susceptible pathogens and lower tract symptoms, it altered the periurethral flora and predisposed to reinfections with resistant *Enterobacteriaceae*. Further studies with smaller doses and shorter duration are needed to determine optimal therapy for bladder infections in women.

ACKNOWLEDGMENTS

This investigation was supported by a grant from Ayerst Laboratories, Division of Ayerst, McKenna, and Harrison Limited, and by the Medical Research Council of Canada, no. MA-3065.

LITERATURE CITED

1. **Bauer, A. W., W. M. M. Kirby, J. C. Sherris, and M. Turck.** 1966. Antibiotic susceptibility testing by a standardized single disc method. Am. J. Clin. Pathol. 45:593–596.
2. **Boutros, P., H. Mourtada, and A. R. Ronald.** 1972. Urinary infection localization. Am. J. Obstet. Gynecol. 112:379–381.
3. **Charlton, C. A. C., A. Crowther, J. G. Davies, M. W. A. Haward, P. G. Mann, and S. Rye.** 1976. Three-day

and ten-day chemotherapy for urinary tract infections in general practice. Br. Med. J. 1:124–126.

4. **Edwards, P. R., and W. H. Ewing.** 1972. Differentiation of Enterobacteriaceae by biochemical reactions, p. 21–47. *In* W. H. Ewing (ed.), Identification of Enterobacteriaceae, 3rd ed. Burgess Publishing Co., Minneapolis.
5. **Gilbert, D. N.** 1974. Comparison of amoxicillin and ampicillin in the treatment of urinary tract infections. J. Infect. Dis. 129:S231–S234.
6. **Miller, G. B., Jr., R. J. Duma, F. G. Middleton, and D. M. Poretz.** 1974. The use of amoxicillin in the treatment of urinary tract infections. J. Infect. Dis. 129:S237–S240.
7. **Ronald, A. R., P. Boutros, and H. Mourtada.** 1976. A simple therapeutic test to diagnose upper urinary tract infection in women with bacteriuria. J. Am. Med. Assoc. 235:1854–1856.
8. **Steers, E., E. F. Foltz, and B. S. Graves.** 1959. An inocula replicating apparatus for routine testing of bacterial susceptibility to antibiotics. Antibiot. Chemother. 9:307–311.
9. **Thomas, T., A. Shelokov, and M. Forland.** 1974. Antibody-coated bacteria in the urine and the site of urinary tract infection. N. Engl. J. Med. 290:588–591.
10. **Turck, M., H. H. Ennsfield, and K. K. Homes.** 1974. Amoxicillin in the treatment of urinary tract infections. J. Infect. Dis. 129:S248–S249.
11. **Vitti, T. G., M. J. Gurwith, and A. R. Ronald.** 1974. Pharmacologic studies of amoxicillin in non-fasting adults. J. Infect. Dis. 129:S149–S153.
12. **Winberg, J., T. Bergstrom, K. Lincoln, and G. Liden-Jonson.** 1973. Treatment trials in urinary tract infection with special reference to the effect of antimicrobials on the fecal and periurethral flora. Clin. Nephrol. 1:142–148.

ANTIMICROBIAL AGENTS AND CHEMOTHERAPY, May 1977, p. 785–790
Vol. 11, No. 5

Beta-Lactamases Produced by a *Pseudomonas aeruginosa* Strain Highly Resistant to Carbenicillin

ROGER LABIA,* MARLÈNE GUIONIE, JEAN-MICHEL MASSON, ALAIN PHILIPPON, AND MICHEL BARTHELEMY

CERCOA-CNRS, 94320 Thiais, France, and Service de Bactériologie CHU Cochin, 75674 Paris, cédex 14, France*

Received for publication 18 November 1976

A *Pseudomonas aeruginosa* strain isolated at Besançon Hospital, France, proved to be highly resistant to carbenicillin and showed a high hydrolytic activity toward this antibiotic. We clearly demonstrated that two β-lactamases were synthetized: one of them, constitutive, has its enzymatic activity directed mainly toward penicillins, and carbenicillin appears to be its best substrate (higher V_{max}); thus, this β-lactamase is a "carbenicillinase" that differs from the well-known "TEM-like" enzymes. The isoelectric point of this carbenicillinase is 5.30 ± 0.03. The other one is an inducible cephalosporinase, very similar to the cephalosporinases usually found in these organisms. Its isoelectric point is 8.66 ± 0.04. These two enzymes have been separated by affinity chromatography and isoelectric focusing. The kinetic constants were measured by computerized microacidimetry.

Pseudomonas aeruginosa resistance to cephalosporins is usually interpreted as the result of the biosynthesis by the bacteria of β-lactamase active toward these antibiotics, an inducible cephalosporinase (29) that seems to be chromosally mediated. As carbenicillin is not a substrate for this enzyme (28, 29), usually *P. aeruginosa* strains are susceptible to this antibiotic, but very early some strains appear to be resistant (2, 9).

P. aeruginosa resistance to carbenicillin is a complex problem: bacterial strains resistant to this antibiotic are frequently encountered, but they do not necessarily show any hydrolytic activity toward this molecule. In these cases, carbenicillin resistance might be related to permeability modifications of the cell wall (1, 14).

Some strains were described where a low hydrolytic activity toward carbenicillin had been shown. This activity did not seem to have much physiological meaning (29).

In 1970 (22), for the first time *P. aeruginosa* strain (Dalgleish) was described that showed an unusually high hydrolytic activity against carbenicillin. A few years later, the enzyme produced by this strain was subjected to more sophisticated investigations (6).

Then the presence of R-factor-determined β-lactamases, active toward carbenicillin, was proved by transfer from *P. aeruginosa* to *Escherichia coli* (5) (31). Transfer occurred with a higher frequency when the recipient strain was another *P. aeruginosa* (3, 8). Some plasmids were isolated (4, 7).

In France (17) a TEM β-lactamase with pI = 5.4 was identified in a *P. aeruginosa* strain. This enzyme is similar to the type I described by Pitton (26).

In this paper, we study a new *P. aeruginosa* strain presenting a high hydrolytic activity toward carbenicillin. This strain has already been subjected to preliminary studies (21).

MATERIALS AND METHODS

Bacterial strain. *P. aeruginosa* strain HL was isolated by Michel Briand at the bacteriology service of Besancon Hospital, France. The carbenicillin minimal inhibitory concentration was approximately 4,000 μg/ml.

Enzymatic extract. To detect the presence of constitutive and/or inducible β-lactamases, uninduced cultures and cultures induced by up to 5 mg of penicillin G per ml added at the last 3 h of exponential phase were used, as described previously (14).

Determination of kinetic constants. Kinetic constants (K_m and V_{max}) were measured by the computerized microacidimetric method (11, 16) with a Mettler pH meter and a Wang 600 computer. Affinity constants (K_m) are given in micromolar concentrations, whereas the V_{max} values are expressed as a percentage of penicillin G maximum rate of hydrolysis.

Enzymatic stability $\tau = K_m/V_{max}$, which reflects the half-life of antibiotics at a low concentration, was also determined for each substrate and expressed as a percentage of enzymatic stability for penicillin G (10).

Enzymatic units. It is convenient to define the β-lactamase unit as the quantity of the enzyme that hydrolyzes 1 μmol of penicillin G per min at pH 7 and 37°C. This unit is almost similar, but not identical, to the one defined by Novick (23). An estimate of total protein concentration was measured either directly by ultraviolet spectrophotometry at 280 nm for concentrated solutions or by the classical Lowry method for diluted solutions. In each case bovine serum albumin was the standard. The specific activity of a bacterial extract is expressed as the number of β-lactamase units per milligram of total protein.

Preparative isoelectric focusing. Preparative isoelectric focusing in sucrose gradients was performed with an LKB 8100 system according to the instructions of the manufacturer, with ampholines of pH range 3.5 to 10 or 4 to 6.

Analytical isoelectric focusing. Analytical isoelectric focusing on polyacrylamide gel sheets was performed with a procedure similar to that of Matthew et al. (19). β-Lactamase revelation was performed with an agar overlay gel containing starch-iodine and penicillin G, as described previously (12). Thus, Fig. 3 is shown as a negative. The samples (20 μl) were applied near the cathode as drops of liquid on the surface of the gel.

Affinity chromatography. For affinity chromatography, Indubiose 4A (Industrie Biologique Française) (100 ml of hydrated form) activated by cyanogen bromide was used, and then cephalosporin C was bound to this activated resin (17). After exhaustive washing of the column with distilled water, the crude enzymatic extract (2 ml) was eluted with a sodium chloride gradient from 0.01 to 2 M.

RESULTS

Enzymatic extracts obtained from uninduced cultures showed a high β-lactamase activity, i.e., 800 to 900 mU/mg of total protein (crude extracts), when measured with penicillin G as substrate. Isoelectric focusing with ampholines of a pH range of 3.5 to 10 gave a single peak of β-lactamase, with a pI of 5.4. This pI can be measured more accurately with ampholines of a pH range of 4 to 6 and was finally found at pH 5.30 ± 0.03.

Table 1 is a summary of the kinetic constants of the enzyme, K_m, V_{max} and τ, at pH 7 and 37°C for 13 β-lactam antibiotics, including carbenicillin and two "carbenicillin-like" compounds, ticarcillin and sulbenicillin. This β-lactamase showed a very low hydrolytic activity toward all the cephalosporins tested, i.e., a very low V_{max} and a high K_m (bad affinity). We therefore looked for a possible inducible cephalosporinase.

Enzymatic extracts prepared from cultures induced with 500 μg of penicillin G per ml showed no significant difference as compared with the first extracts. It was only with penicillin G concentrations as high as 5,000 μg/ml that we induced a good cephalosporinase activity: the specific activity of that cephalosporinase being about 15% of the penicillinase activity (both measured with penicillin G as substrate). We then undertook the separation of these two enzymes by affinity chromatography and isoelectric focusing.

Affinity chromatography. Elution of extracts obtained with highly induced cultures (5 mg of penicillin G per ml) gave two peaks of enzymatic activity (Fig. 1); the enzyme eluted first showed little affinity for the column and is therefore little purified.

Elution with NaCl >0.5 M was needed to obtain the second peak of enzymatic activity, and the enzyme purification was approximately a 100-fold.

Isoelectric focusing of the fractions corresponding to the two peaks gave, respectively,

TABLE 1. *Kinetic constants of the constitutive carbenicillinase from P. aeruginosa strain HL*

Antibiotic	K_m (μM)	V_{max} (relative)[a]	τ (relative)[a]
Penicillin G	11.1	100	100
Penicillin V	9.7	98	89
Ampicillin	20.1	148	122
Amoxicillin	17.0	54	285
Epicillin	33	187	159
Carbenicillin	196	282	626
Ticarcillin	34	104	295
Sulbenicillin	23	88	235
Cephalothin	46	1.1	37,700
Cephaloridine	395	28	12,700
Cephalexin	Very low hydrolysis, if any		
Cefazolin	222	4.5	42,500

[a] Values are expressed as a percentage of the corresponding values for penicillin G.

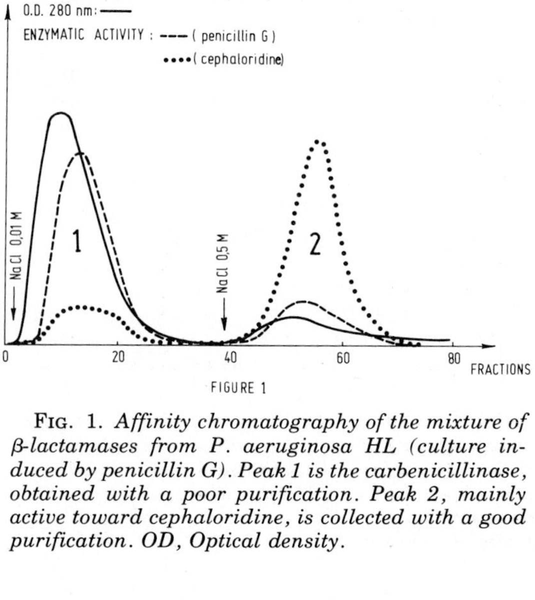

FIG. 1. *Affinity chromatography of the mixture of β-lactamases from P. aeruginosa HL (culture induced by penicillin G). Peak 1 is the carbenicillinase, obtained with a poor purification. Peak 2, mainly active toward cephaloridine, is collected with a good purification. OD, Optical density.*

one band at pH 5.30 for peak 1 and one band at pH 8.66 for peak 2. The two fractions were, thus, not contaminated by each other.

Isoelectric focusing. Preparative isoelectric focusing in sucrose gradients of the crude enzymatic extract (induced by penicillin G) was in good agreement with the preceeding results; it also gave two peaks of enzymatic activity at pH 5.30 and 8.66 (Fig. 2). Analytical isoelectric focusing on polyacrylamide gels gave the same results (Fig. 3).

The fractions obtained from affinity chromatography or preparative isoelectric focusing were suitable for kinetic studies, particularly for the inducible cephalosporinase that must be separated from the constitutive carbenicillinase.

The kinetic constants of the inducible cephalosporinase are given in Table 2; these data and also analytical isoelectric focusing show that this cephalosporinase is very similar to type C (13). This enzyme gives very low, if any, hydrolysis of the ampicillin and carbenicillin groups. The K_i values were measured for ampicillin (K_i = 0.3 μM), carbenicillin (K_i = 0.02 μM), and cloxacillin (K_i = 0.002 μM).

DISCUSSION

P. aeruginosa strain HL produces two lactamases. One of them is a constitutive β-lactamase (pI = 5.30) biosynthetized at a fairly high level, with a specific activity reaching 800 to 900 mU/mg (crude preparation). Kinetic constants (Table 1) show a very good hydrolytic activity against the eight penicillins tested, but a very poor activity against the cephalosporins. Carbenicillin is the antibiotic hydrolyzed at the higher rate, and this enzyme could be named "carbenicillinase."

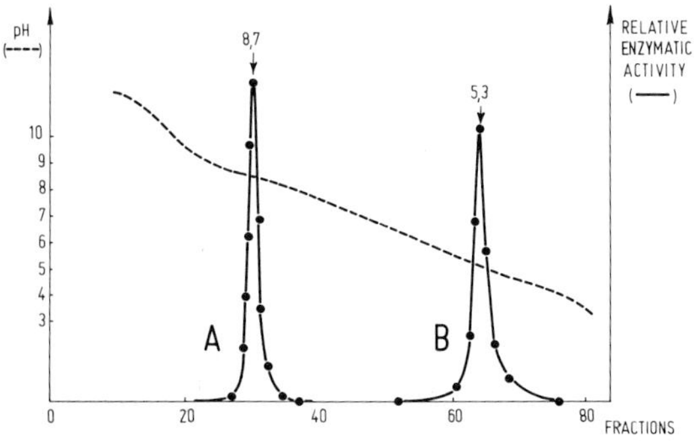

FIG. 2. *Isoelectric focusing of the β-lactamase mixture (crude extracts from culture induced by penicillin G) clearly shows two peaks, peak A (pI then precises at about 8.66) being the cephalosporinase and peak B (pI = 5.30) the carbenicillinase. Enzymatic activity was detected with cephaloridine.*

We previously studied in our laboratory *P. aeruginosa* strain MAR (17), which produced another constitutive penicillinase at a lower level (90 to 100 mU/mg), but showed a very similar isoelectric point of 5.40. This last enzyme had the same pI and kinetic constants as those of the extrachromosomic β-lactamase

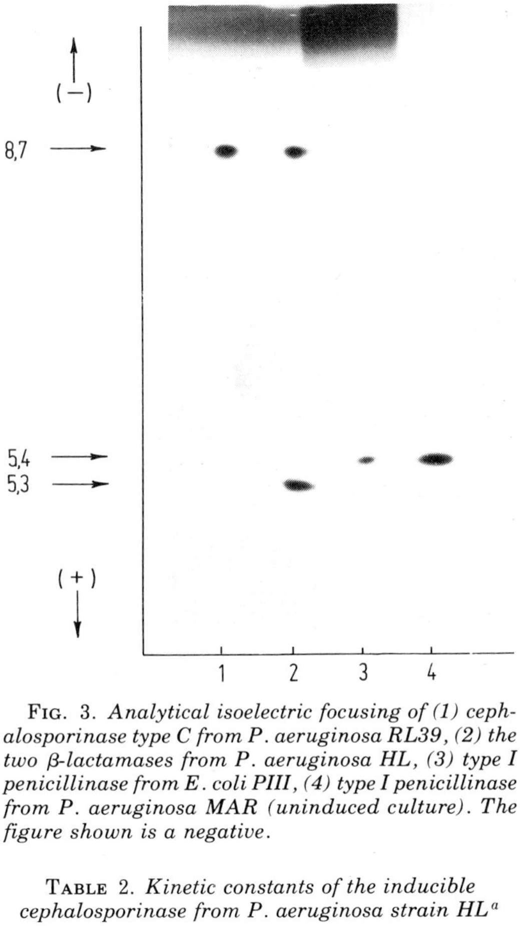

FIG. 3. *Analytical isoelectric focusing of (1) cephalosporinase type C from P. aeruginosa RL39, (2) the two β-lactamases from P. aeruginosa HL, (3) type I penicillinase from E. coli PIII, (4) type I penicillinase from P. aeruginosa MAR (uninduced culture). The figure shown is a negative.*

TABLE 2. *Kinetic constants of the inducible cephalosporinase from P. aeruginosa strain HL*[a]

Antibiotic	K_m (μM)	V_{max} (relative)	τ (relative)
Penicillin G	1.0	100	100
Penicillin V	0.9	60	150
Ampicillin	K_i = 0.3		
Amoxicillin	Low hydrolysis, if any		
Epicillin	Low hydrolysis, if any		
Carbenicillin	Low hydrolysis, if any	(K_i = 0.02 μM)	
Ticarcillin	Low hydrolysis, if any		
Sulbenicillin	Low hydrolysis, if any		
Cephalothin	40	800	500
Cephaloridine	60	540	1,100
Cephalexin	3	30	1,000
Cefazolin	400	6,500	615
Cefamandole	3	4	7,500

[a] Ampicillin and carbenicillin were tested as inhibitors, with penicillin G as substrate.

type I produced by *Escherichia coli* P111 (15, 26), which was also indistinguishable from the well-known R-TEM penicillinase. These are enzymes from class III of Richmond and Sykes (27).

It was possible to study the two β-lactamases from the two *P. aeruginosa* strains HL and MAR by the same techniques in our laboratory, and these two enzymes appear to be clearly different. First, analytical isoelectric focusing showed a clear reproducible difference between β-lactamases HL and MAR (Fig. 3). Another interesting difference was shown in the kinetic constants (K_m and V_{max}) (Tables 1 and 3, essentially with carbenicillin, ticarcillin, sulbenicillin, cephalothin, and cephaloridine. Despite these differences, we can see that the parameter $\tau = K_m/V_{max}$, corresponding to the half-life of the antibiotic at a "low" concentration, is very similar. For example, with HL carbenicillinase, carbenicillin gives $\tau = 626$, and with type I penicillinase $\tau = 450$.

The constitutive β-lactamase of the HL strain looks a little like the one of the Dalgleish strain (6), especially its "profile" defined with maximum rates. But it is very different when the K_m values are considered, which were measured with different techniques: computerized microacidimetry (11) for the HL strain and microiodometry (25) for the Dalgleish strain. The results of Furth (6) unfortunately lack precision concerning the pI of the enzyme she studied, but the value given (5.0 to 5.5) is of the same order as ours. These two enzymes could belong to class Vd of Richmond and Sykes (27).

Table 4 gives some characteristics of a few β-lactamases with high activity against penicillin G (and ampicillin) and low, if any, action against oxacillin and cloxacillin; all of them are constitutive. The TEM-1 β-lactamase (pI = 5.4) is produced by many bacteria, such as *P. aeruginosa* MAR (17) or *E. coli* Rms212 (= R-GN14) (30, 33), and is similar to type I of Pitton (15, 26). A common characteristic of the enzymes of Table 4 is the isoelectric point, which ranges from 5.0 to 5.7. Only one penicillinase, type II of Pitton (15, 26), shows a very different pI, 7.7. Most of these enzymes appear to be R-factor mediated.

Based on the relative rate of carbenicillin hydrolysis, the enzymes from Table 4 may be classified into two groups. One group gives high hydrolysis of carbenicillin (Rms139, Dalgleish, and HL), and the other gives a low hydrolysis (Rms165, RP4, TEM-1, and type II). These values for βL75 are not given (24).

P. aeruginosa HL extracts from cultures induced with 5,000 μg of penicillin G per ml show the presence of an inducible β-lactamase.

One needs to observe that the concentration of inducer needed in this case is much higher than the one used for the cephalosporinase from *P. aeruginosa* MAR (17). This might be related to the fact that the constitutive carbenicillinase of the HL strain is produced at a much higher level than the R-TEM β-lactamase and then destroys the inducer more rapidly.

The induced β-lactamase from the HL strain has a pI of 8.66. The kinetic constants show that it has a good activity toward cephalosporins and a lower one toward penicillins G and V (Table 2). It is therefore a cephalosporinase, with kinetic characteristics very similar to the ones of enzymes already described. To us, this

TABLE 3. *Kinetic constants of the extrachromosomic β-lactamase TEM-1 obtained from P. aeruginosa MAR*

Antibiotic	K_m (μM)	V_{max} (relative)	τ (relative)
Penicillin G	21	100	100
Penicillin V	11.5	59	93
Ampicillin	31.3	94	159
Amoxicillin	24.9	78	152
Epicillin	43.8	127	164
Carbenicillin	10.0	10.6	450
Ticarcillin	9.7	9.6	481
Sulbenicillin	7.4	4.5	783
Cephalothin	230	10	10,900
Cephaloridine	950	170	2,700
Cephalexin	170	0.33	2.5×10^5
Cephradine	115	0.26	2.1×10^5

TABLE 4. *Comparison of some β-lactamases from literature data and the constitutive carbenicillinase produced by P. aeruginosa HL*[a]

Enzyme, bacterial strain, or reference	pI	Penicillin G K_m (μM)	Carbenicillin	
			K_m (μM)	V_{max} (relative)
Dalgleish (6, 22)	5–5.5 (imprecise)	1	2	150
Rms139 (30)	5.7	15	40	110
HL (this paper)	5.30	11.1	196	282
Rms165 (30)	5.25	50	8	10
RP4 (= RP1) (TEM-2)	5.5 (reference 30) Corrected: 5.6 (references 19 and 20)	10	5	9
TEM-1 β-lactamase	5.4	21	10	10
βL75 (24)	5.26	42.8		
Type II (26) (15)	7.7	10.6	6	9

[a] In the case of βL75, the values for carbenicillin are not published. All of them are constitutive.

TABLE 5. *Comparison of a few cephalosporinases from literature data and the inducible cephalosporinase from P. aeruginosa HL*

Enzyme or strain (reference)	pI	Cephalothin K_m (μM)	Cephaloridine K_m (μM)	Penicillin G K_m (μM)	Cloxacillin K_i (μM)
Strain NCTC 8203 (1, 29)	7.5 (reference 18)	450	130	13	0.03
Bobrowski et al. (1)			400		0.18
Yaginuma et al. (32)	8.7	132	156	12	0.023
Type A (16)	9.2	41	51	2.4	0.015
Type B (16)	6.67	8.5	19.8	0.9	0.003
HL and type C (13)	8.66	40	60	1	0.002

cephalosporinase appears to be identical (pI, K_m, V_{max}) to our type C cephalosporinase (13).

Table 5 is a comparison of the five cephalosporinases already known with the one identified in the HL strain. The pI of the type C cephalosporinase is the same as the pI of the cephalosporinase produced by the GN918 strain (32). These two cephalosporinases might be identical; at any rate, they present strong analogies. The pI of the enzyme from strain NCTC 8203 has been measured recently and is different, i.e., 7.5 (18). It can also be observed in Table 2 that the pI values of cephalosporinases from *P. aeruginosa* are mainly basic (Table 4). All of these cephalosporinases belong to the Id group defined by Richmond and Sykes (27).

ACKNOWLEDGMENTS

We thank Y. Michel-Briand for generously providing the *P. aeruginosa* HL strain.

LITERATURE CITED

1. **Bobrowski, M., and E. Borowski.** 1971. Interaction between carbenicillin and β lactamases from Gram negative bacteria. J. Gen. Microbiol. 68:263–272.
2. **Brumfitt, W., A. Percival, and D. A. Leigh.** 1967. Clinical and laboratory studies with carbenicillin, a new penicillin active against *Ps. pyocyanea*. Lancet i:1289–1293.
3. **Bryan, L. E., H. M. Van Den Elzen, and Jui Teng-Tseng.** 1972. Transferable drug resistance in *Pseudomonas aeruginosa*. Antimicrob. Agents Chemother. 1:22–29.
4. **Datta, N., R. W. Hedges, E. Shaw, R. B. Sykes, and M. H. Richmond.** 1972. Properties of an R factor from *Pseudomonas aeruginosa*. J. Bacteriol. **108**:1244–1249.
5. **Fullbrook, P. D., S. W. Elson, and G. T. Slocombe.** 1970. R-factor mediated β-lactamase in *Pseudomonas aeruginosa*. Nature (London) **226**:1054–1056.
6. **Furth, A. J.** 1975. Purification and properties of a constitutive β-lactamase from *Pseudomonas aeruginosa* strain Dalgleish. Biochim. Biophys. Acta 377:431–443.
7. **Ingram, L. C., M. H. Richmond, and R. B. Sykes.** 1973. Molecular characterization of the R factors implicated in the carbenicillin resistance of a sequence of *Pseudomonas aeruginosa* strains isolated from burns. Antimicrob. Agents Chemother. 3:279–288.
8. **Iyobe, S., K. Hasuda, A. Fuse, and S. Mitsuashi.** 1974. Demonstration of R factors from *Pseudomonas aeruginosa*. Antimicrob. Agents Chemother. 5:547–552.
9. **Jones, R. M., and E. J. L. Lowbury.** 1967. Prophylaxis and therapy for *Pseudomonas aeruginosa* with carbenicillin and with gentamicin. Br. Med. J. **III:** 79–92.
10. **Labia, R.** 1974. Comportement enzyme-substrat, introduction de la notion de stabilité enzymatique dans le case des β lactamases. C.R. Acad. Sci. Ser. D **279**:109–112.
11. **Labia, R., J. Andrillon, and F. Le Goffic.** 1973. Computerized microacidimetric determination of a β lactamase Michaelis Menten constant. FEBS Lett. 33:42–44.
12. **Labia, R., M. Barthelemy, and J. M. Masson.** 1976. Multiplicité des β lactamases: un problème d'isoenzymes? C.R. Acad. Sci. Ser. D **283**:1597–1600.
13. **Labia, R., C. Fabre, and M. Guionie.** 1976. Etude cinétique d'une nouvelle céphalosporinase de *Ps. aeruginosa*. Biochimie 58:913–915.
14. **Labia, R., A. Kazmierczak, A. Philippon, F. Le Goffic, J. C. Faye, F. W. Golstein, and J. F. Acar.** 1975. β lactamases de *Pseudomonas aeruginosa* et résistance à la carbenicilline. Ann. Microbiol. (Paris) **126A**:449–459.
15. **Labia, R., F. Le Goffic, and J. Andrillon.** 1974. Etude cinétique de deux β lactamases responsables d'un même phenotype. Biochime **56**:1025–1030.
16. **Labia, R., F. Le Goffic, J. C. Faye, and A. Philippon.** 1974. Deux cephalosporinases de *Pseudomonas aeruginosa*. Biochimie **56**:1333–1337.
17. **Labia, R., A. Philippon, F. Le Goffic, and J. C. Faye.** 1975. Identification de la β lactamase R-TEM chez le *Pseudomonas aeruginosa*. Biochimie **57**:139–143.
18. **McPhail, M., and A. J. Furth.** 1973. Purification and properties of an inducible β-lactamase from *Pseudomonas aeruginosa* NCTC 8203. Biochem. Soc. Trans. 1:260–263.
19. **Matthew, M., A. M. Harris, M. J. Marshall, and G. W. Ross.** 1975. The use of analytical isoelectric focusing for detection and identification of β lactamases. J. Gen. Microbiol. 88:169–178.
20. **Matthew, M., and R. W. Hedges.** 1976. Analytical isoelectric focusing of R factor-determined β-lactamases: correlation with plasmid compatibility. J. Bacteriol. **125**:713–718.
21. **Michel-Briand, Y., and L. Bruant.** 1972. Etude de la production de β lactamase pour la carbenicilline chez trente souches de *Pseudomonas aeruginosa* (mise en évidence d'une souche hautement résistante). C.R. Acad. Sci. Ser. D. **275**:503–506.
22. **Newson, S. W. B., R. B. Sykes, and M. H. Richmond.** 1970. Detection of a β-lactamase markedly active against carbenicillin in a strain of *Pseudomonas aeruginosa*. J. Bacteriol. **101**:1079–1080.
23. **Novick, R. P.** 1962. Micro-iodometric assay for penicillinase. Biochem. J. **83**:236–240.
24. **Ogawara, H., K. Maeda, and H. Umezawa.** 1972. A β-lactamase of *Escherichia coli*. Biochim. Biophys. Acta **289**:203–211.

25. **Perret, J. C.** 1954. Iodometric assay of penicillinase. Nature (London) **174**:1012–1013.
26. **Pitton, J. S.** 1973. β-lactamase à dépendance plasmidique chez les enterobactériacées. Pathol. Microbiol. **39**:3.
27. **Richmond, M. H., and R. B. Sykes.** 1973. The β lactamases of gram-negative bacteria and their possible physiological role. Adv. Microb. Physiol. **9**:31–88.
28. **Sabath, L. D., and M. Finland.** 1967. Resistance of penicillins and cephalosporins to beta lactamases from gram negative bacilli: some correlation with antibacterial activity. Ann. N.Y. Acad. Sci. **145**:237–247.
29. **Sabath, L. D., M. Jago, and E. P. Abraham.** 1965. Cephalosporinase and penicillinase activities of a β lactamase from *Pseudomonas pyocyanea*. Biochem. J. **96**:739–752.
30. **Sawada, Y., S. Yaginuma, M. Tai, S. Iyobe, and S. Mitsuhashi.** 1976. Plasmid-mediated penicillin beta-lactamases in *Pseudomonas aeruginosa*. Antimicrob. Agents Chemother. **9**:55–60.
31. **Sykes, R. B., and M. H. Richmond.** 1970. Intergeneric transfer of a β lactamase gene between *Ps. aeruginosa* and *E. coli*. Nature (London) **226**:952–954.
32. **Yaginuma, S., T. Sawai, H. Ono, S. Yamagishi, and S. Mitsuhashi.** 1973. Biochemical properties of a cephalosporin β lactamase from *Pseudomonas aeruginosa*. Jpn. J. Microbiol. **17**:141–149.
33. **Yamagishi, S., K. O'Hara, T. Sawai, and S. Mitsuhashi.** 1969. The purification and properties of penicillin β lactamases mediated by transmissible R-factors in *Escherichia coli*. J. Biochem. **66**:11–20.

ANTIMICROBIAL AGENTS AND CHEMOTHERAPY, May 1977, p. 791-796
Vol. 11, No. 5

In Vitro Activity of Netilmicin Compared with Gentamicin, Tobramycin, Amikacin, and Kanamycin

THEODORE C. EICKHOFF* AND JOSEPHINE M. EHRET

Division of Infectious Disease, Department of Medicine, University of Colorado Medical Center, Denver, Colorado 80262

Received for publication 23 August 1976

The in vitro activity of netilmicin was compared with that of gentamicin, tobramycin, amikacin, and kanamycin against 636 strains of bacteria recently isolated from clinical sources. Gentamicin was the most active antibiotic, but netilmicin and tobramycin closely paralleled it. Netilmicin was generally four- to eightfold less active than gentamicin against *Serratia* and group A streptococci, and was twofold less active against *Pseudomonas aeruginosa*. When effects of inoculum size and concentration of divalent cations in the media were evaluated, netilmicin was shown to be similar to gentamicin in vitro. Minimum inhibitory concentrations for *P. aeruginosa* were increased as much as 18-fold when the Mg^{2+} and Ca^{2+} concentrations were increased to physiological levels in Mueller-Hinton broth.

The increasing frequency of nosocomial infections caused by gram-negative bacilli has become one of the major infectious disease problems of the 1970s (7). *Escherichia*, *Klebsiella*, *Enterobacter*, *Pseudomonas*, and *Serratia* now account for well over half of all hospital-acquired infections (5). The aminoglycosides are among the most useful drugs currently available for treating serious infections due to these genera, but the problems associated with their use, that is, development of resistant strains (10, 14, 15, 20) and potential toxicity (2, 3, 6, 9, 11, 12, 13, 19, 21), are well known.

Because of its broad spectrum, gentamicin has been particularly useful in the treatment of such infections. One of the most worrisome factors in the use of gentamicin is the narrow margin between an effective dose and a toxic dose. Netilmicin, *O*-2,6-diamino-2,3,4,6,-tetradeoxy-α-D-glycerol-hex-4-enopyranosyl-(1 → 4)-*O*-[3-deoxy-4-*C*-methyl-3-(methylamino)-β-L-arabinopyranosyl-(1 → 6)]-2-deoxy-1-*N*-ethyl-D-streptamine, is a new semisynthetic aminoglycoside antibiotic that, based on subacute toxicity studies done in rats and dogs, may have less nephrotoxic and ototoxic potential than gentamicin (17). The purpose of this study is to compare the in vitro activity of netilmicin with that of gentamicin, tobramycin, amikacin, and kanamycin.

MATERIALS AND METHODS

Bacteria. A total of 636 strains of bacteria were tested. These were distributed as follows: 70 *Escherichia coli*, 35 *Enterobacter*, 52 *Klebsiella*, 35 *Proteus mirabilis*, 46 *Proteus rettgeri*, 17 *Serratia*, 35 *Salmonella*, 10 *Shigella*, 75 *Pseudomonas aeruginosa*, 75 *Staphylococcus aureus*, 52 *Staphylococcus epidermidis*, 26 group D streptococci, 18 alpha-hemolytic streptococci (non-group D), 23 group A beta-hemolytic streptococci, 14 *Streptococcus pneumoniae*, 19 *Neisseria gonorrhoeae*, 18 *Neisseria meningitidis*, and 16 *Haemophilus influenzae*. Most of these organisms were recently isolated from clinical sources and identified in the Clinical Microbiology Laboratory of Colorado General Hospital under the direction of L. Barth Reller. The strains of *N. gonorrhoeae* were supplied by the Colorado General Hospital Venereal Disease Laboratory under the direction of Peter E. Dans. Most of the strains of *Salmonella* and *Shigella* were obtained from the Colorado State Public Health Laboratory. The *P. rettgeri* isolates were provided by F. Marc LaForce of the Denver Veterans Administration Hospital.

Aminoglycosides. Standard laboratory reference powders of netilmicin and gentamicin sulfate were provided by the Schering Corp., amikacin and kanamycin sulfate were donated by Bristol Laboratories, and tobramycin standard solution was provided by Eli Lilly & Co.

Susceptibility testing methods. (i) Broth minimal inhibitory concentration. The minimal inhibitory concentrations (MICs) of *E. coli*, *Enterobacter*, *Proteus*, *Salmonella*, *Shigella*, *Klebsiella*, *Serratia*, *P. aeruginosa*, *S. aureus*, *S. epidermidis*, group D streptococci, and *S. pneumoniae* were determined by a microtiter broth dilution technique. All tests were performed in standard Mueller-Hinton broth (pH 7.4, 7.2 mg of magnesium and 12 mg of calcium per liter), with the exception of group D streptococci and *S. pneumoniae*, which were tested in Trypticase soy broth (pH 7.35). The group D streptococci were also tested in Mueller-Hinton broth supplemented with 2% defibrinated sheep erythrocytes. All strains of

Pseudomonas were additionally tested in Mueller-Hinton broth (pH 7.38) adjusted to contain 31.2 mg of magnesium and 76.0 mg of calcium per liter. Magnesium and calcium levels in both the adjusted and unadjusted broth were determined in the Pediatric Microchemistry Laboratory of the University of Colorado Medical Center by means of atomic absorption spectrophotometry.

Serial twofold dilutions of freshly prepared antibiotics were made in the appropriate broth, and 0.05 ml of each dilution was dropped into the wells of a microtiter plate (Cooke Engineering Co.). With the exception of *S. pneumoniae,* which was diluted 10^{-3}, overnight broth cultures of the organisms were diluted 10^{-5} in the appropriate broth, and 0.05 ml was then added to the diluted antibiotic. The plates were placed on a shaker for 5 min, and then incubated overnight at 35°C in ambient air. The MIC was defined as the lowest concentration of antibiotic in which there was no visible growth. The minimal bactericidal concentration (MBC) was determined by using an adaptation of the Steers replicator (18), which delivered approximately 0.003 ml from each well of the microtiter plates to Mueller-Hinton agar. The strains of group D streptococci and *S. pneumoniae* were subcultured on Mueller-Hinton agar containing 4% defibrinated sheep erythrocytes. Subcultures of *S. pneumoniae* were incubated overnight at 35°C in a 5% CO_2 atmosphere. All other subcultures were incubated overnight at 35°C in ambient air.

(ii) Agar dilution method. The strains of *N. gonorrhoeae, N. meningitidis, H. influenzae,* group A beta-hemolytic streptococci and alpha-hemolytic streptococci (non-group D) were all tested by the twofold agar dilution method with the Steers inocula replicator (18). *Neisseria* and *Haemophilus* were inoculated onto plates containing GC medium base (Difco) supplemented with 1% hemoglobin (BBL) and 1% IsoVitaleX (BBL). Strains of the non-group D alpha-hemolytic streptococci and the group A beta-hemolytic streptococci were tested on Trypticase soy agar containing 4% defibrinated sheep erythrocytes.

As inoculum, a volume of approximately 0.003 ml of an overnight undiluted broth culture was applied to the surface of the antibiotic-containing plates with the Steers replicator. Strains of *Neisseria* and *Haemophilus* were grown overnight in Mueller-Hinton broth supplemented with 1% hemoglobin and 1% IsoVitaleX at 35°C in a 5% CO_2 atmosphere. For *N. gonorrhoeae* this provided an inoculum of approximately 1.5×10^8 colony-forming units (CFU) per ml; for *N. meningitidis,* 1.3×10^6 CFU/ml; and for *H. influenzae,* 1.5×10^8 CFU/ml.

Group A beta-hemolytic streptococci and alpha-hemolytic streptococci were grown overnight in Trypticase soy broth supplemented with 2% defibrinated sheep erythrocytes. For the group A streptococci, this resulted in an inoculum of approximately 5×10^8 CFU/ml and, for the alpha-hemolytic streptococci, an inoculum of 2×10^7 CFU/ml. All of the plates were incubated at 35°C in a 5% CO_2 atmosphere for 24 to 36 h.

RESULTS

There were only rare instances of significant difference between MICs and MBCs; therefore, only MICs are shown. The activity of the five aminoglycosides against members of *Enterobacteriaceae* is shown in the cumulative distribution curves of Fig. 1 and 2. In general, there appears to be little significant in vitro difference among netilmicin, gentamicin, and tobramycin, except in the case of *Serratia,* for which gentamicin demonstrates clearly greater activity. These aminoglycosides were consistently the most active antibiotics against the *Enterobacteriaceae,* with amikacin the next most active and kanamycin the least active. The one striking exception to this was found when 46 strains of *P. rettgeri* were tested. Amikacin was fourfold more active than any of the other aminoglycosides tested, with 100% of strains in-

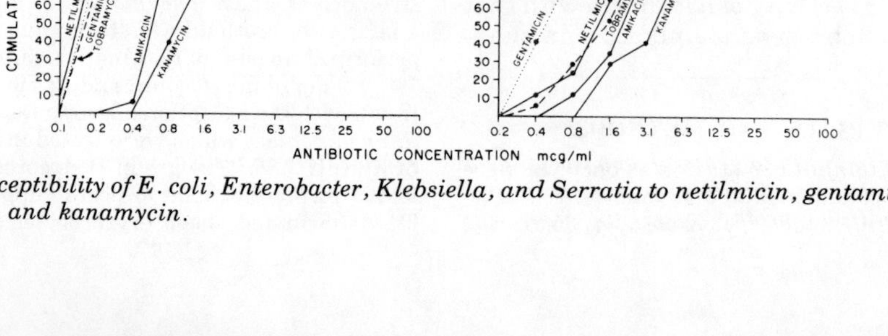

FIG. 1. *Susceptibility of E. coli, Enterobacter, Klebsiella, and Serratia to netilmicin, gentamicin, tobramycin, amikacin, and kanamycin.*

hibited at 6.3 μg/ml. This is particularly worthy of note, since disk susceptibility testing by the Kirby-Bauer method (1) had previously demonstrated that 55% of these strains were resistant to cephalothin, 73% to kanamycin, 100% to nitrofurantoin, 54% to ampicillin, 47% to gentamicin, and 43% to carbenicillin.

Figure 3 demonstrates the activity of the aminoglycosides when tested against 75 strains of *P. aeruginosa* in standard Mueller-Hinton broth and in a calcium- and magnesium-adjusted Mueller-Hinton broth. These strains were divided among two groups; the first consisted of 31 strains reported as susceptible to gentamicin when tested by the Kirby-Bauer method; the second consisted of 44 strains reported as intermediate or resistant by the Kirby-Bauer method. Tobramycin was the most active aminoglycoside against both groups of *P. aeruginosa*. Gentamicin, netilmicin, and amikacin were very similar in their activity. The Ca^{2+} and Mg^{2+} content of the broth was most significant when netilmicin and gentamicin were tested. In Mueller-Hinton broth unadjusted for divalent cation concentration, netilmicin had an activity against *P. aeruginosa* of approximately one dilution less than gentamicin, and was slightly more active than amika-

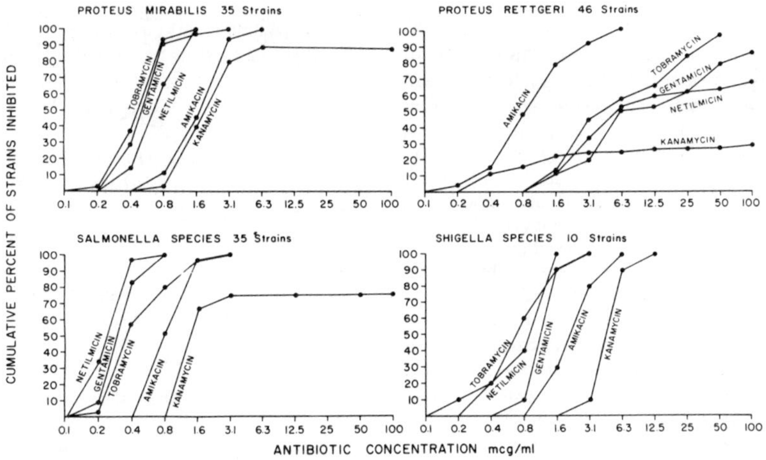

FIG. 2. *Susceptibility of P. mirabilis, P. rettgeri, Salmonella, and Shigella to netilmicin, gentamicin, tobramycin, amikacin, and kanamycin.*

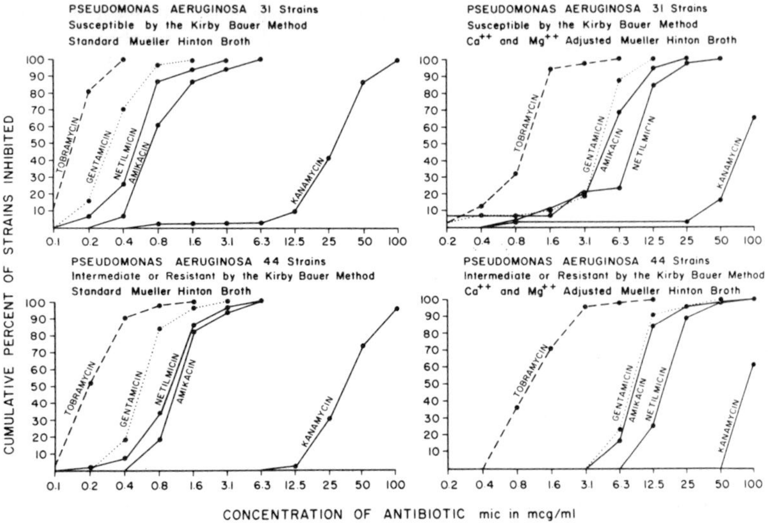

FIG. 3. *Susceptibility to gentamicin-susceptible and intermediate or resistant strains of P. aeruginosa to netilmicin, gentamicin, tobramycin, amikacin, and kanamycin in standard and calcium-magnesium–adjusted Mueller-Hinton broth.*

cin. In broth adjusted to physiological levels of Ca^{2+} and Mg^{2+}, netilmicin remained one dilution less active than gentamicin but showed less activity than amikacin. The geometric mean MIC of netilmicin against *P. aeruginosa* in unadjusted broth was 0.73 μg/ml for gentamicin-susceptible strains and 1.35 μg/ml for gentamicin-resistant strains. In Ca^{2+}- and Mg^{2+}-adjusted broth, the netilmicin MIC for gentamicin-susceptible *P. aeruginosa* was 9.6 μg/ml, and for gentamicin-resistant strains it was 23.1 μg/ml, an 18-fold increase.

Despite the Kirby-Bauer disk susceptibility reports, only a one-dilution difference in the gentamicin MIC was found between those strains of *P. aeruginosa* reported as susceptible and those reported as resistant. The "resistant" group had a geometric mean gentamicin MIC of 0.81 μg/ml, as compared to 0.45 μg/ml for the susceptible group when tested in standard Mueller-Hinton broth. In broth adjusted to physiological levels of Ca^{2+} and Mg^{2+}, geometric mean MICs of gentamicin were 5 μg/ml for the susceptible group and 11.8 μg/ml for the resistant group. In view of the lack of strong correlation between the reported disk susceptibility test results and the broth dilution MICs, the effect of inoculum size was also examined. Table 1 demonstrates that inoculum size has a more significant effect when the divalent cation content of the broth is low. This is more marked with susceptible strains than with resistant ones. The significance of increased cation content of the broth was not as great when tobramycin was tested. In standard Mueller-Hinton broth, tobramycin was approximately twofold more active against *P. aeruginosa* than gentamicin. In Ca^{2+}- and Mg^{2+}-adjusted broth, tobramycin was four- to sixfold more active. Kanamycin was consistently the least active aminoglycoside.

Gentamicin, netilmicin, and tobramycin continued to be the most active aminoglycosides when tested against staphylococci and group D streptococci, as illustrated in Fig. 4. When tested in Trypticase soy broth, group D streptococci continued to demonstrate their characteristic resistance to aminoglycosides. A striking medium effect was found, however, when MICs in Trypticase soy broth were compared with those determined in Mueller-Hinton broth supplemented with 2% defibrinated sheep erythrocytes. The MICs were 7- to 22-fold higher when measured in Trypticase soy broth.

Figure 5 illustrates the results of testing *S. pneumoniae*, alpha-hemolytic streptococci (non-group D), group A beta-hemolytic streptococci, *N. gonorrhoeae*, *N. meningitidis*, and *H. influenzae*. Once again, gentamicin, netilmicin, and tobramycin were consistently more active than amikacin and kanamycin.

DISCUSSION

The results of this study show that, with few exceptions, the in vitro activity of netilmicin closely parallels that of gentamicin. The major

TABLE 1. *Effect of inoculum size on the MIC of four aminoglycoside antibiotics*

Antibiotic (μg/ml)	Gentamicin MIC for *P. aeruginosa* (with given dilution) classified by Kirby-Bauer method as:											
	Susceptible (5 strains)						Intermediate or resistant (5 strains)					
	10^{-2} [a]		10^{-5} [a]		$10^{-2}/10^{-5}$		10^{-2} [a]		10^{-5} [a]		$10^{-2}/10^{-5}$	
	Range	Mean[b]	Range	Mean[b]	Range	Mean[b]	Range	Mean[b]	Range	Mean[b]	Range	Mean[b]
Gentamicin												
MHB-S[c]	6.3–25	12.5	0.4–0.8	0.53	16–62	24	1.6–12.5	5	0.4–1	0.9	2–16	5.7
MHB-A[d]	6.3–25	16.5	3.1–6.3	4.7	3.1–6.3	3.5	12.5–25	22	6.3–25	12.5	1–4	1.8
Netilmicin												
MHB-S[c]	50	50	0.4–1.6	0.6	32–125	72.5	3.1–25	9.9	0.8–3.1	1.8	2–8	5.7
MHB-A[d]	25–50	37.9	6.3–12.5	10.9	2–8	3.5	25–50	39.7	25–50	31.5	0.5–2	1.3
Tobramycin												
MHB-S[c]	25–50	43.5	0.2–0.4	0.26	62.5–250	104	1.6–3.1	2.5	0.2–0.8	0.28	4–16	9
MHB-A[d]	1.6–12	5.5	0.8–1.6	1.1	2–8	4.6	0.4–3.1	1.1	0.8–3.1	1.3	0.3–2	0.9
Amikacin												
MHB-S[c]	25	25	0.8–1.6	1.1	16–32	24.3	6.3–25	8.9	0.8–6.3	1.8	2–8	5
MHB-A[d]	12.5–25	21.8	3.1–12.5	9.2	2–8	3.5	25–50	28	6.3–25	14.1	1–4	2

[a] Dilution of an overnight Mueller-Hinton broth culture containing 10^9 organisms per ml.
[b] Geometric mean.
[c] Unadjusted Mueller-Hinton broth (Difco), pH 7.4, 7.2 mg and 12 mg of calcium per liter.
[d] Adjusted Mueller-Hinton broth (Difco), pH 7.38, adjusted to contain 31.2 mg of magnesium and 76 mg of calcium per liter.

exceptions to this were found when strains of *Serratia* and group A streptococci were tested. In both instances, gentamicin showed approximately a two- to threefold greater activity than netilmicin. Netilmicin was approximately one dilution less active against *P. aeruginosa* than gentamicin. Overall, gentamicin, netilmicin, and tobramycin were the most active antibiotics tested. Amikacin, however, was significantly more active against multi-drug-resistant strains of *P. rettgeri*. Kanamycin was consistently the least active antibiotic against all or-

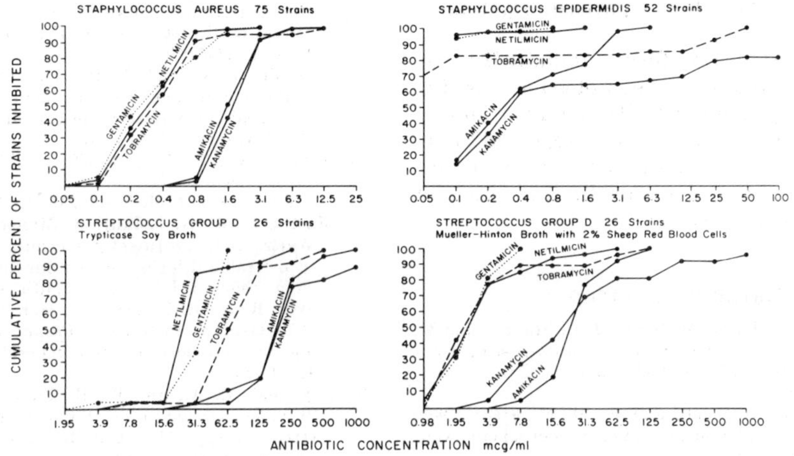

FIG. 4. *Susceptibility of S. aureus, S. epidermidis, and group D streptococci to netilmicin, gentamicin, tobramycin, amikacin, and kanamycin.*

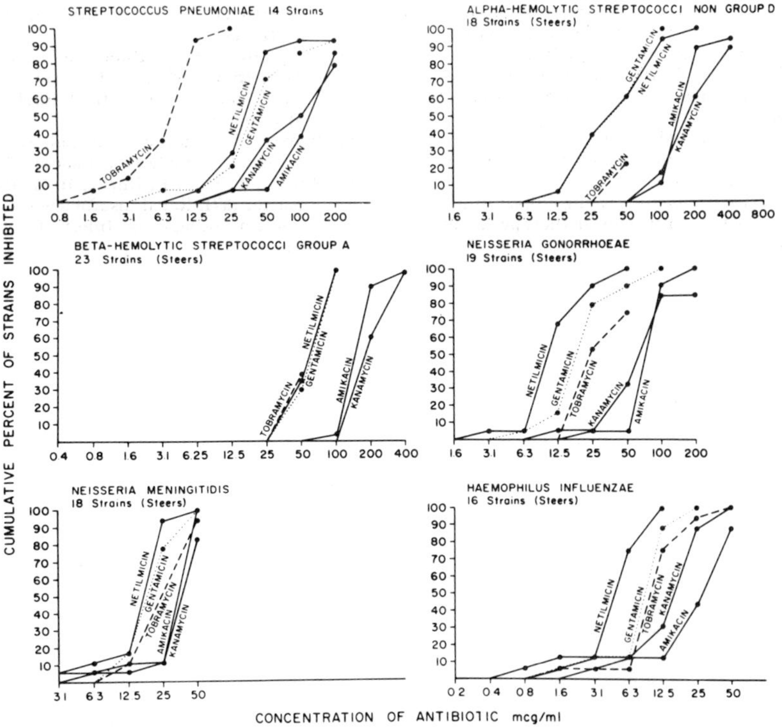

FIG. 5. *Susceptibility of S. pneumoniae, alpha-hemolytic streptococci (non-group D), group A streptococci, N. gonorrhoeae, N. meningitidis, and H. influenzae to netilmicin, gentamicin, tobramycin, amikacin, and kanamycin.*

ganisms tested. As has been reported with other aminoglycoside antibiotics (4, 8), the Ca^{2+} and the Mg^{2+} concentration of the medium was shown to have an important effect on the MIC of netilmicin when *P. aeruginosa* was tested. Our data also demonstrate an increased importance of inoculum size when broth low in Mg^{2+} and Ca^{2+} is used. This is particularly true of susceptible strains.

Another significant effect is found when media supplemented with sheep blood are used to test aminoglycoside activity against enterococci. This has previously been reported to enhance the activity of gentamicin against enterococci (16). Our data confirm this and extend it to other aminoglycosides.

LITERATURE CITED

1. **Bauer, A. W., W. M. M. Kirby, J. C. Sherris, and M. Turck.** 1966. Antibiotic susceptibility testing by a standardized disk method. Am. J. Clin. Pathol. 45:493–496.
2. **Bulger, R. J., S. Sidell, and W. M. M. Kirby.** 1963. Laboratory and clinical studies of gentamicin. Ann. Intern. Med. 59:593–604.
3. **Chang, J. C., and B. Reyes.** 1975. Agranulocytosis associated with gentamicin. J. Am. Med. Assoc. 232:1154–1155.
4. **Davis, S. D., and A. Iannetta.** 1973. Relative antagonism *in vitro* of calcium in serum to the bactericidal activities of gentamicin and tobramycin on *Pseudomonas aeruginosa*. Chemotherapy 19:243–253.
5. **Eickhoff, T. C.** 1975. New antibacterial treatment of nosocomial infections. Bull. N.Y. Acad. Med. 51:1056–1064.
6. **Falco, F. G., H. M. Smith, and G. M. Arcieri.** 1969. Nephrotoxicity of aminoglycosides and gentamicin. J. Infect. Dis. 119:406–409.
7. **Finland, M.** 1970. Changing ecology of bacterial infections as related to antibacterial therapy. J. Infect. Dis. 122:419–431.
8. **Gilbert, D. N., E. Kutscher, P. Ireland, J. A. Barnett, and J. P. Sanford.** 1971. Effect of the concentrations of magnesium and calcium on the *in vitro* susceptibility of *Pseudomonas aeruginosa* to gentamicin. J. Infect. Dis. 124(Suppl.):S37–S45.
9. **Holtzman, J. L.** 1976. Gentamicin and neuromuscular blockade. Ann. Intern. Med. 84:55.
10. **Houang, E. T., and E. McKay-Ferguson.** 1976. Activities of tobramycin and amikacin against gentamicin resistant gram-negative bacilli. Lancet 1:423–424.
11. **Jackson, G. G.** 1967. CCXXXIV.–Gentamicin. Curr. Ther. 198:855–866.
12. **Jackson, G. G., and G. Arcieri.** 1971. Ototoxicity of gentamicin in man: a survey and controlled analysis of clinical experience in the United States. J. Infect. Dis. 124(Suppl.):S130–S137.
13. **Klein, J. O., T. C. Eickhoff, and M. Finland.** 1964. Gentamicin: activity *in vitro* and observations in 26 patients. Am. J. Med. Sci. 248:528–543.
14. **Martin, C. M., N. S. Ikuri, J. Zimmerman, and J. A. Waitz.** 1971. A virulent nosocomial *Klebsiella* with a transferable R factor for gentamicin: emergence and suppression. J. Infect. Dis. 124(Suppl.):S24–S29.
15. **Meyer, R. D., R. P. Lewis, J. Halter, and M. White.** 1976. Gentamicin resistant *Pseudomonas aeruginosa* and *Serratia marcesens* in a general hospital. Lancet 1:580–583.
16. **Raymond, E. A., and W. H. Traub.** 1971. Medium-dependent activity of gentamicin sulfate against enterococci. Appl. Microbiol. 21:192–194.
17. **Schering Corporation.** 1975. Investigational brochure–informational material for the investigational drug Sch 20569. Schering Corp., Bloomfield, N.J.
18. **Steers, E., E. L. Foltz, and E. S. Graves.** 1959. Inocula replicating apparatus for routine testing of bacterial sensitivity to antibiotics. Antibiot. Chemother. 9:307–311.
19. **Tjernstrom, O., G. Banck, S. Belfrage, I. Juhlin, L. Nordstrom, and N. G. Taremalm.** 1973. The ototoxicity of gentamicin. Acta. Pathol. Microbiol. Scand. 81(Suppl.):73–78.
20. **Warren, R. E., and S. O. B. Roberts.** 1976. Gentamicin-resistant staphylococci. Lancet 1:543–544.
21. **Wilfert, J. N., J. P. Burke, H. A. Bloomer, and C. B. Smith.** 1971. Renal insufficiency associated with gentamicin therapy. J. Infect. Dis. 124(Suppl.):S148–S153.

ANTIMICROBIAL AGENTS AND CHEMOTHERAPY, May 1977, p. 797-802 Vol. 11, No. 5

Inhibition of Herpes Simplex Virus Strains Isolated from Herpetic Keratitis by Polyinosinic Acid-Polycytidylic Acid

OFIRA SMETANA, EMANUEL EYLAN,* AND MIRIAM WEINBERG

Department of Human Microbiology, Sackler School of Medicine, Tel-Aviv University, Tel-Aviv, Ramat-Aviv, Israel

Received for publication 13 December 1976

Fifty strains of herpes simplex virus, isolated from patients with herpetic keratitis, were examined in vitro for susceptibility to polyinosinic acid-polycytidylic acid [poly(I:C)] in the presence of a constant concentration of diethylaminoethyl-dextran. The minimal inhibitory concentration of poly(I:C) for 44 of these strains ranged from 0.0001 to 0.1 μg/ml; for the remaining six strains, the minimal inhibitory concentration stood at 1 to 2 μg/ml. Fifteen isolates from primary infections were more susceptible to poly(I:C) than 35 isolates from recurrent infections. Isolates acquired at different points of a given clinical episode showed similar susceptibilities to poly(I:C). In two patients, isolates from consecutive recurrences of infection exhibited reduced susceptibilities. The implications of the above observations for the therapeutic use of poly(I:C) are discussed.

It is known that polyinosinic acid-polycytidylic acid [poly(I:C)], a double-stranded ribonucleic acid complex, is highly active in inducing interferon as well as in resistance to viral infections in animals and in cell cultures (2).

Herpes simplex virus (HSV), the widespread virus of ocular inflammations, has been reported to be only moderately susceptible to the antiviral action of interferon (5). However, Park and Baron (9) found that poly(I:C)-induced interferon was effective in treating herpetic keratoconjunctivitis in rabbits. Guerra et al. (3) reported success in a preliminary study on treatment of human herpetic conjunctivitis by topical poly(I:C). Oosterhuis et al. (8) recently described favorable results in patients with stromal keratitis treated with a combination of poly(I:C) and iododeoxyuridine (IUdR).

Several investigators have evaluated the effect of poly(I:C) in vitro in the hope of using it as an interferon inducer in human ocular herpetic keratitis (4, 6, 11, 14). One such study (14) investigated the ability of poly(I:C)-induced interferon to protect rabbit eye tissue cultures prepared from cornea, conjunctiva, and iris against HSV infection: the degree of protection inversely proportional to the virus challenge was significantly enhanced by addition of neomycin. Other in vitro studies tested susceptibility of HSV to poly(I:C)-induced interferon in different tissue cultures, including HEp-2, rabbit kidney cells, and mouse embryonic cells (4, 6, 11).

In the present study, the effect of poly(I:C) on different HSV strains from human herpetic keratitis was investigated in an attempt to determine the value of this interferon inducer in the treatment of such ocular infections. We selected 50 HSV strains isolated during different stages of the disease from primary or recurrent infections in humans, from recurrences in the same individual, and from different days of the same recurrence.

MATERIALS AND METHODS

Cell cultures. Primary rabbit kidney (PRK) cell cultures were prepared from 3-week-old rabbit kidneys according to the method of Smith and Wagner (13). The cells were dispersed in tissue culture tubes in M-199 medium containing 10% calf serum at a density of 6×10^5 to 8×10^5 cells per ml. Confluent monolayers were obtained after 7 to 10 days of incubation at 37°C. For preparation of Vero cells, a continuous line of African Green Monkey kidney cells was grown in tissue culture tubes in M-199 medium containing 5% calf serum at a cell density of 1.5×10^5 to 2×10^5 cells per ml. The tissue cultures were used after 1 to 2 days, when a confluent monolayer was obtained. M-199 medium contained: penicillin, 200 U/ml; streptomycin, 200 mg/ml; and mycostatin, 50 U/ml. The maintenance media used was M-199 containing 2% calf serum.

Viruses. The 50 HSV strains were isolated from patients with herpetic keratitis from the Department of Ophthalmology of the Haim Sheba Medical Center. The viruses were isolated at various stages of the disease from untreated patients and from patients treated with IUdR, corticosteroids, or poly(I:C). The standard HSV strains used were HSV type 1, VR_3 McIntyre strain, and HSV type 2, Rapp strain. The challenge viruses for interferon determination were vesicular stomatitis virus, Indiana strain, and vaccinia virus.

Isolation and identification of HSV strains. Material for HSV isolation was obtained by gentle swabbing of the corneal epithelium with a sterile cotton swab moistened with M-199 medium containing: 5% fetal calf serum; penicillin, 500 U/ml; streptomycin, 500 mg/ml; and mycostatin, 50 U/ml. The swabs were agitated, inoculated immediately into PRK tissue cultures, and incubated at 37°C until appearance of cytopathogenic effect (CPE). After CPE detection and specific neutralization with anti-HSV serum, the virus stocks were held at −70°C. Before each experiment, the virus titer was determined in PRK cells, and the mean tissue culture infective dose was calculated for each virus stock. All 50 HSV strains isolated from the eyes were found to belong to the type 1 HSV group.

Reagents. Poly(I:C) was obtained from Miles Chemical Co., Elkart, Ind., as a lyophylized preparation. The stock solution was prepared in a concentration of 1,000 μg/ml in phosphate buffer, pH 7 (2), and stored at −70°C. The working solutions were made in M-199 just before the experiments and held in an ice bath until used.

Diethylaminoethyl (DEAE)-dextran was obtained from the Pharmacia Co., Uppsala, Sweden, at a molecular weight of 2×10^6. The stock solution was prepared in phosphate buffer, pH 7, to a concentration of 400 μg/ml and held at 4°C. The working solution was diluted in M-199 to 100 μg/ml.

Trypsin (crystallized two times) and soya bean trypsin inhibitor (crystallized three times) were obtained from Worthington Biochemicals Corp., Freehold, N.J. Actinomycin D was obtained from Sigma Chemical Co., St. Louis, Mo.

Procedure for HSV inhibition by poly(I:C). PRK tissue cultures were incubated for 2 h with 100 μg of DEAE-dextran per ml. The DEAE-dextran was removed, the tissue cultures were washed three times with phosphate-buffered saline, and poly(I:C) was added in dilutions of 2 to 0.0001 μg/ml. Control tissue cultures were incubated with 1 ml of M-199 with 2% calf serum. After 18 to 24 h of incubation at 37°C, the poly(I:C)-treated and control cultures were challenged with 100 mean tissue culture infective doses of each HSV strain tested. The tissue cultures were reincubated at 37°C until the CPE in the virus control tubes was observed, usually after 2 days. Then the poly(I:C)-induced cellular resistance was measured as the percent reduction of the CPE in test cultures as compared with the control.

A 50% CPE reduction was taken as the minimal inhibitory concentration (MIC) of poly(I:C) required by every HSV strain tested.

RESULTS

Comparison of the MICs of poly(I:C) with and without DEAE-dextran. In a preliminary experiment, it was found that DEAE-dextran used alone does not induce interferon or antiviral resistance in PRK tissue cultures treated for 18 to 24 h with 50 to 200 μg of DEAE-dextran per ml (and washed three times with phosphate-buffered saline). When 10 HSV strains were tested to compare the MICs of poly(I:C) required with and without DEAE-dextran (Table 1), the MIC of poly(I:C) with DEAE-dextran was 5 to 20,000 times lower than that without it. Note in Table 1 that HSV strains inhibited by a low MIC of poly(I:C) with DEAE-dextran show a very high ratio of poly(I:C) with DEAE-dextran to poly(I:C) without DEAE-dextran. The results show that for better inhibition of HSV strains, it is important to use poly(I:C) together with DEAE-dextran.

MIC of poly(I:C) with DEAE-dextran required against 50 HSV strains. Once it was established that poly(I:C) together with DEAE-dextran was a better inducer for HSV inhibition, 50 HSV strains were tested for determination of the MIC of poly(I:C) with DEAE-dextran required for inhibition of each strain. The HSV strains were tested against different dilutions of poly(I:C) from 2 to 0.0001 μg/ml. The DEAE-dextran concentration was 100 μg/ml in all the experiments. The results (Fig. 1) show that the 50 HSV strains were distributed into six groups in accordance with the concentration of poly(I:C) required for inhibition of each strain: 1 of the HSV strains was inhibited by the smallest dose of poly(I:C) used, 0.0001 μg/ml; 13 were inhibited by 0.001 μg/ml; nearly half (24) were inhibited by 0.01 μg/ml; and 6 were inhibited by 0.1 μg/ml. The remaining six HSV strains were inhibited by 1 to 2 μg of poly(I:C) per ml, the highest dose used.

To state the data in another way, 88% of the HSV strains were inhibited by a low MIC of poly(I:C), ranging from 0.1 to 0.0001 μg/ml, and only 12% were inhibited by a higher MIC, 1 to 2

TABLE 1. *MIC of poly(I:C) compared to that of poly(I:C) with DEAE-dextran*

HSV strain	MIC of poly(I:C) (μg/ml)	MIC of poly(I:C) with DEAE-dextran[a] (μg/ml)	MIC of poly(I:C)/ MIC of poly(I:C) + DEAE-dextran
1	5.0	1.0	5
2	5.0	0.1	50
3	50.0	2.0	25
4	50.0	1.0	50
5	100.0	2.0	50
6	100.0	1.0	100
7	20.0	0.01	2,000
8	5.0	0.001	5,000
9	10.0	0.001	10,000
10	2.0	0.0001	20,000

[a] The concentration of DEAE-dextran was 100 μg/ml.

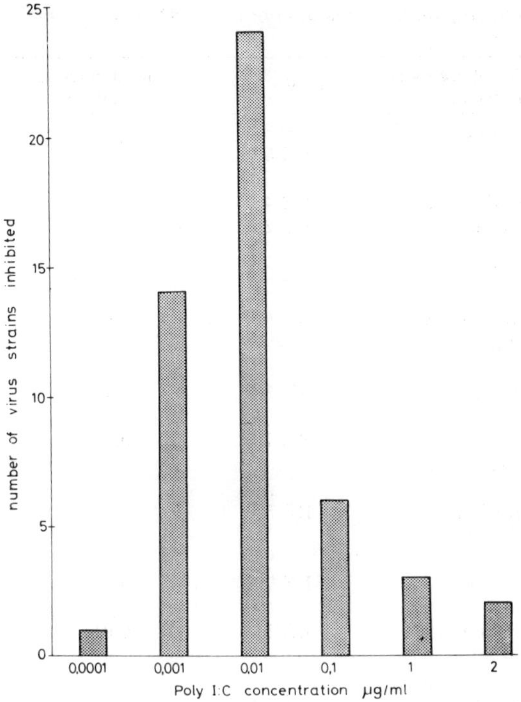

FIG. 1. *Inhibitory effect of poly(I:C) on HSV strains in PRK tissue cultures. The indicated dilutions of poly(I:C) were added to PRK cultures after treatment with 100 µg of DEAE-dextran per ml.*

µg/ml. The MICs of poly(I:C) required for the standard HSV strains were found to be 0.01 µg of poly(I:C) per ml for inhibition of HSV type 1 strain McIntyre and 0.001 µg of poly(I:C) per ml for inhibition of HSV type 2 strain Rapp.

Comparative MIC of poly(I:C) used against HSV strains isolated from primary and recurrent infections. Of the 50 HSV strains tested, 15 were isolated from primary ocular infections and 35 from recurrent infections. A comparison of the resistance of these two groups to poly(I:C) in vitro (Fig. 2) showed that more of the HSV strains isolated from primary infections were inhibited by a MIC of poly(I:C) ranging from 0.001 to 0.1 µg/ml. Under the same conditions, fewer of the HSV strains from recurrent infections were inhibited by this low MIC of poly(I:C). HSV strains isolated from primary infections were slightly more susceptible to poly(I:C) than those isolated from recurrent infections.

Susceptibility to poly(I:C) of HSV strains isolated from the same patient on different days of the same recurrence. Of the 50 HSV strains tested, 4 were isolated more than once in the same patient on different days during the same recurrence: 2 were isolated twice, and 2 were isolated three times (Table 2). These viruses were isolated despite treatment with either IUdR or poly(I:C), which caused a decrease in virus titer but did not affect reisolation. No changes were found in the MIC of poly(I:C) required against the HSV strains isolated from the same patient on different days of the same recurrence. The results were the same in untreated patients and in those who had received IUdR or poly(I:C).

Susceptibility to poly(I:C) of HSV strains isolated from recurrences in the same patient. It was important to determine whether HSV strains isolated from recurrences in the same patient retained their original susceptibility to poly(I:C). This issue was examined in seven patients: in five there were two recurrences; in two cases there were three consecutive recurrences. The HSV isolations were made from recurrences that occurred at 0.5- to 2-year intervals despite the treatment given between and before isolations [UIdR, corticosteroids, or poly(I:C), the latter administered only when IUdR treatment proved unsuccessful]. The seven HSV strains were tested for their resistance to poly(I:C) in vitro (Table 3). No differences were found among five HSV strains isolated in different recurrences. However, for the inhibition of two HSV strains (no. 270 and 195), 10 times the MIC of poly(I:C) was required. HSV 270 was reisolated 1 year after IUdR treat-

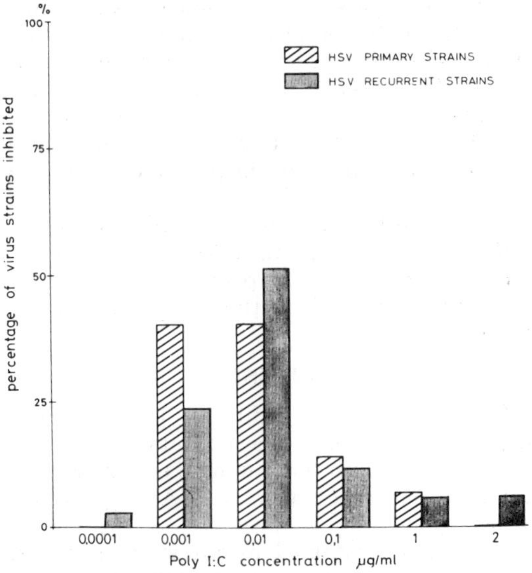

FIG. 2. *Inhibitory effect of poly(I:C) on HSV strains isolated from primary and recurrent infections. The experimental procedures used were the same as in Fig. 1. The comparison of the HSV strains isolated from primary infections and those from recurrent infections are presented as percentages.*

TABLE 2. *Susceptibility to poly(I:C) of HSV strains isolated from patients during different days of same recurrence*

HSV strain	Treatment before virus isolation	Time intervals between virus isolations	HSV titer[a]	MIC of poly(I:C) (μg/ml)
696[b]	None	1st isolation	RE 8.0 LE 5.0	0.1
	IUdR (2 days)	2nd isolation, 2 days later	RE 4.0 LE 2.0	0.1
1000	None	1st isolation	RE 6.5	0.0001
	IUdR (4 days)	2nd isolation, 4 days later	RE 5.0	0.0001
1097	IUdR (3 days)	1st isolation	RE 8.5	0.1
	None	2nd isolation, 1 day later	RE 7.5	0.1
	Poly (I:C) (6,200 μg/ml)	3rd isolation, 7 days later	RE 5.0	0.1
1162	None	1st isolation	LE 7.5	0.01
	None	2nd isolation, 2 days later	LE 7.0	0.01
	Poly(I:C) (2,000 μg/ml)	3rd isolation, 4 days later	LE 4.0	0.01

[a] HSV titer = $\log_{10}$ mean tissue culture infective doses per milliliter. RE, Right eye; LE, left eye.
[b] Bilateral herpetic keratitis.

ment (no change in MIC) and 0.5 year after poly(I:C) treatment, at which time the MIC had risen 10-fold. HSV 195 was isolated from a primary infection and 2 years later from the first recurrence, never having been treated by poly(I:C): the MIC required for the latter was 10-fold that required for the primary strain (Table 3).

It is important to note that this change in MIC of poly(I:C) for strain 195 occurred between the HSV isolated from a primary infection and the HSV isolated from the first recurrence 2 years later.

DISCUSSION

Of the interferon inducers, poly(I:C) was found to be one of the best inhibitors of HSV (11), and the inhibition could be enhanced by a polybasic substance such as DEAE-dextran (1) or neomycin (14).

The results obtained in our study revealed differences in susceptibility to poly(I:C) among the various HSV strains tested; some differences were found between HSV strains from primary and recurrent infections and from recurrences in the same patient. The 50 HSV strains could be divided into six groups according to the MIC of poly(I:C) required for inhibition. Standard HSV strains tested also required a different MIC of poly(I:C): HSV type 1 strain VR_3 McIntyre was inhibited by 0.01 μg/ml, and HSV type 2 strain Rapp was inhibited by 0.001 μg/ml. Our data are in accordance with the findings of Oh (7) and Munk and Frick (6), who showed that genital HSV was better inhibited in vitro by poly(I:C) than oral or corneal HSV strains. It is known that HSV is resistant to inhibition by interferon (5, 7, 11), but there are interstrain differences in addition to intertype differences (7). It is important to note that most of the HSV strains tested (88%) were inhibited by a low MIC of poly(I:C) (0.0001 to 0.1 μg/ml), and few strains (12%) were inhibited by a higher MIC of poly(I:C) (1 to 2 μg/ml). We assumed that this low MIC of poly(I:C) was obtained by the use of DEAE-dextran, which increased the permeability of the infected cells to the inducer (1).

Another reason for this low MIC of poly(I:C) required may be the tissue cultures: PRK cultures are known for their high sensitivity to induction and testing of rabbit interferon. The importance of the appropriate tissue culture system was demonstrated by Person et al. (10),

TABLE 3. *Susceptibility to poly(I:C) of HSV strains isolated from recurrences in the same patient*

HSV strain	Treatment between virus isolations	Time intervals between virus isolations	Treatment before each isolation	HSV titer[a]	MIC of poly(I:C) (μg/ml)
166	IUdR	1st isolation	IUdR	3.7	0.1
	IUdR	2nd isolation, 2 yr	None	3.5	0.1
163	IUdR	1st isolation	IUdR	5.0	0.001
	c.st.[b]	2nd isolation, 1 yr	None	5.2	0.001
139	IUdR + c.st.	1st isolation	c.st.	5.0	1.0
	Poly(I:C) (10,000 μg/ml)	2nd isolation, 2 yr	c.st.	5.7	1.0
525	IUdR	1st isolation	c.st.	6.7	0.01
	Poly(I:C) (5,200 μg/ml)	2nd isolation, 2 yr	c.st.	4.7	0.01
170	IUdR	1st isolation	IUdR	6.5	0.01
	Poly(I:C) (5,000 μg/ml)	2nd isolation, 1 yr	None	6.0	0.01
	IUdR	3rd isolation, 2 yr	None	7.0	0.01
270	IUdR	1st isolation	None	5.5	0.1
	Poly(I:C) (5,300 μg/ml)	2nd isolation, 1 yr	None	4.5	0.1
	Poly(I:C) (5,600 μg/ml)	3rd isolation, 0.5 yr	IUdR	4.5	1.0
195	None	1st isolation	None	4.5	0.001
	IUdR	2nd isolation, 2 yr	None	6.7	0.01

[a] HSV titer from the eye = $\log_{10}$ mean tissue culture infective doses per milliliter.
[b] c.st., Corticosteroids.

who concluded that the variation in susceptibility of different HSV types to antiviral agents resulted from differences in the cell culture system used. We found no significant differences in susceptibility to poly(I:C) among HSV strains isolated from primary and recurrent infections; however, the HSV strains isolated from primary infections were somewhat more susceptible than "recurrent strains." The same results were obtained by testing HSV strains isolated from recurrences in the same patient. In one case a rise in MIC of poly(I:C) was found between the virus strain isolated from the primary infection and the strain isolated 2 years later from the first recurrence of the infection. In another study (12) a high correlation was found between the severity of the patient's herpetic keratitis, the resistance of the isolated HSV in vitro (MIC) to IUdR and poly(I:C), and the virulence of the same virus strain for laboratory animals. In view of our results in vitro and those of the previous study, it is suggested that each HSV strain isolated from patients with herpetic keratitis, especially in those "treatment resistant" to IUdR, may be tested in vitro for the MIC of poly(I:C) required, to determine the efficacy of poly(I:C) treatment of this ocular infection.

ACKNOWLEDGMENTS

We thank A. Romano from the Department of Ophthalmology, Haim Sheba Medical Center, for generously providing us with clinical material used in this study.

LITERATURE CITED

1. **Dianzani, F., S. Baron, C. E. Buckler, and H. B. Levy.** 1971. Mechanisms of DEAE-dextran enhancement of polynucleotide induction of interferon. Proc. Soc. Exp. Biol. Med. **136**:1111–1114.
2. **Field, A. K., A. A. Tytell, G. P. Lampson, and M. R. Hilleman.** 1967. Inducers of interferon and host resistance. II. Multistranded synthetic polynucleotide complexes. Proc. Natl. Acad. Sci. U.S.A. **58**:1004–1010.
3. **Guerra, R., R. Frezzotti, R. Bonanni, F. Dianzani, and G. Rita.** 1970. A preliminary study on treatment of human herpes simplex keratitis with an interferon inducer. Ann. N.Y. Acad. Sci. **173**:823–829.
4. **Hamilton, L. D., V. I. Babcock, and C. M. Southam.** 1969. Inhibition of herpes simplex virus by synthetic double-stranded RNA (polyriboadenylic and polyribouridylic acids and polyribinosinic and polyribocytidylic acids). Proc. Natl. Acad. Sci. U.S.A. **64**:878–883.
5. **Ho, M., and Y. F. Enders.** 1959. Further studies on an inhibitor of viral activity appearing in infected cell cultures and its role in chronic infections. Virology **9**:446–477.

6. **Munk, K., and T. Frick.** 1972. Effect of Poly I:C-induced interferon on herpes virus hominis infection in vitro and in vivo. Z. Naturforsch. Teil B 27:220–222.
7. **Oh, J. O.** 1971. Senstivity of types 1 and 2 *Herpesvirus hominis* to an interferon inducer, poly I:C. Infect. Immun. 3:847–848.
8. **Oosterhuis, J. A., S. M. Sie, W. A. Nolen, J. Versteeg, and I. G. Jeltes.** 1976. Therapy of herpetic keratitis with a combination of Poly I:C and idoxiuridine. Ophthalmic. Res. 8:152–159.
9. **Park, J. H., and S. Baron.** 1968. Herpetic keratoconjunctivitis: therapy with synthetic double-stranded RNA. Science 162:811–813.
10. **Person, D. A., P. J. Sheridan, and E. C. Herrmann.** 1970. Sensitivity of types 1 and 2 herpes simplex virus to S-iodo-2′-deoxyuridine and 9-β-D-arabinofuranosyladenine. Infect. Immun. 2:815–820.
11. **Schachter, N., M. A. Galin, M. Weissenbacher, S. Baron, and A. Billiau.** 1970. Comparison of antiviral action of interferon, interferon inducers and IDU against herpes simplex and other viruses. Ann. Ophthalmol. 2:795–798.
12. **Smetana, O., M. Weinberg, R. Cohen, A. Romano, and E. Eylan.** 1976. Virulence and resistance to idoxuridine and Poly I:C of herpes simplex viruses isolated from herpetic keratitis. Isr. J. Med. Sci. 12:711.
13. **Smith, T., and R. Wagner.** 1967. Rabbit macrophage interferon. Conditions for biosynthesis by virus infected and uninfected cells. J. Exp. Med. 125:559–579.
14. **Weissenbacher, M., M. A. Galin, E. Chowchuvech, N. Schachter, and S. Baron.** 1970. Protection by polyinosinic-polycytidylic acid complex of rabbit eye tissue cultures infected with herpes simplex virus. Invest. Ophthalmol. 9:857–854.

ANTIMICROBIAL AGENTS AND CHEMOTHERAPY, May 1977, p. 803-808
Vol. 1, No. 5

Printed in U.S.A.

Amphotericin B and Filipin Effects on L and HeLa Cells: Dose Response

JANINA KOTLER-BRAJTBURG, GERALD MEDOFF,* DAVID SCHLESSINGER, AND GEORGE S. KOBAYASHI

Divisions of Infectious Diseases and Dermatology, Department of Medicine and Department of Microbiology and Immunology,* Washington University School of Medicine, St. Louis, Misouri 63110*

Received for publication 22 November 1976

Amphotericin B (AmB) and filipin effects on L and HeLa cells were compared by monitoring drug-induced potassium leakage from cells, changes in radioactive uridine incorporation into cellular ribonucleic acid, protein leakage from cells, and cell viability. L cells were much more susceptible to both AmB and filipin than were HeLa cells, but the overall dose response was similar. For AmB, the various effects were easily separable. Potassium leakage occurred at the lowest concentrations of AmB and was reversible. Inhibition of uridine incorporation and loss of viability occurred at intermediate levels, and protein loss occurred at higher levels. In contrast, filipin was much more potent; its effects on potassium leakage were only minimally reversible, and the separation of the permeabilizing effects from complete cell lysis was possible only over a limited concentration range and for a short time.

Amphotericin B (AmB) belongs to the class of polyene antibiotics, which bind to the sterol component of the membranes of all eucaryotic cells (6, 13). At sufficiently high concentrations, the polyene antibiotics cause an increase in membrane permeability, with leakage of metabolites and macromolecules from the cell and resultant cell death. Previous studies with fungi and animal cells in culture have shown that at low concentrations AmB can induce nonlethal permeabilizing changes in cell membranes which enhance uptake of certain small molecules (16) and even macromolecules (9). These properties of AmB have been exploited to achieve the penetration into cells of pharmacologically active compounds (9, 12, 17) that do not penetrate the untreated cell membranes.

We have undertaken the present study to compare the nonlethal and lethal effects of AmB on cultured L and HeLa cells, and to determine under which conditions they can be separated and whether the cell damages can be repaired. Similar studies have also been performed with filipin to determine whether permeability changes induced by this polyene antibiotic are separable from lethality.

MATERIALS AND METHODS

Chemicals. AmB in the form of Fungizone was purchased from E. R. Squibb and Sons, Inc., Princeton, N.J. It was dissolved in sterile water before use. The concentrations of the AmB solutions were calculated on the basis of the amounts of AmB in the Fungizone, as stated by the manufacturer. Filipin, in the form of the unfractionated antibiotic complex, which was 86% pure, was donated by The Upjohn Co., Kalamazoo, Mich. The amounts noted refer to the crude product. Filipin was dissolved in methanol before use.

[5-^{3}H]uridine (specific activity, 8 Ci/mmol) was purchased from Schwarz/Mann, Orangeburg, N.Y. L-[*methyl*-^{3}H]methionine (specific activity, 5.0 mCi/0.071 mg) was purchased from the New England Nuclear Corp., Boston, Mass. Triton X-100 (Triton) was purchased from Packard Instrumental Co., Downers Grove, Ill. Lithium diluent was purchased from Instrumental Laboratory, Inc., Lexington, Mass.

Cell culture. HeLa and L 929 cells were maintained and assayed in monolayer in Eagle minimum essential medium supplemented with 0.2 mM of nonessential amino acids, 2 mM glutamine, 10% fetal calf serum, 100 U of penicillin per ml and 100 μg of Kantrex per ml (medium).

Growth of cells. Cells were removed from a monolayer with 0.25% trypsin, seeded in 3 ml of medium at a density of 4.0×10^5 cells per plastic 35-mm-diameter dish, and grown for 17 h. The medium was then removed, and the cells were rinsed once with 2 ml of fresh medium and incubated at 37°C with 1 ml of medium containing the antibiotic to be assayed. The incubation was terminated by aspiration of the medium, and the specific analyses were performed. The results were expressed as percentages of control values obtained for untreated cells.

Because Fungizone contains 41% sodium deoxycholate by weight, the control cells in the AmB experiments were treated with appropriate amounts of sodium deoxycholate. In the filipin experiments, all cells were treated with methanol at a final concentration of 0.2%.

Determinations of intracellular potassium. A standard curve was obtained for 0 to 15 μg of potassium in 4 ml of solution composed of 3.5 ml of lithium diluent, containing 15 meq of Li per liter, and 0.5 ml of 2% Triton. When these potassium concentrations were assayed with a flame photometer (model 143, Instrumentation Laboratory, Inc., Boston, Mass.), linear dependency of reading on potassium concentration was observed. All of our subsequent measurements were done in this concentration range.

Potassium leakage, determined by the amount of potassium remaining in cells after antibiotic treatment, was measured under two conditions. In the first, we determined the leakage of potassium from cells during the incubation with drug and before rinsing. After cells were incubated for 1 h with AmB or filipin, the medium was removed and the cells were extracted at room temperature with two 400-μl portions of 2% Triton. Of the combined extracts, 0.5 ml was mixed with 3.5 ml of lithium diluent and measured for potassium content. The difference between the potassium content in the extract of untreated, unrinsed cells and the extract from untreated cells additionally rinsed three times with 2-ml portions of 0.15 M NaCl (saline) was the amount of potassium originating from the medium, and this value was subtracted from all results.

In the second part of this experiment, we determined the potassium content remaining in rinsed cells. After aspiration of antibiotic-containing medium, cells were rinsed at room temperature three times with 2-ml portions of saline, and then extracted and assayed as before.

Cell viability. To test the viability of cells after exposure to the antibiotics, the medium was removed and the cells were rinsed twice with 2 ml of Hanks solution and incubated for 10 min at 37°C with 0.1% trypan blue. They were then removed from the monolayer with a rubber policeman and counted in a hemocytometer.

[^{3}H]uridine incorporation into acid-insoluble pool (ribonucleic acid [RNA]). To test changes in radioactive uridine incorporation, the cells were exposed to 0.5 μCi of ml [^{3}H]uridine, and the incorporated radioactivity was measured as previously described (J. Kotler-Brajtburg, G. Medoff, G. S. Kobayashi, D. Schlessinger, and A. Atalach, Biochem. Pharmacol., in press).

Methylation of RNA with radioactive methionine. Methylation of RNA with radioactive methionine was carried out according to Zimmerman and Holler (18). Cells were grown for 1 h with 0.5 μg of radioactive methionine per ml. The RNA was then extracted by a standard procedure (15).

Protein measurements. To measure the amount of protein remaining after incubation of the cells with antibiotics, cells were rinsed twice with Hanks solution, and the protein content was determined by a modified Folin method (14), with bovine serum albumin as standard.

RESULTS

Effect of AmB and filipin as a function of dose. Figure 1 shows dose response curves of L and HeLa cells to AmB and filipin as measured by effects on intracellular potassium content, radioactive uridine incorporation, cell viability, and intracellular protein content.

Potassium leakage from L or HeLa cells pretreated with AmB into potassium-free solution occurred at the lowest AmB concentrations employed. When the AmB concentration was increased, the other effects occurred in the same order in L (A) and HeLa (B) cells, but higher concentrations of AmB were required in the latter. The AmB concentrations (micrograms per milliliter) that caused a 50% decrease in each of the following indexes in L cells were: 4 (intracellular potassium content); 36 (radioactive uridine incorporation); 40 (cell viability); and 65 (intracellular protein content).

In HeLa cells, the corresponding values were 20, 56, 115 and 200 μg/ml. A higher concentration of AmB (20 μg/ml) was required to decrease K^+ content by 50% in unrinsed L cells (data not shown) than in rinsed cells.

The response of L (C^-) and HeLa (D) cells to increasing filipin concentrations showed a different pattern. Below a concentration of 2 μg/ml, no filipin effect was observed. Above this value, potassium content in rinsed and nonrinsed cells (data not shown), protein content, radioactive uridine incorporation, and cell viability all fell at about the same rate. Although the decrease in potassium content in saline-rinsed cells occurred at lower antibiotic concentrations than other effects, the differences were not great and were only apparent in a narrow concentration range. Filipin at 4 μg/ml (for L cells) and 6 μg/ml (for HeLa cells) induced 50% loss of potassium, whereas the other effects were minimal at these concentrations. However, complete loss of potassium occurred at the same concentration as complete cell lysis (20 μg/ml).

Reversibility of potassium leakage. Potassium content was measured in cells preincubated with antibiotics and then washed free of the drugs and allowed to recover by incubation in antibiotic-free medium for a defined time. The cells were then harvested and rinsed with saline, and the potassium content was measured. Figure 2 shows the decrease in potassium content with different antibiotic concentrations, immediately after exposure and after different recovery times in antibiotic-free medium.

L cells preincubated with AmB (A) at a concentration inducing 90% potassium leakage recovered at 0.5 h and 1 h after exposure in fresh medium. They had lost, respectively, 30 and 10% of their content. HeLa cells incubated with AmB (B) at a concentration inducing 90% po-

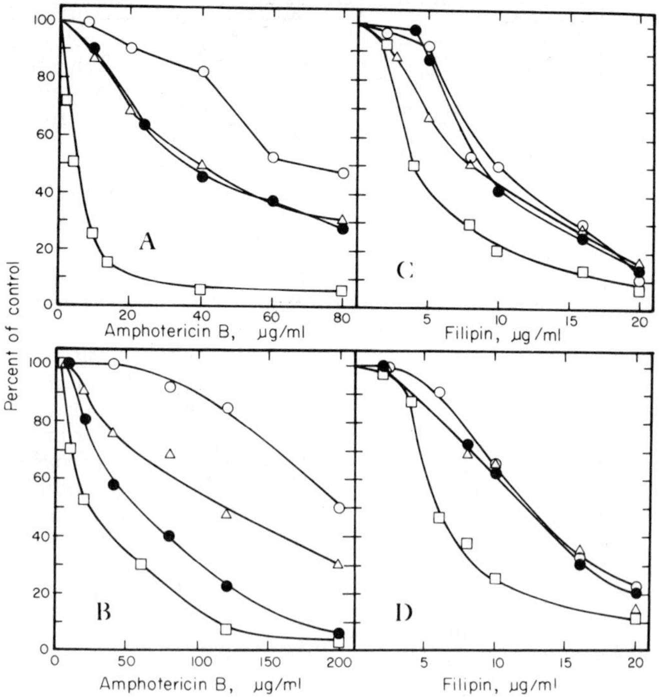

FIG. 1. *Effects of increasing concentration of AmB (A and B) or filipin (C and D) on L (A and C) or HeLa (B and D) cells. After incubation of cells with antibiotic for 1 h, the specific assays were carried out. Symbols:* (□) *potassium remaining in cells rinsed with saline,* (●) *[³H]uridine incorporated,* (△) *number of viable cells,* (○) *protein remaining in cells.*

tassium loss showed a decrease of only 20% from controls after a 1-h recovery period in fresh medium. L cells incubated with filipin (C) at a concentration inducing 85% potassium leakage still had 70% potassium loss after 1 h of recovery and 20% after 3 h. HeLa cells treated with filipin did not recover after incubation for 1 h in fresh medium (data not shown), and after 3 h there was only slight recovery (D).

Therefore, both L and HeLa cells could recover from the permeabilizing effects of both antibiotics. L cells recovered faster and more completely than HeLa, and the recovery occurred faster and over a wider concentration range when cells were pretreated with AmB than with filipin.

Effects of time of exposure to the antibiotics. The effect of the time of exposure of the cells to the antibiotic on changes in permeability to potassium was compared with the effect on incorporation of radioactive uridine (Fig. 3).

Cells preincubated for 8 min with 10 μg of AmB per ml and then rinsed with saline lost 50% of the potassium. After 30 min of incubation, practically all of the potassium had disappeared from the cells. In contrast, the changes in radioactive uridine incorporation induced by the same AmB concentration (10 μg/ml) were more complicated. Initially, an increase in incorporation of radioactivity occurred. An increase of 25% over control values was observed after 20 min, and a maximal increase of 45% was reached after 30 min of incubation with 10 μg of AmB per ml. After this, a gradual decrease in incorporated [³H]uridine followed. When cells were treated with AmB at 20 μg/ml, the increase in [³H]uridine incorporation had a similar pattern, but was present for a shorter time, and the subsequent decrease was more pronounced. The maximal increase in [³H]uridine incorporation observed at 10 and 20 μg of AmB per ml occurred at the same time as when cells were approaching maximal potassium loss. With AmB at 40 μg/ml, no initial increase was observed, and the fall in incorporated radioactivity that occurred later was very marked.

Filipin effects on potassium leakage and [³H]uridine incorporation as a function of incubation time are shown in Fig. 4. L (A) and HeLa (B) cells treated for 15 min with filipin at concentrations of 6 and 8 μg/ml, respectively, released 20% of their potassium. At this time, they incorporated 20 to 30% more radioactive

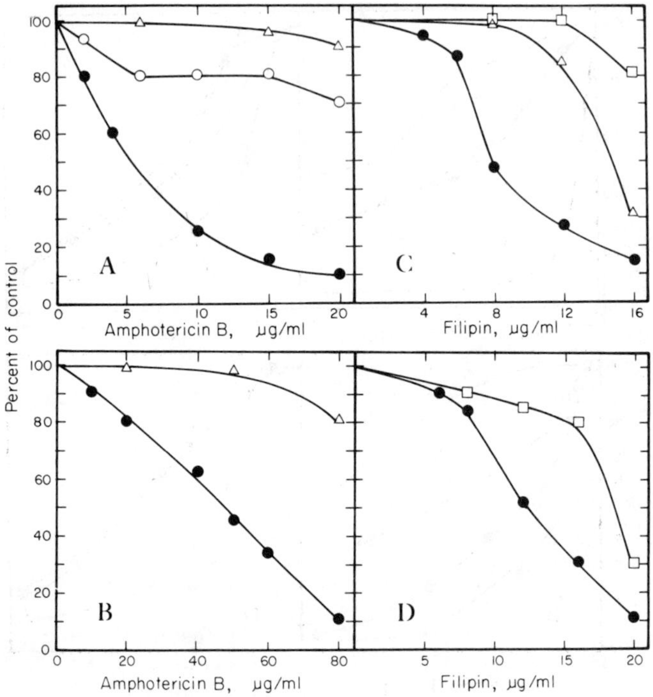

FIG. 2. *Reversibility of the antibiotic-induced permeability to potassium. Cells, L (A and C) or HeLa (B and D), were preincubated for 0.5 h with increasing concentrations of AmB (A and B) or filipin (C and D); they were then rinsed with saline (●) immediately or after additional incubation in antibiotic-free medium for (○) 0.5 h, (△) 1 h, or (□) 3 h. Cells were then extracted with 2% Triton, and the potassium content in the extract was determined.*

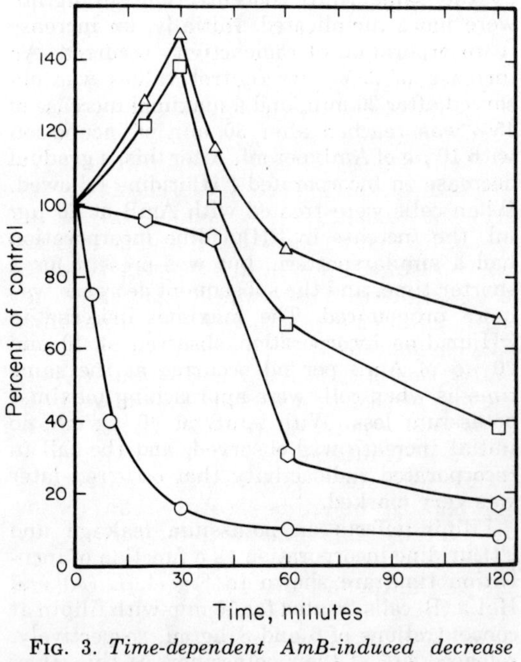

FIG. 3. *Time-dependent AmB-induced decrease in (○) potassium content and in changes of [³H]uridine incorporation into L cells. Potassium content was measured in cells preincubated with 10 μg of AmB per ml and rinsed with saline. [³H]uridine incorporation was measured in cells incubated with the AmB concentrations: (△) 10 μg/ml; (□) 20 μg/ml; and (⬡) 40 μg/ml.*

uridine than control cells. As the time of incubation with filipin increased, there was a decrease in [³H]uridine incorporation.

AmB and filipin effects on pulse labeling of RNA. Table 1 presents the incorporation of radioactivity into RNA of L cells pulsed for 20 min with [³H]uridine. Incorporation increased with time of preincubation with AmB up to 2 h and was lower for 20 μg of AmB per ml than 10 μg/ml. The pulse experiments with L cells and filipin showed small increases over control (10%). HeLa cells preincubated 70 min with filipin and then pulsed for 10 min with radioactive uridine incorporated more radioactivity than control cells. The values were in percentages of control: 116% at 5 μg of filipin per ml and 125% at 10 μg of filipin per ml.

To gain a second measure of RNA synthesis independent of pool effects (5), L cells were

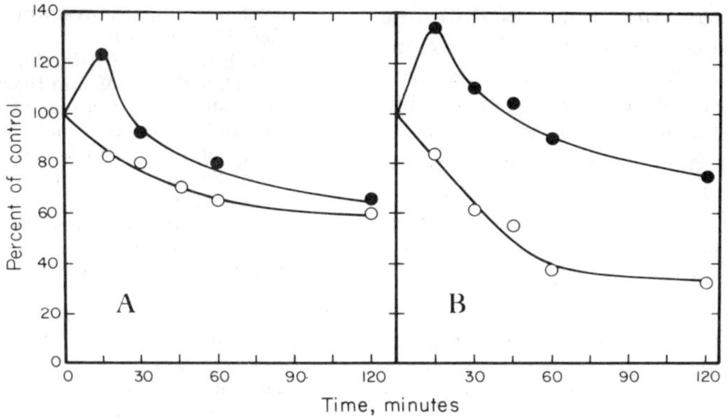

FIG. 4. *Time-dependent filipin-induced decrease in* (○) *potassium content in saline-rinsed cells and in* (●) *changes in [³H]uridine incorporation into L cells incubated with 6 μg of filipin per ml (A) and into HeLa cells incubated with 8 μg of filipin per ml (B).*

TABLE 1. *Incorporation of radioactive uridine into RNA of L cells*

Preincubation time (min)	Incorporation (% of control)[a]	
	A	B
5	124	111
60	154	119
120	186	149

[a] AmB was added at zero time at concentrations of 10 μg/ml (A) or 20 μg/ml (B); cells were preincubated for the times shown and pulsed for 20 min with [³H]uridine.

grown with radioactive methionine in the medium in the absence or in the presence of 10 μg of AmB per ml. The incubation was stopped after 15, 30, 45, or 60 min. The amount of radioactivity in RNA extracted from control cells, grown without AmB, increased linearly, whereas the radioactivity in RNA extracted from cells grown with AmB was equal to control values up to 30 min of incubation and then fell to 50% of controls.

When L cells preincubated for 1 h with 10 μg of AmB per ml were pulsed with radioactive methionine for 20 min, the radioactivity of extracted RNA was 74% of control values.

DISCUSSION

AmB and filipin effects on L and HeLa cells were compared by analyzing potassium leakage, radioactive uridine incorporation, cell viability, and protein leakage. The reversibility of potassium leakage from cells and the responses of potassium leakage and of radioactive uridine incorporation as functions of time were also measured. We found that the different effects of AmB occurred over a wide range of concentrations and were easily separable even at high concentrations of AmB, whereas the filipin effects occurred at lower concentrations and over a narrower range.

The effects of AmB and filipin on cell permeability to potassium were reversible, but recovery was faster and more complete from the changes caused by AmB than by filipin. Cells with the highest AmB-induced permeability to potassium recovered completely, whereas filipin-induced permeability of HeLa cells was closely linked to cell destruction. Other investigators with different experimental systems have also observed the two properties of these polyene antibiotics we have noted: the stepwise reversible changes induced by AmB and the all-or-none irreversible effects of filipin (2–4, 7, 11).

A time study of AmB-induced effects on L cells demonstrated that, at low concentrations of the antibiotic, the change in cell permeability to potassium was correlated with an increase in radioactive uridine incorporation. The pulse-label experiments with radioactive uridine and radioactive methionine exclude the possibility that the increase in uridine incorporation resulted from antibiotic stimulation of RNA synthesis. The simplest explanation for our observation is that the greater permeability of cell membrane to uridine results in increased penetration of radioactive uridine into cells or the loss of pool uridine from cells or both. In both these events, the specific activity of the internal [³H]uridine pool would be higher in antibiotic-treated cells, and the radioactivity incorporated would be greater than in untreated cells. This increase in radioactivity incorporation was induced by both antibiotics, but the AmB effect was more pronounced and lasted longer.

On the basis of previous work (3, 4), we assume that the various indexes of antibiotic action examined by us correspond to different degrees of cell membrane damage. For example, the potassium leakage into potassium-free solution reflects the least perturbing, reversible change in membrane permeability (10). These same changes can also be monitored as increases in radioactive uridine incorporation.

The inhibition of uridine incorporation probably reflects more serious membrane damage. This assumption is in line with work by others (1).

Cell viability was impaired at AmB concentrations equal to or slightly higher than that required to inhibit [^{3}H]uridine incorporation, and finally, protein leakage from cells can be linked to the most severe cell damage equivalent to lysis.

This progressive spectrum of membrane effects was seen with AmB, but not with filipin. With filipin, the separation of the permeabilizing phase from an overall destructive phase was possible only for a short time of incubation and over a narrow range of concentrations.

In regard to clinical applicability of our findings, we conclude that because the toxic and permeabilizing effects of filipin occur over a narrow range, they are not easily separable; and in contrast to AmB, filipin will not be useful to potentiate the action of other pharmacologically active agents. However, it may be that other polyenes maximize the favorable permeabilizing effects without increasing the toxic effects. This would make them even more useful than AmB in potentiating the effects of second agents. It is worthwhile screening other polyene antibiotics for these properties by the methods described in this report.

ACKNOWLEDGMENTS

This work was supported by Public Health Service Program Project CA15665 from the National Cancer Institute and by research grant AI 10622 and training grants AI 00459 and AI 07015 from the National Institute of Allergy and Infectious Diseases.

LITERATURE CITED

1. **Badaracco, B., and G. Cassani.** 1976. Ribonucleic acid synthesis dependent on exogenous triphosphates in nystatin-treated cells of *Kluyveromyces lactis*. Antimicrob. Agents Chemother. 9:748–753.
2. **Cass, A., A. Finkelstein, and V. Krespi.** 1970. The ion permeability induced in thin lipid membranes by the polyene antibiotics nystatin and amphotericin B. J. Gen. Physiol. 56:100–145.
3. **De Kruijff, B., W. G. Gerritsen, A. Oerlemans, R. A. Demel, and L. L. M. van Deenen.** 1974. Polyene antibiotic-sterol interactions in membrane of *Acholeplasma laidlawii* cells and lecithin liposomes. 1. Specificity of the membrane permeability changes induced by the polyene antibiotics. Biochim. Biophys. Acta 339:30–43.
4. **Gent, M. P., and J. H. Prestegard.** 1976. Interaction of the polyene antibiotics with lipid bilayer vesicles containing cholesterol. Biochim. Biophys. Acta 426:17–30.
5. **Greenberg, H., and S. Penman.** 1966. Methylation and processing of ribosomal RNA in HeLa cells. J. Mol. Biol. 21:527–535.
6. **Hamilton-Miller, J. M. T.** 1973. Chemistry and biology of the polyene macrolide antibiotics. Bacteriol. Rev. 37:166–196.
7. **Kinsky, S. C.** 1962. Effect of polyene antibiotics on protoplasts of *Neurospora crassa*. J. Bacteriol. 83:351–358.
8. **Kumar, B. V., G. Medoff, G. Kobayashi, and D. Schlessinger.** 1974. Uptake of *Escherichia coli* DNA into HeLa cells enhanced by amphotericin B. Nature (London) 250:323–325.
9. **Kwan, C. N., G. Medoff, G. S. Kobayashi, D. Schlessinger, and H. J. Raskas.** 1972. Potentiation of the antifungal effects of antibiotics by amphotericin B. Antimicrob. Agents Chemother. 2:61–65.
10. **Lambert, P. A., and S. M. Hammond.** 1973. Potassium flux. First indications of membrane damage in micro-organisms. Biochem. Biophys. Res. Commun. 54:796–799.
11. **Lampen, J. O., and P. M. Arnow.** 1963. Differences in action of large and small polyene antifungal antibiotics. Bull. Res. Counc. Isr. Sect. A 2(4):286–291.
12. **Medoff, G., F. Valeriote, R. G. Lynch, D. Schlessinger, and G. S. Kobayashi.** 1974. Synergistic effect of amphotericin B 1,3-bis (2-chloroethyl-1-nitrosourea against a transplantable AKR leukemia. Cancer Res. 34:974–978.
13. **Norman, A. W., A. M. Spielvogel, and R. G. Wong.** 1976. Polyene antibiotic-sterol interaction, p. 127–170. *In* R. Paoletti and D. Kritchevsky (ed.), Advances in lipid research. Academic Press, New York.
14. **Oyama, V. J., and H. Eagle.** 1953. Measurement of cell growth in tissue culture with a phenol reagent (Folin-Ciocalteau). Proc. Soc. Exp. Biol. Med. 91:305–307.
15. **Penman, S.** 1966. RNA metabolism in the HeLa cell nucleus. J. Mol. Biol. 17:117–130.
16. **Rossomando, E. G., G. Creme, B. Maldonado, M. A. Hesla, and E. E. Golub.** 1976. Effect of amphotericin B on growth and membrane permeability in *Distyostelium discoideum*. Antimicrob. Agents Chemother. 9:618–624.
17. **Shadomy, S., G. Wagner, A. Espinel-Ingrof, and B. A. Davis.** 1975. In vitro studies with combinations of 5-fluorocytosine and amphotericin B. Antimicrob. Agents Chemother. 8:117–121.
18. **Zimmerman, E. F., and B. W. Holler.** 1967. Methylation of 45s ribosomal RNA precursor in HeLa cells. J. Mol. Biol. 23:149–161.

Antimicrobial Agents and Chemotherapy, May 1977, p. 809-812 Vol. 11, No. 2

Effect of Probenecid on the Blood Levels and Urinary Excretion of Cefamandole

R. S. GRIFFITH,* H. R. BLACK, G. L. BRIER, and J. D. WOLNY

Lilly Laboratory for Clinical Research, Wishard Memorial Hospital, and Indiana University School of Medicine, Indianapolis, Indiana 46202*

Received for publication 30 November 1976

Two oral 0.5-g doses of probenecid given 7 and 1 h before a single 1-g intramuscular dose of cefamandole resulted in higher serum levels of cefamandole than when cefamandole was given alone: 37 versus 20 μg per ml of serum, respectively. Cefamandole was not measurable (<0.3 μg/ml) at 8 h when it was given alone, whereas an average 8-h value of 2.9 μg/ml was obtained after pretreatment with probenecid. By prolonging the duration of these high cefamandole levels, probenecid should permit the treatment of more serious clinical infections, including those due to relatively resistant organisms, or permit a reduction in either the dosage of cefamandole or the frequency of administration.

Probenecid has been shown to competitively inhibit the excretion of penicillin and cephalosporins by the tubules of the kidneys (6). In a previous publication, we reported the pharmacokinetics of cefamandole after intramuscular (i.m.) and intravenous injection (3). The data in this paper illustrate the effect of probenecid on the serum levels and urinary excretion of cefamandole.

MATERIALS AND METHODS

Antibiotic. The lithium salt of cefamandole as standard powder was supplied in 20-mg ampoules by Eli Lilly & Co., Indianapolis, Ind. The cefamandole for clinical use, CT-2883-4F, was cefamandole nafate furnished as 1 g of cefamandole activity per ampoule.

Subjects. Twelve male volunteers between the ages of 25 and 55 years were admitted to the study after being screened by history and physical examination and laboratory determination of blood, renal, and liver function. Informed written consent was obtained.

Injection of antibiotic. For i.m. injection, 3 ml of distilled water was added to each 1-g ampoule of cefamandole. The injection was given in the gluteal muscle through a 1.5-inch (ca. 3.8-cm) 20-gauge needle.

Probenecid. Commercially available tablets of probenecid (Benemid, Merck Sharp & Dohme, West Point, Pa.) were administered orally in a dose of 0.5 g 7 and 1 h before the injection.

Serum assays. Blood samples were drawn before and at intervals after the administration of single doses of cefamandole (see Table 1). The blood samples were centrifuged and the sera were frozen until assayed. Serum concentrations were measured using the *Bacillus subtilis* cup plate method (4).

Urine assays. Urine was collected at the intervals shown in Table 2. The urines were assayed by using an Elanco Autoturb (Elanco Products Co., Indianapolis, Ind.) with a *Klebsiella* strain as the indicator organism.

Statistical analysis. A paired *t* test was used to test the hypothesis that the means for both treatment groups are the same versus the hypothesis that these means are different. This pairing was necessary since each patient in this study received each of the study medications.

RESULTS

Figure 1 shows the average cefamandole blood levels achieved after the i.m. injection of 1 g of cefamandole alone compared with those obtained when 1 g of cefamandole was given to the same subjects after they had received probenecid orally. Figure 2 illustrates the alteration of cefamandole excretion by probenecid.

Probenecid administered orally in doses of 0.5 g every 6 h (for two doses) almost doubled the peak blood levels obtained after administration of 1 g of cefamandole: 37 and 20.4 μg/ml, respectively. The half-life was obviously prolonged by probenecid: 1.1 to 2 h; and at 8 h cefamandole could not be assayed in the blood after cefamandole alone, but after cefamandole plus probenecid, 2.9 μg/ml was found.

The higher and more prolonged levels seen with prebenecid plus cefamandole are related to the delay in excretion of cefamandole by the effect of probenecid on the kidney tubules. In Fig. 2 it is apparent that more cefamandole appeared in the urine during the first and second 2-h collection periods after cefamandole

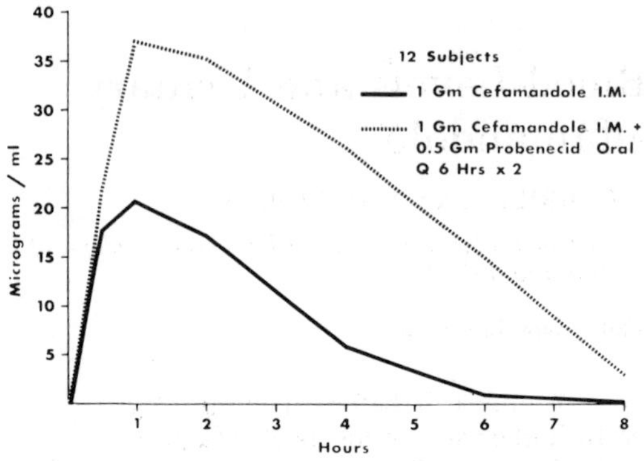

FIG. 1. *Effect of probenecid on cefamandole blood levels.*

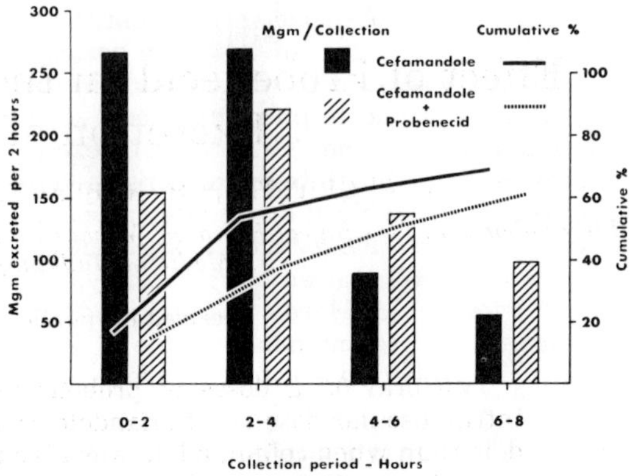

FIG. 2. *Urinary excretion of cefamandole.*

TABLE 1. *Concentrations of cefamandole in serum after i.m. administration*

Subject	Concn (μg/ml) in serum at h:						
	0	0.5	1	2	4	6	8
Cefamandole (1 g)							
AB	0	25	16	10	3.5	1.2	0.4
RD	0	47.6	26.6	14.3	2.5	0.5	<0.3
ME	0	29.3	43.5	21.4	2.5	0.4	<0.3
HG	0	17.1	16.7	17.6	4.9	0.8	<0.3
JH	0	9	9	9.7	6.3	2.2	0.6
TH	0	4.4	12.3	14.4	2.9	0.8	<0.3
RM	0	5.8	14	15.1	6.2	2.2	1.1
AP	0	22.4	40.2	20.4	6.2	1.6	1.2
DW	0	19.5	20.1	13.1	4	0.7	<0.3
RB	0	4.1	7.1	20.1	6	0.9	<0.3
PM	0	23.6	26.2	14.9	2.3	0.5	<0.3
ES	0	5.9	13.3	12.6	25.3	0.6	<0.3
Mean	0	17.8	20.4	15.3	6.1	1	<0.3
SD[a]	0	13	11.7	3.8	6.3	0.6	0.4
Cefamandole (1 g) + probenecid[b]							
AB	0	24.3	45.3	50.4	86.4	26.3	8.3
RD	0	23.8	14.8	6.2	1.5	0.3	<0.3
ME	0	84.2	93.8	54.7	27.1	7	2.5
HG	0	2.3	18.5	24.2	24.9	19	3.6
JH	0	7.9	25.5	28.4	10.8	2.5	<0.3
TH	0	9.5	31.5	32.7	20.2	9.5	2.9
RM	0	9.4	13	13	7.3	2.9	1
AP	0	23.1	62.8	50.9	16.9	2	0.4
DW	0	8.4	21.6	37.3	25.6	11.6	3
RB	0	10.4	19.7	30.9	24.2	10.8	3.3
PM	0	19.7	48.5	37.9	32.1	17.2	5.9
ES	0	28.4	48.6	57.1	67	83	3.8
Mean	0	21	37	35.3	28.7	16	2.9
SD	0	21.6	24	16.2	24.5	22.5	2.4
Paired *t*-value		0.55	3.31	4.29	3.47	2.28	3.33
P-value[c]		0.598	0.007	0.001	0.005	0.043	0.007

[a] SD, Standard deviation.
[b] A 0.5-g dose of probenecid 7 and 1 h before cefamandole injection.
[c] Two-tailed probability value.

alone than when probenecid was present. During the third and fourth 2-h collection periods, the reverse was true: more was excreted in the urine after cefamandole plus probenecid than after cefamandole alone. This delay in excretion may be related both to the prolongation of higher cefamandole blood levels after probenecid and to a progressive reduction in probenecid effect, as it is also removed by the kidney.

The individual blood levels (Table 1) and urinary excretion of cefamandole (Table 2) with and without probenecid are shown for closer scrutiny.

DISCUSSION

Probenecid is an organic acid that has a relatively high affinity for the renal tubular transport system and is readily secreted with subsequent rapid reabsorption. This "recirculation" accounts for the prolonged action of probenecid (6). Since other organic acids, such as the penicillins or cephalosporins, are excreted by the same tubular mechanism, the administration of probenecid competitively blocks their elimination by the kidney tubules (1). Renal clearance values for the penicillins and cephalosporins by the kidney under the influence of probenecid approach the glomerular filtration rate.

Fong et al. showed a half-life of approximately 50 min for cefamandole administered i.m. (2). These same authors reported that the renal clearance of cefamandole was 257 ml/min per 1.73 m^2.

Using the same formula, we found a renal clearance of 229 ml/min per 1.73 m^2 during the 2- to 4-h and 4- to 6-h urine collection periods.

TABLE 2. *Concentrations of cefamandole in urine after i.m. administration*

Subject	0–2 h			2–4 h			4–6 h			6–8 h		
	μg/ml	Total vol (ml)	Total mg	μg/ml	Total vol (ml)	Total mg	μg/ml	Total vol (ml)	Total mg	μg/ml	Total vol (ml)	Total mg
Cefamandole (1 g)												
AB	1,365	230	314	844	250	211	355	210	75	145	180	26
RD	2,973	160	476	2,426	90	218	406	75	30	197	90	18
ME	4,800	80	384	3,876	50	194	344	60	21	251	60	15
HG	1,037	100	104	2,205	120	265	2,139	110	235	1,486	80	119
JH	750	190	143	2,205	150	353	1,564	110	172	392	110	43
TH	3,857	95	366	2,459	90	221	719	50	36	356	80	28
RM	1,780	115	205	1,898	120	228	800	130	104	313	90	28
AP	797	240	191	2,503	100	250	406	160	65	217	160	35
DW	1,520	210	319	3,050	60	183	810	80	65	267	60	16
RB	1,185	100	119	4,153	110	457	1,289	100	129	188	60	11
PM	938	300	281	1,313	260	341	492	170	84	267	60	16
ES	3,234	90	291	3,189	65	207	970	70	68	356	60	21
Mean	2,020	159	266	2,510	122	261	858	110	90	370	91	31
SD[a]	1,356	73	115	958	60	82	546	46	63	360	41	29
Cefamandole (1 g) + probenecid[b]												
AB	63	140	9	438	180	79	500	170	85	500	180	90
RD	813	310	252	500	280	140	1,039	240	249	1,477	150	222
ME	750	220	165	500	240	120	1,297	70	91	1,092	40	44
HG	250	100	25	1,125	160	180	1,799	80	144	1,211	90	109
JH	313	250	78	1,250	180	225	1,053	130	137	1,039	110	114
TH	1,000	180	180	3,749	80	300	1,105	115	127	1,053	65	68
RM	3,550	10	36	938	180	161	1,105	110	122	1,013	90	91
AP	2,179	150	327	1,920	85	163	1,320	100	132	969	80	78
DW	750	190	143	1,680	210	353	1,590	100	159	781	50	39
RB	1,063	110	117	2,511	170	427	1,158	130	151	969	100	97
PM	2,238	120	269	1,000	180	180	1,026	90	92	1,013	130	132
ES	2,961	85	252	2,596	120	312	1,053	150	158	938	100	94
Mean	1,327	155	154	1,517	172	221	1,170	124	137	1,005	99	98
SD	1,130	81	105	1,017	58	105	321	46	44	231	40	47
Paired *t*-value		3.146			1.342			2.088			4.278	
P-value[c]		0.0093			0.2069			0.0608			0.0013	

[a] SD, Standard deviation.
[b] A 0.5-g dose of probenecid 7 and 1 h before cefamandole injection.
[c] Two-tailed probability value.

Probenecid produced a decrease in renal clearance of cefamandole to 57 ml/min per 1.73 m^2 during these same collection periods. No attempt was made to establish the maximal effective dose of probenecid required to block the tubular transport of cefamandole. The usual adult dose of probenecid, 0.5 g every 6 h, has been shown to adequately block penicillin (1). This clearance rate of 57 ml for cefamandole when given with probenecid is similar to the rate of 75 ml reported by Kirby and Regamey for cefazolin without probenecid (5).

When probenecid is used, approximately 2% of the patients will have some noticeable degree of gastrointestinal irritation; hence, caution should be exercised if probenecid is administered to patients with known peptic ulcer (1). In addition, skin rash has been reported in 2 to 4% of those taking probenecid (1). Thus, it is difficult to differentiate the etiology of hypersensitivity should probenecid be given with another medication, a diagnostic dilemma not uncommon with the polytherapy of today.

In conclusion, the administration of probenecid, 0.5 g every 6 h orally, with cefamandole will almost double the blood levels and prolong the duration of therapeutic levels of cefamandole by competitively blocking the renal tubular transport of cefamandole.

The higher and more prolonged blood levels of cefamandole associated with probenecid should permit the treatment of more serious clinical infections, including those due to relatively resistant organisms, or a reduction either in dose or in frequency of administration.

LITERATURE CITED

1. **Brazeau, P.** 1975. Inhibitors of tubular transport of organic compounds, p. 860–866. *In* L. S. Goodman and A. Gilman (ed.), The pharmacological basis of therapeutics, 5th ed. Macmillan Publishing Co., Inc., New York.
2. **Fong, I. W., E. D. Ralph, E. R. Engelking, and W. M. M. Kirby.** 1976. Clinical pharmacology of cefamandole as compared with cephalothin. Antimicrob. Agents Chemother. 9:65–69.
3. **Griffith, R. S., H. R. Black, G. L. Brier, and J. D. Wolny.** 1976. Cefamandole: in vitro and clinical pharmacokinetics. Antimicrob. Agents Chemother. 10:814–823.
4. **Grove, D., and W. A. Randall.** 1955. Assay methods for antibiotics. Antibiot. Monogr., Vol. 2.
5. **Kirby, W. M. M., and C. Regamey.** 1973. Pharmacokinetics of cefazolin compared with four other cephalosporins. J. Infect. Dis. 128:S341–S346.
6. **Weiner, I. M., J. A. Washington, and G. H. Mudge.** 1960. On the mechanism of action of probenecid on renal tubular secretion. Bull. Johns Hopkins Hosp. 106:336–346.

ANTIMICROBIAL AGENTS AND CHEMOTHERAPY, May 1977, p. 813-916
Vol. 11, No. 5

Synergistic Action of Erythromycin and Cefamandole Against *Bacteroides fragilis* Subsp. *fragilis*

R. S. GRIFFITH,* G. L. BRIER, AND J. D. WOLNY

Lilly Laboratory for Clinical Research, Wishard Memorial Hospital, and Indiana University School of Medicine, Indianapolis, Indiana 46202*

Received for publication 30 November 1976

Erythromycin and cefamandole have exhibited synergistic activity against eight strains of *Bacteroides fragilis* subsp. *fragilis*. In concentrations of only 0.25 to 0.5 μg of erythromycin per ml (easily obtainable with oral therapy), less than 0.4 μg (0.015 to 1.0) of cefamandole per ml inhibited the *B. fragilis* strains. In the presence of the erythromycin, the potency of cefamandole was increased more than 100-fold. On the basis of the mechanism of action of these two antibiotics, the synergism may be related to inhibition of beta-lactamase formation by the erythromycin, removal of the bacterial cell wall by the cefamandole permitting erythromycin penetration to the ribosomal level, and decreasing inoculum effect.

The dominant species of bacteria isolated from the intestinal tract of man is *Bacteroides fragilis* (1, 21). These same organisms have been isolated from patients with infection: 437 of 7,500 nonfecal specimens submitted to the hospital laboratory for culture. Only 30 of these anaerobes were present as pure culture (5). In a review of 306 cases of anaerobic infection reported in the literature, 211 or 69% occurred in patients with malignancy. The remainder had some other compromising condition, such as diabetes, steroid therapy, etc. (7). It evolves, therefore, that in antimicrobial programs designed for prevention or treatment of infection, both in the compromised host and severe infections of undetermined etiology, it may be reasonable to include agents that are active against *B. fragilis* subsp. *fragilis* in addition to those antibiotics active against other potential pathogens (3).

Several agents, when studied in combination, have shown synergistic activity against *B. fragilis* subsp. *fragilis* (3). This report describes the results of in vitro tests of eight clinical isolates of *B. fragilis* subsp. *fragilis* against two antimicrobial agents, erythromycin and cefamandole.

MATERIALS AND METHODS

Antibiotics. Stock solutions of 1,000 μg/ml were made by diluting standard powers of lithium cefamandole and erythromycin gluceptate (Eli Lilly and Co., Indianapolis, Ind.) in phosphate buffer, pH 7.2. The final working dilutions were made in supplemented brain heart infusion (Difco Laboratories, Detroit, Mich.) broth.

Antibiotic dilution. The microdilutions for each antibiotic for determination of the minimal inhibitory concentration (MIC) of the anaerobic organisms were made outside the glove box (Coy Manufacturing, Ann Arbor, Mich.) with an Autotiter IV (Ames Co., Division of Miles Laboratory, Elkhart, Ind.), producing a typical "checkerboard" (2, 19). The plates were passed into the glove box and allowed to reduce prior to inoculation. The range of antibiotic concentrations in the checkerboard arrangement, after inoculation, was 32 to 0.015 μg/ml for each antibiotic. Growth and sterility controls were maintained for each assay.

Medium. The medium in the microdilution plate wells consisted of brain heart infusion broth supplemented with yeast extract, 0.5%, plus 1 μg of heme and 5 μg of menadione per ml. L-Cysteine, as the hydrochloride (0.5% final concentration), was added to the medium as a reducing agent. Indigo carmine dye (colorless at an E_h of less than −0.125 mV) was added as a redox indicator to control wells (20, 23). The pH of the medium was adjusted to 8.2 with NaOH before autoclaving. After autoclaving (the indicator dye is now colorless), the medium was stored in the glove box and allowed to cool. The pH stabilized at 7.2 in this controlled atmosphere (10% H_2, 10% CO_2, 80% N_2).

Organisms. The eight strains of *B. fragilis* subsp. *fragilis* were picked at random from 77 clinical isolates recovered from the Indiana University School of Medicine hospitals between 1972 and 1975. The criteria for identification were those described in the literature (13).

Inoculum. The inoculum for the plates consisted of 50 μl per well of a 1:100 dilution of an overnight broth culture, approximately 10^6 organisms per ml. The plates were inoculated using 50-μl plastic, disposable pipettes (no. 22036, Cooke Laboratory Products, Alexandria, Va.). The final inoculum per well of 10^6 organisms per ml was verified by using a du Pont Luminescence Biometer (E. I. du Pont Instruments, Wilmington, Del.). The adenosine 5′-triphosphate produced by bacteria is proportional to the number of bacteria present. Since the luminescence of luciferase enzyme can be quantitated to the amount of adenosine 5′-triphosphate present, luminescence can be used to measure bacteria counts. The Biometer is designed to convert luminescence directly to bacterial count (4, 15).

After inoculation, the plates were sealed with plastic tape and incubated in the anaerobic glove box at 37°C for 24 h. After incubation the plates were read with the Autotray Viewer (Ames Co.) (14, 17). The addition of L-cysteine, prereducing the medium by autoclaving, and storage in the controlled atmosphere of the glove box made it possible to read the results in 24 instead of 48 h.

RESULTS

The susceptibility of the eight *Bacteroides* strains to erythromycin and cefamandole alone is shown in the second and third columns of Table 1. When erythromycin was present in a concentration of 0.5 μg/ml, all eight strains were susceptible to less than 0.015 μg of cefamandole per ml. The lowest concentration for each antibiotic showing synergism, when studied in combination, is underlined in the table. The increase in activity of the erythromycin and cefamandole in combination is illustrated in the last column of Table 1. An average concentration of 0.2 μg of erythromycin and less than 0.4 μg of cefamandole per ml in combination inhibited *B. fragilis* subsp. *fragilis*. The range of concentrations showing activity against the eight strains was 0.125 to 0.25 μg of erythromycin and <0.015 to 2 μg of cefamandole per ml.

Drug interaction was considered to be synergistic when the strain of *Bacteroides* was inhibited by the combination of erythromycin and cefamandole, each at a concentration of less than or equal to 25% of its MIC when tested alone. As shown in the last column of Table 1, six of the eight strains exhibited this degree of synergism. The overall effect of the combination on the eight strains of *Bacteroides* tested was evaluated by constructing an isobologram (Fig. 1). The isobologram for the combination can be compared with the theoretical straight-line isobologram formed by connecting the points representing the mean MIC for each antibiotic. Bowing of the isobologram toward the

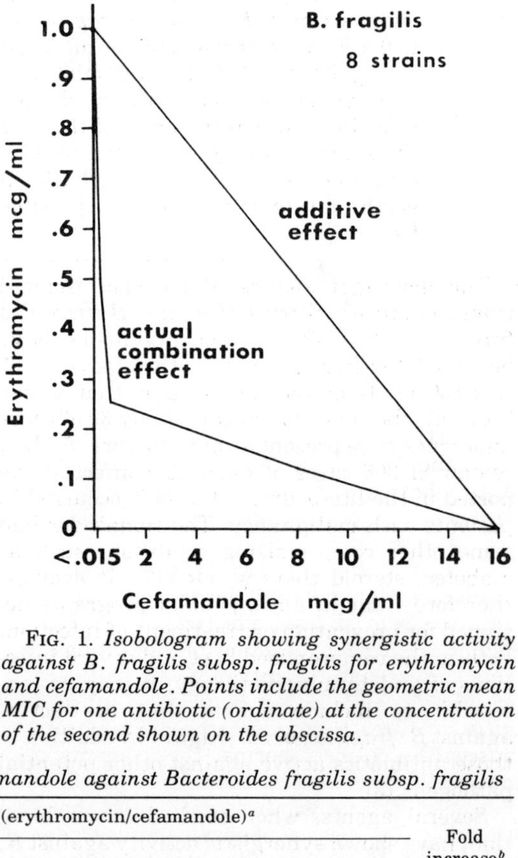

FIG. 1. *Isobologram showing synergistic activity against B. fragilis subsp. fragilis for erythromycin and cefamandole. Points include the geometric mean MIC for one antibiotic (ordinate) at the concentration of the second shown on the abscissa.*

TABLE 1. *Synergistic action of erythromycin and cefamandole against Bacteroides fragilis subsp. fragilis*

Strain	Single[a]		Combined (erythromycin/cefamandole)[a]				Fold increase[b]
	Erythromycin	Cefamandole	Concn 1	Concn 2	Concn 3	Concn 4	
88	0.5	8.0	0.5/<0.015[a]	0.25/<0.015	0.125/<0.015[c]	0.06/8	8/>512
76	1.0	16	0.5/<0.015	0.25/<0.015	0.125/0.06	0.06/8	4/256
83	0.5	8	0.5/<0.015	0.25/<0.015	0.125/8	—[d]	2/>512
72	1.0	16	0.5/<0.015	0.25/<0.015	0.125/8	0.06/16	4/>1024
89	0.5	16	0.5/<0.015	0.25/1	0.125/16	—	2/16
57	1.0	8	0.5/<0.015	0.25/0.06	0.125/8	—	4/128
74	1.0	16	0.5/<0.015	0.25/2	0.125/16	—	4/8
86	2.0	8	0.5/<0.015	0.25/0.125	0.125/8	—	8/64
Average	1.0	12					4/>128

[a] Drug concentrations in micrograms per milliliter.
[b] Erythromycin/cefamandole.
[c] The underlined figures designate the lowest concentration of each antibiotic showing synergism.
[d] —, Indicates no additional effect.

intersection of the vertical and horizontal axes is indicative of synergism (22). Maximal synergistic effect was observed when the average concentration of erythromycin was 0.2 μg/ml and that of cefamandole was 0.4 μg/ml.

DISCUSSION

The only combination of antimicrobial agents that has shown significant synergistic activity in vitro against *B. fragilis* subsp. *fragilis* is clindamycin with metronidazole (3). It would be reassuring to know that the antimicrobial agents being used clinically to treat infections are also effective against anaerobic *Bacteroides*, even though this is considered a relatively rare pathogen causing infection in humans. Our in vitro data, coupled with the blood levels achievable with erythromycin and cefamandole, suggest an alternate combination to use as therapy in selected *Bacteroides* infection. The average peak blood level after the usual oral dose of erythromycin has been shown to be 1.4 μg/ml (10). In concentrations of 0.5 μg/ml or greater of erythromycin, less than 0.015 μg of cefamandole per ml was needed for inhibition of the *Bacteroides* strains studied. Obviously, the peak level of 19 μg/ml obtained after 1 g of cefamandole injected intramuscularly (11) would be more than 1,000-fold greater than the MIC of cefamandole required to inhibit these same *Bacteroides* strains when erythromycin is present in concentrations of 0.5 μg/ml or greater.

It has been suggested that a knowledge of the mechanism of synergy permits antibacterial substances to be used effectively (19). The accepted antibacterial action of the cephalosporins is related to inhibition of cell wall synthesis (8). However, since *B. fragilis* subsp. *fragilis* produces a beta-lactamase that destroys susceptible cephalosporins, these agents may not be effective against these bacteria (5, 6). It has been shown that those antibiotics that lose their activity because of enzymatic degradation show a marked increase in activity as the inoculum is decreased (16). It has been suggested that beta-lactam antibiotics remove the cell wall and permit erythromycin to more easily penetrate the bacterial cell and reach the ribosome (9, 12). This, in turn, slows or stops beta-lactamase synthesis, allowing greater cephalosporin activity. As the viable inoculum is reduced, both agents show greater activity.

Although essentially all strains of *B. fragilis* subsp. *fragilis* can be inhibited by easily obtainable concentrations of several antimicrobial agents, combinations such as cefamandole plus erythromycin may prove useful in the treatment of selected infections, where this organism is implicated as a single or primary pathogen, and for infections due to this organism where maximal antibacterial activity is desired.

In summary, eight clinical isolates of *B. fragilis* subsp. *fragilis* were tested against cefamandole and erythromycin by the microdilution technique. A synergistic effect was observed. No antagonism was noted. For selected *Bacteroides* infections, the combination of cefamandole and erythromycin may be useful.

LITERATURE CITED

1. **Atterbery, H. R., V. L. Sutter, and S. M. Finegold.** 1974. Normal human intestinal flora, p. 91. *In* A. Balows, R. M. DeHaan, V. R. Dowell, Jr., and L. B. Guze (ed.), Anaerobic bacteria. Role in disease. Charles C Thomas, Publisher, Springfield, Ill.
2. **Bourque, M., R. Quintiliani, and R. C. Tilton.** 1976. Synergism of cefazolin-gentamicin against enterococci. Antimicrob. Agents Chemother. **10**:157–163.
3. **Busch, D. F., V. L. Sutter, and S. M. Finegold.** 1976. Activity of combinations of antimicrobial agents against *Bacteroides fragilis*. J. Infect. Dis. **133**:321–328.
4. **Chappelle, E. W.** Use of the firefly bioluminescent reaction for rapid detection and counting of bacteria. Biochem. Med. **2**:41–52.
5. **Davis, C. E., W. J. Hunter, J. L. Ryan, and A. I. Braude.** 1973. Simple method of culturing anaerobes. Appl. Microbiol. **25**:215–221.
6. **Del Bene, V. E., and W. E. Farrar, Jr.** 1972. Antimicrobial therapy of infections due to anaerobic bacteria. Semin. Drug Treat. **2**:295–312.
7. **Finegold, S. M., V. H. Marsh, and J. G. Barlett.** 1970. Anaerobic infections in the compromised host, p. 123–134. *In* P. S. Brachman and T. C. Eickhoff (ed.), Proc. Int. Conf. Nosocomial Infections, Aug. 3–6. Am. Hosp. Assoc., Chicago.
8. **Gale, E. F., E. Cundliffe, P. E. Reynolds, M. H. Richmond, and M. J. Waring.** 1972. The molecular basis of antibiotic action, p. 94. John Wiley & Sons, New York.
9. **Gale, E. F., E. Cundliffe, P. E. Reynolds, M. H. Richmond, and M. J. Waring.** 1972. The molecular basis of antibiotic action, p. 337. John Wiley & Sons, New York.
10. **Griffith, R. S., and H. R. Black.** 1962. A comparison of blood levels after oral administration of erythromycin and erythromycin estolate. Antibiot. Chemother. (Basel) **12**:398–403.
11. **Griffith, R. S., H. R. Black, G. L. Brier, and J. D. Wolny.** 1976. Cefamandole: in vitro and clinical pharmacokinetics. Antimicrob. Agents Chemother. **10**:814–823.
12. **Hewitt, W. L., S. J. Seligman, and R. A. Deigh.** 1966. Kinetics of the synergism of penicillin-streptomycin and penicillin-kanamycin for enterococci and its relationship to L-phase variants. J. Lab. Clin. Med. **67**:792–807.
13. **Holdeman, L. V., and W. E. C. Moore (ed.).** 1972. Anaerobe laboratory manual. Anaerobe Laboratory, Virginia Polytechnic Institute and State University, Blacksburg.
14. **Jones, R. N., and P. C. Fuchs.** 1976. Identification and antimicrobial susceptibility of 250 *Bacteroides fragilis* subspecies tested by broth microdilution methods. Antimicrob. Agents Chemother. **9**:719–721.

15. **Picciolo, G. L., B. N. Kelbaugh, E. W. Chappelle, and A. J. Fleig.** 1971. An automated luciferase assay of bacteria in urine. Goddard Space Flight Center, Greenbelt, Md.
16. **Roberts, C. B., Jr., L. S. Rosenfeld, and W. M. M. Kirby.** 1963. Synergism of erythromycin and penicillin against resistant staphylococci: mechanism and relation to synthetic penicillins, p. 149–155. Antimicrob. Agents Chemother. 1962.
17. **Ritilie, C. A., R. J. Fass, R. B. Prior, and R. L. Perkins.** 1975. Microdilution technique for antimicrobial susceptibility testing of anaerobic bacteria. Antimicrob. Agents Chemother. 7:311–315.
18. **Sabath, L. D.** 1968. Synergy of antibacterial substances by apparently known mechanisms, p. 210–217. Antimicrob. Agents Chemother. 1967.
19. **Sabath, L. D., C. E. McCall, N. H. Steigbigel, and M. Finland.** 1967. Synergistic penicillin combinations for treatment of human urinary-tract infections, p. 149–155. Antimicrob. Agents Chemother. 1966.
20. **Smith, L. DS., and L.V. Holdeman.** 1968. The pathogenic anaerobic bacteria, p. 9. Charles C Thomas, Publisher, Springfield, Ill.
21. **Sonnenwirth, A. C.** 1974. Incidence of intestinal anaerobes in blood cultures, p. 159. *In* A. Balows, R. M. DeHaan, V. R. Dowell, Jr., and L. B. Guze (ed.), Anaerobic bacteria. Role in disease. Charles C Thomas, Publisher, Springfield, Ill.
22. **Weinstein, R. J., L. S. Young, and W. L. Hewitt.** 1975. Comparison of methods for assessing in vitro antibiotic synergism against *Pseudomonas* and *Serratia*. J. Lab. Clin. Med. 86:853–862.
23. **Williams, P. P.** 1966. Dispensing apparatus for controlling E_h, pH, and volume of anaerobic bacterial and protozoal culture media. Appl. Microbiol. 14:1045–1046.

Antimicrobial Agents and Chemotherapy, May 1977, p. 817-820 Vol. 11, No. 5
 Printed in U.S.A.

Antimicrobial Therapy of Experimental Group B Streptococcal Infection in Mice

A. DEVEIKIS,* V. SCHAUF, M. MIZEN, and L. RIFF

Departments of Pediatrics and Medicine, University of Illinois College of Medicine, Chicago, Illinois 60680*

Received for publication 5 January 1977

Group B beta-hemolytic streptococci (GB-BHS) frequently cause severe infection in newborns. Previous in vitro studies showed accelerated killing of GB-BHS by ampicillin plus gentamicin as compared with ampicillin alone. To extend the in vitro observations, mice were infected experimentally with GB-BHS and treated with gentamicin plus ampicillin or ampicillin alone. Untreated mice died within 10 to 48 h. Compared with treatment with ampicillin alone, ampicillin-and-gentamicin therapy resulted in improved survival when the antibiotics were given in established infection or as a single dose at the time of infection. Ampicillin and gentamicin accelerated the clearing of bacteremia as compared with treatment with ampicillin alone. In view of these findings, the therapy of GB-BHS infection in newborns and other patients should be reconsidered in that a combination of ampicillin or penicillin G plus gentamicin might be superior to the use of ampicillin or penicillin G alone.

Group B beta-hemolytic streptococcus (GB-BHS) is a frequent and serious cause of infection in infancy (4, 6), despite susceptibility of GB-BHS to penicillin and ampicillin (5, 13). Penicillin or ampicillin is recommended for the treatment of GB-BHS infection of infants (12). Since these agents act by similar mechanisms, the bactericidal effect of one of these agents, ampicillin, against this organism was measured. The rate of killing of GB-BHS by ampicillin was slower than that observed for group A beta-hemolytic streptococci (13); whereas less than 4 h is required for a 99.99% reduction in bacterial colony counts of group A beta-hemolytic streptococci, up to 48 h is required for the same reduction in GB-BHS. Although GB-BHS are resistant to gentamicin as a single drug, killing was accelerated by the combination of ampicillin with gentamicin (13). To examine the relevance of these in vitro findings, we produced experimental GB-BHS infection in weanling mice. The influence of ampicillin alone and in combination with gentamicin on survival in mice and on the kinetics of bacteremia was studied.

MATERIALS AND METHODS

Organism. GB-BHS reference strain Ia was chosen for these studies because infections with this strain are common and often fatal in newborns (3). GB-BHS reference strain Ia, SS-615, was supplied by R. R. Facklam, Center for Disease Control, Atlanta, Ga. The organism was passaged monthly on 5% blood agar and kept at 4°C. Streptococci were grown in tryptose phosphate broth. The minimal inhibitory concentration (MIC) of ampicillin for the organism was 0.06 μg/ml, and the minimal bactericidal concentration (MBC) was 2.0 μg/ml. The MIC of gentamicin for the organism was 8 μg/ml, and the MBC was 16.0 μg/ml.

Antibiotics. Sodium ampicillin (Omnipen N, Wyeth Laboratories Inc., Philadelphia, Pa.) was diluted in normal saline immediately before each administration. Gentamicin (Garamycin, Shering Corp., Kenilworth, N.J.) was diluted in normal saline and stored at 4°C until injection. The total ampicillin dose was 125 mg/kg; the total gentamicin dose was 25 mg/kg.

Antibiotic assay. Gentamicin and/or ampicillin concentrations in serum were measured 1 h after subcutaneous injection by the agar well diffusion technique (8). For ampicillin assay, *Bacillus subtilis* ATCC 6633 was used; for gentamicin assay, *Staphylococcus epidermidis* ATCC 27626 was used. To assay ampicillin in the presence of gentamicin, 4% sodium chloride was incorporated in the agar. Antibiotic standards of ampicillin (5, 10, 20, and 40 μg/ml) or gentamicin (1.25, 2.5, 5, 10, and 20 μg/ml) diluted in NIH Swiss mouse serum, were included on each assay plate.

Therapeutic evaluations. Female NIH Swiss mice, 16 to 19 g, were obtained from Scientific Small Animal Laboratories (Arlington Heights, Ill.). Mice were injected intraperitoneally with approximately 10^7 colony-forming units (CFU) of GB-BHS in 0.1 ml of an undiluted overnight culture. Inoculation of 10 CFU streptococci per mouse resulted in a mortality of 50%. All mice injected with 10^7 CFU died 10 to 48 h after infection. In one series of experiments, the total dose of antibiotics was divided into three portions and injected 4, 10, and 16 h after infection.

Deaths due to streptococcal infection were tabulated for the following 9 days. In some experiments, mice received the total daily antibiotic dose simultaneously with streptococcal infection. Antibiotics were injected subcutaneously as 0.1 ml of ampicillin or 0.1 ml of ampicillin and 0.1 ml of gentamicin in separate sites.

Quantitative blood cultures. Mice were infected as described above and injected 1 h later with 125 mg of ampicillin per kg or the same dose of ampicillin and 25 mg of gentamicin per kg, or were left untreated. Groups of 20 animals were exsanguinated by cardiac puncture at each of four time points: 1 h after infection (at the time of antibiotic injection) and hourly for the next 3 h. Undiluted blood (0.1 ml) and 10-fold dilutions of blood were plated on blood agar, and CFU per milliliter of blood were counted after overnight incubation.

RESULTS

Survival. The efficacy of ampicillin was compared with that of ampicillin and gentamicin in established GB-BHS infection. Table 1 shows data from three replicate experiments in which mice were infected and treated 4, 10, and 16 h later with ampicillin alone (125 mg/kg divided in three doses) or the same dose of ampicillin plus gentamicin (25 mg/kg divided in three doses). One hour after the first dose of antibiotics, serum levels of ampicillin averaged 18 μg/ml and those of gentamicin averaged 5 μg/ml. Ninety-five animals treated with ampicillin had a survival of 53% at the end of 9 days, whereas 95 animals treated with ampicillin and gentamicin had a survival of 73% ($\chi^2 = 9.06$, $P < 0.01$). Of animals given the same dose of gentamicin alone, none survived.

We attempted to determine whether simultaneous treatment with ampicillin or ampicillin and gentamicin would protect mice from lethal GB-BHS infection. Animals were given either ampicillin alone (125 mg/kg) or ampicillin and gentamicin (125 and 25 mg/kg, respectively) as a single dose at the time of infection. One hour after the antibiotic dose, serum levels of ampicillin averaged 30 μg/ml and those of gentamicin averaged 8 μg/ml. Table 1 shows the data from three replicate experiments. The group of mice treated with ampicillin had a survival of 43% 9 days after inoculation, whereas 98% of the group receiving ampicillin and gentamicin survived ($\chi^2 = 54$, $P < 0.01$). In all experiments, untreated mice had no survivors at 48 h after infection with GB-BHS. Animals treated with gentamicin alone had a 15% survival.

Kinetics of streptococcal bacteremia. The improved survival of mice receiving combined antibiotics compared with those treated with ampicillin alone was investigated by studies of the kinetics of clearing streptococcal bacteremia. One hour after infection, ampicillin (125 mg/kg) or ampicillin (125 mg/kg) and gentamicin (25 mg/kg) were given as a single dose. No deaths occurred in mice receiving antibiotics during the sampling period.

Figure 1a illustrates the incidence of bacteremia among the three groups. Bacteremia was present in 100% of the untreated animals at all times. With ampicillin treatment, 90 to 95% of mice remained bacteremic 1, 2, and 3 h after treatment. In contrast, 52% of mice treated with ampicillin and gentamicin were bacteremic 2 h after treatment, and only 33% were bacteremic 3 h after treatment ($\chi^2 = 12.7$, $P < 0.01$). Figure 1b illustrates the comparative level of bacteremia among the three groups. At each time, the concentration of bacteria in blood was less in mice receiving ampicillin plus gentamicin than in those receiving ampicillin

TABLE 1. *Cumulative survival of GB-BHS-infected mice*

Treatment (total dose in mg/kg)	No. of mice in group	No. of survivors on day after inoculation: 1	2	3	5	7	9	Percent survivors on day 9
Three-dose regimen[a]								
None	20	0						0
Ampicillin (125)	95	93	85	78	59	53	51	53
Gentamicin (25)	20	20	4	0				0
Ampicillin (125) + gentamicin (25)	95	90	90	82	73	72	69	73
Single-dose regimen[b]								
None	20	2	0					0
Ampicillin (125)	117	117	97	80	67	54	51	43
Gentamicin (25)	40	32	23	12	9	6	6	15
Ampicillin (125) + gentamicin (25)	117	117	117	116	115	115	115	98

[a] Treatment given in three divided doses 4, 10, and 16 h after infection.
[b] Treatment given at the time of infection.

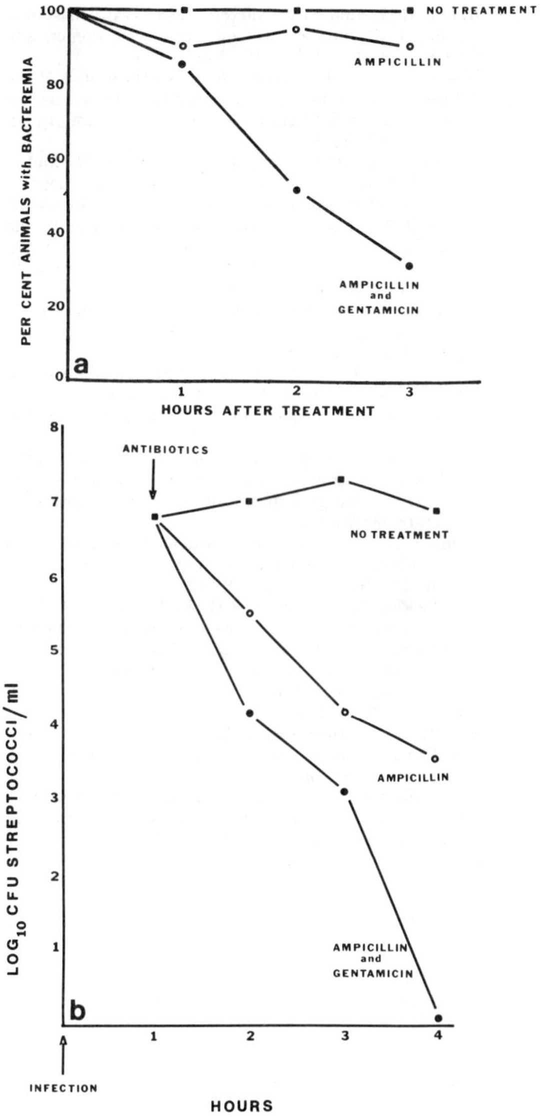

FIG. 1. *Inoculation with 10^7 CFU of streptococci 1 h before treatment with antibiotics. Each point shown is the average of 20 mice. (a) Percentage of animals with bacteremia; (b) quantitation of bacteremia. The variation for each average shown for the last time point was less than 2 log_{10}.*

alone. The average CFU of streptococci per milliliter of blood in all animals in the untreated group varied from 7×10^6 to 2×10^7. In mice treated with ampicillin alone, the average CFU of streptococci per milliliter of blood had decreased to 7×10^3 3 h after therapy. In comparison, 3 h after antibiotic administration, an average of 0.8 CFU per ml of blood was observed in animals that received ampicillin plus gentamicin.

DISCUSSION

The observation that gentamicin accelerates the bactericidal effect of ampicillin for GB-BHS in vitro (13) led to an investigation of the effect of this drug combination in mice after experimental streptococcal infection. Although as few streptococci as 10 CFU produced death in 50% of untreated animals, 10^7 CFU of streptococci were used to establish infection and resulted in bacteremia of approximately 10^6 CFU/ml. The dose of ampicillin and the resultant serum levels of ampicillin were similar to dosages and levels recommended for newborn infants (11). Although these studies were performed with ampicillin, future studies should be carried out to determine whether similar results are observed with penicillin G, as would be expected. The dose of gentamicin was higher than for human use, but was necessary to obtain blood levels similar to the ones recommended in humans (11). Although ampicillin and gentamicin were more effective than ampicillin alone in the treatment regimens reported here as shown in Table 1, a difference between the two groups in a number of other treatment schedules did not occur. A comparable effect of dosing on survival was observed by Andriole (1, 2) and Lumish et al. (10) in experimental pseudomonas infections of normal or neutropenic rodents with carbenicillin and gentamicin or tobramycin.

GB-BHS are susceptible to ampicillin and penicillin with MICs only a fewfold higher than for group A beta-hemolytic streptococci. Nevertheless, the rate of bactericidal effect of ampicillin against GB-BHS is considerably slower than against group A beta-hemolytic streptococci (13). With the increased penicillin concentrations required for effectiveness against a large inoculum size (7) and the slow bactericidal rate of ampicillin alone against GB-BHS (13), it is possible that the presently recommended dosages for penicillin in newborn infants may produce levels in cerebrospinal fluid that are inadequate for eradication of infection. Although GB-BHS are more susceptible to penicillins and less susceptible to gentamicin than are enterococci, the enhanced activity of the combination of the two drugs against GB-BHS is similar to that seen for enterococci (14). Greater activity of the combination is also observed with *Listeria monocytogenes* (9).

In the experiments reported here we have shown that the combination of drugs was more effective than ampicillin alone in the treatment of mice with established infection (Table 1). The combination was also more effective than ampicillin alone in the protection of mice against lethal streptococcal infection (Table 1). Not only was incidence of bacteremia lower

(Fig. 1a), but in the presence of bacteremia the concentration of streptococci was lower (Fig. 1b) in animals given the combination. The differences in ampicillin plus gentamicin compared with ampicillin alone may account for the improved survival observed with the combination. The correlation of these findings with our in vitro observations (13) shows that in experimental infection, the combination of antibiotics produced a more rapid bactericidal effect and beneficially influenced the outcome of infection. Based on our present data and our previous observations in vitro, we suggest that further examination of the benefits of combined therapy with ampicillin or penicillin and gentamicin for patients with GB-BHS infection is indicated.

ACKNOWLEDGMENTS

A.D. was supported by Public Health Service training grant AI 00208 from the National Institute of Allergy and Infectious Diseases. Support was also provided by the Schering Corp.

We acknowledge the helpful advice of George G. Jackson and the assistance of Victoria Zimelis.

LITERATURE CITED

1. **Andriole, V. T.** 1971. Synergy of carbenicillin and gentamicin in experimental infection with pseudomonas. J. Infect. Dis. **124**(Suppl.): S.46–S.55.
2. **Andriole, V. T.** 1974. Antibiotic synergy in experimental infection with *Pseudomonas*. II. The effect of carbenicillin, cephalothin, or cephanone combined with tobramycin or gentamicin. J. Infect. Dis. **129**:124–133.
3. **Baker, C. J., and F. F. Barrett.** 1973. Transmission of group B streptococci among parturient women and their neonates. J. Pediatr. **83**:919–925.
4. **Baker, C. J., F. F. Barrett, R. C. Gordon, and M. D. Yow.** 1973. Suppurative meningitis due to streptococci of Lancefield group B: A study of 33 infants. J. Pediatr. **82**:724–729.
5. **Bergqvist, G., B. Hurvell, A. Malmorg, M. Rylander, and R. Tunnell.** 1971. Neonatal infections caused by group B streptococci. Scand. J. Infect. Dis. **3**:157–162.
6. **Eickhoff, T. C., J. O. Klein, A. K. Daly, D. Ingall, and M. Finland.** 1964. Neonatal sepsis and other infections due to group B beta-hemolytic streptococci. N. Engl. J. Med. **27**:1221–1228.
7. **Feldman, W. E.** 1976. Concentrations of bacteria in cerebrospinal fluid of patients with bacterial meningitis. J. Pediatr. **88**:549–552.
8. **Giamarellou, H., V. M. Zimelis, D. O. Matulionis, and G. G. Jackson.** 1975. Assay of aminoglycoside antibiotics in clinical specimens. J. Infect. Dis. **132**:399–406.
9. **Gordon, R. C., F. F. Barrett, and D. J. Clark.** 1972. Influence of several antibiotics, singly and in combination, on the growth of *Listeria monocytogenes*. J. Pediatr. **80**:667–670.
10. **Lumish, R. M., and C. W. Norden.** 1976. Therapy of neutropenic rats infected with *Pseudomonas aeruginosa*. J. Infect. Dis. **133**:538–547.
11. **McCracken, G. H., Jr., and H. F. Eichenwald.** 1974. Antimicrobial therapy: therapeutic recommendations and a review of newer drugs. J. Pediatr. **85**:297–312.
12. **McCracken, G. H., Jr., and W. E. Feldman.** 1976. Editorial comment. Group B streptococcal infection. J. Pediatr. **89**:203–204.
13. **Schauf, V., A. Deveikis, L. Riff, and A. Serota.** 1976. Antibiotic-killing kinetics of group B streptococci. J. Pediatr. **89**:194–198.
14. **Watanakunakorn, C.** 1971. Penicillin combined with gentamicin or streptomycin: synergism against enterococci. J. Infect. Dis. **124**:581–586.

ANTIMICROBIAL AGENTS AND CHEMOTHERAPY, May 1977, p. 821-825 Vol. 11, No. 5

Printed in U.S.A.

Renal Pharmacology of Netilmicin

PETER J. S. CHIU,* GEORGE H. MILLER, ARTHUR D. BROWN, JAMES F. LONG, AND J. ALLAN WAITZ

Schering Corporation, Research Laboratories Division, Bloomfield, New Jersey 07003

Received for publication 23 December 1976

Netilmicin (Sch 20569), a new semisynthetic aminoglycoside, was studied for its effects on kidney function and mechanisms by which it is handled by the kidneys. Measurements of glomerular filtration rate (GFR) and urinalysis in chronic rat studies indicated that the nephrotoxicity of netilmicin was remarkably less than that of gentamicin. Gentamicin caused a dose-related reduction in GFR in association with glucosuria and elevated fractional excretion of K^+. By contrast, high doses of netilmicin produced only slight reduction in GFR with increased fractional excretion of K^+ but without glucosuria. In separate experiments, rats were shown to excrete 71 to 90% of netilmicin or gentamicin in 24 h after daily intramuscular administration of doses of 20 or 40 mg/kg for 4 days. In acute experiments on anesthetized dogs, GFR and renal plasma flow were unaffected at serum levels of 11.0 ± 0.6 μg/ml maintained by constant infusion of netilmicin for 5 h. The renal clearance of netilmicin was significantly correlated with GFR. The urinary output of netilmicin was 80.0 ± 4.2% of the infusion rate and was independent of urine flow over the range of 0.04 to 0.33 ml/kg per min. Preferential accumulation of netilmicin occurred in the renal cortex; the cortex-serum and medulla-serum ratios were 9.9 ± 1.2 and 4.2 ± 0.6, respectively. In addition, the extraction ratio of netilmicin, which was lower than that of inulin, suggested that netilmicin reabsorption occurs in the proximal tubule and results in cortical accumulation. It is concluded that netilmicin, like gentamicin, is excreted by the dog kidney by glomerular filtration plus limited reabsorption. However, the new drug is characterized by low intrinsic nephrotoxicity in rats.

Netilmicin (Sch 20569) is a newly described semisynthetic aminoglycoside (18). Its effect on kidney function was evaluated in comparison with gentamicin in rats chronically treated with the drugs. In addition, urinary excretion of the drugs was measured after repeated administration. The renal handling of netilmicin was investigated in acute dog experiments to determine the method of drug excretion. The intrarenal distribution was studied to determine the extent and location of drug accumulation in the dog.

(This work was presented in part at the 16th Interscience Conference of Antimicrobial Agents and Chemotherapy, Chicago, 1976.)

MATERIALS AND METHODS

Renal function study in rats. Seventy-eight male Sprague-Dawley rats (180 to 200 g) were divided into 13 groups of six each. They were injected intramuscularly (i.m.) with saline, gentamicin (batch no. GMC-4M-6231), or netilmicin (batch no. 7733-15) according to the dosing schedule listed in Table 1.

Twenty-four hours after administration of the last dose, the animals were anesthetized by intraperitoneal injection of 100 mg of thiobarbital (Inactin) per kg. Body temperature was maintained at 38°C. After tracheostomy, the left jugular vein was cannulated for blood sampling and the right femoral vein was cannulated for fluid infusion. Carotid arterial blood pressure was measured with a Statham pressure transducer. Urine samples were taken by puncture of the urinary bladder for urinalysis with Labstix (Ames Co., Elkhart, Ind.), and the bladder was then cannulated for urine collection. Priming the animals with 0.4 ml of normal saline containing [^{14}C]inulin (2.4 μCi/ml) was immediately followed by continuous infusion of the same solution at 1.2 ml/h. Collection of blood and urine samples began after allowing 1 h for equilibration. The individual experiments consisted of three consecutive 30-min clearance periods. The [^{14}C]inulin activity in plasma and urine was measured in a liquid scintillation counter with external standardization. The channel ratio method was used to account for quenching.

Urinary excretion study in rats. Twenty-four male Sprague-Dawley rats (180 to 270 g) were kept singly in metabolic cages. The animals were divided into four groups of six each. Netilmicin (batch no. 7733-15) and gentamicin (batch no. GMC-4M-6231) were given by a single daily i.m. injection into the hind limb at a dosage of 20 or 40 mg/kg per day for

TABLE 1. *Incidence of glucosuria and FE_K in rats treated with gentamicin and netilmicin*

Treatment[a]	No. of rats	FE_K[b] (%)	Glucosuria[c]
Saline control			
0.2 ml/rat o.d. × 7 days	6	19.1 ± 2.3	0/6
0.2 ml/rat o.d. × 14 days	6	15.8 ± 3.2	0/6
0.2 ml/rat b.i.d. × 7 days	6	20.3 ± 3.7	1/6[d]
Gentamicin			
80 mg/kg o.d. × 7 days	6	27.1 ± 2.8*	1/6
120 mg/kg o.d. × 7 days	5	68.1 ± 18.5*	4/5
160 mg/kg o.d. × 7 days	3	50.7 ± 14.6	3/5
40 mg/kg b.i.d. × 7 days	5	58.4 ± 26.6	3/6
50 mg/kg b.i.d. × 7 days	6	46.1 ± 10.1*	3/6
60 mg/kg b.i.d. × 7 days	6	45.9 ± 6.2*	2/6[e]
Netilmicin			
160 mg/kg o.d. × 14 days	4	27.0 ± 1.8*	0/4[e]
80 mg/kg b.i.d. × 7 days	5	32.5 ± 1.8*	0/6
125 mg/kg b.i.d. × 7 days	4	24.9 ± 5.3	0/5[d]
170 mg/kg b.i.d. × 7 days	4	45.8 ± 4.8*	0/4[e]

[a] The drugs were given i.m. in saline of a volume similar to that of controls. (o.d.) Once daily; (b.i.d.) twice daily.

[b] All values represent mean ± standard error. (*) Indicates significant difference ($P < 0.05$) from appropriate controls.

[c] Glucosuria determined prior to clearance experiments. Numbers signify number of incidences per number of observations.

[d] One of six animals died from acute toxicity.

[e] Two of six animals died from acute toxicity.

four consecutive days. Urine was collected daily during the first 4 h and from 5 to 24 h after administration of drugs to the rats. To ensure accurate and complete recovery, urinary bladders were emptied by manual pressure on the suprapubic area at the beginning and end of each collection period.

Clearance studies in anesthetized dogs. The experimental procedures were the same as described previously (3). Seventeen mongrel dogs of either sex (mean body weight, 11.3 kg; range, 8.1 to 14.1 kg) were fasted overnight and were anesthetized with 30 mg of nembutal per kg intravenously (i.v.). Clearance rates of *para*-aminohippuric acid (PAH) and inulin were used to measure effective renal plasma flow and glomerular filtration rate, respectively. A 20-mg amount of netilmicin (batch no. 5533-156-I) per kg was given i.v. and followed by sustaining infusion at a rate of 3.0 mg/kg per h, the total dose administered being approximately 200 mg per animal over a period of 5 h. Netilmicin and gentamicin from the preceding studies were assayed by the cylinder-plate method with *Bacillus subtilis* (ATCC 6633) as the test organism (3).

RESULTS

Rats. (i) Renal function study. Frequent occurrences of glucosuria were associated with gentamicin (Table 1). By contrast, glucose was not detected in the urine of netilmicin-treated animals. Glucosuria was noted in one control animal.

The effects of gentamicin and netilmicin on glomerular filtration rate (GFR) are shown in Fig. 1. A dose-related reduction in GFR was observed in gentamicin-treated groups. By contrast, moderate decreases in GFR occurred only when high doses of netilmicin were used. On the basis of dose-response curves, 40% reduction in GFR occurred at a 600-mg/kg total dose of gentamicin compared with a 2,400-mg/kg total dose of netilmicin. Elevation in fractional excretion of K^+ (FE_K) tended to accompany reductions in GFR (Table 1). In general, gentamicin seemed to produce greater rises in FE_K than did netilmicin.

Five of 18 rats receiving the higher doses of netilmicin died from acute toxicity (see Table 1). Hypoactivity, ataxia, and irregular respiration were the principal signs of toxicity. Histopathological work on the kidneys was not performed on any of the animals tested.

(ii) Urinary recovery of netilmicin and gentamicin during repeated administration. On the first day after i.m. administration of 20 or 40 mg of netilmicin per kg, 76.6 ± 4.1 and 69.9 ± 4.9% of the total injected dose, respectively, were excreted in the urine during the first 4 h, followed by 6.5 ± 0.9 and 7.7 ± 0.8%, respectively, during the next 20 h. Similar fractions of the injected drug appeared in the urine after daily treatment through day 4, with a mean of 86% excreted over each of the subsequent 3 days at 20 mg/kg and a mean of 84% at the 40-mg/kg dose. Gentamicin demonstrated a similar ex-

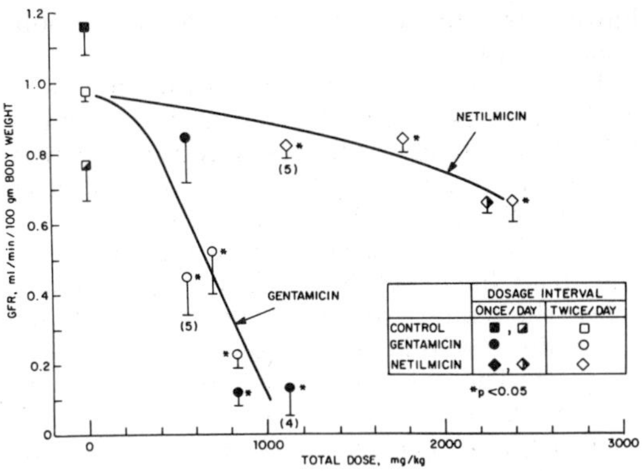

FIG. 1. *Effect of chronic dosing of gentamicin and netilmicin on GFR in rats. Netilmicin and gentamicin are represented by circles and diamonds, respectively. Squares represent appropriate saline controls. Solid symbols denote single daily dose treatment and open symbols represent twice-daily treatment, both for a period of 7 days. The half-open symbols indicate once-daily treatment for 14 days. On the abscissa is the total amount of drug in milligrams per kilogram of body weight given to the animals over the entire treatment period. Each point represents the mean value of individual groups; the vertical bars are standard errors. Control and gentamicin groups consisted of six animals each and netilmicin groups consisted of four animals each, except where indicated by numbers in parentheses.*

cretion pattern, with 24-h excretion of a mean of 79% per day at 20 mg/kg and a mean of 81% at the 40-mg/kg dose.

Dogs. (i) Renal hemodynamics. Fairly steady serum levels of netilmicin (11.0 ± 0.6 μg/ml, $N = 10$) were achieved during the eight consecutive clearance periods (Fig. 2). The inulin and PAH clearances remained stable in the presence of netilmicin. The mean values of the two parameters did not differ from those of controls (Table 2). In addition, the arterial pressure was also found to be stable throughout these acute experiments.

(ii) Renal clearance of netilmicin. The mean clearance value of netilmicin was slightly lower than the mean inulin clearance in the 10 dogs studied ($P < 0.05$, paired comparison) (Table 2). Based on the finding that the ratio of netilmicin clearance to inulin clearance (0.92 ± 0.03) was significantly less than unity ($P < 0.05$), it appeared that a small fraction of netilmicin was reabsorbed by the renal tubule after being filtered. With serum levels maintained at a steady state, the netilmicin appeared in the urine at 80.0 ± 4.2% of the constant infusion rate. Both the fractional excretion and absolute excretion rates were independent of variations in urine flow rate (Fig. 3).

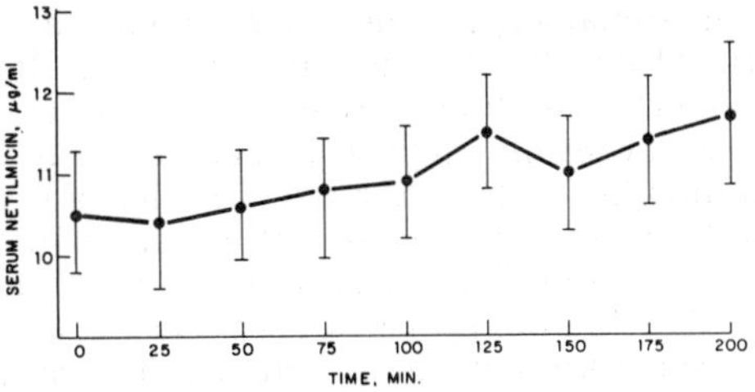

FIG. 2. *Serum levels of netilmicin in anesthetized dogs. Netilmicin was given at 2 mg/kg i.v. and followed by a sustaining infusion at a rate of 3.0 mg/kg per h. Collection of blood and urine samples began 90 min after start of infusion. Each point represents the mean of 10 animals; the vertical bars are standard errors.*

TABLE 2. *Renal handling of netilmicin in anesthetized dogs*[a]

Determination	Saline group (N=7)	Netilmicin group (N=10)
C_N (ml/min)[b]		43.3 ± 2.9
C_{In} (ml/min)[b]	46.7 ± 4.4	47.5 ± 3.8
C_{PAH} (ml/min)[b]	108.0 ± 6.0	121.0 ± 13.0
FE_N (%)[c]		92.4 ± 3.4[d]
U_NV (μg/kg per min)[e]		40.0 ± 2.1
V (ml/kg per min)[e]	0.14 ± 0.03	0.18 ± 0.03

[a] All values represent mean ± standard error.

[b] C_N, C_{In}, and C_{PAH} represent clearance values for netilmicin, inulin, and PAH, respectively.

[c] FE_N represents the percentage of filtered netilmicin being excreted in the urine.

[d] The mean value is significantly ($P < 0.05$) less than 100.

[e] U_NV represents the absolute rate of urinary excretion of netilmicin. V represents the urine flow rate.

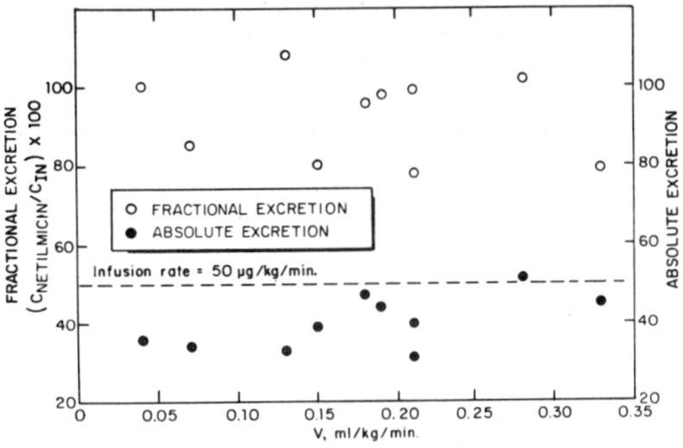

FIG. 3. *Urine flow rate versus urinary excretion of netilmicin in anesthetized dogs. Symbols: (○) Fractional excretion of netilmicin, 8 out of 10 are below 100%. (●) Absolute rate of excretion, of which all except one were less than the sustaining infusion rate (- - -). Each circle represents the mean of eight consecutive clearance values per animal.*

(iii) Renal extraction ratios. The extraction ratio (Table 3) and clearance value of PAH (Table 2) in netilmicin-treated dogs did not differ from controls, indicating that the drug did not interfere with the tubular secretion of PAH. On the other hand, the extraction ratio of netilmicin was significantly lower than that of inulin. This finding provided additional evidence that the drug undergoes tubular reabsorption.

(iv) Renal tissue and urine antibiotic levels. Accumulation of netilmicin occurred in the renal cortex; the mean cortical concentration was 10 times that of the steady-state serum level (Table 4). On the other hand, the renal medulla had a much lower level despite the high values of netilmicin present in the urine.

DISCUSSION

Aminoglycoside antibiotics are promptly excreted in the urine mainly by glomerular filtration in man (5) and experimental animals (2, 16). Close similarity in the excretion patterns of netilmicin and gentamicin was demonstrated in this study. Rapid elimination of the two drugs was consistent with their short serum half-life in rats, i.e., 0.5 h (11; G. Miller, unpublished data).

The urinary excretion of netilmicin is also rapid in dogs. With the serum levels maintained in a steady state, the output of the drug in an active form was 80% of the infused dose. Apparently, disposition of the drug is associated with little metabolism; no metabolites of the drug have yet been identified. Furthermore, the renal clearance of the drug was found to be directly related to glomerular filtration (Fig. 4). The calculations of netilmicin clearance were based on the assumption that the new drug, like gentamicin (6, 13, 14), has negligible plasma binding. Regardless, the significant relationship between netilmicin and inulin clearances would remain unaffected even if protein binding did occur. Variations in urine flow within the ranges found in the present study did not appear to influence the excretion of netilmicin. Gentamicin had previously been shown to exhibit the same behavior in dogs (3) and in man (9).

TABLE 3. *Extraction ratios of netilmicin, inulin, and PAH in anesthetized dogs*[a]

Drug	Saline group (N=7)	Netilmicin group[b] (N=9)
Inulin	0.29 ± 0.05[c]	0.31 ± 0.02
PAH	0.60 ± 0.03	0.76 ± 0.02
Netilmicin		0.16 ± 0.03[d]

[a] Extraction ratio = [Pa − Pv]/Pa, where Pa and Pv are the femoral arterial and renal venous concentrations of the individual compounds, respectively. All values represent the mean ± the standard error.

[b] Due to proximity of the confluence of the renal vein and spermatic or ovarian vein to the inferior vena cava, determinations of extraction ratio were not performed in one of the 10 netilmicin dogs.

[c] Mean value of four animals. Measurements of venous inulin in the other three animals were not done.

[d] Significantly different from the mean extraction ratio for inulin ($P < 0.05$).

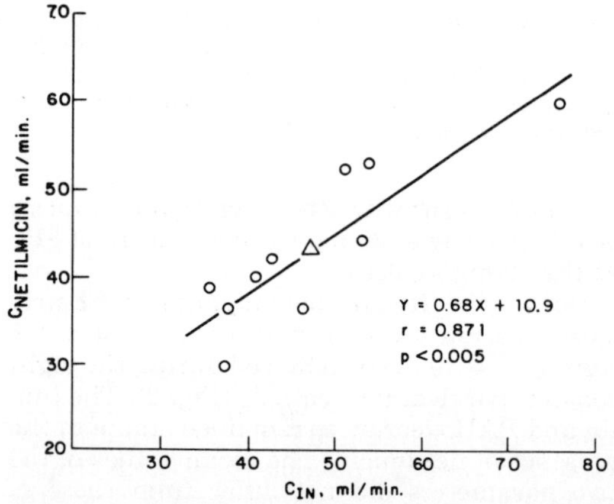

FIG. 4. *Relationship of netilmicin clearance (C_N) to inulin clearance (C_{In}). The linear regression line relates C_N to C_{In}. Each point represents a mean value of eight consecutive clearance values per animal, and the triangle depicts the mean of C_N average in relation to the C_{In} average.*

TABLE 4. *Netilmicin in serum, kidney, and urine of anesthetized dogs*[a]

Concentration				Ratio[b]		
Tissue[c] (μg/g)		Liquid (μg/ml)				
Cortex	Medulla	Serum	Urine	Cortex/serum	Medulla/serum	Cortex/medulla
102.4 ± 7.2	45.9 ± 6.6	11.0 ± 0.6	338.0 ± 87.0	9.9 ± 1.2	4.2 ± 0.6	2.6 ± 0.4

[a] All values represent mean ± standard error of 10 dogs.

[b] Serum concentrations of netilmicin are shown in Fig. 2.

[c] Tissue concentration is based on the wet weight of tissues.

The rat has served as a useful species in studying the potential nephrotoxicity of many compounds including aminoglycosides (10, 12). A. Sugarman et al. (Clin. Res. 24:413A, 1976) demonstrated that gentamicin caused a linear, dose-related decrease in rat GFR. In our study, the renal impairment caused by gentamicin was characterized by a reduction in GFR in association with glucosuria and potassium wasting as reflected by elevation in the fractional excretion of potassium. By contrast, the rat was quite insensitive to netilmicin with reference to kidney function. The daily doses of netilmicin utilized in evaluation of nephrotoxicity were only limited by its relatively high acute toxicity (mean lethal dose, ca. 200 mg/kg, i.m.) in comparison with gentamicin. Nevertheless, our data indicate that the nephrotoxicity of netilmicin was clearly less than that of gentamicin.

High concentrations of netilmicin similar to that described for gentamicin (3) occurred in the renal cortex. Prolonged accumulation in the cortex (11) may be related in some way to the nephrotoxicity typically associated with aminoglycoside nephrotoxicity in experimental animals (8). However, conclusive evidence in support of this view is not yet available. In this regard, cephaloridine also caused similar lesions in the kidney, which suggests that its nephrotoxicity was related to high intracellular concentrations of the drug (17). Despite the similarity of cortical uptake of netilmicin and gentamicin, the former drug has remarkably less effect on kidney function, probably due to its lower intrinsic toxicity or different kinetics in binding to renal tissues.

The renal extraction ratios of netilmicin and gentamicin (3) are similar, and both are lower than those of inulin and PAH. The results indicate that a small fraction of filtered drug is reabsorbed by the proximal tubule since the bulk of drug is recoverable in the urine. Previous clearance studies in man and dogs have indeed shown that limited tubular reabsorption is associated with gentamicin (1, 3, 7), tobramycin (15), and amikacin and kanamycin (4). It appears that the reabsorptive mechanism present in the epithelium of proximal tubules is responsible for the cortical buildup of netilmicin and the other aminoglycosides.

In conclusion, whereas netilmicin demonstrated lower nephrotoxicity than gentamicin, the excretory mechanisms that mediate the renal handling of the two drugs are essentially the same. Rapid excretion can be ascribed to their primary dependence on glomerular filtration with limited tubular reabsorption.

LITERATURE CITED

1. **Bergan, T., E. K. Brodwall, and A. Oyri.** 1971. Renal excretion of gentamicin in chronic pyelonephritis. Acta Med. 189:1-5.
2. **Cabana, B. E., and J. G. Taggart.** 1973. Comparative pharmacokinetics of BB-K8 and kanamycin in dogs and humans. Antimicrob. Agents Chemother. 3:478-483.
3. **Chiu, P. J. S., A. Brown, G. Miller, and J. F. Long.** 1976. Renal extraction of gentamicin in anesthetized dogs. Antimicrob. Agents Chemother. 10:277-282.
4. **Clarke, J., R. Libke, and C. Regamey.** 1974. Comparative pharmacokinetics of amikacin and kanamycin. Clin. Pharmacol. Ther. 15:610-616.
5. **Goodman, L. S., and A. Gilman.** 1970. The pharmacological basis of therapeutics, 4th ed. Macmillan Publishing Co., New York.
6. **Gordon, R. C., C. Regamy, and W. M. M. Kirby.** 1972. Serum protein binding of the aminoglycoside antibiotics. Antimicrob. Agents Chemother. 2:214-216.
7. **Gyselynck, A. M., A. Forrey, and R. Cutler.** 1971. Pharmacokinetics of gentamicin: distribution and plasma and renal clearance. J. Infect. Dis. Suppl. 124:70-76.
8. **Houghton, D. C., M. Hartnett, M. Campbell-Boswell, G. Porter, and W. Bennett.** 1976. A light and electron microscopic analysis of gentamicin nephrotoxicity in rats. Am. J. Pathol. 82:595-599.
9. **Jao, R. L., and G. G. Jackson.** 1964. Gentamicin sulfate, new antibiotic against gram-negative bacilli—laboratory, pharmacological and clinical evaluation. J. Am. Med. Assoc. 189:817-822.
10. **Kosek, J. C., R. I. Mazze, and M. J. Cousins.** 1974. Nephrotoxicity of gentamicin. Lab. Invest. 30:48-57.
11. **Luft, F. C., and S. A. Kleit.** 1974. Renal parenchymal accumulation of aminoglycoside antibiotics in rats. J. Infect. Dis. 130:656-659.
12. **Luft, F. C., V. Patel, M. N. Yum, B. Patel, and S. A. Kleit.** 1975. Experimental aminoglycoside nephrotoxicity. J. Lab. Clin. Med. 86:213-220.
13. **Naumann, V. P., and W. Auwärter.** 1968. Pharmakologische and therapeutische Eigenschaften von Gentamycin. Arzneim. Forsch. 18:1119-1123.
14. **Ramirez-Ronda, C. H., R. K. Holmes, and J. P. Sanford.** 1975. Effects of divalent cations on binding of aminoglycoside antibiotics to human serum proteins and to bacteria. Antimicrob. Agents Chemother. 7:239-245.
15. **Regamey, C., R. C. Gordon, and W. M. M. Kirby.** 1973. Comparative pharmacokinetics of tobramycin and gentamicin. Clin. Pharmacol. Ther. 14:396-403.
16. **Stone, W. J., R. E. Bryant, A. Hoyumpa, and S. Schenker.** 1974. Renal neomycin excretion in the dog. Proc. Soc. Exp. Biol. Med. 145:1074-1080.
17. **Tune, B. M.** 1975. Relationship between the transport and toxicity of cephalosporins in the kidney. J. Infect. Dis. 132:189-194.
18. **Wright, J. J.** 1976. Synthesis of 1-N-ethylsisomicin: a broad-spectrum semisynthetic aminoglycoside antibiotic. J. Chem. Soc. Chem. Commun. 6:206-208.

ANTIMICROBIAL AGENTS AND CHEMOTHERAPY, May 1977, p. 826-843 Vol. 11, No. 5

Printed in U.S.A.

Activities of Various 4-Aminoquinolines Against Infections with Chloroquine-Resistant Strains of *Plasmodium falciparum*[1]

L. H. SCHMIDT,* DENNIS VAUGHAN, DONNA MUELLER, RUTH CROSBY, AND REBECCA HAMILTON

The Kettering-Meyer Laboratory, Southern Research Institute, Birmingham, Alabama 35205

Received for publication 22 December 1976

The studies reported here stemmed from a personal report by Geiman on the capacity of the 4-aminoquinoline amodiaquin to inhibit in vitro maturation of ring stages of the chloroquine-resistant Monterey strain of *Plasmodium falciparum*. This observation, confirmed in owl monkeys infected with this strain, led to a comparison of the activities of chloroquine, amodiaquin, amopyroquin, and dichlorquinazine (12,278 RP) against infections with various chloroquine-susceptible and chloroquine-resistant strains. The results showed that: (i) these 4-aminoquinolines were essentially equally active against infections with chloroquine-susceptible strains and (ii) the activities of amodiaquin, amopyroquin, and dichlorquinazine were reduced significantly in the face of chloroquine resistance, but (iii) well-tolerated doses of these compounds would cure infections with strains that fully resisted treatment with maximally tolerated doses of chloroquine. Two other 4-aminoquinolines, SN-8137 and SN-9584, which also exhibited activity against chloroquine-resistant parasites in vitro, displayed curative activity in monkeys infected with a chloroquine-resistant strain. These observations show that there is cross-resistance among the 4-aminoquinolines, confirming earlier findings, but indicate that the dimensions of this phenomenon are sufficiently limited so that some derivatives are therapeutically effective against infections refractory to maximally tolerated doses of chloroquine.

In early 1961, Moore and Lanier (25) described the events associated with the first recognized infection with a strain of *Plasmodium falciparum* resistant to the 4-aminoquinoline chloroquine. Shortly thereafter, Young and Moore (49) provided unequivocal documentation of the resistance of this strain to the above drug via studies on blood-induced infections in a group of patients with neurosyphilis. Young (45) went on to demonstrate (i) that established infections with this parasite, of Colombian origin, were also refractory to treatment with recommended therapeutic doses of amodiaquin and hydroxychloroquine (two other 4-aminoquinolines) and (ii) that neither chloroquine nor amodiaquin, delivered in conventional suppressive regimens, would prevent evolution of clinical disease in patients bitten by mosquitoes infected with this plasmodium. Based on these observations, it was suggested that strains of *P. falciparum* resistant to chloroquine would probably be cross-resistant to other agents of the same chemical class. This suggestion has been strengthened by numerous observations on individual patients or small numbers of human volunteers infected with various chloroquine-resistant strains of *P. falciparum*, for the most part of southeast Asian origin (3–5, 8, 14, 19, 24, 29, 30, 31, 35, 46, 47). With few exceptions, infections with such strains were not eradicated and in some subjects were not controlled with respect to parasitemia and fever, when treated with the recommended curative doses of amodiaquin, amopyroquin, or hydroxychloroquine, the only 4-aminoquinolines other than chloroquine currently available for patient use. The concept of cross-resistance received further support from results of studies on mice infected with chloroquine-resistant strains of *P. berghei*, showing that infections with these parasites were in no way susceptible to treatment with maximally tolerated doses of amodiaquin and amopyroquin (17, 27, 39; personal communication, 1970, from the late Paul Thompson, University of Georgia, Athens).

The above observations on cross-resistance led those concerned with and responsible for development of new blood schizonticides to accord a very low priority to either synthesis and experimental and clinical evaluations of new 4-

[1] Contribution no. 1436 from the Army Research Program on Malaria.

aminoquinoline derivatives or expanded studies on agents currently available. The results of substantial experimental studies, set forth in the current report, indicate clearly that these negative positions are not fully supportable and should be revised.

The investigations summarized here had their origins in late September 1969 after a discussion with Quentin Geiman (Department of Preventive Medicine, Stanford University, School of Medicine), who was then studying the cultivation of various strains of *P. falciparum* in vitro and the effects of diverse antimalarial drugs on parasite multiplication. Geiman related results of studies, published in detail 3 years later (38), that indicated that there were distinct differences in the capacities of chloroquine and amodiaquin to inhibit development of the chloroquine-resistant Vietnam Monterey strain. Briefly stated, he had found that chloroquine, added to culture medium at concentrations of 0.3 μg or less per ml, was without effect on maturation of parasites of this strain. In striking contrast, addition of amodiaquin, at a concentration of 0.12 μg/ml, inhibited development completely.

Within a week of the above communication, our laboratories initiated an exploratory study aimed at determining whether the interesting observations of Geiman could be duplicated in vivo in owl monkeys infected with the Monterey strain. Ten subjects, used previously in evaluating a new agent for antimalarial activity, with parasitemias partially suppressed, but still readily measurable on thin films, were assigned to the experiment, one as an untreated control, three to treatment with chloroquine, and six to treatment with amodiaquin. Both drugs were administered once daily, via stomach tube, in doses of 20.0 mg of base equivalent per kg of body weight for 7 consecutive days. As in previous evaluations, administration of chloroquine had no significant effect on parasitemia. In contrast, clearance of parasitemia occurred in all six recipients of amodiaquin by the time dose 7 of this drug had been administered. The absence of recrudescences over a 90-day post-treatment follow-up period indicated that the infections had been cured. This in vivo confirmation of the in vitro observations of Geiman led to the sequence of studies summarized below. Some of the more relevant results were set forth previously (L. H. Schmidt, D. Vaughan, D. Mueller, and R. Hamilton, 1970 Annu. Meet. Am. Soc. Trop. Med. Hyg., San Francisco).

MATERIALS AND METHODS

Monkeys – acquisition, husbandry, and handling. Owl monkeys (*Aotus trivirgatus griseimembra*) of northern Colombian origin, subadults of both sexes ranging from 700 to 1,100 g in weight, were used exclusively. All were purchased through the offices of the Tarpon Zoo, Tarpon Springs, Fla., transported via air directly from Barranquilla, Colombia, to Birmingham, with a brief stopover in Miami for customs and quarantine clearance. The housing and caging of these subjects, dietary regimens, conditioning procedures, capture and handling practices, and methods used in obtaining blood specimens for various purposes, parasite inoculation, and drug treatment have been detailed elsewhere (36). All experimental procedures were carried out on hand-caught monkeys, neither tranquilized, sedated, nor anesthetized.

Prior to assignment to experiments, monkeys were screened for the presence of preexisting malarial or filarial infections via examination of thick blood films stained with Giemsa. Searches for plasmodia were uniformly negative. Monkeys with microfilaremias, sometimes infected with two or more filarial species (9), were uncovered. These animals were excluded from the current therapeutic experiments since systematic studies (results to be published) showed that the evolution of *P. falciparum* infections is either blocked completely or retarded markedly in owl monkeys with preexisting filarial disease.

Strains of plasmodia – origins, characteristics, and susceptibilities to standard antimalarial drugs. The strains of *P. falciparum* used in various experiments included the Uganda Palo Alto, Malayan Camp-CH/Q, Vietnam Monterey, Vietnam Oak Knoll, Vietnam Smith, and Malayan IV. The patient origins of these strains have been described by others (2, 6, 21, 38, 41). We are indebted to Quentin Geiman for providing owl monkeys actively infected with the Uganda Palo Alto, Vietnam Monterey, and Vietnam Oak Knoll strains (1968); to Peter G. Contacos (Laboratory of Parasite Chemotherapy. National Institute of Allergy and Infectious Diseases, Chamblee, Ga.) for a monkey infected with the Malayan IV strain (1968); and to Ronald Ward (Walter Reed Army Institute of Research, Washington, D.C.) for a monkey infected with the Vietnam Smith strain (1971). The procedures involved in establishing these strains in the owl monkey have been described by these investigators (7, 38, 41).

We are also indebted to Robin Powell (then of the Department of Medicine, University of Chicago) for providing blood from a volunteer in the Army Medical Research Project actively infected with the Malayan Camp-CH/Q strain (1968). Inoculation of two owl monkeys with this blood evoked low-level infections. Rapid serial transfers brought the strain to full virulence.

When first introduced to our laboratory, the Palo Alto strain was the only strain that produced fatal infections when passed in small numbers (about 10^2 parasites) to owl monkeys with intact spleens. The other five strains had been maintained in splenectomized monkeys and multiplied erratically in intact subjects. Via rapid serial transfers in monkeys with spleens, the virulence of each of these strains was enhanced to a level where intravenous inocula of 10^2 parasites invariably produced fatal disease.

This level of pathogenicity has been maintained by regular passage of each strain from intact monkey to intact monkey approximately every 2 weeks, utilizing an inoculum of 5×10^4 parasites, intravenously.

The strains referred to above were selected for use in the current study because of their diverse responses to standard antimalarial drugs such as chloroquine, quinine, and pyrimethamine. These responses, determined preliminarily to utilizing the strains in the search for new and more effective antimalarial drugs, have been detailed elsewhere (36). Stated briefly, infections with the Uganda Palo Alto and Malayan Camp-CH/Q strains are susceptible to treatment with well-tolerated doses of chloroquine and quinine and fully resistant to treatment with maximally tolerated doses of pyrimethamine. Infections with the Vietnam Monterey strain are resistant to treatment with chloroquine and quinine and susceptible to treatment with high doses of pyrimethamine. Infections with the Vietnam Oak Knoll strain are resistant to treatment with chloroquine and quinine and fully susceptible to treatment with pyrimethamine. Infections with the Vietnam Smith and Malayan IV strains are resistant to treatment with maximally tolerated doses of each of the above drugs. As indicated previously, the responses of infections in owl monkeys to the above drugs paralleled responses in patients from whom the strains were isolated and/or in human volunteers (36).

Experimental drugs and administration. The structures of the seven compounds used in these studies are shown in Fig. 1. The group included six 7-chloro-4-aminoquinoline derivatives, with diverse substituents at position 4, and a single 6-methoxy-4-aminoquinoline (SN-10274), with a 4-substituent identical to that of amodiaquin. All were available as bulk crystalline preparations. Chloroquine diphosphate was provided by Sterling Winthrop Research Institute (1968), amodiaquin dihydrochloride and amopyroquin hydrochloride by Parke Davis Research Laboratories (1969), and dichlorquinazine base (12,278 RP) by Rhone Poulenc (1965). SN-8137 diphosphate, SN-9584 diphosphate, and SN-10274 dihydrochloride were drawn from a stock of active antimalarial drugs that had been maintained in our laboratories since the end of the World War II Malaria Program (1945). The first two agents were prepared (1944) by the late Nathan L. Drake, University of Maryland. The third compound was synthesized (1944) by J. H. Burckhalter, then of Parke, Davis & Co. Prior to use in the current investigations, these old compounds were checked for purity via countercurrent distribution to determine whether they had deteriorated during protracted storage. Results indicated no change in purity. All agents were water soluble, except dichlorquinazine (our personal designation for "12,278 RP"). At the time of use, the latter compound, a base, was converted to the water-soluble dihydrochloride salt by grinding the requisite quantity with the theoretical volume of 1.0 N hydrochloric acid prior to dilution to the appropriate volume.

Stock solutions of all compounds, 5 mg of base equivalent per ml, were prepared weekly and stored at 4°C. Just prior to delivery to infected monkeys, the volumes of these stock drugs required for treatment were measured into Erlenmeyer flasks and diluted to 10 ml with distilled water. These working solutions, followed by 5 ml of distilled water rinses, were administered via stomach tubes to the designated monkeys, utilizing procedures described elsewhere (36). Except as indicated below, drugs were administered once daily for 7 consecutive days, between 8:00 and 9:00 a.m., 3 to 4 h prior to the regular feeding period (probably on a fasting stomach). In situations where doses were utilized that might provoke acute toxic reactions, the total daily dose was administered in two equal fractions at 8:00 a.m. and 8:00 p.m.

Parasitological procedures. All assignees to therapeutic studies were inoculated intravenously with 5×10^6 parasites. This inoculum was derived from a

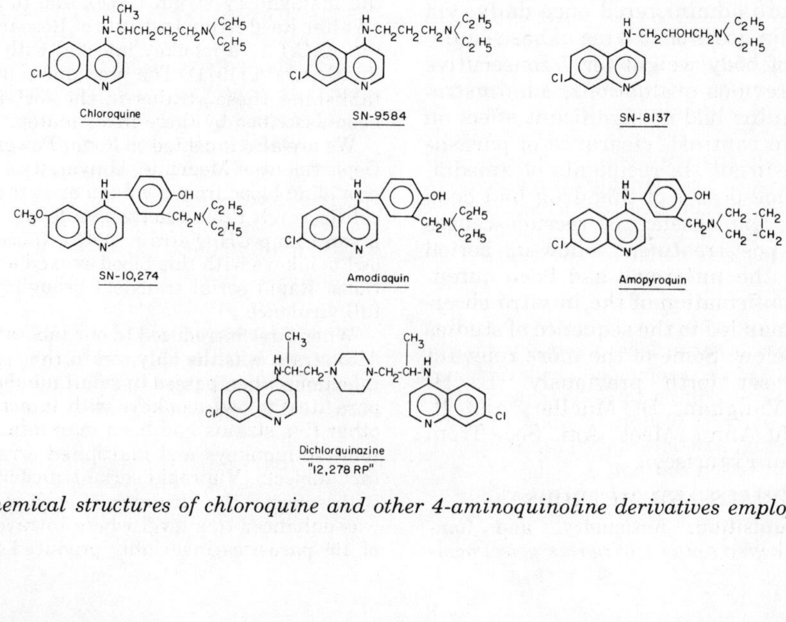

FIG. 1. *Chemical structures of chloroquine and other 4-aminoquinoline derivatives employed in various studies.*

monkey of the appropriate passage series in the midcourse of disease when 8 to 12% of the erythrocytes were parasitized. After precise measurement of parasitemia, via methods described previously (37), 0.3 to 0.5 ml of blood was drawn from the midsaphena of the donor into a 1.0-ml glass tuberculin syringe coated with diluted heparin and transferred to a volume of sterile iced saline such that each milliliter contained 5×10^6 parasites. One-milliliter portions of this diluted blood were injected immediately into the midsaphena of each monkey committed to a given therapeutic study, using a different glass syringe and hypodermic needle for each inoculee. Strict attention was given to maintenance of asepsis during these inoculation procedures. The sterility of the inoculum was always established by culture of 0.2-ml volumes in beef heart infusion broth and liquid thioglycolate medium.

To protect against rare but potentially disastrous transfer of small numbers of β-hemolytic streptococci, *Streptococcus pneumoniae*, *Pasteurella multocida*, and *Haemophilus influenzae* from the blood of donor monkeys to recipients, the latter were routinely injected intramuscularly with procaine penicillin (200,000 U) and streptomycin sulfate (50 mg) once daily for 5 consecutive days, beginning immediately after parasite inoculation. Critical studies have shown that the evolution of parasitemia is not altered by this antimicrobial drug regimen.

Parasitological studies were initiated 48 h after inoculation and repeated daily throughout the pretreatment and treatment intervals. Thick and thin films were prepared with blood obtained from the marginal ear vein and stained with Geimsa, and the numbers of parasites thereon were measured by established procedures (37). Drug treatments were started when parasite densities of 20 to $100/10^4$ erythrocytes were attained. The response to the initial treatment regimen determined the course of subsequent studies.

When treatment had no effect on parasitemia, the monkey was usually transferred out of the current experiment and assigned to evaluation of an agent of a chemical class different from the 4-aminoquinolines. When parasitemia was held near pretreatment levels or persisted at reduced levels, the infection was retreated with either twice the dose of the compound used initially or the same dose of a second 4-aminoquinoline. If such retreatment did not result in parasite clearance, the monkey was reassigned to another ongoing experiment as described above. If retreatment resulted in parasite clearance, parasitological examinations followed the pattern described below.

If blood films became parasite negative during the period of drug delivery or immediately thereafter and remained so for at least 5 consecutive days after treatment had been completed, parasitological examinations were reduced to a schedule of three times weekly (Monday, Wednesday, and Friday or Tuesday, Thursday, and Saturday) for the ensuing 3 weeks. If the infection did not recrudesce in this interval, parasitological examinations were further reduced to a schedule of once weekly and maintained there for 10 to 12 additional weeks. If blood films were consistently negative throughout the total 13- to 15-week post-treatment period, the infection was considered cured and the monkey was transferred to a pool of previously used monkeys reserved for evaluating the activities of new agents against infections with *P. vivax* (36). If the infection recrudesced subsequent to a blood film-negative interval of 7 to 14 days, retreatment was undertaken according to the pattern described above for subjects whose parasitemias had been suppressed by primary treatment. In this situation the schedule of parasitological studies, carried out subsequently to retreatment, was identical with that pursued after primary treatment. In the event of retreatment failure, monkeys were eliminated from the current series of experiments and assigned to pilot evaluations of newly submitted antimalarial agents of diverse chemical classes. This procedure avoided the complications of acquired immunity in the current study, but at the same time made qualified use of the infected subject in our malaria chemotherapy program.

Categorization of therapeutic responses. Impacts of treatment on the course of infection have been categorized in conventional terms. "No effect" implies that evolution of parasitemia in a treated subject differed little, if at all, from the parasitic courses of untreated controls. "Suppressed" implies that parasitemia persisted under treatment, either at approximately the starting level or at a significantly lower level. "Cleared" implies that thick blood films were consistently negative for at least 10 days after completion of treatment. Such a response could be an antecedent to either recrudescence of infection or cure. "Cure" implies the absence of parasitemia for 90 to 105 days after delivery of the last drug dose.

RESULTS

Comparative activities of chloroquine and amodiaquin against infections with the Vietnam Monterey strain of *P. falciparum*. Twenty owl monkeys infected with the chloroquine-resistant Vietnam Monterey strain were used in this comparison. Two of these monkeys served as untreated controls; two subgroups, of three monkeys each, were assigned to treatment with chloroquine in daily doses of 5.0 or 20.0 mg of base equivalent per kg of body weight; four similarly sized subgroups were treated with amodiaquin in daily doses of 2.5, 5.0, 10.0, or 20.0 mg per kg of body weight. The responses of these subjects to the initial treatment course are shown in Fig. 2. Responses of four owl monkeys infected with the chloroquine-susceptible Uganda Palo Alto strain to treatment with this 4-aminoquinoline (experiment of 13 November 1969) have been included in Fig. 2.

A comparison of the data in charts 1 through 3, upper section of Fig. 2, shows that chloroquine, administered in doses of 5.0 mg/kg, had

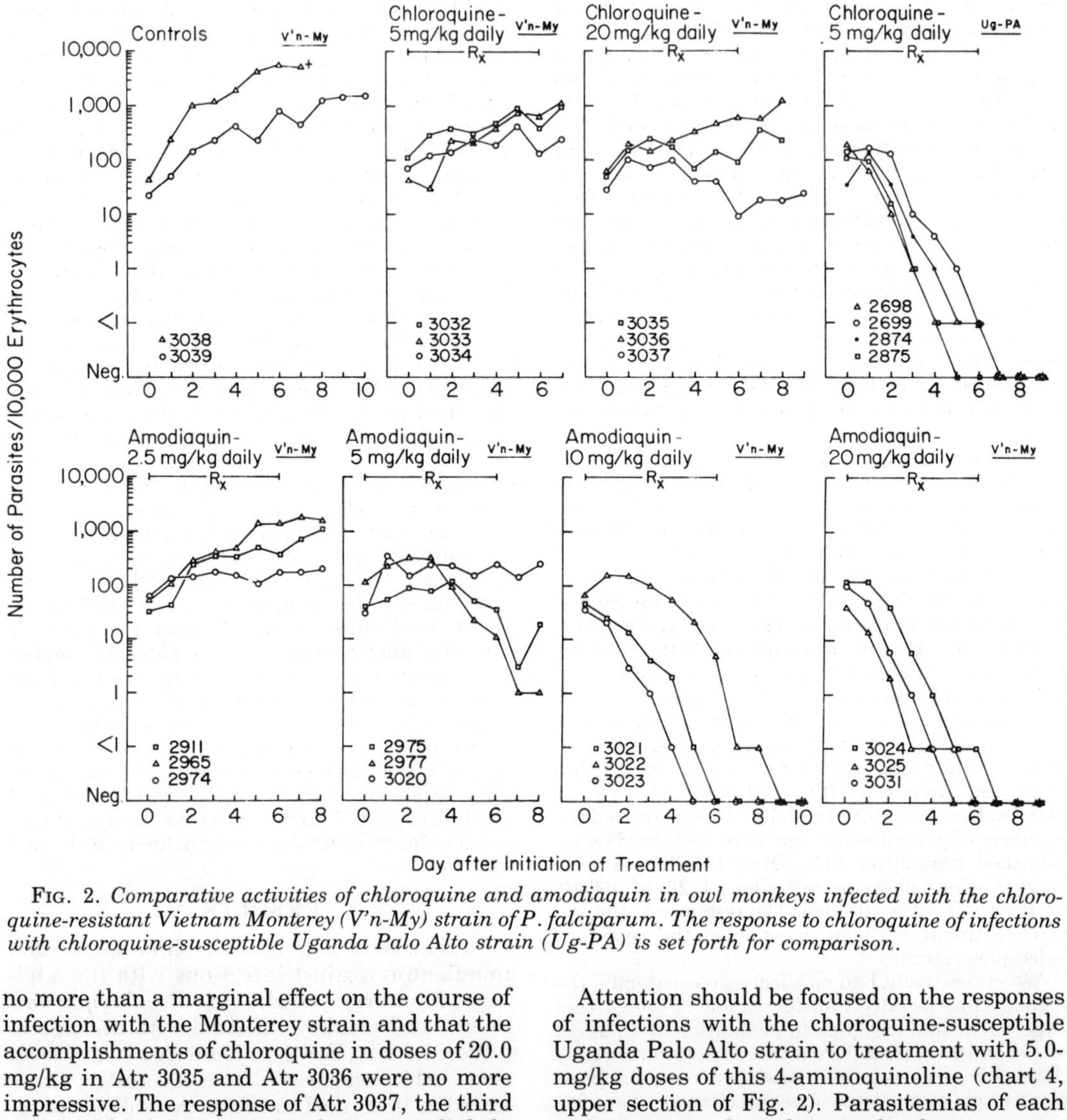

FIG. 2. *Comparative activities of chloroquine and amodiaquin in owl monkeys infected with the chloroquine-resistant Vietnam Monterey (V'n-My) strain of P. falciparum. The response to chloroquine of infections with chloroquine-susceptible Uganda Palo Alto strain (Ug-PA) is set forth for comparison.*

no more than a marginal effect on the course of infection with the Monterey strain and that the accomplishments of chloroquine in doses of 20.0 mg/kg in Atr 3035 and Atr 3036 were no more impressive. The response of Atr 3037, the third recipient of the 20.0-mg/kg dose, was slightly more favorable, parasitemia being maintained at the level that prevailed at the start of treatment.

The responses of infections to amodiaquin in doses of 5.0, 10.0, or 20.0 mg/kg (charts 2 through 4, lower section of Fig. 2) were clearly superior to the responses to 20.0-mg/kg doses of chloroquine. Parasitemias of all three recipients of 5.0-mg/kg doses of amodiaquin were suppressed; parasitemias of the six recipients of 10.0- and 20.0-mg doses were cleared. The infections of Atr 3021 and Atr 3023, both treated with 10.0-mg doses, subsequently recrudesced. The infections of Atr 3022, the third recipient of such doses, and all three recipients of 20.0-mg/kg doses were cured.

Attention should be focused on the responses of infections with the chloroquine-susceptible Uganda Palo Alto strain to treatment with 5.0-mg/kg doses of this 4-aminoquinoline (chart 4, upper section of Fig. 2). Parasitemias of each recipient were cleared promptly; the customary follow-up showed that these infections had been cured. Thus, as would be anticipated from the strain classification, chloroquine has a wholly different level of effectiveness against infections with the Uganda Palo Alto strain than against infections with the Vietnam Monterey strain. It is essential to emphasize, however, that, on a comparable dose basis, the activity of chloroquine against infections with the above chloroquine-susceptible strain is clearly superior to the activity of amodiaquin against infections with the chloroquine-resistant strain. Since amodiaquin and chloroquine have closely comparable activities against infections with susceptible strains, one is forced to conclude that the effectiveness of the former 4-aminoquinoline, although not lost entirely, is compromised by preexisting chloroquine resistance. Thus, there is clear evidence of the existence of cross-resistance insofar as amodiaquin and chloroquine are concerned; however, this cross-resistance is not of a sufficient dimension to destroy the utility of amodiaquin.

Comparative activities of chloroquine, amodiaquin, amopyroquin, and dichlorquinazine (12,278 RP) against infections with various strains of *P. falciparum*. The provocative observations summarized above encouraged an expanded study of the activities of amodiaquin against infections with a variety of strains of *P. falciparum* possessing diverse levels of susceptibility or resistance to chloroquine. Amopyroquin and dichlorquinazine (see structures in Fig. 1) were included in this investigation. The inclusion of amopyroquin was suggested by the late Paul Thompson (University of Georgia, Athens), who had found that this compound was as active as the structurally related amodiaquin against infections with blood schizonts of *P. cynomolgi* in rhesus monkeys, but was better tolerated by these animals (40). Dichlorquinazine, a conjugate of 7-chloro-4-(2-diethylamino-1-methylethyl)-aminoquinoline, was included at the suggestion of the late Jean Schneider (Rhone-Poulenc, Vitry, France), who directed attention to both the published (1) and unpublished (personal communication) results of Benazet that showed that this compound had essentially the same activity against infections with chloroquine-susceptible and chloroquine-resistant strains of *P. berghei* in mice.

Side-by-side comparisons of the activities of amodiaquin, amopyroquin, dichlorquinazine, and chloroquine were carried out in varying sized groups of owl monkeys infected with the chloroquine-susceptible Uganda Palo Alto and Malayan Camp-CH/Q strains and the chloroquine-resistant Vietnam Monterey and Vietnam Oak Knoll strains. Due to restrictions on the availability of owl monkeys, experiments with the chloroquine-resistant Malayan IV and Vietnam Smith strains were limited to a comparison of the activities of amopyroquin and chloroquine.

The results of these comparative studies, compartmentalized with respect to the level of therapeutic achievement (capacity to suppress, clear, or cure), have been detailed in Tables 1 through 3. Since the numbers of infections treated with chloroquine in the current study were not large and the range of doses employed was quite limited (2.5 and 5.0 mg/kg against infections with susceptible strains and 10.0 and 20.0 or 20.0 and 40.0 mg/kg against infections with resistant strains), the results of this comparative study have been supplemented with results obtained in unrelated experiments in which the activity of chloroquine was evaluated over a broader range of doses. This reinforcement was deemed acceptable since both groups of studies were pursued with identical techniques in the same general time period.

Tables 1 through 3 show that the capacities of amodiaquin, amopyroquin, or dichlorquinazine to suppress, clear, or cure infections with the chloroquine-susceptible Uganda Palo Alto or Malayan Camp-CH/Q strains were remarkably similar to the corresponding capabilities of chloroquine. There are suggestions that the curative activity of amopyroquin against infections with the Camp strain is slightly superior to that of chloroquine and that the curative activity of dichlorquinazine is slightly inferior. The dimensions of the current experience would have to be expanded substantially to make these suggestions fully supportable.

As the data in Tables 1 through 3 show, the activities of amodiaquin, amopyroquin, and dichlorquinazine against infections with chloroquine-resistant strains were markedly different from the activities of chloroquine. The former three agents were uniformly and significantly superior to chloroquine in the capacity to suppress and clear parasitemia or cure infections with the chloroquine-resistant Vietnam Monterey and Oak Knoll strains. Amopyroquin exhibited a similar level of superiority over chloroquine against infections with the resistant Malayan IV and Vietnam Smith strains.

By utilizing the data in Tables 1 through 3 and the conventional graphic log of the dose-probit analysis procedure, rough calculations were made of the doses of each compound required to suppress, clear, or cure 90% of the infections with each of the chloroquine-susceptible and chloroquine-resistant strains. The results of these calculations (Table 4) show, as would be expected, that doses required for cure are systematically greater than those required for parasite clearance, which in turn are larger than doses required to suppress parasitemia. Since dose-drug-strain relationships are roughly parallel for these various end points, comments will be limited to data on the 90% effective dose (ED_{90}).

Table 4 shows that the ED_{90} values for chloroquine, amodiaquin, amopyroquin, and dichlorquinazine against infections with the chloroquine-susceptible Uganda Palo Alto strain were essentially the same (7.0 to 7.5 mg/kg). The ED_{90} values of the first three agents against infections with the susceptible Malayan Camp-CH/Q were also essentially identical (8.0 to 8.5 mg/kg). Dichlorquinazine ap-

TABLE 1. *Capacities of various 4-aminoquinolines to suppress parasitemia in established infections with diverse chloroquine-susceptible and chloroquine-resistant strains of P. falciparum*

Strain		Response to treatment				
Designation	Response to chloroquine[a]	Daily dose[b] (mg of base/kg of body wt)	No. of infections suppressed[c]/no. treated			
			Chloroquine	Amodiaquin	Amopyroquin	Dichlorquinazine
Uganda Palo Alto	S	1.25	8/22			
		2.5	18/21	3/3	2/2	2/3
		5.0	70/71	4/4	4/4	5/5
		10.0	17/17	6/6	4/4	3/3
Malayan Camp-CH/Q	S	1.25	1/3			
		2.5	3/3	3/3	8/8	0/3
		5.0	15/15	6/6	12/12	4/4
		10.0	12/12	4/4	6/6	5/5
Vietnam Monterey	R	2.5	0/6	4/5		
		5.0	1/15	9/9	2/2	9/9
		10.0	0/4	12/12	9/9	
		20.0	22/35	24/24	12/12	10/10
		40.0	30/30		8/8	
Vietnam Oak Knoll	R	1.25	0/6			
		5.0	2/6	3/3	7/7	5/5
		10.0		3/3	15/15	6/6
		20.0	15/19	9/9	18/18	6/6
Vietnam Smith	R	5.0	0/4			
		20.0	10/11		22/22	
Malayan IV	R	1.25	1/18			
		5.0	12/28		2/2	
		10.0	1/2		5/5	
		20.0	66/66		6/6	

[a] S, Susceptible to chloroquine; R, resistant to chloroquine.

[b] Doses of 1.25 to 20.0 mg/kg were administered once daily between 8:00 and 9:00 a.m. for 7 consecutive days; doses of 40.0 mg/kg were administered in two equal fractions at 8:00 a.m. and 8:00 p.m. over the same time period.

[c] Infections were categorized as suppressed when parasitemias were consistently positive throughout the course of treatment and for 5 days thereafter, but at no time exceeded twice the levels that existed when therapy was started.

peared to be slightly less active than these compounds against infections with the latter strain. In contrast to the above findings, the ED_{90} values of amodiaquin, amopyroquin, or dichlorquinazine against infections with the chloroquine-resistant Vietnam Monterey and Oak Knoll strains and the ED_{90} values of amopyroquin against infections with the Vietnam Smith and Malayan IV strains were significantly less, by a factor of 2 to 5, than the ED_{90} values of chloroquine. However, the doses of amodiaquin and amopyroquin required for cure of 90% of the infections with these resistant strains were two to three times larger than the doses required for a similar result in infections with the chloroquine-susceptible strains. Surprisingly, the data indicated that dichlorquinazine was equally active against infections with the chloroquine-resistant Vietnam Monterey and Oak Knoll strains and the susceptible Malayan Camp strain. This provocative observation merits confirmation before it is accepted without qualification.

These observations are fully supportive of the conclusion reached during study of the activity of amodiaquin against infections with the Vietnam Monterey strain. They show that there is significant cross-resistance among different 4-aminoquinolines, but that cross-resistance is not solid. As a result, infections that are refractory to treatment with maximally tolerated doses of chloroquine may still be cured by larger-than-normal, but well-tolerated, doses of amodiaquin, amopyroquin, and dichlorquinazine.

Comparative activities of selected 4-amino-

TABLE 2. *Capacities of various 4-aminoquinolines to clear parasitemia in established infections with diverse chloroquine-susceptible and chloroquine-resistant strains of P. falciparum*

Strain		Response to treatment				
Designation	Response to chloroquine[a]	Daily dose[b] (mg of base/kg of body wt)	No. of infections cleared[c]/no. treated: Chloroquine	Amodiaquin	Amopyroquin	Dichlorquinazine
Uganda Palo Alto	S	1.25	0/22			
		2.5	13/21	3/3	2/2	1/3
		5.0	69/71	4/4	4/4	5/5
		10.0	16/17	6/6	4/4	3/3
Malayan Camp-CH/Q	S	1.25	0/3			
		2.5	2/3	2/3	6/8	0/3
		5.0	15/15	6/6	12/12	3/4
		10.0	12/12	4/4	6/6	5/5
Vietnam Monterey	R	2.5	0/6	0/5		
		5.0	0/15	4/9	0/2	9/9
		10.0	0/4	10/12	8/9	
		20.0	6/35	24/24	12/12	10/10
		40.0	27/30		8/8	
Vietnam Oak Knoll	R	1.25	0/6			
		5.0	0/6	1/3	3/7	4/5
		10.0		3/3	15/15	6/6
		20.0	5/19	9/9	18/18	6/6
Vietnam Smith	R	5.0	0/4			
		20.0	3/11		22/22	
Malayan IV	R	1.25	0/18			
		5.0	6/28		0/2	
		10.0	0/2		5/5	
		20.0	66/66		6/6	

[a] S, Susceptible to chloroquine; R, resistant to chloroquine.

[b] Doses of 1.25 to 20.0 mg/kg were administered once daily between 8:00 and 9:00 a.m. for 7 consecutive days; doses of 40.0 mg/kg were administered in two equal fractions at 8:00 a.m. and 8:00 p.m. over the same time period.

[c] Infections were categorized as cleared when thick blood films became parasite negative during the treatment interval or 3 days thereafter and remained so for a minimum of 10 days after therapy had been completed.

quinolines against infections with the chloroquine-susceptible Malayan Camp-CH/Q and chloroquine-resistant Vietnam Oak Knoll strains of *P. falciparum*. The results of the experiments summarized in the preceding sections were reported in early 1970 to the staff of the Walter Reed Army Institute of Research responsible for direction and management of the Department of the Army Malaria Chemotherapy Program. The question was raised promptly as to whether other 4-aminoquinolines might be as effective or more effective than amodiaquin and amopyroquin against infections with chloroquine-resistant strains. The stock of World War II antimalarials, referred to earlier, containing 42 4-aminoquinolines, made it possible to undertake a pilot test of this question without embarking on a new program of chemical synthesis. To keep evaluations in owl monkeys at a manageable level, it was decided to carry out assessments of the activities of type compounds in vitro, limiting in vivo appraisals to derivatives that exhibited the same or relatively similar in vitro activity against parasites of chloroquine-susceptible and chloroquine-resistant strains. Responsibility for the in vitro assessments was assumed by Karl Rieckmann, Army Medical Research Project, University of Chicago, who had adapted a relatively uncomplicated procedure for identifying infections with chloroquine-resistant plasmodia in the field (34) to measurement of drug activities in the laboratory (33).

Samples of 17 derivatives with distinctive chemical characteristics were drawn from the above stock and together with amodiaquin,

TABLE 3. *Capacities of various 4-aminoquinolines to cure established infections with diverse chloroquine-susceptible and chloroquine-resistant strains of P. falciparum*

Strain		Response to treatment				
			No. of infections cured[c]/no. treated			
Designation	Response to chloroquine[a]	Daily dose[b] (mg of base/kg of body wt)	Chloroquine	Amodiaquin	Amopyro-quin	Dichlorquin-azine
Uganda Palo Alto	S	1.25	0/22			
		2.5	7/21	0/3	0/2	1/3
		5.0	53/71	2/4	2/4	3/5
		10.0	16/17	6/6	4/4	3/3
Malayan Camp-CH/Q	S	1.25	0/3			
		2.5	0/3	0/3	4/8	0/3
		5.0	9/15	3/6	11/12	0/4
		10.0	11/12	4/4	6/6	4/5
Vietnam Monterey	R	2.5	0/6	0/5		
		5.0	0/15	0/9	0/2	4/9
		10.0	0/4	2/12	4/9	
		20.0	2/35	21/24	8/12	10/10
		40.0	21/30		8/8	
Vietnam Oak Knoll	R	1.25	0/6			
		5.0	0/6	0/3	3/7	2/5
		10.0		2/3	13/15	5/6
		20.0	4/19	8/9	18/18	6/6
Vietnam Smith	R	5.0	0/4			
		20.0	0/11		22/22	
Malayan IV	R	1.25	0/18			
		5.0	1/28		0/2	
		10.0	0/2		0/5	
		20.0	44/66		6/6	

[a] S, Susceptible to chloroquine; R, resistant to chloroquine.

[b] Doses of 1.25 to 20.0 mg/kg were administered once daily between 8:00 and 9:00 a.m. for 7 consecutive days; doses of 40.0 mg/kg were administered in two equal fractions at 8:00 a.m. and 8:00 p.m. over the same time period.

[c] Infections were categorized as cured when parasite clearance was achieved during or immediately after drug treatment and thick blood films were uniformly parasite negative for at least 12 to 13 consecutive weeks after completion of therapy.

amopyroquin, and dichlorquinazine were forwarded as unknowns to Rieckmann. Each of these agents was evaluated for the capacity to inhibit maturation of the ring forms of the Uganda I and Vietnam Marks strains of *P. falciparum*. The former strain differs from the Uganda Palo Alto strain in being susceptible to pyrimethamine as well as to chloroquine and quinine (33). According to studies in human volunteers (6, 33), the Vietnam Marks strain has the same spectrum of drug resistance as the Vietnam Smith strain used previously in our studies.

The first assessments reported by Rieckmann divided the test compounds clearly into two groups: (i) six agents that inhibited maturation of parasites of the Vietnam Marks strain at concentrations of not more than 2.5 times those required for inhibition of the Uganda I strain and (ii) 14 agents that, like the control chloroquine, inhibited the development of parasites of the Marks strain at concentrations of 10 or more times higher than those required for the inhibition of the Uganda I strain. Breaking of the code showed that amodiaquin, amopyroquin, dichlorquinazine, SN-8137, SN-9584, and SN-10274 comprised the first group referred to above (see Fig. 1 for structures of the latter three agents). The initial appraisals were confirmed subsequently for all 20 agents, except SN-8137, which on repeat testing exhibited the same activity differential as chloroquine against the test strains. Table 5 summarizes the observations on the five derivatives with a high order of activity against parasites of the Marks strain, plus observations on SN-8137.

TABLE 4. *Summary: Calculated ED_{90} values of various 4-aminoquinolines required for suppression and clearance of parasitemias or cure of infections with diverse chloroquine-susceptible and chloroquine-resistant strains of P. falciparum*

Strain		Calculated ED_{90}—daily dose (mg of base/kg of body wt)[b]			
Designation	Response to chloroquine[a]	Chloroquine	Amodiaquin	Amopyroquin	Dichlorquinazine
To effect suppression of parasitemia[c]					
Uganda Palo Alto	S	2.8	<2.5	<2.5	3.5
Malayan Camp-CH/Q	S	2.0	<2.5	<2.5	4.5
Vietnam Monterey	R	30.0	3.0	<5.0	<5.0
Vietnam Oak Knoll	R	30.0	<5.0	<5.0	<5.0
Vietnam Smith	R	20.0		<20.0	
Malayan IV	R	13.0		<5.0	
To effect clearance of parasitemia[c]					
Uganda Palo Alto	S	4.0	<2.5	<2.5	4.0
Malayan Camp-CH/Q	S	3.5	3.5	3.5	7.0
Vietnam Monterey	R	40.0	13.0	13.0	<5.0
Vietnam Oak Knoll	R	ca. 50.0	8.0	8.0	7.0
Vietnam Smith	R	ca. 50.0		<20.0	
Malayan IV	R	17.0		9.0	
To cure infection[c]					
Uganda Palo Alto	S	7.5	7.5	7.5	7.0
Malayan Camp-CH/Q	S	8.5	8.0	8.0	11.0
Vietnam Monterey	R	50.0	21.0	25.0	12.0
Vietnam Oak Knoll	R	ca. 60.0	17.0	12.0	12.0
Vietnam Smith	R	>50.0		<20.0	
Malayan IV	R	28.0		15.0	

[a] S, Susceptible to chloroquine; R, resistant to chloroquine.
[b] Dose, administered once daily for 7 consecutive days, required to suppress or clear parasitemias or cure infections in 90% of the treated subjects.
[c] See Tables 1, 2, and 3, respectively, for definitions of suppression, clearance, and cure.

We are deeply indebted to Rieckmann for permission to present this summary of his evaluations.

In the middle of June 1970, shortly after receipt of Rieckmann's initial assessments, our laboratory embarked on a comparison of the activities of SN-8137, SN-9584, SN-10274, chloroquine, amodiaquin, and amopyroquin against infections with the chloroquine-susceptible Malayan Camp-CH/Q strain and the chloroquine-resistant Vietnam Oak Knoll strain. The latter strain was substituted for the Monterey strain, which had been stored in the frozen state in December 1969 in order to conserve the then short supply of owl monkeys. It was believed that this substitution would not prejudice the results of the current study since the Oak Knoll and Monterey strains have essentially the same levels of resistance to chloroquine and quinine and differ only with respect to susceptibility to pyrimethamine.

Thirty owl monkeys were inoculated with the Malayan Camp-CH/Q strain. Three groups of two subjects each served as untreated and chloroquine- or amodiaquin-treated controls. Four groups, each of six monkeys, were assigned to evaluation of the activities of amopyroquin, SN-8137, SN-9584, or SN-10274, with subgroups of two each treated with 2.5, 5.0, or 10.0-mg/kg doses of the respective compounds. One of the assignees to 10.0-mg/kg doses of SN-9584 died of an overwhelming pneumonia the day prior to scheduled treatment. Thirty-two monkeys were inoculated with the Vietnam Oak Knoll strain. One group of two subjects and two groups of three served, respectively, as untreated and chloroquine- or amodiaquin-treated controls. Four groups of six monkeys were allocated to evaluations of the activities of amopyroquin, SN-8137, SN-9584, or SN-10274, with subgroups of three each receiving 5.0 or 20.0-mg/kg doses of the respective compounds.

As indicated by the early responses to doses of 5.0 mg/kg (Fig. 3), the activities of SN-8137 and SN-9584 against infections with the chloroquine-susceptible Malayan Camp-CH/Q strain compared favorably with the activities of chloroquine, amodiaquin, and amopyroquin. However, it would be an error to conclude that these five compounds have equal antimalarial activ-

TABLE 5. *Capacities of chloroquine and related 4-aminoquinolines to block in vitro maturation of blood schizonts of the chloroquine-susceptible Uganda I strain and the chloroquine-resistant Vietnam Marks strain of P. falciparum*[a]

Compound[b]	Concn required for >90% inhibition of maturation (μg of salt/liter of blood): Uganda I strain	Concn required for >90% inhibition of maturation (μg of salt/liter of blood): Vietnam Marks strain	Ratio of activities (Uganda I vs. Vietnam Marks)
Chloroquine	250	2,500	10
Amodiaquin	50	100	2
Amopyroquin	50	100	2
Dichlorquinazine	250	500	2
SN-8137	100 (100)[c]	1,000 (250)[c]	10 (2.5)[c]
SN-9584	250	500	2
SN-10274	250	500	2

[a] We are indebted to Karl Rieckmann and co-workers of the Army Medical Research Project, The University of Chicago, for making these data available and especially to Rieckmann (Malaria Research Program, University of New Mexico, Albuquerque, N.M.) for permission to present them in this report.

[b] See Fig. 1 for structures of the various compounds.

[c] The result of the initial test, not confirmed.

ity. As Fig. 3 and Tables 1 and 3 show, chloroquine, amodiaquin, and amopyroquin regularly effected suppression of parasitemia at doses of 2.5 mg/kg and cured a high proportion of infections at doses of 5.0 mg/kg. Doses of 5.0 mg of SN-8137 or SN-9584 per kg of body weight were required for suppression of parasitemia (Fig. 3), and doses of 10.0 mg/kg were required for cure of either primary or retreatment infections. These comparative data have led to the conclusion that SN-8137 and SN-9584 have approximately one-half the activity of chloroquine, amodiaquin, or amopyroquin against infections with the chloroquine-susceptible Malayan Camp-CH/Q strain. SN-10274 was clearly less active than SN-8137 or SN-9584. Doses of 10.0 mg/kg were required for suppression of parasitemia, and doses of 20.0 mg/kg were required for cure (Fig. 3).

With respect to activity against infections with the chloroquine-resistant Vietnam Oak Knoll strain, Fig. 4 shows that SN-8137 and SN-9584 occupy a position between that of chloroquine on one extreme and those of amodiaquin and amopyroquin on the other. At daily doses of 20.0 mg/kg of body weight, chloroquine had no significant effect on the evolution of parasitemia; SN-8137 and SN-9584 suppressed parasite development; amodiaquin and amopyroquin effected parasite clearance. Infections in two of three recipients of 20.0-mg/kg doses of amodiaquin and in all three recipients of such doses of amopyroquin were cured.

The above assessments of the relative positions of the five 4-aminoquinolines against infections with the Oak Knoll strain are reinforced by the responses of primary treatment failures to retreatment with the same agent ("+" items in Fig. 4). Retreatment with chloroquine at daily doses of 40.0 mg/kg (20.0 mg/kg twice daily) temporarily reduced the parasitemias of two subjects and cured one infection. Infections of five of six primary treatment failures on SN-8137 and six of six failures on SN-9584 were cured by retreatment with the same 40.0-mg/kg regimen. Retreatment with 10.0-mg/kg doses of amopyroquin effected cure of the three infections that had been suppressed by primary treatment with doses of 5.0 mg/kg.

SN-10274 exhibited less activity than any other agent against infections with the Oak Knoll strain. Doses of 5.0 or 20.0 mg/kg had little effect on parasitemia. Retreatment of each of the six primary treatment failures with doses of 40.0 mg/kg led to no more than a slight suppression of parasitemia.

Although the data are limited, they suffice to show that the decrement in therapeutic activity of either SN-8137 or SN-9584, in the face of chloroquine resistance, is less than that for chloroquine itself, but is substantially greater than the reduction in activity for either amodiaquin or amopyroquin. Although from the practical viewpoint the accomplishments of SN-8137 and SN-9584 were disappointing, they certify to the absence of solid cross-resistance among the 4-aminoquinolines and thereby encourage further study of representatives of this class of drug.

DISCUSSION

The results of the current studies have shown that the 4-aminoquinoline derivatives, amodiaquin, amopyroquin, and dichlorquinazine, are essentially as active as chloroquine against established infections with chloroquine-susceptible strains of *P. falciparum* in owl monkeys, but that each of the aforementioned compounds is less active against infections with chloroquine-resistant strains than against infections with chloroquine-susceptible strains. This finding provides general support for the concept that chloroquine-resistant strains of *P. falciparum* are cross-resistant to other 4-aminoquinolines. More importantly, however, these investigations have shown that infections with such resistant strains, not curable when treated with the maximally tolerated doses of chloroquine, can be cured regularly by treatment with well-tolerated doses of amodiaquin, amopyroquin, and dichlorquinazine. This finding has led to the conclusion that, at least with the strains of *P. falciparum* examined in this study, the dimensions of cross-resistance are limited,

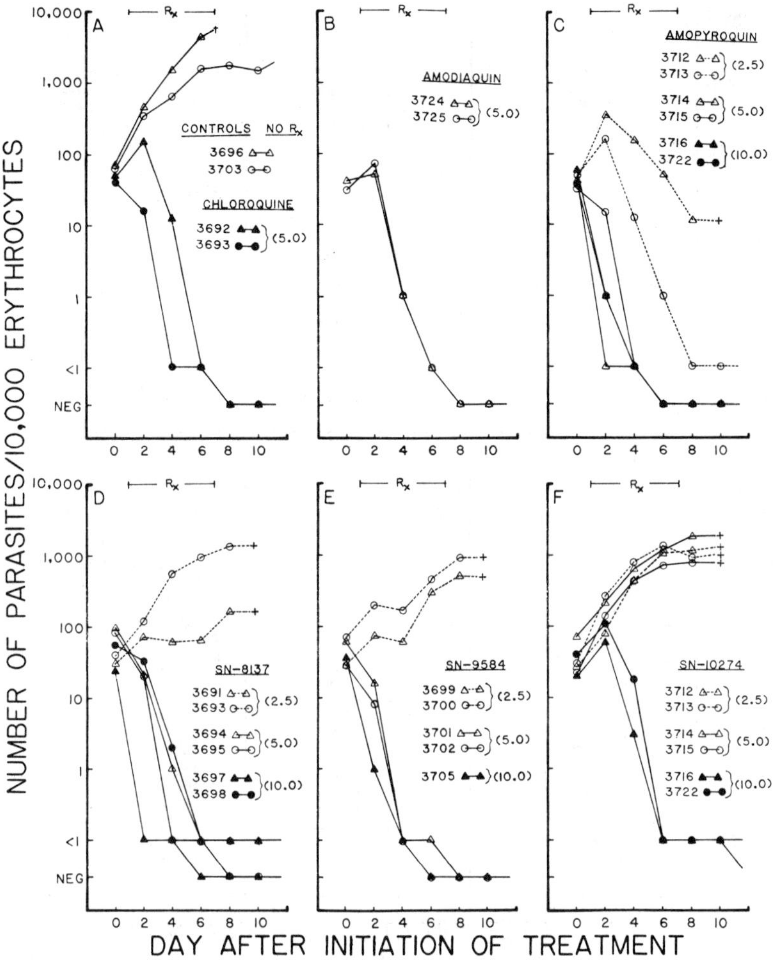

FIG. 3. *Comparative activities of chloroquine, amodiaquin, amopyroquin, SN-8137, SN-9584, and SN-10274 in owl monkeys infected with the chloroquine-susceptible Malayan Camp-CH/Q strain of P. falciparum. +, Point of retreatment with increased dose of same drug; †, death from malaria.*

sufficiently so that some 4-aminoquinolines, including the three derivatives mentioned above, retain substantial levels of therapeutic utility in the face of chloroquine treatment failures. This implies discrete, but nonetheless important, differences in the actions of various 4-aminoquinolines on the malaria parasite.

The foregoing conclusion provokes numerous questions, including the following. (i) Are the demonstrated activities of amodiaquin, amopyroquin, and dichlorquinazine against infections with chloroquine-resistant strains of *P. falciparum* in owl monkeys compatible with published assessments of the activities of these agents against infections with this plasmodium in humans or infections with other plasmodia in experimental animals? (ii) Is there a theoretical basis, or any rational explanation, for the superior activities of amodiaquin, amopyroquin and dichlorquinazine against infections with chloroquine-resistant parasites? (iii) Should attention be directed to both currently available and newly synthesized 4-aminoquinolines in an effort to uncover a derivative or derivatives with greater activity than amodiaquin, amopyroquin, or dichlorquinazine against infections with chloroquine-resistant strains of *P. falciparum*? If so, are there reliable, comparatively simple, and economical approaches to this end? In approaching these questions, it is necessary to rest heavily on experiences with amodiaquin since comparatively few rounded clinical or experimental investigations have been pursued with either amopyroquin or dichlorquinazine.

Before turning to the first question, attention should be directed to the similarity of the doses of amodiaquin (also chloroquine) required to

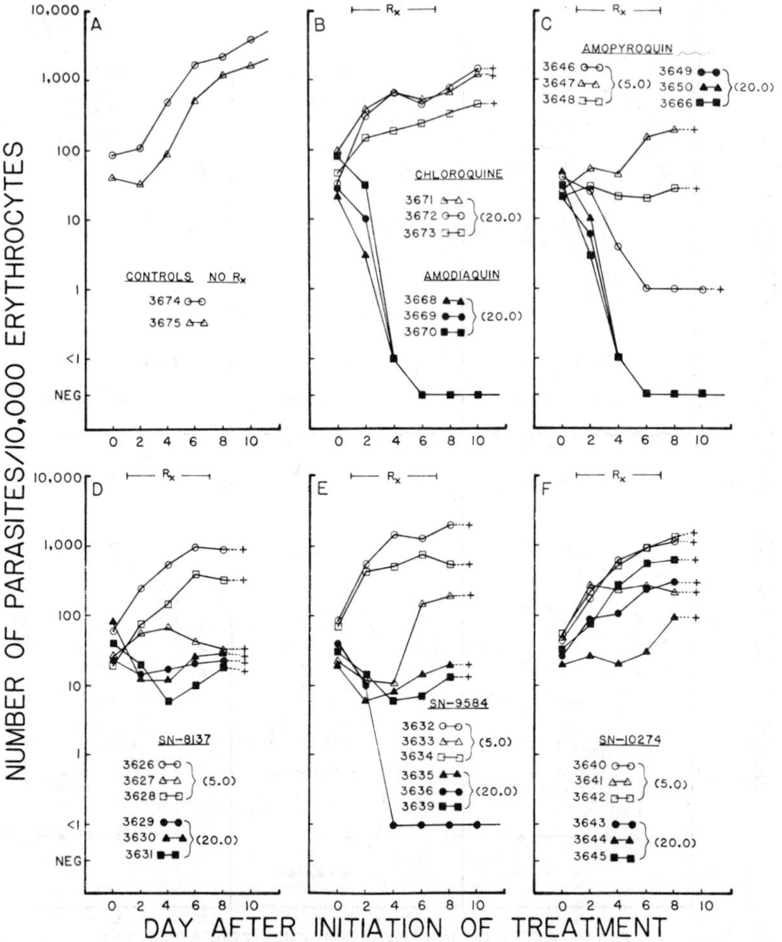

FIG. 4. *Comparative activities of chloroquine, amodiaquin, amopyroquin, SN-8137, SN-9584, and SN-10274 in owl monkeys infected with the chloroquine-resistant Vietnam Oak Knoll strain of P. falciparum. +, Point of retreatment with increased dose of same drug.*

cure infections with chloroquine-susceptible strains of *P. falciparum* in humans and owl monkeys. The total doses for such achievements approximate 20.0 mg/kg of body weight (1.4 g to a 70-kg patient) for humans, and 52.5 mg/kg for owl monkeys (Table 4). These quantities equate (13) to 740 and 630 mg/m². The essential identity of the doses required to achieve a comparable end point in these two dissimilar hosts should engender confidence in use of the owl monkey-human malaria model for resolving some of the problems of chloroquine resistance in the human malarias.

As for the first question, we have been unable to identify any serious incompatibilities between published appraisals of the activity of amodiaquin against human infections with chloroquine-resistant strains of *P. falciparum* and assessments in owl monkeys infected with such strains. The great majority of investigators (3–5, 8, 14, 19, 24, 29, 30, 31, 35, 46–48), all but one of whom (48) have worked with very small groups of subjects infected with a variety of chloroquine-resistant strains, have found that such infections cannot be cured by treatment with 1.4-g doses of amodiaquin, the dosage recommended for cure of infections with sensitive strains. This finding is compatible with observations in owl monkeys that show that doses that cure infections with susceptible strains do not cure infections with resistant strains. However, three other groups of investigators (15, 33, 43), who have pursued the issue of cross-resistance in much greater depth, have reported that amodiaquin, although not regularly curative, is significantly more active than chloroquine in volunteers or patients infected with resistant strains. One of these studies (43) involved work with 30 volunteers of comparable immune status, infected with the highly chloroquine-resistant Vietnam Marks strain. Chloroquine, administered to 10 of these volunteers in total doses ranging from 1.5 to 3.0 g, produced temporary clearance of parasitemia in 3 subjects and suppression of parasite multiplication in 1 and was without effect on the course of disease in 6. In contrast, amodiaquin, administered to 20 volunteers in total doses of 1.5 to 3.6 g, cured 4 infections, produced temporary clearance of parasitemia in 15 subjects, and was without effect in only 1. A second study (15), pursued in Thailand, compared the activities of chloroquine and amodiaquin in 45 patients with naturally acquired infections with chloroquine-resistant strains. Eleven patients were treated with 1.5 g of chloroquine. Temporary clearance of parasitemia was achieved in a single patient; parasitemias persisted in 10 subjects. Thirty-four patients received amodiaquin in doses of 1.5 and 2.0 g. Cure was achieved in 13 subjects, and temporary clearance of parasitemia was achieved in 17. In four subjects, parasitemias persisted. The superiority of amodiaquin in these studies was demonstrable at doses that were relatively less than those found necessary to cure infections with chloroquine-resistant strains in owl monkeys. It would be interesting to know whether the accomplishments of amodiaquin in humans could be improved by administration of doses three- to fourfold greater than those commonly employed, assuming that doses of such magnitude can be delivered without evoking untoward reactions.

The current observations on the activity of amodiaquin, amopyroquin, and dichlorquinazine against infections with chlorquine-resistant strains of *P. falciparum* are not in harmony with published observations (17, 27, 39) on the activities of these 4-aminoquinolines in mice infected with chloroquine-resistant strains of *P. berghei*. The latter are solidly cross-resistant to amodiaquin and amopyroquin (17, 27, 39) and under comparable conditions to dichlorquinazine (42). This dichotomy between the two sets of observations is not surprising, considering that they were based on different plasmodial species, one with a quotidian and the other with a tertian cycle of development, and a variety of other distinguishing features. It is important to emphasize that, apart from their response to the relevant 4-aminoquinolines, chloroquine-susceptible and chloroquine-resistant strains of *P. falciparum* are biologically indistinguishable. They are identical in virulence, exhibit the same morphology, and have the same age of erythrocyte preference and predilection for sequestration in deep vascular loci. Chloroquine resistance is a stable characteristic, persisting unaltered through years of passage through the untreated host (personal observation, manuscript in preparation). On the other hand, the biological features of chloroquine-resistant and chloroquine-susceptible *P. berghei* are quite different. Chloroquine-resistant strains are less virulent than susceptible strains (39), and, unlike the latter strains, produce little pigment (26), multiply selectively in reticulocytes (28), and preferentially localize in deep vascular sites (18). Furthermore, in most strains of *P. berghei*, resistance is an unstable characteristic, with reversal to the susceptible state occurring rapidly upon passage through normal untreated mice (16, 39).

The above broad biological differences between chloroquine-resistant *P. berghei* and *P. falciparum*, although doubtless important, may be less significant than the differences in levels of chloroquine resistance. Resistant strains of *P. berghei* are developed via extended serial transfer of the parasite through mice treated with increasing doses of chloroquine, up to the maximally tolerated level. The resulting strains have a very high level of resistance. The infections that they produce cannot be controlled by treatment with 30 to 200 times the dose of chloroquine required to control infections with the parent susceptible strains (16, 17, 27, 32, 39). Whereas, because of toxicity limitations, the dimensions of chloroquine resistance in *P. falciparum* cannot be fully assessed, our studies in owl monkeys, as well as those of McKelvey and co-workers (20) in patients, suggest that the difference between the susceptibilities of sensitive and resistant strains are at most not more than eightfold and in some strains may be considerably less. Thus, the challenges posed to amodiaquin, amopyroquin, and dichlorquinazine in infections with chloroquine-resistant *P. berghei* are of a different magnitude than those posed by infections with chloroquine-resistant *P. falciparum*. Until studies with the two parasites can be carried out at comparable resistance levels, it would be advisable to postpone concerns with incompatibilities. (Subsequent to preparation of this manuscript, it was learned that a strain of *P. berghei*, designated N-67, is now available which may make such comparison possible. According to a personal communication from F. Benazet, Rhone-Poulenc, Vitry, France, infections with this strain respond to 10 to 20 times the dose of chloroquine required for control of infections with the parent susceptible strain. More importantly, infections with the

N-67 strain respond to treatment with amodiaquin and a relative of dichlorquinazine, designated 12,494-R.P., whereas infections with conventional chloroquine-resistant strains are totally refractory to treatment with these compounds.)

With respect to the second question, there is as yet no adequately supported concept of the mode of action of chloroquine or other 4-aminoquinoline on any plasmodium, although there are numerous provocative hypotheses. Despite this deficit, there are a series of observations that appear to provide a reasonable explanation for the activity of amodiaquin in the face of chloroquine resistance. These observations had their origin in the work of Macomber and coworkers (22), who pursued a complicated, but well-executed, study in groups of mice infected with either chloroquine-susceptible or chloroquine-resistant strains of *P. berghei* and treated with various doses of [^{14}C]quinoline ring-labeled chloroquine at an appropriate time in the infection. At various times after treatment, animals were sacrificed and critical comparisons were made of the concentrations of the label in erythrocytes of noninfected mice and in the parasitized and nonparasitized erythrocytes of mice infected with susceptible and resistant strains. The results showed that the concentrations of the label in erythrocytes (parasitized and nonparasitized) obtained from mice infected with the chloroquine-susceptible strain were 25-fold greater than the concentrations in erythrocytes drawn from noninfected mice. More importantly, under identical dosage and harvesting conditions, the concentrations of the label in erythrocytes derived from mice infected with the chloroquine-resistant strain were only one-tenth of the concentrations in erythrocytes obtained from mice infected with the susceptible strain. Macomber et al. (22) concluded that "The results . . . suggest that chloroquine is selectively toxic because it attains higher concentrations in parasitized cells than in normal tissue cells and that plasmodial resistance to chloroquine is based on an impairment of the mechanism by which such drug levels are accumulated."

Fitch (10) pursued the above suggestion with a simple, but very precise, in vitro procedure based on measuring the uptake of labeled chloroquine by parasitized erythrocytes from medium to which this compound had been added in concentrations well within the range of those found in plasma of patients treated with this drug. He confirmed the essential correctness of Macomber's observations on the difference in chloroquine binding by erythrocytes parasitized with chloroquine-susceptible and chloroquine-resistant strains of *P. berghei* and went on to demonstrate that, although of lesser magnitude, there was also a marked difference in binding of labeled chloroquine by parasitized erythrocytes derived from owl monkeys infected with the chloroquine-susceptible Malayan Camp-CH/Q strain versus those infected with the chloroquine-resistant Vietnam Monterey and Oak Knoll strains (11, 12). On the basis of critical physicochemical measurements, he concluded that the parasites of the chloroquine-resistant strains of *P. falciparum* were deficient in high-affinity binding sites for chloroquine (11). The observations most relevant to the current findings came from a comparison of the uptakes of ^{14}C-labeled chloroquine and ^{14}C-labeled amodiaquin by parasites of the Malayan Camp-CH/Q and Vietnam Oak Knoll strains (12). This comparison showed that although the association constants for binding of the two compounds were identical, the chloroquine-susceptible Malayan Camp-CH/Q parasites bound two to three times as much amodiaquin as chloroquine. More importantly, binding of amodiaquin by parasites of the Malayan Camp-CH/Q and Vietnam Oak Knoll strains was essentially identical, whereas binding of chloroquine by the latter resistant strain amounted to only 30 to 40% of the binding by the susceptible Malayan Camp-CH/Q strain. The resulting differences in localization of chloroquine and amodiaquin in erythrocytes parasitized with susceptible and resistant strains of *P. falciparum* seem to go a long way toward explaining why amodiaquin has activity in the face of chloroquine resistance.

The third and final question posed earlier in this section has two parts, one concerned with the merit of pursuing further investigations with currently available and newly synthesized 4-aminoquinolines and a second pertaining to approaches to such studies, assuming that they are indicated. Before addressing these issues, it should be noted that, on the basis of available data, it is doubtful whether the demonstrated capacities of amodiaquin, amopyroquin, or dichlorquinazine to control infections with chloroquine-resistant strains of *P. falciparum* can be exploited in practice. The best results achieved with amodiaquin (15, 43) were far from optimal. In view of the steep dose-response curves of the relevant 4-aminoquinolines, cures might be attained regularly by doubling the largest dose of amodiaquin employed in the above studies. However, such a dosage increase would probably be pushing the limits of tolerability of amodiaquin, an allowable procedure as a lifesaving measure in a critically ill patient under close observation in a hospital environment, but not acceptable for unsupervised suppressive use in the field or for treatment of developed disease under minimal supervision. The value of the current observations on amodiaquin and related compounds is, therefore, not at the practical therapeutic level, but rather in identifying the limits of cross-resistance and focusing attention on the possibility of developing a 4-aminoquinoline with usable therapeutic activity against infections with chloroquine-resistant plasmodia.

Having arrived at the above conclusion, there would appear to be substantial merit to evaluating the activities of currently available 4-aminoquinolines and to the synthesis and evaluation of new derivatives. To date, only 20 compounds, from what must be a large pool of derivatives remaining from the World War II Malaria Chemotherapy Program, have been examined. The results of this limited exploration, revealing five agents with significant activity against infections with chloroquine-resistant strains, should encourage the release of compounds of this class now being held in diverse "drug repositories." Studies on available agents will doubtlessly have to be supplemented by studies on newly synthesized compounds. Hopefully, these will be prepared on a rational basis. Although not skilled in chemical theory, it seems to us that the investigations of Marquez et al. (23) provide at least one reasonable theoretical approach to the synthesis of amodiaquin congeners.

As for evaluation of various 4-aminoquinolines, it should be emphasized that for reasons set forth earlier, use of infections with chloroquine-resistant strains of *P. berghei* for this purpose is clearly contraindicated. Ideally, the evaluation should be pursued in owl monkeys infected with a chloroquine-resistant strain of *P. falciparum* well established in the laboratory (e.g., the Smith strain), but this may not be possible because of limited availability of these subjects. Even if they were in unlimited supply, it would probably be wise to initiate studies of new derivatives in vitro, starting with culture procedures such as have been developed by Rieckmann et al. (34) and Siddiqui et al. (38). In these systems, groups of test compounds could be compared for activities against parasites of chloroquine-susceptible and chloroquine-resistant strains of *P. falciparum* derived from infected owl monkeys. Agents that exhibited essentially equal activity against both parasites could then be examined for binding to susceptible and resistant parasites, utilizing the basic techniques evolved by Fitch (10), but measuring the concentrations of the compound by fluorometric rather than radiolabel procedures, since preparation of every labeled compound to be studied would not be practical. (This sequence of evaluations would be helpful at all times, but especially so when the supply of a new agent is limited.) Compounds that bind equally well to susceptible and resistant parasites would then be evaluated in infected owl monkeys. The ultimate evaluations for tolerability and therapeutic and suppressive activities would proceed from this point in conventional order.

In concluding this report, it should be emphasized that interest in developing another 4-aminoquinoline as a possible replacement for chloroquine rests on the remarkable worldwide performance of this drug for a period of close to 30 years in suppressing and treating infections with all three human plasmodia. The premier position of chloroquine rests on the fact that it is very well tolerated in recommended doses, that it controls parasitemia and fever more rapidly than any other drug except the related amodiaquin, that it has a steep dose-response curve (making for uniformly reliable activity), and that it is extensively localized in tissues and slowly degraded, even then to a metabolite with essentially the same antimalarial activity as the parent compound (unpublished observation of L. H. Schmidt). Except in those limited regions where chloroquine-resistant strains of *P. falciparum* have appeared, it is still the agent of choice for suppression and treatment of malaria. The pioneering studies (44) on the 4-aminoquinolines showed that most 7-chloro derivatives were endowed with many of the same pharmacological characteristics as chloroquine. It is our opinion that uncovering a compound with the biological properties of chloroquine, but effective in the face of resistance to this agent, would contribute importantly to malaria chemotherapy.

ACKNOWLEDGMENTS

We gratefully acknowledge the assistance of Lee Vogel in preparing this manuscript and Trudie Jerkins, Tarpon Springs, Fla., for facilitating direct importation of owl monkeys from Colombia.

The experimental components of this report were supported by contract DADA 17-69-C-9104 with the U.S. Army Medical Research and Development Command. Manuscript preparation was supported by this contract and by the Southern Research Institute.

LITERATURE CITED

1. **Benazet, F.** 1965. *Plasmodium berghei* et antimalariques à action de longue durée. Ann. Soc. Belge. Med. Trop. 45:459–466.

2. **Chin, W. P., P. G. Contacos, G. R. Coatney, and H. G. King.** 1966. The evaluation of sulfonamides, alone or in combination with pyrimethamine, in the treatment of multi-resistant falciparum malaria. Am. J. Trop. Med. Hyg. **16**:823–829.
3. **Clyde, D. F., H. L. DuPont, R. M. Miller, and V. C. McCarthy.** 1970. Prophylactic and sporontocidal treatment of chloroquine-resistant *Plasmodium falciparum* from Malaya. Trans. R. Soc. Trop. Med. Hyg. **64**:834–838.
4. **Clyde, D. F., V. C. McCarthy, H. L. DuPont, and R. B. Hornick.** 1973. Characterization of a drug resistant strain of *Plasmodium falciparum* from Burma. J. Trop. Med. Hyg. **76**:54–60.
5. **Clyde, D. F., V. C. McCarthy, R. H. Gilman, and R. M. Miller.** 1973. Characterization of a drug resistant strain of *Plasmodium falciparum* from Sabah. J. Trop. Med. Hyg. **76**:226–230.
6. **Clyde, D. F., R. M. Miller, H. L. DuPont, and R. B. Hornick.** 1970. Treatment of falciparum malaria caused by strain resistant to quinine. J. Am. Med. Assoc. **213**:2041–2045.
7. **Collins, W. E., P. G. Contacos, E. G. Guinn, M. H. Jeter, and T. M. Sodeman.** 1968. Monkey to man transmission of *Plasmodium falciparum* by *Anopheles freeborni* mosquitoes. *J. Parasitol.* **54**:1166–1170.
8. **Degowin, R. L., and R. D. Powell.** 1965. Drug resistance of a strain of *Plasmodium falciparum* from Malaya. Am. J. Trop. Med. Hyg. **14**:519–528.
9. **Esslinger, J. H., and C. H. Gardiner.** 1974. *Dipetalonema barbascalensis* Sp. N. (Nematode: filarioidea) from the owl monkey, *Aotus trivirgatus*, with a consideration of the status of *Parlitomosa zakii* Nagaty, 1935. J. Parasitol. **60**:1001–1005.
10. **Fitch, C. D.** 1969. Chloroquine resistance in malaria: a deficiency of chloroquine binding. Proc. Natl. Acad. Sci. U.S.A. **64**:1181–1187.
11. **Fitch, C. D.** 1970. *Plasmodium falciparum* in owl monkeys: drug resistance and chloroquine binding capacity. Science **169**:289–290.
12. **Fitch, C. D.** 1973. Chloroquine-resistant *Plasmodium falciparum*: difference in the handling of ^{14}C-amodiaquin and ^{14}C-chloroquine. Antimicrob. Agents Chemother. 3:545–548.
13. **Freireich, E. J., E. A. Gehan, D. P. Rall, L. H. Schmidt, and H. E. Skipper.** 1966. Quantitative comparison of toxicity of anticancer agents in mouse, rat, hamster, dog, monkey, and man. Cancer Chemother. Rep. **50**:219–244.
14. **Glew, R. H., L. H. Miller, W. E. Collins, W. A. Howard, D. J. Wyler, E. Chaves-Carballo, and F. Neva.** 1974. Response to treatment in man of multidrug resistant *Plasmodium falciparum* from Panama. Am. J. Trop. Med. Hyg. **23**:1–7.
15. **Hall, A. P., H. E. Segal, E. J. Pearlman, P. Phintuyothin, and S. Kosakal.** 1975. Amodiaquine resistant falciparum malaria in Thailand. Am. J. Trop. Med. Hyg. **24**:575–580.
16. **Hawking, F.** 1966. Chloroquine resistance in *Plasmodium berghei*. Am. J. Trop. Med. Hyg. **15**:287–293.
17. **Jacobs, R. L.** 1965. Selection of strains of *Plasmodium berghei* resistant to quinine, chloroquine, and pyrimethamine. J. Parasitol. **51**:481–482.
18. **Jacobs, R. L., and M. Warren.** 1967. Sequestration of schizonts in the deep tissues of mice infected with chloroquine-resistant *Plasmodium berghei*. Trans. R. Soc. Trop. Med. Hyg. **61**:273–275.
19. **Jefferey, G. M., W. E. Collins, and J. C. Skinner.** 1963. Antimalarial drug trials on a multiresistant strain of *Plasmodium falciparum*. Am. J. Trop. Med. Hyg. **12**:844–850.
20. **McKelvey, T. P. H., A. R. T. Lundie, R. M. Vanreenen, E. D. H. Williams, H. S. Moore, M. J. G. Thomas, D. E. Worsley, and I. P. Crawford.** 1971. Chloroquine-resistant falciparum malaria among British service personnel in West Malaysia and Singapore. Trans. R. Soc. Trop. Med. Hyg. **65**:286–309.
21. **McNamara, J. V., K. H. Rieckmann, H. Frischer, T. A. Stockert, P. E. Carson, and R. D. Powell.** 1967. Acquired decrease in sensitivity to quinine observed during studies with a strain of chloroquine-resistant *Plasmodium falciparum*. Ann. Trop. Med. Parasitol. **61**:386–395.
22. **Macomber, P. B., R. L. O'Brien, and F. E. Hahn.** 1966. Chloroquine: physiological basis of drug-resistance in *Plasmodium berghei*. Science **152**:1374–1375.
23. **Marquez, V. E., J. W. Cranston, R. W. Ruddon, L. B. Kier, and J. H. Burckhalter.** 1971. Mechanism of action of amodiaquine. Synthesis of its indoloquinoline analog. J. Med. Chem. **15**:36–39.
24. **Montgomery, R., and D. E. Eyles.** 1963. Chloroquine resistant falciparum malaria in Malaya. Trans. R. Soc. Trop. Med. Hyg. **57**:409–416.
25. **Moore, D. V., and J. E. Lanier.** 1961. Observations on two *Plasmodium falciparum* infections with an abnormal response to chloroquine. Am. J. Trop. Med. Hyg. **10**:5–9.
26. **Peters, W.** 1964. Pigment formation and nuclear division in chloroquine-resistant malaria parasites (*Plasmodium berghei*, Vincke and Lips, 1948). Nature (London) **203**:1290–1291.
27. **Peters, W.** 1965. Drug resistance in *Plasmodium berghei* Vincke and Lips, 1948. I. Chloroquine resistance. Exp. Parasitol. **17**:80–89.
28. **Peters, W.** 1968. The chemotherapy of rodent malaria. II. Host-parasite relationships, part 2: the relationship between sensitivity and the age of the host cell. Ann. Trop. Med. Parasitol. **62**:246–251.
29. **Powell, R. D., G. J. Brewer, and A. S. Alving.** 1963. Studies on a strain of chloroquine-resistant *Plasmodium falciparum* from Colombia, South America. Am. J. Trop. Med. Hyg. **12**:509–512.
30. **Powell, R. D., G. J. Brewer, A. S. Alving, and J. W. Millar.** 1964. Studies on a strain of chloroquine-resistant *Plasmodium falciparum* from Thailand. Bull. W.H.O. **30**:29–44.
31. **Powell, R. D., G. J. Brewer, R. L. Degowin, and A. S. Alving.** 1964. Studies on a strain of chloroquine-resistant *Plasmodium falciparum* from Viet Nam. Bull. W.H.O. **31**:379–392.
32. **Ramakrishnan, S. P., S. Prakash, and D. S. Choudhury.** 1957. Studies on *Plasmodium berghei* Vincke and Lips, 1948. XXIV. Selection of a chloroquine resistant strain. Indian J. Malariol. **11**:213–220.
33. **Rieckmann, K. H.** 1971. Determination of the drug sensitivity of *Plasmodium falciparum*. J. Am. Med. Assoc. **217**:573–578.
34. **Rieckmann, K. H., J. V. McNamara, H. Frischer, T. A. Stockert, P. E. Carson, and R. D. Powell.** 1968. Effects of chloroquine, quinine, and cycloguanil upon the maturation of asexual erythrocytic forms of two strains of *Plasmodium falciparum in vitro*. Am. J. Trop. Med. Hyg. **17**:661–671.
35. **Sandosham, A. A., D. E. Eyles, and R. Montgomery.** 1964. Drug-resistance in falciparum malaria in South-East Asia. Med. J. Malaya **18**:172–183.
36. **Schmidt, L. H.** 1973. Infections with *Plasmodium falciparum* and *Plasmodium vivax* in the owl monkey—model systems for basic biological and chemotherapeutic studies. Trans. R. Soc. Trop. Med. Hyg. **67**:446–474.
37. **Schmidt, L. H., R. N. Rossan, and K. F. Fisher.** 1963. The activity of a repository form of 4,6-diamino-1-

(ρ-chlorophenyl)-1,2-dihydro-2,2-dimethyl-s-triazine against infections with *Plasmodium cynomolgi*. Am. J. Trop. Med. Hyg. 12:494–503.

38. **Siddiqui, W. A., J. V. Schnell, and Q. M. Geiman.** 1972. A model *in vitro* system to test the susceptibility of human malarial parasites to antimalarial drugs. Am. J. Trop. Med. Hyg. 21:392–399.
39. **Thompson, P. E., B. Olszewski, A. Bayles, and J. A. Waitz.** 1967. Relations among antimalarial drugs: results of studies with cycloguanil-, sulfone-, or chloroquine-resistant *Plasmodium berghei* in mice. Am. J. Trop. Med. Hyg. 16:133–145.
40. **Thompson, P. E., K. Weston, A. J. Glazko, R. A. Fisken, T. A. Reutner, A. Bayles, and J. K. Weston.** 1958. Laboratory studies on amopyroquin (Propoquin) an antimalarial compound. Antibiot. Chemother. (Washington, D.C.) 8:450–460.
41. **Ward, R. A., D. E. Hayes, S. C. Hembree, L. C. Rutledge, S. J. Anderson, and A. J. Johnson.** 1972. Infectivity of *Plasmodium falciparum* gametocytes from *Aotus trivirgatus* to anopheline mosquitoes. Proc. Helminthol. Soc. Wash. (Special issue) 39:33–46.
42. **Warhurst, D. C.** 1966. Chloroquine-resistant rodent malaria and the long-acting antimalarial 12,278 R.P. Trans. R. Soc. Trop. Med. Hyg. 60:565–566.
43. **Willerson, D., Jr., L. Kass, H. Fischer, K. H. Rieckmann, P. E. Carson, L. Richard, and J. E. Bowman.** 1974. Chemotherapeutic results in a multidrug-resistant strain of *Plasmodium falciparum* malaria from Vietnam. Mil. Med. 139:175–183.
44. **Wiselogle, F. Y. (ed.).** 1946. A survey of antimalarial drugs 1941–1945, vol. 1, p. 94–107. J. W. Edwards, Ann Arbor, Mich.
45. **Young, M. D.** 1961. Amodiaquine and hydroxychloroquine resistance in *Plasmodium falciparum*. Am. J. Trop. Med. Hyg. 10:689–693.
46. **Young, M. D.** 1962. Failure of chloroquine and amodiaquine to suppress *Plasmodium falciparum*. Trans. R. Soc. Trop. Med. Hyg. 56:252–256.
47. **Young, M. D., P. G. Contacos, J. E. Stitcher, and J. W. Millar.** 1963. Drug resistance in *Plasmodium falciparum* from Thailand. Am. J. Trop. Med. Hyg. 12:305–314.
48. **Young, M. D., and C. M. Johnson.** 1972. *Plasmodium falciparum* malaria in Panama resistant to 4-aminoquinoline drugs. Am. J. Trop. Med. Hyg. 21:13–17.
49. **Young, M. D., and D. V. Moore.** 1961. Chloroquine resistance in *Plasmodium falciparum*. Am. J. Trop. Med. Hyg. 10:317–320.

ANTIMICROBIAL AGENTS AND CHEMOTHERAPY, May 1977, p. 844-847
Vol. 11, No. 5

Antimicrobial Susceptibility of *Haemophilus parainfluenzae*

JOAN B. MAYO AND LAURENCE R. McCARTHY[1]*

Infectious Disease Service, and the Diagnostic Microbiology Laboratory, Memorial Sloan-Kettering Cancer Center, New York, New York 10021, and Cornell University Medical College, New York, New York 10021

Received for publication 22 November 1976

Fifty random clinical isolates of *Haemophilus parainfluenzae* were tested for their susceptibility to 10 antibiotics by a microtiter broth dilution method. Three of the strains tested were resistant to ampicillin, whereas eight were resistant to tetracycline. All strains tested were susceptible to chloramphenicol, kanamycin, gentamicin, cephalothin, and colistin. The ranges of minimal inhibitory concentrations for the three remaining antibiotics were: 0.5 to ≥128 μg of penicillin G per ml, 0.03 to 4 μg of carbenicillin per ml, and 1 to 16 μg of erythromycin per ml. Elevated minimal inhibitory concentrations for penicillin and carbenicillin were noted for the three ampicillin-resistant strains. Tests for beta-lactamase production demonstrated the presence of this enzyme in each of the three ampicillin-resistant strains.

The importance of *Haemophilus influenzae*, especially type b, in human disease is well established (1, 21). As a consequence, a large body of research has focused on this species of the genus *Haemophilus*. It has been generally thought that the other three common species (*H. parainfluenzae*, *H. parahaemolyticus*, and *H. haemolyticus*) are a part of the upper respiratory tract normal flora and rarely cause disease. With increasing frequency, however, *H. parainfluenzae* has been cited as the causative agent of meningitis, epiglottitis, brain abscess, bacteremia, and endocarditis (8, 9, 12). Despite these reports that establish *H. parainfluenzae* as a pathogen, little is known about its susceptibility to antimicrobial agents.

Studies on the antimicrobial susceptibility of *H. influenzae* have been well documented (19, 22). Recently, strains of *H. influenzae* have been isolated that demonstrate resistance to ampicillin (6, 14). As a consequence, ampicillin is no longer recommended as the drug of choice in those areas of the United States where resistant strains have been found (2).

In view of these findings and the increasing role of *H. parainfluenzae* in human disease, this study was undertaken to determine the susceptibility of *H. parainfluenzae* to 10 antibiotics and to determine if ampicillin resistance is also present in this species.

(This work constitutes part of a thesis in the Department of Microbiology, College of Dentistry, in partial fulfillment of the requirements for the Degree of Master of Science at New York University.)

[1] Present address: Department of Hospital Laboratories, North Carolina Memorial Hospital, Chapel Hill, NC 27514.

MATERIALS AND METHODS

Organisms. The 50 strains of *H. parainfluenzae* used in this study represented random clinical isolates recovered from respiratory tract specimens taken from 50 different patients seen at the Memorial Sloan-Kettering Cancer Center between May and November 1974. Identity of the strains was confirmed by their demonstration of a V-factor requirement on Columbia agar (BBL) and their inability to produce hemolysis on 5% defibrinated rabbit blood agar. All isolates were preserved for study by freezing of bacterial suspensions in sterile defibrinated rabbit blood at −70°C.

Preparation of inocula. A standardized inoculum was prepared by first streaking strains of *H. parainfluenzae* onto chocolate agar (BBL). After 24 h of incubation at 35°C in 10% CO_2, colonies of the test bacteria were suspended in 1.0 ml of Mueller-Hinton broth (BBL) enriched with 5% supplement B (Difco). The suspension was adjusted to contain 10^8 colony-forming units per ml by comparison with a 0.5 MacFarland standard and subsequently diluted in the supplemented Mueller-Hinton broth to yield a final inoculum concentration of 10^4 colony-forming units.

Susceptibility tests. Each isolate was tested for its susceptibility to chloramphenicol, tetracycline, gentamicin, kanamycin, erythromycin, colistin, penicillin, ampicillin, carbenicillin, and cephalothin. Techniques used were identical to those described by Thornsberry and Kirven (19) for antibiotic susceptibility testing of *H. influenzae* except that Mueller-Hinton broth was enriched with 5% supplement B rather than 5% Fildes reagent. Stock solutions of the 10 antibiotics were prepared, and 14 serial twofold dilutions were made in sterile flat-bottom 120-well microtiter trays (Ames Co.) using the supplemented Mueller-Hinton broth. The last well in each row of each microtiter tray contained broth without added antibiotic and served as the growth control. All antibiotics except carbenicillin were tested over a concentration range of 0.015 to 128 μg/ml. Carbenicillin concentrations used ranged from 0.03 to 256 μg/ml.

The inoculated trays were sealed with sterile plastic strips (Ames Co.) and incubated at 35°C without CO_2 for 24 h. The minimal inhibitory concentration (MIC) was determined as the lowest concentration of an antibiotic with which there was no macroscopic evidence of growth.

To assure sterility, all preparation of antibiotic dilutions and inoculation of the microtiter trays were performed under a laminar flow hood. Two selected strains of *H. parainfluenzae* were tested simultaneously with each new series of antibiotic dilutions to check the reproducibility of the method.

Beta-lactamase tests. Tests for beta-lactamase production by ampicillin-resistant strains of *H. parainfluenzae* were performed using both a rapid capillary tube method (20) and an iodometric test (4). Positive controls for beta-lactamase activity for both test methods used a penicillinase-producing strain of *Staphylococcus aureus* and two ampicillin-resistant *H. influenzae* strains provided by Clyde Thornsberry of the Center for Disease Control. Ampicillin-susceptible strains of *H. parainfluenzae* served as negative controls.

RESULTS

The MICs of the 10 antibiotics for the strains of *H. parainfluenzae* tested in this study are shown in Table 1. All 50 strains were susceptible to chloramphenicol. MICs ranged between 0.25 and 2.0 μg/ml with a median MIC of approximately 0.5 μg/ml. The results for tetracycline demonstrated that 84% of the isolates were susceptible to 0.5 μg/ml or less, whereas 16% were resistant with MICs of 8 μg/ml.

Gentamicin was the more active of the two aminoglycoside antibiotics tested. All strains of *H. parainfluenzae* yielded MICs of 1 μg or less per ml. Results for kanamycin demonstrated that 94% of the strains were susceptible with MICs less than 6 μg/ml, and 6% were moderately susceptible with MICs of 8 or 16 μg per ml.

MICs for erythromycin ranged between 1 and 16 μg/ml. Using the National Committee for Clinical Laboratory Standards breakpoint of ≤2.0 μg/ml (15) to indicate susceptibility, it appears that only 28% of the strains were susceptible, 70% were moderately susceptible, and 2% were resistant. All strains tested were susceptible to colistin with MICs of 1 μg/ml or less.

MICs for penicillin ranged between 0.5 and 128 μg/ml. Fifty-four percent of the strains of *H. parainfluenzae* were susceptible with MICs less than 1.5 μg/ml; 40% were moderately susceptible; and 6% were resistant with MICs in excess of 32 μg/ml. MICs for ampicillin ranged between 0.25 and 128 μg/ml. Ninety-four percent of the strains were susceptible with MICs less than 1.5 μg/ml, and 6% resistant with MICs of 8 to 128 μg/ml.

All isolates including those demonstrating resistance to ampicillin displayed sensitivity to the beta-lactam antibiotics, carbenicillin and cephalothin. MICs for carbenicillin ranged between 0.03 and 4 μg/ml, whereas MICs for cephalothin ranged between 0.5 and 2 μg/ml. Slightly elevated MICs for carbenicillin were observed with those strains displaying resistance to penicillin and ampicillin.

Correlation between ampicillin resistance and beta-lactamase production. The three ampicillin-resistant strains produced beta-lactamase as determined by both test methods. In contrast, 11 ampicillin-sensitive strains of *H. parainfluenzae*, randomly selected from the strains used in the study, showed no beta-lactamase activity with either method.

TABLE 1. *MICs of 10 antibiotics for 50 strains of Haemophilus parainfluenzae*

Antibiotic	No. of strains inhibited (%)												
	0.03[a]	0.06	0.12	0.25	0.5	1	2	4	8	16	32	64	128
Chloramphenicol				20 (40)	27 (54)	2 (4)	1 (2)						
Tetracycline			4 (8)	33 (66)	5 (10)				8 (16)				
Gentamicin			1 (2)	2 (4)	19 (38)	28 (56)							
Kanamycin					1 (2)	1 (2)	31 (62)	14 (28)	2 (4)	1 (2)			
Erythromycin						1 (2)	13 (26)	29 (58)	6 (12)	1 (2)			
Colistin		6 (12)	23 (46)	16 (32)	4 (8)	1 (2)							
Penicillin					2 (4)	25 (50)	10 (20)	9 (18)	1 (2)			1 (2)	2 (4)
Ampicillin				17 (34)	25 (50)	5 (10)			1 (2)				2 (4)
Carbenicillin	44 (88)	3 (6)			1 (2)			2 (4)					
Cephalothin					3 (6)	36 (72)	11 (22)						

[a] Minimal inhibitory concentration (micrograms per milliliter).

DISCUSSION

The reported pathogenicity of *H. parainfluenzae*, as well as the prevalence of strains of *H. influenzae* resistant to ampicillin, prompted us to examine the antimicrobial susceptibility of 50 strains of *H. parainfluenzae*. All strains were isolates from respiratory specimens of patients admitted to Memorial Sloan-Kettering Cancer Center. All isolates appeared to be a part of the normal respiratory flora for each of these patients and were not related to any disease process.

All strains tested were susceptible to chloramphenicol, gentamicin, kanamycin, colistin, carbenicillin, and cephalothin and demonstrated variable susceptibilities for tetracycline and erythromycin. Three strains of *H. parainfluenzae* demonstrated resistance to ampicillin and penicillin. One of these strains and seven ampicillin-susceptible strains were found to be resistant to tetracycline. These findings correlate with the incidence of tetracycline resistance in *H. influenzae* noted recently (22).

In this study, the enzyme produced by these ampicillin-resistant *H. parainfluenzae* was characterized as a beta-lactamase. Thus, the mechanism of resistance appears similar to the described ampicillin-resistant strains of *H. influenzae* (4, 14, 20). The beta-lactamase produced by strains of *H. influenzae* has been characterized as a constitutive plasmid-mediated enzyme which exhibits high activity against penicillin, ampicillin, and cephaloridine substrates, low activity against penicillins such as oxacillin and methicillin, and intermediate activity against carbenicillin and cephalothin (10, 14, 18). Although oxacillin and methicillin were not tested in our study, all ampicillin-resistant strains of *H. parainfluenzae* demonstrated resistance to penicillin and slightly elevated MICs for carbenicillin and cephalothin. This observation suggests some similarity between the beta-lactamase enzymes of *H. influenzae* and *H. parainfluenzae*. During our study of *H. parainfluenzae*, we also determined the susceptibility of 14 clinical isolates of *H. parahaemolyticus* to ampicillin and found one strain to demonstrate a high level of ampicillin resistance (>128 μg/ml), which was also mediated by a beta-lactamase. Our results and the recent reports of diseases caused by ampicillin-resistant strains of *H. parainfluenzae*, *H. haemolyticus,* and *H. paraphrophilus* (11, 13) suggest that ampicillin resistance occurs throughout the genus.

In the past ampicillin has been the drug of choice for treating meningitis due to *H. influenzae* (3, 17): chloramphenicol and tetracycline have been acceptable alternatives (16, 17). Our results support the recommendation that chloramphenicol is the drug of choice for initial treatment of serious infections due to *Haemophilus* species. However, recent reports of chloramphenicol-resistant strains of *H. influenzae* and *H. parainfluenzae* have appeared (5, 7). Our results indicate that treatment of infections caused by *H. parainfluenzae* with ampicillin ideally should be discouraged until adequate antimicrobial susceptibility studies have been performed using carefully standardized techniques. Further studies of ampicillin resistance in *H. parainfluenzae* as it relates to *H. influenzae* are needed to determine similarities of the beta-lactamase enzyme and whether R-factors are responsible for ampicillin resistance in *H. parainfluenzae*.

ACKNOWLEDGMENTS

We gratefully acknowledge the advice, encouragement, and support of Donald Armstrong, of the Infectious Disease Service, Department of Medicine, Memorial Sloan-Kettering Cancer Center; Heiner Hoffman, of the Microbiology Department, College of Dentistry, New York University; and Clyde Thornsberry, of the Antimicrobic Investigation Unit, National Center for Disease Control.

LITERATURE CITED

1. **Alexander, H. E.** 1965. The *Hemophilus* group, p. 726–740. *In* R. J. Dubos and J. G. Hirsch (ed.), Bacterial and mycotic infections of man. J. B. Lippincott Co., Philadelphia.
2. **American Academy of Pediatrics, Committee on Infectious Disease.** 1975. Ampicillin-resistant strains of *Hemophilus influenzae* type b. Pediatrics 55:145–146.
3. **Barrett, F. F., L. H. Taber, C. R. Morris, W. B. Stephenson, D. J. Clark, and M. D. Yow.** 1972. A 12-year review of the antibiotic management of *Hemophilus influenzae* meningitis. Comparison of ampicillin and conventional therapy including chloramphenicol. J. Pediatr. 81:370–377.
4. **Catlin, B. W.** 1975. Iodometric detection of *Haemophilus influenzae* beta-lactamase: rapid presumptive test for ampicillin resistance. Antimicrob. Agents Chemother. 7:265–270.
5. **Cavanagh, P., C. A. Morris, and N. J. Mitchell.** 1975. Chloramphenicol-resistant *Haemophilus*. Lancet i:696.
6. **Center for Disease Control.** 1975. Ampicillin-resistant *Haemophilus influenzae*. Morbid. Mortal. Weekly Rep. 24:205–206.
7. **Center for Disease Control.** 1976. Chloramphenicol-resistant *Haemophilus influenzae*. Morbid. Mortal. Weekly Rep. 25:385–386.
8. **Chow, A. W., L. L. Bushkell, T. T. Yoshikawa, and L. B. Guze.** 1974. *Haemophilus parainfluenzae* epiglottitis with meningitis and bacteremia in an adult. Am. J. Med. Sci. 267:365–368.
9. **Dahlgren, J., F. P. Tally, G. Brothers, and J. Ruskin.** 1974. *Haemophilus parainfluenzae* endocarditis. Am. J. Clin. Pathol. 62:607–611.
10. **Elwell, L. P., J. Degraaff, D. Seibert, and S. Falkow.** 1975. Plasmid-linked ampicillin resistance in *Haemo-*

philus influenzae type b. Infect. Immun. 12:404–410.
11. **Groves, D. J.** 1976. Ampicillin-resistant *Hemophilus sp*. Can. Med. J. 114:407.
12. **Hable, K. A., G. B. Logan, and J. A. Washington.** 1971. Three *Hemophilus species*. Am. J. Dis. Child. 121:35–37.
13. **Jones, R. N., J. Slepack, and J. Bigelow.** 1976. Ampicillin-resistant *Haemophilus paraphrophilus* laryngo-epiglottitis. J. Clin. Microbiol. 4:405–407.
14. **Khan, W., S. Ross, W. Rodriguez, G. Controni, and A. K. Saz.** 1974. *Haemophilus influenzae* type b resistant to ampicillin. A report of two cases. J. Am. Med. Assoc. 229: 298–301.
15. **National Committee for Clinical Laboratory Standards.** 1975. Performance standards for antimicrobial disc susceptibility tests, p. 1–11. National Committee for Laboratory Standards,
16. **Nelson, K. E., S. Levin, H. W. Spies, and M. H. Lepper.** 1972. Treatment of *Hemophilus influenzae* meningitis: a comparison of chloramphenicol and tetracycline. J. Infect. Dis. 125:459–465.
17. **Schulkind, M. L., W. A. Altemeier, and E. M. Ayoub.** 1971. A comparison of ampicillin and chloramphenicol therapy in *Haemophilus influenzae* meningitis. Pediatrics 48:411–416.
18. **Sykes, R. B., M. Matthew, and C. H. O'Callaghan.** 1975. R-factor mediated beta-lactamase production by *Haemophilus influenzae*. J. Med. Microbiol. 8:437–441.
19. **Thornsberry, C., and L. A. Kirven.** 1974. Antimicrobial susceptibility of *Haemophilus influenzae*. Antimicrob. Agents Chemother. 6:620–624.
20. **Thornsberry, C., and L. A. Kirven.** 1974. Ampicillin resistance in *Haemophilus influenzae* as determined by a rapid test for beta-lactamase production. Antimicrob. Agents Chemother. 6:653–654.
21. **Turk, D. C., and J. R. May.** 1967. *Haemophilus influenzae*: its clinical importance in modern medicine. English University Press, Ltd., London.
22. **Williams, J. D., and J. Andrews.** 1974. Sensitivity of *Haemophilus influenzae* to antibiotics. Br. Med. J. 1:134–137.

Antimicrobial Agents and Chemotherapy, May 1977, p. 848–851 Vol. 11, No. 5
 Printed in U.S.A.

Rapid Microbiological Assay for Chlorhydroxyquinoline That Uses a Cryogenically Stored Inoculum

R. F. COSGROVE

International Development Laboratory, E. R. Squibb & Sons, Moreton, Wirral, Merseyside, L46 1QW, England

Received for publication 29 November 1976

A rapid microbiological assay for chlorhydroxyquinoline is described. It is a turbidimetric procedure that uses *Streptococcus faecalis* as the test organism. Results are available within 5 h. Data are presented to show the advantages of using a cryogenically stored inoculum over an inoculum prepared on a daily basis.

Chlorhydroxyquinoline (CHQ) is a non-antibiotic agent that has reported activity against a variety of bacterial, fungal, and protozoal organisms (2, 4, 7, 9). It is a mixture of three chlorinated oxines in the following proportions: 5,7-dichlor-8-hydroxyquinoline (57 to 74%, wt/wt), 5-monochlor-8-hydroxyquinoline (23 to 40%, wt/wt), and 7-monochlor-8-hydroxyquinoline (3% wt/wt). It is formulated into several pharmaceutical dosage forms for both human and veterinary use.

Current assay methods for CHQ are chemical, e.g., spectrophotometric (10), spectrofluorimetric (3), gas chromatographic (6), and as such do not reflect the antimicrobial potency of the material but simply the total amount present. It was thus felt that an assay capable of determining potency would, on occasions, be useful.

Ideally, an assay should be rapid, sensitive, and readily reproducible. The latter criterion can, on occasion, be a problem with microbiological assays mainly due to the variability of the assay organism used as inoculum. This problem is minimized by the freezing of a large batch of inoculum and its subsequent storage in liquid nitrogen. This enables the use of the same inoculum over long periods of time and consequently increases both the reliability and accuracy of the assay. The advantages of cryogenically stored inocula over conventionally prepared inocula have been summarized by many authors (5, 8, 11–14).

By the use of a turbidimetric procedure using a rapidly growing culture of *Streptococcus faecalis*, an assay result can be obtained within 5 h.

It should be emphasized that the use of a cryogenically stored culture is not an essential feature of this method; it works equally as well with inoculum prepared fresh each day, but the results are then less predictable as regards dose response and incubation time.

MATERIALS AND METHODS

Test organism. The test organism used was *S. faecalis* ATCC 10541, maintained on Trypticase soy agar (BBL).

Assay medium. The assay medium consisted of the following: soya peptone (Oxoid), 9.0 g; glucose, 20.0 g; yeast extract, 5.0 g; trisodium citrate, 10.0 g; dipotassium hydrogen phosphate, 1.0 g; potassium dihydrogen phosphate, 1.0 g; and distilled water to 1 liter. The medium was autoclaved at 121°C for 15 min at pH 6.8 to 7.0.

Preparation of inoculum for noncryogenic storage. A total of 20 ml of assay medium was inoculated with a loop of test organism from an overnight slope. The inoculated broth was incubated for 18 h at 37°C. A 2-ml amount of inoculum was used per liter of assay broth.

Preparation of inoculum for cryogenic storage. An overnight slope of the test organism was washed into 8 liters of antibiotic medium no. 3 (peptone, 5.0 g; yeast extract, 1.5 g; beef extract, 1.5 g; sodium chloride, 3.5 g; glucose, 1.0 g; dipotassium phosphate, 3.68 g; and potassium dihydrogen phosphate, 1.32 g [pH 7.0]). Incubation followed at 37°C with stirring and aeration for 18 h. The cells were harvested by centrifugation, washed once in fresh antibiotic medium no. 3, and finally resuspended in 200 ml of the medium. The concentrated suspension was then immediately divided into 2-ml portions in sterile polypropylene ampoules (Sterilin 506, 2 ml, screw cap). By using the method described by Beezer et al. (1), the ampoules were initially frozen in the vapor phase of liquid nitrogen at a rate of 5°C/min down to −70°C and then plunged into the liquid nitrogen. They were transferred to a cryostat (British Oxygen Co. Ltd, CPV 35) for storage.

Immediately prior to assay, sufficient ampoules (one ampoule per liter of assay broth) were transferred to a 40°C water bath for 5 min. The contents of the ampoule were then washed in prewarmed (37°C) assay broth, which was immediately used for assay.

Preparation of standard CHQ. A total of 25 mg of

CHQ was dissolved in 25 ml of dimethylformamide (DMF). From the initial solution, further dilutions were made in DMF to give final concentrations of 100, 80, 60, 40, and 20 μg/ml.

Sample preparation. Various CHQ (Halquinol *British Pharmacopeia*)-containing products manufactured by E. R. Squibb & Sons have been assayed: a suspension (Quixalin suspension) containing 125 mg of CHQ per ml; tablets (Quixalin tablets) containing 250 mg of CHQ per tablet; a veterinary suspension containing 27.5 mg of CHQ per ml; and a veterinary bolus (Quixalud bolus) containing 1.5 g of CHQ.

It was found that the CHQ present in these formulations dissolved readily in DMF without any preliminary extraction procedures. Hence, the products were assayed as per the standard, but only diluted to levels of 80 and 60 μg/ml.

Assay. After the standards and samples were prepared and the assay broth was inoculated, 0.1 ml of each standard and sample solution was added to each of three sterile test tubes with 9.9 ml of inoculated broth (a Fisons diluter LFA/20 was used). A DMF control (0.1 ml of DMF to 9.9 ml of broth) and a growth control (inoculated broth, no additions) were included with each assay.

The loaded tubes were transferred to a shaking water bath at 37°C and incubated until the growth control gave a reading of 25% transmission. The latter reading was made on a Vitatron photometer UC200S, using a 623-nm filter against a broth blank set at 100% transmission.

Upon completion of incubation, 1 ml of formaldehyde solution (3%) was added to each tube as rapidly as possible. The percent transmission of each tube was then determined as per the growth control above.

RESULTS AND DISCUSSION

Viable cells after cryogenic storage. Viable counts were made on ampoules immediately prior to freezing and at intervals after storage in liquid nitrogen (Table 1). There was a high recovery of viable cells after storage in liquid nitrogen both initially and up to 3 months. Other microorganisms have been stored cryogenically in these laboratories in excess of 12 months without any decline in viability.

Dose-response curves. The dose-response curves for inoculum prepared on a daily basis and for cryogenically stored inoculum are shown in Fig. 1. The data used to prepare the curves are summarized in Table 2 for unfrozen cells and in Table 3 for cryogenically stored cells. These data show that the response with the unfrozen cells at any particular level can vary on different days by as much as 7.8%,

TABLE 1. *Viable counts before and after cryogenic storage*

Time	No. of cells ($\times 10^{10}$)/ml	Recovery from liquid nitrogen (%)
Prior to freeze	4.5	
Immediately after freeze	4.6	102
1 day after freeze	4.2	93
1 week after freeze	4.4	98
1 month after freeze	4.6	102
3 months after freeze	4.3	96

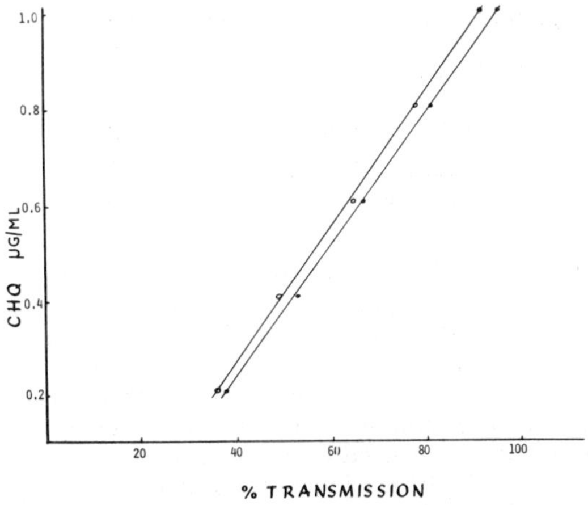

FIG. 1. *Dose-response curves. Symbols: ○, mean result of 5 days of testing with an inoculum prepared daily; ●, result of 5 days of testing with a cryogenically stored inoculum.*

TABLE 2. *Response of assay inocula prepared daily to five standard levels of CHQ over 5 separate days of testing*

Standard concn (μg/ml)	Transmission (%) on day: 1	2	3	4	5	Mean	Standard deviation
1.0	92.8	88.5	93.1	88.3	91.5	90.8	2.308
0.8	80.6	72.0	80.9	78.4	74.9	77.4	3.837
0.6	65.3	59.6	68.9	66.8	59.7	64.1	4.224
0.4	52.5	48.8	49.5	47.0	46.9	48.9	2.288
0.2	38.4	36.0	31.7	36.0	35.3	35.5	2.418
DMF control	31.0	29.4	30.3	31.8	30.9	30.7	0.893
Growth control	26.8	24.7	25.2	25.1	26.6	25.7	0.952

TABLE 3. *Response of a cryogenically stored assay inoculum to five standard levels of CHQ over five separate days of testing*

Standard concn (μg/ml)	Transmission (%) on day: 1	2	3	4	5	Mean	Standard deviation
1.0	94.6	94.8	93.3	94.0	95.5	94.4	0.832
0.8	80.7	81.9	79.2	80.5	78.2	80.1	1.430
0.6	64.9	66.5	65.9	66.6	66.5	66.1	0.716
0.4	52.0	53.8	52.5	51.9	53.0	52.6	0.783
0.2	38.1	36.0	38.0	37.6	36.4	37.2	0.960
DMF control	30.4	30.8	30.3	30.7	29.9	30.4	0.356
Growth control	25.4	25.5	24.8	25.2	25.9	25.4	0.404

TABLE 4. *Assay results, together with their mean and confidence interval (P = 0.05), are shown for five formulated products*

Sample	Dose[a]	Results on day: 1	2	3	Mean result (%)
Quixalin Suspension (125 mg of CHQ per ml)	High	122.8	124.4	125.2	124.2 ± 2.0
	Low	125.2	120.2	127.1	
Quixalud Bolus (1.5 g of CHQ)	High	1.48	1.50	1.41	1.49 ± 3.2
	Low	1.52	1.49	1.55	
Quixalin Tablets A (0.25 g of CHQ)	High	0.25	0.25	0.22	0.237 ± 4.2
	Low	0.22	0.24	0.24	
Quixalin Tablets B (0.25 g of CHQ)	High	0.27	0.24	0.24	0.255 ± 3.8
	Low	0.25	0.27	0.26	
CHQ Veterinary Suspension (27.5 mg/ml)	High	27.0	28.7	28.3	28.0 ± 3.9
	Low	28.8	28.9	26.3	

[a] The "high dose" and "low dose" refer to the sample dilutions described in the text.

whereas with the cryogenically stored cells the response to any particular level varies from one day to another by no more than 3%. Furthermore, the time taken for the assay to reach its end point was repeatedly 4.75 h with the cryogenic inoculum, whereas with the other inoculum the time varied from 4 to 5 h.

Thus, the frozen inoculum provides not only a consistent dose response, but also a standard incubation time that greatly facilitates the carrying out of the assay by junior staff. The inoculum is, of course, readily available and enables the performance of an assay at very short notice.

Effect of DMF on dose-response curve. Tables 2 and 3 show that the growth of the test organism in the DMF controls is marginally less than that in the growth controls. There is, however, a significant difference between the degree of growth in the DMF control and that in the lowest level of standard and, as the DMF concentration in all standards and samples is constant, the assay results are not affected by this slight retardation of growth.

Effect of oxine ratios on standard response. As mentioned above, CHQ is a mixture of three chlorinated oxines. The amounts of two of these oxines can vary significantly between batches of CHQ, and it was thought that this may influence the assay results obtained. Standard response curves were, therefore, determined for different mixtures of the oxines in amounts varying within the proportions stated above. No significant effect on the standard response was detected, and it was concluded that the assay would not be biased by different batches of CHQ.

Sample results. Samples listed earlier were assayed on each of 3 days with the frozen inoculum. Since the dose-response was so consistent, the standard was reduced to three levels. The results, together with their confidence interval ($P = 0.05$), are shown in Table 4.

It is therefore concluded that the method is a reliable and accurate system for measurement of CHQ antibacterial activity in the dosage forms examined.

ACKNOWLEDGMENT

The technical assistance of P. Walton in carrying out some of the assays is gratefully acknowledged.

LITERATURE CITED

1. **Beezer, A. E., R. D. Newall, and H. J. V. Tyrrell.** 1976. Application of flow microcalorimetry to analytical problems: the preparation, storage and assay of frozen inocula of *Saccharomyces cerevisiae*. J. Appl. Bacteriol. **41**:197–207.
2. **Ellenrieder, V. M., and K. H. Sensch.** 1972. The influence of chlorinated oxyquinoline derivatives on anaerobic micro-organisms. Arzneim. Forsch. **22**:908–909.
3. **Fairbrother, J. E., and W. F. Heyes.** 1973. Determination of chlorhydroxyquinoline in medicated pig feeds. Analyst (London) **98**:797–801.
4. **Fiedler, H., and U. Kaben.** 1966. Antimycotic and antibacterial action of 8 quinolinols and nicotinic acid esters. Pharmazie **21**:233–238.
5. **Froud, D. J. R.** 1972. Methods for the preservation of bacteria and fungi in liquid nitrogen. J. Sci. Technol. India **16**:1–6.
6. **Gruber, M. P., R. W. Klein, M. E. Foxx, and J. Campisi.** 1972. Rapid analysis of iodochlorhydroxyquin and related halogenated 8-hydroxyquinolines via GLC (gas-liquid chromotography) of their trimethylsilyl ethers. J. Pharm. Sci. **61**:1147–1152.
7. **Heseltine, W. W., and P. J. Campbell.** 1960. Laboratory studies on chlorhydroxyquinoline. J. Trop. Med. Hyg. **63**:1–3.
8. **Hossack, D. J. N.** 1972. Liquid nitrogen frozen inocula – a year's experience. Proc. Soc. Anal. Chem. **9**:36–38.
9. **Lamy, L.** 1964. A comparative experimental study of the activity of certain hydroxyquinoline derivatives on multiplication of *Entamoeba histolytica* cultures and associated bacteria. Ann. Inst. Pasteur Paris **107**:98–108.
10. **Lubina, B.** 1971. Analysis of 5-chloro-8 hydroxyquinoline in pharmaceutical preparations. Spectrophotometric determinations in the presence of other active compounds. Pharm. Ztg. **116**:1015–1017.
11. **McDaniel, L. E., and E. G. Bailey.** 1968. Liquid nitrogen preservation of standard inoculum: gas-phase storage. Appl. Microbiol. **16**:912–916.
12. **Sokolski, W. T., and E. M. Stapert.** 1964. Liquid nitrogen storage for microbiologic assays. Cryobiology **1**(Suppl. 1):59.
13. **Sokolski, W. T., E. M. Stapert, and E. B. Ferrer.** 1964. Liquid nitrogen freezing in microbiological assay systems. I. Preservation of *Lactobacillus leichmannii* for direct use in the vitamin B_{12} assay. Appl. Microbiol. **12**:327–329.
14. **Stapert, E. M., W. T. Sokolski, W. M. Kaneshiro, and R. J. Cole.** 1964. Liquid nitrogen freezing in microbiological assay systems. II. Preservation of *Sarcina lutea* for antibiotic assays. J. Bacteriol. **88**:532–533.

ANTIMICROBIAL AGENTS AND CHEMOTHERAPY, May 1977, p. 852-857 Vol. 11, No. 5

Printed in U.S.A.

Clavulanic Acid: a Beta-Lactamase-Inhibiting Beta-Lactam from *Streptomyces clavuligerus*

C. READING AND M. COLE*

Beecham Pharmaceuticals Research Division, Brockham Park, Betchworth, Surrey, RH3 7AJ, England

Received for publication 29 December 1976

A novel β-lactamase inhibitor has been isolated from *Streptomyces clavuligerus* ATCC 27064 and given the name clavulanic acid. Conditions for the cultivation of the organism and detection and isolation of clavulanic acid are described. This compound resembles the nucleus of a penicillin but differs in having no acylamino side chain, having oxygen instead of sulfur, and containing a β-hydroxyethylidine substituent in the oxazolidine ring. Clavulanic acid is a potent inhibitor of many β-lactamases, including those found in *Escherichia coli* (plasmid mediated), *Klebsiella aerogenes, Proteus mirabilis,* and *Staphylococcus aureus,* the inhibition being of a progressive type. The cephalosporinase type of β-lactamase found in *Pseudomonas aeruginosa* and *Enterobacter cloacae* P99 and the chromosomally mediated β-lactamase of *E. coli* are less well inhibited. The minimum inhibitory concentrations of ampicillin and cephaloridine against β-lactamase-producing, penicillin-resistant strains of *S. aureus, K. aerogenes, P. mirabilis,* and *E. coli* have been shown to be considerably reduced by the addition of low concentrations of clavulanic acid.

Streptomyces clavuligerus ATCC 27064 (NRRL 3585) has been described as producing several antibiotics structurally related to cephalosporin C, namely, the 3-carbamoyloxymethyl analogue, the 7-methoxy derivative of the latter compound (cephamycin C), and deacetoxy cephalosporin C, as well as penicillin N (8, 9, 12, 16; M. Gorman, M. M. Hoehn, R. Nagarajan, L. D. Boeck, E. A. Presti, J. G. Whitney, and R. L. Hamill, Prog. Abstr. Intersci. Conf. Antimicrob. Agents Chemother., 11th, Atlantic City, N.J., abstr. 14, p. 7, 1971). During an investigation of the metabolites produced by this culture, a pronounced β-lactamase inhibitory activity was detected in the culture filtrate using a special bioassay procedure based on β-lactamase inhibition (4). The substance responsible for the β-lactamase inhibitory activity was named clavulanic acid (4) and has been shown to have the structure given in Fig. 1 (10). We describe below the detection, isolation, and preliminary information on the β-lactamase-inhibitory properties of clavulanic acid.

MATERIALS AND METHODS

Cultural conditions for *S. clavuligerus*. *S. clavuligerus* ATCC 27064 (NRRL 3585) was grown at 26°C on agar slopes containing 1% Yeatex yeast extract, 1% glucose, and 2% Oxoid agar no. 3, pH 6.8. Mycelium and spores from the slope were used to inoculate flasks containing a seed stage medium consisting of (wt/vol) 1% malt extract (Oxoid), 1% bacteriological peptone (Oxoid), and 2% glycerol. The medium was made up using tap water and adjusted to pH 7.0 with sodium hydroxide solution. Inoculated flasks were shaken for 3 days at 26°C.

Production stage flasks containing the DAS medium were inoculated with 5% vegetative inoculum from the seed flasks. The DAS medium consisted of 2% dextrin, 1% Arkasoy 50 soyabean flour (British Arkady Co., Manchester, U.K.), 0.1% Scotasol dried distillers solubles (Thomas Borthwick Ltd, Glasgow, U.K.), and 0.01% $FeSO_4 \cdot 7H_2O$ in deionized water at a final pH of 7.0.

Media for both seed and production stages were dispensed in 100-ml volumes in 500-ml conical flasks which were closed with foam plugs and sterilized by autoclaving at 121°C for 15 min. Seed and production flasks were shaken at 26°C on a rotary shaker with 2-inch (5.08-cm) throw and a speed of 240 rpm.

The cultivation in stainless-steel fermentors was carried out using the DAS medium as described above, except that antifoam was added before steam sterilization. The antifoam was 10% Pluronic L81 (Ugine Kuhlmann Chemicals Ltd, London, U.K.) in soyabean oil and was added to give a final concentration of 0.05% (wt/vol). The seed fermentor containing 50 liters of medium was inoculated with 100 ml of a spore/mycelial suspension prepared by adding a sterile solution of 0.05% Triton X-100 in water to a Yeatex/glucose agar (see above) slope in a roux bottle grown for 10 days at 26°C. The 90-liter baffled seed fermentor was agitated by a 13-cm disk turbine impeller at 240 rpm. Sterile air was supplied at 50 liters/min, and the temperature was 26°C. After 72 h the seed fermentor was used to provide a 5% vegetative inoculum into 150 liters of DAS fermentation medium contained in a 300-liter baffled fermentor. This fermentor was stirred at 210 rpm using a 21-cm

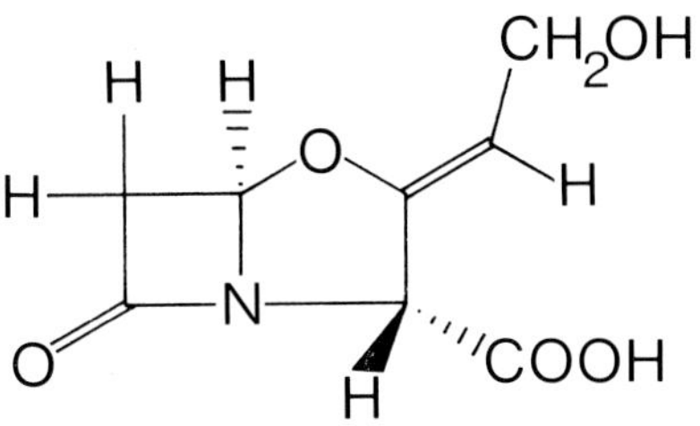

FIG. 1. *Structure of clavulanic acid, Z-(2R,5R)-3-(β-hydroxyethylidene)-7-oxo-4-oxa-1-azabicyclo[3,2,0]heptane-2-carboxylic acid.*

disk turbine impeller. The temperature was maintained at 26°C and the air flow at 150 liters/min. The above-mentioned antifoam was added in 10-ml amounts when required.

Preparation of β-lactamases. The β-lactamase preparations consisted of ultrasonic extracts of bacterial cells and were prepared as follows.

Nutrient agar cultures of the organisms listed in Table 2 were used to inoculate flasks containing the tryptone medium. These flasks were shaken overnight and used to provide a 1% inoculum into further flasks of the same medium. The tryptone medium consisted of 3.2% tryptone (Oxoid), 2% yeast extract (Oxoid), and 0.5% NaCl. The final pH was adjusted to 7.4 with dilute NaOH, and the medium was dispensed in 100-ml volumes in 500-ml conical flasks. The flasks were closed with foam plugs and sterilized at 121°C for 15 min.

All flasks were incubated on a rotary shaker running at 240 rpm and having a 2-inch throw. The temperature was 37°C for all cultures except *Escherichia coli* JT410, JT4, and JT39 and *Proteus mirabilis* C889, which were grown at 30°C. After shaking for 2 h, 6-aminopenicillanic acid was added to cultures of *Pseudomonas aeruginosa* A to give a final concentration of 500 μg/ml. Methicillin was added at 2 h to the *Staphylococcus aureus* cultures to give a final concentration of 1 μg/ml. The total incubation time was about 16 h for all cultures except for the two strains of *P. aeruginosa*, which were grown for 7 h.

The bacterial cells were collected by centrifugation and resuspended in deionized water to give a cell concentration 100 times that in the growth medium. This cell suspension was then disrupted in an MSE ultrasonic disintegrator for 5 min at 6.3-μm amplitude with ice cooling. The cell debris was removed by centrifugation, and samples of the supernatant were deep frozen until required.

The β-lactamase of *Bacillus cereus* was an extracellular enzyme preparation obtained from Whatman Biochemicals Ltd, Maidstone, U.K.

β-Lactamase inhibition assay and determination of I_{50} value. Before use in the assay procedures the β-lactamase preparation was diluted in 0.005 M phosphate buffer (pH 7) until it gave about 75% hydrolysis of a 1-mg/ml solution of substrate (see Table 2) in 30 min at 37°C. Suitable dilutions of the clavulanic acid preparation were mixed with the β-lactamase solution and incubated at 37°C for 15 min because of the progressive nature of the inhibition. A control with buffer in place of clavulanic acid preparation was also incubated. Substrate in pH 7.0 buffer was then added to both inhibitor and control reaction mixtures to give a final concentration of 1 mg/ml, and incubation at 37°C was continued for a further 30 min at 37°C. The residual substrate in each mixture was then estimated using the hydroxylamine assay (3), and the results were used to calculate the percentage of inhibition.

Sodium benzylpenicillin (Beecham) was used as a substrate except for the cephalosporinase-producing cultures *P. aeruginosa* A, *E. coli* JT410, and *Enterobacter cloacae* P99, where cephaloridine (Glaxo) was used. The concentration and assay methods were the same for the two substrates except that the reaction time with the hydroxylamine reagent was reduced from 10 to 3 min for cephaloridine to optimize color formation with the ferric reagent.

The I_{50} for clavulanic acid is defined as the concentration giving 50% inhibition of the β-lactamase as measured by the above procedure, I_{50} values being obtained from a plot of percentage of inhibition against inhibitor concentration.

Chromatography of clavulanic acid. Paper chromatography was carried out on 1-cm-wide paper strips of Whatman grade 1. The solvent systems described in the text were used in the descending fashion at 4°C. The position of clavulanic acid was located using the bioautographic method described below.

Thin-layer chromatography was carried out at 20°C using precoated, glass-backed, thin-layer plates (Merck silica gel 60). Clavulanic acid was detected by spraying with the TTC reagent, which consisted of equal volumes of 4% methanolic solution of 2,3,5-triphenyltetrazolium chloride and aqueous 1 N NaOH.

Special bioautographic detection method for clavulanic acid. Clavulanic acid was located on paper strip chromatograms by contacting the dried strips with agar containing benzylpenicillin and seeded with *Klebsiella aerogenes* A, a variant of *K. aerogenes* NCTC 418. Inoculum was prepared by growing this culture overnight in 2.5% Oxoid nutrient broth CM67 in a test tube at 28°C. A 300-ml amount of 4% blood agar base (Oxoid CM55) was cooled to 50°C after sterilization before addition of 0.8 ml of inoculum and 1 ml of 1.8 mg of sodium benzylpenicillin per ml (final concentration, 6 μg/ml). For ordinary bioautography the benzylpenicillin was omitted and the inoculum level was halved. The agar was poured onto glass plates (13 by 16 inches [ca. 33 by 40 cm], the chromatogram strips were laid on the agar, and the plates were incubated for 16 h at 28°C.

Antibacterial synergy tests. The enhancement of the antibacterial activity of β-lactam antibiotics by clavulanic acid was demonstrated using the microtiter method. All organisms were grown in tryptone soy broth (Lab M. Ltd, Salford, Lancs., England) at 37°C overnight to provide inoculum for tests. Serial dilutions of antibiotics were prepared in tryptone soy broth, with or without the addition of sodium clavulanate, and inoculum was added to give a final dilution of 1/500. The trays were incubated overnight at 37°C, and minimum inhibitory concentrations values were taken as the lowest concentrations producing inhibition of growth.

RESULTS

Detection and isolation of clavulanic acid. *S. clavuligerus* ATCC 27064 was grown for 4 days in shaken conical flasks using the DAS medium. Samples of culture filtrate were tested for β-lactamase inhibitory activity and were found to give a mean inhibition of 56% at a final dilution of 1/2,500 against the R factor-mediated β-lactamase of *E. coli* JT4.

The culture fluid was examined by paper chromatography, the location of β-lactamase-inhibitory material being determined by a special bioautographic procedure based on the fact that the β-lactamase of *K. aerogenes* is readily inhibited by clavulanic acid (Table 2).

The results in Fig. 2 clearly show the presence of a zone of β-lactamase-inhibitory activity. The substance responsible for this zone of activity had an R_f of 0.6 to 0.65 and has been named clavulanic acid. It is quite distinct from cephamycin C and penicillin N, neither of which shows β-lactamase-inhibitory activity in the special bioautographic system used (Table 1, Fig. 2). Furthermore, clavulanic acid has a much higher R_f value than the various naturally occurring, amino adipyl-containing β-lactam antibiotics. It will be noticed in Fig. 2 that chromatograms of fermentation samples showed no antibiotic zones when contacted with *K. aerogenes* seeded agar, the cephamycin C level presumably being just too low to be detected except when added as a marker.

In addition to the above procedure, clavulanic acid can also be detected on thin-layer chromatography plates by spraying with TTC reagent. It appears as a dark red spot after heating the sprayed chromatogram and has an R_f value of 0.44 when using a solvent system consisting of *n*-butanol–ethanol–water (4:1:5, vol/vol/vol, top phase).

To provide culture fluid for the isolation of clavulanic acid, *S. clavuligerus* was grown in a 300-liter fermentor containing 150 liters of the DAS medium for 4 days at 26°C, by which time the clavulanic acid titer was in the region of 150 to 200 μg/ml. Clavulanic acid was isolated as its sodium salt according to the procedure outlined in Fig. 3. During the isolation the metabolite was followed using the enzyme inhibition assay with the β-lactamase from *E. coli* JT4.

β-Lactamase-inhibitory properties of clavulanic acid. The enzyme-inhibitory activity of sodium clavulanate against a range of β-lactamases was determined by measuring the amount required to give 50% inhibition (I_{50}) under the conditions of the test (see Materials and Methods). For all of the β-lactamase preparations it was found that the degree of inhibition of the β-lactamase increased with time. An interaction time of 15 min was arbitrarily chosen for the determination of I_{50} values. The results given in Table 2 show that β-lactamases from both gram-negative and gram-positive organisms are inhibited by very low concentrations of clavulanic acid. The enzymes not so readily inhibited under the test conditions were those with a predominantly cephalosporinase activity and the enzyme preparation from *B. cereus*, which contained both enzymes I and II. Enzymes that are well inhibited include those from clinically important organisms such as *E. coli* harboring the R_{TEM} plasmid. This is exemplified in Table 2 by *E. coli* JT4, which was found to produce a β-lactamase indistinguishable by isoelectric focusing and substrate profile from that found in *E. coli* K-12 pR_{TEM}.

β-Lactamase stability of clavulanic acid. Using paper chromatography and the special bioautographic detection method, no gross destruction of clavulanic acid was observed on incubation with those β-lactamases that were less readily inhibited by clavulanic acid, such as those produced by *P. aeruginosa* A, *E. coli* JT410, and *E. cloacae* P99. The poor inhibitory activity against these β-lactamases thus does not seem to be due to instability of the compound.

The activity of sodium clavulanate was the same against strains of bacteria that produced β-lactamase as against those that did not, reflecting the high stability of the compound to β-lactamase. Thus, the minimum inhibitory concentration for the β-lactamase-producing Russell strain of *S. aureus* was the same as that against the Oxford strain, and the minimum inhibitory concentration for *E. coli* JT39, a potent β-lactamase producer, was the same as that against *E. coli* NCTC 10418, an ampicillin-susceptible strain.

Enhancement of antibacterial activity of β-lactamase-labile antibiotics by clavulanic acid. When low levels of sodium clavulanate were added to β-lactamase-labile compounds, the antibacterial spectrum of the labile compound could be widened to include many previously resistant β-lactamase-producing organisms. Good correlations could be seen between enzyme inhibition data and antibacterial synergy tests. Data in Tables 2 and 3 show that where good inhibition was seen against isolated enzymes the organisms producing those enzymes were rendered susceptible to β-lactam antibiotics in the presence of sodium clavulanate. However, where inhibition was poor against isolated enzymes, such as the chromo-

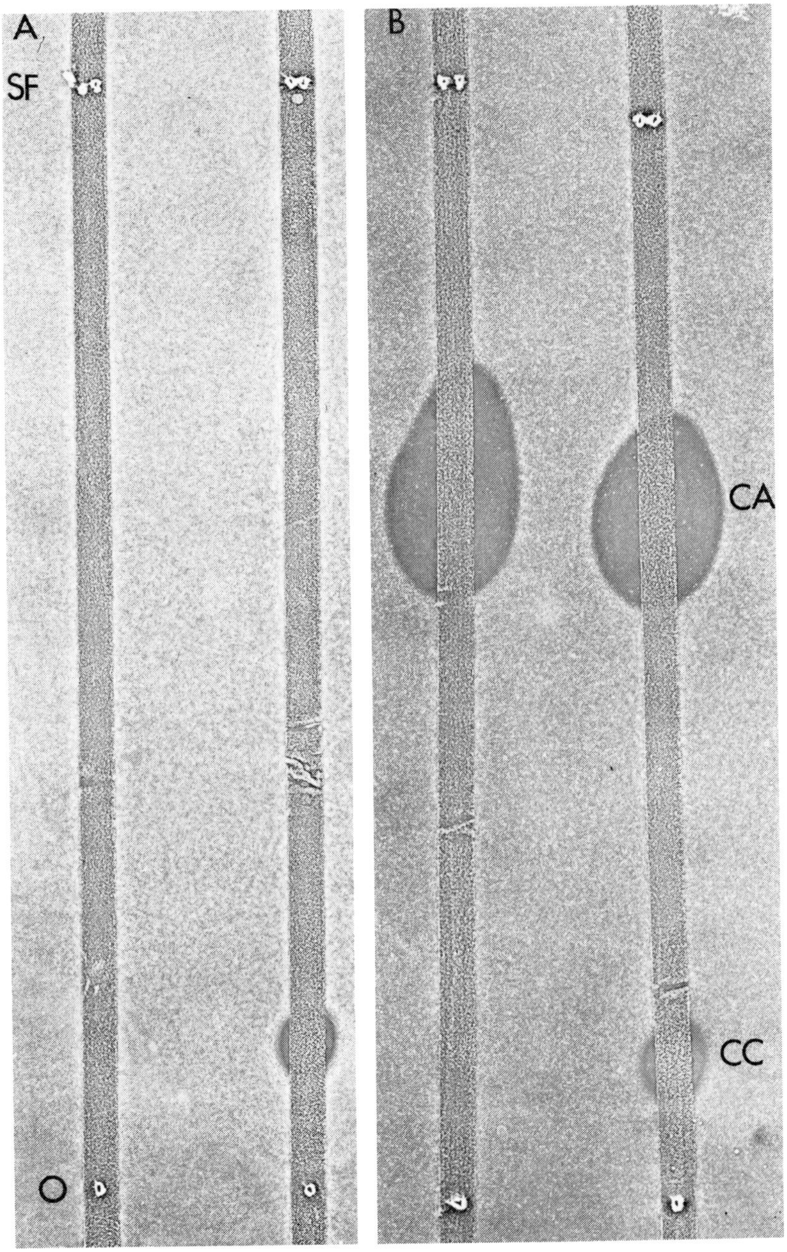

FIG. 2. *Paper chromatographic detection of clavulanic acid in a 4-day fermentation sample of S. clavuligerus grown as described in the text. The chromatograms were contacted with agar seeded with a β-lactamase-producing strain of K. aerogenes without (A) or with (B) the addition of a subinhibitory concentration of benzylpenicillin (6 μg/ml) to the agar. The second chromatogram of each pair was of a fermentation sample supplemented with cephamycin C (10 μl of 1 mg/ml). The solvent system was n-butanol–acetic acid–water (12:3:5, vol/vol/vol), the paper was Whatman grade 1, and the loading was 15 μl of sample. SF, Solvent front; O, origin; CA, clavulanic acid; CC, cephamycin C.*

somal β-lactamase of *E. coli* JT410, no significant change in minimum inhibitory concentration against this organism could be seen when sodium clavulanate was added to cephaloridine or ampicillin.

DISCUSSION

The property of β-lactamase inhibition is well known for certain penicillins and cephalosporins (1). The inhibition exhibited by these compounds is usually restricted to a small num-

TABLE 1. *Paper chromatography of sodium clavulanate*

Solvent system	R_f on Whatman no. 1 paper strips: Sodium clavulanate	Penicillin N	Cephamycin C
n-Butanol–acetic acid–water, 12:3:5 (vol/vol/vol)	0.63	0.3	0.18
n-Butanol–ethanol–water, 4:1:5 (vol/vol/vol, top phase)	0.14	0	0
n-Butanol–pyridine–water, 1:1:1 (vol/vol/vol)	0.56	0.3	0.23

Culture supernatant
↓ HCl to pH 2.0; 3/4 vol of *n*-butanol Extraction at 5°C
n-Butanol extract
↓ 1/15 vol of water to pH 7.0 with 20% (wt/vol) aqueous NaOH
Aqueous back extract
↓ Ion-exchange chromatography; permutit FFIP (SRA 62) resin Cl^-, NaCl 0–0.35 M gradient elution, 5°C; combined active fractions vacuum concentrated
Concentrated active eluate
↓ Desalted on Bio-Rad Bio-Gel P2 column at 5°C and vacuum concentrated combined, active, NaCl-free fractions
Concentrated desalted material
↓ Column chromatography at 5°C on Whatman CC31 cellulose using *n*-butanol–ethanol–water, 4:1:5 (top phase); active fractions combined, evaporated to dryness, dissolved in distilled water and freeze dried
Sodium clavulanate

FIG. 3. *Isolation of clavulanic acid as its sodium salt.*

ber of β-lactamases and is of the competitive and mainly reversible type. Furthermore, the inhibitory properties of these compounds are clearly associated with the side chain (5, 13). Some semisynthetic penicillins have been reported to inactivate *B. cereus* and staphylococcal enzymes, but only at very high concentrations (1, 2, 6). In contrast, clavulanic acid, which has no acylamino side chain, inhibits a wide range of β-lactamases and does so in a progressive fashion at low concentrations. The similarity between the stereochemistry of clavulanic acid and the penicillin nucleus could explain the affinity between clavulanic acid and β-lactamases, whereas the reactivity may in some ways be associated with the hydroxyethylidene in position 3.

The only naturally occurring, low-molecular-weight β-lactamase inhibitors apart from clavulanic acid that have been reported are those from our laboratory, namely, MM 4550, MM 13902 and MM 17880 produced by *Streptomyces olivaceus* (4; Belgian Patent 1,467,413, 16 March 1977, D. Butterworth, M. Cole, and J. D. Hood) and MC696-SY2 A and B described by Umezawa et al. from *Streptomyces fulvoviridis* (15, U.S. Patent 3,928,569, 23 December 1975, H. Umezawa, S. Mitsuhashi, R. Utahara, and T. Ishikawa). Chromatographic and spectral data indicate that clavulanic acid is clearly different from these metabolites. Inhibitors of β-lactamase have been reported by Hata et al. from *Streptomyces gedanensis* (7) and by Miyamura and Ochiai, also from a streptomycete (11), but these were macromolecular substances.

Although clavulanic acid has weak broad-spectrum antibacterial activity, its potential application is as an inhibitor of many clinically important β-lactamases. It is thus possible, by adding clavulanic acid at low concentrations, to demonstrate marked improvement in the activity of β-lactamase-labile penicillins and cephalosporins. This improvement of activity is very marked for strains of bacteria that owe their resistance to the production of β-lactamase but only occurs where this enzyme is readily inhibited by clavulanic acid.

TABLE 2. *β-Lactamase inhibitory activity of sodium clavulanate*

Source of β-lactamase	Substrate[a]	I_{50} (μg/ml)
Pseudomonas aeruginosa A (Sabath type [14])	C	160
Escherichia coli JT410 (chromosomally mediated)	C	56
Enterobacter cloacae P99	C	10.0
Klebsiella aerogenes NCTC 418	P	0.03
Escherichia coli JT4 (R factor mediated)	P	0.08
Escherichia coli JT39 (R factor mediated)	P	0.08
Proteus mirabilis C889	P	0.03
Pseudomonas aeruginosa Dalgleish (preparation contains some Sabath-type enzyme)	P	0.1
Staphylococcus aureus Russell	P	0.06
Bacillus cereus (Whatman Biochemicals Ltd.)	P	17.0

[a] C, Cephaloridine; P, benzylpenicillin.

TABLE 3. *Activity of β-lactamase-labile antibiotics in the presence of sodium clavulanate*

β-Lactam antibiotic plus sodium clavulanate	Minimum inhibitory concn (μg/ml)[a]					
	Staphylococcus aureus Russell	*Klebsiella aerogenes* NCTC 418	*Proteus mirabilis* C889	*Escherichia coli* JT39	*Escherichia coli* JT410	*Pseudomonas aeruginosa* Dalgleish
Sodium clavulanate alone	15	31	62–125	31	31	250
Ampicillin alone	500	250	>2,000	>2,000	250	>2,000[b]
Ampicillin + 1 μg/ml	0.8	0.4	62	31	250	2,000[b]
Ampicillin + 5 μg/ml	0.02	0.1	8	4	250	500[b]
Ampicillin + 20 μg/ml					125	125[b]
Cephaloridine alone	0.6		62	62	62	
Cephaloridine + 1 μg/ml	0.15		8	4	62	
Cephaloridine + 5 μg/ml	0.06		4	2	62	

[a] Microtiter technique using serial dilutions in tryptone soy broth with a 1/500 dilution of overnight broth culture as inoculum. End points read after 18 h at 37°C.
[b] Carbenicillin in place of ampicillin.

It is hoped that clavulanic acid will provide a new aid to the treatment of infections caused by penicillin- and cephalosporin-resistant bacteria.

ACKNOWLEDGMENTS

We thank the following colleagues for their assistance: S. J. Box, A. G. Brown, D. Byrom, S. E. M. Cox, C. J. Davis, G. Hanscomb, P. J. Hepburn, T. T. Howarth, P. A. Hunter, L. R. Jeffries, M. Kenig, A. Lawrence, M. S. Verrall.

We thank D. Hendlin of the Merck Institute of Therapeutic Research for a sample of cephamycin C.

LITERATURE CITED

1. **Abraham, E. P.** 1974. Biosynthesis and enzymic hydrolysis of penicillins and cephalosporins. University of Tokyo Press, Tokyo.
2. **Batchelor, F. R., J. Cameron-Wood, E. C. Chain, and G. N. Rolinson.** 1963. Studies on penicillinase produced by a strain of *Staphylococcus aureus*. Proc. R. Soc. London 158:311–328.
3. **Boxer, G. E., and P. M. Everett.** 1949. Colorimetric determination of benzylpenicillin. Anal. Chem. 21:670–673.
4. **Brown, A. G., D. Butterworth, M. Cole, G. Hanscomb, J. D. Hood, C. Reading, and G. N. Rolinson.** 1976. Naturally occurring β-lactamase inhibitors with antibacterial activity. J. Antibiot. 29:668–669.
5. **Cole, M., S. Elson, and P. D. Fullbrook.** 1972. Inhibition of the β-lactamases of *Escherichia coli* and *Klebsiella aerogenes* by semisynthetic penicillins. Biochem. J. 127:295–308.
6. **Dyke, K. G. H.** 1967. Substrate-specific inactivation of staphylococcal penicillinase. Biochem. J. 103:641–646.
7. **Hata, T., S. Omura, Y. Iwai, H. Ohno, H. Takeshima, and N. Yamaguchi.** 1972. Studies of penicillinase inhibitors produced by microorganisms. J. Antibiot. 25:473–474.
8. **Higgens, C. E., R. L. Hamill, T. H. Sands, M. M. Hoehn, N. E. Davis, R. Nagarajan, and L. D. Boeck.** 1974. The occurrence of deacetoxy cephalosporin C in fungi and streptomycetes. J. Antibiot. 27:298–300.
9. **Higgens, C. E., and R. E. Kastner.** 1971. *Streptomyces clavuligerus* sp. nov., a β-lactam antibiotic producer. Int. J. Syst. Bacteriol. 21:326–331.
10. **Howarth, T. T., A. G. Brown, and T. J. King.** 1976. Clavulanic acid, a novel β-lactam isolated from *Streptomyces clavuligerus*. J. Chem. Soc. Chem. Commun., p. 266–267.
11. **Miyamura, S., and H. Ochiai.** 1974. Inhibitors of β-lactamases from Gram-negative bacilli, p. 218–223. *In* G. K. Daikos (ed.), Progress in Chemotherapy I, Proceedings of the 8th International Congress of Chemotherapy, Athens, 1973. Hellenic Society for Chemotherapy, Athens.
12. **Nagarajan, R., L. D. Boeck, M. Gorman, R. L. Hamill, C. E. Higgens, M. M. Hoehn, W. M. Stark, and J. G. Whitney.** 1971. β-Lactam antibiotics from Streptomyces. J. Am. Chem. Soc. 93:2308–2310.
13. **O'Callaghan, C. H., and A. Morris.** 1972. Inhibition of β-lactamases by β-lactam antibiotics. Antimicrob. Agents Chemother. 2:442–448.
14. **Sabath, L. D., M. Jago, and E. P. Abraham.** 1965. Cephalosporinase and penicillinase activities of a β-lactamase from *Pseudomonas pyocyanea*. Biochem. J. 96:739–752.
15. **Umezawa, H., S. Mitsuhashi, M. Hamada, S. Iyobe, S. Takahashi, R. Utahara, Y. Osato, S. Yamazaki, H. Ogawara, and K. Maeda.** 1973. Two β-lactamase inhibitors produced by a Streptomyces. J. Antibiot. 26:51–54.
16. **Whitney, J. G., D. R. Brannon, J. A. Mabe, and K. J. Wicker.** 1972. Incorporation of labeled precursors into A16886B, a novel β-lactam antibiotic produced by *Streptomyces clavuligerus*. Antimicrob. Agents Chemother. 1:247–251.

ANTIMICROBIAL AGENTS AND CHEMOTHERAPY, May 1977, p. 858-864 Vol. 11, No. 5

Aggregation-Dependent Changes in Susceptibility of *Dictyostelium discoideum* to Amphotericin B

EDWARD F. ROSSOMANDO,* MARY ANN HESLA, MARY ANN HEITZ, AND BARBARA MALDONADO

Department of Oral Biology, The University of Connecticut Health Center, Farmington, Connecticut 06032

Received for publication 3 December 1976

In this study, the polyene antibiotic amphotericin B was used to induce changes in permeability and viability of the eucaryotic microorganism *Dictyostelium discoideum*. The results show that as the cells progress from the growth phase through stationary phase to eventual aggregation, they become increasingly resistant to both permeability changes and lysis. Plasma membranes were prepared from cells harvested at exponential growth, stationary phase, and the aggregation-competent stage, and both the neutral lipid and phospholipid content were determined. An increase in the neutral lipid and a decrease in the phospholipid were observed as the cells progressed from growth into aggregation, with the overall result that the phospholipid-sterol ratio decreased during this period. The extent of amphotericin B binding by cells from the different stages was also determined. Aggregation cells exhibited a small but significant increase in binding compared to cells from either of the other two stages. The permeability changes produced by the drug were measured as a function of temperature. Exponentially growing cells showed a marked temperature dependence for the drug effect, whereas aggregating cells did not. Rates of inactivation by the drug were also determined over a range of temperatures. With exponentially growing cells, the rate of inactivation was temperature dependent, whereas with aggregating cells it was not. Finally, drug binding for both growing and aggregating cells was temperature dependent. Thus, no binding was observed for cells of either type at 4°C. This finding suggests that the differences in the temperature dependence of the permeability changes and inactivation between the cells involve parameters other than drug binding.

Polyene antibiotics, such as amphotericin B, have been shown to produce striking increases in water and solute permeability in both lipid bilayers (4, 6) and intact cells (8), which often leads to cell death by lysis. Although the action of these drugs is dependent upon the binding of the polyene to sterol residues in the membrane (13), the mechanisms underlying the permeability changes and lysis remain to be elucidated. In a previous study in this laboratory, amphotericin B together with the eucaryotic microorganism *Dictyostelium discoideum* were used to study this question, and we showed that lysis is preceded by the formation of an osmotically fragile cell (22). In addition, the results of the previous study suggested that growing cells were more susceptible to the drug than those from the stationary phase (22).

To explore the relationship between growth and drug sensitivity in more detail, we have taken advantage of the fact that *D. discoideum* begins to aggregate only after the cessation of growth. This means that cell populations can be obtained from three separate growth stages: i.e., exponential growth, the stationary growth phase, and the stage of no growth that is found at aggregation. In the present study, cells from all three stages were exposed to amphotericin B, and the effects of the drug on viability and permeability were determined.

Part of the present study necessitated a comparison of the extent of drug binding by cells from the three different stages. Although several chemical procedures for this determination have been reported (10, 14), a bioassay technique of a type similar to one previously described using erythrocyte hemolysis as the indicator was developed for the present study. (12). In the present assay, *D. discoideum* cell lysis is the indicator.

The assay used in the present study is based on the observation that, although cell lysis by the polyenes occurs above a threshold value (11), *D. discoideum* can be induced to lyse below its threshold by dilution into distilled water (22). This bioassay has enabled us to compare the extent of drug binding by cells from the different stages.

MATERIALS AND METHODS

Organisms and growth conditions. Cells of the axenic strain of *D. discoideum* AX-3, a derivative of NC-4 (haploid), were grown as previously described (22). Under these conditions, the cells double in about 10 to 12 h.

Materials. Amphotericin B (Fungizone, E. R. Squibb & Sons) solutions were prepared by the addition of a low-phosphate saline (LPS) buffer (22, 23). [^{14}C]thiourea (25.9 mCi/mmol) was purchased from New England Nuclear Corp. and diluted with water before use. Stigmasterol was purchased from the Sigma Chemical Co.

Aggregation and disaggregation conditions. The synchronous formation of aggregates was accomplished by dispensing cells, at a final concentration of 7×10^7 to 8×10^7 cells/ml, on 42-mm Whatman no. 50 filters resting on absorbant pads in 60-mm plastic petri dishes as previously described (19, 23). Cells, harvested from filter pads, were resuspended in LPS buffer and disaggregated by repeatedly pipetting the solution with a fine-tipped 10-ml pipette (1, 18). This procedure was continued until over 99% of the aggregates had been disrupted to single cells, as confirmed by microscopic examination. No evidence of cell lysis was obtained using the clonal assay procedure.

Preparation of plasma membranes. Plasma membranes were isolated and purified from *D. discoideum* as previously described (21).

Cell viability. The effect of amphotericin B on cell viability was determined using the clonal assay procedure as previously described (22). Cells were harvested from the required stage of growth or development and resuspended in LPS at a density of 1×10^7 cells/ml, and they were further incubated with amphotericin B at 22°C on a gyratory shaker. After 2 h, the drug reaction was terminated by diluting a portion of the incubation solution with protease peptone broth (1:100; 22). The number of viable cells present in portions of the culture was determined. The cells were appropriately diluted and spread on an agar surface together with *Aerobacter aerogenes* as food source. Clones, observed for 3 to 4 days after incubation at 22°C, were counted, and the number was used to calculate the number of viable cells (22).

Thiourea incorporation. Thiourea incorporation into intact cells was determined as previously described (22). [^{14}C]thiourea (2×10^5 cpm) was added to cell cultures harvested from the appropriate stages. After the addition of amphotericin B, the culture was incubated at 22°C with shaking. After 2 h, a 0.2- to 0.5-ml portion was transferred to 2 ml of water, shaken vigorously, and filtered using a glass-fiber circle (Whatman, GF/C.) The filter was dried, and the amount of radioactivity retained on the filter was determined by liquid scintillation counting (22).

Binding of amphotericin B to cells. Cells were harvested from the required stage and resuspended in 10 ml of LPS at a final concentration of 1×10^6 cells/ml in a Corex tube (30 ml). Amphotericin B was added to a final concentration of 400 μg/ml, and the tube was shaken for 5 min at room temperature. The control tubes contained cells but no drug. After the incubation, the cell titer was determined by counting a portion in a hemocytometer (Neubauer Bright Line) under ×200 total magnification. No cell lysis occurred at the drug-cell ratio used under these incubation conditions in this part of the experiment. In separate experiments, it was shown that, although incubation for as long as 1 h did not influence the extent of binding, some (about 10%) of the cells did lyse. After the 5-min incubation, the cells were removed from the solution by centrifugation (5,000 × *g* for 5 min), and the supernatant (S-1) was recovered. In experiments performed without cells, it could be shown that all the drug remained in the S-1 fraction. In addition, to determine if any unbound drug remained with the pellet, it was resuspended in 10 ml of LPS, the centrifugation was repeated, and the supernatant (S-2) was recovered. This washing procedure was repeated twice, yielding supernatant fractions S-3 and S-4. Determinations of the drug concentration in each of the supernatants showed that over 95% of the drug was recovered in the S-1 fraction. The procedure used to measure the concentration of drug in the supernatants is the bioassay technique described below.

Bioassay procedure. The bioassay procedure employed cells from stationary growth phase as the indicator cells. Indicator cells were resuspended at a final concentration of 10^8 cells/ml in 1 ml of LPS in a 10-ml test tube. A 0.1-ml portion was transferred to 0.9 ml of S-1 in a 25-ml beaker, and the solution was incubated at room temperature. After 30 min, a 0.1-ml portion was transferred to 0.9 ml of glass-distilled water, and the number of cells present was determined by counting a portion of this suspension in a hemocytometer.

In the absence of drug, about 10% of the indicator cells were lysed by the dilution into distilled water. To relate the titer of indicator cells to drug concentration, a calibration curve was constructed by incubating indicator cells with drug over a concentration range of 0 to 400 μg/ml. After the 30-min incubation, the indicator cells were diluted into distilled water, and the cell titer was determined as described above. About 90% of the cells lysed at 400 μg/ml, whereas proportional numbers of the cells survived at the intermediate drug concentrations. The log of the cell concentration observed was plotted as a function of drug concentration, and a straight line was obtained. This curve was used to determine the drug concentration present in S-1 (S-2,-3, and -4; see above) after the addition of cells from various stages.

Chemical determinations. Proteins were determined by the Lowry procedure (16), using bovine serum albumin as standard. Neutral lipid content of purified membranes was determined as described (22, 24), using stigmasterol as standard. Control experiments showed that amphotericin B did not interfere with the neutral lipid determination using this procedure. Phospholipids were extracted as described by Bligh and Dyer (5), and phosphorous was determined according to the procedure of Ames (2).

RESULTS

Changes in susceptibility of cells during growth. To determine the effect of amphotericin B on cells during growth, cells were harvested from either the exponential or stationary phase and resuspended at 10^7 cells/ml in LPS buffer together with amphotericin B. After a 2-h incubation, portions were removed, and the concentration of viable cells was determined by the clonal assay. The data obtained shows that a greater number of viable cells are present in the stationary-phase culture (Table 1). In addition, cells harvested after 5 h on filters showed an even greater resistance to drug action (Table 1). These results suggest that growing cells are more susceptible to the drug and are consistent with a previous observation, which suggested that the susceptibility of the cells to the drug decreases with the growth rate (22).

Changes in susceptibility of cells during aggregation. The susceptibility of cells to the drug during aggregation was determined using both viability and thiourea incorporation. For these experiments, cells were harvested from filter pads during the initial 5 h of development and disaggregated by rapid pipetting, and the single cells were resuspended in LPS buffer together with amphotericin B. After a 2-h incubation with the drug, the concentration of viable cells and the amount of thiourea incorporation were determined. In Fig. 1, the fraction of cells remaining viable in the population is shown as a function of developmental time. The results indicate that, as aggregation procedes, there is an increase in the concentration of viable cells. These data also show that, in the absence of the drug, the number of viable cells detected at each developmental time point remains constant. This indicates that the extent of disaggregation at each stage is the same. Therefore, the observed effect is not due to some effect of aggregation. In Fig. 2, the rate of uptake of thiourea is also shown as a function of developmental time. These results show that during aggregation, there is also a decrease in the uptake of thiourea. Thus, the results of both assays suggest that as cells proceed through the aggregation stage of development, there is an increase in resistance of the cells to the drug.

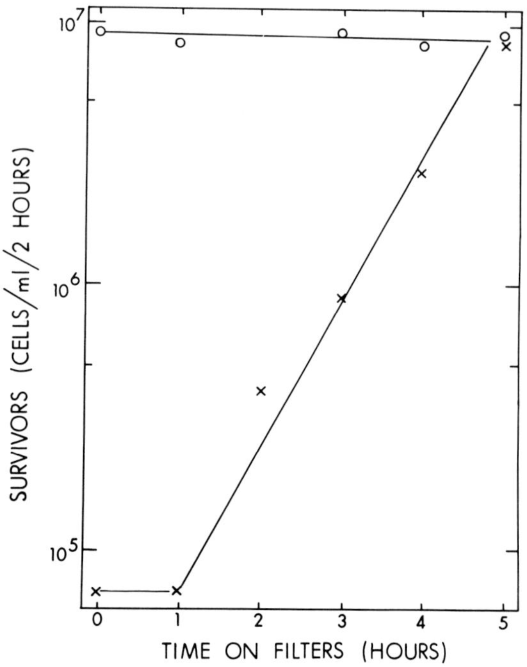

FIG. 1. *Effect of amphotericin B on the viability of cells from different stages of aggregation. Cells were harvested from liquid culture at 2 × 10⁶ to 4 × 10⁶ cells/ml, washed in LPS, and resuspended at a final titer of 1.8 × 10⁸ cells/ml. Portions (0.5 ml) were dispensed on Whatman no. 50 filters (presoaked in LPS) resting on absorbant pads (also soaked in LPS) in 60-mm plastic petri dishes. Cells were harvested from filters at intervals, washed and resuspended in LPS, and dispersed by repeated pipetting as described in Materials and Methods. Disaggregation to single cells could be achieved after a few passes through the pipette. The cells were diluted to 10⁷ cells/ml and incubated with 200 μg of amphotericin B per ml. After 2 h, the reaction was terminated by dilution, and the number of viable cells was determined by the clonal assay. Each point represents the results of three determinations. Symbols: survivors with* (×) *and without* (○) *amphotericin B.*

TABLE 1. *Susceptibility of cells from different stages of growth and development to inactivation by amphotericin B*

Stage	Survivors (%)[a]
Exponential growth, 1×10^6 to 2×10^6 cells/ml	2
Stationary phase, 1×10^7 to 2×10^7 cells/ml	10
Preaggregation, 5 h on filters	90

[a] Cells harvested from the required stage were resuspended at 1×10^7 cells/ml in LPS buffer with amphotericin B at a final concentration of 100 μg/ml. After incubation at room temperature (22°C) for 2 h, a portion was diluted 1:100 into broth, and portions were transferred to an agar plate and spread together with *A. aerogenes*. Plates were incubated 3 days at 22°C, and the number of viable cells was determined by counting clones that were visible on plates.

Lipid content of membranes from growing and aggregating cells. Although the exact mechanism by which amphotericin B induces changes in osmotic permeability has not been determined, available data suggest that the process requires the binding to sterols in the membrane as the first step (13). To determine if the increased drug resistance could be accounted for by a decrease in membrane sterols, the total sterol content of plasma membranes, prepared from cells harvested from exponential growth, stationary phase, and after 5 h on filters, was determined. Values of approximately 7, 9, and 11 μg of protein per ml were obtained

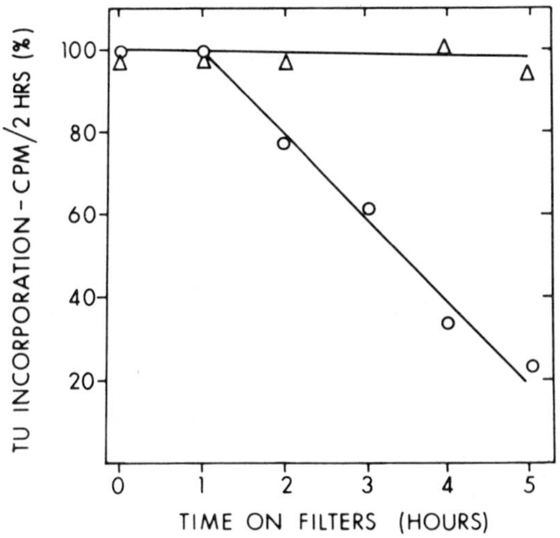

FIG. 2. *Effect of amphotericin B on thiourea (TU) incorporation of cells from different stages of development. Cells were allowed to develop on filters, harvested, and incubated at 22°C with amphotericin B as described in legend to Fig. 1. Thiourea (2 × 10^5 cpm) was added, and after 2 h, the cell-associated radioactivity was determined as described in Materials and Methods. Symbols: incorporation with* (○) *and without* (△) *amphotericin B.*

for cells from exponential growth, stationary growth, and the aggregation stage, respectively (Table 2). These data show that there is a small, but significant, increase in the neutral lipid content of the plasma membrane as the cells progress from exponential growth to aggregation. This finding suggests that the increase in drug resistance observed for aggregating cells is not due to a decrease in the sterol content of the membrane.

Since it has been suggested that increased resistance of cells to polyenes is related to an increase in the phospholipid-sterol ratio (12, 25), both the phospholipid content of *D. discoideum* membranes and this ratio were determined. Table 2 shows these values. In contrast to the neutral lipid values, the phospholipid content of the membrane decreased while the phospholipid-neutral lipid ratio decreased from 8.3 for exponentially growing cells to 4.4 for aggregation-competent cells. This finding suggests that the increased resistance of aggregating cells cannot be explained by this mechanism.

Effect of aggregation on amphotericin B binding. Since polyene action requires the binding of the drug as the first step (13), the extent of binding by cells from the three representative stages was determined using the bioassay procedure described in Materials and Methods.

Table 3 shows the results of this comparison. The titer of indicator cells as well as the concentration of free drug, as determined from a calibration curve (see Materials and Methods), are

TABLE 2. *Lipid content of D. discoideum plasma membranes from different stages*

Stage	Lipid content (μg/mg of protein, ± S.D.)[a]		
	Phospholipid	Neutral lipid	P/S[b]
Exponential growth, 1 × 10^6 to 2 × 10^6 cells/ml	64 ± 10.1	7.7 ± 1.2	8.3
Stationary phase, 1 × 10^7 to 2 × 10^7 cells/ml	54 ± 8.5	8.9 ± 1.6	6.1
Aggregation competent (5 h)	46 ± 11.2	10.5 ± 1.5	4.4

[a] Lipid determinations were performed as described in Materials and Methods.
[b] Ratio of phospholipid to neutral lipid.

TABLE 3. *Extent of amphotericin B binding by cells from different stages*

Stage	Titer of indicator cells (×10^5 cells/ml)	Concn of amphotericin B (μg/ml)	
		Free[a]	Bound[b]
Exponential growth, 1 × 10^6 to 2 × 10^6 cells/ml	1.5 ± 10%	200	200
Stationary phase, 1 × 10^7 to 2 × 10^7 cells/ml	2.5 ± 10%	115	285
Aggregation competent (5 h)	3.1 ± 10%	75	325

[a] The concentration of free drug was determined from the indicator cells titer, and the calibration curve was constructed as described in Materials and Methods.
[b] The bound drug concentration was calculated as the difference between the original (400 μg/ml) and free drug concentrations.

presented in Table 3. Also shown are the values obtained for the concentration of bound drug. Taken together, these data show no decrease in the extent of drug binding as cells progress from growth to aggregation. In fact, there appears to be an increase in the extent of binding, a result which might be explained by the increase in sterol content of the membrane shown in Table 2.

Effect of temperature on permeability changes of cells from different stages. Temperature has been implicated as a factor in polyene action (14, 15). Therefore, the permeability changes produced by the drug were studied as a function of temperature for cells from different stages. For these experiments, exponentially growing and aggregating cells were incubated with amphotericin B over a range of temperatures, and the permeability changes were determined by the amount of thiourea incorporated (23). The results shown in Fig. 3 indicate that for cells from the exponential growth phase, no permeability change occurs until about 6°C. Above this temperature, the permeability increases with increasing temperature until it reaches approximately 28°C, when no further increase occurs. In contrast, with aggregating cells, the increase in temperature results in only a minor increase in a permeability (Fig. 3). These data show that the permeability changes in growing cells are temperature dependent, whereas in aggregating cells they are not.

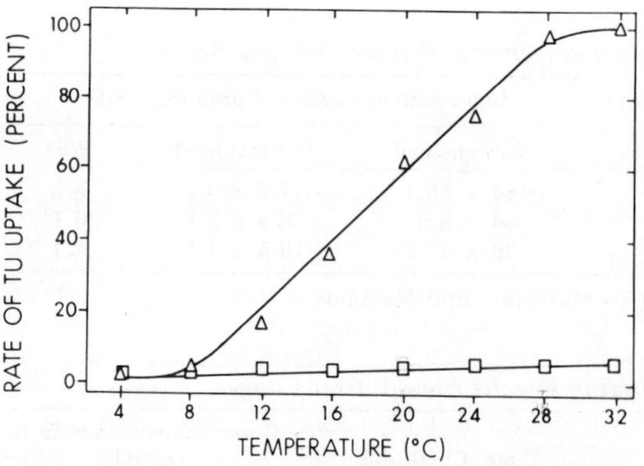

FIG. 3. *Effect of temperature on rate of thiourea (TU) incorporation. Cells were incubated at indicated temperatures with amphotericin B and TU for 2 h as described in the legend to Fig. 2. Amount of cell-associated radioactivity was determined after a 2-h incubation as described in Materials and Methods. Symbols: TU uptake in cells harvested from exponential growth* (△) *and cells after 5 h on filters* (□).

Effect of temperature on inactivation of cells from different stages. The effect of temperature on the ability of the drug to lyse cells from different stages was also studied. The rate of cell lysis, determined at each temperature, normalized to the rate obtained at 30°C (the maximum rate), is shown in Fig. 4 as a function of the reciprocal of temperature. These data show that, for growing cells, the rate of inactivation is temperature dependent, but that the increase in rate between 18 and 22°C is greater than that between 22 and 30°C. In contrast, aggregating cells show only a minor temperature dependence on the effect of the drug. Thus, at 30°C there is only a slight increase in the rate of inactivation as compared to the rate at 18°C, and there is no change in slope. These results show that temperature affects the rate of inactivation of growing cells but not aggregating cells.

Effect of temperature on drug binding. Since we showed above that the extent of drug binding by cells from the different stages at 22°C was similar, it was of interest to compare the binding values at 4°C. Consistent with previous observations (15), we found that the extent of binding at 4°C was about 1% the value obtained at 22°C and, in addition, there were no differences between the cells from the different stages.

DISCUSSION

The results of a previous study on the effects of amphotericin B on *D. discoideum* suggested that exponentially growing cells were one order of magnitude more susceptible to the drug than were cells from the stationary phase (22). The results of the present study confirm this observation and, in addition, show that during the aggregation process the cells become completely resistant to the drug.

Polyene action requires, as a first step, binding of the drug to sterols in the plasma membrane (13). Therefore, one possible explanation for the resistance of the aggregating cells to drug action might be a decrease in the accessibility or number of binding sites. However, direct measurements of amphotericin B binding showed no decrease in drug binding by aggregation-competent cells. In fact, a small, but significant, increase in binding by these cells was observed. This finding is consistent with the results of direct determinations of the sterol content of plasma membranes from the three stages. These results showed a small, but significant, increase in sterol content. These findings suggest that the acquisition of resist-

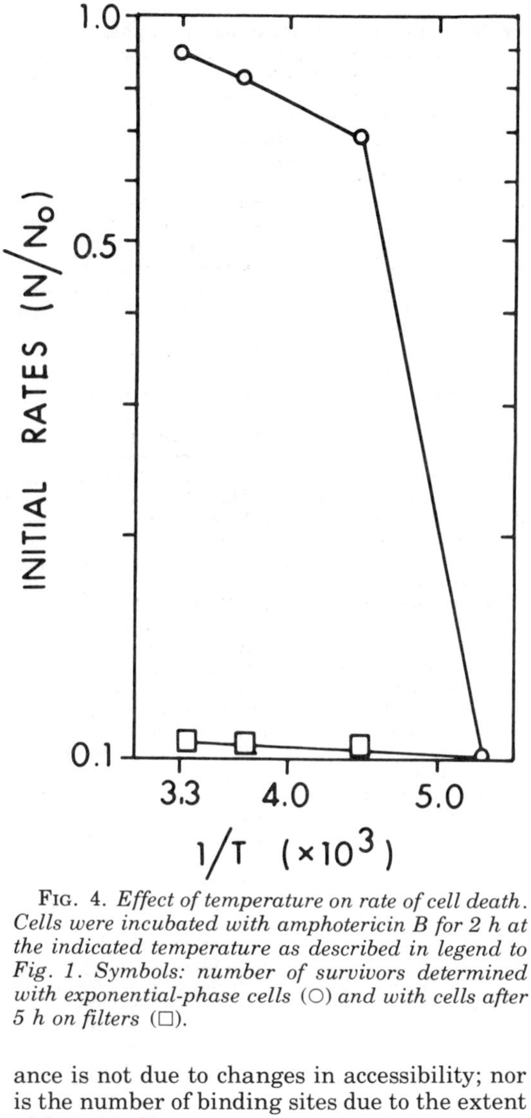

FIG. 4. *Effect of temperature on rate of cell death. Cells were incubated with amphotericin B for 2 h at the indicated temperature as described in legend to Fig. 1. Symbols: number of survivors determined with exponential-phase cells* (○) *and with cells after 5 h on filters* (□).

ance is not due to changes in accessibility; nor is the number of binding sites due to the extent of drug binding.

Although polyene action requires sterols for drug action, some types of sterol-containing cells (20) and organelles (12) are not lysed by this class of drugs. In a previous study, a correlation between cell lysis and the ratio of phospholipids to sterol was found (12). For example, it was shown that erythrocytes with a ratio of approximately 1 were lysed, whereas mitochondria with a ratio of approximately 40 were not (12). On the basis of this correlation, it was suggested that this ratio might be a factor regulating the effect of the drug (12, 25). As part of the present study, this ratio was determined for plasma membranes from *D. discoideum* cells at the three stages. Since we found that this ratio decreased as the cells entered the aggregation stage, we conclude that the increased resistance of *D. discoideum* cannot be explained by changes in the phospholipid-sterol ratio. The results of a study on a lecithin membrane model system are consistent with the idea that polyene-induced permeability alteration is affected by the composition of the membrane phospholipid fatty acyl chains (9). Since we have not analyzed the compositional differences between growing and aggregating cells, we cannot rule out this explanation.

As part of the present study, we examined the effect of temperature on the drug-induced permeability changes using cells from two stages. With cells from the exponential growth stage, we find that decreasing the temperature produces a decrease in permeability. However, since a reduction in temperature also produces a decrease in drug binding, the effect of temperature on permeability might be explained by this result. In contrast, when aggregation-competent cells were studied, we found that temperature produced no significant change in permeability, even though it produces the same change in the extent of binding. This finding suggests that the temperature-dependent changes in permeability are mediated by events occuring after drug binding and that it is these steps at which the aggregation-competent cells are unable to complete. Based on previous studies which have implicated temperature as a factor affecting the rearrangement of sterol residues (7), the present results are consistent with the possibility that the sterol residues in the aggregating cell surface are more restricted in their mobility within the plane of the membrane than are those on the surface of growing cells. This interpretation is similar to one previously suggested to explain permeability changes in lipid bilayers (3).

The effect of temperature on the lytic effects of the drug was also studied. With exponentially growing cells, when the rates obtained are plotted as a function of the reciprocal of the temperature, an abrupt change in slope is observed at 22°C. Since a change in slope, such as that observed here, has been interpreted in terms of phase transitions of membrane components (17), this change could reflect alterations in the physical state of the membrane of exponentially growing cells, a change which apparently cannot occur in aggregating cells.

ACKNOWLEDGMENTS

This research was supported by grants from the National Institutes of Health (DE-03715) and the American Cancer Society (BC-157).

LITERATURE CITED

1. **Alexander, S., R. Brackenbury, and M. Sussman.** 1975. Tryptic destruction of aggregative competence in *Dictyostelium discoideum* and subsequent recovery. Nature (London) 254:698–699.
2. **Ames, B. N.** 1966. Assay of inorganic phosphate, total phosphate and phosphatases. Methods Enzymol. 8:115–118.
3. **Andreoli, T. E.** 1973. On the anatomy of amphotericin B-cholesterol pores in lipid bilayer membranes. Kidney Int. 4:337–345.
4. **Andreoli, T. E., V. W. Dennis, and A. M. Weigl.** 1969. The effect of amphotericin B on the water and nonelectrolyte permeability of thin lipid membranes. J. Gen. Physiol. 53:133–156.
5. **Bligh, E. G., and W. T. Dyer.** 1959. A rapid method of total lipid extraction and purification. Can. J. Biochem. Physiol. 37:911–917.
6. **Dennis, V. W., N. W. Stead, and T. E. Andreoli.** 1970. Molecular aspects of polyene- and sterol-dependent pore formation of thin lipid membranes. J. Gen. Physiol. 55:375–400.
7. **Engelman, D. M.** 1970. X-ray diffraction studies of phase transitions in the membrane of *Mycoplasma laidlawii*. J. Mol. Biol. 47:115–117.
8. **Feingold, D. S.** 1965. The action of amphotericin B on *Mycoplasma laidlawii*. Biochem. Biophys. Res. Commun. 19:261–267.
9. **Hsuchen, C.-C., and D. S. Feingold.** 1973. Selective membrane toxicity of the polyene antibiotics: studies on lecithin membrane models (liposomes). Antimicrob. Agents Chemother. 4:309–315.
10. **Kinsky, S.** 1962. Nystatin binding by protoplasts and a particular fraction of *Neurospora crassa*, and a basis for the selective toxicity of polyene antifungal antibiotics. Proc. Natl. Acad. Sci. U.S.A. 48:1049–1056.
11. **Kinsky, S.** 1963. Comparative responses of mammalian erythrocytes and microbial protoplasts to polyene antibiotics and vitamin A. Arch. Biochem. Biophys. 102:180–188.
12. **Kinsky, S. C., G. R. Gronan, and M. M. Weber.** 1965. Interaction of polyene antibiotics with subcellular membrane system. I. Mitochondria. Mol. Pharmacol. 1:190–201.
13. **Kinsky, S. C., S. A. Luse, and L. L. M. Van Deenen.** 1966. Interaction of polyene antibiotics with natural and artificial membrane systems. Fed. Proc. 25:1503–1510.
14. **Kotler-Brajtburg, J., G. Medoff, D. Schlessinger, and G. S. Kobayasi.** 1974. Characterization of the binding of amphotericin B to *Saccharomyces cerevisiae* and relationship to the antifungal effect. Antimicrob. Agents Chemother. 6:770–776.
15. **Lampen, J. O., E. R. Morgan, A. Slocum, and P. Arnow.** 1959. Absorption of nystatin by microorganisms. J. Bacteriol. 78:282–289.
16. **Lowry, O. H., N. J. Rosebrough, A. L. Farr, and R. J. Randall.** 1951. Protein measurement with the Folin phenol reagent. J. Biol. Chem. 193:265–275.
17. **Melchior, D. L., H. J. Morowitz, J. M. Sturtevant, and T. Y. Tsong.** 1970. Characterization of the plasma membrane of *Mycoplasma laidlawaii*. Biochem. Biophys. Acta 219:114–122.
18. **Newell, P. C., M. Longlands, and M. Sussman.** 1971. Control of enzymes synthesis by cellular interaction during development of the cellular slime mold *Dictyostelium discoideum*. J. Mol. Biol. 58:541–554.
19. **Newell, P. C., A. Telser, and M. Sussman.** 1969. Alternative developmental pathways determined by environmental conditions in the cellular slime mold *Dictyostelium discoideum*. J. Bacteriol. 100:763–768.
20. **Oppenheimer, S. B., R. L. Potter, and M. L. Barber.** 1973. Alteration of sea urchin embryo cell surface properties by mycostatin a sterol binding antibiotic. Dev. Biol. 33:218–223.
21. **Rossomando, E. F., and L. S. Cutler.** 1975. Preparation and biochemical characterizations of cell fractions and isolated plasma membrane vesicles of *Dictyostelium discoideum*. Exp. Cell Res. 95:67–78.
22. **Rossomando, E. F., G. Creme, B. Maldonado, M. A. Hesla, and E. Golub.** 1976. Effect of amphotericin B on growth and membrane permeability in *Dictyostelium discoideum*. Antimicrob. Agents Chemother. 9:618–624.
23. **Rossomando, E. F., A. J. Steffek, D. K. Mujwid, and S. Alexander.** 1974. Scanning electron microscopic observations on cell surface changes during aggregation of *Dictyostelium discoideum*. Exp. Cell Res. 85:73–78.
24. **Searey, R. L., and L. M. Berquist.** 1960. A new color reaction for the quantitation of serum cholesterol. Clin. Chim. Acta 5:192–199.
25. **Van Zutphen, H., L. L. M. Van Deenen, and S. Kinsky.** 1966. The action of polyene antibiotics on bilayer lipid membranes. Biochem. Biophys. Res. Commun. 22:393–398.

ANTIMICROBIAL AGENTS AND CHEMOTHERAPY, May 1977, p. 865-870 Vol. 11, No. 5

Azlocillin: In Vitro Studies of a New Semisynthetic Penicillin

DOROTHY STEWART AND GERALD P. BODEY*

Department of Developmental Therapeutics, The University of Texas System Cancer Center, M. D. Anderson Hospital and Tumor Institute, Houston, Texas 77030

Received for publication 5 November 1976

The activity of azlocillin, a new semisynthetic penicillin, was determined against 582 clinical isolates of gram-negative bacilli and gram-positive cocci. Over 75% of the isolates of *Pseudomonas aeruginosa* were inhibited at a concentration of 12.5 μg or less per ml. Azlocillin is also active against indole-negative and -positive *Proteus* spp., inhibiting 98 and 71%, respectively, at a concentration of 12.5 μg or less per ml. Isolates of *Klebsiella* spp. and *Enterobacter* spp. showed less susceptibility than isolates of *Escherichia coli* and *Serratia* spp. Gram-positive cocci except penicillin G-resistant *Staphylococcus aureus* were susceptible to azlocillin. Azlocillin failed to inhibit the growth of gram-negative bacilli when large inocula were used. It was more active in alkaline pH, but the type of medium used had little effect on its activity. Azlocillin was more active than mezlocillin, ticarcillin, and carbenicillin and as active as BLP-1654 against isolates of *P. aeruginosa*. It was not as active as mezlocillin against the majority of the other gram-negative bacilli.

Gram-negative bacilli, especially *Klebsiella* spp. and *Pseudomonas aeruginosa*, continue to be a major cause of infection among patients with malignant diseases and patients receiving immunosuppressive therapy (6, 7). Some of these patients fail to improve even when an appropriate antibiotic is administered on the basis of in vitro susceptibility testing (2). In general, penicillins have been more effective than other antibiotics against susceptible organisms in the compromised host (1). Since penicillins have been more effective than other classes of antimicrobial agents for the treatment of such infections, new penicillin derivatives with broad-spectrum activity, particularly against gram-negative bacilli, are of special interest. Azlocillin, a new semisynthetic penicillin, is of interest because of its activity against these organisms and especially *P. aeruginosa*. Figure 1 shows the chemical structure of azlocillin (6[D-2-(2-oxoimidazolidine-1-carboxamido)-2-phenylacetamido]-penicillanic acid, sodium salt). This report presents an in vitro evaluation of azlocillin and compares its activity with other semisynthetic penicillins, including another new derivative, mezlocillin.

MATERIALS AND METHODS

Susceptibility tests were conducted on 479 clinical isolates of gram-negative bacilli and 99 clinical isolates of gram-positive cocci, using a dilution technique with an automatic microtiter system (Canalco, *Autotiter Instruction Manual*). All gram-negative bacilli and *Staphylococcus aureus* isolates to be tested were incubated in Mueller-Hinton broth (pH 7.4) for 18 h at 37°C. *Streptococcus pyogenes* and *S. pneumoniae* were incubated in tryptose phosphate broth. Approximately 10^5 colony-forming units (CFU) per ml was used as the inoculum for gram-negative bacilli and *S. aureus*. For the remaining gram-positive cocci, an inoculum of 10^6 CFU/ml was used for the in vitro susceptibility testing.

All gram-negative bacilli used in this study were cultured from blood specimens of patients who were hospitalized at this institution and had underlying malignant diseases. A total of 100 isolates each of *P. aeruginosa*, *Klebsiella* spp., and *Escherichia coli*, 79 isolates of *Proteus* spp., 50 isolates each of *Serratia* spp., and *Enterobacter* spp. were used. All gram-positive cocci used in this study were cultured from specimens obtained from hospitalized patients, most of whom did not have cancer. A total of 40 isolates of *S. pyogenes*, 9 isolates of *S. pneumoniae*, and 50 isolates of *S. aureus* were used. Isolates of *S. aureus* were divided according to their susceptibility to penicillin G. Those isolates that were inhibited by less than 0.10 μg/ml were selected as penicillin G susceptible and those isolates resistant to more than 25 μg/ml were selected as penicillin G resistant.

Organisms used for studies of the effect of inoculum size on the activity of azlocillin were incubated in Mueller-Hinton broth for 18 h at 37°C. It was assumed that approximately 10^8 CFU/ml were present after incubation, which was subsequently confirmed by subculturing 0.1-ml portions on sheep blood agar and performing colony counts after 14 h of incubation at 37°C. Serial 10-fold dilutions of the broth culture were made, with Mueller-Hinton broth, so that 10^7 and 10^5 CFU/ml were used as inocula. An inoculum of 10^5 CFU/ml was used in all other studies of gram-negative bacilli. Studies of the

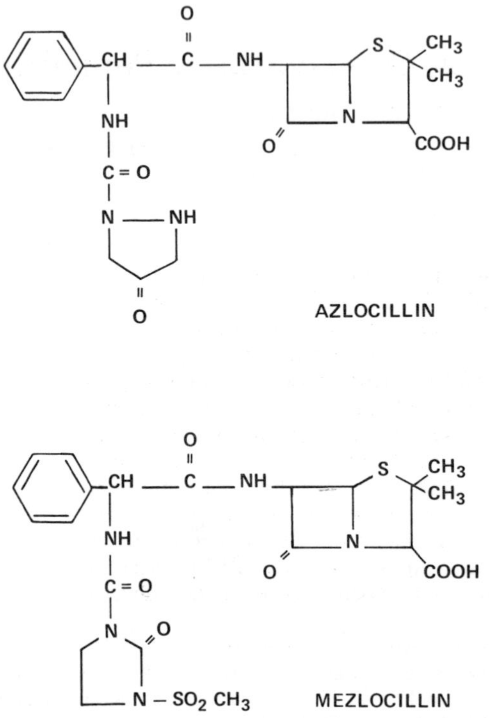

FIG. 1. *Chemical structure of azlocillin and mezlocillin.*

effect of pH on the activity of azlocillin were conducted in Mueller-Hinton broth, and the pH was adjusted to 6.4, 7.2, and 8.2 with phosphate buffer. Studies comparing the activity of azlocillin with mezlocillin, BLP-1654, carbenicillin, and ticarcillin were conducted in Mueller-Hinton broth. Fifty isolates each of *E. coli*, *Klebsiella* spp., *P. aeruginosa*, *Serratia* spp., *Enterobacter* spp., and *P. mirabilis* and 14 isolates of indole-positive *Proteus* spp. were used. Isolates were selected so that organisms with differing susceptibilities to azlocillin were included.

Azlocillin and mezlocillin (Bay 6905 and 1353) were supplied as powders by Delbay Pharmaceuticals Inc., Bloomfield, N.J. Carbenicillin and ticarcillin were supplied by Beecham Pharmaceuticals, Bristol, Tenn. BLP-1654, 6 [D-α(3-guanylureido)-phenylacetamido]-penicillanic acid, was supplied by Bristol Laboratories, Syracuse, N.Y. All antibiotics were diluted serially in Mueller-Hinton broth or tryptose phosphate broth. The minimum inhibitory concentration (MIC) was determined as no visible growth after 18 h of incubation at 37°C. The minimum bactericidal concentration (MBC) was defined as the lowest concentration of drug that yielded less than 5 colonies on subculture to sheep blood agar (99% kill). A 0.01-ml calibrated pipette was utilized to transfer the inoculum. Comparative studies were performed simultaneously in triplicate.

RESULTS

The in vitro susceptibility of azlocillin against gram-positive cocci and gram-negative bacilli is shown in Fig. 2. At a concentration of 12.5 μg/ml, over 75% of the isolates of *P. aeruginosa* were inhibited. Both indole-negative and -positive *Proteus* spp. were susceptible to azlocillin, with 75% of *P. mirabilis* inhibited at 1.56 μg/ml and 71% of indole-positive *Proteus* spp. inhibited at 12.5 μg/ml. Azlocillin exhibited moderate activity against isolates of *E. coli* and *Serratia* spp., inhibiting 63 and 46%, respectively, at a concentration of 12.5 μg/ml. *Klebsiella* spp. and *Enterobacter* spp. showed less activity with only 21 and 26%, respectively, inhibited at the same concentration of 12.5 μg/ml. All isolates of *S. pyogenes* were inhibited by a concentration of 0.10 μg or less per ml. However, only four of nine isolates of *S. pneumoniae* were inhibited at 0.10 μg/ml. The majority of the penicillin G-susceptible *S. aureus* were inhibited by 0.20 μg or less of azlocillin per ml, whereas the penicillin G-resistant *S. aureus* was also resistant to azlocillin. The MBC generally was the same as, or one concentration higher than, the MIC.

The effect of inoculum size on the MIC and MBC was determined for 10 isolates each of *K. pneumoniae*, *E. coli*, and *P. aeruginosa*. All of the isolates of *E. coli* were completely inhibited at 6.25 μg/ml when an inoculum of 10^5 CFU/ml was used. At a concentration of 50 μg/ml or less, 8 of the 10 isolates of *K. pneumoniae* and 8 of the 10 isolates of *P. aeruginosa* were inhibited when an inoculum of 10^5 CFU/ml was used. With the exception of one isolate of *P. aeruginosa*, all the isolates had similar MICs and MBCs. None of the isolates was inhibited at a concentration of 400 μg/ml when an inoculum of 10^7 CFU/ml was used.

The effect of pH on susceptibility of 10 isolates each of *E. coli*, *K. pneumoniae*, and *P. aeruginosa* to azlocillin is shown in Fig. 3. The activity of azlocillin increased against all organisms as the pH became more alkaline. As shown in Fig. 4, media variation had little effect on the activity of azlocillin. However, isolates of *P. aeruginosa* were slightly more susceptible in nutrient broth, whereas isolates of *E. coli* and *K. pneumoniae* were not.

The susceptibility of isolates of Enterobacteriaceae was determined for azlocillin, carbenicillin, mezlocillin, ticarcillin, and BLP-1654 (Fig. 5). Mezlocillin was consistently more active than azlocillin. Mezlocillin was the most active penicillin against *Klebsiella* spp. Azlocillin was as active as BLP-1654 and inhibited 54% of the isolates at a concentration of 25 μg/ml. Azlocillin was the least active penicillin against *Enterobacter* spp.: 70% of the isolates were resistant to 25 μg/ml. Mezlocillin and carbenicillin were the most active penicillins against *Enterobacter* spp., although about half

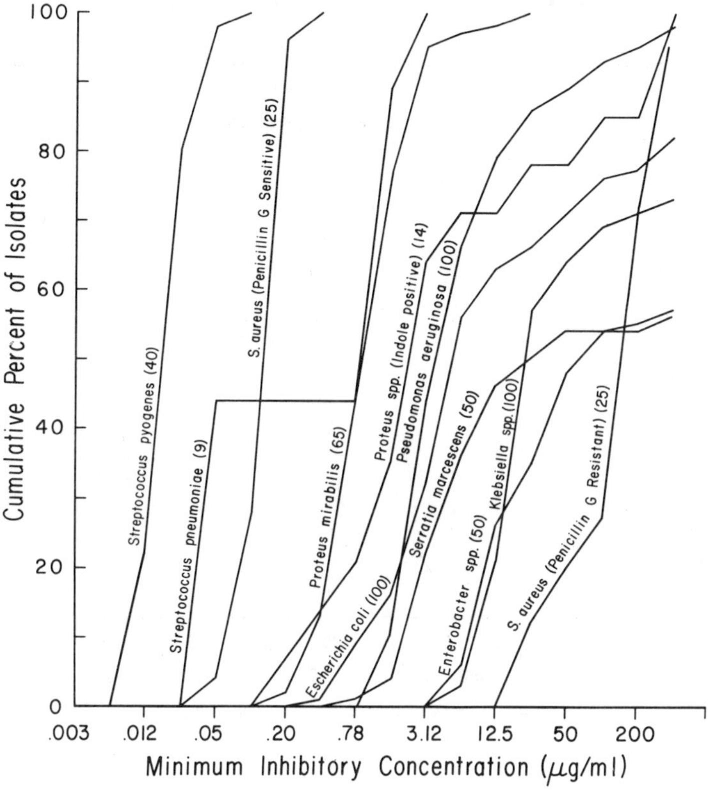

FIG. 2. *In vitro activity of azlocillin.*

of the isolates were resistant to 25 μg of these penicillins per ml. Azlocillin inhibited fewer isolates of *S. marcescens* at a concentration of 12.5 μg/ml than the other penicillins. However, some of the isolates resistant to carbenicillin and ticarcillin were inhibited by azlocillin. Mezlocillin was the most active penicillin against *Serratia* spp., *E. coli*, and *P. mirabilis*. Azlocillin, carbenicillin, BLP1654, and ticarcillin had similar activity against isolates of *E. coli*. All of these antibiotics were active against most of the isolates of *Proteus mirabilis* at a concentration of 3.12 μg/ml. At lower concentrations, azlocillin was the least active penicillin. Azlocillin also was less active than mezlocillin against indole-positive *Proteus* spp., but more active than BLP-1654. It inhibited 64% of these isolates at a concentration of 3.12 μg/ml.

The activity of the five penicillins against isolates of *P. aeruginosa* is shown in Fig. 6. Azlocillin and BLP-1654 were the most active penicillins and were substantially more active than carbenicillin. Mezlocillin and ticarcillin were intermediate in their activity. Eleven isolates of *P. aeruginosa* that were resistant to carbenicillin (MIC, ≥400 μg/ml) were tested for their susceptibility to the other penicillins (Table 1). Five isolates of *E. coli*, five isolates of *S. marcescens*, and four isolates of *Enterobacter* spp. were also tested. Those isolates of *P. aeruginosa*, which were inhibited by 400 μg of carbenicillin per ml, were generally susceptible to the other penicillins, and azlocillin was the most active. Most of the isolates of *P. aeruginosa* resistant to 400 μg of carbenicillin per ml were also resistant to the other penicillins. All of the isolates of other gram-negative bacilli were not inhibited by 400 μg of any of these penicillins per ml.

DISCUSSION

Azlocillin is a new ureido-substituted penicillin with activity against gram-negative bacilli. In general, its spectrum of activity is similar to that of BLP-1654 (5). The only major advantage of azlocillin is its antipseudomonal activity, which is substantially greater than carbenicillin. Against most isolates of *P. aeruginosa*, it is four times more active than ticarcillin. Another new penicillin, mezlocillin, has a broader spectrum of activity than azlocillin, but is not as active against *P. aeruginosa*. A major disadvantage of BLP-1654 was renal damage, which was observed in toxicology studies. Azlocillin

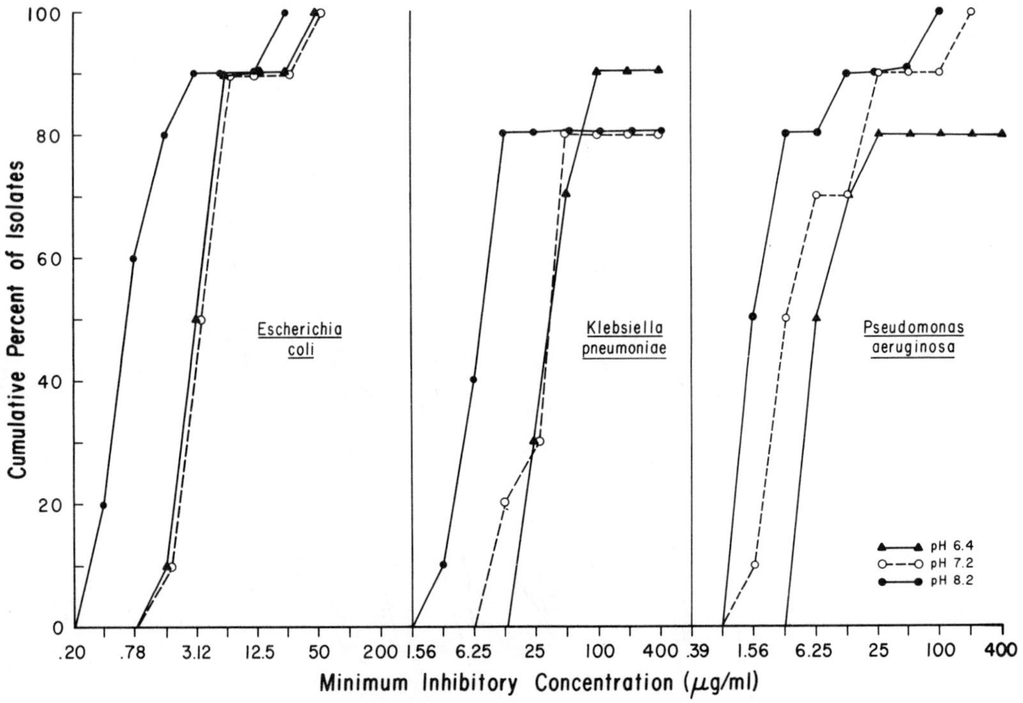

FIG. 3. *Effect of pH on activity of azlocillin.*

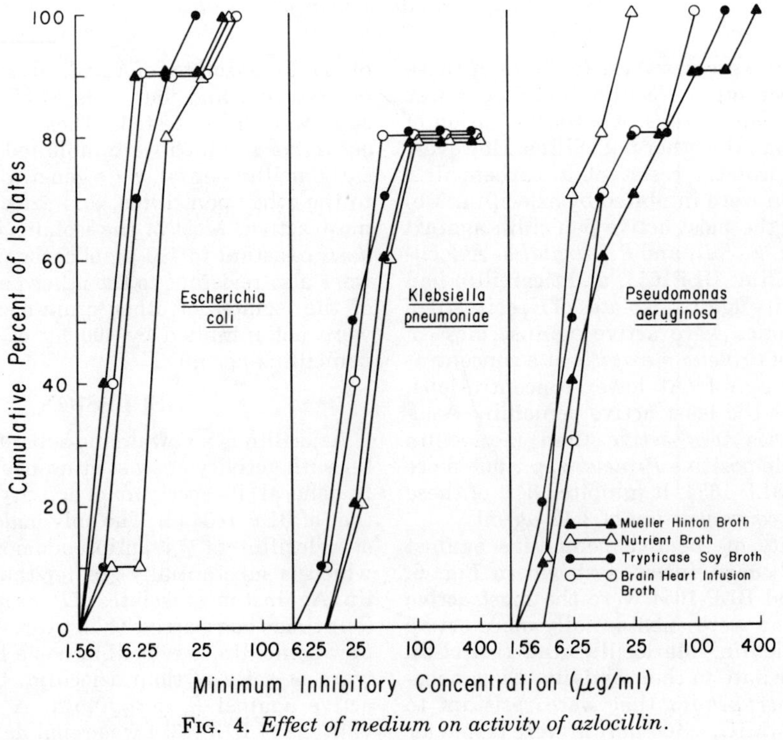

FIG. 4. *Effect of medium on activity of azlocillin.*

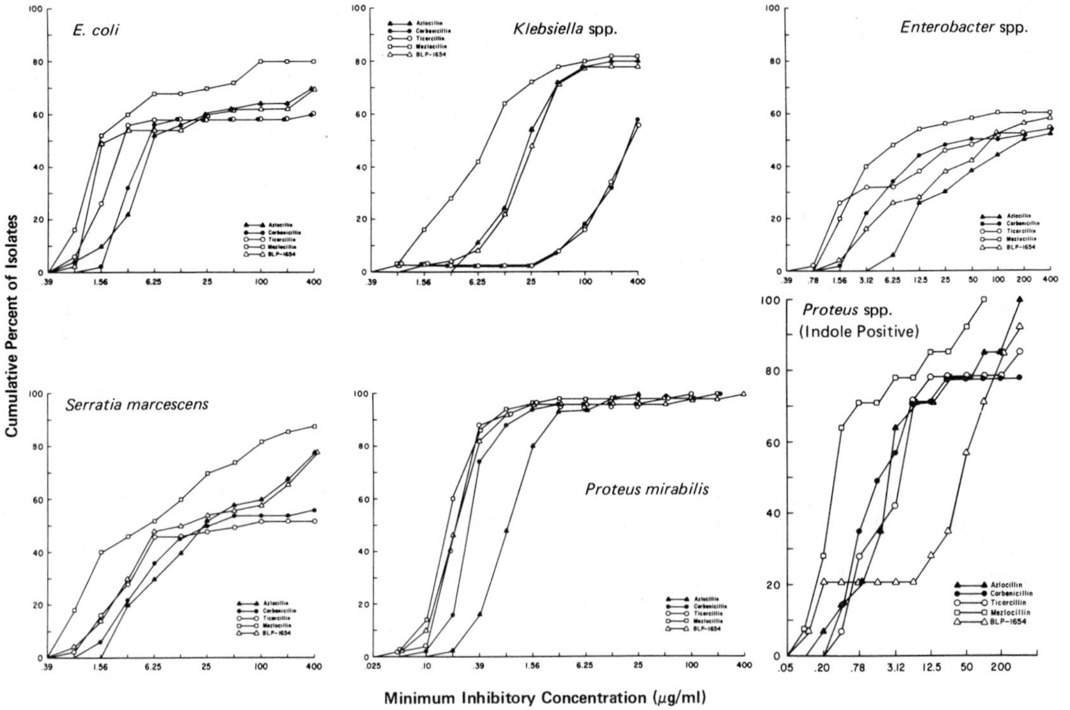

FIG. 5. *Comparative activity of antibiotics against gram-negative bacilli. Fifty isolates each were used except for indole-positive Proteus spp., where only 14 isolates were available.*

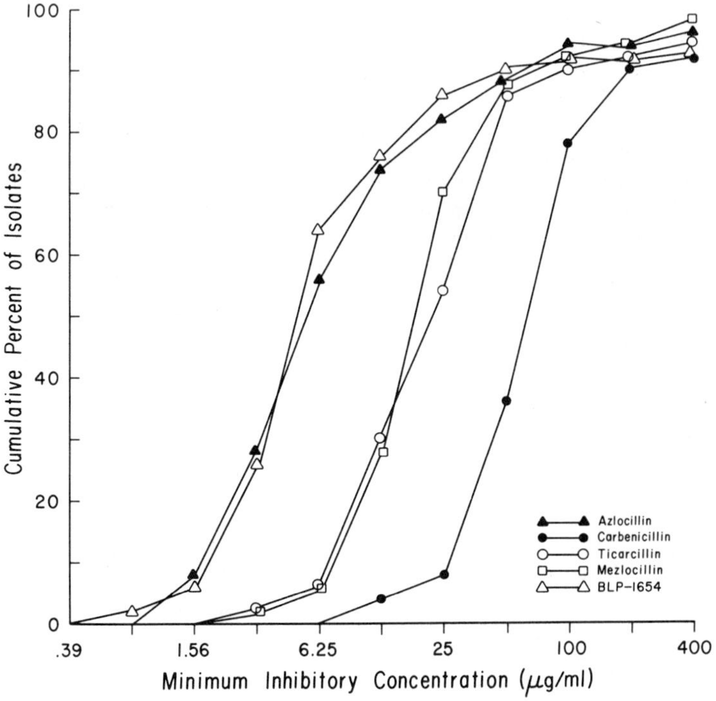

FIG. 6. *Comparative activity of penicillins against P. aeruginosa.*

TABLE 1. *Activity of azlocillin against P. aeruginosa resistant to carbenicillin*

MIC (μg/ml)				
Carbenicillin	Azlocillin	BLP-1654	Mezlocillin	Ticarcillin
400	25	12.5	200	100
400	50	200	200	200
400	50	>400	200	400
400	25	50	50	400
>400	>400	400	>400	>400
>400	>400	>400	>400	>400
>400	50	100	100	>400
>400	>400	400	>400	>400
>400	50	25	100	400
>400	>400	>400	>400	>400
>400	400	>400	>400	>400

does not appear to cause nephrotoxicity (E. F. Murray, personal communication). Our in vitro results are somewhat better than those obtained by Krasemann, who found nearly 60% of isolates of *Klebsiella* spp. and *S. marcescens* resistant to azlocillin (C. Krasemann, Prog. Abstr. Intersci. Conf. Antimicrob. Agents Chemother., 16th, Chicago, Ill., Abstr. 346, 1976).

Unfortunately, most isolates of *P. aeruginosa* and other gram-negative bacilli that were resistant to carbenicillin were also resistant to azlocillin. However, a few carbenicillin-resistant isolates of *P. aeruginosa* were susceptible to azlocillin. This may be explained by the fact that ureido-penicillins are resistant to destruction by the β-lactamase produced by these organisms (B. Wiedemann, V. Kremery, and H. Knothe, International Congress of Chemotherapy, London, Abstr. M366, 1975). Azlocillin was active against those isolates of *P. aeruginosa* that were only marginally susceptible to carbenicillin and ticarcillin. This could be of importance clinically, since it is difficult to achieve serum concentrations of carbenicillin of 400 μg/ml without toxicity.

Inoculum size had a major effect on the activity of azlocillin. It was inactive against all isolates of *E. coli*, *K. pneumoniae*, and *P. aeruginosa* when a large inoculum was used. It has been suggested that a larger inoculum contains a greater number of resistant cells. This effect of inoculum variation has been observed by other investigations with other penicillins, including BLP-1654 and pirbenicillin (4, 5, 8, 9). The clinical relevance of this observation is not clear.

The effect of pH on the activity of azlocillin is similar to the results obtained with other semisynthetic penicillins (3). Its activity increases as the pH increases. Media variation had little effect on the activity of azlocillin. However, the activity of other penicillins, like BLP-1654 and pirbenicillin, is influenced by the type of medium utilized (4, 5).

Azlocillin is an interesting semisynthetic penicillin, because it is more active than carbenicillin and ticarcillin against *P. aeruginosa* and has a somewhat broader spectrum of activity. Pharmacology studies indicate that adequate serum concentrations of this drug can be obtained, and preliminary therapeutic studies have been encouraging (H. Lode, U. Niestrath, P. Koeppe, and H. Langmaack, Prog. Abstr. Intersci. Conf. Antimicrob. Agents Chemother., 16th, Chicago, Ill., Abstr. 348, 1976). It is deserving of further investigation to ascertain its potential value for clinical therapeutic studies.

ACKNOWLEDGMENTS

Supported by Public Health Service grant CA 10042 from the National Cancer Institute.

LITERATURE CITED

1. **Bodey, G. P.** 1972. Antibiotic therapy of infections in patients undergoing cancer chemotherapy, p. 49–88. *In* H. Schonfled, R. W. Brockman, and F. E. Hahn (ed.), Antibiotics and chemotherapy—chemotherapy under special conditions, vol. 18. S. Karger, New York.
2. **Bodey, G. P., E. Middleman, T. Umsawasdi, and V. Rodriguez.** 1972. Infections in cancer patients—results with gentamicin sulfate therapy. Cancer 29:1697–1701.
3. **Bodey, G. P. and T. Pan.** 1977. Mezlocillin: in vitro studies of a new broad-spectrum penicillin. Antimicrob. Agents Chemother. 11:74–79.
4. **Bodey, G. P., V. Rodriguez, and S. Weaver.** 1976. Pirbenicillin, a new semisynthetic penicillin with broad-spectrum activity. Antimicrob. Agents Chemother. 9:668–674.
5. **Bodey, G. P., and D. Stewart.** 1971. In vitro studies of semisynthetic α-(substituted-ureido) penicillins. Appl. Microbiol. 21:710–717.
6. **Eickhoff, T. C.** 1973. Infectious complications in renal transplant patients. Transplant. Proc. 5:1233–1238.
7. **Inagaki, J., Rodriguez, V. and Bodey, G. P.** 1974. Causes of death in cancer patients. Cancer 33:568–573.
8. **Neu, H. C. and E. B. Winshell.** 1971. In vitro studies of a semisynthetic penicillin, 6-[D(-)-α-carboxy-3-thienylacetamido] penicillanic acid (BRL 2288), active against *Pseudomonas*, p. 385–389. Antimicrob. Agents Chemother. 1970.
9. **Standiford, H. C., A. C. Kind, and W. M. M. Kirby.** 1969. Laboratory and clinical studies of carbenicillin against gram-negative bacilli, p. 286–291. Antimicrob. Agents Chemother. 1968.

ANTIMICROBIAL AGENTS AND CHEMOTHERAPY, May 1977, p. 871-876 Vol. 11, No. 5

Inducible Resistance to D-Cycloserine in *Bacillus subtilis* 168

VIRGINIA L. CLARK[1] AND FRANK E. YOUNG*

Department of Microbiology, University of Rochester, School of Medicine and Dentistry, Rochester, New York 14642

Received for publication 22 December 1976

Resistance to D-cycloserine could be induced in *Bacillus subtilis* 168 by sublethal concentrations of D-cycloserine. Sensitivity to the antibiotic could be regained by growth in the absence of D-cycloserine. The bactericidal activity of D-cycloserine apparently was not altered by resistant cells, and peptidoglycan synthesis was still inhibited by D-cycloserine in resistant cells. The D-cycloserine resistance apparently resulted from a decreased uptake of the antibiotic. The decrease in D-cycloserine transport could be prevented by simultaneous treatment of the cells with rifampin and D-cycloserine. D-Cycloserine was transported by the same system as glycine in *B. subtilis*. D-Cycloserine was able to exchange for intracellular glycine in both sensitive and resistant cells, suggesting that D-cycloserine is not excluded from the cell in resistant cultures.

Resistance to antibiotics can be achieved by a variety of mechanisms: destruction or chemical modification of the antibiotic (1, 3), alteration of the target of the antibiotic (1), or decreased intracellular accumulation of the antibiotic (1, 4). Tetracycline, an inhibitor of protein synthesis, is actively transported into the cell. Bacteria resistant to this antibiotic have a markedly reduced rate of uptake of tetracycline (1, 4). The induction of tetracycline resistance by sublethal concentrations of the antibiotic can be prevented by inhibitors of ribonucleic acid or protein synthesis (10). Resistant cells contain a protein not found in sensitive strains (14–16), and this protein can be released from *Escherichia coli* by osmotic shock (4).

D-Cycloserine is an analogue of D-alanine and is therefore an inhibitor of DL-alanine racemase (EC 5.1.1.1) (6) and D-alanine:D-alanine ligase (EC 6.3.2.4) (8). Because of its structural similarity, it is actively transported into the cell by the same system(s) that is responsible for D-alanine, L-alanine, and glycine transport (5, 11) in a variety of bacterial species. Previous reports (12, 13) indicate that D-cycloserine resistance in *E. coli* results from a loss, due to mutation, of the active transport of the antibiotic. Sensitivity to the antibiotic is regained only by reversion of the mutation(s). In this study we shall present evidence for an inducible resistance to D-cycloserine in *Bacillus subtilis* 168. This resistance is more similar to the inducible tetracycline resistance (4) than it is to the D-cycloserine resistance observed in *E. coli* (13).

[1] Present address: Department of Biology, Massachusetts Institute of Technology, Cambridge, MA 02139.

MATERIALS AND METHODS

Materials. The D-[U-^{14}C]cycloserine (specific activity, 51 μCi/mmol) was a generous gift from Roger Harned of Commercial Solvents Corp., Terre Haute, Ind. The [U-^{14}C]glycine (specific activity, 92 mCi/mmol) and Omnifluor were purchased from New England Nuclear. Rifampin and D-alanine were purchased from Sigma Chemical Co., and acid-hydrolyzed casein was from Nutritional Biochemicals Corp. All other chemicals were of reagent-grade purity.

Strains. The strains of *B. subtilis* 168 used in this study were BR151 (*lys-3 trpC2 metB10*) and RUB1402 (*dal hisA1 leu-8 metB10*).

Growth conditions. Cells were grown aerobically on a New Brunswick gyratory shaker at 240 rpm at 37°C in Spizizen minimal salts medium (10) supplemented with 22 mM glucose and 0.5% casein hydrolysate. Additional supplements included 0.5 mM D-alanine for RUB1402 and 40 μg of tryptophan per ml for BR151. Turbidity was determined with a Klett-Summerson colorimeter at 620 nm. The medium was inoculated from an overnight culture of cells grown in the same medium to give an initial turbidity reading of 10 Klett units.

Determination of D-cycloserine resistance. Cells whose D-cycloserine resistance was to be determined were used to inoculate a 10-ml culture to give a final concentration of about 4×10^7 cells per ml. The volume of inoculating culture required was estimated from the Klett reading, with a Klett reading of 40 corresponding to 4×10^7 cells per ml. The viable count was determined immediately after the inoculation of the culture (treated cells). D-Cycloserine was added to a final concentration of 0.5 mM, and the culture was grown aerobically at 37°C for 2 h, at which time the viable count was again determined (survivors). Cycloserine resistance was expressed as survivors per treated cell.

Preparation of cells for transport. In most cases, late-exponential-phase cells (about 150 Klett units) were harvested by filtration (Millipore Corp., 0.45-μm pore size, 45-mm diameter), washed with Spizizen minimal salts, and suspended in a volume of Spizizen minimal salts equal to three times the culture volume. This gave a final cell protein concentration (7) of about 100 μg/ml. Additions were made to this incubation mixture as indicated, and the cell suspension was incubated aerobically at 37°C for the time indicated before transport was measured.

Measurement of transport. Uptake was initiated by the addition of 2.0 ml of cell suspension to 0.5 ml of minimal salts containing the ^{14}C-labeled compound to be transported plus any additions as indicated (uptake mixture). After incubation of the cells at 37°C for the indicated time, transport was terminated by membrane filtration (Millipore Corp., 0.45-μm pore size, 24-mm diameter). The filters were washed with 2 ml of Spizizen minimal salts, placed in scintillation vials, and dried overnight at 45°C; 5 ml of nonaqueous scintillation fluid was added, and the radioactivity was determined in a Beckman LS-230 liquid scintillation spectrometer. The filtration and washing procedures took about 5 s. The sensitivity of transport to inhibition by azide was determined with cells incubated for 30 min at 37°C in Spizizen minimal salts plus 10 mM sodium azide.

Analytical procedures. Protein was determined by the method of Lowry et al. (7) for trichloroacetic acid precipitates, with bovine serum albumin as a standard. Peptidoglycan biosynthesis was measured by incubating cells with 0.09 μmol of *N*-acetyl-D-[1-^{14}C]glucosamine for 2 min at 37°C in complete growth medium. Peptidoglycan was isolated by the fractionation procedure of Park and Hancock (9), and the radioactivity was determined as discussed below.

Determination of radioactivity. The radioactivity of nonaqueous samples was determined with the use of a scintillation fluid consisting of 4 g of Omnifluor per liter of toluene.

RESULTS

Characterization of D-cycloserine resistance in *B. subtilis*. During the study of the effects of inhibition of cell wall biosynthesis by D-cycloserine in *B. subtilis,* we observed that, as a function of time and D-cycloserine concentration, cells were able to recover from inhibition and resume growth. Figure 1 shows the turbidities of cultures treated with various concentrations of D-cycloserine. There was a short time lag before the effect of the antibiotic was evident, which was followed by a decrease in turbidity due to lysis of cells (as determined by phase microscopy and viable count). The cultures were able to recover and resume growth, as a function of the initial concentration of D-cycloserine. This resumption of growth proceeded even if fresh D-cycloserine (0.5 mM) was added (data not shown).

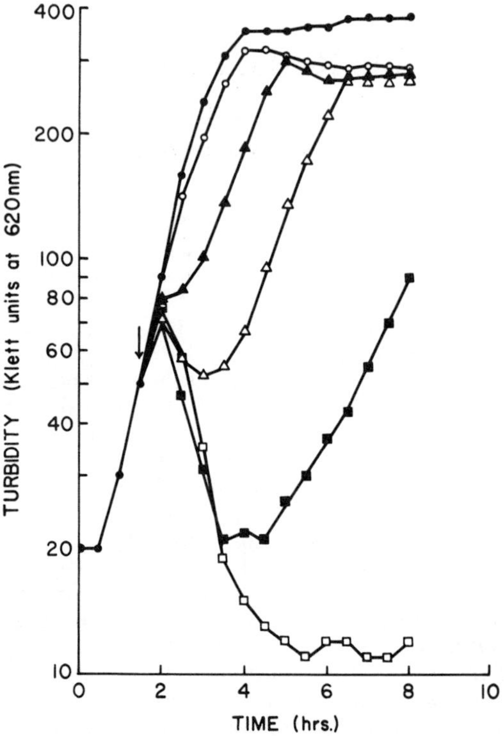

FIG. 1. *Recovery of cells from inhibition by D-cycloserine. Strain BR151 was grown in glucose-minimal salts medium. At the time indicated, D-cycloserine was added to a final concentration of:* (●) *0 mM;* (○) *0.05 mM;* (▲) *0.1 mM;* (△) *0.2 mM;* (■) *0.3 mM; or* (□) *0.5 mM.*

A method of measuring D-cycloserine resistance was devised that was more convenient than monitoring turbidity (see Materials and Methods). The principle is the measurement of viable count before and 2 h after the addition of D-cycloserine. Resistance is then expressed as survivors per treated cell. Figure 2 compares the D-cycloserine resistance of cells not exposed to the antibiotic with that of cells grown in the presence of D-cycloserine for 90 min. At a concentration of D-cycloserine of 0.5 mM, there was almost a 1,000-fold difference in the survival rate of exposed cells.

The resistance to and the transport of D-cycloserine was measured as a function of growth (Fig. 3). Early-logarithmic-phase cells were highly sensitive to killing by the antibiotic, but there was an increase in resistance as growth progressed. The transport of D-cycloserine also

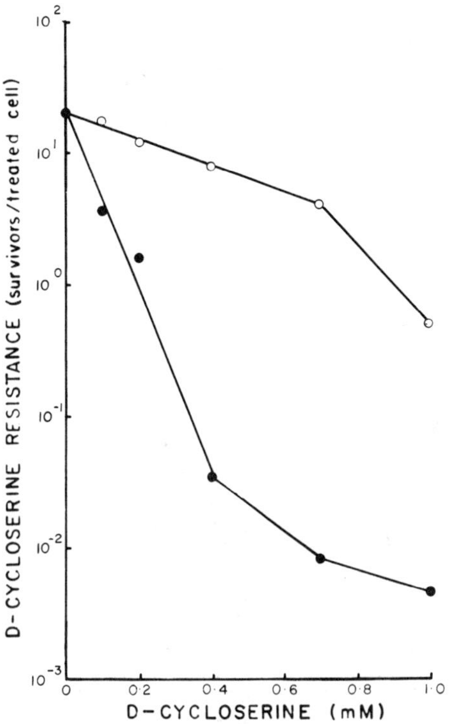

FIG. 2. *D-Cycloserine resistance in sensitive and resistant cells. D-Cycloserine resistance was determined in strain BR151 as described in Materials and Methods in cells not previously exposed to D-cycloserine (●) and in cells grown in the presence of 0.1 mM D-cycloserine for 90 min (○).*

decreased as growth progressed (Fig. 3). If D-cycloserine was added to early-logarithmic-phase cells, the loss of D-cycloserine transport was significantly enhanced (Fig. 4). This loss of transport could be prevented by simultaneous treatment with rifampin.

Induction of D-cycloserine resistance. To demonstrate that D-cycloserine can induce D-cycloserine resistance, early-logarithmic-phase cells were suspended in Spizizen minimal salts medium containing 1 mM glucose, and D-cycloserine resistance was monitored (Fig. 5). After 5 min of incubation, 0.1 mM D-cycloserine was added to one of the two cultures. It can be seen that D-cycloserine resistance in the treated culture increased rapidly compared with the control culture. Under these conditions it is clear that D-cycloserine resistance can be induced by treatment of the cells with D-cycloserine.

Reversibility of D-cycloserine resistance. The acquisition of D-cycloserine resistance was reversible (Fig. 6). D-Cycloserine resistance was induced as described in Fig. 5 for 15 min, and then cells were resuspended in fresh complete growth medium with no antibiotic. The cells were kept in the early logarithmic phase of growth by repeated dilution into fresh medium. The D-cycloserine resistance was monitored as a function of time, and it can be seen that, after a short time lag, sensitivity to the antibiotic was regained.

D-Cycloserine inhibition of peptidoglycan. D-Cycloserine resistance could be attained by the formation of enzymes that would destroy or modify the antibiotic, by the alteration of the target site of the antibiotic such that it is no longer inhibited by the antibiotic, or by a decreased accumulation of the antibiotic. To de-

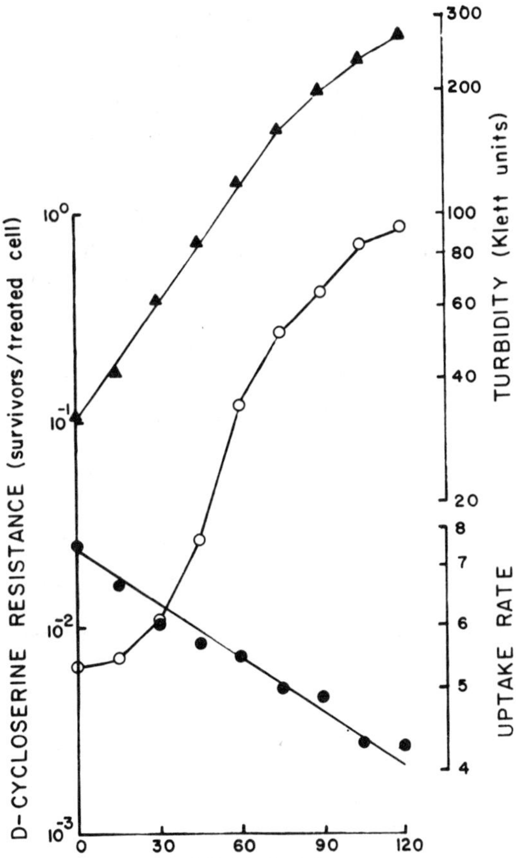

FIG. 3. *Determination of D-cycloserine resistance and transport as a function of growth. Strain BR151 was grown in glucose-minimal salts medium; at appropriate times the turbidity of the culture (▲), D-cycloserine resistance (○), and D-cycloserine transport (●) were determined as described in Materials and Methods. Uptake rate is expressed as nanomoles of D-cycloserine transported per minute per milligram of protein at a D-cycloserine concentration of 0.1 mM.*

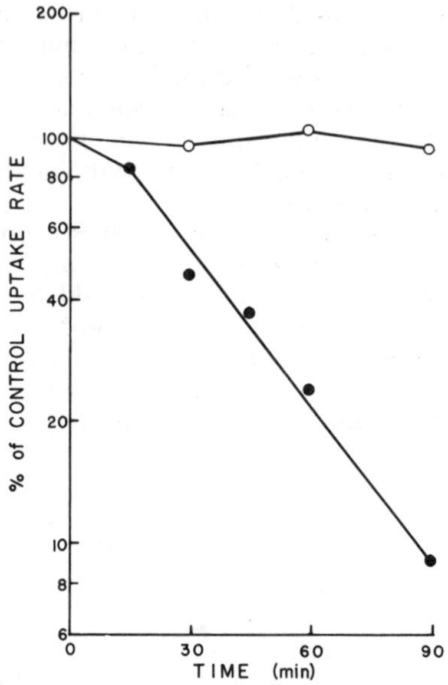

FIG. 4. *Effect of* D-*cycloserine incubation on the transport of* D-*cycloserine. 0.1 mM* D-*cycloserine* (●) *or 0.1 mM* D-*cycloserine plus 5 μg of rifampin per ml* (○) *was added to growing BR151 cells at zero time, and the transport of* D-*cycloserine was measured in washed cell samples at the indicated times. The control uptake rate was that observed at zero time. Transport was measured at a* D-[^{14}C]*cycloserine concentration of 0.1 mM.*

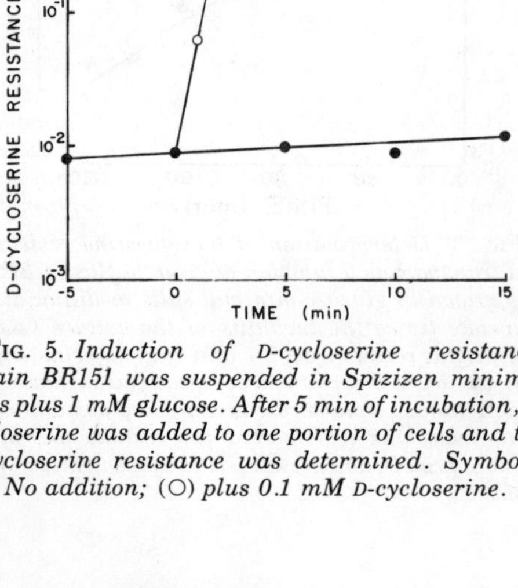

FIG. 5. *Induction of* D-*cycloserine resistance. Strain BR151 was suspended in Spizizen minimal salts plus 1 mM glucose. After 5 min of incubation,* D-*cycloserine was added to one portion of cells and the* D-*cycloserine resistance was determined. Symbols:* (●) *No addition;* (○) *plus 0.1 mM* D-*cycloserine.*

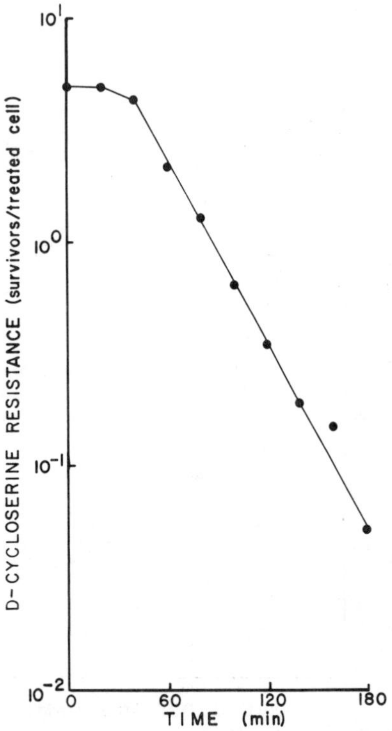

FIG. 6. *Recovery of* D-*cycloserine sensitivity. Strain BR151 was induced for* D-*cycloserine resistance by incubation in Spizizen minimal salts containing 1 mM glucose and 0.1 mM* D-*cycloserine for 10 min. The* D-*cycloserine was removed by membrane filtration (0.65-μm pore size), and cells were suspended in glucose-minimal salts growth medium. Samples were removed at 20-min intervals, and* D-*cycloserine resistance was determined as described in Materials and Methods. Cells were periodically diluted into fresh medium to maintain them in the early logarithmic phase of growth.*

termine whether the D-cycloserine is inactivated, the culture supernatant from resistant cells containing D-cycloserine was obtained by membrane filtration (0.45-μm pore size). When cells unexposed to the antibiotic were added to this culture medium, they were killed, indicating that resistant cells do not inactivate significant quantities of the D-cycloserine (data not shown). To determine whether the target site of the antibiotic is altered, peptidoglycan synthesis in the presence or absence of D-cycloserine was measured in uninduced and induced cells (Table 1). At the concentration of D-cycloserine used, peptidoglycan synthesis was inhibited by 98% in uninduced cells and by 95% in induced cells. The actual rate of synthesis in the presence of the antibiotic was lower in the induced cells than in the uninduced cells, in-

TABLE 1. *Inhibition of peptidoglycan synthesis by D-cycloserine in uninduced and induced cells of B. subtilis 168*[a]

Incubation conditions	Assay conditions	Peptidoglycan synthesis	Inhibition of peptidoglycan synthesis (%)
No addition	No addition	0.371	
	+ D-Cycloserine	0.0088	98
+ D-Cycloserine	No addition	0.113	
	+ D-Cycloserine	0.0051	95

[a] A sample of cells was induced for D-cycloserine resistance by incubation in 0.1 mM D-cycloserine for 10 min as previously described. The D-cycloserine was removed by membrane filtration (0.65-μm pore size). Peptidoglycan synthesis was assayed by incubation of uninduced or induced cells with 0.09 μmol of *N*-acetyl-D-[1-^{14}C]glucosamine for 2 min at 37°C in complete growth medium containing 5 μg of rifampin per ml plus or minus 2 mM D-cycloserine. Peptidoglycan was purified by Park-Hancock fractionation. Peptidoglycan synthesis is expressed as nanomoles of *N*-acetylglucosamine incorporated per minute per milligram of protein.

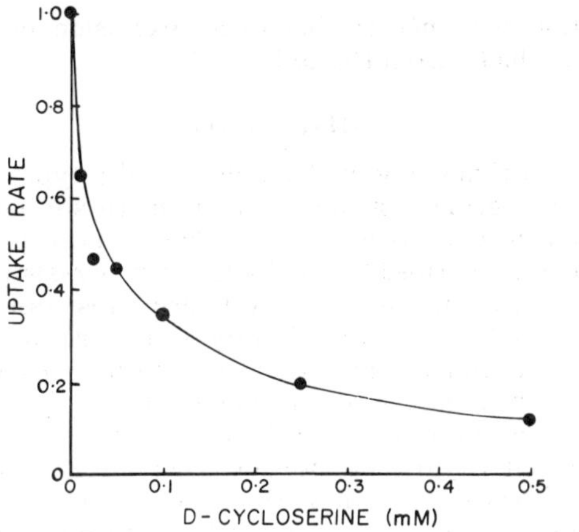

FIG. 7. *Decrease in accumulation of D-cycloserine as a function of the concentration of D-cycloserine used for the induction of resistance. Strain BR151 was induced for D-cycloserine resistance by incubation in Spizizen minimal salts containing 1 mM glucose and the indicated concentrations of D-cycloserine for 10 min. Uptake rate is expressed as nanomoles of D-cycloserine transported per minute per milligram of protein at a D-[^{14}C]cycloserine concentration of 20 μM.*

dicating that the target site of D-cycloserine is not more resistant to inhibition in resistant cells. The lower rate of synthesis in induced cells may have been due to residual D-cycloserine that was not removed during the washing procedure.

Decrease in D-cycloserine transport induced by various concentrations of D-cycloserine. To determine the effect of D-cycloserine on transport, cells were treated with various concentrations of D-cycloserine for 10 min, after which the rate of uptake of D-cycloserine was determined. The apparent mode of D-cycloserine resistance was a reduction of D-cycloserine transport (Fig. 7). The decrease in antibiotic transport was dependent on the incubation concentration of D-cycloserine. Concentrations of D-cycloserine that were subinhibitory (0.1 mM) induced a considerable loss of transport.

Exchange of D-cycloserine for intracellular glycine. It has been proposed (4) that tetracycline resistance is due to the synthesis of a protein that prevents the entry of the antibiotic into the cell. To determine whether D-cycloserine is able to enter D-cycloserine-resistant cells, we investigated the ability of the antibiotic to exchange for preloaded [^{14}C]glycine (Fig. 8). Unexposed and induced cells were allowed to take up [^{14}C]glycine for 8 min, at which time excess glycine or D-cycloserine was added. If D-cycloserine is excluded from the cell in induced cells, D-cycloserine should not be able to cause the loss of [^{14}C]glycine from the cells. However,

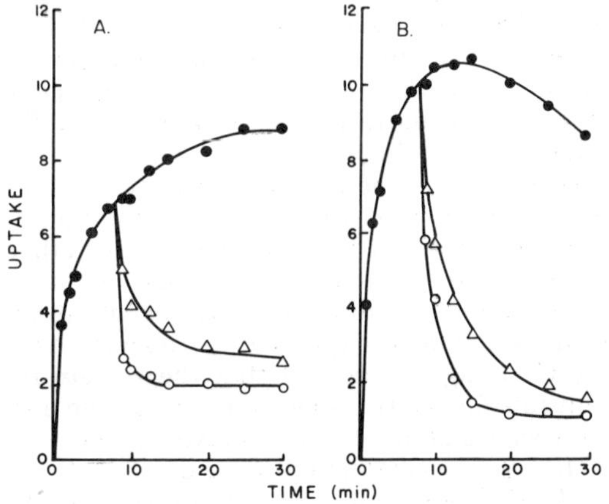

FIG. 8. *Exchange for preloaded [^{14}C]glycine in sensitive and resistant cells. RUB1402 cells unexposed to D-cycloserine (A) or induced to D-cycloserine resistance by incubation in Spizizen minimal salts plus 0.1 mM D-cycloserine for 15 min (B) were allowed to accumulate 20 μM [^{14}C]glycine for 8 min, at which time no addition was made (●), 50 mM glycine was added (○), or 50 mM D-cycloserine was added (△). Uptake is expressed as nanomoles of glycine transported per minute per milligram of protein.*

if it is not excluded in induced cells, the antibiotic should be effective in causing the loss of intracellular [^{14}C]glycine. As can be seen, the latter alternative occurred. It therefore appears that the reduction in D-cycloserine accumulation may not be due to an exclusion of the antibiotic from the cell.

DISCUSSION

In this study we have described a type of D-cycloserine resistance that is more similar to tetracycline resistance (4) than it is to previously described types of D-cycloserine resistance (12, 13). In this case D-cycloserine resistance is inducible by subinhibitory concentrations of the antibiotic, and sensitivity to D-cycloserine can be regained by allowing the cells to grow in the absence of the antibiotic. This recovery of sensitivity to D-cycloserine is not observed in *E. coli* cells resistant to the antibiotic (13), since resistance is due to a mutation(s) in the gene(s) responsible for transport of D-cycloserine, D-alanine, and glycine.

The apparent mode of the inducible resistance is a marked decrease in the accumulation of D-cycloserine. The antibiotic probably is not chemically altered, since the culture supernatant from cells that have become resistant is still able to kill sensitive cells. The target of the antibiotic, cell wall biosynthesis, is not less sensitive to inhibition by D-cycloserine. Cells induced for D-cycloserine resistance rapidly lose the ability to accumulate the antibiotic, and the loss of D-cycloserine transport is dependent upon the concentration of antibiotic used for induction.

Although it is known that tetracycline-resistant cells have decreased rates of accumulation of the antibiotic, it is not established whether this is due to an exclusion of uptake or to an increased rate of efflux (4). This alternative can be investigated for D-cycloserine transport, taking advantage of the fact that the system responsible for the transport of D-cycloserine also transports D-alanine, L-alanine, and glycine (2, 5). If D-cycloserine uptake were decreased, the antibiotic would enter the cell at a slower rate and would be less efficient in exchanging for preloaded [^{14}C]glycine. If efflux is increased, then the D-cycloserine will cause the loss of preloaded [^{14}C]glycine from the cell. The latter case was found to occur, indicating that the decreased accumulation of D-cycloserine may be caused by an active efflux of the antibiotic from the cell.

ACKNOWLEDGMENTS

This work was supported by Public Health Service grants 5TI-GM-00592 from the National Institute of General Medical Science and 5ROI-AI-10141 from the National Institute of Allergy and Infectious Diseases.

LITERATURE CITED

1. **Benveniste, R., and J. Davies.** 1973. Mechanisms of antibiotic resistance in bacteria. Annu. Rev. Biochem. 42:471–506.
2. **Clark, V. L., and F. E. Young.** 1974. Active transport of D-alanine and related amino acids by whole cells of *Bacillus subtilis*. J. Bacteriol. 120:1085–1092.
3. **Davis, J. E., and R. E. Benveniste.** 1974. Enzymes that inactivate antibiotics in transit to their targets. Ann. N.Y. Acad. Sci. 235:130–136.
4. **Franklin, T. J.** 1973. Antibiotic transport in bacteria. Crit. Rev. Microbiol. 2:253–272.
5. **Halpern, Y. S.** 1974. Genetics of amino acid transport in bacteria. Annu. Rev. Genet. 8:103–133.
6. **Lambert, M. P., and F. C. Neuhaus.** 1972. Mechanism of D-cycloserine action: alanine racemase from *Escherichia coli* W. J. Bacteriol. 110:978–987.
7. **Lowry, O. H., N. J. Rosebrough, A. L. Farr, and R. J. Randall.** 1951. Protein measurement with the Folin phenol reagent. J. Biol. Chem. 193:265–275.
8. **Neuhaus, F. C., and J. L. Lynch.** 1964. The enzymatic synthesis of D-alanyl-D-alanine. III. On the inhibition of D-alanyl-D-alanine synthetase by the antibiotic D-cycloserine. Biochemistry 3:471–480.
9. **Park, J. T., and R. Hancock.** 1960. A fractionation procedure for studies of the synthesis of cell wall mucopeptide and other polymers in cells of *Staphylococcus aureus*. J. Gen. Microbiol. 22:249–258.
10. **Reynard, A. M., P. E. Noker, M. E. Beck, and L. F. Nellis.** 1975. Induction of tetracycline resistance in *Escherichia coli*. Microbios 14:157–166.
11. **Spizizen, J.** 1958. Transformation of biochemically deficient strains of *Bacillus subtilis* by deoxyribonucleate. Proc. Natl. Acad. Sci. U.S.A. 44:1072–1078.
12. **Wargel, R. J., C. A. Shadur, and F. C. Neuhaus.** 1970. Mechanism of D-cycloserine action: transport systems for D-alanine, D-cycloserine, L-alanine, and glycine. J. Bacteriol. 103:778–788.
13. **Wargel, R. J., C. A. Shadur, and F. C. Neuhaus.** 1971. Mechanism of D-cycloserine action: transport mutants for D-alanine, D-cycloserine, and glycine. J. Bacteriol. 105:1028–1035.
14. **Wojdani, A., R. R. Avtalion, and D. Sompolinsky.** 1976. Isolation and characterization of tetracycline resistance proteins from *Staphylococcus aureus* and *Escherichia coli*. Antimicrob. Agents Chemother. 9:526–534.
15. **Yang, H. L., G. Zubay, and S. B. Levy.** 1976. Synthesis of an R plasmid protein associated with tetracycline resistance is negatively regulated. Proc. Natl. Acad. Sci. U.S.A. 73:1509–1512.
16. **Young, T. W., and S. J. Hubball.** 1976. R-factor-mediated resistance to tetracycline in *Escherichia coli* K-12: an R-factor with a mutation to temperature-sensitive tetracycline resistance. Biochem. Biophys. Res. Commun. 70:117–124.

ANTIMICROBIAL AGENTS AND CHEMOTHERAPY, May 1977, p. 877-880 Vol. 11, No. 5

Printed in U.S.A.

D-Cycloserine-Induced Alterations in the Transport of D-Alanine and Glycine in *Bacillus subtilis* 168

VIRGINIA L. CLARK[1] AND FRANK E. YOUNG*

Department of Microbiology, University of Rochester, School of Medicine and Dentistry, Rochester, New York 14642

Received for publication 22 December 1976

D-Alanine, L-alanine, and glycine transport was investigated in *Bacillus subtilis* 168 cells that were phenotypically resistant to D-cycloserine. These cells showed enhanced rates of uptake as compared with that observed in sensitive cells. The usual enhancement in D-alanine and glycine transport resulting from treatment of the cells with D-cycloserine could be prevented by the addition of rifampin. Kinetic analyses of the initial rate of glycine transport indicated an increase in the V_{max} for transport in resistant cells, with no alteration in the K_m for glycine. Investigations of the net transport of glycine revealed that resistant cells maintained a higher gradient of glycine than did sensitive cells. Kinetic analyses of the net transport of glycine suggested that a new system for the accumulation of glycine was present in D-cycloserine-resistant cells.

The antibiotic D-cycloserine is actively transported, in various bacterial species, by the same system(s) responsible for the transport of D-alanine, L-alanine, and glycine (3, 5–7, 9, 11). Resistance to D-cycloserine has been reported to result from a decreased accumulation of the antibiotic (1, 4, 5, 12). In *Escherichia coli* there is a concomitant decrease in the transport D-alanine, L-alanine, and glycine in resistant cells (5, 12). We have reported an inducible D-cycloserine resistance in *Bacillus subtilis* 168 (4) that is also a result of a decreased accumulation of the antibiotic. In this paper we will present evidence that D-cycloserine-resistant cells of *B. subtilis* do not transport D-alanine, L-alanine, and glycine at reduced rates. In fact, the transport of D-alanine and glycine is enhanced by treatment of the cell with D-cycloserine.

MATERIALS AND METHODS

Materials. The L-[U-^{14}C]alanine (specific activity, 153 mCi/mmol), L-[U-^{14}C]proline (specific activity, 233 mCi/mmol), and Omnifluor were purchased from New England Nuclear; the D-[U-^{14}C]alanine (specific activity, 37 mCi/mmol) was obtained from Amersham/Searle Corp. Rifampin and D-alanine were purchased from Sigma Chemical Co., and acid-hydrolyzed casein was from Nutritional Biochemicals Corp. All other chemicals were of reagent-grade purity.

Strains and growth conditions. The strains of *B. subtilis* 168 and the growth conditions used were described previously (4).

[1] Present address: Department of Biology, Massachusetts Institute of Technology, Cambridge, MA 02139.

Measurement of transport. The preparation of cells for transport studies and the procedures for analysis of transport were similar to those in the accompanying paper (4).

Protein determination. Protein was determined by the method of Lowry et al. (8) for trichloroacetic acid precipitates, with bovine serum albumin as a standard.

Determination of radioactivity. The radioactivity of nonaqueous samples was determined with use of a scintillation fluid consisting of 4 g of Omnifluor per liter of toluene.

Calculation of intracellular substrate concentration. If it is assumed that *B. subtilis* protein constitutes 50% of the dry weight of the cell, and that the cell is 80% water throughout the growth cycle, then 1 mg of protein is equal to 2 mg of dry weight plus 8 mg of water. Therefore, since 1 mg of water is 1 μl, 1 mg of cell protein is approximately equal to 8 μl of water. To convert the uptake values that are expressed as nanomoles of substrate transported per milligram of protein to millimolar, divide by a factor of 8.

RESULTS

Transport of D-alanine in D-cycloserine-resistant cells. Previous reports of D-cycloserine resistance in *E. coli* (12) indicated a reduction in the transport of the antibiotic as the mechanism of resistance. In this case there is a concomitant reduction in the transport of D-alanine, L-alanine, and glycine. We investigated the rate of transport of D-alanine and glycine in growing cells of *B. subtilis* treated with D-cycloserine (Fig. 1). Under conditions in which D-cycloserine is transported at only 10% of the original rate after 90 min of treatment (data not

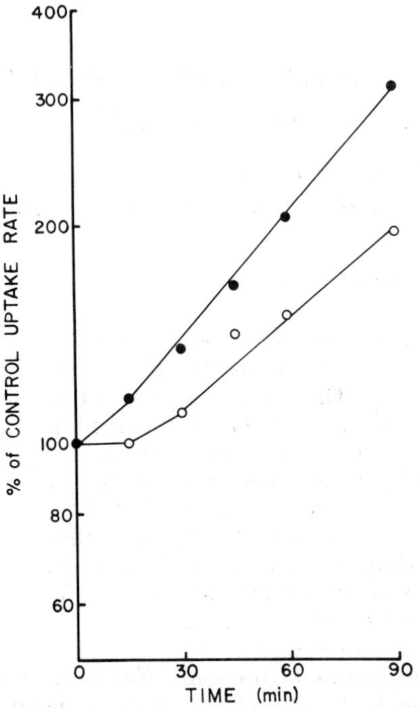

FIG. 1. *Effect of D-cycloserine incubation on the transport of D-alanine and glycine. 0.1 mM D-cycloserine was added to growing BR151 cells at zero time, and the transport of D-alanine (●) and glycine (○) was measured in washed cell samples at the indicated times. The control uptake rate was that observed at zero time. The substrate concentrations were: 1 μM D-[14C]alanine and 20 μM [14C]glycine.*

shown), the transport of D-alanine and glycine was substantially increased. The increase in D-alanine transport could also occur in the glucose-minimal salts medium used for the induction of D-cycloserine resistance (Fig. 2). Uninduced cells were suspended in minimal salts with no addition or plus D-cycloserine. The cells to which the antibiotic was added were initially slightly inhibited, but with time transport of D-alanine by these cells exceeded the level observed in untreated cells. This enhancement could be prevented by simultaneously treating the cells with rifampin (Fig. 2B). Induced cells accumulated D-alanine to a higher degree and showed no further enhancement in the presence of D-cycloserine (Fig. 2C).

Transport of glycine in D-cycloserine-resistant cells. We investigated the effects of D-cycloserine incubation on the initial rates of transport and on the net transport of D-alanine, L-alanine, glycine, and L-proline (Table 1). Transport was investigated at two substrate concentrations, 1 and 20 μM, because of the two transport systems observed in *B. subtilis* (3). L-Proline was included as a control substrate that is not transported by the alanine systems. Incubation in D-cycloserine caused an increased ability by the cells to transport D- and L-alanine and glycine when initial rates were measured. When net transport was measured, however, enhancement was evident only with D-alanine and glycine. The enhanced level of retention was especially pronounced with glycine.

The effect of D-cycloserine incubation on glycine transport was further investigated by determining the kinetic parameters for the initial rate of transport of glycine (Fig. 3). The initial rate of transport by induced cells had the same K_m value for glycine, but a higher V_{max} than was observed in uninduced cells. The net transport of glycine was investigated at various concentrations of glycine in uninduced and induced cells. The intracellular concentration of glycine was calculated from the values of nanomoles glycine transported per 15 min per milligram of protein as described in Materials and Methods and plotted versus the extracellular glycine concentration (Fig. 4). The gradient of glycine retained in induced cells was compared with that in uninduced cells (Fig. 4, insert). It can be seen that the increased retention of glycine by induced cells was more pronounced at higher glycine concentrations. Although the Michaelis-Menten equation was devised to deal with initial rates of reaction, the use of the equation

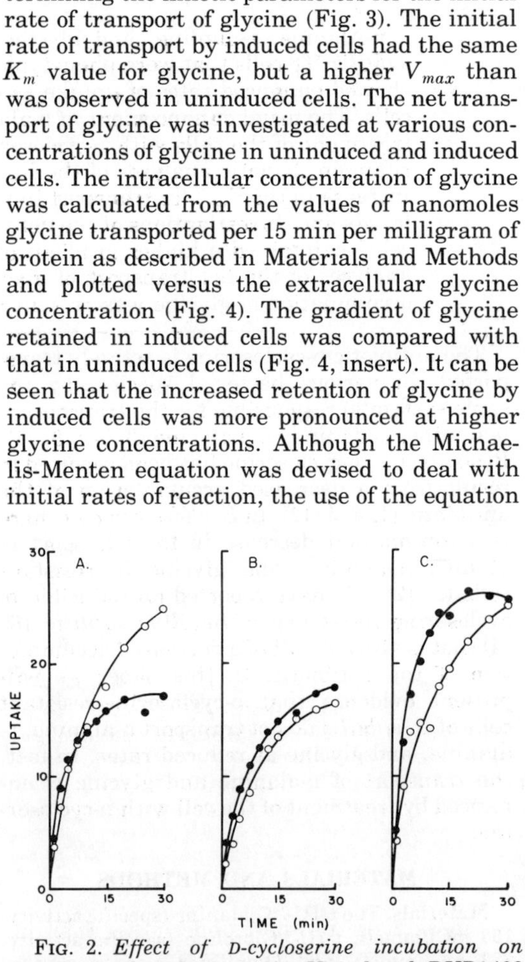

FIG. 2. *Effect of D-cycloserine incubation on transport of D-alanine. (A) Uninduced RUB1402 cells were incubated in Spizizen minimal salts with no addition (●) or plus 0.1 μM D-cycloserine (○). (B) Uninduced RUB1402 cells were incubated in Spizizen minimal salts containing 5 μg of rifampin per ml with no further addition (●) or plus 0.1 mM D-cycloserine (○). (C) RUB1402 cells induced by incubation in Spizizen minimal salts plus 0.1 mM D-cycloserine for 15 min were washed and incubated in Spizizen minimal salts with no addition (●) or plus 0.1 mM D-cycloserine (○). All samples had 1 μM D-[14C]alanine added at zero time. Uptake is expressed as nanomoles of D-alanine transported per milligram of protein.*

TABLE 1. *Enhanced uptake rates for D-alanine and glycine in D-cycloserine-resistant cells*[a]

Compound transported	Concn (μM)	Uptake rate					
		Initial rate			Net transport		
		Uninduced	Induced	% of uninduced	Uninduced	Induced	% of uninduced
D-Alanine	1	0.770	1.03	134	5.44	6.19	114
	20	8.67	9.73	112	46.2	49.2	106
L-Alanine	1	0.289	0.502	174	2.13	2.14	100
	20	4.31	5.03	117	38.7	24.7	64
Glycine	1	0.521	0.712	137	1.77	2.32	131
	20	4.64	8.74	188	6.62	15.9	240
L-Proline	1	0.349	0.384	110	2.71	2.09	77
	20	1.32	0.632	48	16.2	11.6	72

[a] Cells were induced for D-cycloserine resistance as described in Materials and Methods. Initial rates of transport were measured for 30 s and net transport for 15 min as described in Materials and Methods. Rates are expressed as nanomoles transported per minute per milligram of protein and nanomoles transported per 15 minute per milligram of protein for initial rates and net transport, respectively.

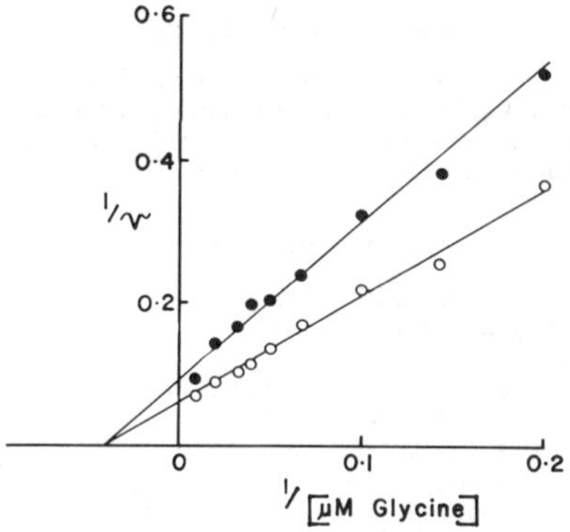

FIG. 3. *Lineweaver-Burk plot of initial rates of glycine transport in uninduced and induced cells. Initial rates of transport (30 s) of glycine were determined in cells unexposed to D-cycloserine (●) and cells induced for 30 min in Spizizen minimal salts plus 0.1 mM D-cycloserine (○). The kinetic parameters were: K_m = 25 μM glycine, V_{max} = 11 nmol of glycine transported per min per mg of protein for uninduced cells, and K_m = 25 μM glycine, V_{max} = 16 nmol of glycine transported per min per mg of protein for induced cells.*

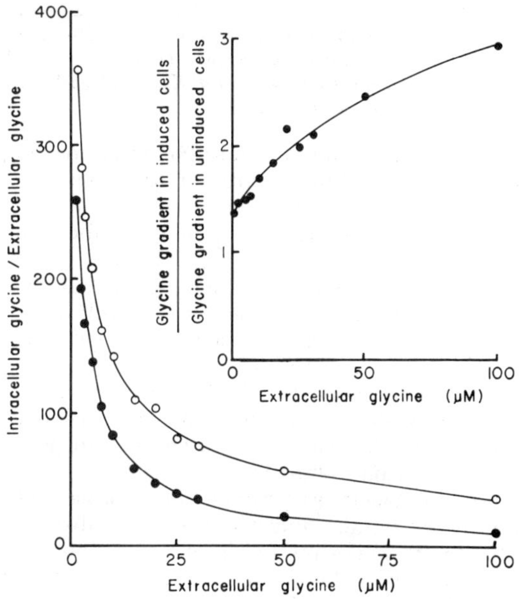

FIG. 4. *Ratio of intracellular to extracellular glycine in uninduced and induced cells. Strain BR151 was induced for D-cycloserine resistance as described in Materials and Methods. Net transport (15 min) of [¹⁴C]glycine was measured in uninduced (●) and induced (○) cells, and the uptake was converted from nanomoles per minute per milligram of protein to millimolar as described in Materials and Methods. The extracellular concentration of glycine was corrected for uptake, and the ratios of intracellular to extracellular [¹⁴C]glycine were determined. Insert: Ratio of intracellular to extracellular glycine in induced cells was divided by that in uninduced cells.*

for measuring transport under other than initial rate conditions has been recognized as providing useful information (2). When this equation was applied to the net transport of glycine (Fig. 5), it appeared that there were two K_m values (4 and 25 μM glycine) for induced cells, rather than the one K_m value (4 μM glycine) observed in uninduced cells.

DISCUSSION

D-Cycloserine resistance in *E. coli* (5, 12) is accompanied by a loss of transport of the antibiotic and a concomitant loss of transport of D-alanine and glycine. We have described an inducible resistance to D-cycloserine in *B. subtilis* (4) that also results from a decreased accumulation of the antibiotic. Under conditions in which D-cycloserine resistance in *B. subtilis* is induced, however, we found that the transport

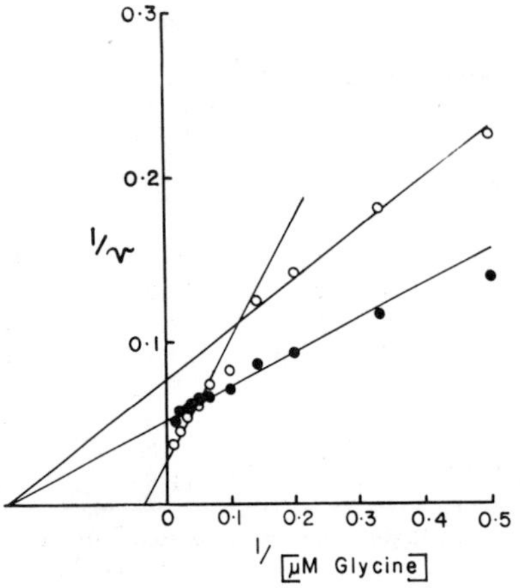

FIG. 5. *Lineweaver-Burk plot of the net transport of glycine in uninduced and induced cells. Net transport (30 min) of glycine determined in cells unexposed to D-cycloserine (●) and in cells induced for 30 min in Spizizen minimal salts plus 0.1 mM D-cycloserine (○). The kinetic parameters were:* K_m *= 4 μM glycine for uninduced cells and* K_m *= 4 μM and* K_m *= 25 μM for induced cells.*

of D-alanine, L-alanine, and glycine is not decreased. When initial rates of transport are measured at 1 μM concentrations of the substrate, the transport of D- and L-alanine and glycine is increased. This may be due to an artifactual example of antiport, such that the transport substrate is pulled into the cell by the efflux of D-cycloserine. When the kinetic parameters for the initial rate of transport of glycine are determined, the K_m for glycine remains constant while the V_{max} for transport increases. This would be consistant with an antiport-driven transport of glycine.

Net transport represents the balance between the uptake and the efflux of substrate (2). In D-cycloserine-resistant cells the net transport of D-alanine and glycine is higher than in sensitive cells. D-Cycloserine-resistant cells maintain a glycine gradient that is two to three times that observed in sensitive cells. This would indicate that in D-cycloserine-resistant cells either the glycine uptake rates is increased or the glycine efflux rate is decreased, causing the retention of a larger portion of the glycine. The kinetic parameters for the net transport of glycine indicate the presence of a high K_m value for glycine transport induced by D-cycloserine which can be prevented by treatment with rifampin. Thus, protein synthesis is required for the alterations to occur.

We propose that D-cycloserine induces a new transport system in *B. subtilis* 168. This new system transports D-alanine and glycine, with glycine the preferred solute. D-Cycloserine-resistant cells would maintain a higher gradient of glycine as a result of the synthesis of this system. We further postulate that this new transport system also transports D-cycloserine, but that the rate of uptake is less than the rate of efflux of the antibiotic. This would cause a net efflux of D-cycloserine, which would render the cells resistant to the antibiotic. These observations suggest that an analysis of the transport of each antimicrobial agent used in combination with D-cycloserine might reveal patterns of illicit transport that could produce inhibition of microbial growth at lower concentrations of antibiotic and thereby reduce toxicity.

ACKNOWLEDGMENTS

This work was supported by Public Health Service grants 5TI-GM-00592 from the National Institute of General Medical Science and 5ROI-AI-10141 from the National Institute of Allergy and Infectious Diseases.

LITERATURE CITED

1. **Benveniste, R., and J. Davies.** 1973. Mechanisms of antibiotic resistance. Annu. Rev. Biochem. **42**:471–506.
2. **Christensen, H. N.** 1975. Biological transport. W. A. Benjamin, Inc., Reading, Mass.
3. **Clark, V. L., and F. E. Young.** 1974. Active transport of D-alanine and related amino acids by whole cells of *Bacillus subtilis*. J. Bacteriol. **120**:1085–1092.
4. **Clark, V. L., and F. E. Young.** 1977. Inducible resistance to D-cycloserine in *Bacillus subtilis* 168. Antimicrob. Agents Chemother. **11**:871–876.
5. **Franklin, T. J.** 1973. Antibiotic transport in bacteria. Crit. Rev. Microbiol. **2**:253–272.
6. **Halpern, Y. S.** 1974. Genetics of amino acid transport in bacteria. Annu. Rev. Genet. **8**:103–133.
7. **Leach, F. R., and E. E. Snell.** 1960. The adsorption of glycine and alanine and their peptides by *Lactobacillus casei*. J. Biol. Chem. **235**:3523–3531.
8. **Lowry, O. H., N. J. Rosebrough, A. L. Farr, and R. J. Randall.** 1951. Protein measurement with the Folin phenol reagent. J. Biol. Chem. **193**:265–275.
9. **Robbins, J. C., and D. L. Oxender.** 1973. Transport systems for alanine, serine, and glycine in *Escherichia coli* K-12. J. Bacteriol. **116**:12–18.
10. **Spizizen, J.** 1958. Transformation of biochemically deficient strains of *Bacillus subtilis* by deoxyribonucleate. Proc. Natl. Acad. Sci. U.S.A. **44**:1072–1078.
11. **Wargel, R. J., C. A. Shadur, and F. C. Neuhaus.** 1970. Mechanism of D-cycloserine action: transport systems for D-alanine, D-cycloserine, L-alanine, and glycine. J. Bacteriol. **103**:778–788.
12. **Wargel, R. J., C. A. Shadur, and F. C. Neuhaus.** 1971. Mechanism of D-cycloserine action: transport mutants for D-alanine, D-cycloserine, and glycine. J. Bacteriol. **105**:1028–1035.

Antimicrobial Agents and Chemotherapy, May 1977, p. 881-887 Vol. 11, No. 5

Energy Coupling Factor as Target of Colicin K: Characterization of a Colicin K-Insensitive *ecf* Mutant of *Escherichia coli*[1]

JEN-SHIANG HONG,* D. LYNNE HAGGERTY, AND MICHAEL A. LIEBERMAN

Department of Biochemistry, Brandeis University, Waltham, Massachusetts 02154

Received for publication 23 February 1977

We isolated a colicin K-insensitive energy uncoupled mutant of *Escherichia coli*. This mutant was presumed to be an *ecf* mutant as evidenced by its similarity to a known *ecf* mutant (M. A. Lieberman and J.-S. Hong, 1974) with respect to the mutational site, reversion pattern, and defects in transport and growth. The mutation conferring the colicin K-insensitivity resided in the *ecf* gene as the majority of the secondary mutations overcoming the *ecf* phenotype reverted the colicin K-insensitive phenotype to colicin K-sensitive. The insensitivity of the mutant to colicin K was not due to either a defect in adsorption or to a lack of the energized membrane state. The defect was most probably due to the inability of colicin K molecules to interact with their target. Our previous studies concerning the role of the *ecf* gene product in energy coupling to active transport and oxidative phosphorylation support the contention that the ECF protein is itself the direct target of colicin K.

The primary action of colicins K and E1 appears to be a de-energization of the cytoplasmic membrane such that active transport and oxidative phosphorylation are abolished (3, 11). This de-energization also contributes to numerous cellular alterations, including the lowering of intracellular adenosine 5'-triphosphate (ATP) levels (2) and the cessation of deoxyribonucleic acid, ribonucleic acid, and protein synthesis (5, 14). Plate et al. (17) showed that the cessation of macromolecular synthesis is largely attributable to the lowering of intracellular ATP levels. They also suggested that the ATP levels decrease because ATP is hydrolyzed by the adenosine 5'-triphosphatase in an effort to re-energize the membrane.

Other cellular alterations brought about by colicin K or E1 include the excretion of glycolytic metabolites (2), the efflux of accumulated potassium ion (20), and an alteration of membrane permeability to Mg^{2+} and Co^{2+} (12; for review see Luria [11]). The biochemical basis for these alterations is not known. Based largely on the observed inhibition of active transport and oxidative phosphorylation, it has been suggested that the primary target of these colicins may be the membrane-bound energy transducing machinery (11).

During the investigation of a novel energy-uncoupled mutant [*metC* ecf*(Ts)] (8) we found that although the mutant was isolated as being defective in active transport, it also exhibited many of the characteristics of cells that have been treated with colicins E1 or K (10). Therefore, we suggested that the ECF protein may be the biochemical target of these colicins (10). In this paper we report the isolation of an *ecf* mutant that is insensitive to the action of colicin K. Genetic evidence is presented showing that the mutation conferring the colicin K-insensitive phenotype resides in the *ecf* gene. We also demonstrate that the insensitivity of the mutant to colicin K is due to a drastically slowed initiation process (the interaction of colicin K with the target molecule; also known as stage 1 [11] of colicin action).

MATERIALS AND METHODS

Bacterial strains and media. Strains used were JSH202 (F^- *thi strA*) and MAL303 (F^- *thi strA metC ilv*). Both are derivatives of *Escherichia coli* K-12. Media used were nutrient broth and minimal salts medium E (19) supplemented with 0.5% glucose and 40 μM vitamin B1. When required, amino acids were added to 0.4 mM. Solid media contained 1.5% agar.

Viability assay. Cultures were aerobically grown in minimal glucose with shaking at 25°C and harvested during mid-log phase. Cells were washed twice with 70 mM potassium phosphate buffer (pH 7.0) containing 1 mM $MgCl_2$ and suspended in the same buffer; sterile conditions were maintained throughout. These cells were used for both transport assays and colicin experiments.

[1] Publication no. 1134 from the Department of Biochemistry, Brandeis University, Waltham, MA 02154.

Standard colicin experiments were carried out as follows. A 1-ml portion of washed cells at an optical density at 660 nm = 3.0 (equivalent to 1.3×10^9 to 1.6×10^9 cells per ml) in a 25-ml flask was preincubated for 3 min with shaking at either 25 or 43°C. At zero time a portion (100 μl) of the cell suspension was withdrawn and added to a tube (13 by 100 mm) containing 20 μl of colicin. Each tube was incubated for a desired length of time after which trypsin (10 μl; 6.6 mg/ml) was added, and the incubation continued for an additional 5 min. Viable cells were determined by diluting in nutrient broth, plating on nutrient broth plates and incubating overnight at 36°C.

Genetic methods. Transductions were performed as described (8).

Colicins. Colicin E2 was a generous gift from M. Nomura, and colicin E3 was from L. Hager. Preparation of colicins E1 and K have been described (3). The number of killing units in the colicin preparation was calculated from the equation $S/So = e^{-m}$, where m is the multiplicity of killing units, and S/So is the survival ratio.

Isolation of colicin K-resistant energy uncoupled mutants. JSH202 cells were mutagenized with diethylsulfate, grown in minimal glucose medium at 25°C, harvested at mid-log phase, washed twice with 70 mM potassium phosphate (pH 7.0), and resuspended at a final density of 2.1×10^9 cells per ml in 70 mM potassium phosphate (pH 7.0) containing 1 mM $MgCl_2$ and 0.5% Casamino Acids. Cells (1 ml) in a test tube (100 by 13 mm) were incubated at 42°C for 30 min after which glucose was added to a final concentration of 0.4 mM. After 5 min, colicin K (m = 10) was added. Ten minutes later trypsin (Sigma) was added to a final concentration of 0.8 mg/ml, and the incubation continued for 5 min. Minimal glucose medium (100 ml) was then inoculated with the colicin K-treated cells (0.2 ml), and the cycle was repeated. After each colicin treatment, survival was determined by plating on nutrient broth plates at 25°C. Nutrient broth plates with 0.2% deoxycholate were used to determine the number of tolerant mutants present (15).

After the second cycle, the cells were diluted, plated on minimal succinate plates, and incubated at 25°C. When the colonies were still small (24 to 48 h), the plates were shifted to 42°C. After 12 to 24 h, small colonies were isolated, purified, and tested for transport ability at 25 or 43°C.

Isolation of Suc$^+$ revertants. These were isolated as described for JSH4 (8).

RESULTS

Isolation of the mutant MAL321. Since colicins K and E1 appear to require the energized membrane state (6; Hong and Haggerty, manuscript submitted for publication) to initiate their lethal activity (initiation process, stage 1), mutants unable to form the energized membrane state should be resistant to colicins K and E1 and therefore could be selected for as uncoupled mutants.

The method we devised is based on an observation made with a previously isolated temperature-sensitive energy uncoupled mutant, MAL300 (10). Basically, when the susceptibility of MAL300 to colicin K was checked after glucose (0.4 mM) addition at the nonpermissive temperature, a loss of trypsin-rescuable viability was observed if colicin K (5 min incubation) was added 2 min after the glucose addition; however, no decrease in cell viability was observed if colicin K was added 5 min after the glucose addition. This result has been related to the finding that MAL300, at 42°C, is capable of establishing and maintaining a membrane potential 2 min after glucose addition, but this potential has been dissipated within 5 min after glucose addition (Lieberman, Simon, and Hong, J. Biol. Chem., in press). The strain is thus colicin-insensitive due to a lack of membrane energy, which is necessary for stage 1 of the colicin attack process (6, 11). Cells were therefore exposed to colicin K and treated with trypsin under the conditions described above. To determine if the procedure is applicable to our cells, a mixture of JSH210 (wild-type) and JSH205 (an energy-uncoupled mutant) (9) at a ratio of 10^6:1 was subjected to two cycles of the selection procedure. The resulting ratio was 67.5:1, representing an enrichment of 1.5×10^4. The selection was then performed on mutagenized JSH202. One mutant that displayed a temperature-sensitive phenotype for transport ability was found. P1 phage were grown on the mutant and MAL303 was transduced to *MetC*$^+$. Three of the eight resulting transductants exhibited an energy-uncoupled phenotype, and one, MAL321, was used for the studies described here.

The mutant is an *ecf* mutant. The mutant MAL321 is capable of utilizing succinate, fumarate, malate or D-lactate as a carbon source at 25 but not at 43°C.

We found by means of P1 phage transduction using JSH210 (*metC*) as a recipient that the mutation conferring the Suc$^-$ and transport$^-$ phenotype is approximately 85% (40/47) linked with *metC*. This linkage is similar to that reported with MAL300 (Lieberman et al., J. Biol. Chem., in press).

The data in Fig. 1 demonstrate that in the absence of an exogenous energy source, the mutant was unable to transport proline and serine at 43°C (compare with wild-type MAL303). The cells could only accumulate the substrate sixfold, whereas the wild-type could do so 300-fold. It was also clear that low levels of glucose (0.4 mM) stimulated the transport of these amino acids, although at 43°C this stimulation was transitory. These results are very

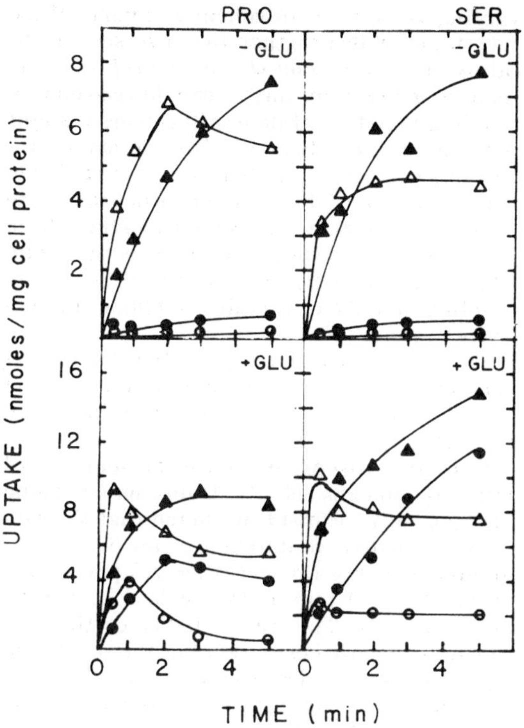

FIG. 1. *Uptake of proline and serine by MAL303 (wild-type) and MAL321 (mutant). Cells were grown in minimal glucose medium at 25°C and transport assayed as described previously (8). Radioactive proline used was L-[U-^{14}C]proline (134.5 Ci/mol) at 7.7 μM. Radioactive serine used was L-[U-^{14}C]serine (159 Ci/mol) at 12.9 μM. Both radioactive compounds were obtained from New England Nuclear Corp. When glucose was used, it was added to the cells immediately after substrate (radioactive amino acid) addition to a final concentration of 0.4 mM. Transport was then assayed as a function of time after the glucose addition. Symbols:* ▲, *MAL303 at 25°C;* △, *MAL303 at 43°C;* ●, *MAL321 at 25°C;* ○, *MAL321 at 43°C.*

similar to the transport results obtained with the *ecf*(Ts) *metC** mutants JSH4 (8) and MAL300 (Lieberman et al., J. Biol. Chem., in press), except that MAL321 exhibited a more severe defect in transport than did the other mutants.

Revertants of MAL321 were selected for their ability to grow on succinate at 43°C. They were found to be of two classes: class I, which is prototrophic, and class II, which is auxotrophic for methionine. The methionine requirement in class II revertants was due to the absence of cystathionase (*metC* gene product) activity (8). This reversion pattern is identical to that observed previously with the *ecf* mutant JSH4. Both classes of revertants grow on succinate and transport normally at 43°C (data not shown).

Since this mutant, MAL321, is similar to MAL300 (or JSH4) with respect to mutational site, reversion pattern, and defects in transport and growth, we tentatively concluded that MAL321 is also an *ecf* mutant. This would give MAL321 the genotype F$^-$: *thi ilv strA metC** *ecf*(Ts). The *metC** notation denotes that the *metC* gene in MAL321, while retaining wild-type levels of cystathionase activity, is different from the wild-type *metC* gene (8; Lieberman et al., J. Biol. Chem., in press).

Insensitivity to colicin K and its relation to *ecf*. We found that, when incubated with colicin K in the presence of 0.4 mM glucose, MAL321 cells were essentially fully rescuable by trypsin against the lethal action of colicin K for at least 10 min (Fig. 2).

To determine if the mutation conferring the colicin K insensitivity in MAL321 is associated with the *ecf* mutation, we isolated 19 independent class I and 7 independent class II revertants. It is important to realize that the reversion events leading to class I and class II revertants occur within different genes: those leading to class II revertants apparently undergo an *metC** to *metC$^-$* transition (8; Lieberman et al., J. Biol. Chem., in press), whereas those leading to class I revertants can occur in either the *ecf*(Ts) gene [*ecf*(Ts) to *ecf*$^+$] or in the *metC**

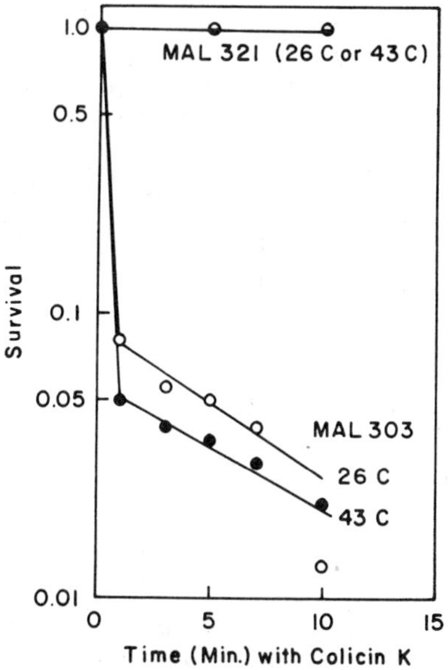

FIG. 2. *Insensitivity of MAL321 to colicin K. Trypsin-rescuable cell viability was determined as described in the text. Glucose was added to 0.4 mM 1 min prior to the addition of colicin K (m = 9.8).*

gene (*metC** to *metC*+). Both classes of revertants occurred at approximately the same frequency (one in 10^5 to one in 10^6), and this frequency suggests that each reversion event was in one gene. Work with both JSH4 (8) and MAL300 (Lieberman et al., J. Biol. Chem., in press) has demonstrated that both the *metC** and *ecf*(Ts) mutations are required for the energy-uncoupled phenotype to be expressed. Thus, if a reversion event occurs in either gene the energy-uncoupled phenotype is lost.

The 26 revertants of MAL321 were examined for their response to colicin K using the same conditions as were used for MAL321 (Fig. 2) except that the incubation with colicin K was for 2 min at 43°C. We found that 17 (17/19) of the class I revertants were sensitive to colicin K; at least 60% of the cells were killed for each revertant under these conditions. The most sensitive of these revertants, 321-I-7 and 321-I-14, were as sensitive to colicin K as was the wild-type MAL303 (Fig. 3). Two class I revertants (321-I-1 and 321-I-13), however, remained insensitive to colicin K (Fig. 3; data for 321-I-13 not shown). All of the class II revertants (7/7) remained as insensitive to colicin K as MAL321 (data not shown).

These results are interpreted as follows: if the reversion event did not occur within the *ecf*(Ts) gene (as in class II revertants) all revertants retained colicin K insensitivity. This strongly suggests that the *metC** gene is not involved in conferring colicin K insensitivity. The data with class I revertants indicate that a single reversion event in the *ecf*(Ts) gene can simultaneously restore the energy-coupling processes as well as the sensitivity to colicin K. The varying sensitivity to colicin K among these revertants indicates that the reversion event can occur at a second site in the *ecf*(Ts) gene rendering a protein capable of wild-type energy coupling activity, while it still confers a slight insensitivity to colicin K. The two class I revertants that remain fully resistant to colicin K (321-I-1 and 321-I-13) could be either *metC** to *metC*+ reversions [which could leave the *ecf*(Ts) gene product unaltered] or could be a second site reversion in *ecf*(Ts) which confers energy coupling activity but retains complete insensitivity to colicin K.

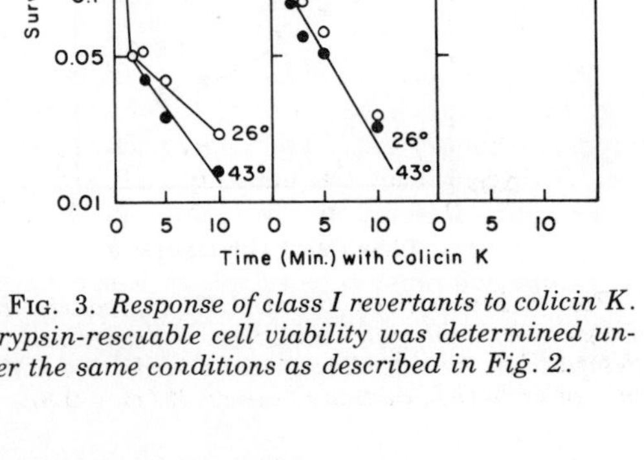

FIG. 3. *Response of class I revertants to colicin K. Trypsin-rescuable cell viability was determined under the same conditions as described in Fig. 2.*

The most consistent explanation for the reversion studies is that the mutation rendering the colicin K-insensitive phenotype is located in the *ecf*(Ts) gene.

Colicin K-insensitive mutation maps at 64 min. By means of P1 transduction using MAL303 as a recipient, we found that the colicin K-insensitive mutation in strain 321-I-1 was greater than 90% linked with *metC*, placing the mutation at 64 min on the revised *E. coli* genetic map (1). This result indicates that the colicin K-insensitive marker has the same linkage with *metC* as does the *ecf*(Ts) marker, and this specific location rules out the possibility that the mutation maps in the gene coding for the colicin K receptor, which is known to map at 12 min (1).

Normal adsorption. To rule out the possibility that the rescuability of cell viability by trypsin seen with the colicin K-insensitive mutant is not due to an adsorption defect, viability tests were carried out in the absence of trypsin. We utilized revertants for this study (321-I-1 and 321-I-7) such that we could be sure that an energized membrane would be established by the cells, since the initiation process appeared to be dependent on the generation of such a state. The extent of killing observed with colicin K-insensitive strains was the same as with the sensitive strains (Fig. 4). This suggests that adsorption is normal. However, the killing could result from readsorption after diluting and plating rather than from adsorption before dilution. To rule this out, an experiment was carried out under the same conditions used in Fig. 4 except that cells and colicin were diluted separately (to 2×10^{-4}), mixed, incubated for 10 min, and then plated. A dilution to 10^{-4} was done in the experiment shown in Fig. 4. Since no killing was observed, we conclude that the killing seen in the absence of trypsin was not due to readsorption. This makes unlikely the possibility that a defect in adsorption is responsible for the trypsin reusability seen with the colicin K-insensitive mutants.

Slowed initiation. The results in Fig. 5 demonstrate that the rate of killing was much slower in the colicin K-insensitive strains. A 1-min incubation of colicin K with sensitive cells was sufficient to kill more than 90% of these cells (Fig. 3). To obtain the same amount of killing with insensitive cells, approximately 70 min of incubation at 43°C or 100 min of incubation at 26°C was required.

Rescuability against colicin K is specific. Under conditions in which they are insensitive to colicin K, 321, 321-I-1, 321-I-7, and two class II revertants were all sensitive to colicins E1, E2, and E3 (Table 1). The colicin K-insensitive mutation is therefore distinct from *tolA* and *tolB*, which map at about 16 min on the *E. coli* genetic map. Both *tolA* and *tolB* mutants are pleiotropically resistant to colicins E2, E3, and K (13, 15). The fact that the colicin K-insensitive strains are sensitive to colicin E1 indicates that the protection observed against colicin K is not due to a lack of energy supplies since colicin E1 also requires an energized membrane state for initiation (6).

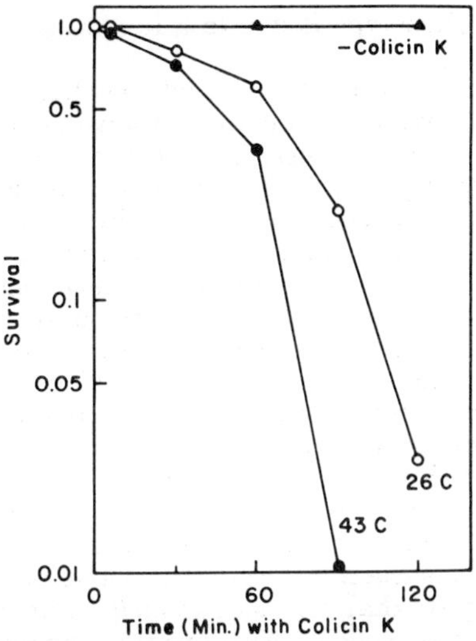

FIG. 5. *Slowed initiation process in colicin K-insensitive strains. Trypsin-rescuable cell viability was determined under the same conditions as those used in Fig. 2 with the exception that glucose was added to 10 mM.*

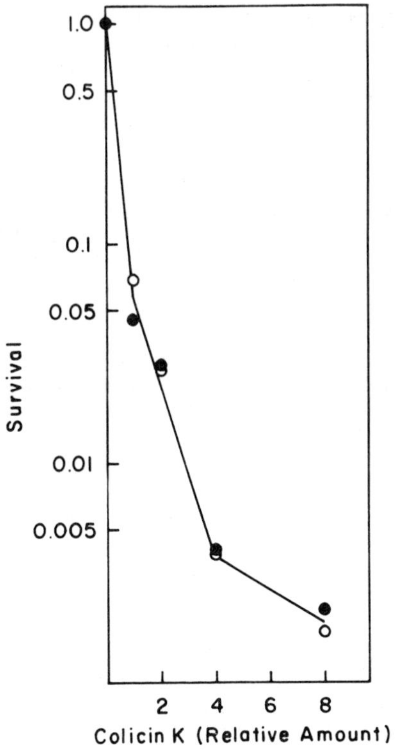

FIG. 4. *Killing by colicin K in the absence of trypsin. The conditions used were exactly the same as those described in the text except that the incubation time with colicin K was 1 min. Glucose was added to 0.4 mM 1 min prior to the addition of colicin K. Temperature was 26°C. Symbols:* ○, *MAL321-I-1;* ●, *MAL321-I-7.*

TABLE 1. *Sensitivity to colicins E1, E2, and E3*[a]

Strain	Trypsin-rescuable survival (%)				
	Control	E1	E2	E3	K
MAL303	100	6.0	2.0	4.7	4.0
MAL321	100	2.4	1.0	2.2	99
MAL321-I-1	100	2.4	6.7	1.6	90
MAL321-I-7	100	8.6	7.4	7.0	4.5
MAL321-II-1	100	8.5	5.1	5.0	100
MAL321-II-2	100	6.0	3.8	3.1	100

[a] The assays were carried out at 43°C under the conditions described in the text. Glucose (0.4 mM) was added to the cells 1 min before the addition of colicin. Incubation time with colicin was 5 min. The colicins were added at the following killing concentrations: E1, $m = 7.4$; E2, $m = 9.2$; E3, $m = 7.4$; K, $m = 8.1$. MAL321-I-1 and 321-I-7 are class I revertants; MAL321-II-1 and 321-II-2 are class II revertants.

DISCUSSION

The results presented in this paper indicate that the colicin K-tolerant mutation probably resides in the *ecf* gene. This conclusion is based on the finding that the majority of the class I revertants [selected to overcome the *ecf*(Ts) phenotype] are capable of reverting the colicin K-insensitive phenotype to colicin K-sensitive. The fact that these revertants occur frequently (10^{-6} to 10^{-5}) indicates that the colicin K-insensitive phenotype is due to a lesion in a single gene.

It is not surprising to find that the class II (*metC*) revertants remained insensitive to colicin K. We previously showed that the mutations giving rise to class II reversion are located in the *metC* gene and concluded that these mutations are intergenic suppressors of the *ecf*(Ts) gene (8). Recent experiments using antiserum prepared against cystathionase (*metC* gene product) indicated that these mutations are structural mutations in the *metC* gene since cross-reacting materials were detected in these *metC* revertants (S. Kagan and J-S. Hong, unpublished data). The mechanism of the *metC* suppression of the *ecf*(Ts) phenotype is not yet understood. The finding that all of the class II revertants examined were insensitive to colicin K suggests that reversion to *metC* cannot suppress the colicin K-insensitive phenotype, whereas it can suppress the *ecf*(Ts) phenotype.

It is apparent that the process leading to cell death is drastically slowed in the colicin K-resistant cells as a result of the colicin K-insensitive mutation. This enables us to observe a full rescuability of cell viability by trypsin during the early stage in the initiation process. It is possible that the colicin K resistance observed may be due to a defect in the adsorption process or a lack of an energized membrane state, which has been shown to be required for the initiation process (6; Hong and Haggerty, manuscript submitted for publication). The first possibility is unlikely because: (i) the colicin K-tolerant mutation does not reside in the colicin K receptor gene; and (ii) in the absence of trypsin no difference is observed in the extent of killing between sensitive and tolerant strains. The second possibility is ruled out since all of the class II revertants (as well as some of those of class I) isolated from MAL321 remain insensitive to colicin K. These Suc^+ revertants transport amino acids and grow on succinate, fumarate, or D-lactate, as do the wild type, at 42°C, which is an indication of the presence of the energized membrane state.

The colicin K insensitivity observed with our mutants is most probably due to a defect in some other aspect of the initiation process, perhaps an inability of colicin K to interact with its target protein. The demonstration that the *ecf* gene product is essential for colicin K-induced cellular damage suggests that the *ecf* gene product is either the target of colicin K or is required for colicin K to reach the target. The following findings strongly support the contention that the *ecf* gene product is itself the direct target of colicin K: (i) the *ecf* gene product is essential for energy coupling in active transport (8) and oxidative phosphorylation (Lieberman et al., J. Biol. Chem., in press), two functions which are altered by colicin K, and (ii) *ecf* mutants exhibit many cellular alterations characteristic of cells that have been treated with either colicin E1 or K (10). It is apparent that the colicin K-insensitive mutation we have studied affects the susceptibility of the ECF to colicin K molecules but not to colicin E1 molecules (Table 1). These two colicins (7, 18) differ considerably in amino acid composition and in isoelectric point and conceivably could have different target proteins or different sites on the same target protein. Therefore, we suggest that the observed insensitivity of the colicin K-insensitive mutants towards colicin K is due to a reduced affinity of the colicin K target protein for colicin K itself.

While this work was in progress, Plate (16) reported the isolation of an energy-uncoupled mutant of *E. coli* also unable to respond to colicin K. It was suggested that the gene product may be the target of colicin K. No mapping of the mutation was reported. If this gene is different from the *ecf* gene, it will raise the question of what is the functional and structural relationship between these two targets.

ACKNOWLEDGMENTS

This work was supported by grant GB40237 from the National Science Foundation and by Public Health Service grant GM22576, training grant GM212, and research career development award KO4-GM-0092, all from the National Institute of General Medical Sciences.

LITERATURE CITED

1. **Bachmann, B. J., K. B. Low, and A. L. Taylor.** 1976. Recalibrated linkage map of *Escherichia coli* K-12. Bacteriol. Rev. **40**:116–167.
2. **Fields, K. L. and S. E. Luria.** 1969. Effects of colicins E1 and K on cellular metabolism. J. Bacteriol. **97**:64–77.
3. **Fields, K. L. and S. E. Luria.** 1969. Effects of colicins E1 and K on transport systems. J. Bacteriol. **97**:57–63.
4. **Fredericq, P.** 1965. Zentralbl. Bakteriol. Parasitenkde. Hyg. Abt. 1: Orig. **196**:142.
5. **Jacob, F., L. Siminovitch, and E. L. Wollman.** 1952. Sur la biosynthése d'une colicine et sur son mode d'action. Ann. Inst. Pasteur Paris 83:295–315.
6. **Jetten, A. M., and M. E. R. Jetten.** 1975. Energy requirement for the initiation of colicin action in *Escherichia coli*. Biochim. Biophys. Acta 387:12–22.
7. **Kunugita, K., and Matsuhashi,** M. 1971. Purification and properties of colicin K. J. Bacteriol. **104**:1017–1019.
8. **Lieberman, M. A., and J-S. Hong.** 1974. A mutant of *Escherichia coli* defective in the coupling of metabolic energy to active transport. Proc. Natl. Acad. Sci. U.S.A. **71**:4395–4399.
9. **Lieberman, M. A., and J-S. Hong.** 1976. Energization of osmotic shock-sensitive transport systems in *Esche-*

richia coli requires more than ATP. Arch. Biochem. Biophys. **172**:312–315.

10. **Lieberman, M. A., and J-S. Hong.** 1976. Changes in active transport, intracellular adenosine-triphosphate levels, macromolecular synthesis, and glycolysis in an energy-uncoupled mutant of *Escherichia coli*. J. Bacteriol. **125**:1024–1031.
11. **Lurai, S. E.** 1973. Colicins, p. 293–320. *In* L. Leive (ed.), Bacterial membranes and walls. Marcel Dekker, Inc., New York.
12. **Lusk, J. E., and D. L. Nelson.** 1972. Effects of colicins E1 and K on permeability to magnesium and cobaltous ions. J. Bacteriol. **112**:148–160.
13. **Nagel de Zwaig, R., and S. E. Luria.** 1967. Genetics and physiology of colicin-tolerant mutants of *Escherichia coli*. J. Bacteriol. **94**:1112–1123.
14. **Nomura, M.** 1963. Mode of action of colicins. Cold Spring Harbor Symp. Quant. Biol. **28**:315–324.
15. **Nomura, M., and C. Witten.** 1967. Interaction of colicins with bacterial cells. III. Colicin-tolerant mutations in *Escherichia coli*. J. Bacteriol. **94**:1093–1111.
16. **Plate, C. A.** 1976. Mutant of *Escherichia coli* defective in response to colicin K and in active transport. J. Bacteriol. **125**:467–474.
17. **Plate, C. A., J. L. Suit, A. M. Jetten, and S. E. Luria.** 1974. Effects of colicin K on a mutant of *Escherichia coli* deficient in Ca, Mg-activated adenosine triphosphatase. J. Biol. Chem. **249**:6138–6143.
18. **Schwartz, S. A., and D. R. Helinski.** 1971. Purification and characterization of colicin E. J. Biol. Chem. **246**:6318–6327.
19. **Vogel, H. J., and D. M. Bonner.** 1956. Acetylornithinase of *Escherichia coli*: partial purification and some properties. J. Biol. Chem. **218**:97–106.
20. **Wendt, L.** 1970. Mechanism of colicin action: early events. J. Bacteriol. **104**:1236–1241.

ANTIMICROBIAL AGENTS AND CHEMOTHERAPY, May 1977, p. 888-896 Vol. 11, No. 5

Printed in U.S.A.

Tolerant Response of *Streptococcus sanguis* to Beta-Lactams and Other Cell Wall Inhibitors

DIANE HORNE AND ALEXANDER TOMASZ*
The Rockefeller University, New York, New York 10021

Received for publication 7 January 1977

In contrast to group A streptococci or *Streptococcus pneumoniae*, cells of *Streptococcus sanguis* (group H) do not exhibit the irreversible effects of penicillin treatment, such as loss of viability or lysis. On the other hand, the same bacteria show typical effects of penicillin, such as morphological alterations, reduction in the rate of cell wall synthesis, and secretion of murein and lipoteichoic acid polymers into the medium. A novel effect of cell wall inhibitors was also noted: treatment with beta-lactams or with fosfomycin, D-cycloserine, or beta-halogeno-D-alanine caused the release of substantial amounts of glycerol lipids into the growth medium. The antibiotic "tolerance" of *S. sanguis* is interpreted in terms of the hypothesis that the activity of bacterial murein hydrolases is essential for the irreversible effects of cell wall inhibitors.

In spite of the major advances made in the understanding of the nature of penicillin-susceptible bacterial enzymes, the mechanism by which antibiotic-treated bacteria lose their viability and disintegrate has remained obscure. Recent studies with pneumococci and with several other species of bacteria have produced strong evidence implicating the central role of bacterial murein hydrolases and their cellular control in the irreversible effects of penicillin and other cell wall inhibitors (3, 9, 15–17). Bacteria with suppressed hydrolase systems were shown to retain their normal susceptibility to penicillin; on the other hand, such cells have become resistant to the lytic effect of penicillin, and their rate of loss of colony-forming ability during drug treatment was also substantially reduced. In an attempt to gain a better understanding of these phenomena, we examined the response of several species of streptococci to penicillin. In the present communication, we describe what appears to be a natural penicillin-tolerant bacterial species: cells of *Streptococcus sanguis* are extremely susceptible to penicillin (minimal growth-inhibitory concentration of benzylpenicillin is 0.013 μg/ml), yet they do not lyse and there is only a minor loss in the colony-forming ability of the cells during treatment with cell wall inhibitors.

MATERIALS AND METHODS

Bacterial strains. Three strains of streptococci were used in these experiments: *Streptococcus pneumoniae* strain R36A (Rockefeller University Laboratory stock); *S. sanguis* strain Wicky, Lancefield group H (obtained from Dennis Perry of Northwestern University Medical School, Chicago); and *Streptococcus pyogenes* strain T4/56, Lancefield group A (obtained from Maclyn McCarty, Rockefeller University).

Antibiotics. Benzylpenicillin (E. R. Squibb & Sons, New York, N.Y.), mecillinam (Leo Pharmaceutical Products, Ballerup, Denmark), and sodium dicloxacillin (Wyeth Laboratories, Philadelphia, Pa.) were commercial products. Cephalexin and cephaloridine were kindly provided by Kenneth Price of Bristol Laboratories, Syracuse, N.Y., and beta-chloro-D-alanine was a gift from James Manning of the Rockefeller University. D-Cycloserine, fosfomycin, 3-fluoro-2-deutero-D-alanine, and D-4-[(2-oxo-3-pentene-4-yl)amino]-3-isoxazolidinone sodium salt (a D-cycloserine derivative) were obtained from Merck Sharp & Dohme Research Laboratories, Rahway, N.J. Mitomycin C was kindly donated by Maria Tomasz of Hunter College, New York, N.Y. All other antibiotics were purchased from Sigma Chemical Co., St. Louis, Mo.

Growth media. The growth media (C medium, containing acid-hydrolyzed casein, and Cden, chemically defined [8; A. Tomasz, Bacteriol. Proc., p. 29, 1964]) were used for both pneumococci and *S. sanguis* strain Wicky. Stock cultures of strain Wicky were, however, maintained in brain heart infusion (Difco Laboratories, Detroit, Mich.) medium. *S. pyogenes* strain T4/56 was routinely grown in Todd Hewitt broth (Difco). All bacteria were grown (10-ml cultures in standard, 18-mm-wide test tubes) at 37°C without aeration.

Growth of the bacteria was determined by measuring the light scattering of the cultures (Coleman nephelometer; 14). Viable titers were determined by routine plating procedures (4, 14). Antibiotics were removed by dilution to concentrations having no detectable effect on bacterial growth in liquid culture or agar-containing medium. With benzylpenicillin, the cells were diluted 1:10 into medium containing a 1,000-fold (wt/wt) excess of penicillinase (Calbiochem, Los Angeles, Calif.) and incubated for 10 min at 37°C.

Assay of incorporation of radioactive precursors into *S. sanguis* and release of radioactively labeled material into the medium. The radioactively labeled precursors used were: [U-^{14}C]glycerol (0.1 Ci/mmol, 1 μCi and 10 μg/ml of medium); [2-^{3}H]glycerol (5 Ci/mmol, 1 μCi and 10 μg/ml of medium); [6-^{3}H]uracil (20 Ci/mmol, 2.5 μCi and 10 μg/ml of medium); L-[5-^{3}H]lysine-4, (60 Ci/mmol, 1 μCi and 9 μg/ml of medium); 1-[G-^{3}H]phenylalanine (10 Ci/mmol, 2.5 μCi and 6 μg/ml of medium); and *N*-acetyl-D-[1-^{3}H]glucosamine (4 Ci/mmol, 1 μCi and 0.05 μg/ml of medium).

Three types of labeling regimes were used in these experiments. (i) In the "old label" type, radioactively labeled precursors were added to the cells at a concentration of approximately 5 × 10^{6} colony-forming units/ml and incubated for 90 min (1.5 generations). The bacteria were then collected and washed with isotope-free medium on membrane filters (0.45 μm; Millipore Corp., Bedford, Mass.). After resuspension in fresh, unlabeled medium, the bacteria were allowed to grow for 30 min before the addition of the antibiotic at a cell density of about 2 × 10^{7} colony-forming units/ml. (ii) In the "nascent label" type of experiment, the label was added at the same time as the antibiotic. (iii) In "continuous labeling," the precursors were added at the same cell density as in (i), but the cells were kept in the isotope-containing medium throughout the time of antibiotic treatment.

Incorporation into macromolecular components was measured as described earlier (18), with some modifications. Amounts of 100 μl of the cell suspension were precipitated with 10% cold trichloroacetic acid and 80 μg of carrier bovine serum albumin (BSA; Armour) for 15 min. The precipitates were collected onto glass fiber filters (GFA; Whatman, Inc., Clifton, N.J.) and washed with 10% trichloroacetic acid. After drying at 100°C for 10 min, the disks were placed in vials containing toluene scintillation fluid with 2,5-diphenyloxazole and counted in a Mark II (Nuclear-Chicago Corp., Des Plaines, Ill.) scintillation counter.

The amount of macromolecular components released into the medium was measured after the removal of the bacteria (0.5 ml) in an Eppendorf microcentrifuge (Brinkmann Instruments Inc., Westbury, N.Y.), and the acid-insoluble material was determined in 100 μl of supernatant as described above.

Polyacrylamide gel electrophoresis. Supernatant fluids from penicillin-treated *S. sanguis*, dialyzed against distilled water and concentrated by lyophilization, were layered on top of 10% acrylamide gels. Electrophoresis in the presence of sodium dodecyl sulfate was done according to the method of Weber and Osborn (20). The gels were sliced (1.2-mm slices), and the slices were added to vials and solubilized in 0.5 ml of 90% (vol/vol) NCS tissue solubilizer (Amersham/Searle Corp., Arlington Heights, Ill.) at 50°C for 2 h. A 10-ml amount of toluene scintillation fluid was added, and the samples were counted as described above.

Sucrose density gradient centrifugation. Supernatant fluids of penicillin-treated *S. sanguis*, di-

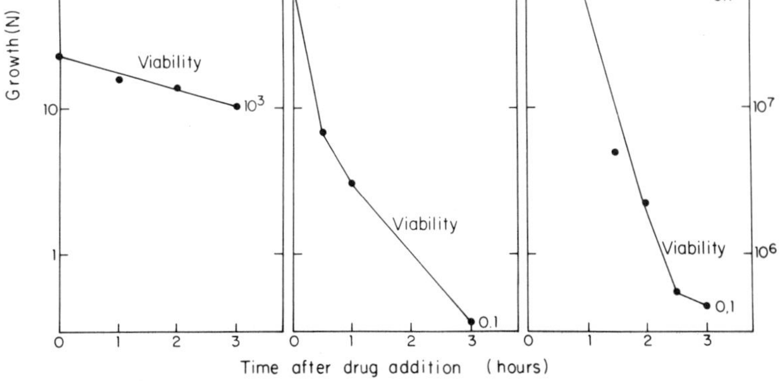

FIG. 1. *Effect of benzylpenicillin on the growth, viability, and lysis of three species of streptococci. Exponentially growing cultures received benzylpenicillin at the concentrations (units per milliliter) indicated. Growth and lysis were monitored by nephelometry (Coleman nephelometer). Viability was determined as described in the text. CFU, Colony-forming units.*

alyzed and concentrated as for electrophoresis, were layered on top of linear sucrose gradients (5 to 25% in saline) with or without the presence of 0.04% sodium dodecyl sulfate throughout the gradient. Centrifugation, collection of fractions, and determination of radioactivity were carried out as described in a recent publication (17).

Lipid extraction and thin-layer chromatography. Lipids were extracted from *S. sanguis* (cells or supernatant fluids) with chloroform and methanol by the method of Arbogast and Henderson (1). Two-dimensional thin-layer chromatography was performed with commercially available Silica Gel G plates (E. Merck, 0.25-mm thickness). The plates were developed in the first dimension with chloroform-methanol-water (65:25:4) and in the second with chloroform-methanol-acetic acid (80:15:8) (13). The lipids located by autoradiography with Cronex $2_C{}^D$ X-ray film (E. I. du Pont de Nemours & Co., Wilmington, Del.) were quantitated by scraping the appropriate areas of gel into vials and counting directly in toluene scintillation fluid. Tentative identification of phospholipids was done by comparison of the R_f values with those of authentic phospholipid standards (Sigma).

RESULTS

Inhibition of growth of *S. sanguis* by penicillin. Figure 1 documents our basic observation: treatment of *S. sanguis* (group H) with benzylpenicillin causes growth inhibition unaccompanied by either lysis or any major loss of viability. For a comparison, the figure also illustrates the response of two other streptococcal species to penicillin treatment: *S. pyogenes* (group A) rapidly loses viability but shows no culture lysis, whereas *S. pneumoniae* loses viability and undergoes culture lysis as well. It is important to note that each one of the three strains is extremely susceptible to benzyl-penicillin, as judged by growth inhibition: the minimum inhibitory concentrations (MICs) are between 0.007 and 0.13 μg/ml for each of the strains.

TABLE 1. *Susceptibility of S. sanguis strain Wicky (group H) to antibiotics*

Antibiotic	MIC (μg/ml)	Survival[a] at: MIC	Survival[a] at: 10× MIC
Benzylpenicillin	0.013	100	63
Cloxacillin	2.5	100	ND[b]
Oxacillin	1.0	ND	67
Mecillinam	10.0	80	ND
Cephalexin	1.0	100	100
Cephaloridine	0.1	93	79
β-Chloro-D-alanine	100.0	100	ND
D-Cycloserine	100.0	ND	95
Fosfomycin	50.0	100	ND
Fluoro-D-alanine[c]	5.0[d]		
+D-cycloserine derivative[e]	10.0[d]	ND	80
Mitomycin C	0.2	ND	0.007

[a] Percentage of surviving cells after 2 h of antibiotic treatment at 37°C.

[b] ND, Not determined.

[c] 3-Fluoro-2-deutero-D-alanine.

[d] The ratio of the antibiotics' concentrations recommended by the Merck Co.

[e] D-4-[(2-Oxo-3-pentene-4-yl)amino]-3-isoxazolidinone, sodium salt.

TABLE 2. *Susceptibility of S. pyogenes strain T4/56 (group A) to antibiotics*

Antibiotic	MIC (μg/ml)	Survival[a] at: MIC	Survival[a] at: 10× MIC
Benzylpenicillin	0.0066	11.0	0.5
Cephalexin	0.5	ND[b]	2.2
Cephaloridine	0.02	ND	2.0
Fluoro-D-alanine[c]	2.0[d]	10.3	4.5
+D-cycloserine derivative[e]	4.0[d]		

[a] Percentage of surviving cells after 2 h of antibiotic treatment at 37°C.

[b] ND, Not determined.

[c] 3-Fluoro-2-deutero-D-alanine.

[d] The ratio of the antibiotics' concentrations recommended by the Merck Co.

[e] D-4-[(2-Oxo-3-pentene-4-yl)amino]-3-isoxazolidinone, sodium salt.

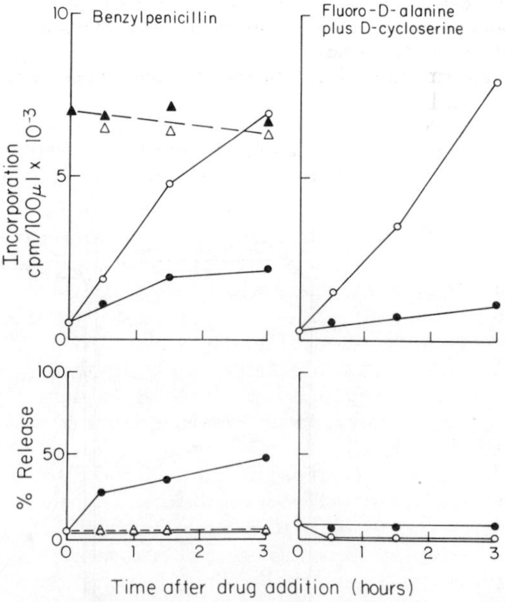

FIG. 2. *Release of N-acetylglucosamine-labeled material from antibiotic-treated S. sanguis. The concentration of benzylpenicillin was 0.66 μg/ml, and those of 3-fluoro-2-deutero-D-alanine and the D-cycloserine derivative were 5 and 10 μg/ml, respectively. Symbols: (○) control (nascently labeled cells); (●) plus antibiotic(s) (nascently labeled cells); (△) control (prelabeled cells); and (▲) plus antibiotic (prelabeled cells).*

The virtually complete lack of irreversible effects in penicillin-treated *S. sanguis* was also found true for other beta-lactams and cell wall inhibitors. Treatment with high doses of these drugs (2 h with 10 times the MICs) gave only a marginal killing effect (loss of viability in a maximum of 40% of the cells) (Table 1). In contrast, treatment of group A streptococci with beta-lactams as well as with inhibitors of early stages in cell wall synthesis (e.g., D-cycloserine) caused extensive loss of viability (Table 2).

Both group A and group H streptococci grow in chains of up to 5 to 15 cells, and this makes a precise quantitation of changes in colony-forming ability difficult. However, the low mortality of *S. sanguis* is not likely to be grossly influenced by chain formation, since the breaking-up of chains (by mechanical shear applied after penicillin treatment) did not substantially decrease the frequency of colony formers, although the average chain size was reduced to 1 to 4. Rapid and extensive loss of viability in mitomycin C-treated *S. sanguis* may be detected without difficulty (see Table 1).

Inhibition of cell wall synthesis. Treatment with benzylpenicillin (0.66 μg/ml) caused an immediate and substantial reduction in the rate of incorporation of radioactive *N*-acetylglucosamine (GlcNAc) into macromolecular material (Fig. 2). The selective use of this label for cell wall synthesis has been documented earlier (4). A significant portion (up to 50%) of the cell wall material synthesized after the addition of penicillin was found to be released into the growth medium in the form of material precipitable with cold trichloroacetic acid and carrier albumin. There was no solubilization of biosynthetically old cell wall label during the penicillin treatment (Fig. 2).

Treatment of the bacteria with a combination of D-cycloserine (10 μg/ml) and fluoro-D-alanine (5 μg/ml) caused about 90% inhibition of cell wall synthesis.

Release of glycerol-labeled material during treatment with cell wall inhibitors. Treatment with benzylpenicillin (0.66 μg/ml) and with fluoro-D-alanine (5 μg/ml) plus D-cycloserine (10 μg/ml) both caused inhibition of glycerol incorporation into macromolecular material; the inhibition was virtually immediate in the case of penicillin, whereas the halt in glycerol incorporation occurred about 1.5 h after the addition of the other drugs (Fig. 3). The drug treatments greatly stimulated the release (into the medium) of glycerol-labeled material that was precipitable with cold trichloroacetic acid in the presence of albumin carrier. A substantial fraction of both biosynthetically new and old

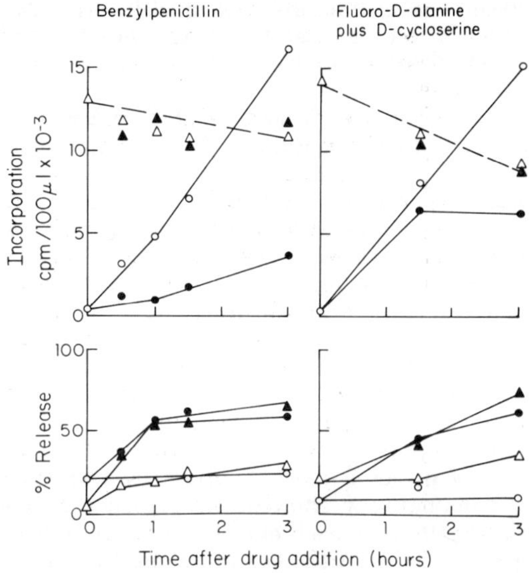

FIG. 3. *Release of glycerol-labeled material from antibiotic-treated S. sanguis. The concentration of benzylpenicillin was 0.66 μg/ml, and those of 3-fluoro-2-deutero-D-alanine and of the D-cycloserine derivative were 5 and 10 μg/ml, respectively. Symbols:* (○) *control (no antibiotic, nascently labeled cells);* (●) *plus antibiotic (nascently labeled cells);* (△) *control (prelabeled cells); and* (▲) *plus antibiotic (prelabeled cells).*

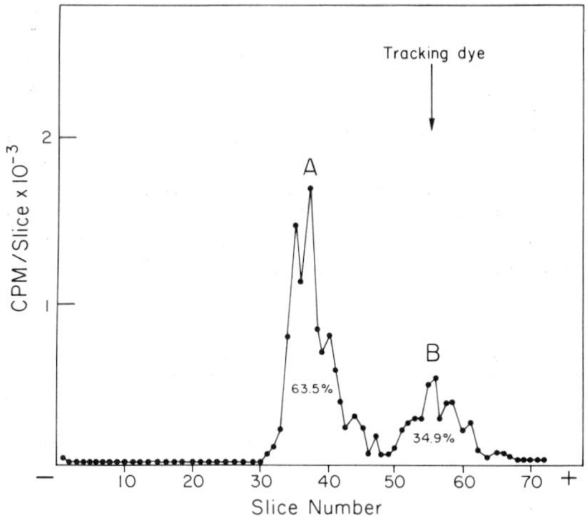

FIG. 4. *Electrophoresis of dialyzed and concentrated supernatant fluids from S. sanguis treated with benzylpenicillin. The sample was derived from the supernatant of a 10-ml streptococcal culture that received 0.66 μg of benzylpenicillin per ml in the exponential phase of growth (2 × 10^7 colony-forming units/ml) and was incubated with the drug for 90 min. The cell-free supernatant was dialyzed against water, freeze-dried, and redissolved in water. A 200-μl sample (containing 3 × 10^5 cpm) was subjected to electrophoresis on 10% acrylamide gels at pH 7.4 in the presence of sodium dodecyl sulfate, according to the method of Weber and Osborn (20).*

glycerol label (i.e., glycerol label incorporated either before or after the drug addition) was found to be released into the growth medium (Fig. 3).

Nature of the glycerol-labeled material released into the medium. The supernatant of penicillin-treated and glycerol-labeled bacteria was dialyzed, concentrated by freeze-drying, and analyzed by several biochemical methods. Gel electrophoresis in the presence of sodium dodecyl sulfate separated the glycerol-labeled materials into two major fractions (Fig. 4A and B). Fraction B, running near the tracking dye and representing about 30% of the radioactivity, was composed of lipids. Extraction of the supernatant of penicillin-treated bacteria with lipid solvents quantitatively removed this fraction of glycerol label. Analysis by thin-layer chromatography showed the presence in the supernatants of each one of the major cellular glycerol-lipids. Although an increase in the relative amount of phosphatidylglycerol was accompanied by a decrease in cardiolipin, all other glycerol-lipids were in virtually the same concentrations as found in normally growing cells (Table 3). Fraction A of the sodium dodecyl sulfate-gel electrophoresis was tentatively identified as lipoteichoic acid-containing material on the basis of the following properties: formation of micellar aggregates, disaggregation by detergents, insolubility in lipid solvents and distribution into the water phase during phenol-water extraction, and positive reaction with antiserum against polyglycerol phosphate (7).

The release of macromolecular cell surface material shows considerable specificity. (i) Release is only caused by inhibitors of cell wall synthesis. (ii) Release is restricted to material labeled with glycerol (and, in the case of cells treated with beta-lactams, to GlcNAc-labeled material), but it does not occur with protein and

TABLE 3. *Lipids extracted from [^{14}C]glycerol-labeled strain Wicky cells and supernatant fluids of penicillin-treated cells*

Lipid[a]	Before addition of antibiotic (% in cells)[b]	After 90 min of incubation (37°C) with:[c] No addition, % in: Cells	No addition, % in: Supernatant	Benzylpenicillin (1 U/ml), % in: Cells	Benzylpenicillin (1 U/ml), % in: Supernatant
Glycolipid A	17.7	30.8	36.8	18.6	28.8
PG	29.1	18.8	35.9	17.0	36.6
CL	19.4	25.3	6.1	39.0	10.1
Glycolipid B	13.8	9.8	10.1	8.4	10.9
Neutral lipids	19.9	14.6	10.9	16.0	11.7

[a] The tentative identification of the phospholipids made by comparison with authentic standards, which include: phosphatidylethanolamine (PE), phosphatidylglycerol (PG), and cardiolipin (CL).
[b] The values listed are the percentages of the total counts chromatographed.
[c] The percent release of total acid-insoluble [^{14}C]glycerol counts per minute into the supernatant was 7.0 before drug addition, 10.0 in the control at 90 min, and 63 in the penicillin-treated sample. Lipid-extractable counts per minute accounted for 65 to 75% of the total counts per minute in the cells and 40 to 50% of that in the supernatants.

TABLE 4. *Selectivity of the antibiotic-induced release of macromolecular material from S. sanguis*

Antibiotic	Concn (μg/ml)	Total incorporation[a] (% of control): Lysine	Phenylalanine	Uracil	Glycerol	Release[b] (% of total): Lysine	Phenylalanine	Uracil	Glycerol
None		100	100	100	100	1.0	2.9	2.8	10.0
Benzylpenicillin	0.066	65	75.7	69.6	36.7	7.0	5.1	4.0	38.5
Fluoro-D-alanine[c]	10.0[d]								
+ D-cycloserine derivative[e]	20.0[d]	80	80.1	85.3	70.3	4.7	4.2	4.9	56.1

[a] Bacteria were labeled with tritiated precursors (nascent labeling, see legend to Fig. 3) plus or minus the drugs for 90 min at 37°C. Incorporation into trichloroacetic acid-precipitable material was determined with BSA carrier as described in the text.
[b] Percentage of total acid-insoluble counts per minute (in the presence of BSA) remaining in the supernatant after centrifugation.
[c] 3-Fluoro-2-deutero-D-alanine.
[d] The ratio of the antibiotics' concentrations recommended by the Merck Co.
[e] D-4-[(2-Oxo-3-pentene-4-yl)amino]-3-isoxazolidinone, sodium salt.

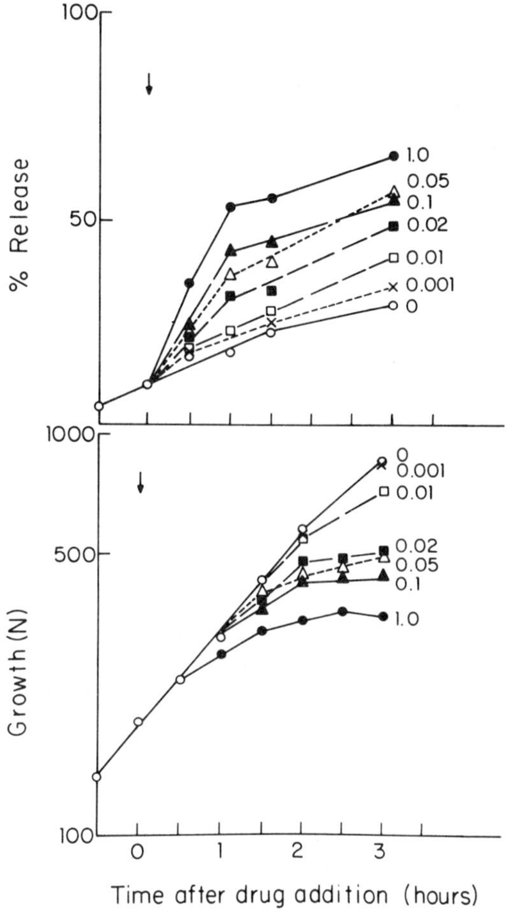

FIG. 5. *Release of prelabeled, macromolecular [^{3}H]glycerol from S. sanguis treated with low doses of benzylpenicillin. The cells were labeled by growth in [^{3}H]glycerol-containing medium (2.5 h), harvested, and allowed to grow in isotope-free medium for an additional 30 min, at which time benzylpenicillin was added (shown by the arrow). The numbers indicate the concentrations of penicillin in units per milliliter. The lower portion of the figure illustrates the effects of these concentrations of penicillin on the growth of the cells.*

nucleic acid material (Table 4). (iii) Stimulation of the release of glycerol label is proportional to the growth inhibition caused by penicillin and is already observable at the minimum growth-inhibitory concentration of the drug (Fig. 5). (iv) In contrast with the case of cell wall inhibitors, inhibition of growth by mitomycin C, rifampin, or chloramphenicol does not cause stimulation of the release of cell surface material (Fig. 6). (v) Release of glycerol label requires both the treatment with cell wall inhibitor and conditions appropriate for growth. Incubation in buffer or at low temperature or exposure of the cells to mechanical shear did not stimulate the release of glycerol-labeled macromolecules (Table 5).

Table 6 summarizes the effects of a large number of inhibitors on the synthesis and release of glycerol- and GlcNAc-labeled material. Inhibitors of both early and late biosynthetic stages of cell wall synthesis greatly stimulated the release of glycerol label into the medium, irrespective of the mode of isotope labeling (nascent, old, or continuous); beta-lactams (but not "early" cell wall inhibitors, such as D-cycloserine and the beta-halogeno alanines) also caused release of nascent GlcNAc-labeled material. Inhibitors of ribonucleic acid (rifampin), deoxyribonucleic acid (mitomycin C), and protein (chloramphenicol) syntheses caused no release of any of the isotope label.

DISCUSSION

S. sanguis is very susceptible to penicillin: 0.013 μg of benzylpenicillin added per ml of culture medium already caused inhibition of growth. In addition, penicillin treatment caused several typical effects of this antibiotic: (i) the rate of cell wall synthesis was reduced; (ii) a substantial fraction of peptidoglycan synthesized after penicillin addition was released into the growth medium, similarly to the case of penicillin-treated bacilli (2, 18); (iii) typical morphological effects of penicillin (formation of "bulges" at the cellular equator and selective inhibition of cell division) could be observed by electron microscopy; and (iv) the bacteria released into the medium lipoteichoic acid-containing macromolecules, similarly to the case described earlier for pneumococci (17). Yet in spite of the presence of these typical phenomena, penicillin had virtually no irreversible antimicrobial effects on this bacterium.

The response of *S. sanguis* to penicillin is reminiscent of that of ethanolamine-grown pneumococci and the mutant pneumococcus defective in murein hydrolase (16). Suppression of the activity of the pneumococcal autolytic system in mutants or physiological variants has been shown to cause resistance to penicillin-induced lysis and a greatly reduced rate in the loss of bacterial viability. Such bacteria nevertheless retain their high susceptibility to penicillin, and their entire dose response to penicillin remains identical to that of the wild-type bacterium (15). The term "antibiotic tolerance" has been suggested for this phenomenon (16). These findings were confirmed in autolysin-defective mutants of *Bacillus licheniformis* (12). More recently, physiological conditions were found for several bacterial species (including

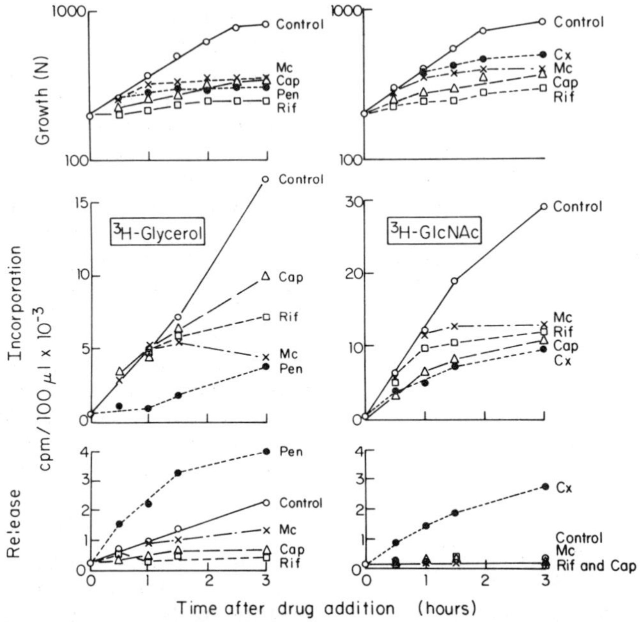

FIG. 6. *Effects of various antibiotics on growth and incorporation and release of macromolecular [³H]glycerol and ³H-labeled GlcNAc in S. sanguis. The isotopic compounds were added at the same time as the antibiotics to exponentially growing cultures. The concentrations used were as follows: benzylpenicillin (Pen), 0.66 µg/ml; mitomycin C (Mc), 1 µg/ml; rifampin (Rif), 1 µg/ml; chloramphenicol (Cap), 20 µg/ml; and cephalexin (Cx), 5 µg/ml.*

TABLE 5. *Effect of experimental conditions on the release of glycerol-labeled macromolecules.*

Experimental conditions during 90 min of incubation	Release of macromolecular glycerol (% of total) with:[a]	
	No antibiotic	Benzylpenicillin (0.66 µg/ml)
In growth medium at:		
37°C	13.4	54.7
30°C	11.2	43.2
0°C	4.0	11.4
37°C, followed by vigorous vortex mixing for 30 s	14.1	60.3
37°C, followed by freezing and thawing[b]	14.4	57.8
In SP buffer at 37°C[c]	1.0	3.7

[a] Bacteria were grown to mid-log phase in medium containing [³H]glycerol, adjusted to the appropriate temperature, and held for 90 min plus or minus penicillin. Total and supernatant trichloroacetic acid-insoluble counts per minute with BSA as carrier was determined as described in the text.

[b] The culture was frozen by immersion into a dry ice-acetone bath (−40°C) for 5 min. Melting was at 37°C.

[c] The labeled bacteria were harvested by centrifugation and resuspended in SP buffer (0.15 M NaCl plus 0.01 M K_2HPO_4).

staphylococci, streptococci, *Bacillus subtilis,* and *Escherichia coli*) that could also reduce or eliminate the lytic and bactericidal effects of penicillin without substantially affecting the MIC and dose response (3, 9). The tolerant response of *S. sanguis* (group H) to penicillin and to other cell wall inhibitors mimics all the typical features of autolysin-defective bacteria. It is important in this respect that extensive attempts to detect murein hydrolase activity (using isologous cell walls as substrates) in *S. sanguis* have been negative so far (unpublished observations). No cell wall turnover could be detected in normally growing (5) or penicillin-treated cultures (see Fig. 2) of this bacterium. On the other hand, it has been reported that *S. sanguis* made "competent" (to undergo genetic transformation with deoxyribonucleic acid) may undergo "lysis" upon incubation in a certain buffer (11). The same incubation conditions did not cause lysis of penicillin-pretreated "incompetent" streptococci (unpublished observation).

It has been suggested recently that the primary physiological response to penicillin and cell wall inhibitors may be a simple, reversible inhibition of growth in all bacteria (A. Tomasz and J. V. Höltje, *Microbiology–1977*, American Society for Microbiology, Washington, D.C., in press). However, this primary response

TABLE 6. *Release of macromolecular material into the growth medium from S. sanguis during treatment with certain antibiotics*

Antibiotic	Concn (μg/ml)	Total incorporation (% of control)[a]		Release (% of total incorporation)[b]	
		Glycerol	GlcNAc	Glycerol	GlcNAc
Nascent label					
None		100.0	100.0	17.7	1.2
Benzylpenicillin	0.66	46.5	48.0	71.0	42.2
Mecillinam	100.0	46.0	61.0	43.5	13.0
Oxacillin	100.0	55.9	26.0	53.0	51.8
Keflin	100.0	58.0	14.5	52.0	45.9
Cephalexin	5.0	51.0	47.9	65.0	17.8
Cephaloridine	1.0	52.0	ND[c]	68.7	ND
Fosfomycin	100.0	69.0	66.0	42.2	4.6
β-Chloro-D-alanine	200.0	70.4	54.8	43.6	3.2
D-Cycloserine	100.0	65.2	42.5	48.3	3.8
Fluoro-D-alanine[d] +	20.0[e]				
D-cycloserine derivative[f]	40.0[e]	55.4	20.8	79.0	2.7
Mitomycin C	1.0	82.9	69.1	11.4	2.1
Rifampin	1.0	87.8	59.3	5.5	2.8
Chloramphenicol	20.0	92.4	48.4	6.3	1.7
Old label					
None		100.0	100.0	23.4	1.2
Benzylpenicillin	0.66	97.0	103.0	55.7	0.7
Fluoro-D-alanine[d]	20.0[e]	93.0	ND	65.5	ND
+ D-cycloserine derivative[f]	40.0[e]				
Continuous label					
None		100.0	100.0	22.9	1.7
Benzylpenicillin	0.66	76.0	86.9	70.6	4.8
Cloxacillin	2.5	84.0	ND	64.6	ND

[a] Bacteria were labeled with radioactive isotopes added to the growth medium at concentrations indicated in the text. Three types of labeling regimes were used. (i) The culture received radioactive isotope at a cell concentration of approximately 5×10^6 colony-forming units/ml; after 90 min (corresponding to 1.5 doublings of cell mass) the cultures were harvested, resuspended in isotope-free growth medium, and incubated at 37°C. Drugs were added to such cultures 30 min after resuspension (old label). (ii) Isotopes and drugs were added simultaneously (nascent label). (iii) In continuous labeling, the regime was similar to that in (i), except the cells were left in the isotope-containing medium during drug treatment. Incorporation into trichloroacetic acid-precipitable material was determined with BSA carrier added, as described in the text.

[b] Percentage of total acid-insoluble counts per minute (plus BSA) remaining in the supernatant after centrifugation.

[c] ND, Not determined.

[d] 3-Fluoro-2-deutero-D-alanine.

[e] The ratio of the antibiotics' concentration recommended by the Merck Co.

[f] D-4[(2-Oxo-3-pentene-4-yl)amino]-3-isoxazolidinone, sodium salt.

can only be observed in autolysin-defective cells, since in most wild-type species the primary response is rapidly followed by secondary effects (triggering of murein hydrolases and, possibly, a separate "killing" event) that constitute the irreversible aspects of penicillin action. In this context *S. sanguis* may represent a bacterial species that is autolysin-defective in the wild type. Alternatively, this bacterium may have an unusually well-controlled (set of) murein hydrolase(s) that would become inhibited whenever cell wall synthesis comes to a halt (e.g., it may require a peptidoglycan precursor for catalytic activity).

Studies by Ward and co-workers (2, 18, 19) have shown that penicillin-treated bacteria may continue peptidoglycan synthesis in such a manner that the products end up in the outside medium. Penicillin-treated penumococci continue synthesis of cell wall teichoic acid and lipid-containing teichoic acid material (Forssman antigen) and secrete these polymers into the growth medium (17). *S. sanguis* seems to exhibit both peptidoglycan release and release of lipoteichoic acid-containing material. In addition, a substantial amount of lipid material also appears in the medium. The exact chemical nature of the polymer containing the lipoteichoic acid-like material is not known yet. Spontaneous release of lipoteichoic acids has been reported in some strains of oral streptococci and lactobacilli (6, 10). It is not clear what the relationship of this phenomenon may be to the antibiotic-induced lipoteichoic acid release described in this communication. Neither is it obvious why and via what exact mechanism lipid and lipoteichoic acid materials are released from this bacterium during inhibition of cell wall synthesis. Release of a lipid-containing teichoic acid (Forssman antigen) with autolysin-inhibitory activity has already been described in pneumococci (17). On the other hand, release of lipid material to the medium during treatment with cell wall inhibitors as it is described in the present communication seems to represent a novel biochemical effect of these antibiotics. The rather limited bactericidal effect of cell wall inhibitors in this bacterium indicates that the release of the glycerol-labeled macromolecules, though specifically stimulated by these drugs, is not in itself sufficient to cause irreversible damage to the bacteria.

S. sanguis, *S. pyogenes*, and *S. pneumoniae* represent a whole spectrum in physiological responses to penicillin treatment. Parallel studies on these three species may provide useful further information concerning the mechanism of the cytocidal and lytic effects of antibiotics.

ACKNOWLEDGMENTS

These investigations have been supported by Public Health Service grant AI 09423 from the National Institutes of Allergy and Infectious Diseases and grant PCM76-11943 from the National Science Foundation.

LITERATURE CITED

1. **Arbogast, L. Y., and T. O. Henderson.** 1975. Effect of inhibition of protein synthesis on lipid metabolism in *Lactobacillus plantarum*. J. Bacteriol. **123**:962–971.
2. **Elliott, T. S. J., J. B. Ward, and H. J. Rogers.** 1975. Formation of cell wall polymers by reverting protoplasts of *Bacillus licheniformis*. J. Bacteriol. **124**:623–632.
3. **Goodell, E. W., R. Lopez, and A. Tomasz.** 1976. Suppression of lytic effect of beta lactams on *Escherichia coli* and other bacteria. Proc. Natl. Acad. Sci. U.S.A. **73**:3293–3297.
4. **Horne, D. S., and D. Perry.** 1974. Effect of competence induction on macromolecular synthesis in a group H streptococcus. J. Bacteriol. **118**:830–836.
5. **Horne, D. S., and D. Perry.** 1975. Relationship of macromolecular synthesis to competence induction in a group H streptococcus. J. Bacteriol. **121**:1014–1021.
6. **Joseph, R., and G. D. Shockman.** 1975. Synthesis and excretion of glycerol teichoic acid during growth of two streptococcal species. Infect. Immun. **12**:333–338.
7. **Knox, K. W., and A. J. Wicken.** 1973. Immunological properties of teichoic acids. Bacteriol. Rev. **37**:215–257.
8. **Lacks, S., and R. D. Hotchkiss.** 1960. A study of the genetic material determining an enzyme activity in Pneumococcus. Biochim. Biophys. Acta **39**:508–517.
9. **Lopez, R., C. Ronda-Lain, A. Tapia, S. B. Waks, and A. Tomasz.** 1976. Suppression of the lytic and bactericidal effects of cell wall-inhibitory antibiotics. Antimicrob. Agents Chemother. **10**:697–706.
10. **Markham, J. L., K. W. Knox, A. J. Wicken, and M. J. Hewett.** 1975. Formation of extracellular lipoteichoic acid by oral streptococci and lactobacilli. Infect. Immun. **12**:378–386.
11. **Ranhand, J. M., C. G. Leonard, and R. M. Cole.** 1971. Autolytic activity associated with competent group H streptococci. J. Bacteriol. **106**:257–268.
12. **Rogers, H. J., and C. W. Forsberg.** 1971. Role of autolysins in killing of bacteria by some bactericidal antibiotics. J. Bacteriol. **108**:1235–1243.
13. **Skipski, V. P., and M. Barclay.** 1969. Thin-layer chromatography of lipids, p. 530–597. *In* S. P. Colowick and N. O. Kaplan (ed.), Methods in enzymology, vol. 1. Academic Press Inc., New York.
14. **Tomasz, A.** 1970. Cellular metabolism in genetic transformation of pneumococci: requirement for protein synthesis during induction of competence. J. Bacteriol. **101**:860–871.
15. **Tomasz, A.** 1974. The role of autolysins in cell death. Ann. N.Y. Acad. Sci. **235**:439–447.
16. **Tomasz, A., A. Albino, and E. Zanati.** 1970. Multiple antibiotic resistance in a bacterium with suppressed autolytic system. Nature (London) **227**:138–140.
17. **Tomasz, A., and S. Waks.** 1975. Mechanism of action of penicillin: triggering of the pneumococcal autolytic enzyme by inhibitors of cell wall synthesis. Proc. Natl. Acad. Sci. U.S.A. **72**:4162–4166.
18. **Tynecka, Z., and J. B. Ward.** 1975. Peptidoglycan synthesis in *Bacillus licheniformis*. The inhibition of cross-linking by benzyl penicillin and cephaloridin *in vivo* accompanied by the formation of soluble peptidoglycan. Biochem. J. **146**:253–267.
19. **Ward, J. B.** 1974. The synthesis of peptidoglycan in an autolysin-deficient mutant of *Bacillus licheniformis* N.C.T.C. 6346 and the effect of beta-lactam antibiotics, bacitracin and vancomycin. Biochem. J. **141**:227–241.
20. **Weber, K., and M. Osborn.** 1969. The reliability of molecular weight determinations by dodecylsulfate. J. Biol. Chem. **244**:4406–4412.

ANTIMICROBIAL AGENTS AND CHEMOTHERAPY, May 1977, p. 897-905
Vol. 11, No. 5

Unusual Susceptibility of *Erwinia amylovora* to Antibacterial Agents in Relation to the Barrier Function of its Cell Envelope

ARUN K. CHATTERJEE, RICHARD F. BUSS, AND MORTIMER P. STARR*
Department of Bacteriology, University of California, Davis, California 95616

Received for publication 5 November 1976

Wild-type strains of the bacterial phytopathogen *Erwinia amylovora* (the cause of fire blight disease of apples and pears) are markedly susceptible to novobiocin, deoxycholate, and sodium dodecyl (= lauryl) sulfate. The inhibitory concentration, expressed as the concentration causing a 99% inhibition of growth, of these three antibacterial agents were 15 to 100, 40 to 800, and 50 to 800 μg/ml, respectively, depending on the *E. amylovora* strain. Growth of strains of other *Erwinia* spp. and *Salmonella typhimurium* is not affected at all, or is only slightly affected, at these concentrations. Introduction of the F'*lac*$^+$, RP1, and R100*drd*-56 (but not E-*lac*$^+$) plasmids into an *E. amylovora* strain results in enhanced susceptibility to novobiocin and sodium dodecyl sulfate but not to deoxycholate. *E. amylovora* wild-type strains spontaneously release a periplasmic enzyme, cyclic phosphodiesterase, but not a cytoplasmic enzyme, glucose-6-phosphate dehydrogenase, into the growth medium. Addition of $MgCl_2$ (20 mM) and NaCl (84 mM) to tryptone broth stimulates the growth of wild-type *E. amylovora* strains and reduces or eliminates leakage of the periplasmic enzyme. Mutant strains of *E. amylovora*, selected for resistance to each separate antibacterial agent (or to all three of them), showed a direct correlation (in all but the novobiocin-resistant mutant) between drug resistance and reduced periplasmic leakiness. The relatively low maximum growth temperature (<37°C) of *E. amylovora* seems unrelated to periplasmic leakage, as judged from the inability of added $MgCl_2$ to raise the maximum growth temperature, although the generation time at 30°C is reduced from 108 to 54 min upon the addition of 20 mM $MgCl_2$. The extensive leakage of periplasmic enzyme and unusual drug susceptibility of *E. amylovora* strains might stem from some defect(s) in some cell envelope component(s) other than the lipopolysaccharide of these bacteria (which contain the usual liposaccharide constituents).

The envelope of gram-negative bacteria is a complex structure made up of three layers: an inner cytoplasmic membrane, a peptidoglycan layer, and an outer membrane (12, 22). The outer membrane, which consists of protein, lipid, and lipopolysaccharide (LPS; 28), is unique to gram-negative bacteria, where it serves as a permeability barrier (22).

Wild-type strains of gram-negative bacteria (notably enterobacteria and pseudomonads) are normally unsusceptible (and possibly impermeable) to numerous drugs and antimetabolites to which gram-positive species are susceptible (14, 32–34, 38). Treatment of gram-negative cells with ethylenediaminetetraacetic acid renders the cells permeable to drugs (such as actinomycin) or to lysozyme (21), and this effect of ethylenediaminetetraacetic acid is believed to result from alterations in the outer membrane (22). Furthermore, mutants with defects in the LPS molecule (heptose-deficient; "deep-rough") are susceptible to a variety of agents; the wild-type ("smooth") strains are not susceptible to these agents, and this differential susceptibility seems to stem from an altered permeability of the mutant strains (32, 38).

In the course of our studies on the genetics and physiology of *Erwinia amylovora*, an enterobacterial species which causes fire blight disease of apples and pears (29, 37), we observed that strains of this species are considerably more susceptible to acridine orange, as compared to strains of other *Erwinia* spp. or to other enterobacteria such as *Escherichia coli* or *Salmonella typhimurium* (19). Here we report our findings to the effect that: (i) wild-type strains of *E. amylovora*, which seem to have a complete LPS molecule in the outer membrane (hence, are smooth strains), are unusually susceptible to various antibacterial agents; (ii) these wild-type strains spontaneously release (i.e., "leak") a periplasmic enzyme (cyclic phosphodiesterase, 3′-nucleotidase) into the growth medium; (iii) this leakage of periplasmic enzyme can be reduced or eliminated entirely by adding 84 mM NaCl or 20 mM $MgCl_2$ to the growth medium; (iv) drug-resistant mutant strains of *E. amylovora* leak less periplasmic enzyme than do drug-susceptible, wild-type strains; (v) *E. amylovora* strains that harbor certain enterobacterial plasmids show enhanced susceptibilities to some of the antibacterial agents; and (vi) the relatively low maximum growth temperature (<37°C) of *E. amylovora* seems unrelated to periplasmic leakiness.

MATERIALS AND METHODS

Bacterial strains. Descriptions of the bacterial strains used in this study are given in Table 1. The strains harboring F′*lac*$^+$, E-*lac*$^+$, or R plasmids were constructed according to the methods of Chatterjee and Starr (7, 8, 10). Mutant strains resistant to antibacterial agents (deoxycholate, novobiocin, and sodium dodecyl sulfate; to avoid cumbersome locutions, we refer to such strains collectively as "drug resistant") were isolated after ethyl methane sulfonate treatment (23). After mutagenesis, and allowing for phenotypic lag, the cultures were inoculated into Luria broth (LB) containing the particular antibacterial agent (or all three of them) in order to enrich the rare mutant that was resistant to that substance (5). After a 12- to 18-h incubation, the cultures that showed visible growth were streaked onto Luria agar (LA) plates containing the particu-

TABLE 1. *Bacterial strains*[a]

Species	Strain designation: ICPB[a]	Strain designation: Other	Characteristics[b]
Erwinia amylovora	EA137	ATCC 15357	WT, *nic*$^-$, virulent
E. amylovora	EA167	Goodman E67HC	WT, *nic*$^-$, virulent
E. amylovora	EA169	ATCC 15580	WT, *nic*$^-$, virulent
E. amylovora	EA177	Goodman E39	WT, *nic*$^-$, virulent
E. amylovora	EA178	ATCC 19381	WT, *nic*$^-$, virulent
E. amylovora	EA212	Goodman E8	Derived from EA213; *nic*$^-$, avirulent
E. amylovora	EA213	Goodman E9	WT, *nic*$^-$, virulent
E. amylovora	EA178-E	AC425	Derived from EA178; *nic*$^-$, contains E-*lac*$^+$ (reference 10)
E. amylovora	EA178-F′	AC426	Derived from EA178; *nic*$^-$, contains F′*lac*$^+$ (reference 7)
E. amylovora	EA178-RP1	AC427	Derived from EA178; *nic*$^-$, contains RP1
E. amylovora	EA178-R100	AC428	Derived from EA178; *nic*$^-$, contains R100*drd*-56 (reference 8)
E. amylovora	EA178-D3	AC416	Derived from EA178; *nic*$^-$, selected for resistance to deoxycholate[c]
E. amylovora	EA178-N2	AC418	Derived from EA178; *nic*$^-$, selected for resistance to novobiocin[c] but also resistant to deoxycholate
E. amylovora	EA178-S1	AC419	Derived from EA178; *nic*$^-$, Arg$^-$; selected for resistance to sodium dodecyl sulfate[c] but also resistant to novobiocin and deoxycholate
E. amylovora	EA178-SDN	AC421	Derived from EA178; *nic*$^-$, selected for joint resistance to sodium dodecyl sulfate, novobiocin, and deoxycholate[c]
E. aroideae	EA144	Dowson 66	Prototrophic, WT, virulent
E. atroseptica	EA153	Shealy 2	Prototrophic, WT, virulent
E. carotovora	EC153	ATCC 15359	Prototrophic, WT, virulent
E. chrysanthemi	EC16	ATCC 11662	Prototrophic, WT, virulent
E. herbicola	EH103	Chatterjee Y46	Prototrophic, WT, plant strain
Salmonella typhimurium	3335	Ingraham LT2	Prototrophic, WT

[a] Bacterial strains maintained in the International Collection of Phytopathogenic Bacteria (ICPB; Department of Bacteriology, University of California, Davis, California 95616; M. P. Starr, Curator).

[b] WT, Wild-type strain; *nic*$^-$, requires nicotinic acid for growth. The R plasmid RP1 specifies resistance to ampicillin, kanamycin, tetracycline, and neomycin; the R plasmid R100*drd*-56 specifies resistance to tetracycline. Refer to Chatterjee and Starr (7–10) for details about the construction of plasmid-bearing *Erwinia* strains.

[c] Refer to the Materials and Methods section for the procedure used in selecting these drug-resistant strains.

lar antibacterial agent. Drug-resistant clones were picked, purified, and studied; only a single drug-resistant clone, originating from one enrichment step in each system, was subjected to further study (Table 1). The identities of these drug-resistant strains were checked by susceptibility to bacteriophages that are specific for *Erwinia amylovora* and by other properties distinctive to this species.

Media and cultural conditions. LB contained (in g/liter of distilled water): tryptone, 10; yeast extract (Difco Laboratories, Detroit, Mich.), 5; NaCl, 10; glucose, 1; pH was adjusted to 7.0 with NaOH before autoclaving; the filter-sterilized glucose was added to the rest of the medium after autoclaving. The corresponding agar medium, LA, was prepared by adding 1.5% agar to LB. Tryptone broth, in which the cultures were grown for enzyme assays, consisted of 1% (wt/vol) tryptone; the pH was adjusted to 7.0 before autoclaving. Other media and procedures were as described previously by us (7–10, 29). Unless otherwise specified, all incubations were at 30°C.

Susceptibility tests. Tests of susceptibility to the antibacterial agents (novobiocin, deoxycholate, and sodium dodecyl sulfate) were carried out in liquid as well as on solid media. The media in each case were LB and LA at pH 7.0. When the test was made in broth, the volume of the separately sterilized stock solution of the antibacterial agent required to yield the final desired concentration was added to 2.0 ml of double-strength LB, and the volume was made up to 4.0 ml with sterile water (the novobiocin solution was sterilized by filtration and the other two solutions by autoclaving). Inoculum consisted of log-phase cells in LB of the strain being tested; 10^5 cells were introduced into each 4-ml portion of medium. The inoculated tubes were incubated on a Gyrotary shaker at 30°C for 18 to 24 h. Growth of cultures was estimated by determining the absorbance at 660 nm with a Klett colorimeter (red filter no. 66). When the test was made on solid media, the required quantities of the sterilized solutions of the antibacterial agents were added to melted LA; the cultures were streaked or spotted on such plates, and growth was scored after 2 days at 30°C.

Enzyme assays. At the desired times, portions of the cultures in tryptone broth destined for enzyme assays were centrifuged (17,000 × *g*). All operations that were subsequent to sampling were carried out at 4°C. The culture supernatant was removed, dialyzed for 16 h against 200 volumes of tris(hydroxymethyl)aminomethane (Tris)-hydrochloride (Sigma Chemical Co., St. Louis, Mo.) buffer (0.005 M, pH 7.0), and assayed for enzyme activity. The cells were resuspended in Tris-hydrochloride buffer (0.01 M, pH 7.0) and assayed for enzyme activity after toluenization (0.02 ml of toluene added to 1 ml of cell suspension, mixed vigorously on a vortex tube shaker, and incubated at 30°C for 30 min) or sonic oscillation (six 10-s bursts, each interrupted by a cooling period of 1 min, using a Biosonik sonicator [Bronwill Scientific, Rochester, N.Y.] at a power output setting of 80%).

Standard published procedures were used for assaying the following enzyme activities: 2′,3′-cyclic phosphodiesterase (3′-nucleotidase; EC 3.1.4.c; 2), with bis-(*p*-nitrophenyl) phosphate as the substrate (27); phosphoglucose isomerase (EC 5.3.1.9), with glucose-6-phosphate as the substrate (30); and glucose-6-phosphate dehydrogenase (EC 1.1.1.49), also with glucose-6-phosphate as the substrate (20). The enzyme units are specified in the footnotes to Table 4.

RESULTS

Susceptibility to antibacterial agents. The results presented in Table 2 reveal that most of the wild-type strains of *Erwinia amylovora* are considerably more susceptible to novobiocin, deoxycholate, and sodium dodecyl (= lauryl) sulfate than are the strains of the other *Erwinia* spp. (*E. aroideae*, *E. atroseptica*, *E. carotovora*, *E. chrysanthemi*, and *E. herbicola*) or *S. typhimurium*.

As determined in the liquid medium (LB), novobiocin at a concentration of 10 to 20 μg/ml markedly inhibits the growth of most of the tested wild-type *E. amylovora* strains; at 50 μg of this antibiotic per ml, there is no growth at all of most of these strains. Similarly, sodium deoxycholate (about 400 μg/ml) and sodium dodecyl sulfate (about 40 to 60 μg/ml, with two exceptions) cause a total cessation of growth of most wild-type *E. amylovora* strains in LB. The growth of the strains of the other *Erwinia* spp. and *S. typhimurium* is only slightly affected, or is completely unaffected, at these concentrations of these antibacterial agents (Table 2). The results were comparable when using the LA solid medium (rather than the LB liquid medium) to determine susceptibility to these antibacterial agents (detailed data not presented here).

Taking into account the relevant literature (13, 31) and our general interest in the plasmid biology of *Erwinia* (7, 8, 10), we determined the susceptibility to these three antibacterial agents of *E. amylovora* strains harboring plasmids belonging to various compatibility groups; results are given in Table 2. The strains harboring a derepressed plasmid (F′*lac*$^+$, R100*drd*-56, or RP1) are more susceptible than the wild-type strain to novobiocin and sodium dodecyl sulfate. The drug susceptibility pattern of the strain harboring the repressed plasmid E-*lac*$^+$ (10) is similar to that of the wild-type strain.

The mutant strain of *E. amylovora* EA178 that was selected for resistance to deoxycholate (AC416) does not show cross-resistance to the other two antibacterial agents tested. The mutant strain (AC418) that was selected for resistance to novobiocin also shows increased resistance to deoxycholate but not to sodium dodecyl sulfate. The mutant strain (AC419) that was selected for resistance to sodium dodecyl sulfate

TABLE 2. *Susceptibility of Erwinia amylovora and other bacterial cultures in LB to NOV, DOC, and SDS*[a]

Species	Strain	LD_{99} (μg/ml)[b] of: NOV	DOC	SDS
Erwinia amylovora (wild-type)	EA137	15	300–500	40
	EA167	15	400–800	40–60
	EA169	15	50	20
	EA177	15	400–800	40
	EA178	15	300–500	40
	EA212	50–100	400–800	200–500
	EA213	50–100	250–500	200–500
E. amylovora (drug-resistant)	EA178-D3 (AC416)	<25	>1,000	<250
	EA178-N2 (AC418)	>100	500–1,000	<250
	EA178-S1 (AC419)	>100	500–1,000	>1,000
	EA178-SDN (AC421)	>100	500–1,000	>1,000
E. amylovora (plasmid-bearing)	EA178-E (AC425)	15	500–1,000	40
	EA178-F′ (AC426)	5–10	250–500	25
	EA178-RP1 (AC427)	5–10	250–500	25
	EA178-R100 (AC428)	5–10	250–500	25
E. aroideae	EA144	50–100	>1,000	>1,000
E. carotovora	EC153	50–100	>1,000	>1,000
E. chrysanthemi	EC16	50–100	>1,000	>1,000
E. herbicola	EH103	50–100	>1,000	>1,000
Salmonella typhimurium	3335	50–100	>1,000	>1,000

[a] Refer to the Materials and Methods section for details of the experimental conditions. Abbreviations: LB, Luria broth; NOV, novobiocin; DOC, deoxycholate; SDS, sodium dodecyl sulfate.

[b] LD_{99}, concentration of the antibacterial agent causing a 99% inhibition of growth in LB as determined by turbidity measurements of the liquid cultures.

shows enhanced resistance (as compared to the wild-type parent strain) to all three of the agents tested (i.e., novobiocin, deoxycholate, and sodium dodecyl sulfate; Table 2).

Spontaneous release of periplasmic enzymes. In light of the relatively high susceptibility of *E. amylovora* to the antibacterial agents shown here, and taking into account an extensive literature that relates enhanced drug susceptibility to defective outer membranes in other enterobacterial systems, it was deemed of interest to determine the periplasmic leakiness of the *E. amylovora* strains. The results summarized in Table 3 reveal that the wild-type strains of *E. amylovora,* grown in 1% (wt/vol) tryptone broth, release about 50 to 69% of the total activity of the periplasmic enzyme, cyclic phosphodiesterase, into the growth medium after an 8-h incubation at 30°C. Such enzymatic activity was undetectable in the culture supernatant from the strains of *E. aroideae, E. atroseptica, E. carotovora,* and *E. herbicola,* although the cell extracts showed this activity (detailed data not presented here). *E. chrysanthemi* strain EC16 shows no cyclic phosphodiesterase activity detectable either in cell extracts or in growth media under the particular conditions of these experiments (cultivation in tryptone broth). There was no detectable activity of glucose-6-phosphate dehydrogenase (a known cytoplasmic enzyme) in any of the *E. amylovora* culture supernatants, although the cell extracts showed this activity (Table 3), thus indicating that substantial cell lysis did not occur under these conditions.

The release of cyclic phosphodiesterase from the mutant strains of *E. amylovora* selected for resistance to deoxycholate (AC416) or to sodium dodecyl sulfate (AC419) or to all three antibacterial agents (AC421) was relatively less (25 to 37% of the total enzyme activity was present in the culture supernatants) than that eventually released by the wild-type strains (in which 50 to 69% of the total enzyme activity was present in the culture supernatants; Table 3). The mutant strain selected for resistance to novobiocin (AC418) behaved in this respect like the wild-type strains.

The results summarized in Table 3 also reveal that the drug-resistant mutants, as compared to the parent wild-type strain (EA178), produce lower levels of cyclic phosphodiesterase under identical conditions; the physiological and genetic bases for this difference are not now known. However, a comparison of the data (Table 3, lines 8, 9, and 11) clearly indicates a lack of correlation between the enzyme levels (total units) and the extent of periplasmic leakage (units present in the supernatant). This behavior leads us to conclude that the decrease in the

TABLE 3. *Spontaneous release of periplasmic (cyclic phosphodiesterase) and cytoplasmic (glucose-6-phosphate dehydrogenase) enzymes by wild-type and drug-resistant strains of Erwinia amylovora during growth for 8 h in 1% (wt/vol) tryptone broth at 30°C*

Strain	Growth (Klett units)	Enzyme activities[a] of: Cyclic phosphodiesterase in:		
		S/C[b]	S(%)[c]	Glucose-6-phosphate dehydrogenase in C[d]
Wild-type strains				
EA167	59	0.7/0.6	54	0.04
EA169	56	1.0/0.9	53	0.07
EA177	48	1.0/0.8	56	0.08
EA178	54	1.1/0.5	69	0.06
EA198	45	0.6/0.6	50	0.11
EA212	31	1.3/0.8	62	0.06
EA213	36	1.1/0.9	55	0.03
Drug-resistant strains				
EA178-D3 (AC416)	98	0.2/0.6	25	0.08
EA178-N2 (AC418)	65	0.4/0.4	50	0.08
EA178-S1 (AC419)	68	0.3/0.5	37	0.10
EA178-SDN (AC421)	30	0.3/0.7	30	0.12

[a] Refer to Materials and Methods section and also to footnotes of Table 4 for details of experimental conditions and definitions of enzyme units. Enzyme activities are expressed here as enzyme units/ml of culture per 100 Klett units; 100 Klett units = about 5×10^8 cells/ml.
[b] S/C = activities of enzyme in supernatants/cells.
[c] S = activities of enzyme in supernatants.
[d] Activities of enzyme in cells; no detectable enzyme activities in culture supernatants.

extent of periplasmic leakiness found in some of the mutants might result from one or more factors that contribute to the drug resistance of the mutants and not from a decrease, relative to the wild-type strain, in the levels of enzyme present in these mutants. This conclusion is further supported by the fact that none of the independently isolated drug-resistant mutants (AC416, AC419, and AC421), all of which spontaneously release lower levels of the enzyme as compared with the wild-type parent strain, was selected for decreased periplasmic leakage (they were selected for drug resistance).

Effects of salts on periplasmic leakage and maximum growth temperature. Since the literature (5) suggests that spontaneous periplasmic leakage in LPS-defective strains of other enterobacteria can be reduced or prevented by the addition of NaCl or $MgCl_2$ to the growth medium, we examined the effects of these salts on the release of a periplasmic enzyme from *E. amylovora* wild-type strain EA178 (Table 4). NaCl (84 mM) or $MgCl_2$ (20 mM) substantially reduced or prevented the leakage of the periplasmic enzyme, cyclic phosphodiesterase; $MgCl_2$ was more effective than NaCl in this regard. There was no detectable phosphoglucose isomerase or glucose-6-phosphate dehydrogenase activity in culture supernatants of *E. amylovora* wild-type strain EA178, regardless of the presence or absence of these salts (Table 4).

Taking into account the relatively low maximum growth temperature (<37°C) of *E. amylovora* (3) and the role that $MgCl_2$ is known to play in increasing the maximum growth temperature in LPS-defective strains of *Salmonella* and *E. coli* (6), we examined the effect of $MgCl_2$ on the growth of *E. amylovora* wild-type strain EA178 at various temperatures and determined the extent of periplasmic leakiness under these conditions. $MgCl_2$ did, in fact, stimulate growth at 30°C (the generation times in the presence and absence of 20 mM $MgCl_2$ were 54 and 108 min, respectively). However, the pattern of growth at 34 and 37°C in the presence or absence of $MgCl_2$ remained unaltered: growth did occur at 34°C, albeit at a very low rate; at 37°C, growth stopped 1 h after the shift to the higher temperature. Leakage of cyclic phosphodiesterase occurred at all three temperatures in the absence of $MgCl_2$, and it was completely prevented by the presence of 20 mM $MgCl_2$ (detailed data not presented here).

DISCUSSION

This study reveals that wild-type strains of *Erwinia amylovora* are unusually susceptible to novobiocin, deoxycholate, and sodium dodecyl (= lauryl) sulfate. These strains also spontaneously release a periplasmic enzyme, cyclic phosphodiesterase, and do not release a cytoplasmic enzyme, glucose-6-phosphate dehydrogenase. Strains of other enterobacteria with

TABLE 4. *Effects of sodium chloride and magnesium chloride on the growth and the spontaneous release of enzymes in wild-type Erwinia amylovora strain EA178 during a growth for 14 h at 30°C in 1% (wt/vol) tryptone broth*[a]

Supplement	Growth (Klett units)[b]	Enzyme activities (U/ml per 5 × 10^8 cells) of: Cyclic phosphodiesterase in S/C[c]	Phosphogluco-isomerase[d] in C[e]	Glucose-6-phosphate dehydrogenase[f] in C
None	92	0.7/0.5 (63.6)	0.11	0.05
NaCl (84 mM)	180	0.11/0.66 (14.3)	0.15	0.06
NaCl (168 mM)	160	0.12/0.70 (14.6)	0.16	0.04
$MgCl_2$ (20 mM)	151	0/0.75 (0)	0.13	0.04

[a] Refer to the Materials and Methods section for details of the experimental conditions.
[b] 100 Klett units = 5 × 10^8 cells.
[c] Activity was measured using bis-(*p*-nitrophenyl)phosphate as the substrate (27); unit of activity = a change of 2.0 U of absorbancy at 410 nm in 30 min at 30°C. S/C = activities of enzyme in supernatants/cells. Figures in parentheses are percentages of total enzymatic activity found in the supernatants.
[d] Activity was measured using glucose-6-phosphate as the substrate (30); unit of activity = micromoles of fructose-6-phosphate formed per minute at 30°C.
[e] C = activities of enzyme in cells; no detectable enzyme activity in culture supernatants.
[f] Activity was measured using glucose-6-phosphate as the substrate (20); unit of activity = micromoles of nicotinamide adenine dinucleotide phosphate reduced per minute at 25°C.

defects in the outer membrane similarly show enhanced susceptibility to antibacterial agents and spontaneously release periplasmic enzymes (17) into the growth medium (5, 18, 24, 25, 32–35, 38).

Our findings and the cited literature suggest, then, that *E. amylovora* might have a defective outer membrane, resulting in an altered permeability. However, our qualitative analysis of the *E. amylovora* LPS molecule has revealed that *E. amylovora* wild-type strains do possess essentially the full complement of LPS components (2-keto-3-deoxyoctonic acid, heptose, glucose, galactose, glucosamine, and rhamnose have been identified to date; A. K. Chatterjee, A. G. Andrewes, and M. P. Starr, unpublished data), the same as is found in other enterobacteria (5, 33). On this basis, these wild-type *E. amylovora* strains are smooth. Thus, the unusual susceptibility of *E. amylovora* strains to the tested antibacterial agents does not result from an obvious qualitative chemical defect in the LPS molecule, though there might be some quantitative peculiarity. It is also possible that *E. amylovora* strains have some defect(s) in lipid and/or protein components of the outer membrane (1, 19, 26) that might contribute to enhanced permeability (leakiness). Comparisons of the outer membrane lipid and protein profiles of the drug-resistant mutant strains with those of the wild-type strains might reveal defects in these lipids and/or proteins, which might in turn relate to the peculiar permeability of these *E. amylovora* strains.

Substances that increase the osmolarity of the growth medium (such as NaCl) or interact in some specific manner with the outer membrane (such as Mg^{2+}) are known to prevent the spontaneous leakage of periplasmic enzymes in LPS-defective (heptose-deficient) strains of *S. typhimurium* (5). The mechanisms by which $MgCl_2$ and NaCl act in preventing periplasmic leakiness in *E. amylovora* are unclear at present, although there is no doubt that these substances do indeed act in this way (Table 4). It is possible that Mg^{2+} stabilizes the outer membrane, and it would have been of interest to determine, explicitly, the effect of Mg^{2+} on the susceptibility of *E. amylovora* to the antibacterial agents. However, in the present state of the art, interpretation of the results of such experiments would not have been unambiguous, since many such antibacterial compounds are known to complex with Mg^{2+}. Such complexed molecules might have an altered antibacterial potency relative to noncomplexed compounds. For example, the formation of a tetracycline-Mg^{2+} complex, and its decreased biological activity, are well documented in the literature (36). In this connection, it is noteworthy that the drug susceptibilities of the *E. amylovora* strains (Table 2) were determined in LB that contained 168 mM NaCl.

That there was no demonstrable phosphoglucose isomerase activity in culture supernatants of *E. amylovora* wild-type strain EA178, regardless of the presence or absence of NaCl or $MgCl_2$ (Table 4), again points up the differences between this phytopathogenic bacterium and other enterobacteria. Phosphoglucose isomerase has been shown to be (at least partly) periplasmic in *E. coli* (15) and in *S. typhimurium* (5); this enzyme is probably not periplasmic, but rather cytoplasmic or possibly membrane-bound, in this *E. amylovora* strain.

We have found that clones of *E. amylovora* harboring derepressed plasmids (F'*lac*$^+$, R100*drd*-56, and RP1) show an enhanced susceptibility to novobiocin and sodium dodecyl sulfate (Table 2). Our results also reveal that the presence in *E. amylovora* of the plasmid E-*lac*$^+$, which is repressed in transfer functions (10), does not alter the susceptibility to these antibacterial agents (Table 2). Riva et al. (31) have demonstrated that some *E. coli* strains harboring derepressed R plasmids are more susceptible (than are strains not harboring these plasmids) to antibiotics such as actinomycin, erythromycin, and rifamycin. These workers hypothesized that some R plasmids might code for functions that alter the LPS backbone of the outer-membrane surface structure and that such alteration might lower the barrier to penetration of some antibiotics. More recently, Derylo et al. (13) have shown that *S. typhimurium* strain Rc902 containing derepressed Col plasmids (ColIb*drd*-2 and ColIb*drd*-7) or a derepressed R plasmid (R64*drd*-11) was considerably more susceptible (as compared to Col$^-$ or R$^-$ strains) to sodium dodecyl sulfate, acriflavin, and deoxycholate. These findings (13) also reveal a decrease in the content of O sidechain sugars in the LPS of *S. typhimurium* strains harboring derepressed Col and R plasmids. It is possible that the enhanced susceptibility to the antibacterial agents of *E. amylovora* strains containing derepressed plasmids, as documented in the present study, also might result from alteration of the LPS molecule. We are presently seeking experimental verification of this notion.

E. amylovora strains are unable to grow at 37°C or higher temperatures (3). In this connection, we note that heptose-deficient (deep-rough) strains of *Salmonella* spp. and *E. coli* fail to grow in a medium of low osmolarity at 42°C or higher temperatures (temperatures and conditions at which the smooth strains do grow) and that this temperature sensitivity in such heptose-deficient strains can be reversed by increasing the osmolarity of the medium with NaCl or by the addition of $MgCl_2$ (the latter at relatively low concentrations) to the growth medium (6). Although $MgCl_2$ does cause more rapid growth of *E. amylovora* wild-type strain EA178 at 30°C, there is no effect of $MgCl_2$ on its slow growth at 34°C or on its total inability to grow at 37°C. $MgCl_2$ does, in fact, eliminate the leakage of the periplasmic enzyme, cyclic phosphodiesterase, from *E. amylovora* at all three temperatures (30, 34, and 37°C). Taking all of our findings (including the preliminary analyses that show no obvious qualitative chemical abnormality in the *E. amylovora* LPS components) and the literature into account, it would appear that the relatively low maximum growth temperature of *E. amylovora* is unrelated to periplasmic leakiness. Nevertheless, it is indeed the case that most wild-type *E. amylovora* strains are unusual with respect to leakiness of their cell envelopes and ordinarily associated properties such as low maximum growth temperature and enhanced susceptibility to antibacterial agents, whatever might be the precise cause(s)!

We turn now to a brief consideration of the possible relationship between the putatively defective (or, better yet, unusually functioning under laboratory conditions) cell envelope of *E. amylovora* and the pathogenicity of this organism for plants. Little is known regarding the mechanisms of pathogenicity by *E. amylovora*, but it seems likely that the presence of a defective cell envelope might play some significant role(s) in its plant pathogenicity. This view stems from the demonstration by Goodman and his associates (16) that *E. amylovora* produces in infected plants a "toxin," a large molecule of polygalactose ("amylovorin"), which they believe is involved in plant pathogenesis. Although it is unclear at present whether amylovorin is the (only) phytotoxic principle of *E. amylovora*, it does seem likely that there is some causal relationship between the production of this substance and occurrence of (some of) the fire blight disease symptoms. Based on this supposition, we have now initiated genetic analyses, using the conjugal gene transmission systems developed by us (9, 29; B. K. Pugashetti, A. K. Chatterjee, and M. P. Starr, manuscript in preparation), regarding the production of amylovorin and other possibly phytotoxic substances by *E. amylovora*.

Assuming that some role(s) of amylovorin in plant pathogenicity can indeed be confirmed, one is then confronted with the problem of how this large amylovorin molecule (molecular weight, about 130,000; 16) might be excreted from the bacterial cells (unless it is somehow assembled extracellularly). A permeable cell envelope might explain the release of this large amylovorin molecule from *E. amylovora* cells. Our preliminary probes (A. K. Chatterjee and M. P. Starr, unpublished data) into the plant pathogenicity of *E. amylovora* strains that are resistant to antibacterial agents (novobiocin, deoxycholate, and sodium dodecyl sulfate) show that necrosis and exudate production caused by *E. amylovora,* as scored on immature pear fruits (4, 29), are markedly reduced in the drug-resistant strains as compared with the drug-susceptible, wild-type strains. In this context, Corwin et al. (11) have found in *Shigella flexneri* a direct correlation between susceptibility to sodium dodecyl sulfate and virulence (in this case, the ability to penetrate intestinal epithelium). If our ongoing studies with *E. amylovora* provide confirmation of (i) the role(s) in plant pathogenicity reported to be played by amylovorin and (ii) the aforementioned direct correlation we have observed between loss of plant pathogenicity and resistance to antibacterial agents, then the exceptional conservation of a presumably defective cell envelope in *E. amylovora* might be explained in terms of the excretion of the large amylovorin molecule.

ACKNOWLEDGMENTS

This study was supported by Public Health Service research grant AI-08426 from the National Institute of Allergy and Infectious Diseases. We acknowledge with thanks the generous help provided by A. G. Andrewes in connection with the analyses of lipopolysaccharide components and competent technical assistance of G. E. Buchanan in other phases of this work.

LITERATURE CITED

1. **Ames, G. F., E. N. Spudich, and H. Nikaido.** 1974. Protein composition of the outer membrane of *Salmonella typhimurium*: effect of lipopolysaccharide mutations. J. Bacteriol. **117**:406–416.
2. **Anraku, Y.** 1964. A new cyclic phosphodiesterase having 3′-nucleotidase activity from *Escherichia coli* B. I. Purification and some properties of the enzyme. J. Biol. Chem. **239**:3412–3419.
3. **Billing, E.** 1974. The effect of temperature on the growth of the fireblight-pathogen, *Erwinia amylovora*. J. Appl. Bacteriol. **37**:643–648.
4. **Billing, E., J. E. Crosse, and C. M. E. Garrett.** 1960. Laboratory diagnosis of fire blight and bacterial blossom blight of pear. Plant Pathol. **9**:19–25.
5. **Chatterjee, A. K., H. Ross, and K. E. Sanderson.** 1976. Leakage of periplasmic enzymes from lipopolysaccharide-defective mutants of *Salmonella typhimurium*. Can. J. Microbiol. **22**:1549–1560.
6. **Chatterjee, A. K., K. E. Sanderson, H. Ross, S. Schlecht, and O. Lüderitz.** 1976. Influence of temperature on growth of lipopolysaccharide-deficient (rough) mutants of *Salmonella typhimurium* and *S. minnesota*. Can. J. Microbiol. **22**:1540–1548.
7. **Chatterjee, A. K., and M. P. Starr.** 1972. Genetic transfer of episomic elements among *Erwinia* species and other enterobacteria: F′*lac*$^+$. J. Bacteriol. **111**:169–176.
8. **Chatterjee, A. K., and M. P. Starr.** 1972. Transfer among *Erwinia* spp. and other enterobacteria of antibiotic resistance carried on R factors. J. Bacteriol. **112**:576–584.
9. **Chatterjee, A. K., and M. P. Starr.** 1973. Gene transmission among strains of *Erwinia amylovora*. J. Bacteriol. **116**:1100–1106.
10. **Chatterjee, A. K., and M. P. Starr.** 1973. Transmission of *lac* by the sex factor E in *Erwinia* strains from human clinical sources. Infect. Immun. **8**:563–572.
11. **Corwin, L. M., S. W. Rothman, R. Kim, and L. A. Talevi.** 1971. Mechanisms and genetics of resistance to sodium lauryl sulfate in strains of *Shigella* and *Escherichia coli*. Infect. Immun. **4**:287–294.
12. **Costerton, J. W., J. M. Ingram, and K.-J. Cheng.** 1974. Structure and function of the cell envelope of gram-negative bacteria. Bacteriol. Rev. **38**:87–110.
13. **Derylo, M., M. Glowacka, Z. Lorkiewicz, and R. Russa.** 1975. Plasmid-determined alterations of *Salmonella typhimurium* lipopolysaccharides. Mol. Gen. Genet. **140**:175–181.
14. **Ennis, H. L., and M. I. Bloomstein.** 1974. Antibiotic-sensitive mutants of *Escherichia coli* possess altered outer membranes. Ann. N.Y. Acad. Sci. **235**:593–600.
15. **Freidberg, I.** 1972. Location of phosphoglucose isomerase in *Escherichia coli* and its relation to the induction of the hexose phosphate transport system. J. Bacteriol. **122**:1201–1205.
16. **Goodman, R. N., J. C. Huang, and P.-Y. Huang.** 1974. Host-specific phytotoxic polysaccharide from apple tissue infected by *Erwinia amylovora*. Science **183**: 1081–1082.
17. **Heppel, L. A.** 1971. The concept of periplasmic enzymes, p. 233–247. *In* L. I. Rothfield (ed.), Structure and function of biological membranes. Academic Press Inc., New York.
18. **Irvin, R. T., A. K. Chatterjee, K. E. Sanderson, and J. W. Costerton.** 1975. Comparison of the cell envelope structure of a lipopolysaccharide-defective (heptose-deficient) and a smooth strain of *Salmonella typhimurium*. J. Bacteriol. **124**:930–941.
19. **Koplow, J., and H. Goldfine.** 1974. Alterations in the outer membrane of the cell envelope of heptose-deficient mutants of *Escherichia coli*. J. Bacteriol. **117**:527–543.
20. **Langdon, R. G.** 1966. Glucose-6-phosphate dehydrogenase from erythrocytes, p. 126–131. *In* W. A. Wood (ed.), Methods in enzymology, vol. 9. Academic Press Inc., New York.
21. **Leive, L.** 1965. A nonspecific increase in permeability in *Escherichia coli* produced by EDTA. Proc. Natl. Acad. Sci. U.S.A. **53**:745–750.
22. **Leive, L.** 1974. The barrier function of the gram-negative envelope. Ann. N.Y. Acad. Sci. **234**:109–129.
23. **Lin, E. C. C., S. A. Lerner, and S. E. Jorgensen.** 1962. A method for isolating constitutive mutants for carbohydrate-catabolizing enzymes. Biochim. Biophys. Acta **60**:422–424.
24. **Lindsay, S. S., B. Wheeler, K. E. Sanderson, J. W. Costerton, and K.-J. Chen.** 1973. The release of alkaline phosphatase and of lipopolysaccharide during the growth of rough and smooth strains of *Salmonella typhimurium*. Can. J. Microbiol. **19**:335–343.
25. **Lopes, J., S. Gottfried, and L. Rothfield.** 1972. Leakage of periplasmic enzymes by mutants of *Escherichia coli* and *Salmonella typhimurium*: isolation of "periplasmic leaky" mutants. J. Bacteriol. **109**:520–525.
26. **Lüderitz, O., C. Galonos, V. Lehmann, M. Nurminer, E. Rietschel, G. Rosenfelder, M. Simon, and O. Westphal.** 1973. Lipid A, chemical structure and biological activity. J. Infect. Dis. **128**:S19–S29.
27. **Neu, H. C.** 1967. The 5′-nucleotidase of *Escherichia coli*. I. Purification and properties. J. Biol. Chem. **242**:3896–3904.
28. **Osborn, M. J., J. E. Gander, E. Parisi, and J. Carson.** 1972. Mechanism of assembly of the outer membrane of *Salmonella typhimurium*. I. Isolation and characterization of cytoplasmic and outer membrane. J. Biol. Chem. **247**:3962–3972.
29. **Pugashetti, B. K., and M. P. Starr.** 1975. Conjugational transfer of genes determining plant virulence in *Erwinia amylovora*. J. Bacteriol. **122**:485–491.
30. **Reithel, F. J.** 1966. Phosphoglucose isomerase. II.

Mammary gland, p. 565-568. *In* W. A. Wood (ed.), Methods in enzymology, vol. 9. Academic Press Inc., New York.

31. **Riva, S., A. M. Fietta, L. G. Silvestri, and E. Romero.** 1972. R factors-determined changes in the permeability of *E. coli* towards rifampicin and other antibiotics, p. 343-348. *In* V. Kreméry, L. Rosival, and T. Watanabe (ed.), Bacterial plasmids and antibiotic resistance. Springer-Verlag, New York.
32. **Sanderson, K. E., T. MacAlister, J. W. Costerton, and K.-J. Cheng.** 1974. Permeability of lipopolysaccharide-deficient (rough) mutants of *Salmonella typhimurium* to antibiotics, lysozyme, and other agents. Can. J. Microbiol. **20**:1135-1145.
33. **Sanderson, K. E., J. Van Wyngaarder, O. Lüderitz, and B. A. D. Stocker.** 1974. Rough mutants of *Salmonella typhimurium* with defects in the heptose region of the lipopolysaccharide core. Can. J. Microbiol. **20**:1127-1134.
34. **Schlecht, S., and O. Westphal.** 1970. Untersuchungen zur Typisierung von *Salmonella*-R-Formen. 4. Mitteilung: Typisierung von *S. minnesota*-R-Mutanten mittels Antibiotica. Zentralbl. Bakteriol. Parasitenkd. Infektionskr. Hyg. Abt. 1 Orig. **213**:356-381.
35. **Singh, A. P., and R. A. F. Reithmeier.** 1975. Leakage of periplasmic enzyme from cells of heptose-deficient mutants of *Escherichia coli* associated with alterations in the protein component of the outer membrane. J. Gen. Appl. Microbiol. **21**:109-118.
36. **Sompolinsky, D., and Z. Samra.** 1972. Influence of magnesium and manganese on some biological and physical properties of tetracycline. J. Bacteriol. **110**:468-476.
37. **Starr, M. P., and A. K. Chatterjee.** 1972. The genus *Erwinia*: Enterobacteria pathogenic to plants and animals. Annu. Rev. Microbiol. **26**:389-426.
38. **Tamaki, S., T. Sata, and M. Matsuhashi.** 1971. Role of lipopolysaccharide in antibiotic resistance and bacteriophage adsorption of *Escherichia coli* K-12. J. Bacteriol. **105**:968-975.

Antimicrobial Agents and Chemotherapy, May 1977, p. 906-908
Vol. 11, No. 5

Printed in U.S.A.

NOTES

Extreme Sensitivity of Staphylococcal Enterotoxin B and C Production to Inhibition by Cerulenin

ROBERT A. ALTENBERN

U.S. Army Medical Research Institute of Infectious Diseases, Frederick, Maryland 21701

Received for publication 21 December 1976

Production of staphylococcal enterotoxins B and C was completely inhibited by concentrations of cerulenin (4 μg/ml and 2 μg/ml, respectively) that did not affect either growth rate or final growth density. Type A toxin formation was not similarly inhibited.

The secretion of bacterial exoproteins has been most extensively investigated by Lampen and collaborators (5, 7) in the case of penicillinase production by *Bacillus licheniformis*. From these studies, it appears that lipid of the cytoplasmic membrane participates in the synthesis and transport of penicillinase to the exterior medium. Kimura and Izui (4) have recently reported that membrane fluidity, which is controlled by the fatty acids in the membrane, plays an important role in induction of alkaline phosphatase in *Escherichia coli*. In this laboratory, there is an ongoing investigation of the role of membrane fatty acids in production of enterotoxin B by *Staphylococcus aureus*. Fatty acid nutrition in *S. aureus* can be directed by exposing cells to the minimal inhibitory concentration (MIC) of cerulenin, an antibiotic which inhibits fatty acid biosynthesis (6), and restoring growth by supplementation with appropriate saturated and unsaturated fatty acids. An unexpected result of these studies was the observation that production of staphylococcal enterotoxins B and C is inhibited by concentrations of cerulenin far too low to affect either the growth rate or final growth density of the strains employed. The present report presents details of this phenomenon.

The strains of *S. aureus* employed were as follows: ATCC 14458, S-6, 137-H2, and 2909. Both strains 14458 and S-6 are wild-type strains that produce enterotoxin B (SEB). Strain 137-H2 is a wild type that elaborates enterotoxin C_1 (SEC). Strain 2909 produces relatively large amounts of enterotoxin A (SEA) and was derived from strain 100 by a multistep mutagenesis procedure (3). Cells were grown in tubes (18 by 150 mm) containing 5 ml of NAK medium (2) prepared in 0.067 M phosphate buffer, pH 7.0, and containing graded concentrations of cerulenin (Makor Chemicals Ltd., Jerusalem, Israel). The tubes were incubated at an angle on a shaker at 37°C. Growth rate was monitored by measuring optical density (absorbance) at 600 nm in a Coleman Junior spectrophotometer. Final growth density (after 21 h of incubation) was assessed by measurement of absorbance at 600 nm of a 1:5 dilution (into water) of the culture. A portion of the final culture was centrifuged to remove cells, and the supernatant was assayed for enterotoxin by the Oudin tube method. Assays for alpha-toxin and coagulase were conducted by microtitration and by conventional serial dilution, respectively.

The MIC of cerulenin for strains 14458, S-6, and 2909 was approximately 100 μg of antibiotic per ml; strain 137-H2 was somewhat more sensitive, with a MIC of about 50 μg/ml (Fig. 1). Concentrations of cerulenin up to at least 10 μg/ml had no demonstrable effect on the final growth density for strain 14458, S-6, or 2909. The final growth density of strain 137-H2 declined gradually above 3 μg of cerulenin per ml.

Pronounced suppression of SEB production by cerulenin concentrations above 1 μg/ml was noted for strains 14458 and S-6 (Fig. 2). Formation of SEC by strain 137-H2 was completely inhibited by a cerulenin concentration (3 μg/ml) that had no effect on final growth density. In contrast, there appeared to be no suppression of SEA production by strain 2909 with concentrations of cerulenin that did not inhibit growth.

Addition of up to 20 μg of cerulenin per ml to preformed enterotoxin B in NAK medium did not alter the assay value by the Oudin method, thus ruling out possible inactivation of SEB or

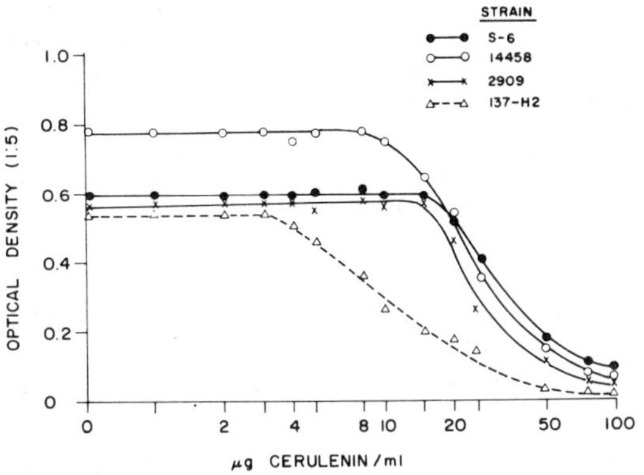

FIG. 1. *Effect of graded concentrations of cerulenin on final growth density of S. aureus strains.*

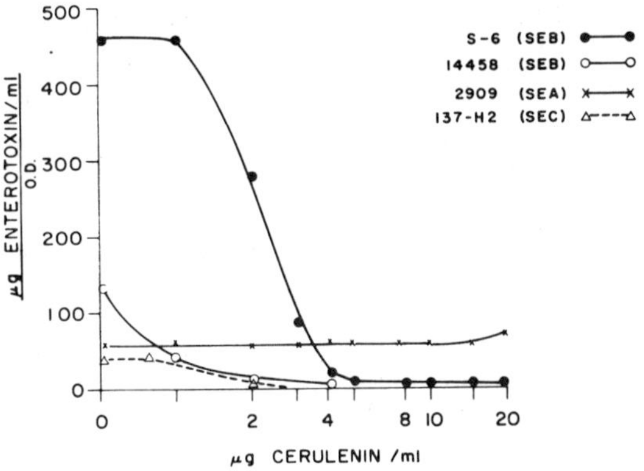

FIG. 2. *Suppression of enterotoxin formation by graded concentrations of cerulenin. Enterotoxin in a concentration of micrograms per milliliter divided by absorbance of 1:5 dilution yields a measure of toxin production per unit of cell mass. Strain number is in parentheses. The lower limit of determination of enterotoxin amounts of all types of Oudin technique is 3 μg/ml.*

inhibition of the antigen-antibody reaction by the antibiotic. Similar tests on SEA and SEC were not performed.

Determinations of mass doubling times from optical density data during exponential growth revealed there was no increase in doubling time for strains 14458, S-6, and 2909 up to at least 10 μg of cerulenin per ml. There was also agreement for strain 137-H2 between the concentration of cerulenin required to induce suppression of final growth density and extension of the mass doubling time (5 μg/ml and above).

Cerulenin is an unsaturated fatty acid amide (6), and it might be expected that other saturated or unsaturated fatty acids would antagonize the inhibition of enterotoxin B production by cerulenin. Accordingly, two sets of tubes of NAK medium were prepared, one set without cerulenin and the other containing 10 μg of cerulenin per ml. Graded concentrations of a mixture of saturated fatty acids were added to each series. The saturated fatty acid mixture (SFA) was composed of equal concentrations (wt/vol) of lauric, myristic, palmitic, stearic, arachidic, behenic, and lignoceric acids. Figure 3 shows that the final growth density of the cultures was affected to the same degree by SFA regardless of the presence or absence of cerulenin in the medium. There was no suppression of SEB formation by the SFA mixture in cerulenin-free medium until final growth density was depressed by the added fatty acids. In contrast, in tubes containing 10 μg of cerulenin per ml, a narrow concentration range of SFA mixture partially reversed the total sup-

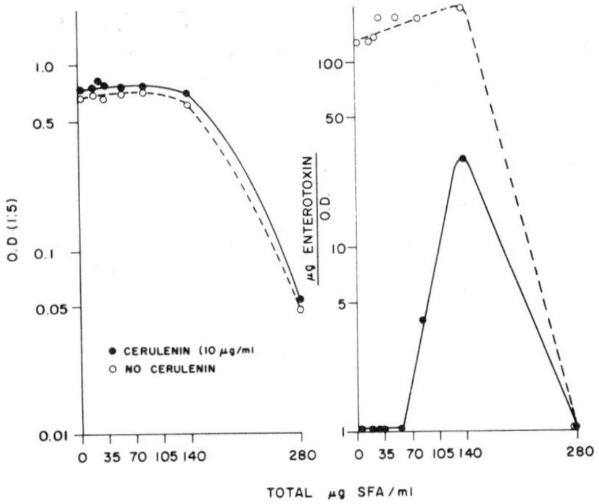

FIG. 3. *Saturated fatty acid-induced reversal of cerulenin suppression of enterotoxin B formation by 14458.*

TABLE 1. *Suppression of production of α-hemolysin and coagulase by strain 14458 with graded concentrations of cerulenin*

Cerulenin (μg/ml)	Titer	
	Alpha-toxin[a]	Coagulase[b]
0	256	4
1	128	2
2	64	2
3	32	0
4	8	0
5	4	0
8	0	0
10	0	0
15	0	0
20	0	0

[a] Reciprocal of highest dilution showing 50% lysis.

[b] Reciprocal of highest dilution displaying any clot.

pression of SEB formation by cerulenin. A mixture of 10 unsaturated fatty acids from C_{16} to C_{24} was unable to reverse cerulenin-induced suppression of SEB production without concomitant severe inhibition of growth (data not shown).

With strain 14458, it was found that low concentrations of cerulenin, which were noninhibitory for growth rate or final growth density, also strongly suppressed production of alpha-toxin and coagulase. It appears that production of SEB, alpha-toxin, and coagulase is severely inhibited by the same concentration of cerulenin (Table 1). It is noteworthy that the inhibition is a general effect, altering production of all three exoproteins in the same manner.

The mechanism of this effect is unknown. The concentration of cerulenin required to suppress production of enterotoxins, α-hemolysin, and coagulase is only a small fraction of the MIC. The effects of cerulenin reported here resemble the inhibition of coagulase release by very low, subinhibitory concentrations of chloramphenicol (1). The observation that strain 2909 is resistant to inhibition of SEA production when growth rate and final density are unaffected is not surprising. Strain 2909 was derived from wild-type strain 100 by a 13-step mutagenesis procedure and is far removed in many of its growth properties from the original wild type. The very low production of SEA by wild-type strains such as strain 100 (less than 3 μg/ml) precluded determination by Oudin assay of the effect of cerulenin in subinhibitory concentrations on formation of this toxin type.

I am grateful to Allen R. Knott for performing Oudin assays for the enterotoxins and to Anna Johnson for conducting α-hemolysin titrations.

LITERATURE CITED

1. **Altenbern, R. A.** 1966. On the nature of albumin-promoted coagulase release by *Staphylococcus aureus*. J. Infect. Dis. 116:593–600.
2. **Altenbern, R. A.** 1976. Enterotoxin B formation by fermentation mutants of *Staphylococcus aureus*. Can. J. Microbiol. 22:182–188.
3. **Friedman, M. E., and M. B. Howard.** 1971. Induction of mutants of *Staphylococcus aureus* 100 with increased ability to produce enterotoxin A. J. Bacteriol. 106:289–291.
4. **Kimura, K., and K. Izui.** 1976. Importance of membrane fluidity in the induction of alkaline phosphatase, a periplasmic enzyme, in *Escherichia coli*. Biochem. Biophys. Res. Commun. 70:900–906.
5. **Lampen, J. O.** 1974. Movement of extracellular enzymes across cell membranes, p. 351–374. *In* M. A. Sleigh and D. H. Jennings (ed.), Transport at the cellular level. Cambridge University Press, Cambridge, England.
6. **Omura, S.** 1976. The antibiotic cerulenin, a novel tool for biochemistry as an inhibitor of fatty acid synthesis. Bacteriol. Rev. 40:681–697.
7. **Yamamoto, S., and J. O. Lampen.** 1976. Membrane penicillinase of *Bacillus licheniformis* 749/C: sequence and possible repeated tetrapeptide structure of the phospholipopeptide region. Proc. Natl. Acad. Sci. U.S.A. 73:1457–1461.

ANTIMICROBIAL AGENTS AND CHEMOTHERAPY, May 1977, p. 909-911
Vol. 11, No. 5

Cephradine Penetration into Cerebrospinal Fluid and Effects of Its Administration into the Cerebral Ventricles of Cats

SAMI I. HARIK,[1]* KAMAL F. AKL, AND MARWAN UWAYDAH[2]

Departments of Medicine, Pediatrics, and Bacteriology and Virology, American University of Beirut, School of Medicine, Beirut, Lebanon

Received for publication 22 November 1976

In cats that had high, sustained serum concentrations of cephradine, penetration of the drug into the cerebrospinal fluid (CSF) was poor. Serum cephradine levels were, on the average, 100-fold higher than the CSF levels. On the other hand, the direct injection of cephradine into the lateral cerebral ventricles of cats yielded high CSF cephradine concentrations without evidence of central nervous system toxicity.

Some organisms that cause meningitis and other central nervous system bacterial infections are demonstrably sensitive, in vitro, to cephalosporin antibiotics. In spite of this, these drugs have proven relatively ineffective, apparently because they fail to penetrate the blood-brain barrier adequately (1-3, 6). In fact, it was documented that cephalothin-sensitive bacteria were responsible for meningitis in patients already receiving therapeutic doses of the drug (5). Intrathecal administration, of course, offers an alternative route, and there is a report that cephaloridine is safe and effective when used in this way to treat meningitis (4).

Cephradine is a newer derivative of this family of drugs. Little information is available regarding its ability to penetrate the central nervous system, nor has its safety when administered intrathecally been assessed. Data along these lines would be of obvious clinical value, and it is to this end that our work was directed.

Adult cats of both sexes, weighing 2.5 to 4.5 kg, were used in all experiments. Unless otherwise stated, cats were anesthetized with pentobarbital sodium (35 mg/kg), paralyzed with gallamine triethiode, and artificially respired. Femoral arterial blood pressure was monitored, and the experiment was stopped if the mean pressure fell below 80 mm of Hg. End-tidal CO_2 was maintained within the physiological range by adjusting the respiratory rate. An electrical heating pad maintained rectal temperature between 37 and 37.5°C. Needle electrodes, inserted into the scalp, recorded a bipolar, two-channel electroencephalogram. Commercial preparations of injectable cephradine (Eskacef, Smith Kline and French; Velosef, Squibb) were dissolved in sterile 0.9% NaCl solution to yield a concentration of 100 mg of cephradine per ml. This was delivered via a catheter in the femoral vein. To attain high, sustained serum cephradine levels, and to avoid uncontrolled variables due to the renal elimination of the antibiotic, bilateral nephrectomy was performed just before the administration of cephradine. Before and at specified intervals after the administration of the antibiotic, arterial blood (2 ml) and cisternal CSF (0.25 to 0.5 ml) samples were collected in sterile tubes for assay of their cephradine content. Cell counts were made on all cerebrospinal fluid (CSF) samples and those containing more than 100 erythrocytes per mm^3 were discarded. Blood samples were allowed to clot and were then centrifuged, and the serum was collected. CSF and serum samples were kept at -20°C until assayed.

In initial experiments (three cats), cephradine was injected intravenously in a single dose of 300 mg per kg of body weight. Blood samples were obtained at 15- to 30-min intervals. One CSF sample was obtained 30 min after cephradine administration. In subsequent experiments (eight cats in which multiple atraumatic CSF samples could be obtained), four doses of cephradine (50 mg/kg) were administered at 30-min intervals. Blood and CSF samples were collected immediately before the administration of each dose and 30 min after the injection of the last dose. In a third type of experiment, cephradine was injected into the right lateral cerebral ventricle of two cats that were lightly anesthetized with ether. Using stereotaxic techniques, a 21-gauge cannula was introduced into the ventricle through a small burr hole in the skull. Over a period of 5 min, one cat re-

[1] Present address: Department of Neurology, University of Miami, School of Medicine, P.O. Box 520875, Biscayne Annex, Miami, FL 33152.

[2] Present address: Division of Infectious Diseases, Boston University Medical Center, Boston, MA 02118.

ceived 40 mg of cephradine dissolved in 0.2 ml of sterile 0.9% NaCl solution, and the other cat received 60 mg dissolved in 0.3 ml of 0.9% NaCl solution. Shortly after the cephradine injection, the cannula was withdrawn, the scalp incision was sutured, and anesthesia was discontinued. The cats were allowed to recover and were not physically restrained. Their gross motor behavior was closely monitored for 3 h. At the end of that time, the cats were deeply anesthetized, and blood and cisternal CSF samples were collected for assay of their cephradine content.

Serum and CSF cephradine concentrations were determined by the cylinder plate bioassay technique, as recommended by one manufacturer (Squibb Institute for Medical Research, N.J., personal communication). Penassay seed agar antibiotic medium no. 1 (Difco) with added sodium chloride (5 g/liter) was used as a single seed layer in the assay petri dishes. The test organism, *Sarcina lutea* ATCC 9341, was grown in Roux bottles containing 300 ml of this medium for 24 h at 37°C. Fifty milliliters of sterile saline solution was used to wash the inoculum from the Roux bottle. One milliliter of the suspension was then diluted in 49 ml of fluid medium that was similar in composition to the first medium but did not contain any agar. One liter of the melted agar medium was inoculated with a previously determined ideal volume of the diluted inoculum (4 to 7 ml). After thorough mixing, 7 ml of the inoculated seed layer was distributed evenly in every plastic petri dish (Falcon). Initial dilution of serum samples was made in 0.1 M phosphate buffer, pH 4.5. Subsequently the diluent contained 1 part normal serum and 4 parts 0.1 M phosphate buffer, pH 4.5. Dilutions of CSF samples were carried out in 0.1 M phosphate buffer, pH 6.0. Samples to be tested were assayed in duplicate plates. After inhibition zone diameters were corrected for, cephradine concentrations were determined by comparison with standard curves prepared in appropriate control fluids. Serum and CSF samples obtained before cephradine administration gave no inhibition zones.

Peak serum cephradine concentrations in nephrectomized cats were well sustained as evidenced by the low rate of decline after a single intravenous injection (Fig. 1). Half an hour after the administration of a 300-mg/kg dose, the mean serum cephradine level was 867 μg/ml (standard deviation, ±117), whereas the

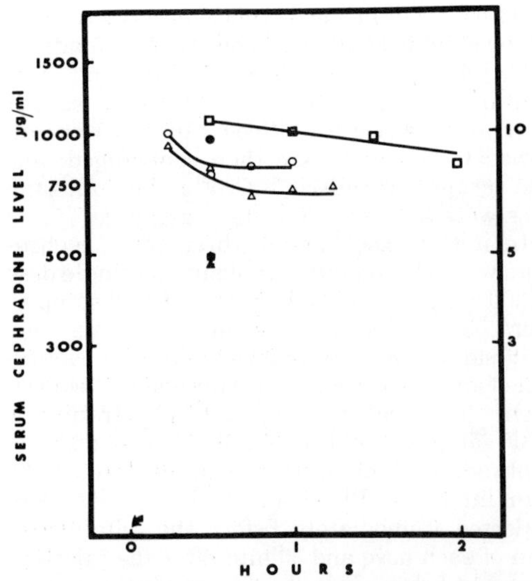

FIG. 1. *Serum and CSF cephradine levels in nephrectomized cats. Cephradine in a dose of 300 mg per kg of body weight was administered intravenously at zero time (arrow) to three cats, and serum and cisternal CSF cephradine levels were determined at intervals. Empty and full symbols indicate serum and CSF levels, respectively.*

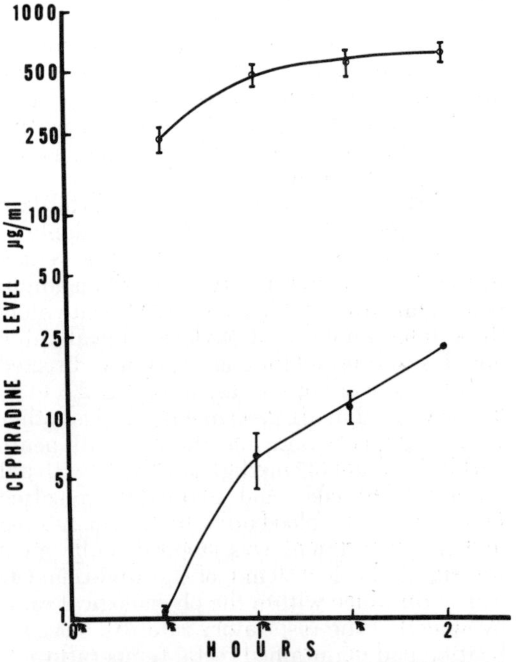

FIG. 2. *Serum (○) and CSF (●) cephradine levels in nephrectomized cats. Cephradine was administered intravenously in repeated doses of 50 mg per kg of body weight every 0.5 h (arrows). Serum and cisternal CSF samples were obtained immediately before the cephradine injections and assayed for their cephradine content. Each point represents the mean of each group of observations ± standard error of the mean.*

mean cisternal CSF cephradine level was 6.4 μg/ml (standard deviation, ±2.7), thus giving a CSF/serum cephradine concentration ratio of only 0.7%. In the group of nephrectomized cats that received repeated doses of cephradine, the serum and CSF antibiotic concentrations increased progressively (Fig. 2). During the 2-h observation period, the cephradine concentrations of serum and CSF both rose, but at different rates. Serum concentrations of cephradine tended to plateau at a time when the CSF cephradine concentrations were steadily increasing. Thus, the CSF/serum cephradine concentration ratio increased from 0.5% at 30 min to 3.6% at 2 h after the initial injection of cephradine. This suggests that the transport of cephradine from blood to CSF is a time-dependent process that does not attain equilibrium quickly. There were no appreciable electroencephalogram (EEG) changes during these experiments. In particular, no abnormal spikes or epileptiform activity was noted even when the CSF cephradine levels exceeded 10 μg/ml.

In the experiments in which cephradine was injected directly into the cerebral ventricle, animals recovered promptly from ether anesthesia and showed no gross behavioral changes. They continued to be alert and to respond normally to a variety of stimuli. In particular, there was no evidence of myoclonic jerks or convulsions. After an observation period of 3 h, the cisternal CSF and serum cephradine concentrations were 410 and 7.2 μg/ml, respectively, in the cat that received 40 mg intraventricularly, and 740 and 10.0 μg/ml in the cat that received 60 mg intraventricularly. These results show that cephradine is distributed widely along CSF pathways after its intraventricular administration and attains high levels in the CSF that are one to two orders of magnitude greater than those achieved after the systemic administration of large doses of cephradine to nephrectomized cats.

Our results suggest that cephradine, like the rest of the cephalosporin antibiotics, does not penetrate the normal blood-brain barrier easily. Only in nephrectomized animals that were given huge doses of cephradine did the CSF antibiotic concentrations reach therapeutic levels. It should be emphasized that the doses of cephradine that were given systematically to nephrectomized cats, as well as those injected into the cerebral ventricles, were dictated by pharmacological considerations and therefore do not represent recommended therapeutic doses for humans. Nevertheless, under the experimental conditions of this study, no apparent encephalotoxic effects were observed. The electroencephalogram remained unchanged despite the relatively high CSF antibiotic concentrations. There were no gross motor or behavioral changes after cephradine was injected into the cerebral ventricles in doses that markedly elevated CSF concentrations. Certainly more work is required before one can draw any final conclusions that may carry therapeutic implications, but as noted earlier, the intrathecal administration of cephaloridine—a compound closely related to cephradine—has been reported safe and effective in the treatment of meningitis (4). Our experimentation suggests that cephradine may be useful in similar ways.

ACKNOWLEDGMENTS

We thank Shaké Albarian for excellent technical assistance and G. Fawaz and S. Jabbur for providing the recording equipment.

LITERATURE CITED

1. **Bassaris, H. P., R. Quintiliani, E. G. Maderazon, R. C. Tilton, and C. H. Nightingale.** 1976. Pharmacokinetics and penetration characteristics of cefazolin into human spinal fluid. Curr. Ther. Res. 19:110–120.
2. **Fisher, L. S., A. W. Chow, T. T. Yoshikawa, and L. B. Guze.** 1975. Cephalothin and cephaloridine therapy for bacterial meningitis. An evaluation. Ann. Intern. Med. 82:689–693.
3. **Lerner, P. I.** 1969. Penetration of cephalothin and lincomycin into the cerebrospinal fluid. Am. J. Med. Sci. 257:125–131.
4. **Love, W. C., P. McKenzie, J. H. Lawson, I. W. Pinkerton, W. M. Jamieson, J. Stevenson, W. Roberts, and A. B. Christie.** 1970. Treatment of pneumococcal meningitis with cephaloridine. Postgrad. Med. J. 46(Suppl):155–159.
5. **Mangi R. J., R. S. Kundargi, R. Quintiliani, and V. T. Andriole.** 1973. Developement of meningitis during cephalothin therapy. Ann. Intern. Med. 78:347–351.
6. **Vianna, N. J., and D. Kaye.** 1967. Penetration of cephalothin into the spinal fluid. Am. J. Med. Sci. 254:216–220.

Antimicrobial Agents and Chemotherapy, May 1977, p. 912-913 Vol. 11, No. 5

Printed in U.S.A.

Susceptibility of Anaerobic Bacteria to Cefoxitin and Related Compounds

VINH TOAN BACH, IRA ROY, AND HARAGOPAL THADEPALLI*

Department of Internal Medicine, Martin Luther King Jr. General Hospital, Charles R. Drew Postgraduate School of Medicine, and University of Southern California School of Medicine, Los Angeles, California 90059*

Received for publication 13 December 1976

Cephalothin, cefazolin, cephradine, and cefoxitin inhibited more than 75% of 326 anaerobic bacteria in vitro, but cefoxitin was the most effective against anaerobes in general and *Bacteroides fragilis* in particular.

Sutter and Finegold (6) reported that only 11% of 124 strains of *Bacteroides fragilis* were inhibited by cephalothin at 32 μg/ml, 13% by cefazolin at 12.5 μg/ml, and 38% by cephaloridine at 25 μg/ml, whereas 86% were inhibited by cefoxitin at 16 μg/ml. Tally et al. (7) observed that 82% of the *B. fragilis* isolates were inhibited by cefoxitin, whereas cephalothin, cephaloridine, and cephalexin were less effective. They concluded that cefoxitin was the most effective among the cephalosporins tested against *B. fragilis*, an important anaerobic pathogen. Our report concerns the in vitro efficacy of cefoxitin compared with that of cephalothin, cefazolin, and cephradine.

(This work was presented in part at the 76th Annual Meeting of the American Society for Microbiology, May 1976.)

Three hundred and twenty-six recent clinical anaerobic isolates, two-thirds of which were from the female genital tract, were tested against cephalothin and cefazolin (Eli Lilly & Co., Indianapolis, Ind.), cephradine (Squibb and Co., Princeton, N.J.), and cefoxitin (Merck Sharp & Dohme, West Point, Pa.) at six different concentrations (2, 4, 8, 16, 32, and 64 μg). The details of identification of the anaerobes and the description of inocula, media, and methods were as reported earlier (5).

The minimal inhibitory concentrations were as shown in Tables 1 and 2. Assuming a serum level of 32 μg/ml as the cutoff point, cefoxitin was the most effective of all four cephalosporins tested against anaerobes in general and *B. fragilis* in particular. Anaerobic cocci were generally susceptible to all four cephalosporins tested. Cephalothin at 32 μg/ml was effective against 75% (55 strains) of *B. fragilis*. Cefazolin inhibited less than 60% of these strains. Cephradine, although effective against 85% of all anaerobes like other cephalosporins, inhibited only 35% of *B. fragilis* subsp. *fragilis* strains.

Tally et al. (7) reported that cefoxitin at 16 μg/ml was effective against 82% of the *B. fragilis* strains tested, but cephalothin, cefazolin, cephaloridine, and cephalexin at 32 μg/ml inhibited only 6, 45, 52, and 24% of strains, respectively. Sutter and Finegold (6) observed that cefoxitin and cephalothin at 32 μg/ml inhibited 100 and 11% of *B. fragilis*, respectively. Cefoxitin, in our study, was found to be effective against 89% of the *B. fragilis* subsp. *fragilis* strains at 32 μg/ml. At this level, cephalothin also inhibited 75% of *B. fragilis* subsp. *fragilis*. In contrast, Martin et al. (2) reported that only 9% of 195 strains of *B. fragilis* tested were susceptible to cephalothin. Nearly two-thirds of our isolates were from the female genital tract, whereas most isolates examined by Sutter and Finegold (6) and Tally et al. (7) were not; this might be why our strains were highly susceptible to cephalothin. Cefazolin is highly effective against anaerobic cocci, but it is not as effective as cefoxitin against the *Bacteroides* group of organisms.

Cephalothin, in a comparative clinical trial, failed to prevent the onset of anaerobic infections associated with abdominal trauma (8). Anaerobic bacterial colonization and anaerobic septicemias predominated to a greater extent among those treated with cephalothin than among those treated with clindamycin. Hackman and Wilkins found that cephalothin was ineffective against an experimental mixed infection containing *B. fragilis* and *Fusobacterium necrophorum* (1). They attributed this to the beta-lactamase susceptibility of cephalothin. In contrast, cefoxitin, a beta-lactamase-resistant cephalosporin, did not inhibit this combination of organisms. Cefoxitin, a cephalosporinase-resistant cephalosporin, is by far the most potent of all cephalosporins tested against anaerobic bacteria in vitro.

Our study confirms the earlier reports (6, 7) that cefoxitin is the most effective of all cephalosporins thus far tested against *B. fragilis*. This, in addition to its resistance to hydrolysis

TABLE 1. *Susceptibility of anaerobic bacteria to cephalosporins*

Organsisms	No. of strains	Organisms inhibited (%) at 32 μg/ml			
		Cephalothin	Cefazolin	Cephradine	Cefoxitin
Gram-negative rods					
Bacteroides fragilis subsp. *fragilis*	28	75	54	53	89
B. fragilis, other subspecies	27	74	59	67	87
Bacteroides sp.	30	84	93	84	97
Bacteroides (all strains)	(85)	(78)	(69)	(68)	(89)
Fusobacterium	10	80	80	80	90
Selanomonas	1	100	100	100	100
Clostridia (all strains)	44	84	91	89	96
Non-spore-forming gram-positive rods					
Eubacterium	36	83	100	100	100
Lactobacillus	12	75	83	83	83
Propionibacterium	5	60	60	60	60
Bifidobacterium	3	100	100	100	100
Actinomyces	6	100	100	100	100
Cocci					
Peptococcus	75	87	91	91	96
Peptostreptococcus	43	93	100	95	93
Veillonella	4	100	50	100	75
Megasphaera elsdenii	2	100	100	100	100

TABLE 2. *Comparison of susceptibility of anaerobic bacteria to cephalosporins*

Organism	Organisms inhibited (%) at 32 μg/ml			
	Cephalothin	Cephradine	Cefazolin	Cefoxitin
Bacteroides (all strains)	78	68	69	95
Other than *B. fragilis*	84	84	83	100
B. fragilis subsp. *fragilis*	75	53	54	89
Other subspecies	74	67	59	81
Clostridia (all)	84	89	91	96
Peptostreptococci	93	95	100	98
Peptococci	87	85	96	97

by beta-lactamases (4) and the spectrum of activity against aerobic and facultative bacteria (3), places cefoxitin in a unique place among the cephalosporins.

LITERATURE CITED

1. **Hackman, A. S., and T. D. Wilkins.** 1975. Comparison of cefoxitin and cephalothin therapy of a mixed *Bacteroides fragilis* and *Fusobacterium necrophorum* infection in mice. Antimicrob. Agents Chemother. 8:224–225.
2. **Martin, W. J., M. Gardner, and J. A. Washington II.** 1972. In vitro antimicrobial susceptibility of anaerobic bacteria isolates from clinical specimens. Antimicrob. Agents Chemother. 1:148–158.
3. **Moellering, R. C., Jr., M. Dray, and L. J. Kunz.** 1974. Susceptibility of clinical isolates of bacteria to cefoxitin and cephalothin. Antimicrob. Agents Chemother. 6:320–323.
4. **Neu, H. C.** 1974. Cefoxitin, a semisynthetic cephamycin antibiotic: antibacterial spectrum and resistance to hydrolysis by gram-negative beta-lactamases. Antimicrob. Agents Chemother. 6:170–176.
5. **Roy, I., V. Bach, and H. Thadepalli.** 1977. In vitro susceptibility of anaerobes to ticarcillin. Antimicrob. Agents Chemother. 11:258–261.
6. **Sutter, V. L., and S. M. Finegold.** 1975. Susceptibility of anaerobic bacteria to carbenicillin, cefoxitin and related drugs. J. Infect. Dis. 131:417–422.
7. **Tally, F. P., N. V. Jacobus, J. G. Bartlett, and S. L. Gorbach.** 1975. Susceptibility of anaerobes to cefoxitin and other cephalosporins. Antimicrob. Agents Chemother. 7:128–132.
8. **Thadepalli, H., S. L. Gorbach, P. W. Broido, J. Norsen, and L. Nyhus.** 1973. Abdominal trauma, anaerobes, and antibiotics. Surg. Gynecol. Obstet. 137:270–276.

ANTIMICROBIAL AGENTS AND CHEMOTHERAPY, May 1977, p. 914-915 Vol. 11, No. 5

Printed in U.S.A.

Gas Chromatographic Determination of 5-Fluorocytosine: a Modified Extraction Method

SIOK-HUI WEE AND JOHN P. ANHALT*

Section of Clinical Microbiology, Department of Laboratory Medicine, Mayo Clinic and Mayo Foundation, Rochester, Minnesota 55901

Received for publication 3 January 1977

A modified procedure for the gas-chromatographic determination of 5-fluorocytosine in serum is described. A more volatile solvent mixture for extraction is used to reduce sample preparation time before chromatography. Comparison of values from assay of 12 serum samples by our method and the reference method gave a correlation coefficient of 0.99.

Harding et al. reported the serum assay of 5-fluorocytosine by a gas-chromatographic method (1), which we shall refer to as the reference method. A lengthy step in that procedure is the evaporation of 1-butanol that is used for extraction of the drug. We have developed a modified procedure that uses a more volatile solvent mixture for extraction.

A gas chromatograph (model 2740, Varian Aerograph, Walnut Creek, Calif.) equipped with a flame ionization detector was used. A glass column (183 cm by 2 mm, internal diameter) packed with 3% OV-17 on 100/120 Gas Chrom Q (Applied Sciences Labs, State College, Pa.) was used for analysis. The operating conditions were as follows: injection port temperature, 185°C; program oven temperature, 100°C (2 min) to 270°C at 20°C/min; detector temperature, 285°C; carrier gas (nitrogen) flow rate, 22 ml/min; hydrogen flow rate, 25 ml/min; and air flow rate, 330 ml/min.

The suppliers for the following reagents were: 5-fluorocytosine, Hoffmann LaRoche, Nutley, N.J.; cytosine, Aldrich Chemical Co., Milwaukee, Wis.; and Regisil, Regis Chemical Co., Morton Grove, Ill.

Method I. A mixture of 200 μl of serum and 1.8 ml of 0.4 M sodium phosphate buffer, pH 7.4, containing 10 μg of internal standard, cytosine, was washed with 5 ml of methylene chloride by shaking for 5 min in a Labquake shaker (Labindustries, Berkeley, Calif.). Phases were separated by centrifuging for 10 min at 1,000 $\times$ g. The aqueous upper layer was then extracted with 5 ml of 2-propanol-methylene chloride (3:1, vol/vol), shaken and centrifuged as above. The organic upper layer was transferred to a conical test tube and evaporated to dryness under a stream of air at 55°C for between 2 and 3 h.

Method II. Serum, 200 μl, was mixed with 2 ml of 0.1 M sodium phosphate buffer, pH 2, containing 10 μg of cytosine. The mixture was then extracted with 5 ml of 2-propanol-methylene chloride (2:1, vol/vol) for 5 min and centrifuged as in method I. The aqueous top layer was neutralized by the addition of 1 ml of 1 M sodium phosphate buffer, pH 7.9. The mixture was extracted with 5 ml of 2-propanol-methylene chloride (2:1, vol/vol), and the organic top layer was removed and evaporated to dryness.

The residue in each case was silylated with

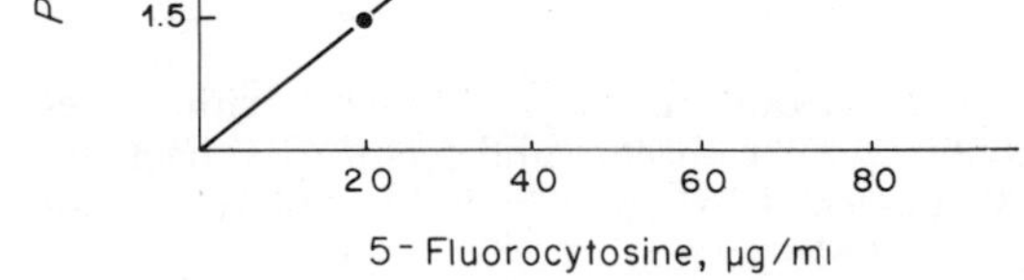

FIG. 1. *Standard curve for 5-fluorocytosine in serum by method I.*

50 μl of acetonitrile-Regisil (2:1, vol/vol) mixture, mixed for 5 min in an ultrasonic vibrator, and allowed to stand at room temperature for 25 min before injection.

Serum standards were prepared as per Harding et al. (1). Typical standard curves are shown in Fig. 1 and 2.

In the recovery study of 5-fluorocytosine from serum, the internal standard was omitted from the buffer but was added to the organic extract before evaporation. The peak height of 5-fluorocytosine was then measured against that of cytosine. Recovery was 74% from method I and 45% from method II.

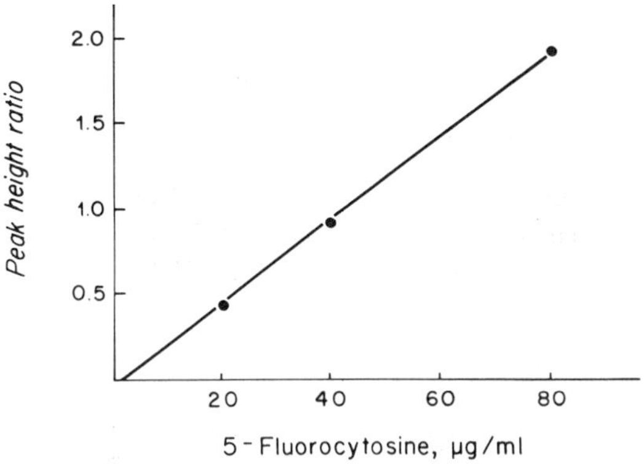

FIG. 2. *Standard curve for 5-fluorocytosine in serum by method II.*

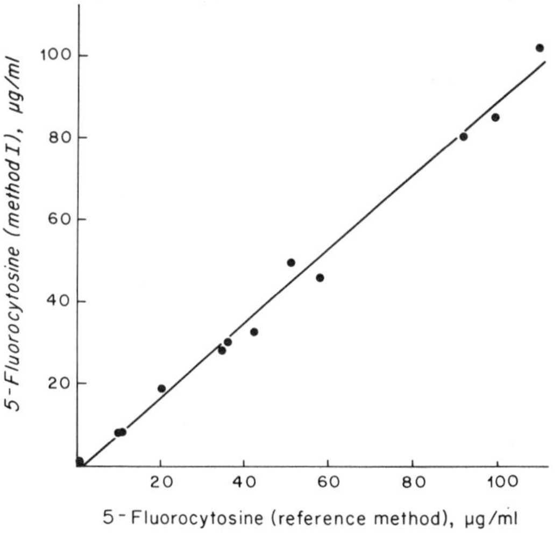

FIG. 3. *Comparison of gas-chromatographic assay of 5-fluorocytosine in serum by reference method and method I.*

Twelve serum samples, which were provided by H. Solomon (Johns Hopkins Hospital, Baltimore, Md.), were analyzed in duplicate by method I and by Solomon, using the reference method. The mean values obtained were regressed against their results. The slope of the linear least squares line was 0.91, the intercept was −1.94, and the correlation coefficient was 0.99 (Fig. 3). Precision was estimated from the differences observed between the duplicate determinations. The mean difference was 4.5%. The maximum difference observed was 10%, which was obtained from a specimen that contained 1.1 μg of 5-fluorocytosine per ml.

Method II was developed after two serum samples were found to contain a peak that could possibly interfere with the accurate measurement of cytosine. This peak was eliminated by acid washing before extraction of 5-fluorocytosine. However, in these two samples, our results with method I still corresponded well with those obtained by the reference method. Duplicate determinations on serum standards by method II showed a mean difference between duplicates of 2.7% ($n = 4$).

The reference method used butanol as an extraction solvent. We found that 2-propanol-methylene chloride effectively reduced the evaporation time from between 4 and 5 h to between 2 and 3 h. Also, method II conveniently resulted with the desired phase in the upper layer, that is, aqueous in the first extraction and organic in the second extraction. This change in solvent also gave a better recovery.

We thank Harvey M. Solomon, Johns Hopkins Hospital, Baltimore, Md., for providing the serum samples for our assay and the data from their assay for the evaluation of our methods.

LITERATURE CITED

1. **Harding, S. A., G. F. Johnson, and H. M. Solomon.** 1976. Gas-chromatographic determination of 5-fluorocytosine in human serum. Clin. Chem. **22**:772–776.

ANTIMICROBIAL AGENTS AND CHEMOTHERAPY, May 1977, p. 916-918
Vol. 11, No. 5

Semiautomated Turbidimetric Bioassay for the Ionophore A23187

J. E. WESTHEAD

The Lilly Research Laboratories, Eli Lilly and Company, Indianapolis, Indiana 46206

Received for publication 14 February 1977

The inhibitory effect of A23187 against *Staphylococcus aureus* was used to quantitate the activity of this ionophore in fermentation samples and in isolation and crystallization samples. The assay was shown to be rapid and reproducible.

A23187 is a divalent cation ionophore obtained from a strain of *Streptomyces chartreusis* (R. L. Hamill et al., Prog. Abstr. Intersci. Conf. Antimicrob. Agents Chemother., 12th, Atlantic City, N.J., Abstr. 65, p. 32, 1972). The biological properties of A23187 were described previously and the structure was determined by X-ray crystallography (1). This ionophore selectively transports divalent cations across artificial or biological membranes (4, 7). It has been used to alter the intracellular Ca^{2+} concentrations in a wide variety of cells, tissues, and subcellular organelles (2, 5, 6). A23187 inhibits the growth of bacteria and fungi. The present study was initiated to quantitate A23187 activity in fermentation extracts and in various solutions derived from its isolation and purification. *Staphylococcus aureus* (H-Heatley strain, NRRL B-314) was used as the test organism. A stock cell suspension of *S. aureus* was prepared by growing the cells in nutrient broth and harvesting during the log phase of growth. The cells were centrifuged, suspended in glycerol-lactose, and maintained in the vapor phase of liquid nitrogen. The inoculum was used at a concentration of 3×10^5 colony-forming units per ml of assay medium.

The medium for the assay of A23187 has the following composition: peptone (Difco), 0.5%; yeast extract (Difco), 0.15%; beef extract (BBL), 0.15%; sodium chloride, 0.35%; K_2HPO_4, 0.37%; and KH_2PO_4, 0.13%. The pH of the medium was 7.0 before sterilization and remained essentially unchanged after the medium was autoclaved for 20 min at 121°C. Prior to use, the medium was chilled and supplemented to contain 0.1% glucose by using a sterile 50% glucose stock solution.

Crystalline A23187 (free acid) was used as the assay standard. A stock standard solution was prepared by dissolving crystalline A23187 in methanol to a final concentration of 1,000 μg/ml. Stock standard solutions were stable for greater than 30 days when refrigerated. On the day of the assay, standard mixtures containing 0.4, 0.6, 0.8, and 1.0 μg of A23187 per ml were prepared by diluting the stock standard solution with a 1:1 water-methanol mixture. Unknown samples were prepared for assay by diluting in a 1:1 water-methanol mixture to ob-

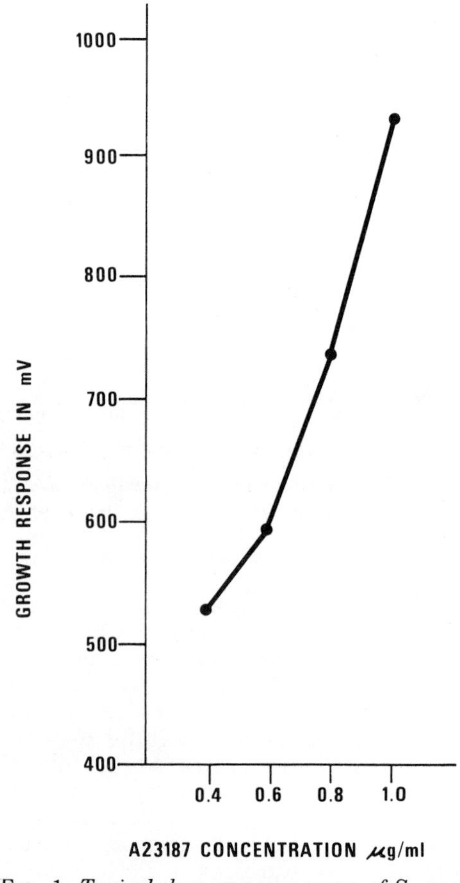

FIG. 1. *Typical dose-response curve of S. aureus to a range of A23187 concentrations.*

TABLE 1. *Precision of turbidimetric assays on seven representative samples of A23187*

Samples	A23187 activity (μg/ml of sample solution) Day 1 Test 1	Day 1 Test 2	Day 1 Test 3	Day 1 Test 4	Day 2 Test 1	Day 2 Test 2	Day 2 Test 3	Day 2 Test 4	Day 3, test 1	Mean[a]	SD[b]	COV[c] (%)
A	92 93	97 102	103 100	101 103	93 94	101 103	99 106	98 107	87 90	98	5.7	5.8
B	91 98	94 95	94 101	99 94	95 97	100 97	92 104	93 96	90 92	96	3.7	3.9
C	87 90	93 89	90 93	93 90	89 91	96 91	90 94	89 91	86 87	90	2.6	2.9
D	234 240	248 274	241 233	239 240	247 244	247 242	243 235	248 236	245 242	242	4.8	2.0
E	80 79	77 82	80 80	72 79	81 80	75 80	81 80	76 79	82 79	79	2.5	3.2
F	50 51	50 54	53 51	49 50	52 51	53 53	52 52	53 53	56 53	52	1.7	3.3
G	158 172	162 162	160 168	164 165	164 167	167 166	162 171	166 169	168 168	166	3.7	2.3

[a] Mean $= \bar{X} = \Sigma \chi_i / n$, where χ_i = individual values, and n = number of individual values.
[b] Standard deviation $= s =$ (SD) $\sqrt{\Sigma(\chi_i - \bar{X})^2/(n-1)}$.
[c] Coefficient of variation (COV) $= (s)\ (100\%)/\bar{X}$.

TABLE 2. *A23187 assay characterization from analysis of variance results*

Assay scheme: No. of days tested	No. of tests per day	Resulting precision: Coefficient of variation (%)	Approximate 95% confidence limits (%)
1	1	2.71	±5.4
1	2	2.12	4.2
1	3	1.88	3.8
1	4	1.75	3.5
2	1	1.93	3.9
2	2	1.51	3.0
2	3	1.34	2.7
2	4	1.24	2.6
3	4	1.02	2.0

tain about 0.75 to 0.85 μg of A23187 activity per ml. The assays were performed by using an Autoturb system, which provides a high order of precision for the microbiological assay of vitamins and antibiotics (3). Test solutions were transferred to an Autoturb Dilutor Carousel, and the dilutor was calibrated to take four 0.15-ml volumes of each solution. The test was incubated in a 37°C constant-temperature water bath. Transmittance was measured by an Autoturb Reader and expressed in terms of millivolts (1,000 mV equals 100% transmittance). Growth of the test organism was monitored by readings taken from control tubes that received the 1:1 water-methanol diluent but no antibiotic. The test was terminated in about 4 h when control tubes had reached 45% transmission measured at 642 nm. The data from the Autoturb Reader were interfaced through an analogue to a digital converter and to a Thomas paper tape punch. The resulting tape was loaded into an external time-sharing computer for data analysis. Data were analyzed point to point by plotting transmittance versus concentration.

An example of the dose-response relationship of A23187 to *S. aureus* by using the described assay is shown in Fig. 1. To test the precision of the assay, representative samples from fermentation extracts and isolation samples were assayed over a period of 3 days. Replications of the tests were made on days 1 and 2, and replications of the samples within the tests were made on days 1, 2, and 3. The same standard dose-response solutions and sample solutions were used in all of the assays. Solutions A, B, and C are partially purified preparations from the isolation, and samples D, E, F, and G are representative extracts from the fermentation.

The test results are presented in Table 1 with summary statistics for each sample. The mean value is the overall average for each sample, and the standard deviation is a measure of the spread of the individual results. The coefficient of variation is the standard deviation expressed as a percentage of the mean (see footnotes of Table 1 for equations).

An analysis of variance was run to determine the sources and magnitude of variation contributing to the overall assay variation. These results were then used to calculate a theoretical coefficient of variation for a given number of tests on a given number of days (the assay scheme). The approximate 95% confidence limits are merely two times the calculated coefficient of variation. The purpose of the results given in Table 2 is to promote an appropriate assay scheme to give a specified level of precision. If, for example, it is desired to detect a 4% change in potency at a 95% confidence level, then it is necessary to use an assay scheme that would yield a result with 95% confidence limits less than or equal to 4%. We can look in Table 2 and see that to achieve this precision we must make at least three assays on 1 day or one assay on each of 2 days to accomplish an overall estimation of potency with the desired precision.

The described assay procedure using semiautomated equipment was successfully used to quantitate A23187 activity in extracts derived from culture development studies and pilot plant fermentations, as well as to evaluate A23187 purification and crystallization procedures. Due to the worldwide research interest in this ionophore, it is felt that the knowledge of the methodology for quantitation of the activity of this compound may be useful to other investigators. Although automated equipment was used in this study, adaptation of the procedure to manual turbidimetric assays would be relatively easy.

I wish to thank D. Smith and L. Simms for supplying the statistical analysis of the assay data.

LITERATURE CITED

1. **Chaney, M. O., P. V. Demarco, N. D. Jones, and J. L. Occolowitz.** 1974. The structure of A23187, a divalent cation ionophore. J. Am. Chem. Soc. **96**:1932–1933.
2. **Foreman, J. C., J. L. Mongar, and B. D. Comparts.** 1973. Calcium ionophores and movement of calcium ions following the physiological stimulus to a secretory process. Nature (London) **245**:249–251.
3. **Kuzel, N. R., and F. Kavanagh.** 1971. Automated system for analytical microbiology. II. Construction of system and evaluation of antibiotics and vitamins. J. Pharm. Sci. **60**:767–773.
4. **Pressman, B. C.** 1973. Properties of ionophores with broad range of cation selectivity. Fed. Proc. **32**:1698–1703.
5. **Prince, W. T., H. Rasmussen, and M. J. Berridge.** 1973. The role of calcium in fly salivary gland secretion analyzed with the ionophore A23187. Biochem. Biophys. Acta **329**:98–107.
6. **Reed, P. W.** 1976. Effects of the divalent cation ionophore A23187 on potassium permeability of rat erythrocytes. J. Biol. Chem. **251**:3489–3494.
7. **Reed, P. W., and H. A. Lardy.** 1972. A23187: a divalent cation ionophore. J. Biol. Chem. **247**:6970–6973.

ANTIMICROBIAL AGENTS AND CHEMOTHERAPY, May 1977, p. 919–922 Vol. 11, No. 5

Printed in U.S.A.

Phosphonoacetic Acid-Resistant Mutants of Herpes Simplex Virus: Effect of Phosphonoacetic Acid on Virus Replication and In Vitro Deoxyribonucleic Acid Synthesis in Isolated Nuclei

YECHIEL BECKER,* YAEL ASHER, YAFFA COHEN, EYNAT WEINBERG-ZAHLERING, AND JOSEPH SHLOMAI

Laboratory for Molecular Virology, Hebrew University-Hadassah Medical School, Jerusalem, 91-000 Israel

Received for publication 16 December 1976

Phosphonoacetic acid (PAA) inhibits the replication of herpes simplex virus in BSC-1 cells and the in vitro synthesis of deoxyribonucleic acid (DNA) in isolated nuclei. Phosphonopropionic acid at a concentration of 100 μg/ml had no effect on herpes simplex virus replication. PAA-resistant mutants were obtained at a rate of 1 in 10^4 plaque-forming units after 5-bromodeoxyuridine mutagenization of the virus. These mutants replicate in BSC-1 cells in the presence of 100 μg of PAA per ml and induce a PAA-resistant DNA polymerase that synthesizes DNA in vitro in the presence of PAA.

The replication of herpes simplex virus (HSV) in mice and rabbits was found to be inhibited by the compound phosphonoacetic acid ($HO{-}P(OH)(=O){-}CH_2C(=O){-}OH$; [PAA]) (12, 13). It was reported (6) that PAA inhibited the replication of cytomegalovirus in WI-38 cells in a reversible fashion: virus replication was resumed after removal of the drug. It was also shown (6) that addition of PAA to a purified cytomegalovirus-induced deoxyribonucleic acid (DNA) polymerase in vitro resulted in the inhibition of the viral enzyme. PAA inhibits the synthesis of HSV DNA in nuclei isolated from infected cells and incubated under in vitro conditions (3) as well as the synthesis of Epstein-Barr virus DNA in Burkitt lymphoblasts and the expression of Epstein-Barr virus late genes (15). In HeLa cells, PAA inhibits the host cell DNA polymerase (3).

These studies suggest that PAA inhibits mainly the virus-induced DNA polymerase in herpesvirus-infected cells, but a host cell DNA polymerase is also affected. It has been demonstrated (9, 10) that the inhibition of a HSV-specified DNA polymerase by PAA involves a specific site on the viral DNA polymerase. Recently, it was shown (7) that PAA molecules interact with the herpesvirus-induced DNA polymerase at the phosphate-binding site and that phosphopropionic acid (PPA) binds more strongly than PAA to the viral DNA polymerase. Hay and Subak-Sharpe (5) reported on the isolation of PAA-resistant virus from HSV types 1 and 2. These resistant virus mutants formed plaques on BHK monolayers in the presence of PAA and induced DNA polymerase activities that were partially resistant to PAA.

In the present study, we determined the effect of PAA and PPA on the replication of HSV in BSC-1 cells and isolated PAA-resistant mutants from virus preparations mutagenized by 5-bromodeoxyuridine (BUdR). The HF strain of HSV type 1 was grown in BSC-1 cell monolayers. To mutagenize the virus, BSC-1 cells were infected with 10 plaque-forming units (PFU) of HSV per ml and treated with 5 μg of BUdR per ml throughout the virus growth cycle. Plaque titration (8) of the BUdR-treated preparation showed a 2-log reduction in infectious virus as compared with the virus yield from untreated infected cells. To isolate PAA^r mutants, 0.2 ml of the BUdR-treated stock virus (about 2×10^4 PFU) was seeded on each BSC-1 culture in 50-mm plastic plates. To each plate was added 100 μg of PAA (Richmond Organics, Va.) per ml, and the cells were covered with an agar overlay. The infected cultures were incubated in a humidified CO_2 incubator for 3 days and screened under an inverted microscope. Plaques that developed in the presence of PAA were removed with a Pasteur pipette, and each plaque was transferred to a BSC-1 culture in a milk bottle. In all experiments, two to three virus plaques were obtained from each plate. After development of complete cytopathogenic effect, which required 2 to 3 days, the bottles

TABLE 1. *Effect of PAA and PPA on the replication of wild-type and PAA-resistant (PAA^r) mutant of HSV*

Virus strain	Drug used (100 μg/ml)	Virus yield (PFU/ml) Expt 1	Expt 2	Expt 3
HSV wild type	None	7×10^7	5.7×10^7	8×10^7
HSV wild type	PAA	6×10^5	4.7×10^5	7×10^4
HSV wild type	PPA	—[a]	10^7	2×10^7
HSV PAA^r	None	2×10^7	5×10^7	4.5×10^7
HSV PAA^r	PAA	7×10^7	1.4×10^7	2×10^7
HSV PAA^r	PPA	—	5.4×10^7	3.1×10^7
HSV PAA^r	BUdR	7×10^5	—	—

[a] —, Not done.

were plugged with rubber stoppers and stored at 4°C. To eliminate revertants sensitive to PAA, the plaque-purified virus isolates underwent an additional passage in BSC-1 cells for 20 h in the presence of 100 μg of PAA per ml. From this culture, stock virus was prepared by seeding each BSC-1 culture in a milk bottle with 5 μl of the homogenate prepared from cells infected with the PAA^r mutant. After incubation at 37°C for 48 h, the infected cultures were stored at 4°C and served as the stock virus for infecting BSC-1 cultures in further experiments.

BSC-1 cells were infected with the wild-type and PAA^r virus strains in the absence or presence of 100 μg of PAA or PPA (Abbott Laboratories, Chicago) per ml. The virus titer was determined by plaque assay on BSC-1 monolayers (8). Table 1 shows that the replication of wild-type virus in BSC-1 cells was inhibited in the presence of PAA. The PAA^r mutant was able to replicate in BSC-1 cells in the presence of 100 μg of PAA per ml but was inhibited by BUdR (Table 1). In contrast, PPA at a concentration of 100 μg/ml did not inhibit the replication of wild-type virus, and the same yield of virus progeny was obtained in the presence of PPA as from the untreated infected control cultures.

The effect of different concentrations of PAA on the synthesis of viral DNA in vitro in nuclei isolated from BSC-1 cells, infected with either the wild-type virus or the PAA^r mutant, was studied. The results presented in Fig. 1 represent a typical experiment and show that DNA synthesis in nuclei isolated from BSC-1 cells infected with the wild-type virus was gradually inhibited by increasing concentrations of PAA. At a concentration of 100 μg/ml of PAA, there was 73% inhibition of DNA synthesis in vitro. Addition of 200 μg of PAA per ml resulted in 80% inhibition of in vitro DNA synthesis. The reason for the incomplete inhibition of in vitro DNA synthesis is not known. DNA synthesis in vitro in nuclei isolated from BSC-1 cells infected with the PAA^r mutant was not affected by the addition of 50 μg of PAA. In the presence of 100 μg of PAA per ml there was 26% inhibition, and in the presence of 200 μg of PAA per ml the inhibition of in vitro DNA synthesis reached 43%.

Higher concentrations of PAA had a similar effect on the kinetics of DNA synthesis in nuclei from cells infected with the wild-type virus or PAA^r mutant. Increasing concentrations of PAA resulted in increased inhibition of DNA synthesis in nuclei from cells infected with wild-type HSV (Fig. 2A). A concentration of 300

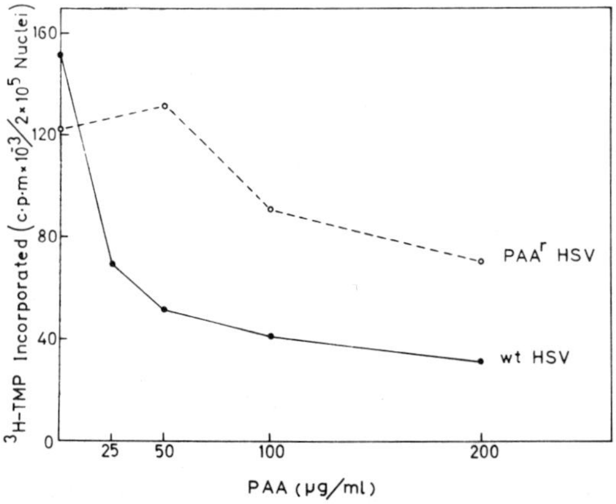

FIG. 1. *Effect of different concentrations of PAA on in vitro DNA synthesis in nuclei isolated from cells infected with wild-type and a PAA^r mutant virus. BSC-1 cells were infected with the wild-type virus and PAA^r mutant at a multiplicity of infection of 10 PFU/ml. After incubation for 12 or 18 h, the infected cells were scraped off the glass and used for the preparation of nuclei for incubation in vitro (1, 14). The reaction mixture contained 0.2 M sucrose (ribonuclease-free; Schwarz/Mann, Orangeburg, N. Y.), 0.04 mM each of deoxyadenosine 5'-triphosphate (dATP), deoxycytidine 5'-triphosphate (dCTP), deoxyguanosine 5'-triphosphate (dGTP), 1 mM dithiothreitol, 5 mM phosphonoenol-pyruvate (PEP), 0.04 mM each of ATP, GTP, CTP, uridine 5'-triphosphate (UTP), 5 mM ethyleneglycol-bis (β-amino ether), N,N'-tetraacetic acid (EGTA), 15 μg of pyruvate kinase per ml (PK) (all from the Sigma Chemical Co., St. Louis, Mo.), 0.002 mM [^{3}H]thymidine 5'-triphosphate (TTP) (specific activity 47 Ci/mmol; The Radiochemical Centre, Amersham, England), 0.4 mM $CsCl_2$, and 6 mM MgCl in a volume of 400 μl in 75 mM potassium phosphate buffer, pH 7.4. To this the nuclei prepared from about 6×10^6 BSC-1 cells were added in a volume of 200 μl of phosphate buffer. The reaction mixtures were incubated for 45 min at 37°C before the reaction was terminated by the addition of trichloroacetic acid. The trichloroacetic acid-precipitable radioactivity was determined. Symbols: ●, wild type; ○, PAA^r.*

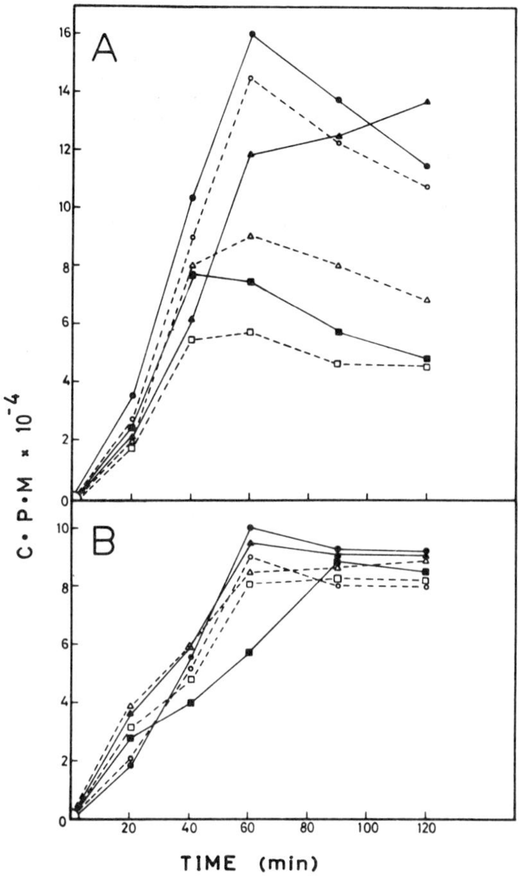

FIG. 2. *In vitro DNA synthesis in nuclei isolated from BSC-1 cells infected with wild-type and PAA^r mutant virus. Nuclei obtained from cultures infected with the wild-type virus (A) and the PAA^r mutant (B) were added to the reaction mixture and incubated at 37°C without PAA (●) and in the presence of 25 (○), 50 (▲), 100 (△), 200 (■) and 300 (□) μg of PAA per ml. Samples were withdrawn at different time intervals, and the trichloroacetic acid-precipitable radioactivity was determined.*

μg/ml of PAA inhibited 75% of the [^{3}H]thymidine incorporation (data not shown). In contrast, the same concentration of PAA only slightly affected DNA synthesis in nuclei from cells infected with the PAA^r mutant (Fig. 2B). These experiments revealed that the PAA^r mutant induces a DNA polymerase activity in infected nuclei that is resistant to high concentrations of PAA.

The present study has shown that HSV mutants resistant to 100 μg of PAA per ml can be isolated from BUdR-mutagenized virus at a frequency of about 1 in 10^4 PFU. The PAA^r mutant virus was able to replicate in infected cells in the presence of 100 μg of PAA per ml, a concentration that completely inhibits the replication of the wild-type virus. PPA had no effect on the wild-type virus. In addition, the mutant virus produced a modified DNA polymerase, since in vitro DNA synthesis was only slightly affected by the addition of 300 μg of PAA per ml to the isolated nuclei. It seems that the PAA^r mutants of HSV code for a DNA polymerase, with a modified amino acid sequence at the site where the PAA molecule binds to the enzyme (9, 10). The appearance of PAA^r mutants at a rate of 1 out of 10^4 PFU indicates that mutagenization by BUdR of the viral genes, which code for the viral DNA polymerase, is a frequent event. This agrees with the demonstration that treatment of HSV-infected cells with BUdR leads to isolated of temperature-sensitive mutants defective in DNA synthesis (2).

It would appear that the viral DNA polymerase activity of the PAA^r mutant studied here is much more resistant to the drug than the mutants described by Hay and Subak-Sharpe (5), which were inhibited at concentrations lower than 10 μg/ml. The reasons for the incomplete inhibition of DNA synthesis by 100 μg of PAA per ml in nuclei isolated from cells infected with the wild-type virus and the partial inhibitory effect on the PAA^r mutants are not known. These may be due to the use of isolated nuclei for DNA synthesis rather than a purified viral DNA polymerase. It is possible that in BSC-1 cells, PAA does not enter easily through the cellular and the nuclear membranes.

The DNA polymerases functioning in infected and uninfected BSC-1 cells are currently under study. Preliminary results (B. Fridlender and Y. Becker, manuscript in preparation) revealed the presence in uninfected cells of two species of the αDNA polymerase, one sensitive and the other resistant to 100 μg PAA per ml, and a PAA-resistant βDNA polymerase. DNA polymerase species different from those of uninfected cells were isolated from HSV-infected cells. DNA polymerases from cells infected with wild-type HSV were highly sensitive to PAA, whereas the DNA polymerase species from cells infected with the PAA^r mutant were resistant to the drug. Further studies are needed to determine the nature of the PAA^r mutation.

Treatment of ocular herpes keratitis with PAA has been shown to cure the disease (4, 11). The findings of Hay and Subak-Sharpe (5) and the present study demonstrate that mutations giving rise to PAA resistance occur quite frequently in HSV. Thus, the use of PAA for treatment of patients could lead to selection of PAA-resistant mutants.

The interest of David Paretsky, on leave from the Department of Microbiology, Kansas University, Kansas, is greatly appreciated.

The study was supported by Public Health Service contract NO1 CP 33310 from the National Cancer Institute, Bethesda, Md.

LITERATURE CITED

1. **Becker, Y., and Y. Asher.** 1975. *In vitro* synthesis of DNA in nuclei isolated from herpes simplex virus-infected cells, untreated and treated with metabolic inhibitors. Virology 63:209–220.
2. **Benyish-Melnick, M., P. A. Schaffer, R. J. Courtney, J. Esparza, and S. Kimura.** 1974. Viral gene functions expressed and detected by temperature-sensitive mutants of herpes simplex virus. Cold Spring Harbor Symp. Quant. Biol. 39:731–746.
3. **Bolden, A., J. Aucker, and A. Weissbach.** 1975. Synthesis of herpes simplex virus, vaccinia virus, and adenovirus DNA in isolated HeLa cell nuclei. I. Effect of viral-specific antisera and phosphonoacetic acid. J. Virol. 16:1584–1592.
4. **Gerstein, D. D., C. R. Dawson, and J. O. Oh.** 1975. Phosphonoacetic acid in the treatment of experimental herpes simplex keratitis. Antimicrob. Agents Chemother. 7:285–288.
5. **Hay, J., and J. Subak-Sharpe.** 1976. Mutants of herpes simplex virus type 1 and 2 that are resistant to phosphonoacetic acid induce altered DNA polymerase activities in infected cells. J. Gen. Virol. 31:145–148.
6. **Huang, E. S.** 1975. Human cytomegalovirus. IV. Specific inhibition of virus-induced DNA polymerase activity and viral DNA replication by phosphonoacetic acid. J. Virol. 16:1560–1565.
7. **Leinbach, S. S., J. M. Reno, L. F. Lee, A. F. Isball, and J. A. Boezi.** 1976. Mechanism of phosphonoacetate inhibition of herpesvirus-induced DNA polymerase. Biochemistry 15:426–430.
8. **Levitt, J., and Y. Becker.** 1967. The effect of cytosine arabinoside on the replication of herpes simplex virus. Virology 31:129–134.
9. **Mao, J. C. H., and E. E. Robishaw.** 1975. Mode of inhibition of herpes simplex virus DNA polymerase by phosphonoacetate. Biochemistry 14:5475–5479.
10. **Mao, J. C. H., E. E. Robishaw, and L. R. Overby.** 1975. Inhibition of DNA polymerase from herpes simplex virus-infected WI-38 by phosphonoacetic acid. J. Virol. 15:1281–1283.
11. **Meyer, R. F., E. D. Varnell, and H. E. Kaufman.** 1976. Phosphonoacetic acid in the treatment of experimental ocular herpes simplex infections. Antimicrob. Agents Chemother. 9:308–311.
12. **Overby, L. B., E. E. Rubishaw, A. Schleicher, N. L. Rueter, N. L. Shipkowitz, and J. C. H. Mao.** 1974. Inhibition of herpes simplex virus replication by phosphonoacetic acid. Antimicrob. Agents Chemother. 6:360–365.
13. **Shipkowitz, N. L., R. R. Bower, R. N. Appell, C. W. Nordeen, L. R. Overby, W. R. Roderick, J. B. Schleicher, and A. A. Von Esch.** 1973. Suppression of herpes simplex virus infection by phosphonoacetic acid. Appl. Microbiol. 26:264–267.
14. **Shlomai, J., and Y. Becker.** 1975. Analysis of herpes simplex virus DNA synthesized *in vitro* in nuclei isolated from infected BSC-1 cells. Virology 68:275–279.
15. **Summers, W. C., and G. Klein.** 1976. Inhibition of Epstein-Barr virus DNA synthesis and late gene expression by phosphonoacetic acid. J. Virol. 18:151–155.

ANTIMICROBIAL AGENTS AND CHEMOTHERAPY, June 1977, p. 925-932
Vol. 11, No. 6

Drug Resistance in Group D Streptococci of Clinical and Nonclinical Origin: Prevalence, Transferability, and Plasmid Properties

J. D. A. VAN EMBDEN,* H. W. B. ENGEL, AND B. VAN KLINGEREN
National Institute for Public Health, Bilthoven, The Netherlands

Received for publication 13 January 1977

Group D streptococci isolated from clinical specimens and from sewage were investigated with regard to resistance to tetracycline (Tc), erythromycin (Em), and chloramphenicol (Cm). The median values of the percentages of resistant strains from sewage were: for Tc, 14%; for Em, 2.8%; and for Cm, 0.1%. For the recent isolates of clinical origin, resistance percentages found were 58% for Tc, 12% for Em, and 14% for Cm, and, in comparison to clinical isolates from 1964, the incidence of drug resistance slightly increased. In strains of both sources, the drug resistance was often found to be transferable to another group D streptococcus, probably by conjugation. Two strains were able to transfer their Em resistance to a streptococcus strain of group B. No transfer of drug resistance to a group A streptococcus and *Escherichia coli* was observed. All beta-hemolytic streptococci were also bacteriocinogenic, and frequently these properties were found to be transferable. The function, size, and base composition of the plasmids of two drug-resistant *Streptococcus faecalis* strains were investigated; strain M439 harbors at least two conjugative plasmids: pRI401, molecular weight 30×10^6, coding for Tc resistance, and pRI402, molecular weight 41×10^6, coding for Em resistance. Strain M403 carries one single conjugative plasmid species, coding for Tc resistance. The molecular weight of this plasmid, pRI404, was 37×10^6. The guanine plus cytosine content of these plasmids was 35 to 36%.

In contrast to the abundance of information on the development of drug resistance in *Enterobacteriaceae* and staphylococci (12), the literature on drug resistance in group D streptococci is scarce. In the period of 1953 to 1968, the occurrence of drug-resistant isolates of group D streptococci increased dramatically (15, 28).

Several authors reported a high incidence of resistance to tetracycline (Tc), chloramphenicol (Cm), and, in a lesser degree, to erythromycin (Em) (14, 18, 20, 21, 24). All isolates of group D streptococci in these studies were of clinical origin. Because of the lack of information on the prevalence of drug resistance in indigenous enterococci from healthy people, we have compared the incidence of drug-resistant group D streptococci from clinical origin with that of group D streptococci in sewage from human origin.

Recently, it was shown that antibiotic resistance in group D streptococci is plasmid mediated (5, 6, 9, 14, 18) and that these plasmids either are self-transferable by conjugation (14) or can be mobilized by conjugative plasmids (9). In this study, the transferability of drug resistance in isolates from clinical and nonclinical origin was investigated, and the molecular properties of some resistance plasmids are reported.

MATERIALS AND METHODS

Bacterial strains. The strains frequently used in this study are listed in Table 1.

Media. Nutrient broth was prepared in this laboratory from fresh meat and contained, in addition, 0.5% NaCl, 1% peptone (Difco), and 0.064% Na_2CO_3, pH 7.5. Nutrient agar contained, in addition, 2% agar (BBL). Unless otherwise stated, these media were used throughout this study. Blood agar was nutrient agar supplemented with 7% horse blood. Burkwall and Hartman medium (BH medium) was used as described (3). Minimal inhibitory concentrations (MICs) were determined on DST medium (Oxoid) supplemented with 7% horse blood.

Determination of MICs. The MICs were determined by inoculating 1:100 diluted overnight cultures by means of a Steers replicator on media supplemented with the appropriate antibiotics. Plates were incubated overnight at 37°C. The antibiotics used were: Tc (Pfizer), Cm (Mycopharm), Em (Abbott), clindamycin (Upjohn), spiramycin (Societé Paris d'Expansion Chemique [SPECIA]), tylosine (Verafarm), lincomycin (Upjohn), oleandomycin (Pfizer), and factor S of virginiamycin (Recherche et Industrie Therapeutiques), pristinamycin Ia (SPECIA).

TABLE 1. *Bacterial strains used*

Strain designation	Relevant properties	Origin
JH2	*Streptococcus faecalis*, susceptible to Tc, Cm, and Em, nonhemolytic	A. E. Jacob (14)
JH2-2	Mutant of JH2, resistant to fusidic acid and rifampin	A. E. Jacob (14)
M434	Mutant of JH2, resistant to streptomycin	This laboratory
M382	*Streptococcus agalactiae,* susceptible to Tc, Cm, and Em	Clinical isolate
M385	Mutant of M382, resistant to rifampin and fusidic acid	This laboratory
M519	Mutant of M382, resistant to streptomycin	This laboratory
M592	*Streptococcus pyogenes,* susceptible to Tc, Cm, and Em	Clinical isolate
M597	Mutant of M592, resistant to rifampin	This laboratory
SC181	*Escherichia coli* K-12, restrictionless	E. Lederberg
M665	Mutant of SC181, resistant to rifampin	This laboratory
M439	*S. faecalis,* resistant to Tc and Em, β-hemolytic	Clinical isolate
M403	*S. faecalis*, resistant to Tc, nonhemolytic	Clinical isolate
M440	*S. faecalis,* resistant to Tc and Em, nonhemolytic	Clinical isolate

Serological grouping and biotyping of streptococci. Group antigens were extracted with hot formamide according to the method described by Fuller (11). Ring precipitation tests were performed in special capillary tubes that have a thicker section where the reaction occurs (8). For recognition of the groups A through U, rabbit antisera prepared in this laboratory were used, with the exception of group D antiserum, which was obtained from Burroughs Wellcome.

The biochemical identification of group D streptococci was done according to the scheme of Facklam (10).

Isolation of streptococci from sewage. One-liter samples of sewage from influent reservoirs were homogenized, and 500 ml was centrifuged at 10,000 × *g* for 10 min. The pellet was suspended in 1 or 2 ml of nutrient broth. The concentrated suspensions and dilutions were plated on BH medium and BH plates containing the appropriate antibiotics (Tc, 8 μg/ml; Cm, 32 μg/ml; Em, 32 μg/ml). In an experiment to test the selectivity of BH medium for streptococci from sewage, all of 58 colonies tested were found to be enterococci, although the group D antigen could be demonstrated in 56 out of the 58 colonies grown on BH medium. Twenty-five belonged to biotype *Streptococcus faecalis*, 13 were of biotype *Streptococcus faecium*, and the other 20 did not belong to an established biotype. The biochemical reaction patterns of these 20 strains differed slightly from those of *S. faecalis* or *S. faecium*. Therefore, the selectivity of BH medium was satisfactory for our purpose.

Transfer of drug resistance and bacteriocin testing. Mating in liquid medium was done as described by Jacob and Hobbs (14). Matings on filters were done by filtering 1 ml of a mixture of equal volumes of overnight cultures of donor and recipient bacteria through a 0.45-μm-pore-size membrane filter (Sartorius). The filter was incubated overnight on a nutrient agar plate and then shaken with 1 ml of nutrient broth to release the bacteria from the filter. Mixtures of streptococcal matings were spread on plates containing the appropriate antibiotics: fusidic acid (LEO Pharmaceutical Products), 25 μg/ml; rifampin (Lepetit), 100 μg/ml; streptomycin (Mycopharm), 2 mg/ml; Em, 5 μg/ml; Tc, 5 μg/ml; and Cm, 25 μg/ml. When matings were done with *Escherichia coli* K-12 as a recipient, the following concentrations of antibiotics were used: rifampin, 50 μg/ml; Tc, 5 μg/ml; and Em, 500 μg/ml. Bacteriocin production was assayed as described by Dunny and Clewell (9), with strain JH2-2 as the indicator strain. Transfer frequencies are expressed as the number of drug-resistant recipients per total number of recipients.

DNA isolation and characterization. Cells were grown in 200 ml of nutrient broth at 37°C under vigorous agitation to an optical density of 0.5 at 600 nm. Deoxyribonucleic acid (DNA) was extracted as described by Clewell et al. (5) with some modifications. Cells were washed in 50 ml of TES buffer [0.01 M tris(hydroxymethyl)aminomethane, 0.001 M ethylenediaminetetraacetic acid (EDTA), 0.01 M NaCl, pH 8.1] at 0°C and resuspended in 5.6 ml of TES, containing 60% sucrose. Lysozyme (10 mg/ml in water), 0.50 ml, was added and the mixture was incubated for 10 min at 37°C. EDTA (0.2 M, pH 8.1), 2.40 ml, was added and the mixture was incubated for 10 min at 37°C. Subsequently, 1.12 ml of Pronase (5 mg/ml in TES, self-digested for 30 min at 37°C) and 10 ml 2% Sarkosyl [in 0.01 M tris(hydroxymethyl)aminomethane, 0.01 M NaCl, and 0.005 M EDTA, pH 8.1] were added, and the mixture was kept at room temperature for 15 min to complete lysis. Ethidium bromide and solid CsCl were added to 800 μg/ml and to 46.5% (wt/wt), respectively. Equilibrium centrifugation, purification, and electron microscopy of circular DNA have been described (30). Guanine plus cytosine (G+C) contents were calculated from the buoyant densities in CsCl as described by Schildkraut et al. (25).

RESULTS

Incidence of drug-resistant group D streptococci from sewage. Samples of influent of two small sewage treatment plants were investigated with regard to the incidence of drug-resistant group D streptococci. The influents originated from the villages Groenekan and Maartensdijk, which have about 900 and 1,400 inhabitants, respectively. According to the local authorities for the maintenance of waterworks, no sewage from animal husbandry farms or industries is discharged into these sewage systems. On 6 days, between March 1976 and June 1976, samples of each of the two installations were collected. The total viable numbers of group D streptococci and the percentages of organisms resistant to Tc, Cm, and Em were determined. The results are summarized in Table 2. The fraction of drug-resistant group D streptococci varied greatly among the various samples. We have no explanation for this variation. Tc resistance was most frequently encountered (median values for the two plants, 13 and 15%), followed by Em resistance with median values of 2.7 and 2.9%. For Cm, resistance median values of 0.1% were found at both plants.

Transferability of drug resistance of strains isolated from sewage. The transferability of drug resistance markers of group D streptococci from sewage samples was investigated. Five colonies grown on BH plates containing Tc, Em, or Cm, respectively, were purified, and the resistance pattern and transferability of the resistance markers were investigated. The results are shown in Table 3. Only one of the 15 strains investigated was found to be beta-hemolytic. The strains selected on Em plates were Tc resistant as well, and three of the five strains selected on Cm resistance plates were also resistant to Em and Tc. Eight strains were able to transfer one or more resistance determinants to *S. faecalis* JH2-2 with a frequency higher than the detection level of 10^{-8} per recipient.

Drug resistance in group D streptococci of clinical origin. Two groups of human clinical isolates of group D streptococci were investigated. One group consisted of a collection of 44 strains isolated in 1964, and the other group included 106 strains isolated in the period between 1974 and 1976. All strains were obtained from hospitals in the Netherlands. The main sources of isolation were urine (40%), mouth and throat (20%), blood (14%), and wounds (8%). The MICs of Tc, Em, Cm, and clindamycin were determined, and the results are presented graphically in Fig. 1. The percentage of Tc-resistant strains (having an MIC >4 μg/ml) was high for both groups of D streptococci: 37 and 58%, respectively. Em, Cm, and clindamycin-resistant strains (having MICs of >16, >16, >8 μg/ml, respectively) were encountered less frequently. Also, for these drugs there was a tendency toward increasing prevalence during the period between 1964 and 1976. The Cm-resistant strains were also found to be resistant to Tc, and the Em-resistant strains were also resistant to Tc and clindamycin.

Transferability of drug resistance of clinical isolates. Thirty-six drug-resistant clinical isolates were mated with the recipient strain JH2-2. Matings were performed in liquid medium and on filters. Twenty-two of thirty-six tested were able to transfer one or more of their resistance markers to JH2-2. The results are summarized in Table 4. The transfer frequencies of filter matings ranged from 10^{-4} to the detection level of 10^{-8} for the different strains tested. In liquid medium, the transfer frequency was generally 10 to 100 times lower than that of matings on filters. About half of the strains were able to transfer the Tc resistance determinant. Cm and Em resistance was transferable in all strains tested. The three Em-resistant donor strains were also resistant

TABLE 3. *Transferability of drug resistance of group D streptococci isolated from sewage to S. faecalis JH2-2*[a]

No. of strains	Biotype	Resistance pattern	Markers transferable[b]
1	*S. faecalis*	Tc	
1	*S. faecium*	Tc	
3	—[c]	Tc	
3	*S. faecalis*	Em, Tc	Em, Tc
1	*S. faecium*	Em, Tc	Tc
1	*S. faecium*	Em, Tc	
2	*S. faecalis*	Cm, Em, Tc	Cm, Em, Tc
2	*S. faecalis*	Cm	Cm
1	*S. faecalis*	Cm, Em, Tc	

[a] All matings were performed on filters.
[b] Detection level of transfer in the mating experiments was 10^{-8} per recipient.
[c] –, Not belonging to an established biotype.

TABLE 2. *Prevalence of drug resistance in group D streptococci isolated from two sewage treatment plants*

Plant	Total viable group D streptococci per ml of influent[a]	Organisms resistant (%) to[a]		
		Tc	Em	Cm
Groenekan	1.7×10^3 (4.2×10^2 – 9.0×10^3)	15 (0.6–24)	2.9 (0.37–5.3)	0.1 (0.003–0.6)
Maartensdijk	4.0×10^3 (3.5×10^2 – 7.2×10^3)	13 (6–55)	2.7 (0.20–2.9)	0.1 (0.01–2)

[a] Median values of six samples taken on different days are presented; values in parentheses are the highest and the lowest observed.

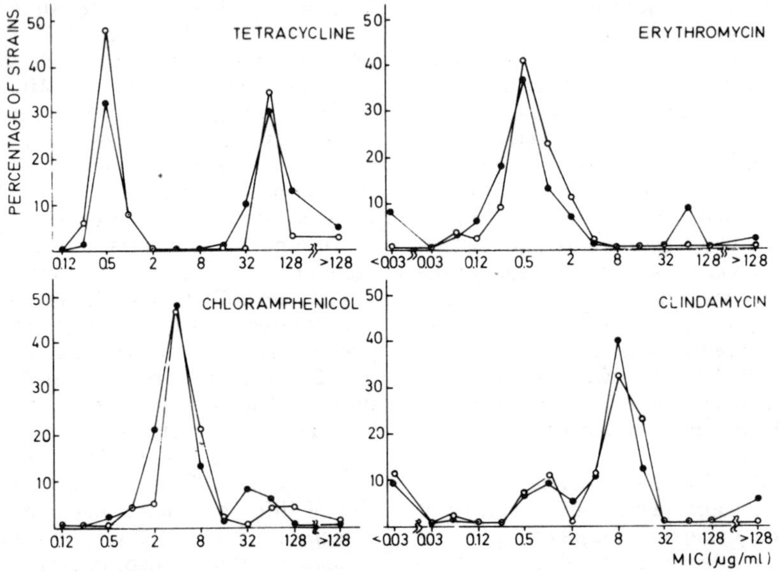

FIG. 1. *Distribution of MICs of four antibiotics. All strains were of clinical origin. Symbols: ●, Strains (106) isolated in the period 1974 to 1976; ○, strains (44) isolated in the year 1964.*

TABLE 4. *Transferability of drug resistance of group D streptococci from clinical sources to S. faecalis JH2-2*

No. of strains	Biotype	Hemolysis	Resistance pattern	Markers transferable
9	*S. faecalis*	γ	Tc	
1	*S. faecium*	γ	Tc	
4	*S. faecalis*	β	Tc	
6	*S. faecalis*	γ	Tc	Tc
7	*S. faecalis*	β	Tc	Tc, β
2	*S. bovis*	γ	Tc	Tc
2	*S. faecalis*	γ	Tc, Em	Tc, Em
1	*S. faecalis*	β	Tc, Em	Tc, Em, β
2	*S. faecalis*	β	Tc, Cm	Cm, β
2	*S. faecalis*	β	Tc, Cm	Tc, Cm, β

to clindamycin, lincomycin, oleandomycin, spiramycin, tylosine (MICs >50 μg/ml), factor S of virginiamycin (MIC >128 μg/ml), and pristinamycin Ia (MIC >32 μg/ml). Em-resistant transconjugants from the matings with the three Em resistance donor strains were also coresistant to all these antibiotics.

One strain transferred its Tc and Cm resistance as one linkage group. In the other double-resistant donor strains, no linkage between the Tc, and the Cm or Em, resistance determinants was observed.

Sixteen of the thirty-six donor strains used were beta-hemolytic, and all these strains were bacteriocinogenic, whereas no bacteriocin production could be demonstrated in the other 20 non-beta-hemolytic strains. In 10 strains, the property of hemolysin production was frequently cotransferred with one of the drug resistance determinants. All hemolytic transconjugants tested acquired the bacteriocinogenic property as well. These observations are in agreement with the view that the hemolysin of group D streptococci is identical to a bacteriocin (1, 2).

Host range of transfer of R-factors in group D streptococci. To learn whether the transfer of drug resistance of group D streptococci is limited to recipients of this serological group, 11 strains were selected that transferred one or more of their resistance markers to JH2-2 with a frequency $>10^{-7}$. These strains were used as donors in filter matings with the following recipients: a group A streptococcus (M597), a group B streptococcus (M385), and a restrictionless *E. coli* (M665).

No transfer of drug resistance to the recipients M597 and M665 was observed. In two matings with the group B streptococcus, M385, transfer frequencies were above the detection level of about 10^{-8} (see Table 5). The Tc- and Em-resistant donor strains M439 and M440 transferred their Em resistance to M385 with frequencies of 5.10^{-8} and 3.10^{-5}, respectively. Once transferred to M385, the Em resistance was transferred more efficiently to another derivative of this group B strain (M519), as is shown in Table 6.

Mechanism of transfer and plasmid properties of strains M439 and M403. Strains M439 and M403 were chosen for further study. Strain M439 is beta-hemolytic and is resistant to Tc and Em. The kinetics of transfer on filters of the drug resistance determinants and the hemolysin character are shown in Fig. 2. The Tc and Em resistance determinants are transferred independently, and 2 h after the beginning of the mating, no significant further increase of transfer was observed. We never observed hemolytic Tc-resistant transconjugants or hemolytic transconjugants that were Em susceptible. Tc- or Em-resistant transconjugants were able to transmit their drug resistance further to strain M434, a streptomycin-resistant derivative of JH2. Once introduced in JH2-2, the hemolysin character was always cotransferred with the Em resistance determinant on further transfer to M434 and, therefore, these two properties seemed to be linked in the transconjugants.

We have been unable to demonstrate any plaque-forming activity on JH2-2 in cell-free filtrates of cultures of M439. Furthermore, when cell-free filtrates of M439 were used instead of bacterial cultures, no transfer of Tc or Em resistance to JH2-2 was observed. Therefore, transduction is not likely to be the mechanism of drug resistance transfer. Also, transformation is highly improbable, because the presence of $MgCl_2$ (0.01 M) and deoxyribonuclease I (300 μg/ml) did not significantly affect the rate of transfer of Tc and Em resistance from M439 to JH2-2.

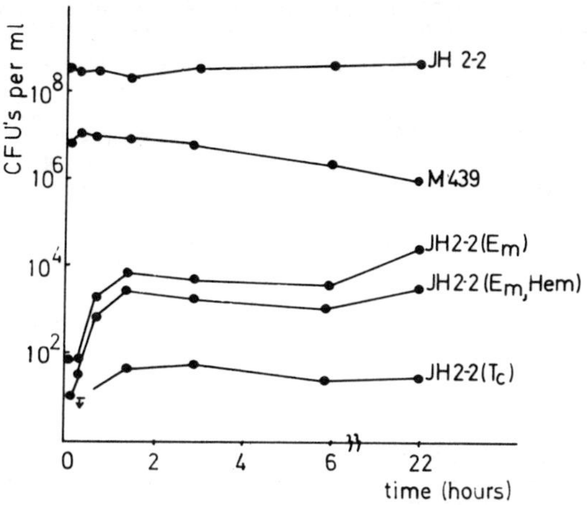

FIG. 2. *Kinetics of transfer of the drug resistance determinants Tc and Em and the hemolysin (Hem) character of strain M439 to strain JH2-2. Donor and recipients were mixed at time zero. The mating was performed in nutrient broth at 37°C. ⊤, Below the level of detection.*

TABLE 5. *Transferability of drug resistance determinants of group D streptococci to strain S. agalactiae M385*

No. of strains tested	Resistance pattern	Hemolysin production	Transferability of resistance: Tc	Em	Cm
3	Tc	+	–		
2	Tc	–	–		
1	Tc, Em	+	–	+	
1	Tc, Em	–	–	+	–
3	Tc, Cm	+	–		
1	Tc, Cm	–	–		–

TABLE 6. *Transfer frequencies of Em resistance of M439 and M440 between streptococci of groups D and B*

Donor strain	Group	Recipient: JH2-2 (group D)	M519 (group B)
M439	D	1 × 10^{-4}	5 × 10^{-8}
M385 (439 EM)[a]	B	3 × 10^{-4}	2 × 10^{-3}
M440	D	1 × 10^{-2}	3 × 10^{-5}
M385 (440 EM)[b]	B	3 × 10^{-5}	2 × 10^{-3}

[a] Em-resistant transconjugant of the mating M439 × M385.

[b] Em-resistant transconjugant of the mating M440 × M385.

To confirm the plasmid nature of the drug resistance of M439, covalently closed circular (CCC) DNA was extracted from this strain and several JH2-2 transconjugants. Jacob and Hobbs (14) showed that strain JH2-2 does not contain any detectable plasmid DNA, and therefore this strain was used as host throughout these studies. It should be noted that in an attempt to find a plasmidless strain of *S. faecalis*, five drug-susceptible, nonhemolytic clinical isolates were examined for the presence of CCC DNA. All five strains, however, contained CCC DNA and, therefore, plasmids seem to be common in this bacterial biotype.

Table 7 shows that strain M439 contains circular molecules with two different contour lengths. In the Tc-resistant transconjugant M510, a species with a mean contour length of 14.5 μm was found, whereas, in the Em-resistant transconjugants M507 and M505, molecules of the larger size class with contour lengths of 19.8 and 18.5 μm, respectively, were mainly found. Occasionally, smaller molecules were observed. The buoyant densities of all plasmid preparations amounted to 1.694 to 1.695. The corresponding guanine plus cytosine (G+C) values of 35 to 36% are close to the G+C values

TABLE 7. *Molecular properties of plasmids in strains M439, M403, and their transconjugants*

Strain	Phenotypic[a] properties	Plasmid sizes[b] observed (μm)	Mol wt	Designation of plasmid	Buoyant density in CsCl	G+C content (%)[c]
M439	Tc, Em, β	14.5 ± 0.7 (*n* = 20)	29.8×10^6		1.6949	35.3
		19.9 ± 0.5 (*n* = 13)	41.0×10^6			
M510[c]	Tc	14.5 ± 0.2 (*n* = 23)	29.8×10^6	pRI401	1.6958	36.5
		6.2 (*n* = 1)	12.8×10^6			
M507[d]	Em	19.8 ± 0.3 (*n* = 21)	40.8×10^6	pRI402	1.6948	35.5
		1.32 (*n* = 1)	2.7×10^6			
		0.50 (*n* = 1)	1.0×10^6			
M505[d]	Em, β	18.5 ± 0.3 (*n* = 21)	38.1×10^6	pRI403	1.6939	36.1
		16.70 (*n* = 1)	34.4×10^6			
		0.76 (*n* = 1)	1.6×10^6			
M403	Tc	17.8 ± 0.5 (*n* = 12)	36.7×10^6	pRI404	1.6939	34.6
M410[e]	Tc	17.0 ± 0.4 (*n* = 13)	35.0×10^6	pRI 404	1.6947	35.4

[a] β, β-hemolytic.
[b] Size and standard deviation; numbers in parentheses show how many molecules were measured.
[c] The G+C content was derived from the buoyant density in CsCl.
[d] Transconjugants of the mating M439 × JH2-2.
[e] Transconjugant of the mating M403 × JH2-2.

of 34.5 and 36.5% as found by Courvalin et al. (6) for Tc and Em resistance plasmids in *S. faecalis* and close to the G+C values of 35 to 38% reported for chromosomal DNA of *S. faecalis* (6, 25).

It is concluded that M439 harbors a Tc resistance plasmid (molecular weight, 30×10^6), designated pRI401, and an Em resistance plasmid (molecular weight, 41×10^6), designated pRI402. It is not clear from our experiments whether M439 also carries the plasmid designated pRI403, which codes for hemolysin production plus Em resistance, as found in the transconjugant M505 and is about the same size as pRI402. Royer-Pokora and Goebel (23) found that hemolysin plasmids from transconjugants originating from the same *E. coli* donor strain may differ considerably in their nucleotide sequences, although they have the same physical sizes. In analogy to these findings, pRI403 may be thought to be formed by a recombination between plasmids present in strain M439 or by translocation of the hemolysin determinant to pRI402.

The nonhemolytic strain M403 was exceptional among the Tc-monoresistant isolates, because the frequency of transfer was high, 10^{-3} to 10^{-4}, whereas in all other Tc-resistant isolates no higher values than 10^{-6} to 10^{-7} were observed. When the same techniques as described above were used, no indication could be found that transformation or transduction was the mechanism of transfer. Strain M403 harbors a plasmid species, homogenous in size, with a molecular weight of 36.8×10^6 and a G+C content of 35%. The transconjugant M410 carried a plasmid with identical molecular properties (Table 7). This plasmid is designated pRI404.

DISCUSSION

The results of the MIC determinations of the group D streptococci isolates of clinical origin show a tendency to increasing antibiotic resistance during the period between 1964 and 1976. The present incidence of Tc-resistant strains, about 50%, is as high as the values of 40 to 70% reported by other authors for group D streptococci (18, 20, 21, 24, 27, 28). However, our observations on resistance to Cm and Em suggest that the incidence of resistance to these drugs (14 and 12%, respectively) is lower than that reported by Toala et al. (28) and Schaal and Rütten (24), who found resistance percentages of around 50%.

The incidence of drug resistance in group D streptococci from sewage of human origin differed highly from sample to sample. We have no explanation for this variation. Although the data of the clinical isolates and isolates from sewage are not fully comparable because of the different methods used, the median values of the percentages of drug-resistant organisms in sewage suggest that drug resistance among the indigenous group D streptococcal flora in healthy people is less common than that found in clinical isolates. Nevertheless, an incidence of 14 and 2.8% for Tc and Em resistance, respectively (Table 2), points to a widespread occurrence. This seems hard to explain by selective pressure solely due to human therapeutic use of these antibiotics.

The frequently observed transferability to JH2-2 of drug resistance of group D streptococci from clinical and nonclinical origin suggests that drug resistance is often plasmid mediated. The experiments with strains M439 and M403 confirm the extrachromosomal nature of drug resistance and indicate that the mechanism of transfer is likely to be conjugation. Conjugal transfer of R-factors in *S. faecalis* has been observed previously (9, 14). In the isolates of clinical origin, we frequently observed cotransfer of hemolysin and bacteriocin production with one of the drug resistance determinants. These observations are consistent with the view that bacteriocin and hemolysin production are linked genetically and mediated by plasmids (9, 13, 19, 29) and that some particular bacteriocins and hemolysins of *S. faecalis* are identical substances (1, 2) or probably coded by the same gene (13).

In this study we have not been able to transfer plasmids of *S. faecalis* to a group A streptococcus strain and to *E. coli* K-12. However, the Em resistance of the strains M439 and M440 was transferable to the group B streptococcus M385. In spite of this, Em resistance in group B streptococci is not frequently encountered. In a pilot study, none of 197 strains of clinical origin tested was found to be Em-resistant, whereas 15% were resistant to Tc (B. van Klingeren, unpublished data).

The molecular sizes of the plasmids in M439 and M403 differ from those found for drug resistance plasmids in other streptococci (4, 5, 6, 14, 17). The conjugative Em resistance plasmids studied here exhibit coresistance to macrolides other than Em and to lincomycin, clindamycin, factor S of virginiamycin, and pristinamycin Ia. With respect to this coresistance, these plasmids are similar to the Em resistance plasmids β (31) and Ero (6, 7) found in *S. faecalis*. Furthermore, pRI402 is expressed constitutively in JH2-2 (J.D.A. van Embden, unpublished observations), similar to the behavior of plasmid β. Yagi et al. (31) showed at least 95% base sequence homology between the plasmid β and a plasmid of the same size (17×10^6 daltons) found in a streptococcus strain of group A. This finding suggests that plasmid exchange between group A and group D streptococci might have taken place. Our results indicate that pRI402 and other conjugative Em resistance plasmids are not easily transferable to the group A strain M597.

In the Netherlands and in other European countries, macrolide antibiotics and virginiamycin (which is partly composed of factor S) are used as feed additives in animal husbandry. Potentially, this might result in a selection of macrolide-resistant organisms. Preliminary studies (J.D.A. van Embden, unpublished observations) indicate that virginiamycin can select in vitro group D streptococci carrying plasmids that code for macrolide resistance. In vivo, such a selection might result in a buildup of a reservoir of macrolide-resistant group D and group B streptococci that are indigenous to animals (16, 26). These organisms could be transferred to humans by consumption of contaminated meat or animal handling (22). Considering the therapeutic value of the macrolide antibiotics lincomycin and clindamycin in human therapy and the transferable, plasmid-borne nature of resistance to these drugs, investigations on the consequences of the use of macrolides and virginiamycin as feed additives are desirable.

ACKNOWLEDGMENTS

We gratefully acknowledge the technical assistance of M. M. M. Meyers-van Nesselrooy, N. Soedirman, and L. J. van Wijngaarden.

LITERATURE CITED

1. **Basinger, S. F., and R. W. Jackson.** 1968. Bacteriocin (hemolysin) of *Streptococcus zymogenes*. J. Bacteriol. **96:**1895–1902.
2. **Brock, T. D., and J. M. Davie.** 1963. Probable identity of a group D hemolysin with a bacteriocine. J. Bacteriol. 86:708–712.
3. **Burkwall, M. K., and P. A. Hartman.** 1964. Comparison of direct plating media for the isolation and enumeration of *Enterococci* in certain frozen foods. Appl. Microbiol. 12:18–23.
4. **Clewell, D. B., and A. E. Franke.** 1974. Characterization of a plasmid determining resistance to erythromycin, lincomycin and vernamycin B_α in a strain of *Streptococcus pyogenes*. Antimicrob. Agents Chemother. 5:534–537.
5. **Clewell, D. B., Y. Yagi, G. M. Dunny, and S. K. Schultz.** 1974. Characterization of three plasmid deoxyribonucleic acid molecules in a strain of *Streptococcus faecalis*: identification of a plasmid determining erythromycin resistance. J. Bacteriol. **117:**283–289.
6. **Courvalin, P. M., C. Carlier, O. Croissant, and D. Blangy.** 1974. Identification of two plasmids determining resistance to tetracycline and erythromycin in group D streptococcus. Mol. Gen. Genet. **132:**181–192.
7. **Courvalin, P. M., C. Carlier, and Y. A. Chabbert.** 1972. Plasmid-linked tetracyclin and erythromycin resistance in group D "streptococcus." Ann. Inst. Pasteur **123:**755–759.
8. **De Moor, C. E.** 1959. Groepering en typering van streptococcen. Versl. Meded. Volksgezond. **2:**500–505.
9. **Dunny, G. M., and D. B. Clewell.** 1975. Transmissible toxin (hemolysin) plasmid in *Streptococcus faecalis* and its mobilization of a noninfectious drug resistance plasmid. J. Bacteriol. **124:**784–790.
10. **Facklam, R. R.** 1972. Recognition of group D streptococcal species of human origin by biochemical and physiological tests. Appl. Microbiol. **23:**1131–1139.
11. **Fuller, A. T.** 1938. The formamide method for the extraction of polysaccharides from hemolytic *strepto-*

cocci. Br. J. Exp. Pathol. 39:130–139.

12. **Falkow, S.** 1976. Infectious multiple drug resistance. Pion Limited, London.
13. **Jacob, A. E., G. J. Douglas, and S. J. Hobbs.** 1975. Self-transferable plasmids determining the hemolysin and bacteriocin of *Streptococcus faecalis* var. *zymogenes*. J. Bacteriol. 121:863–872.
14. **Jacob, A. E., and S. J. Hobbs.** 1974. Conjugal transfer of plasmid-borne multiple antibiotic resistance in *Streptococcus faecalis* var. *zymogenes*. J. Bacteriol. 117:360–372.
15. **Jones, W. F., Jr., and M. Finland.** 1957. Susceptibility of Enterococcus to eleven antibodies in vitro. Am. J. Clin. Pathol. 27:467–481.
16. **Kjellander, J.** 1960. Enteric streptococci as indicators of fecal contamination of water. Acta Pathol. Microbiol. Scand. 48(Suppl. 136):1–123.
17. **Malke, H., H. E. Jacob, and K. Störl.** 1976. Characterization of the antibiotic resistance plasmid ERLl from *Streptococcus pyogenes*. Mol. Gen. Genet. 144:333–338.
18. **Marder, H. P., and F. H. Kayser.** 1974. Epidemiologische und genetische Untersuchungen der Antibiotikaresistenz bei Enterokokken. Pathol. Microbiol. 41:131–132.
19. **Marder, H. P., and F. H. Kayser.** 1975. Genetische Instabilität der Hämolysin/Bacteriocin-Bildung bei *Streptococcus faecalis* var. *zymogenes*. Pathol. Microbiol. 42:282–283.
20. **Matsen, J. M., and C. B. Coghlan.** 1972. Antibiotic testing and susceptibility patterns of Streptococci. *In* L. W. Wannamaker and J. M. Matsen (ed.), Streptococci and streptococcal diseases. Academic Press Inc., New York.
21. **Nord, C. E., and T. Wadstrom.** 1973. Susceptibility of haemolytic oral enterococci to eight antibiotics in vitro. Acta Odontol. Scand. 31:395–399.
22. **Obiger, A.** 1972. Food as vehicle of pathogenic streptococci. Arch. Lebensmittelhyg. 25:236–240.
23. **Royer-Pokora, B., and W. Goebel.** 1976. Plasmids controlling synthesis of hemolysin in *Escherichia coli*. II. Polynucleotide sequence relationship among hemolytic plasmids. Mol. Gen. Genet. 144:177–183.
24. **Schaal, K. P., and D. Rütten.** 1973. Zur Resistenz der Enterokokken gegen penizilline, cephalosporine und klassische Breitbandantibiotika. Med. Welt. 24:402–405.
25. **Schildkraut, C. L., J. Marmur, and P. Doty.** 1962. Determination of the base composition of desoxyribonucleic acid from its buoyant density in CsCl. J. Mol. Biol. 4:430–443.
26. **Smith, H. W., and W. E. Crabb.** 1961. The faecal bacterial flora of animals and man: its development in the young. J. Pathol. Bacteriol. 82:53–66.
27. **Thornsberry, C., C. N. Baker, and R. R. Facklam.** 1974. Antibiotic susceptibility of *Streptococcus bovis* and other group D streptococci causing endocarditis. Antimicrob. Agents Chemother. 5:228–233.
28. **Toala, P., A. MacDonald, C. Wilcox, and M. Finland.** 1969. Susceptibility of group D streptococcus (Enterococcus) to 21 antibiotics in vitro, with special reference to species differences. Am. J. Med. Sci. 258:416–430.
29. **Tomura, T., T. Hirano, T. Ito, and M. Yoshioka.** 1973. Transmission of bacteriocinogenicity by conjugation in group D streptococci. Jpn. J. Microbiol. 17:445–452.
30. **Van Embden, J. D. A., and S. N. Cohen.** 1973. Molecular and genetic studies of an R factor system consisting of independent transfer and drug resistance plasmids. J. Bacteriol. 116:699–709.
31. **Yagi, Y., A. E. Franke, and D. B. Clewell.** 1975. Plasmid-determined resistance to erythromycin: comparison of strains of *Streptococcus faecalis* and *Streptococcus pyogenes* with regard to plasmid homology and resistance inducibility. Antimicrob. Agents Chemother. 7:871–873.

ANTIMICROBIAL AGENTS AND CHEMOTHERAPY, June 1977, p. 933-935 Vol. 11, No. 6

Penetration of Cefamandole into Spinal Fluid

EVAN A. STEINBERG,* GARY D. OVERTURF, LARRY J. BARAFF, AND JEANETTE WILKINS

*Department of Pediatrics, Los Angeles County-University of Southern California Medical Center; and Department of Pediatrics and Hastings Infectious Disease Laboratory, University of Southern California School of Medicine, Los Angeles, California 90033**

Received for publication 7 December 1976

Twelve patients, aged 6 months to 62 years, with proven bacterial meningitis, were given a single intravenous dose of cefamandole (33 mg/kg) 75 to 140 min before a routine lumbar puncture. Infecting organisms included *Haemophilus influenzae* (eight cases), *Streptococcus pneumoniae* (two cases), and *Neisseria meningitidis* and β-hemolytic streptococcus (one each). Cerebrospinal fluid (CSF) was analyzed by microbiological assay for cefamandole. The median concentration was 0.60 μg/ml, ranging from undetectable to 7.4 μg/ml. CSF cefamandole concentrations correlated with CSF protein: in six patients with CSF protein less than 100 μg/dl, the range of drug concentration was 0 to 0.62 μg/ml; and in six patients with CSF protein above 100 mg/dl, the range was 0.57 to 7.4 μg/ml. No significant correlation was noted between severity of illness, type of organism involved, or patient age and concentration of drug achieved.

Cefamandole nafate, 7-D-mandelamido-3 {[(1-methyl-1H-tetrazole-5-yl)-thio]methyl}-3 cephem-4-carboxylic acid, formate (ester), sodium salt, is a semisynthetic cephalosporin antibiotic with broad antibacterial spectrum (4, 14, 15), and is 70 to 80% protein bound (7, 8). It is notably active against β-lactamase-producing *Haemophilus influenzae* type b (9). Therefore, a pilot study was conducted to evaluate achievable antibiotic levels in cerebrospinal fluid (CSF) after the intravenous administration of a single dose of cefamandole to patients with bacterial meningitis.

MATERIALS AND METHODS

Patients. Twelve patients admitted to the Los Angeles County-University of Southern California Medical Center with bacterial meningitis were selected for study. The diagnosis was confirmed by a positive CSF culture on all patients. Informed written consent was obtained from patients or from their parents or responsible guardians. The patients included two adults (62 and 46 years), one adolescent (13 years), and nine children (6 months to 3.5 years with a median age of 10 months). Patients 4 and 5 had *Streptococcus pneumoniae* isolated from CSF; patient 12 had a β-hemolytic streptococcus; patient 10 had *Neisseria meningitidis*. All other patients had *H. influenzae* type b isolated (Table 1).

The severity of meningitis upon admission was graded according to the criteria of Mathies (13). All patients were treated with ampicillin intravenously, 200 mg/kg per day in six divided doses. One dose of cefamandole, 33 mg/kg, was substituted for ampicillin before a routine lumbar puncture within the first 72 h of treatment in all patients, except no. 12, whose dose was given on day 7 of treatment. Infusion times varied from 10 to 25 min. Two serum samples were obtained for cefamandole concentration (micrograms per milliliter): the first at 35 to 135 min, the second at 5 to 9 h. CSF was obtained for cefamandole assay at 75 to 140 min postinfusion, a time interval yielding the highest CSF concentrations of ampicillin and carbenicillin (16).

Antibiotic assay. A modification of the standard microbiological assay of Bennett et al. (2) was used. Test plates were prepared with polystyrene petri dishes (Van-Lab) (150 by 15 mm). The assay agar used nutrient agar (pH 6.8, Difco), in 40-ml portions, seeded with 0.3 ml of a *Bacillus subtilis* spore suspension prepared by the addition of one vial of spores (Difco) to 50 ml of 0.1 M phosphate buffer (pH 7.4). Two thousand units of penicillinase (Difco) was added concomitantly with the spore inoculum. Standard curves, utilizing cefamandole lithium, with CSF or serum as diluent, were run simultaneously by the inclusion of three control wells (0.8, 6.25, and 50 μg/ml). Sera and CSF that were not analyzed immediately were stored at −20°C; no specimen was stored longer than 7 days before analysis.

Susceptibility testing. Minimal inhibitory concentrations (MICs) were determined for cefamandole lithium by standard twofold serial dilution methods: Levinthal broth was used for *H. influenzae*; tryptic soy broth was used for streptococcus. An inoculum of approximately 10^5 organisms was prepared from overnight growth. Minimal bactericidal concentrations (MBCs) were determined by plating broth, with a 3-mm loop, from tubes without growth after 24 h of incubation. Chocolate agar plus supplement B was used for *H. influenzae*; sheep blood agar was used for streptococcus. MBC was defined as the lowest antibiotic concentration which allowed growth of no greater than 10 colonies after

TABLE 1. *Cefamandole concentrations in serum and CSF of patients with bacterial meningitis*[a]

Patient	Age	Day of therapy	Serum: Postinfusion time	Serum: Concn (μg/ml)	Serum: Postinfusion time	Serum: Concn (μg/ml)	CSF: Postinfusion time	CSF: Concn (μg/ml)	CSF: Protein (mg/dl)
1	9 mo	1	60 min	19.20	9 h	0	1 h, 20 min	0	69
2	9 mo	3	1 h, 20 min	36.70	ND[b]	ND	1 h, 50 min	0.24	32
3	2 yr, 1 mo	3	1 h, 55 min	2.60	5 h, 45 min	0	1 h, 35 min	0.30	93
4	13 yr	3	65 min	40.00	6 h	0.33	2 h, 15 min	0.42	37
5	46 yr	3	1 h, 10 min	18.00	5 h, 30 min	0.29	1 h, 25 min	0.54	118
6	6 mo	1	40 min	38.50	ND	ND	1 h, 35 min	0.57	77
7	2 yr, 3 mo	3	1 h, 20 min	6.25	6 h	0	1 h, 15 min	0.62	87
8	10 mo	1	50 min	37.00	5 h	2.60	2 h, 20 min	2.00	196
9	2 yr	3	1 h, 20 min	27.50	6 h, 20 min	0.19	1 h, 35 min	2.55	159
10	3 yr, 9 mo	1	35 min	35.00	6 h	0.93	2 h, 20 min	3.10	120
11	10 mo	3	1 h, 52 min	6.25	6 h, 20 min	0	1 h, 30 min	5.20	1,000
12	62 yr	7	2 h, 15 min	35.00	6 h, 30 min	7.40	2 h, 20 min	7.40	160

[a] Concentrations were measured after single dose of cefamandole, 33 mg/kg, given intravenously.
[b] ND, Not done.

18 h of incubation. All *H. influenzae* isolates were tested for β-lactamase production by the method of Thornsberry (19).

RESULTS

Serum concentrations of cefamandole ranged from 2.6 to 40 μg/ml, with a median of 31.25 μg/ml in 12 patients, at 35 to 135 min after administration (Table 1), and from undetectable to 7.4 μg/ml, with a median of 1.17 μg/ml, in 10 patients, at 5 to 9 h after administration (Table 1). The wide range in serum cefamandole concentrations may be explained by the fact that the rate of antibiotic infusion and the time of serum collection postinfusion were not kept constant. All patients had normal renal function, as indicated by serum urea nitrogen, which was less than 18 mg/dl, or serum creatinine, which was less than 1.1 mg/dl.

CSF concentrations of cefamandole ranged from undetectable in one patient to 7.4 μg/ml, with a median of 0.60 μg/ml, at 75 to 140 min after administration. No correlation was apparent between the concentration attained and type of organism or severity of disease upon admission. Greater CSF concentrations were observed in CSF with higher protein concentrations. In six patients with CSF protein less than 100 mg/dl, concentrations ranged from undetectable to 0.62 μg/ml, with a median of 0.36 μg/ml. In six patients with CSF protein above 100 mg/dl, concentrations ranged from 0.54 to 7.4 μg/ml, with a median of 2.83 μg/ml. (Table 1).

All *H. influenzae* type b isolates were negative for β-lactamase production. Susceptibility studies to cefamandole on five of these yielded an MIC of 0.4 μg/ml and an MBC of 0.4 μg/ml on each organism. The single β-hemolytic streptococcus had an MIC of 0.1 μg/ml and an MBC of 0.8 μg/ml.

Two patients manifested unusual symptoms in association with administration of the drug. One adult developed agitation and a generalized urticarial rash within 15 min. All symptoms resolved within 3 h, after the administration of 50 mg of diphenhydramine intravenously. One child had an increase in temperature from 100⁴°F to 102⁶°F (ca. 37.8 to 38.9°C) at 1 h and 45 min after administration of the drug. This was associated with generalized shaking, but there was no change in other vital signs and no loss of consciousness.

DISCUSSION

The spectrum of cefamandole includes the three organisms responsible for most bacterial meningitis in children and adults. *S. pneumoniae* is highly susceptible; reported MICs have ranged from 97% inhibited at less than or equal to 0.4 μg/ml (4, 14) to 100% inhibited at less than or equal to 0.2 μg/ml (5, 15). *N. meningitidis* has MICs less than or equal to 0.25 μg/ml (12). Reported MICs for *H. influenzae* type b have ranged from 90% susceptible to less than or equal to 2.5 μg/ml (4, 14) to 100% susceptible to 2.0 μg/ml, including ampicillin-resistant strains producing β-lactamase (9).

Concentrations achieved in CSF during treatment of bacterial meningitis have been reported for several antibiotics (18). An antibiotic that fails to achieve measurable CSF concentrations in the presence of meningitis is generally ineffective in treating central nervous system infections. However, neither proof of CSF penetration nor actual concentrations measured, by themselves, assures the efficacy of an antibiotic (6).

Penicillin and ampicillin generally attain CSF concentrations between 0.5 and 10 μg/ml during treatment of meningitis (1, 18, 20, 22), but single random samples may have no detectable concentrations despite clinical evidence of therapeutic efficacy (16, 22). On a daily dosage of 200 mg/kg given in six doses of 33 mg/kg, ampicillin achieved a median concentration of 0.45 μ/ml, with a range of 0.1 to 2.3 μg/ml in 15 patients with CSF protein less than 75 mg/dl. At a similar dosage, in 14 patients with CSF protein greater than 75 mg/dl, ampicillin achieved a median concentration of 2.20 μg/ml, with a range of 0.37 to 30 μg/ml (16). Cephalosporins have also demonstrated penetration of CSF in the presence of meningeal inflammation. Cephalothin (3, 10, 17, 21) and cephaloridine (11) each have attained CSF median concentrations in the range of 0.1 to 6 μg/ml. Yet, despite adequate drug dosage and measured antibiotic concentrations exceeding the MIC of the infecting organism, these cephalosporins have, on occasion, been associated with persistence of bacteria in CSF and poor clinical response (3, 6).

Chloramphenicol is, at present, the most reliable effective antibiotic for infections with *H. influenzae* type b. The documented occurrence of aplastic anemia after the administration of chloramphenicol, although rare, has caused concern about its use. The results of this pilot study show that cefamandole does penetrate inflamed meninges. It is possible that this agent may be useful in the therapy of meningitis, but further in vitro and careful in vivo research is required before cefamandole can be considered as a therapeutic agent for central nervous system infections.

LITERATURE CITED

1. **Barrett, F. F., W. A. Eardley, M. D. Yow, and H. A. Leverett.** 1966. Ampicillin in the treatment of acute suppurative meningitis. J. Pediatr. **69**:343–353.
2. **Bennett, J. V., J. L. Brodie, E. J. Benner, and W. M. Kirby.** 1966. Simplified accurate method for antibiotic assay for clinical specimens. Appl. Microbiol. **14**:170–177.
3. **Brown, J. D., A. W. Mathies, Jr., D. Ivler, W. S. Warren, and J. M. Leedom.** 1970. Variable results of cephalothin therapy for meningococcal meningitis, p. 432–440. Antimicrob. Agents Chemother. 1969.
4. **Eykyn, S., C. Jenkins, A. King, and I. Phillips.** 1973. Antibacterial activity of cefamandole, a new cephalosporin antibiotic, compared with that of cephaloridine, cephalothin, and cephalexin. Antimicrob. Agents Chemother. **3**:657–661.
5. **Finland, M., C. Garner, C. Wilcox, and L. D. Sabath.** 1976. Susceptibility of pneumococci and *Haemophilus influenzae* to anti-bacterial agents. Antimicrob. Agents Chemother. **9**:274–287.
6. **Fisher, L. S., A. W. Chow, T. T. Yoshikawa, and L. B. Guze.** 1975. Cephalothin and cephaloridine therapy for bacterial meningitis. Ann. Intern. Med. **82**:689–693.
7. **Fong, I. W., E. D. Ralph, E. R. Engelking, and W. M. M. Kirby.** 1976. Clinical pharmacology of cefamandole as compared with cephalothin. Antimicrob. Agents Chemother. **9**:65–69.
8. **Griffith, R. S., H. R. Black, G. L. Brier, and J. D. Wolney.** 1976. Cefamandole: in vitro and clinical pharmacokinetics. Antimicrob. Agents Chemother. **10**:814–823.
9. **Kammer, R. B., D. A. Preston, J. R. Turner, and L. C. Hawley.** 1975. Rapid detection of ampicillin-resistant *Haemophilus influenzae* and their susceptibility to sixteen antibiotics. Antimicrob. Agents Chemother. **8**:91–94.
10. **Lerner, P. I.** 1969. Penetration of cephalothin plus lincomycin into the cerebrospinal fluid. Am. J. Med. Sci. **257**:125–131.
11. **Lerner, P. I.** 1971. Penetration of cephaloridine into cerebrospinal fluid. Am. J. Med. Sci. **262**:321–326.
12. **Lilly Research Laboratories.** 1976. Cefamandole nafate clinical investigation manual, p. 6. Lilly Research Laboratories, Indianapolis.
13. **Mathies, A. W., Jr.** 1972. Penicillin in the treatment of bacterial meningitis. J. R. Coll. Physicians London **6**:139–146.
14. **Meyers, B. R., B. Leng, and S. Z. Hirschman.** 1975. Cefamandole: antimicrobial activity in vitro of a new cephalosporin. Antimicrob. Agents Chemother. **8**:737–741.
15. **Neu, H. C.** 1974. Cefamandole, a cephalosporin antibiotic with an unusually wide spectrum of activity. Antimicrob. Agents Chemother. **6**:177–182.
16. **Overturf, G. D., E. A. Steinberg, A. E. Underman, J. Wilkins, J. M. Leedom, A. W. Mathies, Jr., and P. F. Wehrle.** 1977. Comparative trial of carbenicillin and ampicillin therapy for purulent meningitis. Antimicrob. Agents Chemother. **11**:420–426.
17. **Riley, H. D., Jr., E. C. Bracken, and M. Flux.** 1963. Studies of cephalothin in infants and children, p. 716–723. Antimicrob. Agents Chemother. 1962.
18. **Taber, L. H., M. D. Yow, F. G. Nieberg.** 1967. The penetration of broadspectrum antibiotics into the cerebrospinal fluid. Ann. N. Y. Acad. Sci. **145**:473–481.
19. **Thornsberry, C., and L. A. Kirven.** 1974. Ampicillin resistance in *Haemophilus influenzae* as determined by a rapid test for beta-lactamase production. Antimicrob. Agents Chemother. **6**:653–654.
20. **Thrupp, L. D., J. M. Leedom, D. Ivler, P. F. Wehrle, B. Portnoy, and A. W. Mathies, Jr.** 1966. Ampicillin levels in the cerebrospinal fluid during treatment of bacterial meningitis, p 206–213. Antimicrob. Agents Chemother. 1965.
21. **Vianna, N. J., and D. Kaye.** 1967. Penetration of cephalothin into the spinal fluid. Am. J. Med. Sci. **254**:216–220.
22. **Wilson, H. D., and K. C. Haltalin.** 1975. Ampicillin in *Haemophilus influenzae* meningitis. Am. J. Dis. Child. **129**:208–215.

ANTIMICROBIAL AGENTS AND CHEMOTHERAPY, June 1977, p. 936-940 Vol. 11, No. 6

Beta-Lactamase-Directed Barrier for Penicillins of *Escherichia coli* Carrying R Plasmids

TATSUO YAMAMOTO AND TAKESHI YOKOTA*

Department of Bacteriology, School of Medicine, Juntendo University, Hongo 2-1-1, Tokyo 113, Japan

Received for publication 30 August 1976

Strains of *Escherichia coli* and *Salmonella typhimurium* carrying R plasmids, which were obtained from ampicillin-resistant clinical isolates of *E. coli* and *Klebsiella* spp. and specified either the type IIIa (TEM-type) or type Va (oxacillin-hydrolyzing) β-lactamase, are resistant not only to ampicillin but also to carbenicillin and sulbenicillin. The latter two derivatives, however, are poorly hydrolyzed in vitro by the β-lactamases. Although values of K_m of the enzymes are lower for sulbenicillin and carbenicillin than for ampicillin, the ratios of V_{max} to K_m for sulbenicillin and carbenicillin are not high enough to explain the high resistance in *E. coli* bearing the R plasmid. Two mutants of the plasmids conferring a temperature-sensitive ampicillin resistance were induced by nitrosoguanidine treatment. It was confirmed that *E. coli* CSH2, harboring the mutant plasmid, produces a temperature-sensitive β-lactamase and is resistant only at low temperatures (below 33°C), but not at 42°C, to ampicillin, sulbenicillin, and carbenicillin simultaneously. It is thus concluded that β-lactamase itself is responsible for the mechanism of resistance not only to ampicillin but also to sulbenicillin and carbenicillin, even though the enzyme as determined in cell-free extracts hydrolyzes the latter two drugs poorly. An unknown barrier for sulbenicillin and carbenicillin directed by β-lactamase in *E. coli* strains carrying R (*bla*) plasmids is postulated.

Beta-lactamases, which open the β-lactam ring of the penicillins and cephalosporins, have been understood as a major mechanism of resistance to these drugs in both gram-positive and gram-negative bacteria (11). The characteristics of these enzymes, however, are different between gram-positive and gram-negative bacteria. The β-lactamases of gram-negative rods are mainly localized in the periplasmic space between the outer and cytoplasmic membranes and are produced constitutively (or rarely inducibly) in rather small amounts (12). They are specified by either the chromosome or plasmids. In contrast, β-lactamases of gram-positive cocci are predominantly exoenzymes mediated by nontransferable mini-plasmids and are produced in relatively large amounts. They are typical inducible enzymes.

Substrate affinities for both groups of β-lactamases also vary. In general, β-lactamases of gram-positive bacteria often display a high affinity for the "natural penicillins," whereas gram-negative bacteria produce enzymes with a variety of substrate specificities (3, 12).

Carbenicillin and sulbenicillin are broad-spectrum penicillins developed for infections of *Pseudomonas aeruginosa* (1, 8). They are more stable than ampicillin against various types of β-lactamases. This paper deals with the role of β-lactamase in resistance to ampicillin, sulbenicillin, and carbenicillin in *Escherichia coli* strains carrying R (*bla*) plasmids.

MATERIALS AND METHODS

R plasmids. Plasmids of RK1 (*amp cml tet str kan sul*) and RE45 (*amp cml tet str sul*) were employed as representative plasmids specifying the type IIIa (TEM-type) and type Va (oxacillin-hydrolyzing) β-lactamases, respectively (6, 12). They were selected from among 61 R (*amp* ---) plasmids obtained from 92 clinical isolates of *E. coli* and *Klebsiella* spp. in Juntendo Hospital, Tokyo, Japan, resistant to ampicillin.

Bacteria. *E. coli* CSH2 (F^-) *metB* (2), *Salmonella typhimurium* LT2, and *Proteus mirabilis* Pm1 *lac thy nia nal* were employed as host bacteria for the R plasmids.

Chemicals. Ampicillin, sulbenicillin, and cephaloridine were provided by Takeda Chemical Industry Co. Ltd. and Shionogi Pharmaceutical Co. Ltd., Osaka, Japan, respectively. Commercially available carbenicillin (Fujisawa Chemical Industry Co. Ltd., Osaka) was also used.

Media. Heart infusion agar (Eiken Chemical Co. Ltd., Tokyo, Japan) and MacConkey agar containing 1% lactose (Eiken) were used as plating media. L broth (4) was employed as the liquid medium.

Measurement of drug resistance levels. Minimal

growth inhibitory concentrations of β-lactam drugs were measured by the plate dilution method. One-loopful portions of a 100-fold-diluted overnight culture of test bacteria in L broth were streaked onto heart infusion agar plates containing serially increasing amounts of drugs and incubated at 37°C overnight. Fifty percent inhibitory concentrations of the drugs were measured by the liquid dilution method. Cells of test microbes reaching midlogarithmic growth phase at 30°C were inoculated into fresh L broth containing serially increasing amounts of drugs to make a final density of 1×10^5 cells/ml and incubated for 5 h at temperatures ranging from 33 to 45°C. The growth rate in the tubes was measured turbidimetrically with a Klett-Summerson colorimeter with a no. 66 filter.

β-Lactamase assay. Crude extracts of *E. coli* CSH2 carrying the RK1 or RE45 plasmids were prepared by growing the cells in 100 ml of L broth at 37°C with shaking, washing with and suspending in 3 ml of 0.01 M phosphate buffer (pH 7.0), and disrupting by four 15-s bursts of sonic treatment at 10 kc. The sonic extracts were centrifuged at 4°C for 15 min at 40,000 × *g*, and the resulting supernatant fluids were used as the crude enzymes (14). The β-lactamase assay was carried out at 30°C in 0.1 M phosphate buffer (pH 7.0) by either the macroiodometric, microiodometric, or biological method (13). For the biological assay, *Bacillus subtilis* PCI 219 and *E. coli* CSH2 were employed instead of *Staphylococcus aureus* and *Sarcina lutea*. The specific activity of β-lactamase is expressed as micromoles of substrate hydrolyzed per 60 min per milligram of protein. Protein concentrations in the crude extracts were measured by either the biuret method or the method of Lowry et al. (5).

Temperature-sensitive mutants of plasmids. The overnight culture of *E. coli* CSH2 carrying plasmid RK1 in L broth was treated with 150 μg of *N*-methyl-*N'*-nitro-*N*-nitrosoguanidine per ml by the method of Mise and Suzuki (7). The mutagenized bacteria were spread on MacConkey agar plates free from drugs, and more than 1,000 subclones were tested for resistance to ampicillin at 30 and 42°C by replica plating onto heart infusion agar plates containing 100 μg of ampicillin per ml. Mutant plasmids that confer temperature-sensitive ampicillin resistance were confirmed by successive transfer of them from *E. coli* CSH2 (R^+) to R^- strains of *E. coli* AB1157 and then *E. coli* CSH2 by conjugation. A new clone of *E. coli* CSH2 carrying the temperature-sensitive plasmids was used for the experiments.

Assay of temperature sensitivity. Fifty percent inhibitory concentrations for ampicillin and sulbenicillin in *E. coli* CSH2 carrying the mutant plasmids RK117 and RK1051 were measured by the method described previously at various temperatures. For testing temperature sensitivity of the β-lactamases specified by the mutant plasmids, the enzyme was first purified 50-fold by gel filtration with Sephadex G-75 (10). The partially purified enzymes were incubated at 42°C at protein concentrations of 0.02 and 0.4 μg/ml in 0.01 M phosphate buffer (pH 7.0) for 2.5 to 20 min, and residual activities of β-lactamases were measured by either the macroiodometric or the microiodometric method (13), with ampicillin as the substrate both before and after incubation.

RESULTS

Resistance levels of gram-negative bacteria carrying the RK1 or RE45 plasmid to β-lactam drugs. Table 1 shows the resistance levels of *E. coli*, *S. typhimurium*, and *P. mirabilis* bearing plasmids RK1 or RE45 to ampicillin, sulbenicillin, carbenicillin, and cephaloridine. In both *E. coli* and *S. typhimurium*, resistance levels conferred by either plasmid were much higher to sulbenicillin and carbenicillin than to ampicillin, although in *P. mirabilis* resistance levels to the former two drugs were lower than that to ampicillin. This evidence indicates that the same R (*bla*) plasmids specify different resistance levels to various β-lactam drugs in different bacterial species.

Enzymological properties of β-lactamases specified by RK1 and RE45 plasmids. Kinetic parameters of β-lactamases specified by RK1 and RE45 are shown in Table 2. Although the plasmids conferred high resistance levels to sul-

TABLE 1. *Resistance levels to β-lactam antibiotics of E. coli CSH2, S. typhimurium LT2, and P. mirabilis Pm1 carrying the RK1 or RE45 plasmid*

Bacteria	Plasmid present	Minimal inhibitory concentration (μg/ml)			
		Ampicillin	Sulbenicillin	Carbenicillin	Cephaloridine
E. coli CSH2		1.6	1.6	1.6	3.2
	RK1	3,200	25,600	25,600	25
	RE45	400	400	400	3.1
S. typhimurium LT2		0.4	1.6	1.6	1.6
	RK1	6,400	25,600	25,600	200
	RE45	200	400	400	3.1
P. mirabilis Pm1		0.2	0.4	0.4	3.1
	RK1	400	100	100	25
	RE45	50	12.5	25	6.3

TABLE 2. *Kinetic properties of β-lactamases specified by the RK1 and RE45 plasmids in E. coli CSH2*

Plasmid	Substrate	V_{max} [a]	K_m (μM)	V_{max}/K_m [a]
RK1	Ampicillin	100	37	100
	Sulbenicillin	5.2	7.1	27
	Carbenicillin	9.4	14	25
	Cephaloridine	120	714	6.3
RE45	Ampicillin	100	20	100
	Sulbenicillin	7.7	34	4.6
	Carbenicillin	16	59	5.4
	Cephalorodine	28	200	2.8

[a] Expressed as values relative to those for ampicillin taken as 100.

benicillin and carbenicillin on *E. coli* CSH2, V_{max} values of β-lactamases specified by those plasmids for sulbenicillin and carbenicillin were less than 16% of that for ampicillin. The V_{max} for cephaloridine was high in the RK1 β-lactamase, but rather low in the enzyme specified by RE45.

K_m values of β-lactamases for the drugs are also shown in Table 2. Since Pollock (9) reported that values of ratios of V_{max} to K_m might be a better indicator for the resistance levels, those for ampicillin, sulbenicillin, carbenicillin, and cephaloridine have been calculated. The value of V_{max} to K_m for the RK1 enzyme for cephaloridine was low enough to account for the low resistance level for that drug, although those for sulbenicillin and carbenicillin were insufficiently high to explain the high resistance levels.

Competitive inhibition of β-lactamase by sulbenicillin. Figure 1 shows a Lineweaver-Burk plot of the RK1 β-lactamase with ampicillin as the substrate, in the presence or absence of various amounts of sulbenicillin. Sulbenicillin inhibited the enzyme activity competitively, with a K_i value of 6.5 μM. Sulbenicillin, therefore, appears to have a common active site on the enzyme with ampicillin.

Accuracy of the iodometric assay. Since activities of β-lactamase were measured iodometrically, it appeared necessary to establish that the methods were accurate enough not only for ampicillin but also for sulbenicillin and carbenicillin. Values of V_{max} for the RK1 β-lactamase were identical regardless of whether determined by macroiodometry or by the bioassay (Table 3).

Hydrolysis of ampicillin, sulbenicillin, and cephaloridine by intact whole cells of *E. coli* CSH2 carrying RK1 was examined (Table 4). Sulbenicillin was hydrolyzed to a lesser extent than ampicillin, even by whole cells, although the efficiency of the enzyme was lower than with the cell-free extracts.

Temperature-sensitive mutants of plasmid RK1. Two mutants of plasmid RK1, RK117 and RK1051, which confer temperature-sensitive ampicillin resistance on the hosts, were obtained after nitrosoguanidine treatment. New subclones of *E. coli* CSH2 carrying the mutant

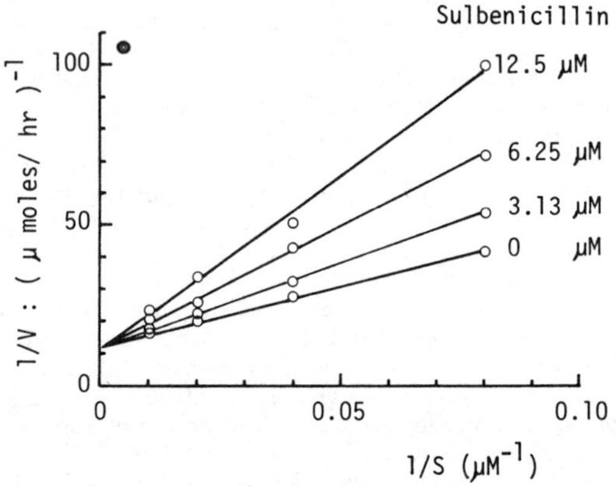

FIG. 1. *Lineweaver-Burk plots of β-lactamase specified by the RK1 plasmid in E. coli CSH2. The reaction was carried out in 2 ml of 0.1 M phosphate buffer, pH 7.0, containing 0.15% gelatin at 30°C with ampicillin as the substrate in the presence of various amounts of sulbenicillin. After 15 min of incubation, the reaction was terminated by chilling and subsequently adding 1 ml of 0.15 M sodium tungstate in 2 M acetate buffer, pH 4.0. Precipitates were removed by centrifugation, and 2 ml of the resulting supernatant was mixed with an equal volume of an aqueous solution containing 0.2% starch, 80 μM I_2, and 1.6 mM KI. The mixtures were kept at room temperature for 15 min and measured spectrophotometrically at 620 nm. The observed values at each point were subtracted by those of blanks processed in the same manner without enzyme during incubation at 30°C.*

TABLE 3. *Comparison of activities of the RK1 β-lactamase[a] measured by different methods*

Substrate	V_{max} values[b] measured by:		
	Macroiodometry	Bioassay with: *B. subtilis* PCI 219	Bioassay with: *E. coli* CSH2
Ampicillin	1,100	1,181	1,100
Sulbenicillin	77	69	61
Carbenicillin	102	134	94

[a] The crude enzyme of *E. coli* CSH2 carrying RK1 was employed.

[b] Expressed as micromoles of substrate hydrolyzed per 60 min per milligram of protein.

TABLE 4. *Hydrolysis of β-lactam antibiotics by whole cells and a cell-free extract of E. coli CSH2 carrying plasmid RK1.*

Enzyme source	μmol of substrate hydrolyzed per 60 min		
	Ampicillin	Sulbenicillin	Cephaloridine
Whole cells[a]	36	9.6	3,228
Extracts of cells[a]	28,800	2,400	30,360

[a] A total of 10^{10} cells.

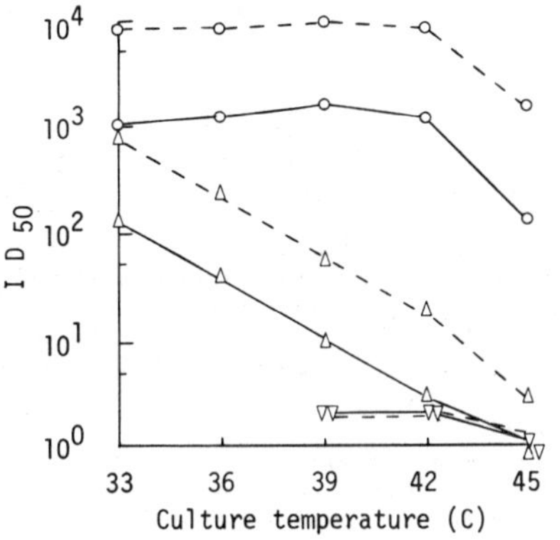

FIG. 2. *Influence of temperature shift on resistance levels to ampicillin and sulbenicillin of E. coli CSH2 harboring or not harboring plasmid RK1 and its temperature-sensitive mutant plasmid RK1051. Bacterial cells grown at 30°C in L broth were diluted with fresh L broth containing serially increasing amounts of ampicillin or sulbenicillin to 1 × 10^5 cells/ml. Portions (2 ml) were incubated at given temperatures for 5 h. Fifty percent inhibitory concentrations (ID_{50}) of antibiotics were determined turbidimetrically and expressed as micrograms per milliliter. Symbols: ——, ampicillin; -----, sulbenicillin; ○, RK1⁺; △, RK1051⁺; ▽, R⁻.*

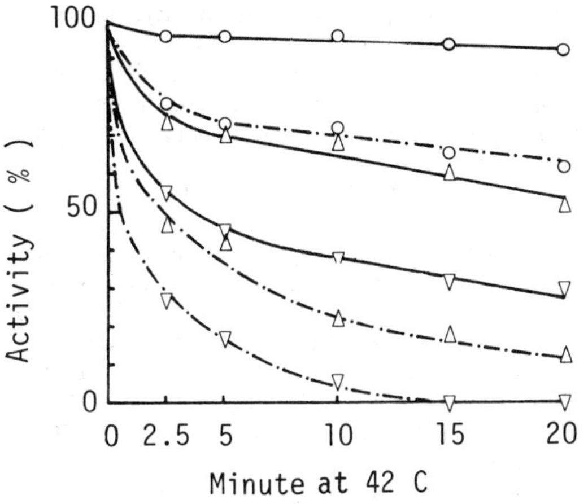

FIG. 3. *Heat stability of β-lactamases from E. coli CSH2 carrying the RK1 plasmid or its temperature-sensitive mutants RK117 and RK1051. Symbols: ○——○, RK1 β-lactamase at a protein concentration of 0.4 μg/ml; ○-·-·-·-○, RK1 β-lactamase at a protein concentration of 0.02 μg/ml; △——△, RK117 β-lactamase at a protein concentration of 0.4 μg/ml; △-·-·-·-△, RK117 β-lactamase at a protein concentration of 0.02 μg/ml; ▽——▽, RK1051 β-lactamase at a protein concentration of 0.4 μg/ml; ▽-·-·-·-▽, RK1051 β-lactamase at a protein concentration of 0.02 μg/ml.*

plasmids were highly resistant to ampicillin only at low temperatures (below 33°C), but the resistance to chloramphenicol, streptomycin, tetracycline, and kanamycin remained unaffected by the mutations. The resistance level to sulbenicillin of cells carrying either RK117 or RK1051 decreased with an increase of culture temperatures, identical to that found for ampicillin (Fig. 2). This fact indicates that the same temperature-sensitive mechanism is responsible for resistance to both ampicillin and sulbenicillin.

Figure 3 shows the influence of incubation at 42°C on the enzymatic activity of the β-lactamases that were partially purified about 50-fold from cell-free extracts of *E. coli* CSH2 harboring RK1 or its mutants, RK117 and RK1051. As shown, more than 90% of the activity of the RK1 β-lactamase remained after 20 min of incubation at 42°C at a protein concentration of 0.4 μg/ml, whereas only 55 and 13% of the activities in the RK117 and RK1051 enzymes were retained, respectively, under the same conditions. When enzyme preparations with lower protein concentration, i.e., 0.02 μg/ml, were incubated at 42°C, loss of enzyme activity was more prominent. Under this condition, more than 95% of the activity of the RK1051 β-lactamase was lost after only 10 min of incubation at 42°C.

Since temperature-sensitive ampicillin resistance of *E. coli* CSH2 carrying the mutant plasmid was confirmed to be based upon a temperature-sensitive β-lactamase, and the sulbenicillin resistance became temperature sensitive simultaneously, the mechanism of resistance to sulbenicillin and ampicillin is considered to be the β-lactamase itself, even though sulbenicillin is poorly hydrolyzed by the cell-free enzyme activity.

DISCUSSION

It appears that *E. coli* and *S. typhimurium* harboring R plasmids that specify the type IIIa

(TEM-type) or type Va (oxacillin-hydrolyzing) β-lactamase are resistant not only to ampicillin but also to sulbenicillin and carbenicillin, even though crude or partially purified enzymes from these strains hydrolyze poorly the latter two drugs.

As pointed out by Pollock (9), the enzyme is never likely to operate under optimum conditions in vivo so that the physiological efficiency of β-lactamase depends upon the values of both K_m and V_{max}. The value of the ratio of V_{max} to K_m is, therefore, a good indicator for the resistance levels to β-lactam drugs. The results obtained have indicated that K_m values of β-lactamases specified by plasmids RK1 and RE45 are lower for sulbenicillin and carbenicillin than for ampicillin, although values of V_{max} to K_m of the enzymes are not high enough for an explanation of the high resistance levels to sulbenicillin and carbenicillin.

Richmond and Curtis (11) have emphasized the importance of the interplay of β-lactamase and intrinsic factors by the recent discovery showing that R plasmid RP1, which was obtained from a strain of *P. aeruginosa*, carries two genetic regions that affect resistance to penicillins. The first is a determinant for the β-lactamase, but the second is a new gene(s) that imparts enhanced intrinsic resistance to bacteria. In contrast, the present results show that, even without the second gene(s), *E. coli* strains carrying R (*bla*) plasmids are resistant not only to ampicillin but also to sulbenicillin and carbenicillin, which are poorly hydrolyzed by the β-lactamases in vitro. This fact was confirmed by isolation of mutant plasmids that specify temperature-sensitive β-lactamases and confer simultaneously temperature-sensitive resistance to three antibiotics. Since the spontaneous reversion frequencies of the mutant plasmids were between 1×10^{-8} and 1×10^{-9}, the mutation in these plasmids was considered to be a point mutation.

It is therefore postulated that resistance to sulbenicillin and carbenicillin in *E. coli* strains carrying R (*bla*) plasmids is based on an unknown barrier directed by β-lactamase itself, which does not effectively hydrolyze these antibiotics, but binds them and prevents their passage through the periplasmic space to the penicillin-sensitive site.

ACKNOWLEDGMENTS

This work was supported by the Scientific Research Fund of the Ministry of Education, Science and Culture of Japan.

We thank N. Kosakai and T. Oguri, Department of Clinical Pathology, Juntendo Hospital, for supplying clinical isolates of *E. coli* and *Klebsiella* spp.

LITERATURE CITED

1. **Acred, P., D. M. Brown, E. T. Knudsen, G. N. Polinson, and R. Sutherland.** 1967. New semisynthetic penicillin active against *Pseudomonas pyocyanea*. Nature (London) **215**:25–30.
2. **Bachmann, B. J.** 1972. Pedigrees of some mutant strains of *Escherichia coli* K-12. Bacteriol. Rev. **36**:525–557.
3. **Dale, J. W., and J. T. Smith.** 1974. R-factor-mediated β-lactamases that hydrolyze oxacillin: evidence for two distinct groups. J. Bacteriol. **119**:351–356.
4. **Lennox, E. S.** 1955. Transduction of linked genetic characters of host by bacteriophage P1. Virology **1**:190–206.
5. **Lowry, O. H., N. J. Rosebrough, A. L. Farr, and R. J. Randall.** 1951. Protein measurement with the Folin phenol reagent. J. Biol. Chem. **193**:265–275.
6. **Matthew, M., and R. W. Hedges.** 1976. Analytical isoelectric focusing of R factor-determined β-lactamases: correlation with plasmid compatibility. J. Bacteriol. **125**:713–718.
7. **Mise, K., and Y. Suzuki.** 1968. Temperature-sensitive chloramphenicol acetyltransferase from *Escherichia coli* carrying mutant R factors. J. Bacteriol. **95**:2124–2130.
8. **Morimoto, S., H. Nomura, T. Fugono, I. Minami, T. Ishiguro, and T. Masuda.** 1973. Semisynthetic β-lactam antibiotics. III. Structure-activity relationships of α-sulfopenicillins. J. Antibiot. **26**:146–152.
9. **Pollock, M. R.** 1965. Purification and properties of penicillinase from two strains of *Bacillus licheniformis*: a chemical, physicochemical and physiological comparison. Biochem. J. **94**:666–675.
10. **Richmond, M. H.** 1975. β-lactamase (*Escherichia coli* R+ TEM). Methods Enzymol. **43**:672–677.
11. **Richmond, M. H., and N. A. Curtis.** 1974. The interplay of β-lactamases and intrinsic factors in the resistance of gram-negative bacteria to penicillins and cephalosporins. Ann. N.Y. Acad. Sci. **235**:553–568.
12. **Richmond, M. H., and R. B. Sykes.** 1973. The β-lactamase of gram-negative bacteria and their possible physiological role, p. 31–85. *In* A. H. Rose and D. W. Tempest (ed.), Advances in microbial physiology, vol. 9. Academic Press Inc., New York.
13. **Ross, G. W., and C. H. O'Callaghan.** 1975. β-Lactamase assay. Methods Enzymol. **43**:69–85.
14. **Yamagishi, S., K. O'Hara, T. Sawai, and S. Mitsuhashi.** 1969. The purification and properties of penicillin β-lactamases mediated by transmissible R factors in *Escherichia coli*. J. Biochem. (Tokyo) **66**:11–20.

ANTIMICROBIAL AGENTS AND CHEMOTHERAPY, June 1977, p. 941-945

Vol. 11, No. 6
Printed in U.S.A.

Mechanism of Accumulation of the Antitumor Protein Antibiotic Neocarzinostatin in Bladder Tissue: Intravenous Administration, Urinary Excretion, and Absorption into Bladder Tissue

HIROSHI MAEDA,* SADAAKI SAKAMOTO, AND JIRO OGATA

Departments of Microbiology and Urology, Kumamoto University Medical School, Kumamoto, Japan 860*

Received for publication 13 December 1976

Some aspects of the absorption, distribution, and excretion of neocarzinostatin (NCS), a proteinous antitumor antibiotic, were studied in rabbits. NCS was given intravenously (i.v.) via the auricular vein, or [^{14}C]NCS was instilled directly into the cavity of the bladder by tubing. In both groups, ureterostomy was performed, so that the drug excreted in the urine did not pass through the bladder. The results showed extremely rapid renal clearance; namely, two-thirds of the total recovered was excreted in the first 5 min. It was also shown that drug infused into the bladder cavity could be recovered in urine from the ureterostomized ureter. Also, the level of biological activity of NCS in bladder tissues after i.v. administration is significantly lower when ureterostomy is performed. Thus, evidence is presented for the absorption of NCS into bladder tissue from the lumen of the bladder. The high levels of NCS in bladder tissue are due to this effect as well as to accumulation via the iliac artery. These data should encourage further trials of NCS in bladder cancer. A study of urine containing NCS derived from i.v. administration showed an increase in antibacterial activity upon incubation, followed by a decrease. These effects are probably due to proteolysis, as shown by the appearance of a low-molecular-weight fragment and by the absence of such an increase in the presence of inhibitors of proteolysis.

Neocarzinostatin (NCS), isolated from the culture filtrate of a *Streptomyces* sp. (4), is the first antibiotic protein to be used in human chemotherapy. NCS is an acidic single-chain polypeptide of 10,700 daltons. The amino acid sequence has been reported by Maeda et al. (11). It contains 109 L-amino acid residues with two disulfide intramolecular cross-linkages, but lacks methionine and histidine residues.

The antibiotic was reported to have a very high chemotherapeutic index in mice bearing ascitic sarcoma S-180 (4). It has been investigated in patients with leukemia and gastric, pancreatic, and other cancers (3, 20). The mechanism of action involves deoxyribonucleic acid metabolism and mitotic inhibition (2, 17). The subcellular site of action appears to be the nucleus of the cell (10).

We have recently reported (15) studies of drug distribution after intravenous (i.v.) administration of [^{14}C]NCS. It was found that NCS accumulates most extensively in kidney and bladder tissues (about 20 to 100 times more than in other organs), and that renal clearance is extremely rapid despite the large molecular size. About 50% of the administered radioactivity was excreted in the first 20 min.

Based on this finding, we have used NCS i.v. for bladder cancer in humans and have obtained unprecedented results (S. Sakamoto, J. Ogata, and H. Maeda, manuscript in preparation). Eleven of 15 patients with bladder cancer responded with a reduction in tumor volume to 1/3 to 1/5 of the original size, based on cystoscopic observation and histological analyses.

So far, systemic chemotherapy of bladder tumors has been unsuccessful. Ogata et al. have devised a method for the treatment of bladder tumors that utilizes catheterization of the internal iliac artery and infusion of a mitomycin C solution through the catheter (16). However, this method is difficult to use successfully. The other alternative is radical cystectomy, with the accompanying inconveniences. Systemic treatment would be more convenient and should also provide a counter measure against micrometastases.

Although we have found high concentrations

of NCS in the bladder tissue after i.v. administration, it is important to determine whether it reaches the tissue via absorption into the tissue from the urine.

MATERIALS AND METHODS

NCS and its ^{14}C derivative. NCS was obtained from Kayaku Antibiotic Research Laboratories, Tokyo, and repurified as described (12). The ^{14}C derivative was prepared by chemical modification using [1,4-^{14}C]succinic anhydride (9, 10). Its specific radioactivity was 5.0×10^6 cpm/mg of protein. The derivative, bis-succinyl NCS, has physicochemical and biological properties similar to the parent compound (molecular weight, water solubility, acidic nature, and in vitro activity [8]) but is more stable to proteolysis (14).

Biological activity assay. NCS was assayed by the cup plate method, with *Sarcina lutea* PCI 1001 as the test organism and purified NCS as standard. The homogenates of assay specimens were prepared with 0.07% each leupeptin, pepstatin, antipain, and *N*-ethylmaleimide to inhibit the proteolytic degradation of the protein antibiotic (14). Each organ specimen was frozen in dry ice and held at −20°C until used. The frozen specimens were sliced into thin sections with a cryostat at −20°C. Two times the specimen weight of 0.01 M phosphate-buffered (pH 7.0) saline (0.15 M) (PBS) containing the inhibitors was added to the frozen sections, which were then homogenized in a glass homogenizer followed by centrifugation at 4°C. The supernatants were used for biological assays. The urine samples were diluted with a 1/10 volume of the inhibitor mixture dissolved in PBS. The standards and samples, placed in the cups on the Mueller-Hinton agar plates, were allowed to diffuse for about 5 h at about 4°C, followed by incubation at 37°C overnight. The assay was sensitive to concentrations of NCS above 0.05 μg/ml.

Animals. Domestic albino male rabbits weighing 2.0 to 3.5 kg were used. For the biological activity measurements, four rabbits were used for one group. Administration i.v. was carried out via the auricular vein. For intrabladder administration, NCS was administered via the urethra using a syringe attached to a Nélaton catheter. Ureterostomy was carried out under anesthesia with pentobarbital sodium, and the urine samples were collected directly from the ureter. Thus, urine flow into the bladder was avoided.

Effect of urine on the biological activity of NCS. A urine specimen obtained from the ureter 5 min after i.v. injection was incubated at 37°C with and without proteolytic inhibitors for various periods of time and then assayed against *S. lutea*. After the incubation periods, the urine samples were stored frozen at −20°C until assayed.

Absorption from epithelium of bladder and recirculation of [^{14}C]NCS. About 2 mg of [^{14}C]NCS per kg of body weight, dissolved in 20 ml of PBS, was administered to the bladder of ureterostomized rabbits by using a syringe and tubing. Excess pressure was avoided during the infusion. Urine samples were obtained at different times, and the radioactivity was determined with a scintillation counter as described (10). During the experiments, the rabbits were infused via the auricular vein with physiological saline at about 40 ml/h to maintain the constant urinary output.

The molecular size profile of the radioactive material in the 90-min urine sample was studied by Sephadex G-50 chromatography. A 4-ml sample was concentrated to 1.5 ml by lyophilization and applied to a 1.5 by 58-cm column. It was eluted with PBS at 75 ml/h, and 3.75-ml fractions were collected. The molecular size of radioactive peaks was estimated by comparison with the reference compounds, purified NCS (molecular weight, 10,700), actinomycin (molecular weight, 1,255), bacitracin (molecular weight, 1,460), and phenol red (molecular weight, 354).

RESULTS

Renal clearance. The urinary recovery of the biological activity of NCS obtained from the data of four rabbits dosed i.v. with 10 mg/kg of body weight is shown in Fig. 1. NCS was almost undetectable (less than 0.05 μg/ml) in serum or urine 20 min after i.v. administration. About 45% of the administered biological activity was recovered in the urine during the 20-min period. Of the total activity recovered, 60 to 70% was excreted in the urine in the initial 5-min period.

Activation and inactivation of NCS in urine. During incubation at 37°C, the biological

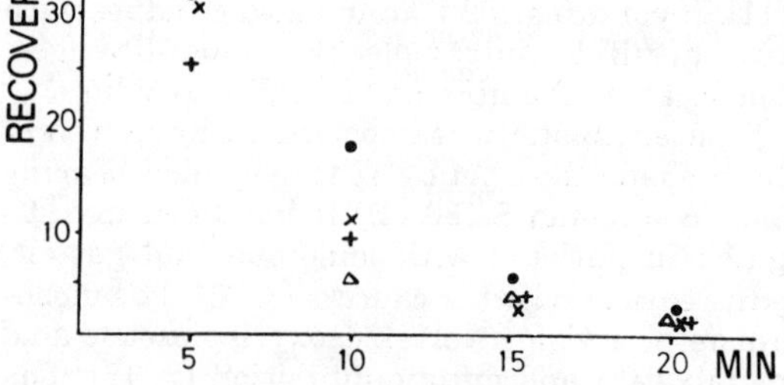

FIG. 1. *Urinary recovery of NCS from the ureter after an i.v. dose of 10 mg/kg in ureterostomized rabbits. The recovery of antibiotic activity was measured every 5 min. The percent recovery relative to the administered dose is shown for the first 20 min. The abscissa indicates time after administration. Four different experiments are shown with different symbols.*

activity measured by *S. lutea* in the urine that was obtained from the ureter increased almost twofold after 2 h, but later decreased to the original level (Fig. 2). Further incubation led to a decrease in activity. However, the incubation of NCS added to urine that was obtained separately from untreated animals showed no activation, but the activity decreased during incubation (Fig. 2). When proteolytic inhibitors were added to the urine sample, the change of activity was less than 10% during the experimental period.

Distribution in tissues. In our previous studies with the ^{14}C derivative, it was found that drug concentrations in various tissues were high shortly after i.v. administration and decreased considerably after 60 min, with the exception of the bladder tissue. Therefore, in the present investigations the tissue levels were studied only at 20 min. The results from the ureterostomized group are compared in Table 1

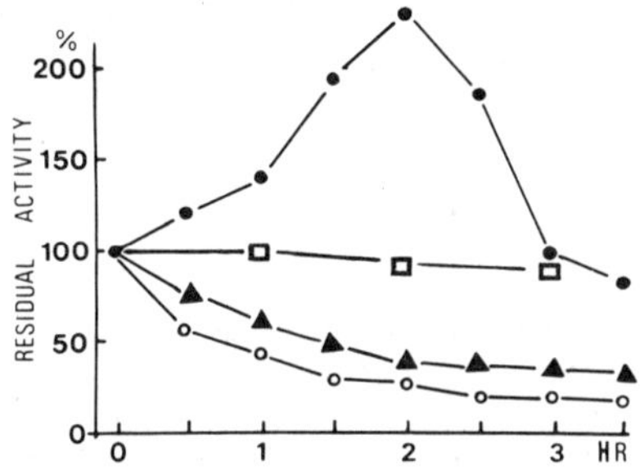

FIG. 2. *Activation and inactivation of NCS by urine of rabbits. The biological activity (percentage) of the drug excreted in urine after intravenous administration (●) and that of an artificial mixture of urine and drug in the test tube (○) were compared with that of the drug (at 50 μg/ml) incubated in 0.01 M phosphate-buffered (pH 7.4) saline alone (▲). All samples were incubated at 37°C at different time intervals. When the urine sample containing drug was incubated in the presence of proteolytic inhibitors, the activation was not observed (□).*

TABLE 1. *Tissue concentration of NCS in rabbits after i.v. administration of 10 mg/kg*

Tissue	μg/g of tissue ± SE[a]	
	Ureterostomized	Control
Bladder	0.53 ± 0.04	1.11 ± 0.05
Kidney	2.89 ± 0.80	3.21 ± 0.68
Stomach	0[b]	0
Large intestine	0.68 ± 0.04	0.77 ± 0.17
Muscle	0	0

[a] Time = 20 min. Biological activity against *S. lutea*. *n* = 4 in each group. SE, Standard error.
[b] 0 = Undetectable.

with those from the control group. The results show that absorption from urine into bladder tissue contributes significantly to the NCS level in bladder tissue. After an i.v. dose of 10 mg/kg, the tissue levels are twice as high ($P <$ 0.001) in normal animals as in those in which urine containing NCS was diverted by ureterostomy before reaching the bladder. Higher doses could not be used because of toxicity, and a dose of 1 mg/kg gave no detectable levels of NCS.

Absorption of NCS from bladder and recovery at ureter. The time course of urinary recovery of [^{14}C]NCS administered into the bladder cavity is shown in Fig. 3. The excretion rate reached a maximum at 90 min after administration and gradually decreased to a low level after 3 h. The total radioactive recovery in urine alone was 0.28% of the total added to the bladder in 3 h, and 56.9% remained in the bladder. The remainder was probably distributed in other tissues or organs throughout the body. A sample of the material recovered from urine at 90 min was examined by Sephadex chromatography. The profile of the radioactive materials showed a major peak near the original NCS and a large peak with a molecular weight of about 1,500 (Fig. 4). These materials showed no antibacterial activity.

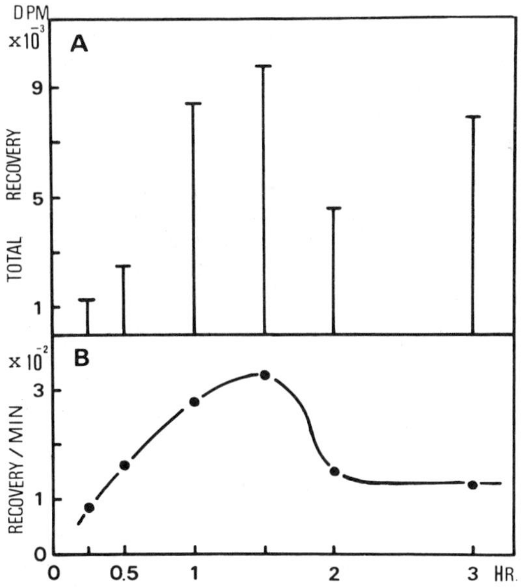

FIG. 3. *Urinary recovery of [^{14}C]NCS from the ureter after intrabladder administration. The recovery is measured by radioactivity. (A) Total activity recovered during each collection period. (B) Rate of excretion (activity excreted per minute) of samples taken at the indicated times.*

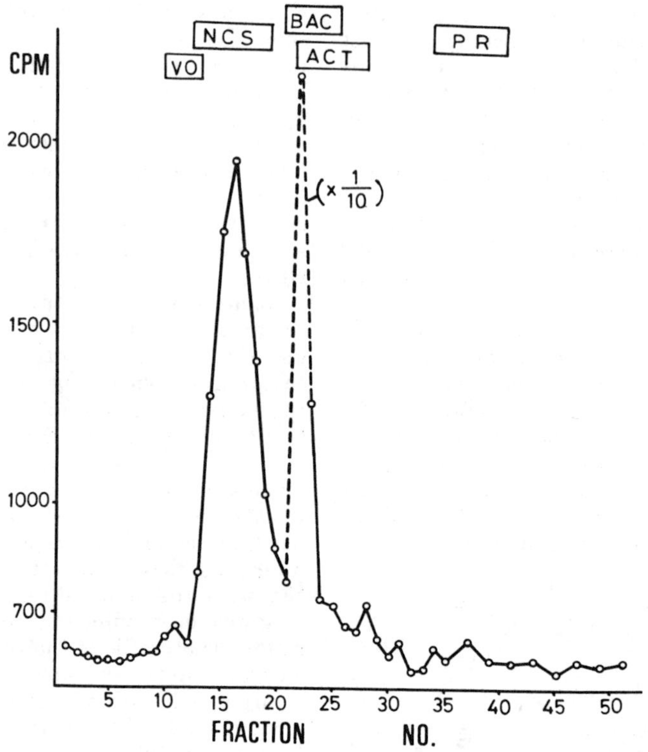

FIG. 4. *Analysis of molecular size distribution of absorbed and metabolized [^{14}C]NCS from urine. The sample was obtained from the ureter of ureterostomized rabbits between 60 and 90 min after intrabladder administration of the drug. It was analyzed on a Sephadex G-50 column. The markers for various molecular sizes are shown at the top. V_0, Void volume (molecular weight, >1.5 × 10^4); NCS, pure neocarzinostatin (ca. 11,000); BAC, bacitracin (1,460); ACT, actinomycin D (1,255); PR, phenol red (354). (× 1/10) indicates the fractions were actually 10 times higher than shown.*

DISCUSSION

The results presented in this study confirmed our earlier finding (15) that NCS administered systemically (i.v.) is excreted with extreme rapidity in urine and accumulates in bladder tissue. When the tissue level of the rabbits of the ureterostomized group and those of the control group are compared, it is clear that half of the biological activity of the bladder tissue in the initial 20-min period is contributed by absorption (diffusion) into the tissue from the urine. The rest, of course, must be from the circulating blood (via the iliac artery). The very rapid excretion of NCS indicates that the toxicity of NCS may be critically influenced by renal function. The subjects with renal malfunction may show toxicity at lower doses of NCS.

The absorption of NCS from the bladder epithelium was further confirmed by identifying [^{14}C]NCS and its fragments in urine when it was administered into the bladder cavity of ureterostomized animals. The time-course study of radioactivity excretion showed that absorption from the bladder was very slow, reaching a maximum between 60 and 90 min, followed by a gradual decline. After 3 h only 57% of the radioactivity remained in the bladder. Examination of the radioactive components in the urine at 90 min showed that the NCS absorbed was extensively degraded by proteolysis, but approximately 30% was recovered with a molecular weight similar to that of NCS. The results help to explain our good results in the treatment of bladder cancer in humans (18).

In vitro incubation of excreted NCS without proteolytic inhibitors at 37°C resulted in activation, as measured by antibacterial activity followed by inactivation. This was not observed for NCS added to urine in vitro. Both activation and inactivation probably result from mild, limited proteolytic breakdown in the blood as noted previously (13, 14). This interpretation is supported by the fact that such changes are minimized in the presence of proteolytic inhibitors.

The present results indicate that metabolism of NCS can occur in urine as well as in liver (15), serum (13), blood (14, 15), and cells (10) and suggest that an active fragment of NCS may be formed. The increase in activity during the incubation of urine containing excreted NCS after i.v. dosing suggests an advantage for i.v. administration over intrabladder administration if the antibacterial activity parallels antitumor activity. Inactivation of NCS in PBS without urine is also seen in Fig. 2. This may be inactivation due to light and temperature, as previously described (5). Another factor is the protein concentration; at a low protein concentration (50 μg/ml), denaturation is more rapid than at a higher concentration (2.5 mg/ml). This has been previously shown for NCS (6). An attempt to isolate and characterize the active fragments is in progress.

Very few antitumor agents are useful for the chemotherapy of bladder cancer by systemic administration. In addition, the systemic administration of a cell cycle-specific drug such as this is, of course, advantageous, particularly for the micrometastases of tumor cells (19).

Uptake of protein molecules from the bladder epithelium was demonstrated for the first time for a protein antibiotic. This phenomenon is not uncommon in physiology, and recent pertinent literature indicates uptake of bovine serum albumin by the lateral line system of trout (1), of the digestive enzymes (chymotrypsin, amylase, and papain) or albumin from the intestine (7, 22; Murachi, Abstr. 10th Int. Congr. Biochem., 16-5-030, 1976), or viral agents or interferon from the epithelial mucous membrane. These materials ultimately reach the systemic circulation.

The present experiments on the protein antibiotic NCS clarify its extremely rapid renal clearance and diffusion from urine into bladder tissue and provide a rationale for the i.v. administration of NCS for the effective treatment of bladder cancer.

ACKNOWLEDGMENTS

We thank Y. Hinuma and K. Ikegami of our departments for their encouragement, and I.R. Hooper of Bristol Laboratories for improving the English.

LITERATURE CITED

1. **Amend, D. F., and D. C. Fender.** 1976. Uptake of bovine serum albumin by rainbow trout from hyperosmotic solution: a model for vaccinating fish. Science 192:793–794.
2. **Ebina, T., K. Ohtsuki, M. Seto, and N. Ishida.** 1975. Specific G2 block in HeLa S_3 cells by neocarzinostatin. Eur. J. Cancer 11:155–158.
3. **Hiraki, K., O. Kamimura, I. Takahashi, T. Nagao, K. Kitajima, and S. Irino.** 1973. Neocarzinostatin, une approche novelle dans la chimiotherapie de leucémies aiguës. Nouv. Rev. Fr. Hematol. 13:445–451.
4. **Ishida, N., K. Miyazaki, K. Kumagai, and M. Rikimaru.** 1965. Neocarzinostatin, an antitumor antibiotic of high molecular weight. Isolation, physicochemical properties and biological activity. J. Antibiot. 18:68–76.
5. **Kono, T., I. Haneda, Y. Koyama, and M. Kikuchi.** 1974. Studies on the stability of an antitumour protein, neocarzinostatin. I. Stability of a solution of neocarzinostatin. Jpn. J. Antibiot. 27:707–714.
6. **Kono, T., F. Ishii, I. Haneda, Y. Koyama, and M. Kikuchi.** 1974. Studies on the stability of an antitumour protein, neocarzinostatin. II. Stability of injection solution of neocarzinostatin. Jpn. J. Antibiot. 27:715–724.
7. **Liebow, C., and S. S. Rothman.** 1975. Enteropancreatic circulation of digestive enzymes. Science 189:472–474.
8. **Maeda, H.** 1974. Chemical and biological characterization of succinyl neocarzinostatin. Alteration in biological and chemical properties. J. Antibiot. 27:303–311.
9. **Maeda, H.** 1974. Preparation of succinyl neocarzinostatin. Antimicrob. Agents Chemother. 5:354–355.
10. **Maeda, H., S. Aikawa, and A. Yamashita.** 1975. Subcellular fate of protein antibiotic neocarzinostatin in culture of a lymphoid cell line from Burkitt's lymphoma. Cancer Res. 35:545–559.
11. **Maeda, H., C. B. Glaser, K. Kuromizu, and J. Meienhofer.** 1974. Structure of the antitumor protein neocarzinostatin. Amino acid sequence. Arch. Biochem. Biophys. 164:379–385.
12. **Maeda, H., K. Kumagai, and N. Ishida.** 1966. Characterization of neocarzinostatin. J. Antibiot. Ser. A 19:253–259.
13. **Maeda, H., and J. Takeshita.** 1975. Degradation of neocarzinostatin by blood sera in vitro and its inhibition by diisopropyl fluorophosphate and N-ethylmaleimide. Gann 66:523–527.
14. **Maeda, H., and J. Takeshita.** 1976. Inhibitors of proteolytic enzymes prevent the inactivation by blood of the protein antibiotic neocarzinostatin and its succinyl derivative. J. Antibiot. 29:111–112.
15. **Maeda, H., N. Yamamoto, and A. Yamashita.** 1976. Fate and distribution of [^{14}C]succinyl neocarzinostatin in rats. Eur. J. Cancer 12:865–870.
16. **Ogata, J., N. Migita, and T. Nakamura.** 1973. Treatment of carcinoma of the bladder by infusion of the anticancer agent (Mitomycin C) via the internal iliac artery. J. Urol. 110:667–670.
17. **Ono, Y., Y. Watanabe, and N. Ishida.** 1966. Mode of action of neocarzinostatin: inhibition of DNA synthesis and degradation of DNA in *Sarcina lutea*. Biochim. Biophys. Acta 119:46–58.
18. **Sakamoto, S., J. Ogata, and H. Maeda.** 1976. Effects of neocarzinostatin on bladder cancer, p. 158. *In* Proceedings of the Japanese Urology Association, Kagoshima, Japan.
19. **Schabel, F. M.** 1975. Concepts for systemic treatment of micrometastases. Cancer 35:15–24.
20. **Takahashi, M., K. Toriyama, H. Maeda, M. Kikuchi, and N. Ishida.** 1969. Clinical trials of a new antitumor polypeptide: neocarzinostatin (NCS). Tohoku J. Exp. Med. 98:273–280.
21. **Toby, R. A.** 1975. Different drugs arrest cells at a number of distinct stage in G2. Nature (London) 245:245–247.
22. **Warshaw, A. L., W. A. Walker, and K. J. Isselbacher.** 1974. Protein uptake by the intestine: evidence for absorption of intact macromolecules. Gastroenterology 66:987–992.

ANTIMICROBIAL AGENTS AND CHEMOTHERAPY, June 1977, p. 946-951
Vol. 11, No. 6

Inhibition of Influenza Virus Ribonucleic Acid Polymerase by Ribavirin Triphosphate

BERTIL ERIKSSON, ERIK HELGSTRAND, NILS GUNNAR JOHANSSON, ALF LARSSON, ALFONS MISIORNY, JAN OLOF NOREN, LENNART PHILIPSON, KJELL STENBERG, GORAN STENING, STIG STRIDH, AND BO ÖBERG*

Research and Development Laboratories, Astra Läkemedel AB, Södertälje, and Department of Microbiology, Biomedical Center, University of Uppsala, Uppsala, Sweden

Received for publication 27 January 1977

Ribavirin 5'-triphosphate (RTP), derived from the broad-spectrum antiviral compound ribavirin (Virazole), can selectively inhibit influenza virus ribonucleic acid polymerase in a cell-free assay. Ribavirin and its 5'-monophosphate have no effect on the polymerase. The inhibition is competitive with respect to adenosine 5'-triphosphate and guanosine 5'-triphosphate. RTP also inhibits ApG- and GpC-stimulated influenza virus ribonucleic acid polymerase. Since ribavirin is phosphorylated in the cell, the inhibition of influenza multiplication in the cell may also be caused by RTP.

The antiviral compound ribavirin (Virazole, 1-β-D-ribofuranosyl-1,2,4-triazole-3-carboxamide) has been shown to inhibit the multiplication of several animal viruses (1a, 17). It can obviously be phosphorylated to the mono-, di-, and triphosphate within mammalian cells (11). The monophosphate inhibits a cellular inosine 5'-monophosphate (IMP) dehydrogenase (EC 2.1.1.14) (19). This effect has been assumed to be the basis for the antiviral activity of ribavirin (11).

On the other hand, it has been demonstrated that the synthesis of influenza virus proteins is inhibited at concentrations of ribavirin that do not suppress cellular protein synthesis (12). This could be explained if influenza virus ribonucleic acid (RNA) polymerase was selectively affected, resulting in a decrease in influenza virus messenger RNA. It has recently been reported that the synthesis of both virion RNA and complementary RNA (cRNA) is suppressed at ribavirin concentrations that do not block cellular RNA synthesis (18).

The present study describes experiments which reveal a selective inhibition of influenza virus RNA polymerase by ribavirin 5'-triphosphate (RTP). An analysis of the kinetics of inhibition and inhibition in the presence of dinucleotides has been carried out.

MATERIALS AND METHODS

Viruses. Influenza virus type A2 strain Aichi 2/68 was obtained as infected allantoic fluid from Statens Bakteriologiska Laboratorium, Stockholm, Sweden, and the virus was purified according to the method of Pons and Hirst (15), except that the purified virus was not treated with ribonuclease. Purified virus, 2 to 3 mg/ml, was kept frozen in aliquots at −70°C.

The Indiana serotype of vesicular stomatitis virus (VSV) was grown in HeLa cells and purified as described by Roy and Bishop (16).

Enzymes. Calf thymus RNA polymerase A and B (EC 2.7.7.6) were prepared according to Kedinger et al. (7), calf thymus deoxyribonucleic acid (DNA) polymerase α (EC 2.7.7.7) was purchased from Worthington, Freehold, N.J., and *Escherichia coli* RNA polymerase type II (EC 2.7.7.6) and *Micrococcus luteus* DNA polymerase (EC 2.7.7.7) were obtained from Sigma, St. Louis, Mo.

Chemicals and isotopes. Activated calf thymus DNA for the *M. luteus* and the calf thymus DNA polymerase assays was prepared according to Fansler and Loeb (4). *E. coli* Q-13 DNA for the *E. coli* RNA polymerase assay was prepared according to Marmur (10). Calf thymus DNA for the calf thymus RNA polymerase A and B assays was from Worthington. Adenosine 5'-triphosphate (ATP), cytidine 5'-triphosphate. (CTP), guanosine 5'-triphosphate (GTP), uridine 5'-triphosphate (UTP), deoxy ATP, deoxy CTP, deoxy GTP, deoxythymidine 5'-triphosphate, ApG, and GpC were from Sigma. Tritiated triphosphates, [^{3}H]GTP (5.6 Ci/mmol), [^{3}H]CTP (26.2 Ci/mmol), and [^{3}H]deoxythymidine 5'-triphosphate (40 Ci/mmol) were from New England Nuclear Corp., Boston, Mass. Samples of ribavirin, ribavirin 5'-monophosphate (RMP), and RTP were kindly supplied by R. Sidwell, ICN Pharmaceuticals Inc., Irvine, Calif.

Assay conditions. The methods for assaying different polymerase activities were essentially as described by the following: by Bishop et al. (2) for influenza virus polymerase, by Baltimore et al. (1) for VSV RNA polymerase, by Kedinger et al. (7) for calf thymus RNA polymerase A and B, by Holmes et al. (6) for calf thymus DNA polymerase α, by Harwood et al. (5) for *M. luteus* DNA polymerase, and by Burgess (3) for *E. coli* RNA polymerase, with minor modifications. Where not otherwise noted, the nucleotide concentrations in the different assays were as indicated in Table 1.

Samples from the assay mixtures were precipitated with trichloroacetic acid on filter paper, washed, and counted in a toluene scintillation solution (Permablend III, Packard). One unit of enzyme activity corresponds to 1 nmol of [^{3}H]GMP, [^{3}H]-CMP, or [^{3}H]dTMP incorporated per h. Zero time incorporation was subtracted.

The specific activities of the enzymes and the amounts used in the assays were: influenza RNA polymerase, 3 U/mg, 100 μg/125 μl; thymus RNA polymerase A, 2.5 U/mg, 100 μg/125 μl; thymus RNA polymerase B, 30.6 U/mg, 100 μg/125 μl; *E. coli* RNA polymerase, 880 U/mg, 1.5 μg/125 μl; *M. luteus* DNA polymerase, 85 U/mg, 8.9 μg/125 μl; thymus DNA polymerase α, 2.5 U/200 μl; VSV RNA polymerase, 37 U/mg, 10 μg/125 μl.

Chromatographic procedures. Two chromatographic systems were used. In system A, silica gel thin-layer plates (Merck) were chromatographed in 2-propanol–concentrated aqueous ammonia–water (7:1:2). The eluted plates were sprayed with methanol containing 10% sulfuric acid and 2% *p*-methoxybenzaldehyde followed by heating at about 110°C. In system B, PEI-cel 200 thin-layer plates (Macherey-Nagel, 20 by 20 cm) were chromatographed in 1.4 M lithium chloride and then sprayed with a mixture of 5 ml of 60% (wt/wt) perchloric acid, 10 ml of 0.1 M hydrochloric acid, 25 ml of 4% (wt/vol) ammonium molybdate, and 60 ml of water.

RESULTS

Purity of the tested inhibitors. Ribavirin (mp, 166 to 168°C, literature mp, 166 to 168°C [20]; system A, R_f = 0.41) and RMP (system B, R_f = 0.70) were chromatographically pure. The sample of RTP contained some minor impurities.

A 1.1-mg (by weight) sample of RTP was purified by chromatography (system B, one plate). The appropriate band (R_f = 0.20) was cut out from the developed and dried plate and was washed with methanol (250 ml). Eluting the band with water and evaporation of the solvent gave a sample containing 0.6 mg of RTP (recovery of 55%, the amount determined by the ultraviolet light absorbance, $\lambda_{max}[H_2O]$ at 206 nm, $\epsilon = 8 \times 10^3$) which was chromatographically pure (system B). Some lingering lithium chloride was washed away from the dry sample with methanol.

No significant difference was found between the inhibitory activities of the crude and the purified samples of RTP. The experiments described below are pertinent to the crude sample.

Selective inhibition of influenza virus RNA polymerase. The polymerase activity of several DNA and RNA polymerases was tested in the presence of ribavirin, RMP, and RTP as shown in Table 2. Influenza virus RNA polymerase was selectively inhibited by the triphosphate. No inhibition was observed with ribavirin or its monophosphate. The triphosphate did not show any significant inhibition of calf thymus RNA polymerase A and B. VSV RNA polymerase, *M. luteus* DNA polymerase, and *E. coli* RNA polymerase were slightly inhibited by 500 μM RTP. Ribavirin and RMP had no inhibitory activity on any of the enzymes tested. A concentration of 100 μM RTP was required to obtain 50% inhibition of influenza virus RNA polymerase. No significant inhibition of any of the other enzymes was observed at this concentration (Table 2). Figure 1 shows the dose-response curve for inhibition of influenza virus RNA polymerase with RTP.

Competitive effect of purine triphosphates. The mechanism of inhibition of influenza virus RNA polymerase by RTP was studied by varying the concentration of nucleoside triphosphates in the polymerase assay system. The Lineweaver-Burk plots obtained for ATP, GTP, CTP, and UTP are presented in Fig. 2. RTP shows a competitive type of inhibition with varying concentrations of the purine triphosphates ATP and GTP (Fig. 2A and B). No competitive inhibition was found when the concentrations of the pyrimidine triphosphates CTP and UTP were varied (Fig. 2C and D).

TABLE 1. *Nucleotide concentrations in the polymerase assays*

Polymerase assay	Nucleotide concn (mM)							
	ATP	GTP	CTP	UTP	dATP[a]	dGTP[a]	dCTP[a]	dTTP[a]
Influenza virus RNA	0.50	0.11	0.10	0.10				
Thymus A RNA	0.50	0.11	0.10	0.10				
Thymus B RNA	0.50	0.11	0.10	0.10				
E. coli RNA	0.40	0.40	0.40	0.40				
M. luteus DNA					0.05	0.05	0.05	0.05
Thymus α DNA					0.10	0.10	0.10	0.10
VSV RNA	1.0	0.07	0.50	0.50				

[a] dATP, Deoxy ATP; dGTP, deoxy GTP; dCTP, deoxy CTP; dTTP, deoxythymidine 5′-triphosphate.

TABLE 2. *Effects of ribavirin, RMP, and RTP on different polymerases*

Polymerase	Inhibition (%)[a]					
	Ribavirin		RMP		RTP	
	100 μM	500 μM	100 μM	500 μM	100 μM	500 μM
Influenza RNA	−10	0, −8	−9	2, −4	50, 40	90, 82
Thymus A RNA	2	−4	−15	−12	−16	5, 3
Thymus B RNA	3	5, 5	9, 8	7, 13	15,9	15, 20, 1
E. coli RNA	4	−4	−1, 3	1, 0	5	20, 17
M. luteus DNA	0	2	1	−4	13	28, 38
Thymus α DNA						22
VSV RNA						36

[a] The different polymerases were assayed as described in Materials and Methods, and the inhibition of polymerase activity is expressed in percent relative to a control without added substance. A negative value refers to the percentage of enhancement observed in the assay. The figures are averages from duplicate incubations. Results from different experiments are given for some enzymes.

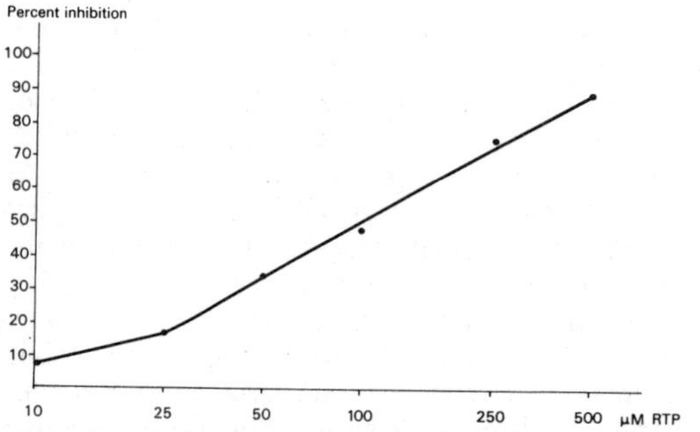

FIG. 1. *Inhibition of influenza virus RNA polymerase by RTP. Inhibition of influenza virus RNA polymerase at different concentrations of RTP was determined as described in Materials and Methods. All samples were in duplicate, and mean values are shown. The incubation time was 1 h, and more than 10^4 cpm was counted in each sample with [^{3}H]GTP as labeled precursor.*

Inhibition of influenza virus RNA polymerase stimulated with dinucleotides. The activity of influenza virus RNA polymerase could be stimulated by ApG or GpC as demonstrated by Plotch and Krug (14) and as also shown in Fig. 3. The polymerase activity in the stimulated system was also inhibited by RTP. The inhibition at 1 h of incubation was more than 80% when equimolar concentrations of RTP and ApG or GpC were used.

The mechanism of inhibition in this system was examined by varying the concentration of ApG and RTP. The result is shown in Fig. 4. When the data were transformed into a Lineweaver-Burk plot, the lines obtained were curved, and no conclusion could be made concerning the type of inhibition.

DISCUSSION

The selective inhibition of viral enzymes without affecting normal cellular functions is a highly desired property of an antiviral compound. Ribavirin has been considered to be a broad-spectrum antiviral substance with activity against several animal DNA and RNA viruses (1a, 17). Earlier reports about the function of ribavirin have indicated that the drug is metabolized to RMP, which inhibits cellular IMP dehydrogenase (10, 11). This inhibition has been shown to result in a decreased GTP pool in leukemic cells (13).

A selective effect on the synthesis of influenza virus proteins was observed by Oxford (12). Scholtissek (18) reported that the synthesis of influenza virus RNA was inhibited at concentrations of ribavirin that did not inhibit cellular RNA synthesis. These findings suggest a mechanism of inhibition that is distinct from the effect on IMP dehydrogenase. It has been reported that ribavirin is phosphorylated intracellularly not only to its monophosphate, but also to the di- and triphosphates (11), and that the intracellular concentration of RTP is of the same magnitude as that of ribavirin (11).

Our results (Table 2) demonstrate that RTP is a selective inhibitor of influenza virus RNA polymerase in a cell-free system. Ribavirin and RMP, on the other hand, do not inhibit the influenza virus RNA polymerase. From Fig. 2 it is evident that RTP shows a competitive inhibition only with ATP and GTP but not with UTP or CTP. The structure of RTP is more closely related to GTP and ATP than to UTP or CTP. It has been suggested that the influenza cRNA initiates with adenosine and guanosine (8). McGeoch and Kitron (9) showed a stimulation of influenza virus RNA polymerase by GpG and GpC, and Plotch and Krug have recently reported (14) that the in vitro initiation of influenza virus cRNA can be stimulated by the dinucleotides ApG and GpG, which are incorporated at the 5′ end of the cRNA. The enhancement of

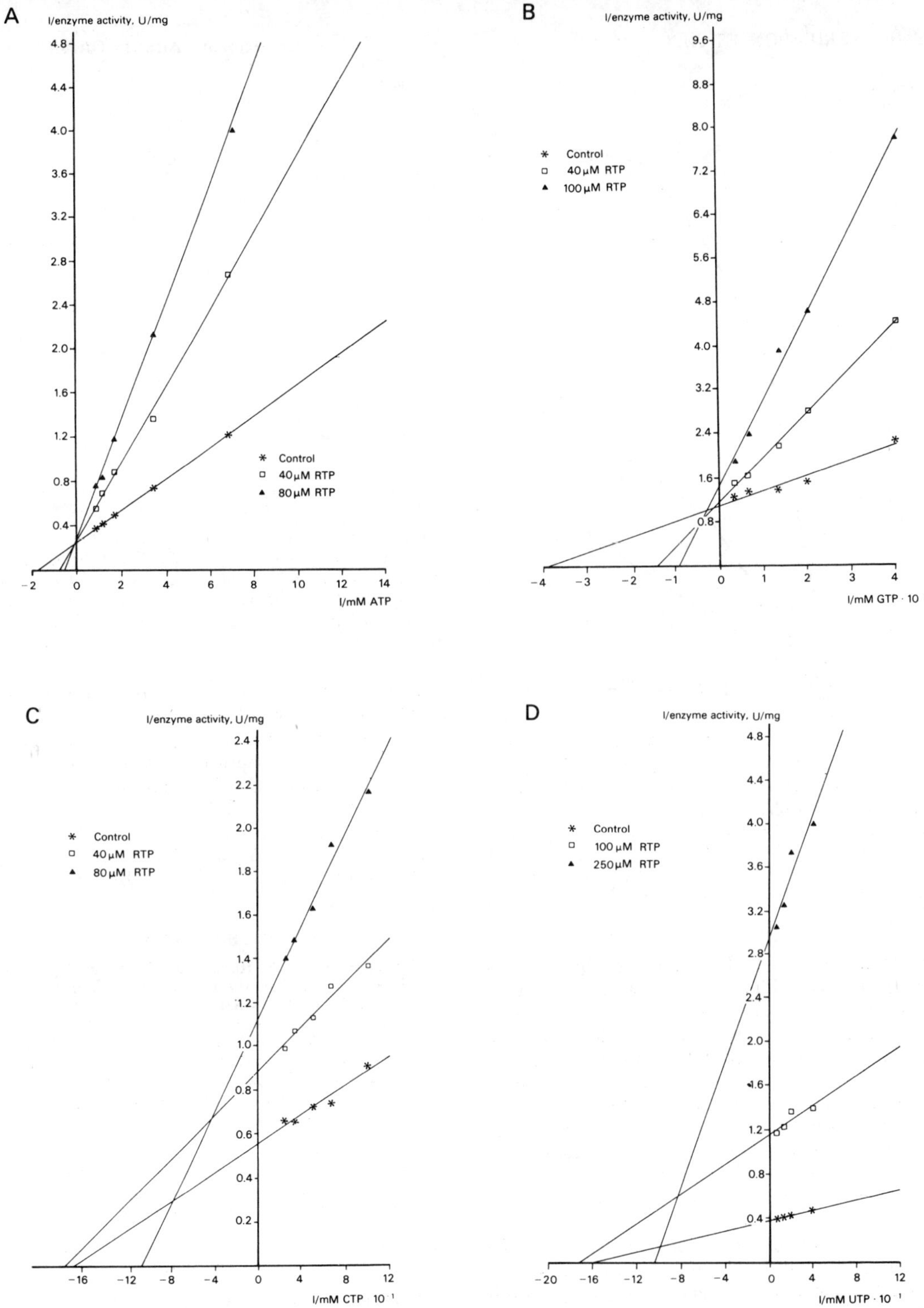

FIG. 2. *Effect of nucleoside triphosphates on the inhibitory activity of RTP. The activity of influenza virus RNA polymerase in the presence of RTP was determined at different concentrations of ATP, GTP, CTP, and UTP. The incorporation of [³H]GTP was measured when the concentration of ATP, CTP, or UTP was varied, and the incorporation of [³H]CTP was determined when the GTP concentration was varied. The data are presented as double reciprocal plots, utilizing a computerized least-squares method for regression analysis. The time of incubation was 1 h, and the nucleotide concentrations were the same as given in Table 1, apart from the one varied. (A) Incorporation at different ATP concentrations with 0, 40, and 80 μM RTP. (B) Incorporation at different GTP concentrations with 0, 40, and 100 μM RTP. (C) Incorporation at different CTP concentrations with 0, 40, and 80 μM RTP. (D) Incorporation at different UTP concentrations with 0, 100, and 250 μM RTP.*

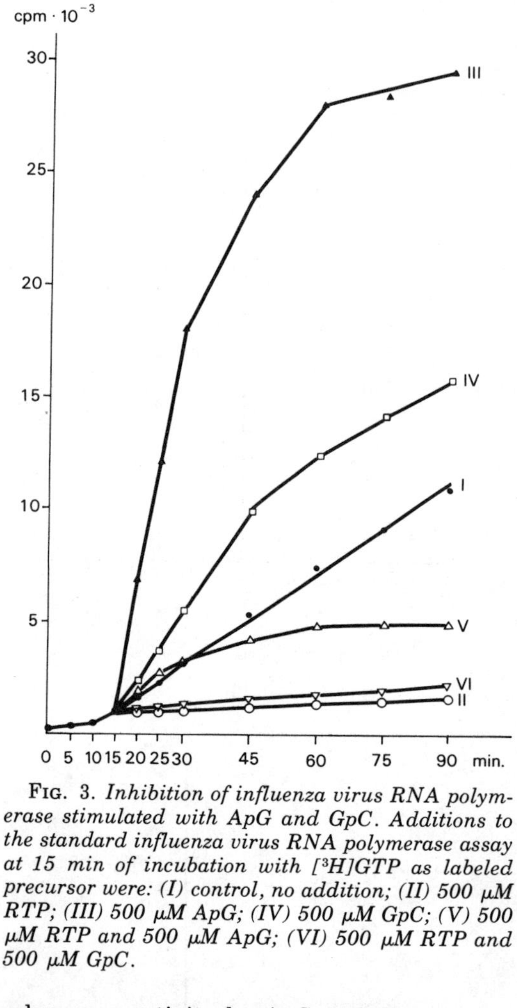

FIG. 3. *Inhibition of influenza virus RNA polymerase stimulated with ApG and GpC. Additions to the standard influenza virus RNA polymerase assay at 15 min of incubation with [³H]GTP as labeled precursor were: (I) control, no addition; (II) 500 μM RTP; (III) 500 μM ApG; (IV) 500 μM GpC; (V) 500 μM RTP and 500 μM ApG; (VI) 500 μM RTP and 500 μM GpC.*

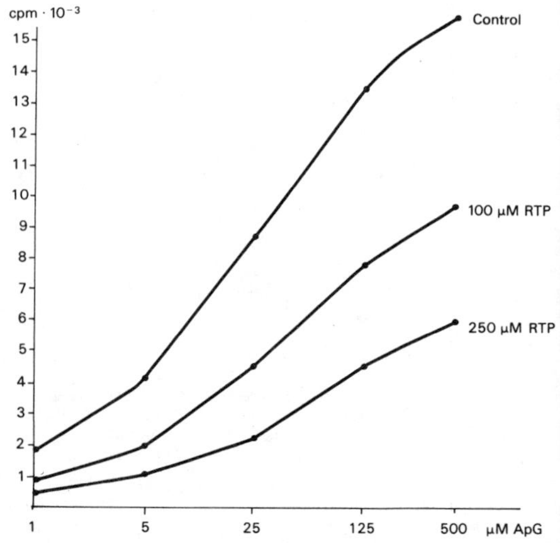

FIG. 4. *Inhibition of ApG-stimulated influenza virus RNA polymerase by RTP. The inhibition of influenza virus RNA polymerase was determined with varying concentrations of both RTP and ApG. The time of incubation was 15 min and [³H]GTP was used to label the product.*

polymerase activity by ApG and GpC can be abolished with RTP (Fig. 4). It could not be established whether the inhibition is competitive with respect to the dinucleotide. This may be due to the fact that the lag period before RNA synthesis assumes a linear rate varies with the concentration of the dinucleotide. It has not yet been determined whether RTP also inhibits the cytoplasmic influenza RNA polymerase synthesizing virion RNA, nor is it known whether the diphosphate has any inhibitory activity.

The lack of inhibition of calf thymus DNA polymerase α and RNA polymerase I and II by RTP has also recently been observed by Müller et al. (13).

It remains to be established whether the inhibition of influenza virus RNA polymerase by RTP also controls influenza virus replication in the infected cell. Considering the facts that both influenza virus RNA and protein synthesis are selectively inhibited by ribavirin (12, 18), it is entirely possible that the prevention of influenza virus multiplication depends on a selective inhibition of the RNA polymerase by the ribavirin metabolite RTP.

The suggested mechanism for inhibition of influenza virus RNA polymerase does not exclude concomitant effects by inhibition of IMP dehydrogenase.

LITERATURE CITED

1. **Baltimore, D., A. S. Huang, and M. Stampfer.** 1970. Ribonucleic acid synthesis of vesicular stomatitis virus. II. An RNA polymerase in the virion. Proc. Natl. Acad. Sci. U.S.A. **66:**572–576.
1a. **Becker, Y.** 1976. Antiviral drugs, p. 57. *In* J. L. Melnick (ed.), Monogr. in virology, vol. II. S. Karger, Basel.
2. **Bishop, D., J. Obijeski, and R. Simpson.** 1971. Transcription of the influenza ribonucleic acid genome by a virion polymerase. I. Optimal conditions for in vitro activity of the ribonucleic acid-dependent ribonucleic acid polymerase. J. Virol. **8:**66–73.
3. **Burgess, R. R.** 1969. A new method for the large scale purification of *E. coli* deoxyribonucleic acid-dependent ribonucleic acid polymerase. J. Biol. Chem. **244:**6160–6167.
4. **Fansler, B. S., and L. A. Loeb.** 1974. Sea urchin nuclear DNA polymerase. Methods Enzymol. **29:**53–70.
5. **Harwood, S. J., P. F. Schendel, and R. D. Wells.** 1970. Micrococcus luteus deoxyribonucleic acid polymerase. J. Biol. Chem. **245:**5614–5624.
6. **Holmes, A. M., I. P. Hesslewood, and I. R. Johnston.** 1976. Evidence that DNA polymerase- α of calf thymus contains a subunit of molecular weight 155000. Eur. J. Biochem. **62:**229–235.

7. **Kedinger, C., F. Gissinger, M. Gniazdowski, J-L. Mandel, and P. Chambon.** 1972. Animal DNA-dependent RNA polymerases. I. Large-scale solubilization and separation of A and B calf thymus RNA-polymerase activities. Eur. J. Biochem. **28**:269–276.
8. **Krug, R. M., M. A. Morgan, and A. J. Shatkin.** 1976. Influenza viral messenger RNA contains internal N^6-methyladenosine and 5′-terminal 7-methylguanosine in cap structures. J. Virol. **20**:45–53.
9. **McGeoch, D., and N. Kitron.** 1975. Influenza virion RNA-dependent RNA polymerase: stimulation by guanosine and related compounds. J. Virol. **15**:686–695.
10. **Marmur, J.** 1961. A procedure for the isolation of deoxyribonucleic acid from microorganisms. J. Mol. Biol. 3:208–218.
11. **Miller, J. P., L. J. Kigwana, D. G. Streeter, R. K. Robins, and L. N. Simon.** 1977. The relationship between the metabolism of ribavirin and its proposed mechanism of action. Ann. N. Y. Acad. Sci., in press.
12. **Oxford, J. S.** 1975. Inhibition of the replication of influenza A and B viruses by a nucleoside analogue (ribavirin). J. Gen. Virol. **28**:409–414.
13. **Müller, W. E. G., A. Maidhof, H. Tashner, and R. K. Zahn.** 1977. Virazole (1-β-D-ribafuranosyl-1,2,4,-triazole-3-carboxamide) a cytostatic agent. Biochem. Pharmacol., in press.
14. **Plotch, S. J., and R. M. Krug.** 1977. Influenza virion transcriptase. The synthesis in vitro of large, poly A-containing complementary RNA. J. Virol. **21**:24–34.
15. **Pons, M. and G. Hirst.** 1968. Polyacrylamide gel electrophoresis of influenza virus RNA. Virology **34**:385–388.
16. **Roy, P., and D. Bishop.** 1972. Genome homology of vesicular stomatitis virus and defective T particles and evidence for the sequential transcription of the virion ribonucleic acid. J. Virol. **9**:946–955.
17. **Sidwell, R. W., J. H. Huffman, G. P. Khare, L. B. Allen, J. T. Witkowski, and R. K. Robins.** 1972. Broad-spectrum antiviral activity of Virazole: 1-β-D-ribofuranosyl-1,2,4-triazole-3-carboxamide. Science **177**:705–606.
18. **Scholtissek, C.** 1976. Inhibition of influenza RNA synthesis by Virazole (ribavirin). Arch. Virol. **50**:349–352.
19. **Streeter, D. G., J. T. Witkowski, G. P. Khare, R. W. Sidwell, R. J. Bauer, R. K. Robins, and L. N. Simon.** 1973. Mechanism of action of 1-β-D-ribofuranosyl-1,2,4-triazole-3-carboxamide (Virazole), a new broad spectrum antiviral agent. Proc. Natl. Acad. Sci. U.S.A. **70**:1174–1178.
20. **Witkowski, J. T., R. K. Robins, R. W. Sidwell, and L. N. Simon.** 1972. Design, synthesis and broad spectrum antiviral activity of 1-β-D-ribofuranosyl-1,2,4-triazole-3-carboxamide and related nucleosides. J. Med. Chem. **15**:1150–1154.

ANTIMICROBIAL AGENTS AND CHEMOTHERAPY, June 1977, p. 952-955
Vol. 1, No. 6

Cyclic Adenylic Acid-Dependent and -Independent Production of Chloramphenicol Acetyltransferase in *Escherichia coli* Carrying R Plasmids

TAKESHI YOKOTA, RIE KUWAHARA, SUMIKO HAGIWARA, AND SHOGO KUWAHARA*

*Department of Bacteriology, School of Medicine, Juntendo University, Toyko 113, and Department of Microbiology, School of Medicine, Toho University, Tokyo 143, Japan**

Received for publication 5 August 1976

A plasmid-specified, inducible, but cyclic adenylic acid (cAMP)-independent resistance to chloramphenicol (CM) is reported. The resistance level to CM was increased two- to fourfold by treatment with a small amount of CM for a short period in *Escherichia coli* strains carrying the R plasmid pJY1, which was obtained from a clinical isolate of *Vibrio cholerae*. Though cAMP was required for production of CM acetyltransferase (CATase) in cAMP-deficient mutants of *E. coli* carrying the R100 plasmid, the same species harboring pJY1 did not require cAMP for production of the enzyme. The possibility of a mechanism other than CATase activity for the CM resistance conferred by R plasmids is discussed.

Cyclic adenosine 3′,5′-monophosphate (cAMP) is an important substance that regulates a variety of phenomena in bacterial physiology. It is known to be an essential component for initiation of transcription of certain bacterial proteins, i.e., inducible enzymes, flagella proteins, etc. (1, 9, 12). Smith and his colleagues (10) reported that cAMP regulates the level of an antibiotic-inactivating enzyme, chloramphenicol acetyltransferase (CATase), produced by *Escherichia coli* harboring R plasmids, even though the enzyme is synthesized constitutively. This evidence was further confirmed by other investigators (2, 3).

Recently, we found that resistance to chloramphenicol (CM) of *E. coli* specified by an R plasmid, pJY1, which was obtained from a clinical isolate of *Vibrio cholerae,* was enhanced by a short period of incubation with a small amount of CM, and therefore appears to be inducible (T. Yokota and S. Kuwahara, Abstr. 11th Jt. Conf. on Cholera, U.S.-Jpn. Coop. Med. Sci. Prog., 1975). It seemed that an investigation of regulation of this inducible CM resistance might provide further insight into the phenotypic expression of R plasmids. This paper deals with cAMP-independent production of CATase in *E. coli* bearing the inducible type of R plasmid.

MATERIALS AND METHODS

R plasmids. R100 (*cat*$^+$*tet*$^+$*aadA*$^+$*sul*$^+$*tra*$^+$) (11) was employed as a representative R plasmid obtained from species of *Enterobacteriaceae*. pJY1 was obtained from a drug-resistant strain of *V. cholerae* (biotype *eltor*) isolated in the Philippines in 1973. This plasmid confers high resistance to streptomycin (SM) and sulfonamide and low resistance to CM. It can be transferred by conjugation not only to *V. cholerae*, but also to derivatives of *E. coli* K-12, *Proteus mirabilis,* and *Serratia marcescens* (14).

Bacteria. Three *cya*$^+$(cAMP-producing) *E. coli* strains, HfrR1 *metB*, CSH2(F$^-$) *metB*, and AB-1157(F$^-$) *argE thi thr leu proC his str lac gal xyl mtl ara*, and two *cya* mutants of *E. coli*, YE100(Hfr) *cya metB* (13) and CA7902 *cya thi* (7), were used as host bacteria for the R plasmids.

Media. MacConkey agar containing 1% lactose or maltose (Eiken Chemical Co. Ltd., Tokyo) was employed as a plating medium. L broth (4) and M9-lactate-casein hydrolysate medium (6) were used as liquid media. The latter medium was supplemented with appropriate vitamins as necessary.

Chemicals. cAMP was provided by Asahi Chemical Industry Co. Ltd. (Tokyo). Acetyl-coenzyme A (acetyl-CoA), 5,5′-dithiobis-2-nitrobenzoic acid (DTN), and crystalline CM were purchased from Sigma Chemical Co. (St. Louis, Mo.), Tokyo Chemical Industry Co. Ltd. (Tokyo), and Sankyo Pharmaceutical Co. Ltd. (Tokyo), respectively.

Induction of CM resistance. cAMP-producing strains of *E. coli*, HfrR1, CSH2, and AB1157, carrying R100 or pJY1, were cultured in L broth at 37°C overnight with shaking. Each culture was divided into two portions, and to one was added one-hundredth of the minimal growth inhibitory concentration (MIC/100) of CM, while the other served as a control. After further incubation at 37°C for 1 to 6 h, with shaking, all cultures were diluted 100-fold with fresh L broth, and 0.1-ml portions were inoculated into 5 ml of L broth containing serially increasing amounts of CM. Resistance levels to CM of each strain treated with and without a small amount of the drug were compared turbidometrically using a Klett-Summerson colorimeter with a no. 66 filter after an incubation at 37°C overnight with shaking. The influence of various amounts of CM at different temperatures for various periods was also tested in the same manner. To confirm that the CM effect on the induced resistance is specific for CM, resistance levels of SM of the bacteria treated with and without an MIC/100 of CM were also measured by the same method. Furthermore, resistance levels to CM, as well as to SM, of bacteria pretreated with and without an MIC/100 of SM were checked.

Effect of cAMP on the induction of CM resistance. The plasmids, R100 and pJY1, were transferred to two strains of cAMP-deficient *E. coli,* YE100 and CA7902, by conjugation. The strains bearing R100 or pJY1 were cultured in L broth with or without 1 mM cAMP at 37°C overnight, with shaking. Each culture was divided into two portions. To one of the cultures grown without exogenous cAMP was added an MIC/100 of CM, while the other served as a control. After further incubation at 37°C for 60 min, with shaking, they were tested for CM resistance level by the method described above. The culture grown with 1 mM cAMP was treated with CM in the same manner, but in the presence of 1 mM cAMP, and then tested for CM resistance levels. Influence of pretreatment with an MIC/100 of SM, instead of CM, on the CM resistance levels was also investigated in the presence or absence of 1 mM exogenous cAMP.

CATase assay. Cell-free extracts were prepared after growing cells of *E. coli* YE100 harboring R100 or pJY1 in M9-lactate-casein hydrolysate medium supplemented with or without 1 mM cAMP to mid-logarithmic phase, and treating with or without CM, 1 μg/ml(MIC/100), in the presence or absence of 1 mM cAMP at 37°C for 60 min. The cells were washed twice with, and resuspended in, cold 0.1 M tris(hydroxymethyl)aminomethane buffer (pH 7.8) and disrupted by three 30-s bursts of sonication at 10 kc (Tomy Seiko Co. Ltd., Tokyo). The sonic extracts were centrifuged at 4°C for 30 min at 30,000 $\times$ *g*, and the resulting supernatant fluids were used as the crude enzymes.

CATase activity was assayed according to the spectrophotometric method of Shaw and Brodsky (8). The reduction of DTN due to the liberation of reduced CoA after acetylation of CM was measured by observing the increase in absorbance at 412 nm. A molar extinction coefficient of 13.6×10^3 was used for calculation of the rate of DTN cleavage that corresponds to acetylation of CM (8). Protein concentrations in crude extracts were measured by the method of Lowry et al. (5). Specific activity of CATase was expressed as micromoles of CM acetylated per minute per milligram of protein. To take an adequate initial velocity, 0.001- to 0.1-mg and 0.2- to 1.0-mg protein concentrations were used for the assay of CATase prepared from *E. coli* YE100 carrying R100 and from the same species carrying pJY1, respectively. For confirmation of the accuracy of the spectrophotometric method, a bioassay of 100 μg of CM per ml was carried out by the cup method with *E. coli* CSH2(R^-) as the assay microbe before and after incubation with 0.4 μmol of acetyl-CoA and 0.5 mg of protein of the crude extracts at 37°C for 30 min in 0.2 M tris(hydroxymethyl)aminomethane buffer (pH 7.8) containing 0.01 M magnesium acetate and 0.06 M potassium chloride.

RESULTS

Inducible CM resistance specified by pJY1. The levels of CM resistance in *cya*$^+$ strains of *E. coli*, HfrR1, CSH2, and AB1157, carrying R100 was 200 μg/ml (MIC) regardless of pretreatment with 2 μg of CM per ml for 60 min. But CM resistance in the same species harboring the other plasmid, pJY1, was increased from 50 to 100 to 200 μg/ml by the CM treatment. As little as 1 μg of CM per ml (approximately an MIC/100 level) was satisfactory for full induction, as shown in Fig. 1, and both lower and higher concentrations were less effective.

Figure 2 indicates the optimal incubation period for the induction. Sixty minutes of incubation with 1 μg of CM per ml at 37°C with shaking resulted in full induction.

Temperatures ranging from 27 to 42°C did not affect the induction of CM resistance. Levels of SM resistance of the bacteria carrying R100 or pJY1 and treated with CM were not changed. Neither CM nor SM resistance levels were affected by treatment with an MIC/100 of SM in the R^+ and R^- strains of *E. coli*. The results are summarized in Table 1.

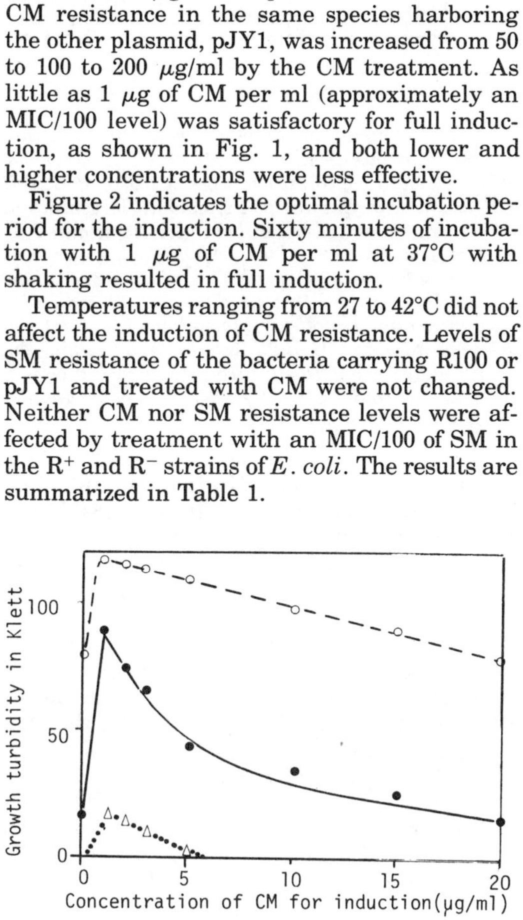

FIG. 1. *Optimal concentration of CM for induction of CM resistance in E. coli CSH2 cya$^+$ carrying the pJY1 plasmid. An overnight culture of E. coli CSH2 cya$^+$ carrying the pJY1 plasmid in L broth at 37°C was divided into eight portions, and to seven were added 1 to 20 µg of CM per ml while the remaining portion served as a control. After further incubation at 37°C for 60 min with shaking, all cultures were diluted 100-fold with fresh L broth, and portions of 0.1 ml were inoculated into 5 ml of L broth containing CM at 25 µg/ml (○), 50 µg/ml (●), or 100 µg/ml (△). Growth turbidity in each tube was measured turbidometrically after 20 h of incubation of 37°C with shaking.*

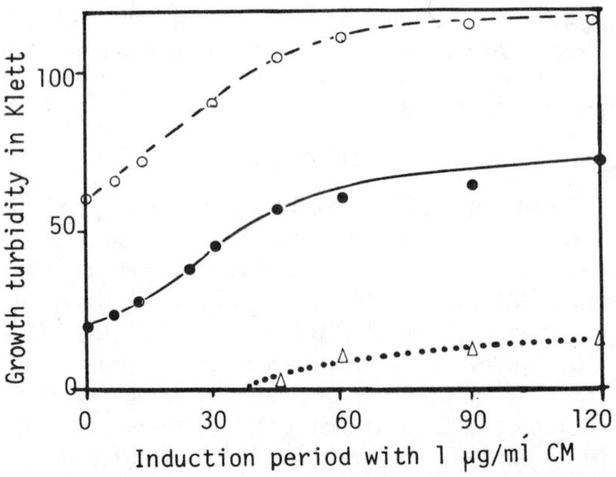

FIG. 2. *Optimal incubation period for induction of CM resistance in E. coli CSH2 cya⁺ carrying the pJY1 plasmid. A 10-ml overnight culture of E. coli CSH2 cya⁺ carrying the pJY1 plasmid in L broth at 37°C with shaking was chilled in ice water and 1 μg of CM per ml was added. After the culture was transferred to a 37°C water bath, 0.1-ml portions were taken at 0-, 5-, 10-, 20-, 30-, 60-, 90-, and 120-min incubation periods and inoculated into 5 ml of L broth containing CM at 25 μg/ml (○), 50 μg/ml (●), or 100 μg/ml (△). Growth turbidity in each tube was measured turbidometrically after 20 h of incubation at 37°C with shaking.*

Role of cAMP in constitutive and inducible CM resistance conferred by R plasmids. It was found that levels of CM resistance of cAMP-deficient strains of *E. coli* carrying R100 were two times higher in the presence of 1 mM exogenous cAMP than in its absence. However, the same bacteria harboring the pJY1 plasmid showed identical CM resistance levels with or without cAMP. This fact indicates a paradoxical phenomenon: cAMP is required for the phenotypic expression of constitutive CM resistance but not for inducible resistance.

Production of CATase by *E. coli* YE100 *cya* was markedly stimulated by the presence of 1 mM cAMP, as shown in Table 2. The activity of CATase in crude extracts of *E. coli* YE100 bearing the plasmid R100 was much higher when cells were cultured in the presence of cAMP than when they were cultured in its absence. Pretreatment with a small amount of CM did not affect enzyme production as much as it affected the level of CM resistance.

On the other hand, CATase activity of the same species carrying the pJY1 plasmid was considerably suppressed by growth in the presence of exogenous cAMP, as indicated in Table 2. It may be noteworthy that CATase activities specified by the pJY1 plasmid are much lower than those mediated by the R100 plasmid under all conditions and that production of CATase by *E. coli* YE100 carrying the pJY1 plasmid is suppressed to some extent not only by exogenous cAMP but also by treatment with CM, which increases the CM resistance level of the species. No CATase activities were confirmed

TABLE 1. *Change of resistance levels of cya^+ strains of E. coli carrying the R100 or pJY1 plasmid by pretreatment with small amounts of antibiotics for a short period*

Strain	Plasmid	Pretreatment at 37°C for 60 min with:	Antibiotic concn (μg/ml)	MICs in L broth (μg/ml): CM	MICs in L broth (μg/ml): SM
HfrR1	R100	None		200	100
		CM	2[a]	200	100
		SM	1	200	100
	pJY1	None		50	500
		CM	1	200	500
		SM	5	50	500
CSH2	R100	None		200	100
		CM	2	200	100
		SM	1	200	100
	pJY1	None		100	500
		CM	1	200	500
		SM	5	100	500
AB1157	R100	None		200	–[b]
		CM	2	200	–[b]
		SM	1	200	–[b]
	pJY1	None		50	–[b]
		CM	1	200	–[b]
		SM	5	50	–[b]

[a] For the pretreatment, MIC/100 levels were employed.

[b] *E. coli* AB1157 carries high resistance to SM that is controlled by the chromosome.

TABLE 2. *Activities of CATase in crude extracts of E. coli YE100 cya carrying the R100 or pJY1 plasmid grown with or without exogenous cAMP and treated with or without CM*

R plasmid present	Grown with 1 mM cAMP	Treated with MIC/100 of CM	Sp act of CATase[a]
R100	–	–	276.7
	+	–	3,272.1
	–	+	397.6
	+	+	3,867.1
pJY1	–	–	10.48
	+	–	1.95
	–	+	4.78
	+	+	0.96

[a] Specific activity of CATase was expressed as micromoles of CM acetylated per minute per milligram of protein, using 13.6×10^3 as an extinction coefficient at 412 nm for DTN cleavage, which corresponds to acetylation of CM (see Materials and Methods).

in an R$^-$ subclone of *E. coli* YE100 grown with or without exogenous cAMP and treated or not treated with CM in the presence or absence of cAMP.

DISCUSSION

Unlike other R plasmids, pJY1 obtained from *V. cholerae* was found to confer inducible, but cAMP-independent, CM resistance on its hosts. Furthermore, it was demonstrated that the presence of an inducible amount of CM considerably suppressed the synthesis of CATase in *E. coli* carrying pJY1. From the results obtained, one can postulate that CATase may not be the only mechanism of CM resistance conferred by the plasmid. Since Smith and his colleagues discovered the requirement of cAMP for production of CATase (10), a question that remains to be answered is why the CM resistance level is not lowered significantly when R plasmids are transferred to cAMP-deficient strains of *E. coli* in which CATase is synthesized at a level less than one-tenth of that in wild strains. If one postulates that mechanisms other than CATase activity are playing roles in CM resistance specified by R plasmids that do not require cAMP, an answer to the question may be possible.

It seems that, in the case of the pJY1 plasmid, such a postulate is necessary. In this case, a small amount of CM, effective for stimulation of the CM resistance specified by the plasmid, considerably suppressed the production of CATase. An explanation of this may require an understanding of the mechanisms of CM resistance other than CATase. It has also been shown that the requirement of cAMP for production of CATase is not a universal phenomenon but depends upon the nature of the plasmid.

ACKNOWLEDGMENTS

This work was supported by the Scientific Research Fund of the Ministry of Education, Science and Culture of Japan, and by the United States-Japan Cooperative Medical Science Program, Cholera Panel.

LITERATURE CITED

1. **deCrombrugghe, B., B. Chen, W. Anderson, P. Nissley, M. Gottesman, I. Pastan, and R. Perlman.** 1971. *lac* DNA, RNA polymerase and cyclic AMP receptor protein, cyclic AMP, *lac* repressor and inducer are the essential elements for controlled *lac* transcription. Nature(London) New Biol. **231**:139–142.
2. **deCrombrugghe, B., I. Pastan, W. V. Shaw, and J. L. Bosner.** 1973. Stimulation by cyclic AMP and ppGpp of chloramphenicol acetyl transferase synthesis. Nature(London) New Biol. **241**:237–239.
3. **Dottin, R. P., S. L. Shiner, and D. I. Hoar.** 1973. Adenosine 3′,5′-cyclic monophosphate regulation of chloramphenicol acetyltransferase synthesis *in vitro* from P1CM DNA. Virology **51**:509–511.
4. **Lennox, E. S.** 1955. Transduction of linked genetic characters of the host by bacteriophage P1. Virology **1**:190–206.
5. **Lowry, O. H., N. J. Rosebrough, A. L. Farr, and R. J. Randall.** 1951. Protein measurement with the Folin phenol reagent. J. Biol. Chem. **193**:265–275.
6. **Nakazawa, T., and T. Yokota.** 1973. Requirement of adenosine 3′,5′-cyclic monophosphate for L-arabinose isomerase synthesis in *Escherichia coli*. J. Bacteriol. **113**:1412–1418.
7. **Schwartz, D., and J. R. Beckwith.** 1970. Mutants missing a factor necessary for the expression of catabolite-sensitive operon in *Escherichia coli*, p. 417–422. *In* The lactose operon. Cold Spring Harbor Laboratory, Cold Spring Harbor, N.Y.
8. **Shaw, W. V., and R. F. Brodsky.** 1968. Characterization of chloramphenicol acetyltransferase from *Staphylococcus aureus*. J. Bacteriol. **95**:28–36.
9. **Silverman, M., and M. Simon.** 1974. Characterization of *Escherichia coli* flagella mutants that are insensitive to catabolite repression. J. Bacteriol. **120**:1196–1203.
10. **Smith, D. H., J. H. Harwood, and F. A. Rubin.** 1972. Studies on the regulation of the chloramphenicol acetyl transferase mediated by R factors, p. 319–335. *In* Bacterial plasmids and antibiotic resistance. Avicenum, Prague, and Springer-Verlag, New York.
11. **Sugino, Y., and Y. Hirota.** 1962. Conjugal fertility associated with resistance factor R in *Escherichia coli*. J. Bacteriol. **84**:902–910.
12. **Yokota, T., and G. S. Gots.** 1970. Requirement of adenosine 3′,5′-cyclic phosphate for flagella formation in *Escherichia coli* and *Salmonella typhimurium*. J. Bacteriol. **103**:513–516.
13. **Yokota, T., and S. Kuwahara.** 1974. Adenosine 3′,5′-cyclic monophosphate deficient mutants of *Vibrio cholerae*. J. Bacteriol. **120**:106–113.
14. **Yokota, T., and S. Kuwahara.** 1977. Temperature-sensitive R plasmid obtained from naturally isolated drug-resistant *Vibrio cholerae* (biotype El Tor). Antimicrob. Agents Chemother. **11**:13–20.

ANTIMICROBIAL AGENTS AND CHEMOTHERAPY, June 1977, p. 956-964
Vol. 11, No. 6

Printed in U.S.A.

Synergy Between Ticarcillin and Tobramycin Against *Pseudomonas aeruginosa* and *Enterobacteriaceae* In Vitro and In Vivo

K. R. COMBER, M. J. BASKER, CHRISTINE D. OSBORNE, AND R. SUTHERLAND*

Beecham Pharmaceuticals Research Division, Brockham Park, Betchworth, Surrey, England

Received for publication 17 January 1977

The antibacterial activities of ticarcillin, carbenicillin, tobramycin, and gentamicin and of combinations of these antibiotics were measured against *Pseudomonas aeruginosa* and other gram-negative bacilli in vitro and in experimental mouse infections. Synergistic effects were produced by the penicillin/aminoglycoside combinations in growth inhibition tests and in bactericidal tests against many of the bacteria tested. Combinations of ticarcillin + tobramycin were more active in vitro than carbenicillin + gentamicin against *P. aeruginosa* but were no more active than the latter against other gram-negative bacilli. Ticarcillin + tobramycin and carbenicillin + gentamicin also demonstrated synergistic activities against *P. aeruginosa, Escherichia coli,* and *Enterobacter cloacae* in experimental mouse infection models. Thus, the penicillin/aminoglycoside combinations produced greater protective effects than the individual antibiotics against lethal intraperitoneal infections and also were more effective in reducing kidney counts of viable bacteria and kidney abscess formation in experimental pyelonephritis infections. As was the case in vitro, ticarcillin + tobramycin was more effective than carbenicillin + gentamicin against the experimental *P. aeruginosa* infections. The results of these in vitro and in vivo studies suggest that combined therapy with ticarcillin and tobramycin may be warranted in the treatment of serious infections due to *P. aeruginosa* and *Enterobacteriaceae*.

Combined therapy with carbenicillin and gentamicin is often recommended for the treatment of serious infections caused by gram-negative bacilli because of the synergy that can be demonstrated in vitro and in vivo against *Pseudomonas aeruginosa* and other gram-negative bacilli (2, 3, 10, 12, 18). A number of newer aminoglycosides with claims to being superior to gentamicin in some respect have become available, and combinations of carbenicillin with tobramycin (2, 7, 9, 21), amikacin (9, 11, 14), sisomicin (9, 14), and netilmicin (14) have been reported to be synergistic against *P. aeruginosa*. Similarly, ticarcillin, a semisynthetic penicillin analogue of carbenicillin, has been shown to produce synergy when combined with gentamicin (1, 15, 20, 21), but no experimental data have been reported for combinations of ticarcillin with the newer aminoglycosides.

The present study was designed to investigate the antibacterial effects produced by combining ticarcillin with tobramycin against *P aeruginosa* and other gram-negative bacilli. The combinations of antibiotics were examined for synergy in growth inhibition and bactericidal tests in vitro and against two experimental mouse infection models. In these tests the activity of ticarcillin + tobramycin was compared with that of carbenicillin + gentamicin.

MATERIALS AND METHODS

Bacteria. Most of the cultures tested in vitro and in vivo were clinical isolates from specimens of blood, urine, and wounds.

Mice. Male and female albino mice, 18 to 22 g, were used for the intraperitoneal infection studies, and female mice, 18 to 20 g, were used for the experimental pyelonephritis. The OLAC strain of mouse (Oxford Laboratory Animal Colony) was employed throughout.

Antibiotics. Dry powder preparations of ticarcillin disodium, 815 μg/mg (Beecham Pharmaceuticals); carbenicillin disodium, 790 μg/mg (Beecham Pharmaceuticals); tobramycin sulfate, 910 μg/mg (Eli Lilly and Co. Ltd., Basingstoke, England); and gentamicin sulfate, 587 μg/mg (Nicholas Laboratories Ltd., Slough, England) were used in the in vitro and in vivo studies. All concentrations were adjusted to penicillin free acid or aminoglycoside free base.

MICs. The activities of the penicillins and aminoglycosides, alone and in combination, were measured by a chess board test using a microtiter broth dilution technique (3). Nutrient broth (Oxoid no. 2) containing the penicillin, the aminoglycoside, or a combination of the penicillin + aminoglycoside was serially diluted by twofold steps in 0.05-ml volumes per well to produce the desired range of antibiotic concentrations. Each well was inoculated with a replicating device (Denley-Tech Ltd., Billingshurst, Sussex, England), using stainless-steel pins delivering 0.001 ml of a 1/10 dilution of an 18-h broth culture of the test organism, an inoculum of approximately 5×10^4 cells per well, equivalent to approximately 10^6 cells per ml. Minimum inhibitory concentrations (MICs) were read after 18 h of incubation at 37°C.

MBCs. Samples of culture (0.001 ml) were removed from each well of the microtiter plates by means of the inoculating device described above, after the MIC values had been read, and subcultured in 0.05-ml volumes of sterile, antibiotic-free nutrient broth in each well of a microtiter plate. The wells were examined for growth after overnight incubation at 37°C, and the minimum bactericidal concentration (MBC) was taken as the concentration of antibiotic or combination of antibiotics from which there was no visible growth.

Viable count experiments. Nutrient broth (10 ml) containing selected concentrations of the antibiotics, alone and in combination, was inoculated with 0.02 ml of an overnight culture of the test strain of *P. aeruginosa*, an inoculum of about 10^6 cells per ml. In one test, the compounds were added to 10-ml volumes of pooled human serum that were inoculated with the test strain of pseudomonas, and the cultures were incubated in a GasPak jar (Baltimore Biological Laboratory, Cockeysville, Md.) in an atmosphere of 10% CO_2/90% air to maintain the pH value of the serum at about 7.4. The cultures were incubated at 37°C, samples were taken at 3, 6, and 24 h, and 0.02-ml volumes of suitable dilutions were pipetted onto the surface of antibiotic-free agar plates. In tests where it was thought that the viable counts had fallen to low levels, 0.1-ml volumes of undiluted culture were spread over the surfaces of the plates. Colonies were counted after overnight incubation at 37°C, and the numbers of viable bacteria were calculated.

Intraperitoneal infections. Mice were injected by the intraperitoneal route with 0.5 ml of a suspension in 5% hog gastric mucin (1701-W, Wilson Laboratories, Chicago, Ill.) of a dilution of an overnight broth culture of the test organism, standardized to give an infective inoculum of approximately 100 median lethal doses. Three clinical isolates of *P. aeruginosa* and one strain of *Enterobacter cloacae* were tested in this model. The antibiotics were administered by the subcutaneous route to groups of 10 mice 1, 3, 5, 7, and 9 h after infection, 0.2 ml/20 g for each dose, as solutions in phosphate-buffered saline. The combinations of a penicillin plus an aminoglycoside were mixed immediately before dosing. The numbers of animals surviving 4 days after infection were recorded, and the percentage of survivors per treatment group was calculated. The data were subjected to a binomial test of proportions for the assessment of statistically significant differences (19).

Bactericidal activity in vivo. Mice were infected intraperitoneally with *P. aeruginosa* 4 and dosed with either ticarcillin or tobramycin alone or with a combination of ticarcillin + tobramycin 1, 3, 5, 7, and 9 h after infection. Groups of three mice were killed by dislocation of the neck at intervals during the 24-h period after infection. The abdomen was swabbed with 70% alcohol, and 4.5 ml of sterile phosphate-buffered saline was injected forcefully into the peritoneum. The abdomen was carefully massaged to ensure adequate mixing, a small incision was made into the peritoneum, and a sample of the washings was collected with a sterile Pasteur pipette. The samples were diluted in 0.2% yeast extract (Difco Laboratories, Detroit, Mich.), 0.02-ml volumes were plated on predried nutrient agar plates, and viable colonies were counted after overnight incubation at 37°C.

Pyelonephritis infections. Mice were infected intravenously with 0.2 ml of a culture of the test organism suitably diluted in double-strength veal infusion broth (Difco). The mice were injected with approximately 10^8 cells of *Escherichia coli* JT415 or 2×10^6 to 5×10^6 cells of *P. aeruginosa* 11. Iron sorbitol citrate (Jectofer, Astra Chemicals Ltd., Watford, England) was administered by the intramuscular route 18, 42, 66, and 90 h after infection to promote the growth of the organism in the kidney (4). Treatment with subcutaneous injection of the ticarcillin and tobramycin was started 20 h after infection and continued four times a day at 2-h intervals for 4 days. Groups of five mice were killed between days 7 and 11 for the pseudomonas infection, and on days 7 and 15 for the *E. coli* infection. After infection, kidneys were examined for macroscopic abscesses, and bacterial counts were performed on homogenates of the infected kidneys.

RESULTS

In vitro studies. Combinations of penicillins and aminoglycosides were considered to be synergistic when one-quarter the MIC or MBC of each antibiotic inhibited growth or killed the test organism and to be partially synergistic when the effective combination contained one-quarter the MIC or MBC of one antibiotic combined with half the MIC or MBC of the other. An indifferent effect was recorded when the concentration of both compounds was only twice as effective in combination as each alone or when the MIC or MBC of one drug did not change when in combination with the other.

(i) MICs. Examples of the synergistic effects obtained with ticarcillin and tobramycin or carbenicillin and gentamicin are illustrated in Table 1, showing typical MIC values obtained with the antibiotics alone and in combination. It can be seen that the higher activities of the new compounds, ticarcillin and tobramycin, against *P. aeruginosa*, compared with carbenicillin and gentamicin, respectively, were reflected also in their combined effects. Synergy was demonstrated not only against strains of *P. aeruginosa* that were susceptible to the penicillins but also against strains that were moderately resistant, but β-lactamase-producing strains with a high level of resistance to carbenicillin and ticarcillin, e.g., Dal and FR11, were always indifferent to the combinations. The pseudomonas strains with a moderate level of resistance to gentamicin usually showed increased susceptibility to ticarcillin + tobramycin and sometimes to carbenicillin + gentamicin, but the former combination was notably more active.

The penicillin/aminoglycoside combinations also showed enhanced activity against gram-negative bacilli other than *P. aeruginosa,* and both combinations were equally active against these organisms, reflecting the activities of the individual antibiotics (Table 1). In general, synergy was most pronounced against bacteria that were susceptible or only moderately resistant to the penicillins and aminoglycosides. Enhancement of activity was never seen with β-lactamase-producing strains of bacteria with a high level of resistance to the penicillins. Synergy was demonstrated against two tobramycin/gentamicin-resistant strains of *Providencia stuartii* tested, but the concentrations of aminoglycosides in the synergistic combinations make the clinical relevance of such synergism doubtful.

The numbers of strains against which synergistic effects were demonstrated by the penicillin/aminoglycoside combinations are shown in Table 2. Ticarcillin + tobramycin showed enhanced activity against 27 of 34 strains of *P. aeruginosa* and against 17 of 20 enterobacteria. Only β-lactamase-producing strains highly resistant to ticarcillin were indifferent to the combination. Essentially similar results were obtained with the combination of carbenicillin + gentamicin, synergistic effects being observed against 24 of 34 strains of pseudomonas and 16 of 20 other gram-negative bacteria. There was no evidence of antagonism in any of these tests.

(ii) MBCs. Table 2 also shows that both ticarcillin + tobramycin and carbenicillin + gentamicin produced enhanced bactericidal activity against most of the strains of *P. aeruginosa* tested. As was the case in the MIC tests, the combination of ticarcillin + tobramycin was two- to fourfold more effective in the MBC tests than was the carbenicillin + gentamicin combination.

(iii) Viable count tests. The bactericidal synergism shown by the ticarcillin + tobramycin combination in MBC tests was reproduced also in viable count experiments against *P. aeruginosa*. For example, Fig. 1a shows that a combination of 100 μg of ticarcillin per ml + 0.1 μg of tobramycin per ml was rapidly bactericidal against *P. aeruginosa* PU4 and caused a 99.99% kill by 6 h, whereas the antibiotics alone were ineffective or only moderately effective. Increasing the tobramycin concentration to 1.0 μg/ml resulted in increased bactericidal activity, and the compound alone caused a 99% kill of the culture, but when combined with ticarcillin (100 μg/ml) the culture was sterilized within

TABLE 1. *Examples of responses of P. aeruginosa and other gram-negative bacilli to combinations of ticarcillin + tobramycin and carbenicillin + gentamicin*

Organism	MIC (μg/ml)					
	Ticarcillin	Tobramycin	Ticarcillin + tobramycin	Carbenicillin	Gentamicin	Carbenicillin + gentamicin
P. aeruginosa R2	31	0.12	8.0 + 0.03	62	0.5	16 + 0.12
R4	62	0.25	8.0 + 0.06	125	1.0	16 + 0.25
R139	16	0.25	8.0 + 0.06	31	1.0	16 + 0.25
Dal	>500	0.25	>500 + 0.25	>500	1.0	>500 + 1.0
PMG-1	31	0.25	8.0 + 0.12	62	12.5	31 + 6.2
WM627	31	6.2	4 + 1.6	125	25	16 + 6.2
PA100	31	>100	8.0 + 25	62	>100	31 + >100
FR11	>500	31	>500 + 31	>500	500	>500 + 500
E. coli JT1	8.0	0.5	2.0 + 0.12	8.0	0.5	2.0 + 0.12
Proteus mirabilis 977	4.0	1.0	1.0 + 0.25	8.0	1.0	2.0 + 0.5
Proteus rettgeri I	4.0	0.5	1.0 + 0.12	4.0	0.5	1.0 + 0.12
Klebsiella aerogenes A	125	0.5	31 + 0.12	250	0.25	62 + 0.06
E. coli JT4	>500	0.5	>500 + 0.5	>500	1.0	>500 + 1.0
P. stuartii	500	50	125 + 25	500	250	250 + 50

6 h. The bactericidal effects produced by the combination were measured also in tests carried out in human serum, and Fig. 1b compares the relative bactericidal activities of ticarcillin and tobramycin against *P. aeruginosa* NCTC 10662 in nutrient broth and in serum. In this test neither antibiotic was particularly effective in broth, whereas the combination demon-

TABLE 2. *Synergy of ticarcillin + tobramycin and carbenicillin + gentamicin combinations against P. aeruginosa and other gram-negative bacilli*[a]

Test	Organism	Combination	No. of strains: Synergy	No. of strains: Partial synergy	No. of strains: Indifference
Bacteriostatic (MIC)	*P. aeruginosa* (34 strains)	Ticarcillin + tobramycin	12	15	7
		Carbenicillin + gentamicin	9	15	10
	Other gram-negative bacilli (20 strains)	Ticarcillin + tobramycin	9	8	3
		Carbenicillin + gentamicin	10	6	4
Bactericidal (MBC)	*P. aeruginosa* (18 strains)	Ticarcillin + tobramycin	7	10	1
		Carbenicillin + gentamicin	8	7	3

[a] See text for definition of synergy.

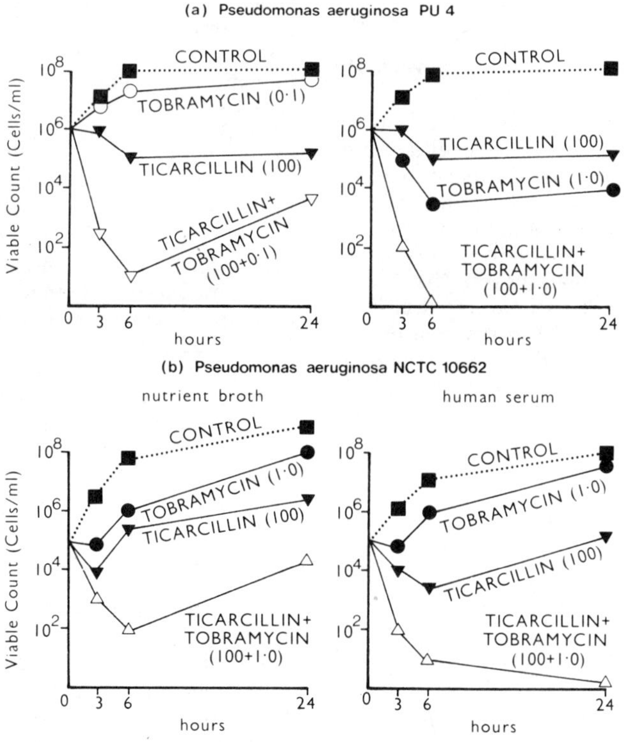

FIG. 1. *Bactericidal activities of ticarcillin and tobramycin, alone and in combination, against two strains of P. aeruginosa (a) in nutrient broth and (b) in nutrient broth and human serum. Figures in parentheses show antibiotic concentrations (micrograms per milliliter).*

strated pronounced bactericidal activity in the early part of the test, causing a 99.9% reduction in the viable count by 6 h, although regrowth of the culture occurred between 6 and 24 h. Ticarcillin showed greater activity in human serum than in broth and caused a 99.9% kill by 6 h but failed to prevent subsequent regrowth. Tobramycin was relatively ineffective, as was the case in broth, but the combination of ticarcillin + tobramycin was rapidly bactericidal, producing a 99.9% kill at 6 h and reducing the 24-h count to a very low level.

Increased bactericidal activity was demonstrated also by ticarcillin + tobramycin against a strain of *P. aeruginosa* resistant to gentamicin (MIC, 15.6 μg/ml). In this experiment, carbenicillin at 100 μg/ml was bactericidal and caused a 99.9% kill in 6 h, gentamicin (10 μg/ml) had little effect, and a combination of the two antibiotics (100 + 10 μg/ml) was no more effective than was carbenicillin itself (Fig. 2). In contrast, ticarcillin (100 μg/ml) showed bactericidal activity slightly greater than that of carbenicillin, and tobramycin (1.0 μg/ml) was markedly bactericidal, reducing the viable count 99.9% by 6 h. The combination of ticarcillin plus tobramycin (100 + 1.0 μg/ml) showed an enhanced rate of bactericidal activity during the first 6 h of the test, although there was some regrowth of the culture during overnight incubation.

Activity against experimental infections. (i) Intraperitoneal infections. The results of parenteral treatment of mouse intraperitoneal infections are shown in Tables 3, 4, and 5. In all these tests the doses of the individual antibiotics were chosen so as to produce only small numbers of survivors (usually less than 20%). Table 3 shows that combinations of ticarcillin + tobramycin produced significantly greater protective effects against the three test strains of *P. aeruginosa* than were produced by the individual antibiotics. Thus, doses of the compounds that were ineffective on their own produced significant increases in the numbers of survivors when the compounds were administered in combination. Similarly, ticarcillin + tobramycin was notably more active against an infection due to *E. cloacae* than when either ticarcillin or tobramycin was administered alone (Table 4).

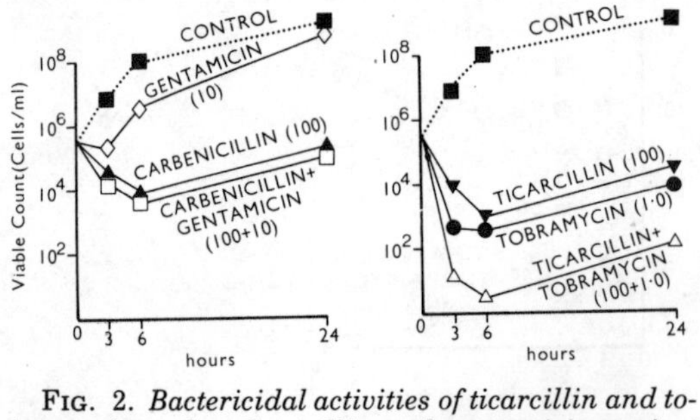

FIG. 2. *Bactericidal activities of ticarcillin and tobramycin and carbenicillin and gentamicin against a gentamicin-resistant strain of P. aeruginosa, PMG1. Figures in parentheses show antibiotic concentrations (micrograms per milliliter).*

TABLE 3. *Synergy between ticarcillin and tobramycin against three intraperitoneal pseudomonas infections in mice*

Treatment	Total dose[a] (mg/kg)	% Survivors[b]		
		P. aeruginosa 4	*P. aeruginosa* 11	*P. aeruginosa* 31
Ticarcillin	78	15	5	20
	39	5	5	0
Tobramycin	6.3	10	5	5
	3.1	0	0	0
Ticarcillin + tobramycin	78 + 6.3	80[c]	85[c]	100[c]
	39 + 6.3	55[d]	45[d]	100[c]
	78 + 3.1	75[c]	55[c]	95[c]
	39 + 3.1	30[e]	5[f]	55[c]

[a] Dosed at 1, 3, 5, 7, and 9 h after infection.
[b] Mean of two tests, 20 mice per group.
[c] $P < 0.001$.
[d] $P < 0.01$.
[e] $P < 0.05$.
[f] P is not significant.

The activity of ticarcillin + tobramycin was also compared with that of carbenicillin + gentamicin against the pseudomonas infections (Table 5). Ticarcillin and tobramycin were relatively ineffective when administered alone, and carbenicillin and gentamicin were, if anything, less effective than the newer compounds against these infections. As before, the combinations of ticarcillin + tobramycin usually resulted in a marked increase in protection of the infected mice, whereas carbenicillin + gentamicin was relatively ineffective, and it was evident that combined therapy with ticarcillin + tobramycin was significantly more effective.

(ii) Bactericidal activity in vivo. The effects of subcutaneously administered ticarcillin, tobramycin, and a combination of ticarcillin + tobramycin on the proliferation of bacteria in the peritoneal cavity of mice after intraperitoneal injection with *P. aeruginosa* 4 are illustrated in Fig. 3. In untreated mice the bacterial peritoneal count fell from the initial inoculum of 7×10^5 cells to 4.9×10^4 cells over the first 3 h and then increased to a count in excess of 10^8 cells at 14 h. Administration of tobramycin had little effect, and the bacterial counts were not significantly different from those of the untreated mice. Treatment with ticarcillin resulted in a reduction of the viable count to 5×10^4 cells for up to 14 h, after which time the count increased to a level of 7.8×10^7 cells. A combination of ticarcillin (78 mg/kg) + tobramycin (6.3 mg/kg) resulted in a notably greater reduction in the viable counts in the peritoneal

TABLE 4. *Synergy between ticarcillin and tobramycin against an intraperitoneal mouse infection caused by E. cloacae T753*

Treatment	Total dose[a] (mg/kg)	% Survivors[b]	
		Test 1	Test 2
Ticarcillin	312	10	10
	156	0	0
Tobramycin	1.6	0	0
	0.8	0	0
Ticarcillin + tobramycin	312 + 1.6	90[c]	90[c]
	156 + 1.6	70[c]	100[c]
	312 + 0.8	30[d]	20[d]
	156 + 0.8	0[d]	0[d]

[a] Dosed at 1, 3, 5, 7, and 9 h after infection.
[b] Ten mice per group.
[c] $P < 0.001$.
[d] P is not significant.

TABLE 5. *Comparative activities of ticarcillin and tobramycin and carbenicillin and gentamicin against intraperitoneal pseudomonas infections in mice*

Treatment	Total dose[a] (mg/kg)	% Survivors[b]		
		P. aeruginosa 4	*P. aeruginosa* 11	*P. aeruginosa* 31
Ticarcillin	78	30	10	30
	39	10	10	0
Tobramycin	6.3	20	10	0
	3.1	0	0	0
Ticarcillin + tobramycin	78 + 6.3	100	100	100
	39 + 6.3	80	70	100
	78 + 3.1	100	90	90
	39 + 3.1	50	0	60
Carbenicillin	78	0	10	0
	39	0	0	0
Gentamicin	6.3	0	0	0
	3.1	0	0	0
Carbenicillin + gentamicin	78 + 6.3	10	10	20
	39 + 6.3	0	0	0
	78 + 3.1	10	0	20
	39 + 3.1	30	0	0

[a] Dosed at 1, 3, 5, 7, and 9 h after infection.
[b] Ten mice per group.

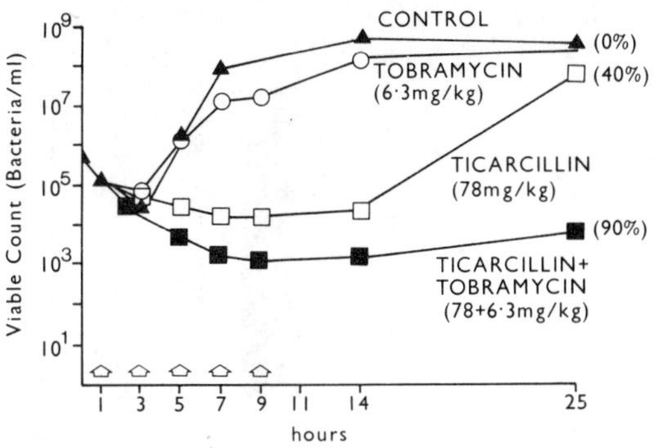

FIG. 3. *Bactericidal effects of a combination of ticarcillin and tobramycin on the growth of P. aeruginosa 4 in the peritoneal cavity of mice. The animals were dosed subcutaneously 1, 3, 5, 7, and 9 h after infection, and the percentages in parentheses show survivors from control groups.*

cavity than either antibiotic alone. Thus, more than 99% of the bacterial cells were killed by 9 h; there was little increase in the bacterial count from then up to 25 h after infection, and at 25 h it was evident that the combination was notably more effective than the individual antibiotics.

The efficacy of treatment of this infection in reducing the mortality of the infected mice in this experiment is also shown in Fig. 3, and it can be seen that the combination of ticarcillin + tobramycin increased the amount of protection afforded. In untreated mice and mice treated with tobramycin, there were no survivors; ticarcillin produced 40% survivors, but half of these were moribund up to 48 h after infection. However, treatment with the combination provided 90% protection of infected animals.

(iii) Experimental pyelonephritis. The effects of therapy with ticarcillin, tobramycin, and ticarcillin + tobramycin in reducing bacterial kidney counts and kidney abscess formation in mice surviving from 7 to 15 days after intravenous infections with *P. aeruginosa* or *E. coli* are illustrated in Fig. 4 and 5. In both infections, some 80% of the untreated control mice had significant kidney bacterial counts, and there was a high incidence of visible kidney lesions.

Interpretation of the results of therapy of the pseudomonas infection was complicated by the fact that a number of mice had to be killed during the experiment because of central nervous system toxicity. This was particularly evident in groups treated with tobramycin, where 33 to 58% of the animals were affected, and was also seen, albeit to a lesser extent, in untreated animals. Also, several deaths occurred within

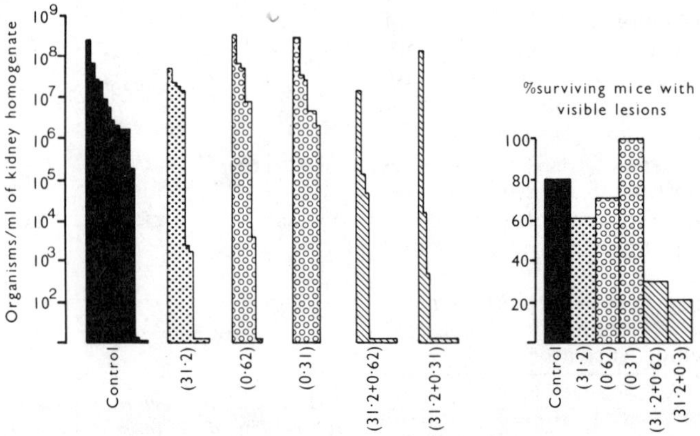

FIG. 4. *Efficacy of ticarcillin and tobramycin, alone and in combination, against an experimental pyelonephritis in mice infected with P. aeruginosa 11. Each bar in the histograms representing the bacterial kidney counts shows the counts measured in an individual animal. Symbols: (dots) ticarcillin; (circles) tobramycin; (stripes) ticarcillin + tobramycin.*

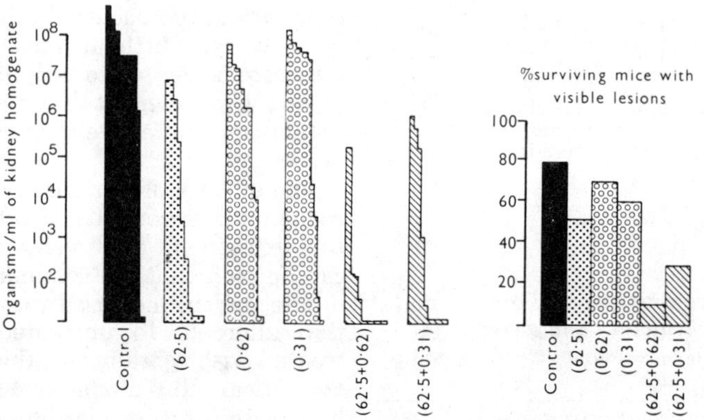

FIG. 5. *Efficacy of ticarcillin and tobramycin, alone and in combination, against an experimental pyelonephritis in mice infected with E. coli JT415. Each bar in the histograms representing the bacterial kidney counts shows the counts measured in an individual animal. Symbols: (dots) ticarcillin; (circles) tobramycin; (stripes) ticarcillin + tobramycin.*

48 h in these groups. Interestingly, central nervous system toxicity was not observed in the groups receiving ticarcillin or combined therapy, although the dose of tobramycin administered to the latter animals was the same, and none of the mice died within 48 h.

In both infections, treatment with the individual antibiotics was relatively ineffective in reducing kidney bacterial counts or in preventing visible abscess formation, whereas ticarcillin + tobramycin produced a much greater degree of protection of the infected animals. Thus, in both experiments the combination of antibiotics was notably more effective than either ticarcillin or tobramycin alone in the treatment of this experimental pyelonephritis, and these results would appear to provide further evidence for synergy between ticarcillin and tobramycin in vivo.

DISCUSSION

The extent of synergy produced by ticarcillin + tobramycin was generally of the same order as that demonstrated by carbenicillin + gentamicin, and consequently the ticarcillin + tobramycin combination was usually four times more effective than the carbenicillin + gentamicin combination against *P. aeruginosa* in the MIC and MBC tests. The greatest differences in activity between the combinations were seen against the gentamicin-resistant, tobramycin-susceptible strains, and these were notably more susceptible to ticarcillin + tobramycin.

Against gram-negative bacilli other than *P. aeruginosa* there was little difference between the combinations in any of the tests. Synergy was observed most often in tests with bacteria susceptible to both the penicillin and the aminoglycoside constituents of the combinations but was also seen on occasion against strains with a moderate level of resistance to the antibiotics. In general, synergistic effects were not seen with bacteria with a high level of resistance to either or both of the antibiotics in the test combinations.

In the in vivo studies described here, the combination of ticarcillin + tobramycin demonstrated a significant enhanced antibacterial activity not only against *P. aeruginosa* but also against *E. coli* and *E. cloacae,* the two organisms tested as examples of nonpseudomonads. Thus, in the intraperitoneal infection model the combination was significantly more effective against all three pseudomonas infections and against the enterobacter infection than either ticarcillin or tobramycin alone. The viable count study of the effect of the antibiotics on the growth of *P. aeruginosa* in the peritoneal cavity of infected animals showed that the combination of ticarcillin + tobramycin produced greater bactericidal effects than either antibiotic alone and that the bactericidal activity correlated with the degree of protection produced. Moreover, ticarcillin + tobramycin was more efficacious than carbenicillin + gentamicin against all three pseudomonas infections, reflecting the superior activities of the newer compounds in this infection model.

Enhancement of activity was also observed against the experimental mouse pyelonephritis when ticarcillin was combined with tobramycin at doses that, alone, showed only little effect in reducing the counts of viable bacteria in the kidneys of infected animals or in preventing visible kidney abscess formation. It was not possible to make a direct comparison of the effect of ticarcillin + tobramycin with that of carbenicillin + gentamicin in this model because of the size of the study involved, but comparison with earlier (unpublished) studies with carbenicillin + gentamicin suggest that the ticarcillin + tobramycin combination would be the more effective of the two combinations. The results of treatment of the experimental pyelonephritis described here might be more significant than those obtained with the intraperitoneal infection, as in this infection model dosing is delayed for 20 h after infection, by which time there is substantial lodgment of the bacteria in the kidney (4). Thus, therapy is not started until the infection is established, as is normally the case in clinical practice.

The observations of McLaughlin and Reeves (13) of the inactivation of gentamicin by carbenicillin caused concern, but it is now generally agreed that the interaction is likely to be of clinical importance only under special circumstances, notably, in patients with renal failure (17). Recent studies by Davies et al. (5) and Holt et al. (6) have shown that there is no significant difference between ticarcillin and carbenicillin with respect to inactivation of aminoglycosides, in agreement with results (unpublished) obtained in this laboratory. The results of the present study, showing evident synergy in vitro and in vivo with ticarcillin + tobramycin, support the view that inactivation of tobramycin by ticarcillin is only rarely likely to be of clinical significance.

In clinical studies, Klastersky et al. (8) have reported better responses in cancer patients treated with combinations of antibiotics, including ticarcillin + tobramycin, that were synergistic than with nonsynergistic combinations. More recently, Parry and Neu (16) found that ticarcillin + tobramycin compared favorably with ticarcillin alone, or with ticarcillin + gentamicin, in eradicating *P. aeruginosa* from the sputum of patients with cystic fibrosis. The results of the in vitro and in vivo studies described in this report support these preliminary clinical observations that combined therapy with ticarcillin and tobramycin may be advantageous in the treatment of infections due to *P. aeruginosa* and other gram-negative bacilli.

ACKNOWLEDGMENTS

We wish to thank Julie King and Carol Pierce for skilled technical assistance and G. Kimber for his assistance with statistical evaluation of the data. We also thank Eli Lilly and Co. Ltd. for a generous gift of tobramycin.

LITERATURE CITED

1. **Acred, P., P. A. Hunter, L. Mizen, and G. N. Rolinson.** 1971. α-Carboxy-3-thienylmethylpenicillin (BRL 2288), a new semisynthetic penicillin: in vivo evaluation, p. 396–401. Antimicrob. Agents Chemother. 1970.
2. **Anderson, E. L., P. K. Gramling, P. R. Vestal, and W. E. Farrar, Jr.** 1975. Susceptibility of *Pseudomonas aeruginosa* to tobramycin or gentamicin alone and combined with carbenicillin. Antimicrob. Agents Chemother. 8:300–304.
3. **Andriole, B. T.** 1971. Synergy of carbenicillin and gentamicin in experimental infection with Pseudomonas. J. Infect. Dis. 124 (Suppl.):S46–55.
4. **Comber, K. R.** 1976. Pathogenesis of an experimental pyelonephritis model in the mouse and its use in the evaluation of antibiotics, p. 311–316. *In* J. D. Williams and A. M. Geddes (ed.), Chemotherapy, vol. 2. Plenum Publishing Corp., New York.
5. **Davies, M., J. R. Morgan, and C. Anand.** 1975. Interactions of carbenicillin and ticarcillin with gentamicin. Antimicrob. Agents Chemother. 7:431–434.
6. **Holt, H. A., J. M. Broughall, M. McCarthy, and D. S.**

Reeves. 1976. Interactions between aminoglycoside antibiotics and carbenicillin or ticarcillin. Infection 4:107–109.

7. **Klastersky, J., A Henri, and L. Vandenborre.** 1973. Antimicrobial activity of tobramycin and gentamicin used in combination with cephalothin and carbenicillin. Am. J. Med. Sci. **266:**13–21.
8. **Klastersky, J., C. Hensgens, and L. Debusscher.** 1975. Empiric therapy for cancer patients: comparative study of ticarcillin-tobramycin, ticarcillin-cephalothin, and cephalothin-tobramycin. Antimicrob. Agents Chemother. **7:**640–645.
9. **Klastersky, J., B. Nyamubeya, and L. Vandenborre.** 1974. Antimicrobial effectiveness of kanamycin, aminosidin, BB-K8, sisomicin, gentamicin and tobramycin combined wtih carbenicillin or cephalothin against gram-negative rods. J. Med. Microbiol. **7:**465–472.
10. **Klastersky, J., G. Swings, and D. Daneau.** 1970. Antimicrobial activity of the carbenicillin/gentamicin combination against gram-negative bacilli. Am. J. Med. Sci. **260:**373–380.
11. **Kluge, R. M., H. C. Standiford, B. Tatem, V. M. Young, W. H. Greene, S. C. Schimpff, F. M. Calia, and R. B. Hornick.** 1974. Comparative activity of tobramycin, amikacin, and gentamicin alone and with carbenicillin against *Pseudomonas aeruginosa*. Antimicrob. Agents Chemother. **6:**442–446.
12. **Konickova, L., and W. Prat.** 1971. Effect of carbenicillin, gentamicin and their combination on experimental *Pseudomonas aeruginosa* urinary tract infection. J. Clin. Pathol. **24:**113–116.
13. **McLaughlin, J. E., and D. S. Reeves.** 1971. Clinical and laboratory evidence for inactivation of gentamicin by carbenicillin. Lancet **1:**261–264.
14. **Marks, M. I., S. Hammerberg, G. Greenstone, and B. Silver.** 1976. Activity of newer aminoglycosides and carbenicillin, alone and in combination, against gentamicin-resistant *Pseudomonas aeruginosa*. Antimicrob. Agents Chemother. **10:**399–401.
15. **Neu, H. C., and E. B. Winshell.** 1971. In vitro studies of a semisynthetic penicillin, 6-[D(−)-α-carboxy-3-thienylacetamido] penicillanic acid (BRL 2288), active against *Pseudomonas,* p. 385–389. Antimicrob. Agents Chemother. 1970.
16. **Parry, M. F., and H. C. Neu.** 1976. Tobramycin and ticarcillin therapy for exacerbations of pulmonary disease in patients with cystic fibrosis. J. Infect. Dis. **134** (Suppl.):S194–197.
17. **Riff, L. J., and G. G. Jackson.** 1972. Laboratory and clinical conditions for gentamicin inactivation by carbenicillin. Arch. Intern. Med. **130:**887–891.
18. **Smith, C. B., J. N. Wilfert, P. E. Davis, T. A. Kurrus, and M. Finland.** 1970. In vitro activity of carbenicillin and results of treatment of infections due to *Pseudomonas* with carbenicillin singly and in combination with gentamicin. J. Infect. Dis. **122** (Suppl.):S14–25.
19. **Snedecor, G. W., and W. G. Cochran.** 1967. Statistical methods, 6th ed. Iowa State University Press, Ames.
20. **Sutherland, R., J. Burnett, and G. N. Rolinson.** 1971. α-Carboxy-3-thienylmethylpenicillin (BRL 2288), a new semisynthetic penicillin: in vitro evaluation, p. 390–395. Antimicrob. Agents Chemother. 1970.
21. **Wald, E. L., H. C. Standiford, B. A. Tatem, F. M. Calia, and R. B. Hornick.** 1975. BL-P1654, ticarcillin and carbenicillin: in vitro comparison alone and in combination with gentamicin against *Pseudomonas aeruginosa*. Antimicrob. Agents Chemother. **7:**336–340.

ANTIMICROBIAL AGENTS AND CHEMOTHERAPY, June 1977, p. 965-967
Vol. 11, No. 6

Nafcillin Entry into Human Cerebrospinal Fluid

BYRON E. FOSSIECK, JR.,* JAMES G. KANE, CARLOS R. DIAZ, AND RICHARD H. PARKER

Section of Infectious Diseases and Medical Oncology, Medical Service, Veterans Administration Hospital, Washington, D.C. 20422

Received for publication 5 January 1977

The entry of nafcillin into the cerebrospinal fluid (CSF) of humans was studied in the absence of meningeal inflammation. Twenty studies were performed in 18 patients receiving 40 mg of sodium nafcillin per kg intravenously over 30 min. The CSF specimens were obtained at 1, 2, 3, and 4 h postinfusion, and sera were obtained at 5 min and 1, 2, 3, and 4 h. Nafcillin was uniformly detected in the lumbar CSF at 1 h, peaked at 2 h postinfusion, and was still detectable in the CSF of three of four patients studied at 4 h.

Meningitis caused by *Staphylococcus aureus* is relatively rare, but presents a major therapeutic problem because of a mortality rate approximating 50% (1). Currently the semisynthetic penicillinase-resistant penicillins are the urugs of choice for the therapy of staphylococcal meningitis (1, 4). However, minimal data exist regarding the passage of these agents into the cerebrospinal fluid (CSF) of humans (4). As a result, very large doses of these antimicrobials are empirically recommended for treatment of staphylococcal meningitis (1).

This paper reports the results of a prospective study undertaken to define the degree of entry of a particular penicillinase-resistant penicillin, sodium nafcillin, into the CSF of patients without meningeal inflammation.

MATERIALS AND METHODS

Patients. The study group was composed of patients admitted to the Medical Oncology ward who underwent lumbar puncture as part of a staging evaluation for malignancy. The subjects were eligible for the study if they were not receiving antimicrobial therapy and had no history of penicillin allergy. After informed consent was obtained, the patients were skin tested for sensitivity to nafcillin before intravenous infusion of the drug. Patients with a clinical history of penicillin allergy were not administered nafcillin, but a portion of their CSF specimen was obtained for assay of intrinsic antimicrobial activity. Twenty studies were performed on 18 patients. Six patients were women and 12 were men. They ranged in age from 36 to 69 years, with a mean age of 57.7 years. Seventeen patients had carcinoma of the lung, and one patient had mycosis fungoides.

Method of study. On the day the lumbar puncture was performed, intravenous access was obtained with a 20-gauge butterfly needle and normal saline. A prestudy blood sample was drawn to assay serum intrinsic antimicrobial activity. Sodium nafcillin, 40 mg/kg in 100 ml of normal saline, was administered by a constant-infusion pump over a 30-min period, after which the intravenous line was removed. The total dose of drug administered ranged from 1.8 to 3.8 g, with an average dose of 2.5 g. A single lumbar puncture was performed on each patient at time intervals varying from 1 to 4 h after the infusion of drug had ceased, and simultaneous CSF and blood specimens were obtained for bioassay of nafcillin concentration. Several patients permitted more than one blood sample to be collected during the 4-h postinfusion period. CSF specimens were obtained at 1, 2, 3, or 4 h after cessation of the nafcillin infusion. Eight CSF specimens were obtained from patients who did not receive nafcillin. Serum specimens were obtained before nafcillin from all patients and 5 min and/or 1, 2, 3, or 4 h after the infusion ended. Table 1 shows the temporal distribution of the CSF and serum specimens.

All CSF specimens were plated on Columbia sheep blood agar, Fildes peptic digest of blood agar, and MacConkey agar in addition to being inoculated into thioglycolate and Trypticase soy broths. The agar plates were placed in a 10% CO_2 atmosphere and examined after 24 and 48 h of incubation. In addition, the leukocyte count with differential cell count and the glucose and protein concentrations were determined for all CSF specimens. The concentration of glucose in the blood at the time of the lumbar puncture was also measured. All specimens were kept frozen at −20°C until assayed.

Antimicrobial assay. Bioassay of CSF and serum nafcillin concentrations were performed using the basic method of Grove and Randall by Wyeth Laboratories, Philadelphia, Pa. (3). CSFs were diluted with pH 7.0 phosphate buffer and assayed, using *Staphylococcus aureus* ATCC 6538P as the test microorganism. Sera were diluted in pooled antibiotic-free human serum and assayed, using *Sarcina lutea* ATCC 9341 as the test microorganism. All specimens from a given patient were assayed simultaneously.

RESULTS

CSF could not be obtained from one patient, and another patient had hemorrhagic CSF

TABLE 1. *Concentration of nafcillin in the cerebrospinal fluid (CSF) and serum of patients before infusion and after intravenous administration of 40 mg/kg*

Time (min)	Nafcillin concn in: CSF			Serum		
	No. of specimens[a]	Range (μg/ml)	Mean (μg/ml)	No. of specimens[b]	Range (μg/ml)	Mean (μg/ml)
Preinfusion	8	0.00–0.00	0.00	20	0.00–0.00	0.00
Postinfusion						
5	0			6	85–125	103.0
60	7	0.02–0.09	0.05	7	24–57	34.4
120	4	0.03–0.17	0.12	6	8–19	12.7
180	3	0.06–0.12	0.09	3	2.4–8.9	4.9
240	4	0.00–0.07	0.03	5	0.7–6.6	2.7

[a] One specimen excluded due to presence of blood.
[b] In some patients, more than one serum specimen was obtained for assay.

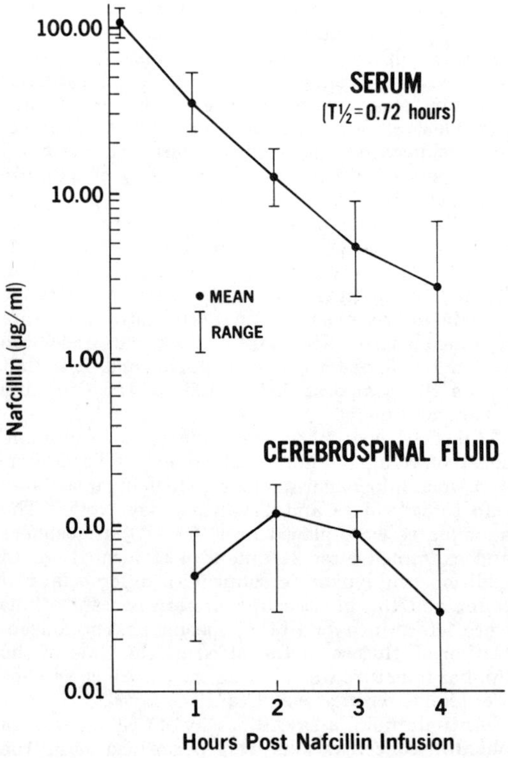

FIG. 1. *Serum and cerebrospinal fluid concentration of nafcillin in patients without meningeal inflammation after a single 40-mg/kg intravenous dose.*

which precluded CSF studies; however, serum studies were carried out for both subjects.

None of the CSF specimens showed changes of meningeal inflammation as shown by the results of biochemical determinations and cell counts. The glucose concentration in the CSF ranged from 20 to 88 mg/dl. It was equal to or greater than 50 mg/dl in all but two CSF specimens, which had values of 20 and 38 mg/dl. The CSF/serum glucose ratio ranged from 0.16 to 0.85 and was greater than 0.4 in all but one case. The CSF protein concentration ranged from 10 to 96 mg/dl and exceeded 43 mg/dl in five cases; the latter values were 50, 60, 69, 94, and 96 mg/dl. The CSF leukocyte count was always 4 cells/mm^3 or less. All CSF specimens were sterile. None of the patients were found to have central nervous system metastases. The serum creatinine was 1.4 mg/dl or less in all subjects, and serum bilirubin concentration did not exceed 1.1 mg/dl.

Five minutes after the end of infusion, the mean serum nafcillin concentration for six studies was 103 μg/ml (Table 1). This concentration fell to a mean of 2.7 μg/ml by 4 h. The mean CSF concentration detectable at 1 h postinfusion was 0.05 μg/ml. A mean peak CSF nafcillin concentration of 0.12 μg/ml occurred 2 h after the end of infusion, and the 4-hour mean concentration reached a nadir of 0.03 μg/ml. The eight CSF specimens from the control patients receiving no drug, and the 20 preinfusion serum samples showed no detectable antimicrobial activity. The relationships between serum and CSF nafcillin concentrations are depicted in Fig. 1.

DISCUSSION

The results of the study indicate that sodium nafcillin enters the CSF of humans in detectable amounts even in the absence of meningeal inflammation. The drug was uniformly present at the first time interval of 1 h in the lumbar CSF of all seven patients studied. The mean peak CSF nafcillin concentration of 0.12 μg/ml occurred at 2 h after the infusion, and nafcillin was still detectable in the CSF of three of four patients studied at 4 h after the end of drug administration.

No prior reports describing the entry of nafcillin into the CSF of humans in the absence of meningeal inflammation have been published. However, Ruiz and Warner have reported serum and CSF nafcillin levels in a patient with staphylococcal meningitis (4). In their patient, who received nafcillin, 200 mg/kg per 24 h, administered as a 3.0-g intravenous bolus every 4 h, the 5- and 60-min postinfusion serum levels of 104 and 26 μg/ml, respectively, closely approximated the results of the current study. Lumbar CSF assay for nafcillin from the same patient revealed no detectable drug at 5 min after the dose. In the current study, nafcillin was present in the CSF in low but detectable concentrations at 4 h after a single dose, 1.8 to 2.4 g, in three of four patients. In contrast, the CSF nafcillin concentration 45 min after the dose in the meningitis patient was 190 times greater than the mean 1 h postdose CSF concentration of 0.05 μg/ml in the patients currently reported.

The dose of antimicrobials used for both prophylaxis and therapy of staphylococcal meningitis is largely empiric (1). Previous studies of the susceptibility of penicillinase-producing staphylococci to nafcillin have revealed minimum inhibitory concentrations ranging from 0.1 to 1.6 μg/ml, with medians of 0.4 to 0.8 μg/ml (2, 5). The concentration of nafcillin in the CSF equaled or exceeded 0.1 μg/ml in five of the patients reported here, and the highest concentration achieved was 0.17 μg/ml. This information and the data reported previously in a patient with meningitis support the concept that large doses of nafcillin are appropriate when used for both prophylaxis and therapy of staphylococcal meningitis.

ACKNOWLEDGMENTS

We wish to thank George H. Warren, Sanford B. Rosenman, Lester S. Weber, and Lawrence Gordon at Wyeth Laboratories for performing the bioassays and Frank Pelsor, research pharmacist, for assistance in analysis of data. We are indebted to the nursing and house staffs of the Medical Oncology Unit for their technical assistance.

This study was supported in part by the Medical Research Service of the Veterans Administration and a grant from Wyeth Laboratories, Philadelphia, Pa.

LITERATURE CITED

1. **Benner, J. E., and P. D. Hoeprich.** 1972. Acute bacterial meningitis, p. 932–942. *In* P. D. Hoeprich (ed.), Infectious diseases. Harper & Row Publishers, Inc., Hagerstown, Md.
2. **Eickhoff, T. C., J. W. Kislak, and M. Finland.** 1965. Clinical evaluation of nafcillin in patients with severe staphylococcal disease. N. Engl. J. Med. 272:699–708.
3. **Grove, D. C., and W. A. Randall.** (ed.). 1955. Assay methods of antibiotics. A laboratory manual. Medical Encyclopedia, Inc., New York.
4. **Ruiz, D. E., and J. F. Warner.** 1976. Nafcillin treatment of *Staphylococcus aureus* meningitis. Antimicrob. Agents Chemother. 9:554–555.
5. **Sabath, L. D., C. Garner, C. Wilcox, and M. Finland.** 1976. Susceptibility of *Staphylococcus aureus* and *Staphylococcus epidermidis* to 65 antibiotics. Antimicrob. Agents Chemother. 9:962–969.

ANTIMICROBIAL AGENTS AND CHEMOTHERAPY, June 1977, p. 968-973 Vol. 11, No. 6

Inhibition of Amino Acid Transport in *Escherichia coli* by Some Beta-Lactam Antibiotics

SCOTT V. ANDERSON[1] AND CLAIRE M. BERG*

Biological Sciences Group (U-131), The University of Connecticut, Storrs, Connecticut 06268

Received for publication 8 March 1977

Among 10 antibiotics tested, cephaloridine and cephalothin showed the greatest inhibition of proline active transport. Ethylenediaminetetraacetate pretreatment of the cells did not enhance inhibition by any of these 10 antibiotics. The inhibition of active transport of 10 additional amino acids by cephaloridine and cephalothin was studied. Both antibiotics inhibited transport of three amino acids which, like proline, have transport systems resistant to osmotic shock; neither antibiotic inhibited transport of the remaining amino acids, including three with shock-resistant and four with shock-sensitive systems.

Escherichia coli can concentrate proline several 1,000-fold against a concentration gradient (5, 9, 12). The proline transport system is highly stereospecific for L-proline (19) and displays biphasic kinetics with a high-affinity (K_m, 0.44 μM) and a low-affinity (K_m, 40 μM) component (12). The transport system is tightly bound to the cytoplasmic membrane: proline-binding activity is not normally released into the medium when cells are subjected to osmotic shock (2), and active transport activity is retained in membrane vesicle preparations (8).

Amino acid transport systems in bacteria have been classified into two categories: osmotic shock resistant (e.g., proline, phenylalanine, alanine, aspartic acid, glycine, serine, and tyrosine) and osmotic shock sensitive (e.g., leucine, arginine, histidine, and glutamine) (13, 16). Unlike the shock-resistant transport systems, the shock-sensitive systems are not tightly bound to the membrane; they are released upon osmotic shock and are generally absent from membrane vesicle preparations.

As a part of our studies of the effects of antibiotics that inhibit the synthesis of cell walls upon proline metabolism in *Escherichia coli* (3, 17, 18), we investigated their effect on proline transport. Several different β-lactam antibiotics that had been reported to bind specific components of the bacterial cell wall (20) were tested. Several that were found to inhibit proline transport were further tested for their effects on the transport of a number of other amino acids.

MATERIALS AND METHODS

Bacterial strain. *E. coli* K-12 W3110 (*thy*$^-$) was used throughout (17).

[1] Present address: Box HC 380, The University of Connecticut Health Center, Farmington, CT 06032.

Media and growth conditions. Vogel and Bonner medium E plus glucose (0.5%), thymine (10 μg/ml), and thiamine (1 μg/ml) was used as the growth medium (17). Overnight cultures were grown in the same medium with limiting (0.05%) glucose.

Chemicals. The antibiotics employed were: potassium penicillin G (citrate buffered or unbuffered) (Squibb); mecillinam (FL1060) (Leo); ampicillin and 6-aminopenicillanic acid (Bristol); D-cycloserine (Sigma); and cephaloridine, cephalothin, cephalexin, cephazolin, and cephalosporin C (Lilly). Stock solutions in water were made just before use at 200 mM.

[U-^{14}C]proline, [U-^{14}C]phenylalanine, [U-^{14}C]-arginine, [U-^{14}C]leucine, [U-^{14}C]histidine, and [U-^{14}C]glutamine were obtained from New England Nuclear Corp. These were diluted in water with unlabeled amino acid (Sigma) to 10^{-5} M at a specific activity of 200 Ci/mol. [U-^{14}C]alanine, [U-^{14}C]aspartic acid, [U-^{14}C]glycine, [U-^{14}C]serine, and [U-^{14}C]tyrosine were obtained from Amersham/Searle. These were diluted in water to 10^{-5} M with specific activities ranging from 50 to 225 Ci/mol, depending on the amino acid. L-Amino acids were used throughout. [5-^{3}H]uridine was obtained from Schwarz/Mann.

Actinomycin D was from Sigma. Ethylenediaminetetraacetate (EDTA), methylethyl ketone, propionic acid, pyridine, and tris(hydroxymethyl)-aminomethane (Tris) were from Fisher Scientific. Econofluor was from New England Nuclear Corp.

Transport assay. Overnight cultures were centrifuged, resuspended at about 5×10^8 cells/ml in fresh growth medium, incubated for 30 to 60 min, and harvested in logarithmic growth by quick chilling to 0°C. Cell titer was determined by optical density measurement at 420 nm in a spectrophotometer (Bausch and Lomb Spectronic 20).

From a logarithmically growing culture, 1.7 ml was incubated for 2 min at 25°C in a shaking water bath, followed by addition of 0.1 ml of antibiotic solution (10 mM, final concentration), pyridine (1 mM, final concentration), or distilled water. Thirty seconds later, the transport reaction was initiated by addition of 0.2 ml of labeled amino acid solution (final concentration, 1×10^{-6} M, except where noted). Samples, 0.2 ml, were withdrawn at 10-s intervals and vacuum-filtered on 0.45-μm-pore-size nitrocellulose membrane filters (1). These were immediately washed with four 0.5-ml volumes of medium at room temperature. Filters were dried and counted in an Isocap 300 (Nuclear Chicago) scintillation counter.

EDTA treatment. Approximately 2×10^{10} cells were washed twice at room temperature with 10-ml volumes of 0.12 M Tris buffer, pH 8.0 (adjusted with HCl), centrifuged, resuspended in 4 ml of 0.5 mM EDTA in the same buffer, and incubated for 2 min at 37°C with shaking. EDTA treatment was stopped by addition of 30 ml of medium at 37°C. The cells were then centrifuged and resuspended at approximately 5×10^8 cells per ml in fresh medium. They were kept for up to 2 h at 0°C for use in the transport assay. Permeability changes were monitored by actinomycin D inhibition of ribonucleic acid synthesis as described by Leive (10), except that [5-^{3}H]uridine was used in place of [1-^{14}C]uracil.

Thin-layer chromatography of cephaloridine with proline and phenylalanine. [^{14}C]proline or [^{14}C]phenylalanine (1×10^{-5} M) was incubated for 1 h at 37°C with or without 10 mM cephaloridine, and then 0.55 ml was spotted on an oven-dried silica gel Chromagram sheet (Kodak) and developed for 3.5 h with a methylethyl ketone-propionic acid-water solvent system (6). The sheet was air-dried and cut into 1-cm squares, and the radioactivity in the squares was counted.

RESULTS

Screening of antibiotics. In screening for inhibition of initial rate of proline active transport, 6-aminopenicillanic acid, D-cycloserine, buffered penicillin G, unbuffered penicillin G, and ampicillin were found to cause little or no inhibition (0, 8, 7, 8, and 14%, respectively), whereas cephalexin caused 24%, mecillinan caused 34%, and cephaloridine caused 71% inhibition of proline transport (Fig. 1).

Because the most significant inhibition of proline transport was found with cephaloridine, three additional cephalosporin antibiotics were

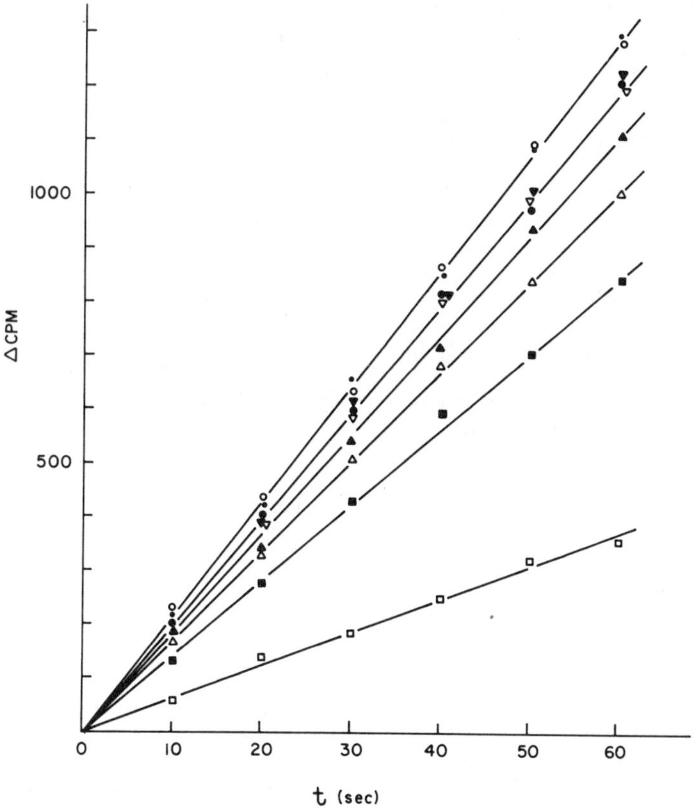

FIG. 1. *Effect of various antibiotics on the initial rate of proline active transport. Additions:* (·) *water,* (○) *6-aminopenicillanic acid,* (●) *unbuffered penicillin G,* (▼) *buffered penicillin G,* (▽) *D-cycloserine,* (▲) *ampicillin;* (△) *cephalexin,* (■) *mecillinam,* (□) *cephaloridine. Ampicillin and 6-aminopenicillanic acid were added as suspensions because they were not completely dissolved at the stock concentrations. Counts extrapolated to zero time were between 120 and 200.*

tested. Cephazolin, cephalosporin C, and cephalothin inhibited the initial rate of proline transport 14, 22, and 40%, respectively.

Kinetics of transport inhibition by cephaloridine. The Dixon plot (7) of cephaloridine inhibition of proline active transport yields a K_i of approximately 5 mM (Fig. 2), indicating that cephaloridine is a very weak inhibitor of proline transport. Nevertheless, the double reciprocal plots suggest a competitive type of inhibition of the high-affinity transport system (Fig. 3).

Basis of transport inhibition. Since the outer membrane of gram-negative bacteria is permeable to cephaloridine and cephalothin but not to many other antibiotics (15), inhibition of proline transport by various antibiotics in cells treated with EDTA (which increases the permeability of the outer membrane) was compared with that obtained in untreated cells. The results indicate that EDTA treatment does not significantly enhance transport inhibition by penicillin G, ampicillin, mecillinam, cephaloridine, cephalothin, cephalexin, cephalosporin C, or cephazolin (data not shown). Therefore, the pattern of inhibition is not due to differences in permeability.

It has been suggested (G. Hite, personal communication) that proline might be acylated by cephaloridine, thus lowering the effective proline concentration in the medium and reducing the apparent initial rate of proline transport. To test this, labeled proline and cephaloridine were incubated together, and the presence of a reaction product was assayed by thin-layer chromatography. All of the radioactivity remained in the proline peak, indicating that there is no direct reaction between cephaloridine and proline.

The primary decomposition product of cephaloridine is pyridine (R. Hosley, personal communication). Pyridine at 1 mM was found to have no effect upon the initial rate of proline transport (data not shown). To test the possibility that some other cephalosporin breakdown product is responsible for the inhibition of proline transport, stock solutions were incubated at 37°C for 68 h before use in proline transport assays (Table 1). The inhibition by cephalosporin C, cephalothin, and cephazolin increased,

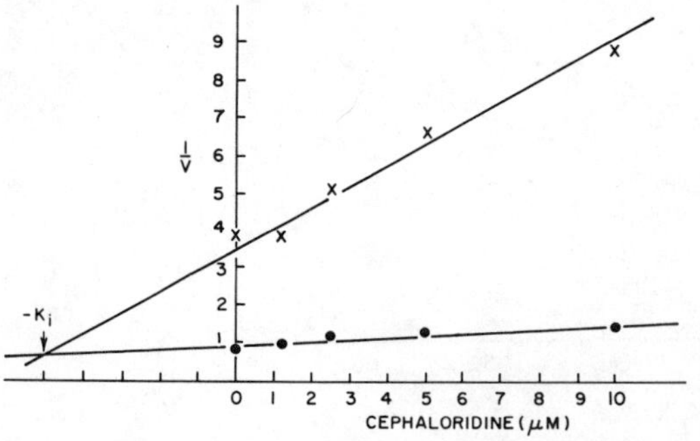

FIG. 2. *Dixon plot of cephaloridine inhibition of initial rate of proline active transport. [¹⁴C]proline was used at 10^{-5} M (●) and 10^{-6} M (×) final concentrations.*

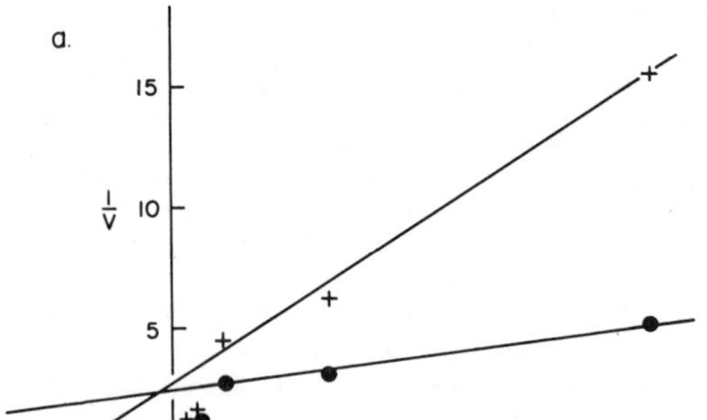

FIG. 3. *Double reciprocal plots of cephaloridine inhibition of initial rate of proline active transport. Symbols: (+) with cephaloridine (10^{-2} M), (●) without cephaloridine. (a) High-affinity system (10^{-6} to 10^{-5} M); (b) low-affinity system (10^{-5} to 10^{-4} M).*

TABLE 1. *Inhibition of initial rate of proline active transport by heat-treated cephalosporin antibiotics*

Antibiotic	Inhibition (%)		Treated/fresh
	Fresh	Treated	
Cephaloridine	72.5	70.5	0.97
Cephalothin sodium	39.8	57.8	1.45
Cephalexin	27.4	27.6	1.01
Cephalosporin C	22.2	52.0	2.34
Cephazolin sodium	13.9	22.3	1.60

indicating that a breakdown product is involved. The inhibition by cephaloridine and cephalexin was, however, not affected by heat treatment. Since an assay (provided to us by R. Hosley) of the batch of cephaloridine we used revealed no contaminant other than acetone (0.12%), cephaloridine itself appears to inhibit proline transport.

Specificity of inhibition. The inhibition by cephaloridine and cephalothin of the initial rates of active transport of proline and 10 other amino acids was assayed (Table 2). Cephaloridine inhibited proline transport, and, to a lesser extent, tyrosine, phenylalanine, and glycine transport. Six other amino acid systems were not significantly inhibited, and aspartic acid transport was marginally stimulated. The pattern for cephalothin inhibition is generally similar, although there is less inhibition of proline and of glycine transport, and aspartic acid transport is unaffected.

DISCUSSION

The active transport system for proline is highly stereospecific for L-isomers. In addition, structural features essential for a compound to inhibit proline transport include both a secondary amine and the carbonyl portion of the carboxyl group at position 2 on the pyrrolidine ring (19). These constraints would seem to rule out any direct effect of the β-lactam antibiotics on proline transport since the antibiotics contain an amide rather than a secondary amine, and, in penicillins, the configuration alpha to the carboxyl group is D, whereas in cephalosporins there is no comparable center of asymmetry. However, the competitive-type inhibition of proline active transport by cephaloridine suggests that either the antibiotic itself competes, with a low affinity, directly with proline transport, or there is an undetected impurity structurally analogous to proline.

Structural comparison of the cephalosporins (Fig. 4) suggests that the thiophene-acetyl group (R_1) shared by both cephaloridine and cephalothin and the pyridine group (R_2) of cephaloridine might both contribute to inhibition of proline transport. Unfortunately, we were unable to assay the effect on proline transport of a third thiophene-acetyl R_1-substituted cephalosporin (cephalonium) because it was too poorly soluble in water to be tested under the conditions employed. We were unable to obtain any other thiopheneacetyl R_1-substituted nor any pyridine R_2-substituted cephalosporins (such as cephalosporin C_A-pyridine). Consequently, the relative roles of the thiopheneacetyl and the pyridine substituents upon the inhibition of proline transport could not be tested further.

Although inhibition by cephaloridine is not affected by prolonged incubation at 37°C, inhibition by several other cephalosporin antibiotics is increased (Table 1) and may be due, at least partially, to a decomposition product.

When the effect of cephaloridine and cephalothin upon the transport of 10 additional amino acids was tested, we found that there was substantial inhibition of only tyrosine, phenylalanine, and glycine (Table 2). It is noteworthy that these three amino acids, like proline, all

TABLE 2. *Effects of cephaloridine and cephalothin on the initial rate of amino acid active transport*

Amino acid	No. of determinations	Initial rate[a]: Additions: None	Cephaloridine	Cephalothin	% Inhibition by: Cephaloridine	Cephalothin
Shock resistant						
Proline	9	0.443 ± 0.048	0.139 ± 0.019	0.285 ± 0.023	68.6	35.7
Tyrosine	2	0.888 ± 0.078	0.440 ± 0.035	0.376 ± 0.057	50.5	57.7
Phenylalanine	3	0.806 ± 0.038	0.434 ± 0.027	0.465 ± 0.017	46.2	42.3
Glycine	2	0.480 ± 0.045	0.283 ± 0.020	0.388 ± 0.033	41.0	19.2
Serine	3	1.604 ± 0.107	1.480 ± 0.072	1.482 ± 0.030	7.7	7.6
Alanine	2	0.674 ± 0.080	0.630 ± 0.105	0.618 ± 0.067	6.5	8.3
Aspartic acid	2	0.619 ± 0.003	0.695 ± 0.029	0.616 ± 0.030	−12.3	0.4
Shock sensitive						
Arginine	2	0.676 ± 0.010	0.599 ± 0.002	0.638 ± 0.020	11.4	5.6
Glutamine	4	0.962 ± 0.157	0.862 ± 0.099	0.941 ± 0.091	10.4	2.2
Histidine	4	0.224 ± 0.026	0.204 ± 0.007	0.199 ± 0.025	8.9	11.2
Leucine	2	1.556 ± 0.044	1.552 ± 0.037	1.545 ± 0.073	0.3	0.7

[a] Picomoles per minute per 10^9 cells.

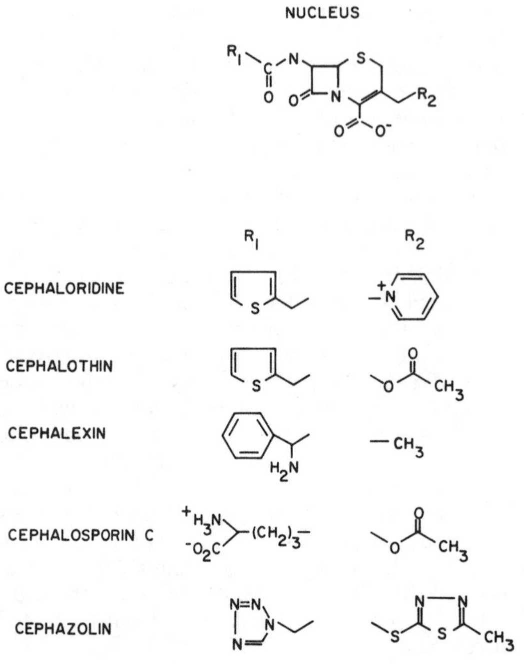

FIG. 4. *Structures of the cephalosporins used (cephalothin and cephazolin were obtained in the form of sodium salts).*

have shock-resistant transport systems (16) and that transport of the four amino acids tested which have shock-sensitive transport systems was not significantly inhibited by either antibiotic. The correlation between shock-resistant transport and antibiotic inhibition is not, however, perfect since transport of three additional amino acids with shock-resistant transport systems was not significantly inhibited by the antibiotics.

E. coli K-12 possesses a low β-lactamase-cephalosporinase activity (11), which is probably responsible for its resistance to low levels of β-lactam antibiotics (4). Although we have not directly tested the effect of this enzyme upon the observed inhibition of amino acid transport, it does not appear that β-lactamase activity can account for our results. For, if antibiotic hydrolysis products were inhibitory, the inhibitor would accumulate during the assay period, and nonlinear transport kinetics would be expected. Similarly, antibiotic inactivation by a β-lactamase would cause nonlinear kinetics. Since we observed linear inhibition of proline transport (Fig. 1), the inhibitory species appears to be present before exposure of the antibiotic to any cellular β-lactamase.

Although some efforts have been directed to finding new antibiotics capable of selective inhibition of bacterial transport systems (21), this represents the first report of bacterial amino acid transport inhibition by any β-lactam antibiotic. Since these antibiotics are not obvious structural analogues of any of the amino acids whose transport was tested, our results were unexpected. It is possible that proline, tyrosine, phenylalanine, and glycine belong to a transport subclass whose membrane recognition site possesses some feature(s) in common with the cephalosporin recognition site.

ACKNOWLEDGMENTS

This work was supported by Public Health Service grant AI-10862 from the National Institutes of Allergy and Infectious Diseases and a grant from The University of Connecticut Research Foundation to C.M.B.

We are indebted to Bristol Laboratories (Syracuse), Leo Laboratories (Ballerup, Denmark), Lilly Laboratories (Indianapolis), and Squibb Laboratories (Princeton) for their generous gifts of antibiotics. In addition, we thank R. Hosley of Lilly Laboratories for technical information. Many helpful discussions with G. Hite, J. Knox, J. Rossi, F. Vasington and J. Vender are also gratefully acknowledged.

LITERATURE CITED

1. **Anderson, S. V., C. M. Berg, and J. J. Rossi.** 1975. An inexpensive membrane filtration manifold. Anal. Biochem. 69:655–656.
2. **Anraku, Y.** 1971. Studies on amino acid binding proteins of *Escherichia coli*. J. Biochem. 69:243–245.
3. **Berg, C. M., and S. V. Anderson.** 1976. Penicillin-induced lysis of *Escherichia coli* in medium that does not support sustained growth. Antimicrob. Agents Chemother. 9:713–715.
4. **Boman, H. G., K. Nordström, and S. Normark.** 1974. Penicillin resistance in *E. coli* K-12: synergism between penicillinases and a barrier in the outer part of the envelope. Ann. N.Y. Acad. Sci. 235:569–586.
5. **Britten, R. J., and F. T. McClure.** 1962. The amino acid pool in *Escherichia coli*. Bacteriol. Rev. 26:292–335.
6. **Clayton, R. A., and F. M. Strong.** 1954. New solvent system for separation of amino acids by paper chromatography. Anal. Chem. 26:1362–1363.
7. **Dixon, M., and E. C. Webb.** 1964. Enzymes, 2nd ed. Academic Press Inc., New York.
8. **Kaback, H. R., and T. F. Deuel.** 1969. Proline uptake by disrupted membrane preparations from *Escherichia coli*. Arch. Biochem. Biophys. 132:118–129.
9. **Kaback, H. R., and E. R. Stadtman.** 1966. Proline uptake by an isolated cytoplasmic membrane preparation of *Escherichia coli*. Proc. Natl. Acad. Sci. U.S.A. 55:920–927.
10. **Leive, L.** 1968. Studies on the permeability change produced in coliform bacteria by ethylenediaminetetraacetate. J. Biol. Chem. 243:2373–2380.
11. **Lindstrom, E. B., H. G. Boman, and B. B. Steele.** 1970. Resistance of *E. coli* to penicillins. J. Bacteriol. 101:218–231.
12. **Morikawa, A., H. Suzuki, and Y. Anraku.** 1974. Transport of sugars and amino acids in bacteria. VIII. Properties and regulation of the active transport reaction of proline in *Escherichia coli*. J. Biochem. 75: 229–241.
13. **Neu, H. C., and L. A. Heppel.** 1965. The release of enzymes from *Escherichia coli* by osmotic shock and during the formation of spheroplasts. J. Biol. Chem. 240:3685–3692.
14. **O'Callaghan, C., and P. W. Muggelton.** 1972. Biologi-

cal reactions of cephalosporins and penicillins, p. 438–495. *In* E. H. Flynn (ed.), Cephalosporins and penicillins—chemistry and biology. Academic Press Inc., New York.
15. **Richmond, M. H., and R. B. Sykes.** 1973. The β-lactamases of gram-negative bacteria and their possible physiological role, p. 31–85. *In* A. H. Rose and D. W. Tempest (ed.), Advances in microbial physiology, vol. 9. Academic Press Inc., New York.
16. **Rosen, B. P., and L. A. Heppel.** 1973. Present status of binding proteins that are released from gram-negative bacteria by osmotic shock, p. 209–239. *In* L. Leive (ed.), Bacterial membranes and walls. Marcel Dekker Inc., New York.
17. **Rossi, J. J., and C. M. Berg.** 1971. Differential recovery of auxotrophs after penicillin enrichment in *Escherichia coli*. J. Bacteriol. **106**:297–300.
18. **Rossi, J. J., and C. M. Berg.** 1975. Effect of enrichment procedure upon auxotroph recovery in *Escherichia coli* K-12. Antimicrob. Agents Chemother. **7**:110–112.
19. **Rowland, I., and H. Tristram.** 1975. Specificity of the *Escherichia coli* proline transport system. J. Bacteriol. **123**:871–877.
20. **Spratt, B.** 1975. Distinct penicillin binding proteins involved in the division, elongation, and shape of *Escherichia coli* K-12. Proc. Natl. Acad. Sci. U.S.A. **72**:2999–3003.
21. **Walsh, C. T., and H. R. Kaback.** 1974. Membrane transport as a potential target for antibiotic action. Ann. N.Y. Acad. Sci. **235**:519–541.

ANTIMICROBIAL AGENTS AND CHEMOTHERAPY, June 1977, p. 974–977
Vol. 11, No. 6

Distribution of Gentamicin and Amikacin in Rabbit Tissues

MARGARET L. KORNGUTH* AND CALVIN M. KUNIN

Veterans Administration Hospital and the Department of Medicine, University of Wisconsin School of Medicine, Madison, Wisconsin 53706.*

Received for publication 24 January 1977

Rabbits were injected intramuscularly with gentamicin and amikacin (15 mg of base per kg), and the antibiotic levels in tissues were determined 20 h after either a single or multiple injections. Disk diffusion assays, with *Bacillus subtilis* ATCC 6633, were carried out both on homogenates and on supernatants deproteinized with trichloroacetic acid. Both assays indicated that the kidney is the major site of antibiotic deposition. Antibiotic levels increased after multiple doses. Gentamicin levels in other tissues were higher than those of amikacin. The assay of trichloroacetic acid-treated material was more sensitive than the assay of the total homogenate.

Aminoglycoside antibiotics are used extensively for the treatment of severe bacterial infections. Several studies have indicated that these antibiotics reach peak levels in serum within several hours of administration and subsequently decline, whereas high levels in the kidney persist much longer (1–4, 9–11).

Usually, tissue aminoglycoside levels are assayed by disk diffusion techniques. The amount of drug in the tissue is extrapolated from the standard curve of the drug in buffer or in control tissue homogenate. Since aminoglycosides become partially bound to tissue macromolecules and thus inactivated (7), the assay with the standard curve in buffer measures only the free drug. The assay with the standard in the homogenate presumably corrects for the bound portion of the drug in tissue and thus gives a better estimate of the total drug. An alternative method is to dissociate the bound antibiotic by a chemical method and subsequently assay the total drug.

The present study reports on the assay of two aminoglycosides, gentamicin and amikacin, in rabbit tissues after a single and multiple injections. The antibiotics were assayed in tissue homogenates directly and in the homogenate supernatants after trichloroacetic acid precipitation of protein. A comparison of the results from these two methods is presented as well as data regarding the binding of these antibiotics by the tissue homogenates in vitro.

MATERIALS AND METHODS

Materials. Gentamicin sulfate (Garamycin, injectable; 40 mg/ml) was obtained from Schering Corp., Kenilworth, N.J. Amikacin (BB-K8) was obtained from Bristol Laboratories, Syracuse, N.Y. (lot no. 76F 1598 and 76F 439). It was dissolved in sterile saline to give 40 mg of amikacin base per ml.

Administration of antibiotics in vivo. Male and female white rabbits (Klubertanz, Edgerton, Wis.), varying in weight from 1.6 to 2.4 kg, were divided in groups of three rabbits each. They had free access to water and were fed Purina Rabbit Chow Checkers W. The rabbits in each group received either a single injection or seven daily injections of gentamicin or amikacin, 15 mg/kg, in the hind leg muscle. The control group received an equivalent volume of saline. Sterile techniques were used throughout these manipulations. In experiments in which antibiotic levels in tissues other than kidney were measured, one experimental group and the controls were injected. In kidney experiments, both gentamicin and amikacin groups, as well as the controls, were injected simultaneously.

Preparation of tissue homogenates. Twenty hours after the last injection, blood was removed from each rabbit by cardiac puncture, and the animal was sacrificed by cervical dislocation. The following tissues were removed and placed on ice in sterile cups: kidney, liver, lung, heart, brain, and hind leg skeletal muscle from the side opposite the injection. The tissues were minced and homogenized in 3 volumes of 0.25 M sucrose-0.01 M tris(hydroxymethyl)aminomethane buffer, pH 7.4 (25%, wt/vol, homogenate), with a Potter-Elvehjem homogenizer. The homogenates were filtered through cheesecloth and then used in the microbiological assay. Three additional dilutions of the experimental kidney homogenates were made with control kidney homogenates. One additional dilution of experimental urine with control urine was also made. Blood samples were allowed to clot at room temperature for 2 h. Sera were obtained after centrifugation at 1,000 × g for 20 min. Urine was withdrawn from rabbit bladders after sacrifice. Most of the urine samples were alkaline and required the addition of 1 N HCl to lower the pH to 7.4. Protein in tissue homogenates was determined by the Lowry procedure (8).

Trichloroacetic acid precipitation. To 2-ml portions of tissue homogenates, 0.2 ml of concentrated trichloroacetic acid (Sigma, St. Louis, Mo.) was added. The tubes were mixed vigorously on a Vortex mixer and then centrifuged at 1,000 × *g* for 15 min. Portions, 1 ml each, of the supernatants were transferred to a new set of tubes, and each sample was adjusted to pH 7 to 8 (Beckman Zeromatic pH meter, model SS-3, equipped with a combination electrode) by the addition of NaOH. Assay of control samples at pH 7 and 8 indicated that there was no significant difference in antimicrobial activity at these two pH values.

Tissue homogenates from control rabbits were incubated with four different concentrations of either gentamicin or amikacin (2.5 to 20 μg/ml; twofold dilutions) at 25°C for 30 min and then treated with trichloroacetic acid as described above. The microbiological assay of these samples provided the standard curves from which the antibiotic levels of the experimental trichloroacetic acid-treated samples were extrapolated. No correction was made for the small increase in volume caused by the addition of trichloroacetic acid and base, because all the samples, experimental as well as standards, were treated identically.

Microbiological assay. Disk diffusion assays were carried out as described by Grove and Randall (6). *B. subtilis* ATCC 6633 was the assay organism, and antibiotic medium no. 5 (BBL, Div. of Becton, Dickinson & Co., Cockeysville, Md.) was used to prepare the bilayered plates. The top layer was prepared from 5 ml of the seeded inoculum. Disks were saturated with the test solution, placed on the agar, and incubated overnight at 37°C. The zones of inhibition were recorded the following morning. All assays for each experiment were carried out simultaneously, and the agar plates were prepared on the day of the experiment.

Each experiment included the following test solutions: (i) tissue homogenates from each of the injected rabbits; (ii) four concentrations (2.5, 5, 10, and 20 μg/ml) of gentamicin or amikacin or both in tissue homogenates from control rabbits for the construction of standard curves; (iii) trichloroacetic acid-treated homogenate supernatants from each of the injected rabbits; (iv) trichloroacetic acid-treated homogenates containing gentamicin and amikacin for standard curves (see Trichloroacetic acid precipitation); (v) control samples of homogenates, trichloroacetic acid supernatants, urine, and sera from uninjected rabbits; (vi) dilutions of gentamicin and amikacin in homogenization buffer and in trichloroacetic acid-treated buffer for standard curves.

The antibiotic level of an experimental homogenate or trichloroacetic acid supernatant was extrapolated from the standard curve (zone size versus the log of antibiotic concentration) corresponding to that particular tissue and treatment. All dilutions of kidney homogenates and of urine were assayed, and the mean values were calculated. Standard curves in homogenization buffer and in trichloroacetic acid-treated buffer were included in each experiment to provide reference points for the other standard curves in which homogenates and trichloroacetic acid supernatants were used as diluents. The percent activity was calculated from these data.

RESULTS

Tissue levels of antibiotics after in vivo administration. Gentamicin and amikacin levels in tissues from injected rabbits were assayed both in the homogenates and in trichloroacetic acid-deproteinized supernatants. The data, derived by either method, indicated that kidney was the major site of antibiotic deposition and that the drug levels increased after multiple injections (Table 1). After a single injection, amikacin was found only in kidney and in urine; gentamicin concentrations in kidney and

TABLE 1. *Antibiotic levels in rabbit tissues after a single and repeated injections*

Tissue	Concn in tissues (μg/g of tissue)[a]							
	Single injection				Seven daily injections			
	Gentamicin		Amikacin		Gentamicin		Amikacin	
	Homogenate	Trichloroacetic acid supernatant	Homogenate	Trichloroacetic acid supernatant	Homogenate	Trichloroacetic acid supernatant	Homogenate	Trichloroacetic acid supernatant
Kidney	70 ± 11	110 ± 54	56 ± 41	50 ± 19	135 ± 65	214 ± 70	84 ± 36	169 ± 74
Liver	0	10 ± 5	0	0	18 ± 5.5	24.5 ± 14	1.7 ± 3	9 ± 3
Heart	0	3 ± 3	0	0	5.8 ± 0.3	22 ± 14	1 ± 2	4.3 ± 2
Lung	5 ± 1.4	6 ± 5	0	0	7.2 ± 1	23 ± 10	0.4 ± 0.7	3 ± 2
Brain	0	0	0	0	0	15 ± 10	0	0
Muscle	0	0	0	0	0	6 ± 4	0	2 ± 4
Serum	0.8 ± 0.9		0		0.5 ± 0.7		0.2 ± 0.3	
Urine	26 ± 14		8.0 ± 8.5		36 ± 7		10.3 ± 2	

[a] Numbers represent the mean antibiotic concentration ± standard deviation. In kidney experiments nine rabbits were used, except for gentamicin, single injection, in which there were eight rabbits. For all other tissues the data are presented for three rabbits.

urine were higher than those of amikacin, and in addition it was detected in lung, heart, and liver by the trichloroacetic acid procedure. After seven daily injections, the kidney levels of both antibiotics were not significantly different; however, again higher amounts of gentamicin were present in the other tissues.

The trichloroacetic acid supernatant procedure was more sensitive than the homogenate procedure in detecting small amounts of antibiotics in tissues other than kidney; in addition, it indicated significantly higher levels of both antibiotics in kidney after multiple injections (gentamicin, $P < 0.05$; amikacin, $P < 0.001$). The difference in the two methods with respect to the kidney was not observed after a single injection.

Effect of tissue homogenates on antimicrobial activity. Homogenates of the rabbit tissues inhibited the activity of amikacin and gentamicin as compared with the homogenization buffer alone (Table 2). This is consistent with the aminoglycoside-binding capacity of homogenates previously reported from this laboratory (7). With liver and kidney homogenates, the lowest percentage of remaining antimicrobial activity was observed. Considering the inhibitory effect in relation to the protein content, it was apparent that no one tissue was more effective than another in binding these drugs in vitro. Serum, on a unit protein basis, was less effective as a binder than the other tissues.

Urine as a diluent consistently augmented the activity of gentamicin and amikacin. Control urine samples did not produce any zones of inhibition, thus eliminating the possibility that endogenous antibacterial compounds were responsible for this enhancement. The careful pH adjustment of all samples before assay eliminated this factor as a variable.

Addition of trichloroacetic acid to the homogenates previously incubated with the antibiotics resulted in the precipitation of protein and in the recovery of the antimicrobials in the supernatant solution (Table 2). Full recovery was obtained with kidney and most other homogenates. Reduced recovery of amikacin was observed with heart and skeletal muscle tissue, which may be related to difficulties of homogenizing these fibrous tissues.

DISCUSSION

The present study indicates that kidney is the site of amikacin as well as gentamicin deposition in rabbits. This is similar to data previously reported for gentamicin in dogs, rats, and man (1, 3, 9) and more recently for amikacin in man (5).

The mode of deposition of aminoglycoside antibiotics is of particular interest because of their nephrotoxic potential. They are excreted mainly by glomerular filtration, but some reabsorption takes place in the proximal tubule, the major portion of which is located in the cortex (3). Thus, a certain cell population is exposed to high levels of the antibiotics. As this process continues, more subcellular organelles and more binding sites may be affected, finally leading to alteration of morphology and function. The identification of the subcellular organelles and the specific macromolecules responsible for binding of the aminoglycosides would be helpful in understanding their mode of accumulation and their potential toxicity.

Amikacin at equal doses tended to accumu-

TABLE 2. *Effect of rabbit tissue homogenates on antimicrobial activity of gentamicin and amikacin*

Diluent	Remaining antimicrobial activity (%)[a]: Homogenates		Remaining antimicrobial activity (%)[a]: Trichloroacetic acid supernatants		Protein in 25% homogenates (mg/ml)
	Gentamicin	Amikacin	Gentamicin	Amikacin	
Buffer	100	100	100	100	0
Kidney	59.0 ± 19.1	66.5 ± 13.9	100.9 ± 25.4	100.6 ± 16.8	42
Liver	41.0 ± 4.7	45.0 ± 17.3	95.5 ± 5.2	87.2 ± 19.0	48
Heart	82.0 ± 7.9	68.3 ± 0.6	87.0 ± 9.6	72.7 ± 17.0	21
Lung	75.0 ± 1.0	68.7 ± 31.5	101.0 ± 9.0	91.0 ± 15.7	28
Brain	68.0 ± 10.7	72.5 ± 20.7	94.8 ± 18.6	86.5 ± 31.7	31
Muscle	77.7 ± 4.5	68.7 ± 22.5	94.7 ± 6.4	69.3 ± 20.5	25
Serum	77.0 ± 20.5	74.6 ± 20.1	109.2 ± 23.4	85.6 ± 11.8	57
Urine	288.0 ± 102	138.4 ± 40.3			

[a] Results are expressed as percentage of antimicrobial activity in each diluent ± standard deviation; for kidney, $n = 8$; serum, $n = 5$; liver, brain, and urine, $n = 4$; heart, lung, brain, and muscle, $n = 3$. Antimicrobial activity in buffer, 0.25 M sucrose–0.01 M tris(hydroxymethyl)aminomethane-hydrochloride, pH 7.4, or in trichloroacetic acid-treated, neutralized buffer was set at 100% in each experiment.

late less than gentamicin in kidney after a single injection and in other tissues both after single and multiple injections. It is difficult, however, to extrapolate these findings to toxicity in man because of species differences, lack of direct information that tissue binding is related to toxicity, and the fact that higher doses of amikacin are recommended for treatment of infection.

This report also compares the utility of two assay procedures. Antibiotic deposition in tissues is most frequently determined with the aid of standard curves in the corresponding diluent, i.e., tissue homogenates. The assumption underlying this method is that even if part of the drug is tissue bound, this effect will be corrected by the standard curve, and a quantitative assessment of the total antibiotic will be obtained. In the present study we have used this method for the determination of gentamicin and amikacin levels in tissues, but in addition we have used trichloroacetic acid to obtain protein-free supernatants. Since most of drug-protein interactions are noncovalent in character and reversible, denaturation and precipitation of protein lead to release of the bound drug into the supernatant. This method is particularly applicable to aminoglycosides because of their stability.

Theoretically, both methods should give identical results, assuming that the addition of the drug in vitro to the homogenates (used for standard curves) is equivalent to drug-tissue interactions in vivo (experimental homogenates). In the present study, similar drug levels in the kidney were found by either method after a single injection. After multiple injections, the trichloroacetic acid method gave significantly higher results, suggesting the possibility that, after prolonged administration, both gentamicin and amikacin become sequestered in a manner such that the in vitro standard curves did not correct for the in vivo binding.

ACKNOWLEDGMENTS

This work was supported by the Medical Research Service of the Veterans Administration and by Bristol Laboratories, Syracuse, N.Y.

We wish to thank Christine Gordon, James Stephens, and Ann Bugg for excellent technical assistance.

LITERATURE CITED

1. **Alfthan, O., O. V. Renkonen, and A. Sivonen.** 1973. Concentration of gentamicin in serum, urine and urogenital tissue in man. Acta Pathol. Microbiol. Scand. Sect. B 81(Suppl. 241):S92–S94.
2. **Bodey, G. P., M. Valdivieso, R. Feld, and V. Rodriguez.** 1974. Pharmacology of amikacin in humans. Antimicrob. Agents Chemother. 5:508–512.
3. **Chiu, P. J. S., A. Brown, G. Miller, and J. F. Long.** 1976. Renal extraction of gentamicin in anesthetized dogs. Antimicrob. Agents Chemother. 10:227–282.
4. **Clarke, J. T., R. D. Libke, C. Regamey, and W. M. M. Kirby.** 1974. Comparative pharmacokinetics of amikacin and kanamycin. Clin. Pharmacol. Ther. 15:610–616.
5. **Edwards, C. Q., C. R. Smith, K. L. Baughman, J. F. Rogers, and P. S. Lietman.** 1976. Concentrations of gentamicin and amikacin in human kidneys. Antimicrob. Agents Chemother. 9:925–927.
6. **Grove, D. C., and W. A. Randall.** 1955. Assay methods of antibiotics: a laboratory manual, p. 34–36. Medical Encyclopedia, Inc., New York.
7. **Kunin, C. M.** 1970. Binding of antibiotics to tissue homogenates. J. Infect. Dis. 121:55–64.
8. **Lowry, O. H., N. J. Rosebrough, A. L. Farr, and R. J. Randall.** 1951. Protein measurement with the Folin phenol reagent. J. Biol. Chem. 193:265–275.
9. **Luft, F. C., and S. A. Kleit.** 1974. Renal parenchymal accumulation of aminoglycoside antibiotics in rats. J. Infect. Dis. 130:656–659.
10. **Luft, F. C., V. Patel, M. N. Yum, and S. A. Kleit.** 1976. Nephrotoxicity of cephalosporin-gentamicin combinations in rats. Antimicrob. Agents Chemother. 9:831–839.
11. **Winters, R. E., K. D. Litwack, and W. L. Hewitt.** 1971. Relation between dose and levels of gentamicin in blood. J. Infect. Dis. 124(Suppl.):S90–95.

ANTIMICROBIAL AGENTS AND CHEMOTHERAPY, June 1977, p. 978-983 Vol. 11, No. 6

Printed in U.S.A.

Altered Surface Properties of *Escherichia coli* Associated With a Specific Amino Acid Change in the S12 Ribosomal Protein of Streptomycin-Resistant Mutants

SIDNEY PESTKA,* HARRY WALTER, AND LAWRENCE G. WAYNE

Roche Institute of Molecular Biology, Nutley, New Jersey 07110; and Veterans Administration Hospital, Long Beach, California 90822

Received for publication 14 January 1977

Escherichia coli mutants resistant to streptomycin exhibited differences in countercurrent distribution from the parental strains. The degree of difference from the parental strain correlated with the degree of restriction of translation and thus the particular *strA* allele. The changes in countercurrent distribution in the phase systems used probably resulted predominantly from surface charge alterations. The differences in countercurrent distribution in these and other mutants may be a useful selective technique to obtain different types of mutants for which specific selective techniques may not be available. In addition, it appears that the surface properties of cells, which determine their position in countercurrent distribution, are a function of the translational efficiency and fidelity, and that the surface of cells consists of a mosaic that is an expression of this translational fidelity.

Alterations in ribosome structure have been shown to influence the fidelity of translation (5, 7). Specifically, alterations in ribosomal protein S12, which is modified in streptomycin-resistant strains, modify translational fidelity. Although numerous studies suggested that translational fidelity is altered physiologically in these strains, only few studies presented evidence that miscoded amino acids were incorporated into proteins as substitutions for the proper amino acids (3, 4, 19, 23).

The surface properties of *Escherichia coli* cells represent a product of the contributions of numerous proteins and other cell components. Thus, it might be expected that a systematic alteration in translational fidelity might be magnified and expressed as a change in surface properties. Modifications in this multicomponent system (cell surface) may therefore be detectable, whereas alterations in the individual components themselves may be small or negligible. In addition, if alterations of some ribosomal proteins are reflected in changes in surface properties, the surface differences might provide a useful, convenient, and potentially valuable selective technique to obtain a variety of mutants. A practical method for detecting subtle differences in surface charge of cells and for separating populations of cells with such differences is based on differential partition of cells betweeen two-polymer aqueous phases (27). Such a technique has already been employed to detect and separate an erythromycin-resistant mutant of *E. coli* from its sensitive parent by exploiting differences in surface charges (29). The studies described in this report were specifically designed to determine if mutants in ribosomal protein S12 exhibited altered surface properties detectable by partition in two-polymer aqueous phases.

MATERIALS AND METHODS

Bacterial strains. Parental and streptomycin-resistant strains of *E. coli* were generously supplied by L. Gorini and D. Elseviers (L44, L44-1, L44-2, L44-4, L44-6, L1, L1-401 and L1-431) and by H. Wittman (SM-1, SM-5, and SM-10). The parental and mutant strains used in this study are listed in Table 1.

Preparation of bacteria for countercurrent distribution. Cultures were grown overnight at 36°C in 7 ml of brain heart infusion broth prepared from the Difco product. A 2- to 3-ml amount of these cultures was inoculated into 60 ml of brain heart infusion broth in 500-ml nephelometric flasks and incubated at 36°C with occasional shaking. When the cultures were in mid-log growth, as determined by optical densities, they were rapidly chilled in an ice bath and centrifuged at 1,300 × g for 30 min at 5°C. The supernatant solution was discarded, and the cell pellet was suspended in a salt solution corresponding to that of the phase system to be used for countercurrent distribution (CCD). The suspension was centrifuged again, and the packed cells were taken up in a small volume of salt solution and transferred to graduated centrifuge tubes. After a third centrifugation, the cells were resuspended in the top phase of the system to be used and centrifuged once more. The packed cell volume was now noted and the cells were resuspended in the top phase as noted below.

Phase systems. Phase systems used were composed of dextran T500 (lot no. 5996, Pharmacia Fine Chemicals, Piscataway, N. J.) and polyethylene glycol (Carbowax 6000, Union Carbide, N. Y.) and appropriate buffer. Phase system I, used for *E. coli* K-12 strains, contained 5% (wt/wt) dextran, 4% (wt/wt) polyethylene glycol, and 0.08 M sodium phosphate buffer (composed of equimolar concentrations of mono- and dibasic sodium phosphates). Phase system II, used for *E. coli* B, contained 5% (wt/wt) dextran, 3.5% (wt/wt) polyethylene glycol and 0.01 M sodium phosphate buffer, pH 6.8. The phases were selected as described by Walter (27) so the partition coefficient of the cells would fall between 0.5 and 2.0. The need for a phase system with higher polymer and phosphate buffer concentrations for *E. coli* K-12 as compared with *E. coli* B indicates that the former has a higher surface charge than does the latter (27). The phases were mixed at 4 to 5°C and equilibrated in a separatory funnel overnight at 4 to 5°C. The top (polyethylene glycol-rich) and bottom (dextran-rich) phases were then separated.

Loading of thin-layer countercurrent apparatus. A thin-layer countercurrent distribution apparatus as described by Albertsson (1) with 120 cavities and a bottom-phase capacity of 0.7 ml was used (Incentive Research and Development AB, Bromma, Sweden). Approximately 0.05 to 0.07 ml of washed, packed *E. coli* was suspended in 1.9 ml of the top phase (load-mix) of the system to be used in CCD (either system I or II). Two mutants of *E. coli* to be compared by CCD were run simultaneously by loading the cells on opposite sides of the 120 cavity plates. Cavities 0 and 1 received 0.5 ml of the bottom phase and 0.9 ml of the load-mix containing the one mutant; cavities 60 and 61 similarly received 0.5 ml of bottom phase and 0.9 ml of the load-mix containing the second mutant. All other cavities received 0.6 ml of bottom phase and 0.8 ml of top phase. Cells were loaded in this manner to obtain a stationary interface (see reference 2 for further discussion). The cycle of operation consisted of shaking for 25 s and a settling time of 6 min, which was followed by a transfer. Sixty or 120 transfers were completed. Since the cells had a partition coefficient between 1.1 and 1.8, 120 transfers could be completed without overlap of the two mutants loaded on opposite sides of the CCD apparatus. Countercurrent distribution was performed at 4 to 5°C.

Collection of cells after CCD. The cells from each cavity of the countercurrent plates were collected directly into plastic centrifuge tubes. To convert the two-phase system into a single phase, 0.35 ml of water was added to each tube and, usually, two adjacent tubes were pooled, one skipped, two pooled, etc. The cell concentration in each tube was then determined by reading the absorbance of the cell suspensions at 540 nm with a Gilford spectrophotometer. The CCD distribution curves of mutants to be compared in a given run were normalized for better comparison of the data.

RESULTS

CCD curves obtained with parental and mutant strains run simultaneously for 60 to 120 transfers are illustrated in Fig. 1. It is apparent that there was a significant difference in the

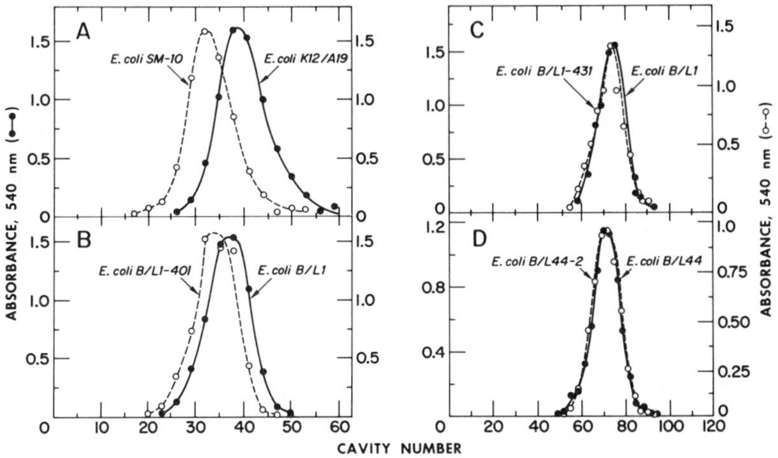

FIG. 1. *CCD patterns of selected E. coli parental strains (●) and mutants (○). E. coli depicted in A were run in phase system I; those shown in B, C, and D were run in phase system II. All CCDs were performed at 4 to 5°C. Sixty transfers were completed on cells shown in A and B and 120 transfers on those in C and D. The E. coli strains shown in each graph were run separately but simultaneously as described in the text. (A) E. coli K-12/A19 and SM-10; (B) E. coli B/L1 and L1-401; (C) E. coli B/L1 and L1-431; (D) E. coli B/L44 and L44-2. For other details see text.*

position of the parent *E. coli* K-12/A19 and *strA* mutant *E. coli* SM-10 curves (Fig. 1A), and parent *E. coli* B/L1 and *strA* mutant *E. coli* B/L1-401 (Fig. 1B). In each case the *strA* mutant had a lower partition coefficient than did the parent strain (that is, it is displaced to the left of the parent strain). Illustrated in Fig. 1C and D are parental and mutant strains showing no detectable differences in the position of the CCD curves even though the number of CCD transfers was increased to 120 to amplify any possible difference not readily seen after 60 transfers (*E. coli* B/L1 versus *E. coli* B/L1-431, Fig. 1C; *E. coli* B/L44 versus *E. coli* B/L44-2, Fig. 1D). It is noteworthy that the two parental strains (*E. coli* K-12/A19 and B/L1) had different surface properties, as reflected in the need to use different phase systems to center them in the CCD. The calculated, apparent partition coefficients for each of the *E. coli* parental strains and mutants are presented in Table 1.

All the *strA* mutants SM-1, SM-5, and SM-10 significantly differed from the parental *E. coli* K-12/A19 strain in apparent partition coefficient *G* (Table 1). Analogous *E. coli* B strains were examined. Of the four streptomycin-resistant mutants of *E. coli* B/L44 examined, none differed significantly in apparent partition coefficient from the parental strain. In addition, L1-401 had a different partition coefficient from the parent *E. coli* B/L1, whereas the streptomycin-resistant mutant L1-431 was not significantly different from the parental strain.

It is apparent that the same mutational alteration is not always reflected in the surface alterations of the cell. For example, the partition coefficients of mutants SM-10 and L1-401 (*strA1*) were markedly different from their respective parental strains. The alteration involves a replacement of lysine with asparagine in amino acid position 42 of the S12 protein (Table 1). In contrast, the same alteration in *E. coli* B/L44-1 produced no detectable change in the surface properties of this streptomycin-resistant mutant compared with the parental *E. coli* B/L44 strain. In addition, the interchange of lysine with arginine in position 87 as manifested in streptomycin-resistant mutants L44-4 and L1-431 produced no detectable alteration in their partition coefficients relative to that of the parental strains. In contrast to this, however, the same mutation in strain SM-1 produced an appreciable difference in the partition coefficient compared with that of the parental *E. coli* K-12/A19. The partition difference between mutant SM-5 and parent was smaller than that between the other mutations (SM-1 and SM-10). In general, the differences in apparent partition coefficient between mutant and parent strains were greater in the K-12 strains than in

TABLE 1. *Strains of E. coli subjected to countercurrent distribution and the G values observed*

Parental strain	Mutant	*strA* allele[a, b]	Amino acid position[b]	Amino acid exchange	Phase system[c]	*G* value[d]
E. coli K-12/A19		*strA*+			I	1.87
E. coli K-12/A19	SM-1	*strA40*	87	LYS → ARG	I	1.58
E. coli K-12/A19	SM-5	*strA60*	42	LYS → ARG	I	1.72
E. coli K-12/A19	SM-10	*strA1*	42	LYS → ASN	I	1.24
E. coli B/L44		*strA*+			II	1.59
E. coli B/L44	L44-1	*strA1*	42	LYS → ASN	II	1.53
E. coli B/L44	L44-2	*strA2*	42	LYS → THR	II	1.57
E. coli B/L44	L44-4	*strA40*	87	LYS → ARG	II	1.53
E. coli B/L44	L44-6	*strA60*	42	LYS → ARG	II	1.49
E. coli B/L1		*strA*+			II	1.62
E. coli B/L1	L1-401	*strA1*	42	LYS → ASN	II	1.31
E. coli B/L1	L1-431	*strA40*	87	LYS → ARG	II	1.61

[a] Data from Breckenridge and Gorini (5).

[b] Data from Funatsu and Wittmann (8) and Funatsu et al. (7).

[c] For details, see text.

[d] *G*, the apparent partition coefficient, is calculated from the distribution curves according to the following formula: $G = [r_{max}/(n - r_{max})]$, where r_{max} is the number of the peak cavity of the distribution curve and n is the total number of transfers. The *G* values for the L44 strains were standardized so that the ΔG between parent and mutant strains reflected the average ΔG observed rather than the actual *G* value. This was necessary since the actual *g* value was strongly dependent on the lot of dextran T-500 used and since a new lot (3936) was used for one determination. Differences in partition coefficient of ≥ 0.15 are considered significant.

the *E. coli* B strains. Thus, it is possible that similar differences exist between mutants (L44-4 and L1-431) and parent, but they were not detectable under the CCD conditions.

DISCUSSION

Bacterial mutants selected for resistance to streptomycin often exhibit characteristics with no obvious relationship to the streptomycin resistance or dependence character (6, 11, 13–18, 20–22, 25, 26). After analysis of some of these properties, four classes of *strA* alleles were described in *E. coli* B based on their patterns of phenotypic suppression by streptomycin and bluensomycin (5), and in *E. coli* K on the basis of restriction of suppression of amber and ochre *T4rII* mutants (9). In order of increasing incompetence for phenotypic suppression these classes are *strA60, strA40, strA2,* and *strA1*. In the same order, these four classes of alleles similarly restrict to an increasing degree the efficiency of genetic suppression of nonsense and missense codons (5, 12). Thus, the *strA* mutations produce a general restriction of translation and result in impairment of translational efficiency, possibly at the level of transfer ribonucleic acid-ribosome binding (12, 24). This impairment is evident in missense and nonsense mutants, whose phenotype is positive or leaky in *strA*$^+$ cells, but becomes negative in cells containing an *strA* mutation.

These observations suggest that surface changes should correlate with the allowable degree of restriction of suppression and increasing incompetence for phenotypic suppression. That is, those cells with the greatest degree of impairment of translation and the greatest degree of restriction of suppression should exhibit the greatest differences from *strA*$^+$ (streptomycin-sensitive) cells, where the translational efficiency is best and restriction is least. Thus, we would predict that increasing differences in partition coefficient should occur in the order *strA60* < *strA40* < *strA2* < *strA1*. This is precisely the order determined for the A19 mutants: *strA60* (SM-5) < *strA40* (SM-1) < *strA1* (SM-10). The results that L1-401 (*strA1*) shows a greater difference than L1-431 (*strA40*) is also consistent with the above order.

Although both *E. coli* B. parental strains have a similar partition coefficient, they differ very significantly from the K-12 parent since different phase systems were required to center these parental strains within the countercurrent apparatus. *E. coli* K-12/A19 is a ribonuclease I$^-$ derivative of AB301 (*Hfr met*$^-$ λ^+). During mutagenesis with *N*-methyl-*N*^{1}-nitro-*N*-nitrosoguanidine, the A19 strain acquired some additional undefined mutations (10). Thus, A19 differs in some unknown ways from its K-12 parent.

All of the K-12 streptomycin-resistant mutants altered in protein S12 expressed differences in their partition coefficient from the parental strain. In addition, it appears that each of the streptomcyin-resistant K-12 mutants represents a different class of surface property alterations, so the partition coefficient reflects the streptomycin-resistant mutant allele. Thus, it is conceivable that the partition coefficient of the streptomycin-resistant mutant could be used to help define the *strA* allele in these strains.

The streptomycin-resistant mutants L44-1, L44-2, L44-4, and L44-6, reflecting the *strA* alleles *strA1, strA2, strA40,* and *strA60*, respectively, showed no significant differences in partition coefficients from the parent *E. coli* B/L44 (Table 1). In contrast, however, the *strA1* mutation (L1-401), which was not expressed as a surface alteration in *E. coli* B/L44, exhibited a markedly different partition coefficient from the parent when expressed in *E. coli* B/L1. Thus, there is a definite difference in the expression of the mutation in the two strains. At present we have no explanation for this difference.

To conclude that the *strA* alterations cause the surface changes, it is necessary to assume that additional unknown mutations in these strains cannot account for the observed differences. It is impossible to exclude completely the presence of other mutations; however, this is delimited somewhat by their genetic history. Since the *strA* markers were introduced into the L1 and L44 strains by transduction of the appropriate *strA* allele into the L1 and L44 parents (5), it is unlikely that the difference in partition coefficients between the mutant (L1-401) and the parental strain (L1) was due to the presence of a second mutation. Nevertheless, it is impossible to exclude entirely a closely linked additional silent mutation in this *strA1* mutant. Since the *strA1* allele was introduced into the L44 parent also by transduction, it was surprising that there was no difference in partition coefficient between the L44-1 streptomycin-resistant mutant and this parent. It appears then that the expression of the surface difference is dependent on other factors in the genetic background. *E. coli* B/L1 (*argF40 argR11 leu*$^+$) and L44 (*argF40 argRII leu*) differ essentially in the *leu* locus. Possibly, however, although all of the strains used contained the appropriate *arg, leu,* and *str* markers, other differences have been introduced inadvertently into these strains during passage. Since the SM strains were selected directly from the parent A19 as streptomcyin-resistant clones (8), the presence of possible additional mutations in these strains is not confined to the vicinity of the *strA* locus.

In genetic studies it is often useful to have methods of selection for mutations. Although it is relatively easy to obtain antibiotic-resistant organisms, antibiotic-sensitive revertants are often difficult to obtain because of a lack of a simple general selection technique. Variations in the surface properties of streptomycin mutants can provide such a selective technique. For example, it could be possible to obtain streptomcyin-sensitive revertants from -resistant strains by CCD and isolation of appropriate fractions corresponding to the revertant strains. In this way it might be possible to enrich for antibiotic-sensitive revertants. Clearly, the direct countercurrent partition of cells would permit the isolation of surface mutants and revertants.

Previously, it was shown that the surface properties of some erythromcyin-resistant mutants of *E. coli* differed from erythromycin-sensitive parental strains (29). By partition of one erythromycin-resistant ribosomal mutant of *E. coli* and its parental strain, we found no difference from the erythromycin-sensitive parent in surface properties. However, *E. coli* strain AB-301 ($met^- \lambda^+$), which is a lambda lysogen, differed significantly in surface properties from *E. coli* AB-301-1 ($met^- \lambda^-$) which is cured of lambda.

Partition of cells in aqueous two-phase systems has been thought to depend predominately on surface charge (27). Recently, however, surface properties other than charge have been shown to contribute to the partition of cells in phase systems of particular salt composition and polymer concentration (28). Partition in the phase systems used in the present experiments primarily reflects surface charge. It is noteworthy that the charge differences produced by the replacement of Lys by Asn in protein S12 of the *strA1* mutants are the reverse of the surface charge changes. Thus, direct expression of the S12 protein alteration as a cell surface-charge change is not likely. Furthermore, it is noteworthy that the degree of restriction of translation and the surface changes are greatest when the charge alterations in position 42 of protein S12 are greatest (Table 1).

We conclude that the surface alterations in the *strA* strains reflect an alteration in translational fidelity produced by the amino acid replacement in ribosomal protein S12. Precisely how the surface properties are altered by the alteration in translational fidelity remains to be elucidated. Furthermore, whether additional types of mutations other than ribosomal mutations will be expressed as surface alterations remains to be explored. Clearly, however, mutations or physiological alterations that directly alter the cell surface may be manifested as differences in CCD. In addition, the alterations in surface properties and CCD of the strain might be used for confirming or establishing the particular *strA* allele present in the K-12 strain and in some of the B strains.

Although the *E. coli* strains were always compared in mid-log phase, it was previously found that strains of *E. coli* isolated at different points in their growth curves exhibited identical CCD patterns (L. Wayne and H. Walter, unpublished data). In addition, strain K-12/A-19 and mutants grown in nutrient broth with shaking yielded the same CCD patterns as those obtained with cells grown in brain heart infusion broth without shaking. Thus, growth rate changes do not account for the differences in the CCD patterns.

Finally, the prediction that misreading would be greatest in those *strA* strains with the least translational restriction of suppression and, therefore, greatest in $strA^+$ strains (see reference 12) correlated well with our CCD data. The surface alterations reflect a mosaic of translational modulations. Additionally, *strA* mutations generally produce a reduction in growth rate. It is very likely, therefore, that a certain level of misreading or translational infidelity provides for optimal growth and survival of cells. Why this should be remains an enigma.

ACKNOWLEDGMENTS

We thank D. Elseviers and L. Gorini as well as H. Wittmann for providing the bacterial strains, and H. Sramek for technical assistance.

This work was supported by Veterans Administration projects 1683-01 and 1695-01.

LITERATURE CITED

1. **Albertsson, P. Å.** 1971. Partition of cell particles and macromolecules, 2nd ed., p. 323. Wiley-Interscience. New York.
2. **Albertsson, P. Å., and G. D. Baird.** 1962. Countercurrent distribution of cells. Exp. Cell Res. 28:296–322.
3. **Bissell, D. M.** 1965. Formation of an altered enzyme by *E. coli* in the presence of neomycin. J. Mol. Biol. 14:619–622.
4. **Bodley, J. W., and E. W. Davie.** 1966. A study of the mechanism of ambiguous amino acid coding by poly U: the nature of the products. J. Mol. Biol. 18:344–355.
5. **Breckenridge, L., and L. Gorini.** 1970. Genetic analysis

of streptomycin resistance in *Escherichia coli*. Genetics 65:9–25.
6. **Couturier, M., L. Desmet, and R. Thomas.** 1964. High pleiotropy of streptomycin mutations in *E. coli*. Biochem. Biophys. Res. Commun. 16:244–248.
7. **Funatsu, G., K. Nierhaus, and H. G. Wittmann.** 1972. Ribosomal proteins. XXXVII. Determination of allele types and amino acid exchanges in protein S12 of three streptomycin-resistant mutants of *Escherichia coli*. Biochim. Biophys. Acta 287:282–291.
8. **Funatsu, G., and H. G. Wittmann.** 1972. Ribosomal proteins. XXXIII. Location of amino acid replacements in protein S12 isolated from *Escherichia coli* mutants resistant to streptomycin. J. Mol. Biol. 68:547–550.
9. **Gartner, T. K., and E. Orias.** 1966. Effects of mutations to streptomycin resistance on the rate of translation of mutant genetic information. J. Bacteriol. **91:** 1021–1028.
10. **Gesteland, R. F.** 1966. Isolation and characterization of ribonuclease I mutants of *Escherichia coli*. J. Mol. Biol. 16:67–84.
11. **Gorini, L.** 1966. The action of streptomycin on protein synthesis *in vivo*. Bull. N. Y. Acad. Med. 42:633–637.
12. **Gorini, L.** 1969. The contrasting role of *strA* and *ram* gene products in ribosomal functioning. Cold Spring Harbor Symp. Quant. Biol. 34:101–111.
13. **Gorini, L., W. Gundersen, and M. Burger.** 1961. Genetics of regulation of enzyme synthesis in the arginine biosynthetic pathway of *Escherichia coli*. Cold Spring Harbor Symp. Quant. Biol. 26:173–182.
14. **Gorini, L., R. Rosset, and R. A. Zimmerman.** 1967. Phenotypic masking and streptomycin dependence. Science 157:1314–1317.
15. **Kuwano, M., and H. Endo.** 1969. Phenotypic suppression by streptomycin of amber mutants in the ribonucleic acid bacteriophage coat protein cistron. J. Virol. 4:252–255.
16. **Kuwano, M., M. Ishizawa, and H. Endo.** 1968. *Su-II*-specific restriction of amber suppression by mutation to streptomycin resistance. J. mol. Biol. 33:513–516.
17. **Lederberg, E. M., L. Cavalli-Sforza, and J. Lederberg.** 1964. Interaction of streptomycin and a suppressor for galactose fermentation in *E. coli* K-12. Proc. Natl. Acad. Sci. U.S.A. 51:678–682.
18. **Lederberg, J.** 1957. Suppression of the multiplication of heterologous bacteriophages in lysogenic bacteria. Virology 3:496–513.
19. **Old, D., and L. Gorini.** 1965. Amino acid changes provoked by streptomycin in a polypeptide synthesized *in vitro*. Science 150:1290–1292.
20. **Otsuji, N., and H. Aono.** 1968. Effect of mutation to streptomycin resistance on amber suppressor genes. J. Bacteriol. 96:43–50.
21. **Reale-Scafati, A.** 1967. Streptomycin suppression of ambivalent phage mutations. Virology 32:543–552.
22. **Rosenkranz, H. S., A. J. Bendich, and H. S. Carr.** 1964. The isolation of two types of streptomycin-resistant mutants of *Escherichia coli* ML_{35} differing in constitutive enzymes . Biochim. Biophys. Acta 82:110–117.
23. **Schwartz, J. H.** 1965. An effect of streptomycin on the biosynthesis of the coat protein of coliphage f2 by extracts of *E. coli*. Proc. Natl. Acad. Sci. U.S.A. 53:1133–1140.
24. **Stringini, P., and L. Gorini** 1970. Ribosomal mutations affecting efficiency of amber suppression. J. Mol. Biol. 47:517–530.
25. **Thomas, R., and L. Lambert.** 1962. On the occurrence of bacterial mutations permitting lysogenization by clear variants of temperate bacteriophages. J. Mol. Biol. 5:373–374.
26. **Valentine, R. C., and N. D. Zinder.** 1964. Phenotypic repair of RNA-bacteriophage mutants by streptomycin. Science 144:1458–1459.
27. **Walter, H.** 1975. Partition of cells in two-polymer aqueous phases: a method for separating cells and for obtaining information on their surface properties, p. 25–50. *In* D. M. Prescott, (ed.), Methods in cell biology, vol 9. Academic Press Inc., New York.
28. **Walter, H., E. J. Krob, and D. E. Brooks.** 1976. Membrane surface properties other than charge involved in cell separation by partition in polymer, aqueous two-phase systems. Biochemistry 15:2959–2964.
29. **Wayne, L. G., and H. Walter.** 1974. Separation of erythromycin-resistant and -susceptible subpopulations of *Escherichia coli* 15 by partition in two-polymer aqueous phases. Antimicrob. Agents Chemother. 5:203–209.

ANTIMICROBIAL AGENTS AND CHEMOTHERAPY, June 1977, p. 984-992 Vol. 11, No. 6

Printed in U.S.A.

Comparation Interferon-Inducing and Antiviral Properties of 2-Amino-5-Bromo-6-Methyl-4-Pyrimidinol (U-25,166), Tilorone Hydrochloride, and Polyinosinic-Polycytidylic Acid

DALE A. STRINGFELLOW

Experimental Biology, The Upjohn Company, Kalamazoo, Michigan 49001

Received for publication 29 December 1976

2-Amino-5-bromo-6-methyl-4-pyrimidinol (U-25,166), polyinosinic acid-polycytidylic acid [poly(I:C)], and tilorone HCl induced high levels of serum interferon in mice. Each consequently protected mice against infection with several viruses. After daily injection of inducer, mice developed a reduced interferon response (hyporeactivity) to each compound. However, hyporeactivity developed more slowly to U-25,166 and poly(I:C) than to tilorone HCl. After onset of hyporeactivity, 5 to 6 days without each inducer were required before normal serum interferon levels could be stimulated. Animals also developed a hyporeactive state as a consequence of Semliki Forest or encephalomyocarditis virus infections. By day 2 of either infection, mice had a suppressed interferon response to tilorone HCl, but remains responsive to poly(I:C) or U-25,166 until day 4. In vivo, poly(I:C) stimulated interferon production in a variety of cells and organs, whereas the tilorone HCl and U-25,166 responses involved a nonlymphoid component of the reticuloendothelial system. In vitro, poly(I:C) induced interferon in a variety of murine cells, U-25,166 was active in murine thymus and spleen organ cultures, and tilorone was inactive. These data indicate that U-25,166 is an interesting low-molecular-weight interferon inducer.

Several synthetic substances have now been demonstrated to be active interferon inducers in various animal species (4, 8, 10, 11, 14). Two of these, polyriboinosinic-polyribocytidylic acid [poly(I:C)] and bis-diethylaminoethylfluorenone (tilorone HCl), have been the object of considerable research and speculation concerning eventual use as antiviral agents (1, 7, 10, 17). Therefore, both represent compounds against which any new interferon inducer might be compared in terms of interferon-inducing and antiviral properties.

In the studies described in this report, a new low-molecular-weight interferon inducer (2-amino-5-bromo-6-methyl-4-pyrimidinol, [U-25,166]) first reported in 1976 by Nichol et al. (13) was compared with poly(I:C) and tilorone HCl. These studies were undertaken to determine the spectrum of antiviral activity and evaluate parameters that might effect eventual clinical utility, including the state of hyporeactivity that develops secondary to virus infection or as a consequence of repeated doses of inducer.

MATERIALS AND METHODS

Mice. Female ICR strain mice (Upj:tuc-ICR) were provided by Upjohn Rearing and Procurement and were housed under conditions of constant temperature and a 12-h light cycle, with food and water provided ad libitum. After being received from the breeder, mice were housed as described for at least 1 week to allow them to adjust to the new environment before being used.

Cells. Murine interferon assays were carried out in a cloned continuous line of mouse L-cell fibroblasts (L_{929}) originally obtained from the American Type Culture Collection (ATCC) Cell Repository.

Media. Eagle minimum essential medium (MEM; Microbiological Associates) containing 10% fetal calf serum (Reheis Chemical Co., Phoenix, Ariz.), 100 U of penicillin per ml, and 50 μg of streptomycin per ml was used to propagate and maintain all tissue cultures.

Viruses. Vesicular stomatitis virus (VSV), Indiana strain, was obtained from the ATCC (Rockville, Md.). Pools of VSV were propagated in primary chicken embryo cell monolayers. The stock preparation of VSV used in these studies had a titer of 2 × 10^7 plaque-forming units (PFU)/ml when assayed in L_{929} mouse cells.

The strain of encephalomyocarditis (EMC) virus used in these studies was obtained from the ATCC. Young adult mice (16 ± 2 g) were infected by the intranasal route. Brains were removed after onset of paralysis and were homogenized as a 10% suspension in MEM. The pool had a titer of 9.5 × 10^6 PFU/ml on L_{929} cells.

A_2 influenza virus (A_2/AA/2160, H_2N_2), obtained from H. E. Renis (Upjohn), had previously been mouse adapted, and the pool used in these studies was prepared by intranasal inoculation of the virus. Lungs were harvested 48 h after infection, homogenized as a 10% suspension in MEM, and stored at −70°C.

The HWC strain of *Herpesvirus hominis* type 1 (HVH-1) was propagated in primary rabbit kidney cells and titered 10^7 PFU/ml on these cells.

Semliki Forest virus (SFV) was obtained originally from S. Baron (National Institutes of Health [NIH]) and was propagated on primary chicken embryo cells. The pool used in these studies titered 2 × 10^8 PFU/ml on primary chicken embryo cells.

West Nile virus was obtained through the NIH (ATCC VR82, catalog no. V554-001-552). Suckling ICR mice were injected intracerebrally, and 48 h later mice were sacrificed and brains were removed and homogenized as a 10% suspension in MEM. The pool titered 5 × 10^8 PFU/ml on primary chicken embryo cells.

Friend leukemia virus (FLV) originally obtained from the ATCC (ATCC 245) was injected intraperitoneally (i.p.) into 25- to 30-g ICR mice. Spleens were removed 21 days later and homogenized as a 10% suspension in MEM. After clarification (2,000 × *g* for 15 min), supernatant fluid was removed and stored at −70°C.

Inducers. Tilorone HCl (bis-diethylaminoethylfluorenone) was generously furnished by Richardson-Merrell (Cincinnati, Ohio) and was dissolved in phosphate-buffered saline at a concentration permitting an inoculum of 250 mg/kg orally (p.o.).

Poly(I:C), prepared by P. L. Laboratories (Milwaukee, Wis), was dissolved in phosphate-buffered saline and was administered i.p. at 100 μg/mouse.

U-25,166, purchased from Aldrich Chemical Co. (Milwaukee, Wis.), was suspended in aqueous 1% carboxymethylcellulose and unless otherwise noted was adminstered at 1,000 mg/kg p.o.

X-irradiation. Mice received 650 R of whole-body irradiation from a Van de Graaff accelerator.

WBC counts. Total leukocyte (WBC) counts were determined by collecting 0.02 ml of blood from the orbital sinus with heparinized capillary tubes. Blood was diluted in a Unipette (Becton-Dickinson) containing 1.1% ammonium oxalate, and cells were counted microscopically in a Neubauer hemacytometer. Thin-layer blood smears were also prepared for differential WBC counts after staining with Wright stain.

Interferon assay. Confluent monolayers of L_{929} cells grown in 35-mm plastic petri dishes (Falcon Plastics) were treated with 1 ml of an appropriate interferon dilution overnight at 37°C. The plaque reduction assay used VSV as the challenge virus and has been previously described (17). An internal laboratory reference murine interferon standard was included with each interferon assay, and the sensitivity of our assay was compared with the International Murine Standard obtained from the NIH. In our system, the International Standard had a mean titer of approximately 4,200 U/ml compared with its accepted titer of 6,500 U/ml.

RESULTS

Interferon response in vivo. Initially, the circulating interferon response induced in mice after a single injection of U-25,166 (1,000 mg/kg, p.o.), tilorone HCl (250 mg/kg, p.o.), or poly(I:C) (100 μg, i.p.) was determined. Doses of compounds used represent the optimal amount of inducer needed to stimulate maximal interferon levels as determined previously (13, 17). At the time periods indicated (Fig. 1), five mice from each treatment group were sacrificed, blood was collected and pooled, and serum was assayed for interferon. The results illustrate that the kinetics of the U-25,166- and poly(I:C)-induced responses were similar, with peak interferon titers being observed 4 to 6 h after poly(I:C) and 6 to 8 h after U-25,166 injections. The U-25,166-induced response remained high through 12 h, and both were clear by 24 h. Tilorone induced a comparably late response, with peak interferon levels being observed 12 to 24 h after injections.

Antiviral spectrum. To measure the antiviral activity of each inducer, mice received a single dose of U-25,166 (1,000 mg/kg, p.o.), poly(I:C) (100 μg, i.p.), or tilorone HCl (250 mg/kg, p.o.) and 18 h later were infected with EMC virus (100 PFU, intranasally), SFV (20 PFU,

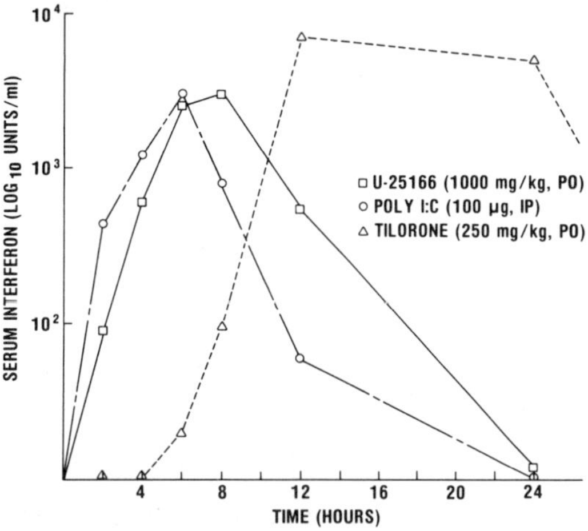

FIG. 1. *Serum interferon response of mice to U-25,166, poly(I:C), and tilorone HCl.*

i.p.), West Nile virus (100 PFU, i.p.), VSV (1×10^4 PFU, i.n.), A_2 influenza virus (10 mean lethal doses, i.n.), or HVH-1 (100 PFU, i.p.). Mice infected with FLV (10 mean lethal doses, i.p.) received inducer at the concentrations listed once a week beginning 5 days after infection for a total of 5 weeks. In each infection mice were checked daily for mortality, and the results in Table 1 present the mean day of death and percent mortality using 30 mice per group. Each inducer protected mice against the lethal consequences of EMC, SFV, and West Nile virus infections. However, although each induced high interferon levels, the antiviral activity observed in VSV, A_2 influenza, FLV, and HVH-1 virus infections varied with inducer. For example, mice infected with VSV were protected from the lethal consequences of infection by poly(I:C) and tilorone but not U-25,166, whereas FLV-infected mice were protected by tilorone and U-25,166 but not poly(I:C). HVH-1-infected mice were protected by poly(I:C) and U-25,166 but not tilorone.

Hyporeactivity due to multiple doses of inducer. To determine the ability of mice to respond to repeated injections of inducer, groups of ICR female 20-g mice received a single injection of tilorone (250 mg/kg, p.o.), poly(I:C) (100 μg, i.p.), or U-25,166 (1,000 mg/kg, p.o.) daily for 5 consecutive days. Five mice from each group were bled daily by cardiac puncture at a time when serum interferon levels were anticipated to be at a maximum as determined previously (4 h post-poly(I:C), 6 h post-U-25,166, or 24 h post-tilorone). The results presented in Fig. 2 illustrate that with each additional injection of inducer mice progressively became hyporeactive or lost their ability to respond. Tilorone HCl was the most severely affected, with extremely low levels (150 U/ml) of serum interferon being induced by the second injection of compound. Poly(I:C) and U-25,166, however, stimulated fairly high interferon levels through the third dose of inducer.

Length of hyporeactivity. Since each compound induced the development of hyporesponsiveness, the following study was undertaken to determine how long the hyporeactive state lasted. Groups of 20-g female ICR mice were injected with an initial dose of each inducer at the concentrations listed in the previous study, followed by a second injection of the same compound 1, 2, 3, 4, 5, or 6 days later. Animals were bled as indicated previously. Serum was collected and stored at $-20°C$ until assayed for interferon. The results represent a mean from two separate experiments (Fig. 3). As illustrated, 5 to 6 days without inducer were required before mice regained a normal interferon response to any of the compounds. Again, tilorone appeared to be the most severely affected, whereas mice regained their response to U-25,166 slightly faster than to poly(I:C).

Hyporeactivity due to infection. To determine the effect of virus infection on the ability of mice to respond to interferon induction, 20-g ICR mice were injected i.p. with a 100% lethal inoculum of SFV or EMC virus (1,000 PFU). Then, 24, 48, 72, or 96 h later, groups of uninfected or virus-infected mice (five animals per group) received a single injection of poly(I:C) (100 μg, i.p.), tilorone HCl (250 mg/kg, p.o.), or U-25,166 (1,000 mg/kg, p.o.). After injection of inducer, blood was drawn when interferon levels were maximal. Blood samples were pooled by group, and serum was collected and stored at

TABLE 1. *Antiviral activity of poly(I:C), tilorone, and U-25, 166 in vivo*[a]

Virus	Route	Treatment[b]										
		PBS		Poly(I:C)			Tilorone			U-25, 166		
		% M[c]	MDD	% M	S[d]	MDD	% M	S	MDD	% M	S	MDD
EMC	i.n.	100	4.6	10	+	4.0	10	+	12.0	20	+	5.0
SFV	i.p.	100	4.8	20	+	11.0	0	+		40	+	6.8
WNV	i.p.	80	11.0	0	+		0	+		30	+	12.4
VSV	i.n.	90	10.5	50	+	9.2	40	+	7.8	80	−	10.1
A_2	i.n.	90	8.5	90	−	8.5	55	+	9.9	50	+	8.7
FLV	i.p.	100	70	70	−	78	10	+	70	30	+	74
HVH-1	i.p.	95	6.2	40	+	6.8	66	−	7.5	32	+	8.3

[a] Abbreviations: PBS, phosphate-buffered saline; MDD, mean day of death; i.n., intranasal; WNV, West Nile virus.

[b] Poly(I:C) (100 μg/mouse, i.p.), tilorone (250 mg/kg, p.o.), and U-25,166 (1,000 mg/kg, p.o.) were administered 18 h before infection, except in FLV-infected mice where animals were treated once every 7 days beginning 5 days after infection for a total of 5 weeks.

[c] Percent mortality, 30 mice per group.

[d] Significance of percent mortality at the $\geq 95\%$ level using chi-square analysis of variance.

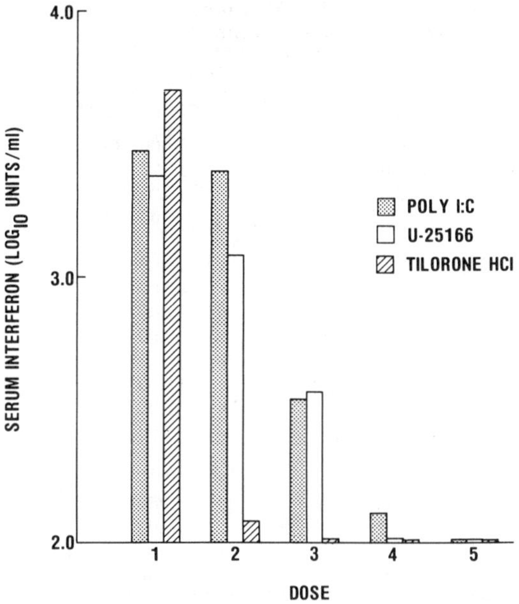

FIG. 2. *Serum interferon levels in mice after daily injection of poly(I:C) (100 μg, i.p.), tilorone HCl (250 mg/kg, p.o.) or U-25,166 (1,000 mg/kg, p.o.).*

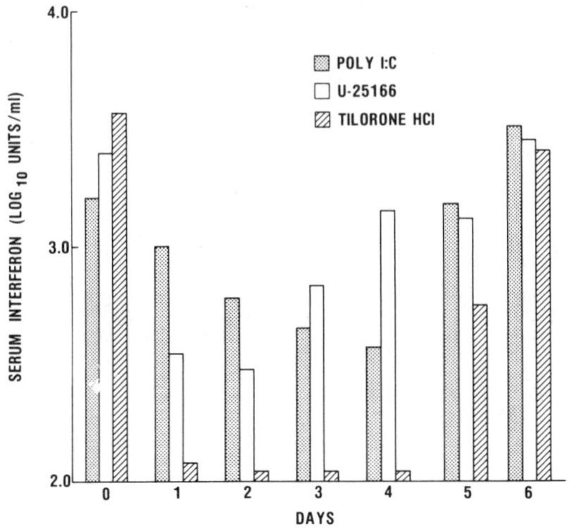

FIG. 3. *Serum inteferon levels in mice that received an initial injection of U-25,166 (1,000 mg/kg, p.o.), poly(I:C), (100 μg, i.p.), or tilorone (250 mg/kg, p.o.) on day 0 and a single injection of the same inducer 1, 2, 3, 4, 5, or 6 days later.*

−20°C until assayed for interferon. Results from two separate experiments with each virus are presented in Table 2, where the mean serum interferon titers at each time period are summarized.

The development of hyporeactivity was most striking in virus-infected mice injected with tilorone. As early as 24 h after infection mice produced only 15% of control interferon levels. At 48 and 72 h the ability of infected mice to respond to tilorone was reduced by 95% and greater than 98%. The ability of mice to produce interferon in response to poly(I:C) or U-25,166 remained high through the first 72 h of infection, but became suppressed by 96 h.

Effect of X-irradiation and antilymphocyte serum of in vivo response. To further explore the basic properties of each inducer, the tissues responsible for the in vivo interferon response were investigated. Initially the effect of antilymphocyte serum and X-irradiation on the ability of mice to produce interferon was evaluated. Animals received 650 R of whole-body X-irradiation or four daily doses (0.5 ml i.p.) of horse anti-mouse lymphocyte serum (ALS; Microbiological Associates, Bethesda, Md.). Four days after X-irradiation or on day 4 of ALS treatment, mice were injected with inducers at the concentrations listed in Table 3 and were bled as described. At the time of inducer injection, five mice treated with normal horse serum, ALS, or 650 R of whole-body X-irradiation were sacrificed. Total and differential WBC counts were determined, and spleen weights were recorded to document the effect of each treatment on the lymphoreticuloendothelial system.

Results from three separate studies with each inducer are summarized in Table 3. ALS treatment suppressed the poly(I:C)- and Newcastle disease virus-induced responses but had no effect on the tilorone or U-25,166 response. X-irradiation suppressed all but the poly(I:C) response. Irradiated mice had suppressed total WBC counts and spleen weights, indicating a severe effect on the entire reticuloendothelial system. ALS, on the other hand, appeared to have a more selective effect, with the decrease in total WBC counts being reflected mainly in a decrease in the number of lymphocytes observed. These results indicate that U-25,166 and tilorone stimulated a non-lymphoid component of the reticuloendothelial system to produce interferon.

Tissue interferon levels in vivo. To further explore which cells participated in the response induced by each compound, mice were injected with poly(I:C) (100 μg, i.p.), U-25,166 (100 mg/kg, p.o.), or tilorone (250 mg/kg, p.o.), and 1, 2, 3, 4, 6, 8, 12 or 24 h later five mice from each group were sacrificed. Blood and subsequent serum was collected by cardiac puncture; spleens, livers, thymuses, and lungs were removed. Each organ was divided into two equal parts, and one-half of each organ from five mice was pooled. One-half was minced with

TABLE 2. *Serum interferon levels induced by poly(I:C) (100 μg, i.p.), U-25,166 (1,000 mg/kg, p.o.), or tilorone HCl (250 mg/kg, p.o.) in EMC- or SFV-infected or uninfected control mice*[a]

Inducer	Days post-infection	Serum interferon response (U/ml)		
		Uninfected control	EMC infected (%)[b]	SFV infected (%)[b]
Poly(I:C)	1	3,500	9,500 (270)	5,000 (140)
	2	4,300	4,300 (100)	2,100 (49)
	3	2,100	850 (40)	720 (34)
	4	2,900	270 (9)	300 (10)
U-25,166	1	5,500	9,500 (170)	4,200 (76)
	2	4,300	4,500 (104)	1,500 (35)
	3	3,700	1,100 (30)	900 (24)
	4	4,800	120 (2)	250 (5)
Tilorone HCl	1	10,000	1,500 (15)	1,200 (12)
	2	6,500	350 (5)	190 (3)
	3	7,000	150 (2)	<100 (<1)
	4	6,500	100 (1.5)	<100 (<1)
PBS (uninduced)	1	<50	150	350
	2	<50	100	100
	3	<50	<50	<50
	4	<50	<50	<50

[a] Animals received a single injection of inducer 24, 48, 72, or 96 h after infection. Blood and subsequent serum samples were collected 4 h post-poly(I:C), 6 h after U-25,166 or phosphate-buffered saline (PBS), and 18 h after tilorone HCl.

[b] Number in parentheses is percentage of uninfected control response.

TABLE 3. *Effect of ALS and X-irradiation on the serum interferon response of mice to U-25,166, poly(I:C), and tilorone HCl*

Inducer	Serum interferon response (U/ml)[a]			
	PBS	NHS	ALS	X-irradiation
U-25,166	2,300	2,100	2,600	260*[b]
Poly(I:C)	1,200	1,300	200*	1,100
NDV[c]	1,200	840	85*	160*
Tilorone HCl	1,200	1,500	1,690	<50*
PBS	<50	<50	<50	<50
Total WBC/mm^3[d]	7,200	7,100	3,300*	200*
Lymphocytes	5,100	4,760	1,452*	
Monocytes	1,100	920	825	
Granulocytes	1,000	1,420	1,023	
Avg spleen wt (g)[d]	0.15	0.16	0.14	0.02*
Avg total body wt (g)[d]	21.2	21.5	21.2	15.2*

[a] Each value represents a mean of three separate experiments. PBS, Phosphate-buffered saline; NHS, normal horse serum.

[b] Asterisk indicates significantly different ($P < 0.05$) from PBS-treated controls using one-way t-test.

[c] NDV, Newcastle disease virus.

[d] Represents a mean of 18 animals.

scalpels, and approximately 0.1 g of tissue was transferred to 16-mm culture dishes containing 1 ml of MEM plus 5% fetal calf serum. These tissues were incubated at 37°C for 24 h, at which time growth medium was collected for interferon assay. The other organ halves were ground as a 10% suspension in MEM. After centrifugation, supernatant fluid was collected and stored frozen until assayed for interferon. Using the tissue in this manner, it was possible to determine the levels of interferon in each organ at each time period and also how early inducer reached each organ after injection. Results summarized in Table 4 suggest that

TABLE 4. *Serum and organ interferon level after in vivo administration of inducer*

Inducer	Time (h)	Interferon response (U/ml)								
		Spleen		Liver		Thymus		Lungs		Serum
		Super[a]	Culture	Super	Culture	Super	Culture	Super	Culture	
U-25,166	0	—[b]	—	—	—	—	—	—	—	—
	1	—	—	—	—	—	—	—	—	—
	2	—	—	—	—	30	—	—	—	90
	3	—	—	—	—	350	21	—	—	100
	4	200	35	—	—	250	38	150	26	600
	6	250	—	—	—	1,000	90	90	25	2,500
	8	100	—	—	—	1,200	160	95	45	3,000
	12	—	—	—	—	400	71	—	—	550
	24	—	—	—	—	80	—	—	—	—
Poly(I:C)	0	—	—	—	—	—	—	—	—	—
	1	—	1,000	—	—	—	300	—	2,000	20
	2	130	350	13	—	—	300	20	1,500	440
	3	190	1,000	18	—	40	480	60	640	2,500
	4	300	680	54	—	24	50	40	800	1,100
	6	250	500	—	—	27	40	17	300	790
	8	130	100	—	—	37	40	13	75	590
	12	200	100	—	—	40	—	18	60	140
	24	—	—		—	—	—	—	—	20
Tilorone HCl	0	—	—	—	—	—	—	—	—	—
	1	—	—	—	—	—	—	—	—	—
	2	—	—	—	—	—	—	—	—	—
	3	—	—	—	—	—	—	—	—	—
	4	—	—	—	—	—	—	—	—	—
	6	—	—	—	—	—	—	—	—	200
	8	290	100	55	—	65	—	—	53	1,000
	12	1,600	620	130	—	540	200	480	180	7,700
	24	670	50	70	65	1,400	890	120	—	3,300
PBS[c]	0	—	—	—	—	—	—	—	—	—
	12	—	—	—	—	—	—	—	—	—
	24	—	—	—	—	—	—	—	—	—

[a] Organs were removed from mice at times indicated after administration of inducer. Organs were split into two equal parts and pooled. Half was homogenized as a 10% suspension, and the other half was minced and incubated at 37°C for 24 h. The supernatant (super) fluid from homogenized organs and growth medium from organ cultures were collected and assayed for interferon.

[b] Titer less than 10 U/ml.

[c] PBS, Phosphate-buffered saline.

U-25,166 induced little, if any, interferon in the lung or liver, whereas relatively high levels were induced in the spleen and thymus. Of particular interest was the thymus interferon response in that it correlated with serum interferon levels and suggested that cells in this organ might be primarily responsible for the U-25,166-induced interferon response.

Although poly(I:C) induced a serum interferon response similar to U-25,166, a much different pattern of organ interferon production was seen. The levels of interferon in lung tissues after poly(I:C) injection were particularly interesting. At no time were levels observed in supernatant fluids from homogenized lungs higher than 60 to 70 U/ml, yet the half of these same lungs incubated in vitro for 24 h at 37°C produced high (1,500 to 2,000 U/ml) interferon levels. These results suggest that poly(I:C) had been delivered to lung tissues as early as 1 h after i.p. injection. The low levels of interferon in homogenized lung tissues are puzzling and suggest that interferon may have been produced locally in lung tissue but was absorbed, distributed systemically, or catabolized in some fashion. A similar interferon resonse was also observed in spleen and thymus tissue where organs taken 1 h after poly(I:C) injection had no or low levels of interferon, yet after incubation for 24 h this same tissue yielded high levels of interferon. These data suggest that poly(I:C) was rapidly distributed and induced several cell types to produce interferon.

Tilorone HCl induced interferon production primarily in the spleen and thymus, although after organ removal these tissues did not appear to produce more interferon, as had been the case with poly(I:C)-induced mice.

Response of tissue induced in vitro. The previous studies suggest that spleen and thymus tissues were primarily responsible for the U-25,166- and tilorone HCl-induced responses, whereas poly(I:C) stimulated a wide variety of cells to produce interferon. To further evaluate these findings, normal mice were sacrificed and thymuses, spleens, and livers were removed and minced with sterile scalpels. Approximately 0.1 g of tissue was suspended in 1 ml of MEM plus 5% fetal calf serum in 16-mm petri dishes. Inducers were prepared in phosphate-buffered saline and added to plates (in duplicate) to give the final concentration listed in Table 5. Plates were returned to 37°C for 24 h, and growth medium was then collected for interferon assay. Only poly(I:C) and U-25,166 induced detectable levels of interferon in vitro. Both inducers stimulated thymus and spleen tissue to produce interferon.

DISCUSSION

Interferon and its inducers have been successfully used in the treatment of experimental virus infections (1, 4, 7, 8, 10, 11, 17). Recent reports suggest that interferon was successful in treating humans infected with a rhinovirus (12) and in patients suffering from osteogenic sarcoma (15) and reduced the Dane particle marker carrier rate during naturally occurring hepatitis B virus infection (6). Interferon inducers have also shown promise, protecting volunteers from rhinovirus infections (14).

TABLE 5. *Interferon response of murine tissue induced in vitro*[a]

Inducer	Concn (μg/ml)	Interferon (U/ml)	
		Thymus	Spleen
Tilorone	10	—[b]	—
	5	—	—
Poly(I:C)	50	156	147
U-26,166	500	240	360
	100	30	80

[a] Minced organ tissues were incubated for 24 h with inducer before growth medium was collected and assayed for interferon.

[b] —, Indicates a titer of less than 10 U/ml.

These data suggest that interferon and its inducers may be clinically useful antiviral agents. For this reason, a great deal of interest has been focused upon identifying agents that might be used to induce interferon and consequently antiviral resistance in humans. During 1976, Nichol et al. (13) reported that U-25,166 induced interferon in mice and protected them from a lethal virus infection. The studies described in this report were initiated to determine the potential of U-25,166 as an interferon inducer and antiviral agent by comparing its biological characteristics and properties with two widely used inducers, poly(I:C) and tilorone HCl.

Each of the inducers stimulated high circulating levels of serum interferon in mice, with peak levels being reached 4 to 6 h after poly(I:C), 6 to 8 h after U-25,166, and 12 to 24 h after tilorone administration. Poly(I:C) stimulated a number of cells and tissues to produce interferon in vivo and in vitro, whereas the U-25,166- and tilorone HCl-induced responses appeared to involve a nonlymphoid component of the reticuloendothelial system. This was reflected in mice treated with ALS having a normal response to U-25,166 or tilorone but a suppressed response to Newcastle disease virus. The interferon response, however, was obliterated when mice received 650 R of total-body X-irradiation 4 days before inducer adminstration. These results are in agreement with previously reported studies where ALS suppressed the poly(I:C) and Newcastle disease virus but not the tilorone response, whereas X-irradiation suppressed the response of mice to Newcastle disease virus and tilorone but not poly(I:C) (2, 3, 5, 9, 17). In vivo, U-25,166 and tilorone induced interferon in high levels in the thymus and spleen, but in vitro tilorone was inactive whereas U-25,166 induced interferon in both thymus and spleen organ cultures. These results suggest, as we have previously postulated (17), that tilorone may be metabolized or altered in some fashion in vivo and that a cell of the reticuloendothelial system is either involved in this process or is the cell consequently induced by the altered tilorone form. It is of interest that U-25,166 is an active interferon inducer in vitro, since many low-molecular-weight interferon inducers, for example, tilorone, are essentially inactive (1, 17). Although not reported, U-25,166 induced no detectable interferon in a number of murine cell lines (i.e., L_{929} or mouse embryo fibroblast cells), further reinforcing the involvement of the reticuloendothelial system in the interferon response. Poly(I:C), however, induced interferon in a number of fibroblast cell cultures, suggesting a ubiquitous ability to stimulate interferon production.

Each of the inducers protected mice from a variety of virus infections. The pattern of protection observed when inducers were administered 18 h before infection, however, varied. U-25,166 was ineffective against intranasal VSV infection, whereas poly(I:C) and tilorone were active. Tilorone was ineffective against HVH-1 infectiona and poly(I:C) had no effect on A_2 influenza virus or FLV infections, whereas both of the other inducers in each case were effective. It should be emphasized that under other circumstances, using different treatment regimens, each inducer could effectively protect mice from each infection and that the differences seen occurred specifically when inducers were given 18 h before infection. However, the interferon response and subsequent antiviral resistance induced by each compound should have reached a maximum by 18 to 24 h. These data suggest that mechanisms other than interferon-mediated antiviral resistance may have been responsible for some of the protection seen.

One of the problems associated with the use of interferon inducers is that animals progressively lose their ability to respond when agents are given in multiple-dose regimens. For example, in this study mice were injected once daily with poly(I:C), U-25,166, or tilorone HCl, and with each additional injection of inducer animals progressively became hyporeactive or lost their ability to respond. The rate of onset and severity of the hyporeactive state was, however, inducer dependent. Mice lost their ability to respond to tilorone HCl by the second dose of compound, whereas U-25,166 and poly(I:C) each induced fairly high serum interferon levels through the third dose of compound. The rate of recovery of a normal interferon response was essentially the same with each inducer. After the initial injection of inducer, 5 to 6 days were required before each animal fully responded to a second dose of the same compound. Animals also develop hyporeactivity as a consequence of virus infection (16, 18). For example, in this study animals infected with SFV or EMC virus progressively developed a depressed ability to respond to each inducer. Development of hyporeactivity was, however, inducer dependent, with tilorone being the most severely affected. Mice responded normally to U-25,166 or poly(I:C) through the first 72-h infection but had a suppressed response to tilorone as early as 24 h. These results are significant in that they suggest that judicious selection of inducers and treatment regimens may minimize the obvious limitations associated with development of hyporeactivity to interferon induction that results as a consequence of multiple doses of inducer or secondary to virus infection.

The results presented indicate that U-25,166 is a broad-spectrum antiviral agent, appears to stimulate a nonlymphoid component of the reticuloendothelial system to produce interferon, is one of few synthetic inducers active in vitro, and compares favorably with poly(I:C) and consistently better than tilorone in terms of sensitivity to the onset of hyporeactivity. Based upon these data, U-25,166 appears to be an interesting low-molecular-weight interferon inducer worthy of further investigation.

ACKNOWLEDGMENTS

The expert technical assistance of H. C. Vanderberg and F. T. Maida and statistical support of P. Good are appreciated.

LITERATURE CITED

1. **DeClercq, E., and T. C. Merigan.** 1971. Bis-DEAE-fluorenone: mechanism of antiviral protection and stimulation of interferon production in the mouse. J. Infect. Dis. **123**:190–199.
2. **DeMaeyer, E., J. DeMaeyer-Guignard, and P. Jullien.** 1969. Interferon synthesis in x-irradiated animals. III. The high radiosensitivity of myxovirus-induced circulating interferon production. Proc. Soc. Exp. Biol. Med. **131**:36–41.
3. **DeMaeyer-Guignard, J., and E. DeMaeyer.** 1971. Effect of antilymphocytic serum on circulating interferon in mice as a function of the inducer. Nature (London) New Biol. **229**:212–214.
4. **Field, A. K., A. A. Tytell, G. P. Lampson, and M. R. Hilleman.** 1968. Inducers of interferon and host resistance: V. *In vitro* studies. Proc. Natl. Acad. Sci. U.S.A. **61**:340–346.
5. **Glasgow, L. A.** 1971. Immunosuppression, interferon, and viral infections. Fed. Proc. **30**:1846–1851.
6. **Greenberg, H. B., R. B. Polland, L. I. Lutwick, P. B. Gregory, W. S. Robinson, and T. C. Merigan.** 1976. Effect of human leukocyte interferon on hepatitis B virus infection in patients with chronic active hepatitis. N. Engl. J. Med. **295**:517–522.
7. **Hilleman, M. R.** 1969. Toward control of viral infections of man. Science **164**:506–514.
8. **Hoffman, W. W., J. J. Korst, J. F. Niblack, and T. H. Cronin.** 1973. *N,N*-dioctadecyl-*N',N'*-bis(2-hydroxyethyl)propanediamine: antiviral activity and interferon stimulation in mice. Antimicrob. Agents Chemother. **3**:498–502.
9. **Jullien, P., J. DeMaeyer-Guignard, and E. DeMaeyer.** 1974. Interferon synthesis in X-irradiated animals. V. Origin of mouse serum interferon induced by polyinosinic-polycytidylic acid and encephalomyocarditis virus. Infect. Immun. **10**:1023–1028.
10. **Krueger, R. F., and G. D. Mayer.** 1970. Tilorone hydrochloride: an orally active antiviral agent. Science **169**:1213–1214.
11. **Mayer, G. D., and R. F. Krueger.** 1970. Tilorone hydrochloride: mode of action. Science **169**:1214–1215.
12. **Merigan, T. C., T. S. Hall, S. E. Reed, and D. A. Tyrrell.** 1973. Inhibition of respiratory virus infection by locally applied interferon. Lancet **1**:563–567.
13. **Nichol, F. R., S. D. Weed, and G. E. Underwood.** 1976. Stimulation of murine interferon by a substituted pyrimidine. Antimicrob. Agents Chemother. **9**:433–

439.

14. **Panusarn, C., E. D. Stanley, V. Oirda, M., Rubenis,and G. G. Jackson.** 1974. Prevention of illness from rhinovirus infection by a topical interferon inducer. N. Engl. J. Med. 291:57–61.
15. **Strander, H., K. Cantell, P. A. Jakobsso, U. Nilsonne, and G. Soderberg.** 1975. Exogenous interferon therapy of osteogenic sarcoma. Acta Orthop. Scand. 45:958–961.
16. **Stringfellow, D. A., and L. A. Glasgow.** 1972. Hyporeactivity of infection: potential limitation to therapeutic use of interferon-inducing agents. Infect Immun. 6:743–747.
17. **Stringfellow, D. A., and L. A. Glasgow.** 1972. Tilorone hydrochloride: an oral interferon-inducing agent. Antimicrob. Agents Chemother. 2:73–78.
18. **Stringfellow, D. A., E. R. Kern, D. K. Kelsey, and L. A. Glasgow.** 1977. Suppressed response to interferon induction in mice infected with encephalomyocarditis, Semiliki Forest, A_2 influenza, Herpes hominis type 2 or murine cytomegalo viruses. J. Infect. Dis. **135:** 540–551.

Antimicrobial Agents and Chemotherapy, June 1977, p. 993-998 Vol. 11, No. 6

Printed in U.S.A.

Evaluation of Three Newer Methods for Investigating Protein Interactions of Penicillin G

LANCE R. PETERSON,* DALE N. GERDING, HORACE H. ZINNEMAN, and BARBARA M. MOORE

Infectious Disease Section, Department of Medicine, Minneapolis Veterans Administration Hospital; and University of Minnesota Medical School, Minneapolis, Minnesota 55417

Received for publication 20 December 1976

The interaction of penicillin G with human serum proteins was evaluated by three different techniques: rate of dialysis, cross-linked dextran exclusion, and ultracentrifugation. The rate-of-dialysis technique demonstrated that penicillin G binding to serum was immediate but incompletely reversible. Cross-linked dextran adsorbed or trapped significant amounts of penicillin G, necessitating correction factors of more than 10%. Ultracentrifugation was found to be the most reliable method for quantitative protein-binding determinations of penicillins.

The binding of penicillin G (pen G) to serum and tissue proteins has aroused much interest since the early work of the 1940s (10, 15, 40). Recent reviews have discussed the various methods used for evaluation of protein binding and have questioned current methodology for quantitative binding determinations and demonstration of binding reversibility (9, 33, 36).

The concept of using a semipermeable membrane for evaluating large- and small-molecule interactions was first proposed by Thomas Graham in 1861 (12). Criticism of this method primarily involves the nature of the cellulose membrane (5 to 7, 9, 12, 20, 38). A new method using the cellulose dialysis membrane was described by Colowick and Womack, who used rate-of-dialysis measurements with radioactive ligands (11, 42). This method has recently been reviewed, and despite the need for radiolabeled compounds of high specific activity, it was felt to be the best cellulose membrane method available for evaluation of small-molecule–protein interactions (7, 9).

Cross-linked dextran gel columns have been widely used for study of ligand-protein interaction with a variety of separatory methods (1, 14, 19, 21, 23 to 25, 37). However, problems may be encountered with this material because of adsorption of aromatic, heterocyclic, and basic substances onto the dextran polymer and rejection of some acidic compounds from the gel matrix (14). Cross-linked dextran exclusion, proposed by Pearlman and Crépy (35), is a novel application of the use of dextran gel in the study of ligand-protein binding.

Finally, the use of ultracentrifugation to sediment protein has been suggested; the major disadvantage of this method is the high cost of equipment (9). High-speed centrifugation has been available for 40 years (3, 4, 31), and the method of standardization for study of ligand-protein interactions has been described (39) and used in non-antibiotic-containing systems (18). However, the ultracentrifuge has only occasionally been used, and its use has never been standardized for the study of antibiotic-protein binding (8, 17, 32, 37, 38).

The present study compares and evaluates these three newer methods for determining protein binding of pen G: rate of dialysis (11, 42), cross-linked dextran exclusion (35), and ultracentrifugation (39).

MATERIALS AND METHODS

Rate of dialysis. The method used was a modification of that reported by Colowick and Womack (11, 42). Studies of quantitative binding and immediate reversibility were performed in a 37°C water bath using a Bio-Rad minibeaker (Bio-Fiber 50 Minibeaker, Bio-Rad Laboratories, Richmond, Calif.). This minibeaker consisted of a chamber into which a radioactive test solution can be added, and contained numerous small Visking tubes (Visking Co., Chicago, Ill.) passing through the chamber, through which a protein-free solution was infused. An ultrafiltrate of human serum at pH 7.3 to 7.5 was passed through the tubing system at a rate of 3 ml/min as the protein-free side of the membrane into which the radioactive pen G (benzyl[^{14}C]penicillin, potassium, 43.5 μCi/mg; Amersham/Searle Corp.) diffused from the sample chamber. Fractions were collected on a drop counter fraction collector in 0.6-ml volumes. Radioactivity was determined on a Beckman LS-100C liquid scintillation counter (Beckman Instruments, Inc., Palo Alto, Calif.), using Aquasol (New England Nuclear, Boston, Mass.) as the scintillation solution.

The control sample consisted of 6 ml of an ultrafiltrate of human serum containing 60 U of pen G and 0.5 μCi of ^{14}C-pen G. This sample was introduced into the chamber, which contained a magnetic stir bar to insure mixing, and eight fractions were collected for radioactive determinations from the effluent passing through the fiber system. During collection of the eighth fraction, 2 ml of ultrafiltrate containing 800,000 U of pen G was added to the sample chamber, and an additional nine effluent fractions were collected.

This procedure was repeated, using serum instead of ultrafiltrate in the sample chamber. Serum was mixed with pen G and ^{14}C-pen G and either immediately introduced into the minibeaker chamber or incubated at 37°C for 1 h before being placed in the chamber. Eight fractions of the ultrafiltrate passing through the fibers were collected, and then an additional 2 ml of serum containing 800,000 U of pen G was added to the chamber to release protein-bound ^{14}C-pen G. The radioactivity in each collected fraction was then measured.

Additionally, studies were performed to evaluate any delayed release of ^{14}C-pen G bound to protein. Unlabeled pen G was added to serum containing 10 U of pen G and 0.1 μCi of ^{14}C-pen G per ml to bring the final concentration of pen G to 100,000 U/ml. This mixture was incubated for 1, 5, 15, and 30 min at 37°C, and 8 ml was then pipetted into a minibeaker chamber. Eight effluent fractions were collected, and the radioactivity in each fraction was compared with that obtained from an ultrafiltrate control sample containing 100,000 U of pen G and 0.1 μCi of ^{14}C-pen G per ml.

Cross-linked dextran exclusion. Determination of pen G binding to protein was performed by the method described by Pearlman and Crépy (35). When cross-linked dextran (Sephadex, Pharmacia Fine Chemicals, Inc., Piscataway, N.J.) is added to a solution containing known amounts of protein and ligand (1), the protein will be concentrated in the external phase (V_e) of the Sephadex, and this external phase will also contain both free (F) and protein-bound (B) ligand. Only free ligand will be allowed into the internal (V_i) compartment of the Sephadex. After equilibration of Sephadex with the starting solution, the concentration of ligand in the external phase ($[t]$) can be measured, and the concentration of free ligand ($[F]$) can be calculated from:

$$[F] = (1 - [t]\cdot V_e)/V_i \quad (1)$$

Once the concentration of free drug is known, the protein binding of the ligand is easily determined.

The internal volume of the Sephadex G-25 (fine) was determined by placing 300 mg of Sephadex in 1.5 ml of human serum ultrafiltrate containing 2.5 g of albumin per 100 ml. After 3-h swelling time in a 37°C shaking water bath, the equilibration of Sephadex was complete and 0.2 ml of clear supernatant was removed for albumin determination. Initial ($[A_s]$) and final ($[A_f]$) albumin concentrations were determined by the method of Lowry et al. (30), and the external volume (V_e) for 300 mg of Sephadex was determined from the following:

$$V_e = 1.5\ \text{ml}\cdot[A_s]/[A_f] \quad (2)$$

Internal volume of 300 mg of Sephadex in this system is then:

$$V_i = 1.5\ \text{ml} - V_e \quad (3)$$

Serum protein-binding determinations were performed by adding 300 mg of Sephadex G-25 (fine) to small disposable tubes (Falcon 2054 tube, Becton-Dickinson and Co., Oxnard, Calif.) containing a mixture of 0.9 ml of pooled human serum, 0.6 ml of human serum ultrafiltrate, 0.03 μCi of ^{14}C-pen G, and known quantities of cold (unlabeled) pen G. Determinations were performed at 10, 100, 1,000, 10,000, and 50,000 U of pen G per ml. Control solutions containing pen G in serum ultrafiltrate were also evaluated. The tubes were then placed in a shaking water bath for 3 h at 37°C to swell the Sephadex. After 3 h, 0.2 ml of supernatant was removed from each tube, and radioactivity in this sample was compared with that of the starting solutions. Serum protein binding was calculated from equation 1.

Ultracentrifugation. Ultracentrifugation was standardized according to the method of Steinberg and Schachman (39). Sedimentation velocity experiments (high-speed centrifugation) were compared with sedimentation equilibrium studies (low-speed centrifugation) in order to validate the high-speed method.

Sedimentation equilibrium studies were performed by mixing 80 U of pen G and 0.25 μCi of ^{14}C-pen G with 8 ml of human serum ultrafiltrate containing 5.0 g of human serum albumin (Cutter Laboratories, Berkeley, Calif.) per 100 ml in an ultracentrifuge cell (Beckman 335349 polycarbonate ultracentrifuge tube, Beckman Instruments, Inc., Palo Alto, Calif.). Centrifugation was performed for 16 h at 14,000 $\times g$ (center of the cell forces) at 3°C on a Beckman L2-65B preparative ultracentrifuge (Beckman Instruments, Inc.), using a type 65 fixed-angle centrifuge rotor (Beckman Instruments, Inc.). Four samples were taken at 1.5-cm intervals throughout the cell and assayed for protein (30) and radioactivity. A control solution containing pen G and ^{14}C-pen G in ultrafiltrate only was also evaluated. Radioactivity was plotted against protein concentration, and the amount of free ^{14}C-pen G was determined by extrapolating to zero protein.

Sedimentation velocity experiments were performed on similar samples with centrifugation for 3 h at 295,000 $\times g$ (center of the cell forces) at 3°C on the Beckman L2-65B centrifuge. The top 0.5 ml of sample from each centrifuge cell was removed and assayed for radioactivity. Three hours at 295,000 $\times g$ was necessary to achieve a 100-fold increase in protein from the top to the bottom of the centrifuge cell (18). Preliminary sedimentation velocity studies to compare serum binding at 3°C and 30 to 35°C were performed at a pen G concentration of 10 U/ml.

Serum samples containing 10, 100, 1,000, 10,000, and 100,000 U of pen G per ml plus 0.03 μCi of ^{14}C-pen G per ml were evaluated by the sedimentation velocity method at 30 to 35°C. The top 0.5 ml from each centrifuge cell was assayed for both radioactive and biological activity. The levels of "free" or unbound pen G determined by both the sedimentation equilibrium and sedimentation velocity methods were compared with levels of pen G in the appropriate starting solution to calculate albumin and serum protein binding.

Specimens and assays. Human serum was obtained from a pool of at least 10 normal fasting volunteers. Serum ultrafiltrate was obtained by passing pooled serum twice through a 90-mm ultrafiltration system (Millipore Corp., Bedford, Mass.) to yield a filtrate containing 0.2 g of protein per 100 ml but no albumin. All sera, filtrates, and other solutions were brought to pH 7.3 to 7.5 with either sodium bicarbonate or carbon dioxide before use. Scintillation counting was performed on a Beckman LS-100C scintillation counter, using Aquasol as a scintillation solution.

Radioactive pen G was determined to be 95 to 97% bioactive drug by paper chromatography and by Sephadex G-10 column chromatography, using a pH 7.0 saline buffer system.

Antibiotic assays were performed in triplicate, using a microbiological disk-plate method with a 24-h incubation at 37°C (29). *Bacillus subtilis* ATCC 6633 was used as the test organism, and standard curves were prepared in the same solution as samples to be tested.

RESULTS

Rate of dialysis. Results of radioactivity determined in each fraction collected are corrected for differences in radioactivity in the starting samples, and then results from the quantitative binding and immediate reversibility experiments are normalized to mean activity found in fractions 13 to 15 of the albumin-free control sample and plotted. There were no differences between incubated and unincubated serum samples, indicating that complete binding occurred in seconds or less (Fig. 1). Also, upon addition of excess nonradioactive pen G there was immediate release of protein-bound ^{14}C-pen G; however, the concentration of free drug only attained 77.2% of that in the non-protein-containing ultrafiltrate control, suggesting that the initial release was not 100%. The drop in radioactivity of the control solution was due to dilution of radioactive drug upon addition of the 2 ml of unlabeled pen G. Comparison of serum to ultrafiltrate control radioactivity in fractions 6 to 8 showed 51.5% binding of pen G at 10 U/ml (Table 1).

Results from the delayed-release protein-binding experiments are normalized to mean activity found in fractions five to seven of the ultrafiltrate control solution and plotted. Binding of ^{14}C-pen G after addition of a concentration of 100,000 U of cold pen G per ml was 9% at 1 min, 5% at 5 min, 5% at 15 min, and 13% at 30 min, with an overall mean of 8%. Therefore, although 22.8% of pen G was not immediately released from serum protein-binding sites, an additional 14.8% appeared to be released within the first minute after additions of excess cold pen G.

Cross-linked dextran exclusion. The V_i (equation 2) found for Sephadex G-25 (fine) was 0.63 ml for 300 mg. Results of binding experiments are shown in Table 1. Pen G activity was significantly reduced by Sephadex, and this was not altered by prewashing the Sephadex with pooled serum. It is also important to note that variation in humidity during storage of the Sephadex altered the V_i and thereby changed the value of pen G binding obtained with the method.

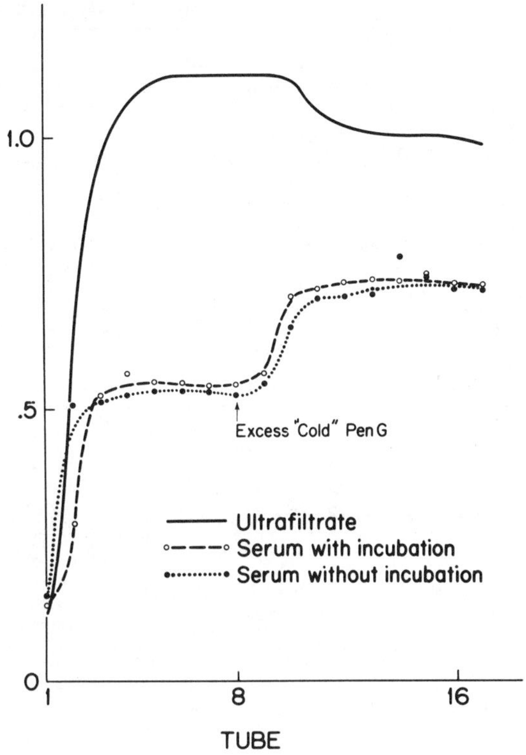

FIG. 1. *Binding and release of ^{14}C-pen G to human serum as determined by a rate-of-dialysis method. Ordinate is a normalization of values based on the mean of tubes 13 to 15 for the protein-free control solution (——). (●) Unincubated serum; (○) 1-h-incubated serum. Concentration of pen G in serum was 10 U/ml initially and was increased to 100,000 U/ml after addition of excess cold pen G (arrow). The drop in activity diffusing from control solution after addition of excess cold pen G was due to dilution of ^{14}C-pen G. Each curve represents the mean of three experiments.*

Ultracentrifugation. Comparisons of sedimentation equilibrium studies and sedimentation velocity studies are shown in Table 2. There was no difference in binding to human albumin between the two methods. Preliminary studies also demonstrated equivalent pen G binding to human serum at 3°C and 30 to 35°C.

Binding to human serum determined by sedimentation velocity is shown in Table 1. Results

TABLE 1. *Serum protein binding of* [14]*C-pen G*

Pen G concn (U/ml)	Method												
	Rate of dialysis				Dextran exclusion					Ultracentrifugation			
	Mean % bound	Range (%)	Mol of pen G/mol of albumin[a]	No. of determinations	Mean % bound	Range (%)	Percent pen G bound to Sephadex	Mol of pen G/mol of albumin	No. of determinations	Mean % bound	Range (%)	Mol of pen G/mol of albumin	No. of determinations
10	51.5	49.3–60.6	0.014	6	52.5	49.7–58.8	14.7	0.015	9	52.8	50.9–55.8	0.015	7
100	NT[b]				45.6	44.2–47.3	13	0.13	3	51.7	49.4–55.6	0.15	7
1,000	NT				39.6	36.7–41.2	12.4	1.15	9	47.6	46.6–48.3	1.38	6
10,000	NT				15.9	13.4–17.4	17.2	4.61	6	26.9	24.3–28.5	7.80	6
50,000	NT				3.5	3.0–3.8	12.3	5.08	3	NT			
100,000	8[c]	0–16.4	23.2	11	NT		NT			12.9	11.9–16.1	37.4	6

[a] Calculation based on human serum containing 4.0 g of albumin per 100 ml with a molecular weight of 68,000 and potassium pen G with a molecular weight of 374.
[b] NT, Not tested.
[c] Results having at least a 1-min incubation of 100,000 U of pen G per ml with ^{14}C-pen G.

TABLE 2. *Pen G binding to human serum albumin*

Method	Mean % bound at 10 U/ml	Range (%)	No. of determinations
Sedimentation equilibrium	31.6	21.6–35.8	12
Sedimentation velocity	29.2	26.3–31.2	15

are the same in both radioactive and bioassay determinations. Sedimentation of pen G in ultrafiltrate alone was small, and the reduction at the top of the ultracentrifuge cell from the starting solution concentration was less than 5%, a difference not detectable by bioassay methods.

DISCUSSION

Continuing interest in serum and tissue binding of antibiotics is manifested in recent reviews of the subject (2, 13, 22). We have evaluated three newer methods for investigating drug-protein interactions and have standardized ultracentrifugation for use in protein-binding determinations of the penicillins. The rate-of-dialysis technique appears well suited for investigations of the rapidity and reversibility of antibiotic protein binding. Table 1 demonstrates good comparability between this method and the others tested for quantitative binding of pen G to serum proteins at 10 U/ml. The finding of 8% pen G bound to serum albumin at 100,000 U of pen G per ml agrees with the ultracentrifuge data and suggests a large number of binding sites available at high antibiotic concentrations (Table 1). The reason for the 14.8% difference in ^{14}C-pen G binding observed immediately (22.8%) and after more than 1 min of incubation (8%) with 100,000 U of pen G per ml is unexplained. We are unable to determine whether this is an artifact in the system or whether a portion of the binding is slowly reversible.

Sephadex exclusion is possibly a reliable technique if all experimental conditions are carefully controlled. However, there is significant binding or trapping of penicillin by Sephadex, which necessitates the large correction factors presented in Table 1. The binding of various penicillins to Sephadex has been shown to have a linear relationship to the serum protein binding of these antibiotics (34). This problem coupled with the variation of Sephadex V_i observed with changes in humidity reduces the usefulness of cross-linked dextran in antibiotic protein-binding studies.

Ultracentrifugation appears to be a reliable technique for determinating static penicillin binding to serum proteins. The lower binding of pen G to purified human albumin and the stability of binding at various temperatures is comparable to results reported by others (26, 36). Results obtained using the sedimentation velocity method are in good agreement with previous reports (28, 41), as are the comparable results obtained with both the radioactive and bioassay determinations (27). This method could easily be extended to tissue-binding studies, and because of the similarity of their structure and molecular weight, this technique should be valid for all the penicillins (16). The advantages of a short centrifugation time (3 h) and absence of extraneous materials to which the antibiotic might bind are obvious. The single disadvantage of this technique is high cost of original equipment in comparison with other methods for antibiotic protein-binding studies.

The demonstration of serum protein binding

at 100,000 U of pen G per ml argues in favor of a large number of binding sites available on human serum albumin or other serum proteins. Although this may be an artifact induced by interaction between the penicillin molecules themselves at high concentrations, this is not demonstrable in saline or ultrafiltrate controls. All three methods demonstrated that at least five binding sites are involved with pen G interaction at concentrations over 10,000 U/ml. Finally, there is good agreement in numbers of binding sites and percentage of binding between the three methods in the range of clinically achievable blood levels (less than 1,000 U of pen G per ml).

With continued interest in the significance of antibiotic binding to serum and tissue proteins, we would recommend use of the ultracentrifuge for quantitative determinations of the binding properties of penicillins and use of a rate-of-dialysis technique for the investigation of dynamic antibiotic-protein interactions when a radiolabeled drug is available.

ACKNOWLEDGMENTS

A special acknowledgment is extended to Evelyn Glatt for assistance in preparation of this manuscript.

LITERATURE CITED

1. **Acred, P., D. M. Brown, T. L. Hardy, and K. R. L. Mansford.** 1963. A new approach to studying the protein-binding properties of penicillins. Nature (London) **199**:758-759.
2. **Barza, M., and L. Weinstein.** 1976. Pharmacokinetics of the penicillins in man. Clin. Pharmacokinetics **1**:297-308.
3. **Bauer, J. H., and E. G. Pickels.** 1936. A high speed vacuum centrifuge suitable for the study of filterable viruses. J. Exp. Med. **64**:503-528.
4. **Beams, J. W., F. W. Linke, and P. Sommer.** 1938. A vacuum type air-driven centrifuge for biophysical research. Rev. Sci. Instr. **9**:248-252.
5. **Bennet, J. V., and W. M. M. Kirby.** 1965. A rapid, modified ultrafiltration method for determining serum protein binding and its application to new penicillins. J. Lab. Clin. Med. **66**:721-732.
6. **Blatt, W. F., S. M. Robinson, and H. J. Bixler.** 1968. Membrane ultrafiltration: the diafiltration technique and its application to microsolute exchange and binding phenomena. Anal. Biochem. **26**:151-173.
7. **Bush, M. T., and J. D. Alvin.** 1973. Characterization of drug-protein interactions by classic methods. Ann. N.Y. Acad. Sci. **226**:36-43.
8. **Büttner, V. H., and F. Portwich.** 1961. Bestimmung der Bindung von Sulfonamiden an Serumeiweiss mit der Ultrazentrifuge. Arzneim. Forsch. **11**:1133-1137.
9. **Chignell, C. F.** 1972. Application of physiochemical and analytical techniques to the study of drug interactions with biological systems. Crit. Rev. Toxicol. **1**:413-465.
10. **Chow, B. F., and C. M. McKee.** 1945. Interaction between crystalline penicillin and human plasma proteins. Science **101**:67-68.
11. **Colowick, S. P., and F. C. Womack.** 1969. Binding of diffusible molecules by macromolecules: rapid measurement by rate of dialysis. J. Biol. Chem. **244**:774-777.
12. **Craig, L. C.** 1965. Differential dialysis. Adv. Anal. Chem. Instr. 4:35-74.
13. **Craig, W. A., and C. M. Kunin.** 1976. Significance of serum protein and tissue binding of antimicrobial agents. Annu. Rev. Med. **27**:287-300.
14. **Gelotte, B.** 1960. Studies on gel filtration sorption properties of the bed material sephadex. J. Chromatogr. **3**:330-342.
15. **Goldstein, A.** 1949. The interactions of drugs and plasma proteins. Pharmacol. Rev. **1**:102-165.
16. **Goodman, L. S., and A. Gilman.** 1970. The pharmacological basis of therapeutics, 4th ed., p. 1220. Macmillan Publishing Co., Riverside, N.J.
17. **Griffith, R. S., H. R. Black, G. L. Brier, and J. D. Wolny.** 1976. Cefamandole: in vitro and clinical pharmacokinetics. Antimicrob. Agents Chemother. **10**:814-823.
18. **Hirsch-Kolb, H., H. J. Kolb, and D. M. Greenberg.** 1970. Determination of binding properties of low molecular weight substances to proteins using ultracentrifugation. Anal. Biochem. **34**:517-528.
19. **Hummel, J. P., and W. J. Dreyer.** 1962. Measurement of protein-binding phenomena by gel filtration. Biochim. Biophys. Acta **63**:530-532.
20. **Karush, F.** 1952. Heterogenicity of the binding sites of bovine serum albumin. J. Am. Chem. Soc. **72**:2705-2718.
21. **Keresztes-Nagy, S., R. F. Mais, Y. T. Oester, and J. F. Zaroslinski.** 1972. Protein binding methodology. Anal. Biochem. **48**:80-89.
22. **Koch-Weser, J., and E. M. Sellers.** 1976. Binding of drugs to serum albumin. N. Engl. J. Med. **294**:311-316, 526-531.
23. **Kornguth, M. L., and C. M. Kunin.** 1976. Binding of antibiotics to the human intracellular erythrocyte proteins hemoglobin and carbonic anhydrase. J. Infect. Dis. **133**:185-193.
24. **Kornguth, M. L., R. A. Monson, and C. M. Kunin.** 1974. Binding of antibiotics to a soluble protein from rat liver. J. Infect. Dis. **129**:552-558.
25. **Kornguth, M. L., R. A. Monson, and C. M. Kunin.** 1976. The binding of penicillin antibiotics to a human liver protein. Arch. Biochem. Biophys. **174**:339-343.
26. **Kunin, C. M.** 1965. Inhibitors of penicillin binding to serum proteins. J. Lab. Clin. Med. **65**:416-431.
27. **Kunin, C. M.** 1966. Clinical pharmacology of the new penicillins. Clin. Pharmacol. Ther. **7**:166-179.
28. **Kunin, C. M.** 1967. Clinical significance of protein binding of the penicillins. Ann. N.Y. Acad. Sci. **145**:282-289.
29. **Lilly Research Laboratories.** 1970. Paper disc or cup plate antibiotic assay procedures. Eli Lilly and Co., Indianapolis, Ind.
30. **Lowry, O. H., N. J. Rosebrough, A. L. Farr, and R. J. Randall.** 1951. Protein measurement with the Folin phenol reagent. J. Biol. Chem. **193**:265-275.
31. **Masket, A. V.** 1941. A quantity type rotor for the ultracentrifuge. Rev. Sci. Instr. **12**:277-279.
32. **Mattie, H., W. R. O. Goslings, and E. L. Noach.** 1973. Cloxacillin and nafcillin: serum binding and its relationship to antibacterial effect in mice. J. Infect Dis. **128**:170-177.
33. **Meyer, M. C., and D. E. Guttman.** 1968. The binding of drugs by plasma proteins. J. Pharm. Sci. **57**:895-918.
34. **Murakawa, T., Y. Wakai, and M. Nishida.** 1970. Studies on the relationship of protein binding and gel-affinity of antibiotics including penicillins. J. Antibiot. **23**:481-487.
35. **Pearlman, W. H., and O. Crépy.** 1967. Steroid-protein interaction with particular reference to testosterone binding by human serum. J. Biol. Chem. **242**:182-189.
36. **Rolinson, G. N., and R. Sutherland.** 1965. The binding of antibiotics to serum proteins. Br. J. Pharmacol. **25**:638-650.

37. **Scholtan, V. W.** 1965. Die Bindung der Sulfonamide an Eiweisskörper. Arzneim. Forsch. **15**:1433–1441.
38. **Scholtan, W.** 1964. Bestimmungsmethoden und Gesetzmässigkeiten der Eisweissbindung von Sulfonamiden und Penicillinen. Antibiot. Chemother. **12**:103–134.
39. **Steinberg, I. Z., and H. K. Schachman.** 1966. Ultracentrifugation studies with adsorption optics. V. Analysis of interacting systems involving macromolecules and small molecules. Biochemistry **5**:3728–3747.
40. **Tompsett, R., S. Shultz, and W. McDermott.** 1947. The relation of protein binding to the pharmacology and antibacterial activity of the penicillins X, G, dihydro F, and K. J. Bacteriol. **53**:581–595.
41. **Warren, G. H.** 1965/66. The prognostic significance of penicillin serum levels and protein binding in clinical medicine. A review of current studies. Chemotherapia **10**:339–358.
42. **Womack, F. C., and S. P. Colowick.** 1973. Rapid measurement of binding of ligands by rate of dialysis. Methods Enzymol. **27**:464–471.

ANTIMICROBIAL AGENTS AND CHEMOTHERAPY, June 1977, p. 999-1003
Vol. 11, No. 6

Mercury Resistance and R Plasmids in *Escherichia coli* Isolated from Clinical Lesions in Japan

HIDEOMI NAKAHARA,[1] TOMOAKI ISHIKAWA,[2] YASUNAGA SARAI,[3] ISAMU KONDO, HIROYUKI KOZUKUE,* AND SUSUMU MITSUHASHI

Departments of Hygiene and Microbiology, The Jikei University School of Medicine, Tokyo 105, Japan; and Department of Microbiology, School of Medicine, Gunma University, Maebashi 371, Japan.*

Received for publication 26 October 1976

The mercury and antibiotic resistance of 338 strains of *Escherichia coli* isolated from hospital patients was determined. Resistance to mercury was found in 58.6% of the isolates. The frequencies of resistance to streptomycin (Sm), tetracycline (Tc), chloramphenicol (Cm), kanamycin (Kan), cephaloridine (Cer), and gentamicin (Gm) were 66.3, 60.3, 56.5, 42.9, 32.1, and 1.5%, respectively. Among the above, 198 mercury- and antibiotic-resistant isolates were selected and tested for their ability to transfer the resistance to susceptible strains of *E. coli* K-12 and *Klebsiella pneumoniae* JK5. R plasmids carrying mercury resistance were demonstrated in 89.9% of the mercury-resistant strains of *E. coli*. Furthermore, R(Hg,Sm,Tc,Cm) plasmids were demonstrated most frequently, followed by R(Hg,Sm,Tc,Cm,Kan), R(Hg,Cm,Kan), and R(Hg,Sm,-Tc,Cm,Kan,Cer) plasmids.

Resistance of bacteria to mercury has been described by several authors from the viewpoints of morphology (23), genetics, and biochemistry. In many bacteria, resistance to mercury is associated with a plasmid (7, 8, 13, 14, 16, 17, 19). Generally, microorganisms have been shown to detoxify mercurial compounds metabolically by forming either volatile mercury derivatives (1, 12, 16, 19, 22) or mercury mercaptides (5, 15, 18, 25). There are also many bacteria that are resistant to other metallic ions such as cadmium, arsenate, lead, zinc, cobalt, and nickel (8–10, 13, 17).

It is of interest that resistance to these metals is mediated by the same plasmid that determines resistance to antibiotics. Also, most of these metals have recently been listed as established or possible causes of environmental pollution. For example, methyl mercury is known to cause Minamata disease (6, 20), and cadmium is the causative agent of Itai-Itai disease in Japan.

The role of R plasmids in drug resistance has been widely studied (2–4, 11, 21, 24), and extrachromosomal determinants are a main cause of the increase in numbers of drug-resistant bacteria. However, the factors selecting for these metal-resistant bacteria have not yet been identified. We believe that metal-resistant microorganisms do not arise by chance, but that there must be selection factors beyond mere drug resistance. One of these selection factors may be environmental contamination by these heavy metals.

We previously investigated the distribution of the resistance to several metallic ions such as Hg, Cd, As, and Pb among 415 strains of *Staphylococcus aureus* (*S. aureus*) isolated from hospital patients (9). Recently, we also demonstrated 198 R plasmids with Hg resistance in *Escherichia coli* isolated from clinical specimens. This paper deals with the genetic properties of these R plasmids carrying Hg resistance.

MATERIALS AND METHODS

Bacterial strains. A total of 338 strains of *E. coli* were isolated from the Clinical Laboratory of The Jikei University Hospital and tested for their resistance to mercury and six antibiotics. Mating experiments were carried out with a total of 198 Hg- and antibiotic-resistant strains as donors to examine the presence of conjugally transferable R plasmids. *E. coli* K-12 ML1410 and *Klebsiella pneumoniae* JK5 were used as recipient bacteria. *E. coli* K-12 ML1410 was kindly supplied by Matsuhisa Inoue, Department of Microbiology, School of Medicine, Gunma University. It is a nalidixic acid- and rifampin (Rif)-resistant mutant of *E. coli* K-12. *K. pneumoniae* JK5 was isolated at our laboratory.

Drug resistance tests. Minimal inhibitory concentrations of the six antibiotics tested against all *E. coli* strains were determined by the agar dilution method using nutrient agar. Antibiotics used were streptomycin (Sm), tetracycline (Tc), chlorampheni-

[1] Present address: Department of Biology, Washington University, St. Louis, MO 63130.

[2] Present address: Department of Internal Medicine, The Third Hospital, The Jikei University School of Medicine, Izumi, Komae, Tokyo 182, Japan.

[3] Present address: Department of Pediatrics, National Medical Center Hospital of Japan, Tokyo 162, Japan.

col (Cm), kanamycin (Kan), cephaloridine (Cer), and gentamicin (Gm). Those cultures not inhibited by 25 μg of Sm, Tc, Cm, or Kan per ml or by 12.5 μg of Cer or Gm per ml were regarded as resistant to each of the antibiotics.

Mercury resistance tests. As the mercury derivative, we used $HgCl_2$. $HgCl_2$ was dissolved in distilled water, sterilized by membrane filtration (Millipore Corp.; pore size, 0.45 μm), and added to agar medium in the designated concentrations.

Conjugation experiments. Donor strains of *E. coli* were cultivated for transfer in nutrient broth (Difco) with shaking for 5 h. One milliliter of a culture containing about 10^6 bacteria was mixed with 1 ml of a similarly prepared recipient culture. The mixture was statically incubated for 4 to 8 h, and then about 0.01 ml was plated on Simmons citrate agar (Eiken) or nutrient agar (Difco) containing 100 μg of Rif per ml plus one of the following substances: 25 μg of Sm, 25 μg of Tc, 25 μg of Cm, or 10 μg of $HgCl_2$ per ml. The plates were incubated overnight at 37°C and then compared with control plates with individual antibiotics and the parental strains, and also with Rif plates plus single-antibiotic or Hg additions.

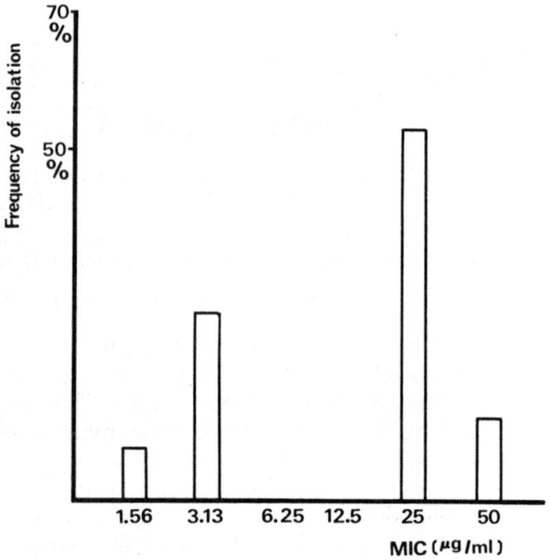

FIG. 1. *Distribution pattern of resistance to Hg in 338 strains of E. coli. The Hg resistance revealed a clear-cut bimodal distribution. From this pattern, those cultures not inhibited by 10 μg of Hg per ml were regarded as resistant to Hg.*

RESULTS

Distribution of Hg- and antibiotic-resistant strains of *E. coli*. Figure 1 shows the distribution curve of Hg resistance obtained by the agar dilution method from 338 clinical isolates of *E. coli*. The bimodal distribution curve of susceptibility to Hg showed a clear-cut distinction between susceptible and resistant populations, and it can be seen that the resistance was differentiated by concentrations of $HgCl_2$ above 10 μg/ml.

The frequency of resistance to Hg was 58.6% among the 338 isolates. On the other hand, the frequencies of resistance to Sm, Tc, Cm, Kan, Cer, and Gm were 66.3, 60.3, 56.5, 42.9, 32.1, and 1.5%, respectively.

Transfer of plasmids carrying Hg resistance. In the first cycle of transfer, the first five strains of *E. coli*, i.e., JE504, JE456, JE333, JE335, and JE224, transferred the whole complex pattern of resistance at a frequency of about 10^{-3} to *K. pneumoniae* JK5 (Table 1). However, exconjugants from crosses of the remaining strain, JE117, were resistant to Hg and all of the antibiotic markers except Kan, the latter apparently segregating out.

These exconjugants were also tested for transfer of their resistance to *E. coli* K-12 ML1410-Rif as the recipient. The resulting exconjugants were selected on nutrient agar with 100 μg of Rif per ml plus a single selecting drug or Hg in the concentrations given above. After 3 h or more of mating, a high frequency of transfer of virtually the total resistance pattern to the *E. coli* K-12 recipient was observed. Some data concerning this second cycle of transfer are given in Table 1. This pattern of resistance was then well transferable in further cycles from and to the recipient strains described.

Resistance patterns of Hg-resistant *E. coli* strains. Resistance patterns of *E. coli* strains possessing Hg resistance are shown in Table 2. Triple-drug resistance appeared most frequently (37.9%) among the strains carrying Hg resistance, followed by quadruple (26.8%)-, double (24.2%)-, and quintuple (7.6%)-drug resistance. In contrast, among these strains, those carrying single- and sextuple-drug resistance were 2 and 1.5%, respectively. Strains carrying only Hg resistance have not been isolated as yet from *E. coli*.

Genetic properties of the R plasmids carrying Hg resistance. Among the 338 isolates of *E. coli*, 198 strains resistant to Hg were selected, and conjugal transferability of their resistance was examined. Among these 198 Hg-resistant strains, 178 R plasmids carrying Hg resistance (89.9%) could be demonstrated (Table 2). With reference to resistance to Hg and/or six antibiotics, R plasmids with (Hg; Sm,Tc,Cm) resistance were isolated most frequently, followed by R(Hg; Tc,Cm,Kan), R(Hg; Sm,Kan), and R(Hg; Sm,Tc,Cm,Kan,Cer), in that order.

The frequencies of strains with resistance to Sm, Tc, Cm, Kan, Cer, and Gm mediated by R plasmids carrying Hg resistance were 88.8, 86.0, 82.6, 51.1, 10.7, and 1.7%, respectively.

DISCUSSION

It is well known that R plasmids in *E. coli* carry genes determining resistance to several metallic ions such as Hg, Co, and Ni (17). Also, penicillinase plasmids mediating resistance to Hg, Cd, As, Pb, and Zn have been observed in *S. aureus* (13, 14). We have reported that the resistances to Hg and Cd mediated by a penicillinase plasmid were found to be controlled by quite different mechanisms (8).

Numerous studies of drug-resistant bacteria have clarified the close relationship between the appearance of drug-resistant bacteria and usage of the drug. However, the nature of the selection factor for these metal-resistant bacteria has not yet been fully explained from the epidemiological and genetic viewpoints. We have assumed that these metallic ions themselves could be the selection factor because of environmental contamination by these metals.

TABLE 1. *Transfer of R plasmids from E. coli (first and second cycles)*

Donor	Resistance pattern	1st cycle			2nd cycle			Resistance spectrum
		Recipient	Selected for:	Frequency	Recipient	Selected for:	Frequency	
JE504	Hg Sm, Tc, Cm Kan, Cer, Gm	JK5	Hg + Cit[a] Sm + Cit	10^{-3} 10^{-2}	ML1410-Rif ML1410-Rif	Hg + Rif[b] Sm + Rif	10^{-4} 10^{-3}	Hg; Sm, Tc, Cm, Kan, Cer, Gm Hg; Sm, Tc, Cm, Kan, Cer, Gm
JE456	Hg Sm, Tc, Cm Kan, Cer	JK5	Hg + Cit Sm + Cit	10^{-2} 10^{-2}	ML1410-Rif ML1410-Rif	Hg + Rif Sm + Rif	10^{-2} 10^{-3}	Hg; Sm, Tc, Cm, Kan, Cer Hg; Sm, Tc, Cm, Kan, Cer
JE333	Hg Sm, Tc, Cm	JK5	Hg + Cit Sm + Cit	10^{-2} 10^{-2}	ML1410-Rif ML1410-Rif	Hg + Rif Sm + Rif	10^{-4} 10^{-3}	Hg; Sm, Tc, Cm Hg; Sm, Tc, Cm
JE335	Hg Tc, Cm	JK5	Hg + Cit Tc + Cit	10^{-3} 10^{-4}	ML1410-Rif ML1410-Rif	Hg + Rif Tc + Rif	10^{-2} 10^{-4}	Hg; Tc, Cm Hg; Tc, Cm
JE224	Hg Cm, Kan	JK5	Hg + Cit Cm + Cit	10^{-3} 10^{-4}	ML1410-Rif ML1410-Rif	Hg + Rif Cm + Rif	10^{-3} 10^{-4}	Hg; Cm, Kan Hg; Cm, Kan
JE117	Hg Sm, Tc, Cm Kan, Cer	JK5	Hg + Cit Sm + Cit	10^{-3} 10^{-4}	ML1410-Rif ML1410-Rif	Hg + Rif Sm + Rif	10^{-3} 10^{-3}	Hg; Sm, Tc, Cm, Cer Hg; Sm, Tc, Cm, Cer

[a] Cit, Simmons citrate agar containing 10 μg of $HgCl_2$ per ml.
[b] Nutrient agar containing 100 μg of Rif plus 10 μg of $HgCl_2$ per ml.

TABLE 2. *Demonstration of R plasmids carrying Hg resistance from E. coli and their resistance patterns of antibiotics*

Resistance pattern	No. of resistant strains	Resistance pattern of R plasmid transferred	No. of strains with R plasmid
Hg; Sm, Tc, Cm, Kan, Cer, Gm	3	Hg; Sm, Tc, Kan, Cer, Gm	3
Hg; Sm, Tc, Cm, Kan, Cer	15	Hg; Sm, Tc, Cm, Kan, Cer	13
		Hg; Sm, Tc, Cm, Cer	2
Hg; Sm, Tc, Cm, Kan	52	Hg; Sm, Tc, Cm, Kan	47
Hg; Sm, Tc, Kan, Cer	1	Hg; Sm, Tc, Kan, Cer	1
Hg; Sm, Tc, Cm	62	Hg; Sm, Tc, Cm	58
Hg; Sm, Tc, Kan	8	Hg; Sm, Tc, Kan	6
Hg; Tc, Cm, Kan	5	Hg; Tc, Cm, Kan	4
Hg; Sm, Tc	6	Hg; Sm, Tc	6
Hg; Sm, Cm	6	Hg; Sm, Cm	5
Hg; Sm, Kan	19	Hg; Sm, Kan	15
Hg; Cm, Kan	2	Hg; Cm, Kan	2
Hg; Tc, Cm	15	Hg; Tc, Cm	12
Hg; Sm	2	Hg; Sm	2
Hg; Tc	1	Hg; Tc	1
Hg; Cm	1	Hg; Cm	1

We have reported the distribution of resistance to Hg, Cd, As, and Pb among 415 isolates of *S. aureus*. The results were as follows. (i) The frequency of the metal-resistant strains was actually higher than that of drug-resistant strains. (ii) Most of metal-resistant strains were found to be multiple-metal resistant and also multiple-drug resistant. (iii) About 10% of the total isolates were found to be metal resistant but drug susceptible. (iv) *S. aureus* MS1396 and JS76 were found to contain a new plasmid that controls only metal resistance (9).

The distribution curve of Hg resistance clearly revealed two peaks, and as a result of this we could isolate Hg-resistant *E. coli* strains as well as antibiotic-resistant strains. From the viewpoint of the origin of Hg- and drug-resistant bacteria and their selection, spread, and prevalence, it should be noted that the frequency of Hg resistance was same as or higher than that of drug resistance. A similar result was found in *S. aureus*.

Among the strains possessing Hg resistance, those carrying triple-drug resistance were isolated most frequently, followed by quadruple-, double-, and quintuple-drug resistance. Furthermore, most of the Hg-resistant strains had joint resistance to Sm, Tc, and Cm, and it would seem that the gene for Hg resistance in these *E. coli* strains is on the same R plasmid as the Sm, Tc, and Cm resistance genes.

From the mating experiments with a total of 198 Hg-resistant strains as donors, 178 with R plasmids (89.9%) with Hg resistance could be demonstrated. In addition, among the above, 5 Hg- and antibiotic-resistant isolates were selected and tested for the elimination of Hg and antibiotic resistance. All Hg and antibiotic resistance determinants in five strains were coeliminated at high frequency by treatment with acriflavine and growth at 43°C (about 2.4 to 15.2%).

The resistance patterns of R plasmids were quite similar to those of the resistant strains that were isolated frequently, indicating that Hg and antibiotic resistances in *E. coli* strains are mainly due to the presence of R plasmids.

ACKNOWLEDGMENTS

We are grateful to S. Silver and R. R. Colwell for their valuable and helpful discussions. We thank K. Kurosaka, K. Machida, T. Sawahata, and K. Itoh for supplying the clinical isolates.

This work was supported by a Grant-in-Aid for Scientific Research of the Japanese Ministry of Education (no. 177156).

LITERATURE CITED

1. **Ben-Bassat, D., G. Shelef, N. Gruner, and H. Shuval.** 1972. Growth of Chlamydomonas in a medium containing mercury. Nature (London) **240**:43–44.
2. **Curtiss, R., III.** 1969. Bacterial conjugation. Annu. Rev. Microbiol. **23**:69–136.
3. **Curtiss, R., III, L. J. Charamella, D. R. Stallions, and J. A. Mays.** 1968. Parental functions during conjugations in *Escherichia coli* K-12. Bacteriol. Rev. **32**:320–348.
4. **Datta, N., and R. W. Hedges.** 1971. Compatibility groups among fi$^-$ R factors. Nature (London) **234**:222–223.
5. **Hamdy, M. K., and O. R. Noyes.** 1975. Formation of methyl mercury by bacteria. Appl. Microbiol. **30**:424–432.
6. **Hirayama, K., and H. Takahashi.** 1970. Studies on the treatment for methyl mercury poisoning "lowing of the methyl mercury content in the poisoned animal brain". Kumamoto Med. J. **23**:56–64.
7. **Iyobe, S., K. Hasuda, H. Sugai, and S. Mitsuhashi.** 1975. Drug resistance and R factors in *P. aeruginosa*, p. 321–327. *In* S. Mitsuhashi and H. Hashimoto (ed.), Microbial drug resistance. University of Tokyo Press, Tokyo.
8. **Kondo, I., T. Ishikawa, and H. Nakahara.** 1974. Mercury and cadmium resistances mediated by the penicillinase plasmid in *Staphylococcus aureus*. J. Bacteriol. **117**:1–7.
9. **Kondo, I., H. Nakahara, and T. Ishikawa.** 1975. The possibility of a specific plasmid mediating metal resistances, p. 145–152. *In* S. Mitsuhashi and H. Hashimoto (ed.), Microbial drug resistance. University of Tokyo Press, Tokyo.
10. **Mitra, R. S., R. H. Gray, B. Chin, and I. A. Bernstein.** 1975. Molecular mechanisms of accommodation in *Escherichia coli* to toxic levels of Cd^{2+}. J. Bacteriol. **121**:1180–1188.
11. **Mitsuhashi, S.** 1971. Drug-resistance of gram-negative bacteria isolated in Japan, p. 7–16. *In* S. Mitsuhashi (ed.), Transferable drug resistance factor R. University of Tokyo Press, Tokyo.
12. **Nelson, J. D., Jr., W. Blair, F. E. Brinckman, R. R. Colwell, and W. P. Iverson.** 1973. Biodegradation of phenylmercuric acetate by mercury-resistant bacteria. Appl. Microbiol. **16**:321–326.
13. **Novick, R. P., and C. Roth.** 1968. Plasmid-linked resistance to inorganic salts in *Staphylococcus aureus*. J. Bacteriol. **95**:1335–1342.
14. **Richmond, M. H., and M. John.** 1964. Co-transduction by a staphylococcal phage of the genes responsible for penicillinase synthesis and resistance to mercury salts. Nature (London) **202**:1360–1361.
15. **Ross, I. S., and K. M. Old.** 1973. Thiol compounds and resistance of *Pyrenophora avenae* to mercury. Trans. Br. Mycol. Soc. **60**:301–310.
16. **Schottel, J., A. Mandal, D. Clark, S. Silver, and R. W. Hedges.** 1974. Volatilisation of mercury and organomercurials determined by inducible R-factor systems in enteric bacteria. Nature (London) **251**:335–337.
17. **Smith, D. H.** 1967. R factors mediate resistance to mercury, nickel and cobalt. Science **156**:1114–1116.
18. **Stutzenberger, F. J., and E. O. Bennett.** 1965. Sensitivity of mixed populations of *Staphylococcus aureus* and *Escherichia coli* to mercurials. Appl. Microbiol. **13**:570–574.
19. **Summers, A. O., and S. Silver.** 1972. Mercury resistance in plasmid-bearing strains of *Escherichia coli*. J. Bacteriol. **112**:1228–1236.
20. **Takizawa, Y., T. Kosaka, and R. Sugai.** 1972. Studies on the cause of Niigata episode of Minamata disease outbreak. Acta Med. Biol. (Niigata) **19**:193–206.
21. **Tanaka, T., A. Kobayashi, K. Ikemura, H. Hashimoto, and S. Mitsuhashi.** 1974. Drug resistance and distri-

bution of R factors among *Escherichia coli* strains. Jpn. J. Microbiol. 18:343-347.

22. **Tonomura, K., K. Maeda, F. Futai, T. Nakagami, and M. Yamada.** 1968. Stimulative vaporization of phenylmercuric acetate by mercury-resistant bacteria. Nature (London) **217**:644-646.
23. **Vaituzis, Z., J. D. Nelson, Jr., L. W. Wan, and R. R. Colwell.** 1975. Effects of mercuric chloride on growth and morphology of selected strains of mercury-resistant bacteria. Appl. Microbiol. **29**:275-286.
24. **Watanabe, T.** 1963. Infective heredity of multiple drug resistance in bacteria. Bacteriol. Rev. **27**:87-115.
25. **Wood, J. M., F. S. Kennedy, and C. G. Rosen.** 1968. Synthesis of methylmercury compounds by extracts of a methanogenic bacterium. Nature (London) **220**:173-174.

ANTIMICROBIAL AGENTS AND CHEMOTHERAPY, June 1977, p. 1004-1006
Copyright © 1977 American Society for Microbiology
Vol. 11, No. 6
Printed in U.S.A.

Transfer of Beta-Lactamase Genes of *Neisseria gonorrhoeae* by Conjugation

LINDA A. KIRVEN* AND CLYDE THORNSBERRY

Center for Disease Control, Atlanta, Georgia 30333

Received for publication 9 February 1977

Recent isolates of *Neisseria gonorrhoeae* have been shown to be resistant to penicillin because they produce β-lactamase. In this study, conjugal transfer of the β-lactamase gene to a recipient *N. gonorrhoeae* strain occurred in one of the two strains studied but not in the other. The transconjugant could also conjugally transfer the β-lactamase gene to an *Escherichia coli* strain.

β-lactamase-producing strains of *Neisseria gonorrhoeae,* which have recently been reported in this country and others, cause cases of gonorrhea that have been generally resistant to treatment with penicillin (1, 3, 7, 8). In our laboratory, we recently characterized the β-lactamase activity of the first two of these strains isolated in the United States; the enzyme resembles those present in some species of gram-negative bacilli, particularly those of the ampicillin-resistant, β-lactamase-producing *Haemophilus influenzae* (unpublished data). Synthesis of β-lactamases in most gram-negative bacilli is mediated by plasmids. Our study was undertaken to determine whether the penicillin resistance (i.e., β-lactamase production) could be transferred from strain to strain of *N. gonorrhoeae* by conjugation.

MATERIALS AND METHODS

Bacterial strains. The donor strains of *N. gonorrhoeae* (61782 and 73389) were cultures received in our laboratory for determination of minimal inhibitory concentrations (MICs) and were from patients who failed to respond to treatment with penicillin. When tested by the agar-dilution method, these strains had penicillin MICs of 4 and 8 μg/ml with an inoculum of between 10^3 to 10^4 colony-forming units (CFU)/ml. When the inoculum was increased, the MICs greatly increased. β-Lactamase production was detected by a test with chromogenic cephalosporin 87/312 and by the acidometric and iodometric techniques (10). The recipient (*N. gonorrhoeae* F-28) was a penicillin-susceptible strain resistant to greater than 2,048 μg of spectinomycin per ml; it was made resistant to greater than 50 μg of rifampin per ml with *N*-methyl-*N*-nitroso-*N'*-nitroguanidine (Pfaltz & Bauer, Inc.). The second chromosomal marker, which would not be selected for (i.e., rifampin would not be used in the selective medium), would be useful in identifying the transconjugant and would aid in the determination of direction of transfer. The recipient, *Escherichia coli,* was restrictionless and susceptible to ampicillin (β-lactamase negative) and spectinomycin, but resistant to rifampin. Stock cultures were suspended in small volumes of defibrinated rabbit blood and stored at −70°C.

Media. The *N. gonorrhoeae* were grown on proteose no. 3 agar (Difco), supplemented with 1% bovine hemoglobin and 1% IsoVitaleX (PHI agar). The selective medium used in the transfer studies consisted of the above medium supplemented with 32 μg of penicillin and 100 μg of spectinomycin per ml. Mueller-Hinton broth (BBL) was used as the suspending medium in the membrane-transfer studies. Columbia broth supplemented with 1% IsoVitaleX was used in the broth-transfer and donor, cell-free filtrate studies. In the transfer studies with the *E. coli,* the selective medium was Schaedler agar containing 40 μg of ampicillin per ml. This medium supported the growth of *E. coli* but not of gonococci.

Antibiotics. Potassium penicillin G was supplied by Bristol Laboratories, spectinomycin sulfate by the Upjohn Co., and rifampin by the Ciba Pharmaceutical Co.

Transfer studies. Donor and recipient strains were grown on PHI agar for 18 h. Some of the resulting growth was suspended in 4.5 ml of Mueller-Hinton broth to a concentration of approximately 5×10^8 CFU/ml. One milliliter of the donor culture and 1.5 ml of the recipient culture were mixed and immediately filtered through a sterile membrane filter (0.45 μm, Millipore Corp.). The filter, with bacteria side up, was placed on a drug-free PHI agar plate and incubated in candle extinction jars for either 6 or 24 h at 35°C. The cells were then recovered by placing the filter in 1 ml of Mueller-Hinton broth and then agitating the mixture vigorously (Vortex) for 1 min. One-tenth milliliter of this suspension was spread on the selective PHI agar medium, which contained both penicillin (32 μg/ml) and spectinomycin (100 μg/ml). After incubation for 3 days at 35°C in a candle jar, the selective media were flooded with chromogenic cephalosporin 87/312. Colonies with β-lactamase-producing bacteria turned red and were presumed to be transconjugant colonies. These colonies were subcultured on PHI agar and incubated for 48 h at 35°C in a candle jar. Single colonies were again subcultured on PHI agar and incubated for 18 h at 35°C in a candle jar. The transconjugant cultures were then tested by a disk-agar-diffusion technique for susceptibility to penicillin, spectinomycin, and rifampin. An inoculum of approximately 10^8 CFU/ml was spread on a PHI plate. A 10-μg penicillin disk, a 100-μg spectinomycin disk, and a 5-μg rifampin disk were then placed on the surface of the plate, which was then incubated for 24 h at 35°C in a candle jar. MICs were also determined for these three antimicrobics with an agar-dilution technique (5). β-Lactamase activity was confirmed with the chromogenic cephalosporin 87/312 test.

The same membrane method was also used with the following differences: (i) a cell-free filtrate of the donor was substituted for donor cells, (ii) recipient cells only were used, and (iii) the transfer was performed in the presence of deoxyribonuclease (DNase) (Sigma). In the DNase experiment, the cells were collected on the membrane filters, which were placed, bacteria side up, on fresh, drug-free PHI agar plates and flooded with DNase at a concentration of 1,000 μg/ml in 0.25 M $MgSO_4$.

Transfer studies were also carried out in broth (i.e., no membrane filter was used). The donor and recipient cells were placed in separate tubes of Columbia broth supplemented with IsoVitaleX to a concentration of approximately 10^8 CFU/ml. One milliliter of the donor suspension was mixed with 1.5 ml of the recipient suspension. This mixture was incubated in a candle jar for 6 h at 35°C. Transconjugants were identified on selective medium as described for the membrane studies.

In a final transfer experiment, a restrictionless strain of *E. coli* was the recipient and the 73389 transconjugant gonococcus was the donor. The membrane technique was used, and the conjugation time was 6 h.

RESULTS

The MICs for the recipient, donor, and transconjugant strains are shown in Table 1. The recipient strain, F-28, which did not produce β-lactamase, was very susceptible to penicillin but was quite resistant to spectinomycin and rifampin. The two donor strains, however, were resistant to penicillin and were susceptible to spectinomycin and rifampin. Transconjugants from 73389 produced β-lactamase and were resistant to all three antibiotics.

Results obtained in transfer experiments are shown in Table 2. In studies with donor 61782, we were unable to select any recipient strains that had acquired β-lactamase activity. However, by using donor 73389 and the membrane filter technique for either 6 or 24 h, we could readily select recipient strains that produced β-lactamase and had high penicillin MICs. These transconjugant strains also had high MICs to spectinomycin and rifampin, indicating that they were recipient strains that had acquired β-lactamase activity. The transfer was not affected by DNase. When a cell-free filtrate of the donor was substituted for the donor cells, no transfer of β-lactamase activity occurred, and when the recipient cells were incubated without the donor cells, no β-lactamase-producing cells could be isolated. Six different 73389 transconjugant strains readily transferred the β-lactamase activity to the *E. coli* recipient.

In the transfer studies carried out in broth (i.e., not collecting the cells on a membrane filter) transfer occurred rarely. We were able to isolate only one colony of a recipient strain that had acquired β-lactamase activity.

In this study, as with other studies on the transfer of a β-lactamase gene (e.g., with *H. influenzae*), it was difficult to determine the frequency of transfer. The β-lactamase-producing gonococci on the selective medium (this includes large numbers of donor organisms in addition to the transconjugant organisms) actively inactivate one of the selective agents, penicillin, which permits the β-lactamase-negative organisms (these are the recipient organisms) to grow. It is for this reason that the quantity of penicillin per milliliter of selective medium is much higher than the penicillin MIC of the donor strain. Although we chose not

TABLE 1. *β-Lactamase (βlac) production by and MICs of recipient, donor, and transconjugant strains of N. gonorrhoeae*

Strain	βlac	MIC (μg/ml)[a]		
		Pen	Spec	Rif
Recipient F-28	−	0.03	>128	>50
Donor 61782	+	>32	16	0.25
Donor 73389	+	32	16	0.50
73389 transconjugants	+	16− >32	>128	>50
73389 transconjugants (DNase experiment)	+	16− >32	>128	>50

[a] MICs to penicillin (Pen), spectinomycin (Spec), and rifampin (Rif) with an inoculum of between 10^4 and 10^5 CFU/ml.

TABLE 2. *Transfer experiments with the two β-lactamase-producing strains of N. gonorrhoeae and a transconjugant of one of these strains*

Donor	Recipient	Transfer expt		
		MF[a]	CFF[b]	DNase[c]
61782	F-28[d]	−	−	−
73389	F-28	+	−	+
73389–F-28[e], transconjugant	*E. coli*	+	ND[f]	ND[f]

[a] MF, Donor and recipient cells mixed and incubated on a membrane filter.

[b] CFF, Cell-free filtrate of donor mixed with recipient cells and incubated on membrane filter.

[c] DNase, Tests performed as with MF but in the presence of DNase.

[d] Non-β-lactamase-producing *N. gonorrhoeae*.

[e] F-28 received β-lactamase gene from 73389.

[f] ND, Not done.

to specifically quantitate the frequency of transfer, we could conclude, through the use of the chromogenic cephalosporin on the selective plate, that with the membrane technique, the frequency was relatively high, and with the broth technique it was extremely low.

DISCUSSION

These data suggest that the transfer of genetic material from donor 73389 to the recipient strain was by conjugation. The transfer occurred on the membrane filter when 73389 (β-lactamase positive) and F-28 (β-lactamase negative) were incubated together, but transfer did not occur if a cell-free filtrate of 73389 was incubated with F-28. This suggests that cell-to-cell contact was necessary for transfer to occur. In addition, transfer occurred when 73389 and F-28 were incubated on a membrane filter in the presence of DNase. In this study, the DNase was 100× as concentrated as that used by Thorne and Farrar in their studies with *H. influenzae* (9). Since this large amount of DNase had no effect on the transfer, it is unlikely that transformation occurred. Subsequently, the recipient and transconjugant strains were examined for plasmids by gel electrophoresis. The transconjugant strains had the β-lactamase plasmid, whereas the recipient strain did not have this plasmid (L. Elwell, personal communication). The transfer of only the β-lactamase property from the transconjugant to the *E. coli* (the transconjugant *E. coli* remained susceptible to spectinomycin) showed that the direction of transfer was from the gonococcus to the *E. coli*. Since no β-lactamase-producing cells could be isolated when the recipient cells alone were tested in the same manner, it is unlikely that mutation occurred. These results suggest that the mechanism of transfer was by conjugation and that the direction of transfer was from the β-lactamase-producing gonococcus to the β-lactamase-negative gonococcus.

The gene for β-lactamase production in both these organisms is borne on a plasmid of 4.5 megadaltons (Mdal) (L. Elwell and S. Falkow, personal communication). Strain 73389 also has a larger plasmid of 24.5 Mdal, which 61782 does not have. Although we could transfer the β-lactamase gene from 73389 by conjugation, we could not from 61782. Elwell et al. (personal communication) report that most of the β-lactamase-producing strains they have examined by gel electrophoresis contain the larger plasmid in addition to the smaller β-lactamase plasmid. These observations strengthen the probability that the larger plasmid in 73389 is a conjugative plasmid and mobilizes the transfer of the nonconjugative 4.5-Mdal plasmid carrying the β-lactamase gene (6). Gonorrhea is currently epidemic in the United States, with approximately 1 million cases reported for 1976 (4), and probably even more cases not reported. The Public Health Service recommends that uncomplicated gonorrhea be treated with penicillin (2). Therefore, any change in susceptibility of gonococci to penicillin, such as β-lactamase production, has serious implications regarding the control of this sexually transmitted disease. It may also be important that the β-lactamase plasmid can be transferred from strain to strain by conjugation, since this method is more efficient than transfer by transformation, the method that would prevail if the resistance were due to a chromosomal mutation.

Most β-lactamase-producing *N. gonorrhoeae* have originated in the Far East (3), including the strains that have been isolated in the United States. There is insufficient epidemiological evidence to determine the source of the strains isolated in England (7, 8). Cases of gonorrhea that are not cured by penicillin treatment, as well as any associated with the Far East, should be thoroughly investigated for the presence of β-lactamase-producing *N. gonorrhoeae*. Patients in whom such a strain is detected should be treated with spectinomycin rather than penicillin.

LITERATURE CITED

1. **Ashford, W. A., R. G. Galash, and V. G. Hemming.** 1976. Penicillinase-producing *Neisseria gonorrhoeae*. Lancet 2:657–658.
2. **Center for Disease Control.** 1974. Gonorrhea – CDC recommended treatment schedules. Morbidity Mortality Weekly Rep. 23(40):341.
3. **Center for Disease Control.** 1976. Follow-up on penicillinase-producing *Neisseria gonorrhoeae*. Morbidity Mortality Weekly Rep. 25:331.
4. **Center for Disease Control.** 1977. Gonorrhea and early syphilis cases – United States, 1976. Morbidity Mortality Weekly Rep. 26(1):1.
5. **Jaffee, H. W., J. W. Biddle, C. Thornsberry, R. E. Johnson, R. E. Kaufman, G. H. Reynolds, and P. J. Wiesner.** 1976. National gonorrhea therapy monitoring study. In vitro antibiotic susceptibility and its correlation with treatment results. N. Engl. J. Med. 294:5–9.
6. **Novick, P., R. C. Clowes, S. N. Cohen, R. Curtiss III, N. Datta, and S. Falkow.** 1976. Uniform nomenclature for bacterial plasmids: a proposal. Bacteriol. Rev. 40:168–189.
7. **Percival, A., J. E. Corkill, O. P. Arya, J. Rowlands, C. D. Allergant, E. Rees, and E. H. Annels.** 1976. Penicillinase-producing gonococci in Liverpool. Lancet 2:1379–1382.
8. **Phillips, I.** 1976. β-Lactamase producing penicillin-resistant gonococcus. Lancet 2:656–657.
9. **Thorne, G. M., and W. E. Farrar, Jr.** 1975. Transfer of ampicillin resistance between strains of *Haemophilus influenzae* type B. J. Infect. Dis. 132:276–281.
10. **Thornsberry, C.** 1976. Antimicrobial susceptibility tests for *Haemophilus influenzae*, p. 79–84. Technical Improvement Service no. 25. American Society for Clinical Pathology, Chicago, Ill.

ANTIMICROBIAL AGENTS AND CHEMOTHERAPY, June 1977, p. 1007-1009
Vol. 11, No. 6
Printed in U.S.A.

Absorption of Orally Administered Nafcillin in Normal Healthy Volunteers

CHATRCHAI WATANAKUNAKORN

Infectious Disease Division, Department of Internal Medicine, University of Cincinnati College of Medicine, Cincinnati, Ohio 45267

Received for publication 14 February 1977

The absorption of orally administered nafcillin sodium monohydrate buffered with calcium carbonate was studied in 10 healthy human volunteers. Dosages of 500 mg and 1 g were studied in fasting and nonfasting states. There was considerable individual variation in the absorption of nafcillin, although measurable serum concentrations were obtained in all subjects. With few exceptions, peak serum concentrations were reached faster and were more predictable in the fasting state than in the nonfasting state. In the majority of subjects, food interfered with nafcillin absorption. Measurable serum concentrations persisted for 4 h in almost all subjects, but there were no or negligible serum concentrations at 6 h. The mean serum concentrations obtained in the present study were higher than those reported in an earlier study.

Nafcillin, a semisynthetic penicillinase-resistant penicillin, is a valuable anti-staphylococcal antibiotic when it is given parenterally. However, it has been shown during clinical investigation of nafcillin that after oral administration of nafcillin, absorption was erratic in both fasting and nonfasting subjects, resulting in poor and unpredictable serum concentrations (7, 11). Consequently, oral nafcillin therapy is not usually recommended (1, 5, 8). There has been no recent study on oral nafcillin. The present investigation was designed to study the serum concentrations of nafcillin after oral ingestion of this antibiotic in a group of healthy human volunteers.

MATERIALS AND METHODS

Antibiotic. The nafcillin preparation used in this study was in the form of film-coated tablets containing nafcillin sodium as the monohydrate, equivalent to 500 mg of nafcillin, buffered with calcium carbonate. Wyeth Laboratories, Inc., Philadelphia, Pa., kindly provided the entire supply needed for this study.

Volunteers. Eight male and two female healthy adults volunteered for the study. The research protocol was approved by the Committee on Human Research, University of Cincinnati College of Medicine. Written informed consent was obtained from all subjects.

Experimental designs. The study was divided into four phases, and all 10 volunteers participated in all four phases of the study. Each phase of the study was performed in weekly intervals.

During phase 1, all subjects received no food from midnight until noon of the day of the study. One tablet of nafcillin (500 mg) was ingested by each subject in the morning. Six milliliters of blood was withdrawn immediately prior to the administration of nafcillin and at 0.5, 1, 1.5, 2, 4, and 6 h after the drug was given.

Phase 2 was similar to phase 1, except that the subjects were allowed to eat breakfast and the nafcillin tablet was ingested within 1 h of breakfast.

In phase 3, the procedure of phase 1 was followed, except two tablets of nafcillin (1 g) were ingested instead of one.

Phase 4 was similar to phase 3, except that the subjects were allowed to eat breakfast and the study was performed within 1 h of breakfast.

Nafcillin assay. The blood was allowed to clot and the serum was separated. The serum samples were immediately frozen at −20°C until tested. In most instances, the samples were tested within 48 h of collection. Nafcillin assay was performed by the cylinder cup-plate agar diffusion method of Bennett et al., using *Sarcina lutea* as the test organism (2). Antibiotic standards were diluted in pooled human serum. Antibiotic standards as well as samples were assayed in triplicate, and the average measurements were used. All serum samples from each subject during the same phase of study were assayed in the same plate.

RESULTS

Results of the study are shown in Tables 1 and 2. In the fasting subjects, measurable but markedly variable concentrations of nafcillin were obtained in all but one subject at 0.5 h. In all but one subject in each of the two fasting studies, peaked serum concentrations were attained at 1 h. One subject in each study attained peak serum concentrations at 1.5 h. There was marked variation in the individual peak serum concentration among the subjects.

TABLE 1. *Serum concentration after oral administration of 500 mg of nafcillin sodium monohydrate buffered with calcium carbonate*

Subject	Serum concn (μg/ml)													
	Fasting							Postprandial						
	0 h	0.5 h	1 h	1.5 h	2 h	4 h	6 h	0 h	0.5 h	1 h	1.5 h	2 h	4 h	6 h
1	0	1.80	2.30[a]	1.60	1.10	0.63	<0.10	0	0	0.69	1.35[a]	1.19	0.88	0
2	0	0	0.47	0.68[a]	0.60	<0.10	0	0	0	0.68	0.97	1.70[a]	0.70	0.23
3	0	0.15	1.82[a]	1.80	1.35	<0.10	0	0	0	0.58	0.80	0.96[a]	0.59	0.24
4	0	2.80	3.50[a]	2.05	1.15	0.18	0	0	0	0.98	3.50[a]	2.30	0.88	0
5	0	0.83	4.30[a]	3.30	1.70	0.68	0	0	0	0.29	1.18	2.70[a]	0.84	0.26
6	0	0.39	2.00[a]	1.70	1.23	0.62	0	0	4.80[a]	3.50	2.20	1.10	0.29	<0.10
7	0	0.41	0.98[a]	0.75	0.58	0.20	0	0	1.18[a]	1.10	0.72	0.29	0	0
8	0	3.90	6.80[a]	4.30	2.30	0.71	0.25	0	5.10[a]	4.00	2.90	2.20	0.40	0
9	0	1.50	5.10[a]	3.10	1.60	0.68	0.22	0	0	0.72	3.20[a]	2.60	0.44	0
10	0	2.00	4.50[a]	1.90	1.20	0.49	0.42	0	0	0	0.11	0.28	0.76[a]	0.10
Mean	0	1.378	3.177	2.118	1.281	0.429	0.094	0	1.108	1.254	1.693	1.532	0.578	0.083

[a] Peak concentration.

TABLE 2. *Serum concentration after oral administration of 1 g of nafcillin sodium monohydrate buffered with calcium carbonate*

Subject	Serum concn (μg/ml)													
	Fasting							Postprandial						
	0 h	0.5 h	1 h	1.5 h	2 h	4 h	6 h	0 h	0.5 h	1 h	1.5 h	2 h	4 h	6 h
1	0	0.52	1.80	5.20[a]	4.60	2.70	0.46	0	0.43	3.00[a]	2.49	1.80	0.36	<0.10
2	0	6.40	9.00[a]	7.80	6.70	1.30	0.15	0	2.80	6.00[a]	4.40	2.49	0.87	0.21
3	0	0.48	5.10[a]	3.50	2.00	0.36	0	0	0	0	<0.10	0.51	1.90[a]	0.25
4	0	2.80	11.50[a]	6.20	2.90	0.41	<0.10	0	0.17	6.00[a]	4.90	3.80	0.45	<0.10
5	0	0.13	9.20[a]	6.70	2.45	0.71	<0.10	0	<0.10	0.33	1.60	6.70[a]	1.40	<0.10
6	0	2.60	7.90[a]	4.80	2.10	0.64	0	0	6.80	7.60[a]	3.70	3.00	0.61	<1.10
7	0	3.70	5.40[a]	2.80	1.50	<0.10	0	0	3.10	5.00[a]	1.30	0.52	<0.10	0
8	0	8.10	11.50[a]	5.40	3.30	0.64	<0.10	0	4.20	4.80[a]	3.40	2.80	0.62	<0.10
9	0	5.60	6.60[a]	4.00	2.80	2.10	0.50	0	2.10	6.40[a]	4.40	2.15	0.80	0.23
10	0	0.92	8.80[a]	6.40	3.50	1.50	<0.10	0	0	<0.10	3.00[a]	1.80	0.34	0
Mean	0	3.125	7.680	5.280	3.115	1.041	0.131	0	1.965	3.918	2.924	2.557	0.740	0.94

[a] Peak concentration.

At 6 h, no or negligible serum concentrations were found.

In the nonfasting studies, the serum concentrations were even more unpredictable. In the 500-mg study, no antibiotic activity was found in the 0.5-h specimens in seven subjects. However, in the remaining three subjects, peak serum concentrations were attained at 0.5 h. Peak serum concentrations were at 1.5 h in three subjects, at 2 h in three subjects, and at 4 h in the remaining subject. Again, the individual peak serum concentration varied markedly among the subjects. The peak serum concentration was the same in one, higher in three, and lower in six subjects as compared with the values obtained in the fasting state. At 6 h, no or negligible serum concentrations were found. In the nonfasting 1-g study, peak serum concentration was attained at 1 h in seven, and in one subject each at 1.5, 2, and 4 h. Marked variation in individual peak concentration also prevailed. In all subjects, the peak serum concentration was lower than that obtained in the fasting state. No or negligible serum antibiotic activity was found at 6 h.

DISCUSSION

The results of this study confirm the previous finding that there was considerable individual variation in the absorption of nafcillin administered orally (7, 11), although measurable serum concentrations were obtained in all subjects. Even in the same individual, the absorption was not predictable. For example, subject no. 2 absorbed poorly in the 500-mg experiments, but had good absorption in the 1-g studies. With few exceptions, peaked serum concentrations were reached faster and were more predictable in the fasting state than in the nonfasting state. In the majority of subjects, food interfered with nafcillin absorption.

It is not clear to what extent individual vari-

TABLE 3. *Mean serum concentration after oral administration of 1 g of nafcillin sodium monohydrate buffered with calcium carbonate*

Study	No. of sub-jects	Condition	Mean serum concn (μg/ml) at h:						
			0.5	1	1.5	2	4	6	8
Klein and Finland (7)	8	Fasting	2.18	6.59		2.01	0.38	0.14	0.003
Present	10	Fasting	3.125	7.680	5.280	3.115	1.041	0.131	
Klein and Finland (7)	8	Nonfasting	0.80	1.64		1.10	0.30	0.07	0.01
Present	10	Nonfasting	1.965	3.918	2.924	2.557	0.740	0.094	

ation in absorption occurs with other orally administered antibiotics since usually only the mean values from a group of experimental subjects are reported. However, in a recent report on josamycin and erythromycin stearate, in which values from individual volunteers were reported, there was also considerable individual variation in the serum concentrations after oral administration of either josamycin or erythromycin stearate (9). The finding of individual variation was not emphasized when the authors only discussed the mean values. Wide individual variation in absorption also occurs with the orally administered isoxazolyl penicillins. Although only mean values from a group of experimental subjects were usually given in the published reports, the wide ranges of serum concentrations obtained in volunteers after the same oral dose of any one of the isoxazolyl penicillins were evident (3, 4, 6, 10), and authors of three of these reports commented specifically on these findings (4, 6, 10).

There is only one report on oral nafcillin in the literature comparable to the present study, using the same oral preparation (1 g of nafcillin sodium monohydrate buffered with calcium carbonate) and the same antibiotic assay technique (cylinder cup-plate agar diffusion method using *S. lutea* as the test organism). Only mean values were given in that particular study, although in the summary and conclusion the authors commented that the serum activity varied widely in different individuals (7). A comparison of the mean nafcillin serum concentrations from that and the present studies is given in Table 3. In both studies, absorption of oral nafcillin was much better in fasting than nonfasting subjects. In both the fasting and nonfasting experiments, the mean serum concentrations from the present study were higher than those from the earlier study that was published in 1963. The significance of this finding is not known. It may be due to the mere fact that the results were from two different laboratories at two different times, or the formulation of the drug may not be exactly the same.

On the basis of the results of this and previous studies (7, 11), it is concluded that the use of nafcillin orally is not warranted.

ACKNOWLEDGMENTS

I am indebted to the volunteers, whose participation made this study possible. Thomas Bannister provided excellent technical assistance. Wyeth Laboratories, Inc., Philadelphia, Pa., supplied the nafcillin tablets used in this study.

This investigation was supported by a grant from Wyeth Laboratories, Inc., and the Morton Hamburger Memorial Fund.

LITERATURE CITED

1. **Abramowicz, M. ed.** Handbook of antimicrobial therapy. 1976. The Medical Letter on Drugs and Therapeutics, New Rochelle, N.Y.
2. **Bennett, J. V., J. L. Brodie, E. J. Benner, and W. M. M. Kirby.** 1966. Simplified, accurate method for antibiotic assay of clinical specimens. Appl. Microbiol. 14:170–177.
3. **Bodey, G. P., C. Vallejos, and D. Stewart.** 1972. Flucloxacillin: a new semi-synthetic isoxazolyl penicillin. Clin. Pharmacol. Ther. 13:512–515.
4. **Bunn, P. A., and S. Milicich.** 1964. Laboratory and clinical studies with cloxacillin, p. 220–226. Antimicrob. Agents Chemother. 1963.
5. **Gardner, P., and H. T. Provine (ed.).** 1975. Manual of acute bacterial infections. Little, Brown and Co., Boston.
6. **Hammerstrom, C. F., F. Cox, M. C. McHenry, and E. L. Quinn.** 1967. Clinical, laboratory, and pharmacological studies of dicloxacillin, p. 69–74. Antimicrob. Agents Chemother. 1966.
7. **Klein, J. O., and M. Finland.** 1963. Nafcillin: antibacterial action in vitro and absorption and secretion in normal young men. Am. J. Med. Sci. 246:10–26.
8. **Kucers, A., and N. McK. Bennett (ed.).** 1975. The use of antibiotics, 2nd ed. J. B. Lippincott Co., Philadelphia.
9. **Strausbaugh, L. J., W. K. Bolton, J. A. Dilworth, R. L. Guerrant, and M. A. Sande.** 1976. Comparative pharmacology of josamycin and erythromycin stearate. Antimicrob. Agents Chemother. 10:450–456.
10. **Sutherland, R., E. A. P. Croydon, and G. N. Rolinson.** 1970. Flucloxacillin, a new isoxazolyl penicillin, compared with oxacillin, cloxacillin, and dicloxacillin. Br. Med. J. 4:455–460.
11. **Whitehouse, A. C., J. G. Morgan, J. Schumacher, and M. Hamburger.** 1963. Blood levels and antistaphylococcal titers produced in human subjects by a penicillinase-resistant penicillin, nafcillin, compared with similar penicillins, p. 384–392. Antimicrob. Agents Chemother. 1962.

ANTIMICROBIAL AGENTS AND CHEMOTHERAPY, June 1977, p. 1010–1016

Vol. 11, No. 6
Printed in U.S.A.

Bactericidal Activity of Macromomycin, an Antitumor Antibiotic

FRANCIS L. A. BUCKMIRE* AND JEFFREY L. WINKELHAKE

Department of Microbiology, The Medical College of Wisconsin, Milwaukee, Wisconsin 53233

Received for publication 1 February 1977

Susceptibility testing by the broth dilution method showed that all the gram-positive but only some of the gram-negative bacteria tested were susceptible to the antitumor antibiotic, macromomycin (MCR; NSC 170105). The minimal inhibitory concentration for the susceptible organisms was less than 3 μg/ml. The action of MCR was bactericidal; however, at very high concentrations (50 μg/ml and above) some organisms occasionally escaped death. None of the escaped organisms was resistant to MCR. In combination with other commonly used antibiotics, MCR displayed partial synergy for *Pseudomonas aeruginosa* (from a minimal inhibitory concentration of >100 to 12.5 μg/ml with 100 μg of chloramphenicol per ml) and for *Bacillus pumilus* and *Staphylococcus aureus* (from 1.6 to 0.4 μg/ml and below) with polymyxin B. As with mammalian cells, ^{125}I-labeled MCR was irreversibly bound to both gram-positive and -negative bacteria. Treatment with trypsin of the ^{125}I-labeled MCR-exposed cells did not release the bound MCR or reverse its lethal effect. When in solution in a protective buffer at 4°C, MCR was stable for up to 45 days; at 37°C, however, 25% of its bactericidal activity was lost in 72 h. Loss of activity was enhanced 16-fold in the presence of both heated and unheated pooled human sera. Urine had no effect on the activity of MCR.

Macromomycin (MCR; NSC 170105) is an unstable, antitumor (7, 9–12) polypeptide antibiotic discovered in 1968 by Chimura et al. (3). Recently, Yamashita et al. (16) have shown that its activity can be stabilized by certain substances, in particular the disaccharides, lactose and maltose. This has facilitated the purification of MCR to homogeneity (J.L. Winkelhake and F.L.A. Buckmire, Cancer Res., in press).

As with other antitumor antibiotics recently isolated, the mode of action of MCR has not been studied in detail. Kunimoto et al. (6) and Winkelhake and Buckmire (Cancer Res., in press) have shown that radioiodine (^{125}I)-labeled MCR readily binds to mammalian cell surfaces and, presumably from that location, causes cessation of deoxyribonucleic acid (DNA), but not ribonucleic acid or protein, synthesis. Kunimoto et al. (7) have hypothesized that the interaction between MCR and the mammalian cells is analogous to the interaction between certain colicins and bacterial cells (4).

Since the initial published data (3), there have been no other studies on the effect of MCR on bacteria. This communication compares the antimicrobial action of purified MCR on some gram-positive and -negative bacteria with several commonly used antibiotics.

MATERIALS AND METHODS

Organisms. The bacteria used in this study were: *Escherichia coli* ATCC 25922 and another clinical isolate, *Pseudomonas aeruginosa* ATCC 27853 and five other clinical isolates, *Staphylococcus aureus* ATCC 25923 and two clinical isolates, *Bacillus pumilus* ATCC 172, two laboratory strains of *Bacillus subtilis*, three strains of *Haemophilus influenzae* type b, and four strains of *Spirillum serpens*. With the exception of *H. influenzae* and *S. serpens*, the cultures were cultivated on Trypticase soy agar (TSA) (Baltimore Biological Laboratories, Inc.) plates. *H. influenzae* was grown on TSA supplemented with oxidized nicotinamide adenine dinucleotide (P-S Biochemicals, Milwaukee, Wis.), recrystallized hemin (Nutritional Biochemicals Corp., Cleveland, Ohio), and glucose (Calbiochem, La Jolla, Calif.) (1, 5), and *S. serpens* was cultivated on a Casamino Acids-salt medium containing agar (Difco Laboratories, Detroit, Mich.) (2). For all experiments, cultures were grown at 37°C for 8 to 14 h, harvested, and suspended in either the growth medium or HEPES (*N*-2-hydroxyethyl piperazine-*N*′-2-ethanesulfonic acid) buffer. Cultures (excluding *H. influenzae*) were maintained by bimonthly transfers on solid agar media, incubated overnight at 37°C, and stored at 4°C. *H. influenzae* was stored at −70°C in Trypticase soy broth (TSB) containing 20% glycerol after 9 h of growth at 37°C.

MCR. MCR was purified by sequential salt precipitation, ultrafiltration, ion exchange and molecular sieve chromatographies, and stabilized during lyophilization in 1% lactose-phosphate-buffered saline (Lac-PBS), pH 7.2, by a modification (Winkelhake and Buckmire, Cancer Res., in press) of the procedure of Yamashita et al. (16). During purification, fractions were monitored for activity by an agar-plate bacteriocidal technique, with *B. pumilus* as the test organism. Preparation homogeneity was determined by sodium dodecyl sulfate-polyacrylamide slab-gel electrophoresis, using 12.5% gel by the method of Laemli (8). A single protein band, which migrated between ribonuclease (13,700 daltons) and lysozyme (11,400 daltons) standards, was obtained. Since the electrophoresis technique employed is sensitive to about 10 μg of protein, our preparation was estimated to be >97% pure. Drug concentrations were determined spectrophotometrically with an 11.6 absorbancy value at 280 nm equivalent to 1%. Purified MCR was stored lyophilized in Lac-PBS at −70°C with no apparent loss of activity.

MCR was radioiodinated with cellulose-immobilized lactoperoxidase (15; Winkelhake and Buckmire, Cancer Res., in press). Gamma radiation was monitored by a Beckman GM100 gamma counter with a data computer. The specific activity of ^{125}I-labeled MCR was $4 \pm 0.5 \times 10^6$ cpm/mg. Iodination did not cause loss of bactericidal activity.

Other antibiotics. Actinomycin D, bacitracin, chloramphenicol, penicillin G, polymyxin B, and tetracycline were obtained from Calbiochem, La Jolla, Calif.; streptomycin sulfate came from E. R. Squibb & Sons, New York, N.Y.; gentamicin reagent was obtained from Schering Laboratories, Bloomfield, N.J.; and bleomycin sulfate (Blenoxane) was from Bristol Laboratories, Syracuse, N.Y.

Stock solutions (1 to 2.5 mg/ml) of all antibiotics were prepared in sterile glass with distilled water (weight corrected for potency) and then sterilized by membrane filtration (pore size, 0.2 μm; Gelman Instrument Co., Ann Arbor, Mich.). Appropriate dilutions were made in sterile TSB to yield 100 or 250 μg of each drug per ml.

Broth dilution susceptibility tests. Serial twofold broth dilution tests were performed in the growth medium in a volume of 1 ml per tube. Cultures for these experiments were grown on agar plates, harvested in the growth medium without agar, adjusted to an optical density of between 0.4 and 0.55 at 600 nm, and diluted 100- to 1,000-fold to produce a final bacterial population in each tube of 10^6 to 10^7 colony-forming units (CFU) per ml.

The minimal inhibitory concentration (MIC) was defined as the lowest concentration of drug that prevented macroscopic growth after incubation of 18 to 24 h at 37°C. Minimal bactericidal concentration (MBC) was determined by subculturing 1 μl (calibrated loop) from each clear tube onto a TSA plate. The MBC was defined as the lowest drug concentration preventing all growth on subculture.

Kill curves. Side arm flasks containing MCR in TSB were inoculated with an appropriate dilution of *B. pumilus* suspension to produce a final bacterial population of approximately 10^7 CFU/ml and incubated at 30°C while shaking. Samples were removed at various time intervals, diluted in TSB, and plated in triplicate on TSA plates.

Antibiotic inactivation test. HEPES buffer (0.01 M, pH 7.55) containing MCR was inoculated with approximately 10^8 CFU/ml of *B. pumilus* and incubated for 30 min at 37°C. After centrifugation at $7,500 \times g$ for 10 min, the pelleted cells were washed twice and plated. The supernatant obtained after initial centrifugation was filter sterilized (pore size, 0.2 μm; Gelman Instrument Co., Ann Arbor, Mich.), reinoculated with 10^8 CFU/ml, and, after incubation at 37°C for 30 min, plated on TSA plates. As a control, the above procedure was simultaneously performed on cells suspended in buffer without MCR.

Synergy. To test for synergy, serial twofold tube dilutions of MCR were made as described above, and, to each dilution, the same concentration of a second antibiotic was added. Three different concentrations of the second antibiotic were used. Synergy was defined as a reduction of the MIC values of both antibiotics by fourfold or more. Partial synergy was defined as a fourfold or greater reduction in the MIC value of one compound but less than fourfold reduction in the MIC value of the second antibiotic. Indifference to combined antibiotics was defined as a twofold or less reduction in MIC values. Antagonism was defined as a fourfold increase in the MIC value of either antibiotic.

^{125}I-labeled MCR binding experiments. Bacterial cell suspensions in HEPES buffer with and without ^{125}I-labeled MCR were incubated either at 4 or 37°C for various time intervals. After incubation, the suspensions were centrifuged at $7,500 \times g$ for 10 min, and the pelleted cells, washed twice with cold HEPES buffer to remove unbound MCR, were resuspended to the original volume in HEPES buffer. These suspensions were again incubated at either 4 or 37°C in the presence and absence of 1% trypsin for up to 30 min and centrifuged, and the pellet was resuspended to the original volume in HEPES buffer. Both the supernatants and cell suspensions were quantitatively analyzed for radioactivity. In cases where CFU determinations were to be made, sterile materials were used throughout. Serial dilutions were made in TSB, and the CFU values were determined on TSA plates.

Chemicals and buffers. All chemicals were of reagent grade. The HEPES buffer concentration throughout this study was 10 mM, pH 7.55. PBS contained 10 mM Na_2HPO_4, 150 mM NaCl, 1 mM $CaCl_2$, and 0.5 mM $MgCl_2 \cdot 6H_2O$, pH 7.2. Lac-PBS contained 1% lactose in PBS.

RESULTS

Antibacterial effects of MCR. MCR displayed strong antibacterial effects against some gram-positive and -negative bacteria (Table 1). It was, however, much more effective against the gram-positive bacteria. The MIC was below

TABLE 1. *Comparative activity of MCR and various other antibiotics against selected species of bacteria*[a]

Antibiotics	Bacteria					
	E. coli	*P. aeruginosa*	*S. serpens*[b]	*B. pumilus*	*S. aureus*	*H. influenzae* type b[c]
MCR	>100/>100	>100/>100	1.3/1.3	1.6/1.6	1.6/12.5	2.5/2.5
Streptomycin	12.5/12.5	100/100	1.6/1.6	25/50	50/100	–[d]
Gentamicin	6.3/6.3	6.3/6.3	0.4/0.4	<0.1/1.6	0.8/6.3	–
Penicillin G	100/>100	>100/>100	1.6/1.6	12.5/100	<0.2/3.1	–
Bacitracin	>100/>100	>100/>100	>100/>100	>100/>100	>100/>100	–
Tetracycline	0.8/>100	25/>100	0.8/25	0.2/>100	0.8/>100	–
Chloramphenicol	6.3/>100	>100/>100	3.1/3.1	12.5/>100	6.3/>100	–
Actinomycin D	>100/>100	>100/>100	50/50	0.4/12.5	1.6/>100	–
Polymxyin B	25/25	1.6/3.1	0.4/25	50/100	>100/>100	–
Bleomycin	<1.3/<1.3	>637/>637	–	159.3/159.3	19.9/79.6	–

[a] The numbers refer to MIC/MBC in micrograms per milliliter.
[b] The medium used for *S. serpens* was Casamino Acids + Ca^{2+} + CB (see Materials and Methods).
[c] Nicotinamide adenine dinucleotide, hemin, and glucose were added to the medium.
[d] –, Not tested.

2 μg/ml for *S. aureus* and *B. pumilus*, the two gram-positive organisms tested by the tube dilution method, as well as for two clinical strains of *S. aureus* and two *B. subtilis* strains tested by a plate dilution method. With the gram-negative organisms, on the other hand, MIC values ranged from 2.5 μg/ml, for organisms such as *H. influenzae* type b (three strains) and *S. serpens* (four strains), to greater than 100 μg/ml, for *E. coli* (two strains) and *P. aeruginosa* (six strains).

When compared with some other commonly used antibiotics, the MIC of MCR was lower than the majority against the gram-positive organisms tested (Table 1). Although its activity compared favorably with the other antibiotics tested against the gram-negative bacterium *S. serpens*, it was not as effective as gentamicin, streptomycin, tetracycline, chloramphenicol, polymyxin B, and bleomycin against *E. coli* or gentamicin, tetracycline, and polymyxin B against *P. aeruginosa*. Additionally, the MBC of MCR was the same as the MIC for most organisms tested. *S. aureus* was the notable exception. MBC and MIC values were generally the same for all the bactericidal antibiotics.

Upon prolonged incubation at 37°C, macroscopic culture growth occasionally occurred at concentrations higher than the MIC of MCR. Such growth may be explained (a) by the spontaneous mutation to resistant cells, (b) by inactivation of the antibiotic, or (c) by a prozone-like effect similar to that seen during antibody-complement-mediated bactericidal activity (14). Cells, isolated from growth at these higher MCR concentrations (50 to 100 μg/ml) and subcultured once, were as susceptible as the original culture, thus indicating they were not resistant mutants.

To determine whether the presence of other antibiotics could enhance the antibacterial activity of MCR, the MIC of MCR for two gram-negative and two gram-positive organisms was determined in the presence of various concentrations of other antibiotics. Table 2 shows that, for *P. aeruginosa* with the chloramphenicol concentration at 100 μg/ml, the MIC of MCR was reduced from >100 to 12.5 μg/ml. No similar synergistic or antagonistic effect was observed with the other antibiotics against either *P. aeruginosa* or *E. coli*. With gram-positive organisms, partial synergy was observed between polymyxin B and MCR. With *B. pumilus*, the MIC of MCR was reduced to 0.1 μg/ml in the presence of 20 μg of polymyxin B per ml, and with *S. aureus*, the MIC was reduced to 0.4 μg/ml in the presence of 100 μg of polymyxin B per ml.

Bactericidal activity of MCR. Table 3 shows the effect of exposure time on the ability of MCR to kill bacteria suspended in a nongrowth medium (HEPES buffer). At effective concentrations (1 μg/ml and above), the bactericidal effect of MCR was immediate on *B. pumilus*, whereas on *S. aureus* and *S. serpens* the effect was time dependent. This time-dependent effect varied with the concentration of the antibiotic used. For example with *S. serpens*, at a concentration of 1 μg/ml (about one-half of the MIC), there was no immediate killing; however, after 20-min of incubation in the presence of the antibiotic, approximately 98% of the cells were killed. At 10 μg/ml (four times the MIC), immediate killing of 80% of the cells, increasing to about 99% within 20 min, occurred.

TABLE 2. *MIC values of MCR for various bacteria in the presence of other antibiotics*[a]

Antibiotics[b] (μg/ml)	MIC of MCR (μg/ml) for:			
	P. aeruginosa	*E. coli*	*B. pumilus*	*S. aureus*
Gentamicin				
(6.5)	*[c]	*	–[d]	–
(1.3)	>100	>100	–	–
(0.3)	>100	>100	–	–
Chloramphenicol				
(100.0)	12.5	–	*	–
(20.0)	>100	–	*	–
(2.0)	>100	–	1.6	–
Penicillin G				
(100.0)	>100	*	–	–
(20.0)	>100	>100	–	–
(2.0)	>100	>100	–	–
Streptomycin				
(100.0)	*	*	–	–
(20.0)	>100	*	–	–
(2.0)	>100	>100	–	–
Polymxyin B				
(100.0)	–	–	*	0.4
(20.0)	–	–	0.1	1.6
(2.0)	–	–	1.6	1.6

[a] MIC values of the various antibiotics for the cultures are given in Table 1.

[b] Parenthetical numbers are antibiotic concentrations added to MCR-treated bacterial cultures.

[c] *, This concentration of the second antibiotic was either greater than or equal to its MIC for the organism tested, and in those cases no growth occurred.

[d] –, Not tested.

Tested organisms always left a residual percentage of surviving cells, even after extensive exposure to the antibiotic. These surviving organisms did not form colonies when plated at the higher antibiotic concentrations (50 μg/ml and above), but as the MCR concentration decreased during serial dilutions to below the MIC for the culture growth occurred. Susceptibility tests on some of the surviving cells indicated that their resistance to the antibiotic had not changed. Microscopic observations also indicated no obvious qualitative or quantitative morphological differences in the treated and untreated cells.

To determine the influence of the suspending medium on bacteriostasis, growth media containing MCR were inoculated with *B. pumilus*, and the CFU was determined at various time intervals. After 5 min of exposure to MCR, the CFU had decreased to approximately 0.2% at the two concentrations (1 and 10 μg/ml) tested (Fig. 1). At 10 μg/ml, the CFU continued to decrease, as a function of time, to approximately 0.02% in 24 h. At 1 μg/ml, however, there was a rapid recovery of cells, such that by 2 h the CFU was approximately 5% of the initial inoculum. Between 2 and 24 h, the growth rate was similar to that of the control culture.

Table 4 shows that the action of MCR was bactericidal, since cells plated directly from a suspension containing MCR (5 μg/ml) gave the same number of CFU as cells removed from the suspension and washed prior to plating. To determine the fate of MCR in the reaction mixture, the cell suspension containing MCR was centrifuged, and the sterile supernatant was inoculated with fresh, untreated cells, incubated at 37°C, and plated. No loss in viability of these cells occurred, thus indicating that the MCR was either adsorbed or inactivated by the original cells.

Binding of ^{125}I-labeled MCR to bacterial cells. To test the possibility that MCR was adsorbed, cells suspended in HEPES buffer were exposed to ^{125}I-labeled MCR and washed free of excess antibiotic, and the amount of bound MCR was determined. When *B. pumilus* was exposed to ^{125}I-labeled MCR, the antibiotic was adsorbed to the cells (Table 5). The amount bound was time independent, since similar amounts of ^{125}I-labeled MCR were absorbed at all time intervals tested (from 0 to 15 min). Similar results were obtained with the gram-negative organism, *S. serpens*. The table also shows that significant amounts of bound MCR (over 20%) were released after incubation at 37°C. Incubation at 4°C reduced the amount released to about 9%. Neither the release of

TABLE 3. *Effect of drug concentration and time of exposure on antimicrobial action of MCR*

Organism	MCR concn (μg/ml)	Length of exposure (min)	CFU/ml	Survival (%)
B. pumilus	0	0	6.5×10^8	100
	0.01	15	6.7×10^8	103.1
	0.1	15	6.0×10^8	92.3
	1.0	0	6.7×10^7	10.3
	1.0	15	6.3×10^7	9.7
	5.0	15	9.0×10^6	1.4
	10.0	0	1.1×10^6	0.2
	10.0	30	1.4×10^6	0.2
	10.0	60	8.6×10^5	0.1
	20.0	15	1.2×10^6	0.2
S. aureus	0	0	4.6×10^8	100
	10	0	4.6×10^8	100
	10	30	1.0×10^6	0.2
	10	60	8.6×10^5	0.2
S. serpens	0	0	1.6×10^8	100
	1	0	1.7×10^8	106.3
	1	20	2.8×10^6	1.8
	10	0	2.9×10^7	18.1
	10	20	1.2×10^6	0.8

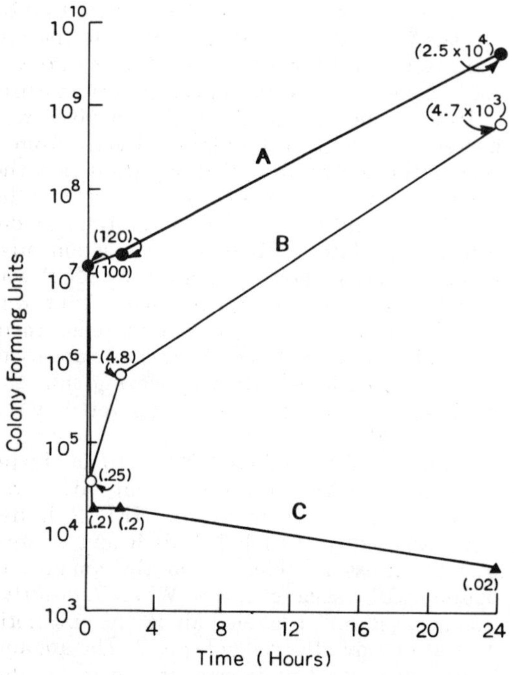

FIG. 1. *Growth of B. pumilus in the presence of MCR. Side arm flasks with TSB containing 0, 1, and 10 μg/ml (A, B, and C, respectively) of MCR were inoculated with B. pumilus and incubated while shaking at 37°C. At various time intervals, samples were removed and plated for viability. The numbers in parentheses are the percentages of the original inoculum.*

cell-bound MCR at 37°C nor its antibacterial action was affected by treating the MCR-adsorbed cells with trypsin.

Influence of cell concentration on the MIC. As other studies (13) on the influence of bacterial cell concentration on MIC show, inoculum size profoundly affected the MIC of MCR (Table 6). Whereas an inoculum of 10^7 CFU/ml gave an MIC of 1.6 μg/ml, 10- and 100-fold decreases in cell concentration gave MIC values of 0.39 and 0.1 μg/ml, respectively, and 10- and 100-fold increases gave 12.5 and 50 μg/ml, respectively.

Stability of MCR in body fluids. Other workers (16) have shown that when MCR suspended in PBS was lyophilized it lost activity. This activity loss was enhanced by increasing the temperature. However, when certain divalent cations and disaccharides were added prior to lyophilization, the rate of inactivation was retarded. At 35°C, for example, there was a 10% activity loss in 31 days when maltose was added, whereas almost all activity was lost in the absence of the protective agent (16). Table 7 presents the effect of certain body fluids on the stability of MCR in solution. At 4°C, no activity loss of MCR stabilized in Lac-PBS occurred for up to 45 days, the longest interval tested. At 37°C, however, there was a 16-fold loss in activity by 96 h. The addition of urine to solubilized MCR had no effect on its activity. When serum (heated or unheated) was added, however, the inactivation rate greatly increased (Table 7). The logarithm plot of MCR residual activity yielded straight lines as a function of time for each of the suspending fluids, indicating a first-order inactivation.

DISCUSSION

MCR used in this study was purified to homogeneity, which allowed us to unequivocally determine the antibacterial action of the drug. Homogeneity was facilitated with lactose as a stabilizing agent (Winkelhake and Buckmire, Cancer Res., in press) during purification.

Stability studies on purified MCR dissolved in Lac-PBS buffer clearly indicate that the drug was unstable in solution at 37 but not at 4°C (Table 7). However, since there was no significant reduction in MCR activity within 24 h at 37°C, the MIC values we obtained are considered valid. Inactivation of MCR at 37°C was also enhanced, and to the same degree (at least 16-fold in 72 h), by both heated and unheated pooled human sera, thus indicating that this inactivation was probably not due to serum-related enzymatic cleavage of the polypeptide. In their thermal inactivation studies on purified MCR, Yamashita and co-workers (16) calculated that the lyophilized powder in maltose would lose 10% of its activity in 31 days and 17 months at 35 and 4°C, respectively.

Although the spectrum of the bacterial gen-

TABLE 4. *Irreversible killing of B. pumilus by MCR*

Sample[a]	MCR concn (μg/ml)	CFU/ml	Survival (%)
A	0	9.8×10^8	100
B	5	5.0×10^6	0.5
C	5	4.8×10^6	0.5
D	S from sample A	2.8×10^8	100
E	S from sample C	2.7×10^8	96.4
F	W from sample C	3.0×10^8	107.1

[a] Samples A and B were plated by serial dilutions directly from the reaction mixtures. For sample C, cells in the reaction mixture were pelleted, washed, suspended in fresh buffer, and then plated by serial dilutions. For samples D, E, and F, untreated cells were suspended in supernatant (S) from sample A and supernatant (S) and washings (W) from sample C, respectively, and then plated by serial dilutions. All samples were incubated for 10 min at 25°C prior to plating for viability.

era used was limited, our data confirm the preliminary studies of Chimura et al. (3) that gram-positive bacteria are susceptible to MCR. In fact, MCR was as effective on gram-positive organisms as most of the other commonly used antibiotics with which it was compared (Table 1). In addition, our data show that certain gram-negative bacteria were also susceptible. In all cases, MCR was bactericidal.

Despite the lethal action of MCR, a population of residual cells that were not killed always remained. For these, high MCR concentrations (more than 30 times the MIC for the culture) were bacteriostatic, since these cells were able to divide (form colonies) only when the concentrations of MCR were reduced below the MIC for the culture. Repeated exposure of these surviving cells to high concentrations of MCR, however, did not lead to resistant cells.

Although the commonly encountered gram-negative bacteria such as *E. coli* and *P. aeruginosa* were resistant to MCR, partial synergy was obtained against *P. aeruginosa* with chloramphenicol, and this lower concentration of MCR (MIC of 12.5 μg/ml) was lethal. A similar additive bactericidal effect was also observed between polymyxin B and MCR against the gram-positive bacteria. No antagonism was encountered between MCR and any of the other antibiotics used. Indifference was generally the rule.

As with mammalian cells (6; Winkelhake and Buckmire, Cancer Res., in press), small quantities of MCR bound irreversibly to bacterial cells within 10 to 20 min, and the adsorption was temperature independent. However, in contrast to mammalian cells, treatment of bacteria with trypsin either before or after exposure to MCR did not release the bound MCR or alter the lethal effect of the drug. Thus it seems that the mechanism governing the association between MCR and bacterial cells may be different from the surface receptor-specific association of mammalian cells postulated by Kunimoto et al. (7) and demonstrated by Nussey and Winkelhake (personal communication). The fundamental mode of action of MCR on mammalian cells (inhibition of DNA synthesis, [6; Winkelhake and Buckmire, Cancer Res., in press]) and bacterial cells (not as yet determined) may well be the same, however.

The time taken for the bactericidal effect of MCR to manifest varied with the organism used. With *B. pumilus* the effect was immediate, whereas with *S. aureus* and *S. serpens* at least a 10-min lag took place. This time difference in responses may represent a difference in the degree of surface control of DNA synthesis or in the cell wall porosity of the organisms, rather than a difference in the mode of antibiotic action.

There have been only a few studies on MCR antitumor effects (7, 9–12) and possible modes of action (6, 7). These studies suggested to Ku-

TABLE 5. *Binding of ^{125}I-labeled MCR to B. pumilus cells*[a]

Time of exposure to MCR (min)	Amount of ^{125}I-labeled MCR adsorbed (cpm)	Trypsin treated	^{125}I-labeled MCR released	CFU (% survival)
0[b]				7.4×10^8 (100)
0	5,557	Yes	1,520	1.2×10^6 (0.2)
15	6,328	Yes	1,747	0.9×10^6 (0.1)
15	6,154	No	2,080	1.0×10^6 (0.1)

[a] Cell suspensions in 0.01 M HEPES buffer were incubated at 37°C with MCR for the indicated time periods and washed three times with cold buffer by centrifugation at 7,500 × *g* for 10 min. After washing, the suspensions were incubated at 37°C for 20 min with and without 1% trypsin, centrifuged as before, and the amount of MCR released as well as viability CFU were determined.

[b] Control culture.

TABLE 6. *Effect of cell concentration on the MIC of MCR for B. pumilus*

Cell concn	MIC of MCR (μg/ml)
1.3×10^9	50
4.2×10^8	12.5
1.3×10^8	3.1
4.2×10^7	1.6
1.3×10^7	0.8
4.2×10^6	0.4
4.2×10^5	0.1

TABLE 7. *Time- and temperature-dependent inactivation of MCR in solution*[a]

Time (h)	Temp °C	MIC (μg/ml)			
		Lac-PBS	Urine	Serum	Heated serum
0	4	1.6	–[b]	–	–
1,080	4	3.1	–	–	–
1	37	1.6	1.6	1.6	1.6
24	37	3.1	3.1	6.3	6.3
48	37	3.1	6.3	25	25
72	37	6.3	12.5	>200	>200
96	37	25	25	>200	>200

[a] Portions of MCR were preincubated with equal volumes of the respective reagents for the times and temperatures indicated. After incubation, the MIC of MCR was determined as described in Materials and Methods. *B. pumilus* was the indicator organism.

[b] –, Not tested.

nimoto et al. (7) that MCR may inhibit DNA synthesis while attached to eucaryotic cell surfaces by a mechanism analogous to that postulated for the interactions between certain colicins and *E. coli* (4). The data presented so far, however, have not been unequivocal. The recent developments of a sensitive-specific assay for detection of minute quantities of the drug (Winkelhake and Buckmire, Cancer Res., in press) and the methodology to stabilize it (16) will undoubtedly stimulate more definite studies in these areas.

ACKNOWLEDGMENTS

We wish to thank B. Houghton for technical assistance and W. T. Bradner, Bristol Laboratories, for the generous gifts of MCR.

LITERATURE CITED

1. **Buckmire, F. L. A.** 1976. Identification and quantitation of capsular antigen in capsulated and noncapsulated strains of *Haemophilus influenzae* type b by crossed-immunoelectrophoresis. Infect. Immun. **13**:1733–1742.
2. **Buckmire, F. L. A., and R. G. E. Murray.** 1970. Studies on the cell wall of *Spirillum serpens*. I. Isolation and partial purification of the outermost cell wall layer. Can. J. Microbiol. **16**:1011–1022.
3. **Chimura, H., M. Ishizaka, M. Hamada, S. Hori, K. Kimura, J. Iwanga, T. Takeuchi, and H. Umezawa.** 1968. A new antibiotic, macromomycin, exhibiting antitumor activity and antimicrobial activity. J. Antibiot. **21**:44–49.
4. **Hardy, K. G.** 1975. Colicinogeny and related phenomena. Bacteriol. Rev. **39**:464–515.
5. **Herriott, R. M., E. Y. Meyer, M. Vogt, and M. Modan.** 1970. Defined medium for growth of *Haemophilus influenzae*. J. Bacteriol. **101**:513–516.
6. **Kunimoto, T., M. Hori, and H. Umezawa.** 1971. Reversible binding of macromomycin, a macromolecular peptide antibiotic, to cell membranes. J. Antibiot. **24**:203–205.
7. **Kunimoto, T., M. Hori, and H. Umezawa.** 1972. An inhibitor of membrane function of tumor cells. Cancer Res. **32**:1251–1256.
8. **Laemli, V. K.** 1970. Cleavage of structural proteins during the assembly of the head of bacteriophage T4. Nature (London) **227**:680–685.
9. **Lippman, M. M.** 1974. Mechanism of action of macromomycin (NSC 170105), an antitumor polypeptide. In Vitro **9**:370.
10. **Lippman, M. M.** 1974. In vitro studies of macromomycin (NSC 170105)L effects on cultured TA3Ha and L1210 cells. Cancer Chemother. Rep. **58**:181–187.
11. **Lippman, M. M., and B. J. Abbot.** 1973. Modification of transplantability and tumor growth following treatment of L1210 and TA3Ha cells with macromomycin (NSC 170105). Cancer Chemother. Rep. **57**:501–503.
12. **Lippman, M. M., W. R. Laster, B. J. Abbot, J. Venditti, and M. Baratta.** 1975. Antitumor activity of macromomycin B (NSC 170105) against murine leukemias, melanoma, and lung carcinoma. Cancer Res. **35**:939–945.
13. **Sanders, C. C., and W. E. Sanders, Jr.** 1975. Effects of procedural variations on the activity of aminoglycosides in vitro. Am. J. Clin. Pathol. **63**:438–445.
14. **Winkelhake, J. L., and D. L. Kasper.** 1972. Affinity chromatography of anti-meningococcal antiserum. J. Immunol. **109**:824–833.
15. **Winkelhake, J. L., and G. L. Nicolson.** 1976. Aglycosylantibody: effects of exoglycosidase treatments on autochthonous antibody survival time in the circulation. J. Biol. Chem. **251**:1074–1080.
16. **Yamashita, J., N. Naoi, K. Watanabe, T. Takeuchi, and H. Umezama.** 1976. Further purification and characterization of macromomycin. J. Antibiot. **29**:415–423.

Antimicrobial Agents and Chemotherapy, June 1977, p. 1017-1020
Vol. 11, No. 6

In Vitro Studies of Netilmicin, a New Aminoglycoside Antibiotic

DOROTHY STEWART, GERALD P. BODEY,* and BARBARA LeBLANC

Department of Developmental Therapeutics, The University of Texas System Cancer Center, M. D. Anderson Hospital and Tumor Institute, Houston, Texas 77030

Received for publication 29 December 1976

Netilmicin, a semisynthetic derivative of sisomicin, was tested in vitro against 600 clinical bacterial isolates. At a concentration of 1.56 μg/ml, over 90% of gram-negative bacilli were inhibited. Netilmicin was substantially more active against isolates of *Serratia marcescens* and *Enterobacter* spp. than gentamicin, sisomicin, tobramycin, or amikacin. Isolates of *Staphylococcus aureus* (both penicillin G susceptible and resistant) were quite susceptible to netilmicin. Most isolates of *Klebsiella* spp. and *Serratia* spp. and some of the isolates of *Pseudomonas aeruginosa* that were resistant to gentamicin proved to be susceptible to netilmicin.

Gram-negative bacilli are responsible for an increasing number of infections in hospitalized patients (2). Aminoglycoside antibiotics, such as gentamicin, amikacin, and tobramycin, have been quite successful in the treatment of gram-negative infections. However, increased resistance to these antibiotics has developed in recent years (6, 7). Recently, a new aminoglycoside, netilmicin, has been synthesized from sisomicin, which is produced by *Micromonospora inyoensis*. It has a spectrum of in vitro activity that is similar to gentamicin sulfate. We determined the activity of netilmicin against clinical bacterial isolates and compared its activity with that of gentamicin, sisomicin, tobramycin, and amikacin. The activity of netilmicin was also determined against gentamicin-resistant isolates of gram-negative bacilli.

MATERIALS AND METHODS

Susceptibility tests were conducted on 497 gram-negative bacilli and 103 gram-positive cocci, using the dilution technique with an automatic microtiter system (*Autotiter Instruction Manual*, Canalco). All isolates of gram-negative bacilli and *Staphylococcus aureus* were inoculated into Mueller-Hinton broth (Difco) and incubated at 37°C for 18 h. Other gram-positive cocci were inoculated into tryptose phosphate broth. An inoculum of approximately 10^5 colony-forming units/ml was used to test isolates of gram-negative bacilli and *S. aureus*. For the other gram-positive cocci, an inoculum of 10^6 colony-forming units/ml was used for susceptibility testing.

All gram-negative bacilli used in this study were cultured from blood specimens obtained from patients hospitalized at The University of Texas M. D. Anderson Hospital between the years 1967 and 1976. The majority of these patients had underlying malignant diseases. A total of 100 isolates each of *Pseudomonas aeruginosa*, *Escherichia coli*, *Klebsiella* spp., and *Enterobacter* spp., 64 isolates of *Proteus* spp., and 50 isolates of *Serratia marcescens* were utilized. All gram-positive cocci used in this study were cultured from hospitalized patients, most of whom did not have underlying malignant diseases. A total of 41 isolates of *Streptococcus pyogenes*, 12 isolates of *S. pneumoniae*, and 50 isolates of *S. aureus* were studied. The susceptibility of isolates of *S. aureus* to penicillin G was determined by means of the broth dilution technique. Those isolates inhibited by less than 0.10 μg/ml were considered to be penicillin G susceptible, and those isolates resistant to more than 25 μg/ml were considered to be resistant to penicillin G. Isolates of gram-negative bacilli that had minimum inhibitory concentrations (MIC) of 12.5 μg or greater per ml were considered to be resistant to gentamicin.

Netilmicin, sisomicin, and gentamicin were supplied by Schering Corp., Bloomfield, N.J. Tobramycin and amikacin were supplied by Eli Lilly & Co., Indianapolis, Ind., and Bristol Laboratories, Division of Bristol-Myers Co., Syracuse, N.Y., respectively. Twofold serial dilutions of the antibiotics were made with appropriate broth, and the MIC was determined after incubation at 37°C for 18 h. The minimum bactericidal concentration (MBC) was defined as the lowest concentration of drug that yielded less than 25 colonies when 0.01 ml was subcultured onto sheep blood agar (less than five colonies per 0.001 ml of inoculum). A calibrated pipette was used to transfer the inoculum. All studies were performed in triplicate, and comparative studies were done simultaneously.

RESULTS

The in vitro activity of netilmicin against gram-negative bacilli and gram-positive cocci is

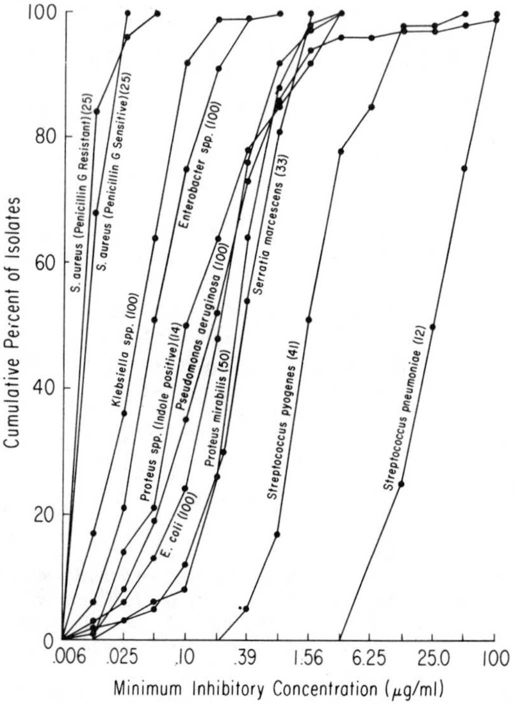

FIG. 1. *In vitro activity of netilmicin.*

shown in Fig. 1. The MIC of netilmicin was 1.56 μg or less per ml against all isolates of *Klebsiella* spp., *S. marcescens*, and *Enterobacter* spp., 97% of *E. coli*, 97% of *Proteus mirabilis*, 92% of indole-positive *Proteus* spp., and 94% of *P. aeruginosa*. All penicillin G-susceptible and penicillin G-resistant isolates of *S. aureus* strains were susceptible to netilmicin at a concentration of 0.05 μg or less per ml. Netilmicin inhibited 78% of the isolates of *S. pyogenes* at a concentration of 3.12 μg/ml, whereas against *S. pneumoniae* it had no activity at this concentration.

In general, the MBC of most of the clinical isolates, with the exception of the *S. marcescens* isolates, equaled the MIC or was a twofold dilution greater. For example, the MBC was 1.56 μg/ml against 94% of isolates of *E. coli*, whereas the MIC was 0.78 μg/ml against 92%. For isolates of *S. marcescens*, the MBC was six times greater than the MIC.

Figure 2 shows a comparison of the in vitro activity of netilmicin with that of four other aminoglycosides: gentamicin sulfate, tobramycin, sisomicin, and amikacin against *Enterobacteriaceae*. The activity of netilmicin was similar to that of gentamicin sulfate. Against isolates of *S. marcescens* and *Enterobacter*

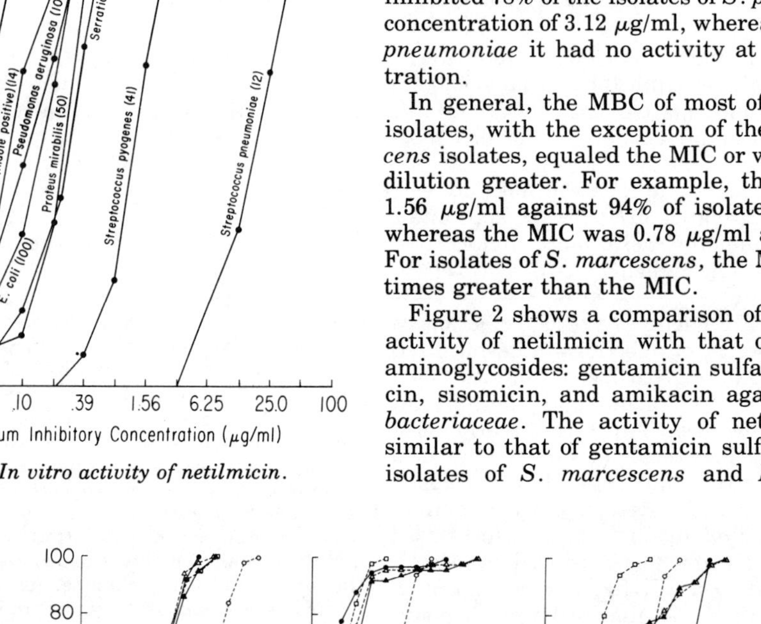

FIG. 2. *Comparative activity of aminoglycosides against gram-negative bacilli.*

spp., it was substantially more active than the other aminoglycosides. At a concentration of 1.56 μg/ml, netilmicin inhibited all isolates of *S. marcescens*, whereas amikacin, sisomicin, gentamicin, and tobramycin inhibited 87, 84, 78, and 72%, respectively. All isolates of *Enterobacter* spp. were susceptible to netilmicin at a concentration of 0.78 μg/ml. Amikacin and sisomicin showed the least activity against *Enterobacter* spp. Sisomicin, gentamicin, tobramycin, and netilmicin had similar activity against *Klebsiella* spp. All isolates were inhibited by netilmicin at a concentration of 0.20 μg/ml. Netilmicin inhibited 92% of the isolates of indole-positive *Proteus* spp. at a concentration of 1.56 μg/ml, whereas sisomicin and tobramycin inhibited 100% of these isolates at the same concentration. Netilmicin was slightly more active against isolates of *P. mirabilis*, inhibiting 98% at this concentration.

The in vitro susceptibility of 50 isolates of *P. aeruginosa* to the five aminoglycosides is shown in Fig. 3. At a concentration of 0.20 μg/ml, sisomicin and tobramycin were the most active, both inhibiting 88% of the isolates. At the same concentration, netilmicin, gentamicin, and amikacin inhibited 70, 78, and 12%, respectively. All of the aminoglycosides inhibited over 90% of the isolates at a concentration of 3.12 μg/ml.

Twenty-three isolates of gram-negative bacilli known to be resistant to gentamicin, tobramycin, or sisomicin were tested for their susceptibility to netilmicin (Table 1). All six isolates of *Klebsiella* spp. were susceptible to netilmicin and amikacin. Some of these isolates were considerably more susceptible to netilmicin than to amikacin. Netilmicin was active against 80% of the isolates of *Serratia* spp. Two isolates of *Serratia* spp. were susceptible only to amikacin. Of the seven *Pseudomonas* isolates tested, four were equally susceptible to netilmicin and amikacin, two were resistant to

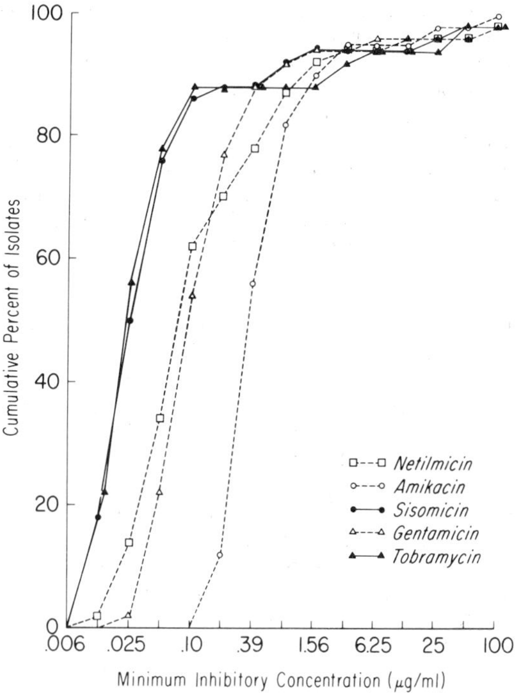

FIG. 3. *Comparative activity of antibiotics against P. aeruginosa.*

netilmicin but susceptible to amikacin, and one was resistant to all five aminoglycosides.

DISCUSSION

Netilmicin is an aminoglycoside antibiotic with a broad-spectrum of activity against gram-negative bacilli and some gram-positive cocci. The in vitro activity of this antibiotic against gram-negative bacilli is similar to that of gentamicin sulfate. However, netilmicin was more active than other aminoglycosides against isolates of *Klebsiella* spp., *Enterobacter* spp., and

TABLE 1. *Activity of aminoglycosides against gram-negative bacilli resistant to gentamicin sulfate*

Organism	No. of isolates	MIC (μg/ml) for:									
		Amikacin		Sisomicin		Gentamicin		Tobramycin		Netilmicin	
		Median	Range	Median	Range	Median	Range	Median	Range	Median	Range
Klebsiella spp.	6	0.20	0.10–0.39	3.12	3.12–6.25	12.5	12.5–25	12.5	12.5–50	0.025	0.012–0.39
P. aeruginosa	7	0.39	0.10–100	>100	50–>100	>100	100–>100	50	50–>100	0.39	0.20–>100
S. marcescens	10	1.56	0.78–12.5	25	6.25–50	50	25–100	50	25–100	1.56	1.56–100

S. marcescens. Also, it was as active as gentamicin and tobramycin against *E. coli* isolates. It was not as active as sisomicin or tobramycin against isolates of *P. aeruginosa*.

Our results are in general agreement with other investigations (3, 5). However, most of our isolates of *Pseudomonas* spp. were equally susceptible to netilmicin and gentamicin. Miller et al. found netilmicin to be twofold less active than gentamicin. This difference could be explained by the different methods used in determination of the MIC (5). We found most isolates of gentamicin-resistant strains of *Pseudomonas* spp. to be susceptible to netilmicin. Some isolates of *Klebsiella* spp. resistant to gentamicin were more susceptible to netilmicin than to amikacin. Most isolates of *S. marcescens* were equally susceptible to both antibiotics. Miller et al. also found that some of their strains of *Enterobacteriaceae* were considerably more susceptible to netilmicin.

Netilmicin appears to have some advantages over other aminoglycoside antibiotics, such as gentamicin, tobramycin, amikacin, and sisomicin. Because of its greater in vitro activity against some clinical isolates of gram-negative bacilli, it deserves further investigation.

ACKNOWLEDGMENTS

This work was supported by Public Health Service grant CA 05831 from the National Cancer Institute and a grant-in-aid from Schering Corp., Bloomfield, N.J.

LITERATURE CITED

1. **Bridis, S. J., and H. G. Robson.** 1976. Comparative activity of netilmicin, gentamicin, amikacin, and tobramycin against *Pseudomonas aeruginosa* and *Enterobacteriaceae*. Antimicrob. Agents Chemother. **10**:592–597.
2. **Dupont, H. L., and W. W. Spink.** 1969. Infections due to gram-negative organisms. Medicine **48**:307–332.
3. **Kabins, S. A., C. Nathan, and S. Cohen.** 1976. In vitro comparison of netilmicin, a semisynthetic derivative of sisomicin and four other aminoglycoside antibiotics. Antimicrob. Agents Chemother. **10**:139–145.
4. **Meyer, R. D., L. L. Kraus, and K. A. Posiecznik.** In vitro susceptibility of gentamicin-resistant *Enterobacteriaceae* and *Pseudomonas aeruginosa* to netilmicin and selected aminoglycoside antibiotics. Antimicrob. Agents Chemother. **10**:677–681.
5. **Miller, G. H., G. Arcieri, M. J. Weinstein, and A. Waitz.** 1976. Biological activity of netilmicin, a broad-spectrum semisynthetic aminoglycoside antibiotic. Antimicrob. Agents Chemother. **10**:827–836.
6. **Shulman, J. A., P. M. Terry, and C. E. Hough.** 1971. Colonization with gentamicin-resistant *Pseudomonas aeruginosa*, pyocine type 5, in a burn unit. J. Infect. Dis. **124** (Suppl.):S18–S23.
7. **Snelling, C., A. A. Ronald, C. Y. Cales, and W. C. Forsythe.** 1971. Resistance of gram-negative bacilli to gentamicin. J. Infect. Dis. **124**(Suppl.):S264–S270.

Antimicrobial Agents and Chemotherapy, June 1977, p. 1021-1026 Vol. 11, No. 6

Printed in U.S.A.

Manner and Meaning of Susceptibility Testing of Ampicillin-Resistant *Haemophilus influenzae*

BARRY M. GRAY, CAROL A. HUBBELL, and HUGH C. DILLON, JR.*

Department of Pediatrics, University of Alabama in Birmingham, School of Medicine, Birmingham, Alabama 35294

Received for publication 31 January 1977

We examined ampicillin-resistant strains of *Haemophilus influenzae* to compare the percentage of resistant organisms in each strain with the susceptibility to ampicillin by an agar dilution method. Using an inoculum of 10^4 colony-forming units, the minimal inhibitory concentration (MIC) increased with the percentage of resistant organisms in the strain. Laboratory-manipulated strains composed of different proportions of a susceptible and a resistant strain behaved similarly. The survival of isolated colony-forming units (colony MIC) was then determined by spreading inocula over the surface of a set of MIC plates, resulting in separation of individual colonies. This modification of the susceptibility test to the colony level gave end points that were clear and reproducible and that did not vary with changes in incubation time or temperature. True differences in susceptibility among strains were demonstrated by this method, whereas results of the conventional MIC test may reflect only the number of resistant organisms present in the inoculum.

Since the emergence of ampicillin-resistant strains of *Haemophilus influenzae*, reliable susceptibility testing of this organism has become a matter of grave importance. Reports concerning susceptibility patterns, as well as case reports, often describe ampicillin-resistant *H. influenzae* in terms of a minimal inhibitory concentration (MIC) as though this were a standard and meaningful laboratory measure. In fact, the fastidious nature of *H. influenzae* necessitates the modification of standard methods merely to obtain growth adequate for testing purposes. Variables such as inoculum size, media, and incubation conditions may all influence results. Among ampicillin-resistant strains, the important factor appears to be the size of inoculum used, regardless of whether agar or broth dilution techniques are used (3, 12). Inoculum size refers to the total number of colony-forming units (CFU) placed into a broth or spotted onto an agar plate. A larger inoculum yields a higher MIC. Cultures of ampicillin-resistant *H. influenzae*, however, are not homogeneous. Resistance is conferred by a plasmid coding for a β-lactamase (10). A resistant strain may contain individuals that do not bear the plasmid and are consequently susceptible to ampicillin at the usual concentrations. Spontaneous loss of the plasmid may occur frequently under laboratory conditions (1). We have also observed this phenomenon and found it to affect the MIC result.

We hypothesized that, inoculum size and other conditions being equal, the MIC of a strain depends on the proportion of β-lactamase-producing individuals in that strain at the time of testing. Our experiments show this to be the case; furthermore, true differences among strains were demonstrated by a method that tests the susceptibility of individual CFU.

MATERIALS AND METHODS

Organisms. We have recently examined 271 strains of *H. influenzae* by agar dilution and disk diffusion tests for susceptibility to ampicillin and two cephalosporins (B.M. Gray, C.A. Hubbell, and H.C. Dillon, Jr., manuscript in preparation). All were clinical isolates recovered from patients at The Children's Hospital, Birmingham, Ala., in 1971, 1975, and 1976. Twenty-six strains were ampicillin resistant, of which 14 were selected for further study. Seven were type b (strains 3, 4, 6, 7, 8, 9, and 13); the remainder were nontypable. Strains were preserved in skim milk at −60°C.

Agar dilution techniques. (i) Strains were recovered from storage on Levinthal agar made with washed human erythrocytes (6, 13). Five to six colonies were incubated until growth appeared (3 to 6 h) in brain heart infusion broth (Difco) supplemented with 8 μg of hemin (type 1, bovine; Sigma Chemical Co.) per ml and 5 μg of nicotinamide adenine dinucleotide (β-NAD, grade III; Sigma Chemical Co.) per ml. Samples (0.1 and 0.2 ml) of this culture were inoculated into prewarmed broths and grown for 2 to 3 h to ensure log-phase growth. Growth was monitored by colony count and optical density; broth cultures of optical density 0.07 at 590 nm yield 10^7 to 10^8 CFU/ml.

(ii) MIC plates were prepared according to the ICS recommendations (4), using ampicillin (anhydrous standard; Wyeth Laboratories) in Levinthal agar poured in 150-mm petri dishes. Plates were used within 24 h.

(iii) The conventional agar dilution method was done using a replicator like that of Steers et al. (11); the bacterial concentration was adjusted such that each pin delivered 10^4 CFU to 5-mm spots on the MIC plates. Plates were incubated in candle jars at 37°C for 18 h. The MIC was read as the lowest dilution of antibiotic to completely inhibit growth.

(iv) The MIC of CFU, hereafter referred to as the "colony MIC," differs from the conventional MIC in that rather than inoculating multiple strains as discrete spots of 10^4 CFU on the plates, the inoculum of each strain tested is spread over the entire surface of a set of MIC plates, resulting in separation of individual colonies. An inoculum of 10^3 CFU in 0.1 ml, spread with a bent glass rod and turntable, proved suitable. Duplicate sets of MIC plates were incubated in candle jars, one set at 37°C and the other at 35°C. The colony MIC was read as the lowest dilution of ampicillin to inhibit growth (see also Fig. 6). One to 10 colonies (less than 1% of the inoculum) on the last plate exhibiting growth were disregarded. Plates with few or no colonies were reincubated and examined at 24 and 36 h.

Determination of percentage of resistant organisms. Ten clinical isolates were grown in broth and diluted to 10^4 CFU/ml in 10% brain heart infusion broth-physiological saline. Samples of 0.1 ml were spread, as above, on Levinthal medium (to grow the total population) and on Levinthal medium containing 2 μg of ampicillin per ml (to select the resistant organisms). The percentage of resistant organisms was calculated from colony counts of the two plates (in duplicate) (Fig. 1). The conventional MIC was determined from the same initial broth cultures.

RESULTS

In the course of testing nearly 300 *H. influenzae* strains for ampicillin susceptibility, we observed several phenomena prompting further investigation. The effect of β-lactamase production by a resistant strain on reducing local ampicillin concentrations, thereby allowing neighboring susceptible colonies to grow (Fig. 2), was one such observation. We also noted that the disk diffusion test, which correlated with resistance by MIC in all cases, exhibited a discontinuous or "double" inhibition zone with many resistant strains (Fig. 3). These observations illustrate two important features of ampicillin-resistant *H. influenzae* strains: resistant strains are composed of both susceptible and resistant individuals; and the presence of resistant organisms permits the growth of susceptible organisms in their immediate vicinity. By spotting a large number of organisms as a unit, the conventional MIC is subject to these influences, collectively called the "inoculum effect."

The proportion of resistant organisms in 10 wild strains ranged from 7 to 100% and the MIC increased correspondingly (Fig. 4). Most strains had 70% or more resistant organisms and gave MICs of 64 μg/ml or greater. The same relationship was reproduced artificially with the nine laboratory-manipulated strains, whose MIC also increased with the percentage of resistant organisms (Fig. 5). Since these nine strains

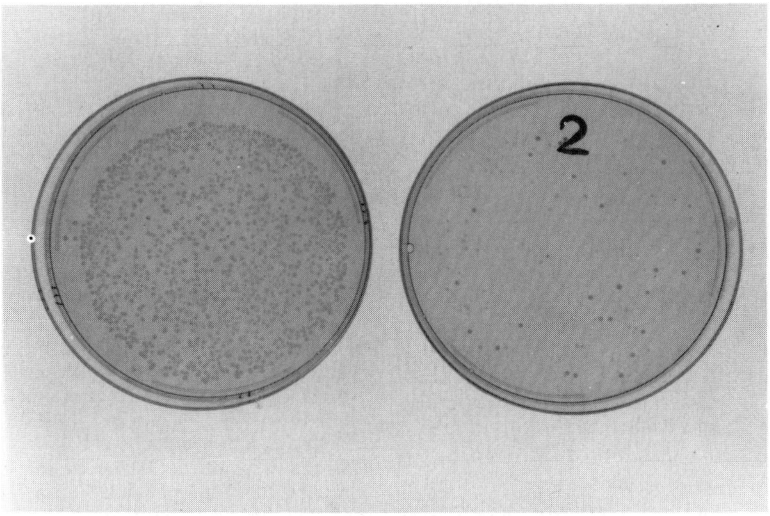

FIG. 1. *Percentage of resistant organisms is calculated from the colony counts of inocula spread on plain agar (left, 1,332 colonies) and on agar containing 2 μg of ampicillin per ml (right, 92 colonies)—for this strain, 7%.*

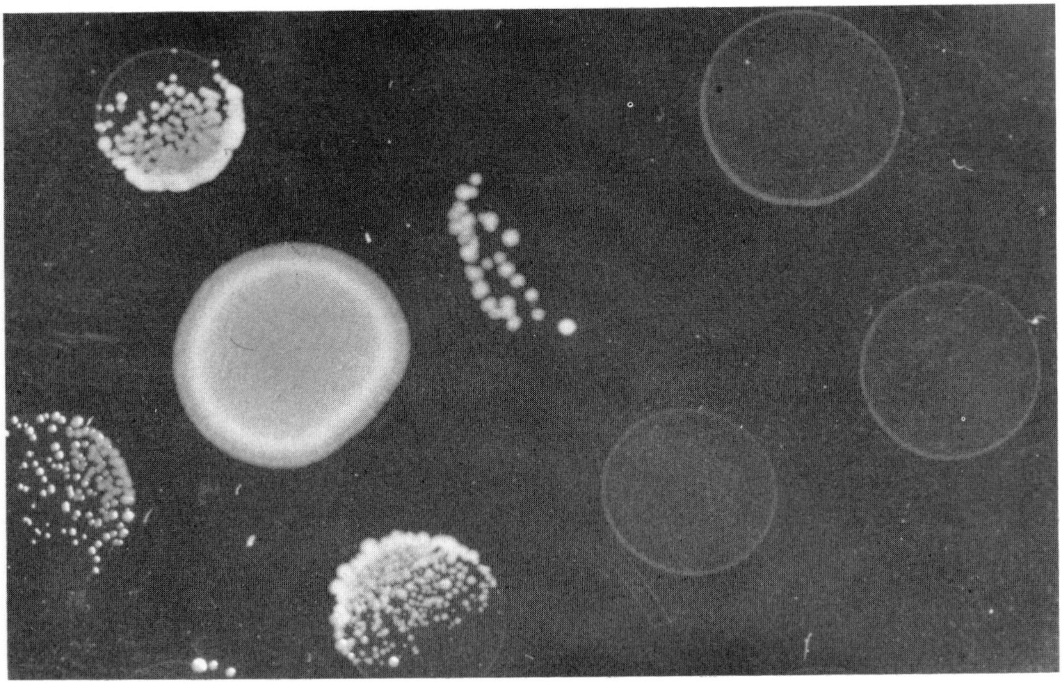

FIG. 2. *Inoculation spots on this 8-μg/ml MIC plate show no growth of susceptible strains to the far right; susceptible colonies adjacent to the resistant strain are capable of growth.*

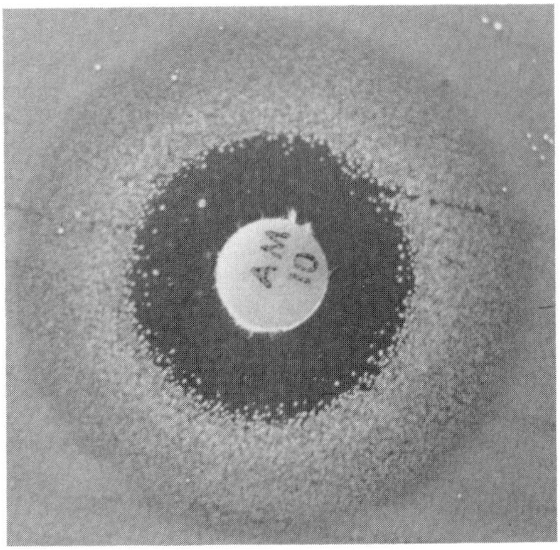

FIG. 3. *Inner ring shows growth of only a few resistant colonies; outer ring approximates the usual susceptibility zone, outside of which all organisms are capable of growth; between these two rings resistant organisms predominate. This effect may not be apparent on opaque media.*

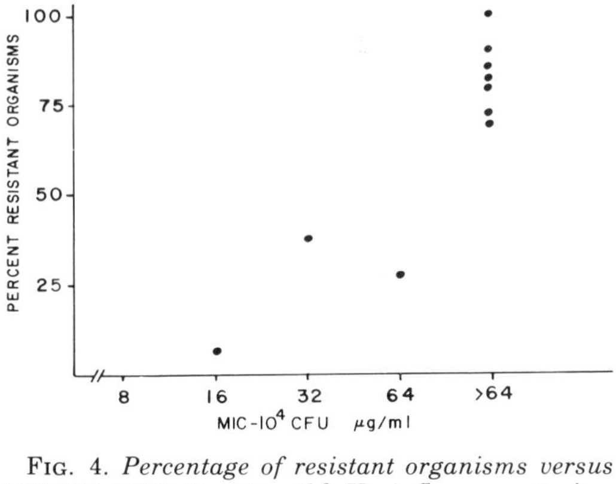

FIG. 4. *Percentage of resistant organisms versus MIC/10⁴ CFU for 10 wild H. influenzae strains.*

were derived from the same parent populations, the effect of inherent strain differences was eliminated in this experiment.

Table 1 summarizes results of conventional MIC and colony MIC determinations and percentage of resistant organisms. Colony MIC values for 12 clinical isolates ranged from 4 to 32 μg/ml. Typical colony MICs are pictured for two strains in Fig. 6. The inhibition of growth on the 4-μg/ml plate clearly marks the end point. Corresponding colony counts displayed graphically showed some decrease at 2 μg/ml. Other strains showed a similar pattern; some had no diminution of growth at the dilution before the end point. End points were all plainly discernible, usually with complete ab-

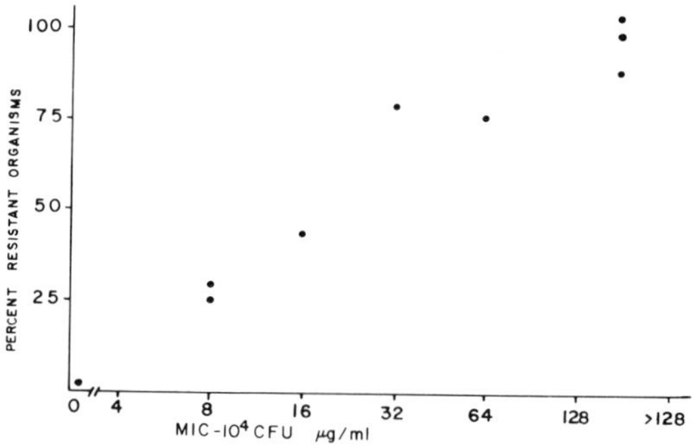

FIG. 5. *Percentage of resistant organisms versus MIC/10⁴ CFU for nine laboratory-manipulated strains.*

sence of growth at the colony MIC; surviving colonies at the end point never exceeded 1% of the inoculum. Reincubation for an additional 6 to 18 h neither increased the number of survivors nor revealed survivors at higher antibiotic dilutions. Colony counts were similar and end points were identical for plates incubated at 35 and 37°C. End points were not altered by preparing inocula from colonies grown on ampicillin-containing agar, and strains retested on different occasions yielded identical results.

DISCUSSION

Ampicillin-resistant *H. influenzae* are now widely distributed. Chloramphenicol is thus recommended in addition to ampicillin for serious *H. influenzae* infections pending susceptibility tests (2). Clinical laboratories usually perform disk susceptibility testing, which, if properly done, is reliable and provides sufficient information for making clinical therapeutic decisions. Chloramphenicol is discontinued only when *H. influenzae* is unequivocally susceptible to ampicillin. MIC determinations as usually performed serve principally to confirm disk susceptibility results and to ensure quality control in the laboratory. The magnitude of the MIC value may characterize the strain in regard to the size of its resistant population, but does not add clinically useful information or guide decisions on antibiotic dosage. Resistance in any degree demands another antibiotic, such as chloramphenicol, not more ampicillin.

Adequate disk and MIC testing of *H. influenzae* requires modification of standard methods (4). Because of excellent growth, we have found Levinthal agar most suitable. Other media have been used (3, 7, 9, 12), including supplemented Mueller-Hinton agar, which we found unsatisfactory because of lot-to-lot variability and generally poorer growth. Factors such as incubation time (12), atmosphere (4, 8, 12), and temperature (4) also contribute to the result; in general, the MIC is increased by improved growth conditions.

The colony MIC measures the susceptibility of single CFU, thus eliminating the effect of inoculum size and minimizing the influence of environmental factors. This technique is not intended to replace the disk or MIC methods. Rather, it serves to characterize a strain in terms of the susceptibility of its individual colonies. Reasons for differences in colony MIC may be speculated upon. As suggested in the work of Medeiros and O'Brien (10), *H. influenzae* has, to a lesser extent than *Escherichia coli*, a barrier that impedes entry of penicillin into the cell; ampicillin permeability may vary among strains. Another possibility is that strains acquire different β-lactamases or elaborate them in varying quantities.

The colony MIC provides a starting point for examining susceptibility differences at the microbial level, but it is not directly applicable to the situation in vivo, where the inoculum size and constitution of the strain vary considerably. The cerebrospinal fluid may contain 10^5 to 10^8 organisms per ml in *H. influenzae* meningitis (5). If a small percentage were resistant, ampicillin might kill some isolated resistant organisms along with the susceptible majority, leaving the remainder to the patient's natural defenses. This may explain anecdotal reports of cures with ampicillin in the face of "resistant" strains. On the other hand, when susceptible organisms are in the minority, they may be protected by their β-lactamase-producing neighbors. In either case, the essential infor-

TABLE 1. *Susceptibility of 14 ampicillin-resistant H. influenzae strains*

Source	MIC/CFU	MIC/10^4 CFU	Resistant organisms (%)
Middle ear aspirate	32	>64	84
Lung aspirate	32	>64	
Knee aspirate	16	16	7
Cerebrospinal fluid	8	>64	72
Sputum	8	>64	
Throat	8	>64	100
Lung aspirate	4	>64	69
Cerebrospinal fluid	4	32	38
Blood	4	>64	80
Tracheal aspirate	4	64	26
Sputum	4	>64	
Middle ear aspirate	4		
Blood		>64	81
Middle ear aspirate		>64	87

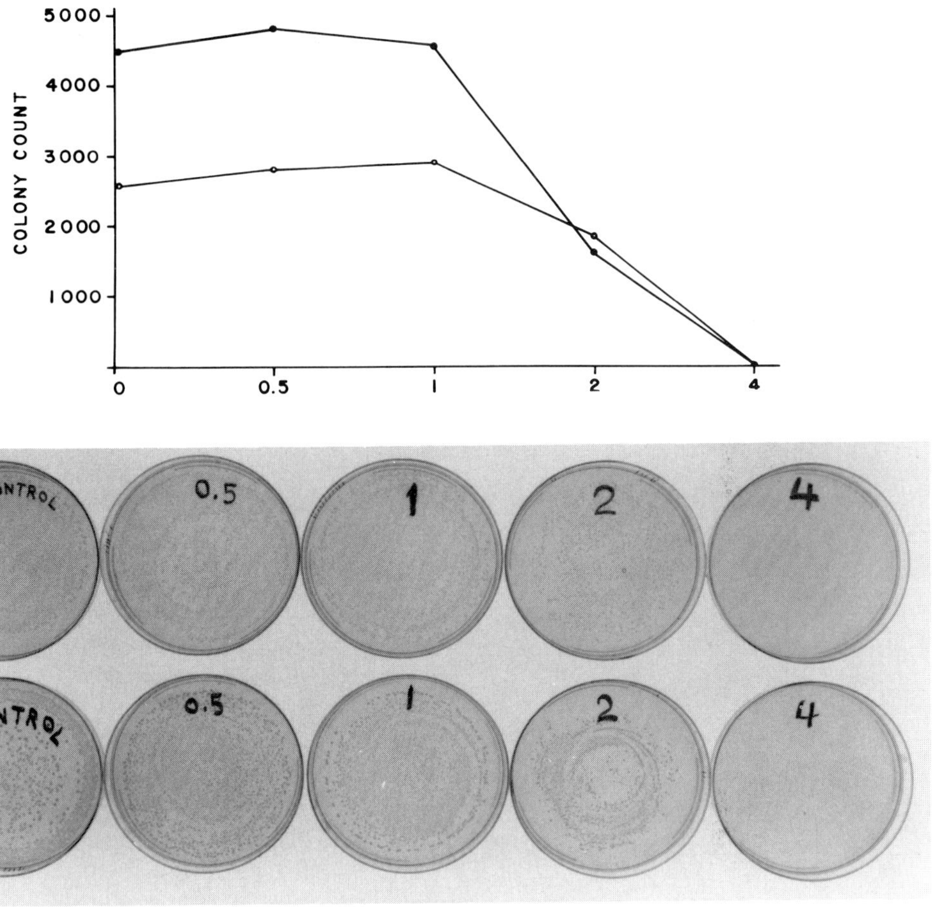

FIG. 6. *MIC of single CFU is determined by spreading inocula of 10^3 CFU over agar containing serial dilutions of ampicillin. Two strains are pictured with a graph of their respective colony counts (●, upper set; ○, lower set). The MIC is thus 4 μg/ml.*

mation is the presence of resistant organisms, not their proportion or their individual susceptibility, since antibiotic therapy is directed against the entire population. The interaction of resistant and susceptible organisms may alter both laboratory results, as shown by our data, and therapeutic outcome, as evidenced by clinical experience.

ACKNOWLEDGMENTS

We are grateful to Ann Kimsey and Marcia McCord for preparation of the manuscript, and to Richard Colan and Richard Gunthorpe for the photography.

B.M.G. was supported by Public Health Service postdoctoral fellowship PO 1 HD 00413 from the National Institute of Child Health and Human Development.

LITERATURE CITED

1. **Caltin, B. W.** 1975. Iodometric detection of *Haemophilus influenzae* beta-lactamase: rapid presumptive test for ampicillin resistance. Antimicrob. Agents Chemother. 7:265–270.
2. **Committee on Infectious Diseases.** 1976. Current status of ampicillin-resistant *Hemophilus influenzae* type b. Pediatrics 57:417.
3. **Emerson, B. B., A. L. Smith, A. L. Harding, and D. H. Smith.** 1975. Hemophilus influenzae type B susceptibility to 17 antibiotics. J. Pediatr. 86:617–620.
4. **Ericson, H. M., and J. C. Sherris.** 1971. Report of the international collaborative study. Acta Pathol. Microbiol. Sect. B, Suppl. 219.
5. **Feldman, William E.** 1976. Concentrations of bacteria in cerebrospinal fluid of patients with bacterial meningitis. J. Pediatr. 88:549–552.
6. **Holt, L. B.** 1961. The growth-factor requirements of *Haemophilus influenzae*. J. Gen. Microbiol. 27:317–322.
7. **Jorgensen, J. H., and P. M. Jones.** 1975. Simplified medium for ampicillin susceptibility testing of *Haemophilus influenzae*. Antimicrob. Agents Chemother. 7:186–190.
8. **Kamme, C.** 1969. Susceptibility in vitro of *Haemophilus influenzae* to penicillin G, penicillin V and ampicillin. Incubation of strains from acute otitis media in air and in CO_2-atmosphere. Acta Pathol. Microbiol.

Scand. 75:611–621.
9. **Marks, M. I., and G. Weinmaster.** 1975. Influence of media and inocula on the in vitro susceptibility of *Haemophilus influenzae* to co-trimoxazole, ampicillin, penicillin, and chloramphenicol. Antimicrob. Agents Chemother. 8:657–663.
10. **Medeiros, A. A., and T. F. O'Brien.** 1975. Ampicillin-resistant Haemophilus influenzae type b possessing a tem-type β-lactamase but little permeability barrier to ampicillin. Lancet i:716–719.
11. **Steers, E., E. L. Foltz, B. S. Graves, et al.** 1959. An inocula replicating apparatus for routine testing of bacterial susceptibility to antibiotics. Antibiot. Chemother. (Basel) 9:307–311.
12. **Thornsberry, C., and L. A. Kirven.** 1974. Antimicrobial susceptibility of *Haemophilus influenzae*. Antimicrob. Agents Chemother. 6:620–624.
13. **Turk, D. C., and R. L. May.** 1967. *Hemophilus influenzae*: its clinical importance, p. 114. English Universities Press, London.

Antimicrobial Agents and Chemotherapy, June 1977, p. 1027-1032
Vol. 11, No. 6

Printed in U.S.A.

Effects of Gestational Age, Birth Weight, and Hypoxemia on Pharmacokinetics of Amikacin in Serum of Infants

MARTIN G. MYERS,* ROBERT J. ROBERTS, AND NAJWA J. MIRHIJ

Divisions of Infectious Diseases and Clinical Pharmacology, the Department of Pediatrics, University of Iowa Hospitals and Clinics, Iowa City, Iowa 52242

Received for publication 21 December 1976

The serum pharmacokinetics of amikacin were studied in 36 infants treated for suspected bacterial infection. A prolonged serum half-life was associated with the related variables of birth at an early gestational age, low birth weight, and hypoxemia. A postnatal age effect was not apparent when hypoxemic infants were excluded.

Gram-negative bacilli represent a serious problem among hospitalized patients of all ages. The aminoglycosides have proven active against most strains of *Enterobacteriaceae*, and gentamicin has been found inhibitory for most strains of *Pseudomonas aeruginosa*. For this reason, an aminoglycoside, such as gentamicin, in combination with a penicillin, has formed the treatment basis for suspected septicemia in neonates. As a consequence, the emergence of gentamicin-resistant organisms has become increasingly more commonplace (7, 21, 27, 29, 30), and so the emergence of multiply resistant organisms in neonates at the University of Iowa Hospitals in 1975 was not surprising.

Amikacin is a new semisynthetic aminoglycoside antibiotic derived by acetylation from kanamycin A that is active in vitro against most strains of *Staphylococcus aureus*, *Enterobacteriaceae*, and *P. aeruginosa*, including strains resistant to gentamicin (14, 15, 19, 22, 23, 33). The serum pharmacokinetics of amikacin and kanamycin are very similar in both adults and children (2, 13). Mean peak serum levels of amikacin, which are approximately three times the minimal inhibitory concentrations of most commonly encountered pathogens, are achievable in adults (1, 2, 13, 32) and newborns (12, 13, 26). The present communication reports our experience with amikacin in newborn infants.

MATERIALS AND METHODS

Amikacin assay. Amikacin levels were determined by a radioenzymatic assay similar to that described by Haas and Davies (11). *Escherichia coli* 21218, from which the acetylating enzyme was derived, was kindly provided by A. L. Smith, Children's Hospital Medical Center, Boston. This assay requires small sample volumes and is unaffected by the presence of antibiotics other than aminoglycosides. Ten freshly prepared amikacin standard solutions containing 0 to 25 μg/ml in human serum were included in each assay procedure. A single lot of amikacin sulfate (Bristol Laboratories, 74-K 590) was used as a standard throughout the study. All samples were assayed in duplicate.

Study population. The study protocol was approved by the appropriate institutional research review committees, and written-informed parental consent was obtained for each study patient.

Thirty-seven newborns with suspected bacterial infection were selected from the neonatal intensive care unit of the University of Iowa Hospitals. One infant, treated for suspected septicemia, was excluded from analysis because of incomplete pharmacokinetic data. Sixteen had roentgenographic pneumonitis (one meconium aspiration; in two, group B streptococcus and, in one, *Staphylococcus epidermidis* were cultured from the blood. No isolate was recovered from the blood or tracheal aspiration cultures in 13 patients). Ten had suspected septicemia from an unknown source (one group B streptococcus, one *E. coli*, one *S. epidermidis*, one *Pseudomonas maltophilia*, and six with no isolate). Four infants suffered chorioamnionitis (one bacteremic from *Peptostreptococcus* and no identified organism from three). Two had cellulitis at an intravenous site (one bacteremic from *Enterobacter agglomerans* and one with no isolate). Two children showed pustular eruptions (one containing gram-positive cocci on Gram stain, but both cultured no organisms). One patient had contracted a urinary tract infection due to *Streptococcus faecalis*, and one had intestinal perforation with peritonitis.

Except in one patient, with an organism known to be sensitive to amikacin prior to antibiotic therapy, initial treatment included 100 mg of ampicillin per kg every 12 h, administered intravenously, in addition to 7.5 mg of amikacin per kg every 12 h, administered by the intramuscular route. Fifteen infants also received a single dose of amikacin, given intravenously over a 30-min period by a constant rate infusion pump (Sage Instruments, Inc.). Intravenous antibiotics were not administered concurrently. Most infants received amikacin for 10 days, and none took it for longer than 14 days. None of these infants had received prior antibiotic therapy, and none had evidence of renal functional impairment as judged by blood urea nitrogen, creatinine, and creatinine clearance determinations.

Prior to the initiation of antibiotic therapy, a complete blood count, serum glutamic oxaloacetic transaminase, bilirubin, urea nitrogen, and creatinine plus a chest roentgenogram, a urinalysis, and blood, urine, and cerebrospinal fluid cultures were obtained on each infant. When possible, creatinine clearance determinations were performed within the first several days of therapy. Response to 3,000 Hz at 88-deciBell sound pressure level was assessed by a Cribogram (Telesensory Equipment) during and after amikacin therapy and, at 90-deciBell sound pressure level, by a Neonatal Meter (Zenith) at the 6- and 12-month follow-up examinations. Estimation of gestational age, performed by the physician caring for the child, was by the Dubowitz method (4).

Blood for determination of PO_2, PCO_2, and pH (Instrument Laboratories, model 3013) was obtained from the radial or umbilical arteries and, on occasion, from arterialized capillary blood. Infants were considered hypoxemic if their P_aO_2 was less than 50 mm of Hg.

Capillary blood for serum amikacin levels was obtained by heel stick prior to antibiotic administration, at 15 min, 30 min, 1 h, 2 h, 4 h, and 8 h after the intramuscular injection of amikacin or after the completion of a timed 30-min intravenous infusion. Serum amikacin determinations were performed during the first two days, in the middle, and at the end of therapy in most infants. Comparative studies of intravenous and intramuscular administration were performed within 48 h of each other during the first 4 days of antibiotic therapy. Peak serum amikacin levels occurred 30 to 60 min after intramuscular injection or completion of intravenous infusion. The line of best fit, derived from a computerized linear regression analysis of the serial serum amikacin levels, was utilized to determine the serum half-life. Statistical analyses included the analysis of covariance and Student t tests (28).

RESULTS

The 36 study infants were 10 days of age or younger at the beginning of therapy; their mean age was 2.2 days. Their gestational age ranged from 30 to 42 weeks, with a mean of 36 weeks. Birth weights ranged from 780 to 4,495 g and the mean birth weight was 2,499 g. The amikacin serum half-life for the 36 newborns ranged from 1.0 to 13.5 h with a mean ± standard deviation (SD) of 5.4 ± 2.0 h, and the mean peak serum level ± SD was 17.7 ± 5.4 μg/ml, with a range from 9.0 to 36.0 μg/ml. The amikacin dosage was reduced for two infants whose peak serum levels exceded 30 μg/ml.

Fifteen infants had serum amikacin pharmacokinetics performed after intramuscular and intravenous administrations. These comparative studies were performed within 2 days of each other. After intravenous administration, the mean peak serum level ± SD was 17.9 ± 3.7 μg/ml, with a mean serum half-life ± SD of 5.7 ± 2.9 h. The mean peak serum level ± SD after intramuscular injection was 18.5 ± 3.3 μg/ml, and the serum half-life ± SD was 5.7 ± 1.8 h. These mean peak serum and half-life values were not statistically different by the paired t test ($P > 0.10$).

While the hemoglobin concentrations in the 36 infants varied from 8.5 to 21.0 g/100 dl and the serum bilirubin varied from 1.5 to 12.5 mg/100 dl, no correlation could be made between the amikacin serum pharmacokinetics and either hemoglobin or serum bilirubin concentrations. Also, no effect of amikacin on either bilirubin or hemoglobin concentrations was apparent.

Twenty-three infants had amikacin serum pharmacokinetics performed on more than one occasion. In most of these infants, the peak amikacin serum level and the amikacin serum half-life were reproducible over time. However, two infants, who had severe respiratory distress with associated hypoxemia, experienced prolonged serum half-lives that subsequently shortened with the resolution of the hypoxic episode. In these two infants, the serum half-life decreased from 13.5 and 12 h to 5.0 and 3.5 h, respectively, as the hypoxic episodes resolved. Nine additional infants were identified as being hypoxemic at the time of pharmacokinetic testing, and seven of these had subsequent serum pharmacokinetics during periods of normoxemia. A prolonged serum amikacin half-life in association with hypoxemia was apparent in these infants (Table 1). The mean serum half-life ± SD for the 11 hypoxemic infants was 7.3 ± 3.4 h (range, 3.0 to 13.5 h) as compared with a mean serum half-life ± SD of 4.8 ± 1.8 h (range, 1.0 to 9.0 h) for the normoxemic infants. These mean half-lives differed significantly when examined by the group t test

TABLE 1. *Hypoxia and serum amikacin pharmacokinetics*

Condition of infant	Serum peak level (μg/ml)[a]	Serum half-life (h)[a]	No. of infants
Normoxemic (P_aO_2 > 50 mm of Hg)	17.9 ± 5.7	4.8 ± 1.8[b]	25
Hypoxemic (P_aO_2 < 50 mm of Hg)	16.6 ± 4.5	7.3 ± 3.4	11

[a] Mean ± SD.

[b] Significantly different from hypoxemic serum half-life value ($P < 0.01$).

($P < 0.01$). There was no difference between the mean peak serum levels for each group ($P > 0.10$). The normoxemic infants had a mean peak amikacin serum level ± SD of 17.9 ± 5.7 μg/ml, and the hypoxemic infants showed 16.6 ± 4.5 μg/ml.

The relationships between postnatal age, hypoxemia, and amikacin serum half-life are outlined in Table 2. Infants in each postnatal age category were evaluated by grouped *t* tests, and those infants on whom values were available for both postnatal age categories were compared by paired *t* tests. The mean gestational ages and birth weights of the 1 to 3 days and older infants were similar. A longer amikacin serum half-life was apparent when values from infants 1 to 3 days and more than 3 days of age were compared ($P < 0.05$, grouped and paired *t* tests). However, no postnatal age differences in serum half-lives were seen when values from hypoxemic infants were excluded. Examination of the data from infants more than 3 days of age showed no significant difference between the mean serum half-lives ± SD of 4.5 ± 2.1 and 5.2 ± 1.9 for the 11 infants 4 to 7 days old and the 7 infants older than 7 days, respectively.

The mean serum half-life ± SD for low-birth-weight infants (≤2,500 g) was 5.9 ± 2.3 h as compared with 4.5 ± 1.6 h for term-birth-weight infants (>2,500 g) (Table 3). Although the mean birth weights of these two groups of infants were significantly different ($P < 0.01$), there was no statistical difference between the respective serum half-lives when only normoxemic infants were considered ($P > 0.10$). The longest amikacin serum half-life occurred in hypoxemic infants of low birth weight ($P < 0.05$).

Preterm infants (<37-week gestation) had a longer mean serum amikacin half-life than full-term infants (≥37-week gestation) ($P < 0.01$) (Table 4). The mean gestational ages as well as the respective mean birth weights were significantly different for the two groups ($P < 0.01$). The gestational age difference in serum amikacin half-life remained statistically significant ($P = 0.02$) even when hypoxemic infants were excluded.

All but 2 of the 37 infants improved clinically. No adverse effects, relatable to amikacin, were observed, and the drug appeared to be tolerated well in all 37 infants. Failures of therapy included one infant with suspected but undocumented septicemia, who continued to be symptomatic, and a second child whose cellulitis responded to therapy but who expired after a pulmonary hemorrhage on day 7. One infant with bacteremia due to *P. maltophilia* resistant

TABLE 2. *Amikacin serum half-life related to postnatal age and hypoxia*

Condition of infant	Postnatal age[a]			
	1–3 days		More than 3 days	
	Serum half-life (h)[b]	No. of infants	Serum half-life (h)[b]	No. of infants
Unpaired comparison				
All infants	6.4 ± 2.7[c]	17	4.8 ± 1.8	19
Normoxemic infants	5.7 ± 2.5	10	4.3 ± 1.1	15
Hypoxemic infants	7.5 ± 2.7	7	7.5 ± 4.5	4
Paired comparison				
All infants[d]	7.1 ± 2.5	10	5.1 ± 2.3	10
Normoxemic infants	6.9 ± 2.0	4	6.1 ± 2.6	4
Hypoxemic infants	6.9 ± 1.5	4	6.0 ± 2.4	4

[a] For the unpaired comparisons, the mean gestational ages ± SD were 36.7 ± 4.1 and 36.4 ± 3.7 weeks with mean birth weights ± SD of 2,565 and 2,417 g for 1- to 3-day and >3-day age groups, respectively.

[b] Mean ± SD.

[c] Significantly different from value for infants more than 3 days of age ($P < 0.05$).

[d] Includes two infants initially hypoxemic who were normoxemic at the time of reevaluation.

TABLE 3. *Amikacin serum half-life in relation to birth weight and hypoxemia*

Condition of infant	Birth weight[a]			
	Low birth weight		Term birth weight	
	Half-life (h)[b]	No. of infants	Half-life (h)[b]	No. of infants
All infants	5.9 ± 2.3[c]	19	4.5 ± 1.6	17
Normoxemic infants	5.0 ± 2.0	12	4.6 ± 1.7	13
Hypoxemic infants	9.0 ± 3.1[d]	7	4.5 ± 1.5	4

[a] Low-birth-weight infants (≤2,500 g) weighed ± SD 1,806 ± 516 g, whereas term-weight infants (>2,500 g) weighed 3,248 ± 476 g ($P < 0.01$). The mean gestational ages ± SD were 34.1 ± 3.0 and 39.4 ± 2.6 weeks, respectively ($P < 0.01$).

[b] Mean ± SD.

[c] Significantly different than values from term-birth-weight infants ($P < 0.05$).

[d] Significantly different from low-birth-weight normoxemic values ($P < 0.01$) and from term-birth-weight values of hypoxemic infants ($P < 0.05$).

TABLE 4. *Amikacin serum half-life in relation to gestational age and hypoxia*

Condition of infant	Gestational age[a]			
	Preterm		Full-term	
	Half-life (h)[b]	No. of infants	Half-life (h)[b]	No. of infants
All infants	6.2 ± 2.2[c]	20	4.1 ± 1.2	16
Normoxemic infants	5.7 ± 2.1[d]	12	4.0 ± 1.2	13
Hypoxemic infants	8.2 ± 3.5[e]	8	5.0 ± 1.5	3

[a] Preterm infants (<37-week gestation) had 33.7 ± 2.4 weeks of gestation as compared with full-term infants (≥37-week gestation) whose mean gestational age ± SD was 40.3 ± 1.5 ($P < 0.01$). The mean birth weights ± SD were 1,960 ± 661 g and 3,135 ± 667 g, respectively ($P < 0.01$).

[b] Mean ± SD.

[c] Significantly different from value for full term ($P < 0.01$).

[d] Significantly different from value for full term ($P = 0.02$).

[e] Not significantly different from value for full term ($p > 0.10$).

to 30 μg of amikacin per ml responded to removal of an umbilical arterial catheter. Ototoxicity during therapy was not apparent in any infant by Cribogram and has not been demonstrated by Neonatal Meter examination of the 20 infants available for reevaluation at 6 and 12 months of age.

DISCUSSION

The volume of aminoglycoside distribution appears to approximate the extracellular fluid volume (10). Excretion is almost entirely through the kidney by glomerular filtration, with the clearance of gentamicin (3), kanamycin (2), and amikacin (2, 17) paralleling that of creatinine. An age-related dose requirement for gentamicin has been reported (6), with children under 5 years of age requiring almost twice as much gentamicin as an adult to obtain similar peak serum concentrations.

Newborn infants have longer serum half-lives than older infants, presumably because of less effective renal function in the early newborn period (12). Similarly, the mean serum amikacin half-life in our infants was approximately twice that reported in adults (1) and, when data from all infants were considered, was longer in the first several days of life than subsequently.

Effects of postnatal age on aminoglycoside pharmacokinetics have also been reported by others (18, 26), including longer half-lives during the first week of life. These data are consistent with renal functional maturation, but other factors such as hypoxemia were not separately examined. Though an effect of postnatal age on amikacin clearance is suggested by both unpaired and paired data, this effect was not apparent when data from hypoxemic infants were excluded (Table 2). Similarly, a relationship of birth weight to amikacin serum half-life may, in part, be due to an inclusion of infants with hypoxemia (Table 3). Interestingly, while low birth weight appeared to have little effect on the amikacin pharmacokinetics of normoxemic infants, a prolongation of the amikacin serum half-life in hypoxemic infants of small birth weight seemed to occur. The amikacin serum half-life was consistently longer in early-gestational-age infants (Table 4). In early-gestational-age infants, hypoxemia was associated with the longest serum half-life.

The related variables of low birth weight, early gestational age, and hypoxemia appear from this data to be associated with prolonged amikacin serum half-lives. Adjusting for birth weight and gestational age, the effect of hypoxemia is not significant in infants less than 4 days of age when examined by analysis of covariance ($P = 0.33$), which may reflect the small sample size.

The renal blood flow in newborns is lower than in adults particularly if considered as a percentage of the cardiac output (31), and anoxic stimulation of the aortic chemoreceptors results in renal vasoconstriction (16). This response to anoxia seems independent of the reflex increase in systemic blood pressure associated with decreased apical heart rate and increased peripheral vascular resistance. For example, when a fetal lamb's umbilical cord is clamped, a momentary increase in renal blood flow associated with an increase in systemic blood pressure followed by a decrease in renal blood flow concomitant with a decrease in arterial PO_2 takes place (5). Guignard et al. (8) reported increases in the inulin and *para*-aminohippuric acid (PAH) clearances during the neonatal period. Subsequently, they showed that the inulin and PAH clearances were markedly depressed in neonates with idiopathic respiratory distress syndrome as compared with control infants (9). The impairment of inulin and PAH clearances correlated with the severity of pulmonary disease, and improvement in inulin and PAH clearances paralleled an improvement in respiratory distress.

The effect of hypoxemia upon newborns' amikacin serum pharmacokinetics and the similar effect observed in adult rats (20) may thus be due to decreased renal blood flow in response to hypoxia, with a concomitant decrease in glomerular filtration rate. Though reported differences in intravenous and intramuscular pharmacokinetics (13) have not been reproducible by us or others (2), it is possible that a difference in absorption from intramuscular sites or alterations in tissue distribution might account for part of the serum half-life prolongation observed in hypoxemic infants. Additional studies will be necessary to clarify the mechanism for this effect.

Shorter aminoglycoside half-lives have been associated with fever and anemia (6); both are factors that may be associated with an increased glomerular filtration rate and could, therefore, affect the half-life of the aminoglycoside by increasing renal clearance. We, however, have been unable to demonstrate a variation in amikacin serum half-life in association with hemoglobin concentration in newborn infants. Since individual patients tend to be consistent in their aminoglycoside response over time (Table 2) (3, 6, 25), these data do not support the recommendation (12) for a loading dose of amikacin in newborn infants. Because multiple variables affect aminoglycoside pharmacokinetics in neonates, monitoring of serum levels is recommended.

A diminished in vitro antimicrobial activity of gentamicin has been demonstrated under anaerobic and hypercapnic conditions (24). That report together with the observations reported here point out the need to examine the effect of hypoxemia upon the pharmacokinetic and pharmacodynamic parameters of the aminoglycoside antibiotics. Such studies in animal models are currently under way in our laboratories.

ACKNOWLEDGMENTS

We were supported by a grant from Bristol Laboratories and a Public Health Service grant (NIGMS 12675) from the National Institute of General Medical Sciences.

Darlene Danney assisted with specimen and data collection. Michael Reeves provided technical assistance. The assistance and enthusiasm of the Pediatric residents for all aspects of this study are gratefully acknowledged.

LITERATURE CITED

1. **Bodey, G. P., M. Valdivieso, R. Feld, and V. Rodriguez.** 1974. Pharmacology of amikacin in humans. Antimicrob. Agents Chemother. 5:508–512.
2. **Clarke, J. T., R. D. Libke, C. Regamey, and W. M. M. Kirby.** 1974. Comparative pharmacokinetics of amikacin and kanamycin. Clin. Pharmacol. Ther. 6:610–616.
3. **Cox, C. E.** 1970. Gentamicin. Med. Clin. North Am. 54:1305–1315.
4. **Dubowitz, L. M., V. Dubowitz, and C. Goldberg.** 1970. Clinical assessment of gestational age in the newborn infant. J. Pediatr. 77:1–10.
5. **Dunne, J. T., J. E. Milligan, and B. W. Thomas.** 1972. Control of renal circulation in the fetus. Am. J. Obstet. Gynecol. 112:323–329.
6. **Echeverria, P., G. R. Siber, J. Paisley, A. L. Smith, D. H. Smith, and N. Jaffe.** 1975. Age-dependent dose response to gentamicin. J. Pediatr. 87:805–808.
7. **Franco, J. A., D. V. Eitzman, and H. Baer.** 1973. Antibiotic usage and microbial resistance in an intensive care nursery. Am. J. Dis. Child. 126:318–321.
8. **Guignard, J. P., A. Torrado, O. DaCunha, and E. Gautier.** 1975. Glomerular filtration rate in the first three weeks of life. J. Pediatr. 87:268–272.
9. **Guignard, J. P., A. Torrado, S. M. Mazouni, and E. Gautier.** 1976. Renal function in respiratory distress syndrome. J. Pediatr. 88:845–850.
10. **Gyselynck, A., A. Forrey, and R. Cutler.** 1971. Pharmacokinetics of gentamicin: distribution and plasma and renal clearance. J. Infect. Dis. 124(Suppl.):70–76.
11. **Haas, M. J., and J. Davies.** 1973. Enzymatic acetylation as a means of determining serum aminoglycoside concentrations. Antimicrob. Agents Chemother. 4:497–499.
12. **Howard, J. B., and G. H. McCracken, Jr.** 1975. Pharmacological evaluation of amikacin in neonates. Antimicrob. Agents Chemother. 8:86–90.
13. **Howard, J. B., G. H. McCracken, Jr., H. Trujillo, and E. Mohs.** 1976. Amikacin in newborn infants: comparative pharmacology with kanamycin and clinical efficacy in 45 neonates with bacterial diseases. Antimicrob. Agents Chemother. 10:205–210.
14. **Karney W., K. K. Holmes, and M. Turck.** 1973. Comparison of five aminocyclitol antibiotics in vitro against *Enterobacteriaceae* and *Pseudomonas*. Antimicrob. Agents Chemother. 3:338–342.
15. **Kluge, R. M., H. C. Standiford, B. Tatem, V. M. Young, W. H. Greene, S. C. Schimpff, F. M. Calia, and R. B. Hornick.** 1974. Comparative activity of tobramycin, amikacin, and gentamicin alone and with carbenicillin against *Pseudomonas aeruginosa*. Antimicrob. Agents Chemother. 6:442–446.
16. **Korner, P. I.** 1963. Effects of low oxygen and of carbon monoxide in unanesthetized rabbits. Circ. Res. 12:361–374.
17. **Levy, J., and J. Klastersky.** 1975. Correlation of serum creatinine concentration and amikacin half-life. J. Clin. Pharmacol. 15:705–707.
18. **McCracken, G. H., Jr., and L. G. Jones.** 1970. Gentamicin in the neonatal period. Am. J. Dis. Child. 120:525–533.
19. **Marks, M. I., S. Hammerberg, G. Greenstone, and B. Silver.** 1976. Activity of newer aminoglycosides and carbenicillin, alone and in combination, against gentamicin-resistant *Pseudomonas aeruginosa*. Antimicrob. Agents Chemother. 10:399–401.
20. **Mirhij, N., M. D. Reeves, R. J. Roberts, and M. G. Myers.** 1976. Effects of hypoxia on amikacin pharmacokinetics. Pediatr. Res. 10:333.
21. **Overturf, G. D., J. Wilkins, and R. Ressler.** 1974. Emergence of resistance of *Providencia stuartii* to multiple antibiotics: speciation and biochemical characterization of *Providencia*. J. Infect. Dis. 129:353–357.
22. **Price, K. E., D. K. Chilsholm, M. Misiek, F. Leitner, and Y. A. Tsai.** 1972. Microbiological evaluation of BB-K8, a new semi-synthetic aminoglycoside. J. Antibiot. 25:709–731.
23. **Price, K. E., T. A. Pursiano, M. D. DeFuria, and G. E. Wright.** 1974. Activity of BB-K8 (amikacin) against clinical isolates resistant to one or more aminoglycoside antibiotics. Antimicrob. Agents Chemother. 5:143–152.
24. **Reynolds, A. V., J. M. T. Hamilton-Miller, and W. Brumfitt.** 1976. Diminished effect of gentamicin un-

der anaerobic or hypercapnic conditions. Lancet 1:447–449.

25. **Riff, L. J., and G. G. Jackson.** 1971. Pharmacology of gentamicin in man. J. Infect. Dis. 124(Suppl.):98–105.
26. **Sardeman, H., H. Colding, J. Hendel, J. P. Kampmann, E. F. Hvidberg, and R. Vejlsgaard.** 1976. Kinetics and dose calculations of amikacin in the newborn. Clin. Pharmacol. Ther. 20:59–66.
27. **Shulman, J. A., P. M. Terry, and C. E. Hough.** 1971. Colonization with gentamicin resistant *Pseudomonas aeruginosa*, pyocine type 5, in a burn unit. J. Infect. Dis. 124(Suppl.):18–23.
28. **Snedecor, G. W., and W. G. Cochran.** 1967. Statistical methods. Iowa State University Press, Ames.
29. **Snelling, C. F. T., A. R. Ronald, C. Y. Gates, and W. C. Forsythe.** 1971. Resistance of gram-negative bacilli to gentamicin. J. Infect. Dis. 124(Suppl.):264–270.
30. **Stone, H. H., and L. D. Kolb.** 1971. The evolution and spread of gentamicin-resistant *Pseudomonas*. J. Trauma 11:586–589.
31. **Thurau, K.** 1964. Renal hemodynamics. Am. J. Med. 36:698–719.
32. **Valdivieso, M., R. Feld, V. Rodriguez, and G. P. Bodey.** 1975. Amikacin therapy of infections in neutropenic patients. Am. J. Med. Sci. 270:453–463.
33. **Young, L. S., and W. L. Hewitt.** 1973. Activity of five aminoglycoside antibiotics in vitro against gram-negative bacilli and *Staphylococcus aureus*. Antimicrob. Agents Chemother. 4:617–625.

ANTIMICROBIAL AGENTS AND CHEMOTHERAPY, June 1977, p. 1033-1035
Copyright © 1977 American Society for Microbiology

Vol. 11, No. 6
Printed in U.S.A.

Penetration of Cefazolin into Pleural Fluid

DONALD R. COLE[1]* AND JUANITO PUNG

Department of Surgery, New York University School of Medicine, New York, N. Y. 10016

Received for publication 10 December 1976

Single doses of cefazolin, 500 mg intramuscularly and 1 g intravenously, were administered to 16 patients having lung pathology who were scheduled for thoracic fluid aspiration. Pleural fluid and serum samples were taken at intervals of 30 to 240 min for determination of cefazolin levels. The levels obtained were variable; however, the levels of cefazolin in pleural fluid generally exceeded the reported minimal inhibitory concentration values for *Staphylococcus pneumoniae* and *Staphylococcus*, and group A beta-hemolytic streptococcus. In addition, the pleural fluid levels exceeded the minimal inhibitory concentration for cefazolin against most of the *Klebsiella* and *Haemophilus influenzae* strains. These data show that cefazolin, despite its comparative high protein binding, produces levels in the pleural fluid capable of inhibiting the organisms commonly found in respiratory tract infections.

Cephalosporins such as cefazolin and cephalothin are used effectively to treat infections of the respiratory tract caused by *Streptococcus pneumoniae*, *Klebsiella* species, *Staphylococcus aureus*, group A beta-hemolytic streptococcus, and *Haemophilus influenzae*. Cefazolin and cephalothin have a similar broad spectrum of activity; however, cefazolin produces higher and longer-lasting blood levels than does cephalothin. On the other hand, cefazolin is more highly protein bound than cephalothin—86% compared with 65%—and some investigators have questioned whether this might be a disadvantage to the use of cefazolin in that it might not penetrate the tissue in adequate doses (5). The clinical significance of protein binding, if any, is highly controversial, particularly as in the case of cefazolin, when the antibiotic has been found to be effective in eradicating the causative organisms and producing the desired clinical response in patients with respiratory tract infections (2, 7, 8, 11). However, levels of cefazolin in the pleural fluid have not been reported, and, therefore, the purpose of this study was to determine simultaneous serum and pleural fluid levels of cefazolin following single doses given intravenously or intramuscularly.

(Presented at the Sixteenth Interscience Conference on Antimicrobial Agents and Chemotherapy, Chicago, Ill. October 27-29, 1976).

[1] Address reprint requests to: 8 Reimer Road, Scarsdale, NY 10583.

MATERIALS AND METHODS

The study group consisted of 16 patients, 11 women and 5 men, aged 43 to 77 years; all had carcinoma with pleural effusion and were scheduled for thoracic fluid aspiration as part of their routine treatment. Informed consent was obtained from all. Single doses of cefazolin were administered, and then serum and pleural fluid samples, each at intervals of 30 min to 4 h, were taken from three patients (two patients participated on two different occasions). Serum and pleural fluid samples were frozen and sent in the frozen condition to Smith Kline & French Laboratories. The concentration of cefazolin was determined microbiologically by disk agar-diffusion technique, with *Bacillus subtilis* as the test organism.

All standards were prepared in pooled human serum for serum and pleural fluid assays. All samples of serum or pleural fluid that required diluting prior to assay were diluted with pooled human serum by using the same lot in which the standards had been prepared. Each of the four to five standards were replicated 12 to 18 times, whereas each sample was replicated 12 times, i.e., 12 to 18 disks per standard concentration with three disks per plate. Although the protein content and pH of the pleural fluid were not known, the samples were evaluated versus a serum curve; therefore, the cefazolin concentration estimates are conservative rather than optimistic, assuming that the serum protein (albumin) content of pleural fluid is less than that of serum, especially with regard to serum albumin.

RESULTS AND DISCUSSION

A total of 18 samples of serum and pleural fluid were obtained. Table 1 shows the serum and pleural fluid levels of cefazolin at each sampling time, the mean inhibitory concentrations (MIC) of cefazolin, and the standard errors. The serum and pleural fluid levels of cefazolin were variable, but this was not unexpected in single sampling. In spite of the variability, the levels of cefazolin in pleural fluid in all patients regardless of dose, route of administration, or sampling time interval, generally

TABLE 1. *Cefazolin levels in pleural fluid and serum*

Cefazolin dose in subject no.:	Sampling time (min)	Cefazolin levels (μg/ml)					
		Serum	Mean	Standard error	Pleural fluid	Mean	Standard error
1 g intravenously							
1	30	48.9			13.9		
2		68.0			83.0		
3		112.0			13.0		
4	60	51.6	76.30	18.68	28.2	36.63	23.18
5		57.0			17.8		
6		111.2			9.1		
7[a]		72.8			5.2		
8[a]	120	36.0	73.15	13.46	6.7	15.08	5.11
9		95.3			18.2		
			65.65	29.65		12.45	5.75
0.5 g intramuscularly							
10	60	89.0			10.0		
11		112.0			16.2		
12		47.0			2.0		
13	120	57.0	82.67	19.03	2.9	9.40	4.11
14		30.7			6.5		
15		40.4			34.5		
16	240	31.2	42.70	7.68	23.4	14.63	9.99
17		31.8			91.8		
18		42.5			43.3		
			35.17	3.67		52.83	20.31

[a] Inadvertently, four samples were taken at 60 min and only two were taken at 120 min.

TABLE 2. *In vitro activity of cefazolin against organisms frequently involved in respiratory infections*

Organism	No. of isolates	MIC (μg/ml)		Isolates inhibited (%)	Source
		Median	~90% inhibition		
S. pneumoniae	20	<0.05	0.1	100	1[a]
	12	0.05	0.2	100	10[b]
S. pyogenes (group A beta-hemolytic streptococcus)	25	0.125	0.25	100	9[c]
	25	0.125	0.25	100	9[d]
	8	0.10	0.10	100	1[a]
S. aureus (includes penicillin-susceptible and -resistant isolates)	25	1.0	2.0	100	9[c]
	25	0.5	1.0	100	9[d]
	28	0.2	0.2	94	1[a]
	32	0.2	0.8	100	10[b]
Klebsiella	25	4.0	16	84	9[c]
	25	2.0	32	88	9[d]
	26	1.6	12.5	93	1[a]
	31	1.6	3.1	90	10[b]
H. influenzae	15	1.6	6.2	93	1[a]
	101	3.1	0.4->6.3	100	3[e]

[a] Minimal bactericidal concentration values in broth dilution assay.
[b] Broth dilution assay.
[c] Broth dilution assay.
[d] Agar dilution assay.
[e] Agar dilution assay.

exceeded the reported MICs of all organisms commonly associated with respiratory tract infections, with the exception of a small number of isolates of *Klebsiella* and *H. influenzae*. The MICs of those in Table 2 were reported by various investigators by a different methodology; however, there is general agreement among investigators (1, 3, 9, 10).

Cephalothin also penetrates the pleural fluid in therapeutic levels (4, 6). Unfortunately, it is not possible to make direct comparisons between these data and ours, since cephalothin was administered in a dosage of 12 g/day, and the serum and pleural fluid samples were taken after 24 or 48 h of dosing. The cephalothin levels reported are of interest, however, in that they show great variability, as did the cefazolin levels. The level of cephalothin in the pleural fluid of one patient, after 2 days of a 12-g/day dosing schedule, was 5.4 μg/ml; the pleural fluid level of cephalothin in the other patient 2 h after dose 11 was 40.8 μg/ml, and it was 70.6 μg/ml 1 h after dose 24.

As was mentioned, cefazolin has been used successfully to treat respiratory tract infections. In our previous study, cefazolin produced satisfactory clinical and bacteriological responses in 22 out of 23 patients having infections such as pneumonia or bronchitis associated with malignant disease; beta-hemolytic streptococcus and *S. pneumoniae* were the most frequently isolated organisms (2). Turck et al. reported that 64 of his 68 patients with pneumonia due to *S. pneumoniae* improved on cefazolin (11). Madhavan et al. obtained good results in all 24 patients having pneumonia caused by *S. pneumoniae*, *Staphylococcus*, or *H. influenzae* (7). Similarly, Mogabgab obtained good results in 54 patients having pneumonococcal pneumonia or pneumonococcal bronchitis; all had severe pulmonary or other diseases (8). It would seem, therefore, that any clinical significance of its protein-binding properties is highly questionable, since cefazolin penetrates the pleural fluid in therapeutic levels and produces the desired clinical and bacteriological responses in pneumonia, bronchitis, and other pulmonary tract infections caused by cephalosporin-susceptible organisms.

ACKNOWLEDGMENTS

We would like to thank Smith Kline & French Laboratories for providing supplies of Ancef and a grant to support the study. We also want to thank Donald H. Pitkin of their Research and Development Department for analyzing the serum and pleural fluid specimens.

LITERATURE CITED

1. **Bergeron, M. G., J. L. Brusch, M. Barza, and L. Weinstein.** 1973. Bactericidal activity and pharmacology of cefazolin. Antimicrob. Agents Chemother. 4:396–401.
2. **Cole, D. R.** 1973. Pulmonary and genitourinary infections in hospitalized patients with malignant disease: response to cefazolin. Presented as a Scientific Exhibit at the Meeting of the Southern Medical Association, November 11–14, 1973, San Antonio, Texas.
3. **Emerson, B. B.,** 1975. *Hemophilus influenza* type B susceptibility to 17 antibiotics. J. Pediatr. 6:617–620.
4. **Gump, D. W., and R. L. Lipson.** 1968. The penetration of cephalothin into synovial and other body fluids. Curr. Ther. Res. Clin. Exp. 10:583–591.
5. **Kirby, W. M. M., and C. Regamey.** 1973. Pharmacokinetics of cefazolin compared with four other cephalosporins. J. Infect Dis. 128(Suppl.):S341–S346.
6. **Klein, J. O.** 1964. Cephalothin: activity *in vitro* absorption and excretion in normal subjects and clinical observations in 40 patients. Am. J. Med. Sci. 52: 640–656.
7. **Madhavan, T., E. L. Quinn, E. Freimer, E. J. Fisher, F. Cox, K. Burch, and D. Pohlod.** 1973. Clinical studies of cefazolin and comparison with other cephalosporins. Antimicrob. Agents Chemother. 4:525–531.
8. **Mogabgab, W. J.** 1973. Treatment of acute infections in hospitalized patients with cefazolin. Clin. Med. 80:27–30.
9. **Motley, M., and S. Shadomy.** 1974. In vitro studies with cefazolin. Antimicrob. Agents Chemother. 6:856–861.
10. **Ries, K., M. E. Levison, and D. Kaye.** 1973. Clinical and in vitro evaluation of cefazolin, a new cephalosporin antibiotic. Antimicrob. Agents Chemother. 3:168–174.
11. **Turck, M.** 1973. Cefazolin in the treatment of bacterial pneumonia. J. Infect. Dis. 128(Suppl.):S382–S385.

ANTIMICROBIAL AGENTS AND CHEMOTHERAPY, June 1977, p. 1036-1041 Vol. 11, No. 6

In Vitro Synergism Between Carbenicillin and Aminoglycosidic Aminocyclitols Against *Acinetobacter calcoaceticus* var. *anitratus*

RICHARD H. GLEW,* ROBERT C. MOELLERING, JR., AND KAREN R. BUETTNER

Department of Medicine and Infectious Disease Unit, Washington University School of Medicine and St. Louis City Hospital, St. Louis, Missouri 63104; and Department of Medicine and Infectious Disease Unit, Harvard Medical School and Massachusetts General Hospital, Boston, Massachusetts 02114*

Received for publication 14 February 1977

Acinetobacter caleoaceticus var. *anitratus* is a nonfermentative, gram-negative bacillus that has been demonstrated to cause severe infections, usually in hospitalized patients. Since mild to moderate resistance of *A. calcoaceticus* to one or more aminoglycosidic aminocyclitols has been noted to occur, a study was undertaken to evaluate the activity of combinations of carbenicillin with either kanamycin, tobramycin, or gentamicin against 28 isolates of *A. calcoaceticus* obtained from clinical sources. Synergism (defined as at least 100-fold-increased killing at 24 h by the combination as compared with the most efficacious of the individual antibiotics) was demonstrated against 26 of 28 strains of *A. calcoaceticus* with carbenicillin plus kanamycin and carbenicillin plus tobramycin and against 25 of 28 strains with carbenicillin plus gentamicin. The median increased killing for the 28 strains was 4.2 $\log_{10}$ with carbenicillin plus kanamycin and with carbenicillin plus tobramycin and 3.1 $\log_{10}$ with carbenicillin plus gentamicin. The most important determinant of synergistic potential of each combination was the level of resistance of each strain of *A. calcoaceticus* to the aminoglycoside component of the combination.

Acinetobacter calcoaceticus var. *anitratus* (*Herellea vaginicola*) is a nonfermentative, gram-negative bacillus that has been associated with infrequent but often serious and life-threatening infections in man (7, 9, 24, 25). This organism usually demonstrates in vitro resistance to ampicillin, cephalothin, and chloramphenicol (7, 9, 17, 21). Although it is usually susceptible to commonly used aminoglycosidic aminocyclitol antibiotics, resistance to gentamicin has been noted to occur (9). Furthermore, infections involving *A. calcoaceticus* are often mixed and commonly involve additional organisms, particularly other gram-negative bacteria (9). Since infections due to acinetobacter are usually nosocomial and frequently occur in patients who have received antecedent therapy with broad-spectrum antibiotics (7, 9), one or more of the infecting organisms is likely to be resistant to commonly used antibiotics. Accordingly, treatment regimens in such cases often involve combination antimicrobial therapy.

Preliminary in vitro studies in our laboratories suggested that combinations of carbenicillin plus one of several aminoglycosides possess synergistic bactericidal activity against certain strains of *A. calcoaceticus* (9). This report describes the results of extensive in vitro studies on the interaction between kanamycin, gentamicin, and tobramycin with carbenicillin against 28 strains of acinetobacter.

(This paper was presented in part at the 16th Interscience Conference on Antimicrobial Agents and Chemotherapy, 27-29 October 1976, Chicago, Ill.)

MATERIALS AND METHODS

Gram-negative coccobacilli isolated from clinical specimens submitted to the Bacteriology Laboratories of the Massachusetts General Hospital were identified as *A. calcoaceticus* var. *anitratus* according to standard criteria (9). All strains failed to ferment lactose (1%) on MacConkey agar plates. Oxidative utilization of dextrose but not maltose was demonstrated. Acid was produced from 10% lactose, nitrates were not reduced, oxidase was absent, and the organisms were nonmotile.

Antibiotics used in these studies included disodium carbenicillin (Roerig, New York, N.Y.), kanamycin sulfate (Bristol Laboratories, Syracuse, N.Y.), gentamicin sulfate (Schering Corp., Bloomfield, N.J.), and tobramycin sulfate (Eli Lilly and Co., Indianapolis, Ind.).

Antimicrobial susceptibility data were obtained

from earlier studies (9) and had been determined by a microdilution technique in Mueller-Hinton broth (BBL, Baltimore, Md.). Of 102 strains of *A. calcoaceticus* tested, 96% were inhibited by carbenicillin at a concentration 62.5 μg/ml, 95% were inhibited by kanamycin at a concentration of 8 μg/ml, 81% were inhibited by tobramycin at a concentration of 2 μg/ml, and 57% were inhibited by gentamicin at a concentration of 2 μg/ml.

The in vitro interaction between carbenicillin and three aminoglycosides was evaluated by the method of "time-kill" curves in Mueller-Hinton broth as described previously (9, 20). An inoculum of 10^7 organisms/ml was prepared by appropriate dilution of an overnight culture grown in broth. The concentrations of antibiotics in the flasks were selected to be within a clinically achievable range for each drug and similar to (usually less than) the minimal inhibitory concentration (MIC) for each drug. The culture flasks (final volume, 20 ml) were incubated without agitation at 37°C, and samples (0.5 ml) were removed at 0, 4, and 24 h for determination of colony counts by a series of 10-fold serial dilutions. Synergism is herein defined as a decrease of 100-fold or more in the number of viable organisms after 24 h of incubation in the presence of the combination as compared with the most effective of the antibiotics alone. "Killing curves" were determined for a total of 28 selected isolates of *A. calcoaceticus*. Approximately one-half of the isolates were selected for study because of nonsusceptibility to either carbenicillin or one or more of the aminoglycosides; preliminary results of studies in seven of these organisms have been reported previously (9). The remainder of the strains were selected at random from the rest of the 102 clinical isolates. To ensure that the 28 strains selected for study represented unique isolates, organisms were selected from different patients at various times and from diverse clinical areas. Furthermore, the patterns of susceptibility (MICs) to eight antibiotics were distinctly different among these 28 strains.

RESULTS

The interaction of carbenicillin with the three aminoglycosides was evaluated against 28 strains of *A. calcoaceticus* (Table 1). Synergism, defined as at least 100-fold (2 $\log_{10}$)-increased killing at 24 h by the combination as compared with the most efficacious of individual drugs, was obtained against 26 of 28 strains with carbenicillin plus kanamycin and with carbenicillin plus tobramycin and in 25 of 28 strains with carbenicillin plus gentamicin (Fig. 1). Overall, the bactericidal effect was slightly greater with the combination of either kanamycin or tobramycin plus carbenicillin than with gentamicin plus carbenicillin: the median increased killing was 4.2 $\log_{10}$ with kanamycin-carbenicillin and with tobramycin-carbenicillin and 3.1 $\log_{10}$ with gentamicin-carbenicillin. Furthermore, increased killing of at least 5

Table 1. *Effectiveness of carbenicillin plus aminoglycosides against 28 strains of Acinetobacter calcoaceticus*

Drug combination	Magnitude of increased killing by combination (cumulative no. of strains)								Median
	0	10^1	10^2	10^3	10^4	10^5	10^6	10^7	
Kanamycin + carbenicillin	1	2	4	9	13	17	25	28	4.2
Tobramycin + carbenicillin	1	2	3	8	13	19	26	28	4.2
Gentamicin + carbenicillin	1	3	5	13	20	24	27	28	3.1

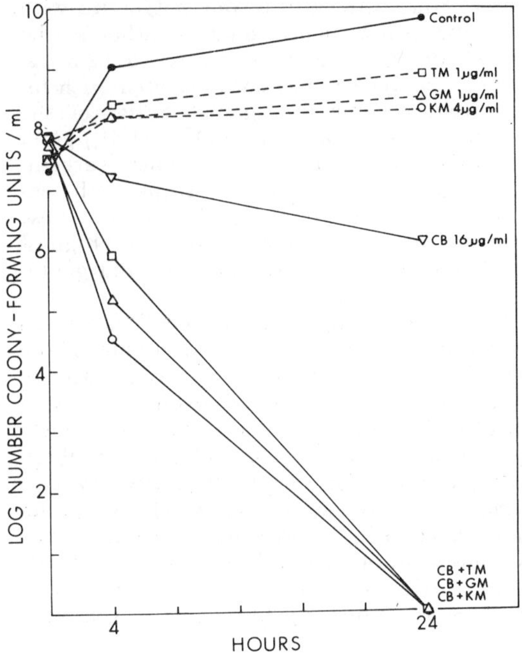

Fig. 1. *Effect of three aminoglycosides alone and in combination with carbenicillin against A. calcoaceticus strain H-7, which is susceptible to carbenicillin (MIC = 31 μg/ml), kanamycin (MIC = 8 μg/ml), tobramycin (MIC = 1 μg/ml), and gentamicin (MIC = 0.5 μg/ml). The starting concentration of each antibiotic (alone and in combination) is listed on the right side of the figure. Abbreviations: CB, carbenicillin; KM, kanamycin; TM, tobramycin; GM, gentamicin.*

$\log_{10}$ by the combination was seen with 15 strains of *A. calcoaceticus* in the presence of either kanamycin-carbenicillin or tobramycin-carbenicillin and with eight strains in the presence of gentamicin-carbenicillin. Antagonism was not seen with any of the combinations against any of the 28 strains of *A. calcoaceticus*.

Synergism could be demonstrated even against most strains of *A. calcoaceticus* that were relatively resistant to the antibiotics used (Table 2). For example, of the 13 strains with kanamycin MICs ≥8 μg/ml, synergistic killing was obtained with kanamycin-carbenicillin in 11; of 11 strains with tobramycin MICs ≥4 μg/ml, synergism with tobramycin-carbenicillin was seen in 9; of 14 strains with gentamicin MICs ≥4 μg/ml, synergism was obtained with gentamicin-carbenicillin in 11 (Fig. 2). However, high-level resistance to an aminoglycoside generally was associated with poor bactericidal activity of the respective aminoglycoside-carbenicillin combination against the isolate. Thus, synergistic killing did not occur with kanamycin-carbenicillin against either of the two strains with kanamycin MICs of 62.5 μg/ml; synergism was not demonstrated with tobramycin-carbenicillin against either of the two strains with tobramycin MICs of 31 μg/ml; synergism occurred with gentamicin-carbenicillin against only two of four strains with gentamicin MICs of ≥62.5 μg/ml (Fig. 3). These represented the strains having the highest MICs for kanamycin, tobramycin, and gentamicin.

The susceptibility of *A. calcoaceticus* strains to carbenicillin was not a determinant of the bactericidal interaction of this drug with the three aminoglycosides. In all seven strains with carbenicillin MICs >62.5 μg/ml, synergism was seen with all three combinations. Similarly, examination of the susceptibility patterns of the five strains in which synergism failed to occur in the presence of various combinations shows that in all but one instance the strain exhibited moderate resistance (i.e., MICs = 31 μg/ml for gentamicin and tobramycin, 62.5 μg/ml for kanamycin) to the aminoglycoside (Table 3). Except for the aminoglycoside-resistant strains, there was no relationship between the degree of synergistic bactericidal activity and the degree of susceptibility to carbenicillin or the aminoglycoside.

TABLE 2. *Effectiveness of carbenicillin plus aminoglycosides against resistant strains of Acinetobacter calcoaceticus*

Strains resistant to:	Gentamicin + carbenicillin	Tobramycin + carbenicillin	Kanamycin + carbenicillin
Gentamicin (≥4)[a]	11/14[b]		
Tobramycin (≥4)		9/11	
Kanamycin (≥8)			11/13
Carbenicillin (≥62.5)	7/7	7/7	7/7

[a] Numbers in parentheses indicate MIC (in micrograms per milliliter).

[b] Number of strains showing synergism/total number of strains tested.

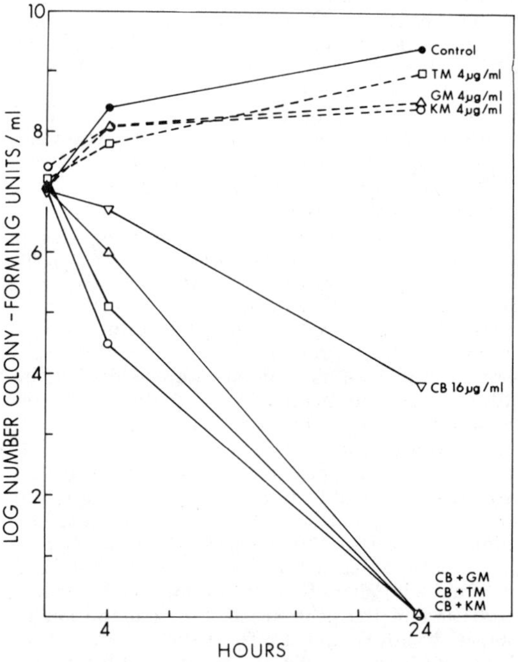

FIG. 2. *Effect of three aminoglycosides alone and in combination with carbenicillin against A. calcoaceticus strain H-106, which is sensitive to carbenicillin (MIC = 62.5 μg/ml) and kanamycin (MIC = 8 μg/ml), moderately resistant to tobramycin (MIC = 8 μg/ml), and resistant to gentamicin (MIC = 31 μg/ml).*

DISCUSSION

Synergistic interaction of several antibiotic combinations has been demonstrated against a variety of gram-negative organisms. In 1962, Plotz and Davis demonstrated synergism between penicillin and streptomycin for *Escherichia coli*, and presented evidence that the basis of this interaction was the increased penetration into the bacterial cell by the aminoglycoside as a result of penicillin-induced, sublethal damage to the bacterial membrane (23). Other investigators have demonstrated synergistic interaction between penicillin, ampicillin, and carbenicillin or other semisynthetic penicillins plus various aminoglycosides against several *Enterobacteriaceae*, including species of *Proteus*, *Klebsiella*, *Enterobacter*, and *Serratia* (5, 6, 10, 14, 29, 30).

Clinically, however, combination therapy of

gram-negative infections is most commonly used in patients infected with *Pseudomonas aeruginosa* (18). In vitro studies have demonstrated synergism between carbenicillin or ticarcillin and either gentamicin, tobramycin, or amikacin against many strains of *P. aeruginosa* (4, 13, 15, 16, 22, 26–28). In addition, animal studies have demonstrated in vivo synergistic efficacy of these combinations against lethal experimental *Pseudomonas* infections in rodents (2, 3). Furthermore, several reports by Klastersky and associates have demonstrated apparent clinical efficacy of such combinations in the therapy of life-threatening infections due to *P. aeruginosa* in immunocompromised patients; concomitant in vitro studies with the organisms from these cases suggested that clinical success was significantly more likely to occur when the combination of drugs was synergistic in vitro for the infecting organism (11–13).

Of the many indications proposed for administration of multiple antibiotics to patients with infections (18), several can be invoked in cases of infection due to *A. calcoaceticus*. First, infections with this organism are often mixed and involve a variety of gram-negative bacteria (9).

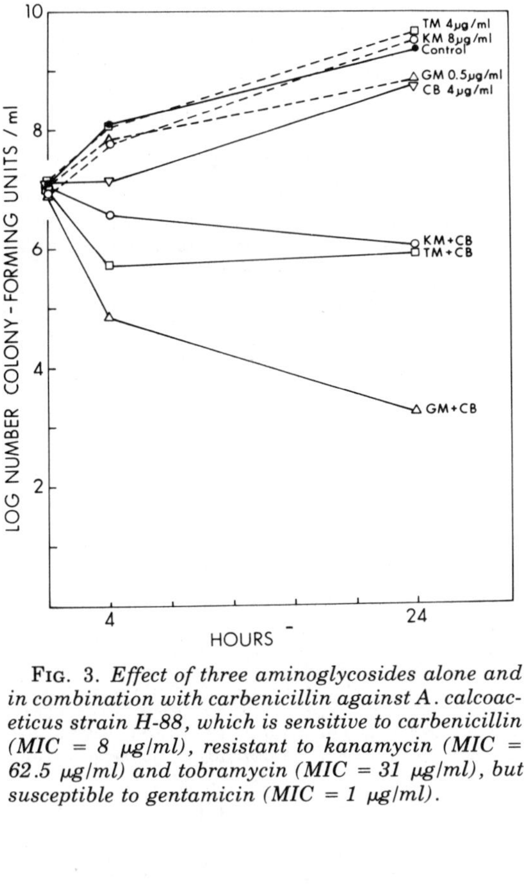

Fig. 3. *Effect of three aminoglycosides alone and in combination with carbenicillin against A. calcoaceticus strain H-88, which is sensitive to carbenicillin (MIC = 8 μg/ml), resistant to kanamycin (MIC = 62.5 μg/ml) and tobramycin (MIC = 31 μg/ml), but susceptible to gentamicin (MIC = 1 μg/ml).*

Table 3. *Antibiotic susceptibility of strains of Acinetobacter calcoaceticus not killed synergistically by carbenicillin plus aminoglycosides*

Drug combination	Strain	MIC (μg/ml)	
		Aminoglycoside	Carbenicillin
Gentamicin + carbenicillin	H-13	8	4
	H-130	31	16
	H-136	31	4
Tobramycin + carbenicillin	H-20	31	31
	H-88	31	8
Kanamycin + carbenicillin	H-20	62.5	31
	H-88	62.5	8

Since these infections are most often acquired in-hospital, these organisms frequently demonstrate resistance to commonly used antibiotics. Second, infections with acinetobacter frequently occur in patients with significant underlying medical and surgical disorders and carry a mortality rate of up to 35% (9). Finally, in nosocomial gram-negative infections, the most commonly used agents that would be active against *A. calcoaceticus* are the aminoglycosides, which possess a relatively small therapeutic/toxic ratio.

In light of these factors, we felt it was important to evaluate the interaction between carbenicillin and aminoglycosides against *A. calcoaceticus*. Studies with 28 strains of *A. calcoaceticus* obtained from clinical sources indicated that combinations of carbenicillin with either kanamycin, tobramycin, or gentamicin were bactericidal in a synergistic fashion against most strains of this organism. Only among strains exhibiting aminoglycoside resistance (MIC ≥31 μg/ml for gentamicin or tobramycin and MIC ≥62.5 μg/ml for kanamycin) was synergism not demonstrable. The combination of carbenicillin with either kanamycin or tobramycin was slightly more active than the combination of carbenicillin plus gentamicin.

With our strains of *A. calcoaceticus*, the level of resistance to the aminoglycoside component of each combination was the primary determinant of synergistic interaction between carbenicillin and the aminoglycosides. Thus, synergistic killing was unlikely to occur with the respective combination if the MIC was ≥31 μg/ml in the case of gentamicin or tobramycin and ≥62.5 μg/ml in the case of kanamycin. In other laboratories, similar studies on the interaction of carbenicillin and aminoglycosides against *P. aeruginosa* have produced conflicting results. Kluge and associates concluded that strains of *P. aeruginosa* with "high-level resistance" to gentamicin or tobramycin (MICs ≥80 μg/ml) were not synergistically inhibited by carbenicillin plus the respective aminoglycoside (15, 16). However, Anderson and co-workers (1) and Marks and associates (19) found no correlation between the level of aminoglycoside resistance and synergistic potential of carbenicillin-aminoglycoside combinations against their isolates of *P. aeruginosa*. Although there were slight differences in experimental techniques between these groups, these variant results are not easily reconciled. However, in some of these studies, criteria for synergism were based on changes in inhibitory activity rather than on bactericidal data such as are provided by killing curves. Although Weinstein and associates have demonstrated good qualitative correlation between inhibitory and bactericidal methods for evaluating antibiotic interaction (30), more standardized studies in this area are needed. Because killing curves are too laborious and time consuming to be used in most clinical microbiology laboratories, it is important to determine the reliability of using levels of resistance to components in antibiotic combinations as predictors of the synergistic killing potential of such combinations.

ACKNOWLEDGMENTS

We thank John Vavra for critical review of the manuscript and Patti Lyles for secretarial assistance.

LITERATURE CITED

1. **Anderson, E. L., P. K. Gramling, P. R. Vestal, and W. E. Farrar, Jr.** 1975. Susceptibility of *Pseudomonas aeruginosa* to tobramycin or gentamicin alone and combined with carbenicillin. Antimicrob. Agents Chemother. 8:300–304.
2. **Andriole, V. T.** 1971. Synergy of carbenicillin and gentamicin in experimental infection with Pseudomonas. J. Infect. Dis. 124 (Suppl.) S46–S55.
3. **Andriole, V. T.** 1974. Antibiotic synergy in experimental infection with Pseudomonas. II. The effect of carbenicillin, cephalothin, or cephanone combined with tobramycin or gentamicin. J. Infect. Dis. 129:124–133.
4. **Brumfitt, W., A. Percival, and D. A. Leigh.** 1967. Clinical and laboratory studies with carbenicillin. A new penicillin active against *Pseudomonas pyocyanea*. Lancet i:1289–1293.
5. **Bulger, R. J., and W. M. M. Kirby.** 1963. Gentamicin and ampicillin: synergism with other antibiotics. Am. J. Med. Sci. 246:717–726.
6. **Bulger, R. J., and U. Roosen-Runge.** 1969. Bactericidal activity of the ampicillin/kanamycin combination against *Escherichia coli*, *Enterobacter-Klebsiella* and *Proteus*. Am. J. Med. Sci. 258:7–13.
7. **Daly, A. K., B. Postic, and E. H. Kass.** 1962. Infections due to organisms of the genus Herellea. Arch. Intern. Med. 110:86–97.
8. **Gardner, P., W. B. Griffin, M. N. Swartz, and L. J. Kunz.** 1970. Nonfermentative gram-negative bacilli of nosocomial interest. Am. J. Med. 48:735–749.
9. **Glew, R. H., R. C. Moellering, Jr., and L. J. Kunz.** 1977. Infections with *Acinetobacter calcoaceticus* (*Herellea vaginicola*): clinical and laboratory studies. Medicine 56:79–97.
10. **Kaye, D., M. G. Koenig, and E. W. Hook.** 1961. The action of certain antibiotics and antibiotic combinations against *Proteus mirabilis* with demonstration of in vitro synergism and antagonism. Am. J. Med. Sci. 242:320–330.
11. **Klastersky, J., R. Cappel, and D. Daneau.** 1972. Clinical significance of in vitro synergism between antibiotics in gram-negative infections. Antimicrob. Agents Chemother. 2:470–475.
12. **Klastersky, J., R. Cappel, and D. Daneau.** 1973. Therapy with carbenicillin and gentamicin for patients with cancer and severe infections caused by Gram-negative rods. Cancer 31:331–336.
13. **Klastersky, J., C. Hensgens, and J. Debusscher.** 1975. Empiric therapy for cancer patients: comparative study of ticarcillin-tobramycin, ticarcillin-cephalothin, and cephalothin-tobramycin. Antimicrob. Agents Chemother. 7:640–645.
14. **Klastersky, J., G. Swings, and D. Daneau.** 1970. Antimicrobial activity of the carbenicillin/gentamicin combination against Gram-negative bacilli. Am. J. Med. Sci. 260:373–379.
15. **Kluge, R. M., H. C. Standiford, B. Tatem, V. M. Young, W. H. Greene, S. C. Schimpff, F. M. Calia, and R. B. Hornick.** 1974. Comparative activity of tobramycin, amikacin, and gentamicin alone and with carbenicillin against *Pseudomonas aeruginosa*. Antimicrob. Agents Chemother. 6:442–446.
16. **Kluge, R. M., H. C. Standiford, B. Tatem, V. M. Young, S. C. Schimpff, W. H. Greene, F. M. Calia, and R. B. Hornick.** 1974. The carbenicillin-gentamicin combination against *Pseudomonas aeruginosa*. Ann. Intern. Med. 81:584–587.
17. **Kuck, N. A.** 1976. In vitro and in vivo activities of minocycline and other antibiotics against *Acinetobacter* (*Herellea-Mima*). Antimicrob. Agents Chemother. 9:493–497.
18. **Levin, S., and A. Harris.** 1975. Principles of combination therapy. Bull. N.Y. Acad. Med. 51:1020–1038.
19. **Marks, M. I., S. Hammerberg, G. Greenstone, and B. Silver.** 1976. Activity of newer aminoglycosides and carbenicillin, alone and in combination, against gentamicin-resistant *Pseudomonas aeruginosa*. Antimicrob. Agents Chemother. 10:339–401.
20. **Moellering, R. C., Jr., C. Wennersten, and A. N. Weinberg.** 1971. Studies on antibiotic synergism against enterococci. I. Bacteriologic studies. J. Lab. Clin. Med. 77:821–828.
21. **Pedersen, M. M., E. Marso, and M. J. Pickett.** 1970. Nonfermentative bacilli associated with man. III. Pathogenicity and antibiotic susceptibility. Am. J. Clin. Pathol. 54:178–192.
22. **Phair, J. P., C. Watanakunakorn, and T. Bannister.** 1969. In vitro susceptibility of *Pseudomonas aeruginosa* to carbenicillin and the combination of carbenicillin and gentamicin. Appl. Microbiol. 18:303–306.
23. **Plotz, P. H., and B. D. Davis.** 1962. Synergism between streptomycin and penicillin: a proposed mechanism. Science 135:1067–1068.
24. **Reynolds, R. C., and L. E. Cluff.** 1963. Infection of man with Mimeae. Ann. Intern. Med. 58:759–767.
25. **Robinson, R. G., R. G. Garrison, and R. W. Brown.** 1964. Evaluation of the clinical significance of the genus *Herellea*. Ann. Intern. Med. 60:19–27.
26. **Smith, C. B., J. N. Wilfert, P. E. Dans, T. A. Kurrus, and M. Finland.** 1970. In vitro activity of carbenicillin and results of treatment of infections due to Pseudomonas with carbenicillin singly and in combination with gentamicin. J. Infect. Dis. 122 (Suppl.):S14–S25.
27. **Sonne, M., and E. Jawetz.** 1969. Combined action of

carbenicillin and gentamicin on *Pseudomonas aeruginosa* in vitro. Appl. Microbiol. **16**:893–896.

28. **Standiford, H. C., A. C. Kind, and W. M. M. Kirby.** 1969. Laboratory and clinical studies of carbenicillin against gram-negative bacilli, p. 286–291. Antimicrob. Agents Chemother. 1968.

29. **Tauchnitz, C. V., and I. Bauer.** 1974. Synergistische Antibiotikakombinationen gengenuber Klebsiellakeimen. Z. Gesamte Inn. Med. **29**:796–799.

30. **Weinstein, R. J., L. S. Young, and W. L. Hewitt.** 1975. Comparison of methods for assessing in vitro antibiotic synergism against *Pseudomonas* and Serratia. J. Lab. Clin. Med. **86**:853–862.

ANTIMICROBIAL AGENTS AND CHEMOTHERAPY, June 1977, p. 1042–1048 Vol. 11, No. 6

Exudate Levels and Bactericidal Activity of Cefazolin in a New Local Infection System Using Rat Granuloma Pouches

MINORU NISHIDA* AND TAKEO MURAKAWA

Research Laboratories, Fujisawa Pharmaceutical Co., Ltd., Osaka 532, Japan

Received for publication 10 December 1976

An experimental local infection system has been developed in which exudates are induced with croton oil in granuloma pouches of rats. This system provided a suitable model for the evaluation of the therapeutic effect of two antibiotics, cefazolin and cephalothin. Exudate levels of cefazolin were found to be higher than those of cephalothin, and these levels correlated with the higher serum level of cefazolin. The therapeutic effect of cefazolin, after intramuscular injection of 20 mg of each antibiotic per kg, was superior to that of cephalothin in eradicating both *Staphylococcus aureus* and *Escherichia coli*.

Evaluation of a new antibiotic usually includes measurements of the levels of its agent in the blood, urine, and tissue homogenates and in vivo estimates of activity against systemic infections in experimental animals. Such studies provide an overall assessment of efficiency and pharmacokinetic characteristics. Their results may or may not be pertinent to the levels of the antimicrobial agent attained at the site of infection and the activity of the drug against the local lesions.

In the present study, we investigated the penetration of cefazolin and cephalothin into exudates in granuloma pouches induced by croton oil in rats. Exudate levels and bactericidal activities of the test antibiotics after parenteral administration were studied to assess the activity of these drugs against local lesions

MATERIALS AND METHODS

Drugs. The following drugs were used: cefazolin (Fujisawa Pharmaceutical Co., Ltd.), cephalothin (Eli Lilly and Co.), and other reagents of guaranteed grade.

Animals. Sprague-Dawley strain rats aged 5 to 6 weeks were used.

Organisms. A standard strain of *Staphylococcus aureus* 209P JC-1 (minimum inhibitory concentration [MIC]–cefazolin, 0.1 μg/ml; cephalothin, 0.05 μg/ml) and a clinical isolate of *Escherichia coli* 312 (MIC–cefazolin, 1.56 μg/ml; cephalothin, 12.5 μg/ml) were used.

Procedure for formation of granuloma pouches and determination of antibiotic levels. Granuloma pouches were induced in rats by the following procedure: 25 ml of air was injected deep into the loose connective tissue between the shoulders with a 27-gauge needle. This was immediately followed by injection of 1 ml of 1% croton oil solution in olive oil into the resulting air space with the same needle (7). Seven days after formation of the granuloma pouch, with or without infection induced by the test organisms, rats were given a single intramuscular (i.m.) injection of cefazolin or cephalothin (20 mg/kg), and levels of the two antibiotics were measured in the sera and exudates. Analytical values of the exudates were obtained with a Technicon Autoanalyzer (Table 1). The antibiotic levels were assayed by the disk method using *Bacillus subtilis* ATCC 6633 as the test organism (5). Standard solutions for bioassay were prepared with the serum for serum levels and with the exudate for exudate levels.

Inoculation of test organisms into the granuloma pouch. The test organisms were cultured overnight at 37°C on heart infusion agar slants. A cell suspension (about 10^4 to 10^8 colony-forming units [CFU]/ml) in 0.9% saline or 5% mucin solution was prepared from the culture, and 0.5 ml of the cell suspension was injected into the granuloma pouch with a 27-gauge needle. At regular intervals, 0.5 ml of the exudate was withdrawn from the granuloma pouch to count viable cells. The test groups consisted of four or five rats, and the results are presented as the mean value of each group.

Determination of viable cells. Viable organisms in the exudates or medium were enumerated by performing colony counts: 10-fold dilutions in 0.9% saline were made. For *S. aureus*, 0.05 ml of each dilution was spread over the surface of staphylococcal agar medium no. 110 (Nissui), and for *E. coli* 1 ml of each dilution was mixed with melted deoxycholate agar medium (about 40°C) in a petri dish; the agar media were incubated for 18 to 24 h at 37°C before colony counting.

RESULTS

Cefazolin and cephalothin levels in exudates and sera of rats with granuloma pouches. Cefazolin and cephalothin levels in the exudates of the rat granuloma pouches after a single i.m. injection of 20 mg/kg were compared with those in the sera. Exudate levels of the two antibiotics were also investigated in the rat granuloma

TABLE 1. *Analytical values of exudates in granuloma pouches*[a]

Exudate no.[b]	Erythrocytes ($\times 10^4/mm^3$)	Leukocytes ($\times 10^3/mm^3$)	Total protein (g/dl)	Albumin (g/dl)	Glucose (mg/dl)	Al-P (mU/ml)	sGPT (mU/ml)	sGOT (mU/ml)
1	25	1.1	3.7	2.2	46	130	35	126
2	38	1.2	4.0	2.5	40	190	32	215

[a] Pouches were analyzed on day 7 after forming. Al-P, Alkaline phosphatase; sGPT, serum glutamic pyruvic transaminase; sGOT, serum glutamic oxaloacetic transaminase.

[b] Specific gravity for exudate no. 1, 1.035; for no. 2, 1.037.

pouches without infection and in those with infection due to *S. aureus* or *E. coli*.

Serum levels of cefazolin in rats after i.m. injection of 20 mg/kg peaked at 68.9 μg/ml at 15 min and were 33.0 μg/ml at 1 h and 6.4 μg/ml at 2 h (Fig. 1a). Exudate levels of cefazolin in the granuloma pouches without infection were 4.9 μg/ml at 2 h, 5.7 μg/ml at 4 h, and 3.1 μg/ml at 8 h. Exudate levels of cefazolin did not increase as much as serum levels, but persisted long after disappearing from the blood. No significant differences in exudate levels were observed between the granuloma pouches without infection and those with infection due to *S. aureus* when cefazolin was given i.m. in a dose of 20 mg/kg 30 min after challenge. Exudate levels of cefazolin in the granuloma pouches with infection, however, were about one-half those without infection when cefazolin was given i.m. 24 h after infection with *S. aureus* 209P. Figure 1b shows the exudate levels of cefazolin in the granuloma pouches infected with *E. coli* 312. The patterns of the exudate levels were almost the same as those obtained from the granuloma pouches infected with *S. aureus* 209P.

Figure 2a and b shows the serum and exudate levels of cephalothin in rats after i.m. injection of 20 mg/kg. Serum levels of cephalothin in rats after i.m. injection were 14.1 μg/ml at 15 min, 6.4 μg/ml at 30 min, 1.6 μg/ml at 1 h, and not more than 0.5 μg/ml at 2 h. Exudate levels of cephalothin in the granuloma pouches without infection were 1.8 μg/ml at 2 h and 0.79 μg/ml at 6 h after administration and were lower than those of cefazolin. Exudate levels of cephalothin in the granuloma pouches with infection were almost the same as those without infection when the drug was given i.m. 30 min after infection with *S. aureus* 209P, but were lower than those without infection when the drug was given i.m. 24 h after infection (Fig. 2a). Exudate levels of cephalothin in the granuloma pouches with infection due to *E. coli* 312 were almost the same as those with infection due to *S. aureus* (Fig. 2b).

Bactericidal effect of cefazolin and cephalothin on *S. aureus* 209P in rat granuloma pouches. (i) Establishment of a local infection system. Figure 3 shows the influence of 5% mucin on the growth of *S. aureus* 209P in rat granuloma pouches. On day 7 after forming, the granuloma pouches were injected with 0.5-ml saline suspensions containing the test organisms, *S. aureus* 209P, in concentrations of 10^4, 10^6, and 10^8 CFU/ml. The exudates in the pouches were examined after 24 and 48 h for viable bacteria. Viable bacteria decreased with all inoculum sizes. However, when 5% mucin was inoculated into the pouches containing 10^6 and 10^8 CFU/ml, there was no decrease in viability at 24 and 48 h. To further examine these in vivo findings, pouch exudates and rat sera were inoculated with *S. aureus* 209P to investigate the effect of mucin in vitro. The results of this study are shown in Fig. 4. When the exudates without mucin were inoculated with *S. aureus* 209P at the initial count of 5×10^5 CFU/ml, the viable bacterial count did not change for 8 h after inoculation. The bacteria in serum without mucin were killed rapidly under the same conditions.

When 3 ml of 5% mucin was added to 7 ml of exudate, the viable bacterial counts increased during the 8 h after inoculation. The bactericidal effect of the serum was significantly inhibited by the addition of mucin, with proliferation of the organisms from 4 to 8 h after inoculation. In heart infusion broth the growth of *S. aureus* 209P was not influenced by the addition of 5% mucin. These results show that mucin reduced the bactericidal activity of sera and exudates.

The above results confirmed that a local infection utilizing granuloma pouches in rats was suitable for evaluating these antibiotics.

(ii) Bactericidal effect. Rat pouches were inoculated with *S. aureus* 209P in 3 ml of 5% mucin in a final concentration of 10^6 CFU/ml. Thirty minutes after inoculation the animals were given 20 mg of either cefazolin or cephalothin per kg i.m., and the viable bacteria in the exudates were determined. In the control group without cephalosporins, the viable bacterial count in the exudates was maintained at 10^6 CFU/ml for 48 h (Fig. 5). In both antibiotic groups the count decreased to approximately 10^4 CFU/ml at 5 h and approximately 10^3 CFU/ml at 24 h. In the cefazolin group, however, the viable bacterial count decreased further to 10^2 CFU/ml at 48 h, whereas in the cephalothin group the count returned to the 5-h level of 10^4 CFU/ml and thereafter tended to increase.

Bactericidal effect of cefazolin and cepha-

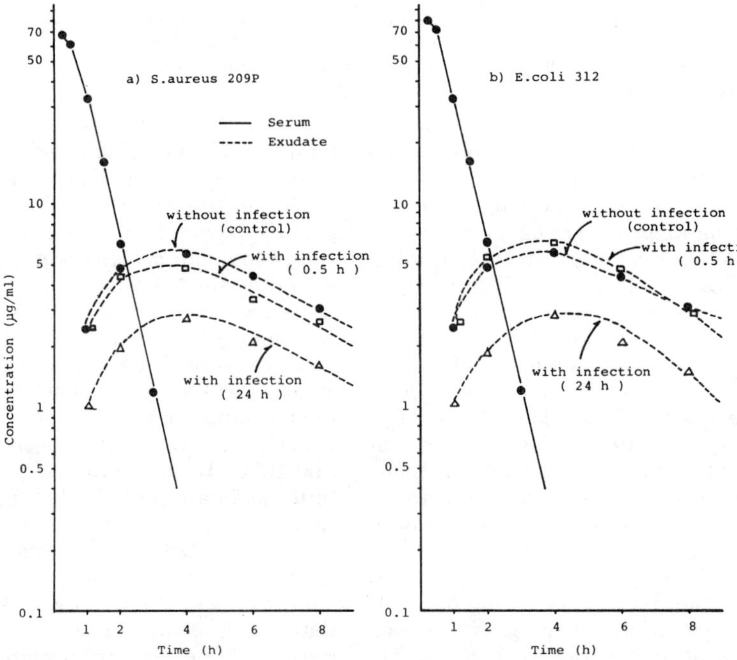

FIG. 1. *Cefazolin levels in exudate and serum after i.m. injection of 20 mg/kg in rats with granuloma pouch (day 7 after forming).*

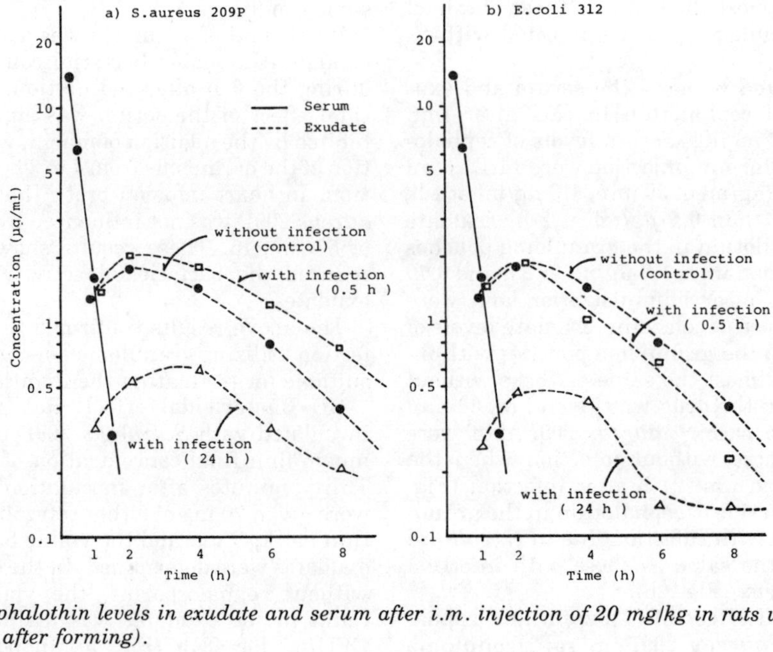

FIG. 2. *Cephalothin levels in exudate and serum after i.m. injection of 20 mg/kg in rats with granuloma pouch (day 7 after forming).*

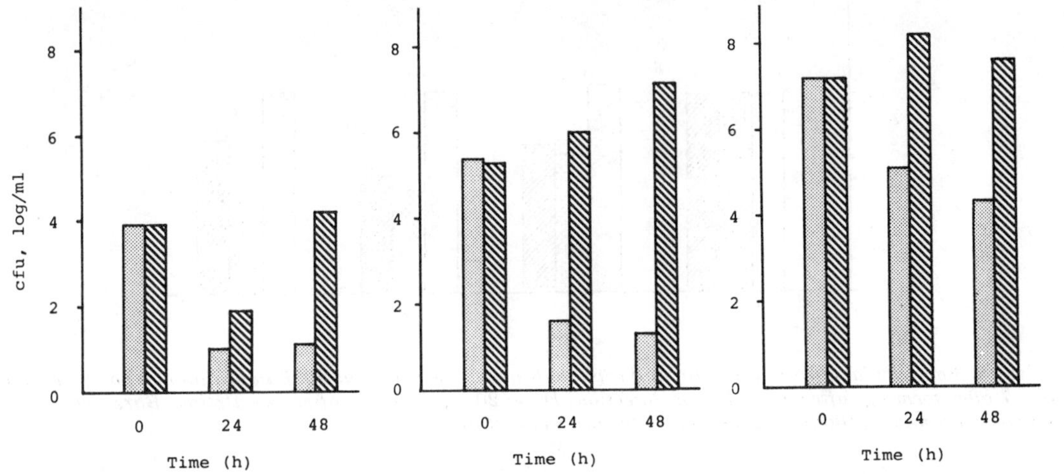

FIG. 3. *Effect of inoculum size on growth of S. aureus 209P in the granuloma pouch (day 7 after forming). Inoculum size: (left) 10^4 cells/ml; (middle) 10^6 cells/ml; (right) 10^8 cells/ml. Bars: (stippled) without mucin (control); (hatched) with mucin.*

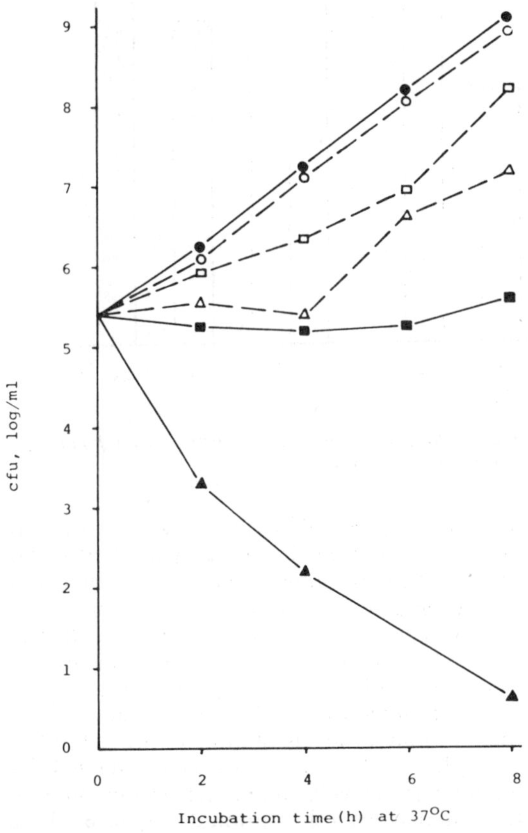

FIG. 4. *Effect of mucin on growth of S. aureus 209P in heart infusion (HI) broth, exudate, and serum. Symbols: (●) HI broth + saline; (○) HI broth + mucin; (□) exudate + mucin; (△) serum + mucin; (■) exudate + saline; (▲) serum + saline.*

lothin on *E. coli* 312 in granuloma pouches in rats. (i) Experimental conditions. Rat pouches were inoculated with various inoculum sizes of *E. coli* 312, and the viable cells in the exudates were counted. The results of this experiment are shown in Fig. 6. Although the viable bacterial counts of *E. coli* 312 in the exudates were lower than those of *S. aureus* at the time of inoculation, there was an increase to 10^8 CFU/ml or greater at 24 h for all inoculum sizes. Mucin was not necessary for the growth of *E. coli* 312, although it was needed for the growth of *S. aureus* 209P.

(ii) Bactericidal effect. Rat pouches were inoculated with *E. coli* 312 in a concentration of approximately 10^5 CFU/ml. Thirty minutes later the animals were given 20 mg of either cefazolin or cephalothin per kg i.m., and the pouch exudates were examined for viable bacteria at 5 and 24 h. Viable bacterial counts of *E. coli* 312 increased in the pouch exudates of the control group untreated with antibiotics and of the cephalothin group at 5 h, but decreased in the cefazolin group at 5 h (Fig. 7). At 24 h viable bacterial counts of 10^8 CFU/ml or greater were found in both drug groups. No satisfactory inhibitory effect of either cephalosporin was obtained under these conditions.

Figure 8 shows the results of two i.m. injections of cefazolin (20 mg/kg) given 30 min and 5 h after inoculation with *E. coli* 312. In the untreated control group, viable bacterial counts in the exudates increased to greater than 10^8 CFU/ml at 24 h, whereas in the cefazolin group viable bacterial counts decreased to less than 10^2 CFU/ml. In the cephalothin group, how-

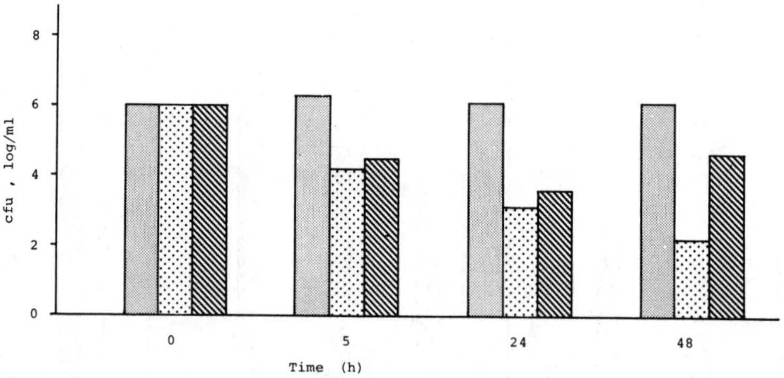

FIG. 5. *Bactericidal effect of cefazolin and cephalothin against S. aureus 209P in granuloma pouch in rats (day 7 after forming) after a single i.m. injection. Dose: 20 mg/kg 0.5 h after inoculation. Bars: (stippled) control, with mucin; (dotted) cefazolin; (hatched) cephalothin.*

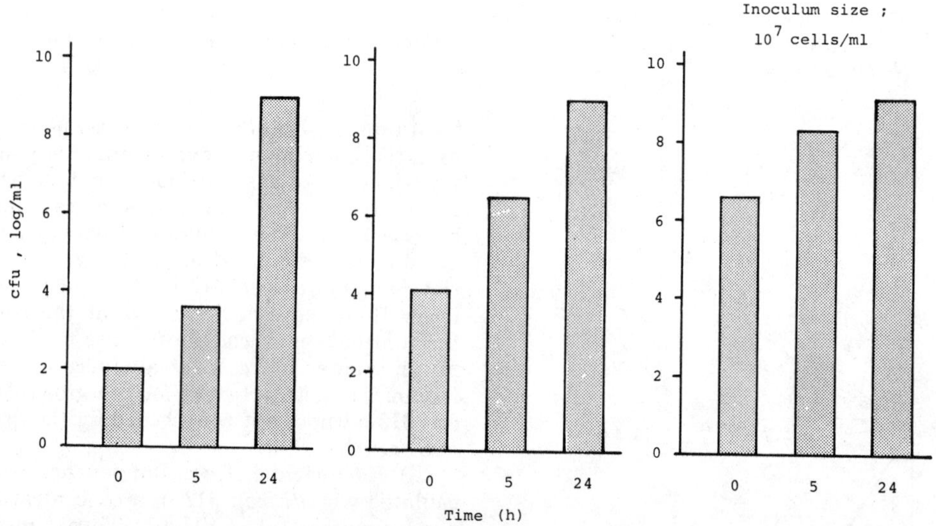

FIG. 6. *Effect of inoculum size on growth of E. coli 312 in the granuloma pouch (day 7 after forming). Inoculum size: (left) 10^2 cells/ml; (middle) 10^4 cells/ml; (right) 10^7 cells/ml.*

ever, no bactericidal effect was obtained after two injections of the test drug.

DISCUSSION

In the laboratory evaluation of an antibiotic, in vivo activity is usually assessed by studying the protective effect in systemic infection in mice. The therapeutic effect, however, should be evaluated on the basis of efficacy in the treatment of established infection. In local infection systems, the effect of an antibiotic depends upon the drug concentrations that reach the site of infection. Therefore, the therapeutic effect in experimental local infections should be assessed on the basis of both in vitro activity and the antibiotic concentration achieved at the infection site. For this reason, we have modified the local infection system of Smith and Wood (9) in granuloma pouches in rats and have compared the therapeutic effect of cefazolin and cephalothin against *S. aureus* 209P and *E. coli* 312 in this system. The therapeutic effect of cefazolin was found to be greater than that of cephalothin, which correlated with the higher exudate levels obtained with cefazolin. Cefazolin is known to be characterized by higher serum levels and higher protein binding in humans and other animals (2, 5, 8). It is generally believed that the high serum levels are due to the high serum protein binding of this antibiotic. It is also conjectured that the high protein binding may inhibit the distribution of this drug into tissue or tissue fluids (3,

6). The tissue distribution of cefazolin in healthy animals, however, is not lower than that of other cephalosporins, as has been reported in a previous paper (5). Likewise, in the present study, exudate levels of cefazolin in granuloma pouches were higher than those of cephalothin. Monti et al. (4) have also reported that cephalosporin concentrations in peritoneal and subcutaneous fluids are unaffected by the degree of protein binding but are better correlated with blood levels achieved and the duration of such levels.

In the local infection system provided in this study, viable cell counts of *S. aureus* 209P, which has a low MIC of 0.1 μg/ml, markedly decreased with a single i.m. injection of 20 mg of cefazolin per kg. In the case of *E. coli* 312, for which the MIC is 1.56 μg/ml, however, two i.m. injections of 20 mg/kg each were required to reduce the viable cell count, even though the

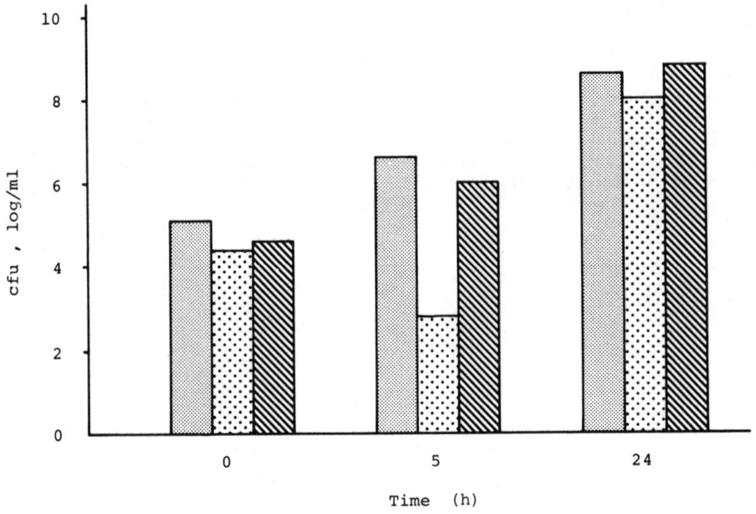

FIG. 7. *Bactericidal effect of cefazolin and cephalothin against E. coli 312 in granuloma pouch (day 7 after forming) in rats after a single i.m. injection. Dose: 20 mg/kg 0.5 h after inoculation. Bars: (stippled) control; (dotted) cefazolin; (hatched) cephalothin.*

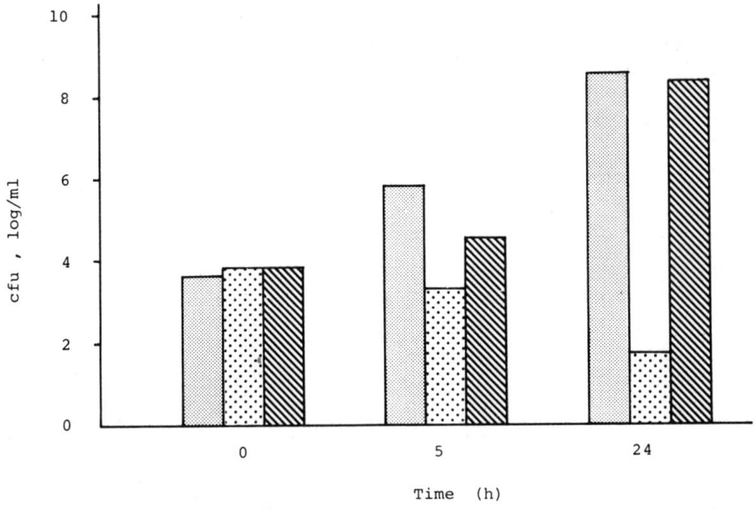

FIG. 8. *Bactericidal effect of cefazolin and cephalothin against E. coli 312 in granuloma pouch (day 7 after forming) in rats after two i.m. injections. Dose: 20 mg/kg each 0.5 and 5 h after inoculation. Bars: (stippled) control; (dotted) cefazolin; (hatched) cephalothin.*

peak concentration of cefazolin in the exudate exceeded the MIC. These results suggest that the duration of antibiotic levels in an exudate and the bacterial species studied are important factors in determining the therapeutic effect of an antibiotic. For the relation between the duration of levels and bactericidal activity of antibiotics, Eagle et al. (1) reported the importance of the aggregate time, when penicillin remains at effective bactericidal levels. These relationships will be evaluated in future studies.

LITERATURE CITED

1. **Eagle, H., R. Fleischman, and A. Musselman.** 1950. Effect of schedule of administration on the therapeutic efficacy of penicillin. Am. J. Med. 9:208–299.
2. **Kirby, W. M. M., and R. Claude.** 1973. Pharmacokinetics of cefazolin compared with four other cephalosporins. J. Infect. Dis. 128(Suppl.):341–346.
3. **Kunin, C. M.** 1965. Effect of serum binding on the distribution of penicillins in the rabbit. J. Lab. Clin. Med. 65:406–415.
4. **Monti, G., A. Bianchi, G. Meinardi, and I. Carneri.** 1975. Relationship between protein binding, blood levels and intraperitoneal and subcutaneous concentrations of cephalosporins in mice and rats. 9th International Congress of Chemotherapy, London.
5. **Nishida, M., T. Matsubara, T. Murakawa, Y. Mine, and Y. Yokota.** 1970. Cefazolin, a new semisynthetic cephalosporin antibiotic. III. Absorption, excretion and tissue distribution in parenteral administration. J. Antibiot. 23:184–194.
6. **Rolinson, G. N.** 1967. The significance of protein binding of antibiotics in vitro and in vivo, p. 254–283. *In* A. P. Waterson (ed.), Recent advances in medical microbiology. J. & A. Churchill Ltd., London.
7. **Selye, H.** 1953. Use of granuloma pouch technic in the study of antiphlogistic corticoids. Proc. Soc. Exp. Biol. Med. 82:328–333.
8. **Shimizu, T.** 1974. Studies on protein binding of cefazolin and other antibiotics. Jpn. J. Antibiot. 27:296–301.
9. **Smith, M., and W. Wood.** 1956. An experimental analysis of the curative action of penicillin in acute bacterial infections. III. The effect of suppuration upon the antibacterial action of the drug. J. Exp. Med. 103:509–525.

Antimicrobial Agents and Chemotherapy, June 1977, p. 1049–1055
Vol. 11, No. 6

Printed in U.S.A.

Uniform Susceptibility of Various Strains of *Coccidioides immitis* to Amphotericin B

M. S. COLLINS AND D. PAPPAGIANIS*

Department of Medical Microbiology, School of Medicine, University of California, Davis, California 95616

Received for publication 23 February 1977

The susceptibility of 12 strains of *Coccidioides immitis* to amphotericin B (amB) was studied in vitro and in vivo. The minimal inhibitory concentration (MIC) of the mycelial phase of these strains was 0.078 to 0.16 μg/ml after 3 days of incubation, but by 15 days all strains were inhibited by 2.5 μg/ml. Mice infected intraperitoneally with these strains were sucessfully treated with 0.5 mg of amB per kg per day. These strains included several studied by others and which reportedly varied widely in susceptibility (MIC from 0.24 to 24.01 μg/ml) to amB. Four of these strains representing this putative broad range of susceptibility were used to infect mice intranasally. Regardless of infecting strain, mice were sucessfully treated with 0.38, 0.75, and 1.5 mg/kg, but 0.19 mg/kg was only partially effective. Thus, in vivo as well as in vitro there was a uniform response of *C. immitis* strains to amB.

Amphotericin B (amB) has for approximately 20 years been the mainstay of chemotherapy of coccidioidomycosis, though recent work has indicated that miconazole may assume a position of some importance (5, 17, 31, 32). The effectiveness of amB in treating various forms of disseminated coccidioidomycosis of humans has been difficult to assess precisely, though it has proved lifesaving in coccidioidal meningitis. There has been little to suggest that variation in susceptibility of various strains of *Coccidioides immitis* to amB influenced the outcome of those cases treated with amB.

Halde et al. (9) reported that three strains of *C. immitis* were inhibited by amB at 0.5 μg/ml (the lowest dose tested) in synthetic asparagine broth after 10 days at 37°C. Littman (18) treated a patient with chronic coccidioidal osteomyelitis with intravenous amB. The strain of *C. immitis* isolated by Littman, when tested in its arthrospore-mycelial phase in vitro, was inhibited by 0.5 μg of amB per ml for at least 4 days at 37°C in Penassay glucose broth to which was added 10% sterile serum (horse, rabbit, or human). Similar testing by Littman et al. (19) showed the minimum inhibitory concentration (MIC) of amB for an additional seven strains of *C. immitis* to be 0.5 μg/ml at 4 days and up to 1.5 μg/ml for some strains when incubation was extended to 11 days. Seabury and Dascomb (25, 26) reported the MIC for one strain of *C. immitis* to be 0.4 μg/ml when incubated at 27°C for 5 days. This approximate level of susceptibility in vitro has been noted for *C. immitis* by others (6, 27). For example, the mycelial phase of *C. immitis* strain Silveira (ATCC 28868) (Silv) was inhibited by 0.25 to 1.0 μg of amB per ml in synthetic medium (2). The spherule-endospore phase of *C. immitis* strain Silv cultured in synthetic medium was inhibited by an even lower concentration, 0.03 to 0.15 μg/ml (2, 3, 14). Despite this level of susceptibility to a dose that can apparently be exceeded in the blood of humans after intravenous administration of amB (19, 20), patients have died of their coccidioidal infections even though treated with this polyene antibiotic.

Seabury and Dascomb (25) reported that a strain of *C. immitis* isolated from a patient before and after 1 year of treatment with amB was unchanged in susceptibility (MIC = 0.4 μg/ml). Sorensen et al. (30) reported that two strains of *C. immitis* were made more resistant to amB by repeated transfer in media containing "increased increments" of amB. This resistance, however, appeared to necessitate no more than (approximately) 1 to 3 μg/ml for inhibition. From a study of several strains of *C. immitis* isolated from patients with various forms of coccidioidomycosis, Hoeprich and Huston (10, 12, 13) concluded that there was marked variability in the susceptibility to amB in vitro. Thus, the MIC of amB for 17 strains of *C. immitis* ranged from 0.24 to 24.01 μg/ml after 48 h and from 0.48 to 24.01 μg/ml after 96 h of incubation, and it was concluded by these authors that 20 to 80% of clinical isolates of *C. immitis* are resistant to amB, requiring >1.0 μg/ml for inhibition (13). The inference from this was that the clinical outcome in patients treated with amB was correlated with the varying susceptibility of the infecting strains.

Because previous work had not indicated such a significant variation of strains of *C. immitis,* we undertook a reexamination of this by studying the response of several strains to amB both in vitro and in vivo.

MATERIALS AND METHODS

Strains of *C. immitis*. The isolates of *C. immitis* were obtained from patients with various forms of coccidioidomycosis, ranging from acute primary pulmonary to chronic focalized (cavitary) or extensively disseminated disease. One strain (Wood) isolated from the soil (35) was also included. Four of these strains (And, Graz, Nel, and Stow) were derived from cultures studied by Hoeprich and Huston (13) and were from their patients 3, 17, 6, and 1, all of whom had received considerable intravenous amB before recovery of the isolates tested. Some of the remaining eight strains had not been exposed to amB.

Testing of susceptibility to amB in vitro. Assessment of susceptibility to amB was determined by an agar dilution method similar to one previously used (4). Sterile amB (Fungizone, Squibb) was suspended in sterile distilled water, then added to sterile cooled (50°C) Sabouraud glucose agar. The medium was poured into plastic petri dishes (150 by 15 mm). Duplicate plates were prepared for each concentration of amB. The medium was solidified with 0.85% ionagar no. 2 (Colab) because of the earlier demonstration that bacteriological-grade agar abrogated the inhibitory action of polymyxin B on *C. immitis* (1).

The inoculum consisted of 1,200 arthrospores in 0.03 ml. These had been rinsed with sterile distilled water from the surface of 2% glucose-1% yeast extract agar slants. The 12 strains were pipetted in a pattern onto the surface of the amB plates. The plates were incubated at 34°C. The MIC of amB was considered to be the concentration of drug that prevented detection of growth when the plates were viewed with the unaided eye. In addition, the spherule-endospore phase of *C. immitis* Silv was grown in modified Converse synthetic medium (16) to which various concentrations of amB were added. The inoculum consisted of endospores derived from cultures in the same synthetic medium. The MIC was noted at 7 days.

Effectiveness of amB against various strains of *C. immitis* in vivo: intraperitoneal inoculation. Initial assessment of the in vivo effectiveness of amB against 12 strains of *C. immitis* was carried out by infection of 10 mice with each strain. Twenty-five hundred arthrospores were inoculated intraperitoneally into 6- to 8-week-old female Namru mice (average weight, 32.7 to 35.0 g). Five days later treatment was begun, using 0.5 mg of amB per kg daily for 8 days and then every second day for an additional 12 days. The drug was adminstered intraperitoneally. Control animals were similarly challenged but treated only with injections of sterile water. The average weight of surviving mice was determined on days 1, 10, and 30. Mice surviving for 56 days were sacrificed, and the approximate fractions indicated of the lungs (1/4), liver (1/6), and spleen (1/3) were cultured to ascertain the presence of viable *C. immitis*.

Intranasal inoculation. Six- to 8-week-old female Namru mice (average weight, 26.7 to 29.4 g) were inoculated intranasally with approximately 2,500 arthrospores of strains And, Graz, Silv, and Stow by the method previously described (22). Each strain of *C. immitis* was inoculated into five groups of ten mice. At 4 days after challenge, treatment was begun, with amB administered intraperitoneally at doses of 0.19, 0.38, 0.75, and 1.50 mg/kg. Mice were treated on days 5 through 12 and on days 14, 16, 19, 21, 23, 26, and 28. Infected controls received 0.1 ml of sterile water. Surviving mice were killed on day 41 after challenge, and portions of their lungs, liver, and spleen were cultured as described above.

RESULTS

Susceptibility of 12 strains of *C. immitis* in vitro. The 12 strains were nearly uniform in susceptibility to amB (Table 1), with MICs ranging from 0.078 μg/ml at 3 days to 2.50 μg/ml at 15 days. A pattern of similar susceptibility to amB was evident throughout the 15-day period of incubation and varied by no more than a twofold dilution. The four isolates of *C. immitis* that had previously been reported by Hoeprich and Huston (13) to vary widely in susceptibility to amB were found by us to be similar in susceptibility to amB (Table 1). The inhibitory level for the spherule-endospore phase of strain Silv was four- to eightfold lower

TABLE 1. *In vitro susceptibility of 12 strains of Coccidioides immitis to amphotericin B*

Strain	MIC[a] (μg/ml) at day:				
	3	5	7	11	15
Abb	0.078[b]	0.16	0.63	1.25	2.50
And (24.01)[c]	0.078	0.16	0.63	1.25	2.50
Clar	0.078	0.16	0.63	1.25	2.50
Graz (0.96)[c]	0.078	0.16	0.31	1.25	2.50
Lee	0.16	0.31	0.63	1.25	2.50
Lund	0.078	0.16	0.63	1.25	2.50
Nel (2.40)[c]	0.16	0.31	0.63	1.25	2.50
Rob	0.078	0.31	0.63	1.25	2.50
Silv (0.08–0.16)[d] (ATCC 28868)	0.078	0.31	0.63	1.25	2.50
Stow (0.48)[c]	0.078	0.31	0.63	1.25	2.50
Turn	0.078	0.31	0.63	1.25	2.50
Wood	0.078	0.31	0.63	1.25	2.50

[a] MIC is the concentration that prevents any visible growth.

[b] All strains grew at 0.039 μg/ml.

[c] MIC at 4 days reported by Hoeprich and Huston (13).

[d] MIC of spherule phase at 7 days.

than that of the mycelial phase at 7 days (Table 1).

AmB susceptibility in vivo: intraperitoneal challenge. The 12 strains of *C. immitis* varied in virulence for mice. Three of the 12 strains, And, Nel, and Tur, were of low virulence and caused no death in untreated controls by day 56; 2 strains, Graz and Wood, were of intermediate virulence and caused 70 and 30% mortality, respectively; the remaining 7 strains caused greater than 80% mortality (Table 2). Despite the high virulence of the majority of *C. immitis* strains, the brief course of treatment with a fairly low cumulative dose of amB prevented death in all 12 groups of challenged animals (Table 3). Despite the administration of amB also intraperitoneally, infection extended to the lungs (Table 3). Moreover, this regimen was not effective in clearing the mice of *C. immitis,* which could still be recovered from the majority of treated animals. Although *C. immitis* was present in most of the treated mice, the animals nonetheless appeared to be in good health throughout the experiment and did not lose weight (Table 4).

TABLE 2. *Comparative virulence of 12 strains of Coccidioides immitis in mice after intraperitoneal challenge*

Strain	Cumulative mortality (%) at day: 20	40	56
Abb	50	100	
And	0	0	0
Clar	40	80	90
Graz	20	50	70
Lee	80	90	90
Lund	90	100	
Nel	0	0	0
Rob	50	60	80
Silv (ATCC 28868)	100	100	
Stow	90	100	
Turn	0	0	0
Wood	20	20	30

AmB susceptibility in vivo: intranasal challenge. In contrast to the variations in virulence seen after challenge of mice intraperitoneally, strains And, Graz, Silv, and Stow were similarly lethal to mice when administered intranasally (Fig. 1). The 70 to 80% mortality seen in the untreated infected controls was markedly reduced by each of the doses of amB used. None of the dose levels of amB cleared the *C. immitis* completely from all mice in a treatment group; however, higher doses of amB reduced the incidence of dissemination of *C. immitis* from the lungs to other organs (Table 5). Although mortality was similar at each amB treatment level, morbidity was less evident at higher doses; thus, mice treated with large doses of amB tended to show the greatest increase in weight (Table 6).

DISCUSSION

The present study indicated that there was little difference in susceptibility of several strains of *C. immitis* to amphotericin B in vitro and in vivo. The level of susceptibility varied

TABLE 3. *Presence of Coccidioides immitis in organs of mice alive 56 days after intraperitoneal challenge with 2,500 arthrospores*

Group	0.5 mg of amB/kg per day: Mice surviving at 56 days	Lung	Liver	Spleen	Percentage of mice with 1 or more infected organs	Water only: Mice surviving at 56 days	Lung	Liver	Spleen	Percentage of mice with 1 or more infected organs
Abb	10/10	6	7	8	100		No survivors			
And	10/10	1	1	0	10	11/11	7	8	10	100
Clar	10/10	4	4	9	90	1/10	1	1	1	100
Graz	10/10	1	2	0	20	3/10	3	3	2	100
Lee	10/10	7	9	8	100	1/10	1	1	1	100
Lund	10/10	2	3	8	100		No survivors			
Nel	10/10	0	0	0	0	10/10	0	3	6	70
Rob	10/10	6	7	5	100	2/10	1	1	1	50
Silv (ATCC 28868)	10/10	3	4	5	60		No survivors			
Stow	10/10	4	5	9	90	0/10	No survivors			
Turn	10/10	1	1	1	10	10/10	4	6	10	100
Wood	9/9	0	0	4	44	7/10	6	6	6	86

with time, but ranged from 0.078 μg/ml after 3 days of incubation to 2.50 μg/ml after 15 days. Thus, cultivation on Sabouraud glucose agar did not appear to counter the antifungal action of amB though some loss in activity of amB can be expected with incubation over several days. The spherule-endospore phase of *C. immitis* strain Silv grown in synthetic medium did have a lower MIC (0.08 to 0.16 μg/ml) when compared at 7 days with the mycelial phase (MIC = 0.63 μg/ml) grown on the more complex Sabouraud medium. However, a previous assessment of the susceptibility of the mycelial phase of strain Silv had been carried out in the synthetic yeast nitrogen base (Difco) medium and yielded an MIC of 0.25 μg/ml at 5 days, increasing to a maximum of 1.0 μg/ml from day 9 to day 23 (2). In that previous study, the spherule-endospore phase was partially inhibited hy 0.03 μg/ml and markedly inhibited by 0.15 μg/ml at 6 days. Thus, morphological form appeared to influence the MIC more than did the culture medium. Huppert and Walker (15) and Hoeprich and Huston (12, 13) concluded that the endospore-sperule phase derived from homogenized infected mouse tissues showed the same susceptibility to amB as did the arthrospore form. Unfortunately, this is not likely to provide clear-cut information on the susceptibility of spherule-endospore forms, since the latter are known to germinate to hyphal forms within 5 h when removed from mouse tissues (23). Furthermore, appropriate tissue extracts would have to be included in controls when comparing endospore-spherule inocula derived from infected mice with the mycelial phase in vitro. Therefore, cultivation in a medium designed to maintain the spherule-endospore form would yield more specific information on susceptibility of this morphological phase.

From the work of several investigators (18, 19, 25, 27, 28) as well as our own data, the antifungal action of amB versus *C. immitis* was not inhibited by complex, ill-defined organic media. The inhibitory action of amB at 0.5 μg/ml noted by Halde et al. (9) was achieved in synthetic broth containing asparagine, glucose, citrate, glycerol, and several salts (29); Huppert (personal communication) has noted MICs for 18 strains of *C. immitis* grown on synthetic yeast morphology agar (pH approximately 4.5) to be between 0.15 and 1.25 μg/ml. Thus, the MICs were in the same range with both the well-defined synthetic media and the complex organic media. This contrasts with the broad spread of MICs noted by Hoeprich and Huston in their defined synthetic medium (11, 13). Moreover, in preparing dilutions of amB, water or glucose in water is recommended. Hoeprich and Huston (13) utilized phosphate-buffered saline (containing additional salts; 11) to prepare dilutions of amB. In our hands, phosphate-buffered saline led to precipitation of the amB.

It is evident from the present study that all strains tested by us, including some of those used in the study by Hoeprich and Huston (13), showed susceptibility to amB in vivo such that one could not discern a significant difference in susceptibility. Treatment of infected mice with 0.5 mg/kg protected virtually all mice that had been inoculated intraperitoneally with strains virulent by this route and reduced the frequency of recovery of *C. immitis* from mice infected with strains of lower virulence. However, because of the need to obtain an appropriate end point to discern possible differences among the strains, we selected four strains to be used for the more rigorous intranasal challenge. These four strains included three that represented the extremes in MIC to amB among those studied by Hoeprich and Huston (13). One, Silv, was a strain long maintained in the laboratory. All four showed similar susceptibility to amB in mice infected intranasally. Thus, 0.19 mg/kg was not sufficient to protect the mice, whereas amB was protective at doses of 0.38, 0.75, and 1.5 mg/kg.

The latter doses approximate the intravenous dose (about 1.0 mg/kg) of amB that has been used for many years in treating coccidioidomycosis in humans. Littman (18), in treating a patient with disseminated coccidioidomycosis with amB, initially used a dose of 0.8 mg/kg and gradually increased this to 2.6 mg/kg. Because of increasing blood urea nitrogen, Littman subsequently reduced the dosage to 1.6

TABLE 4. *Average weight of mice in groups challenged intraperitoneally with 2,500 arthrospores*

Group	Avg wt (g) after treatment with:					
	0.5 mg of amB/kg per day			Water only		
	Day 1	Day 10	Day 30	Day 1	Day 10	Day 30
Abb	34.5	34.7	37.4	35.0	35.1	–[a]
And	34.1	33.4	37.4	34.2	34.3	36.4
Clar	34.4	34.5	37.8	34.7	31.9	–
Graz	33.6	33.3	36.3	33.7	34.4	31.2
Lee	33.6	33.6	36.8	33.9	31.2	–
Lund	33.8	33.7	36.8	34.3	30.0	–
Nel	35.0	34.7	38.2	34.4	35.2	38.7
Rob	35.0	34.2	37.5	34.1	32.5	–
Silv (ATCC 28868)	34.5	34.1	38.6	34.6	28.6	–
Stow	33.3	33.1	36.6	33.7	23.6	–
Turn	32.7	32.2	35.8	33.2	33.0	35.8
Wood	33.0	33.0	37.5	33.6	33.2	33.8

[a] –, Mice not weighed if 50% or less were alive.

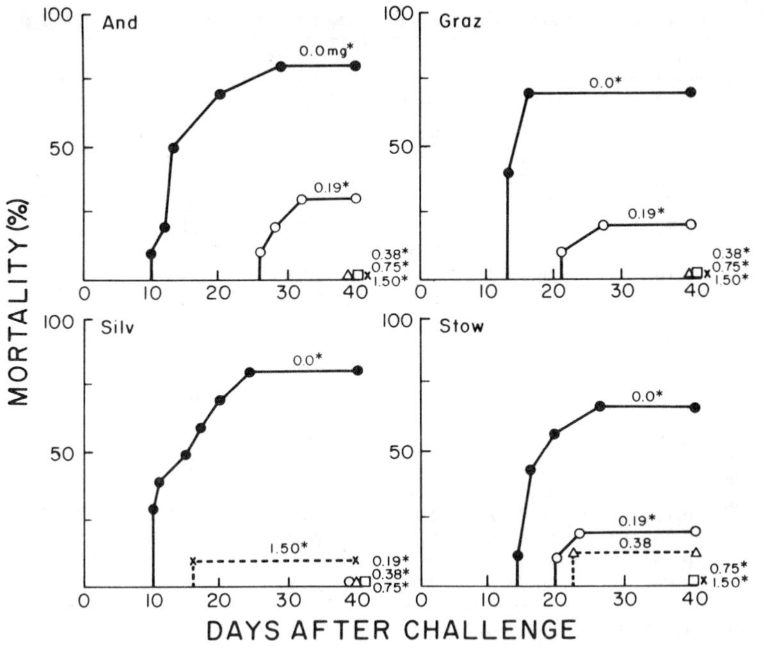

FIG. 1. *Comparative efficacy of amB in treatment of mice infected intranasally with four strains of Coccidioides immitis. Numbers with asterisk represent dose (in milligrams) of amB per kilogram per day.*

TABLE 5. *Presence of Coccidioides immitis in organs of mice alive 41 days after intranasal challenge with 2,500 arthrospores*

Group	Treatment (mg of amB/kg per day)	Surviving mice	Organ		
			Lungs	Liver	Spleen
And	0	2/10	1	1	0
	0.19	7/10	6	6	3
	0.38	10/10	7	2	0
	0.75	10/10	5	0	0
	1.50	10/10	3	0	0
Graz	0	3/10	2	1	1
	0.19	8/10	5	1	0
	0.38	10/10	3	3	1
	0.75	10/10	9	3	1
	1.50	10/10	7	2	0
Silv	0	2/10	2	1	1
(ATCC	0.19	10/10	5	4	2
28868)	0.38	10/10	7	0	1
	0.75	10/10	6	0	0
	1.50	9/10	4	1	2
Stow	0	3/10	3	2	1
	0.19	8/10	5	4	2
	0.38	7/9	4	3	2
	0.75	10/10	7	2	1
	1.50	10/10	6	1	0

mg/kg, administered on alternate days. At doses of 2.4 and 1.6 mg/kg, intravenous amB produced blood serum levels of 1.8 and 0.9 μg/ml, respectively, the latter being detected 12 and 18 h after discontinuation of the infusion, but not at 38 h.

Louria (20) detected average peak blood levels of amB of 0.5 to 2.6 μg/ml after intravenous administration of 0.5 to 1.0 mg/kg. Winn (34) advised the use of intravenous amB at doses of 1.0 mg/kg in adults and 1.25 to 1.50 mg/kg in children or infants in order to maintain a desired serum level of 0.5 to 1.0 μg/ml, though he reported the presence of 1.0 to 12.0 μg/ml at 24 to 48 h after the infusion. Sanford et al. (24) emphasized the toxicity of intravenous amB given daily at 1.0 mg/kg, but felt that it was necessary to use such a dose to maintain therapeutic serum levels, advising, however, that alternate-day therapy might be desirable to ameliorate the nephrotoxicity.

Seabury and Dascomb (25) indicated that at 24 h after administration of 0.6 to 0.8 mg/kg, they detected 0.5 to 1.0 μg/ml in the serum. In treating disseminated mycotic infections other than coccidioidomycosis, Drutz et al. (7) detected up to 12.5 μg/ml in the serum of a patient who received 1.5 mg/kg of amB intravenously. These authors emphasized the need to adjust the dose of intravenous amB to the individual patient to achieve an appropriate serum level. In their studies, 1.56 μg/ml was regarded as the appropriate level inasmuch as this was twice the dose needed to inhibit any of the infecting fungi in their patients. Fields et al. (8) demon-

TABLE 6. *Average weight of mice in groups challenged intranasally with 2,500 arthrospores*

Group	Treatment (mg of amB/kg per day)	Avg wt (g)					Percent wt change from days 1 to 37
		Day 1	Day 5	Day 10	Day 21	Day 37	
And	0	29.4	28.8	26.4	—[a]	—	—
	0.19	28.6	28.9	27.7	26.5	27.1	− 5.2
	0.38	28.7	29.1	29.1	28.7	31.0	8.3
	0.75	29.0	29.7	29.3	29.5	31.3	7.9
	1.50	27.6	28.4	28.1	28.5	30.3	9.8
Graz	0	28.6	29.4	27.2	—	—	—
	0.19	28.2	28.5	26.3	25.1	29.0	2.8
	0.38	27.5	27.5	27.1	26.5	28.3	2.9
	0.75	26.7	27.0	25.9	26.5	27.8	4.1
	1.50	28.1	28.8	28.1	27.9	31.0	10.3
Silv (ATCC 28868)	0	28.5	29.3	25.7	—	—	—
	0.19	28.6	28.9	28.8	28.0	29.7	3.8
	0.38	27.8	28.4	27.9	26.7	28.5	2.5
	0.75	28.9	29.7	29.5	29.5	31.6	9.3
	1.50	27.4	26.8	27.0	28.5	30.3	10.6
Stow	0	27.8	28.1	26.7	—	—	—
	0.19	28.9	29.3	28.1	26.3	29.6	2.4
	0.38	29.4	28.9	28.4	25.0	29.7	1.0
	0.75	28.9	29.1	28.9	29.4	31.5	5.5
	1.50	26.7	26.6	26.4	26.4	38.1	5.2

[a] Mice not weighed if 50% or less were alive.

strated peak levels of amB in the serum in the range of 0.42 to 2.0 μg/ml (mean, 1.21 μg/ml) 1 h after infusion of 50 mg of amB intravenously. The mean serum level was 0.62 μg/ml (0.27 to 1.38 μg/ml) 18 h later and 0.32 μg/ml (0.13 to 0.79 μg/ml) at 42 h after the infusion. These levels all exceed the MIC noted for the 12 strains studied by us at 5 days of incubation and are well above the MIC noted for the spherule-endospore phase of strain Silv. The results of Taylor et al. (33), on the other hand, differed from those of most others in that they detected only 0.05 to 0.4 μg/ml after intravenous doses of 0.5 to 1.0 mg/kg.

From our studies in mice, 0.25 and 0.5 mg/kg appeared to provide adequate therapeutic levels against four different strains of *C. immitis*. Although caution is necessary in extrapolating from these data to human patients, it seems likely that the use of 1.0 mg/kg in humans would yield serum levels needed to inhibit at least the many strains tested in the present study. Thus far there appears to be no serious justification for assessing the susceptibility to amB of *C. immitis* from each patient. Should such an assessment be desired, it may best be carried out by testing the patient's strain in comparison with a reference strain, e.g., *C. immitis* strain Silveira (ATCC 28868), that has been used in many previous studies (2, 14, 17). However, it is reasonable to monitor periodically the serum levels of amB in patients with coccidioidomycosis so that the intravenous dosage can be adjusted to provide serum levels of 1.0 to 2.0 μg/ml, which appears to suffice for inhibition of *C. immitis*. This of course does not necessarily assure that adequate penetration of all infected sites will occur. Indeed, experience to date indicates that cavitary coccidioidomycosis is not likely to respond to intravenous amB. This is more likely due to inadequate levels of amB at the site of the cavity than to inordinate resistance of the mycelial phase that may be found in the walls of such cavities.

ACKNOWLEDGMENTS

We thank Philip Cabasso for his laboratory assistance.

M.S.C., a Bank of America-Giannini Foundation Fellow, is grateful for the support of the Foundation. This work was supported in part by the U.S. Army Medical Research and Development Command under research contract no. DADA 17-69-C-9061 and by the Valley-Lode Lung Association.

LITERATURE CITED

1. **Collins, M. S.** 1975. Inhibition of growth of *Coccidioides immitis* on Sabouraud medium containing polymyxin B. J. Clin. Microbiol. 1:335–336.
2. **Collins, M. S., and D. Pappagainis.** 1974. Lysozyme-enhanced killing of *Candida albicans* and *Coccidioides immitis* by amphotericin B. Sabouraudia 12:329–340.
3. **Collins, M. S., and D. Pappagianis.** 1975. Inhibition of *Coccidioides immitis* in vitro enhancement of anticoccidioidal effects of amphotericin B by polymyxin B. Antimicrob. Agents Chemother. 7:781–787.
4. **Collins, M. S., and D. Pappagianis.** 1976. Treatment of murine coccidioidomycosis with polymyxin B. Antimicrob. Agents Chemother. 10:318–321.
5. **Deresinski, S. C., R. B. Lilly, H. B. Levine, J. N. Galgiani, and D. A. Stevens.** 1976. Treatment of fun-

gal meningitis with miconazole. Am. Rev. Respir. Dis. 113:71.

6. **Drouhet, E.** 1967. Some biological activities of antifungal antibiotics and their mode of action, p. 206–241. *In* G. E. W. Wolstenholme and R. Porter (ed.), Systemic mycoses. Little, Brown and Co., Boston.
7. **Drutz, D. J., A. Spickard, D. E. Rogers, and M. G. Koenig.** 1968. Treatment of disseminated mycotic infections. A new approach to amphotericin B therapy. Am. J. Med. 45:405–418.
8. **Fields, B. T., Jr., J. H. Bates, and R. S. Abernathy.** 1970. Amphotericin B serum concentrations during therapy. Appl. Microbiol. 19:955–959.
9. **Halde, C., V. D. Newcomer, E. T. Wright, and T. H. Sternberg.** 1957. An evaluation of amphotericin B *in vitro* and *in vivo* in mice against *Coccidioides immitis* and *Candida albicans*, and preliminary observations concerning the administration of amphotericin B to man. J. Invest. Dermatol. 28:217–231.
10. **Hoeprich, P. D.** 1973. Susceptibility of *Coccidioides immitis in vitro*. Clin. Res. 21:215.
11. **Hoeprich, P. D., and P. D. Finn.** 1972. Obfuscation of the activity of antifungal antimicrobics by culture media. J. Infect. Dis. 126:353–361.
12. **Hoeprich, P. D., and A. C. Huston.** 1974. Relevance of susceptibility testing of *Coccidioides immitis*. Clin. Res. 22:104A.
13. **Hoeprich, P. D., and A. C. Huston.** 1975. Susceptibility of *Coccidioides immitis, Candida albicans*, and *Cryptococcus neoformans* to amphotericin B, flucytosine, and clotrimazole. J. Infect. Dis. 132:133–141.
14. **Huppert, M., D. Pappagianis, S. H. Sun, I. Gleason-Jordan, M. S. Collins, K. R. Vukovich.** 1976. Effect of amphotericin B and rifampin agains *Coccidioides immitis* in vitro and in vivo. Antimicrob. Agents Chemother. 9:406–413.
15. **Huppert, M., and L. J. Walker.** 1959. The sensitivity of different cell types of *Coccidioides immitis* to amphotericin B (Fungizone), p. 297–301. *In* Conference on Chemotherapy of Tuberculosis, Transactions of the 18th Conference U.S. Veterans Administration.
16. **Levine, H. B., J. M. Cobb, and C. E. Smith.** 1960. Immunity to coccidioidomycosis induced in mice by purified spherule, arthrospore and mycelial vaccines. Trans. N.Y. Acad. Sci. 22:436–449.
17. **Levine, H. B., D. A. Stevens, J. M. Cobb, and A. E. Gebhardt.** 1975. Miconazole in coccidioidomycosis. I. Assays of activity in mice and in vitro. J. Infect. Dis. 132:407–414.
18. **Littman, M.** 1957. Preliminary observations on the intravenous use of amphotericin B, an antifungal antibiotic, in the therapy of acute and chronic coccidioidal osteomyelitis, p. 86–94. *In* Proceedings of Symposium on Coccidioidomycosis, Public Health Service Publ. no. 575. U.S. Government Printing Office, Washington, D.C.
19. **Littman, M. L., P. L. Horowitz, and J. G. Swadey.** 1958. Coccidioidomycosis and its treatment with amphotericin B. Am. J. Med. 24:568–592.
20. **Louria, D. B.** 1957. Some aspects of the absorption, distribution, and excretion of amphotericin B in man. Antibiot. Med. Clin. Ther. 5:295–301.
21. **Pappagianis, D., and G. S. Kobayashi.** 1960. Approaches to the physiology of *Coccidioides immitis*. Ann. N.Y. Acad. Sci. 89:109–121.
22. **Pappagianis, D., H. B. Levine, C. E. Smith, R. J. Berman, and G. Kobayashi.** 1961. Immunization of mice with viable *Coccidioides immitis*. J. Immunol. 86:28–34.
23. **Pappagianis, D., C. E. Smith, and G. S. Kobayashi.** 1956. Relationship of the in vivo form of *Coccidioides immitis* to virulence. J. Infect. Dis. 98:312–319.
24. **Sanford, W. G., J. R. Rasch, and R. B. Stonehill.** 1962. A therapeutic dilemma. The treatment of disseminated coccidioidomycosis with amphotericin B. Ann. Intern. Med. 56:553–563.
25. **Seabury, J. H., and H. E. Dascomb.** 1958. Experience with amphotericin B for the treatment of systemic mycoses. Arch. Intern. Med. 102:960–976.
26. **Seabury, H., and H. E. Dascomb.** 1960. Experience with amphotericin B. Ann. N.Y. Acad. Sci. 89:202–220.
27. **Shadomy, S.** 1971. In vitro antifungal activity of clotrimazole (Bay b 5097). Infect. Immun. 4:143–148.
28. **Shadomy, S., and A. Espinel-Ingroff.** 1974. Susceptibility testing of antifungal agents, p. 569–574. *In* E. H. Lennette, E. H. Spaulding, and J. P. Truant (ed.), Manual of clinical microbiology, 2nd ed. American Society for Microbiology, Washington, D. C.
29. **Smith, C. E., E. G. Whiting, E. E. Baker, H. G. Rosenberger, R. R. Beard, and M. T. Saito.** 1948. The use of coccidioidin. Am. Rev. Tuberc. 57:330–360.
30. **Sorensen, L. J., E. G. McNall, and T. H. Sternberg.** 1959. The development of strains of *Candida albicans* and *Coccidioides immitis* which are resistant to amphotericin B, p. 920. *In* Antibiotics annual 1958–1959. Medical Encyclopedia, Inc., New York.
31. **Stevens, D. A., H. B. Levine, and S. C. Deresinski.** 1976. Miconazole in coccidioidomycosis. II. Therapeutic and pharmacologic studies in man. Am. J. Med. 60:191–202.
32. **Sung, J. P., J. G. Grendahl, and H. B. Levine.** 1977. Intravenous and intrathecal miconazole therapy for systemic mycoses. West. J. Med. 126:5–13.
33. **Taylor, R. L., H. P. Lynch, R. R. Taylor, and O. L. Weiser.** 1958. The determination of serum concentrations of amphotericin B in man. Am. Rev. Tuberc. 77:1023–1025.
34. **Winn, W. A.** 1959. The use of amphotericin B in the treatment of coccidioidal disease. Am. J. Med. 27:617–635.
35. **Winn, W. A., H. B. Levine, J. E. Broderick, and R. W. Crane.** 1963. A localized epidemic of coccidioidal infection. N. Engl. J. Med. 268:867–870.

ANTIMICROBIAL AGENTS AND CHEMOTHERAPY, June 1977, p. 1056-1063
Vol. 11, No. 6

Novel Actinomycins Formed by Biosynthetic Incorporation of *cis*- and *trans*-4-Methylproline

E. KATZ,* W. K. WILLIAMS, K. T. MASON, AND A. B. MAUGER

Department of Microbiology, Georgetown University, Schools of Medicine and Dentistry, Washington, D.C. 20007, and Research Foundation of the Washington Hospital Center, Washington, D.C. 20010*

Received for publication 8 March 1977

Streptomyces parvulus (*Streptomyces parvullus*) normally produces actinomycin D; in the presence of *cis*-4-methylproline, this species synthesizes two additional actinomycins, designated K_{1c} and K_{2c}, in which one and two proline sites, respectively, are occupied by *cis*-4-methylproline. Analogously, actinomycins K_{1t} and K_{2t} are formed in the presence of *trans*-4-methylproline. Both mixtures were separated chromatographically, and the four novel actinomycins were obtained in crystalline form. Their biological activities were compared with that of actinomycin D in respect to inhibition of ribonucleic acid, deoxyribonucleic acid, and protein synthesis and antimicrobial potency. In all cases examined, the order of activity $D > K_{1t} > K_{1c} > K_{2t} > K_{2c}$ was observed, and the same sequence prevailed in a spectroscopic measure of their binding to deoxyribonucleic acid. In addition, proton nuclear magnetic resonance studies revealed that the replacement of proline by *cis*-4-methylproline alters the conformation of the antibiotic molecule.

In an earlier study of the effects of 3-, 4-, and 5-methylproline upon actinomycin biosynthesis by *Streptomyces antibioticus*, it was reported that new actinomycins were formed in the presence of 4-methylproline (isomeric mixture) (39, 40). Hydrolysis of the actinomycin mixture, which was too complex to separate, demonstrated that the 4-methylproline had been incorporated into the peptide moieties of the antibiotic. Similar observations were made with pipecolic acid and azetidine-2-carboxylic acid (17), and, more recently, various novel actinomycins containing the latter proline analogues have been isolated and characterized (10, 11, 18). The present study was designed to furnish individual actinomycins containing *cis*- and *trans*-4-methylproline for characterization and for comparisons of their biological activities with that of actinomycin D. For this purpose, *Streptomyces parvulus* (*Streptomyces parvullus*) was used with a modified culture medium (37). The advantages of using this species include higher yields of antibiotic and the fact that relatively few actinomycin analogues are synthesized since, under normal conditions, only one component (actinomycin D) is elaborated. *cis*- and *trans*-4-Methylproline were used in separate experiments; as each isomer was incorporated into one or both proline sites of the actinomycin molecule, a total of four new actinomycins (Fig. 1) was obtained.

cis- and *trans*-Methylproline have both been described as normal constituents of other peptide antibiotics. Thus, *cis*-4-methyl-L-proline occurs in antibiotic ICI 13,959 (22), whereas *trans*-4-methyl-L-proline is a component of griselimycin (35) and the monamycins (13). In addition, the free *trans* isomer has been detected in apples (15). *cis*-3-Methylproline is a component of the peptide antibiotic bottromycin A (32), whereas *trans*-3-methylproline occurs in roseotoxin B (9). *cis*-5-Methylproline has been identified as a component of actinomycin Z_5 (7, 19), and 2,3-*trans*-2,5-*cis*-3-hydroxy-5-methylproline (20, 30) and 4-keto-5-methylproline (6) occur in actinomycin Z_1. A related example is 2,3-*trans*-3,4-*cis*-3-hydroxy-4-methylproline, which is a constituent of echinocandin B (3). The potent inhibitory effect of actinomycins upon deoxyribonucleic acid (DNA)-dependent ribonucleic acid (RNA) synthesis and their resulting antitumor activity have prompted the production and evaluation of numerous analogues (31). The present study with *cis*- and *trans*-4-methylproline is an example of the directed biosynthesis approach. Comparisons of the biological activities of these modified actinomycins with that of actinomycin D were made, and the Sobell model (16) for intercalation of the actinomycin chromophore between the DNA base pairs was considered in attempting to explain the structure-activity relationships observed in this series.

MATERIALS AND METHODS

Radioisotopes. L-[U-^{14}C]valine (270 mCi/mmol),

[2-^{14}C]uridine (60 mCi/mmol), [2-^{14}C]thymidine (57 mCi/mmol), and [U-^{14}C]adenosine-5'-triphosphate (555 mCi/mmol) were purchased from Amersham/Searle Corp., Des Plaines, Ill.

Actinomycins. Actinomycin D (IV) was provided by Merck Sharp & Dohme Research Laboratories, Rahway, N. J. Actinomycins K_{1c}, K_{1t}, K_{2c}, and K_{2t} were purified from cultures of *S. parvulus* supplemented with *cis*- or *trans*-4-methylproline in the medium as described below. For biological studies, the antibiotics were dissolved in 50% ethanol (1 mg/ml). Dilutions were prepared in water or tris-(hydroxymethyl)aminomethane-NaCl buffer and pasteurized at 70°C for 20 min before use.

4-Methylproline isomers. Syntheses of *cis*-4-methyl-DL-proline-hydrochloride · H_2O (95% *cis* + 5% *trans*) and of a mixture (1:1) of the *trans*-L and *cis*-D isomers will be described elsewhere. It was established that use of the latter material resulted in incorporation of only the *trans* isomer into actinomycins.

Chromatographic materials. Silicic acid (Sil B-200, 60 to 200 mesh) for column chromatography was purchased from the Sigma Chemical Co., St. Louis, Mo. Thin-layer chromatography sheets (Gelman ITLC) containing silicic acid (20 by 20 cm, 250 μm thick) were obtained from the Gelman Instrument Co., Ann Arbor, Mich. Acid-washed alumina was prepared from alumina (Brockmann activity no. 1, 80 to 200 mesh; Fisher Scientific Co., Pittsburgh, Pa.) by a published procedure (1).

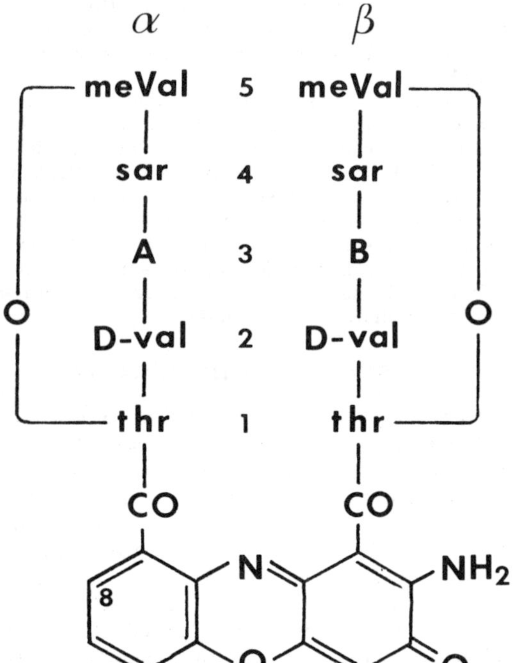

FIG. 1. *Structures of actinomycins. Abbreviations: thr = L-threonine; val = D-valine; sar = sarcosine; meVal = N-methyl-L-valine. In actinomycin D, A = B = L-proline; in k_{1c}, A/B = L-proline/cis-4-methylproline; in K_{2c}, A = B = cis-4-methylproline; in K_{1t}, A/B = L-proline/trans-4-methylproline; in K_{2t}, A = B = trans-4-methylproline.*

Nucleic acids, nucleotides, and enzymes. *Micrococcus lysodeikticus* DNA and calf thymus DNA were obtained from Miles Laboratories, Inc., Elkhart, Ind. Crude *Bacillus subtilis* (Marburg strain) DNA was provided by O. Landmann, Department of Biology, Georgetown University, and purified by the Marmur procedure (26). Salmon sperm DNA (for DNA assays) and yeast RNA (for RNA assays) were obtained from the Sigma Chemical Co. *Escherichia coli* K-12 DNA-dependent RNA polymerase and guanosine-, uridine- and adenosine-5'-triphosphate were procured from Miles Laboratories. Cytidine-5'-triphosphate was from Boehringer Mannheim Biochemicals, Indianapolis, Ind., and bovine serum albumin (for protein assays) was purchased from Schwarz/Mann, Div. of Becton, Dickinson & Co., Orangeburg, N.Y.

Organisms and conditions of cultivation. *S. parvulus* (ATCC 12434) was employed for the synthesis of actinomycins. The organisms were maintained on slants of a glucose-yeast extract-malt extract agar medium (14), and were stored at 4°C. The procedure for preparation of vegetative mycelium (NZ-Amine liquid medium) as inoculum for actinomycin synthesis (glutamic acid-histidine-fructose-mineral salts medium) has been described previously (37). *Micrococcus luteus* (ATCC 15307), *Sarcina subflava*, *Staphylococcus aureus* (penicillin susceptible), and *B. subtilis* (Marburg strain, wild type) were employed for investigation of the biological properties of the actinomycins. The bacterial cultures were grown on nutrient agar slants at 37°C, except *M. luteus* which was incubated at 26°C.

Production of actinomycins. All experiments were carried out at 30°C on a gyratory shaking incubator (New Brunswick Scientific Co., New Brunswick, N.J.) at 250 rpm. For the production of actinomycins containing *cis*- or *trans*-4-methylproline, the proline analogue was added to the chemically defined medium (37) after 24 h of incubation (i.e., at the onset of actinomycin biosynthesis). The cultures were then reincubated for 5 days. The mycelium was separated from the culture medium by filtration and washed twice with an equal volume of water. After extraction of the filtered medium and washings with ethyl acetate, the extracts were evaporated under reduced pressure, and the residual actinomycin mixtures were separated into their components.

Separation of actinomycins containing *cis*-4-methylproline. Separation of actinomycins containing *cis*-4-methylproline was effected by descending preparative paper chromatography on paper sheets (Whatman 3MM, 18 by 20 inches [about 45.7 by 50.8 cm]) impregnated with 5% aqueous sodium *o*-cresotinate. The antibiotic mixture (15 mg) in acetone was applied as a streak to each paper, and the chromatograms were developed with amyl acetate for 10 to 12 h. Three zones were distinguished, corresponding to actinomycins D (R_D = 1.00), K_{1c} (R_D = 2.13), and K_{2c} (R_D = 3.73). The zones were cut out, chopped into small pieces, and blended with water and ethyl acetate in a Waring blender for 3 to 5 min.

The paper pulp was filtered off, and the ethyl acetate layer was washed with aqueous sodium bicarbonate (to remove *o*-cresotinate) and water and then evaporated to dryness. Actinomycin K_{1c} was rechromatographed by the same procedure to remove traces of K_{2c}.

Separation of actinomycins containing *trans*-4-methylproline. Separation of actinomycins containing *trans*-4-methylproline was accomplished by preparative thin-layer chromatography on Gelman ITLC silicic acid-impregnated glass-fiber sheets (20 by 20 cm), using ethyl acetate. Three zones were distinguished, which corresponded to actinomycins D (R_D = 1.00), K_{1t} (R_D = 1.24), and K_{2t} (R_D = 1.42). The zones were cut out and extracted with methanol-ethyl acetate (1:1), and the extracts were filtered and evaporated. Actinomycin K_{1t} was rechromatographed by the same procedure to remove traces of K_{2t}.

Purification of separated actinomycins. Individual actinomycin preparations obtained as described above were chromatographed on columns of silicic acid with 10% methanol in ethyl acetate and finally purified on columns of acid-washed alumina (1), using chloroform. They were then recrystallized from chloroform-ethanol, with the exception of K_{2t}, which crystallized from chloroform-benzene. Melting points were obtained using a Thomas micro hot-stage Kofler-type apparatus.

Circular paper chromatography. Homogeneity of the individual actinomycins described above was established by circular paper chromatography (11), using the solvent systems (i) di-*n*-butyl ether–*sym*-tetrachloroethane–10% aqueous sodium *o*-cresotinate (3:1:4 and 5:1:6), (ii) isopropyl ether–chloroform–10% sodium *o*-cresotinate (3:2:5), and (iii) amyl acetate–5% sodium *o*-cresotinate. In each case the paper was impregnated with the aqueous phase prior to chromatography.

Amino acid analysis. Each actinomycin (5 to 10 mg) was hydrolyzed in 5 ml of 6 N HCl for 3 h at 121°C. The hydrolysates were decolorized with Norit A charcoal (neutral), filtered, evaporated under reduced pressure, and redissolved twice in water and evaporated. The amino acid content of the residue was evaluated by using the following procedures.

(i) Quantitative amino acid analysis was carried out on a Beckman-Spinco automatic amino acid analyzer, model 120C, as described previously (38). The data were normalized to D-valine = 2.00 residues per actinomycin molecule.

(ii) Two-dimensional paper electrophoresis and paper chromatography (38) were effected on sheets of Whatman 3MM paper. The first dimension involved high-voltage (3,000 V) paper electrophoresis (Gilson Medical Electronics, Inc., Middleton, Wis.) with a 4% formate buffer at pH 1.9 for 3 h at 180 mA. For the second dimension, solvent system (i) 1-butanol–acetic acid–water (4:1:5, upper layer) or (ii) methanol-pyridine-water (20:1:5) were employed. Amino acids were visualized with 0.2% ninhydrin in acetone; cyclic imino acids were detected with 0.2% isatin in acetone.

(iii) In gas-liquid chromatography, the hydrolysates were evaporated in vacuo, and the residual amino acids were derivatized to their *N*-trifluoroacetyl methyl esters as described previously (29). Chromatography was effected on a gas chromatograph (Shimadzu, model 4BM) containing a column (6 feet [about 1.83 m] by 3 mm) of ethylene glycol adipate (0.5% on Chromosorb W, 60 to 80 mesh) at 100°C with argon (40 ml/min) as carrier gas.

NMR. Proton nuclear magnetic resonance (NMR) spectra were obtained in $CDCl_3$ solution (0.05 M) at 220 MHz using a Varian HR220 instrument, with tetramethylsilane as internal reference.

Biological activities. Determination of minimal inhibitory concentrations and of 50% inhibition of the exponential growth and biopolymer synthesis of *B. subtilis* (RNA, DNA, and protein) by the various actinomycins was accomplished by procedures that have been described in previous publications (12, 27). The inhibitory effect of different concentrations of the various actinomycins on the *E. coli* K-12 DNA-dependent RNA polymerase reaction was also studied (8).

Difference spectra. Difference spectra (12, 27) were obtained manually with a Gilford model 2000 spectrophotometer.

Actinomycin concentration. The actinomycin concentration in culture filtrates was carried out spectrophotometrically at 443 nm in ethyl acetate (21). In the case of pure actinomycins, determinations were effected in methanol at the same wavelength.

Radioactive measurements. Radioactive measurements on portions of solubilized protein, RNA, and DNA were made in 10 ml of Bray's liquid scintillation fluid (4). For the DNA-dependent RNA polymerase-catalyzed reaction, the acid-insoluble product was collected on a Whatman glass-fiber filter and counted in 10 ml of Omnifluor (New England Nuclear Corp., Boston, Mass.). Measurements were effected in a Mark I Nuclear-Chicago refrigerated liquid scintillation spectrometer.

RESULTS AND DISCUSSION

Synthesis of 4-methylproline-containing actinomycins. Preliminary experiments to determine the levels of *cis*- and *trans*-4-methylproline suitable for maximum production of modified actinomycins revealed that 250 and 200 μg/ml, respectively, represented the optimum concentrations. Furthermore, no significant inhibition of synthesis occurred with the *cis* isomer, whereas a moderate reduction (30 to 40%) was noted with the *trans* isomer relative to control cultures (550 to 600 μg of actinomycin D per ml). A total of 2.9 g of actinomycin mixture was obtained after supplying the *cis* isomer; correspondingly, 2.7 g of crude actinomycin mixture was obtained after supplementation with the *trans* isomer.

Separation and purification of modified ac-

tinomycins. The individual components of each of the above-mentioned actinomycin complexes were separated and purified by the chromatographic procedures described in Materials and Methods. Four novel actinomycins were obtained in crystalline form (red prisms) and designated K_{1c} and K_{2c} (from *cis*-4-methylproline) and K_{1t} and K_{2t} (from *trans*-4-methylproline). Their melting points were: actinomycin K_{1c}, 244 to 246°C; K_{2c}, 236 to 237°C; K_{1t}, 248 to 250°C; K_{2t}, 245 to 247°C.

Amino acid analysis. The quantitative data obtained with the amino acid analyzer are summarized in Table 1, and typical elution profiles are shown in Fig. 2. These results correlate with the outcome of the two-dimensional paper electrophoresis-paper chromatography separations; details of the mobilities and R_f values of these amino acids have been published (19, 29). Since these two methods make no distinction between *cis*- and *trans*-4-methylproline, gas-liquid chromatography (29) was used to identify the isomer present in each hydrolysate. The retention times (minutes) of standards were: proline, 12.3; *trans*-4-methylproline, 13.5; *cis*-4-methylproline, 15.0. In the hydrolysate chromatograms the following results were obtained: actinomycin K_{1c} contained proline, *cis*-4-methylproline, and a trace of *trans*-4-methylproline; K_{1t} contained proline, *trans*-4-methylproline, and a trace of *cis*-4-methylproline; K_{2c} contained *cis*-4-methylproline plus a trace of *trans*-4-methylproline; K_{2t} contained *trans*-4-methylproline and a trace of *cis*-4-methylproline. Some interconversion of *cis*- and *trans*-4-methylprolines occurs during hydrolysis of the actinomycins. These results form the basis for the designations given in Table 1.

NMR. The NMR data indicate that actinomycins K_{1c} and K_{1t} are both single entities, as distinct from mixtures of two possible isomers having the α- and β-peptide moieties interchanged. However, the question of which isomer is present in each case is not yet resolved. Spectra of K_{1t} and K_{2t} were remarkably similar to those of actinomycin D (2, 23, 24, 36), except for the presence of doublets at δ 1.17 and 1.12, respectively, which were assigned to the *trans*-4-methylprolyl methyl groups. On the other hand, spectra of K_{1c} and K_{2c}, especially the latter, displayed small but important differences in chemical shifts, revealing that conformational adjustments occur when proline is replaced by *cis*-4-methylproline, but not by *trans*-4-methylproline. The most striking example is that of the β-peptide threonine NH signal of K_{2c}, which occurs at δ 6.94 in $CDCl_3$. In other actinomycins, this resonance covers the range δ 7.50–7.86. The threonine NH coupling constants ($J_{NH,C\alpha H}$) are somewhat larger (7.0 and 7.5 Hz) than those of other actinomycins (typically, 6.2 and 6.8 Hz), reflecting slightly altered NH-CαH dihedral angles. The chromophoric 8-proton of K_{2c} is at higher field (δ 7.50) than in actinomycin D (δ 7.65), revealing a slight adjustment in the angle between the chromophoric plane and that of the actinocyl-threonine (α-peptide) amide bond. A fundamental difference in pyrrolidine ring conformation is evident from the 4-methylprolyl α-proton splittings. The latter, in the case of *trans*-4-methylproline (in K_{1t} and K_{2t}), resemble those of proline in actinomycin D (approximate doublet), whereas in the case of *cis*-4-methylproline (in K_{1c} and K_{2c}) a triplet pattern is observed. The latter formation (actually an overlapping doublet of doublets) results from two nearly equal $J_{\alpha,\beta}$ coupling constants, whereas the doublet situation arises when one $J_{\alpha,\beta}$ approximates to 0, due to a *trans*-α,β dihedral angle close to 90°. This conformational difference in the case of *cis*-4-methylproline in turn affects the peptide backbone conformation of K_{1c} and K_{2c}, with the result that, especially in K_{2c}, a noticeable de-

TABLE 1. *Quantitative amino acid analyses of actinomycins*

Actinomycin	Amino acid[a]						
	Valine	Sarcosine	Threonine[b]	*N*-Methylvaline	Proline	*cis*-4-Methylproline	*trans*-4-Methylproline
D	2.0	2.1	1.0	1.7	2.0	0.0	0.0
K_{1c}	2.0	2.0	0.9	1.8	0.9	1.0	0.0
K_{2c}	2.0	1.9	0.9	1.8	0.0	2.0	0.0
K_{1t}	2.0	1.8	0.9	1.6	0.7	0.0	1.0
K_{2t}	2.0	1.7	0.9	1.7	0.0	0.0	2.0

[a] Residues per molecule normalized to valine = 2.0.

[b] The low yields of threonine are due to destruction of the amino acid during acid hydrolysis of an actinomycin molecule.

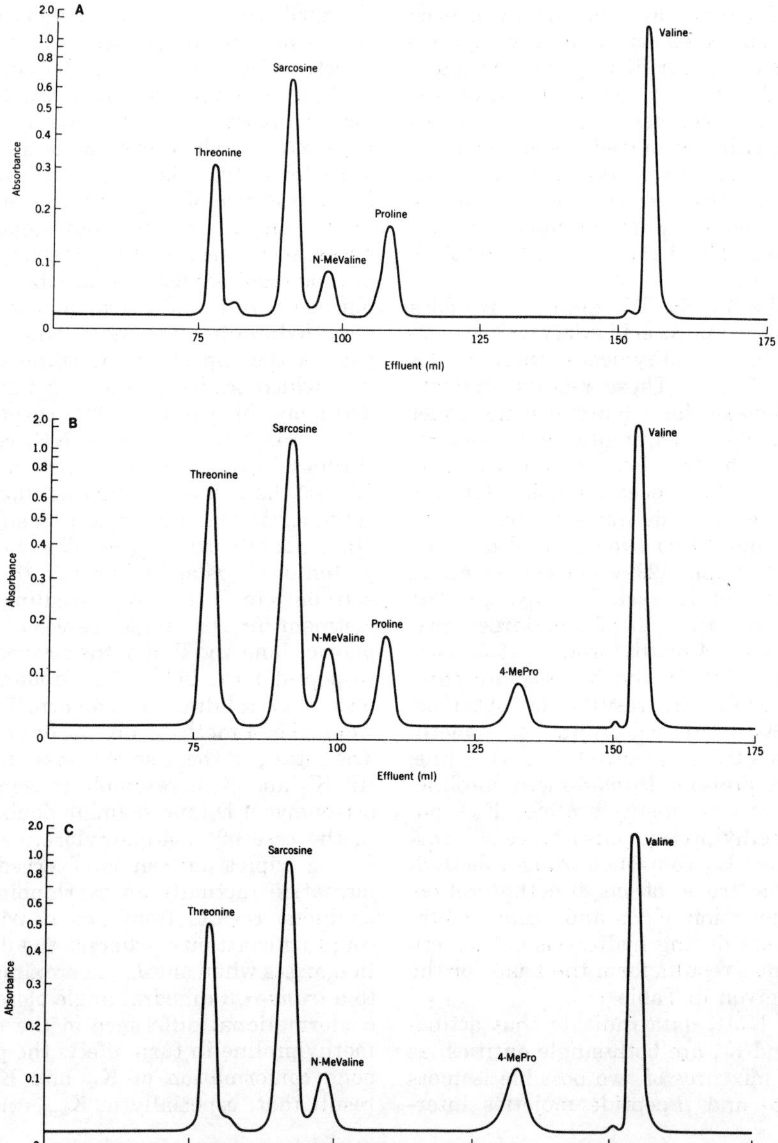

FIG. 2. *Separation of amino acid hydrolysates from a crystalline actinomycin component: (A) actinomycin D; (B) actinomycin* K_{1c}*; (C) actinomycin* K_{2c}*. The amino acids were eluted with 0.2 sodium citrate buffer at pH 3.05 and 4.25 from the column (0.9 by 69 cm). Flow rate of both the buffer and ninhydrin solutions were 34 ml/h. Absorbance was measured at 570 nm, except for the imino acids, which were measured at 440 nm (38). N-MeValine = N-methyl-L-valine.*

parture from the uniform conformation observed for various other actinomycins (25, 28) ensues. This conclusion, which is also supported by ^{13}C NMR studies (W. A. Thomas and A. B. Mauger, unpublished data), will be described in detail elsewhere.

Biological activities. In qualitative aspects, the biological activities of these modified actinomycins in vivo and in vitro resemble that of actinomycin D. However, an exception is seen in the inhibition of DNA synthesis in vivo (Table 2), where markedly reduced activity was exhibited by the modified actinomycins. In the other studies (difference spectroscopy with DNA, antibacterial activity, and inhibition of RNA and protein synthesis) a uniform trend was observed: D > K_{1t} > K_{1c} > K_{2t} > K_{2c}. The parallel behavior of these compounds under various experimental conditions is noteworthy. For example, the minimal inhibitory concentrations obtained with *B. subtilis* (Table 3) relate favorably to the 50% inhibition of the exponential growth of this organism and to the inhibition of its RNA and protein synthesis (Table 4). This uniform trend even extends to the difference spectra with DNA, strongly suggesting that differences in biological activity in this series of actinomycin analogues are directly related to the differences in their complexing with DNA (Fig. 3). Similar spectral data, although not presented here, were obtained with preparations of *B. subtilis* DNA. A comparable correlation between physicochemical and biological data was observed in the case of a series of actinomycins produced in the presence of pipecolic acid (12, 18). In contrast, there is a less direct comparison between these two criteria in the case of actinomycin Z components (27).

In comparison with actinomycin D, replacement of both proline residues by *cis*- or *trans*-4-methylproline resulted in greater loss of biological potency than replacement of one proline moiety. A similar effect was noted in the replacement by pipecolic acid (12, 18), but not by azetidine-2-carboxylic acid (10). It was also observed that substitution of proline by *cis*-4-methylproline reduced potency more than in the case of the *trans* isomer, i.e., $K_{1t} > K_{1c}$ and $K_{2t} > K_{2c}$. This effect may be related to the conclusions drawn from the NMR data, particularly, that the replacement of proline by *cis*-4-methylproline in actinomycin is accompanied by a conformational change that is not so apparent in the case of the *trans* isomer. It should also be noted, however, that the proline sites in actinomycin are in a critical location in respect to the interaction of the molecule with DNA, such that a substituent can exert a steric effect (16, 34). Thus, in the case of replacement of proline by *trans*-4-hydroxyproline (actinomycin $X_{0\beta}$) or *cis*-4-(allo)-hydroxyproline ($X_{0\delta}$) biological activities were considerably higher in the latter case (5, 33); the hydroxyl group of the imino acid (in the case of $X_{0\beta}$) may sterically hinder complexing between the actinomycin molecule and DNA. In terms of the Sobell model (16, 34), an analogous difference (*cis* > *trans*) was expected in the case of the 4-methylproline substitution. The methyl groups of *trans*-4-methylproline in actinomycins K_{1t} and K_{2t} are located so that they contact the DNA

TABLE 2. *Inhibition of DNA synthesis in B. subtilis by actinomycins*

Actinomycin (5 μg/ml)	DNA synthesis (% of control)	
	Expt 1[a]	Expt 2[b]
D	15	4
K_{1t}	58	69
K_{1c}	77	85
K_{2t}	65	74
K_{2c}	79	77

[a] Ten milliliters of an exponentially growing culture of *B. subtilis* was added to a flask containing [2-^{14}C]thymidine (1 μCi, 17.5 nmol) and actinomycin and incubated for 15 min at 37°C in a Dubnoff metabolic shaking incubator.

[b] Ten milliliters of an exponentially growing culture of *B. subtilis* was preincubated with an actinomycin preparation for 10 min, and then [2-^{14}C]thymidine (1 μCi, 17.5 nmol) was added. Incubation was then resumed as described in experiment 1.

TABLE 3. *Antimicrobial activity of actinomycins*

Species	Minimal inhibitory concentration (μg/ml)				
	D	K_{1t}	K_{1c}	K_{2t}	K_{2c}
M. luteus[a]	0.03	0.06	0.08	0.11	0.16
S. subflava[a]	0.04	0.08	0.11	0.12	0.20
S. subflava	0.03	0.06	0.10	0.10	0.18
B. subtilis	0.09	0.25	0.45	0.60	0.90
S. aureus	0.2	0.6	1.2	3.5	4.0
Relative activity (%)	100	33–50	17–36	5–33	5–20

[a] Incubation at 26°C for 40 h; all other incubations at 37°C for 20 h.

TABLE 4. *Inhibition (50%) of bacterial growth and macromolecular synthesis by actinomycins*

Expt	Actinomycin (μg/ml)				
	D	K_{1t}	K_{1c}	K_{2t}	K_{2c}
Exponential growth[a]	0.045	0.13	0.24	0.32	0.47
RNA synthesis[a]	0.10	0.28	0.52	0.68	1.08
Protein synthesis[a]	0.21	0.56	1.09	1.28	2.2
DNA-dependent RNA polymerase-catalyzed reaction[b]	0.25	0.60	0.97	1.65	2.0

[a] *B. subtilis*; procedures used are described in a previous publication (27).

[b] *E. coli* DNA-dependent RNA polymerase; calf thymus DNA (6.7 μg) was used as template. All other procedures used have been described (8, 27).

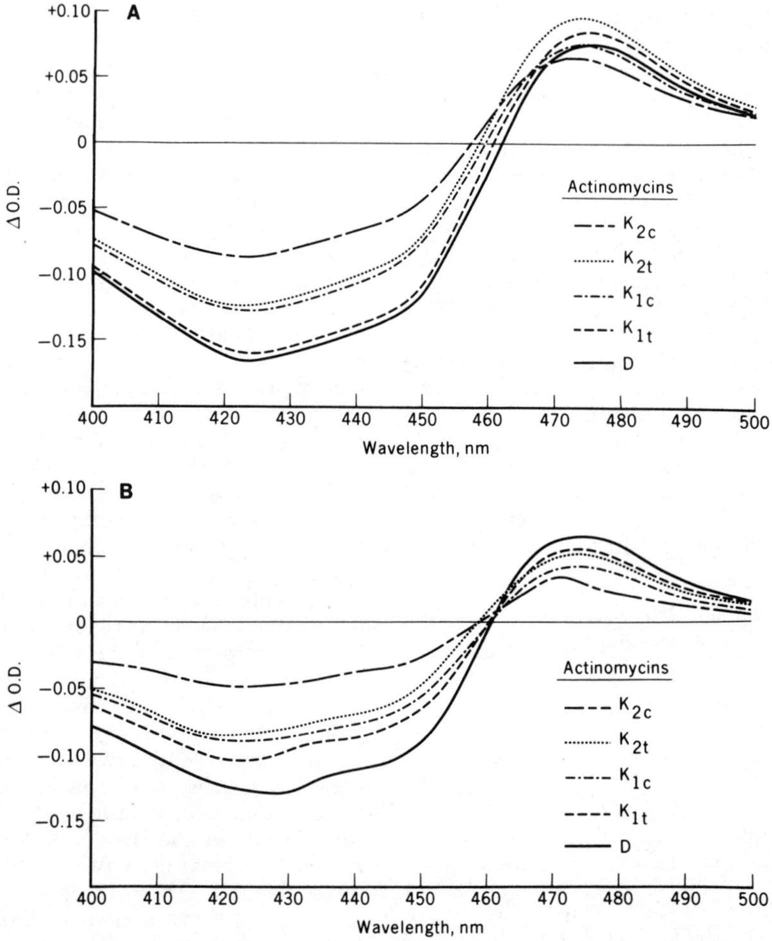

FIG. 3. *Difference spectra obtained with: (A) M. lysodeikticus DNA (36.4 μg) and (B) calf thymus DNA (36.6 μg), using actinomycins D, K_{1t}, K_{2t}, K_{1c}, and K_{2c} in 0.001 M tris(hydroxymethyl)aminomethane-hydrochloride–0.005 M NaCl buffer, pH 7.4.*

bases during intercalation, whereas the corresponding methyl groups in K_{1c} and K_{2c} extend away from the chromophore and, hence, the intercalation site. The fact that the *trans*-4-methylproline-substituted actinomycins were more active than the corresponding *cis* compounds could be explained by hydrophobic interactions as well as the conformational differences observed.

ACKNOWLEDGMENTS

This investigation was supported by Public Health Service Research Grants no. CA-06926 (to E. K.) and CA-11627 (to A. B. M.) and contract no. NO1-CM-43732 from the National Cancer Institute.

We thank R. Esperanza for technical assistance and E. Becker and R. Bradley (National Institutes of Health) for the use of a 220-MHz NMR instrument. We are also grateful to Jerome Birnbaum (Merck Sharp & Dohme Research Laboratories) for a generous supply of actinomycin D.

LITERATURE CITED

1. **Angyal, S. J., E. Bullock, W. G. Hanger, W. C. Howell, and A. W. Johnson.** 1957. Actinomycin. Part III. The reaction of actinomycin with alkali. J. Chem. Soc., p. 1592–1602.
2. **Arison, B. H., and K. Hoogsteen.** 1970. Nuclear magnetic resonance spectral studies on actinomycin D. Preliminary observations on the effect of complex formation with 5′-deoxyguanylic acid. Biochemistry **9:**3976–3983.
3. **Benz, F., F. Knüsel, J. Nüesch, H. Treichler, W. Voser, R. Nyfeler, and W. Keller-Schierlein.** 1974. Echinocandin B, ein neuartiges Polypeptid-Antibioticum aus *Aspergillus nidulans* var. *echinulatus*: Isolierung und Bausteine. Helv. Chim. Acta **57:**2459–2477.
4. **Bray, G.** 1960. A simple efficient liquid scintillator for counting aqueous solutions in a liquid scintillation counter. Anal. Biochem. **1:**279–285.
5. **Brockmann, H., and J. H. Manegold.** 1960. Überführung von Actinomycin X_2 in die Actinomycine C_1, $X_{0\beta}$ und $X_{0\delta}$. Chem. Ber. **93:**2971–2982.

6. **Brockmann, H., and J. H. Manegold.** 1965. Actinomycin Z_1. Zur quantitativen Aminosäureanalyse der Actinomycine. Hoppe-Seyler's Z. Physiol. Chem. **343**:86–100.
7. **Brockmann, H., and E. A. Stähler.** 1973. Zur Konstitution des Actinomycins Z_5. Tetrahedron Lett., p. 2567–2570.
8. **Burgess, R. R.** 1969. A new method for the large scale purification of *Escherichia coli* deoxyribonucleic acid-dependent ribonucleic acid polymerase. J. Biol. Chem. 244:6160–6167.
9. **Engstrom, G. W., J. V. DeLance, J. L. Richard, and A. L. Baetz.** 1975. Purification and characterization of roseotoxin B, a toxic cyclodepsipeptide from *Trichothecium roseum*. Agric. Food Chem. 23:244–253.
10. **Formica, J. V., and M. A. Apple.** 1976. Production, isolation, and properties of azetomycins. Antimicrob. Agents Chemother. **9**:214–221.
11. **Formica, J. V., and E. Katz.** 1973. Isolation, purification and characterization of pipecolic acid-containing actinomycins, Pip 2, Pip 1α and Pip 1β. J. Biol. Chem. 248:2066–2071.
12. **Formica, J. V., A. J. Shatkin, and E. Katz.** 1968. Actinomycin analogues containing pipecolic acid: relationship of structure to biological activity. J. Bacteriol. **95**:2139–2150.
13. **Hassall, C. H., R. B. Morton, Y. Ogihara, and D. A. S. Phillips.** 1971. The molecular structures of the monamycins, cyclodepsipeptide antibiotics. J. Chem. Soc. C, p. 526–532.
14. **Hook, D. J., and L. C. Vining.**1973. Biosynthetic precursors of etamycin, a peptidolactone antibiotic from *Streptomyces griseoviridus*. Can. J. Biochem. **51**: 1630-1637.
15. **Hulme, A. C., and W. Arthington.** 1954. Methylproline in young apple fruits. Nature (London) 173:588–589.
16. **Jain, S. C., and H. M. Sobell.** 1972. Stereochemistry of actinomycin binding to DNA. I. Refinement and further structural details of the actinomycin-deoxyguanosine crystalline complex. J. Mol. Biol. 68:1–20.
17. **Katz, E.** 1960. Biogenesis of the actinomycins. Ann. N.Y. Acad. Sci. **89**:304–322.
18. **Katz, E.** 1974. Controlled biosynthesis of actinomycins. Cancer Chemother. Rep. 58:83–91.
19. **Katz, E., K. T. Mason, and A. B. Mauger.** 1973. Identification of *cis*-5-methylproline in hydrolysates of actinomycin Z_5. Biochem. Biophys. Res. Commun. 52:819–826.
20. **Katz, E., K. T. Mason, and A. B. Mauger.** 1975. 3-Hydroxy-5-methylproline, a new amino acid identified as a component of actinomycin Z_1. Biochem. Biophys. Res. Commun. 63:502–508.
21. **Katz, E., and H. Weissbach.** 1963. Incorporation of C^{14}-labeled amino acids into actinomycin and protein by *Streptomyces antibioticus*. J. Biol. Chem. **238**:666–675.
22. **Kenner, G. W., and R. C. Sheppard.** 1958. α-Aminoisobutyric acid, β-hydroxyleucine and γ-methylproline from the hydrolysis of a natural product. Nature (London) 181:48.
23. **Lackner, H.** 1971. Synthesen von selektiv deuterierten Pentapeptidlactonen und stellungsspezifisch im (α)-oder (β)-peptidring markierten Actinomycinen. Chem. Ber. **104**:3653–3678.
24. **Lackner, H.** 1971. Zur Sekundär- und Tertiarstruktur der Actinomycine, III. Selektiv im (α)- oder (β)-Peptidlactonring deuterierte Actinomycine C_1 (D). Tetrahedron Lett., p. 2221–2226.
25. **Lackner, H.** 1975. Three-dimensional structure of the actinomycins. Angew. Chem. **14**:375–386.
26. **Marmur, J.** 1961. A procedure for the isolation of deoxyribonucleic acid from microorganisms. J. Mol. Biol. 3:208–218.
27. **Mason, K. T., E. Katz, and A. B. Mauger.** 1974. Studies on the biological activities of actinomycins Z_1 and Z_5. Arch. Biochem. Biophys. **160**:402–411.
28. **Mauger, A. B.** 1975. NMR conformational studies of actinomycins containing sarcosine in place of proline. p. 181–186. *In* R. Walter and J. Meienhofer (ed.), Peptides: chemistry, structure and biology, Proceedings of the 4th American Peptide Symposium. Ann Arbor Science Publishers Inc., Ann Arbor, Mich.
29. **Mauger, A. B., E. Katz, and K. T. Mason.** 1973. Chromatographic procedures for the identification of isomeric methylprolines. J. Chromatogr. 85:167–170.
30. **Mauger, A. B., O. A. Stuart, E. Katz, and K. T. Mason.** 1977. Synthesis and stereochemistry of 3-hydroxy-5-methylproline, a new naturally occurring imino acid. J. Org. Chem. **42**:1000–1005.
31. **Meinhofer, J., and E. Atherton.** 1973. Structure-activity relationships in the actinomycins. Adv. Appl. Microbiol. **16**:203–300.
32. **Nakamura, S., T. Chikaike, H. Yonehara, and H. Umezawa.** 1965. Isolation, characterization and structural elucidation of new amino acids from bottromycin A. Chem. Pharm. Bull. 13:599–602.
33. **Reich, E., I. H. Goldberg, and M. Rabinowitz.** 1962. Structure-activity correlations of actinomycins and their derivatives. Nature (London) **196**:743–748.
34. **Sobell, H. M., S. C. Jain, T. D. Sakore, G. Ponticello, and C. E. Nordman.** 1971. Concerning the stereochemistry of actinomycin binding to DNA: an actinomycin-deoxyguanosine crystalline complex. Cold Spring Harbor Symp. Quant. Biol. **36**:263–270.
35. **Terlain, B., and J.-P. Thomas.** 1971. Constitution de la grisélimycine, antibiotique polypeptidique extrait de cultures de streptomyces. II. Structure de la grisélimycine. Bull. Soc. Chim. Fr., p. 2357–2362.
36. **Victor, T. A., F. E. Hruska, C. L. Bell, and S. S. Danyluk.** 1969. A nuclear magnetic resonance study of the structure and interaction of actinomycin D: analysis and conformational properties. Tetrahedron Lett., p. 4721–4724.
37. **Williams, W. K., and E. Katz.** 1977. Development of a chemically defined medium for the synthesis of actinomycin D by *Streptomyces parvulus*. Antimicrob. Agents Chemother. **11**:281–291.
38. **Yajima, T., M. A. Grigg, and E. Katz.** 1972. Biosynthesis of antibiotic peptides with isoleucine stereoisomers. Arch. Biochem. Biophys. **151**:565–575.
39. **Yoshida, T., A. Mauger, H. Weissbach, and E. Katz.** 1968. Effect of structural and stereochemical methylproline isomers on actinomycin biosynthesis. J. Bacteriol. **95**:952–958.
40. **Yoshida, T., A. Mauger, B. Witkop, and E. Katz.** 1966. Influence of methylproline isomers upon actinomycin biosynthesis. Biochem. Biophys. Res. Commun. **25**:66–72.

ANTIMICROBIAL AGENTS AND CHEMOTHERAPY, June 1977, p. 1064-1066
Vol. 11, No. 5
Printed in U.S.A.

NOTES

Five-Hour Minimal Inhibitory Concentration Test of Four Antimicrobial Agents for *Pseudomonas aeruginosa*

W. J. BROWN* AND R. L. SAUTTER

Hutzel Hospital and Wayne State University School of Medicine, Detroit, Michigan 48201

Received for publication 15 February 1977

A rapid 5-h minimal inhibitory concentration procedure and a minimal bactericidal concentration procedure are described for testing *Pseudomonas aeruginosa* against gentamicin, tobramycin, amikacin, and carbenicillin. The rapid test results were demonstrated to correlate with the conventional tube dilution procedure.

Automated susceptibility testing has proven a useful method for measuring the activity of antimicrobial agents on clinical isolates of bacteria (6). The instrumentation of susceptibility testing contributes several advantages to the testing procedure, among which is the more rapid determination of results. However, the instrument available has not been described by the manufacturer for doing minimal inhibitory concentration (MIC) testing. Semiquantitation tests were reported by McGowan et al. (2) with the Autobac 1 instrument (Pfizer Inc.), and recently Ryan and Tilton have described an MIC procedure using this instrument for MIC testing of ampicillin for *Haemophilus influenzae* (4).

This study reports on our using the Autobac 1 for a rapid (5 h) MIC measurement of commonly used antibiotics for treating *Pseudomonas aeruginosa* infections. Thirty-six strains of *P. aeruginosa* were used in this study. The ATCC strain 27853 of *P. aeruginosa* and 35 blood culture isolates from patients with *P. aeruginosa* endocarditis were tested. Four antibiotics were used: gentamicin (Schering Corp., Bloomfield, N.J.), tobramycin (Eli Lilly and Co., Indianapolis, Ind.), amikacin (Bristol Laboratories, Syracuse, N.Y.), and carbenicillin (Pfizer, Inc., New York, N.Y.). The base powders with known biological activity were supplied by the manufacturers. Stock solutions were prepared in water and frozen at -30°C until used, except for tobramycin which was supplied in suspension. The stock solutions were used within 2 weeks.

Tube macrodilution MIC and minimal bactericidal concentration (MBC) tests were performed by a conventional method (1). The organism to be tested was inoculated into a tube containing Trypticase soy broth (BBL) and incubated for 4 to 6 h until the turbidity was greater than the turbidity standard (McFarland number 0.5). The culture was then diluted until it equaled the turbidity standard, and an additional dilution of 1:100 was made in Mueller-Hinton broth (Difco) (10 mg of Ca^{2+} per liter and 5 mg of Mg^{2+} per liter) or in Eugonic broth (Pfizer) (71 mg of Ca^{2+} per liter and 33 mg of Mg^{2+} per liter) to produce a final concentration of approximately 10^6 bacteria/ml. The bacterial suspensions were added to antibiotic dilutions made in Mueller-Hinton broth, and all tubes were incubated to 35°C in air for 16 to 18 h. The MIC value was read as the greatest dilution (least concentration) of antibiotic that completely inhibited any visible growth. The MBC value was considered the greatest dilution of the antibiotic that had 99% less bacteria in subcultures than were inoculated into the tubes.

The rapid MIC and MBC tests were performed in the Autobac 1. The procedure used is a modification of that previously described for operation of the Autobac 1 (6). For the rapid MIC tests, blank sterile disks (Difco) were impregnated with 20 μl of various concentrations of the antibiotics. The Autobac 1 cuvette wells contain 1.5 ml of Eugonic broth, and, therefore, the amount of antibiotic added to each elution disk was 1.5 times the amount desired per ml. Six different concentrations of each antibiotic were prepared in elution disks so that two antibiotics could be tested in each cuvette, which contained 12 test wells and 1 growth control well. Inoculum for the rapid test was prepared by transferring growth from a 16- to 18-h-old sheep blood agar plate to "inoculum standardization solution" (Pfizer, phosphate-buffered saline). The inoculum was standardized in the Autobac 1 according to the manufacturer's instructions, so that the saline suspension contained between 1.5×10^7 to 3.0×10^7 bacteria/ml. An additional dilution of 1:5 was made in the saline and a further 1:10 dilution in Eugonic broth, so that the final concentration of the inoculum was between 3×10^5 and 6×10^5 bacteria/ml. A 0.001-ml sample of the inoculum was cultured to a sheep blood agar plate to confirm the inoculum size and purity as well as to serve as a measurement of the inoculum size, which is used in the MBC test. The inoculated cuvettes were incubated in a shaker incubator for 5 h. After incubation, the cuvettes were placed in the Autobac 1 and readings were taken in the background mode setting. This method provided a numerical value for each well in the cuvette regardless of the growth in the control well. Therefore, any well with good growth was detected by a marked increase in numerical value. The MIC was read as the greatest dilution (lowest concentration) of antibiotic that inhibited growth of the organism as determined by the instrument reading.

The MBC from the rapid MIC tests were determined by subculturing from the cuvette wells that had low numerical readings after a 5-h incubation. A biological assay technique was made to measure the antibiotic concentration eluted from the disks after a 45-min incubation (5). All measured values were very close to the theoretical concentrations, demonstrating that the desired concentration of antibiotics was eluted from the disks.

Tube dilution MIC tests were done in duplicate for gentamicin, tobramycin, amikacin, and carbenicillin. The results of these conventional tests were compared with the values obtained by testing the same organisms and antibiotics in the Autobac 1. The Autobac 1 results were available after a 5-h incubation, whereas the conventional tube test required a 16- to 18-h incubation. A comparison of the results of the two methods can be seen in Table 1. The 18-h MIC tube results and the 5-h Autobac MIC results had 100% correlation as follows: carbenicillin within 2 dilutions, tobramycin within 1 dilution, amikacin with 2 dilutions, and gentamicin (tube test in Eugonic broth) within 1 dilution.

The MBC results from the tube test and the Autobac 1 procedures are also compared in Table 1. Good correlation was obtained, with greater than 90% agreement within two dilutions for all four antibiotics.

Mueller-Hinton broth of low calcium and magnesium content was used in the tube test, since this medium has been used for MIC tests in our laboratory for several years. However, the effect of divalent cations on the MIC of *P. aeruginosa* tested against gentamicin is well recognized (3). Therefore, the discrepancy in results between the low cation concentration of Mueller-Hinton broth and the higher levels of cations in the Eugonic broth is not surprising. When the *P. aeruginosa* were retested against gentamicin in Eugonic broth in the conventional tube system and these results were compared with those of the cuvette system performed in Eugonic broth, there was very good agreement between the two procedures. Comparison of the rapid test with the conventional procedure demonstrated that accurate MIC results were produced by the rapid method. For all 36 strains and the four antibiotics all results were within one dilution, with the exception of one strain with amikacin and two strains with carbenicillin, which had a two-dilution difference.

Our data show that MBC values can be obtained from the rapid MIC procedure, but the

TABLE 1. *Comparison of the MIC and MBC end points from the rapid 5-h tests with the end points obtained by the conventional macrotube tests for 36 strains of P. aeruginosa*

Antibiotic	Macrodilution medium	Dilution differences[a]										
		MIC						MBC				
		+3	+2	+1	0	−1	−2	+3	+2	+1	0	−1
Gentamicin	MH[b]	4	9	18	5	—[c]	—	—	7	15	14	—
Gentamicin	EB[d]	—	—	3	20	13	—	—	—	4	19	13
Tobramycin	MH	—	—	11	18	7	—	2	9	11	11	3
Amikacin	MH	—	1	4	18	13	—	1	6	10	13	6
Carbenicillin	MH	—	1	6	16	12	1	1	6	9	19	1

[a] 0, Both rapid and conventional tests had the same end point; +1, rapid-procedure end point was one tube higher (more antibiotic); +2, two tubes higher; +3, three tubes higher; −1, one tube lower; −2, two tubes lower.

[b] MH, Mueller-Hinton broth.

[c] None at this dilution.

[d] EB, Eugonic broth.

MBC values do not correlate as accurately as those of the MIC procedures. A possible explanation for this observation may be that the time of contact between the antimicrobial agents and the organisms was not sufficient in the rapid procedure to cause the 99% killing effect. However, there was a 94% or greater correlation within two dilutions and 100% within three dilutions between the two procedures.

Our results indicate that the 5-h rapid semiautomated MIC values for *P. aeruginosa* tested against gentamicin, tobramycin, amikacin, and carbenicillin correlate with the conventional 18- to 24-h tube dilution MIC procedure. However, a poorer correlation was obtained with MBC values. Additional work with other organisms and antimicrobial agents seems to be warranted from these results.

LITERATURE CITED

1. **Ericsson, H. M., and J. C. Sherris.** 1971. Antibiotic sensitivity testings, report of an international collaborative study. Acta Pathol. Microbiol. Scand. Sect. 13. **217**(Suppl):1–90.
2. **McGowan, J. E., Jr., C. Ayres, and L. D. Sabath.** 1975. Rapid semiquantitative testing of antibiotic susceptibility: use of a multicell disk elution system. Antimicrob. Agents Chemother. **7**:543–548.
3. **Reller, L. B., F. D. Schoenknecht, M. A. Kenny, and J. C. Sherris.** 1974. Antibiotic susceptibility testing of *Pseudomonas aeruginosa*: selection of a control strain and criteria for magnesium and calcium content in media. J. Infect. Dis. **130**:454–463.
4. **Ryan, R., and R. C. Tilton.** 1977. Rapid method for determining the minimum inhibitory concentration of ampicillin for *Haemophilus influenzae*. Antimicrob. Agents Chemother. **11**:114–117.
5. **Sabath, L. D., J. I. Casey, P. A. Ruch, L. L. Strumpf, and M. Finland.** 1971. Rapid microassay of gentamicin, kanamycin, neomycin, streptomycin, and vancomycin in serum or plasma. J. Lab. Clin. Med. **78**:457–467.
6. **Thornsberry, C., T. L. Gaven, J. C. Sherris, A. Balows, J. M. Matsen, L. D. Sabath, F. Schoenknecht, L. D. Thrupp, and J. A. Washington II.** 1975. Laboratory evaluation of a rapid, automatic susceptibility testing system: a review of a collaborative study. Antimicrob. Agents Chemother. **7**:466–480.

ANTIMICROBIAL AGENTS AND CHEMOTHERAPY, June 1977, p. 1067-1068

Vol. 11, No. 6
Printed in U.S.A.

Induction of Bacteriocins from *Clostridium perfringens* by Treatment with Mitomycin C

D. E. MAHONY

Department of Microbiology, Faculty of Medicine, Dalhousie University, Halifax, Nova Scotia, B3H 4H7 Canada

Received for publication 4 February 1977

Six of ten bacteriocinogenic strains of *Clostridium perfringens* were inducible by treating the cultures with mitomycin C. Induction did not occur in the continued presence of mitomycin C but only when excess mitomycin C was removed. Cell death was associated with induction of bacteriocin.

Some bacteriocins of *Clostridium perfringens* are inducible by ultraviolet light (2, 3, 5), and there is one report (1) of induction by mitomycin C. In this latter report, a fourfold increment in bacteriocin titer resulted from a 2-h treatment of *C. perfringens* cultures with 2 μg of mitomycin C per ml. We (4) previously described a typing scheme for *C. perfringens* based on the susceptibility of various strains of the species to 10 bacteriocins. This paper describes the inducibility of these 10 bacteriocins and the technique that was found valuable for detecting induction.

The 10 bacteriocin-producing strains of *C. perfringens*, their origin, and their cultivation have been described (4). Mitomycin C was obtained from Sigma Chemical Co., St. Louis, Mo. This antibiotic was suspended in brain heart infusion (BHI) broth (Difco) as a stock solution of 400 μg per ml. A range of mitomycin C concentrations was tested for induction capability as follows. One hundred milliliters of BHI broth was inoculated with 6 ml of an 18-h cooked-meat culture of the bacteriocinogenic strain to be tested. This 100-ml culture was referred to as the "primary culture." After this culture was incubated for 2 h at 37°C, mitomycin C was added (final concentrations ranging from 0.25 to 8 μg per ml). The culture was incubated for 1 more h and then centrifuged at 6,000 $\times$ *g* in an International B-20 centrifuge for 10 min. The bacterial pellet was resuspended in 5 ml of BHI broth and added to 100 ml of freshly boiled and cooled BHI broth. This culture, referred to as the "secondary culture," was incubated for up to 24 h, and 2-ml samples were removed for the assay of bacteriocin titer or other characteristics of growth at various times. Viable counts of bacteria were done by plating duplicate 0.1-ml volumes of serially diluted samples onto blood agar plates. These were incubated anaerobically at 37°C for 18 h. The remainder of the samples were centrifuged to remove bacteria, and the supernatant fluids were titrated against indicator strain no. 2 in our collection. The method of assay has been described (4), but, essentially, it involves spotting 16 μl of serially diluted bacteriocin onto blood agar plates that have been seeded with a 1:100 dilution of a 3-h culture of strain no. 2.

Six of the ten bacteriocinogenic strains were inducible with mitomycin C (strains 28, 43, 55, 63, 73, and 78). The usual inducing dose was 2 to 4 μg/ml, although strain 43 was more efficiently induced with 1 μg/ml. Higher concentrations inhibited growth and bacteriocin production. Exposure of bacteria to mitomycin C for less than 1 h decreased the final yield of bacteriocin, whereas exposures of more than 1 h did not increase the yield obtained.

C. perfringens strain no. 28 was further studied as a model for the induction phenomenon. Bacteriocin production by strain no. 28 is shown in Fig. 1. These results are representative of at least four such experiments. The time scale refers to time after the centrifugation step and subculturing to the second 100-ml volume of broth (secondary culture). There was a 32- to 64-fold increment in bacteriocin titer in mitomycin C-induced cultures compared with that of control cultures treated exactly the same way but without the addition of mitomycin C. The somewhat lower titer shown for the control culture at time zero in Fig. 1 is not a consistent finding and probably represents differences in bacteriocin carryover from the primary to the secondary culture. The titer of the induced culture rapidly increased 15 to 30 min after subculturing, until 2 h, when the maximum titer was achieved. No increase in bacteriocin titer beyond control values was observed in the pri-

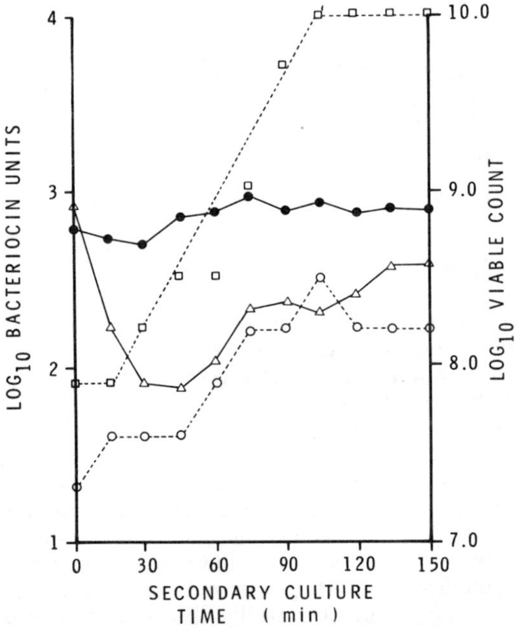

FIG. 1. *Mitomycin C induction of bacteriocin 28 and the effect upon viability of the induced culture. Viable count of the control culture (●), viable count of the induced culture (△), bacteriocin titer of the control culture (○), and bacteriocin titer of the induced culture (□).*

mary culture in the continued presence of mitomycin C, even after several hours of incubation. Therefore, the centrifugation and subculturing steps were required for the expression of induction.

The viabilities of induced and control cultures were compared to determine whether bacteriocin production or release or both resulted in death of the producing bacteria (Fig. 1). The mitomycin C-induced secondary culture showed a rapid 1-log drop in viability during the first 30 min, which was followed by a recovery of growth and survival throughout the rest of the experiment. Control cultures showed a slight decline in viability during the first few minutes of the secondary culture, after which the count increased slightly and then remained stationary. The production and/or release of bacteriocin in induced cultures would, therefore, seem to be related to cell death.

The effect of mitomycin C on alpha- and theta-toxin production was briefly examined, and there was no marked difference in toxin titers obtained in induced or control cultures during the primary culture. In the secondary culture, toxin levels were either slower appearing or generally lower in induced cultures when compared with control cultures. Table 1 relates these data with respect to the period of incubation when the highest bacteriocin level is achieved in both the primary and secondary cultures. Rescuing the induced bacteriocin at 2 h in the secondary culture provided high bacteriocin titers with relatively low amounts of the two toxins assayed.

TABLE 1. *Comparison of toxin and bacteriocin titers obtained in C. perfringens strain 28 treated with mitomycin*

Substance produced	Titer: Primary 3-h culture (before centrifugation step)	Titer: Secondary 2-h culture (after centrifugation step)
Alpha-toxin	1/16	1/16
Theta-toxin	1/256	1/32
Bacteriocin	1/320	1/10,240

In conclusion, we have shown that some bacteriocin-producing strains of *C. perfringens* are inducible by treating with mitomycin C and that mitomycin C must be removed from the culture for the subsequent expression of induction.

I would like to acknowledge the technical assistance of K. A. Patrick and the financial support of the Medical Research Council of Canada (grant no. MA5581).

LITERATURE CITED

1. **Clarke, D. J., R. M. Robson, and J. G. Morris.** 1975. Purification of two *Clostridium* bacteriocins by procedures appropriate to hydrophobic proteins. Antimicrob. Agents Chemother. 7:256–264.
2. **Ionesco, H., A. Wolff, and M. Sebald.** 1974. Production induite de bactériocine et d'un bactériophage par la souche BP6K-N_5 de *Clostridium perfringens*. Ann. Microbiol. Inst. Pasteur 125B:335–346.
3. **Mahony, D. E.** 1973. Antibiotic sensitivity of *Clostridium perfringens* and L-forms of *C. perfringens* induced by bacteriocin. Can. J. Microbiol. 19:735–739.
4. **Mahony, D. E.** 1974. Bacteriocin susceptibility of *Clostridium perfringens*: a provisional typing schema. Appl. Microbiol. 28:172–176.
5. **Tubylewicz, H.** 1966. Experimental studies on bacteriocinogeniety in *Clostridium perfringens* type A. 1. Isolation of bacteriocines and their antibacterial spectrum. Bull. Acad. Pol. Sci. Ser. Sci. Biol. 14:31–36.

Antimicrobial Agents and Chemotherapy, June 1977, p. 1069-1070
Vol. 11, No. 6

Response of Influenza Virus-Infected Mice to Selected Doses of Ribavirin Administered Intraperitoneally or by Aerosol

R. F. BERENDT,* J. S. WALKER,[1] J. W. DOMINIK, AND E. L. STEPHEN

U.S. Army Medical Research Institute of Infectious Diseases, Frederick, Maryland 21701

Received for publication 24 January 1977

The effects of graded doses of ribavirin administered either by aerosol or intraperitoneally were compared in influenza virus-infected mice. The median effective dose values (based upon percent survival) were 3.3 and 15.8 mg/kg per day for the aerosol and intraperitoneal routes, respectively. Lung lesion scores and titer of virus were lower after aerosol than intraperitoneal therapy.

Recently, ribavirin (1-β-D-ribofuranosyl-1,2,4-triazole-3-carboxamide) was found to be effective for the treatment of type A influenza virus infections in mice (1, 3-5). These experiments indicated that small-particle aerosols (mass median diameter, 1.4 μm) of ribavirin were more effective in reducing mortality, lesions in the lung, and virus concentrations in the lungs than approximately equivalent doses of drug given intraperitoneally (i.p.) (4). However, the data did not indicate how much better aerosol administration was than i.p. in terms of dosage required to achieve the same effect, i.e., how much ribavirin was required to achieve an effective dose that would allow >50% of the mice to survive (ED_{50}). This information would be helpful when considering the possible administration of ribavirin by aerosol for the treatment of humans, especially if a significant therapeutic advantage was gained by using the aerosol route.

The objective of this research was to determine the response of influenza virus-infected mice to selected doses of ribavirin given either by aerosol or i.p.

The procedures employed for housing, infecting, and treating mice [Tac:(SW)fBR] have been described by Stephen et al. (4). Four selected doses of ribavirin were administered by each route. Doses ranged from 2.5 to 20 mg/kg per day by aerosol and from 5.0 to 40.0 mg/kg per day by the i.p. route. Treatment was initiated at 6 h after exposure to the virus and was repeated daily for a total of 5 days. i.p. injections were given once daily at the same time as the aerosols. A virus control group received no treatment. The degree of gross pathology in the lungs (lung lesion score) was evaluated in three mice on day 4 and in five mice on day 7 by methods that have been described previously (4). The concentration of virus in the lungs was also determined on day 4 by previously described methods (5). Survival was recorded daily for 21 days in 25 mice that were randomly allocated for this purpose from each treatment group. Survival data from five replicate experiments were analyzed by probit analysis (2), and the dose of ribavirin yielding 50% survival (ED_{50}) was calculated together with 95% confidence limits. Lung lesion scores and lung virus concentration data were evaluated by analysis of variance.

The results are shown graphically in Fig. 1. The ED_{50} values after aerosol and i.p. administration of ribavirin were 3.3 mg/kg per day (95% confidence limits, 2.5 to 4.3) and 15.8 mg/kg per day (95% confidence limits, 12.7 and 19.5), respectively. The slopes (data not shown) for the regression of probits of percent survival on log dose were approximately the same, i.e., 2.65 and 2.66 for aerosol and i.p. treatments, respectively. Significantly lower lung virus titers ($P < 0.001$) and less extensive lung lesions (at 10 and 20 mg/kg, $P < 0.001$) were seen after aerosol than after i.p. administration. Especially noteworthy was the relatively small decrease in virus concentration in the lungs that accompanied marked increase in survival. Even in the case of aerosol therapy, survival increased from 33 to 99% with only a 0.5 $\log_{10}$ decrease in viral concentration.

We have shown that about one-fifth the amount of ribavirin is required to prevent most mortality in influenza virus-infected mice when the drug is administered by aerosol than when it is administered i.p. Aerosol therapy was also significantly more effective in reducing the amount of virus and extent of lesions in the lungs than was i.p. treatment when equivalent doses were compared. Our observation of the superiority of aerosol over i.p. therapy, there-

[1] Present address: Plum Island Animal Disease Center, P.O. Box 848, Greenport, NY 11944.

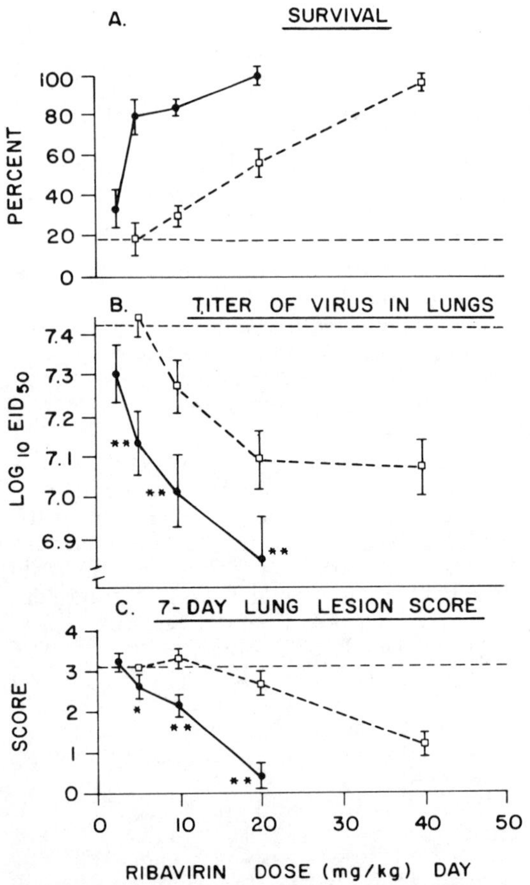

FIG. 1. *Survival (A), virus titer in lungs (B) and lung lesion scores (C) of influenza virus-infected mice. Statistical comparisons were carried out between comparable aerosol and i.p. doses. Symbols: ---, untreated virus control; ○, aerosol; □, i.p.; *, P < 0.005; **, P < 0.001. EID$_{50}$, mean egg infective dose.*

fore, confirms and extends those reported earlier by Stephen et al. (4) and Walker et al. (5).

Our observation of the effect of ribavirin on the concentration of virus in lungs is consistent with those of Stephen et al. (4) and Walker et al. (5). Although the effect of aerosol treatment differed significantly from that of the same dosage given i.p. ($P < 0.001$), the magnitude of difference was very small, and 90% survival was achieved despite the presence of almost 10^7 mean egg infective doses of virus in the lungs. Although we have not attempted to delineate growth curves, it seems unlikely that the activity of ribavirin (in vivo) is based primarily upon its antiviral properties.

The importance of the anti-inflammatory effect of ribavirin claimed by several authors (1, 4, 5) is not clear. A dramatic decrease in lung lesion scores was seen with increasing dose, particularly in aerosol-treated mice, but it is noteworthy that >80% of the mice survived with lung consolidation of 55 to 87.5% (lesion scores of 2.2 and 2.7, respectively). Further investigation with pathological examination at frequent periods after treatment would be necessary to resolve this point.

Although ribavirin was significantly more effective after aerosol administration than after i.p. administration, the question of the effect of more frequent administration by the i.p. and other routes must be addressed before recommendations can be made concerning the utility of aerosol therapy with this particular drug. Also, the i.p. route of administration is a good one for routine screening, but attention must be given to the routes that are commonly employed in clinical situations, e.g., oral or intramuscular. Also, pharmacokinetic studies must be carried out to provide information on the dosage schedules that would maintain optimum drug levels in the lungs.

LITERATURE CITED

1. **Durr, F. E., H. F. Lindh, and M. Forbes.** 1975. Efficacy of 1-β-D-ribofuranosyl-1,2,4-triazole-3-carboxamide against influenza virus infections in mice. Antimicrob. Agents Chemother. 7:582–586.
2. **Finney, D. J.** 1971. Probit analysis, 3rd ed., p. 50–99. Cambridge University Press, London.
3. **Khare, G. P., R. W. Sidwell, J. T. Witkowski, L. N. Simon, and R. R. Robins.** 1973. Suppression by 1-β-D-ribofuranosyl-1,2,4-triazole-3-carboxamide (Virazole, ICN 1229) of influenza virus-induced infections in mice. Antimicrob. Agents Chemother. 3:517–522.
4. **Stephen, E. L., J. W. Dominik, J. B. Moe, and J. S. Walker.** 1976. Therapeutic effects of ribavirin given by the intraperitoneal or aerosol route against influenza virus infections in mice. Antimicrob. Agents Chemother. 10:549–554.
5. **Walker, J. S., E. L. Stephen, and R. O. Spertzel.** 1976. Small-particle aerosols of antiviral compounds in treatment of type A influenza pneumonia in mice. J. Infect. Dis. 133 (Suppl.):S140–S144.

ANTIMICROBIAL AGENTS AND CHEMOTHERAPY, June 1977, p. 1071-1073
Vol. 11, No. 6
Printed in U.S.A.

In Vitro Antibiotic Susceptibility of Salmonellae

FACELUCIA BARROS, OKSANA M. KORZENIOWSKI, MERLE A. SANDE,* KATIA MARTINS, LUIZ CARLOS SANTOS, AND HEONIR ROCHA

Department of Medicine, University of Virginia School of Medicine, Charlottesville, Virginia 22901, Department of Medicine, Federal University of Bahia, Salvador, Bahia, Brazil, and Couto Maia Hospital, Salvador, Bahia, Brazil.*

Received for publication 27 January 1977

In vitro antibiotic susceptibilities were determined for 101 strains of salmonellae. Resistance to chloramphenicol and ampicillin was low. Cefamandole was active against the majority of strains and deserves further evaluation.

The recent identification of chloramphenicol and multiple drug-resistant salmonella epidemics has generated increased interest in the overall drug sensitivities of these organisms in various localities as well as a search for alternate drug therapy when such resistant strains are identified (4, 5). Cefamandole, a new parenteral cephalosporin prepared by substitution of heterocyclic groups on 7-aminocephalosporanic acid, has been shown to have a marked effect on a small number of strains of *Salmonella typhi* in vitro. To evaluate the potential usefulness of this antibiotic, 101 strains of salmonella, isolated in Salvador, Brazil, were tested in vitro to a variety of antibiotics currently in use or under investigation.

Strains studied. The 101 strains of salmonella used in our evaluations were isolated from patients at the Hospital Professor Edgard Santos and the Hospital Couto Maia from 1972 to 1975. Both hospitals are referral centers for patients with suspected or proven typhoid fever and other infectious diseases. The salmonella strains were collected randomly in an area where typhoid fever is endemic, and no epidemic outbreak was documented during the period of collection. Serotyping was performed on isolation and reconfirmed prior to antibiotic susceptibility testing. Of 59 strains of group D *S. typhi*, 53 were recovered from blood, 4 from stools, and 2 from cerebralspinal fluid. Of the remaining 42 "non-typhi" salmonella strains, 22 were recovered from blood, and 20 were isolated from stool, cerebralspinal fluid, urine, or synovial fluid.

Antimicrobial testing. The minimum inhibitory concentration for each drug was determined by serial twofold dilutions in Trypticase soy broth with freshly prepared solutions of chloramphenicol, ampicillin, carbenicillin, tetracycline, tobramycin, gentamicin, cefamandole (Eli Lilly and Co., Indianapolis, Ind.), and BLP-1761 (an ester of hetacillin, Bristol Laboratories, Syracuse, N.Y.). An inoculum of 10^4 organisms was added to each tube. After 24 h of incubation, samples were taken from all tubes with no visible growth and were plated on Trypticase soy agar to determine minimum bactericidal concentrations. Strains of *S. typhi* (Fig. 1) were, in general, more susceptible to the antimicrobial agents tested than the "non-typhi" strains (Fig. 2). Cefamandole was the most active drug by weight, with 100% of *S. typhi* strains inhibited by 1.56 μg/ml or less (Fig. 1a). This is in contrast to other cephalosporins previously tested (1, 2). Ninety-seven percent of *S. typhi* strains was inhibited by BLP-1761 at a concentration of 3.1 μg/ml as opposed to 90% for ampicillin. Carbenicillin was the least active of the penicillin derivatives.

Chloramphenicol inhibited 97% of *S. typhi* strains with concentrations of less than 12.5 μg/ml (Fig. 1b). Ninety-three percent of the strains was inhibited by 12.5 μg of tetracycline per ml. Gentamicin and tobramycin had similar activity with 93% of strains inhibited by a concentration of less than 12.5 μg/ml.

In contrast to *S. typhi*, the "non-typhi" salmonella strains exhibited in vitro resistance of 30 to 40% to most antibiotics tested. Cefamandole and BLP-1761 again appeared to be quite active, each inhibiting 70% of strains with concentrations of 1.6 μg/ml (Fig. 2a).

In this evaluation of 101 strains of salmonella, only a minor emergence of resistant strains to the antibiotics currently utilized in the community was noted. High-level resistance to chloramphenicol and ampicillin remains in the 2 to 3% range, comparable to the data of Finland et al. (2), but much less than the 16 to 33% range reported in other areas not involved in an epidemic of chloramphenicol-resistant strains.

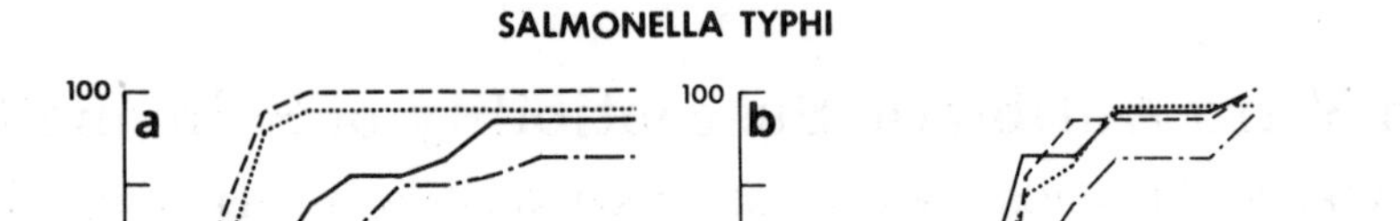

FIG. 1. *(a) and (b) show antibiotic susceptibilities of 59 strains of S. typhi.*

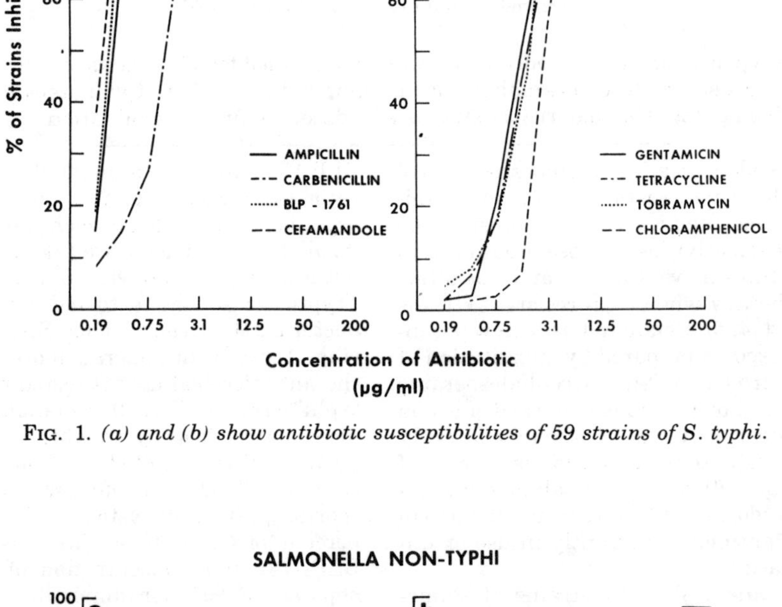

FIG. 2. *(a) and (b) show antibiotic susceptibilities of 42 strains of "non-typhi" salmonellae.*

Of note is the emergence of aminoglycoside resistance (7%), which has not been seen by other investigators (1–3). This decreased susceptibility to aminoglycosides is also found in the group of "non-typhi" strains, which showed up to 30% resistance to the maximum achievable serum levels.

LITERATURE CITED

1. **Bissett, M. L., S. L. Abbott, and R. M. Wood.** 1974. Antimicrobial resistance and R factors in *Salmonella* isolated in California (1971–1972). Antimicrob. Agents Chemother. 5:161–168.
2. **Finland, M., C. Garmer, C. Wilcox, and L. Sabath.** 1974. Salmonellosis and shigellosis at Boston City Hospital. J. Am. Med. Assoc. 229:1309–1312.
3. **Marks, M. I., M. Kazemi, and E. MacKay.** 1973. In vitro sensitivity of *Salmonella* to ten antimicrobial agents including sulfamethoxazole and trimethoprim, alone and in combination. Antimicrob. Agents Chemother. 4:555–559.
4. **Olarte, J., and E. Galindo.** 1973. *Salmonella typhi* resistant to chloramphenicol, ampicillin, and other antimicrobial agents: strains isolated during an extensive typhoid fever epidemic in Mexico. Antimicrob. Agents Chemother. 4:597–601.
5. **Overturf, G., K. I. Marton, and A. W. Mathies, Jr.** 1973. Antibiotic resistance in typhoid fever. N. Engl. J. Med. 289:463–465.

ANTIMICROBIAL AGENTS AND CHEMOTHERAPY, June 1977, p. 1074-1076 Vol. 11, No. 6
 Printed in U.S.A.

Double-Osmotic-Shock Procedure to Prepare Gentamicin Adenine Mononucleotide Transferase for the Enzymatic Assay of Gentamicin

J. DANKERT* AND J. WOLTJES

Laboratory of Medical Microbiology, Division of Hospital Infections, University of Groningen, A.Z.G., Groningen, The Netherlands

Received for publication 27 January 1977

The release of gentamicin adenine mononucleotide transferase during single, cold, osmotic-shock treatment of *Escherichia coli* K-12 W677/HJR66 is not always maximal. The quantity of gentamicin adenine mononucleotide transferase in osmotic extracts could be significantly increased when a double-shock procedure was performed.

The enzymatic assay for gentamicin based upon the adenylylation of this aminoglycoside has been reported (1, 4, 7, 8). The enzyme required for the adenylylation is usually prepared from *Escherichia coli* W677/HJR66 by using the osmotic-shock procedure (6). Technical problems concerning the assay procedure have been described (2, 4, 9) and may be related to a low yield of the enzyme (gentamicin adenine mononucleotide transferase [GAdT]) in the osmotic extracts. We report increased yields of GAdT activity in extracts obtained after a double osmotic shock.

E. coli K-12 W677/HJR66 (kindly provided by D. H. Smith, Children's Hospital Medical Center, Boston, Mass.) was grown overnight in 25 ml of Trypticase soy broth (Baltimore Biological Laboratory, Cockeysville, Md.) supplemented with gentamicin (100 μg/ml). A sample (5 ml) from this culture was diluted to 1 liter with Trypticase soy broth and incubated in a rotary shaker at 37°C (New Brunswick Scientific Co., New Brunswick. N.J.) for 90 to 120 min until optical density at 490 nm of 0.3 was reached. Gentamicin was not added to this last medium to avoid high background activity in the assay (4). Shock extracts were prepared using the technique reported previously (4, 6, 7). The supernatants obtained at the end of the procedure were supplemented with reduced dithiothreitol (Sigma Chemical Co., St. Louis, Mo.) in a final concentration of 0.01 M. Small samples of the isolates (1 ml) were frozen quickly in liquid N_2 and stored at −20°C. Protein content of the extracts was measured by the method of Lowry et al. (5).

GAdT activity was determined by using the procedures previously described (4, 7). To a standard reaction mixture containing 0.5 M tris(hydroxymethyl)aminomethane (Tris)-chloride, pH 8.5 at 36°C (25 μl), 0.08 M $MgCl_2 \cdot 6H_2O$ (25 μl), and [^{14}C]adenosine 5′-monophosphate (5 nmol) from a stock solution (45 μCi/μmol; New England Nuclear Corp., Boston, Mass.), 30 μl of an extract and 30 μl of gentamicin standards were added. Standard solutions of gentamicin sulfate (Schering Corp., Essex Co., The Netherlands) were prepared in pooled human sera (0, 1, 3, 5, 10, and 12.5 μg/ml).

Using the assay procedure for each osmotic extract, a standard curve was drawn. In the assay, 1 unit of GAdT is defined as that amount that produces 1 pmol of gentamicin adenylylate in 1 min at 36°C.

Only one out of six shock extracts contained a satisfactory GAdT activity (5.67 U/ml; specific activity, 4.73 U/mg of protein). The enzymatic activity of the remaining extracts varied from 0.07 to 2.60 U/ml of extract, whereas the specific activity ranged from 0.13 to 2.60 U/mg of protein. The protein content of the extracts ranged from 500 to 1,200 μg/ml in all cases, suggesting that the shock treatment was sufficient but not fully adequate to release the adenylylating enzyme.

We decided to subject the pellet remaining after the shock procedure to a second osmotic shock performed in a similar manner. The pellet was resuspended immediately in 20% (wt/vol) sucrose with 0.003 M ethylenediaminetetraacetate and 0.033 M Tris-chloride (pH 7.3), gently stirred (for 10 min at 20°C), and centrifuged (12,000 × *g* for 10 min at 4°C). The packed cells were quickly resuspended in ice-cold 0.0005 M $MgCl_2 \cdot 6H_2O$ and stirred at 0°C for 10 min. After centrifugation at 26,000 × *g* at 4°C for 10 min, the supernatant was collected and designated as the "double-shock" extract.

The treatment yielded extracts with significantly higher GAdT activity than in single-

TABLE 1. *Yield of protein and GAdT activity in four extracts from E. coli K-12 W677/HJR66 obtained with the first osmotic-shock treatment and subsequently with the second osmotic-shock treatment*

Osmotic extract	Single-shock extract			Double-shock extract		
	Protein (μg/ml)	Activity (U/ml)	Sp act (U/mg of protein)	Protein (μg/ml)	Activity (U/ml)	Sp act (U/mg of protein)
I	650	0.07	0.10	600	10.00	16.67
II	400	0.50	1.25	750	8.33	11.00
III	500	3.00	10.00	450	0.67	1.48
IV	700	0.70	0.95	500	6.67	13.33

shock extracts (Table 1). The protein content was similar in both single- and double-shock extracts, but specific activities were increased in the latter except on one occasion (extract III), due to the fact that a high enzymatic activity was already present in the single-shock extract.

The viability of *E. coli* cells after a double shock was in agreement with that reported after a single shock (6). Viability studies performed by using the pour plate method showed that the number of cells was lowered from 1.90 $\times 10^8$ to 2.0 $\times 10^8$ (initial count) to 1.80 $\times 10^8$ to 1.85 $\times 10^8$ cells per ml after the single shock and to 1.60 $\times 10^8$ to 1.70 $\times 10^8$ cells per ml after the double shock.

The double-shock extract was assayed for adenylylation of gentamicin and sisomicin (Schering Corp., Essex Co., The Netherlands), tobramycin and kanamycin (Bristol Laboratories and Eli Lilly & Co., The Netherlands), and streptomycin and neomycin. Optimal activity was found for gentamicin, whereas intermediate activity occurred with sisomicin and tobramycin (Fig. 1). The reproducibility of the assay for gentamicin was estimated. For concentrations of 3, 5, and 10 μg/ml of serum, the values within two standard deviations differed from the mean by ≤18%.

In assays using single-shock extracts, low background activity was reported when osmotic extracts were prepared from *E. coli* cells grown in gentamicin-free medium (4). We have had similar results with double-shock extracts and dialyzed (double) shock extracts (Tris-chloride buffer at 4°C for 4 h).

The instability of the enzymatic activity in the double-shock extracts is comparable to that in the single-shock extracts (4, 7).

The osmotic-shock procedure was described originally as a method for the release of hydrolytic enzymes from the periplasmic gap (6), where GAdT has been suggested to be situated (7). Since the activity profiles of periplasmic hydrolytic enzymes and GAdT showed differences, Goldman and Northrop (3) suggested that there are large differences in their periplasmic location. It is possible that the release of GAdT as compared with other enzymes is more difficult because of this location difference. The binding of GAdT to an unknown component in the periplasmic region, thereby hindering its release after a single shock, must also be considered. Our experiments show that high GAdT activity is always obtained with the double-shock procedure, whereas with the single-shock procedure high GAdT activity only occasionally occurs.

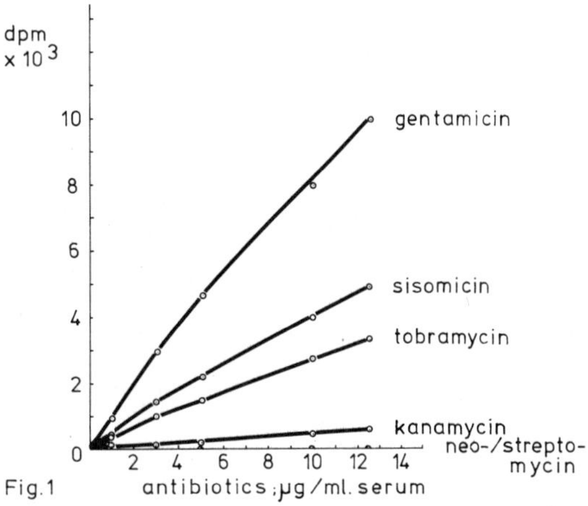

FIG. 1. *Adenylylation of different aminoglycosides in standard solutions using a double-shock extract in a standard assay procedure.*

We gratefully acknowledge the help of Kees Beenakker with the measurements.

LITERATURE CITED

1. **Benveniste, R., and J. Davies.** 1971. R-factor mediated gentamicin resistance: a new enzyme which modifies aminoglycoside antibiotics. FEBS Lett. 14:293–296.
2. **Forrey, A. W., A. Blair, M. O'Neil, R. E. Cutler, and T. G. Christopher.** 1973. Enzymatic assay for gentamicin. N. Engl. J. Med. 288:108.
3. **Goldman, P. R., and D. B. Northrop.** 1975. Preparation of stable gentamicin adenylyl transferase of high specific activity. Biochem. Biophys. Res. Commun. 66:1408–1413.
4. **Holmes, R. K., and J. P. Sanford.** 1974. Enzymatic assay for gentamicin and related aminoglycoside antibiotics. J. Infect. Dis. 129:519–527.
5. **Lowry, O. H., N. J. Rosebrough, A. L. Farr, and R. J. Randall.** 1951. Protein measurement with the Folin phenol reagent. J. Biol. Chem. 193:265–275.

6. **Nossal, N. G., and L. A. Heppel.** 1966. The release of enzymes by osmotic shock from Escherichia coli in exponential phase. J. Biol. Chem. 241:3055–3062.
7. **Smith, A. L., and D. H. Smith.** 1974. Gentamicin: adenine mononucleotide transferase: partial purification, characterization, and use in the clinical quantitation of gentamicin. J. Infect. Dis. 129:391–401.
8. **Smith, D. H., B. van Otto, and A. L. Smith.** 1972. A rapid chemical assay for gentamicin. N. Engl. J. Med. 286:583–586.
9. **Tilton, R. C., J. R. Murphy, and E. Mallett.** 1972. Assay for gentamicin. N. Engl. J. Med. 287:1100.

ANTIMICROBIAL AGENTS AND CHEMOTHERAPY, June 1977, p. 1077-1078
Vol. 11, No. 6

Printed in U.S.A.

Effect of Anaerobiosis on Antimicrobial Susceptibility of Staphylococci[1]

LIZZIE J. HARRELL AND JAMES B. EVANS*

Department of Microbiology, North Carolina State University, Raleigh, North Carolina 27607

Received for publication 29 December 1976

The minimum inhibitory concentration (MIC) of 12 antibiotics was determined for four strains of staphylococci (representing the three major species) under aerobic and anaerobic conditions by using the broth dilution method. Nine of the antibiotics showed no significant difference between aerobic and anaerobic MIC for any of the four cultures. Gentamicin and kanamycin showed a small, but significant, increase in MIC for at least two strains under anaerobic conditions. Trimethoprim was less effective against all strains under anaerobic conditions.

It has long been known that anaerobiosis brings about changes in nutritional requirements and metabolic pathways of staphylococci (3). Recent reports indicate that the susceptibility of staphylococci to some antibiotics also may be altered drastically by anaerobic conditions. Virtanen (6) reported that up to 100 times as much antibiotic may be needed for inhibition of anaerobic growth of several strains of *Staphylococcus aureus* when the minimum inhibitory concentration (MIC) of sulfamethoxazole, trimethoprim, and Septra was compared at the surface (aerobic environment) and in the depth (anaerobic environment) of semisolid Wellcotest medium. Reynolds et al. (4) reported that the MIC of gentamicin was 20-fold higher when some strains of *S. aureus* were tested by using the agar dilution technique and Oxoid Sensitest agar under anaerobic conditions as compared with aerobic conditions. Resistance to kanamycin was also increased under anaerobic conditions. Stalons and Thornsberry (5) employed the standard reference strain of *S. aureus* (ATCC 25923) as a control while investigating a method for determining the antibiotic susceptibility of obligately anaerobic bacteria. They found little difference between the aerobic and anaerobic MIC of five of the antibiotics tested (chloramphenicol, clindamycin, erythromycin, lincomycin, and vancomycin). However, in modified Schaedler broth there was an eightfold increase in MIC of gentamicin anaerobically and a fourfold increase in MIC of penicillin and tetracycline aerobically. In Mueller-Hinton broth these differences were not found.

We have conducted a systematic investigation of the aerobic and anaerobic MIC of 12 antibiotics (cephalothin, chloramphenicol, clindamycin, erythromycin, gentamicin, kanamycin, methicillin, oxacillin, penicillin, tetracycline, trimethoprim, and vancomycin) for four strains of staphylococci. The cultures tested included three isolates from human skin (*S. aureus* AW 151, *S. epidermidis* MK 214, and *S. saprophyticus* TW 111) and the standard reference strain of *S. aureus* (ATCC 25923).

Two test media were used: a semisynthetic medium containing vitamin-free, acid-hydrolyzed casein (CH broth) that supports good anaerobic growth of staphylococci (1) and brain heart infusion (BHI) broth. Mueller-Hinton broth was not used because it did not support good anaerobic growth of the test organisms.

The inoculum was prepared by diluting an overnight CH or BHI broth culture to 10^5 colony-forming units/ml in the test medium. The conventional tube dilution method (2, 7) was employed, with a duplicate set of tubes incubated in GasPak (BBL) anaerobic jars. Three independent experiments were conducted with each antibiotic against each culture.

Nine of the antibiotics showed no significant difference between their aerobic and anaerobic MIC for any of the four cultures. In most instances there was less than one-dilution (twofold) difference between the average aerobic and anaerobic MIC values. Both gentamicin and kanamycin had a significantly higher MIC anaerobically for two or more cultures in one or both media. The results with these two antibiotics are summarized in Table 1. Somewhat greater differences were generally observed in the CH broth than in the BHI broth.

Trimethoprim had a significantly higher MIC for all four cultures under anaerobic conditions in CH broth. It could not be tested in BHI

[1] Paper no. 5156 of the Journal Series of the North Carolina Agricultural Experiment Station, Raleigh, N.C.

TABLE 1. *MIC of gentamicin and kanamycin for the four test strains of staphylococci*

Test strain	MIC (μg/ml)[a]							
	Gentamicin				Kanamycin			
	CH broth		BHI broth		CH broth		BHI broth	
	Aerobic	Anaerobic	Aerobic	Anaerobic	Aerobic	Anaerobic	Aerobic	Anaerobic
S. aureus 25923	0.83	2.70	0.42	0.92	12.0	34.7	5.3	3.3
S. aureus AW151	1.70	4.70	1.00	2.17	21.3	37.3	6.0	12.0
S. epidermidis MK214	0.42	1.70	0.17	0.25	7.3	34.7	4.0	7.3
S. saprophyticus TW111	0.08	0.14	0.12	0.11	1.0	1.3	1.3	3.3

[a] Results are the average of three independent experiments.

broth, perhaps because of the presence of sufficient thymidine to interfere with the action of this antibiotic.

Our results fall far short of the dramatic differences reported by some other authors (4, 6) and probably are not of clinically significant magnitude. However, they do confirm the reported reduction in effectiveness of gentamicin, kanamycin, and trimethoprim under anaerobic conditions. The tube dilution technique is probably less aerobic than conditions encountered on body surfaces or in the disk diffusion method of determining susceptibility, and the GasPak system falls short of the level of anaerobiosis that might be achieved by more vigorous techniques or in some infection sites. Thus, the differences reported here may indicate potentially greater differences under other circumstances.

ACKNOWLEDGMENTS

This investigation was supported by Public Health Service Biomedical Sciences Support grant no. RR7071.

Special thanks are extended to Robert J. Monroe for advice and guidance in the statistical analysis of our data. The antibiotics were kindly supplied by Burroughs Wellcome Co., Eli Lilly & Co., Schering Laboratories, Parke Davis & Co., Upjohn Co., Bristol Laboratories, and Sigma Chemical Co. W. E. Kloos provided three of the cultures used in these studies.

LITERATURE CITED

1. **Evans, J. B.** 1976. Uracil and pyruvate requirements for anaerobic growth of staphylococci. J. Clin. Microbiol. 2:14–17.
2. **Gerlach, E. H.** 1974. Microdilution I: a comparative study, p. 63–76. *In* A. Balows (ed.), Current techniques for antibiotic susceptibility testing. Charles C Thomas, Publishers, Springfield, Ill.
3. **Lascelles, J.** 1974. Anaerobic growth requirements of staphylococci and the enzymes of pyrimidine synthesis. Ann. N.Y. Acad. Sci. 236:96–104.
4. **Reynolds, A. V., J. M. T. Hamilton-Miller, and W. Brumfitt.** 1976. Diminished effect of gentamicin under anaerobic or hypercapnic conditions. Lancet i: 447–449.
5. **Stalons, D. R., and C. Thornsberry.** 1975. Broth-dilution method for determining the antibiotic susceptibility of anaerobic bacteria. Antimicrob. Agents Chemother. 7:15–21.
6. **Virtanen, S.** 1974. Antibacterial activity of sulphamethoxazole and trimethoprim under diminished oxygen tension. J. Gen. Microbiol. 84:145–148.
7. **Washington, J. A., and A. L. Barry.** 1974. Dilution test procedures, p. 410–417. *In* E. H. Lennette, E. H. Spaulding, and J. P. Truant (ed.), Manual of clinical microbiology, 2nd ed. American Society for Microbiology, Washington, D.C.

Antimicrobial Agents and Chemotherapy, June 1977, p. 1079–1080
Vol. 11, No. 6

Incidence and Elimination of R Plasmids in *Vibrio cholerae*

SUJATA G. DASTIDAR, ROMA PODDAR, RANAJIT KUMAR, AND A. N. CHAKRABARTY*

Division of Microbiology, Jadavpur University, and Division of Microbiology, Indian Institute of Experimental Medicine, Calcutta 700 032, India*

Received for publication 14 December 1976

Of 124 strains of *Vibrio cholerae*, 32 were multiply resistant to antibiotics. This resistance appeared to be determined by R plasmids on the basis of their effective elimination by sodium dodecyl sulfate, acridine orange, ethidium bromide, and ultraviolet radiation.

Naturally occurring R plasmids in vibrios generally appear to be stable, although some transferred R plasmids have been reported to be unstable (5, 6, 8, 9). The present study was undertaken to examine the incidence and elimination of naturally occurring R plasmids after treatment with several "curing" agents in vibrios. In this study, 124 human isolates were examined for multiple resistance to penicillin, cloxacillin, chloramphenicol, erythromycin, polymyxin, kanamycin, streptomycin, and tetracycline as well as for bacteriocinogeny. Resistance to each antibiotic was determined by spotting 10^5 colony-forming units of a culture on nutrient agar containing 0 (control), 10, 25, 50, 100, 200, 400, or 800 μg of an antibiotic per ml and examining for growth up to 48 h. Thirty-two strains exhibited resistance to at least three of these antibiotics (Table 1). The results showed that, whereas resistance to cloxacillin and polymixin was encountered most often and was highest in comparison with all other antibiotics tested (200 to 800 and 100 to 200 μg/ml, respectively), resistance to chloramphenicol and tetracycline was lowest (<10 μg/ml for 115 and 120, respectively, of 124 strains tested). Resistance to other antibiotics varied between 25 and 100 μg/ml.

Five multiply resistant strains representing five different combinations of antibiotic resistance and belonging to different bacteriocin types (3; Table 2) were chosen for studying the effects of sodium dodecyl sulfate, acridine orange, ethidium bromide, and ultraviolet radiation on these resistances and bacteriocinogeny. The minimum inhibitory concentrations of sodium dodecyl sulfate, acridine orange, and ethidium bromide were first determined. Other procedures were as described (2, 4), and the "curing" effects with ultraviolet radiation were as in reference 6. The treated clones were tested for loss of antibiotic resistance as well as bacteriocinogeny (4). The effects of these agents on the antibiotic resistance and bacteriocinogeny are described in Table 2. Only one colony each of *Vibrio cholerae* 1369 treated with sodium dodecyl sulfate and ethidium bromide lost bacteriocinogeny. These elimination studies suggest that the antibiotic resistance determinants in *V. cholerae* are probably plasmid linked, like

Table 1. *Distribution pattern of multiple resistance among strains of V. cholerae*

Multiple resistance pattern[a]	No. of strains[b]	Multiple resistance pattern[a]	No. of strains[b]
$Pe_{25}Cx_{400}Cm_{25}Ka_{25}$	1	$Pe_{25}Cx_{200}Po_{100}$	2
$Pe_{25}Cx_{400}Er_{50}Po_{50}Ka_{25}Sm_{50}$	1	$Pe_{50}Cx_{200}Ka_{50}$	1
$Pe_{100}Cx_{400}Er_{25}Ka_{25}Sm_{100}$	2	$Cx_{200}Cm_{25}Er_{100}Ka_{100}$	1
$Pe_{25}Cx_{400}Er_{50}Po_{100}Ka_{50}$	1	$Cx_{400}Er_{25}Po_{100}Ka_{25}Sm_{25}$	1
$Pe_{100}Cx_{400}Er_{50}Po_{100}$	3	$Cx_{400}Er_{100}Ka_{100}$	2
$Pe_{50}Cx_{400}Er_{100}Po_{100}Tc_{50}$	1	$Cx_{400}Po_{100}Ka_{25}Sm_{25}$	2
$Pe_{100}Cx_{400}Er_{25}$	6	$Cx_{400}Po_{100}Sm_{25}$	1
$Pe_{100}Cx_{400}Po_{100}Ka_{25}Sm_{25}$	2	$Cx_{400}Ka_{25}Sm_{25}$	2
$Pe_{100}Cx_{400}Po_{100}Ka_{50}$	3		

[a] Pe, Penicillin; Cx, cloxacillin; Cm, chloramphenicol; Er, erythromycin; Po, polymyxin; Ka, kanamycin; Sm, streptomycin; Tc, tetracycline; subscripted numbers denote levels of corresponding antibiotic resistance in micrograms per milliliter.

[b] When more than one strain belonged to a particular resistance pattern, resistance described belong to a representative strain.

TABLE 2. *Co-elimination of antibiotic resistances in V. cholerae resulting from the action of several agents*

V. cholerae	Wild-type resistance pattern[a]	Curing agent	Resistances eliminated
K-23	$Pe_{25}Cx_{400}Er_{50}Po_{50}Ka_{25}Sm_{50}B^5$	SDS	PePo(1)[b], Pe(44)
		AO	PePo(2), PeEr(1), Pe(47)
		UVR	PeEr(1), Pe(43)
		EB	PePo(1), Pe(49)
601	$Pe_{100}Cx_{400}Po_{100}Ka_{50}B^{2A}$	SDS	Pe(46)
		AO	PePo(31), Pe(16)
		UVR	Pe(50)
		EB	Pe(48)
805	$Pe_{100}Cx_{400}Er_{50}Po_{100}B^3$	SDS	PeCxPo(10), PeCxEr(9), CxPo(5), Er(7)
		AO	PeCxEr(50)
		UVR	PeCxPo(14), PeCx(36)
		EB	Pe(50)
824	$Pe_{25}Cx_{400}Er_{50}Po_{100}Ka_{50}B^6$	SDS	PePo(2), PeEr(1), Pe(46)
		AO	
		UVR	
		EB	Pe(49)
1369	$Pe_{50}Cx_{400}Er_{100}Po_{100}Tc_{50}B^8$	SDS	PeCxErPoB^8(1), Pe(27)
		AO	Pe(47)
		UVR	Pe(39)
		EB	PeErPoB^8(1), PeEr(46), Pe(2)

[a] Pe, Penicillin; Cx, cloxacillin; Er, erythromycin; Po, polymyxin; Ka, kanamycin; Sm, streptomycin; Tc, tetracycline; subscripted numbers denote levels of resistance (micrograms per milliliter) to respective antibiotics; B^5, B^{2A}, B^3, B^6, and B^8 represent bacteriocin types 5, 2A, 3, 6, and 8, respectively (3); SDS, sodium dodecyl sulfate; AO, acridine orange; UVR, ultraviolet radiation; EB, ethidium bromide.

[b] Numbers within parentheses indicate number of colonies "cured" of resistance(s) of 50 colonies tested; broth cultures after treatment with one of the "curring" agents were plated out for isolated colonies, which were then transferred to different antibiotic-agar and nutrient agar plates. Antibiotic(s) in these plates contained 25% of the original level of resistance.

that of bacteriocinogeny (1, 4), and that independent elimination of each plasmid for antibiotic resistance and bacteriocinogeny occurs; this is most readily interpreted on the basis that each of these is determined by an independent plasmid.

LITERATURE CITED

1. **Bhaskaran, K.** 1964. Segregation of genetic factors during recombination in *Vibrio cholerae* strain 162. Bull. W.H.O. 30:845–853.
2. **Bounchaud, D. H., M. R. Scavizzi, and Y. A. Chabbert.** 1969. Elimination by ethidium bromide of antibiotic resistance in Enterobacteria and Staphylococci. J. Gen. Microbiol. 54:417–425.
3. **Chakrabarty, A. N., S. Adhya, J. Basu, and S. G. Dastidar.** 1970. Bacteriocin typing of *Vibrio cholerae*. Infect. Immun. 1:293–299.
4. **Chakrabarty, A. N., and S. G. Dastidar.** 1974. Paradoxical inhibition in bacteria. Characterization of the phenomenon and nature of the genetic process. J. Gen. Microbiol. 80:339–361.
5. **Chakrabarty, A. N., S. N. Sarkar, S. Chaudhuri, M. Ganguli, and S. G. Dastidar.** 1977. Transformation of vibrios with R-factors from enterobacteria. Indian J. Med. Res. 65:992–1000.
6. **Kuwahara, S., T. Akiba, K. Koyama, and T. Arai.** 1963. Transmission of multiple drug-resistance from *Shigella flexneri* to *Vibrio comma* through conjugation. Jpn. J. Microbiol. 7:61–67.
7. **Siccardi, A. G.** 1966. Colicin resistance associated with resistance factors in *Escherichia coli*. Genet. Res. 8:219–228.
8. **Watanabe, T., and Y. Ogata.** 1970. Genetic stability of various R-factors in *Escherichia coli* and *Salmonella typhimurium*. J. Bacteriol. 102:363–368.
9. **Yokota, Y., T. Kasuga, M. Kaneko, and S. Kuwahara.** 1972. Genetic behavior of R factors in *Vibrio cholerae*. J. Bacteriol. 109:440–442.

Antimicrobial Agents and Chemotherapy, June 1977, p. 1081-1083
Vol. 11, No. 6

Distribution of Amikacin in Serum, Muscle, and Fat in Children After a Single Intramuscular Injection

F. DASCHNER,[1]* E. REISS, and JÜRGEN ENGERT

Division of Antimicrobial Therapy, Children's Hospital, and Department for Pediatric Surgery, University of Munich, 8000 Munich 2, Federal Republic of Germany

Received for publication 26 October 1976

Amikacin concentrations in serum, muscle, and fat were determined in 41 children after intramuscular administration of 7.5 mg/kg of body weight. At 1.5 h amikacin reached peak concentrations in serum (mean value, 14.9 μg/ml) as well as in muscle (2.2 μg/g) and fat (1.89 μg/g) tissue; from then on all concentrations declined. Amikacin concentrations exceeded 1 μg/g in muscle for at least 3 h and in fat for at least 4 h.

One of the parameters for evaluating a new antibiotic is the determination of its ability to penetrate into various tissues. Most studies concerning tissue concentrations of antibiotics have been done in either laboratory animals or humans, whose pharmacokinetic behavior often varies greatly from that of children. Almost no data have been accumulated on concentrations of aminoglycoside antibiotics in the tissues of children, although these drugs are frequently and sometimes unsuccessfully used for treatment of various deep tissue infections in children.

An unusually high incidence of postoperative wound infections due to a gentamicin-resistant strain of *Klebsiella pneumoniae* offered us the opportunity to study the deportment of amikacin in a small group of children at risk. Amikacin was highly effective in reducing the incidence of these postoperative wound infections.

The distribution of amikacin was studied in tissue having a good or a relatively poor blood supply, i.e., in muscle or in fat, respectively, in relation to the corresponding drug concentrations in serum. The cooperation of the pediatric surgeon enabled us to obtain data covering the whole range of a usual 12-h administration period.

Amikacin (kindly supplied by Bristol-Myers GmbH, Germany) was given intramuscularly to 41 children (mean age, 7 years) in a dose of 7.5 mg/kg of body weight at various intervals before inguinal hernia or undescended testes operations. All children were premedicated with atropine and received a 1:5 mixture of 5% dextrose in Ringer solution at an average rate of 7 ml/kg per h at the time of the operation.

All children had normal renal function, and none of the serum specimens drawn from the children before administration of amikacin showed any antibacterial activity. None of the children experienced any local or systemic side effects.

Blood (obtained by venipuncture), muscle from the abdominal wall, and subcutaneous fat (obtained electrosurgically) were taken at a single time from each patient during the operation; time intervals are indicated in Table 1. Blood was removed from the tissue specimen (mean weight 200 mg) by gently touching with sterile gauze. Blood was centrifuged, and the serum and tissue specimens were frozen at −22°C and assayed within 1 week.

Tissue fluid in a 1:3 dilution (wt/vol) with 0.15 M phosphate buffer, pH 8, was obtained by use of a Colworth Stomacher no. 80. Two paddles in the machine alternately pounded a plastic bag with the tissue specimen and compressed its contents against the door (A. J. Seward Ltd., Bury St. Edmunds, Suffolk, England). The method correlates well with extraction methods using tissue grinders or automated mixing devices (4). The amikacin content of serum and tissue was assayed with an agar diffusion method using punched holes according to Grove and Randall (2). *Bacillus subtilis* ATCC 6633 was the test organism used (spore suspension, BBL; antibiotic agar no. 5, Merck AG, Darmstadt, Germany).

Standard curves for determination of amikacin concentrations in serum (amikacin dissolved in phosphate-buffered pooled human serum, pH 8) or in tissue (amikacin dissolved in phosphate buffer, pH 8) were obtained from the mean of nine single values for each concentra-

[1] Present address: Klinikhygieniker des Universitätsklinikums Freiburg, 7800 Freiburg, Federal Republic of Germany.

tion. A standard curve of amikacin dissolved in muscle tissue fluid obtained from an amputated leg of an adult patient paralleled standard curves in phosphate buffer, giving values for muscle concentrations that deviated by no more than ±5%.

All serum and tissue specimens were assayed twice, on two different days, each time at least in triplicate. The lowest detectable amikacin concentration in serum was 0.15 μg/ml, and in tissue it was 0.1 μg/g. The average hemoglobin concentration in fluid obtained from muscle was 1.5 g/100 ml, and from fat it was 1.1 g/100 ml.

Informed consent was obtained from all parents before administering the antibiotic and collecting the specimens.

The number of specimens, range of values, and standard deviations for amikacin levels in serum, muscle, and fat are given in Table 1 for each time interval after a single dose of 7.5 mg/kg. For technical reasons specimens could be taken no earlier than 1.5 h after amikacin application in this group of patients. At 1.5 h the mean peak serum level of amikacin was 14.9 μg/ml, with a range from 7 to 19.3 μg/ml. Serum levels then declined slowly but constantly to 0.44 and 0.18 μg/ml, respectively, at 12 and 13 h after administration.

The muscle and fat content of amikacin, as with serum, reached concentration peaks at 1.5 h, thereafter declining to lower values. The concentrations in muscle exceeded those in fat only at 1.5 and 2.5 h and were almost identical to those in fat at 3.5 h and from 6 to 13 h. At 4 and 5 h amikacin content of fat was higher than that of muscle. The differences, however, were not statistically significant.

Percentages of amikacin content of fat and muscle in relation to the corresponding level in serum at various time intervals are given in Table 2. Percentages increased progressively to a maximum of 77% at the end of the usual 12-h administration interval.

In this study amikacin concentrations in muscle and fat had their peak at the same time as in serum. Peak amikacin concentrations in serum were somewhat lower than those found by Howard and McCracken (3) 1 h after administration in neonates, which in that study might be due to the older age group as well as time of assay after intramuscular injection of the drug.

The increasing percentage of amikacin tissue content as opposed to the corresponding serum levels towards the end of the administration interval seems to indicate that higher concentrations in tissue might be reached with repeated doses (1).

TABLE 2. *Distribution of amikacin in serum and muscle tissue*

No. of specimens	Time interval (h)	Mean serum concn (μg/ml)	Tissue concn (μg/g)	
			Muscle	Fat
19	1.5–3.5	11.64	1.8 (16%)[a]	1.47 (13%)
9	4–6	3.66	0.68 (19%)	0.98 (27%)
9	7–9	1.07	0.54 (51%)	0.5 (47%)
4	10–13	0.35	0.27 (77%)	0.25 (71%)

[a] Percentage of corresponding serum level.

TABLE 1. *Mean values, ranges, and standard deviations of the concentrations of amikacin in serum, muscle, and fat at given times after intramuscular administration to 41 children*

Specimen	Amikacin concn (μg/ml; μg/g) at:											
	1.5 h (6)[a]	2.5 h (5)	3.5 h (8)	4 h (4)	5 h (2)	6 h (3)	7 h (3)	8 h (3)	9 h (3)	11 h (1)	12 h (2)	13 h (1)
Serum	14.88	11.72	8.33	5.60	3.40	2.08	1.50	1.08	0.63	0.45	0.44	0.18
	4.39[b]	3.95	2.73	1.59	ND	1.00	0.7	1.28	0.39		ND	
	19.3[c]	15.4	11.4	7.0	4.3	1.8	2.04	2.56	0.9		0.72	
	7.0[c]	5.5	2.9	3.3	2.3	1.25	1.78	0.2	0.18		0.16	
Muscle	2.20	1.95	1.24	0.98	0.50	0.57	0.62	0.50	0.52	0.33	0.26	0.24
	1.28	0.73	1.13	0.01	ND	0.43	0.46	0.44	0.28		ND	
	4.45	2.9	4.16	1.1	0.75	0.85	1.0	0.85	0.75		0.52	
	0.8	1.06	0.6	0.9	0.25	<0.1	0.1	0.67	0.2		<0.1	
Fat	1.89	1.24	1.29	1.20	1.21	0.53	0.59	0.56	0.36	0.35	0.21	0.20
	0.73	0.57	0.55	0.41	ND	0.47	0.33	0.34	0.25		ND	
	2.81	1.82	2.1	1.60	1.62	0.89	0.98	0.88	0.65		0.42	
	1.0	0.4	0.6	0.7	0.8	<0.1	0.39	0.2	0.18		<0.1	

[a] Number in parentheses indicates number of specimens.
[b] ±1 standard deviation. ND, Not done.
[c] Ranges.

To the best of our knowledge there are only three studies of tissue concentrations of amikacin: two were in animals (K. E. Price, personal communication), and one was in humans as well as in other animals (W. Fry, J. P. Menezes, J. Ximenes, and J. Mimica, Prog. Abstr. Intersci. Conf. Antimicrob. Agents Chemother-apy, 15th, Washington, D.C., abstr. 87, 1975).

Comparison of our results with those reported from these studies is difficult since the amikacin doses were significantly larger in animals, and the amikacin tissue content in adult humans was not determined beyond the 3rd h after intramuscular administration of the drug. According to these studies, however, the amikacin content in muscle in children seems to be higher than that in adults and in beagle dogs; in adults none of 10 muscle specimens assayed 1, 2, and 3 h after 500 mg of amikacin administered intramuscularly showed drug concentrations greater than the least detectable amount (0.6 μg/g) in tissue. In dogs the amikacin content of muscle did not exceed 10% of the corresponding serum concentration.

So far fat has not been assayed in any study. The amikacin content in fat was found to be almost identical to that in muscle, whose blood supply is substantially superior to that of fat. Thus, amikacin does seem to have some affinity to fat.

This investigation was supported by a grant from Bristol-Myers GmbH, Germany.

LITERATURE CITED

1. **Barza, M., J. Brusch, M. G. Bergeron, and L. Weinstein.** 1974. Penetration of antibiotics into fibrin loci in vivo. III. Intermittent vs. continuous infusion and the effect of probenecid. J. Infect. Dis. **129**:73–78.
2. **Grove, D. C., and W. A. Randall.** 1955. Assay methods of antibiotics: a laboratory manual. Medical Encyclopedia, New York.
3. **Howard, J. B., and G. H. McCracken, Jr.** 1975. Pharmacological evaluation of amikacin in neonates. Antimicrob. Agents Chemother. 8:86–90.
4. **Sharpe, A. N., and A. K. Jackson.** 1972. Stomaching: a new concept in bacteriological sample preparation. Appl. Microbiol. 24:175–178.

Antimicrobial Agents and Chemotherapy, June 1977, p. 1084-1086
Vol. 11, No. 6

Printed in U.S.A.

Production of an Antibiotic by an Organism from Human Feces

WALLACE J. IGLEWSKI

Department of Microbiology and Immunology, University of Oregon Health Sciences Center, Portland, Oregon 97201

Received for publication 4 April 1977

An antibiotic-producing, gram-positive, rod-shaped bacterium was isolated from an individual who often lacked coliforms and fungi in fecal samples. The cell-free antibiotic is 1,200 daltons and Pronase sensitive and was shown to have activity against some coliforms and yeast.

Fecal samples from a healthy individual on a normal diet were found to lack or have low numbers of coliforms over a 19-month period (3). The absence of coliforms in fecal samples was always accompanied by the absence of fungi. Further examination of fecal flora from this individual revealed the presence of an antibiotic-producing bacterium. The isolation and partial characterization of the antibiotic are presented in this report. The cell-free antibiotic is effective against coliforms and a number of fungi when assayed in vitro, suggesting that the presence of the antibiotic-producing organism in the intestinal tract could account for the absence of coliforms and fungi in the fecal samples described in the previous report (3). The depressed level of resident coliforms, together with the repetitive isolation of an antibiotic-producing bacillus over a period of a year, also suggests that this microbe may be a member of the resident flora of this individual.

An antibiotic-producing organism was isolated from the subject's feces by dispersing 1 g of feces in 10 ml of phosphate-buffered saline, clarifying the extract by centrifuging the extract at 2,000 in the Sorvall SS-34 rotor, pelleting the bacterium from the extract at 10,000 rpm in the Sorvall SS-34 rotor, resuspending the pellet in phosphate-buffered saline, and streaking the resulting inoculum of intestinal flora onto MS coliform agar (5) freshly inoculated with an *Escherichia coli* 3000 lawn. After the lawns had grown, several 1-mm turbid plaques were observed. Inocula were taken from the turbid areas and streaked onto MS coliform and blood agar for isolation of pure cultures. Twenty-one distinct colony types were observed after incubation at 37°C for 24 h. Each of the bacterial isolates was streaked onto MS coliform agar plates and incubated 48 h at 37°C, and then *E. coli* 3000 was streaked 5 mm from each isolate in a parallel manner and incubated for an additional 24 h. One of the isolates, a gram-positive rod designated WWR, caused complete inhibition of *E. coli* growth. Isolate WWR produced grayish-white membranous colonies on MS agar and white, powdery undulant colonies surrounded by a slight hemolytic area on blood agar. This isolate tends to spread on MS coliform agar during the initial 48 to 72 h of incubation but forms discrete colonies on blood agar, 3 to 4 mm in diameter. A subsequent series of physiological and morphological tests indicated that WWR was a nonsporulating strain of *Bacillus subtilis* (manuscript in preparation).

As the number of subcultures on MS agar increased, the ability of WWR to inhibit growth of *E. coli* diminished. A number of media were examined for their ability to enhance the inhibitory effect. Sabouraud agar was found to be superior to MS agar, presumably because Neopeptone was preferred for antibiotic production (Table 1). Maximum inhibition of the *E. coli*

Table 1. *Inhibition of Escherichia coli growth by cocultivation with the WWR strain of Bacillus subtilis on agar media*

Incubation of WWR before inoculation of *E. coli* (h)	Zone of inhibition of *E. coli*[a] (mm)		
	MS agar (pH 6.8)	Sabouraud agar	
		pH 5.6	pH 7.0
24	0	±[b]	±
48	0	11	10
72	±	25	23
96	10	30	29
120	22	30	27

[a] Isolate was inoculated as a single streak across the agar medium and incubated for various periods of time at 37°C before inoculating a perpendicular streak of *E. coli* 3000. The zone of inhibition is defined as the distance between WWR and *E. coli* growth.

[b] ±, Reduced *E. coli* growth near WWR.

test strain occurred when WWR was preincubated on Sabouraud for 72 to 96 h at 37°C. In addition, subculturing WWR on blood agar was adopted since WWR occasionally produces colony variants on repeated subculture. Culturing on blood agar allows detection of these colony variants and subsequent selection and maintenance of the original colony type.

The isolate WWR was grown under a variety of broth culture conditions in attempts to produce a cell-free antibiotic. Growing WWR in MS or Sabouraud broth in deep or shallow stationary cultures at temperatures ranging from 22 to 37°C did not result in antibiotic production detectable by the antibiotic disk method. In addition, an antibiotic could not be detected in the cell-free media of cultures incubated under various degrees of aeration on reciprocating or rotary shakers. However, a cell-free antibiotic was recovered from Sabouraud agar plates only after growth of WWR. Sephadex gel filtration of the cell-free antibiotic activity indicated a single active component of approximately 1,200 daltons (Fig. 1). The antibiotic from the Sephadex gel produced a clear zone of inhibition of *Proteus vulgaris* UOMS-1-WI growth around the antbiotic-containing paper disk. An inoculum taken from the zone of inhibition did not grow in nutrient broth, indicating that the antibiotic has a bactericidal effect on the *P. vulgaris* used in the assay. The isolated antibiotic is similar in size to polymyxin B but does not bind to the heterogenous population of peptides in the media as does polymyxin B. In addition, the spectrum of action of the isolated antibiotic is different from the spectrum of action of polymyxin B (Table 2). Polymyxin B is effective against *Pseudomonas aeruginosa* but is not effective against *P. vulgaris* or fungi (2), whereas the reverse spectrum of action is observed for the newly isolated antibiotic. The antibiotic from WWR was also unusual in being equally effective against certain gram-negative bacteria and yeasts (Table 2). The cell-free antibiotic was dialyzable and was inactivated by treatment with Pronase (Table 3).

An antibiotic-producing organism with the same characteristics and antimicrobial spectrum of action as WWR has been isolated from the feces of the subject on three separate occasions over a 12-month period. The repeated isolation of an antibiotic-producing organism suggests that it may be a part of the intestinal flora of this individual and may cause the lack of coliforms and fungi in the individual's fecal samples (3). This mechanism assumes that the WWR strain of *Bacillus* can grow in the environment of the intestinal tract. This assumption appears reasonable since species of *Bacillus* are capable of in vitro growth under anaerobic conditions in complex media containing glucose (4). In addition, human stool samples have been shown to contain a mean value of 10^7 colony-forming units of *Bacillus* species per g of feces with a range of 10^4 to 10^{11} (1). The isolation of large numbers of *Bacillus* in feces suggests they may have the potential to grow in certain regions of the intestinal tract. The aerobic

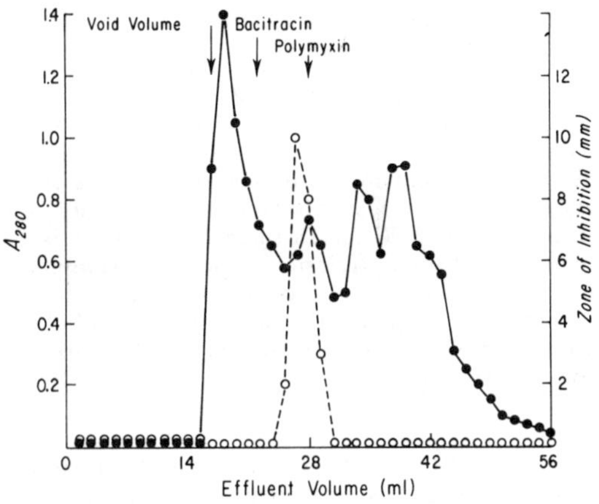

FIG. 1. *Molecular sieve chromatography of the cell-free antibiotic solution. The bacterial isolate was streaked onto Sabouraud agar and incubated at 37°C for 72 h. Eight milliliters of Sabouraud broth was added to the culture and incubated for 24 h at 5°C to allow diffusion of the antibiotic from the agar. The fluid was decanted, sterilized by membrane filtration (Millipore) and applied to a Sephadex G-15 column (0.9 by 30 cm) equilibrated with 15 mM tris(hydroxymethyl)aminomethane-hydrochloride buffer, pH 7.5. A flow rate of 16 ml/h was set, 1.4-ml fractions were collected, and the absorbance (A) at 280 nm of each fraction was measured. A 75-µl portion of each fraction was applied to a 13-mm paper disk (Schleicher and Schuell, Inc., Keene, N.H.) and placed on Sabouraud agar plates freshly inoculated with a lawn of Proteus vulgaris UOMS-1-WI. Cultures were incubated for 24 h at 37°C prior to recording the zone of inhibition of bacterial growth. The zone of inhibition was recorded as the diameter (millimeters) of the zone of inhibition of bacterial growth minus the diameter of the paper disk. The bacitracin marker (molecular weight = 1,411) was mixed with the isolated antibiotic before chromatography, and a 75-µl portion of each of the fractions was assayed for bacitracin activity on Sabouraud agar plates with Staphylococcus aureus UOMS-10 lawns. Since polymyxin B interacts with other proteins, it was chromatographed on the same bed of Sephadex after the isolated antibiotic had been eluted. Polymyxin B activity (molecular weight = 1,150) was assayed on Mueller-Hinton agar on a lawn of Escherichia coli 3000.*

TABLE 2. *Spectrum of action of the isolated antibiotic*

Organism tested	MIC titer[a]
Proteus vulgaris UOMS-1-WI	62
Escherichia coli 3000	2
Salmonella typhimurium UOMS-7	2
Shigella flexneri UOMS-8	4
Klebsiella pneumoniae UOMS-5	2
Pseudomonas aeruginosa UOMS-6	No effect
Candida albicans UOMS-2	128
Candida stellatoidea UOMS-3	8
Candida tropicallis UOMS-4	No effect
Saccharomyces cerevisiae UOMS-9	8
Aspergillus niger UOMS-1	No effect

[a] MIC titer was determined by making twofold serial dilutions of the sterile antibiotic solution in Sabouraud broth, inoculating with 0.1 ml of a 1:20 dilution of an exponentially growing culture of test organism having a turbidity at 610 nm of 0.1, and incubating at 37°C for 18 to 24 h. The titer is the reciprocal of the antibiotic dilution that completely lacked visual turbidity after the incubation period. A control for growth of the test organism in Sabouraud broth and a sterility control for the antibiotic solution were included.

sporeformers isolated from our subject ranged from 10^3 to 10^4 colony-forming units per g of feces (3).

ACKNOWLEDGMENTS

This investigation was supported by the University of Oregon Health Sciences Center, Portland, Oreg. I thank L. Smith and D. Ohman for technical assistance.

TABLE 3. *Effect of proteolytic enzymes on the antibiotic activity*[a]

Enzyme	Zone of inhibition (mm)	
	Enzyme + Sabouraud broth	Enzyme + antibiotic
Trypsin	0	19
Pronase	2	2

[a] Antibiotic produced by growth of the organism on Sabouraud agar and extracted with Sabouraud broth was filter-sterilized and incubated with trypsin or Pronase (1 mg/ml) for 8 h at 37°C. A 75-μl portion of each sample was applied to paper disks and assayed as described in the legend of Fig. 1. The untreated antibiotic produced a zone of inhibition of 19 mm.

LITERATURE CITED

1. **Attebery, H. R., V. L. Sutter, and S. M. Finegold.** 1974. Normal human intestinal flora, p. 81–97. *In* A. Borlows, R. M. DeHaan, V. R. Dowell, and L. B. Guye (ed.), Anaerobic bacteria – role in disease. Charles C Thomas, Springfield, Ill.
2. **Garrod, L. P., H. P. Lambert, F. O'Grady, and P. M. Waterworth.** 1973. Peptides, p. 179–195. *In* Antibiotic and chemotherapy. Churchill Livingstone, Edinburgh and London.
3. **Gerhardt, N. B., and W. G. Iglewski.** 1976. Alterations in the fecal flora of an individual frequently lacking coliforms. J. Infect. Dis. 134:490–494.
4. **Gibson, T., and R. E. Gordon.** 1974. Endospore-forming rods and cocci, p. 529–573. *In* R. E. Buchanan and N. E. Biggson (ed.), Bergey's manual of determinative bacteriology. Williams & Wilkins Co., Baltimore.
5. **Spangler, V. I., and W. J. Iglewski.** 1972. Effect of R17 bacteriophage-specific proteins on ribosomal ribonucleic acid synthesis of *Escherichia coli*. J. Virol. 9:792–799.

ANTIMICROBIAL AGENTS AND CHEMOTHERAPY, June 1977, p. 1087-1088
Vol. 11, No. 6

Rapid Penicillinase Paper Strip Test for Detection of Beta-Lactamase-Producing *Haemophilus influenzae* and *Neisseria gonorrhoeae*

JAMES H. JORGENSEN,* JEAN C. LEE, AND GARY A. ALEXANDER

Departments of Pathology and Microbiology, The University of Texas Health Science Center, and the Bexar County Hospitals, San Antonio, Texas 78284*

Received for publication 18 February 1977

A modified 1-min iodometric paper strip test for penicillinase activity was developed for detection of beta-lactamase-producing isolates of *Haemophilus influenzae* and *Neisseria gonorrhoeae*. The test is simple to perform and uses reagent-impregnated strips that may be stored for 1 year or more prior to use.

The emergence of ampicillin resistance in *Haemophilus influenzae* has caused considerable interest in rapid, reliable techniques for recognition of resistant isolates. Several new media formulations and procedures have been described for performance of reliable antimicrobial drug susceptibility tests (3, 4, 5, 9). However, all of these have been modifications of conventional susceptibility test methods that require an additional 18- to 24-h period for completion after the organism is isolated on primary growth media. More recently, penicillinase-producing strains of *Neisseria gonorrhoeae* have been isolated from at least 11 different countries, including the United States (Morbidity Mortality Weekly Rep. vol. 26, no. 5, p. 29, 4 February 1977). Like the ampicillin-resistant *Haemophilus* isolates, penicillin-resistant strains of gonococci may occur sporadically in widely separated geographic areas in the future.

Several rapid penicillinase tests have recently been described which allow recognition of beta-lactamase-producing (and thus penicillin- and ampicillin-resistant) bacteria as soon as growth is apparent on initial media (1, 2, 7, 8). The present report describes an even more rapid, simplified procedure for detection of penicillinase activity in *H. influenzae* and *N. gonorrhoeae* that is based on a method originally described by Shaefler (Abstr. Annu. Meet. Am. Soc. Microbiol. 1972, M209, p. 114).

Strips of Whatman no. 3 filter paper (approximately 5 by 1 cm) are immersed in a solution of 0.2% soluble starch (BBL) and 1% penicillin (potassium penicillin G for injection). The strips are then allowed to dry at room temperature for approximately 2 h on a perforated metal rack. Dried strips are then stored at −20°C, which ensures their stability for at least 1 year.

To perform the test, a strip is removed from the freezer and placed in a disposable plastic petri dish. The strip is thoroughly moistened with either Gram or Lugol iodine, producing a deep purple color, and excess liquid is then poured off. Approximately 10 colonies of the primary growth of the test organism on chocolate agar or Thayer-Martin medium are then applied to the center of the moistened strip by rubbing it with an inoculating loop in a circular fashion, describing a circle approximately 5 mm in diameter. For purposes of quality control, stock strains of *H. influenzae* or *N. gonorrhoeae* showing both ampicillin (or penicillin) resistance and susceptibility are likewise immediately applied to either end of the paper strip. If penicillinase is produced, the deep purple color of the strip becomes white within 1 min in the area where the organisms were applied. If penicillinase is not produced, the strip remains purple or becomes slightly yellow at the immediate site of inoculation. A completed test is considered valid only if the resistant control produces a large white zone, and the susceptible control strain does not.

The mechanism of the test involves a preliminary positive starch test as evidenced by the strip turning purple when iodine solution is added. The test area of the strip becomes white if penicilloic acid produced by the action of penicillinase converts the iodine to idoide, which is then no longer available to form the purple starch-iodine complex.

Parallel agar dilution ampicillin susceptibility tests (3) and penicillinase tests performed on a group of 100 isolates (68 susceptible, 32 resistant) of *H. influenzae* showed agreement between the two procedures in 99 of 100 instances. One strain had an ampicillin minimal inhibitory concentration (MIC) of 8 μg/ml, but consistently gave negative penicillinase tests by the present method and two previously described techniques (1, 7). This strain would seem to be unique in prossessing a resistance mechanism other than penicillinase production, and it bears further investigation.

Twenty-seven strains of *N. gonorrhoeae* were examined for penicillinase production and susceptibility to penicillin by an agar dilution procedure that uses Mueller-Hinton agar supplemented with 1% IsoVitaleX. Seventeen isolates were penicillinase test negative and had penicillin MICs of $\leq$0.5 U/ml, whereas 10 isolates with MICs of $\geq$2 U/ml yielded positive penicillinase tests.

The current policy in our hospital laboratory is to perform rapid penicillinase tests on all clinically significant *Haemophilus* isolates and all isolates of *N. gonorrhoeae*. These are followed by confirmatory conventional susceptibility testing of *H. influenzae* with ampicillin and chloramphenicol (3). This assures that ampicillin-resistant, but non-penicillinase-producing, strains, as well as the recently described chloramphenicol-resistant strains of *Haemophilus*, (6) may be detected. Likewise, any penicillinase-producing isolate of *N. gonorrhoeae* is verified by a conventional agar dilution susceptibility test. The method that we have described is a simpler, more rapid modification of the iodometric technique for detection of penicillinase activity. We have found it to be superior to previously described methods with respect to technical simplicity, time required, and stability of reagents.

LITERATURE CITED

1. **Catlin, B. W.** 1975. Iodometric detection of *Haemophilus influenzae* beta-lactamase: rapid presumptive test for ampicillin resistance. Antimicrob. Agents. Chemother. 7:265–270.
2. **Escamilla, J.** 1976. Susceptibility of *Haemophilus influenzae* to ampicillin as determined by use of a modified, one-minute beta-lactamase test. Antimicrob. Agents. Chemother. 9:196–198.
3. **Jorgensen, J. H., and P. M. Jones.** 1975. Simplified medium for ampicillin susceptibility testing of *Haemophilus influenzae*. Antimicrob. Agents. Chemother. 7:186–190.
4. **Jorgensen, J. H., and J. C. Lee.** 1975. Microdilution technique for antimicrobial susceptibility testing of *Haemophilus influenzae*. Antimicrob. Agents. Chemother. 8:610–611.
5. **Khan, W., S. Ross, W. Rodriguez, G. Controni, and A. K. Saz.** 1974. *Haemophilus influenzae* type B resistant to ampicillin. J. Am. Med. Assoc. 229:298–301.
6. **Manten, A., B. Van Klingersen, and Dessens-Kroon.** 1976. Chloramphenicol resistance in *Haemophilus influenzae*. Lancet 1:702.
7. **Scheifele, D. W., V. P. Syriopoulou, A. L. Harding, B. B. Emerson, and A. L. Smith.** 1976. Evaluation of a rapid B-lactamase test for detecting ampicillin-resistant strains of *Haemophilus influenzae* type b. Pediatrics 58:382–387.
8. **Thornesberry, C., and L. A. Kirven.** 1974. Ampicillin resistance in *Haemophilus influenzae* as determined by a rapid test for beta-lactamase production. Antimicrob. Agents. Chemother. 6:653–654.
9. **Thornesberry, C., and L. A. Kirven.** 1974. Antimicrobial susceptibility of *Haemophilus influenzae*. Antimicrob. Agents. Chemother. 6:620–624.
10. **Tomeh, M. O., S. E. Starr, J. E. McGowan, Jr., P. M. Terry, and A. J. Nahmias.** 1974. Ampicillin-resistant *Haemophilus influenzae* type B infection. J. Am. Med. Assoc. 229:295–297.

ERRATUM

Microassay for Amphotericin B

ROBERT M. BANNATYNE,* ROSE CHUENG, AND HANNA R. DEVLIN

Department of Bacteriology, The Hospital for Sick Children, Toronto, Ontario M561X8, Canada

Volume 11, no. 1, p. 44, column 2, line 8: "containing 100 mg/ml" should read "containing 1,000 mg/ml."

Page 44, column 2, line 18: "serum (heat inactivated and filtered) and 5 μg/ml" should read "serum (heat inactivated and filtered) to 5 μg/ml."

AUTHOR INDEX

VOLUME 11

Abedallah, Nadia, 373
Abreu, Sergio L., 521
Actor, P., 760
Afzelius, H., 388
Akl, Kamal F., 909
Alford, Robert H., 84
Allen, Norris E., 661, 669
Altenbern, Robert A., 574, 906
Alexander, Gary A., 1087
Allison, Richard G., 251
Anderson, Raymond J., 411
Anderson, Scott V., 968
Andrews, Fred A., 615
Anhalt, John P., 651, 914
Arnold, Keith, 645
Arroyo, Julio, 21, 760
Asher, Yael, 919
Atkinson, Barbara, 541
Azuma, Keizo, 743

Bach, Vinh, 258
Bach, Vinh Toan, 912
Bak, A. Leth, 388
Ballard, Charles A., 688
Bannatyne, Robert M., 44
Barabas, G., 392
Baraff, Larry J., 933
Baron, S., 80
Barros, Facelucia, 1071
Barthelemy, Michel, 785
Basker, M. J., 956
Becker, Yeichiel, 919
Beggs, William H., 615
Berech, John, Jr., 234
Berendt, R. F., 1069
Berg, Claire, M., 968
Bernard, Betty, 688
Bill, Nancy J., 470
Birnbaum, Jerome, 725
Black, H. R., 809
Bodey, Gerald P., 74, 865, 1017
Booth, S. J., 712
Borgers, M., 500
Brier, G. L., 809, 813
Brion, Nils, 594
Britt, Michael R., 240
Brown, Arthur D., 821
Brown, W. J., 1064
Bryson, Yvonne J., 299
Buck, R. E., 324
Buckmire, Francis L. A., 1010
Buettner, Karen R., 1036
Burke, John P., 240
Busch, David F., 427
Buss, Richard F., 897
Butler, Thomas, 645
Byrd, Daniel M., 312

Calia, Frank M., 441
Carbon, Claude, 594
Carreira, José, 38
Cesario, Thomas C., 291
Chakrabarty, A. N., 1079
Chao, Lee, 161
Chao, Lian-Yu, 451
Chatterjee, Arun K., 897
Cheung, Rose, 38
Chiu, Peter J. S., 821
Cho, Dong Tåek, 209
Chow, Anthony W., 679
Chun, Doki, 209
Ciak, Jennie, 176
Clark, Virginia L., 871, 877
Clough, D. W., 307
Cohen, Yaffa, 919
Colding, Hanne, 214
Cole, M., 852
Cole, Donald R., 1033
Collins, M. S., 1049
Comber, K. R., 956
Contrepois, Alain, 594
Cosgrove, R. F., 31, 848
Counts, George W., 708
Courvalin, Patrice, 619
Craig, William A., 462
Crenshaw, R. R., 571
Crosa, Jorge H., 553
Crosby, Ruth, 826
Cundliffe, Eric, 491

Dankert, J., 1074
Darland, Gary, 725
Daschner, F., 1081
Dastidar, Sujata G., 1079
Davies, Julian, 491, 619
Dean, Evelyn, 171
De Clercq, Erik, 756
de Menezes, Jairo Perche, 331
De Nollin, Sonja, 500
Dessens-Kroon, M., 383
Deveikis, A., 817
Devlin, Hanna R., 47
Dhawan, Vijay, 64
Diaz, Carlos R., 965
Dillion, Hugh C., Jr., 1021
Dolak, L., 569
Dominik, J. W., 1069
Donoghue, Helen D., 34
Dougherty, Paula F., 225
Dowding, J. E., 47
Dowling, John N., 656
Duncan, I. B. R., 179

Ehret, Josephine M., 791
Eickhoff, Theodore C., 791
Elwell, Lynn P., 528
Engel, H. W. B., 925
Engel, Robert, 147
Engert, Jurgen, 1081
Espinel-Ingroff, Ana, 365
Eriksson, Bertil, 946
Evans, James B., 1077
Everett, E. Dale, 171
Eylan, Emanuael, 797

Fairbrother, J. E., 31
Falkow, Stanley, 528
Fanning, W. Lee, 712
Fathy, Shadia, 373
Faulkner, D. John, 411
Feldman, Rhoda I., 359
Felix, Haya, 202
Finegold, Sydney M., 427
Fisher, John F., 365
Flodström, Anders, 185
Foglesong, M. A., 174
Forsgren, Arne, 580
Fossieck, Byron E., Jr., 965
Frame, Peter T., 244
Freeman, K. B., 563
Fukuda, Shigemi, 51

Garcia-Cazares, Salvador J., 688
Garibaldi, Richard A., 240
Gerding, Dale N., 993
Glew, Richard H., 1036
Glotzbecker, Cheryl, 88
Goodwin, C. S., 26
Goossens, F., 500
Gordon, N., 773
Goyer, S., 638
Gray, Barry M., 1021
Greenberg, Joseph, 534
Gregory, David, 708
Griffith, R. S., 809, 813
Griffiths, A., 599
Gröschel, Dieter, 277
Guionie, Marlene, 785
Gump, Dieter W., 712
Gurwith, M., 780
Guze, Lucien B., 679

Haggerty, D. Lynne, 881
Hagiwara, Sumiko, 952
Hahn, Fred E., 176, 251
Hallander, Hans O., 185
Hamilton, Rebecca, 826
Hammerberg, S., 566
Harding, G., 780
Harik, Sami I., 909
Harrell, Lizzie J., 1077
Hasegawa, Mitsuto, 376
Hebertson, Richard M., 240
Hedges, R. W., 585
Heitz, Mary Ann, 858
Helgstrand, Erik, 946
Helsa, Mary Ann, 858

Henderson, David K., 679
Heseltine, Peter N. R., 427
Hewitt, William L., 768
Highsmith, Anita K., 449
Hill, Gale B., 625
Hill, Joyce P., 26
Hilmas, D. E., 80
Hirschman, Shalom Z., 118, 248, 369
Hoban, S., 780
Hoeprich, Paul D., 7
Hong, Jen-Shiang, 881
Hopfer, Roy L., 277, 248
Horne, Diane, 888
Hornick, Richard B., 441
Hubbell, Carol A., 1021
Huber, F. M., 455
Hui, J., 773

Iglewski, Wallace J., 1084
Isenberg, Henry D., 271
Ishikawa, Tomoaki, 999

Jackson, Andre, 331
Jackson, Roger T., 84
Jagdis, F., 780
Janik, Borek, 756
Jensen, Herluf, 214
Johansson, K. Nils Gunnar, 946
Johnson, J. K., 718
Johnson, Marcia, 171
Jones, P. M., 415
Jordan, George W., 7
Jorgensen, James H., 1087
Jorgensen, J. H., 415
Jouvenot, M., 581

Kajioka, R., 773
Kamimura, Toshiaki, 51
Kampmann, Jens P., 214
Kane, James G., 965
Kantor, Robert J., 126
Katz, Edward, 281
Katz, E., 1056
Katz, Ehud, 202
Kauffman, Carol A., 244
Keith, Alex, 98
Keller, Gregory, 98
Kilburn, James O., 534
Kirven, Linda A., 1004
Klein, Richard D., 559
Kobayashi, George S., 21, 154, 803
Koch, Patricia A., 462
Kondo, Isamu, 999
Kono, Yoko, 51
Kornguth, Margaret L., 974
Korzeniowski, Oksana M., 1071
Kotler-Brajburg, Janina, 803
Kozukue, Hiroyuki, 999
Kronenberg, L. H., 299
Kuehne, Ralph W., 92, 683
Kundsin, Ruth B., 267
Kumar, Ranajit, 1079
Kunin, Calvin M., 974

Kuwahara, Rie, 952
Kuwahara, Shogo, 13, 952

Labia, Roger, 785
Lamotte-Barrillon, Suzanne, 594
Larsson, Alf, 946
Lau, Curtis C., 462
LeBlanc, Barbara, 1017
Lee, Jean C., 1087
Lee, J. C., 415
Lee, Lanfong H., 753
Levy, H. B., 80
Levy, Louis, 122
Lieberman, Michael A., 881
Lin, Hsiu-san, 132
Linh, Nguyen Ngoc, 645
Leedom, J. M., 420
Long, James F., 821
Lopez, Carlos E., 441
Lorian, Victor, 541
Lucas-Lenard, Jean, 521
Luginbuhl, G. H., 559
Luthrop, Linda K., 553

MacGregor, Rob Roy, 110
Madsen, Paul O., 262
Maeda, Hiroshi, 941
Mahon, W. A., 359
Mahony, David E., 1067
Maldonado, Barbara, 858
Marks, M. I., 566
Marso, Eugene, 64
Martin, R. Russell, 407
Martin, William J., 64
Martins, Katia, 1071
Mason, K. T., 1056
Masson, Jean-Michel, 785
Masuda, Gohta, 376
Mata, Leonardo J., 553
Mathies, A. W., Jr., 420
Mathies, Allen W., 688
Matthews, Thomas R., 225
Matusiak, P. M., 735
Mauger, A. B., 1056
Mayer, Leonard W., 528
Mayo, Joan B., 844
McCarthy, Laurence R., 844
Medoff, Gerald, 21, 154, 760
Mellin, Hans-Eberhard, 262
Merati, Wilma, 396
Merigan, Thomas C., 122
Meyer, Richard D., 427
Meyers, Burt R., 118, 248, 369
Michel-Briand, Y., 589
Miller, Albert, 369
Miller, George H., 821
Miller, William A., 240
Mirhij, Najwa, 1027
Misiorny, Alfons, 946
Mitsuhasi, Susumu, 999
Mizak, S., 569
Mizen, M., 817
Moellering, Robert C., Jr., 1036
Moffatt, John G., 191, 198

Mogyoros, M., 362
Mogyoros, Miguel, 750
Møller, J. K., 388
Moore, Barbara A., 993
Moreschi, Gail, 609
Morgan, J. R., 362
Morgan, John R., 750
Mueller, Donna, 826
Muir, P., 780
Muñoz, Emilio, 38
Murakawa, Takeo, 1, 51, 1042
Murray, Patrick, R., 605
Myers, Martin G., 1027

Nakahara, Hideomi, 999
Nakamoto, Shoji, 51
Nakazawa, Atsushi, 219
Neuhaus, D. W., 638
Neuhaus, F. C., 638
Nishida, Minoru, 51, 1042
Nishiyama, Shinya, 198
Nitzan, Dorrit, 435
Nomura, Akio, 191
Norden, Carl W., 126
Nórén, Jan Olof, 946

Oberg, Bo, 946
O'Brien, William M., 132
Ogata, Jiro, 941
O'Grady, F., 585
Okada, Naohiko, 51
Olarte, Jorge, 553
Osborne, Christine D., 956
Overturf, G. D., 420, 933

Pan, Theresa, 74
Pannier, Wallace L., 92, 683
Pappagianis, D., 1050
Parenti, Francesco, 396
Parker, Richard H., 965
Parkhurst, J. Rodney, 307
Pato, Martin L., 318
Pearson, N. J., 585
Penaranda, Maria E., 553
Person, Stanley, 98
Peterson, Lance R., 993
Pestka, Sidney, 978
Pfeffer, Morris, 331
Phillipippon, Alain, 785
Phillips, Ian, 402
Philipson, Lennart, 946
Pieper, R. L., 455
Pitkin, D. H., 760
Poddar, Roma, 1079
Postic, Bosko, 656
Price, K. E., 324
Prusoff, William H., 312
Pugsley, Anthony P., 345
Pung, Juanito, 1033
Putman, Margaret, 407

Reading, C., 852
Reeves, Peter, 345
Regeur, Lisbeth, 214
Reib, E., 1081

Reiss, E., 1081
Renis, Harold E., 701
Rennie, R. P., 179
Riff, Louise J., 609
Riff, L., 817
Roberts, Marilyn, 528
Roberts, Robert J., 1027
Robertson, R. G., 735
Rocha, Heonir deJ., 1071
Ronald, A. R., 780
Rosenblatt, Jon E., 605
Rossomando, Edward F., 858
Roy, Ira, 258, 912
Rubinstein, Ethan, 577
Rugloski, Raymond J., 132
Ryan, D. M., 599
Ryan, Raymond, 114

Sabath, L. D., 1
Sachs, C., 760
Sakamoto, Hiroshi, 51
Sakamoto, Sadaaki, 941
Salstrom, Sara Jane, 698
Salyers, A. A., 142
Sammons, M. L., 80
Sande, Merle A., 1071
Santos, Luiz Carlos, 1071
Sarai, Yasunaga, 999
Sarosi, George A., 615
Sato, Kosaburo, 191, 198
Saunders, J. R., 339
Saunders, Priscilla P., 451
Sautter, R. L., 1064
Schaberg, Dennis R., 449
Schauf, V., 817
Scherr, George H., 459
Schimpff, Stephen C., 441
Schlessinger, David, 783
Schmeling, David, 580
Schmidt, L. H., 826
Schoen, Howard F., 234
Schryer, Patricia J., 291
Schwartzman, Joseph D., 695
Sebek, O. K., 569
Seno, E. T., 455
Seol, Sung Yong, 209
Shadomy, Smith, 229, 365
Shainberg, Bracha, 577
Shannon, Kevin, 402
Shimi, Ibrahim R., 373
Shlomai, Joseph, 919
Siegel, E. B., 675
Siminoff, Paul, 571
Sjövall, Jan, 185
Smetana, Ofire, 797
Smith, Anne, 402
Smith, J. A., 362
Smith, John A., 750
Snipes, Wallace, 98

Snyder, Merrill J., 441
Sofferman, Robert A., 712
Sokolski, W. T., 569
Somma, Sergio, 396
Sommer, Ronald G., 756
Sorger, S., 566
Sottile, William, II, 482
Spaepen, Moniek S., 267
Spratt, Bryan G., 161
Spyker, Daniel A., 132
Standiford, Harold C., 441
Stanisich, Vilma A., 589
Starr, Mortimer P., 897
Steinberg, Evan A., 933
Steinberg, E. A., 420
Stenberg, Kjell, 946
Stenderup, A., 388
Stening, Göran, 946
Stephen, E. L., 80, 1069
Stephen, Edward L., 92, 683
Stevens, Paul, 768
Stewart, Dorothy, 865, 1017
Stridh, Stig, 946
Stringfellow, Dale A., 984
Stroman, D. W., 569
Sutherland, R., 956
Suzuki, Nobuo, 219
Sykes, R. B., 339, 529
Szabo, G., 392

Tak, Ryonbin, 209
Tamada, Terumi, 219
Tan, James S., 698
Tang, Chu-Tay, 147
Tatem, Beverly A., 441
Taylor, William, 98
Thadepalli, Haragopal, 258, 912
Thomas, Frank E., 84
Thoné, F., 500
Thornsberry, Clyde, 1004
Thrupp, Lauri D., 688
Tilles, Jeremiah G., 291
Tilton, Richard C., 114, 271
Tomasz, Alexander, 888
Tomioka, Susumu, 376
Tropp, Burton E., 147
Turck, Marvin, 708

Uchica, Hiroshi, 376
Underman, A. E., 420
Underwood, Gerald E., 765
Uwaydah, Marwan, 909

Van Belle, H., 500
van Embden, J. D. A., 383, 925
van Klingeren, B., 925
van Klingeren, V., 383
Vann, Robert L., 132
Vaughn, Dennis, 826

Venezia, Richard A., 735
Vialard, J. L., 585

Wachsmuth, Ina K., 449
Wagner, Gerald E., 229
Waitz, J. Allan, 821
Walker, Clay B., 435
Walker, J. S., 1069
Walter, Harry, 978
Wang, Ching Yung, 753
Wang, Wen Lan Lou, 171
Wang, Wen-Lan L., 695
Washington, John A., II, 470
Watanakunakorn, Chatrchai, 88, 1007
Wayne, Lawrence G., 978
Wee, Siok-Hui, 914
Weed, Sheldon D., 765
Wehrle, P. F., 420
Wehrle, Paul F., 688
Weinberg, Miriam, 797
Weinberg-Zahlering, Eynat, 919
Welling, Peter G., 262, 462
Westhead, Jack E., 919
Wilkins, Jeanette, 933
Wilkins, J., 420
Wilkins, Tracy D., 435
Wilkins, T. D., 142, 718
Williams, J. A., 514
Williams, Jimmy C., 475
Williams, W. Kenneth, 281
Williams, W. K., 1056
Wilson, Samuel Z., 407
Winkelhake, Jeffrey L., 1010
Wold, John S., 105
Wolfe, Margaret S., 411
Wolny, J. D., 809, 813
Woltjes, J., 1074
Wong, J., 142
Woodman, Daniel R., 475
Wratten, Stephen J., 411
Wüst, Jürg, 631

Ximenes, Jose, 331

Yamada, Yasuo, 743
Yamamoto, Tatsuo, 936
Yamanaka, Toshihiko, 198
Yokota, Takeshi, 13, 936, 952
Yokota, Yoshiko, 51
Yotter, David W., 225
Young, Frank E., 871, 877
Young, Lowell S., 768

Zabransky, R. J., 482
Zachariae, H., 388
Zajac, I., 760
Zeleznik, Dolores, 708
Zinneman, Horace H., 993

SUBJECT INDEX

VOLUME 11

Acinetobacter calcoaceticus
carbenicillin and aminocyclitols, 1036
Actinomycin D
S. parvulus, 281
Actinomycins
cis- and *trans-*4-methylproline incorporation, 1056
Adenine arabinoside
antiviral effects, 299
with interferon, 299
Adenine arabinoside 5-monophosphate
antiviral effects, 299
with interferon, 299
Allicin
antifungal activity, 743
6β-Amidinopenicillanic acid, 161
Amikacin
aminoglycoside phosphotransferase, 619
compared with netilmicin, 64
dialysis, 214
distribution in rabbit tissue, 974
interstitial fluid, 698
in vitro activity 126, 791
penetration into exudate fluid, 110
pharmacokinetics, 214
pharmacokinetics in infants, 933
tissue distribution in children, 1081
2-Amino-5-bromo-6-methyl-4-pyrimidinol (U-25, 166)
antiviral properties, 984
interferon induction, 984
Aminoglycoside phosphotransferase
amikacin, 619
Aminoglycosidic amino cyclitols
synergy with carbenicillin, 1036
A. calcoaceticus, 1036
6-Aminopenicillanic acid
P. mirabilis, 541
E. coli, 541
S. aureus, 541
Amoxicillin
acute urinary infection, 780
dose dependence, 132
Amphotericin B
antioxidants, 615
aspergillosis, 21
Bactec system, 277
bioactivity, 615
bioassay method, 31
C. immitis, 1049
dose response, 803
effects on macrophages, 154
filipin, 803
HeLa cells, 803
microassay, 44
yeasts, 277
Ampicillin
anti R-plasmid compounds, 176
H. influenzae, 559
H. influenzae MICs, 114
resistance 553, 1021
Salmonella (nontyphoid), 577
S. dysenteriae, 553
Shigella, 577
S. typhimurium, 176
Anaerobe growth
four commonly used media, 482
Anaerobes
cefoxitin susceptibility, 912
ticarcillin, 258
2,2′-Anhydro-1-β-D-arabinofuranosylcytosine
acyl derivatives, 191
antiviral activity, 191
encephalitis, 198
Antibiotic susceptibility test device
performance parameters, 271
Anti-R-plasmid compounds
ampicillin, 176
S. typhimurium, 176
Antiviral compounds
indirect mouse model, 683
Venezuelan equine encephalomyelitis virus, 603
1-β-D-arabinofuranosyl cytosine
acyl derivatives, 191
antiviral activity, 191
Aspergillosis
amphotericin B therapy, 21
5-fluorocytosine, 21
rifampin therapy, 21
Atebrin
effect on bacterial membrane ATPases, 38
Autobac-1 susceptibility testing
evaluation, 750

Bacillus subtilis
D-cyloserine resistance, 871
transport of D-alanine and glycine, 877
Bactec system
amphotericin B, 277
yeasts, 277
Bacteriocin production
Bacteroides, 718
feces, 718
Bacteriophage T4*td*8*r*II
5-iodouracil, 312
Bacteriuria
catheter-associated, 240
Bacteroides
bacteriocin production, 718
Bacteroides fragilis
chemotherapy, 435
Bacteroides fragilis subsp. *fragilis*
synergy between cefamandole and erythromycin, 813
Bacteroides melaninogenicus
β-lactamase,142
penicillin resistance, 605

penicillinase production, 605
Bacteroides oralis
β-lactamase, 142
BL-20803
analogues, 571
interferon, 571
leukocytes, 571
BL-P1624
P. aeruginosa, 441
Bioassay method
for polyene antibiotics, 31
Bone marrow toxicity
5-fluorocytosine, 244
Broad-spectrum penicillin
mezlocillin,74

Cairomycin B, 373
Carbenicillin
anaerobes, 258
interstitial fluid, 698
meningitis, 420
P. aeruginosa, 1, 441, 589
serum, 698
versus ampicillin, 420
versus ticarcillin, 258
Catheter-associated bacteriuria
prophylaxis, 240
Cefaclor
in vitro activity, 470
versus cephalexin and cephradine, 470
Cefadroxil
broad-spectrum cephalosporin, 324, 331
versus cephalexin and cephadrine, 331
Cefamandole
B. fragilis subsp. *fragilis*, 813
erythromycin synergy, 813
interstitial fluid penetration, 594, 698
pharmacokinetics, 248, 262
probenecid, 809
renal failure, 248, 262
serum, 698
spinal fluid penetration, 933
S. typhi, 369
Cefazaflur
in vitro studies, 708
Cefazolin
analysis of serum levels, 105
bactericidal activity, 1037
exudate levels, 1037
interstitial fluid, 594, 698
liquid chromatography (high pressure), 105
pleural fluid, 1033
rat granuloma system, 1037
serum, 698
Cefazolin sodium
distribution in rabbit tissues, 760
Cefoxitin
anaerobe susceptibility, 679, 912
B. fragilis, 725
clinical evaluation, 427
K. pneumoniae, 84
β-lactamase resistance, 725
lysis of enterobacteria, 26
Cefuroxime
H. influenzae, 599
Cephadrine
in vitro activity, 470
penetration into cerebrospinal fluid, 909
versus other cephalosporins, 331, 470
Cephalexin
in vitro activity, 470
versus other cephalosporins, 331, 470
Cephaloridine
interstitial fluid penetration, 594
Cephalosporin
cefadrozil, 324
cefazaflur, 708
cephadrine, 331
cephalexin, 331
FR 10024, 51
horse serum, 174
stability, 174
Cephalothin
interstitial fluid, 698
serum, 698
Cerulenin
cell inhibition, 574
inhibition of staphylococcal enterotoxin A and B, 906
S. aureus, 574
Chemotaxis
antibiotics, 580
leukocytes, 580
Chloramphenicol
H. influenzae, 383
nontyphoid *Salmonella*, 577
plasmid-mediated resistance, 383
Shigella, 577
Chloramphenicol acetyltransferase
cyclic adenylic acid, 952
E. coli, 952
D-chloramphenicol
N-trifluoroacetyl analogue, 563
Chlorhydroxyquinoline
rapid microbiological assay, 848
Cinoxacin
nontyphoid *Salmonella*, 577
Shigella, 577
Clavulanic acid
β-lactamase-inhibiting β-lactam, 852
S. clavuligerus, 852
Closed circular deoxyribonucleic acid
anti-R-plasmid drugs, 251
intercalation, 251
primaquine, 251
superhelical density, 251
Clostridium perfringens
bacteriocins, 1067
mitomycin, 1067
susceptibility to twenty antibiotics, 695
Coccidioides immitis
amphotericin B, 1049
Colicin B-K260
characterization, 345
purification, 345
Colicin D-CA23
characterization, 345
purification, 345
Colicin E1 induction
glucose requirements, 219

Colicin K
  ecf mutant, 881
  E. coli, 881
  energy-coupling factor, 881
Cyclic adenylic acid
  chloramphenicol acetyltransferase, 952
  E. coli, 952
D-Cycloserine
  B. subtilis, 871
  inducible resistance, 871
  transport of D-alanine and glycine, 877
Cytomegalovirus
  susceptibility to human interferon, 656

3-Deazauridine
  Japanese B encephalitis virus, 475
  with 3-deoxy-D-glucose, 475
2-Deoxy-D-glucose
  Japanese B encephalitis virus, 475
  with 3-deazauridine, 475
5,6-Dihydro-5-azathymidine
  herpes simplex virus, 765
Doxycycline
  bioavailability, 462
Drug resistance plasmids
  in *S. typhi,* 209

Encephalitis
  2,2′-anhydro-1-β-D-arabinofuranosylcytosine, 198
  HSV-1, 307
  trifluoromethyl-2′-deoxyuridine, 307
Enterobacteria
  lysis by cefoxitin, cefuroxime, and cephalothin, 26
Equine encephalitis virus
  tilorone hydrochloride, 92
Erwinia amylovora
  barrier function of cell envelope, 897
Erythrocyte damage
  measurement, 675
  polyene antibiotics, 675
Erythromycin
  B. fraglis subsp. *fragilis,* 813
  cefamandole synergy, 813
  S. aureus, 407
Escherichia coli
  altered surface properties, 978
  6β-amidinopenicillanic acid derivatives, 161
  amino acid transport, 968
  6-aminopenicillanic acid, 541
  cephalosporins, 933
  colicin K, 881
  ecf mutant, 881
  energy-coupling factor, 881
  inhibition by D-norvalyl-D-alanine, 638
  β-lactam antibiotics, 968
  β-lactamase-directed barrier, 936
  mecillam, 541
  mercury resistance, 999
  morganocin, 514
  nalidixic acid, 167
  penicillins, 936
  protein alterations, 167
  R-plasmids, 936
  streptomycin-resistant mutants, 978
Ethanbutol
  M. smegmatis, 534

Filipin
  dose response, 803
  HeLa cells, 803
  L cells, 803
5-Fluorocytosine
  aspergillosis, 21
  bone marrow toxicity, 244
  gas chromatographic determination, 914
5-Fluorouracil
  growth inhibition of *S. fimicola,* 234
FR 10024
  cephalosporin derivative, 51

Gardimycin
  peptidoglycan synthesis inhibitor, 396
Genital HSV-2
  chemotherapy, 701
L-Glyceraldehyde 3-phosphate
  bactericidal agent, 147
Gentamicin
  assay by high-pressure liquid chromatography, 651
  compared with netilmicin, 64
  distribution in rabbit tissue, 974
  hemagglutination inhibition assay, 359
  interstitial fluid, 698
  in vitro activity, 126, 791
  new assay procedure, 1074
  P. aeruginosa, 441
  penetration into exudate fluid, 110
  serum, 698
  versus netilmicin, 118, 402, 609
  with pirbenicillin, 441
  with tobramycin, 88
Gentamicin resistance
  Klebsiella, 179
  S. aureus, 47
Haemophilus influenzae
  ampicillin, 114, 559, 599
  ampicillin-resistant, 1021
  bactericidal factor, 735
  cefuroxime, 599
  chloramphenicol, 383
  penicillinase paper strip test, 1087
  plasmid, 383
  plasmid-specified β-lactamase gene, 339
  susceptibility testing, 1021
Haemophilus parainfluenzae
  antimicrobial susceptibility, 844
HeLa cells
  amphotericin B, 803
  filipin, 803
Hemagglutination inhibition assay
  gentamicin, 359
Herpes simplex virus
  cutaneous, 765
  5,6-dihydro-5-azathymidine, 765
  herpetic keratitis, 797
  inhibition by polyinosinic acid-polycytidylic acid, 797
Herpes simplex virus type 1
  encephalitis, 307
  5-trifluoromethyl-2′-deoxyuridine, 307
Herpes simplex virus type 2
  chemotherapy, 701
  genital, 701

High-pressure liquid chromatography cefazolin analysis, 105
Horse serum
cephalosporins, 174
Hydroxamic acids
antibacterial activity, 753
mutagenicity, 753
Hypoxanthine arabinoside
antiviral effect, 299
with interferon, 299

Influenza virus
Ribavirin triphosphate, 946
RNA polymerase, 946
Interferon
antiviral effects, 299
BL 20803 analogues, 571
cytomegalovirus, 656
human, 291
human fibroblast cultures, 299
5-Iodouracil
phage T4*td*8*r*II, 312
Ionenes
interferon induction, 756
poly(inosinic acid)·poly(cytidylic acid), 756
Isatin β-thiosemicarbazone
HeLa cells, 202
vaccinia viral antigens, 202

Japanese B encephalitis virus
3-deazauridine, 475
2-deoxy-D-glucose, 475
Josamycin
S. aureus, 407

Kanamycin
in vitro activity, 791
Klebsiella pneumoniae
cefoxitin activity, 84
multiple resistance, 84
Klebsiella
gentamicin resistance, 179

β-Lactam antibiotics
amino acid transport, 968
bactericidal activity, 376
bacteriostatic activity, 376
E. coli, 968
β-Lactamase
barrier for penicillins and cephalosporins, 936
B. melaninogenicus, 142
B. oralis, 142
carbenicillin-resistant, 785
E. coli, 936
gene transfer by *N. gonorrhoeae,* 1004
H. influenzae, 339
N. gonorrhoeae, 528
P. aeruginosa, 785
plasmid-specified, 399
R plasmids, 936
β-lactamase production
N. gonorrhoeae, 528
β-Lactams
S. sanguis, 888
L cells
amphotericin B, 803
filipin, 803
Leukocytes
antibiotics, 580
chemotaxis, 580
Lipid-containing viruses
inactivation by long-chain alcohols, 98

Macrolide resistance
S. aureus, 661, 669
Macromycin
bactericidal activity, 1010
Macrophages
amphotericin B, 154
Marine pseudomonad
antibiotic metabolites, 411
Mecillam
P. mirabilis, 541
E. coli, 541
S. aureus, 541
Megacin C, 34
Megacin Cx, 34
Membrane ATPases
effect of atebrin, 38
Mercury resistance
E. coli, 999
R-plasmids, 999
Methicillin
against enterococci, 88
combined with gentamicin and tobramycin, 88
3-Methyleneoxindole
cellular protein synthesis, 521
viral protein synthesis, 521
Metronidazole
anaerobes, 631, 679
Mezlocillin
broad-spectrum penicillin, 74
Miconazole
bioassay, 365
yeasts, 500
Minocycline
mixed anaerobic infection, 625
side effects, 712
Mitomycin C
bacteriocins, 1067
C. perfringens, 1067
Morganocin
E. coli, 514
plasmid, 514
production, 514
Proteus, 514
Mycobacteria
rifampin, 773
Mycobacterium chelonei
radiometric susceptibility test, 763
Mycobacterium leprae
polyinosinic-polycytidylic acid, 122
Mycobacterium smegmatis
ethambutol, 534

Nafcillin
absorption, 965
cerebrospinal fluid, 965
enterococci, 88
with gentamicin and tobramycin, 88
Nalidixic acid
E. coli

protein alterations, 167
Neisseria gonorrhoeae
β-lactamase production, 528, 1004
Neocarzinostatin
accumulation in bladder tissue, 941
Netilmicin
antibacterial activity, 402
^{125}I radioimmunoassay, 768
in vitro activity, 126, 791, 1017
renal pharmacology, 821
versus amikacin, 64
versus gentamicin, 64, 118, 402, 609
versus gisomicin, 118
versus tobramycin, 64, 118, 609
D-Norvalyl-D-alanine
inhibition of *E. coli,* 638
Nystatin
Bioassay method, 31

Ornidazole
anaerobes, 631
Oxacillin
combined with gentamicin and tobramycin, 88

Penicillin
anaerobes, 258
mezlocillin, 74
S. griseus, 392
streptomycin production, 392
versus ticarcillin, 258
Penicillinase paper strip test
H. influenzae, 1087
Penicillinase production
B. melaninogenicus, 605
Penicillin G
pentration into exudate fluid, 110
protein interactions, 993
Penicillin resistance
B. melaninogenicus, 605
Peptidoglycan synthesis
gardinycin, 396
inhibition, 396
Pirbenicillin
P. aeurginosa, 1, 441
versus carbenicillin, 441
with gentamicin, 441
Polyene antibiotics
bioassay method, 31
erythrocyte damage, 675
Polyinosinic-polycytidylic acid
M. leprae, 122
Poly(inosinic acid)·poly(cytidylic acid)
antiviral properties, 984
interferon induction, 756, 984
ionenes, 756
Probenecid
cefamandole, 809
Propionibacterium acnes
susceptibility to seventeen antibiotics, 171
Proteus
morganocin, 514
Proteus mirabilis
6-aminopenicillanic acid, 54
mecillam, 541
Pseudomonas aeruginosa
carbencillin resistance plasmid, 589
carbenicillin-resistant, 785
five-hour minimal inhibitory concentration test, 1064
in vitro activity of antibiotics, 1
β-lactamase, 785
susceptibility test medium, 415
ticarcillin, 956
tobramycin, 956

Radiometric susceptibility test
M. chelonei, 763
Renal failure
cefamandole, 248, 262
Ribavirin
influenza virus, 1069
intraperitoneal versus aerosol administration, 1069
Ribavirin triphosphate
inhibition of influenza virus RNA polymerase, 1069
Rifampin
aspergillosis, 21
permeability barrier in mycobacteria, 773
R plasmids
E. coli, 936
temperature-sensitive, 13
V. cholerae, 13, 585, 1079
Rubidium efflux
bioassay method for polyene antibiotics, 31

Salmonellae
in vitro antibiotic susceptibility, 1071
Salmonella (nontyphoid)
ampicillin, 577
chloramphenicol, 577
cinoxacin, 577
Salmonella typhi
cefamandole, 369
Salmonella typhi
drug resistance plasmids, 209
Salmonella typhimurium
ampicillin, 176
anti-R-plasmid compounds, 176
Serratia mercescens
resistance plasmids, 449
urine, 449
Shigella
ampicillin, 577
chloramphenicol, 577
cinoxacin, 577
Shigella dysenteriae type 1
ampicillin resistance, 553
R-plasmid, 553
Sisomycin
versus netilmicin, 118
Sordaria fimicola
5-fluorouracil inhibition, 234
Staphylococcal enterotoxin B and C
cerulenin inhibition, 906
Staphylococci
effect of anaerobiosis on antimicrobial susceptibility, 1077

Staphylococcus aureus
6-aminopenicillanic acid, 541
cerulenin inhibition, 574
erythromycin, 407
gentamicin, 47
josamycin, 407
macrolide resistance, 661, 669
mecillam, 541
nasal carriage, 407
susceptibility to newer antibiotics, 7
Streptococcal infection
antimicrobial therapy, 817
group B, 817
Streptococci (group B)
antimicrobial therapy, 817
Streptococci (group D)
drug resistance, 925
Streptococcus sanguis
β-lactams, 888
Streptomyces clavuligerus
clavulinic acid, 852
β-lactamase-inhibiting β-lactam, 852
Streptomyces griseus
penicillin effect, 392
streptomycin production, 392
Streptomyces parvulus
actinomycin D, 281
Streptomycin
S. griseus production, 392
penicillin, 392
resistant *E. coli*, 978
Susceptibility test medium
P. aeruginosa, 415
Synergy of antimicrobials
microdilution transfer plate technique, 225

Temperature-sensitive R plasmid
from drug-resistant *V. cholerae*, 13
Tetracycline
bioavailability, 462
DNA replication, 318
membrane properties, 318
mixed anaerobic infection, 265
plasmid-mediated drug resistance, 338
4-Thiouracil
microbial formation, 569
Ticarcillin
anaerobic susceptibility, 258, 679
Enterobacteriaceae, 956
interstitial fluid, 698
P. aeruginosa, 1, 956
serum, 698
versus carbenicillin, 258
versus penicillin, 258
Tilorone hydrochloride
antiviral properties, 984
evaluation of analogues, 92
interferon induction, 984
Venezuelan equine encephalitis virus, 92
Tinidazole
anaerobes, 631
Tobramycin
Enterobacteriaceae, 956
interstitial fluid, 698
in vitro activity, 791
maternal-fetal pharmacology, 688
P. aeruginosa, 956
serum, 698
synergy with ticarcillin, 956
versus netilmicin, 118
Trichothecene fungal toxins
eukaryotic protein synthesis, 491
5-Trifluoromethyl-2′-deoxyuridine
encephalitis, 307
HSV-1, 307
Tylosin
biosynthesis, 455
Typhoid fever
antimicrobial resistant, 645

Ureaplasma urealyticum
susceptibility testing, 267
Urinary infection
anoxicillin, 780

Vaccinia viral antigens
HeLa cells, 202
isatin β-thiosemicarbazone, 202
synthesis, 202
Venezuelan equine encephalomyelitis virus
indirect mouse model, 683
tilorone hydrochloride, 92
Vibrio cholerae
Asian strains, 585
R plasmids, 585, 1079
Vibrio cholerae (El Tor)
temperature-sensitive drug plasmid, 13

Yeasts
amphotericin B, 277
Bactec system, 277
miconazole, 500
Yersinia enterocolitica biotype 4, serotype O:3
microbial susceptibility, 566

INDEX TO DATE OF ISSUE

Month	Date of Issue	Pages
January	24 January 1977	1–178
February	22 February 1977	179–372
March	29 March 1977	373–576
April	5 May 1977	577–771
May	26 May 1977	773–923
June	20 June 1977	925–1089